MEASURE	SI	CONVENTIONAL (C)	CONVERSION FACTOR (CF) C × CF = SI
Gonadal Steroids, plasma			
Androstenedione			
Women	3.5–7.0 nmol/L	1–2 ng/mL	3.492
Men	3.0–5.0 nmol/L	0.8–1.3 ng/mL	3.492
Estradiol			
Women: Basal	70–220 pmol/L	20–60 pg/mL	3.671
Ovulatory surge	>740 pmol/L	>200 pg/mL	3.671
Men	<180 pmol/L	<50 pg/mL	3.671
Dihydrotestosterone			
Women	0.17–1.0 nmol/L	0.05–0.3 ng/mL	3.467
Men	0.87–2.6 nmol/L	0.25–0.75 ng/mL	3.467
Progesterone			
Women: Luteal phase	6–64 nmol/L	2–20 ng/mL	3.180
Follicular phase	<6 nmol/L	<2 ng/mL	3.180
Men	<6 nmol/L	<2 ng/mL	3.180
Testosterone			
Women	<3.5 nmol/L	<1 ng/mL	3.467
Men	10–35 nmol/L	3–10 ng/mL	3.467
Prepubertal boys and girls	0.2–0.7 nmol/L	0.05–0.2 ng/mL	3.467
Gonadotropins, plasma			
Women, basal			
FSH	5–20 IU/L	5–20 mIU/mL	1.0
LH	5–25 IU/L	5–25 mIU/mL	1.0
Women, ovulatory peak			
FSH	12–30 IU/L	12–30 mIU/mL	1.0
LH	25–100 IU/L	25–100 mIU/mL	1.0
Men			
FSH	5–20 IU/L	5–20 mIU/mL	1.0
LH	5–20 IU/L	5–20 mIU/mL	1.0
Prepubertal boys and girls			
FSH	<5 IU/L	<5 mIU/mL	1.0
LH	<5 IU/L	<5 mIU/mL	1.0
Growth Hormone (GH), plasma			
After 100 g glucose orally	<5 μg/L	<5 ng/mL	1.0
After insulin-induced hypoglycemia	>9 Ug/L	>9 ng/mL	1.0
Human chorionic gonadotropin, beta subunit, plasma			
Men and nonpregnant women	<3 IU/L	<3 mIU/mL	1.0
Insulin, plasma			
Fasting	35–145 pmol/L	5–20 μU/mL	7.175
During hypoglycemia (plasma glucose <2.8 nmol/L [<50 mg/dL])	<35 pmol/L	<5 μU/mL	7.175
Insulin-like Growth Factor I (IGF-1, somatomedin-C)	123–463 ng/ml	123–463 μg/L	1
Osmolality, plasma	285–295 mmol/kg	285–295 mOsm/kg	1.0
Oxytocin, plasma			
Random	1–4 pmol/L	1.25–5 ng/L	0.80
Ovulatory peak in women	4–8 pmol/L	5–10 ng/L	0.80
Parathyroid hormone, serum	10–65 ng/L	10–65 pg/mL	1.0
Phosphorus, inorganic, serum	1–1.5 mmol/L	3.0–4.5 mg/dL	0.3229
Potassium, serum	3.5–5.0 mmol/L	3.5–5.0 mEq/L	1.0
Prolactin, serum	2–15 μg/L	2–15 ng/mL	1.0
Renin activity, plasma, normal-sodium diet			
Supine	3.2 ± 1 μg/L/h	3.2 ± 1.1 ng/mL/h	1.0
Standing	9.3 ± 4.2 μg/L/h	9.3 ± 4.3 ng/mL/h	1.0
Sodium, serum	136–145 mmol/L	136–145 mEq/L	1.0
Thyroid Function Tests			
Free thyroxine estimate	9–26 pmol/L	0.7–2.0 ng/dL	12.87
Radioactive iodine uptake, 24 h	0.05–0.30	5–30%	—
Reverse triiodothyronine (rT_3), serum	0.15–0.61 nmol/L	10–40 ng/dL	0.01536
Thyrotropin (TSH), highly sensitive assay, serum	0.6–4.6 mU/L	0.6–4.6 μU/mL	1.0
Thyroxine (T_4), serum	51–42 nmol/L	4–11 μg/dL	12.87
Thyroxine-binding globulin, serum (as thyroxine)	150–360 nmol/L	12–28 μg/mL	12.87
Triiodothyronine (T_3), serum	1.2–3.4 nmol/L	75–220 ng/dL	0.01536
Triiodothyronine resin uptake, serum	0.25–0.35	25–35%	—
Triglycerides, plasma	<1.80 mmol/L	<160 mg/dL	0.01129
Uric acid, serum	120–420 μmol/L	2–7 mg/dL	59.48
Vitamin D (as vitamin D_3, cholecalciferol), pl			
1,25-Dihydroxycholecalciferol (1,25$(OH)_2D$			2.400
25-Hydroxycholecalciferol (25-OHD)			2.496

Updated from Ann Intern Med 106:114–128, 1987

Reproductive Endocrinology

Reproductive Endocrinology

Physiology, Pathophysiology, and Clinical Management

4th Edition

Samuel S.C. Yen, M.D., D.Sci.
W.R. Persons Professor of Reproductive Medicine
University of California, San Diego
School of Medicine
La Jolla, California

Robert B. Jaffe, M.D.
Fred Gellert Professor of Reproductive Medicine and Biology
Director, Reproductive Endocrinology Center
Department of Obstetrics, Gynecology and Reproductive Sciences
University of California, San Francisco
School of Medicine
San Francisco, California

Robert L. Barbieri, M.D.
Kate Macy Ladd Professor of Obstetrics and Gynecology
Chairman, Department of Obstetrics, Gynecology and Reproductive Biology
Brigham & Women's Hospital
Harvard Medical School
Boston, Massachusetts

W.B. SAUNDERS COMPANY
A Division of Harcourt Brace & Company
Philadelphia London Toronto Montreal Sydney Tokyo

W.B. SAUNDERS COMPANY
A Division of Harcourt Brace & Company

The Curtis Center
Independence Square West
Philadelphia, Pennsylvania 19106

Library of Congress Cataloging-in-Publication Data

Reproductive endocrinology: physiology, pathophysiology, and clinical management / [edited by] Samuel S.C. Yen, Robert B. Jaffe, Robert L. Barbieri.—4th ed.

p. cm.

Includes bibliographical references and index.

ISBN 0-7216-6897-6

1. Generative organs—Diseases—Endocrine aspects. 2. Human reproduction—Endocrine aspects. 3. Endocrine gynecology. I. Yen, Samuel S.C. II. Jaffe, Robert B. III. Barbieri, Robert L. [DNLM: 1. Reproduction—physiology. 2. Endocrine Glands—physiology. 3. Endocrine Diseases—physiopathology. WQ 205 R4287 1998]

RC877.R457 1999
612.6—dc21
DNLM/DLC 97-36836

Cover: Logo

The three-dimensional structure of IGF based on x-ray of rhombohedral 2-Zn insulin crystals and proposed confirmation based on model building for IGF. (Redrawn from ER Froesch, J Zapf, E Rinderknecht, et al. *Cold Spring Harbor Conf. Cell Proliferation* 6:62, 1979.)

REPRODUCTIVE ENDOCRINOLOGY: Physiology, Pathophysiology, and Clinical Management ISBN 0-7216-6897-6

Printed in the United States of America.

Last digit is the print number: 9 8 7 6 5 4 3 2 1

This book is dedicated to our families
and to all those investigators and clinicians
who have contributed to the advances
in the understanding of reproductive processes and disorders.

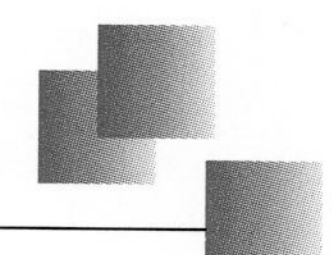

Contributors

Eli Y. Adashi, M.D.
John A. Dixon Presidential Endowed Chair; Professor of Obstetrics/Gynecology and Pediatrics, University of Utah Health Sciences Center, Salt Lake City, Utah
The Ovarian Life Cycle

Aydin Arici, M.D.
Associate Professor and Coordinator, Reproductive Endocrinology Fellowship Program, and Director, Yale Recurrent Pregnancy Loss Program, Department of Obstetrics and Gynecology, Yale University School of Medicine, New Haven, Connecticut
Prostaglandins and Prostaglandin-like Products in Reproduction: Eicosanoids, Peroxides, and Oxygen Radicals; Reproductive Immunology and Its Disorders

Robert L. Barbieri, M.D.
Kate Macy Ladd Professor of Obstetrics and Gynecology, Chairman, Department of Obstetrics, Gynecology and Reproductive Biology, Brigham & Women's Hospital, Harvard Medical School, Boston, Massachusetts
The Breast; Infertility; Assisted Reproduction; Endocrine Disorders in Pregnancy

Harold R. Behrman, Ph.D.
Professor of Obstetrics and Gynecology and Pharmacology and Director, Endocrine Laboratory, Department of Obstetrics and Gynecology, Yale University School of Medicine, New Haven, Connecticut
Prostaglandins and Prostaglandin-like Products in Reproduction: Eicosanoids, Peroxides, and Oxygen Radicals

Henry G. Burger, M.D., FRACP
Professor of Medicine, Monash University; Director, Prince Henry's Institute of Medical Research, Monash Medical Centre, Clayton, Melbourne, Victoria, Australia
Inhibin, Activin, and Neoplasia

Gerard N. Burrow, M.D.
Special Advisor and Professor of Medicine and Obstetrics and Gynecology (David Paige Smith), Yale University School of Medicine, New Haven, Connecticut
The Thyroid Gland and Reproduction

William W. Chin, M.D.
Professor of Medicine and of Obstetrics, Gynecology, and Reproductive Biology, Harvard Medical School. Chief, Division of Genetics, Brigham & Women's Hospital, Boston, Massachusetts
Gonadotropic Hormones: Biosynthesis, Secretion, Receptors, and Action

Christos Coutifaris, M.D., Ph.D.
Associate Professor and Director, Division of Human Reproduction, Department of Obstetrics and Gynecology, University of Pennsylvania Medical Center. Director, Center for Reproductive Medicine and Surgery, Department of Obstetrics and Gynecology, University of Pennsylvania Health System, Philadelphia, Pennsylvania
The Endometrium and Myometrium: Regulation and Dysfunction

Lisa M. Halvorson, M.D.
Assistant Professor of Obstetrics and Gynecology, Tufts University School of Medicine. Assistant Endocrinologist, New England Medical Center, Boston, Massachusetts
Gonadotropic Hormones: Biosynthesis, Secretion, Receptors, and Action

Silvio E. Inzucchi, M.D.
Assistant Professor of Medicine, Yale University School of Medicine, New Haven. Attending Physician, Yale-New Haven Hospital, New Haven, Connecticut
The Thyroid Gland and Reproduction

Robert B. Jaffe, M.D.
Fred Gellert Professor of Reproductive Medicine and Biology, Director, Reproductive Endocrinology Center, Department of Obstetrics, Gynecology and Reproductive Sciences, University of California, San Francisco School of Medicine, San Francisco, California
Prolactin in Human Reproduction; Menopause and Aging; Disorders of Sexual Development; Neuroendocrine-Metabolic Regulation of Pregnancy

David L. Keefe, M.D.
Associate Professor, Department of Obstetrics and Gynecology, Brown University School of Medicine. Director, Division Director of Reproductive Endocrinology, Women's and Infant's Hospital, Providence, Rhode Island
Prostaglandins and Prostaglandin-like Products in Reproduction: Eicosanoids, Peroxides, and Oxygen Radicals

Harvey J. Kliman, M.D., Ph.D.
Research Scientist, Department of Obstetrics and Gynecology, Yale University School of Medicine, New Haven, Connecticut
Reproductive Immunology and Its Disorders

Paul G. McDonough, M.D.
Professor, Departments of Obstetrics & Gynecology, Pediatrics, Endocrinology and Physiology, Medical College of Georgia, Augusta, Georgia
Molecular Biology and the Reproductive Sciences

Walter L. Miller, M.D.
Professor, Department of Pediatrics and The Metabolic Research Unit; Director, Child Health Research Center, and Director, Pediatric Endocrine Training Program, University of California, San Francisco, San Francisco, California
Female Puberty and Its Disorders

Patricia Miron, Ph.D.
Wellesley, Massachusetts
Cytogenetics in Reproduction

Daniel R. Mishell, Jr., M.D.
The Lyle G. McNeile Professor and Chairman, Department of Obstetrics and Gynecology, University of Southern California, Los Angeles, School of Medicine. Chief of Professional Services, Los Angeles County and University of Southern California Medical Center; Women's and Children's Hospital, Los Angeles, California
Contraception

Cynthia C. Morton, M.D., Ph.D.
William Lambert Richardson Professor of Obstetrics, Gynecology and Reproductive Biology and Professor of Pathology, Harvard Medical School. Director of Cytogenetics, Brigham & Women's Hospital, Boston, Massachusetts
Cytogenetics in Reproduction

David L. Olive, M.D.
Professor, Division of Reproductive Endocrinology/ Department of Obstetrics and Gynecology, Yale University School of Medicine. Chief of Obstetrics and Gynecology, Yale-New Haven Hospital, New Haven, Connecticut
Reproductive Immunology and Its Disorders

Bert W. O'Malley, M.D.
Professor and Chairman, Department of Cell Biology, Baylor College of Medicine, Houston, Texas
Steroid Hormones: Metabolism and Mechanism of Action

Robert W. Rebar, M.D.
Professor and Director, Department of Obstetrics and Gynecology, University of Cincinnati College of Medicine. Chief, Obstetrics and Gynecology, University Hospital, Cincinnati, Ohio
Practical Evaluation of Hormonal Status

Richard J. Santen, M.D.
Professor of Medicine, University of Virginia School of Medicine. Oncology Division, University of Virginia Health Sciences Center, Charlottesville, Virginia
The Testis: Function and Dysfunction

Jerome Strauss III, M.D., Ph.D.
Luigi Mastroianni Jr. Professor, Director, Center for Research on Reproduction and Women's Health, and Associate Chair, Department of Obstetrics and Gynecology, University of Pennsylvania Medical Center. Staff, Hospital of the University of Pennsylvania, Philadelphia, Pennsylvania
The Endometrium and Myometrium: Regulation and Dysfunction

Charles A. Strott, M.D.
Head, Section on Steroid Regulation, Endocrinology and Reproduction Research Branch, National Institute of Child Health and Human Development, National Institutes of Health, Bethesda, Maryland. Adjunct Professor of Medicine, Division of Endocrinology and Metabolism, Georgetown University Medical Center, Washington, D.C.
Steroid Hormones: Metabolism and Mechanism of Action

Dennis M. Styne, M.D.
Professor, Department of Pediatrics, University of California, Davis, School of Medicine, Davis. Chief, Pediatric Endocrinology, University of California, Davis, Medical Center, Sacramento, California
Female Puberty and Its Disorders

Johannes D. Veldhuis, M.D.
Professor of Medicine, University of Virginia School of Medicine. Division of Endocrinology, University of Virginia Health Sciences Center, Charlottesville, Virginia
Male Hypothalamic-Pituitary-Gonadal Axis

John Yeh, M.D.
Professor of Obstetrics and Gynecology, University of Minnesota School of Medicine, Minneapolis. Head, Department of Obstetrics and Gynecology Health Partners, and Chairman, Department of Obstetrics and Gynecology, Regions Hospital, St. Paul, Minnesota
The Ovarian Life Cycle

Samuel S.C. Yen, M.D., D.Sci.
W.R. Persons Professor of Reproductive Medicine, University of California, San Diego School of Medicine, La Jolla, California
Neuroendocrinology of Reproduction; The Human Menstrual Cycle: Neuroendocrine Regulation; Prolactin in Human Reproduction; Polycystic Ovary Syndrome: (Hyperandrogenic Chronic Anovulation); Chronic Anovulation Caused by Peripheral Endocrine Disorders; Chronic Anovulation Due to CNS-Hypothalamic-Pituitary Dysfunction

Preface to the Fourth Edition

It has been over twenty years since the first edition of Reproductive Endocrinology appeared. Since that time, the face of the discipline has changed remarkably. We have attempted to keep pace with these advances with each edition. In this fourth edition, we have incorporated recent developments in the molecular, genetic, cellular and clinical aspects of the endocrinology and neuroendocrinology of reproduction in a comprehensive, lucid, and readable manner, without becoming encyclopedic. The fourth edition continues the tradition of having world-recognized experts present the most up-to-date overviews of the areas of their expertise in a comprehensive yet comprehensible manner.

There have been a number of significant changes to the fourth edition which we feel will make it more attractive and useful to our readers. New chapters and authors have been added, in part reflecting new areas of major interest in reproductive endocrinology. Additionally, the format has changed in several respects for ease of reading and comprehension. For example, each chapter is introduced by a series of Key Points to highlight the major areas addressed. This will allow the reader to keep in focus the major themes of each chapter. In addition, the typeface and illustrations have been improved over the previous editions. When review articles are available, they have been referenced to allow the reader to seek further detail in a particular area.

We have not shied away from controversy. When there are differing views concerning a particular topic, these have been included, rather than presenting a dogmatic, unifocused perspective. If we have provided our readers with a useful, readable, encompassing perspective of this dynamic, rapidly changing, and exciting field, we will have achieved our objective.

With this fourth edition, we welcome Robert L. Barbieri as a co-editor. Dr. Barbieri is a well known investigator in reproductive endocrinology and an effective communicator. He has contributed some of the key chapters in the present edition. Our task as editors was greatly facilitated by the help and cooperation of the contributing authors. We also wish to express our appreciation to Deidre Dolan (R. Barbieri), Lee Hillman (R. Jaffe), and Dawn Nye/Gail Laughlin (S. Yen) for the excellent assistance and dedication. Finally, we extend our thanks to Janice Gaillard, Lisette Bralow, and the staff at W.B. Saunders Company, whose capable assistance helped overcome some of the trying problems we met.

Samuel S.C. Yen
Robert B. Jaffe
Robert L. Barbieri

Preface to the First Edition

Among those biomedical fields in which a virtual explosion of new knowledge and understanding has occurred over the past decade, the physiology and pathophysiology of reproductive processes are prime examples. The neural and endocrine regulation of reproduction has been explored with new and sophisticated methods and with increasing comprehension of the important factors involved in the control of this important function. By extrapolation from animal models, as well as by direct investigation involving humans, new light has been shed on the operation of the human reproductive system in both health and disease.

The planning of a book embodying these advances began in July, 1976, when the author-editors were Visiting Scholars at the Villa Serbelloni, an elegant conference and study center operated under the auspices of the Rockefeller Foundation in the picturesque environment of Lake Como, Italy. An outline of this book was completed there, contributing authors were identified, and the writing of several chapters was begun.

Our overall purpose is to provide contemporary factual information and new understanding of human reproductive processes. We attempted to keep in mind the needs of students and investigators in reproductive endocrinology and biology, as well as the needs of clinicians who face the problem of diagnosing and treating reproductive dysfunction. To accomplish these purposes, our authors' expert knowledge ranges from the clinical and systemic to the cellular and molecular. Thus, whenever possible, cellular or molecular mechanisms for normal or disturbed function are presented.

The elements of the reproductive system with which we deal most extensively are various parts of the brain, the pituitary gland, and the gonads. Each of these obviously is a separate and distinguishable component of the system. However, not only are they intimately associated to form an integrated system for periodically releasing germ cells and hormones but, in addition, they have a number of common mechanistic features. We hope that these similarities and integrated modes of action will impress the reader as they have impressed us, and that some readers will be provoked into continued, deeper study of this intriguing field.

The contributing authors were chosen for recognized authority in their respective areas and for their ability to transmit information in a manner we think is lucid and interesting. The lists of references are not intended to be exhaustive but do include key articles and reviews.

Our task as editors was greatly facilitated by the help and cooperation of the contributing authors. We also wish to express our appreciation to Marcia Finkle, Leslie Muga, Alana Schilling, and Rae Feinstein, our secretaries, whose capable assistance helped overcome the few trying problems we met. My (S.Y.) special thanks to Dr. Allen Lein for his critical review of and suggestions for several of my chapters. The editors are grateful to the staff of the W.B. Saunders Company, particularly John Hanley for his confidence, encouragement, and courtesies, which made the preparation of this book a satisfying experience.

The information in this book is at the cutting edge of contemporary reproductive endocrinology. If the book assists the clinician, excites and teaches the student and investigator, and lends deeper understanding of the control of reproductive processes, it will have served its purpose.

S. S. C. Yen
R. B. Jaffe

Contents

NOTICE

Medicine is an ever-changing field. Standard safety precautions must be followed, but as new research and clinical experience broaden our knowledge, changes in treatment and drug therapy become necessary or appropriate. Readers are advised to check the product information currently provided by the manufacturer of each drug to be administered to verify the recommended dose, the method and duration of administration, and contraindications. It is the responsibility of the treating physician, relying on experience and knowledge of the patient, to determine dosages and the best treatment for the patient. Neither the publisher nor the editors assume any responsibility for any injury and/or damage to persons or property.

THE PUBLISHER

Part I

Endocrine Regulation of the Reproductive System

Chapter 1

MOLECULAR BIOLOGY AND THE REPRODUCTIVE SCIENCES

Paul G. McDonough

CHAPTER OUTLINE

KEY POINTS

- The numbers of mutations in genes that affect reproductive disorders and the technology to identify them are expanding greatly. This windfall has been spearheaded by conceptual and experimental advances made possible by the polymerase chain reaction.
- The multiple uses of this technique to amplify DNA, RNA, and the whole genome are clarified. Many of the other techniques described in this chapter for disease diagnosis are increasingly important in identification of molecular mutation in humans.
- The use of transgenic animals as in vivo analytical models of human reproductive disorders is a prime example of the innovative power of this new and ever-changing technology. All these promising advances are being tested in many laboratories and within the Human Genome Project.
- These new, evolving techniques help us to understand the biochemical basis for disease, the etiology of fundamental developmental aberrations, and individual genomic variation.

MOLECULAR GENETICS

In the several years since the previous edition of this book, direct examination of a patient's deoxyribonucleic acid (DNA) has emerged as a definitive means of establishing the presence of specific genetic changes that cause disease. The analysis of human genomic DNA (nucleated cells in blood or other nucleated cells) for disease-associated mutations has become an increasingly important part of clinical reproductive medicine. One can anticipate that all monogenic disorders related to reproductive endocrinology will have molecular determinants by the year 2000. The identification of these molecular determinants for monogenic disorders and the development of further insights into polygenic diseases will radically alter the approach to clinical diagnosis in humans. The ambiguity of clinical criteria for disease, phenotypic similarities between different disorders, and the latent period for disease onset can be largely avoided by molecular diagnosis. In addition, the high specificity of molecular diagnosis makes it possible with some diseases to screen populations for the carrier state. The precise structural alteration in DNA will be the final arbitrator of phenotypic and biochemical variations of the same disease in different subjects. A knowledge of the precise pathologic process at the molecular level has provided important insights into the biochemical basis for many diseases of humans. It is apparent that a firm knowledge of the DNA alterations in disease will also provide more directed therapeutic strategies to modify or limit the expression of these mutant nucleotides.

The remarkable advances in DNA diagnostics have been expedited by development of the polymerase chain reaction (PCR) and the ability to isolate DNA from many different sources such as blood, saliva, hair roots, microscopic slides, paraffin-embedded tissue sections, clinical swabs, and even cancellous bone. These technical advances have been bolstered by the development of an increasing number of effective screening techniques to scan genomic DNA for unknown point mutations. At the same time, unique sequence DNA probes and probes for simple sequence repeat polymorphisms are being generated at an exponential rate. In late 1995, the first physical map of the human genome based on 15,000 specific sequence markers distributed over all the human chromosomes was completed.[1] These human genome markers consist of short sequences of 200 to 500 base pairs (bp) approximately 200 kilobases (kb) apart. These markers, referred to as sequence-tagged sites, do not need to be stored as DNA. Given the sequence of the marker DNAs, one can simply use this information to design the appropriate primers to amplify the intervening segment of DNA with PCR. The amplification product will give the investigator a stretch of DNA that comes from a specific location in the genome. One of the objectives of the Human Genome Project is to provide DNA markers that cover the human genome at approximately 50- to 100-kb intervals. These closely spaced markers are important, but the ultimate target of the project is to sequence the entire genome. The continued development of technology for this purpose will ultimately result in automated DNA diagnosis for the practicing clinician.

This chapter is designed to acquaint the reader with recent concepts of DNA structure, current techniques of testing at the DNA level, prototype mutations in the reproductive sciences, new concepts in the molecular mechanisms of disease, and several important transgenic models of disorders of human reproduction. Finally, the most vital use of this new science, understanding the biochemical basis for disease, is outlined along with the broader applications of recombinant technology. Understanding the physical and biochemical properties of nucleic acids is crucial to the development and implementation of clinical assays that test for diseases at the gene level.

Biochemistry of the DNA Molecule

Genetic information is carried in DNA, the helix or "spiral staircase" molecule described by Watson and Crick[2] in 1953. In its natural state, DNA consists of two linear strands that are wound helically around each other. The backbone of the strands or staircase is made of simple sugar and phosphate molecules. The rungs consist of four bases or nucleotides: adenine (A), guanine (G), cytosine (C), and thymine (T). The molecule is held together by hydrogen bonds between the four specific nucleotide bases on each of the rungs or strands. The single strands are complementary, meaning that thymine is always linked with adenine (A–T) and guanine with cytosine (G–C). As a result, the two strands are mirror images of each other and will not fit together in any other way. The use of DNA probes centers on the process of molecular hybridization, which depends on the mutual attraction of the paired bases. Individual strands of double-stranded DNA can be artificially separated by heating or by the addition of chemical agents to produce a single-stranded DNA. This process is referred to as denaturation. Under controlled conditions, cooling will force the single strands to reassociate or reanneal but only with complementary sequences. The constrained requirement for complementary pairing is the reason for the great specificity of DNA probe assays. This specificity is put to use in a wide spectrum of techniques used to identify different forms of human mutations that alter the function of the resulting protein. Similar techniques are used for detecting the presence of pathogenic bacteria, fungi, parasites, or viruses.

Basic Structure of Human Genes

Genes encode information that specifies functional products, either ribonucleic acid (RNA) molecules or proteins that are used for various cellular functions. A gene itself is a defined unit of DNA that determines the structure of a string of amino acids that form the building blocks of all enzymes and proteins. Each naturally occurring amino acid is coded for by a trio of bases called a codon or triplet. Because there are 64 possible ways to arrange four bases in unique sets of three, there is a degeneracy in the genetic code, that is, there is more than one way of coding for a particular amino acid. Genes, with their regulatory machinery, ensure that their products are synthesized in cells in precisely the right amounts in the appropriate tissues and at the correct time during development. Each cell contains the genetic information to make an entire human being. Certain genes encoding proteins that are vital to every cell in the organism are called "housekeeping genes." Other genes encode proteins that have tissue-specific or temporal-specific patterns of expression.

A structural gene consists of several regions, referred to as exons, that encode proteins. These exons are separated by DNA sequences, referred to as intervening sequences or introns, that do not encode proteins. Figure 1–1 is a theoretical mammalian gene that encodes a structural protein with 200 amino acids for which these features can be demonstrated. This gene has three coding regions, now termed exons, and two intervening sequences or introns. Even though only 600 nucleotides are necessary to encode the protein (three nucleotides per amino acid), because of introns the gene contains roughly 1000 nucleotides.[3] The polarity of a DNA strand is conventionally marked according to the phosphodiester bond from the fifth carbon atom on a deoxyribose subunit to the third carbon atom on the adjacent deoxyribose. In a double helix (or duplex) of DNA, one strand runs in the 5′ to 3′ direction, whereas the complementary strand runs in the 3′ to 5′ direction (i.e., the two strands are antiparallel). At the 5′ end of the gene, there is a specific triplet (ATG) that determines the initiation of protein synthesis on messenger RNA (mRNA);

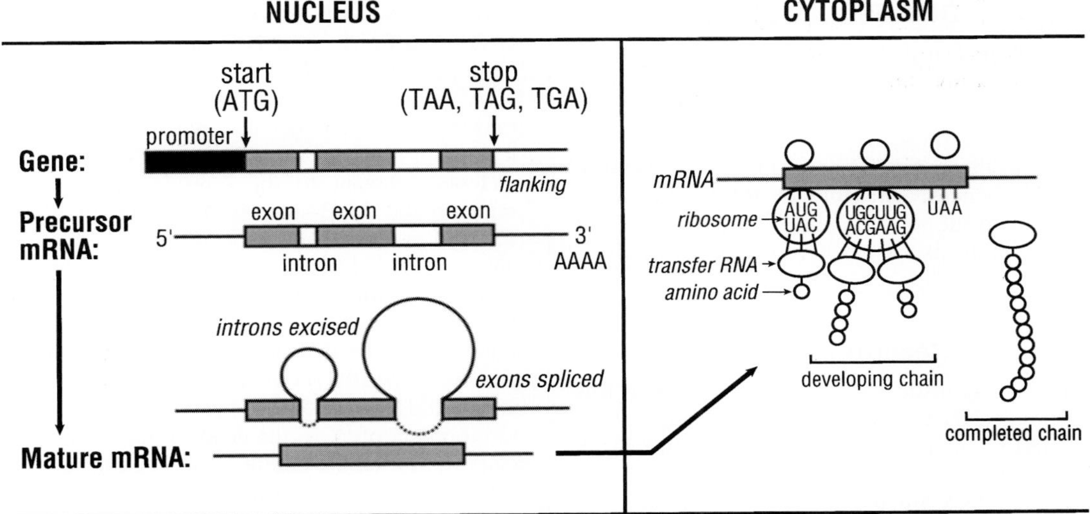

Figure 1–1 ■ Depiction of a typical mammalian gene and mechanism of gene expression. Messenger RNA (mRNA) is synthesized on its DNA template in a 5′ → 3′ direction by the action of the enzyme RNA polymerase II. The primary transcript is a large mRNA precursor, which is processed by cutting out introns and splicing the remaining exons together before delivery to the cell cytoplasm. In the cell cytoplasm, mRNA acts as a template for protein synthesis. ATG indicates the initiation codon for transcription, codon to codon, until a specific termination codon (TAA, TAG, or TGA) is reached. The polyadenylate (poly A) tail is added to the 3′ end of the mRNA to direct its exit from the nucleus for translation. The promoter elements act to localize the exact start site for transcription, control the quantity of RNA, and regulate tissue-specific expression of the gene.

at the 3′ end, there is a termination triplet (TAA, TAG, or TGA). Sequences that are upstream (to the left in a DNA strand reading left to right) are of particular importance in the regulation of the level of transcription of mRNA. These upstream regulatory regions or promoters are important in initiating and controlling the rate of gene transcription. Elements such as proteins produced by other genes that may regulate genes may be on the same chromosome (called *cis*-acting elements) or on a different chromosome (called *trans*-acting factors). Those regulatory nucleotide sequences that lie in the regions of DNA upstream to the transcription start site may undergo mutation and silence the structural gene or cause it to act inappropriately. In contrast to promoters, other DNA regulatory elements may occur in unpredictable locations, often at a considerable distance from the transcription start site. These "enhancers" augment transcription from the gene promoter. The promoter regions of genes tend to have common motifs, whereas enhancer regions do not share many sequences.

Gene Expression

The first step in gene expression is the transcription of a full-length RNA copy of the DNA. These RNA transcripts then serve as templates or messengers for protein synthesis. For a gene to be expressed, an enzyme, RNA polymerase II, slides along a DNA strand and splices free ribonucleotides into an mRNA chain based on the DNA template. The strand of DNA that is copied or transcribed into mRNA is then decoded or translated by the protein synthesis machinery of the cytoplasm. The mRNA comprises a single-stranded polynucleotide chain with a sugar phosphate backbone in which the order of bases is the complement of the transcribed DNA strand of the gene. In RNA, thymine (T) is replaced by a closely related base, uracil (U), which will also base pair with adenine (A). The gene for gonadotropin-releasing hormone (GnRH) is unique in that one strand of the DNA encodes for GnRH, whereas the other strand encodes a different protein.[4] There are now several other examples of mammalian genes in which two different genes are transcribed from opposite strands of the same DNA locus.[5] The expression of eukaryotic protein coding genes can be regulated at a variety of levels from transcription to translation.

Gene Expression

$$\text{DNA} \xrightarrow{\text{Transcription}} \text{RNA} \xrightarrow{\text{Processing} \qquad \text{Translation}} \text{Protein}$$

Transcription is regulated by a variety of factors mediated through the promoter sequences that are upstream or 5′ to the structural gene. These regulatory sequences have specific regions that direct the enzyme RNA polymerase II to the correct site to initiate transcription. The initial RNA transcript must undergo a highly regulated process called splicing in which the introns are removed to create the mature mRNA (see Fig. 1–1). The process by which introns are removed and the flanking exons (expressed regions) are stitched back together is called pre-mRNA splicing. This process of splicing depends on a large molecular apparatus containing RNA and protein molecules, called the spliceosome. Spliceosomes are biochemical machines similar to ribosomes in size and complexity. Sometimes the same mRNA may be spliced differently in different cells to produce entirely different transcripts. The gene for calcitonin is a good example in which differential splicing or processing will generate different mRNAs in different tissues.[6] The best example of post-translational modification is the pro-opiomelanocortin gene or protein.[7]

TECHNIQUES OF DNA-RNA ANALYSIS

Insights into the molecular pathology of reproductive disorders require a firm knowledge of the techniques to analyze DNA for the detection of mutants. The purpose of this segment is to describe those techniques of analyses with special reference to those gene systems that are relevant to the reproductive sciences. The role of RNA analysis is discussed briefly with future applications of these and other techniques to the diagnosis and study of reproductive disorders.

Polymerase Chain Reaction

Almost all of the diagnostic techniques discussed in this chapter use genomic DNA isolated from nucleated cells in blood as the starting material. The next step after DNA isolation is the amplification of specific nucleic acid segments in genomic DNA by the technique of PCR (Fig. 1–2). This amplification technique has been incorporated into virtually all mutation detection strategies. PCR is an in vitro method for producing large amounts of a specific DNA fragment of defined length and sequence from small amounts of a complex template (see Fig. 1–2). This procedure enables one to generate millions of copies of a specific genomic fragment of DNA by exponential amplification without cloning in host cells. In fact, many cloning methods can be complemented or entirely circumvented by using PCR. The range of applications of PCR includes the molecular diagnosis of inherited disorders (prenatal and carrier screening), screening for susceptibility to disease, identification of viral and bacterial pathogens, and single-cell diagnosis. Almost all of the diagnostic techniques discussed in this chapter start by first amplifying the DNA target and then subjecting the PCR-amplified product to differential analysis. Alternatively, the amplified product itself can be labeled and used as a probe for the analysis of other DNAs. PCR can be carried out with either an RNA (total RNA or mRNA) or a DNA template. DNA can be amplified from RNA by synthesizing the first strand of DNA by reverse transcription with the enzyme reverse transcriptase and either a downstream primer, oligo (dT), or random hexamers.

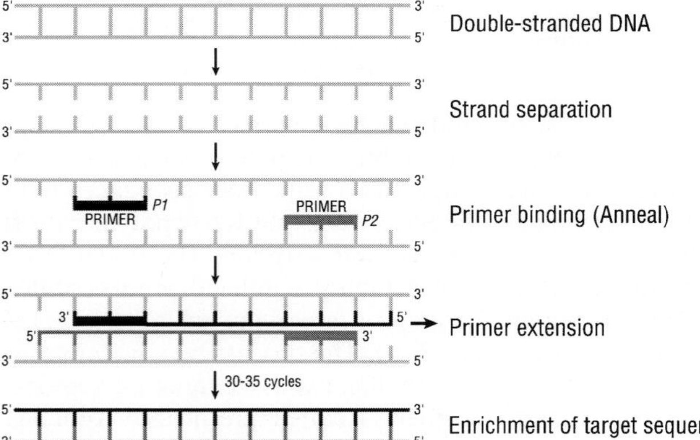

Figure 1–2 ■ A cycle of polymerase chain reaction. The double-stranded DNA is first denatured by heating (94°C) to separate the strands. The temperature is then lowered (55°C), and the primers (P1, P2) are added. The primers are complementary to the 3′ ends of each piece of the double-stranded DNA to be amplified. In the fourth step, the temperature is again raised (72°C), and the primers with the help of the "copying enzyme" (Taq polymerase) copy their respective templates in a 3′ to 5′ direction. After 30 to 35 cycles, the gene of interest may be amplified more than 1 million times, such that it can be easily visualized on an agarose gel as a discrete band without the need for DNA probes.

Genes relevant to the reproductive sciences, such as prolactin and the β-subunit of follicle-stimulating hormone (FSH-β), are usually present as one copy (single-copy DNA). The analysis of single-copy genes by standard techniques of Southern blotting and hybridization with radioactive probes requires 5 to 10 μg of DNA. If the target sequences to be detected are repeated many times in the genome (repetitive-copy DNA), then smaller amounts of extracted DNA (0.5 to 3 μg) are adequate. Before the development of PCR, the need for large amounts of starting material limited the potential applications of DNA diagnostics. A solution to the sample size problem was developed in 1985 when Saiki and colleagues[8] reported this brilliantly conceived method of DNA amplification called PCR. In the PCR procedure, a specific gene region of interest is amplified enzymatically in vitro by DNA polymerase. A DNA segment of up to approximately 6000 bp in length can be amplified exponentially by this method. This approach requires sufficient knowledge of the gene or segment of DNA to develop short DNA primers flanking the region of interest. The primers are short synthetic single-stranded oligonucleotides that are designed to be complementary to the ends of opposite DNA strands and frame the gene or region of interest. Each primer is complementary to one of the original DNA strands, to either the left (5′) or right (3′) side of the region that has been defined for amplification. These short primers will, under appropriate conditions, direct the DNA polymerase to synthesize new complementary DNA strands corresponding to the intervening region (see Fig. 1–2). With this technique, the DNA of even a single oocyte, blastomere, or sperm can be denatured and incubated with the two synthetic oligonucleotide primers corresponding to the opposite ends of the gene of interest. The primers are present in such vast molar excess that they are more likely to anneal to the dissociated strands than the strands are to reanneal with each other. The annealing of the primers is followed by the synthesis of new strands of DNA that are extensions of the primer nucleotides. The synthesis of new complementary strands of DNA is catalyzed by a DNA polymerase that adds nucleotides complementary to those in the dissociated unpaired strand onto the annealed primer. The enzyme used in this reaction is the DNA polymerase of *Thermus aquaticus* (Taq polymerase). The use of this remarkable heat-stable enzyme has permitted automation of PCR because all reaction components, nucleic acid from the specimen of interest, primers, buffers, nucleotides, and enzyme, can be combined at the beginning of the reaction. The number of target DNA strands doubles on completion of each reaction cycle. After 30 cycles, a single copy of DNA can be increased up to 1,000,000 (10^6) copies. Each replication cycle is controlled by simply varying the temperature to permit denaturation of the DNA strands, annealing of the primers, and synthesizing new DNA strands. PCR allows the replication of a discrete segment of DNA to be manipulated in a tube under controlled conditions. After 30 or 60 cycles of replication, the reaction product is electrophoresed on a polyacrylamide gel, stained with ethidium bromide, and inspected under ultraviolet light. The elapsed time from the initiation of PCR to direct visualization of the amplified DNA is usually 4 to 6 hours[9] (see Fig. 1–2).

A striking example of the clinical utility of PCR was provided in 1989 when, starting with a single blastomere from each of 25 human embryos, Handyside and colleagues[10] were able to amplify by PCR a 149-bp segment of Y DNA and correctly sex 15 of the embryos. The amplified 149-bp segment was part of a 3.4-kb repeat localized to Yq11–12 and was easily seen with ethidium bromide staining alone (Fig. 1–3). A prime example of the sensitivity, selectivity, and fidelity of the amplification technique was demonstrated by Witt and Erickson.[11] PCR was used to specifically amplify a series of repeat sequences in the pericentromeric regions of the human X and Y chromosomes. Two oligonucleotide primers (Y^1 and Y^2) flanking a 170-bp fragment of alphoid repeats on the Y chromosome were synthesized. A pair of primers (X^1 and X^2) flanking a 130-bp fragment of alphoid repeats in the pericentromeric region of X were similarly synthesized. When the Y^1–Y^2 pair of primers were used to amplify male DNAs, they selectively amplified the Y-specific 170-bp fragment (Fig. 1–4*A*, lanes 1, 3, 5). Using only the primers designed to amplify the alphoid sequences on X, one observes that male DNAs also generate the 130-bp band (Fig. 1–4*A*, lanes 2, 4, 6). The same primers (X^1–X^2) used to amplify female DNAs generate the 130-bp X-localized band. When the Y^1–Y^2 primers are used with female DNA as the template, no bands are seen (Fig. 1–4*B*, lanes 1, 3, 5). These results were obtained with use of dried blot spots as the starting material for amplification and without the benefit of hybridization to centromeric-specific Y or X DNA probes. Amplification of these specific alphoid sequences affords a sensitive, rapid, and accurate method for sex determination through PCR.[11] Another approach to sex determination is to identify a DNA sequence that is common to X and Y (i.e., *ZFY, ZFX,* or amelogenins) and amplify both targets simultaneously with a pair of specifc primers. One can use a postamplification restriction enzyme digest to differentiate between X- and Y-specific bands. The X-specific band pattern provides an internal control for amplification failures.

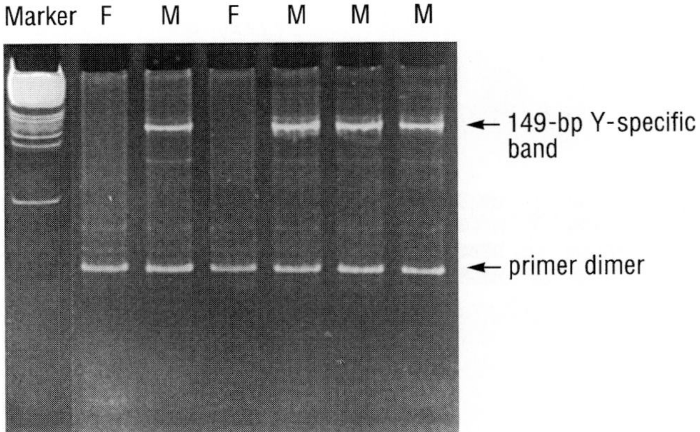

Figure 1–3 ■ The DNA of a single *human* blastomere was amplified for a segment of 149 bp within a 3.4-kb repeat sequence on the long arm of the Y chromosome. A strong 149-bp band is present in male blastomeres and absent in female blastomeres. The low-molecular-weight band on the gel represents the "primer dimer." Marker lane is at left. M, male; F, female. (From Handyside AH, Penketh RJA, Winston RML, et al. Biopsy of human preimplantation embryos and sexing by DNA amplification. Lancet I:347–349, 1989. © by The Lancet Ltd.)

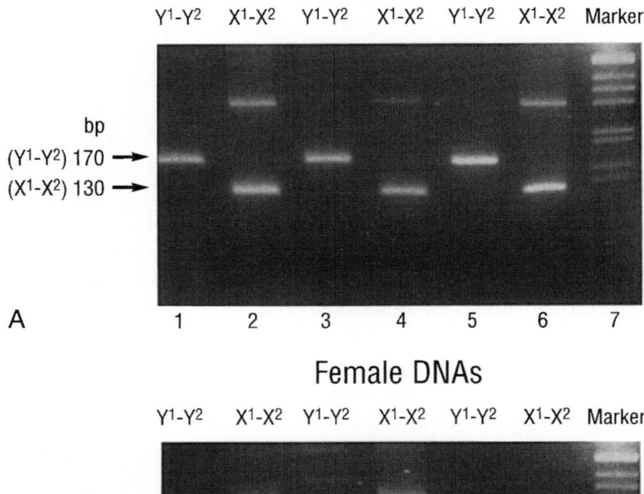

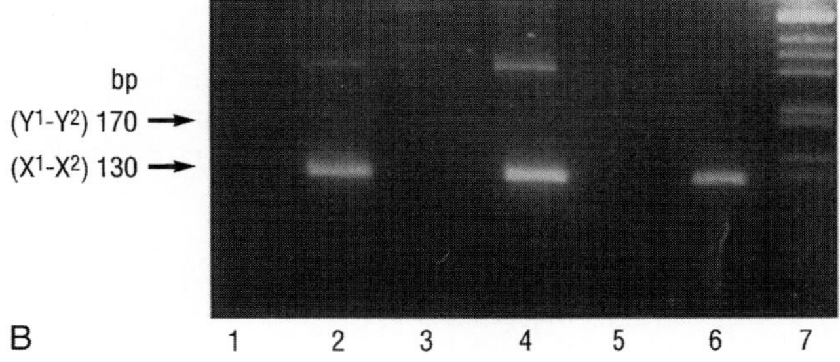

Figure 1–4 ■ *A,* DNA from three different males (lanes 1 and 2, 3 and 4, 5 and 6) used as a template. In lanes 1, 3, and 5, the primers were for centromeric alphoid repeats on the Y chromosome (Y^1–Y^2). In lanes 2, 4, and 6, the primers were for centromeric alphoid repeats on the X chromosome (X^1–X^2). The 170-bp fragment is Y specific, and the 130-bp fragment is X specific. Lane 7 is a size marker. *B,* DNA from three different females (lanes 1 and 2, 3 and 4, 5 and 6) used as a template. In lanes 1, 3, and 5, the primers were for centromeric alphoid repeats on the Y chromosome (Y^1–Y^2). In lanes 2, 4, and 6, the primers were for centromeric alphoid repeats on the X chromosome (X^1–X^2). The 170-bp fragment is Y specific, and the 130-bp fragment is X specific. Lane 7 is a size marker. (*A* and *B* from Witt M, Erickson RP. A rapid method for the detection of Y chromosomal DNA from dried blood specimens by the polymerase chain reaction. Hum Genet 82:271–274, 1989. Courtesy of Springer-Verlag.)

The ability to amplify a single region of a gene in a diploid cell opened the way for preimplantation embryonic diagnosis. Any disease for which the molecular defect is known at the molecular level is amenable to this approach. PCR can be used to amplify specific regions of single-copy genes for identification of a mutation as well as to demonstrate the presence or absence of a particular gene sequence. PCR can generate sufficient product to permit the use of restriction fragment length polymorphism (RFLP) analysis or the use of allele-specific oligonucleotide (ASO) probes to detect point mutations. In many instances, definitive identification of the PCR product is usually performed with an ASO probe. King and Wall[12] amplified by PCR the single-copy bovine luteinizing hormone β-subunit (LH-β) gene in purified bovine genomic DNA representing as few as 25 embryonic cells. After electrophoresis of the amplification product, the gels were hybridized to the radiolabeled bovine LH-β DNA probe for definitive identification of the PCR product. In this case, the extremely small quantity of the target sequence (single-copy gene) could lead to amplification of nonspecific sequences and yield too little specific DNA to be visualized. Final detection assays usually rely on hybridization of a portion of the amplified product to specific synthetic DNA probes representing a portion of the amplified sequences. For overall purposes of gene analysis, PCR offers the advantage of increased signal intensity for any subsequent detection system, including some of the newer techniques to scan the amplified product for single-base substitutions (denaturing gradient gels, heteroduplex analysis). Another major advantage of PCR is that sufficient quantities of the segment or gene of interest are usually available for direct nucleotide sequencing. An RNA sequence can be similarly amplified, but a DNA copy of it (cDNA) must be initially synthesized by using reverse transcriptase before the PCR is begun.[13]

Multiplex Genomic Analysis

Innovative PCR has made possible many new and different approaches to problems in molecular genetics, evolutionary biology, forensic medicine, and development. For example, it is possible with PCR to amplify and screen multiple segments of a gene for deleted regions. This rapid and simple technique known as multiplex genomic DNA amplification permits the detection of deletions (X-linked locus) over megabase regions in a hemizygous gene. This technique does require sequence data over the gene or region of interest to synthesize oligonucleotide primers for PCR. Multiple primers homologous to sequences flanking a number of exons over a large region of interest are used to amplify five or six different segments of the region with PCR. Lack of signal for any of these segments flanked by the primers would indicate a deletion. This technique can be performed in less than 5 hours and is amenable to automation. It is especially practical for X-localized genes.[14]

Reverse Transcription–Polymerase Chain Reaction

PCR can be carried out with either an RNA (total RNA or mRNA) or a DNA template. DNA can be amplified from RNA by synthesizing the first strand of DNA by reverse transcription with the enzyme reverse transcriptase and either a downstream primer, oligo (dT), or random hexamers. In this way, PCR in conjunction with reverse transcriptase (RT-PCR) provides a convenient and highly sensitive method for examining gene expression. This is important in reproductive endocrinology because many occasions arise in which accurate quantitative information concerning the level of gene expression is desirable. RT-PCR is often the only way to analyze RNA when it is produced in exceedingly low numbers. Various modifications of the RT-PCR method to accomplish this goal have been introduced. Starting with the mRNA, they all have in common the first step with reverse transcriptase to convert the mRNA into a DNA-RNA double-stranded hybrid and then a step to convert that hybrid into double-stranded cDNA. A standard PCR reaction is then performed on the synthesized cDNA.

Primer-Extension Preamplification

One of the important byproducts of PCR technology that has important implications for preimplantation diagnosis is primer-extension preamplification (PEP). PEP is an in vitro procedure developed to duplicate a large fraction or entire genome from limited amounts of DNA, such as that derived from a single haploid cell. PEP involves repeated primer extensions using a mixture of 15-base random oligonucleotides (Fig. 1–5). The diversity of the oligonucleotide sequence helps to ensure amplification of segments throughout the genome. It is estimated that at least 78 percent of the genome sequence in a single haploid cell can be copied no less than 30 times. Through PEP, it is possible to perform multiple genotyping experiments on DNA from a single sperm, oocyte, or blastomere cell. PEP is a valuable adjunct to single-cell diagnosis.[15]

Amplification Strategies and Automation

PCR is also a powerful and practical research tool. In time, it will assume a prominent place in the clinical laboratory and will afford a simple and rapid means to increase signal to noise ratios in many types of DNA analysis. Machines capable of performing the PCR technique in 48 DNA

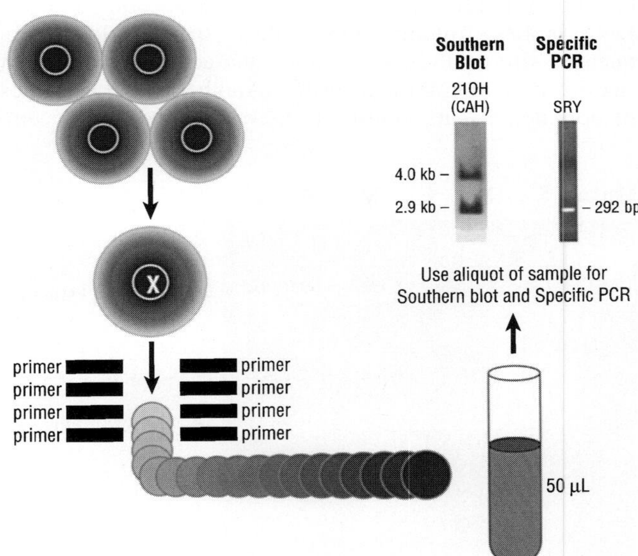

Figure 1–5 ■ Illustration of the use of primer-extension preamplification to amplify the whole genome of a single cell many times. A series of degenerate oligonucleotide primers, approximately 15 bp in size, are developed to amplify the entire genome of the cell by use of a standard PCR reaction. Multiple copies of the single cell's genome provide a generous amount of material (50 µl) for multiple diagnostic tests. The genes for congenital adrenal hyperplasia (21-hydroxylase) and sex-related Y (*SRY*) are analyzed in a Southern blot and a specific PCR reaction using an aliquot of the original 50-µl product.

samples simultaneously, amplifying individual DNA segments 10^6-fold in 4 hours and then sequencing, are available.[16] In addition to automation, the ability to start with a small sample size also makes PCR a practical approach to the diagnosis of a wide range of viral, bacterial, and parasitic infections. Mitochondrial DNA from single hairs has been amplified by PCR and characterized for use as a distinct genome marker in forensic medicine.[17] Short segments of old (sperm stains) or ancient DNA (mummies) can be amplified by PCR. In summary, PCR has become one of the most frequently used techniques in DNA diagnostics.[17, 18]

Other amplification techniques have been developed to circumvent the patent protection for PCR. These other methods include ligase chain reaction, ribosomal RNA amplification, transcription-mediated amplification, Qβ replicase amplification, branched DNA signal amplification, self-sustained sequence replication, and nucleic acid sequence–based amplification. Because of its simplicity, sensitivity, and specificity, the prototype PCR technique has many factors driving its use even in cases in which adequate DNA samples are available and conventional Southern blotting procedures may be performed. One of the principal advantages of PCR is that fully intact DNA is not an absolute prerequisite to perform the genetic analysis. Many of the diagnostic techniques that follow are usually used in conjunction with the initial PCR amplification reaction. The subsequent detection steps that follow amplification of the target DNA range from simple visualization of the amplified product to direct sequencing.

Analysis of Extracted and Amplified DNA

Southern Blot

For analysis, DNA can be extracted from any cell that contains a nucleus, and the target sequence of interest can be amplified by PCR. Platelets contain mitochondrial DNA but do not have a nuclear genome for study. Apart from this exception, DNA can be extracted from peripheral blood leukocytes, tissue, amniocytes, sperm, oocytes, and even mummified ancient tissue samples.[18] The most common source is a peripheral blood sample collected in a heparinized or EDTA tube. After extraction, DNA (with or without prior PCR) is restricted or cut into pieces by specific enzymes (restriction enzymes). These restriction endonucleases that cut double-stranded DNA at specific sequences are the most important tools for handling DNA in a reproducible manner. Each of the restriction enzymes used for this purpose is unique in that it recognizes a specific base sequence (e.g., GAG, ATAG) where it cuts the DNA. Some restriction enzymes consistently cut every six base pairs, others every eight, and so on, to generate DNA fragments of different sizes. Few diagnostic problems are solved by simply testing for the presence or absence of hybridization. The main application of probes is to detect changes in the pattern of fragments produced by restriction enzyme digestion (restriction analysis). If the DNA being analyzed has been changed or "mutated" so that there is a gain or loss of a restriction enzyme cut site, then the size of the fragments generated by enzymatic digestion will be altered. These changes in fragment size are diagnostic of a change in the nucleotide sequence of the gene or its flanking regions. Restriction enzymes are named after the bacterium from which they were isolated. The restriction enzyme *Hae*III is named after the bacterium *Haemophilus aegyptius*.

After the DNA has been cut or restricted into millions of fragments, the pieces (1- to 30-kb) are separated on the basis of molecular weight. This is achieved by running the pieces of DNA on an agarose gel through an electrical field. The smaller, low-molecular-weight fragments migrate quickly down the gel, whereas the larger, less mobile fragments remain at the top of the gel. Fragments of 500 to 30,000 base pairs (500 bp to 30 kb) are readily resolved, and the technique of pulsed-field or field inversion gel electrophoresis can extend the upper limits of resolution to several megabases or fragments greater than 50 kb. Electrophoresis results in a smear on the agarose gel of many fragments, whose position on the gel is a measure of their size. To test for hybridization, the smear of linearized fragments is next transferred to a nitrocellulose membrane or nylon filter without disturbing their pattern. This is the purpose of the Southern blot, named after its inventor, E. M. Southern.[19] After denaturing with alkali, the fragments are drawn from the gel and deposited on the filter by capillary action. A similar technique can be used to transfer RNA (Northern blotting) or proteins (Western blotting) from an electrophoretic gel onto a nitrocellulose filter.[20] At this juncture, it is usually not possible to visualize any of the fragments as discrete bands. To detect or capture the fragment or gene of interest, one must have a piece of DNA corresponding to or complementary to the gene of interest. This piece of DNA or probe is a small fragment of single-stranded DNA that usually represents all or part of a single gene sequence. The nucleic acid sequence is unique for that gene and that organism. Because single-stranded DNA will recombine only with a nucleic acid strand whose sequence is homologous, a probe identifies a specific gene because it binds to a segment of DNA in the organism or on the gel that is complementary to the gene of interest. Normally double-stranded in form, specimen DNA can be denatured to form single strands. Specially designed single-stranded probes can then seek out and bind to complementary sequences on the specimen DNA (Fig. 1–6). Hybridization formats are not limited to DNA-DNA. It can also occur between RNA and DNA strands that contain complementary sequences. In general, the nucleotide homology, temperature, and salt concentrations form the conditions of stringency for hybridization. More stringent conditions permit hybridization only between highly homologous sequences. A single base mismatch in a stretch of 20 bases may be sufficient to prevent hybridization under the most stringent conditions. Another factor influencing duplex stability is the sugar moiety in the backbone of the nucleic acid. Thus, RNA-RNA duplexes are more stable than RNA-DNA ones, which are more stable than DNA-DNA. This property may be exploited in hybridization experiments in which strong binding is desired and in which high stringency can be used.

A nucleic acid probe is a reagent that is typically labeled to permit detection of whether it has hybridized to target nucleic acids in a sample undergoing analysis. DNA probes can be prepared or obtained in many different ways. For example, a target sequence can be amplified by PCR,

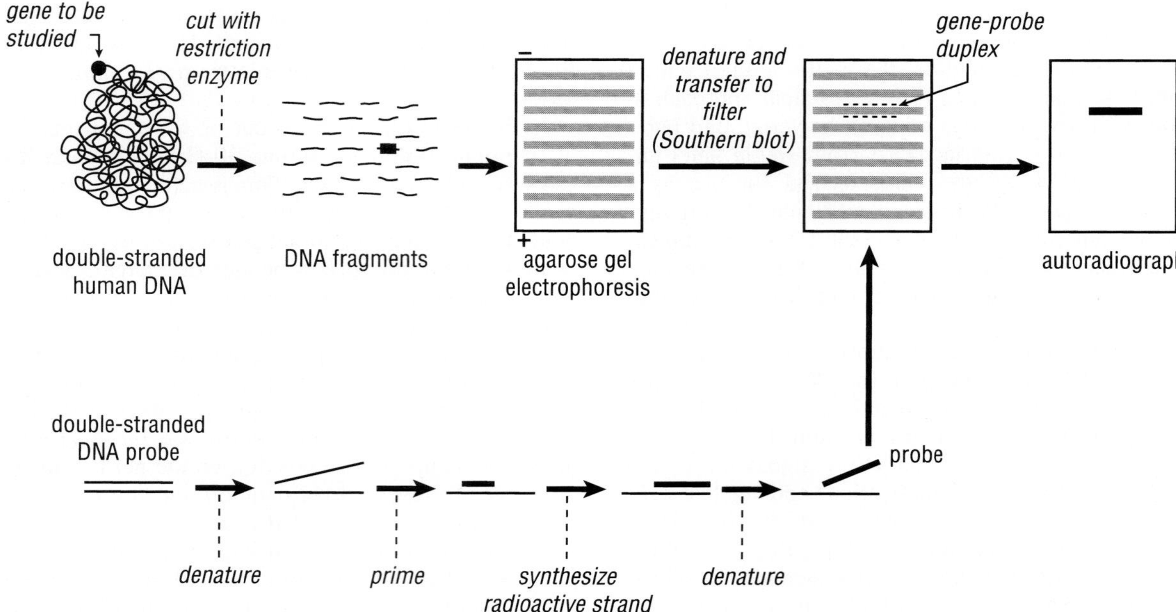

Figure 1–6 ■ Technique of Southern blotting. Extracted DNA is exposed to an appropriate restriction enzyme, and the resultant fragments are subjected to electrophoresis on an agarose gel. The denatured DNA fragments are transferred and permanently fixed to a nitrocellulose filter. The filter is placed in a solution of an appropriate probe of labeled DNA or RNA for hybridization to occur. Hybridization with the radioactively labeled probe is detected by autoradiography.

labeled, and used as a DNA probe. Other DNA probes can be obtained from portions of human DNA that are cloned into bacteriophages or plasmids and propagated in bacterial culture systems. Many DNA probes are the product of the direct chemical synthesis of DNA sequences from the nucleotides one by one in the correct order. Synthesis of oligonucleotides (about 20 nucleotides long) is routine and can be contracted through various service laboratories. Another example is the preparation of probes for the Y chromosome. One can isolate the Y chromosome by chromosome sorting, digest it into small fragments, and put each of the Y fragments into a vector DNA such as a plasmid. The plasmids containing these Y fragments or inserts can be amplified or cloned in bacteria. After cloning, the individual Y inserts can be cut out of the plasmid vector and used as probes for Y DNA. Once a probe is constructed and refined, it can be used in a variety of ways. The DNA probe corresponding to the gene or sequence of interest must first be labeled or tagged so that its capture or hybridization with the target DNA can be easily detected. The probe DNA is first made single stranded by boiling and is radiolabeled by replacing the phosphorus atoms with ^{32}P. Two of the procedures to radiolabel probes to a high degree of specific activity are "nick translation" and "random primers." The nitrocellulose or nylon membrane is soaked in a solution containing the radioactive probe at appropriate temperature and washed to eliminate the unbound probe. The presence of hybridized probe is detected by autoradiography. The probe or gene of interest will hybridize to its complementary strand that is immobilized on the nitrocellulose or nylon membrane. This hybridization must take place under controlled conditions of temperature and salt concentration (stringency). After the membrane is baked and exposed to x-rays, the autoradiograph will reveal the precise fragments of DNA corresponding to the gene probe being used. An analysis of these fragments will reveal information concerning the presence and structure of the gene.

Allele-Specific Oligonucleotide (ASO) Probes

In most instances, the mutation in the gene does not ablate or create a new restriction enzyme cut site. It becomes necessary to have alternative approaches to the detection of DNA mutations. As more genes are sequenced and mutations recognized, an even more direct approach to diagnosis can be used. Oligonucleotide probing depends on the development of two DNA probes, one corresponding to the normal gene and one complementary to the known mutant sequence. In practice, a sequence of 20 to 30 bp (oligomers) corresponding to the normal gene is manufactured. A similar series of 20 to 30 bp corresponding to the mutant gene is developed. Each of these oligomers can now be radiolabeled and used to probe the DNAs of normal subjects and of heterozygotes and homozygotes for the mutation in question. The DNA of an individual with two normal genes will hybridize to the normal probe but not to its mutant counterpart. The DNA of an individual who is homozygous for the mutation will hybridize only to the mutant probe. A heterozygous carrier will reveal bands with both the normal and mutant probes (Fig. 1–7).

Oligonucleotide probing in which there are two short pieces of DNA complementary to the normal and mutant allele obviously requires sequence information on the normal and mutant gene. Genes that are known to have many different mutations are not so amenable to this approach. In such situations, one would need to know the spectrum of mutations and develop ASO probes for each of them.

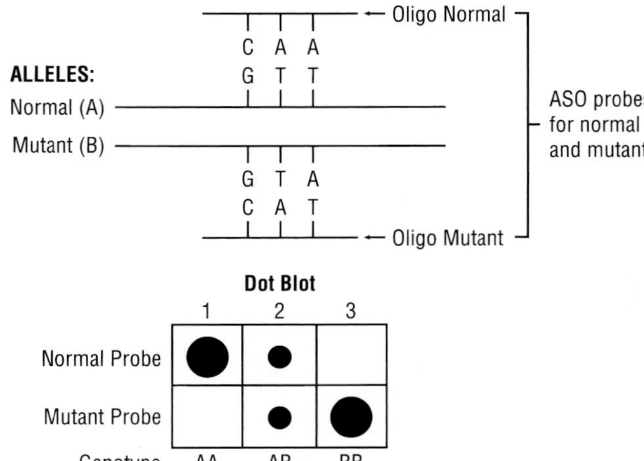

Figure 1–7 ■ The use of allele-specific oligonucleotide (ASO) probes with dot blots to identify the specific genotype of an individual's DNA. The ASO probes are synthesized to detect the normal (A) and mutant (B) alleles for a given gene. The DNA, obtained by cell lysis, is denatured in high-salt solution, fixed to a solid surface (nitrocellulose filters or blots), and exposed to the normal and mutant probes. DNAs that are homozygous normal (AA) will hybridize only with the normal probe (lane 1) and DNAs from homozygous mutants (BB) only with the mutant probe (lane 3). DNAs from individuals that are heterozygous (AB) will hybridize with both probes (lane 2).

Fortunately, certain mutations tend to be more prevalent in specific ethnic groups or geographic areas, which can simplify the process. In addition, the hybridization conditions of ASO probing must be carefully controlled and are usually stringent. In the technique of reverse ASO screening, the various wild-type and mutant DNAs are spotted to the filter and the labeled, amplified DNA is used as a probe. ASO screening is more suitable for screening samples of many patients for one or only a few possible missense mutations. Reverse ASO is better suited for screening one patient at a time for many different possible missense base pair substitutions. More recently, the ability to amplify a target gene and sequence it directly has reduced some of the need for oligonucleotide probing. Nevertheless, by itself or in adjunct with gene amplification, it is an important approach to DNA diagnosis at this time.

There are many examples in reproductive medicine in which the use of ASOs is valuable. For example, there are six human chorionic gonadotropin β-subunit (hCG-β) genes and one LH-β gene that pose a problem at the diagnostic level.[21] Using sequence data, one can develop an oligonucleotide probe for the LH-β gene that carries sequences specific for LH-β to avoid cross-hybridization with hCG-β nucleotides.[22] An oligonucleotide has been developed that is specific for the single LH-β gene.

In their search for a genomic fragment containing the GnRH gene, Seeburg and Adelman[23] used synthetic oligonucleotides coding for GnRH alone and for GnRH plus putative post-translational processing sites to screen genomic DNA. These synthetic oligonucleotides were constructed on the basis of the known amino acid sequence of GnRH and the predicted DNA sequences inferred from the genetic code. A 600-bp genomic fragment was obtained in this way and used as a highly specific probe to screen a cDNA library for the corresponding recombinant, from which the structure of the precursor protein could be determined. One can currently synthesize any oligonucleotide probe in a synthesizer apparatus provided that one knows the sequence of the gene or gene region of interest.

The final sequencing of the human genome will facilitate the continued development of synthetic oligonucleotides to probe for gene normalcy. Automated techniques for screening for mismatches between probe and target suggestive of mutation will be part of the future technology of ASO probing.

Dot Blot (Slot Blot)

The use of standard Southern blotting as described for gene analysis is specific but requires restriction digestion of the DNA sample, electrophoresis, and hybridization. A more rapid method used especially in microbiology is a technique called slot or dot blotting of DNA or RNA (see Fig. 1–7). This variation of hybridization on a membrane eliminates the electrophoretic step and is used to detect the presence, absence, or amount of a genetic element. In this technique, isolated, unrestricted DNA or RNA that is denatured in high-salt concentration is spotted onto nitrocellulose filters in a vacuum apparatus, baked, and hybridized to the labeled probe of interest. The technique is rapid and may be used to screen multiple samples. With radiolabeled probes of high specific activity, the resulting sensitivity (i.e., the smallest detectable amount) is about 0.2 to 0.5 pg. Although the technique is highly sensitive and rapid, it may not be as specific as the Southern blot. The signal generated from the hybridization in a slot blot may be nonspecific because appropriate band size is not determined. It has the weakness of not knowing the molecular size of the reacting nucleic acid target (equivalent to loss of specificity). Dot blotting must be standardized and controlled for each probe and appropriate stringency conditions determined. Nevertheless, it is a valuable technique for use with microgram quantities of samples and for the detection of specific DNA or RNA sequences in a sample.

In Situ Hybridization

The in situ hybridization method for DNA analysis can be performed on chromosomal preparations, frozen sections, cytologic specimens, or formalin-fixed paraffin-embedded sections. Its utility results from its ability to localize relevant DNA sequences within larger structures, thus linking biochemistry with cytogenetics or histochemistry. Genes can be localized to specific chromosomes by radioactive (autoradiography) or fluorochrome-labeled (fluorescence in situ hybridization) probes. Important information about gene expression can be obtained in relation to the development of specific tissues by identifying the presence of mRNA in histologic sections by autoradiography or fluorescence microscopy. Viral genomes can be specifically localized within tissues with this technique.

In situ hybridization is similar to blot methods in that the probe is placed directly on the specimen that has the DNA sequences immobilized in a solid substrate. The tissue on the slide is treated with a protease to allow the probe access to the nuclear DNA, which is denatured by heating. The probe is added in an overlying hybridization buffer, and hybridization occurs if the target DNA complementary to the probe is present. Extensive washing after the hybridization reaction removes unbound labeled probe and mismatched sequences. The probe is then detected with a variety of reporting systems ranging from avidin-biotin enzyme reactions to fluorescence or autoradiography. Once the duplex DNA strand forms between the target and the probe, the duplex can be quantitated or visualized on the basis of the label used. To date, these techniques have been primarily used to detect viral sequences in tissues. Alternatively, mRNA, which may be present in more copies than DNA, may be the target of the probe in tissue specimens.[24] In this way, the DNA is detected and localized within individual chromosomes or in cells in tissues.

Restriction Fragment Length Polymorphisms (RFLPs)

In the early years of DNA diagnostics, the most frequently employed technique to follow the transmission of a genetic disease is the use of RFLPs. The first step in this type of indirect gene analysis depends on the identification of a fragment or piece of DNA that is so closely linked to the gene of interest that they are invariably transmitted together during meiosis. The tight linkage between this DNA fragment and the gene of interest makes the segregating fragment a clear signpost or road sign for the presence of the gene itself. This unique, close relationship could be disrupted only by a crossover between chromosomal homologues during meiosis that might transfer the marker or RFLP to the other homologue. In general, the smaller the physical distance between the gene of interest and the RFLP, the less likelihood that crossover or recombination might occur. To use this DNA marker to follow the gene, it is necessary that the restriction fragment generated be polymorphic, or at least dimorphic in the family under consideration. This is crucial because the RFLP enables one to follow the gene of interest only if it can distinguish one member of a chromosomal pair from the other. Polymorphic simply indicates that a given segment of DNA may have extensive sequence length variation or polymorphism without affecting the organism. This type of variation in the structure of DNA is seen particularly in regions that do not code for proteins and regions that are not involved in important regulatory functions. Nevertheless, these differences or polymorphisms can affect any type of DNA sequence. A benign alteration in DNA producing an RFLP may occur within a noncoding sequence of a gene (intron), sequences between genes, repetitive DNA, and even a coding sequence of a gene. These variations between sequences at the same loci on two homologous chromosomes can be detected by observing fragments of different size generated by cutting with a restriction enzyme. Pairs of variation or dimorphisms or alleles are inherited as traits and segregate in a mendelian manner. These inherited variations in the size of DNA fragments after restriction enzyme digestion are referred to as RFLPs. Figure 1–8 is a hypothetical or drawing board example of the use of this technique for disease diagnosis. The theoretical family under study is from Kenya and has three female children. The oldest child is 22 years old and has been diagnosed with Kallmann's syndrome due to an absence of GnRH; the two younger children are 5 and 7 years. The parents would like to know if either or both of their younger girls will have Kallmann's syndrome. The gene for GnRH has been isolated, cloned, and mapped to the short arm of chromosome 8 in humans as indicated previously.[25] A reasonable approach to diagnosis would be to study the DNA of the affected child with use of standard Southern analysis with the GnRH gene as the probe. However, this approach reveals identical Southern blots in all family members including the child affected with GnRH deficiency. Now one wonders whether the mutation in the GnRH gene is at a site that is not recognized by a restriction enzyme and requires ASO probing. The second approach is a possibility, especially because the entire nucleotide sequence encoding the normal human GnRH gene and its flanking sequences has been determined.[26] The synthesis

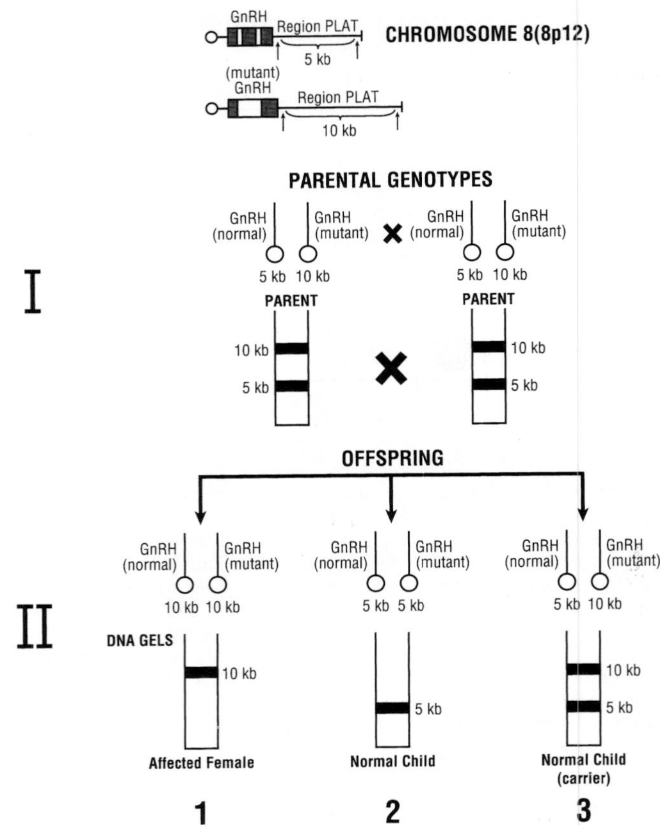

Figure 1–8 ■ Hypothetical illustration of the use of a restriction fragment length polymorphism to follow the segregation of a mutant allele, pedigree of family with three female offspring. The eldest daughter (II-1) has hypogonadotropic hypogonadism due to a deficiency of GnRH. The parents request to know whether their two prepubertal daughters (II-2, II-3) will be similarly affected. The gene for GnRH is mapped to 8p but is not polymorphic. A closely linked gene for tissue plasminogen activator *(PLAT)* is dimorphic, demonstrating two different alleles, one 10 kb and the other 5 kb. Extracted DNAs from the parents probed with *PLAT* demonstrate that they are heterozygous for these two different alleles. The affected daughter (II-1) is homozygous for the 10-kb band, indicating that the mutant GnRH gene is segregating in this family with this *PLAT* allele. One younger daughter (II-2) is homozygous for the 5-kb band (normal), and the other child (II-3) is a heterozygous carrier demonstrating both bands similar to the parents.

of an ASO probe for the normal gene is technically easy. The different types and numbers of mutations affecting the mutated gene obfuscate the development of an ASO mutant probe. It might be difficult to synthesize and test a series of ASOs, each carrying a different mutant for the GnRH gene. It is possible that the mutation producing GnRH absence in Kenya may be different from that of the rest of the world. This lack of knowledge concerning the molecular pathology of the gene under study limits the first two approaches for analysis of the mutant gene. The analysis of gene pathology by use of RFLP analysis does not require any presumptive information concerning the gene of interest or the pathology of that gene. Diagnosis instead is based on a neighboring DNA marker that can be used to follow the inheritance of a putative gene (GnRH) as it segregates through a family. A gene that is closely linked to the gene for GnRH on chromosome 8 is the *PLAT* gene encoding tissue plasminogen activator (t-PA).[27] Noncoding sequences in (introns) and around (flanking) the *PLAT* gene are known to be polymorphic. Differences in the nucleotide sequence for a given locus on homologous chromosomes create dimorphisms that are unique for an individual or within members of the same family. These DNA polymorphisms or markers are sometimes called alleles. To date, these alleles do not demonstrate a recognizable function like those alleles or genes coding for a protein, but they are transmitted in mendelian fashion. In the family under study, the DNAs of both parents are cut with a restriction enzyme and probed with the linked *PLAT* gene. On a Southern blot, each parent has two bands, two polymorphisms or alleles. The parents are informative because their DNAs contain two different bands, one at 10 kb and a lower molecular weight 5-kb band. They are heterozygotes for the t-PA polymorphism. Because the t-PA probe hybridized with this gene on chromosome 8, we can infer that one band is linked to one chromosome 8 and the other to its homologue. This benign variation in an intron or noncoding flanking sequence at this locus now enables us to follow the segregation of these two chromosome 8 homologues. Because each parent has two alleles, or is dimorphic for this sequence, they are said to be *informative*. To be homozygous for GnRH deficiency, the affected child must have received one copy of the mutant gene from each parent. The only information we are lacking is whether the mutant gene is linked to and segregating with the 10-kb RFLP or the 5-kb RFLP. This linkage or "phase" can be determined by analyzing the DNA of an affected individual in the family. Southern analysis of the DNA of the affected adult female with use of the t-PA probe reveals only the intense 10-kb band. This indicates that the mutant phenotype is segregating with the 10-kb band. Each parent has contributed one 10-kb allele to make the child homozygous for the deficiency of GnRH. This can be inferred without any knowledge of the precise mutation affecting the GnRH gene or even regulatory regions of the gene. The diagnosis and phase are further corroborated by similar analysis of the DNAs of the other two children. One child is homozygous for the 5-kb allele, whereas the other has received a 10-kb allele from one parent and a 5-kb allele from the other parent. The former child is normal phenotypically and genotypically, whereas the latter is phenotypically normal but a carrier like her parents. It is apparent now that the use of RFLPs for diagnosis requires the DNA of at least one affected individual in the pedigree to establish phase. This is a strong argument for extracting and freezing DNA of everyone for future comparative studies and diagnosis. Before specific gene isolation, RFLPs have been used for the diagnosis of Huntington's disease, factor VIII and factor IX deficiencies, some cases of β-thalassemia, cystic fibrosis, and phenylketonuria. There is an RFLP linked to the *C4A* complement gene on chromosome 6, which is closely linked to the gene for 21-hydroxylase. Potentially, this fragment or polymorphism could also be used to diagnose and follow the inheritance of the mutant gene for 21-hydroxylation. The versatility of DNA technology is enormous because a disease like congenital adrenal hyperplasia might potentially be diagnosed by any one of the three described techniques, specific restriction enzyme, ASO probing, or RFLP analysis.

The same restriction fragment polymorphisms can be used to determine the parental origin of the extra chromosome in aneuploidic situations such as trisomy 21. As more and more of these polymorphisms are recognized and RFLPs are identified to cover the entire human genome, every monogenic disorder is potentially diagnosable by this linkage technique.

The overall advantage of the technique of RFLP is that a gene can be linked with one of its flanking DNA polymorphisms. In humans with about 3×10^9 bp in the genome, calculations indicate that there would be several million detectable differences in the DNA between any two individuals. This would appear to be more than sufficient DNA variation to be used to establish linkage of any defective gene to an RFLP. By following an RFLP that cosegregates with a mutant phenotype, it should be possible to recognize recessive carriers, the nonpenetrant dominant carrier, and delayed-onset mutant phenotypes such as Kallmann's syndrome that generally do not express themselves until adolescence. The ultimate goal is to map the human genome with a series of overlapping RFLPs or at the least no greater distance apart than 1 cM.* It has been estimated that 2500 markers would be needed to construct a 1-cM RFLP map. At that point, every gene of interest in the genome would be linked to one of these polymorphic loci. The recent identification of simple sequence repeat polymorphisms distributed randomly throughout the genome has rapidly expanded the numbers of DNA markers available to track disease.

Northern Blot

The gene under analysis is a unique sequence of nucleotides that are transcribed into mRNA. It is the sequence of nucleotides that determines gene function. Both exons and introns are transcribed into a pre-mRNA, but the exon sequences are translated into protein, whereas the intron sequences are processed or spliced out of the pre-mRNA and are not translated. The sequences at the intron-exon junctions, called splice sites, are crucial for mRNA processing and important potential sites of mutation.

*Centimorgan, a unit for expressing the relative distance between genes on a chromosome; 1 cM indicates that recombination between that gene and another marker gene occurs in 1 percent of meiosis.

RNA molecules are analyzed either to assess the quantitative level of expression of particular genes or to identify structural mutations. Specific RNA molecules may be separated in gels according to size, transferred onto a membrane, and detected with a complementary probe (Northern blot). The study of RNA affords one the opportunity to study the mRNA or tissue-specific expression and regulation of a given structural gene. Opportunities to study the mRNA or gene transcripts are not frequent in clinical reproductive medicine because one must have available for study the tissue where the gene is most likely to be expressed. The identification and study of factors regulating transcription for the genes encoding FSH-β, LH-β, dopamine receptor, and aromatase, for instance, require the presence of pituitary tissue and ovary to isolate total RNA and ultimately mRNA for study.

At a practical level, to analyze whether a gene is being expressed (whether the DNA template is being transcribed into mRNA), whether an mRNA transcript has the appropriate size, whether a gene is expressed at an appropriate level compared with the control, and whether mRNA is intact or degraded, RNA hybridization may be performed by the Northern procedure. In this method, RNA is isolated from cells or tissue samples and electrophoresed through agarose gels under denaturing conditions. Although mRNA is naturally single stranded, the mRNA molecule may fold back on itself and form base pairs internally over short segments of complementary nucleotides, creating an extensive secondary structure within the molecule. Thus, the mRNA electrophoresed through a gel must be denatured with gentle heating and electrophoresed in the presence of a denaturant such as formaldehyde, methyl mercury, or glyoxal so that the mRNA species migrate through the agarose according to their true linear size. Agarose-denaturant gels may be stained with ethidium bromide after electrophoresis and visualized in a manner similar to Southern DNA gels.

Ninety-eight to 99 percent of the mass of total RNA is ribosomal RNA (predominantly the 28S and 18S subunits) and transfer RNA. When total RNA is electrophoresed through denaturing gels, only the ribosomal RNA bands are visualized because the mass of mRNA (1 to 2 percent of the total) is too small to be directly visualized after ethidium bromide staining. Transfer of RNA fragments from a denaturing gel to nylon membrane may be performed by electroblotting. The solid support system or nylon membranes are hybridized with a solution containing the single-stranded radiolabeled probe of the gene of interest. The probe binds to appropriate complementary RNA sequences, and subsequent autoradiography of the nitrocellulose membrane after hybridization reveals DNA transcripts complementary to the labeled probe. One determines the kilobase size of the transcripts from RNA size standards run simultaneously in the original denaturing gel.

Analysis of the mRNA enables us to consider questions related to tissue- and temporal-specific expression of genes and the factors involved in their regulation. Studies of RNA frequently provide confirmatory and new insights into reproductive biology. The isolation of a large number of homeotic genes in *Drosophila* permitted a study of their patterns of expression during human development.[28] The homeotic gene Hu-2 studied in human trophoblast is seen on Northern analysis to have a temporal-specific pattern of expression during early pregnancy (Fig. 1–9). Similarly, the isolation and cloning of the gene for bovine and human müllerian duct–inhibiting hormone (MIH) provided the opportunity to study the expression of this important gene.[29] Northern blot analysis revealed transcripts for MIH in newborn calf testis as anticipated, but surprisingly, transcripts are clearly seen in mature human granulosa cells. The former was confirmatory but the latter raised interesting biologic questions as to the possible function of the mRNA transcripts for MIH. One might speculate that MIH may play some role in initiating or suppressing the process of meiosis. The homology between transforming growth factor-β (TGF-β) and MIH is of particular interest because both are capable of inhibiting the cell cycle and normal cellular growth. Structural comparison of the MIH and TGF-β genes may provide insight into the regions of these proteins responsible for their antitumor activity and improve our understanding of the regulation of cell growth. The homologies between TGF-β, MIH, and the β-subunits of inhibin have led to speculation that the three proteins may be members of a single gene family.[30]

The technique of Northern blotting has also been helpful in confirming the relative role of the three different subunits of inhibin. Inhibin purified from porcine follicular fluid consists of two forms; each form is composed of one α-subunit and one of two possible β-subunits, β_A or β_B. Furthermore, inhibin consisting of either $\alpha\beta_A$ or $\alpha\beta_B$ chains inhibits release of pituitary FSH, whereas combinations of the two β chains ($\beta_A\beta_A$ or $\beta_B\beta_B$) induce FSH release. These proteins have been termed FSH-releasing protein ($\beta_A\beta_A$) or activin ($\beta_A\beta_A$).[31, 32] Northern blotting with the DNA probes for these three subunits indicates that concentrations of α-subunit precursor mRNA are at least 10-fold higher than those of the β_A-subunit precursor mRNA and 20-fold higher than those of the β_B-subunit precursor mRNA. The larger amount of α-subunit precursor mRNA

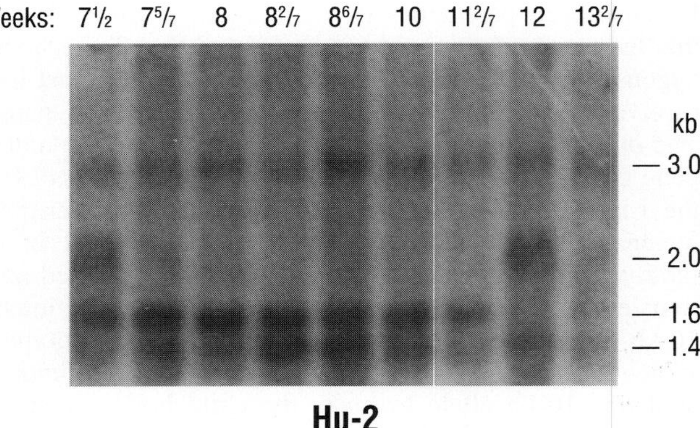

Figure 1–9 ■ Northern blot hybridization pattern of gene Hu-2 to poly(A) + RNA isolated from human fetal trophoblast (7½ to 13²⁄₇ weeks). The Hu-2 gene probe hybridized strongly to a 1.6-kb transcript (7½ to 11²⁄₇ weeks), and a smaller 1.4-kb transcript showed a similar pattern of expression. A 3-kb transcript was detected throughout the period. Two samples hybridized to a 2.0-kb transcript at 7½ weeks (one sample) and 12 weeks (one sample). (From Su BC, Strand D, McDonough PG, McDonald JF. Temporal and constitutive expression of homeobox-2 gene [Hu-2], heat shock gene [hsp-70] and oncogenes c-*sis* and N-*myc* in early human trophoblast. Am J Obstet Gynecol 159:1195–1199, 1988.)

is consistent with the need for this subunit; however, the quantity of different transcripts in different tissue might reflect the functional role of that tissue in FSH inhibition or stimulation.

The identification of RNA molecules in tissue sections by means of in situ hybridization with a labeled probe has important applications in pathology. RNA molecules may also be converted into more stable DNA molecules by reverse transcriptase and then studied by the techniques available for DNA analysis. Tissue and cell localization of mRNA transcripts is a rapidly evolving technology and now includes techniques to amplify the target DNA or RNA. The presence of specific mRNAs has been examined in preimplantation mouse embryos by first converting mRNA to cDNA, followed by DNA amplification with PCR.[33] This level of sensitivity will further our understanding of gene expression during embryogenesis.

Techniques to Screen for Mutations in Genomic DNA

To date, molecular genetics has made substantial progress in identifying disease-causing genes and characterizing the mutations that disrupt them. However, the detection and characterization of single nucleotide variations in genomic DNA still represent a common technical obstacle in the genetic analysis of human inherited disorders. There are still many factors that limit the science of mutation detection. Before 1985, it was possible to screen for gross deletions, insertions, and rearrangements in genes as described by Southern blotting. Small alterations including single-base changes could be detected only if they were present in the recognition sequence of restriction enzymes. To scan for small deletions, insertions, and single-base changes not found in enzyme recognition sites, it was necessary to laboriously sequence long stretches of DNA. Identification of previously characterized mutations was possible using selective oligonucleotide hybridization to genomic DNA. The first effective scanning methods for unknown point mutations were published in 1985, and the current methods of mutation detection can be broadly categorized into either diagnostic or scanning methods.[34] Diagnostic or specific methods are devised to detect previously defined and usually well characterized mutations in specific genes. A good example of the diagnostic category is the detection of the 3-bp deletion in cystic fibrosis. More frequently, one is dealing with a disorder in which there are 50 to 100 known disease-causing mutations or no mutations identified to date. These situations require techniques in which hundreds or thousands of base pairs can be screened or scanned for a mutation before definitive sequencing. The following scanning methods are designed to screen hundreds or thousands of base pairs of DNA for a previously unidentified mutation. The majority of these scanning techniques start with the amplification by PCR of a DNA fragment or overlapping PCR-amplified fragments to establish where the putative nucleotide variant or mutation is located. The pieces of the gene that are amplified are usually exon-sized pieces of DNA. The DNA scanning methods that are designed for use in the clinical diagnosis of certain genetic disorders fall into the following categories. Some of the methods that are used for scanning exon-sized pieces of DNA are as follows.

Single-Stranded Conformation Polymorphisms

The single-stranded conformation polymorphism (SSCP) method is the most simple and most widely used technique to detect sequence differences between DNA fragments. This technique is based on the observation that the migration of short, single-stranded fragments in nondenaturing gels is a function of their length and sequence. Single-stranded DNA or RNA molecules will assume different secondary structures depending on their sequence. A single-base change can result in altered structure and changed mobility in the gel. The original sample of PCR-amplified genomic DNA or reverse-transcribed cDNA is first denatured to separate the DNA strands and run on a nondenaturing gel. In this nondenaturing environment, the single strands of DNA that differ by as little as a single base pair take up different conformations and migrate at different speeds in the gel compared with normal wild-type controls (Fig. 1–10).[34] The sensitivity of SSCP analysis decreases with increasing fragment size, or alternatively, the shifts in mobility are decreasingly apparent in a fragment of increasing size. For this reason, the technique favors the scanning

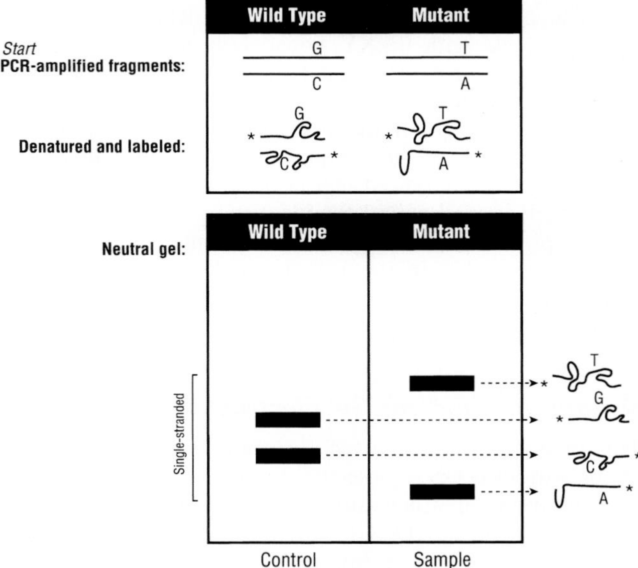

Figure 1–10 ■ Illustration of the technique of detecting previously unidentified mutations by single-stranded conformation polymorphism. The gene of interest in the control (wild) and sample (mutant) DNA is first amplified by PCR. The PCR products are denatured to convert them into single-stranded DNA. The single-stranded DNAs are run on a nondenaturing gel. The single strands will form conformations consistent with their specific base pair sequence. The assumption of these specific "snap back" configurations will alter the migration of the mutant strand in the gel compared with the control. Samples that have migration patterns different from the control are then sequenced to identify specific mutations. (Modified from Prosser J. Detecting single-base mutations. Trends Biotechnol 11:238–246, 1993.)

SSCP for SRY

M F 46,XY Swyer's

1 2 3* 4 5 6 7

Sequencing Gel of DNA from Lane 3*

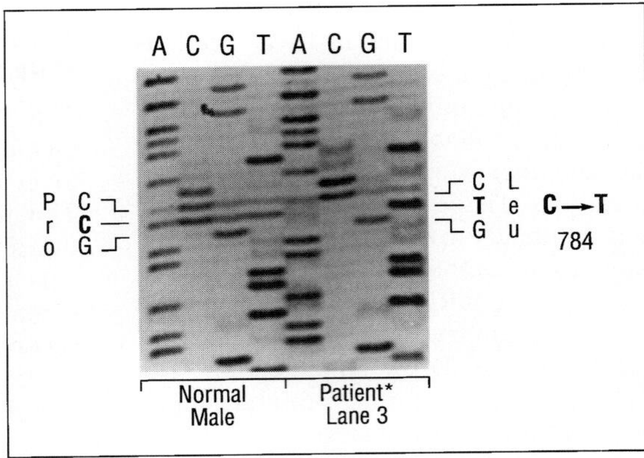

Figure 1–11 ■ Technique of single-stranded conformation polymorphism (SSCP) to identify previously unidentified mutations in the sex-related Y gene (*SRY*). The *SRY* gene in the DNAs of control subjects (male and female) and subjects with Swyer's syndrome (n = 7) was amplified by use of PCR and specific primers for the conserved region of *SRY*. The amplified products were denatured and run on a nondenaturing gel. The DNA of one of the 46,XY sex-reversed females (Swyer's syndrome), lane 3(*), has a distinctive migration pattern compared with that of the control male. Sequencing of the DNA from the subject in lane 3 revealed a single missense mutation (C → T), changing a proline to a leucine and inactivating the *SRY* gene.

of short segments of DNA. In general, SSCP works best with PCR products that are 100 to 250 bp in length. In Figure 1–11, the PCR product of the conserved region of the mammalian *SRY* has been denatured to separate the DNA strands and then electrophoresed on a nondenaturing gel. The DNA samples in each of the lanes come from seven subjects with 46,XY gonadal dysgenesis (Swyer's syndrome). Control male and female DNAs are placed to the extreme right and left. The sample in lane 3 migrates differently from all of the other samples. Elution of the sample from the gel and sequencing revealed a missense mutation in the conserved region of the *SRY* gene. Overall, PCR-SSCP is well suited for identifying the presence but not the precise identity of new mutations. The technique has obvious value in the genetic analysis of families in which members carry a spontaneously arising mutation that has not been previously characterized.

Denaturing Gradient Gel Electrophoresis

This method is based on the electrophoretic mobility of a double-stranded DNA molecule through linearly increasing concentrations of a denaturing agent. Denaturing gradient gel electrophoresis (DGGE) literally separates fragments according to their denaturing properties. Consequently, the success of DGGE depends on the careful choice of denaturing conditions. Foramide and urea are mainly employed as the denaturing agents, but increasing temperature gradients are frequently used by many investigators. A DNA duplex with a mismatched pair denatures more rapidly than does a perfectly matched duplex. If denaturation occurs, it will be accompanied by a decrease in migration on the gel and will appear at a higher molecular weight than the perfectly matched control duplex. The mismatched duplex can be eluted off the gel and sequenced to characterize the specific mutation. The PCR-DGGE technique is extremely powerful when it is applied to the detection of heterozygous nucleotide variants. The continuous denaturation and reannealing of single-stranded molecules during PCR allow the formation of homoduplexes as well as hybrid heteroduplex molecules. The presence of a single mismatch within the heteroduplexes greatly decreases their melting temperature, allowing separation from the homoduplexes and an easier visual detection of the mutants. With DNA fragments up to 500 bp, DGGE has high sensitivity and will detect 99 percent of the sequence changes if gel conditions are optimized. This scanning technique detects approximately 50 percent of all single-base changes.[16] Although this is a rapidly evolving field, the technique of DGGE has withstood the test of time.

Heteroduplex Method

This technique is virtually identical to SSCP in concept, but instead of separating single-stranded molecules on the basis of molecular shape, it separates double-stranded heteroduplex molecules. Particular mismatches and their location in the double-stranded fragment distort the usual shape and alter the mobility of the fragment. In a nondenaturing gel, a heteroduplex with a single mismatch will have a different mobility from the corresponding duplex without the mismatch, allowing the separation of the two. Initially, a special acrylamide matrix (Hydrolink) was used, but normal acrylamide has been substituted more recently. Heteroduplex analysis probably detects 80 percent of the mutations and like SSCP is an easy technique to perform. It has been suggested that a combination of SSCP and heteroduplex analysis might detect close to 100 percent of mutations. If this were the case, the same PCR-amplified fragment could be prepared for electrophoresis in two ways.

Automated Sequencing

DNA sequencing is the ultimate technique for detecting and identifying mutations. In routine diagnostic use, it is not an attractive tool because it involves a number of demanding technical and interpretative procedures. In cases in which mutations have been identified, one of the preceding techniques is often sufficient for detection. However, DNA sequencing is a powerful technique that is useful when the nature of the mutation is not known. The DNA sequence information obtained from new mutation analysis provides the basis for designing simpler strategies for mutation detection as illustrated before in SSCP, DGGE, heteroduplex analysis, and ASO probing. Obviously, the ultimate tool for detecting DNA sequence variants is DNA sequence analysis. Automated DNA sequencing techniques are likely to replace other scanning techniques because they are able to provide precise information about a mutation that can be used in simpler tests to follow the inheritance of the mutation in an affected family. One can anticipate that future studies will reveal that susceptibility to most diseases is affected not by a single gene but by several. Conversely, each disease-related gene can have one or more possible mutations. Sometimes the sheer numbers of analyses are beyond the scope of the techniques that have been discussed. It is hoped that the solution to this technical challenge will be provided by so-called DNA chip technology.

In the past 5 years, there has been much research devoted to extending blot techniques for DNA sequencing by attaching a large array of DNA probes to a substrate and exposing these arrays to a patient's single-stranded DNA sample. By recording the locations where hybridizations occur and using appropriate software, it is possible to sequence a large length of DNA in a single parallel operation. This technology, when refined, essentially allows large numbers of genetic mutations to be identified simultaneously. The arrays are short segments of synthesized nucleic acids that correspond to the gene under investigation. The DNA probe arrays are bound directly onto small squares of wafer-thin glass or silicon chips. The chips with their attached probes are incubated together with the copies of the patient's gene being tested. If the patient's gene has the same sequence as the probe, it will bind exactly and be detected. Mismatching sequences indicating mutations can be identified automatically by advance software. The power of DNA chip technology over conventional sequencing techniques lies in the large number of probes that can be squeezed onto a single chip. Currently, 16,000 different oligonucleotides can fit onto a chip with an area of less than 1.5 cm^2. In the future, it is anticipated that arrays of oligonucleotides can be immobilized in clusters on solid supports to perform large sets of reactions in a single DNA sample. A silicon chip with its special array of DNA probes could check for drug resistance, cystic fibrosis, a spectrum of sexually transmitted diseases, or even a multigene disorder. One might develop profiles of gene expression rather than look directly for gene mutations by using chips that contain oligonucleotides complementary to mRNA rather than DNA. The applications of sequencing by hybridization are myriad and extend to everything from the Human Genome Project, to DNA fingerprinting, to drug development and evaluation. Streamlining this technology in the next decade will be a major interdisciplinary project in science.

TECHNICAL ADVANCES

Analyte Detection with DNA Labels and Reporter Systems

The easy amplification of DNA targets through techniques such as PCR and techniques to screen for molecular mutations (i.e., SSCP, DGGE, heteroduplex analysis) have helped to rapidly identify a wide spectrum of functionally significant human mutations. The enormous versatility in DNA diagnostics and its use in combination with other systems is illustrated by the detection of minute amounts of antigens by means of antibody-DNA conjugates and recombinant cell assay.

Immuno-PCR

In this technique, a linker molecule with bispecific binding affinity for DNA and antibodies is used to attach a DNA molecular marker specifically to an antigen-antibody complex.[35] This results in the formation of a specific antigen-antibody–DNA conjugate. The attached marker DNA can then be amplified by PCR with the appropriate primers (Fig. 1–12). In principle, the extremely high sensitivity of immuno-PCR should permit this technology to be applied to the detection of single antigen molecules. No method is currently available with this level of sensitivity. Immuno-PCR demonstrates that current antigen detection systems can be enhanced by many orders of magnitude simply by the introduction of PCR or recombinant DNA technology. The controllable sensitivity and the simple procedure of

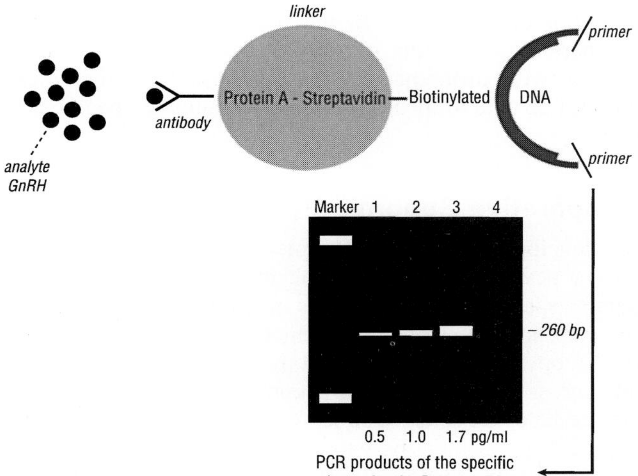

Figure 1–12 ■ Illustration of the principle of the technique of immuno-PCR. This figure demonstrates the antibody to a specific analyte (e.g., GnRH) linked to an intermediary linker (protein A–streptavidin). The streptavidin portion of the linker protein is biotinylated so that it can be linked in turn to an anonymous piece of DNA. Primers that are designed specifically to amplify this segment of reporter DNA increase the sensitivity of the assay by several orders of magnitude over standard radioimmunoassays. In this illustration, increasing amounts of GnRH are quantitated by the intensity of the 260-bp band (lanes 1 to 3).

immuno-PCR should allow the development of fully automated assay systems without loss in sensitivity and with a great potential promise for applications in clinical diagnostics. It also illustrates how hybridoma and recombinant DNA technology can be combined to enhance the detection of specific low-level analytes such as GnRH. This approach extends the detection limits of immunoassay by a factor of two to three orders of magnitude over the detection limits achieved with conventional enzyme-linked immunosorbent assays.[36] In the future, one can anticipate that the development of new families of coamplifiable DNA labels should increase the potential for the simultaneous detection of multiple analytes. Given the enormous amplification advantages of DNA and the existing means to differentiate DNA on the basis of size and sequence differences, immuno-PCR could provide the basis for a new generation of sensitive multianalyte immunoassays.

Recombinant Cell Assay

A novel but still experimental approach to increase the sensitivity of hormone assays is the use of a gene reporter system with the human estrogen receptor cDNA to quantitate levels of estradiol. The regulatory elements of the reporter system include two tandemly arranged estrogen response elements. The reaction of the estradiol analyte with the estrogen response elements stimulates transcription of the reporter gene β-galactosidase. The activity of the reporter gene is quantitated by the conversion of an enzyme substrate using a colorimetric detection system. Galactosidase activity was converted to estradiol equivalent units by linear interpolation from the standard curve constructed by adding known amounts of estradiol to charcoal-stripped plasma samples. This recombinant cell assay was able to detect estradiol with a sensitivity of less than 0.02 pg/ml. Most commercial assays are able to detect down to 20 pg/ml of estradiol.[37] In the next few years, one will see increasing numbers of similar recombinant cell assay systems with different reporter genes such as luciferase that will be able to measure minute amounts of specific analytes.

Comparative Genomic Hybridization

The development of fluorochrome-labeled probes has provided a new dimension for cytogenetics with the ability to identify specific DNA sequences in resting interphase cells. These techniques, when complemented with confocal laser microscopy, permit the resolutions of intervals on a chromosome as small as 150 kb. If one uses a series of fluorochrome-labeled probes such as for the Y chromosome, one can literally "paint" the entire metaphase chromosome in the color of the specific fluorochrome. Deletions, duplications, or amplifications of DNA can be seen by variations in the intensity of the fluorochrome signal. Comparative genomic hybridization is a novel outgrowth of this technology in which total tumor DNA and normal genomic reference DNA are simultaneously hybridized to normal metaphase spreads. Hybridization of tumor DNA is detected with green-fluorescing fluorescein isothiocyanate–labeled avidin, and the reference DNA is detected with red-fluorescing rhodamine-labeled antidigoxigenin. The relative amounts of tumor and reference DNA bound at a given chromosomal locus are dependent on the relative abundance of those sequences in the two DNA samples and can be quantitated by measurement of the ratio of green to red fluorescence.[38] Amplification of a specific oncogene (e.g., N-*myc*) in the tumor DNA will produce an elevated green to red ratio, whereas deletions of antioncogenes (e.g., *p53, Rb*) or chromosome loss will cause a reduced ratio. The ability to survey the whole genome in a single hybridization is a distinct advantage over allelic loss studies by RFLPs that target only one locus at a time. Using comparative genomic hybridization, one can generate a complete copy number karyotype for a given tumor or tumor cell line. Comparative genomic hybridization can be used to screen DNA samples from solid tumors to identify and map physical deletions that may uncover mutant suppressor genes. Once these regions have been identified, further studies will be required to determine which loci contain novel oncogenes and which represent coincidental, random DNA amplification characteristic of general genomic instability.

Differential Display Assay for mRNAs

Differential display analysis (DDA), first described by Liang and Pardee,[39] is a procedure for quantitative detection of differentially expressed genes. The advantage of DDA is that it permits simultaneous identification of genes that are up- or down-regulated under different conditions. The procedure is based on the PCR amplification of mRNAs of cells or tissues, using a short 5′ arbitrary primer, an oligo (dT)–NN 3′ primer, and radiolabeled deoxyribonucleotide triphosphate. Differential gene expression is visualized by autoradiography after electrophoretic separation (Fig. 1–13). The cDNA bands are then recovered from the gel, reamplified by PCR, and molecularly cloned for sequencing

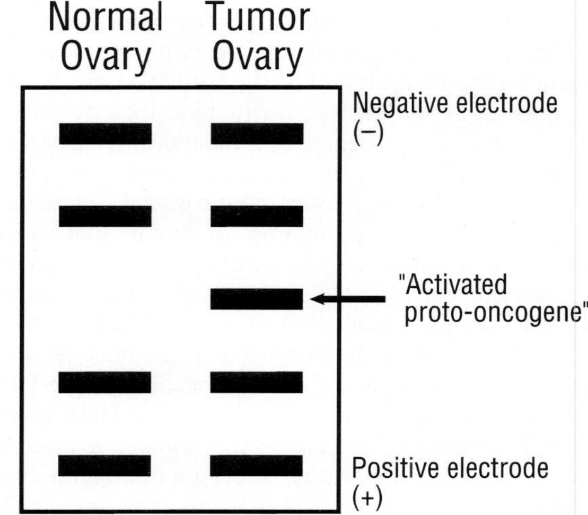

Figure 1–13 ■ The principle of differential display of eukaryotic mRNA. Differential display of mRNAs enables one to isolate those genes that are differentially expressed in different tissues (normal versus tumor) and under different conditions (i.e., stimulated versus nonstimulated). Arbitrary primers are designed to amplify the cDNAs after reverse transcription. The different mRNA subpopulations are resolved on a DNA sequencing gel.

and further identification. The DDA has several technical advantages over subtractive and differential hybridization. With DDA, the band patterns are obtained in 2 to 3 days and the clones in 5 days. DDA allows the simultaneous detection of both groups of differentially expressed genes (i.e., tumor suppressors and oncogenes) and requires only 1 μg of mRNA per 100 lanes of the gel. This PCR-based method has important uses in reproductive endocrinology, cancer, and developmental biology.

Microsatellite Regions

The continued analysis of polymorphisms within the human genome has generated more and more RFLPs that can be used in following the inheritance pattern of human disease. The source of polymorphic markers has increased with the observation that short interspersed tandem repeats or microsatellites are frequently highly polymorphic and can be analyzed by use of PCR techniques. Microsatellites composed of mononucleotide, dinucleotide, trinucleotide, and tetranucleotide repeats are more random in their distribution and can be scored by PCR. These polymorphisms can be detected even within simple sequence repeats, such as dinucleotides. The search for these polymorphisms has been facilitated by the advent of yeast artificial chromosomes technology, which has made it possible to isolate large, contiguous segments of DNA from a specific locus that can then be screened for segments detecting RFLPs and simple sequence repeat polymorphisms. In fact, Weissenbach and colleagues[40] have used microsatellite markers on a large scale combined with a multiplex genotyping procedure to construct a genomic map with greater than 0.7 heterozygosity and covering a linkage distance spanning 90 percent of the genome with an average distance between adjacent markers of about 5 cM. These dinucleotide and trinucleotide polymorphisms can be analyzed in single cells (e.g., sperm, polar body, blastomeres, forensic samples, ancient DNA).[41] A specific example of the value of this technology is in the area of the autosomal dominant endocrine cancer syndromes, multiple endocrine neoplasia type IIA, multiple endocrine neoplasia type IIB, and familial medullary thyroid carcinoma. In the past, predictive testing for the inheritance of mutant alleles in individuals at risk for these disorders has been limited by the availability of highly informative and closely linked linking markers. However, this technology has enabled the development of accurate linkage-based genetic testing by use of highly informative linking markers that are tightly linked to each of these disease loci. The genotyping for these polymorphisms is performed by PCR, thus requiring relatively small amounts of genomic DNA, and results can be obtained within a matter of days compared with several weeks for Southern hybridization procedures (Fig. 1–14). The value of linkage-based testing systems such as RFLPs and simple sequence repeat polymorphisms will depend on the number and complexity of mutations that are identified in a specific gene. If, as in the case of cystic fibrosis, these mutations turn out to be heterogeneous (i.e., about 130 have been identified) or if a number of mutations are not readily found, linkage-based studies may continue to play an important role in predictive testing for many genetic disorders well into the future.[42] At a practical level, the

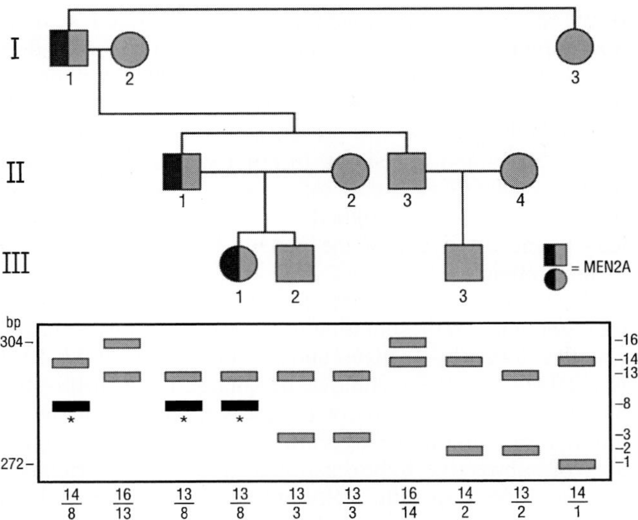

Figure 1–14 ■ The use of microsatellite DNA markers or simple sequence repeat polymorphisms to follow the segregation of multiple endocrine neoplasia type IIA (MEN2A). The gene responsible for MEN2A was mapped to the proximal part of the long arm of chromosome 10 (10q). A locus on 10q close to the centromere was found to contain 16 different microsatellite repeats. These dinucleotide repeats ranged in size from 272 to 304 bp. A single individual at a given genetic locus carries only two variations of these polymorphic simple sequence repeats. This figure illustrates a family with MEN2A in which three family members are affected (I-1, II-1, III-1). For simplicity, the different alleles at this locus are numbered 1 to 16, corresponding to the actual sizes of the alleles (272 to 304 bp). It is clear that the three individuals within the family who have MEN2A and medullary carcinoma of the thyroid all have the numbered 8 allele. The specific gene causing this disorder has been isolated by positional cloning. The gene called *ret* is a proto-oncogene, encodes a tyrosine kinase–type receptor, and maps close to this polymorphic locus on 10q. Current studies rely on the direct detection of activating mutations in the *ret* proto-oncogene. The principal value of microsatellite loci is the high degree of polymorphisms associated with these simple sequence repeats (trinucleotides, dinucleotides, or tetranucleotides). (Modified from Howe JR, Lairmore TC, Mishra SK, et al. Improved predictive test for MEN2, using flanking dinucleotide repeats and RFLPs. Am J Hum Genet 51:1430–1442, 1992.)

development of these high-density microsatellite-based maps will help in the mapping of genes causing less common genetic disorders, allowing prenatal diagnosis and eventual gene cloning. A high-resolution map of this sort is also required for identifying the genetic components of complex common diseases such as heart disease and behavioral disorders. These brute force accomplishments point out that not all science needs to be "curiosity driven."

Representational Difference Analysis

One of the most challenging areas in DNA diagnostics is the identification of sequence differences between individuals or, as in the case of cancer, differences between tumor and genomic DNA in the same individual. This type of comparative analysis involves whole genomes and would include the identification of polymorphic variation between individuals. The applications of this type of technology might include differences due to foreign DNA segments from an infecting pathogen that has integrated into the host genome, induced and naturally occurring mutations producing genetic disease, and genomic rearrangements in cancer cells. The last would have to be highly purified cancer cells to avoid the presence of normal stroma from the cancer biopsy specimen. In other words, a single technology that defines small differences between two DNA populations could be applied to these problems and could lead to the discovery of the genetic basis for many types of phenomena.

The technique for cloning the differences between complex genomes, representational difference analysis (RDA), was developed by Lisitsyn and coworkers[43] in 1993. RDA is a takeoff on the technique of subtractive hybridization but uses PCR to enrich for differences that are identified initially by subtractive hybridization. One of the original uses of subtractive hybridization without PCR enrichment was to clone Y-specific DNA probes. In this approach, an excess of denatured sheared DNA from a female (driver DNA) was denatured and allowed to hybridize with restriction enzyme–cleaved male DNA (tester DNA). Y chromosome–specific DNA that was free after the hybridization reaction was allowed to self-anneal and was cloned after ligation into the acceptor site of a plasmid. RDA is fundamentally a similar process except that special adapters are linked to the fractionated Y DNA sample (tester sample) so that only self-reannealed Y molecules have these adapters at their 5′ ends. These Y-specific molecules can be amplified at an exponential rate by using primers that are specific for these adapters. Using this modification, one is able to enrich for the unique sequences in the target DNA to a magnitude of 10^6 compared with only 100 or 1000 times with standard subtraction hybridization. The application of RDA should provide an economical route to the solution of many problems in reproductive biology.

Genomic Mismatch Scanning

Genomic mismatch scanning is also a technique that compares whole genomes, but rather than trying to identify differences, the strategy is to identify regions that are shared in common by individuals with a diseased phenotype. This technique is obviously designed to decipher the etiology of more complex, multigenic disorders such as polycystic ovarian disease. The technique of genomic mismatch scanning also involves DNA hybridization and starts out similarly by treating the two genomes with restriction enzymes to produce DNA fragments of varying size. In contrast to RDA, one sample is treated so that methyl groups are tacked on at intervals all along the DNA fragments. Once altered in this way, the two samples are melted to produce single-stranded DNA, then mixed together and allowed to hybridize. The result is a mixture of double-stranded DNA fragments, some containing two methylated strands from the first sample, some containing two unmethylated strands from the second sample, and some containing one strand from each. The next chemical step eliminates those duplexes that are derived from only one sample, and the last step eliminates those strands from different samples that contain mismatches. This leaves only those hybrids in which each strand is derived from a different sample, and the strands from the different samples are identical for the two genomes being compared. With this technique, it would be possible to compare the genomes of two individuals with polycystic ovary syndrome from the same or different families to identify common regions that might be inherited from a distant ancestor. Both RDA and genomic mismatch scanning offer the prospect of comparing whole genomes for similarities or differences in one single analysis. The theoretical resolution of these techniques is just beginning to be explored.[44]

PROTOTYPE MUTATIONS IN THE REPRODUCTIVE SCIENCES

The practical applications of DNA technology to the clinical reproductive sciences are gradually increasing in number. At this time, it is the insights concerning human gene structure and regulation that have been most enlightening. These insights continue to enhance our knowledge about the cellular basis for human disease. In this section, certain diseases are mentioned for their interest to reproductive biologists and others because they constitute unique examples of the cellular mechanisms underlying human disease or reflect the practical applications of recombinant DNA technology.

Detection of Covert Y DNA

It is of crucial clinical importance to detect cryptic Y DNA in 45,X subjects who have low-level mosaicism for 46,XY cell lines and subjects carrying structurally abnormal chromosomes that are thought to be Y derivatives. This combination is associated with a high risk of gonadal tumors and virilization. Conventional cytogenetic studies are limited by the numbers of cells that can be examined and the numbers of tissues that can be studied. PCR-based analysis for the presence of Y chromosome sequences and the development of fluorescence in situ hybridization permit the identification of covert Y DNA in 45,X subjects (Fig. 1–15). This can be done most simply by amplifying centromeric repeat sequences (alphoid satellite DNA) on both the Y and X chromosome. Alternatively, the amplification of *ZFY* and *ZFX* provide a similar set of homologous targets on the Y and X chromosomes, respectively. The simultaneous amplification of the *ZFX* target provides an internal control for amplification failures. The use of fluorescence in situ hybridization techniques in 45,X subjects with low-level Y mosaicism is not as sensitive as a PCR-based approach. The precise portion of the Y chromosome involved in oncogenesis is still unknown; however, the Yq11 region is under suspicion at this time.[45] A family of genes from the Yq11 region of Y have been found to be expressed in a small number of subjects with gonadoblastoma. The portion of the Y chromosome identified by deletion mapping and shared in common among subjects who develop gonadal tumors has been called the *GBY* gene for the gonadoblastoma locus on the Y chromosome. It is still uncertain whether there is a specific gene involved in the etiology of these dysgenetic tumors or whether they arise secondarily owing to continued pituitary stimulation of a primitive, immature gonad. The sex-related Y gene *(SRY)* does not appear to play a direct role in oncogenesis because it is not consistently present in subjects with gonadal tu-

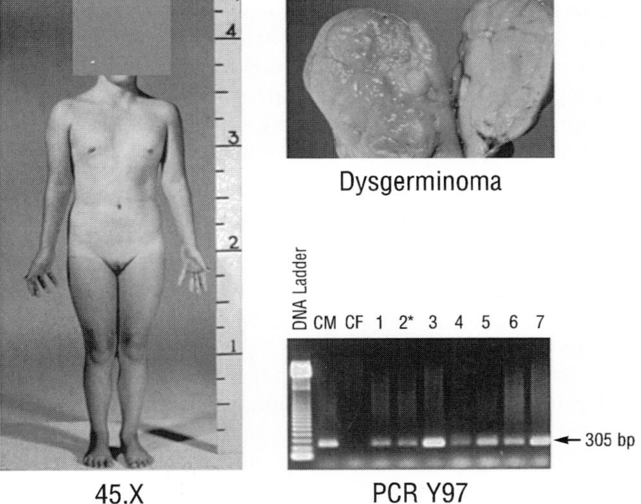

Figure 1–15 ■ This composite figure depicts a 15-year-old female with sexual infantilism who had a peripheral blood karyotype of 45,X. She developed an ipsilateral dysgerminoma and a contralateral gonadoblastoma in her rudimentary streak gonads. Subsequent analysis of 150 metaphase chromosomes revealed two 46,XY cells. Amplification of Y-specific centromeric sequences (Y97) was positive for Y DNA. The first and second lanes are control male (CM) and female (CF) DNAs in which the Y-specific centromeric sequences (alphoid satellite DNA) have been amplified (305 bp) by use of Y-specific primers. The DNA from the patient (mos. 45,X/46,XY) is seen in lane 2(*). The remainder of the DNAs are from individuals with varying degrees of 45,X/46,XY cell lines with morphologically normal or abnormal Y chromosomes.

mors (gonadoblastoma, dysgerminoma).[46] The report of gonadal stromal tumors in mice that are homozygous deleted for α-inhibin adds further speculation as to the relative role of genes versus endocrine environment in the predisposition to dysgenetic tumors.[47] The clinical importance of a low number of Y-positive cells in 45,X patients and the risk of neoplasia with or without virilization require continued inquiry.

Peptide Hormones

The growth hormone (hGH) and human placental lactogen (hPL) genes were two of the first peptide hormone genes in which human mutations were detected. Deletions of the active hGH gene located on the long arm of chromosome 17 (17q22–24) produce a type of growth hormone–deficient phenotype categorized as type IA (Ilig)[48] (Fig. 1–16). Deletions in the active portion of the hPL gene appear to have no functional significance. Individuals who are homozygous deleted for the active hPL gene make no protein, and there is no evidence of any physiologic compensations during pregnancy for its absence.[49] This is an example in which precise knowledge of a human mutation provides instructive insights concerning the physiologic role of a specific pregnancy hormone. There is some evidence from studies of mutations in the hGH gene that individuals with larger deletions are more likely to develop antibodies when growth hormone therapy is initiated. The hGH-hPL gene cluster is a good example of a gene family that has undergone considerable change over eons of time.

A combined pituitary hormone deficiency in humans has been shown to be due to a mutation in the Pit-1 gene, which encodes a transcription factor that is necessary for the development and generation of somatotrophs and two other pituitary cell types (lactotrophs and thyrotrophs). It appears that Pit-1 activates the receptor for growth hormone–releasing hormone and the receptors for both thyroid-releasing factor and dopamine.[50] In the absence of these receptors during early development, there is lack of pituitary cell stimulation and proliferation. Pit-1 is therefore a pituitary-specific transcription factor whose protein product has the genes encoding the receptors for growth hormone–releasing hormone, thyroid-releasing factor, and dopamine as its target. A mutation in Pit-1 that was present in dwarfed mice (Snell dwarf) provided the clue to search for a similar mutation in humans.[51, 52] These studies provided clear evidence for cell-specific transcription factors such as Pit-1 that function as developmental regulators and ensure the proliferation and survival of cells such as somatotrophs, lactotrophs, and thyrotrophs during mammalian organogenesis. In short, Pit-1 is a model for the coordinate control of cell proliferation and differentiation phenotype by tissue-specific transcription factors during organogenesis.[53] The Pit-1 mutation in humans is one of the first involving a transcription factor. Weiss and colleagues[54] described a single nucleotide substitution in the LH-β gene changing a wild-type amino acid glutamine to arginine at position 54. This was present in the homozygous state in a male with sexual infantilism, low testosterone, and elevated immunoactive LH. The hormone profile of the proband was consistent with testicular failure, but responsiveness to hCG in terms of testicular secretion was normal. The analysis of the proband and his family pointed out that functionally active LH is not critical for the production of the male phenotype. These studies also pointed out that the mutations affecting pituitary trophic hormones in humans will prove to be heterogeneous in causation. This should

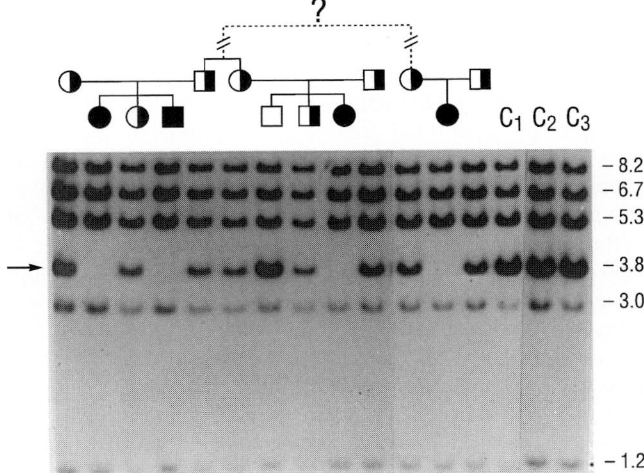

Figure 1–16 ■ This Southern blot illustrates the deletion of the active growth hormone gene in Ilig type IA growth hormone deficiency. The 3.8-kb band (*arrow*) is absent in affected individuals and reduced in intensity in heterozygous deleted carriers. (From Phillips JA III, Hjelle BL, Seeburg PH, et al. Molecular basis for familial isolated growth hormone deficiency. Proc Natl Acad Sci USA 78:6372–6375, 1981.)

not come as any surprise to the astute clinical observer of growth disorders in mice and humans.

Steroid Pathway Mutations

The correlations between steroid pathway mutations and clinical phenotypes, although exciting, are too numerous to cover within the context of this presentation. All of the human steroid pathway genes have been isolated, cloned, and mapped to specific chromosomes. Mutations have been identified in the majority of these genes. The spectrum of mutation points out on one hand the simplicity of these mutations and, on the other hand, the complexities involved in understanding the specific biochemical basis for a single phenotype. The gene encoding the active 21-hydroxylase gene that maps to the short arm of chromosome 6 has a wide spectrum of known mutants ranging from simple deletions, which are present in the more classical forms of congenital adrenal hyperplasia, through gene conversions to single-base substitutions, which have been described in two or three instances of late-onset congenital adrenal hyperplasia. The paucity of functionally documented mutations in late-onset congenital adrenal hyperplasia raises the question of whether this is a real entity.[55] There is considerable versatility in the prenatal diagnosis of 21-hydroxylase deficiency, because a combination of a 21-hydroxylase probe, a C_4B probe, an HLA-B probe, and an HLA-DRβ probe constitutes a useful panel for diagnosis in that more than 95 percent of families with a surviving affected child are informative for at least one of these probes.[56] Studies of steroid pathway genes have revealed that the activities of 17-hydroxylation and 17,20-lyase are catalyzed by a single 17-hydroxylase gene (P45017α) that is mapped to chromosome 10 (10q24.3) in humans.[57] The steroid pathway enzymes are extremely complex because those localized in the endoplasmic reticulum, such as P45017α, require the assistance of NADPH for reduction through the microsomal flavoprotein NADPH–cytochrome P450 reductase; whereas the mitochondrial steroid hydroxylases P450scc and P45011β are reduced by NADPH through an electron transport chain involving a flavoprotein, adrenodoxin reductase, and an iron-sulfur protein, adrenodoxin, to function properly. One can even suspect that other proteins encoded by additional genes are required to put these enzymes in the proper orientation with respect to their specific substrates. The complexity of this process raises the question of whether the precise cellular pathology of certain diseases will ever be completely understood. It is also interesting to note that deletions of the 21-hydroxylase gene and C_4B gene in the mouse appear to be embryonic lethals.[58] Studies of the 5α-reductase gene responsible for the conversion of testosterone to dihydrotestosterone indicate that two genes are involved rather than one. It appears that one of these genes encodes a protein that is active at a more acidic pH and is expressed specifically in genital tissues. The other gene is active at an alkaline pH and is expressed in extragenital somatic tissues. These insights have furthered our understanding of the biochemical basis for the various forms of undermasculinization syndromes that have a genetic basis in 46,XY subjects.[59] Finally, mutations have been identified in the aromatase gene that lead to in utero masculinization of female fetuses.[60] The aromatase gene has turned out to be under the control of many different types of tissue-specific promoters and subject to regulation by diverse *cis-* and *trans-*acting elements. Investigations into the regulation of this important gene should prove to be interesting and important to our understanding of many disorders in reproductive medicine.

Peptide and Steroid Receptors

Mutations in the growth hormone receptor gene lead to the clinical phenotype known as Laron dwarfism. The majority of the mutations in the growth hormone receptor gene to date have been deletions. Homozygous inactivating mutations have been described in the LH receptor gene (*LHR*) within two different families leading to testicular and ovarian resistance to LH.[61] The mutation in the family with multiple affected members is a nonsense mutation and truncates the protein for the LH receptor. Compound heterozygous inactivating mutations in the LH receptor have been described in males with Leydig cell hypoplasia and testicular failure.[62]

The FSH receptor has received considerable attention, but it was only recently that a C–T transition (alanine to valine substitution) at residue 189 in the extracellular ligand binding domain of the receptor was found to segregate with the phenotype of ovarian failure.[63] The receptors for both FSH and LH map close to each other on 2p.

Mutations in the more recently cloned cDNA for the GnRH receptor have not been identified to date.[64] The cloning of this receptor provides a reagent with which to search for genetic linkage to particular disorders that involve hypothalamic signaling, such as hypothalamic amenorrheas (inactivating mutations) or disturbances in regulation such as polycystic ovary syndrome (activating mutations).

Because these receptors are G protein–coupled receptors, it will also be interesting to continue to look for mutations in the receptors and coupled G proteins in the DNAs of a variety of subjects. The first example of a genetic defect in a G protein–coupled hormone receptor is a frame shift deletion in the antidiuretic hormone (arginine vasopressin) V_2 receptor that results in X-linked congenital nephrogenic diabetes insipidus.[65] Genetic defects have been found in the G protein–coupled photoreceptor rhodopsin. Individuals with such defects are affected by autosomal dominant retinitis pigmentosa.[66] Mutations have now been described in a wide range of G protein–coupled receptors and in the genes encoding the G protein itself. Mutations have now been described in a wide range of steroid receptors ranging from the androgen receptor through the glucocorticoid receptor and thyroid receptor to the receptor for vitamin D.[67] The majority of these mutations lead to syndromes that involve resistance to the specific ligand. Mutations in the glucocorticoid receptor lead to increased serum levels of cortisol and increased stimulation of the adrenal cortex by adrenocorticotropic hormone, leading to mild degrees of adrenal androgen overproduction and clinical hirsutism. Mutations in the gene for the androgen receptor have now been identified in a wide range of phenotypes from complete androgen resistance to males with azoospermia.[68] The latter, of which three have been described, do not appear to have any distinctive phenotype or characteristic spermiogram, except for oligospermia or azoospermia. Mutations in the gene encoding the receptor for thyroid hormone (v-*erb A*) leading to thyroid resistance have been described in several kindreds and are transmitted in a mendelian manner. In addition to mutations in gene-encoding receptors, many orphan receptors for which the ligands are unknown have been identified. These receptors have been euphemistically called orphan or receptoroids.

Miscellaneous Mutations

Genes that have been involved in spermatogenesis have been a source of intense interest during the past several years. The tentative mapping of a gene involved in spermatogenesis to the proximal portion of the long arm of the Y chromosome has culminated in the detection of several mutations in this region in a small series of azoospermic males. These mutations described by Ann Chandley and her group in Edinburgh appear to represent spontaneous germ mutations.[69] David Page and his group studied the DNAs of 89 infertile, azoospermic males and found overlapping de novo deletions spanning a common region of about 500 kb within Yq11. Using the technique of exon trapping, they were able to identify a novel gene called *DAZ1* (deleted in azoospermia) that is expressed specifically in the testis. A similar type of deletion was identified by the same group in two males with oligospermia.[70, 71] The father of one of the males is mosaic for this mutation. This work has been confirmed in a much larger group of azoospermic and oligospermic subjects by Peter Vogt[72] from Heidelberg. Further analysis is necessary to identify mutations in *DAZ1* in nondeleted azoospermic patients. Finally, the cDNA for the long-sought gene for H-Y antigen has been isolated by deletion mapping and microcapillary liquid chromatography with electrospray mass spectrometry. Other than a minor histocompatibility locus, the function of the H-Y antigen protein remains unknown.[73]

Although the majority of genotype-phenotype studies have involved the analysis of a candidate gene, the detection of mutations in Kallmann's syndrome followed a somewhat different course. For many years, it was known that there are a series of contiguous genes on the short arm of the X chromosome that may produce syndromes involving ichthyosis, anosmia, and hypogonadotropic hypogonadism. Studies of this region led to the isolation of a gene that appears to encode a cell adhesion molecule that is in part responsible for a migration of the GnRH neurons from the region of the olfactory placode to the hypothalamus. Mutations in this gene or region on Xp lead to Kallmann's syndrome with anosmia.[74] On the other hand, studies of the human GnRH gene itself, which is mapped to the long arm of chromosome 8, have not revealed any mutations to date. Interestingly, the hypogonadal (*hpg*) mouse is the result of a large truncation in the GnRH gene resulting in the failure to synthesize GnRH.

IMPORTANT NEW CONCEPTS IN THE MOLECULAR MECHANISM OF DISEASE

Disease-Causing Mutations in Cell-Signaling Proteins

Within the last year, there has been an exponential increase in the numbers of identified mutations that affect cell-signaling proteins. Many of these mutations involve oncogenes and tumor suppressor genes, but there are others that cause some of the well-recognized phenotypes associated with endocrine disease. The majority of these are discussed with their specific diseases, but a few prototypes are discussed here.

Inactivating Mutations

Inactivating mutations literally destroy the activity of the protein product that is encoded by the specific gene. Many such mutations have been described to date that involve the steroid hormone receptors and to a lesser degree the receptors for polypeptide hormones. More interesting is the identification of both germ line and somatic mutations in signaling proteins that are downstream from the initiating receptor. Many receptors activate second messenger systems by coupling with G proteins. G proteins are heterotrimeric proteins that consist of α-, β-, and γ-subunits. The α-subunit protein appears to be important in signal transduction and in the resting state is coupled with guanosine diphosphate. Activation of the G protein by the activated receptor causes disassociation of the α-subunit from the other subunits and displacement of guanosine diphosphate with guanosine triphosphate. The α-subunit coupled with guanosine triphosphate is now in its active state prepared to activate adenylate cyclase or phospholipase A, depending on the nature of the second messenger system. Mutations that inactivate the α-subunit G protein have been identified in Albright's hereditary osteochondrodystrophy, leading to resistance (complete or partial) to parathyroid hormone, thyroid hormone, and occasionally gonadotropins.[75] The G protein mutations that occur in Albright's hereditary osteochondrodystrophy are unique in that they are vertically transmitted within families who have this disorder.

Activating Mutations

On the other hand, somatic mutations have been described in G proteins in which the G protein is turned on in a constitutive manner, leading to continuous stimulation of cyclic adenosine monophosphate. In ordinary circumstances, the α-subunit of the G protein has the ability to hydrolyze guanosine triphosphate back to the inactive resting guanosine diphosphate state. Mutations in the G protein that are responsible for this activity lead to perpetual activation of guanosine triphosphate and uninterrupted stimulation of the second messenger system. These activating mutations, which have been described in 30 percent of growth hormone–producing pituitary tumors and in a syndrome known as the McCune-Albright syndrome, provide interesting clinical phenotypes.[76, 77] Somatic mutations in G protein have been described in the ovary and skin of individuals with McCune-Albright or gonadotropin-independent precocious puberty syndrome. Spontaneously occurring mutations of this type in this or other structurally related receptor genes in vivo may therefore *subvert* the normal function of these receptors and result in human disease states associated with uncontrolled cell growth, including neoplasia and atherosclerosis. In addition, the identification of such mutant receptors may provide specific disease markers and pharmacologic targets for therapeutic interventions.

These mutations probably represent the tip of the iceberg in terms of mutations that are and may potentially be present in signaling or transduction systems. Genetic mutation or mutations in signaling systems could involve the nucleotide sequences encoding the regulatory G proteins or specific domains of the ionic channel, as shown in the case of the chloride channel in cystic fibrosis. Detailed analysis of these mutations not only holds out promise for treatment, but it also continues to provide deep and general insights into cell biology, biochemistry, and physiology. It is anticipated in the next several years that further investigations of the genes encoding the proteins in these signaling systems will produce a myriad of mutations as the basis for certain diseases, including certain types of cancer, aging, and immunologic impairment. The cycle of searching for germ line and somatic mutations in signaling system proteins as the basis for many human afflictions is just beginning. Expectations are high. The emphasis to date has been on receptor and G protein genes. It is just as likely that mutations producing polycystic ovary syndrome could be farther downstream in protein kinase C or an ion channel gene, which could uncouple the protein products of these genes from their normal upstream regulator phospholipase C. The possibility of genetic defects within ion channel genes as causative agents in hypothalamic signaling disturbances is exciting to imagine. Studies of more subtle mutations or variations in GnRH signaling proteins should provide insights into a wide variety of hypothalamic pulsing abnormalities.

Uniparental Disomy (Genomic Imprinting): Prototype Prader-Willi Syndrome

Prader-Willi syndrome appears to be due to a microdeletion on the proximal long arm of chromosome 15 in humans. This phenotype is manifested when this deletion occurs in the chromosome 15 that is inherited from the father. The normal Prader-Willi gene, because of imprinting, is expressed predominantly from only the paternal chromosome. The current candidate gene is the γ-aminobutyric acid receptor, β_3-subunit *(GABRB3)*. In fact, if the deletion is present on the chromosome inherited from the mother, an entirely different syndrome known as the Angelman syndrome is present.

Studies of Prader-Willi syndrome led to the discovery that some individuals with Prader-Willi syndrome had inherited both chromosomes 15 from the mother without any paternal contribution.[78] This phenomenon of uniparental disomy occurred also, but rarely, in cystic fibrosis for chromosome 7 and in the aniridia–Wilms' tumor complex syndrome. From these observations evolve concepts concerning genomic imprinting and the differential functional effect of a mutation, depending on which parent transmitted the mutation. One of the suspected causes of uniparental disomy in Prader-Willi syndrome is the initial formation of a 47, + 15 embryo in which two of the three 15 homologues are derived from the mother. In a subsequent mitotic division of the embryo, the chromosome 15 derived from the father is lost, and the resultant embryo now has two chromosomes 15 that are maternally derived. For people in obstetrics and gynecology, it raises the question of investigating normal disomic individuals who demonstrate tissue mosaicism either in chorionic villus or amniotic fluid sampling.

Gene Expansions and Unstable DNA

One of the most interesting and disturbing developments in the last 2 years has been the observation that the expansion of certain trinucleotide repeats is responsible for disease. Diseases caused by this genetic phenomenon include fragile X syndrome (*FMR1*), which causes mental retardation; spinal and bulbar atrophy (*SBMA*), which involves muscle weakness and neural degeneration; and myotonic dystrophy (*DM*), which is characterized by cardiac arrhythmias, cataracts, testicular failure, and rarely ovarian failure.[79] The amplification of these short sequences of DNA was first demonstrated in the fragile X syndrome, in which affected individuals carry more than 200 copies of the trinucleotide repeat CGG within the *FMR1* gene compared with 6 to 54 (mean, 29) in the normal population. Subsequent studies of these triple repeat mutations in the fragile X syndrome indicated that large CGG expansions or amplifications appear to be a predominantly female meiotic event. A similar situation is present in myotonic dystrophy (*DM*), and more recently a similar phenomenon has been found in the first exon of the gene for the androgen receptor (*AR*). Myotonic dystrophy develops in conjunction with the expansion of a $(CTG)^n$ repeat situated in the 3′ untranslated region of the DM kinase gene (myotonin protein kinase gene). Sometimes the expansion may reach 6 kb. Expansion of these trinucleotide repeats (CAG) within the first exon of the *AR* gene leads to the clinical syndrome of spinal and bulbar atrophy (Kennedy's syndrome). In addition to the neurologic findings, male individuals with Kennedy's syndrome may have gynecomastia and azoospermia. Common among the three disorders are four features: (1) the site of the expansion in affected individuals is a GC-rich repeat; (2) the repeat is present within the mature transcript; (3) the repeat is polymorphic in length among normal individuals; and (4) in affected families, the mutant alleles exhibit meiotic instability leading to the triplet expansion, not encountered with their respective normal although polymorphic alleles.

These trinucleotide repeat elements are clearly premutations and are unstable with the potential to expand from one generation to the next. At present, it is not known precisely what the mechanism of this threshold level of repeats is relative to the inception of these disease phenotypes. Several investigators are at work trying to identify a specific dysfunctional protein that may be produced as a result of the expansion of these repeat elements. The identification of such a protein may help to understand the mental retardation that occurs in the fragile X syndrome and the relationships between these expansions and gonadal function in myotonic dystrophy and Kennedy's disease. Investigators are relishing the prospects of uncovering genes that contain similar repeats prone to expansion that may be at the root of other hereditary defects. Approximately 40 human genes have been identified that contain polymorphic trinucleotide repeats within the transcribed unit.[80] All of these loci have the potential to undergo this novel type of mutagenesis giving rise to human disease.

Gene Insertions and Their Role in Oncogenesis

It has become apparent in the last year that DNA viruses such as human papillomavirus may alter cell cycle control by interfering with certain antioncogenes. In the ordinary cell cycle, antioncogenes such as the retinoblastoma gene or *p53* are negative regulators of the cell cycle. The products of tumor suppressor genes normally act as negative regulators of the cell cycle. This group of genes now includes *p53*, *WT1* (Wilms' tumor), *DCC* (deleted in colon cancer), *NF1* (neurofibromatosis), and *APC* (adenomatosis polyposis coli). In the ordinary cell cycle, they maintain the cell in a G_0 state but when phosphorylated they release this hold on the cell and permit cycling to occur. In the case of the human papillomavirus, the *E7* gene in the virus couples with the retinoblastoma gene and maintains the cell in a constant state of mitotic activity.[81] Similarly, the *E6* gene of the human papillomavirus couples with the *p53* antioncogene and creates the same dysfunction. It is clear that antisense technology may be helpful in ameliorating the impact of the human papillomavirus and its potential role in cervical cancer.

Developmental Systems

In the past year, it is clear from work in *Drosophila* that a large number of genes, approximately 35, are expressed specifically by the oocyte and are crucial for early embryonic development. These genes encoding specific proteins are responsible for localization of these proteins within the oocyte and for the activation of embryonic genes. A large number of well-characterized mutations have been described in these genes leading primarily to fundamental defects in axis formation and embryonic lethality.[82] Clearly the time has come to take this "rogues' gallery" of probes that have been developed in *Drosophila* and apply these to the study of mammalian oocyte-specific gene expression.

ANALYTICAL MODELS OF HUMAN DISEASE

Transgenic animals carry experimentally introduced foreign DNA that has become stably integrated into the animals' genome. For both practical and experimental purposes, one usually strives to have appropriate tissue-specific expression of the foreign gene; this may not predictably occur as evidenced by the first transgenic mouse expressing the growth hormone gene inappropriately in liver rather than mouse pituitary. Pituitary expression of the gene was achieved in subsequent experiments. These accidents of gene integration and inappropriate expression frequently provide opportunities to further analyze gene-protein function in this transgenic system that has become a remarkable analytical model to study many facets of developmental biology.[83] Attempts to have foreign genes stably integrated into the early embryo or to inactivate specific genes to better understand their function are being carried out by many different groups around the world and in many different species. The species used range from *Caenorhabditis elegans* and *Drosophila* to mouse, rat, fish, amphibians, porcine species, bovine species, and subhuman primate. The objectives of different investigators vary considerably; however, the techniques are relatively constant from species to species. The following discussion provides a brief résumé of the two most common techniques to create transgenic animals and some of the interesting murine models of human reproductive disorders.

Techniques

Microinjection

The microinjection of foreign DNA into the pronuclear zygote or rarely in some species into the mature oocyte is one of the most frequently used techniques to generate transgenic animals. In the mouse, this injection is usually made into the male pronucleus simply because it is larger and easier to visualize than is the female pronucleus. Bovine pronuclei are obscured by the cytoplasm, and prior centrifugation is necessary to displace this material to the opposite pole of the zygote. DNA injected at this early stage of development will be propagated to all embryonic and extraembryonic cell lineages of the developing embryo. Integration of the foreign gene into the genome usually occurs at one random chromosomal site before the first cleavage division. This integration site usually harbors multiple copies of the injected sequence. Experience in the transgenic mouse indicates that the level of expression of a given gene from one transgenic mouse to another varies considerably and does not bear a direct relationship to copy number. The efficiency of integration and appropriate tissue expression even in the mouse is still low because 10 to 30 percent of the injected and transferred eggs survive to term. Among the live born, 20 to 30 percent are expected to carry the injected sequences stably integrated in their genome.

Use of Embryonic Stem Cells as Gene Vectors

This technique provides the opportunity to inject into the embryo only those cells that have been shown to have integrated the normal or modified foreign gene. In this technique, primitive, totipotential embryonic cells are removed from a mouse embryo. These cells are cultured further on a fibroblast feeder cell line to maintain their undifferentiated state. In this state, the gene of interest is transfected into these stem cells by any one of several different in vitro gene transfer techniques. Those cells that have incorporated the gene of interest are selected, further cloned, and then injected into the blastocyst stage of a second mouse embryo. The adult mouse will be a chimera containing two different somatic and germ line cell populations, one of which will contain the foreign insert. Breeding of this chimeric mouse with normal animals will result in some offspring that are hemizygous for the foreign gene. Breeding of these hemizygous individuals will produce mice homozygous for the original foreign gene that was inserted into the embryonic stem cells. This system allows one to select for the gene of interest, normal or mutant. It provides the opportunity to create mice mutants or gene "knockouts" for study that are similar to known mutations in humans. Male mice carrying the X-linked mutation for Lesch-Nyhan disease were produced by creating the mutation in embryonic stem cells and injecting the mutant cells into mouse blastocyst to create a chimera. Mating of the chimeric mice resulted in the female's carrying the X-linked *HPRT* mutation. When these carrier females were mated with normal males, half of the male offspring were hypoxanthine phosphoribosyltransferase deficient.[84]

Embryonic stem line transfer may have application to human germ line therapy in that correction of a genetic defect probably does not require a large amount of the normal protein product. The gene known to be deficient in the embryo could be transfected into embryo stem cells from another embryo. Cells expressing the gene appropriately could then be injected into a later stage (blastocyst) human embryo.

Spontaneous and Transgenic Models of Human Reproductive Disorders

To date, there have been some interesting and important murine models of human reproductive diseases. Some of these analytical in vivo models of human disease occur spontaneously, and others are the result of genetic manipulation.

Transgenic Mouse with Polycystic Ovary Syndrome

This is an interesting experimental model in which a chimeric LH-β gene has been used to create a mouse that hypersecretes LH. A unique feature of the gene construct was the addition of the gene for the C-terminal peptide of hCG-β. The expression of this transgene with the addition of the carboxyl portion of hCG-β prolonged the half-life of the LH protein and produced mice with elevated levels of LH, increased testosterone, and cystic ovaries.[85]

Transgenic Mouse with Gonadal Stromal Tumors

Mice that are α-inhibin deficient have been created by targeted deletion of the α-inhibin gene in murine embryonic stem cells. Mice that are homozygous deleted for the null allele (inhibin deficient) develop normally, but every mouse ultimately develops mixed or incompletely differentiated gonadal stromal tumors.[47] The relative role of elevated FSH levels versus α-inhibin deficiency in the etiology of these tumors is still uncertain.

Transgenic Mouse with Ovarian Teratomas

In *Xenopus,* the c-*mos* proto-oncogene product (Mos) is essential for the initiation of oocyte maturation, for the progression from meiosis I to meiosis II, and for the second meiotic metaphase arrest acting as an essential component of the cytostatic factor. The expression of the gene that encodes the c-*mos* protein appears to be oocyte-specific in the mouse and in humans. It is interesting that c-*mos*–deficient mice generated by gene targeting in embryonic stem cells develop ovarian teratomas at a high frequency and have reduced fertility.[86, 87] The role of the c-*mos* gene is probably to prevent parthenogenetic activation of the primary oocyte leading to ovarian teratoma formation. This type of mouse model would be useful in studying the mechanisms of oogenesis, teratogenesis, and infertility in humans.

Obese Female Mice (ob/ob) with Infertility

The recent cloning of a gene (*ob/ob*) that may be involved in human obesity has catalyzed a number of studies to clarify the role of its protein product (leptin) in energy homeostasis.[88] It appears that the *ob* gene product leptin is secreted predominantly by adipose tissue and acts on receptors in the hypothalamus. Mice that are homozygous deleted for the gene that encodes leptin are massively obese and infertile. Their fertility can be restored temporarily by using appropriate hormone replacement (FSH, LH). Exogenous leptin replacement therapy in addition to reducing body mass restores fertility to these genetically obese *ob/ob* females. Weight loss alone induced by food restriction in leptin-deficient mice does not restore fertility without leptin replacement. Fertility can be restored in knockout mice homozygous deleted for the *ob* gene (*ob/ob*) by repeated administration of recombinant leptin. This treatment corrects their ovulatory disorder and leads to successful pregnancy and parturition.[89] All of this suggests a more primary role for leptin in reproduction.

Mice with Implantation Failure

Mice that are homozygous deleted for leukemia inhibitory factor gene *(LIF)* are fertile, but their blastocysts fail to implant and do not develop. The blastocysts are viable and can develop if they are transferred to wild-type pseudopregnant recipients. Under such circumstances, they can implant and carry to term. It appears that the uterine expression of *LIF* is essential for implantation in the mouse. It will be interesting to see whether other mammals share this requirement.[90]

In addition to these transgenic models, there are numerous transgenic models of embryonic lethality and sterility. Several of these models have occurred through the accidental disruption of an endogenous gene at the time of insertion of a foreign gene (insertional mutagenesis).[91] As our knowledge of the spectrum of lethal molecular mutations increases in mice, we can begin to search for defects involving similar critical genes such as connexin 37 in humans.[92] Potentially, one could screen DNA from euploidic abortuses for normalcy or abnormalcy of critical genes for collagen, actin, and so on. Parents could then be studied for molecular heterozygosity. At that point, in vitro fertilization and gene therapy become therapeutic options.

FUTURE

The isolation of new genes, the rapid detection of unknown mutations in human DNA, and the identification of differences between genomes require the continued development of many of the techniques mentioned in this chapter (genomic mismatch scanning, differential expression of mRNAs, representational difference analysis, and others). It is clear, however, that the precise nature and location of a mutation must ultimately be defined by DNA sequencing and functional analysis. Many different strategies are being developed to make direct sequencing of DNA from the amplified PCR product rapid, accurate, and efficient. These automated methods for sequencing use fluorescence detection technology. Although they are expensive, they represent the "ideal" mutation scanning technique.

The pace of improvements in gene isolation and mutation detection techniques has been extremely rapid during the past few years. Many promising advances are being tested in many laboratories and within the Human Genome Project. A rapid, accurate, sensitive, and inexpensive method of direct sequencing from the amplified PCR product will be the ultimate in automated mutation analysis. The refinement of this direct sequencing technique will be upon us in a short time and will be the catapult for more widespread preclinical DNA diagnosis.

These new, evolving techniques are helping us to understand the biochemical basis for disease and the etiology of fundamental developmental aberrations. The applications of these techniques to clinical medicine will change the way that medicine is practiced in the future. Diagnosis will become presymptomatic. At present, the clinical sciences are largely an inferential science in which one reasons from a phenotype to a genotype. In the future, physicians will have to identify individuals who are at risk for specific diseases and suggest DNA analysis. Some of us may have preneoplastic or precardiac genotypes, and appropriate measures need to be put in place to limit the expression of these deleterious genes. Obviously, there is still a large hiatus between diagnosis and therapy. As the second-generation biotechnology products develop, one will see techniques and maneuvers such as antisense technology that are developed to control the expression of inappropriate genes. These techniques include blocking the genetic code by use of novel classes of molecules to block receptors and designing organic molecules to interfere with signaling pathways. The importance of animal models for disease created by altering specific genes and the importance of animal models for testing gene therapy cannot be underestimated. Overall we can look forward to an exciting decade that will bring about revolutions in our conceptual knowledge of biology and provide us with unifying principles to compare and analyze the evolution of species.

General Reading

Adolph KW. Gene and Chromosome Analysis (Methods in Molecular Genetics). San Diego, Academic Press, 1993.

Alberts B, Bray D, Lewis J, et al. Molecular Biology of the Cell, 3rd ed. New York, Garland Publishing, 1994.

Costantini F, Jaenisch R (eds). Genetic Manipulation of the Early Mammalian Embryo. Cold Spring Harbor, NY, Cold Spring Harbor Laboratory, 1985.

Emery AEH, Malcolm S. An Introduction to Recombinant DNA in Medicine, 2nd ed. New York, John Wiley & Sons, 1995.

Freifelder D. Molecular Biology, 2nd ed. Boston, Jones & Bartlett, 1987.

Keller GH, Manak MM. DNA Probes, 2nd ed. New York, Stockton Press, 1996.

King RC, Stansfield WD. A Dictionary of Genetics, 3rd ed. New York, Oxford University Press, 1985.

Lewin B. Genes V. New York, Oxford University Press, 1994.

Stine GJ. The New Human Genetics. Dubuque, IA, William C. Brown Publishers, 1989.

Watson JD, Hopkins NH, Roberts JW, et al. Molecular Biology of the Gene, 4th ed. Menlo Park, CA, Benjamin/Cummings Publishing Company, 1987.

Watson JD, Tooze J, Kurtz DT. Recombinant DNA: A Short Course. New York, Scientific American Books, 1983.

Weatherall DJ. The New Genetics and Clinical Practice, 3rd ed. Oxford, UK, Oxford University Press, 1991.

References

1. Hudson TJ, Stein LD, Gerety SS, et al. An STS based map of the human genome. Science 270:1945–1954, 1995.
2. Watson JD, Crick FHC. Molecular structure of nucleic acids: A structure for deoxyribose nucleic acid. Nature 171:737–738, 1953.
3. Kazazian HH Jr. Globin gene structure and the nature of mutation. Birth Defects 23:77–92, 1987.
4. Adelman JP, Bond CT, Douglass J, et al. Two mammalian genes transcribed from opposite strands of the same DNA locus. Science 235:1514–1517, 1987.
5. Speek M, Miller WL. Hybridization of the complementary mRNAs for P450c21 (steroid 21-hydroxylase) and tenascin-X is prevented by sequence-specific binding of nuclear proteins. Mol Endocrinol 9:1655–1665, 1995.
6. Emeson RB, Hedjran F, Yeakley JM, et al. Alternative production of calcitonin and CGRP mRNA is regulated at the calcitonin-specific splice acceptor. Nature 341:76–80, 1989.
7. Nakanishi S, Inoue A, Kita T, et al. Nucleotide sequence of cloned cDNA for bovine corticotropin-β-lipotropin precursor. Nature 278:423–427, 1979.
8. Saiki RK, Scharf S, Faloona F, et al. Enzymatic amplification of β-globin genomic sequences and restriction site analysis for diagnosis of sickle cell anemia. Science 230:1350–1354, 1985.
9. Layman LC, McDonough PG. Molecular genetics in reproductive endocrinology. *In* Wallach EE, Zacur HA (eds). Reproductive Medicine and Surgery. St. Louis, Mosby–Year Book, 1995, p 18.
10. Handyside AH, Pattinson JK, Penketh RJA, et al. Biopsy of human preimplantation embryos and sexing by DNA amplification. Lancet 1:347–349, 1989.
11. Witt M, Erickson RP. A rapid method for detection of Y chromosomal DNA from dried blood specimens by the polymerase chain reaction. Hum Genet 82:271–274, 1989.
12. King D, Wall JR. Identification of specific gene sequences in preimplantation embryos by genomic amplification: Detection of a transgene. Mol Reprod Dev 1:57–62, 1988.
13. Rappolee DA, Wang A, Mark D, et al. Novel method for studying mRNA phenotypes in single or small numbers of cells. J Cell Biochem 39:1–11, 1989.
14. Chamberlain JS, Gibbs RA, Ranier JE, et al. Deletion screening of the Duchenne muscular dystrophy locus via multiplex DNA amplification. Nucleic Acids Res 16:11141–11156, 1988.
15. Zhang L, Cui X, Schmitt K, et al. Whole genome amplification from a single cell: Implications for genetic analysis. Proc Natl Acad Sci USA 89:5847–5851, 1992.
16. Myers RM, Lumelsky N, Lerman LS, et al. Detection of single base substitutions in total genomic DNA. Nature 313:495–498, 1985.
17. Higuchi R, von Beroldingen CH, Sensabaugh GF, et al. DNA typing from single hairs. Nature 332:543–546, 1988.
18. Paabo S, Gifford JA, Wilson AC. Mitochondrial DNA sequences from a 7000-year old brain. Nucleic Acids Res 16:9775–9787, 1988.
19. Southern EM. Detection of specific sequences among DNA fragments separated by gel electrophoresis. J Mol Biol 98:503–517, 1975.
20. Alwine JC, Kemp DJ, Stark GR. Method for detection of specific RNAs in agarose gels by transfer to diazobenzyloxymethyl-paper and hybridization with DNA probes. Proc Natl Acad Sci USA 74:5350–5354, 1977.
21. Policastro PF, Daniels-McQueen S, Carle G, et al. A map of the hCGβ-LH-β gene cluster. J Biol Chem 261:5907–5916, 1986.
22. Julier C, Weil D, Couillin P, et al. The beta chorionic gonadotropin–beta luteinizing gene cluster maps to human chromosome 19. Hum Genet 67:174–177, 1984.
23. Seeburg PH, Adelman JP. Characterization of cDNA for precursor of human luteinizing hormone releasing hormone. Nature 311:666–668, 1984.

24. Fenoglio-Preiser CM, Willman CL. Molecular biology and the pathologist. Arch Pathol Lab Med 111:601–619, 1987.
25. Yang-Feng TL, Seeburg PH, Francke U. Human luteinizing hormone–releasing hormone gene (LHRH) is located on short arm of chromosome 8 (region 8p11.2–p21). Somat Cell Mol Genet 12:95–100, 1986.
26. Hayflick JS, Adelman JP, Seeburg PH. The complete nucleotide sequence of the human gonadotropin-releasing hormone gene. Nucleic Acids Res 17:6403–6404, 1989.
27. Yang-Feng TL, Opdenakker G, Volckaert G, et al. Human tissue-type plasminogen activator gene is located near chromosomal breakpoint in myeloproliferative disorders. Am J Hum Genet 36:79–87, 1986.
28. Su BC, Strand D, McDonough PG, et al. Temporal and constitutive expression of homeobox-2 gene (Hu-2), human heat shock gene (hsp-70) and oncogenes c-*sis* and N-*myc* in early human trophoblast. Am J Obstet Gynecol 159:1195–1199, 1988.
29. Cate RL, Mattaliano J, Hession C, et al. Isolation of the bovine and human genes for Mullerian inhibiting substance and expression of the human gene in animal cells. Cell 45:685–698, 1986.
30. Massague J. The TGF-β family of growth and differentiation factors. Cell 49:437–438, 1987.
31. Vale W, Rivier J, Vaughan J, et al. Purification and characterization of an FSH releasing protein from porcine ovarian follicular fluid. Nature 321:776–779, 1986.
32. Ling N, Ying S-Y, Ueno N, et al. Pituitary FSH is released by a heterodimer of the β-subunits from the two forms of inhibin. Nature 321:779–782, 1986.
33. Rappolee DA, Brenner CA, Schultz R, et al. Developmental expression of PDGF, TGF-α, and TGF-β genes in preimplantation mouse embryos. Science 241:1823–1825, 1988.
34. Prosser J. Detecting single-base mutations. Trends Biotechnol 11: 238–246, 1993.
35. Sano T, Smith CL, Cantor CR. Immuno-PCR: Very sensitive antigen detection by means of specific antibody-DNA conjugates. Science 258:120–122, 1992.
36. Joerger RD, Truby TM, Hendrickson ER, et al. Analyte detection DNA-labeled antibodies and polymerase chain reaction. Clin Chem 41:1371–1377, 1995.
37. Klein KO, Baron J, Colli MJ, et al. Estrogen levels in childhood determined by an ultrasensitive recombinant cell bioassay. J Clin Invest 94:2475–2480, 1994.
38. Kallioniemi A, Kallioniemi OP, Sudar D, et al. Comparative genomic hybridization for molecular cytogenetic analysis of solid tumors. Science 258:818–821, 1992.
39. Liang P, Pardee AB. Differential display of eukaryotic messenger RNA by means of the polymerase chain reaction. Science 257:967–971, 1992.
40. Weissenbach J, Gyapay G, Dib C, et al. A second-generation linkage map of the human genome. Nature 359:794–801, 1992.
41. Hubert R, Weber JL, Schmitt K, et al. A new source of polymorphic DNA markers for sperm typing: Analysis of microsatellite repeats in single cells. Am J Hum Genet 51:985–991, 1992.
42. Howe JR, Lairmore TC, Mishra SK, et al. Improved predictive test for MEN2, using flanking dinucleotide repeats and RFLPs. Am J Hum Genet 51:1430–1442, 1992.
43. Lisitsyn NA, Lisitsyn NM, Wigler MH. Cloning the difference between complex genomes. Science 259:946–951, 1993.
44. Brown PO. Genome scanning methods. Curr Opin Genet Dev 4:366–373, 1994.
45. Tho SPT, Layman LC, Lanclos KD, et al. Absence of the testicular determining factor gene SRY in XX true hermaphrodites and presence of this locus in most subjects with gonadal dysgenesis caused by Y aneuploidy. Am J Obstet Gynecol 167:1794–1802, 1992.
46. Tsuchiya K, Reijo R, Page D, et al. Gonadoblastoma: Molecular definition of the susceptibility region of the Y chromosome. Am J Hum Genet 57:1400–1407, 1995.
47. Matzuk MM, Finegold MJ, Su J-GJ, et al. α-Inhibin is a tumour-suppressor gene with gonadal specificity in mice. Nature 360:313–319, 1992.
48. Phillips JA III, Hjelle BL, Seeburg PH, et al. Molecular basis for familial isolated growth hormone deficiency. Proc Natl Acad Sci USA 78:6372–6375, 1981.
49. Walker WH, Fitzpatrick SL, Barrera-Saldãna HA, et al. The human placental lactogen genes: Structure, function, evolution and transcriptional regulation. Endocr Rev 12:316–328, 1991.
50. Lin C, Lin S-C, Chang C-P, et al. Pit-1–dependent expression of the receptor for growth hormone releasing factor mediates pituitary cell growth. Nature 360:765–768, 1992.
51. Radovick S, Nations M, Du Y, et al. A mutation in the POU-Homeodomain of Pit-1 responsible for combined pituitary hormone deficiency. Science 257:1115–1118, 1992.
52. Pfäffle RW, DiMattia GE, Parks JS, et al. Mutation of the POU-specific domain of Pit-1 and hypopituitarism without pituitary hypoplasia. Science 257:1118–1121, 1992.
53. Voss JW, Rosenfeld MG. Anterior pituitary development: Short tales from dwarf mice. Cell 70:527–530, 1992.
54. Weiss J, Axelrod L, Whitcomb RW, et al. Hypogonadism caused by a single amino acid substitution in the β subunit of luteinizing hormone. N Engl J Med 326:179–183, 1992.
55. Speiser PW, New MI, White PC. Molecular genetics analysis of nonclassic steroid 21-hydroxylase deficiency associated with HLA-B14, DR1. Obstet Gynecol Surv 43:693–695, 1988.
56. Strachan T. Molecular pathology of congenital adrenal hyperplasia. Clin Endocrinol (Oxf) 32:373–393, 1992.
57. Yanase T, Simpson ER, Waterman MR. 17α-Hydroxylase/17,20-lyase deficiency: From clinical investigation to molecular definition. Endocr Rev 12:91–108, 1991.
58. Gotoh H, Sagai T, Hata J-I, et al. Steroid 21-hydroxylase deficiency in mice. Endocrinology 123:1923–1927, 1988.
59. Thigpen AE, Davis DL, Gautier T, et al. Brief report: The molecular basis of steroid 5α-reductase deficiency in a large Dominican kindred. N Engl J Med 327:1217–1219, 1992.
60. Harada N, Ogawa H, Shozu M, et al. Genetic studies on the origin of the mutation in placental aromatase deficiency. Am J Hum Genet 51:666–672, 1992.
61. Latronico AN, Anasti J, Arnhold IJP, et al. Brief report: Testicular and ovarian resistance to luteinizing hormone caused by inactivating mutations in the luteinizing hormone receptor gene. N Engl J Med 334:507–512, 1996.
62. Laue LL, Wu SM, Kudo M, et al. Compound heterozygous mutations of the luteinizing hormone receptor in Leydig cell hypoplasia. Mol Endocrinol 10:987–997, 1966.
63. Aittomäki K, Lucena JLD, Pakarinen P, et al. Mutation in the follicle-stimulating hormone receptor gene causes hereditary hyper-gonadotropic ovarian failure. Cell 82:959–968, 1995.
64. Reinhart J, Mertz LM, Catt KJ. Molecular cloning and expression of cDNA encoding the murine gonadotropin-releasing hormone receptor. J Biol Chem 267:21281–21284, 1992.
65. Rosenthal W, Seibold A, Antaramian A, et al. Molecular identification of the gene responsible for congenital nephrogenic diabetes insipidus. Nature 359:233–235, 1992.
66. Sung C-H, Schneider BG, Agarwal N, et al. Functional heterogeneity of mutant rhodopisms responsible for autosomal dominant retinitis pigmentosa. Proc Natl Acad Sci USA 88:8840–8844, 1991.
67. Jenster G, van der Korput HAGM, van Vroonhoven C, et al. Domains of the human androgen receptor involved in steroid binding, transcriptional activation, and subcellular localization. Mol Endocrinol 5:1396–1404, 1991.
68. Akin JW, Behzadian A, Tho SPT, et al. Evidence for a partial deletion in the androgen receptor gene in a phenotypic male with azoospermia. Am J Obstet Gynecol 165:1891–1894, 1991.
69. Vogt P, Chandley AC, Hargreave TB, et al. Microdeletions in interval 6 of the Y chromosome of males with idiopathic sterility point to disruption of *AZF*, a human spermatogenesis gene. Hum Genet 89:491–496, 1992.
70. Reijo R, Lee T-Y, Salo P, et al. Diverse spermatogenic defects in humans caused by Y chromosome deletions encompassing a novel RNA-binding protein gene. Nat Genet 10:383–393, 1995.
71. Reijo R, Alaqappan RK, Patrizio P, et al. Severe oligospermia from deletions of the azoospermia factor gene on Y chromosome. Lancet 347:1290–1293, 1996.
72. Vogt PH, Edelmann A, Kirsch S, et al. Human Y chromosome azoospermia factors (AZF) mapped to different subregions in Yq11. Hum Mol Genet 5:933–943, 1996.
73. Wang W, Meadows LR, den Haan JMM, et al. Human H-Y: A male specific histocompatibility antigen derived from the SMCY protein. Science 269:1588–1590, 1995.

74. Hardelin J-P, Levilliers J, Castillo ID, et al. X chromosome–linked Kallmann syndrome: Stop mutations validate the candidate gene. Proc Natl Acad Sci USA 89:8190–8194, 1992.
75. Patten JL, Johns DR, Valle D, et al. Mutation in the gene encoding the stimulatory G protein of adenylate cyclase in Albright's hereditary osteodystrophy. N Engl J Med 322:1412–1419, 1988.
76. Lyons J, Landis CA, Harsh G, et al. Two G protein oncogenes in human endocrine tumors. Science 249:655–659, 1990.
77. Weinstein LS, Shenker A, Gejman PV, et al. Activating mutations of the stimulatory G protein in the McCune-Albright syndrome. N Engl J Med 325:1688–1695, 1991.
78. Cassidy SB, Lai L-W, Erickson RP, et al. Trisomy 15 with loss of the paternal 15 as a cause of Prader-Willi syndrome due to maternal disomy. Am J Hum Genet 51:701–708, 1992.
79. Caskey CT, Pizzuti A, Fu Y-H, et al. Triplet repeat mutations in human disease. Science 256:784–789, 1992.
80. Riggins GJ, Lokey LK, Chastain JL, et al. Human genes containing polymorphic trinucleotide repeats. Nat Genet 2:186–191, 1992.
81. Nevins JR. A closer look at E2F. Nature 358:375–376, 1992.
82. Manseau LJ, Schüpbach T. The egg came first, of course! Trends Genet 5:400–405, 1989.
83. Palmiter RD, Brinster RL, Hammer RE, et al. Dramatic growth of mice that develop from eggs microinjected with metallothionein–growth hormone fusion genes. Nature 300:611–615, 1982.
84. Hooper M, Hardy K, Handyside A, et al. HPRT-deficient (Lesch-Nyhan) mouse embryos derived from germ line colonization by cultured cells. Nature 326:292–295, 1987.
85. Risma RA, Clay CM, Nett TM, et al. Targeted overexpression of luteinizing hormone in transgenic mice leads to infertility, polycystic ovaries, and ovarian tumors. Proc Natl Acad Sci USA 92:1322–1326, 1995.
86. Hashimoto N, Watanabe N, Furuta Y, et al. Parthenogenetic activation of oocytes in c-*mos* deficient mice. Nature 370:68–71, 1994.
87. Furuta Y, Shigetani Y, Takeda N, et al. Ovarian teratomas in mice lacking the proto-oncogene c-*mos*. Jpn J Cancer Res 86:540–545, 1995.
88. Zhang Y, Proenca R, Maffei M, et al. Positional cloning of the mouse obese gene and its human homologue. Nature 372:425–432, 1994.
89. Chehab FF, Lim ME, Ronghua L. Correction of the sterility defect in homozygous obese female mice by treatment with the recombinant human ob protein. Nat Genet 12:318–320, 1996.
90. Stewart CL, Kaspar P, Brunet LJ, et al. Blastocyst implantation depends on maternal expression of leukaemia inhibitory factor. Nature 359:76–79, 1992.
91. McDonough PG. Molecular biology in reproductive endocrinology. *In* Yen SSC, Jaffe RB (eds). Reproductive Endocrinology, 3rd ed. Philadelphia, WB Saunders, 1991, p 59.
92. Li E, Goodenough DA, Simon AM, et al. Female infertility in mice lacking connexin 37. Nature 385:525–528, 1997.

Chapter 2

NEUROENDOCRINOLOGY OF REPRODUCTION

S. S. C. Yen

■ CHAPTER OUTLINE

KEY POINTS

- The hypothalamus and its neuroendocrine communications that control pituitary hormone secretion form the basis of the neuroendocrinology of reproduction.
- Several classes of putative chemical messengers have been identified: monoamines, amino acids, neuropeptides, growth factors, and oncogenes. These biochemical messengers perform numerous functions in target cells, including *endocrine, neuroendocrine, paracrine* (affecting neighboring cells), *autocrine* (affecting the cell of origin), and *intracrine* (within the cell) mechanisms of action.
- Astrocytes are paracrine cells that play an important role in neuronal function, particularly that of GnRH neurons, by virtue of the presence of growth factors, thyroid hormone enzymes, LH/hCG receptors, neurosteroids, CRF-binding protein, and immunomodulatory molecules.
- Neuroendocrine regulation of reproductive homeostasis involves *circadian* rhythmicity and *sleep-wake* cycles within the 24-hour biologic clock. These dynamic processes are properties of a hypothalamic pacemaker *(the suprachiasmatic nucleus),* and they invoke cyclic changes of almost all clinically discernible physiologic variables such as body temperature, blood pressure, and pituitary hormone release.
- *Neurosteroids* are synthesized in the brain and modify the activity of *GABA (inhibitory)* and *glutamate (excitatory)* neurotransmitters, which may have important implications in the deterioration of memory and cognitive function with aging.
- New evidence suggests that GnRH neurons are endowed with receptors for neurotransmitters, GnRH, catecholamines, steroid and thyroid hormones, and growth factors. Pulsatile GnRH release is an intrinsic property of the GnRH neurons; thus, GnRH neurons may constitute the pulse generator.
- The recently discovered GH secretagogues and receptor contribute a new level of complexity to the central control of GH pulsatility in concert with GHRH and somatostatin.
- The high-affinity CRF-binding protein may play a role in the timing of parturition as well as in modulating the availability of "free CRF" in the brain to interact with its receptor.
- Urocortin, a new member of the CRF family of peptides, selectively binds to the CRF type 2 receptor and exerts a potent stimulatory action on ACTH secretion and an inhibitory effect on LH release, thus providing another link between reproductive dysfunction and stress.

THE HYPOTHALAMUS AND NEUROENDOCRINE ORGANIZATION

Neuroendocrinology seeks to understand the neuronal mechanisms regulating peripheral endocrine tissues through the pituitary gland and feedback influence on the operation of the neuronal system. The field represents one

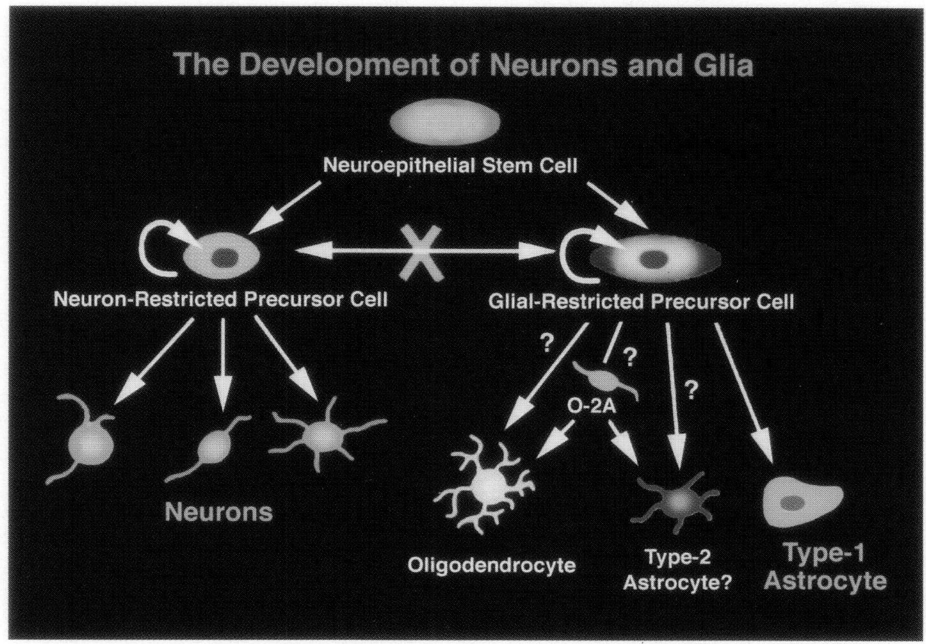

Figure 2–1 ■ The development of neurons and glia from a neuroepithelial progenitor (stem cell). Neuron-restricted precursor cells yield various types of *neurons*. Glia-restricted precursor cells are to yield astrocytes and oligodendrocytes. The *type 1 astrocyte* is the most extensively studied astrocyte population, and it appears that all the functions of astrocytes (see text) can be carried out by type 1 astrocytes. The process of development of *type 2 astrocytes* and their function are not well understood. That *oligodendrocytes* provide myelination is well established. (Reproduced from Mayer-Pröschel M, Rao MS, Noble M. Progenitor cells of the central nervous system: A boon for clinical neuroscience. J NIH Res 9:31–36, 1997.)

of the major series of accomplishments[1] in basic biomedical research during the past quarter century with *major ramifications for reproductive endocrinology,* as the remainder of this text illustrates.

Cells and Function of Hypothalamic Nuclei

Structure and Function of Neurons and Glia

The brain is composed of two cell types; neurons constitute 10 percent of brain cells, and the other 90 percent is made up by glia—astrocytes and oligodendrocytes. The development of neurons and glia is derived from a neuroepithelial progenitor—the stem cell. The first step is the generation of two cell lines (Fig. 2–1): the *neuron-restricted precursor* cells, which yield various types of *neurons;* and the *glia-restricted precursor* cells, which give rise to *astrocytes* and *oligodendrocytes.*

NEURONS

Neurons are highly differentiated cells with distinctive sizes, shapes, and intracellular organelles. Like virtually all other cells except erythrocytes, neurons have a cell body in which a centrally placed nucleus is surrounded by varying volumes of cytoplasm. Distinct for neurons are the cell-specific forms of cytoplasmic extensions, or cellular processes, which may range from a single process in a unipolar neuron to multiple extensions in a multipolar neuron.

The processes extending from the neuronal surface are *receiving processes*, termed *dendrites*, and a single main transmitting process, *the axon*, which may vary considerably in the length to which it extends to its specific synaptic target cells (Fig. 2–2). The synthetic machinery of the neuron is concentrated selectively in the cytoplasm of the cell body (also termed the *perikaryon)*; its products are transported to axon and dendrites. The integrity of a neuron's function thus depends on efficient intracellular cytoplasmic transport. Two-way *transport between compartments* of the cell body and the distal processes occurs continuously through an energy-dependent process operating in concert with microtubules.

GLIA

Glia, meaning glue, were thought to be the supporting cells of the brain, but advances made in recent years have identified an important functional role for glia as regulators

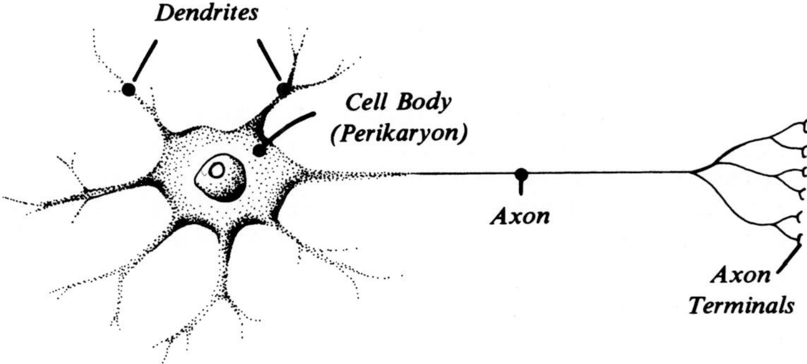

Figure 2–2 ■ A nerve cell, or neuron. Multiple branching processes extending from the cytoplasm of the neuron cell body are termed *dendrites*. A single *axon* also extends from the cell body, and this may terminate at a distance from the cell body in numerous axon terminals.

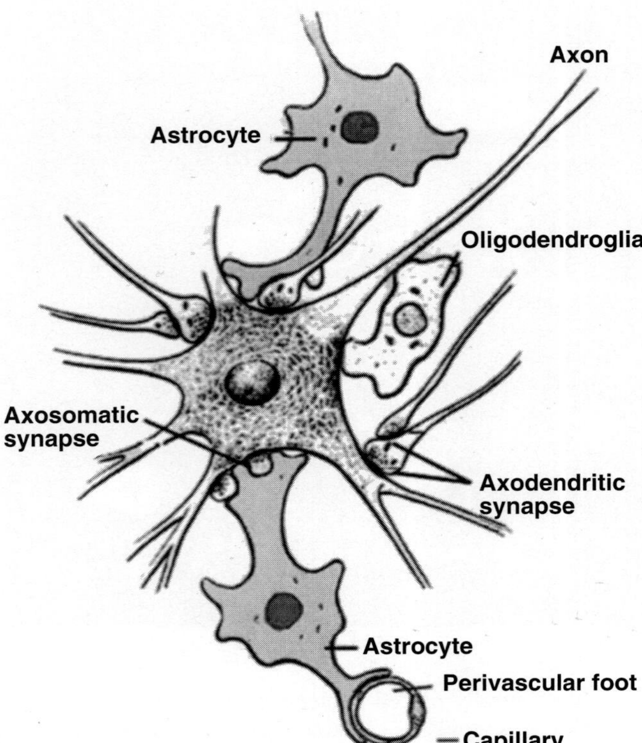

Figure 2–3 ■ Relation of neuron, astrocyte, oligodendroglia, and synapses. Astrocyte processes extend from *neurons* to *capillaries* where they form *perivascular feet.* The perineuronal oligodendrocytes are also glial cells with thick, stubby processes (see text).

of neurons. This class of non-neuronal cellular elements, estimated at nine times the number of neurons, actually interacts with the neurons. The most numerous of the glia are termed *astrocytes* for their multiprocessed shapes. These cells are identified by their unique expression of *glial fibrillary acidic protein (GFAP)* and are spatially placed between the external surfaces of the vasculature and the neurons and their connections (Fig. 2–3). The capillary feet of astrocytes cover about 85 percent of capillaries in the human brain and are instrumental in the development of the blood-brain barrier.[2, 3] Their properties are extensive and some of them are not well established, although it is clear that they possess functions that allow them to respond to transmitters released by neurons and provide substrates to the neurons. Using GFAP as a specific immunochemical marker, studies of glial function have revealed neuroendocrine roles within the hypothalamus and posterior lobe of the pituitary gland. Attributes of astrocytes as paracrine cells to neurons are the following:

- *Insulin-like growth factor (IGF) type I* immunoreactivity is present in astrocytes; its density increases with *puberty* and with *estrogen* treatment in the arcuate nucleus of the rat hypothalamus.[4]
- *Pituicytes*, as a type of astrocyte (positive for GFAP), are the main non-neuronal cellular element in the neurohypophysis and play a role in the *control of oxytocin and vasopressin* release from neurosecretory nerve terminals.[5]
- Astrocytes of hypothalamic origin *secrete transforming growth factors* α *and* β, which stimulate the gene expression of gonadotropin-releasing hormone (GnRH) neurons (GT-1 cells).[6–8]
- The presence of luteinizing hormone/human chorionic gonadotropin (LH/hCG) receptors suggests that LH/hCG may influence glial cell function for brain development and function.[9]
- *Angiotensin receptors (AT-1a)* are expressed in hypothalamic astrocytes and are directly up-regulated by growth hormone (GH), but not by IGF-I, supporting a role for the renin-angiotensin system in the brain.[10]
- *Prolactin* induces mitogenesis and cytokine expression in astrocytes,[11, 12] and astrocytes are capable of producing many immunomodulatory molecules such as interleukin-1 (IL-1), IL-3, IL-6, tumor necrosis factor-α, transforming growth factor-α, interferon, and prostaglandin E.[12–15]
- *Corticotropin-releasing factor–binding protein (CRF-BP),* a 37-kDa protein with a high binding affinity for corticotropin-releasing factor (CRF), is widely distributed in the brain.[16] Both astrocytes and neurons are capable of producing CRF-BP and express CRF-BP messenger ribonucleic acid (mRNA), and a robust increase in CRF-BP levels occurs after treatments with protein kinase C activators. Steroids, such as dexamethasone, hydrocortisone, and to a lesser extent dehydroepiandrosterone (DHEA), inhibit the stimulated release of CRF-BP from astrocytes.[17, 18]
- *Astrocytes and thyroid hormone status in the brain*: Conversion from thyroxine (T_4) to triiodothyronine (T_3) is catalyzed only by *type 2 deiodinase* in the brain. Conversely, removal of iodine from the tyrosyl ring of T_4 or T_3 leads to degradation of T_4 and T_3 into the inactive metabolites rT_3 and T_2, a process catalyzed by *type 3 deiodinase* in the brain.[19, 20] *Astrocytes contain both type 2 and type 3 deiodinases,* and their relative abundance is regulated by thyroid hormone status; *hyperthyroidism* increases type 3 and decreases type 2 deiodinase activities (enhance degradation), and *hypothyroidism* decreases type 3 and increases type 2 deiodinase activities (enhance T_3 production). Thus, modulation of thyroid hormone metabolism by astrocytes may contribute to the maintenance of optimal T_3 concentrations essential for neuronal functions.[21, 22]
- *Astrocytes and neurosteroids:* Steroidogenic enzymes are found in brain tissue, and the biosynthesis and secretion of neuroactive steroids are greater in astrocytes than in oligodendrocytes and neurons (see Neurosteroids).[23–25] Hypothalamic astrocytes are about four times more active than cortical astrocytes in the formation of DHEA.
- Astrocytes may also participate in the regulation of neurotransmitter levels of *glutamate (excitatory)* and γ-aminobutyric acid (GABA, inhibitory) by virtue of the presence of *glutamine synthetase* in the astrocyte.[26]

A second major class of glia are the *oligodendrocytes* (a cell with few processes), which form the myelinated covering of axons that permits neurons to conduct their action potentials rapidly and nondecrementally over long distances within the nervous system. These cells also *express P450scc* and produce pregnenolone from cholesterol.[23]

■ TABLE 2–1
Small-Molecule Transmitters in the Brain*

γ-Aminobutyric acid (GABA)	Dopamine
Glutamate/aspartate	Norepinephrine
Serotonin	Epinephrine
Acetylcholine	Histamine
Glycine	Nitric oxide

*The small-molecule neurotransmitters are listed in the general order of the number of neurons in the central nervous system that produce each. Adenosine, not yet established as neuronally made or released, can modulate transmitter release and responses.

SYNAPTIC TRANSMISSION

There are three main chemical forms of transmitter: *amino acids*, *monoamines*, and *neuropeptides*. Table 2–1 contains a listing of all currently considered central transmitter substances. The criteria for identification of synaptic transmitters rely heavily on the demonstration that a substance contained in a neuron is secreted by that neuron to transmit information to its postsynaptic target.[1, 27] A variety of well-known transmitters that mediate target cell actions are shown in Figure 2–4.

Amino Acids as Transmitters. Amino acids act as transmitters through both excitation and inhibition. At excitatory junctions within autonomic ganglia, *acetylcholine* is the accepted transmitter substance. The transmitter receptor molecule is a multimeric ion channel positioned across the hydrophobic planes of the plasma membrane. Occupation of the ligand recognition site by acetylcholine leads to allosteric shifts in the ion channel, permitting the influx of cations and the reversible depolarization of the membrane potential. The depolarizing overshoot (more positive than

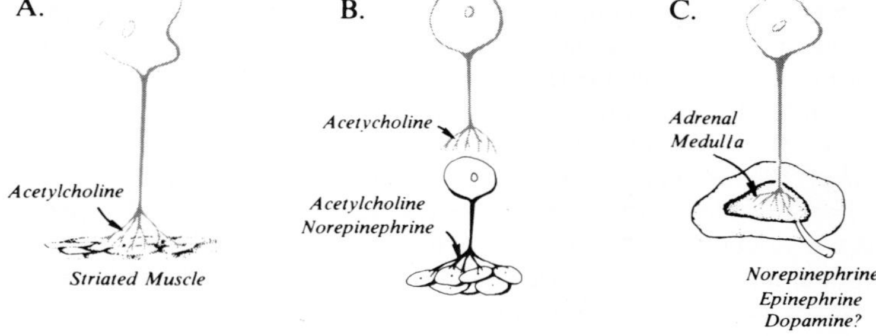

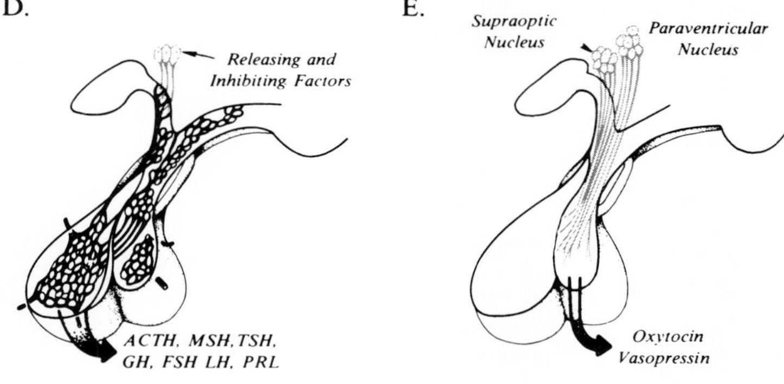

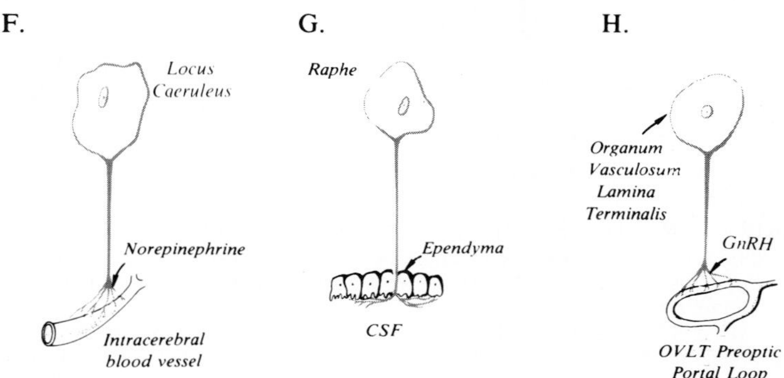

Figure 2–4 ■ The variety of relationships between a neuron producing a transmitter or hormone and the tissue on which the substance acts.

A, Motor neuron innervating striated muscle in the classical synapse, in which acetylcholine is the transmitter.

B, Sympathetic nervous system, in which acetylcholine is released by preganglionic axons and either acetylcholine or norepinephrine is released by the postganglionic axons.

C, Sympathetic nervous system innervating the adrenal medulla. The preganglionic axons release acetylcholine, which stimulates the adrenal medullary cells to secrete epinephrine, norepinephrine, and, perhaps, dopamine as neurohormones into the systemic circulation.

D, Hypothalamic neurons produce releasing or inhibiting factors that are secreted into the portal circulation to effect the release of pituitary hormones (ACTH, MSH, TSH, GH, FSH, LH, PRL) into the systemic circulation.

E, Neurosecretion of the classical type; oxytocin and vasopressin are produced by neurons of the supraoptic and paraventricular nuclei and released in the neural lobe of the pituitary into the systemic circulation.

F, Norepinephrine-producing neurons of the pontine nucleus, the locus caeruleus, innervate cerebral blood vessels, providing a central control of brain vasculature.

G, Serotonin-producing neurons of the midbrain raphe nuclei extend axonal branches through the ependymal lining of the ventricles to secrete serotonin directly into the cerebrospinal fluid.

H, The organum vasculosum of the lamina terminalis (OVLT) has a separate portal circulation into which its neurons secrete GnRH.

the normal resting membrane potential) then triggers subsequent functional events in the target cell (such as muscle contraction or, in other cases, glandular secretion) (see Fig. 2–4). *Central excitation* is also transmitted by the amino acids *glutamate* and *aspartate*. Their receptor-ionophore complexes are similar to the multimeric nicotinic cholinergic receptor.

At inhibitory synaptic junctions operated by the amino acids *GABA* or *glycine*, the presynaptic processes are similar, as is the nature of the transmembrane, multimeric receptor–ionophore molecules. The main differences are in the nature of the *ion channels*, in this case permitting only the *influx of chloride ions*, thus shifting the membrane potential to more polarized levels (termed *hyperpolarization*), which decreases the probability of activation by a subsequent excitatory transmission.[28]

Monoamines as Transmitters. Monoamine-containing neuronal pathways consist of catecholaminergic (epinephrine, norepinephrine, and dopamine) and serotonergic transmitters. Their biosynthesis, release, and metabolic processes are shown in Figure 2–5. Although their effects as transmitters may be superficially similar to the qualities of an inhibitory transmitter, their mechanisms of operation differ, exhibiting hyperpolarizing effects associated with a *decrease in ionic permeability*. In the case of central *noradrenergic systems*, these postsynaptic actions have been associated with the generation of the intracellular second messenger, cyclic adenosine monophosphate (cAMP), and the cascade of intracellular protein phosphorylations that are its consequence.[27, 29–31]

Receptors for monoamines are monomeric proteins, which exhibit *seven putative transmembrane domains* that show a surprising degree of sequence similarity regardless of the ligand (acetylcholine muscarinic, α- and β-noradrenergic receptors, serotonin [5-hydroxytryptamine] receptors, and dopamine receptors as well as receptors for the peptides of the tachykinin family) to which they respond.[32–34] Similarly, electrophysiologic and biochemical effects have been established for the central dopaminergic system within the basal ganglia. In principle, a similar second messenger–mediated transduction involving breakdown of inositol triphosphate underlies responses to cholinergic muscarinic and tachykinin neuropeptide signals.

Studies focused on the longer term biochemical effects of signals transduced by specific neurotransmitter receptors coupled to second messenger intracellular mediators have revealed that some amines could serve as growth-regulatory factors and perhaps, through such actions, as the mediators of short-term functional adaptations.[35, 36] In these cases, the data indicate that transmitter receptor–regulated second messenger mediators can activate the phosphorylation or dephosphorylation as well as the de novo expression of special *phosphoproteins*. These intracellular proteins were originally termed oncogenes because of their increased abundance in cells infected by oncogenic viruses. The natural counterparts of some of these genes and gene products, termed *cellular proto-oncogenes*, have been found to be abundantly expressed in the nervous system both during terminal differentiation and in some locations in the mature brain, especially after intensive increases in neuronal activity.

Peptide Transmitters. Peptide-containing neurons of the hypothalamus were originally described as "neurosecretory" neurons, but it became apparent that virtually all hypothalamic neuropeptides are projecting to many regions of the brain. They perform neurotransmitter functions in the regulation of food intake, mood-behavior, and sexual behavior (Table 2–2). These peptides are thyrotropin-releasing hormone (TRH), CRF, somatostatin, GnRH, arginine vasopressin (AVP), and oxytocin. Moreover, these

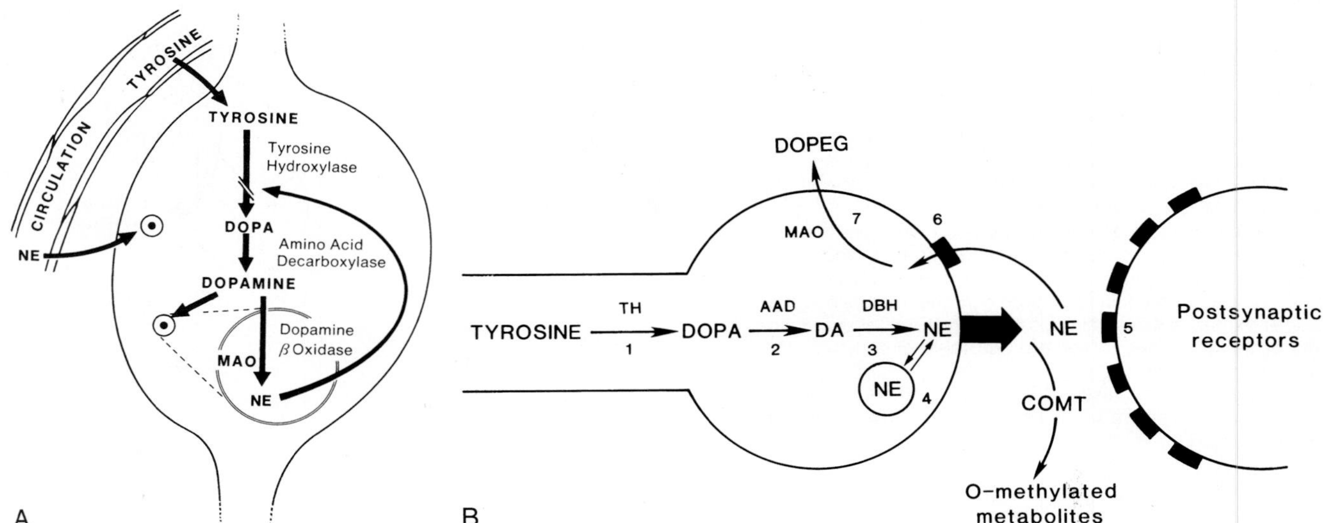

Figure 2–5 ■ *A*, The biosynthesis of dopamine (DA) and norepinephrine (NE) is depicted. Tyrosine derived from the blood stream serves as substrate inside the catecholamine neurons. Tyrosine hydroxylase catalyzes the formation of dopa from tyrosine. Dopa transformation to dopamine is catalyzed by amino acid decarboxylase (AAD). Dopamine β-oxidase in noradrenergic neurons transforms dopamine to norepinephrine.

B, DA and NE are released into the synaptic cleft where they rapidly bind to postsynaptic receptors. Excess transmitters undergo either metabolic inactivation by catechol-*O*-methyltransferase (COMT) or reuptake into the terminal by presynaptic receptors where they undergo metabolic degradation by monoamine oxidase (MAO). DBH, dopamine β-hydroxylase; DOPEG, 3,4-dihydroxyphenylethylglycol.

■ TABLE 2–2
Peptides in the Central Nervous System

Hypophysiotropic Hormones	Gastrointestinal Peptides
Thyrotropin-releasing hormone	Vasoactive intestinal polypeptide
Gonadotropin-releasing hormone	Peptide histidine isoleucine
Corticotropin-releasing hormone and urocortin	Cholecystokinin
Growth hormone–releasing hormone	Gastrin
Somatostatin	Substance P
Neurohypophysial Hormones	Neurotensin
Vasopressin	Methionine enkephalin
Oxytocin	Leucine enkephalin
Neurophysin I and II	Dynorphin
Others	Neoendorphin
Neuropeptide Y	Insulin
Angiotensin I	Glucagon
Bradykinin	Bombesin
Carnosine	Secretin
Sleep peptides	Somatostatin
Calcitonin gene–related peptide	Motilin
Interleukin-1	**Pituitary Peptides**
Inhibin	Adrenocorticotropic hormone
Pancreastatin	β-Endorphin
Amylin	α-Melanocyte–stimulating hormone
Parathormone-related peptide	Prolactin
Activin	Luteinizing hormone
	Growth hormone
	Thyrotropin

Modified from Krieger DT. Brain peptides: What, where, and why? Science 222:975–985, 1983. © 1983 by the AAAS.

peptides are also distributed to many other neurons where they coexist with classic amino acid and amine transmitters.[1, 37, 38] Furthermore, neurons projecting to the posterior pituitary also give off additional axonal branches directed to neuronal targets within and beyond the hypothalamus.[39] All existing data are pharmacologic actions of exogenously administered peptides or of synthetic fragments designed to simulate or antagonize their effects in model endocrine systems. However, at this point in the emergence of peptide molecular analyses at both the protein and gene levels, at least three structural types of family relationships may be distinguished:

1. those in which a common genetic or peptidic precursor can give rise to multiple different agonists with little similarity in their structures, such as pro-opiomelanocortin (POMC), somatostatin, or the brain calcitonin gene–related peptide;
2. those in which a strong structural similarity relates long domains of peptides, which are individually expressed either in different species (the tachykinin family, the CRF/urotensin/urocortin family, and the oxytocin/vasopressin/vasotocin family) or in different neurons and endocrine tissues of the same species (the glucagon/secretin/vasoactive intestinal polypeptide family, the gastrin/cholecystokinin family, and the pancreatic polypeptide family); and
3. those with short domains of structural similarity in which the prohormone may contain several copies of identical or highly similar agonists (such as the pro-enkephalins or the pro-dynorphins and, possibly, the pro–vasoactive intestinal polypeptide).

Nitric Oxide and Carbon Monoxide as Neurotransmitters (stimulate GnRH release). The discovery of the role of *nitric oxide* in the central and peripheral nervous system has radically altered our thinking regarding synaptic transmission. Although there is considerable evidence that nitric oxide functions as a neurotransmitter, it is an unusual transmitter in that it is a labile free radical gas that is not stored in the synaptic vesicles. Nitric oxide is synthesized by nitric oxide synthase from L-arginine (Fig. 2–6) and simply diffuses from the nerve terminals as opposed to the exocytosis by which conventional neurotransmitters are released. Moreover, nitric oxide does not undergo reversible interactions with receptors, as do the conventional neurotransmitters, but forms covalent linkages with several potential targets, which include enzymes such as guanylate cyclase and other molecules. The action of conventional neurotransmitters is terminated by *presynaptic uptake* or *enzyme degradation*, whereas the action of nitric oxide is terminated by *diffusion away from its targets* or by formation of covalent linkages with the superoxide anion or scavenger proteins. A similar mode of action and disposal for *carbon monoxide* have been described.[40] A special neurotransmitter function has been demonstrated for nitric oxide in peripheral autonomic nerves; nitric oxide neurons are prominent in penile tissue, specifically in pelvic plexus and axonal processes that form the cavernous nerve as well as the nerve plexus in the adventitia of the deep cavernosal arteries and the sinusoids in the periphery of the corpora cavernosa. Intravenous injection of *nitric oxide synthase inhibitor blocks the penile erection* elicited by electric nerve stimulation.[41]

In the hypothalamus, both nitric oxide and carbon monoxide have been clearly demonstrated to stimulate GnRH release by activating guanylate cyclase in both hypothalamic explants and an immortalized neuronal cell line (GT-1 cells).[42, 43]

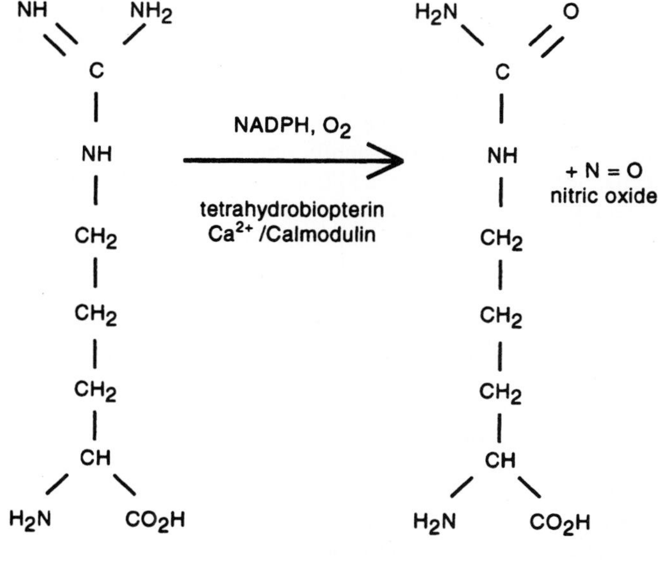

Figure 2–6 ■ The formation of nitric oxide from arginine in the brain is catalyzed by nitric oxide synthase. This process requires oxygen with NADPH as a coenzyme and tetrahydrobiopterin as a cofactor.

A growing list of combinations of peptides and smaller molecular weight transmitters is evolving. It seems clear that this molecular interrelatedness will become increasingly important in the unraveling of the complex control of neuroendocrine specificity.

Hypothalamic Nuclei

The hypothalamus is a phylogenetically old and stable component of the central nervous system (CNS) and shows few changes throughout mammalian evolution in its general organization or its connections with other brain areas. In humans and other primates, the growth of cortical structures reduces the relative brain volume represented by the hypothalamus to approximately 10 gm in a 1200- to 1400-gm brain. Although no sharp boundaries exist, the *hypothalamus is defined* as being ventral to the ventral thalamus, forming the lateral walls of the ventral part of the third ventricle. Its rostral boundary, the lamina terminalis, represents the equally ill-defined junction between the diencephalon and the telencephalon. Its most clear-cut boundary is caudally, at the caudal perimeter of the mamillary complex, at the junction with the mesencephalon. Laterally, the hypothalamus is delimited by its prominent landmark, the medial forebrain bundle—the major pathway by which all medial hypothalamic nuclei are interconnected with the rest of the brain. Hypothalamic neurons are formed from the ventral portion of the embryonic diencephalon, predominantly during the second to third month of human gestation and during the second week of rodent embryogenesis.[44]

ORGANIZATION OF HYPOTHALAMIC NUCLEI

By anatomic custom, the hypothalamus is generally split into three major subdivisions or zones: the medial, lateral, and periventricular zones (the last being just medial to the third ventricular ependyma). The lateral zone may be viewed as the relay through which connections are made out of the hypothalamus and received from more rostral brain structures. The medial and periventricular zones contain the majority of structures and fiber systems pertinent to central regulation of the endocrine system. The neurons here show the most consistently clustered groups of nerve cells, termed *nuclei;* in addition, less clustered and less distinctly demarcated neurons within the hypothalamus are designated *areas.* The major hypothalamic nuclei are shown in Figure 2–7. Each of the three zones of the hypothalamus is also conveniently subdivided further into three groups of nuclei or areas: (1) a rostral (anterior) group; (2) a tuberal group, so named because of its association with the tuber cinereum (infundibulum); and (3) a posterior group.[39]

Anterior Group. The anterior group includes the medial *preoptic area*, the *anterior hypothalamic area*, the *suprachiasmatic nucleus*, the *supraoptic nucleus*, and the *paraventricular nucleus* (see Fig. 2–7).

Tuberal Group. The tuberal hypothalamus includes three prominent nuclei: the ventromedial nucleus, the dorsomedial nucleus, and the *arcuate nucleus—located immediately above the median eminence and adjacent to the third ventricle* (see Fig. 2–7). The tuberal area together with the paraventricular nucleus contains most of the neurons

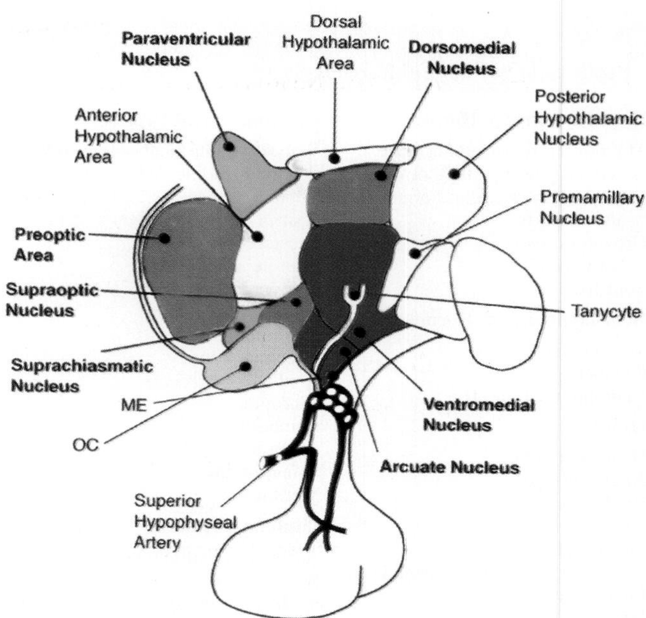

Figure 2–7 ■ Nuclear organization of the hypothalamus shown diagrammatically in the sagittal plane as it would appear from the third ventricle. Rostral is to the left and caudal to the right. The pituitary is shown ventrally. ME, median eminence; OC, optic chiasm. See text for description.

producing hypothalamic hormones, which regulate the endocrine output of the anterior pituitary and can thus be considered the *hypophysiotropic* zone. Surgical isolation of this zone from the rest of the brain was shown to maintain most aspects of pituitary function, although the regulatory influences normally imposed by other brain areas were lost.

Posterior Group. Caudal to the tuberal area, the posterior hypothalamic area contains the mamillary complex, the posterior hypothalamic nucleus, the supramamillary nucleus, and the tuberomamillary nucleus. With the exception of the tuberomamillary nucleus, it is unlikely that the other nuclei of this region participate significantly in the direct regulation of endocrine function.

NEURAL CONNECTIONS OF HYPOTHALAMIC NUCLEI

Ascending Input to the Hypothalamus. Neurons innervating the hypothalamus are present at all levels of the brain stem, from the caudal medulla to the rostral mesencephalon. Typical of such connections are those of the monoamine neuron groups.[45–47]

Noradrenergic Projections. There are two principal norepinephrine projections to the hypothalamus. *One* set of afferents arises from the medulla and pons, ascends, and eventually forms dense terminal plexuses in the medial preoptic area, the anterior hypothalamic area, the paraventricular nucleus, the ventral tuberal area, the dorsomedial nucleus, the tuberomamillary nucleus, *the entire periventricular system including its arcuate nucleus*, and the *internal and subependymal layers of the median eminence.* The *second* noradrenergic hypothalamic input is relatively minor, arising from the pontine *nucleus locus caeruleus* to innervate more restricted target neurons in the periventricular system, the dorsomedial nucleus, the paraventricular nucleus, and the supraoptic nucleus.

Serotonergic Projections. Neurons of the *midbrain raphe* also project rostrally through the ventral tegmental area into the medial forebrain bundle to provide widespread innervation of the medial hypothalamus, which is most dense in the mamillary complex, the periventricular nucleus, the arcuate nucleus, and the suprachiasmatic nucleus. In addition, the median eminence receives a moderate serotonin neuron input to the internal and subependymal layers with a sparse input to the palisade zone.[46]

Dopaminergic Projections. Dopaminergic neurons project across varying distances:

1. Ultrashort systems are dopamine neurons located in the retina and olfactory bulb.
2. Intermediate systems are tuberohypophysial dopamine cells that project from arcuate to periventricular nuclei into the intermedian lobe of the pituitary and into the median eminence. This system is important in the regulation of GnRH and prolactin secretion.
3. Long systems—long projections of dopamine neurons are *mesocortical* and *mesolimbic* systems, with the latter targeted to the limbic neurons.

Descending Input to the Hypothalamus. The most dense projections arise from the basal forebrain structures, the olfactory tubercle, the septum, the piriform cortex, the *amygdala*, and the *hippocampus*. Afferents from the amygdaloid complex project to the anterior hypothalamic area and the region surrounding the ventromedial nucleus. A projection from the hippocampal formation leaves the fornix system in the septum and descends through the medial hypothalamus to terminate in the *arcuate nucleus*. A particularly noteworthy afferent pathway is the *retinohypothalamic projection,* a direct projection from the retina to the *suprachiasmatic nucleus* of the hypothalamus that contributes to the mediation of visual influences on neuroendocrine rhythms,[48] particularly melatonin synthesis and secretion (see later).

EFFERENT CONNECTIONS OF THE HYPOTHALAMUS

Perhaps most significant of the efferent connections are the *projections of hypothalamic neurons on the neurohypophysis,* including the median eminence, the infundibular stalk, and the neurointermediate lobe of the pituitary. This group consists of the classic *magnocellular neurosecretory system,* originating largely in the cells of the supraoptic and paraventricular hypothalamic nuclei producing the hormones *oxytocin* and *vasopressin*. The *parvicellular neurosecretory system*[39, 49] arises mainly from the mediobasal hypothalamus. The parvicellular system includes *two components directly related to reproduction*: the *gonadotropin-releasing hormone neurons (GnRH system)* and the *tuberohypophysial dopamine neurons*.

Circumventricular Organs

The circumventricular organs[50] represent a series of unpaired structures adjacent to the ventricular system (Fig. 2–8). The important attribute of these organs is the *lack of a blood-brain barrier;* thus, they may serve as "windows" for transport of substances from blood to the brain. The development of a blood-brain barrier in the CNS capillaries appears to be directed by astrocytes.[3] The five circumventricular organs associated with the third ventricle consist of the (1) median eminence, (2) pineal gland, (3) organum vasculosum of lamina terminalis (OVLT), (4) subfornical organ, and (5) subcommissural organ.

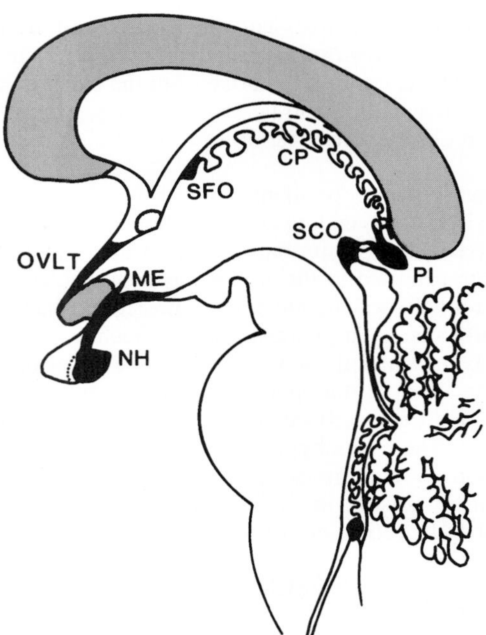

Figure 2–8 ■ The circumventricular organs of the brain *(black areas)*. These structures are highly vascularized and characterized by the *lack* of a blood-brain barrier. ME, median eminence; NH, neurohypophysis; SCO, subcommissural organ; SFO, subfornical organ; OVLT, organum vasculosum of the lamina terminalis; PI, pineal.

MEDIAN EMINENCE

The median eminence is a midline prominence progressively shaped by a lateral and ventral invagination into the infundibular stalk that also forms as its termination the neural lobe of the pituitary. It consists of five layers: ependymal, subependymal, fibrous, reticular, and palisade. Within the subependymal layer, axons of hypophysiotropic neurons form synaptic-like contacts on the ependymal or glial elements through which they gain access to the pituitary portal circulation as well as making axoaxonic contacts with each other. The palisades on the outer zone of the median eminence consist of a more or less continuous row of terminals of neural and non-neural elements lying opposed to the basement membrane surrounding the portal capillaries. A modified population of ependymal cells (the tanycyte, with each exhibiting numerous microvilli on its ventricular surface) extends through the entire width of the median eminence, and they may serve as a transporter cell between the third ventricle and the portal circulation[51] (see Fig. 2–7).

PINEAL GLAND

The pineal gland is composed of a parenchymal organ attached to the roof of the diencephalon by a stalk. The pineal gland in mammals has three major cellular components: the *pineal cell*, or pinealocyte; *glial cells*; and *nerve endings*. The nerve endings arise from the superior cervical sympathetic ganglion and lie predominantly in perivascular spaces in close approximation to processes of the pinealocytes.

The basic stimuli regulating pineal function are environmental light and endogenous rhythm-generating mechanisms (see later). Information concerning environmental light is transmitted to the suprachiasmatic nucleus by way of the retinohypothalamic tract. The suprachiasmatic nucleus projects to the paraventricular nucleus. Neurons of the paraventricular nucleus project to the superior cervical ganglion. This is the putative pathway by which light inhibits and dark activates pineal melatonin synthesis and secretion. The retinohypothalamic projection appears to serve and to entrain the endogenous rhythm-generating mechanisms arising in the suprachiasmatic nuclei, which then drive the remainder of the pathway (see later).[52]

ORGANUM VASCULOSUM OF LAMINA TERMINALIS

The OVLT is a neurovascular specialization lying at the rostral end of the third ventricle in the ventral portion of the lamina terminalis. Within the OVLT, a layer of nerve cells surrounds glial cells, axons, axon terminals, and a capillary network that is part of a *separate portal plexus*. In the rat, the OVLT and the medial preoptic area also contain GnRH-producing neurons.[53]

SUBFORNICAL ORGAN

The subfornical organ protrudes into the roof of the third ventricle, where the columns of the fornix join. It is covered by nonciliated ependyma, is intensely vascularized, and contains both classic neurosecretory neurons and glia. This organ also receives a dense innervation from serotonin-containing neurons of the midbrain raphe and has been implicated in the *mediation of angiotensin-induced drinking*.

SUBCOMMISSURAL ORGAN

Located immediately below the posterior commissure at the caudal surface of the third ventricle, the subcommissural organ shows a close topographic relationship to the pineal complex. The subcommissural organ contains an ependymal layer consisting of highly specialized, secretory, ependymal cells that release an apical secretory product into the ventricular fluid to form Reissner's fiber and a subependymal layer composed of glial cells, vasculature, and nerve endings. Many of the nerve endings are serotonin neuron terminals arising from the midbrain raphe. However, its functional significance remains obscure.

Pituitary-Portal Circulation

The blood supply of the basal hypothalamus, the infundibulum, the infundibular stalk, and the pituitary gland arises from the superior hypophysial arteries. The posterior median eminence receives blood through separate vessels, and the most ventral portion of the infundibular stalk receives its blood supply from a pair of vessels termed trabecular arteries. The neural lobe obtains arterial blood from the inferior hypophysial arteries, which have anastomoses with the trabecular arteries.

The arteries supplying the median eminence and the infundibular stalk empty into a dense network of heavily innervated capillaries and drain into the portal venous plexus. The portal vessels lead directly from the median eminence and the upper stalk to the anterior lobe. In the human, approximately *80 to 90 percent of the blood supply of the anterior lobe is provided by the long portal vessels*, with the remainder provided by short portal veins. The portal vessels distribute blood into the sinusoids of the anterior lobe, which are drained by veins that empty into the cavernous sinus.

Steroid Hormones and Neurosteroids

Responsiveness of CNS targets to blood-borne steroid hormones provides for the feedback regulation of hypophysiotropic releasing and inhibiting factors, an essential link in the coordinated regulation of neuroendocrine operations and behavioral functions. Steroid binding to neurons is similar to that of peripheral tissues. Steroid hormones enter the target cells and bind stereospecifically to discrete, soluble cytoplasmic receptor proteins normally concentrated at or near the plasma membrane. After steroid binding, the hormone-receptor complex moves to the nucleus, where cellular function is ultimately regulated through modifications in gene transcription and protein synthesis.[54]

Sites of Steroid Hormone Actions

ESTROGEN-RESPONSIVE TARGETS (Fig. 2–9)

The pattern of estrogen-binding neurons is virtually identical among various mammalian species, being concentrated in the preoptic and hypothalamic areas. Estrogen receptor binding and its mRNA are most dense in the periventricular area between the preoptic region and the arcuate nucleus. There is also dense labeling and estrogen receptor mRNA in the anterior hypothalamic area and the ventrolateral portion of the ventromedial hypothalamic nucleus. In the telencephalon, dense labeling is found in both the rat and the monkey in the interstitial nucleus of the stria terminalis and the medial amygdaloid nucleus. Other areas in both the forebrain and the brain stem show less dense and more variable labeling.[54–57] However, these findings were described before the recent discovery of the *second estrogen receptor (ERβ)*. The transactivation property of the two estrogen receptors, *ERα and ERβ,* showed opposite ways when complexed with ligand, 17β-estradiol, from the AP-1 site: with ERα, estradiol-activated transcription, whereas with ERβ, estradiol-inhibited transcription. Thus, ERα and ERβ may play different roles in gene regulation.[55] Moreover, distribution of these two estrogen receptors in brain regions differs, with ERα found in the arcuate nucleus and ERβ in the paraventricular nucleus.[58] Undoubtedly, functional and expression studies of both ERα and ERβ in the brain are forthcoming.

ANDROGEN TARGETS IN THE BRAIN

The distribution of labeled cells after injection of a castrated male rat with tritiated testosterone is similar to the

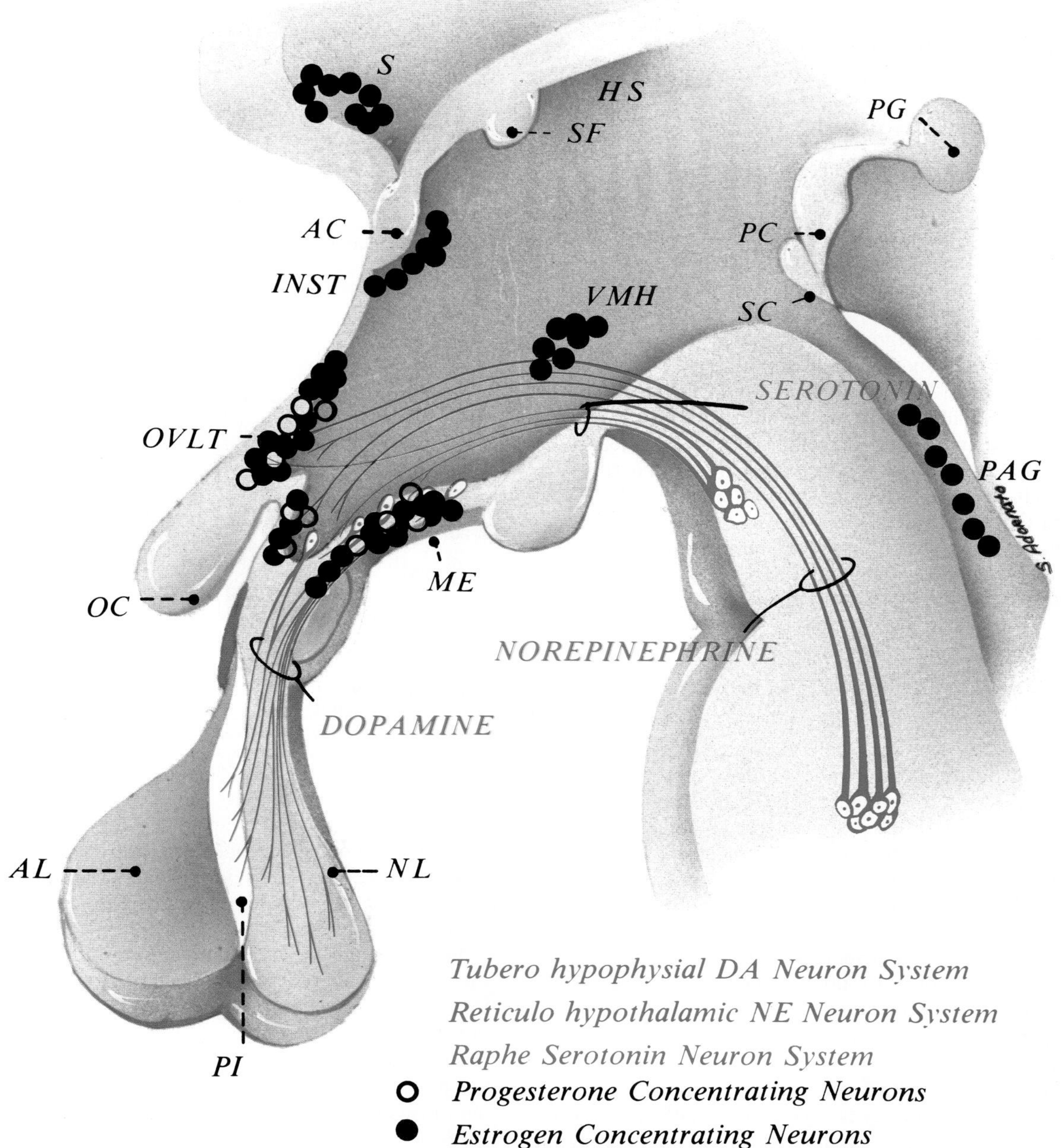

Figure 2–9 ■ Distribution of estrogen-binding *(closed circles)* and progesterone-binding *(open circles)* neurons in the primate brain in relation to the ascending monoamine-neuron systems innervating the hypothalamus and adjacent areas. See text for description.

distribution of cells labeled with tritiated estradiol. These cells are found with greatest density in the hypothalamus, the amygdala, and, to lesser extent, the septum and the hippocampus. The binding of testosterone differs from that of estradiol, however, in three significant ways: (1) the concentration of labeled testosterone in various brain regions, relative to the amount of labeled hormone in blood, is lower in all areas than estradiol; (2) the proportion of testosterone bound to the nuclear fraction is less than 25 percent of the total; and (3) a significant proportion of testosterone bound to the nuclear fraction in the brain has been converted to estradiol.[59] These factors make the interpretation of any experiment using labeling of brain with testosterone difficult. In the newborn rat brain, the specific uptake, binding, and capacity for aromatization of testosterone to estrogen may play a role in the sexual differentiation of the brain. Some workers suggest that the morphologic differentiation of the male brain is dependent, at least in part, on the formation of estrogens and their actions on neuronal development in the hypothalamus and the basal forebrain.[59]

PROGESTERONE TARGETS IN THE BRAIN (see Fig. 2–9)

Progesterone receptor mRNA has been found in the medial basal hypothalamus in the region around the median eminence in the monkey brain.[57, 60] However, progesterone receptor density is highly dependent on estrogen priming, which increases progesterone receptor mRNA. This estrogen-dependent induction of progesterone receptor is similar to that observed in the primate and human endometrium. However, it differs from the endometrium in that progesterone treatment down-regulates estrogen receptor in the ventromedial nucleus without having an impact on the expression of progesterone receptor.[60]

ADRENAL GLUCOCORTICOID TARGETS IN THE BRAIN

The regional distribution of glucocorticoid receptor mRNA in the brain differs markedly from that described for sex steroid hormones. High density of glucocorticoid receptor mRNA expression was *found in the hippocampus*, the septum, and the amygdala, with much lower levels of expression in the hypothalamus, including the preoptic area and the midbrain. The proportion of nuclear mRNA in the cytosol in the hippocampus is similar to that for estrogens—greater than 80 percent.[61, 62] The significance of the *high binding in the hippocampus* in comparison with the hypothalamus is now known, particularly with respect to its participation in feedback regulation of CRF production, response to stress, or circadian rhythms in adrenal function. Hypercorticalism induced by chronic stress has been implicated in the development of Alzheimer's disease.[63]

Neurosteroids: Formation and Function

The discovery of in situ formation of estrogen in the hypothalamus by Naftolin and colleagues[64] opened the possibility that the brain may have steroidogenic function. In 1981, the presence of pregnenolone and pregnenolone sulfate (PREG-S) and DHEA and its sulfate ester (DHEA-S) were found in the brain of the adult male rat. This finding was unforeseen because rodent steroidogenic glands, including adrenals, do not secrete significant amounts of DHEA. This led to the discovery of a steroid biosynthetic machinery in the CNS responsible for producing "neurosteroids." The amount of pregnenolone and DHEA-S in rodent brains is 10 times higher than in peripheral circulation, supporting the proposal of de novo synthesis of neurosteroids.[23] Thus, the brain is capable of de novo synthesis of steroids independent of gonads and adrenals.[23]

The mitochondrial enzyme cytochrome P450scc responsible for cholesterol side-chain cleavage and the formation of neurosteroids with 3β-hydroxy-Δ^5 structures, such as pregnenolone and DHEA, was found throughout the rat brain. Production of pregnenolone was found in type 1 astrocytes and oligodendrocytes, but *not in neurons*. The biosynthesis of DHEA and DHEA-S from pregnenolone requires the enzyme complex 17α-hydroxylase/17,20-lyase (P450c17), which was only recently identified in the fetal, neonatal, and adult rat brain[24, 25, 65] (Fig. 2–10).

In the brain, PREG-S and DHEA-S are metabolized to other neurosteroids. Pregnenolone can be converted to progesterone by 3β-hydroxysteroid dehydrogenase primarily in the *glia*. Brain tissue also contains steroid 5α-reductase and 3α-oxidoreductase, which can convert progesterone to tetrahydroprogesterone. Similarly, DHEA can be converted in CNS to androstenedione and subsequently reduced to androsterone. Also, synthesis of 7α- and 7β-hydroxylated metabolites of DHEA in the brain was found, leading to the formation of the metabolites androstenediol and androstenetriol. Because glia (astrocytes and oligodendrocytes) seem to be the primary site of synthesis of neurosteroids, they can be regarded as a "neuroparacrine gland" (see earlier, Glia).[66]

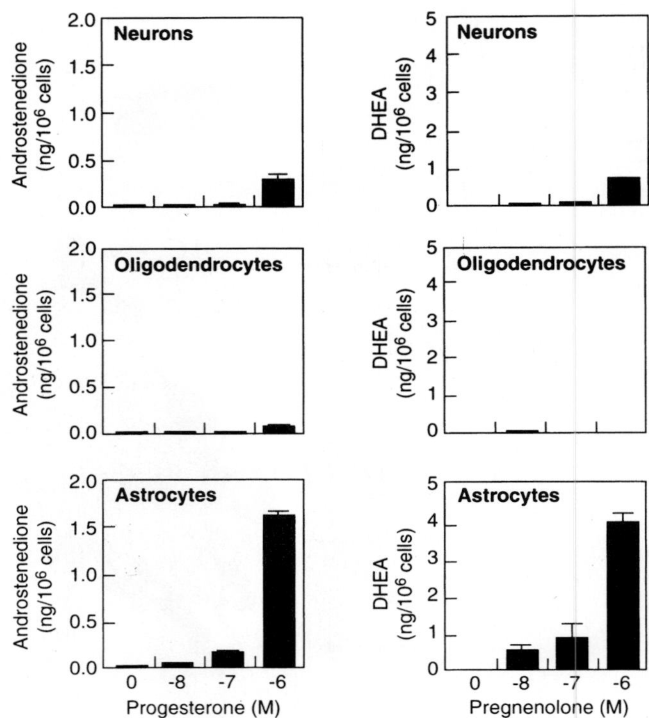

Figure 2–10 ■ Conversions of pregnenolone to DHEA and progesterone to androstenedione, reflecting the presence of P450c17 (17α-hydroxylase/17,20-lyase activities), occurring mainly in the astrocytes, compared with oligodendrocytes and neurons, from neonatal rat brain. (From Zwain I, Yen SSC. Unpublished data.)

In the *human brain*, neurosteroids were also found in men and women older than 60 years.[67, 68] DHEA, pregnenolone, and progesterone are present in all regions of the brain at concentrations severalfold higher than those in plasma. Both DHEA sulfotransferase and sulfatase activities have been identified in monkey and human brain. Thus, the formation of DHEA-S occurs directly in the brain, particularly because DHEA-S does not cross the blood-brain barrier and the enzymatic system to perform sulfation and desulfation of DHEA is present.[23] Steroidogenic factor 1 (SF-1), a tissue-specific orphan nuclear receptor, regulates the genes of several steroidogenic enzymes. SF-1 mRNA expression is widespread in human brain including several components of the limbic system. Thus, SF-1 may play a role in neurosteroid biosynthesis in human brain.[69]

NEUROMODULATORY FUNCTION OF NEUROSTEROIDS

It has been shown that neurosteroids are able to modify $GABA_A$ and glutamate receptor activities. The physiologic significance of these observations may include effects on memory and recall and modulation of neuronal activities.[70]

$GABA_A$ Receptors (Fig 2–11). The effects of DHEA-S and PREG-S on the ligand binding and functional properties of $GABA_A$ receptor have been examined.[71–73] PREG-S displays mixed GABA agonistic/antagonistic activities,

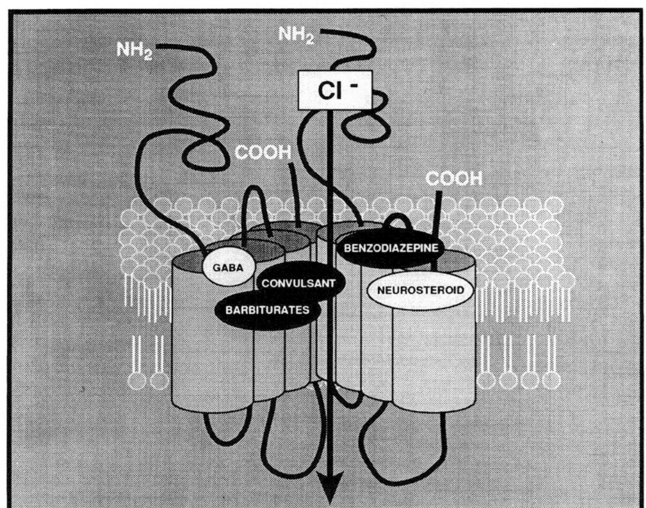

Figure 2–11 ■ Diagrammatic depiction of $GABA_A$ receptor complex with multiple binding sites for several ligands including neurosteroids-DHEA.

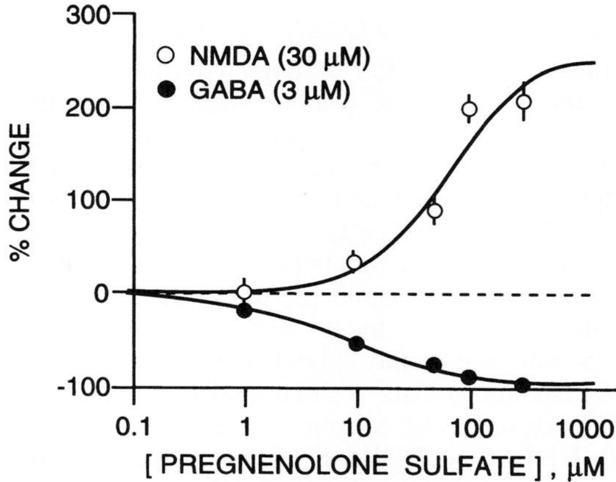

Figure 2–13 ■ Dose-response curves for modulation of NMDA- and GABA-induced currents by pregnenolone sulfate. Data are displayed as percentage change in peak current in the presence of varying concentrations of pregnenolone sulfate. (Reproduced from Wu FS, Gibbs TT, Farb DH. Pregnenolone sulfate: A positive allosteric modulator at the *N*-methyl-D-aspartate receptor. Mol Pharmacol 40:333–336, 1991.)

whereas DHEA-S functions as an antagonist (Fig. 2–12). The affinity of the DHEA-S–blocked receptor for GABA is reduced approximately 50 percent. DHEA-S does not alter the chloride currents and the duration of opening of the channels. Most remarkable was the finding that one molecule of DHEA-S is sufficient to block the GABA receptor.[72] DHEA, although less potent, mimics the effect of DHEA-S, whereas pregnenolone is totally inactive.[73]

Glutamate Receptors. PREG-S functions as a positive allosteric modulator at the *N*-methy-D-aspartate (NMDA) receptor; it enhances NMDA-gated currents in rat spinal cord neurons with 197 percent potentiation, whereas PREG-S inhibited GABA-gated currents (Fig. 2–13). In contrast, DHEA-S is weakly active, potentiating NMDA receptor–mediated responses by only 29 percent.[71] This action of PREG-S may have important implications because the NMDA receptor is believed to play a major role in learning and excitotoxic neuronal damage.

Sigma Receptors. Recent evidence suggests that DHEA-S and PREG-S regulate the NMDA response through sigma receptors. NMDA (200 μmol/L) evokes the *release of [^{3}H]norepinephrine* from rat hippocampal slides. This effect is potentiated by DHEA-S but it is inhibited by PREG-S at concentrations of 100 nmol/L. Thus, opposite neuromodulatory effects of these two steroid sulfates have been uncovered. Progesterone (100 nmol/L) mimicked the antagonist effects. These findings suggested that DHEA-S acts as a sigma agonist, that PREG-S acts as a sigma inverse agonist, and that progesterone may act as a sigma antagonist.[23]

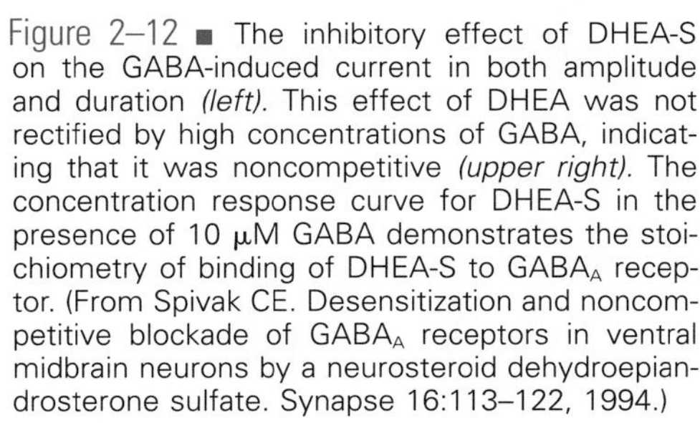
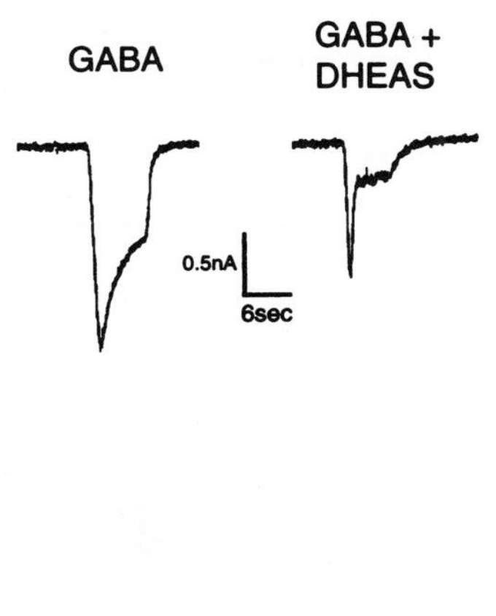

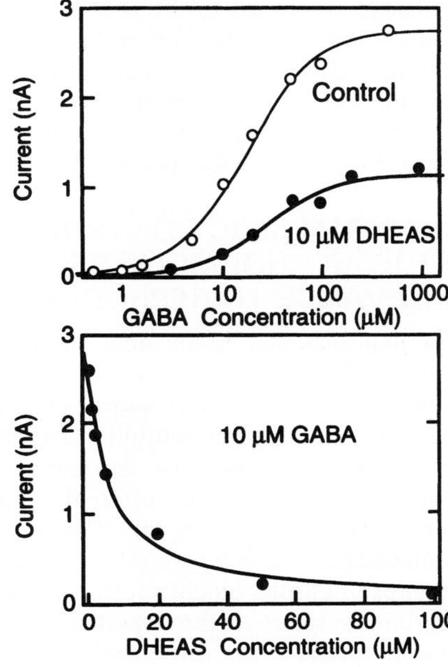

Figure 2–12 ■ The inhibitory effect of DHEA-S on the GABA-induced current in both amplitude and duration *(left)*. This effect of DHEA was not rectified by high concentrations of GABA, indicating that it was noncompetitive *(upper right)*. The concentration response curve for DHEA-S in the presence of 10 μM GABA demonstrates the stoichiometry of binding of DHEA-S to $GABA_A$ receptor. (From Spivak CE. Desensitization and noncompetitive blockade of $GABA_A$ receptors in ventral midbrain neurons by a neurosteroid dehydroepiandrosterone sulfate. Synapse 16:113–122, 1994.)

NEUROSTEROIDS AND COGNITIVE FUNCTION

Memory. Deterioration of cognitive function typically accompanies aging. The role of GABA in learning and memory is evidenced by the fact that GABA antagonists facilitate long-term potentiation in hippocampal neurons,[74] a synaptic process mediated through excitatory neurotransmitters and believed to be fundamental to long-term memory. Because inhibitory inputs provided by the GABAergic interneurons set a threshold for postsynaptic modification of excitatory inputs,[74] the GABAergic neurosteroids are likely to influence memory. DHEA, DHEA-S, and PREG-S as GABA antagonists are expected to enhance learning and memory, and GABA agonist to impair these functions. Indeed, DHEA and DHEA-S improved memory in aging mice and prevented pharmacologically induced amnesia.[75] The memory-enhancing property of PREG-S has also been reported.[76–79] Further, this effect of PREG-S in aged rats depends on endogenous PREG-S levels in the hippocampus, with responses more evident in rats with reduced levels. Moreover, PREG-S administered intraventricularly stimulated acetylcholine release in adult rat hippocampus. These data suggest that the hippocampal content of PREG-S plays a physiologic role in preserving or enhancing cognitive abilities in aging rats possibly through interaction with the central cholinergic system.[79]

In humans, the mood-elevating and pro-memory effects of oral ingestion of DHEA have been observed in middle-aged healthy men and women[80] and in patients with depression.[81] In addition, DHEA administration augmented *rapid eye movement (REM) sleep in men* and events believed to be involved in the consolidation of memory.[82] In contrast to the memory-enhancing properties of DHEA-S, GABA-agonist progesterone may impair automatized memory tasks in humans.[83]

Trophic Action: Myelination. Myelin repair in a damaged peripheral nerve responded to progesterone. Pregnenolone is present in the sciatic nerve of humans with a mean concentration more than 100-fold the circulating level.[83, 84] The formation of progesterone from pregnenolone occurs in oligodendrocytes and Schwann cells. During regeneration after cryolesion of the sciatic nerve (rats), remyelinization is markedly enhanced in the presence of progesterone, and the effect can be negated by the addition of RU 486 through blockade of the progesterone receptor in the Schwann cells. These data strongly suggest that neurosteroids also partake a functional role in the peripheral nerve.[85]

HYPOTHALAMIC CONTROL OF PITUITARY HORMONE SECRETION: RELEVANCE TO REPRODUCTION

The hypothalamus is the final pathway between the brain and the pituitary gland. The secretion of adenohypophysial (anterior pituitary gland) hormones is controlled by hypothalamic releasing and inhibiting factors. The pituitary hormones, released into the peripheral circulation, in turn regulate cellular growth, differentiation, and functional activities of the target organs. The maintenance of internal homeostasis and adaptation to the external environment requires multiple biochemical signals converging on the neuronal systems of the hypothalamus. This, in turn, leads to appropriate endocrine-metabolic responses through release of pituitary hormones.

Such a neuro-(hypothalamus)–endocrine (adenohypophysis) chemotransmitter system was originally suggested by the pioneering work of Green and Harris.[86] In recent decades, several classes of putative chemical messengers have been identified: monoamines, amino acids, neuropeptides, growth factors, and oncogenes. These biochemical messengers perform numerous functions in target cells, including *endocrine, neuroendocrine, paracrine* (affecting neighboring cells), *autocrine* (affecting the cell of origin), and *intracrine* (within the cell) mechanisms of action (Fig. 2–14). The neurohypophysis (posterior pituitary), in contrast, is an extension of the hypothalamus and conveys the neurosecretory neurons of the paraventricular nucleus and the supraoptic nucleus for the release of oxytocin, vasopressin, and their associated neurophysins.

To date, five hypophysiotropic hormones have been isolated: (1) TRH, (2) GnRH, (3) somatostatin, (4) CRF, and (5) growth hormone–releasing hormone (GHRH). The amino acid sequences of each of these neuropeptides are shown in Figure 2–15. Most recently, *urocortin*, a new member of the CRF family with 95 percent identity to the rat urocortin, was cloned and localized to human chromosome 2. It binds with high affinity to CRF receptors and induces adrenocorticotropic hormone (ACTH) release in pituitary cells in culture.[87] These peptidergic neuronal systems, originally thought to be unique to the hypothalamus, are now found in many regions of the brain, brain stem, and spinal cord. Further, they are present in the peripheral and central autonomic nervous systems; in exocrine and endocrine glands; in the diffuse endocrine tissues of the gastrointestinal, respiratory, and reproductive tracts; and in

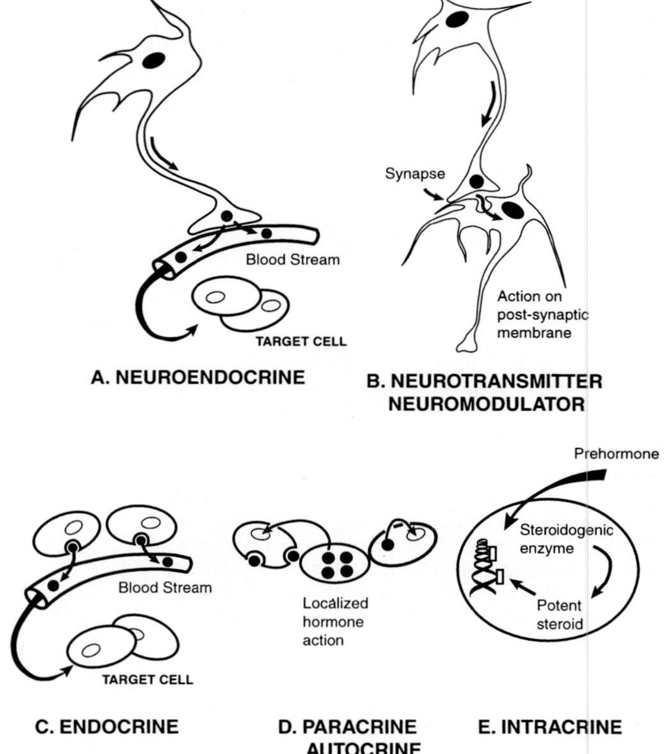

Figure 2–14 ■ Schematic illustration of various modes of neuroendocrine communications between and within cells.

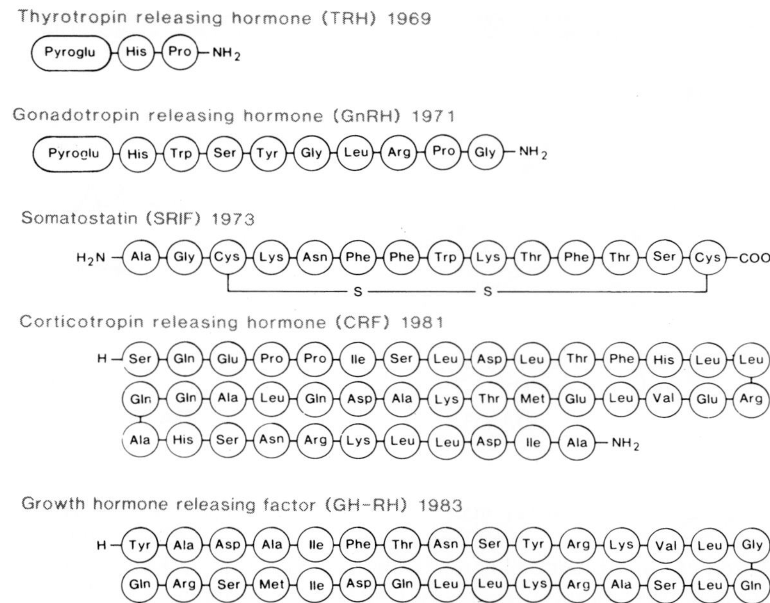

Figure 2–15 ■ The amino acid sequence of the hypophysiotropic peptides that have been isolated, characterized, and synthesized. The GHRH molecule was derived from pancreatic tumors. An identical or similar structure of hypothalamic origin remains to be isolated.

the placenta. The identification of genes encoding each of the hypothalamic hormones and their receptors has been accomplished.

In contemporary reproductive endocrinology, an understanding of hypothalamic control of *metabolic* as well as of *reproductive hormones* is required. For example, reproductive dysfunction may be associated with GH excess (acromegaly), with ACTH excess (Cushing's syndrome), and with thyroid deficiency and excess. Further, neuroendocrine regulation of reproductive homeostasis has been recognized to involve *circadian* rhythmicity and *sleep-wake* cycles within the 24-hour biologic clock. These dynamic processes are properties of a hypothalamic pacemaker (the suprachiasmatic nucleus), and they invoke cyclic changes of almost all clinically discernible physiologic variables such as body temperature, blood pressure, and pituitary hormone release.[88] Frequent sequential measurement of plasma hormones has led to the recognition that most hormones are secreted episodically *(ultradian* rhythm); several have prominent circadian rhythmicity; some are linked to the sleep-wake cycle; and others are synchronized with food ingestion and the dark-light cycle.[88–91] These entrained neuroendocrine rhythms have emerged as crucial indices of "glandular" function of the brain with growing appreciation that desynchronization of these rhythms may underlie a number of important reproductive disorders.[90, 92]

This section describes the control of adenohypophysial function by all of the established hypothalamic hormones and the regulation and function of neurohypophysial hormones. The hypothalamic control of neuroendocrine rhythms relevant to reproductive function is also covered.

Hypothalamic GnRH/Gonadotropin System

The elucidation of the structure of the 10–amino acid hypothalamic GnRH in 1971[93] and the cloning of genes for GnRH and human GnRH receptors[94] have led to rapid advances in the understanding of central regulation of reproductive function. Moreover, the recent development of immortal GnRH cell lines (GT-1 cells) derived from GnRH neurons by genetic targeting of oncogene expression in transgenic mice[95] has permitted studies to identify factors that regulate GnRH neuronal activities (see later). The pulsatile nature of hypothalamic GnRH release is now known to determine episodic pituitary gonadotropin secretion. The periodicity and amplitude of the pulsatile rhythm of GnRH/gonadotropin secretion are crucial in regulating gonadal activities and therefore the entire reproductive axis. The attributes of the self-priming effect of GnRH on its receptors on the gonadotroph are expressed only at the physiologic periodicity (60 to 90 minutes) by way of *upregulation* of GnRH receptors; slower frequency causes anovulation and amenorrhea, and higher frequency or constant exposure to GnRH induces refractory gonadotropin responses resulting in a state of *down-regulation* (Fig. 2–16). The activation of gene expression for gonadotropin subunits (α- and β-subunits of luteinizing hormone [LH] and β-subunit of follicle-stimulating hormone [FSH]), dimerization of αβ-subunits, and glycosylation are also governed by intermittency of GnRH inputs to the gonadotroph (for details, see Chapter 3).

Potent agonistic and antagonistic analogues of the decapeptide not only provide a reversible means of "medical castration" for potential use in contraception, endometriosis, leiomyomas, and hormone-dependent cancers but also serve as unique probes for the study of GnRH regulation of gonadotropin synthesis and secretion (see later).

GnRH Neuronal System and Gene Expression

GnRH NEURONAL SYSTEM

The GnRH neuronal system has been mapped in detail by use of immunocytochemical methods. GnRH neurons are

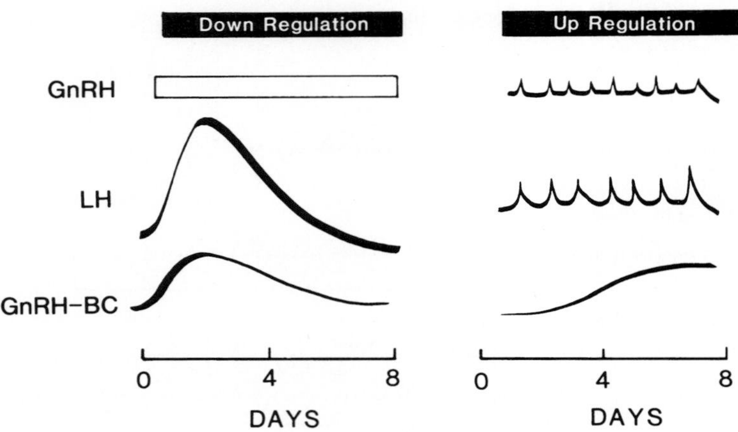

Figure 2–16 ■ Diagrammatic representation of down-regulation and up-regulation of luteinizing hormone (LH) secretion by inputs of continuous and pulsatile modes of gonadotropin-releasing hormone (GnRH) delivery, respectively. The GnRH binding capacity (GnRH-BC) represents the fundamental basis for down-regulation and up-regulation of gonadotropin release.

not grouped into distinct nuclei but appear as loose networks spread through several anatomic divisions. The population of GnRH neurons is relatively limited and is in the range of 1000 to 3000. There are considerable differences in the distribution of GnRH neurons among mammalian species. *In primates, including humans, GnRH neurons are located mainly in the arcuate nucleus* of the medial basal hypothalamus and the preoptic area of the anterior hypothalamus,[95] whereas in rodents, few GnRH neurons have been detected in the arcuate nucleus. The most prominent network in the rodent is composed of neurons forming a loose continuum of the *septopreoptic-infundibular pathway.*[96]

Axons from GnRH neurons project to many sites within the brain. One of the most distinct projections is from the medial basal hypothalamus to the median eminence,

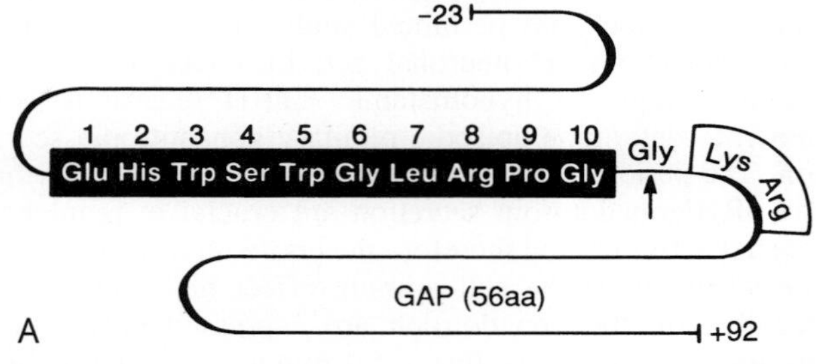

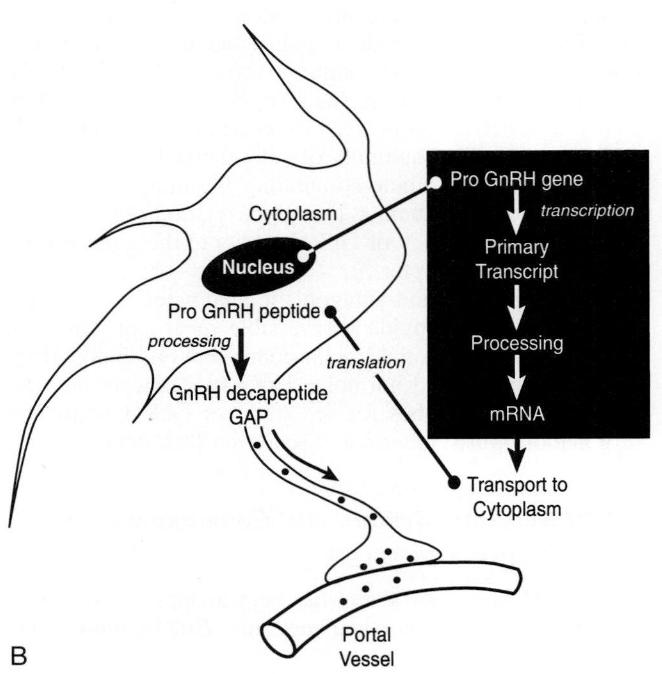

Figure 2–17 ■ The GnRH gene and processing of pre-pro-GnRH.

A, Diagrammatic representation of the structure and the 92–amino acid sequence of pre-pro-GnRH. The decapeptide (amino acids 1 to 10) is sandwiched between the signal peptide and the Gly-Lys-Arg sequence. The arrow indicates the site of proteolytic processing and C-terminal amidation of the GnRH molecule.

B, Molecular processing of GnRH decapeptide. In the nucleus, the pro-GnRH gene is processed to mRNA after transcription; mRNA is transported to the cytoplasm of the cell body (soma), where pro-GnRH peptide is generated after translation. Further processing leads to the generation of GnRH decapeptide and GnRH-associated peptide (GAP). GnRH and GAP are then transported to the nerve terminals and secreted in tandem into the portal circulation.

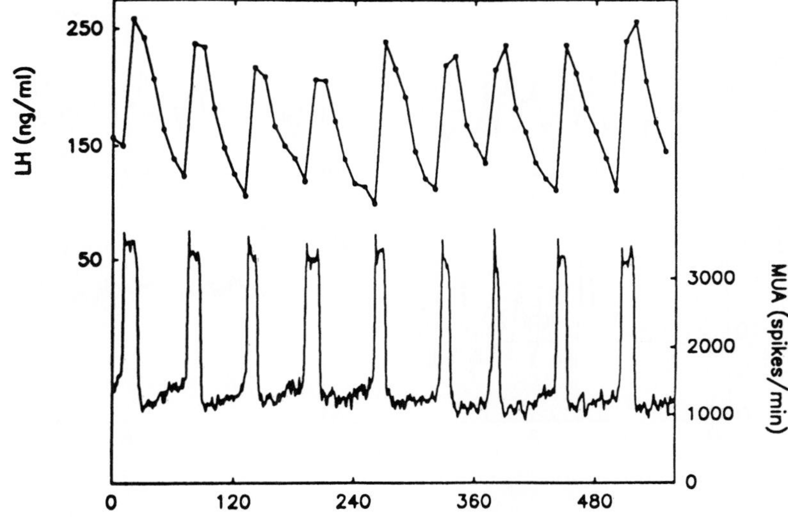

Figure 2–18 ■ Characteristic volleys of electrical multiunit activity (MUA) recorded from the medial basal hypothalamus in relation to LH pulses in peripheral circulation in an ovariectomized monkey. (From Knobil E. The electrophysiology of the GnRH pulse generator. J Steroid Biochem 33:669–671, 1989.)

terminating in an extensive plexus of boutons on the primary portal vessel, which delivers GnRH to its target cell—the gonadotroph. Axons of GnRH neurons also project to the limbic system and circumventricular organs other than the median eminence, such as the OVLT and neurohypophysis in humans and other mammals.[97, 98] These projections appear to serve a neuroendocrine role as neurotransmitters or modulators and may thereby regulate reproductive behavior.[99]

GnRH GENE AND ITS EXPRESSION

GnRH gene sequences were first isolated in 1984 from a human genomic deoxyribonucleic acid (DNA) library.[100] Analysis of the nucleotide sequence of mRNA reveals that the GnRH decapeptide is derived from the post-translational processing of a large precursor molecule, pre-pro-GnRH (Fig. 2–17*A*). The pre-pro-GnRH consists of 92 amino acids with a tripartite structure: the decapeptide is preceded by a signal peptide of 23 amino acids and followed by a Gly-Lys-Arg sequence (positions 11 to 13) essential for proteolytic processing and C-terminal amidation of GnRH molecules. The last 56 amino acid residues are designated GnRH-associated peptide *(GAP)*, which may have prolactin-inhibiting properties.[101] GnRH is encoded from a single gene located on the *short arm of chromosome 8*. The human gene contains four exons: exon 2 encodes pro-GnRH; exon 3 and a part of exon 2 and 4 encode the GAP protein; and a long 3′ untranslated region is also encoded in exon 4. *Placental pro-GnRH mRNA is longer* than hypothalamic pro-GnRH mRNA because of an encoded 900–base pair intron, which may modify or be regulated by tissue-specific promoters.[101]

With use of nucleic acid probes for in situ hybridization of pre-pro-GnRH mRNA as well as precursor-specific and GAP-specific antisera, the molecular processing within the GnRH neurons is found to occur primarily in the nucleus of the cell body (soma). After transcription and processing of the pro-GnRH gene, the mRNA is transported to the cytoplasm where translation takes place with the generation of GnRH decapeptide (Fig. 2–17*B*). The cleavage products, GnRH and GAP, are then transported to the nerve terminals and secreted in tandem into the portal circulation.[101–104] Within the brain, GAP is invariably colocalized with GnRH, but the functional significance of this tight association is unclear.[102]

GnRH Pulse Generator and Modulators

In a series of elegant experiments conducted in the rhesus monkey by Knobil and associates,[105] it was firmly established that the GnRH neuronal system within the medial basal hypothalamus exhibits rhythmic behavior with acute and short-lasting volleys of electrical multiunit activity. These volleys occur at approximately hourly intervals and have their origin in the vicinity of the arcuate nucleus within the medial basal hypothalamus. This mode of GnRH secretion occurs in all mammalian species studied. There is a remarkable synchrony between pulses of GnRH in the portal blood and LH pulses in the peripheral blood[105–108] (Fig. 2–18). Thus, an ultradian rhythm within the medial basal hypothalamus, which governs the pulsatile discharge of GnRH from the nerve terminals at the median eminence, represents the key controller of pituitary gonadotropin secretion and hence the entire reproductive process.

In humans, the patterns of hypothalamic pulsatile GnRH secretion and the site of the putative GnRH pulse generator have been largely inferred by characteristics of LH pulses determined in high-intensity blood sampling. To explore this functional-anatomic relationship in humans, the pulse generator has been studied in isolated human medial basal hypothalamus. Discrete pulsatile GnRH release from the medial basal hypothalamus of the human fetus (at 20 to 23 weeks of gestation) and adult can be observed in an in vitro perfusion system (Fig. 2–19). The periodicity of GnRH pulses is approximately 60 minutes for the fetal medial basal hypothalamus and 60 to 100 minutes for the adult medial basal hypothalamus.[109] Thus, in humans, as in monkeys, the hypothalamic GnRH pulse-generating system is located within the medial basal hypothalamus. However, it remains to be determined whether this "GnRH pulse

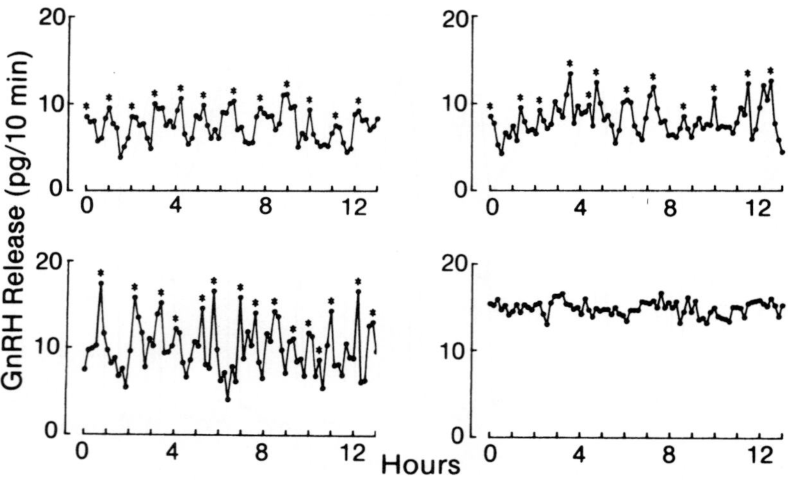

Figure 2–19 ■ Pulsatile release of GnRH from the human mediobasal hypothalamus (fetal and adult) in a perfusion system. The right lower panel represents medium control. (From Rasmussen DD, Gambacciani M, Swartz W, et al. Pulsatile gonadotropin-releasing hormone release from the human mediobasal hypothalamus in vitro: Opiate receptor–mediated suppression. Neuroendocrinology 49:150–156, 1989.)

generator" is an intrinsic property of the GnRH neuron itself or is influenced by electrical and chemical coupling to other neurons. This critical issue appears to be resolved by the observations of spontaneous pulsatile GnRH release of GT-1 neuronal cells in culture. Thus, GT-1 cells are endowed with rhythmic activities and pulsatile GnRH release is an intrinsic property of GnRH neurons, and *GnRH neurons per se* constitute the GnRH pulse generator.[110]

THE GT-1 CELLS

The development of immortalized GnRH-secreting GT-1 neurons by Mellon and colleagues[111] has afforded the analysis of mechanisms underlying the pulsatile secretion of GnRH and its regulation. These cells carry neuronal, but not glial, markers and contain extensive endoplasmic reticulum, Golgi apparatus, and neurosecretory granules. These cells proliferate and secrete GnRH, and the processing of pro-GnRH to GnRH and GAP has been clearly demonstrated.[110, 112] The most remarkable biologic effect of these cells is their ability to *reverse the hypogonadism of mutant hpg mice* (GnRH deficiency due to mutation of GnRH gene) after intrahypothalamic injection.[113] GT-1 cells express a wide variety of receptors and ligand-regulated channels and synthesize GnRH and its associated GAP peptide (see Fig. 2–16). Thus, modulation of GnRH release by a variety of neurotransmitters, hormones, and growth factors may be mediated *not* by connected neurons but by a direct action on receptors and channels expressed in the GnRH neurons.[114, 115]

MODULATORS OF GnRH NEURONS (GT-1 CELL MODEL)

Extensive studies using GT-1 cells have provided much needed information in regard to modulators acting on GnRH neurons as highlighted in the following (Fig. 2–20).

1. GT-1 neurons have been found to *express GnRH receptor*, activation of which is associated with rapid, prominent, and dose-dependent elevation of cytoplasmic calcium concentrations ([Ca^{2+}]i) and GnRH release, indicating *autocrine regulation of GnRH release by GnRH*[116] as also suggested by in vivo studies.[117]
2. *Opioids* are well-known inhibitors of GnRH neuronal activity as demonstrated both in vitro and in vivo.[118, 119] Using GT-1 cells, it was found that opioids have a direct effect on GnRH neurons that attenuate the stimulatory action of α-adrenergic and dopaminergic inputs. Thus, the inhibitory effect of opioids on GnRH release in vivo is by way of reducing the responsiveness to GnRH secretagogues and may not require an interneuron.[120]
3. The identification of *β_1-adrenergic* and *D_1-dopaminergic receptors* on GT-1 GnRH neurons provides evidence that the effect of norepinephrine and dopamine on gonadotropin release is mediated by *direct synapses* on GnRH neurons. β_1-Adrenergic and D_1-dopaminergic receptors are positively coupled to adenylate cyclase.[121, 122]
4. *Tyrosine kinase receptors* including IGF-I and IGF-II, insulin, epidermal growth factor, basic fibroblast growth factor, and prolactin are expressed in GT-1 cells. The presence of the insulin receptor family in GT-1 cells has allowed the demonstration of mitogenic effects of both insulin and IGF-I, but not of IGF-II. In contrast, IGF-II has a biphasic effect on GnRH release, but IGF-I and insulin are without effect.[123] The potent neurotropic effects of basic fibroblast growth factor[124] together with the ability of IGFs and insulin to stimulate mitogenesis and GnRH secretion suggest that these growth factor receptors may be important regulators of GnRH neuron expansion, survival, migration, and connectivity. It remains to be determined that these receptor mRNAs are expressed in native hypothalamic GnRH neurons as well as GT-1 cells.
5. *The ionotropic family of receptors*: Glutamate is one of the dominant *excitatory transmitters* in the hypothalamus and functions as a critical central mediator in neuroendocrine regulation of diverse processes such as cognition, memory, puberty, menstrual cyclicity, and reproductive behavior.[28] The synthesis of glutamate from glutamine appears to occur in glial cells because the biosynthetic enzyme *glutamine synthetase* is found only in the glial cells.[125] Once released into the synaptic cleft, glutamate can

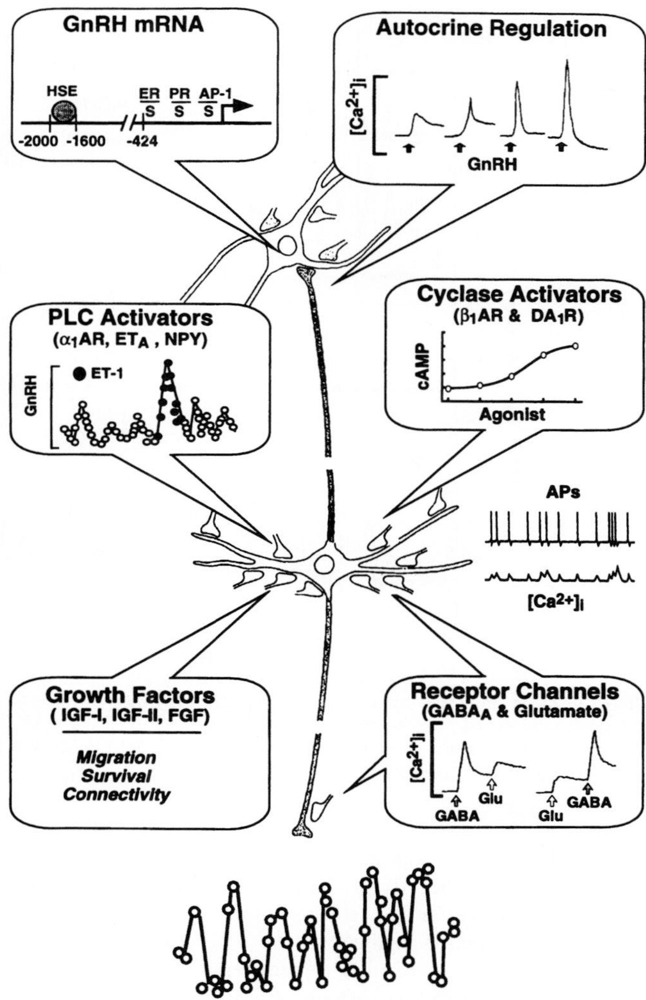

Figure 2–20 ■ The GnRH neuron and its regulation (data generated from GT-1 cell model). The three panels on the left and the three panels on the right indicate regulatory and modulatory processes of pulsatile GnRH secretion.

Left top panel, Transcriptional regulation of GnRH biosynthesis by multiple factors. HSE, hypothalamic enhancer element; S [SCIP], suppressed cAMP-induced POU (Pit-1, Oct-1, Unc-1) transcription factors; ER, estrogen receptor; PR, progesterone receptor; AP-1, transcriptional regulatory site for fos:jun and jun:jun dimer. Note: the T_3 *receptor* is also expressed on GnRH neurons (see text).

Left middle panel, Control of GnRH secretion by G protein–coupled receptors that activate phospholipase C (PLC) and adenylate cyclase, and receptor channels that influence ion fluxes and cytoplasmic calcium levels. α_1AR, α_1-adrenergic receptor; ET-1, endothelin 1; ET_A, endothelin A receptor; NPY, neuropeptide Y. Note that addition of ET-1 enhances GnRH pulse amplitude.

Left lower panel, Influences of tyrosine kinase receptor growth factors on GnRH neuronal activities. IGF-I and IGF-II, insulin-like growth factors I and II; FGF, fibroblast growth factor; PRL receptor not shown.

Right top panel, Autocrine action of GnRH on its neurons of origin. GnRH neurons express GnRH receptor, activation of which is associated with rapid, prominent, and dose-dependent elevation of intracellular calcium concentration ($[Ca^{2+}]$i).

Right middle panel, Adenylate cyclase–coupled receptors such as β_1-adrenergic receptor (β_1AR) and dopaminergic receptor (DA_1R). These receptors are also Ca^{2+}-mobilizing and cAMP-generating receptors. APs, action potentials as related to $[Ca^{2+}]$i flux.

Right lower panel, Receptor channels: NMDA (*N*-methyl-D-aspartate), kainate, and $GABA_A$ and $GABA_B$ receptor channels.

Bottom panel, Intrinsic pulsatile GnRH release of GT-1 GnRH neurons—the majority of hormones and growth factors that can influence the GnRH neurons are not essential for generating pulsatile release. (Modified from Turgeon JL. Gonadotropin-releasing hormone neuron cell biology. TEM 7:55, 1996.)

bind to NMDA receptors on presynaptic or postsynaptic neurons, or it can be cleared from the synaptic cleft by either glial or neuronal transporter protein. Agents that can inhibit glutamate exocytosis by acting at presynaptic receptors include GABA agonists and opioids.[126, 127]

In GT-1 GnRH neuronal cells, receptors for glutamate (NMDA), $GABA_A$, and $GABA_B$ have been identified.[128] The nitric oxide–cyclic guanosine monophosphate pathway is also operative in these cells modulating GnRH release in vitro.[42] It has been proposed that a potential interaction of glutamate neurons, *nitric oxide,* and opioid neurons occurs in the control of GnRH secretion.[28]

6. *Steroid and thyroid hormone receptors*: Intranuclear receptor proteins, which function as ligand-modulated transcription factors and are members of a large family of related hormone-dependent nuclear proteins, include the steroid, thyroid, and retinoid receptors that share common functional domains.[129, 130] Because estrogen receptors (ERα and ERβ) (unpublished results), progesterone receptors, glucocorticoid receptors, and T_3 receptor are all identified in the GT-1 cells as well as in the GnRH neurons,[131–135] steroid feedback sites and T_3 targets in the brain now include GnRH neurons. Potential interactions of estrogen and thyroid hormone receptors on a progesterone receptor estrogen response element sequence may occur and suggest a neuroendocrine-metabolic integration that is important for reproductive behavior.[136]

IN VIVO STUDIES

Experiments conducted in rhesus monkeys and humans have shown that GnRH pulse generator activities and associated LH pulses are subject to adrenergic modulation. Blockade of α_1-adrenergic receptor by phentolamine and the dopamine antagonist metoclopramide inhibits the frequency of pulse generation or arrests it altogether in rhesus monkeys, suggesting that central catecholaminergic systems exert modulating inputs to GnRH neurons.[137, 138] In contrast to findings with the rhesus monkey, α-adrenergic blocking agents have been ineffective in altering LH pulsatile frequency in humans. Acute administration of dopamine and dopamine agonists has been shown to decrease mean LH levels.[139–141] Morphine or endogenous opioids have an inhibitory effect, which can be reversed by the

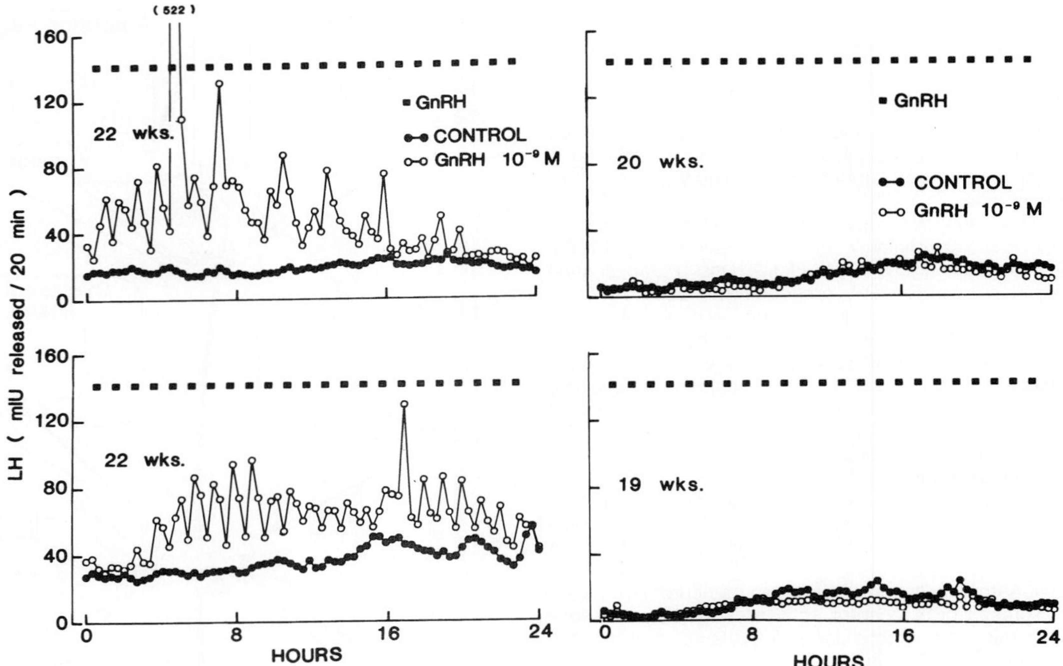

Figure 2–21 ■ Pulsatile LH release by human fetal pituitary (19 to 22 weeks) in response to pulses of GnRH stimulation (black squares) in a perfusion system. Note the marked differences in LH release between female *(left)* and male *(right)* fetuses. (From Rossmanith WG, Swartz WH, Tueros VS, et al. Pulsatile GnRH-stimulated LH release from the human fetal pituitary in vitro: Sex-associated differences. Clin Endocrinol [Oxf] 33:719–727, 1990.)

administration of the opiate antagonist naloxone.[142–144] CRF administered peripherally promptly suppresses GnRH pulse generator activity in the rhesus monkey, an effect that appears to be mediated through the activation of endogenous opiates.[105, 106, 145] Similar experiments in humans failed to discern an inhibitory effect of CRF on LH pulsatile secretion.[146] The presence of a high-affinity CRF-BP unique to humans may account for disparate results by a rapid binding of CRF to CRF-BP, thereby reducing free CRF at the receptor site (see CRF section for details).

Neuropeptide Y, galanin, and aspartate are putative excitatory neuromodulators of GnRH release in primates and rodents. Although aspartate appears to exert its effect directly by increasing the activity of the GnRH pulse generator, neuropeptide Y and galanin require gonadal steroids for their action.[147, 148]

Ontogeny of the GnRH Neuronal System

MIGRATION OF GnRH NEURONS FROM OLFACTORY PLACODE

During early development, neurons expressing GnRH immunoreactivity are found in the epithelia of the olfactory pit. Cords of GnRH cells course across the nasal septum and traverse the nervus terminalis into the forebrain. Thereafter, most GnRH cells form an arch through the developing forebrain into the anlagen of the septum and hypothalamus, extending into the preoptic area by embryonic day 14. This migratory route of GnRH neurons, studied in mice, supports the notion of an olfactory pit origin, in that increasing numbers of GnRH cells are found in the septopreoptic-hypothalamic area, with a concomitant decrease in the number of GnRH cells in the olfactory pit and nasal septum as gestation advances.[149] With the use of immunocytochemistry and in situ hybridization, a similar migratory pattern of GnRH neurons from the nasal region to the basal hypothalamus is found in fetal rhesus monkeys.[150] It is likely that the full set of signals guiding GnRH neuronal migration from the nose to the brain includes both mechanical and chemical forces. A *neuronal cell adhesion molecule*, a cell surface glycoprotein that mediates cell to cell adhesion, appears to be an important migratory force.[151] An olfactory epithelial origin for GnRH neurons provides an explanation for the anosmia associated with isolated gonadotropin deficiency in patients with *Kallmann's syndrome* (see Chapter 19). This link was confirmed in a 19-week-old fetus with a complete deletion of X-linked Kallmann locus; postmortem studies revealed that GnRH neurons had failed to migrate into the brain. They appeared to have been hooked up with numerous GnRH cells along the early migration route but were totally absent in the brain beyond the meninges.[152] This is the only hypothalamic neuronal system with its origin outside the brain.

DURING FETAL LIFE

LH-containing cells develop in the human fetal anterior pituitary as early as 10 weeks of gestation, and GnRH has been found in the human hypothalamus at 14 to 16 weeks.[153] Furthermore, isolated medial basal hypothalamus from the midgestational (20 to 23 weeks) human fetus releases GnRH in a pulsatile manner in vitro,[109] and the fetal gonadotroph has the capacity to respond in vivo and in vitro to GnRH stimulation with the release of LH.[154] Thus, by midgestation in the human fetus, the hypothalamic

GnRH pulse generator and the pituitary gonadotroph constitute a functional unit for maintaining LH and FSH secretion.

Concentrations of immunoreactive LH in serum and the pituitary are significantly greater in the female than in the male human fetus at midgestation.[155, 156] Because GnRH secretion at this time is quantitatively similar in the male and female medial basal hypothalamus,[157, 158] this sex-associated difference in LH secretion may reflect a negative feedback action by factors from the fetal testis that attenuate the pituitary sensitivity to GnRH stimulation. Indeed, during repetitive GnRH pulse administrations, LH responses are six times greater in pituitary tissue from female than male fetuses[154] (Fig. 2–21).

DURING SEXUAL MATURATION

The onset of puberty is brain driven by way of an increase in pulsatile release of hypothalamic GnRH. It is initiated in the absence of gonads, as observed in patients with gonadal dysgenesis,[159] and in the infantile monkey, puberty can be activated prematurely by exogenous pulses of GnRH.[160]

The ontogeny of pulsatile GnRH/gonadotropin secretion appears to conform to a U-shaped curve (Fig. 2–22); the elevated gonadotropin levels found during the first year of life are followed by a progressive decline, reaching a quiescent hypogonadotropic state at the age of 6 to 8 years with a parallel decrease in pituitary responsiveness to exogenous GnRH. Because the gonadotropin nadir occurs in the absence of ovarian function,[159] this prepubertal restraint on gonadotropin secretion can be attributed to the central inhibition of hypothalamic GnRH secretion. Although endogenous opioids are a most attractive candidate as a central inhibitor on GnRH neuronal activities, studies in monkeys[161] and humans[162] have failed to support this hypothesis. Instead, evidence suggests that the onset of puberty, but not the prepubertal gonadotropin nadir, is associated with increased opioidergic tone[162] and enhanced POMC gene expression in the arcuate nucleus.[163] The role of the putative excitatory neurotransmitters aspartate and glutamate in the activation of GnRH neuronal secretion during puberty should be considered. Glutamate enhances GnRH release from arcuate nucleus–median eminence fragments in vitro,[164] and prolonged intermittent intravenous injection of an analogue of aspartate, NMDA, results in onset of precocious puberty in immature monkeys.[165]

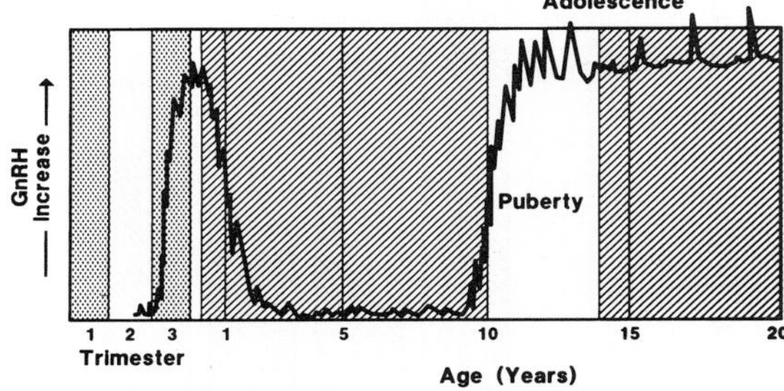

Figure 2–22 ■ Diagrammatic representation of the ontogeny of GnRH secretion from fetal life to adolescence. Note the prepubertal nadir and upswing of GnRH secretory activity at the onset of puberty. This is followed by irregular LH surges during adolescence in girls. (Redrawn from Yen SSC. Reproductive strategy in women: Neuroendocrine basis of endogenous contraception. *In* Roland R [ed]. Neuroendocrinology of Reproduction. Amsterdam, Excerpta Medica, 1988, pp 231–239.)

The pubertal activation of the GnRH secretory program (the upswing of the U-shaped curve) implies a decline in hypothalamic inhibitors or an increase of stimulators, either of which would permit a progressive increase in GnRH/LH pulse amplitude without changing frequency.[159] In addition, the sleep-entrained amplification of GnRH/LH pulsatility occurs at puberty that is critical to the activation of pituitary-gonadal function.[166] Before the hypothalamic-pituitary-ovarian axis is synchronized, luteal-phase defects and anovulatory cycles are common occurrences in adolescent girls.[167]

GnRH ACTION: RECEPTOR UP- AND DOWN-REGULATION (see Fig. 2–16)

The first step in GnRH action is its recognition by specific receptors localized exclusively on the plasma membrane of the gonadotroph. GnRH receptors are initially distributed evenly on the cell surface, but coupling with GnRH induces dimerization of receptors and formation of clusters, which then become internalized. Subsequent to their internalization, there is a substantial degradation of hormone-receptor complex in the lysosomes. A significant fraction of GnRH receptors is rapidly shuttled back to the cell surface. This recycling process is causally related, in part, to the *up-regulation* of GnRH receptors by GnRH.[168]

The GnRH receptor is a 60-kDa glycoprotein that contains sialic acid residues, with the oligosaccharide portion essential for the functional expression of the receptor on the cell surface of the gonadotrophs. A negatively charged domain interacts predominantly with arginine at position 8 of the GnRH molecule. GnRH induces and maintains a state of receptor cross-linking (microaggregation), thereby triggering subsequent events of hormone action. Prolonged or continuous exposure to GnRH or its agonists results in profound suppression of gonadotropin release, known as *down-regulation.* A GnRH antagonist, on the other hand, is capable of binding to the receptor but is unable to induce dimerization of receptors; thus, it reduces gonadotropin secretion by occupying the receptor without triggering hormone action.[168]

Physiologic regulation of LH and FSH biosynthesis and secretion by appropriate pulses of GnRH involves the interaction of inhibin, activin, and *follistatin* within the gonadotroph and influences by ovarian steroids (estradiol and progesterone) (for details, see Chapters 3 and 17).

GnRH and GnRH Analogues

AGONISTIC ANALOGUES

Native GnRH is degraded by peptidases in the hypothalamus and pituitary gland; these peptidases cleave the molecule at the Gly^6-Leu^7 bond and at position 10.[169] These degradation processes account for the short half-life of GnRH of 2 to 4 minutes.[170] The increased biologic activity of agonistic peptides has been attributed to the high binding affinity to GnRH receptors and to their reduced susceptibility to enzymatic degradation resulting in a plasma half-life 2.5 times longer than for native GnRH. Numerous

■ TABLE 2–3
GnRH Agonists Available for Clinical Use

NAME	STRUCTURE	MODE OF ADMINISTRATION
GnRH decapeptide	pGlu-His-Trp-Ser-Tyr-Gly-Leu-Arg-Pro-Gly-NH_2	Pulsatile pump
Leuprolide (Lupron)	pGlu-His-Trp-Ser-Tyr-DLeu-Leu-Arg-Pro-NHEt	Subcutaneous, depot implant
Buserelin (Suprefact, Suprecur, Suprefact depot)	pGlu-His-Trp-Ser-Tyr-DSer(O^tBu)-Leu-Arg-Pro-NHEt	Subcutaneous, nasal, depot
Nafarelin (Synarel)	pGlu-His-Trp-Ser-Tyr-D2Nal-Leu-Arg-Pro-GlyNH_2	Subcutaneous, nasal
Goserelin (Zoladex)	pGlu-His-Trp-Ser-Tyr-DSer(O^tBu)-Leu-Arg-Pro-AzaglyNH_2	Subcutaneous, depot
Histrelin (Supprelin)	pGlu-His-Trp-Ser-Tyr-DHis(Bzl)-Leu-Arg-Pro-AzaglyNH_2	Subcutaneous
Triptorelin pamoate (Decapeptyl)	pGlu-His-Trp-Ser-Tyr-DTrp-Leu-Arg-Pro-GlyNH_2	Subcutaneous, depot

superactive agonistic analogues of GnRH have been synthesized (Table 2–3); a D–amino acid *substitution at position 6* leads to metabolic stability, and the replacement of the C-terminal glycinamide residue by an *ethylamide group* leads to 10 times the affinity for the receptors.[169] Agonists such as leuprolide (Abbott), buserelin (Hoechst), and nafarelin (Syntex) are up to 200-fold more effective in stimulating gonadotropin release than is native GnRH. Down-regulation of the gonadotropin-gonadal axis can be achieved by the administration of a depot formulation of GnRH agonists, but it is preceded by a period of stimulation of gonadotropin secretion during the first 2 weeks of treatment.[171] At the moment, the Food and Drug Administration has approved the use of these agonists for the treatment of precocious puberty (see Chapter 15), endometriosis (see Chapter 20), and prostate cancer.

The side effects of long-term GnRH agonist–induced down-regulation of gonadal function are consequences of resulting sex hormone deficiency. In women, it induces menopausal-type hot flushes and vaginal dryness, and prolonged hypoestrogenism may result in bone resorption and osteopenia. This potentially serious complication, fortunately, is reversible in young women if treatment is maintained for no more than 6 months.[172, 173] Thus, in young patients with benign disease such as endometriosis, the risk-benefit ratio must be considered before GnRH agonist therapy is extended for longer duration. Currently, *"add back" regimens*, in which synthetic sex steroids are administered along with the agonists, have provided a means to overcome these side effects and permit extending the duration of agonist treatment.

GnRH ANTAGONISTS

In contrast, GnRH antagonists are characterized by modification of the pyroglutamic and glycine termini (positions 1 and 10) or deletion and substitution of hydrophobic D–amino acids at positions 2 and 3.[169] GnRH antagonists bind to the GnRH receptor without affecting gonadotropin synthesis, suggesting the N-terminal region is involved in the postreceptor mechanisms necessary for GnRH actions. GnRH antagonists have the distinct advantage of inducing an immediate decrease in circulating gonadotropin levels with rapid reversal.[174] Investigations using the earlier generation of these analogues have already demonstrated the crucial dependency of pulsatile gonadotropin secretion, bioactivity, and gonadal function in women and in men receiving GnRH.[175–177] However, because of a relatively low bioactivity and the induction of histamine release by mast cells, the clinical application of GnRH antagonists has been limited. New generations of GnRH antagonists are currently undergoing clinical trials.

Nal-Glu Antagonist (Salk Institute). Studies in women and men have demonstrated that Nal-Glu is a long-acting GnRH antagonist in the suppression of gonadotropin secretion.[178, 179] The absence of the initial flare associated with agonist treatment and the rapid recovery represent distinct advantages. These advantages are clearly illustrated by the rapid reduction of leiomyoma by 50% after 4 weeks of treatment (Fig. 2–23) and by the rapid recovery of gonadotropins after suppression of the midcycle surge in the induction of multiple follicular growth during ovulation induction in assisted reproduction programs.

In postmenopausal women, 50 μg/kg of Nal-Glu induces a suppression of 51 to 63 percent in 5 to 8 hours lasting for 24 hours. With a larger dose (300 μg/kg), the duration of action extends to 72 hours but does not alter the degree of suppression. The absence of dose-response relationship in the degree of gonadotropin suppression is similar to that observed with the first-generation "4F-antagonist" in postmenopausal women and in men, suggesting that suppression of gonadotropin secretion beyond 50 to 60 percent cannot be achieved with Nal-Glu antagonists. Histamine release occurred only at the site of injection. There is,

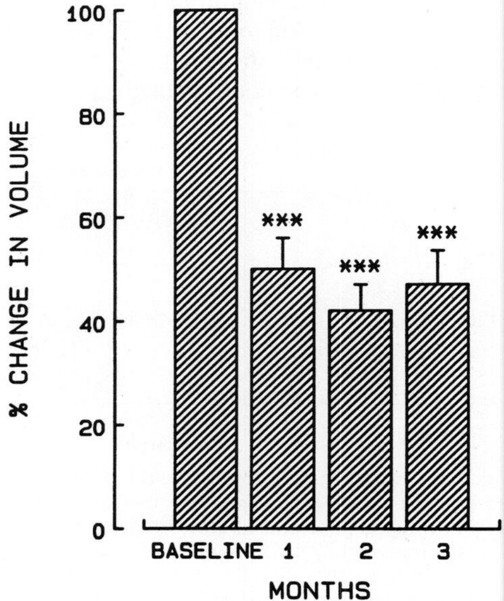

Figure 2–23 ■ Percentage change (±SE) in uterine leiomyoma volume after treatment with Nal-Glu GnRH antagonist (50 μg/kg/day, subcutaneously) for 3 months. ***$P < .0001$.

■ TABLE 2–4
Clinical Applications of GnRH and its Agonists

Activation of Pituitary-Gonadal Function (GnRH)

Delayed puberty
Cryptorchidism
Functional hypothalamic amenorrhea
Hypogonadotropic hypogonadism (Kallmann's syndrome)

Pituitary-Gonadal Inhibition (agonists)

Precocious puberty
Hormone-dependent tumors
  Endometriosis
  Uterine leiomyoma
  Breast cancer
  Prostatic cancer
Suppression of ovarian function in polycystic ovary syndrome and in vitro fertilization
Suppression of testicular function in men with severe paraphilia*
Premenstrual syndrome
Dysfunctional uterine bleeding including clotting disorders

Contraception

Suppression of spermatogenesis
Ovulation inhibition

*Data from Rösler A, Witztum E. Treatment of men with paraphilia with a long-acting analogue of gonadotropin-releasing hormone. N Engl J Med 338:416, 1998. Copyright by the Massachusetts Medical Society.

however, a greater reduction of bioactive forms for both LH and FSH than in their respective immunoreactive levels, thus yielding a significant reduction of the biologic to immunologic ratio.

Antide Antagonist (Serono). In monkeys receiving Antide intramuscularly, gonadotropin suppression lasts for 40 to 50 days. This surprisingly long duration of action may be due to formation of a depot at the site of injection by the Antide because of its extreme hydrophobicity. This low water solubility represents a major obstacle in the progress of clinical studies.[180]

Cetrorelix (Asta Pharma). This antagonist is currently undergoing clinical studies. The median effective dose of cetrorelix for histamine release is similar to that of Nal-Glu. In normal men, a single 6-mg dose suppressed testosterone levels for 12 hours.[181] A daily dose of 10 mg effectively and uniformly suppressed gonadotropin and testosterone. In a recent report, suppression of gonadotropin and testosterone was achieved by an initial high dose of the antagonist (10 mg/day × 5 days) followed by a maintenance dose (1 to 2 mg/day) with satisfactory outcome.[182]

Ganirelix (Syntex). This GnRH antagonist is also in clinical studies. The modification of the amino acid sequence has reduced the histamine reaction by 72 times, rendering this compound sufficiently safe for clinical trial. In phase I studies, a single dose of 1, 3, 6 or 12 mg of ganirelix administered subcutaneously to men and women showed only local erythema at the site of injection. At a 3-mg daily dose for 21 days, testosterone levels were suppressed by more than 90 percent in healthy men and remained suppressed until the end of the study.[183] With use of intranasal administration, similar results in the suppression of the gonadotropin-ovarian axis were reported in cycling women.[184]

Detirelix (Syntex). Administration of detirelix in doses of 5, 10, or 20 mg at weekly intervals to normal men showed approximately 50 percent suppression of gonadotropin with a greater decline in testosterone (~85 percent).[185] In postmenopausal women, suppression of LH is greater than FSH with decrease in androgen levels in response to doses of 1, 5, or 20 mg.[186] These acute studies did not encounter side effects. Long-term studies are not available.

CLINICAL APPLICATIONS

The induction of ovulation with pulses of GnRH in patients with ovulatory disorders and the suppression of the pituitary-gonadal axis with long-acting potent agonists in sex hormone–dependent disorders have had major impacts on clinical management (Table 2–4). A brief overview is given.

Activation of Pituitary-Gonadal Function. By means of an automatic portable pump designed to deliver a pulse of GnRH every 60 to 120 minutes, a large body of data has been collected that has shown this mode of ovulation induction to be effective and safe, particularly in patients with endogenous GnRH deficiency, such as Kallmann's syndrome and functional hypothalamic amenorrhea[187–190] (Fig. 2–24). The response to the intravenous route of administration is more predictable than to the subcutaneous route.[191] The usual frequency of delivery is one pulse per 90 minutes.

In male hypogonadotropic hypogonadism, long-term (30

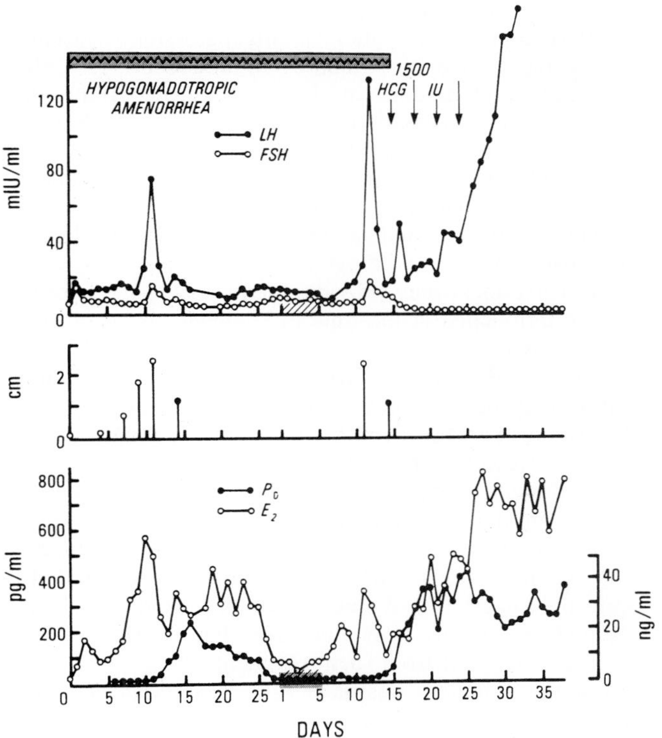

Figure 2–24 ■ Effect of pulsatile GnRH administration (1 μg every 96 minutes; shaded bar in top panel) during a period of 40 days on plasma gonadotropin levels *(top panel)* and ovarian steroid levels *(bottom panel)* and on follicular development *(middle panel)*. Note the occurrence of an LH surge on two occasions, with the second surge (followed by luteal support with human chorionic gonadotropin) resulting in pregnancy. Follicular size was measured by ultrasonography. Closed circles *(middle panel)* signify ovulation; shaded hatched areas *(top and bottom panels)* indicate menses.

to 60 weeks) pulsatile subcutaneous delivery of GnRH has been successful in inducing puberty and stimulating sustained testosterone secretion and spermatogenesis, with the ability to impregnate in some patients.[192–194] Thus, the use of pulsatile GnRH in the activation of pituitary-gonadal function in hypogonadotropic women and men represents an important advance in the management of hypothalamic GnRH disorders.

Pituitary-Gonadal Inhibition. Because of the ability of GnRH agonists to reversibly suppress the pituitary-gonadal axis without discernible side effects, the clinical use of these synthetic peptide analogues in the treatment of disease mediated by gonadal steroids represents a novel therapeutic measure in several endocrine disorders (see Table 2–4). Clinical uses of GnRH agonist for the treatment of *precocious puberty, endometriosis,* and *polycystic ovary syndrome* and as a potential modality for contraception are covered in their respective chapters. GnRH agonist down-regulation also offers promise of greater control over timing and avoiding cancellation during in vitro fertilization therapy.

Other Sex Hormone–Dependent Conditions May Benefit from GnRH Agonist Therapy

Uterine Leiomyoma (Fibroids). Uterine leiomyoma is an estrogen-dependent benign tumor occurring in up to 20 percent of women older than 30 years. GnRH agonist administration is the only medical treatment available at present. In a substantial number of patients, a rapid regression of the tumor occurs, with a maximal decrease in size of 30 to 80 percent at 3 months; this regression is sustained during the course of 6 months of treatment.[195–198] More than half of leiomyomas are likely to regrow within a few months after the cessation of treatment. Thus, GnRH agonist therapy may be most effective in reducing the non-myoma uterine volume more than the tumor size,[199] thereby decreasing mechanical interference with tubal function (improving fertility)[196] and facilitating myomectomy. In perimenopausal women with symptomatic leiomyomas, GnRH agonist treatment may provide a temporizing measure that can be terminated at the time of spontaneous cessation of ovarian function.

Hormone-Dependent Cancers. GnRH agonist administration may be an effective alternative to ovariectomy for the palliative treatment of breast cancer in premenopausal women. However, the attainment of complete pituitary-gonadal suppression requires sufficiently large dosages of GnRH agonists, and breast cancer develops in many women after menopause, that is, when spontaneous cessation of endogenous estrogen secretion has occurred. Despite the suggestion of direct antitumor effects of GnRH agonist treatment, it is doubtful that postmenopausal women will profit from such treatment.[200]

For the palliative treatment of prostatic cancer, GnRH agonist therapy induces a transient rise in plasma testosterone levels during the first week of treatment and a flare-up of disease. In a multicenter controlled study, the addition of an androgen receptor blocker, flutamide, prevented this adverse consequence of GnRH agonist treatment.[201] The efficacy of GnRH agonists is comparable to surgical castration and stilbestrol treatment, with fewer side effects. However, progression of tumor growth despite castration or stilbestrol is not likely to be improved by GnRH agonist therapy alone. Because of adrenal contributions to circulating androgens, the addition of an antiandrogen, nilutamide, has been reported to provide an increase in the median length of survival.[202–204]

Hypothalamic CRF/ACTH System

The isolation of CRF from ovine hypothalamus in 1981 by Vale and colleagues[204] represents a major milestone in the understanding of stress and adaptation. CRF has the capacity to stimulate pituitary ACTH and β-endorphin release in vitro and in vivo.[204] The CRF peptide consisting of 41 amino acid residues has been sequenced in several species including humans and has remarkable interspecies homology. Rat and human CRF is identical. The CRF gene, isolated from sheep, rats, and humans, also shows striking interspecies homology.[205] The human CRF gene is located on the long arm of chromosome 8.[206]

On the basis of extensive clinical and experimental studies, CRF is acknowledged as the primary hypothalamic player driving stress-induced ACTH-cortisol secretion.[204, 207] It is also clear that the action and distribution of CRF and its receptors extend beyond hypophysiotropic neurosecretory neurons in the paraventricular nucleus. Indeed, CRF is recognized as a crucial neuropeptide mediator of stress-related *endocrine*, *autonomic*, *behavioral,* and *immune responses.*[208, 209] Further, CRF has been implicated in the pathophysiology of a variety of diseases associated with dysregulation of stress responses and autoimmunity.[208, 210]

During the past 5 years, major advances have been made in the disclosure of the molecular identity and function of *CRF receptors* and *CRF-BP,* and alternative *endogenous ligands* in addition to CRF have been discovered. This section describes these advances and their functional role as well as the CRF system within and outside the brain.

CRF Pathways (Fig. 2–25)

The CRF neuronal system is extensively distributed in hypothalamic and extrahypothalamic sites as well as outside the brain. Three major systems have been identified in the brain.[211, 212]

1. The CRF pathway that controls pituitary ACTH secretion originates in the paraventricular nucleus and terminates in the median eminence (Fig. 2–25*A*). The concentration of CRF in the portal blood of the rat approximates 10^{-10} mol/L, which is in the range required to induce ACTH and β-endorphin release from human adenohypophysial tissue in vitro.[213] The presence of CRF cell bodies, together with oxytocin and vasopressin within the paraventricular nucleus, has opened a new understanding of their functional interactions (see later). The paraventricular nucleus contains more CRF cells than either oxytocinergic or vasopressinergic cells (Fig. 2–25*B*).
2. The paraventricular nucleus contains an autonomic division that projects to the brain stem and spinal cord. The CRF-rich part of the paraventricular nucleus contains adrenergic receptors and is densely innervated by noradrenergic and adrenergic fibers from the brain

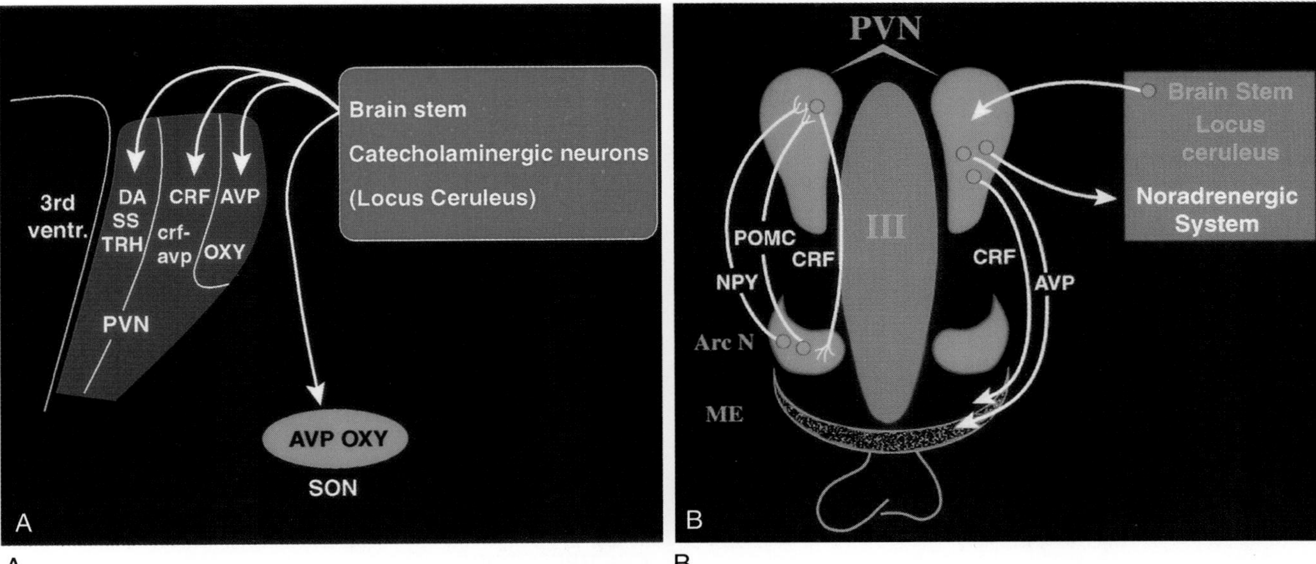

A B

Figure 2–25 ■ *A*, Anatomic depiction of multiple neuronal distributions within the paraventricular nucleus (PVN). Each of the PVN has three divisions; referenced from the third ventricle, the most lateral portion of the PVN contains arginine vasopressin (AVP) and oxytocin (OXY) neurons. In the middle portion of the PVN, the corticotropin-releasing factor (CRF) neuronal system is located with a small population of neurons that produce both CRF and AVP (crf/avp), and the innermost portion (nearest to the third ventricle) contains neurons producing thyrotropin-releasing hormone (TRH), somatostatin (SS), and dopamine (DA). The supraoptic nucleus (SON) contains neurons producing arginine vasopressin and oxytocin. Neurons of both paraventricular and supraoptic nuclei are innervated by adrenergic and noradrenergic terminals from the brain stem. (Based on the data from Sawchenko PE, Swanson LW. Immunohistochemical identification of neurons in the paraventricular nucleus of the hypothalamus that project to the medulla or to the spinal cord in the rat. J Comp Neurol 205:260–272, 1982; and Swanson LW, Kuypers HGJM. The paraventricular nucleus of the hypothalamus: Cytoarchitectonic subdivisions and organization of projections to the pituitary, dorsal vagal complex, and spinal cord as demonstrated by retrograde fluorescence double-labeling methods. J Comp Neurol 194:555–570, 1980.)

B, CRF and AVP from the PVN project to the median eminence (ME) and are secreted into portal circulation where they synergistically stimulate pro-opiomelanocortin (POMC)–containing neurons in the arcuate nucleus (Arc N) with the release of ACTH and β-endorphin by the pituitary. The lateral portion of the PVN also contains adrenergic neurons that project to the brain stem as well as receiving adrenergic input from the brain stem (see Fig. 2–25*A*). POMC and neuropeptide Y (NPY) in the arcuate nucleus project their fibers to the PVN. When activated, both POMC and NPY inhibit the secretion of CRF and norepinephrine such as occurs with leptin feedback to the arcuate nucleus.

stem.[214] Thus, the paraventricular nucleus has emerged as a site for integrating autonomic and neuroendocrine responses as occur in stress (Fig. 2–25*A).*

3. A scatter of CRF neurons is found in the cerebral cortex and in regions of the limbic system, including the amygdala, and in the nucleus of the stria terminalis. It is also found in the preoptic area of the hypothalamus that does not project to the median eminence. These scattered CRF interneurons may *act as excitatory neurotransmitters*. The widespread distribution of CRF within the CNS may serve to integrate neuroendocrine activation of the brain-pituitary-adrenal axis and stress-related autonomic reflexes and behavior (e.g., pain perception, arousal, and motivation).

Outside the brain, CRF immunoreactivity, CRF, and CRF receptor mRNAs have been found in the human placenta,[215, 216] endometrial stromal cells,[217, 218] ovary,[219, 220] T lymphocytes,[221] and adrenal medulla.[222] A variety of tumors also express CRF, such as carcinoids, pheochromocytomas, and neuroblastomas. CRF production at these ectopic sites may account for the development of Cushing's syndrome (see Chapter 18).[223]

Placental CRF may play a role in the regulation of ACTH secretion and processing of the POMC peptides within the fetal-placental and maternal-placental units. Circulating levels of CRF increase during pregnancy, reaching a peak at term with parallel increases in placental CRF content and CRF mRNA levels. Circulating CRF disappears rapidly after delivery of the placenta. CRF in blood is bound to a high-affinity CRF-BP that may mask the ACTH-releasing activity of CRF. However, the increase in CRF in late pregnancy is associated with a rapid decline in CRF-BP, thereby increasing free CRF, and may account for increased cortisol levels near term. Interestingly, cortisol exerts a *positive feedback effect on placental CRF secretion*.[224] It is suggested that these events may have significance in the initiation of parturition (see later, CRF-Binding Protein).[225]

Regulation of CRF

The release of CRF is mediated by multiple extrahypothalamic and intrahypothalamic neuronal pathways converging on both the paraventricular nucleus and the median eminence (axoaxonic interactions). On the basis of studies of CRF content, immunocytochemistry, and gene expression (mRNA) under a variety of experimental conditions, the regulation of CRF neuronal activities can be summarized as follows[226] (Table 2–5):

■ TABLE 2–5

Actions of CRF Involved in the Integrated Response to Stress

Activation of the pituitary-adrenal axis
Increased sympathetic nervous system activity after central injection, including increased blood glucose, oxygen consumption, cardiac output, and blood pressure
Diminished reproductive function
  Suppression of GnRH release
  Decreased sexual activity
Decreased growth hormone release (in animals)
Decreased gastrointestinal function
  Anorexia
  Decreased gastric acid secretion
Stimulation of respiration
Altered immune/inflammatory responses
  Response to interleukins
  Antipyretic effect
Behavioral activation (arousal, locomotor activity)

1. CRF secretion is under negative feedback regulation by circulating cortisol. Adrenalectomy depletes hypothalamic CRF initially and is followed by a subsequent rise to steady-state levels with parallel changes in CRF mRNA levels in the paraventricular nucleus but not other brain areas.[227]
2. Activation of CRF neurons occurs under stress conditions through a number of pathways:
   - Catecholaminergic inputs to the paraventricular nucleus from ascending brain stem pathways; the stimulatory nature of this system has been conclusively identified[211, 228] (see Fig. 2–25*A*).
   - The amygdala–stria terminalis (the limbic system) CRF pathway may function in concert with other neurotransmitters to modulate mood and behavior.[209]
   - IL-1, a cytokine, acts as a link between CRF and immune responses to stress.[210]
   - Hypoglycemic stress induced by insulin in rats causes a rise in CRF mRNA in the paraventricular nucleus, reaching a peak (180 percent) 2 hours after the onset of the stress. This is accompanied by increases in POMC mRNA levels in the anterior pituitary gland without affecting cerebrocortical CRF mRNA levels.[229, 230] *In humans*, insulin-induced hypoglycemia activates both ACTH secretagogues, with an acute increase in *both CRF and vasopressin* levels occurring after 30 to 120 minutes through activation of α-adrenergic input.[231, 232]
3. Other pathways that regulate CRF activity include the:
   - arcuate nucleus–paraventricular nucleus POMC pathway: opioidergic pathways from the arcuate nucleus to the paraventricular nucleus exert an inhibitory effect on CRF release, and this effect is reversible by naloxone, suggesting an opioid receptor–mediated event[233] (see Fig. 2–25*B);*
   - angiotensinergic pathway from the subfornical organ to the paraventricular nucleus, which may function to regulate water-salt metabolism;
   - neuropeptide Y pathway from the arcuate nucleus to the paraventricular nucleus, which stimulates CRF release independent of catecholaminergic inputs,[234] a pathway that may have an appetite-suppressive effect (see Fig. 2–25*B);*
   - suprachiasmatic nucleus–paraventricular nucleus pathway, which may partake in regulating the circadian rhythm of the CRF-ACTH-adrenal axis.

These findings demonstrate that CRF mRNA is under transcriptional regulation not only by glucocorticoids but also by other neural pathways, even in the face of rising glucocorticoid levels such as occur with stress. Thus, the ability of CRF to release ACTH and β-endorphin as well as to exert direct actions in the brain implicates CRF as a key signal in mediating and integrating endocrine, visceral, behavioral, and immune responses to stress[209, 210] (see Table 2–4).

CRF Mode of Action on Corticotrophs

CRF RECEPTORS

The initial step in CRF action on target cells or neurons is binding to the CRF receptors. The first CRF receptor gene to be identified encodes *CRF-R1*, a receptor that is expressed in the CNS, the pituitary, and the gonads. A second CRF receptor gene was cloned that encodes two isoforms, *CRF-2*α and *CRF-2*β. In the rat, CRF-2α is found mainly in the CNS, whereas CRF-2β is expressed predominantly in peripheral tissues. Both CRF receptors are members of a seven-transmembrane domain receptor family.[235] Type 1 CRF receptors are present in all regions of the brain known to contain CRF cell soma and fibers.[236, 237] In the hypothalamus, CRF-R1 are also present in the preoptic and arcuate nucleus, areas in which CRF may impinge on GnRH or GHRH terminals to affect their secretion.[238, 239] The CRF receptors are coupled to guanyl nucleotide proteins (G_s), which are linked to the adenylate cyclase–cAMP system. In the pituitary, activation of CRF-R1 induces rapid ACTH secretion (minutes) and POMC synthesis (hours).[240] The effects of cAMP are dependent on the transmembrane flux of Ca^{2+}. AVP, a cosecretagogue for ACTH, is less dependent on extracellular calcium, and its actions are mediated by the phosphoinositide–protein kinase C system. Further, the AVP target corticotrophs are distinct from CRF target corticotrophs, in that AVP target cells do not contain ACTH but act in a paracrine fashion to influence ACTH secretion.[241] Other secretagogues that may influence CRF action on ACTH secretion, such as oxytocin, epinephrine, and angiotensin II, are also mediated by cAMP-independent pathways.

Studies investigating the regulation of the expression of CRF receptor subtypes in the pituitary have thus far been limited to CRF-R1. In anterior pituitary cells in culture, CRF-R1 mRNA levels are decreased after treatment with glucocorticoids. Similar effects have been observed with in vivo glucocorticoid administration[242, 243] and in response to acute or chronic stress[244] and endotoxin.[245] In the paraventricular nucleus, CRF-R1 mRNA is markedly *up-regulated* by CRF, stress, and inflammatory responses and down-regulated by glucocorticoids.[235] In contrast, CRF-R2α mRNA levels in the paraventricular nucleus are not altered by any of these treatments.[246]

CRF-BINDING PROTEIN

In addition to interacting with its cognate receptors, CRF is bound by a high-affinity CRF-BP that inhibits the biologic activity of CRF. CRF-BP was originally identified, isolated, and purified from human plasma.[247] Human and rat CRF-BP cDNA display a high degree of sequence homology and encode a precursor protein 322 amino acids in length with one putative glycosylation site.[248] *In humans*, CRF-BP has been localized in the liver, brain, and placenta, but it is present only in the brain and pituitary in rodents. The absence of *circulating CRF-BP* in other species *except humans* indicates a unique biologic function for CRF-BP in humans.[247] Plasma CRF-BP concentrations are similar in men and women and during the first 8 months of pregnancy (~1 to 2 nmol/L). However, a precipitous drop in CRF-BP concentration occurs about 30 days before delivery, and this is accompanied by a rapid rise in serum CRF concentrations of placental origin reaching a peak at delivery.[249] These dynamic events should render an increased bioavailability of free CRF in late pregnancy (Fig. 2–26). It is proposed that this process is analogous to a "placental clock" that triggers the onset of parturition. This hypothesis holds that CRF stimulates the release of prostaglandins from decidua and amnion in vitro through CRF receptors present in the myometrium and fetal membranes, and CRF promotes the synthesis of prostaglandins and glucocorticoids, which in turn stimulate further CRF secretion by the placenta, resulting in a positive feedback loop between compartments[249] (see also Chapter 27).

Within the brain, CRF-BP is synthesized in, and secreted by, both neurons and astrocytes.[17] CRF-BP immunoreactivity is present in several regions of the cerebral cortex in human and rat brains.[250] The expression of CRF-BP in the hypothalamus is limited to the ventral premamillary and dorsomedial nuclei. In the pituitary, it is expressed exclusively within the corticotrophs, and it is inhibited by stress and adrenalectomy.[16] Whereas the exact function of CRF-BP under normal and pathologic conditions remains uncertain, substantial data have clearly demonstrated the ability of CRF-BP in the brain to modulate the availability of "free CRF" to interact with its receptor.[235]

UROCORTIN (THE PUTATIVE CRF RECEPTOR LIGAND)

Vaughan and colleagues[251] have recently identified and cloned a putative alternative CRF receptor ligand in rats named urocortin. The human counterpart has also been cloned and localized in human chromosome 2. The mature 40–amino acid human urocortin shares 95 percent sequence homology with rat urocortin.[87]

Human urocortin is a potent ligand for all three functional receptors (CRF-R1, CRF-R2α, and CRF-R2β). The affinity of human urocortin for CRF-R1 is comparable to that of rat urocortin. Whereas CRF-R1 does not appear to discriminate between CRF and urocortin, CRF-R2α and CRF-R2β show definite selectivities; urocortin exhibits much greater affinity than CRF *for CRF-R2β*, and urocortin has approximately 10-fold higher affinity than CRF *for CRF-R2α*. Thus, *type 2 CRF receptors favor urocortin* over CRF and may prove to be the endogenous ligand for type 2 receptors. Moreover, human urocortin, like rat urocortin, is *more potent than CRF* in its ability to stimulate ACTH release in vitro[87] and in its appetite-suppressing effect.[252]

Urocortin immunoreactivity and mRNA have been found in rat pituitary[253] and human pituitary and placenta. Within the pituitary, urocortin is colocalized with cells expressing GH (~75 percent) and prolactin (~22 percent), whereas ACTH-expressed cells contain only 1 percent or less of urocortin. Thus, urocortin is synthesized in the pituitary gland and may play a role as an autocrine and a paracrine regulator.[254] In the placenta, decidua, and fetal membranes, urocortin mRNA and peptide are expressed independent of gestational age.[255] The physiologic role of placental urocortin versus placental CRF remains to be determined.

In addition to interacting with CRF receptors, urocortin is also bound by CRF-BP. The binding coefficient of urocortin is twofold lower than for CRF,[251] and urocortin displaces CRF bound to CRF-BP, thereby elevating "free" CRF levels in the brain.[256] When administered directly into the rat brain, urocortin elicits endocrine responses resembling those of stress, increasing plasma ACTH and decreasing circulating LH concentrations (Fig. 2–27).

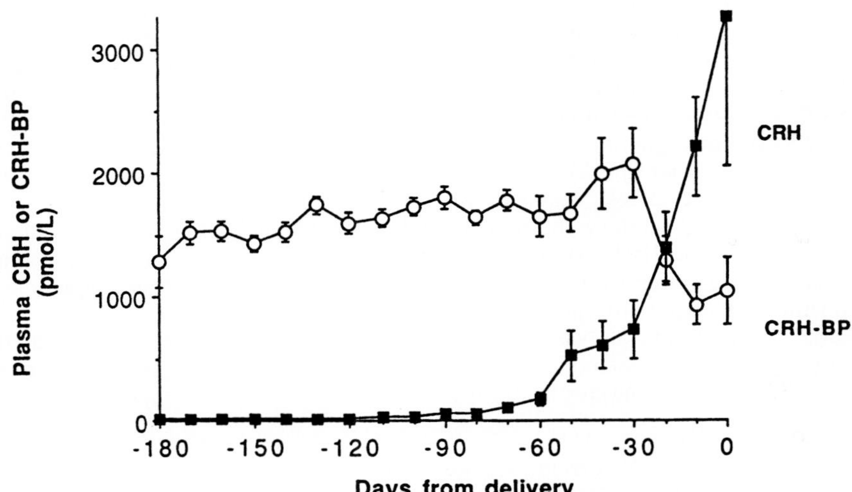

Figure 2–26 ■ Comparison of the molar concentrations of corticotropin-releasing hormone (CRH, ■) and CRH-binding protein (CRH-BP, ○) in maternal plasma during the final 180 days of gestation in pregnancies ending in spontaneous term labor (37 to 42 weeks gestation). Each point represents the mean (±SEM) of samples grouped by 10-day intervals calculated retrospectively from the day of delivery (mean of 59 samples at each point). CRH and CRH-BP concentrations are significantly different *(P* < .002) at all points except at the intersection of the two curves, 20 days before delivery. (From McLean M, Bisits A, Davies J, et al. A placental clock controlling the length of human pregnancy. Nat Med 1:460–463, 1995.)

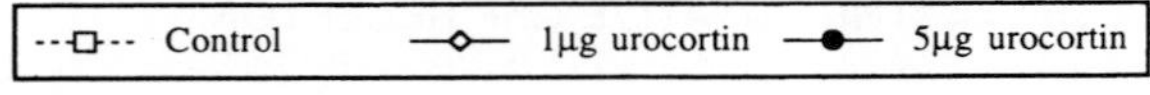

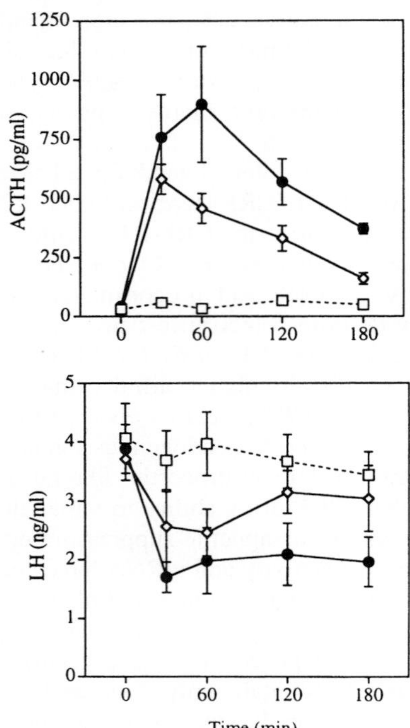

Figure 2–27 ■ Effects of urocortin administered intraventricularly on circulating levels of ACTH and LH in conscious castrated male rats. (From Turnbull AV, Rivier C. Corticotropin-releasing factor [CRF] and endocrine response to stress: CRF receptors, binding protein, and related peptides. Soc Exp Biol Med 215:1–10, 1997.)

CRF and Stress/Immune System

STRESS

Stress constitutes an essential stimulus for learning. The hypothalamic-pituitary-adrenal (HPA) axis and the systemic sympathetic/adrenomedullary system are the peripheral components of the stress system. The main function of the system is to maintain homeostasis during stress.[257] The central components of the system are located in the paraventricular nucleus, arcuate nuclei, and brain stem (see Fig. 2–25). CRF and noradrenergic neurons of the central stress system innervate and stimulate each other; CRF stimulates norepinephrine release, and norepinephrine stimulates the secretion of CRF through α_1-noradrenergic receptors.[257, 258] CRF, AVP, and noradrenergic neurons are *stimulated by serotonergic and cholinergic systems* and *inhibited by GABAergic and opioidergic systems* in the brain. This system is active at rest, responding to distinct circadian, ultradian, neurosecretory, hormonal, and limbic signals. Activation of the HPA axis heightens arousal, accelerates motor reflexes, improves cognitive function, suppresses appetite and sexual arousal, and increases the tolerance of pain.[257] In addition, activation of this system also alters cardiovascular and metabolic function and cytokine release in response to immune-mediated inflammation.[259]

CRF AND GnRH

Using synthetic CRF, several studies have demonstrated the inhibitory role of CRF in reproductive function. When cortisol is in excess, such as in anorexia nervosa,[260] depression,[261] psychogenic hypothalamic amenorrhea,[262–265] and exercise-associated amenorrhea,[266, 267] CRF administration results in a blunted ACTH response.[266, 268] This is best explained by endogenous hypersecretion of CRF and increased feedback inhibition of cortisol on the pituitary corticotroph. Elevated cerebrospinal fluid levels of CRF in anorexia[269] and depression[270] are consistent with this proposition. The link of CRF and reproductive dysfunction may involve its inhibitory effect on GnRH release. CRF infusion inhibits gonadotropin release in primates[271] and promptly suppresses the electrophysiologic activity of the GnRH pulse generator.[106] Central CRF administration in rats decreases GnRH levels in portal blood,[272] and stress-mediated suppression of gonadotropins is blocked in rats by a CRF antagonist.[239] The inhibition of GnRH release by CRF appears to be dose dependent, as shown in perfused medial basal hypothalamus.[273]

THE IMMUNE SYSTEM

It is now well established that activated immune/inflammatory cells synthesize a spectrum of peptides classically associated with the neuroendocrine system, which include the components of the CRF/ACTH–POMC system and their respective receptors.[221, 274–278] The concentrations of CRF in inflammatory sites are as high as those in the hypophysial portal system, but in plasma obtained concurrently, CRF is undetectable.[275] Rapid catabolism, uptake, or quenching by CRF-BP may prevent the appearance of CRF peptide in systemic circulation.[275, 279]

Several cytokines released from the immune cells may mediate the activation of the HPA axis during inflammatory stress. Tumor necrosis factor-α, IL-1, and IL-6 are the major players in stimulating the HPA axis.[259] All three cytokines can stimulate their own secretion by immune cells. This autocrine mode of regulation together with their ability to act synergistically in the activation of the HPA axis constitutes a novel interaction between immune cells and the neuroendocrine system in response to inflammation. In humans, IL-6 elevates plasma concentrations of ACTH and cortisol well above those achieved with maximal stimulating doses of CRF. IL-6, therefore, may induce the release of cosecretagogues, AVP,[280] or the newly identified potent secretagogue urocortin.[87]

IL-1 has been shown to be present within neurons in the human hypothalamus and is produced in the brain by astroglial and microglial cells as well as by macrophages.[281, 282] In the brain, IL-1 can stimulate CRF secretion,[283] and CRF can function to elicit IL-1 release by immune cells.[284–286] Thus, a two-way communication between IL-1 and CRF appears to be operative. Furthermore, an increase in cortisol secretion, consequent to CRF/ACTH activation, would exert a negative feedback on the synthesis and secretion of both IL-1 and CRF. It is suggested that such a neuroimmune feedback loop may serve to coordinate adaptations to inflammatory stress.[259, 287]

Hypothalamic GHRH/Somatostatin/ Growth Hormone System

GH Regulation and Gene Expression

GH REGULATION

The GH molecule, a 191–amino acid single-chain polypeptide hormone, is synthesized, stored, and secreted by soma-

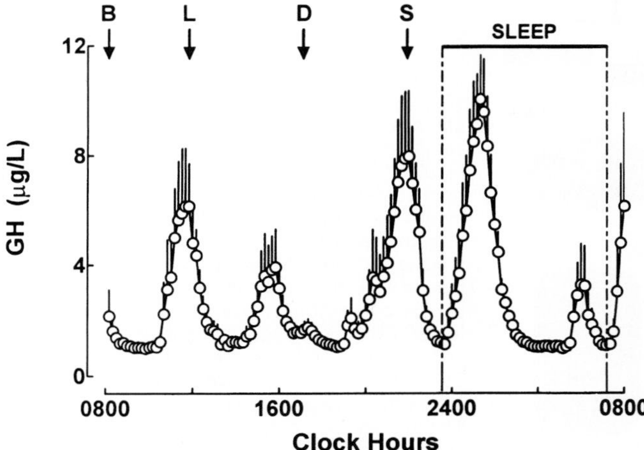

Figure 2–28 ■ Mean ±SE growth hormone pulsatile secretory pattern during the 24-hour sleep-wake cycle in healthy women. Arrows denote mealtimes. Note the large episode of release at sleep onset and the striking uniformity of the pattern of GH pulses when the timing, content, and duration of meals, as well as sleep time, are controlled. (From Laughlin GA, Dominguez DE, Yen SSC. Nutritional and endocrine-metabolic aberrations in women with functional hypothalamic amenorrhea. J Clin Endocrinol Metab 83:25–32, 1998. © The Endocrine Society.)

totroph cells, located predominantly in the lateral wing of the anterior pituitary gland. As a metabolic hormone, pituitary GH secretion is influenced by a variety of external stimuli and by endogenous neural rhythms. GH release is triggered by a host of activities, such as exercise, physical and emotional stress, a high-protein meal, hypoglycemia, and sleep. The 24-hour pattern of GH secretion is characterized by episodic release, and the number of GH surges increases from four to six to as frequent as eight episodes per 24 hours around puberty, with the highest amplitude pulse occurring about 1 hour after sleep onset during slow-wave sleep (stages III and IV)[292, 293] (Fig. 2–28). The daily secretory rate of GH is age dependent, being 90 μg in prepubertal children, increasing to 700 μg in adolescents, and decreasing to 380 μg in young adults,[292] with a further decline in age-advanced postmenopausal women.[294] This decline of GH as well as of IGF-I levels is primarily due to a diminished GH pulse amplitude (Fig. 2–29). The circulating half-life of GH is between 17 and 45 minutes. GH secretion by the pituitary is enhanced by exercise, physical stress, emotional stress, and sepsis; augmented by estrogen, testosterone, and thyroid hormones; and suppressed by free fatty acids and factors related to adiposity. GH secretion appears to be stimulated by central dopaminergic input: apomorphine, a central dopamine receptor agonist, stimulates GH secretion, and the administration of L-dopa for 6 months to GH-deficient children increases their growth velocity.[295] Norepinephrine increases GH secretion through α-adrenergic pathways and inhibits GH secretion through β-adrenergic pathways.[296] Activation of α-adrenergic activity by clonidine, arginine, exercise, L-dopa, and antidiuretic hormone facilitates GH secretion. The clinical significance of these responses remains to be clarified. Jet lag transiently increases the amplitude of GH peaks, resulting in an increase in 24-hour GH secretion. Further, jet lag is associated with a circadian shift of the maximal GH peak from the early to late sleep period.[297]

The actions of GH are numerous and include stimulation of skeletal and muscle growth, regulation of lipolysis, and promotion of cellular uptake of amino acids. GH induces insulin resistance and thus is diabetogenic but also exerts insulin-like effects. Most of the effects of GH on growth are mediated indirectly through the production of insulin-like growth factors (IGF-I and IGF-II) at multiple tissue sites.[298] Serum GH is bound to GH-binding protein, and circulating IGF-I and IGF-II are also bound to specific binding proteins (IGFBPs) that are critically important in modulating IGF action at target tissues. In addition, IGF-I exerts a negative feedback effect on GH secretion.[299] The functional activities, target sites, and multilevels of regulation of the GH–IGF-I axis are depicted in Figure 2–30.

GH GENE EXPRESSION

The GH gene, consisting of a cluster of five highly conserved regions, spans approximately 66 kilobases on the long arm of chromosome 17 at bands q22–24.[300] These genes are arranged 5′ to 3′ as follows: *hGH-N*, *hCS-A*, hGH variant (*hGH-V*), and *hCS-B*. The hCS-A, hCS-B, and hGH-V are expressed in human placental tissue; *hGH-N* codes a 22-kDa protein consisting of 191 amino acids and is exclusively *expressed in somatotrophs*.[301]

Hypothalamic Control: GHRH/Somatostatin/GHRP

The episodic secretion of pituitary GH is under the dual control of two hypothalamic peptides; somatostatin inhibits its release, and GH-releasing factor (GHRH) stimulates its

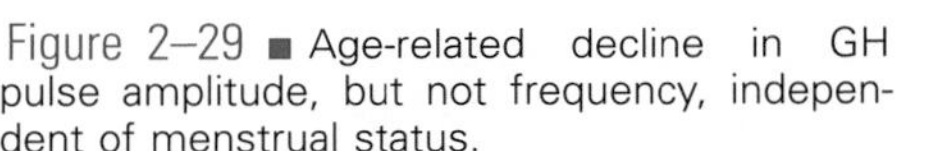
Figure 2–29 ■ Age-related decline in GH pulse amplitude, but not frequency, independent of menstrual status.

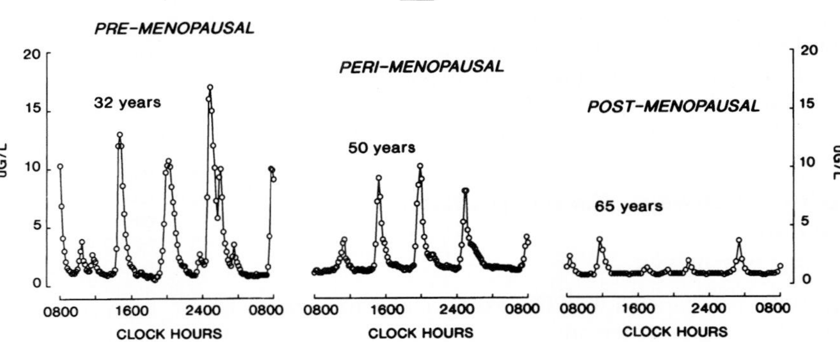

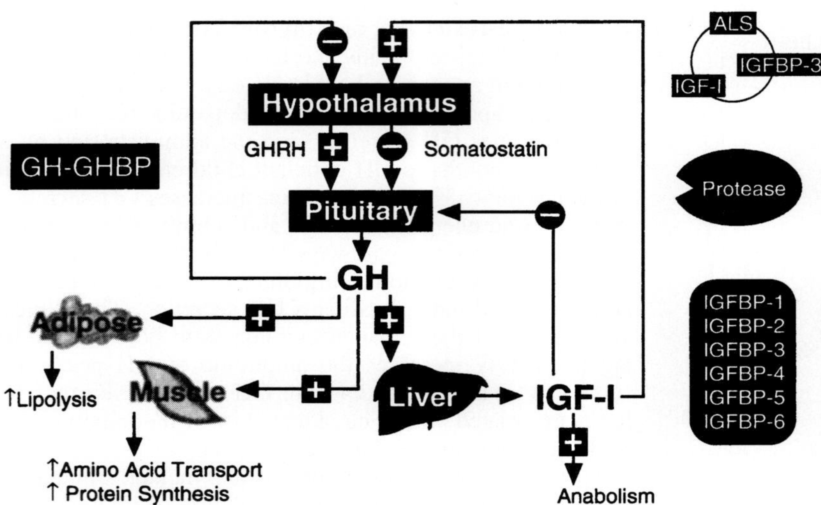

Figure 2–30 ■ The GH–IGF-I axis. This figure depicts the sites of production of GH and IGF-I, the feedback loops regulating their secretion, binding proteins, and main metabolic actions. The hypothalamic hormones GHRH and somatostatin control GH secretion from the pituitary. GH circulates in the blood, in part bound to a GH-binding protein (GHBP), and acts to inhibit its own secretion and to stimulate the production of insulin-like growth factor I (IGF-I) in the liver. IGF-I circulates in the blood bound primarily to IGF-binding protein 3 (IGFBP-3), which is in turn complexed to a third protein, the acid-labile subunit (ALS), but a total of six IGFBPs are known. IGFBP-IGF complexes are subject to protease attack, which induces the dissociation of IGF-I. The actions of GH are exerted either directly or indirectly, through the generation of IGF-I. (From Clark R. The somatogenic hormones and insulin-like growth factor-I: Stimulators of lymphopoiesis and immune function. Endocr Rev 18:157–178, 1997. © The Endocrine Society.)

secretion. In portal blood, GHRH is secreted episodically and induces pulsatile release of pituitary GH. However, the regulation of GH secretion has been dramatically modified by the recent disclosure of an important class of *GH secretagogues,* which include GH-releasing peptide 6 (*GHRP-6*) and several synthetic peptides such as MK-0677. These secretagogues stimulate GH release in vivo by acting at both pituitary and hypothalamic sites. Moreover, the receptor that mediates the action of secretagogues has recently been cloned, although the specific endogenous ligands for this receptor are currently unknown.[302] Interestingly, continuous exposure to elevated levels of GH secretagogues is accompanied by a striking and prolonged enhancement of the pulsatile pattern of GH secretion.[302]

The action of these secretagogues, and in particular their interaction with GHRH and somatostatin neurons, assumes a major significance for a full understanding of the physiologic regulation of GH release. Although this additional level of central regulation of GH secretion is under vigorous investigation, the concise interpretation of available data suggests that an unknown endogenous ligand for the GH secretagogue receptor will soon be discovered that may prove to govern the GHRH-mediated self-entrainment of GH pulsatility (Fig. 2–31). In fact, oral administration of a GH secretagogue (MK-0677) in healthy aging subjects has demonstrated an enhancement of preexisting pulsatile secretion with amplification of both pulse height and interpulse nadir concentrations without changes in pulse number. With a 25-mg daily dose, IGF-I concentrations increased into the young adult range.[303] This remarkable effect of MK-0677 offers important medical significance. In this setting, the increased circulating IGFs exert a feedback action at the pituitary and hypothalamic levels by inhibiting the action of GHRH on the somatotroph and stimulating the release of hypothalamic somatostatin.[304–306]

GHRH Pathways, Gene Expression, and Action

GHRH PATHWAYS

In 1981, two patients with GH excess and acromegaly were found to have pancreatic islet cell adenomas secreting "ectopic" GHRH, which led to the rapid isolation and sequencing of GHRH. Subsequent studies of human hypothalami confirmed that the 44–amino acid C-terminal amide peptide $hGHRH_{1-44}NH_2$ is the authentic GHRH.[307] GHRH from several other species showed nearly complete homology with hGHRH. The ability of hGHRH to elicit GH release is both rapid and brief in humans and resembles spontaneous pulses of GH secretion (Fig. 2–32).

In the CNS of humans and rats, most of the GHRH is located in the medial basal hypothalamus, specifically the posterior part of the arcuate nucleus. These neurons project primarily to nerve endings in the median eminence. GHRH-containing neurons are also found in the ventromedial nucleus of the hypothalamus and within the parvicellular (small cell) zone of the paraventricular nucleus. Most of these neurons project not to the median eminence but, rather, to the anterior hypothalamus, where they may partic-

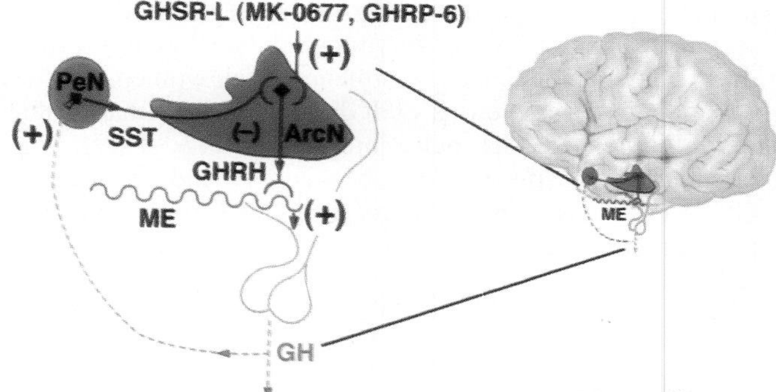

Figure 2–31 ■ A schematic model of GH-mediated feedback regulation through somatostatin (SST) subtype 2 in the hypothalamus. *The GH secretagogue receptor* ligands (GHSR-L) such as MK-0677 and GHRP-6 activate neurons in the arcuate nucleus (ArcN). GHRH is released into the median eminence (ME) to stimulate GH release from the somatotroph. GH, in turn, feeds back by interacting with GH receptors on neurons of the periventricular nucleus (PeN) to cause the release of SST. SST, by interacting with the SST type 2 receptor, inhibits arcuate GHRH neurons, thereby decreasing GHRH release. (Adapted from Zheng H, Bailey A, Jiang M-H, et al. Somatostatin receptor subtype 2 knockout mice are refractory to growth hormone–negative feedback on arcuate neurons. Mol Endocrinol 11:1709–1717, 1997.)

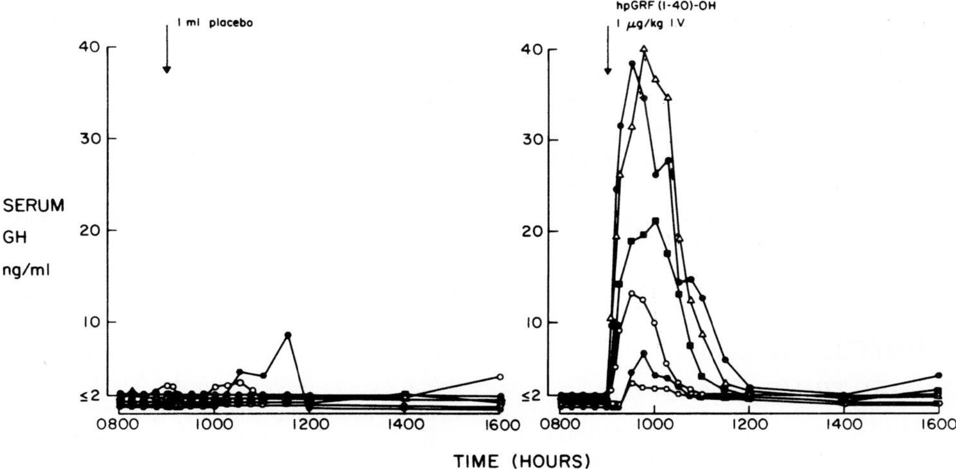

Figure 2–32 ■ Circulating growth hormone (GH) levels after a placebo and after human pancreatic growth hormone–releasing factor (hpGRF) administration to six normal men. (From Thorner MO, Spiess J, Vance ML, et al. Human pancreatic growth-hormone-releasing factor selectively stimulates growth-hormone secretion in man. Lancet 1:24–28, 1983. © by The Lancet Ltd.)

ipate in a stimulatory role on somatostatinergic neurons.[308–310] This anatomic-functional relationship may account for the presence of pulsatile GH secretion in humans during continuous GHRH infusion or subcutaneous injection.[311, 312] Thus, GH pulses are the result, in part, of somatostatin withdrawal that is associated with a release of GHRH.

Among the hypothalamic hormones, GHRH is most circumscribed in its hypothalamic localization. Apart from ectopic GHRH-producing tumors and GHRH in the human placenta and immune cells, *no other extrahypothalamic GHRH sites have been identified.* In peripheral blood, GHRH is detectable at levels of about 10 pg/ml or less in humans. Thus, the presence of elevated plasma levels of GHRH in a patient with acromegaly is presumptive evidence of an ectopic GHRH-producing tumor.[313]

REGULATION OF GHRH GENE EXPRESSION

The structure of the GHRH gene includes five exons and four introns. Exons 1 and 2 encode the 5′ untranslated sequences; exons 2 to 4 encode most of the 107- or 108–amino acid pre-pro-hormone, with exon 3 encoding almost all of the bioactive portion of mature GHRH.[314] The short-loop feedback by GH and the long-loop feedback by IGF-I also reciprocally act on hypothalamic somatostatin and GHRH secretion.[304, 315] Further, a direct feedback regulation of GHRH gene expression by GH has been demonstrated; hypophysectomy in the rat produces a sixfold rise in GHRH mRNA within 3 days, increasing to maximal levels at 7 days without changes in somatostatin mRNA levels. Thyroidectomy and adrenalectomy have no discernible effect on GHRH mRNA levels.[316]

GHRH MODE OF ACTION ON SOMATOTROPHS

After binding of GHRH to membrane receptors on the pituitary somatotroph, the ligand-receptor complex is coupled directly to the stimulatory (guanosine triphosphate) binding protein (G_s), which in turn activates the catalytic subunit of adenylate cyclase to form cAMP. Calcium influx occurs independently and may be further enhanced by cAMP-mediated phosphorylation of calcium channels.[317] GH release and synthesis in response to GHRH are independently regulated: the release of GH may be mediated by calcium influx, and the cAMP-dependent protein kinases may stimulate GH gene transcription and synthesis. Similarly, binding of somatostatin to its receptor induces inhibition of GHRH-stimulated release of GH through activation of an inhibitory G_i protein, which directly inhibits the calcium channel as well as the adenylate cyclase catalytic subunit.[317] Thus, the interaction of two opposing hypothalamic regulators on GH secretion and synthesis may prevent down-regulation of the GH response to prolonged GHRH stimulation.[318, 319]

Somatostatin and Pathways

Somatostatin, a 14–amino acid cyclic peptide with GH release–inhibiting activity, was isolated and sequenced by Brazeau and coworkers[320] in 1973. The somatostatin pathway regulating pituitary GH secretion arises in the anterior region of the *periventricular nuclei* and a well-defined *subdivision of the paraventricular nuclei.* As indicated before, episodic GH secretion is coordinated by a decrease of somatostatin and an associated increase in GHRH release. The constant presence of somatostatin, both in vivo and in vitro, exerts potent inhibition on GH release in all species studied, regardless of the stimulus used to induce GH secretion. Somatostatin also serves a physiologic role as a thyroid-stimulating hormone (TSH) release–inhibiting factor.[317]

Somatostatin was the first hypothalamic hormone found to be widely distributed. It is present in the CNS outside the hypothalamus as well as in the gastrointestinal tract, pancreas, and placenta and possesses a diversity of functions. Somatostatin functions as a neurotransmitter in CNS neurons and has an inhibitory role on pituitary and gastrointestinal hormone secretion, on gut blood flow and motility, and on nutrient absorption; it may also have a suppressive effect on the immune system. Thus, somatostatin has endocrine, paracrine, and neurotransmitter modes of action within and outside the brain.[317]

Synthetic somatostatin analogues that possess longer half-life and selective target sites (i.e., pituitary, pancreas, and gastrointestinal tract) have been partially successful in treatments of GH excess of specific organ sources. Octreotide, a somatostatin analogue, appears to inhibit pituitary GH secretion preferentially. Subcutaneous administration of a 50-μg dose of octreotide lowers GH levels in both normal subjects and acromegalics.[317]

Hypothalamic TRH/TSH System

Hypothalamic Control: TRH/Somatostatin

The hypothalamic control of the pituitary TSH-thyroid axis is exerted by the stimulatory action of TRH and the inhibitory action of somatostatin. TRH, a tripeptide (pyroglutamyl-histidyl-proline-amide), was the first hypothalamic hormone to be chemically identified (1969). TRH cell bodies in the hypothalamus are aggregated *in a discrete area of the paraventricular nucleus*, and their fibers project to the neurovascular zone of the median eminence. Electrolytic lesioning of the paraventricular nucleus results in tertiary (hypothalamic) hypothyroidism. TRH-containing neurons in the paraventricular nucleus are densely innervated by catecholaminergic axons, which exert a stimulatory effect on TRH secretion (see Fig. 2–25*A*). TRH neurons also receive a dense innervation by neuropeptide Y that may function to antagonize the facilitatory influence of norepinephrine.[321] Perhaps most important is the innervation of TRH neurons by somatostatin-containing axons within the paraventricular nucleus. Somatostatin is known to inhibit TRH secretion (see Fig. 2–25*A*).

In addition, TRH is present throughout the brain, spinal cord, pancreas, and gastrointestinal tract. The function of TRH in other CNS regions is largely unknown. TRH- and pro-TRH–containing neurons are present in the olfactory lobe and limbic structures. A prominent group of cell bodies is present in the raphe nucleus (serotonin neurons) and projects to the spinal cord, where fibers terminate on anterior horn alpha motor neurons. In this location, TRH may serve a neurotrophic role for the motor neuron.[322] This raphe nuclei projection of TRH fibers is colocalized with serotonin and substance P. Another group of TRH neurons is in the dorsal motor nucleus of the vagus, where TRH may modulate vagal input in the control of gastric secretion.[323]

TRH Gene and Regulation

The mRNA and gene structure of human TRH were characterized by Yamada and coworkers,[324] and the gene has been assigned to chromosome 3. The gene consists of three exons and two introns. Exons 1 and 2 encode untranslated mRNA and peptide leader sequences respectively; exon 3 encodes the remainder of the peptide, *including all five copies of TRH*. This is analogous to prepro-enkephalin, in which a single exon encodes the pentapeptide with multiple copies.[325]

Thyroid hormones exert a negative feedback on TRH mRNA and secretion: hypothyroidism causes a substantial increase in pro-TRH mRNA in the paraventricular nucleus, whereas hyperthyroidism inhibits its expression and secretion, establishing the feedback relationship between thyroid hormone and TRH gene expression and synthesis.[326] As expected, T_3 implanted directly into the paraventricular nucleus completely inhibits TRH mRNA expression.[326] As with CRF, hormone-related changes in TRH mRNA expression occur specifically in the paraventricular nucleus and not in other areas of the hypothalamus or brain. The stimulatory inputs to TRH neurons are the ascending catecholaminergic fibers from the locus caeruleus and other brain stem nuclei (see Fig. 2–25*A*). However, the negative feedback regulation of TRH gene expression by thyroid hormone occurs directly on the TRH neurons and is independent of catecholaminergic inputs.[327] Thus, thyroid hormones may be the most important regulators of hypothalamic TRH biosynthesis.

TRH Mode of Action

Binding of TRH to its membrane receptor activates the phosphoinositide pathway similar to the mechanism described for GnRH action (see Chapter 3 for details).[328] However, unlike other hypothalamic hormones, TRH has only a minor effect on TSH-β mRNA transcription. On the other hand, TRH does have important effects on post-translational TSH synthesis and glycosylation.[329] In addition, TRH has a distinct property in that it stimulates the release of prolactin at the pituitary level (for details, see Chapter 9).

HYPOTHALAMIC CONTROL OF THE NEUROHYPOPHYSIAL SYSTEM

The neurohypophysial hormones oxytocin and AVP are of historical significance in that the neural lobe of the pituitary was found to possess oxytocic activity in 1906 and the posterior pituitary extract was already being used for labor induction in 1911. Soon after, the milk ejection property of oxytocin and the pressor and antidiuretic effects of AVP were revealed. In the recent decade, the genes for oxytocin and AVP have been cloned in several species, including humans, and oxytocin and AVP have been found to be widely distributed both within and outside the brain. Their functions have been extended to include, among others, learning, behavior, and stress responses.

Oxytocin, Arginine Vasopressin, and Neurophysins

Oxytocin and AVP are hormones secreted by the axonal terminals of the neurohypophysis (posterior pituitary) emanating from the neurosecretory neurons of the supraoptic and paraventricular nuclei. The identification and synthesis of oxytocin (1950) and AVP (1954) by du Vigneaud and coworkers[330] from the posterior lobe of the pituitary represented the *first concrete evidence of an endocrine function of the hypothalamus*.

Oxytocin and AVP and their respective neurophysin carrier proteins are processed by endopeptidase cleavages of a large glycoprotein molecule called pro-pressophysin (for AVP) and pro-oxyphysin (for oxytocin)[331] (Fig. 2–33*A*).

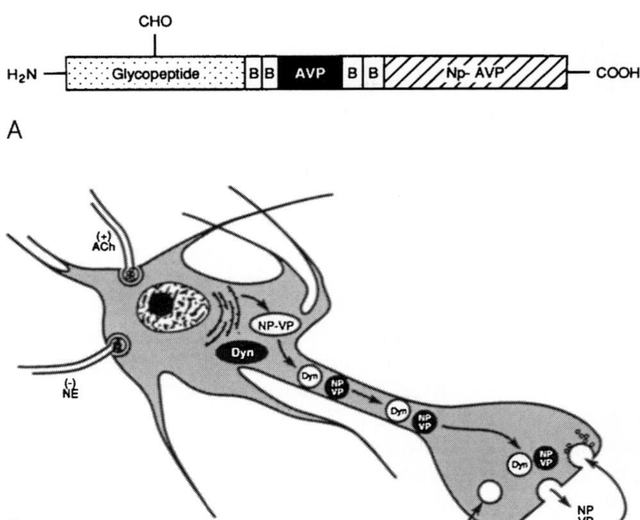

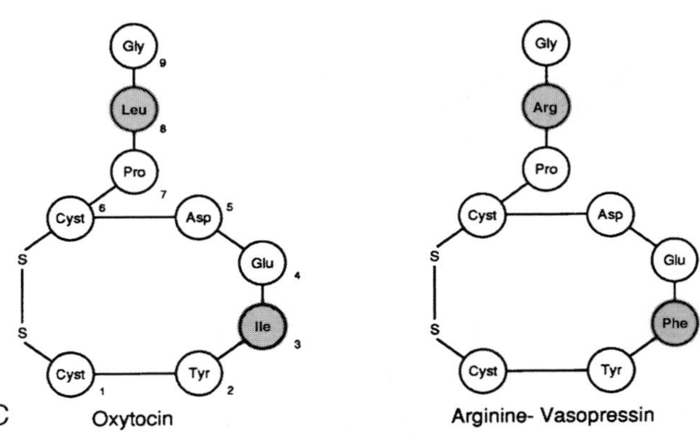

Figure 2–33 ■ Neurohypophysial hormones.

A, Proposed structure of the pro-hormone (pro-pressophysin), a glycopeptide that gives rise to arginine vasopressin (AVP) and vasopressin-associated neurophysin (Np-AVP). An identical arrangement exists for the oxytocin pro-hormone pro-oxyphysin. (Modified from Land H, Schutz G, Schmale H, Richter D. Nucleotide sequence of cloned cDNA encoding bovine arginine vasopressin–neurophysin II precursor. Nature 295:299–303, 1982. Copyright 1982, Macmillan Magazines Ltd.)

B, Biosynthesis, translocation, processing, and release of oxytocin and vasopressin. The cell body (soma) produces a pro-peptide in the rough endoplasmic reticulum, and the secretory granules are packaged in the Golgi body. Dynorphin (Dyn) is also synthesized in the soma of AVP neurons, but not oxytocin neurons, and it is coreleased with AVP during exocytosis. The post-translational processing to oxytocin and AVP occurs in the soma as well as in the axon during transport. The granules are exocytosed (released) when nerve terminals are depolarized, a calcium-dependent process. The stimulatory role of acetylcholine (ACh) and inhibitory action of norepinephrine (NE) are also depicted. (Modified from Brownstein MJ, Russell JT, Gainer H. Synthesis, transport, and release of posterior pituitary hormones. Science 207:373–378, 1980. © 1980 by the AAAS.)

C, The structures and amino acid compositions of oxytocin and AVP.

The primary structure of pro-pressophysin was determined with use of cloned cDNA from bovine hypothalamic mRNA.[332] These precursors are present in human neurohypophysial tissue and are processed into biologically active molecules while being transported along the axon and stored in the nerve terminals in the neurohypophysis.[333] The neurophysins are large peptides with no known biologic action other than in the axonal transport of oxytocin and AVP. They are secreted together with oxytocin and AVP in a fixed ratio by exocytosis of the neurosecretory granule from the axon terminals (Fig. 2–33*B*). To date, oxytocin and AVP are the only peptides known to be cosynthesized, copackaged in granules, and cosecreted with specific carrier proteins.

Both oxytocin and AVP are cyclic nonpeptides consisting of nine amino acid residues. The molecular weights of oxytocin and AVP are 1007 and 1084, respectively. Both have an identical cys-cys bridge in the 1 and 6 position, linked by disulfate bonds. They differ by only two amino acids *at positions 3 and 8* (Fig. 2–33*C*).

Several secretory pathways designated for oxytocin and AVP neuronal systems have been identified (see Fig. 2–25*A* and *B*).

Hypothalamic Pathways

1. The *paraventricular nucleus–neurohypophysial* system: Neurons from the paraventricular nucleus descend toward the neurohypophysis where oxytocin and AVP are secreted into the general circulation, with peripheral targets being the reproductive system for oxytocin and the kidney for AVP (see later).
2. The *paraventricular nucleus–median eminence* pathway secretes into the portal circulation and posterior pituitary where concentrations of oxytocin and AVP are 50-fold higher than in peripheral plasma and may play a role in regulating pituitary hormone secretion.
3. AVP neurons are found in the *suprachiasmatic nucleus*, where they may be involved in the regulation of circadian rhythms (see later).

Extrahypothalamic Pathways

Within the CNS, an extensive network of oxytocin and AVP fibers is found throughout the brain. In general, AVP fibers dominate the forebrain areas, whereas oxytocin fibers are predominant in the caudal brain stem and spinal cord, where they may mediate the autonomic nervous system responses to stress and the suckling reflex.[334]

In the Reproductive Tract

Oxytocin and AVP have been found in the human ovary, follicular fluid, and oviductal tissue. The concentrations in these tissues and in follicular fluids are approximately 4000- and 30-fold higher, respectively, than in peripheral plasma. The concentration of oxytocin, but not AVP, in the corpus luteum is six times higher than in ovarian tissue with no corpus luteum.[335, 336] Remarkably, the level of oxytocin mRNA in the corpus luteum is 250 times greater than in the hypothalamus.[337]

It has been shown that oxytocin inhibits basal and human chorionic gonadotropin–stimulated progesterone production by dispersed human luteal cells in vitro[336] and that both oxytocin and AVP are potent inhibitors of androgen

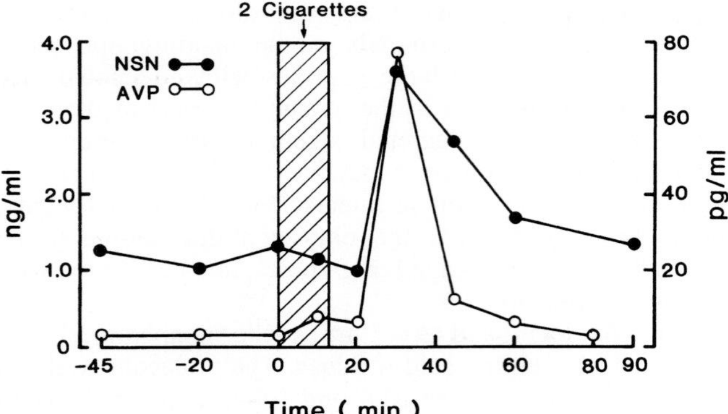

Figure 2–34 ■ Concomitant release of vasopressin and nicotine-stimulated neurophysin (NSN) in a subject who smoked two cigarettes during a 12-minute period beginning at time 0. (Modified from Husain MK, Frantz AG, Ciarochi F, Robinson AG. Nicotine-stimulated release of neurophysin and vasopressin in humans. J Clin Endocrinol Metab 41:1113–1117, 1975. © The Endocrine Society.)

biosynthesis in the rat testis.[338] Oxytocin induces uterine prostaglandin $F_{2\alpha}$ release, which in turn can cause an increase in ovarian oxytocin levels. Thus, a self-propagating system may play a role in oviductal contractility and luteolysis. Further, the well-known vasoconstrictive properties of AVP may participate with other vasoactive peptides and growth factors (e.g., fibroblast growth factor) in the control of ovarian microcirculation. The vascular endothelial growth factor, produced by the luteal cells, is involved in the process of corpus luteum angiogenesis.[339] Additional studies are needed to define the regulation and functional role of oxytocin and AVP produced within the reproductive tract.

Control of Secretion of Neurohypophysial Hormones

The release of neurohypophysial hormones involves multiple regulatory sites and mechanisms. Central or hypothalamic control involves cholinergic and noradrenergic neurotransmitters as well as several neuropeptides.

Acetylcholine. Acetylcholine stimulation releases AVP and oxytocin through nicotinic cholinergic receptors. Application of acetylcholine onto supraoptic neurons markedly accelerates their firing rate, and nicotine or tobacco smoking induces antidiuresis by acute increments of AVP and neurophysin in plasma[340, 341] (Fig. 2–34). This response is abolished or attenuated by prior ingestion of ethanol, which is well known for its inhibitory effect on AVP secretion.

Noradrenergic Influence. The noradrenergic influence on the secretion of oxytocin and AVP involves a stimulatory α-adrenergic and an inhibitory β-adrenergic pathway. There is direct innervation of magnocellular neurons by adrenergic fibers arising from the locus caeruleus.[342] The firing rate of magnocellular neurons is reduced by exposure to an α-adrenergic antagonist and enhanced by a β-adrenergic antagonist, such as propranolol. The latter facilitates milk "let-down"; thus, it is likely that the stress-induced inhibition of the milk let-down reflex in nursing mothers is due to inhibition of oxytocin release mediated through β-adrenergic activation.[334] A similar mechanism of AVP release may be responsible for stress-induced diuresis.

Opioid Peptides. Opioid peptides are also involved in the regulation of AVP and oxytocin. The neurohypophysis receives opioid peptide–containing nerve fibers from the arcuate nucleus and the nucleus tractus solitarius; it also possesses opiate receptors of kappa subtype.[343, 344] Dynorphin, a kappa receptor agonist, inhibits oxytocin release by an action on axonal terminals within the neurohypophysis. Naloxone, a mu receptor antagonist, markedly enhances the release of oxytocin induced by electrical stimulation.[345, 346] Dynorphin A is localized within the AVP neurons, colocalized with AVP in common neurosecretory vesicles, and *released in tandem with AVP*.[347] The local release of AVP and dynorphin, therefore, may exert a direct paracrine inhibitory effect on oxytocin neurons.[347, 348] Stress, such as fear, anger, or dehydration (by water deprivation), induces an increase in AVP-dynorphin release, thereby inhibiting oxytocin secretion through the kappa receptor at the nerve terminal of oxytocin neurons as demonstrated in the rat (Fig. 2–35). Thus, the corelease of a neuromodulator (dynorphin) and a neurohormone (AVP) could attenuate oxytocin release and may also account for stress-mediated inhibition of milk let-down in lactating women.

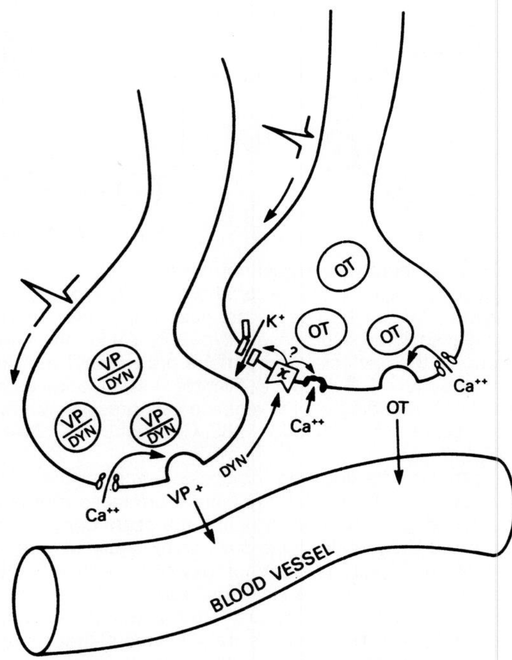

Figure 2–35 ■ A model illustrating the paracrine inhibition of oxytocin (OT) secretion by dynorphin (DYN) coreleased with vasopressin (VP). Dynorphin, binding to kappa receptors on oxytocin terminals, causes a decrease in calcium entry through voltage-dependent calcium channels by acting either directly to modify the calcium channels or indirectly on potassium channels to cause an increase in repolarizing potassium conductance, thereby foreshortening the action potential and limiting the degree of voltage-dependent calcium channel opening. The net effect, in either case, would be a reduction in terminal calcium entry, hence a decrease in oxytocin secretion. (From Bondy CA, Gainer H, Russell JT. Dynorphin A inhibits and naloxone increases the electrically stimulated release of oxytocin but not vasopressin from the terminals of the neural lobe. Endocrinology 122:1321–1327, 1988. © The Endocrine Society.)

Activin-Containing Neurons. Activin is localized in the nucleus of the tractus solitarius, a major recipient of visceral sensory information with projections to the paraventricular nucleus. That activin conveys inputs to oxytocinergic neurons is suggested by the finding that oxytocin secretion is elicited by infusion of femtomolar quantities of purified activin into the paraventricular nucleus, and infusion of antiactivin sera into the paraventricular nucleus attenuates suckling-induced oxytocin secretion. Thus, the nucleus tractus solitarius serves as an ascending somatosensory pathway and may represent the circuitry involving activin-mediated oxytocin secretion.[349]

Estrogen. Oxytocin-producing cells in the paraventricular nucleus contain estrogen-binding sites, and estrogen induces an increased sensitivity to oxytocin by augmenting oxytocin receptors.[350] The elevated immunoreactive oxytocin and neurophysin in women or men treated with estrogen is not authentic oxytocin but an oxytocin precursor intermediate, oxytocin-glycine.[351] The physiologic role, if any, of this estrogen-induced change in processing precursor hormone remains to be determined. The reported increase in serum "oxytocin" levels during the follicular phase to a peak at midcycle and then decrease early in the luteal phase[352] is also oxytocin-glycine.[351] Thus, the role of estrogen in the regulation of oxytocin secretion and processing requires further studies.

Angiotensin II. A product of the renin-angiotensin system, angiotensin II plays an important role in the control of AVP secretion. All components of the system, including specific angiotensin II receptors, are found in the brain. A large body of evidence suggests the involvement of central angiotensin receptors in the osmotic control of AVP secretion.[353]

Peripherally generated angiotensin II also participates in the regulation of AVP release through an efferent neuronal connection from the subfornical organ and the OVLT to the supraoptic nuclei.[354] Both the subfornical organ and the OVLT are anterior circumventricular organs and are outside the blood-brain barrier (see earlier, Circumventricular Organs). They serve as windows for the central action of peripheral angiotensin II, which is excluded by the blood-brain barrier. The signals generated by circulating angiotensin II to effect AVP release and water retention are transmitted to the supraoptic nuclei through subfornical organ and OVLT neural projections. Thus, both central and peripheral angiotensin II play regulatory roles in the physiologic control of body fluid homeostasis by controlling AVP secretion.[355]

Cholecystokinin (CCK). A gastrointestinal hormone, CCK has been localized in the paraventricular and supraoptic nuclei as well as in the posterior lobe of the pituitary.[356] Exogenous administration of CCK is known to decrease food intake, to slow gastric emptying in humans, and to cause a dose-related increase in AVP secretion and induction of emesis. Nausea is a potent stimulus of AVP secretion in humans.[357] Thus, CCK-mediated AVP release in humans may reflect the activation of the brain stem emetic center and serves as a link between brain and gut.[358]

Thyrotropin-Releasing Hormone. Injected intraventricularly, TRH produces a rapid elevation of both plasma AVP and oxytocin. A much slower time course for the increments of these two hormones occurs after intravenous administration of TRH.[359] The site of action of TRH with regard to AVP and oxytocin release is probably the neurohypophysis, but a direct action of TRH on the oxytocinergic and vasopressinergic neurons within the paraventricular nucleus cannot be excluded. The physiologic role is unclear.

Physiologic Functions of Neurohypophysial Hormones

Arginine Vasopressin

Osmolality and Volume Regulation. The major homeostatic functions of AVP operate through several mechanisms, responding to both rising osmotic pressure and decreasing hydrostatic pressure of the blood. AVP serves as a powerful vasoconstricting agent, and as an *antidiuretic hormone (ADH)* it acts on the kidney to increase water retention. These actions of AVP are mediated through tissue-specific G protein–coupled receptors and are classified into V_1 *vascular* (V_1R), V_2 *renal* (V_2R), and V_3 *pituitary* (V_3P).[360, 361]

Blood osmolality is carefully monitored and adjusted over a relatively narrow range (± 1.8 percent) with a mean of 285 mOsm/kg.[362] Release of AVP-ADH increases promptly when plasma osmolality rises (such as by infusion of hypertonic saline) and is inhibited by water loading, leading to antidiuresis and diuresis, respectively.[363] The central detector for this remarkably sensitive system appears to be an osmoreceptor system in the anterior hypothalamus.[362]

Blood Volume Reductions. Decreased blood volume, from any cause, is followed by release of AVP. With acute changes in intravascular volume of more than 10 percent, AVP release and water retention occur.[362, 363] The mechanism for this homeostatic control involves a complex sequence of communication between peripheral sensors and central responses: a decrease in blood pressure due to the reduction of blood volume activates baroreceptors (located in the left atrium, vena cava, and pulmonary veins); their signals are transmitted to the hypothalamus, ultimately causing release of AVP. Lowering blood pressure activates the renin-angiotensin system and provides an increase in circulating angiotensin II, which causes vasoconstriction. Angiotensin II enters the brain through the anterior circumventricular organs (outside the blood-brain barrier) and activates supraoptic neurons for AVP release.[355] Moreover, angiotensin stimulates the secretion of aldosterone and induces thirst. Thus, the major neuroendocrine mechanism for maintaining homeostasis of blood pressure and blood osmotic pressure is by an integrated *release of AVP-ADH and angiotensin II*. The possibility that the recently characterized *adrenomedullin* may also play a role in controlling volume and osmotic homeostasis should be considered.[364]

Atrial Natriuretic Hormones. Atrial natriuretic hormones, 24- to 33–amino acid peptides secreted by the cardiac atria, are important regulators of salt and water metabolism. These hormones exert a direct, short-lasting effect on aldosterone secretion as well as an indirect effect through suppression of the renin-angiotensin system. They may also influence the AVP system in the overall control of water and salt metabolism through diuresis and natriuresis.[365]

ACTH Release. AVP also plays a role in regulating ACTH release. Although AVP has intrinsic ACTH-releasing activity, the combination of AVP and CRF augments ACTH release fivefold more than that of CRF alone and exceeds the sum of the separate ACTH responses to CRF and AVP in women.[366]

Oxytocin

Identification of human oxytocin receptors has been accomplished. The encoded receptor is a 388–amino acid polypeptide with serum transmembrane loops typical of G protein–coupled receptors. Messenger RNAs have been isolated from human ovary, endometrium, and myometrium.[367]

Parturition. Although the prevailing view is that oxytocin is not involved in the initiation of labor in humans, oxytocin is important as a stimulator of myometrial contraction late in labor and in hemostasis at the placental site after delivery. Plasma oxytocin levels are unchanged until the expulsive phase of labor[368] (Fig. 2–36). The primary stimulus for release of maternal oxytocin during labor appears to be vaginal distention or the Ferguson reflex (Fig. 2–37). Estrogen induces an increase in oxytocin receptors in myometrial and decidual tissue of pregnant women, *and oxytocin receptors* in both of these tissues reach maximal concentrations near term.[369] This may account for the increase in spontaneous myometrial contraction and the increased sensitivity to oxytocin during late pregnancy even in the absence of increased plasma oxytocin levels. During the second stage of labor, oxytocin

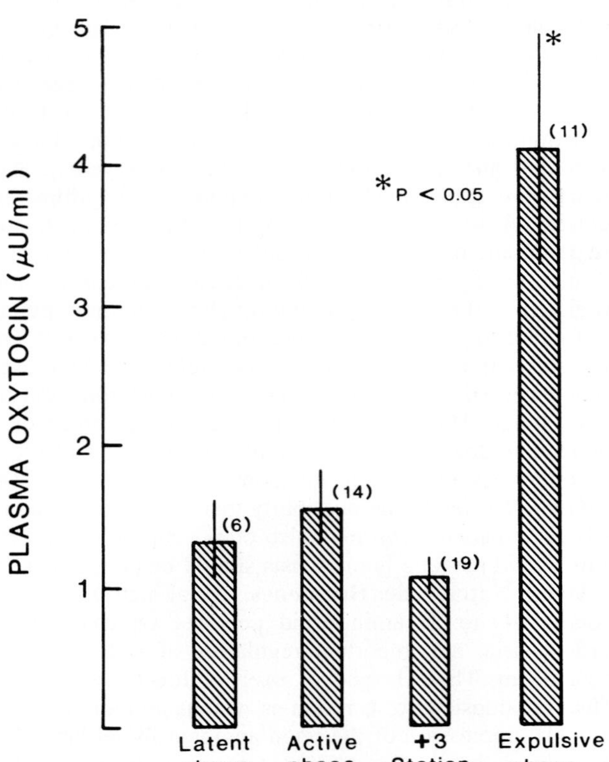

Figure 2–36 ■ Plasma oxytocin levels during different stages of labor. (From Fisher DA. Maternal-fetal neurohypophyseal system. Clin Perinatol 10:695–707, 1983.)

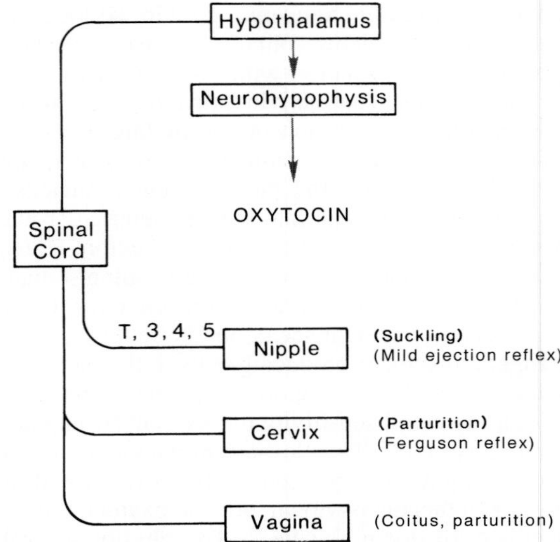

Figure 2–37 ■ Diagrammatic portrayal of neural pathways of reflexes for the release of oxytocin by the hypothalamic-neurohypophysial system.

release may play a synergistic role in the expulsion of the fetus by virtue of its ability to stimulate prostaglandin release.[368]

Milk Let-down. Milk release involves the action of oxytocin. Myoepithelial cells of the mammary gland possess binding sites for oxytocin, and oxytocin induces myoepithelial contraction as well as contraction of mammary duct smooth muscle. Myoepithelial cells are arranged longitudinally on the lactiferous ducts and around the alveoli. During nursing, stimulation of nerve endings in the nipple induces oxytocin release. This neurogenic reflex is transmitted through the spinal cord, midbrain, and hypothalamus, where it triggers oxytocin release from the neurohypophysis[334] (see Fig. 2–37). Of particular significance is the episodic release of oxytocin even in anticipation of suckling[370] (Fig. 2–38). This psychogenic reflex is suppressed when fear, anger, or other stresses are encountered, thereby inhibiting oxytocin release and suppressing milk outflow.[334]

Sexual Behavior. During sexual arousal in men, there is a marked elevation in plasma AVP levels and return to baseline value by the time of ejaculation. Although there is no change in plasma oxytocin at the time of arousal, a rapid increase in plasma oxytocin does occur at the moment of ejaculation[371] (Fig. 2–39, *left*). Because AVP is colocalized and coreleased with dynorphin, which suppresses oxytocin release (see earlier), it is suggested that AVP release during arousal is associated with specific inhibition of oxytocin release until ejaculation. In women, tactile genital stimulation leads to oxytocin secretion, with further rise during orgasm.[372] The function of oxytocin release may be related to smooth muscle contractions of the reproductive tract at orgasm (Fig. 2–39, *right*).

Learning and Behavior. Learning and behavior are known to be influenced by AVP and oxytocin. These neurohypophysial hormones have been shown to influence memory in rats.[373] AVP plays a role in consolidating information in memory and facilitates its retrieval, whereas oxytocin has a reverse effect and is regarded as an endogenous

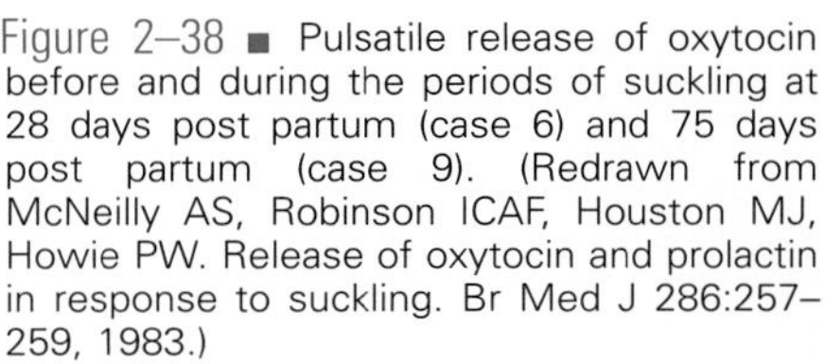

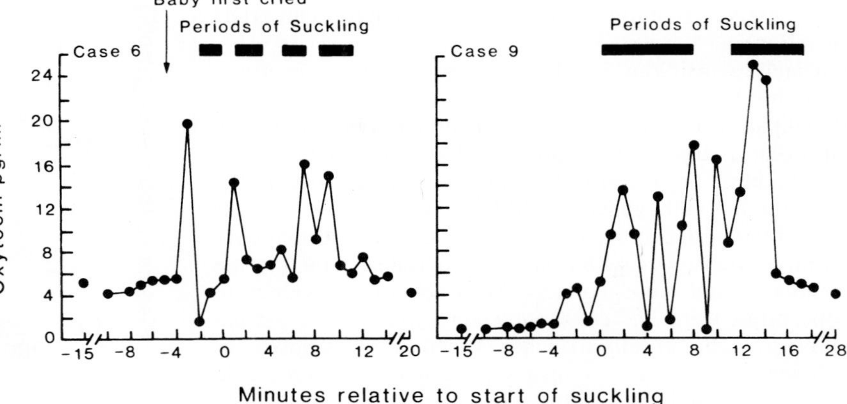

Figure 2–38 ■ Pulsatile release of oxytocin before and during the periods of suckling at 28 days post partum (case 6) and 75 days post partum (case 9). (Redrawn from McNeilly AS, Robinson ICAF, Houston MJ, Howie PW. Release of oxytocin and prolactin in response to suckling. Br Med J 286:257–259, 1983.)

amnesic peptide. Studies performed in *humans* have confirmed these experimental data. With the use of an analogue of AVP, enhancement of learning and memory has been observed. The determinants of this enhancement include effects on consolidation processes, organization of memories, and "strengthened" trace events in memory (as measured by increased consistency in recall). Tests of memory after the intranasal or intravenous administration of large doses of oxytocin to human subjects show that even though learning does not appear to be affected, subsequent recall is impaired. This effect, which is transient, is opposite to that caused by AVP.[374, 375]

Maternal behavior can also be linked to a central action of oxytocin. Intracerebroventricular administration of oxytocin to ovariectomized, estrogen-primed, virgin female rats evokes rapid onset of full maternal behavior. This behavior, lasting for 5 hours, includes grouping and regrouping of pups, licking of pups, crouching over grouped pups, nest building, and retrieval of pups. Estrogen priming is required for these responses.[376]

Diabetes Insipidus

As described in a previous section, AVP-ADH release and the subsequent regulation of fluid balance occur primarily in response to alterations of blood volume and osmotic pressure, so that relative constancy of the values of these two variables is maintained. This sensitive regulatory system can be disrupted by disease states in which inappropriate ADH release occurs in response to the usual normal inputs. The resulting clinical disturbance is an imbalance of body water and may be characterized by hypernatremia or hyponatremia and by excessive loss (diabetes insipidus)

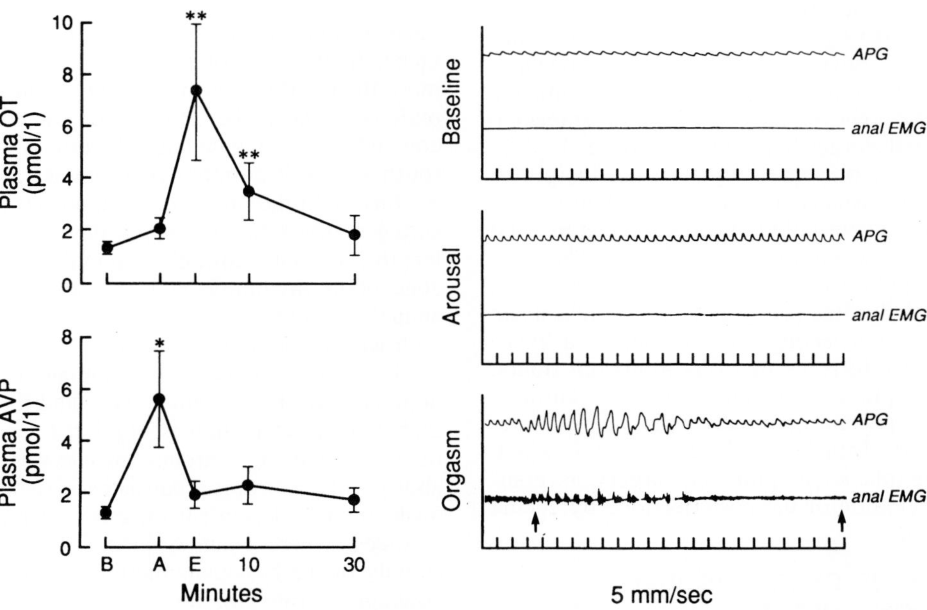

Figure 2–39 ■ *Left,* Acute and sequential release of arginine vasopressin (AVP) and oxytocin (OT) (mean ± SE) during sexual arousal (A) and at the time of ejaculation (E) in normal men. *Right,* Polygraph recording in one woman before and during sexual self-stimulation and at the moment of orgasm. Arrows indicate the onset and offset of orgasmic sensation. Oxytocin levels, systolic blood pressure, and pulse rates were significantly increased during arousal and orgasm (not shown). B, baseline value; APG, anal blood pulse amplitude; anal EMG, anal electromyographic activity. (Modified from Murphy MR, Seckl JR, Burton S, et al. Changes in oxytocin and vasopressin secretion during sexual activity in men. J Clin Endocrinol Metab 65:738–741, 1987; and Carmichael MS, Humbert R, Dixen J, et al. Plasma oxytocin increases in the human sexual response. J Clin Endocrinol Metab 64:27–31, 1987. © The Endocrine Society.)

or excessive retention of body water (inappropriate ADH secretion).

Diabetes insipidus involves the loss of water resulting from failure of adequate tubular reabsorption by the kidney. Polydipsia and polyuria are characteristic symptoms. The basic defect lies in the neurohypophysial neuronal system for synthesis or secretion of AVP-ADH. Receptors on the renal tubular cells generate cAMP, which in turn increases membrane permeability to water. Thus, under normal conditions, when ADH secretion is appropriate for the plasma osmolality and blood volume, ADH acts on the kidney to concentrate urine and conserve water by enhancing permeability of tubular cells to water. When ADH is absent or deficient, as in diabetes insipidus, a marked decrease in water resorption and increased urinary flow ensue. The ADH mechanism normally maintains plasma osmotic pressure within narrow limits. Normal average osmotic pressure may be defined as about 285 mOsm/kg; when osmolality is lowered to about 282 mOsm/kg with the administration of an excessive water load, complete inhibition of ADH release occurs and maximal diuresis is observed. On the other hand, an osmolality of 287 mOsm/kg, achieved by infusion of hypertonic saline, induces rapid ADH release and antidiuresis. Thus, the osmolar excursion from full diuresis to detectable antidiuresis is only about 5 mOsm/kg, representing 3 percent of the total normal osmolality. Diabetes insipidus can be treated effectively by replacement of a long-acting synthetic analogue of AVP-ADH. DDAVP (1-desamino-8-D-AVP) in doses of 10 to 20 μg, intranasally, given at 12- to 24-hour intervals reverses the diuresis and excessive water intake.[362, 377]

Diabetes insipidus can result from a congenital defect caused by a failure of normal development of the AVP neurons of the neurohypophysial system. Failure to transport ADH to the site of release can occur as a result of a number of disease processes; hypothalamic or posterior pituitary lesions that disrupt the neurohypophysial pathway are common causes. Most patients with *hypothalamic diabetes insipidus* do not have detectable or low concentrations of plasma AVP in response to hypertonic infusion (Fig. 2–40). They do, however, have a normal thirst mechanism as demonstrated during hypertonic infusion (Fig. 2–40). Because thirst is preserved in diabetes insipidus, plasma osmolality is usually maintained within normal range, and hypernatremia usually indicates a defect in thirst mechanism rather than severe renal water loss.[377] The presence of diabetes insipidus together with visual disturbances, hypopituitarism, and elevated prolactin levels represents an *important combination reflecting* the presence of a hypothalamic lesion that interrupts neurohypophysial tracts. Compression of the optic chiasm causes visual impairment and disrupts the hypophysiotropic factors that control anterior pituitary function. Transient diabetes insipidus, which develops after transsphenoidal pituitary surgery, is commonly due to compression of the posterior lobe by edema of the pituitary gland.

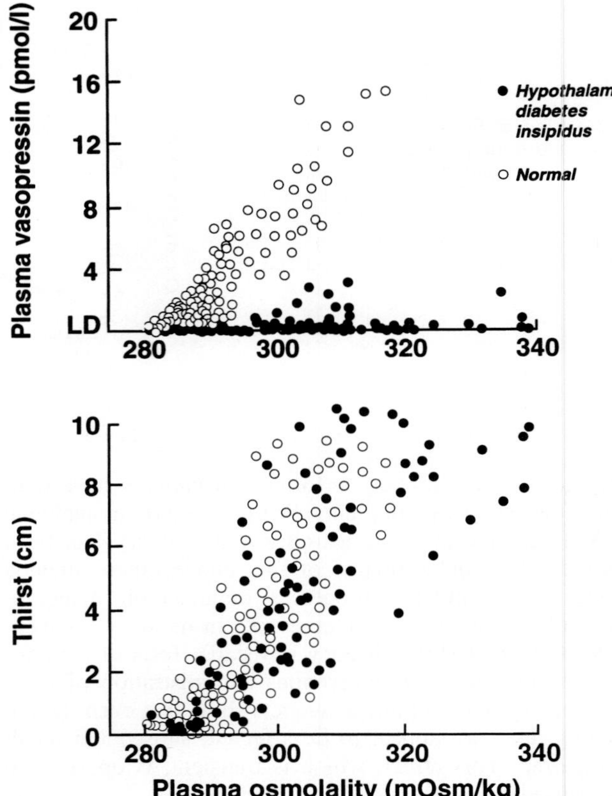

Figure 2–40 ■ The relationships between plasma osmolality and plasma vasopressin *(upper panel)* and thirst *(lower panel)* during infusion of hypertonic saline in patients with hypothalamic diabetes insipidus (●) and healthy control subjects (○). (From Baylis PH, Thompson CJ. Osmoregulation of vasopressin secretion and thirst in health and disease. Clin Endocrinol [Oxf] 29:549–576, 1988.)

NEUROENDOCRINE RHYTHMS AND SEASONALITY OF HUMAN REPRODUCTION

Annual Rhythm of Human Reproduction

Reproduction shows an obvious seasonality throughout the animal kingdom. This annual timing of reproduction reflects a high selective pressure for an appropriate seasonal niche. In the case of the human birth rhythm, analyzing more than 3000 years of monthly birth rates covering 166 regions of the globe, Roenneberg and Aschoff[378, 379] have concluded that the annual rhythm of human conception (birth minus 9 months) is a characteristic of geographic regions, with the onset of maximal rates lying close to the spring equinox (a time when day and night are of equal length). The data strongly support a biologic basis for the conception rhythm. However, the maximal and minimal annual conception rates have been attenuated in parallel with worldwide industrialization.[378]

The biologic basis for this human conception rhythm is dominated by food availability[380] and the photoperiod on a global scale. Ovulation is regulated seasonally in populations experiencing a strong seasonal variation in food availability, such as tropical subsistence societies in which adequate food is dependent on seasonal rainfall.[380] At higher latitudes, where changes in day length are pronounced, activity of the hypothalamic-pituitary-ovarian axis and the conception rate are decreased during the dark winter months and a steep increase in conceptions coincides with the vernal equinox (springtime).[381] Temperature extremes also decrease the probability of conceptions. Recent evidence suggests that deterioration in *sperm quality* during the hot summer months in subequatorial areas may result in a lower conception rate.[382] In the last century, the ability of humans to control food availability and modify both temperature (by heating and air conditioning) and photoperiods (by indoor work) has resulted in specific changes of several features of the annual conception rhythm.[378, 383] Thus, the biologic rhythm of human conceptions is influenced primarily by seasonal environmental cues, and social changes have an indirect influence in the human microenvironment. The endogenous annual timing system in humans, as in other mammals, uses photoperiod (dark-light cycle) as a synchronizing signal to predict an optimal time favorable for survival of both parent and offspring.[378, 379, 384]

Circadian Rhythms

The vital functions of the body change from day to night with a periodicity of about 24 hours. These changes constitute the human circadian system, which is governed by environmental cues. Among the most evident markers of circadian pacemaker activity are the magnitude, duration, and timing of pineal melatonin secretion.[385]

Melatonin Synthesis and Secretion

Melatonin (*N*-acetyl-5-methoxytryptamine) represents the index of pineal function. It is synthesized from the *circulating substrate tryptophan to serotonin* in the pinealocytes. Subsequent steps involve two sequential enzymatic activities: *N*-acetyltransferase (NAT, the rate-limiting enzyme) and hydroxyindole-*O*-methyltransferase (HIOMT). NAT is responsible for the *N*-acetylation of serotonin, and HIOMT is responsible for the *O*-methylation of the indole ring (Fig. 2–41). There is a large nocturnal increase in NAT activity,

Tryptophan: CH_2-CH($COOH$)(NH_2)

tryptophan hydroxylase

5-Hydroxytryptophan: HO, CH_2-CH($COOH$)(NH_2)

aromatic l-amino acid decarboxylase

Serotonin (5-hydroxytryptamine): HO, CH_2-CH_2-NH_2

N-acetyltransferase

N-acetylserotonin: HO, CH_2-CH_2-NH-C(=O)-CH_3

Hydroxyindole-O-methyltransferase

Melatonin (5-methoxy N-acetylserotonin): CH_3O, CH_2-CH_2-NH-C(=O)-CH_3

Figure 2–41 ■ The biosynthesis of melatonin from tryptophan and the enzymatic systems involved.

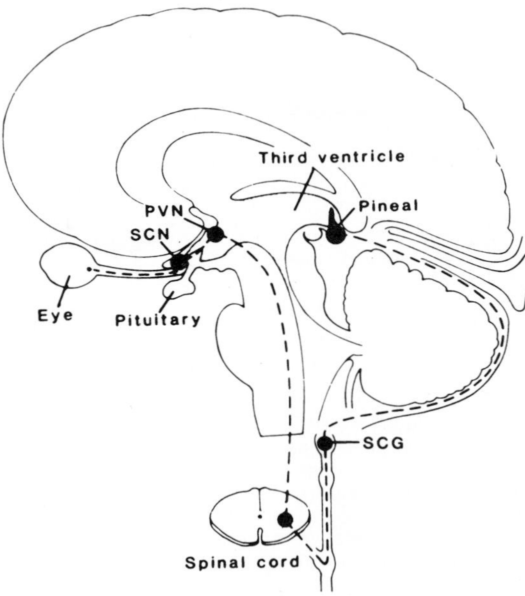

Figure 2–42 ■ Diagram of the human brain (midsagittal section) showing the neural pathway *(dotted line)* from the retina to the pineal gland by way of suprachiasmatic nuclei (SCN), paraventricular nuclei (PVN), spinal cord, and superior cervical ganglia (SCG). (Modified from Tamarkin L, Baird CJ, Almeida OFX. Melatonin: A coordinating signal for mammalian reproduction? Science 227:714–720, 1985. © 1985 by the AAAS.)

which governs melatonin synthesis, and in HIOMT activity, which determines the amplitude of the nocturnal rise in melatonin.[386] Concentrations of melatonin have been found to increase at night in the pineal, blood, cerebrospinal fluid, and urine in all mammalian species studied to date, including humans,[387–389] and account for 40 percent of the nocturnal decline in core body temperature in humans.[390]

The daily rhythm of melatonin secretion is governed by the dark-light cycle: activated by darkness and inhibited by light. This environmental cue (photoperiodic information) is transmitted to the pineal gland by a circuitous neural pathway (Fig. 2–42). The light signal is conveyed through the retinohypothalamic tract to the *circadian oscillator*, the suprachiasmatic nuclei, and then to the paraventricular nuclei. These impulses pass along nerve fibers that traverse the medial forebrain bundle and reticular formation to the intermediolateral nucleus of the spinal cord. From there, signals are transmitted to preganglionic adrenergic fibers and then pass to the superior cervical ganglion. The postganglionic sympathetic input represents the final neural pathway to the pineal gland.[391]

The release of norepinephrine at the nerve terminals on the pinealocytes converts the neural signal into endocrine output; coupling of norepinephrine to β-adrenergic receptors is followed by the activation of cAMP and NAT activity, thereby enhancing synthesis of melatonin.[386, 391, 392] The β-adrenergic receptors on the pinealocyte membrane exhibit a 24-hour rhythm with an increasing number of receptors near the end of the light phase and peak density during darkness.[391, 393–396] Noradrenergic stimulation is initiated in the dark phase and is followed by a decrease (downregulation) of β-receptors during the second half of the night.[397] The α_1-adrenergic receptor binding is less signifi-

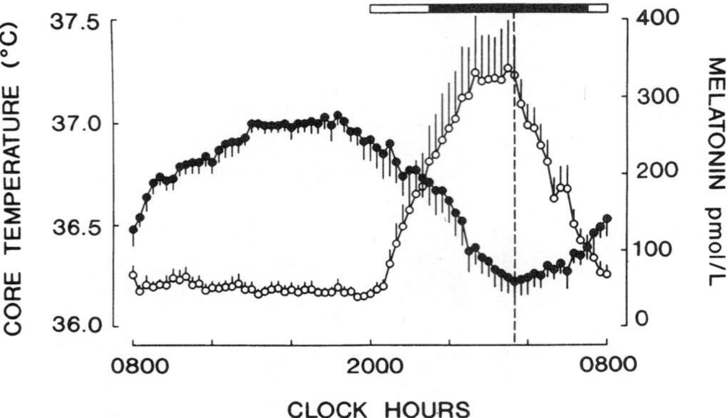

Figure 2–43 ■ Time course and 24-hour patterns of mean (±SE) serum melatonin levels (○) and core body temperature values (●) in 12 early follicular–phase women. The bar depicts duration of nocturnal melatonin secretion *(open area)* and sleep time *(black area)*. Close temporal correlations are evident between the onset or offset of melatonin secretion and the decline or rise in core body temperature. The initial events precede the onset of sleep by about 3 hours. (From Cagnacci A, Elliott JA, Yen SSC. Melatonin: A major regulator of the circadian rhythm of core temperature in humans. J Clin Endocrinol Metab 75:447–452, 1992. © The Endocrine Society.)

cant in mediating nocturnal production of melatonin, but it potentiates the β-adrenergic stimulation.[398, 399] Under direct neural control, melatonin is secreted into the general circulation and delivered to the ventricular system and other target sites. Nocturnal melatonin secretion is associated with several important physiologic changes, such as enhanced sleep propensity, decreased core body temperature and heart rate, and increased distal skin temperature (hands and feet) (Fig. 2–43). Alterations of melatonin secretion may have important implications in psychobiologic illnesses that impinge on the reproductive axis.[387, 392, 400] Two *unexpected but important new findings are an additional circadian clock found in the retina*[401] *and extraocular circadian phototransduction in humans* (i.e., light transmitted from the skin to suprachiasmatic nuclei).[402] Future development in both findings may have significance in the search for more effective treatments of sleep and circadian rhythm disorders.

Melatonin Rhythm Ontogeny. Assessments of melatonin levels during both daytime and nighttime have revealed major age-related changes in nocturnal serum melatonin levels.[403] During the first 6 months of life, melatonin levels are low, and the circadian rhythm of melatonin secretion does not become apparent until after 3 months of age.[404] The highest nocturnal melatonin concentrations are found in children aged 1 to 3 years (325 pg/ml or 1400 pmol/L), followed by a rapid decrease of approximately 80 percent by the age of 15 to 20 years with daytime levels and nocturnal peak of 10 and 60 pg/ml (40 and 260 pmol/L), respectively. The decrease in melatonin levels during puberty and adolescence is correlated with an increase in body weight and body surface area.[403] Similar data obtained from longitudinal studies in rhesus monkeys have been reported.[405] Although the timing of sexual maturation is inversely related to the nocturnal melatonin levels, these findings by themselves are insufficient to prove a causal relationship. Further, neither delayed puberty nor precocious puberty is associated with inappropriate melatonin secretion for age.[406, 407] Aging is associated with a progressive decline in nocturnal melatonin secretion (see later).[403, 408]

Menstrual Cycle. Despite marked ovarian steroid excursions characteristic of ovulatory cycles, variations in 24-hour plasma melatonin patterns by menstrual phase are not found. Daytime levels are at or below 43 pmol/L and display prominent nocturnal elevations in all phases of the menstrual cycle studied.[409, 410] Thus, the secretory profile of melatonin is unaltered by fluctuations of ovarian steroids. The immunohistochemical localization of receptors for LH, FSH, androgen, and estrogen in human pineal gland from infancy to old age is of interest.[411] However, these preliminary findings do not by themselves implicate the presence of *functional receptors* in the pineal gland.

Melatonin concentrations in ovarian follicular fluid, obtained from spontaneous cycles or at the time of oocyte retrieval in women undergoing in vitro fertilization, are three times higher than the serum levels.[412, 413] Further, follicular fluid melatonin levels in the early morning hours are higher than daytime levels and are higher in dark seasons than in light seasons.[413] These variations of follicular fluid melatonin levels are consistent with the circadian and seasonal contrast of luminosity and its inverse relationship to melatonin secretion.[414] Because the ovary lacks the capacity of synthesizing melatonin,[387] the higher concentration of melatonin found in follicular fluids suggests an active uptake mechanism and retention by maturing follicles. The putative role of melatonin in the regulation of ovarian function in humans remains to be defined.[415]

Nocturnal Melatonin Secretion Interrupted by Light. That light is the synchronizer for the circadian activity of pineal melatonin secretion in humans is demonstrated by the rapid suppression of the nocturnal melatonin rise on exposure to different intensities of light (lux = unit of light) at nighttime (Fig. 2–44) with a concomitant rise in core body temperature, suggesting the role of melatonin in the regulation of core body temperature.[390, 416, 417] The β_1-adrenergic pathways that convey the light signal in humans appear to be identical to those in other mammalian species, and blockade of β_1-adrenergic receptor by atenolol is capable of completely suppressing melatonin production in humans.[387] Thus, melatonin secretion serves as a circadian rhythm marker and reflects the functional status of the pinealocyte noradrenergic synapse. Desynchronization of the melatonin rhythm occurs in conditions of shifting dark-light cycle (i.e., jet lag), nightshift work, and blindness.[418]

Mechanism of Action

Melatonin Receptors. The molecular cloning of a family of G protein–coupled receptors for melatonin represents the major advance in understanding melatonin actions.[419] The first melatonin receptor cloned in 1994 was designated the *Mel_{1a} melatonin receptor*, which is coupled to G_i. The gene is expressed in the rodent suprachiasmatic nuclei and pars tuberalis, the presumed sites of the circadian and reproductive actions of melatonin, respectively. The Mel_{1a} receptor may account for all the ^{125}I-Mel binding observed by in vitro autoradiography in mammals. However, the extremely low mRNA expression has prevented a firm assessment of ^{125}I-Mel binding in some sites such as blood vessels. The second receptor subtype, designated the *Mel_{1b}*

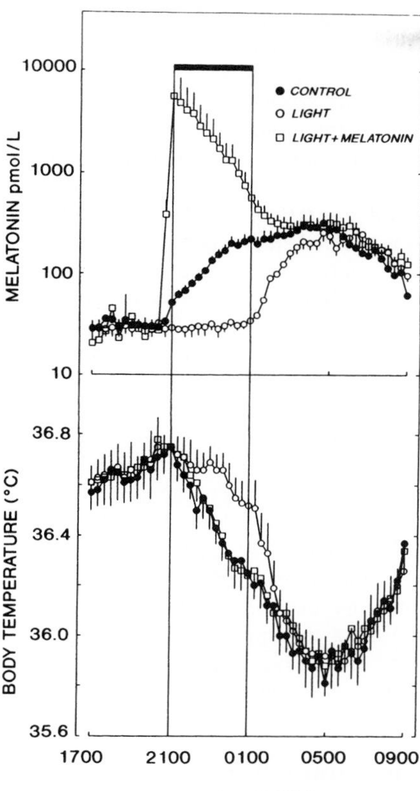

Figure 2–44 ■ Mean (±SE) melatonin *(top)* and core body temperature *(bottom)* values in seven women before, during *(box),* and after bright light (3000 lux) or bright light plus melatonin (1 and 0.75 mg at 2030 and 2300 hours). A delay in the onset of nocturnal melatonin secretion *($P < .001$)* and a contemporaneous slowing of the nocturnal temperature decline *($P < .01$)* were evident during bright light. Exogenous melatonin, by obviating the suppressive effect of light on circulating melatonin, completely counteracted *($P < .01$)* the hyperthermic effect of bright light.

receptor, was cloned in the human. The human Mel_{1b} receptor is 60 percent identical to the human Mel_{1a} receptor. The expression of Mel_{1b} receptor exhibits ligand binding characteristics that are similar to those of the Mel_{1a} receptor. The Mel_{1b} receptor is also coupled to G_i, and Mel_{1b} receptor mRNA is expressed in human retina and brain, suggesting that the Mel_{1b} receptor may mediate the reported action of melatonin in the retina in some mammals. The two human melatonin receptor genes are located on different chromosomes: Mel_{1a} on 4q35.1 and Mel_{1b} on 11q21–22. A third *Mel_{1c} receptor subtype* was recently cloned in zebra fish with pharmacologic and functional properties similar to those of Mel_{1a} and Mel_{1b} receptors. However, a Mel_{1c} receptor orthologue has not yet been cloned in mammals. It is possible that mammals have evolved without the Mel_{1c} receptor gene.

Melatonin Targets. Pineal melatonin has been implicated in the regulation of the circadian clock and of core body temperature and in photoperiodic control of reproduction. The suprachiasmatic nuclei appear to be one of the sites of melatonin action. The Mel_{1a} receptor has been localized in the human suprachiasmatic nuclei, where melatonin inhibits metabolic activity.[420] In addition to the suprachiasmatic nuclei, the pars tuberalis Mel_{1a} receptor implicates the role of melatonin in the induction of prolactin release,[421] in lowering core body temperature,[390] in the sleep-promoting effect,[422, 423] and in its resynchronization properties in alleviating jet lag.[424]

NEUROENDOCRINOLOGY OF AGING

Recent studies have provided cogent evidence that deterioration of pituitary hormone secretion occurs during the process of aging. Alterations of ultradian and circadian rhythms appear to be accountable for the diminished functional activities of neuroendocrine axes and sleep (Fig. 2–45). Chief among them are (1) diminished output of nocturnal melatonin secretion with fragmentation of sleep, (2) decline in activity of the GH–IGF-I axis (somatopause), (3) decline in activity of the gonadotropin–gonadal axes (menopause/andropause), (4) decreased levels of the adre-

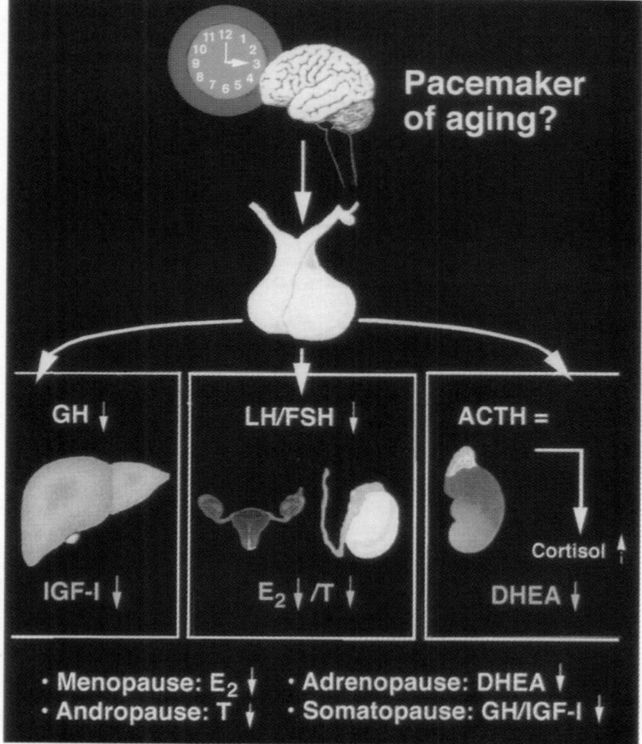

Figure 2–45 ■ During aging, a decline in the activities of a number of hormonal systems occurs. *Left,* A decrease in growth hormone (GH) release by the pituitary gland causes a decrease in the production of insulin-like growth factor I (IGF-I) by the liver and other organs (somatopause). *Middle,* A decrease in release of gonadotropin luteinizing hormone (LH) and follicle-stimulating hormone (FSH) together with a decreased secretion at the gonadal level (from the ovaries, decreased estradiol [E_2]; from the testicle, decreased testosterone [T]) causes menopause and andropause, respectively. *Right,* The adrenocortical cells responsible for the production of DHEA decrease in activity (adrenopause) without clinically evident changes in corticotropin (ACTH) and cortisol secretion. A central pacemaker in the hypothalamus or higher brain areas (or both) is hypothesized, which together with changes in the peripheral organs (the ovaries, testicles, and adrenal cortex) regulates the aging process of these endocrine axes. (From Lamberts SWJ, van den Beld AW, van der Lely AJ. The endocrinology of aging. Science 278:419–424, 1997. Copyright I997 by the AAAS.)

nal sex steroid precursors (adrenopause), and (5) increased levels of the catabolic steroid cortisol.[288, 425, 426] Understanding of neuroendocrine aspects of aging would facilitate the rendering of effective medical advice and care to aged postmenopausal women and men. The processes of aging are multifactorial, and their negative impacts are frequently interrelated.

Menopause/Andropause

Menopause represents the most dramatic and rapidly occurring change in women around the age of 50 years. The acute decline in ovarian production of estrogen (estradiol)—the "estrogen withdrawal syndrome"—triggers a host of symptoms with long-term consequences.[427] For decades, the prevailing view was that menopause resulted from a depletion of ovarian follicles. Recently, however, compelling evidence suggests that both the ovary and the brain are key pacemakers in the initiation of menopause.[428] Changes in the activity of the hypothalamic-pituitary-testicular axis in males are slower and more subtle—during aging, a gradual decline in serum total and free testosterone levels occurs (see Chapter 23 for details). This so-called *andropause* is characterized by a decrease in testicular Leydig cell numbers and in their secretory capacity for testosterone as well as an age-related decline in episodic gonadotropin secretion.[429]

Adrenal Function

Circulating DHEA-S levels in healthy adults are more than 10 times higher than those of cortisol.[430] DHEA and DHEA-S decline after age 25 years to levels about 10 percent of those of young adults.[431] In this regard, DHEA-S has been used as a biomarker of aging. This event has been referred to as *adrenopause* and may be related to the reduced mass of the *zona reticularis* of the adrenal cortex with aging.[432] In contrast to DHEA, circulating cortisol levels remain relatively stable until age 60 years. Thereafter, 24-hour integrated cortisol levels are elevated, and the level of the nocturnal nadir increases progressively and its timing is phase advanced in both men and women.[288] It is estimated that 24-hour mean cortisol levels increase by 20 to 50 percent between 20 and 80 years of age. There is good evidence to suggest that the elevation of cortisol in human aging is due, in part, to a reduced sensitivity to cortisol feedback inhibition.[433] The decline of DHEA-S and the increase in cortisol levels results in a marked increase in the cortisol to DHEA ratio and, thereby, enhanced catabolism from young to old age. Chronic cortisol excess in aging individuals may be linked to the development of senile dementia and Alzheimer's disease.[434] A study has shown that an increase in urinary cortisol levels is associated with memory decline.[435] These observations together with the decline of the antiglucocorticoid effects of DHEA and DHEA-S may have important implications for age-related alteration of cognitive function and catabolism.[425, 436]

Growth Hormone–IGF-I

As noted before, a parallel decline of GH–IGF-I levels occurs with aging. This event has been referred to as *somatopause*. Human aging is accompanied by an increase in fat body mass with decreased muscle strength. These

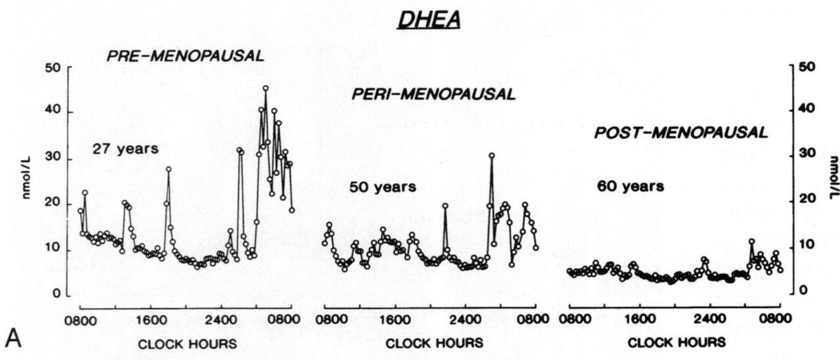

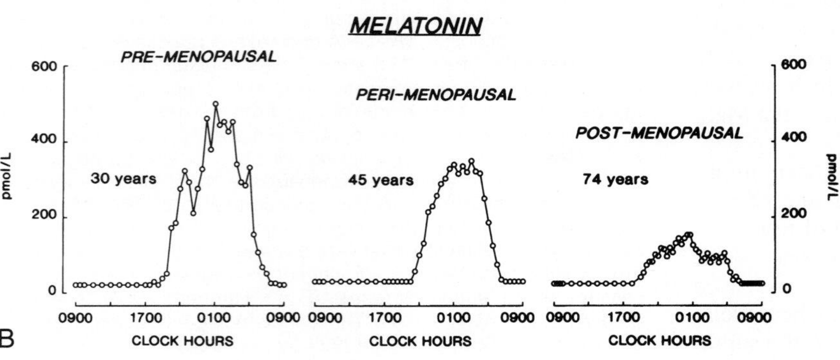

Figure 2–46 ■ *A,* Decline of DHEA pulse amplitude but not frequency during aging. *B,* Decline of melatonin amplitude during nocturnal hours during aging.

changes are associated with a progressive shift from an anabolic to a catabolic state, an event that may involve multiple neuroendocrine-metabolic impairments. Mechanisms contributing to this shift with aging include the functional decline of the GH–IGF-I axis[437] and its mitogenic-anabolic properties as well as of the adrenal sex steroid precursors (DHEA). Serum IGF-I levels decline approximately 40 percent in both genders by age 60 years.[438]

These findings have provided a rationale for recent clinical trials with the aim of restoring the anabolic state by "replacement" of rhGH. Treatment with rhGH reversed the unfavorable changes in body composition,[439] but its effects in older women were equivocal.[440] Administration of rhGH-I (0.060 mg/kg) twice a day for 4 weeks to elderly women results in a significant decrease in fat body mass and an increase in lean body mass and nitrogen retention.[441] These anabolic changes in response to rhGH and rhIGF-I were accompanied by significant negative side effects, particularly in women.[440, 441] However, a preliminary clinical trial with GHRP (MK-0677) administered orally to healthy aging subjects has demonstrated an enhancement of preexisting pulsatile secretion with amplification of both pulse height and interpulse nadir concentrations and increases in serum IGF-I concentrations to the young adult range.[303] This remarkable effect of MK-0677 offers important medical significance.

The results of clinical trials for DHEA have also shown promising results, but large-scale trials are required to confirm the beneficial effects of DHEA replacement in aging.[80]

Circadian Rhythmicity

The *circadian rhythm* of hormone secretion in aging individuals is impaired.[426] Daytime and nighttime levels of TSH and GH are diminished, whereas melatonin and prolactin concentrations are decreased only in the nighttime. Declines in pulsatile hormone secretion in aging are related to reductions in pulse amplitude and not frequency, as displayed in Figure 2–46 (see also Fig. 2–29). In addition, the circadian rise of cortisol, TSH, and melatonin occurs 1 to 1.5 hours earlier (phase advanced), and the distribution of REM sleep stage is likewise advanced. Further, the decline of core body temperature is attenuated in aging men and women.[442] Collectively, these alterations suggest that circadian timekeeping (the biologic clock) is modified during normal senescence and is likely to account, in part, for aging-related alterations of neuroendocrine function.

References

1. Guillemin R. Peptides in the brain: The new endocrinology of the neuron. Science 202:390, 1978.
2. Virgintino D, Monaghan P, Robertson D, et al. An immunohistochemical and morphometric study on astrocytes and microvasculature in the human cerebral cortex. Histochem J 29:655, 1997.
3. Janzer RC, Raff MC. Astrocytes induce blood-brain barrier properties in endothelial cells. Nature 325:253, 1987.
4. Dueñas M, Luquin S, Chowen JA, et al. Gonadal hormone regulation of insulin-like growth factor-I–like immunoreactivity in hypothalamic astroglia of developing and adult rats. Neuroendocrinology 59:528, 1994.
5. McQueen JK. Glial cells and neuroendocrine function. J Endocrinol 143:411, 1994.
6. Melcangi RC, Galbiati M, Piva MF, et al. Type 1 astrocytes influence luteinizing hormone–releasing hormone release from the hypothalamic cell line GT1-1: Is transforming growth factor-β the principle involved? Endocrinology 136:679, 1995.
7. Galbiati M, Zanisi M, Messi E, et al. Transforming growth factor-β and astrocytic conditioned medium influence luteinizing hormone–releasing hormone gene expression in the hypothalamic cell line GT1. Endocrinology 137:5605, 1996.
8. Ma YJ, Berg–von der Emde K, Rage F, et al. Hypothalamic astrocytes respond to transforming growth factor-α with the secretion of neuroactive substances that stimulate the release of luteinizing hormone–releasing hormone. Endocrinology 138:19, 1997.
9. Al-Hader AA, Lei ZM, Rao CV. Novel expression of functional luteinizing hormone/chorionic gonadotropin receptors in cultured glial cells from neonatal rat brains. Biol Reprod 56:501, 1997.
10. Wyse B, Sernia C. Growth hormone regulates AT-1a angiotensin receptors in astrocytes. Endocrinology 138:4176, 1997.
11. DeVito WJ, Avakian C, Stone S, et al. Prolactin-stimulated mitogenesis of cultured astrocytes is mediated by a protein kinase C–dependent mechanism. J Neurochem 60:835, 1993.
12. DeVito WJ, Avakian C, Stone S, et al. Prolactin induced expression of interleukin-1 alpha, tumor necrosis factor-alpha and transforming growth factor-alpha in cultured astrocytes. J Cell Biochem 57:290, 1995.
13. Chung IY, Benveniste EN. Tumor necrosis factor α production by astrocytes. Induction by lipopolysaccharide, IFN-γ and IL-Iβ. J Immunol 144:2999, 1990.
14. Frei K, Bodmer S, Schwerdel C, et al. Astrocytes of the brain synthesize interleukin 3–like factors. J Immunol 135:4044, 1985.
15. Tedeschi B, Barrett JN, Keane RW. Astrocytes produce interferon that enhances the expression of H-2 antigens on a subpopulation of brain cells. J Cell Biol 102:2244, 1986.
16. Potter E, Behan DP, Linton EA, et al. The central distribution of a corticotropin-releasing factor (CRF)–binding protein predicts multiple sites and modes of interaction with CRF. Proc Natl Acad Sci USA 89:4192, 1992.
17. Behan DP, Maciejewski D, Chalmers D, et al. Corticotropin releasing factor binding protein (CRF-BP) is expressed in neuronal and astrocytic cells. Brain Res 698:259, 1995.
18. Maciejewski D, Crowe PD, DeSouza EB, et al. Regulation of corticotropin-releasing factor–binding protein expression in cultured rat astrocytes. J Pharmacol Exp Ther 278:455, 1996.
19. Visser TJ, Leonard JL, Kaplan MM, et al. Kinetic evidence suggesting two mechanisms for iodothyronine 5′-deiodination in rat cerebral cortex. Proc Natl Acad Sci USA 79:5080, 1982.
20. Kaplan MM, Visser TJ, Yaskoski KA, et al. Characteristics of iodothyronine tyrosyl ring deiodination by rat cerebral cortical microsomes. Endocrinology 112:35, 1983.
21. Leonard JL, Siegrist-Kaiser CA, Zuckerman CJ. Regulation of type II iodothyronine 5′-deiodinase by thyroid hormones. Inhibition of actin polymerization blocks enzyme inactivation in cAMP-stimulated glial cells. J Biol Chem 265:940, 1990.
22. Esfandiari A, Courtin F, Lennon A-M, et al. Induction of type III deiodinase activity in astroglial cells by thyroid hormones. Endocrinology 131:1682, 1992.
23. Baulieu E-E. Neurosteroids: Of the nervous system, by the nervous system, for the nervous system. Recent Prog Horm Res 52:1, 1997.
24. Stromstedt M, Waterman MR. Messenger RNAs encoding steroidogenic enzymes are expressed in rodent brain. Mol Brain Res 34:75, 1995.
25. Zwain IH, Yen SSC. Characterization of cellular origin and biosynthesis of neurosteroids in neonatal rat brain. Unpublished work, 1998.
26. Norenberg ND, Martinez-Hernandez A. Fine structural localization of glutamine synthetase in astrocytes in rat brain. Brain Res 161:303, 1979.
27. Bloom FE. Neurotransmitters: Past, present, and future directions. FASEB J 2:32, 1988.
28. Brann DW, Mahesh VB. Excitatory amino acids: Evidence for a role in the control of reproduction and anterior pituitary hormone secretion. Endocr Rev 18:678, 1997.

29. Bloom FE. General features of chemically identified neurons. *In* Bjorklund A, Hokfelt T (eds). Handbook of Chemical Neuroanatomy, Vol 2. Amsterdam, Elsevier, 1984, pp 1–22.
30. Siggins GR, Gruol DG. Synaptic mechanisms in the vertebrate central nervous system. *In* Bloom FE (ed). Handbook of Physiology, Section I. The Nervous System, Vol IV. Bethesda, American Physiological Society, 1986, pp 1–114.
31. Nestler EJ, Greengard P. Protein phosphorylation in the nervous system. New York, John Wiley & Sons, 1984, pp 1–398.
32. Kobilka BK, Mutsui H, Kobilka TS, et al. Cloning, sequencing and expression of the gene coding for the human platelet α-2 receptor. Science 238:650, 1987.
33. Vitale ML, Chiocchio SR. Serotonin, a neurotransmitter involved in the regulation of luteinizing hormone release. Endocr Rev 14:480, 1993.
34. Lubbert H, Hoffman BJ, Snutch TP, et al. cDNA cloning of a serotonin 5-HT1c receptor by electrophysiological assays of mRNA-injected *Xenopus* oocytes. Proc Natl Acad Sci USA 84:4332, 1987.
35. Hanley MR. Mitogenic neurotransmitters [news]. Nature 340:97, 1989.
36. Mocchetti I, DeBernardi MA, Szekely AM, et al. Regulation of nerve growth factor biosynthesis by β-adrenergic receptor activation in astrocytoma cells: A potential role of c-Fos protein. Proc Natl Acad Sci USA 86:3891, 1989.
37. Hokfelt T, Fuxe K, Pernow B. Coexistence of neuronal messengers—a new principle in chemical neurotransmission. Prog Brain Res 68:380, 1986.
38. Kreiger DT. Brain peptides: What, where and why? Science 222:975, 1983.
39. Swanson LW. The hypothalamus. *In* Bjorklund A, Hokfelt T, Swanson LW (eds). Handbook of Chemical Neuroanatomy. Amsterdam, Elsevier, 1987, pp 1–125.
40. Dawson TM, Snyder SH. Gases as biological messengers: Nitric oxide and carbon monoxide in the brain. J Neurosci 14:5147, 1994.
41. Burnett AL, Lowenstein CJ, Bredt DS, et al. Nitric oxide: A physiologic mediator of penile erection. Science 257:401, 1992.
42. Moretto M, Lopez FJ, Negro-Vilar A. Nitric oxide regulates luteinizing hormone–releasing hormone secretion. Endocrinology 133:2399, 1993.
43. Lamar CA, Mahesh VB, Brann DW. Regulation of gonadotropin-releasing hormone (GnRH) secretion by heme molecules: A regulatory role for carbon monoxide? Endocrinology 137:790, 1996.
44. Palkovits M, Zaborsky L. Neural connections of the hypothalamus. *In* Morgane PJ, Panksepp J (eds). Anatomy of the Hypothalamus. New York, Marcel Dekker, 1979, pp 379–509.
45. Moore RY, Bloom FE. Central catecholamine neuron systems: Anatomy and physiology of the norepinephrine and epinephrine system. Annu Rev Neurosci 2:113, 1979.
46. Steinbusch HWM, Nieuwenhuys R. The raphe nuclei of the brainstem: A cytoarchitectonic and immunohistochemical study. *In* Emson P (ed). Chemical Neuroanatomy. New York, Raven Press, 1983, pp 380–383.
47. Bjorklund A, Lindvall O. Dopamine-containing neuron systems in the CNS. *In* Bjorklund A, Hokfelt T (eds). Handbook of Chemical Neuroanatomy, Vol 1. Amsterdam, Elsevier, 1984, pp 55–122.
48. Moore RY. Organization and function of a CNS circadian oscillator: The suprachiasmatic hypothalamic nucleus. Fed Proc 42:783, 1983.
49. Szentagothai J. The parvicellular neurosecretory system. *In* Bargmann W, Schade JP (eds). Lectures on the Diencephalon. Amsterdam, Elsevier, 1967, pp 135–146.
50. Weindl A. Neuroendocrine aspects of circumventricular organs. *In* Ganong WF, Martini L (eds). Frontiers in Neuroendocrinology. New York, Oxford University Press, 1973, pp 3–32.
51. Knigge KM, Silverman AJ. Anatomy of the endocrine hypothalamus. *In* Knobil E, Sawyer WH (eds). Handbook of Physiology. Endocrinology, Vol IV. Washington, DC, American Physiological Society, 1974, pp 1–32.
52. Moore RY. The innervation of the mammalian pineal gland. *In* Reiter RJ (ed). The Pineal Gland and Reproduction. Basel, S Karger, 1978, pp 1–29.
53. Jennes L. Prenatal development of the gonadotropin-releasing hormone–containing systems in rat brain. Brain Res 482:97, 1989.
54. Pfaff DW, McEwen BS. Actions of estrogens and progestins on nerve cells. Science 219:808, 1983.
55. Paech K, Webb P, Kuiper GGJM, et al. Differential ligand activation of estrogen receptors ERα and ERβ at AP1 sites. Science 277:1508, 1997.
56. Pelletier G, Liao N, Follea N, et al. Mapping of estrogen receptor–producing cells in the rat brain by in situ hybridization. Neurosci Lett 94:23, 1988.
57. Romano GJ, Krust A, Pfaff DW. Expression and estrogen regulation of progesterone receptor mRNA in neurons of the mediobasal hypothalamus: An in situ hybridization study. Mol Endocrinol 3:1295, 1989.
58. Shughrue PJ, Komm B, Merchenthaler I. The distribution of estrogen receptor-β mRNA in the rat hypothalamus. Steroids 61:678, 1996.
59. Roselli CE, Klosterman SA, Fasasi TA. Sex differences in androgen responsiveness in the rat brain: Regional differences in the induction of aromatase activity. Neuroendocrinology 64:139, 1996.
60. Bethea CL, Brown NA, Kohama SG. Steroid regulation of estrogen and progestin receptor messenger ribonucleic acid in monkey hypothalamus and pituitary. Endocrinology 137:4372, 1996.
61. McEwen BS, DeKloet ER, Rostene W. Adrenal steroid receptors and actions in the nervous system. Physiol Rev 66:1121, 1986.
62. Sousa RJ, Tannery NH, Lafer EM. In situ hybridization mapping of glucocorticoid receptor messenger ribonucleic acid in rat brain. Mol Endocrinol 3:481, 1989.
63. Sapolsky RM, Packan DR, Vale WW. Glucocorticoid toxicity in the hippocampus: In vitro demonstration. Brain Res 453:369, 1988.
64. Naftolin F, Ryan KJ, Davie KJ, et al. The formation of estrogens by central neuroendocrine tissues. Recent Prog Horm Res 31:95, 1975.
65. Compagnone NA, Bulfone A, Rubenstein JR, et al. Steroidogenic enzyme P450c17 is expressed in the embryonic central nervous system. Endocrinology 136:5212, 1995.
66. Majewska MD. Neuronal actions of dehydroepiandrosterone: Possible roles in brain development, aging, memory, and affect. Ann N Y Acad Sci 774:111, 1995.
67. Lanthier A, Patwardhan VV. Sex steroids and 5-en-3β-hydroxysteroids in specific regions of the human brain and cranial nerves. J Steroid Biochem 25:445, 1986.
68. Lacroix C, Fiet J, Benais JP, et al. Simultaneous radioimmunoassay of progesterone, androst-4-enedione, pregnenolone, dehydroepiandrosterone and 17-hydroxyprogesterone in specific regions of human brain. J Steroid Biochem 28:317, 1987.
69. Ramayya MS, Zhou J, Kino T, et al. Steroidogenic factor 1 messenger ribonucleic acid expression in steroidogenic and nonsteroidogenic human tissues: Northern blot and in situ hybridization studies. J Clin Endocrinol Metab 82:1799, 1997.
70. Harrison NL, Majewska MD, Meyers DER, et al. Rapid actions of steroids on CNS neurons. *In* Galveston Neuroscience Symposium. Neural Control of Reproductive Function. New York, Alan R Liss, 1989, pp 137–166.
71. Wu FS, Gibbs TT, Farb DH. Pregnenolone sulfate: A positive allosteric modulator at the *N*-methyl-D-aspartate receptor. Mol Pharmacol 40:333, 1991.
72. Spivak CE. Desensitization and noncompetitive blockade of $GABA_A$ receptors in ventral midbrain neurons by a neurosteroid dehydroepiandrosterone sulfate. Synapse 16:113, 1994.
73. Majewska MD. Neurosteroids: Endogenous bimodal modulators of the $GABA_A$ receptor. Mechanism of action and physiological significance. Prog Neurobiol 38:379, 1992.
74. Wigstrom H, Gustafsson B. Facilitation of hippocampus long-lasting potentiation by GABA-antagonists. Acta Physiol Scand 125:159, 1985.
75. Flood JF, Roberts E. Dehydroepiandrosterone sulfate improves memory in aging mice. Brain Res 448:178, 1988.
76. Flood JF, Morley JE, Roberts E. Pregnenolone sulfate enhances post-training memory processes when injected in very low doses into limbic system structures: The amygdala is by far the most sensitive. Proc Natl Acad Sci USA 92:10806, 1995.
77. Isaacson RL, Varner JA, Baars J-M, et al. The effects of pregnenolone sulfate and ethylestrenol on retention of a passive avoidance task. Brain Res 689:79, 1995.

78. Frye CA, Sturgis JD. Neurosteroids affect spatial/reference, working, and long-term memory of female rats. Neurobiol Learn Mem 64:83, 1995.
79. Vallée M, Mayo W, Darnaudéry M, et al. Neurosteroids: Deficient cognitive performance in aged rats depends on low pregnenolone sulfate levels in the hippocampus. Proc Natl Acad Sci USA 94:14865, 1997.
80. Morales AJ, Nolan J, Nelson G, et al. Effects of replacement dose of dehydroepiandrosterone (DHEA) in men and women of advancing age. J Clin Endocrinol Metab 78:1360, 1994.
81. Wolkowitz OM, Reus VI, Roberts E, et al. Dehydroepiandrosterone (DHEA) treatment of depression. Biol Psychiatry 41:311, 1997.
82. Friess E, Trachsel L, Guldner J, et al. DHEA administration increased rapid eye movement sleep and EEG power in the sigma frequency range. Am Physiol Soc 268:E107, 1995.
83. Sanders SA, Reinisch JM. Behavioral effects on humans of progesterone related compounds during development and in the adult. *In* Ganten D, Pfaff D (eds). Actions of Progesterone on the Brain. Berlin, Springer-Verlag, 1995, pp 175–206.
84. Morfin R, Young J, Corpéchot C, et al. Neurosteroids: Pregnenolone in human sciatic nerves. Proc Natl Acad Sci USA 89:6790, 1992.
85. Koenig HL, Schumacher M, Ferzaz B, et al. Progesterone synthesis and myelin formation by Schwann cells. Science 268:1500, 1995.
86. Green JD, Harris GW. Observation of the hypophyseal-portal vessels in the living rat. J Physiol 108:359, 1949.
87. Donaldson CJ, Sutton SW, Perrin MH, et al. Cloning and characterization of human urocortin. Endocrinology 137:2167, 1996.
88. Aschoff J. The circadian system in man. *In* Krieger DT, Hughes JC (eds). Neuroendocrinology. Sunderland, MA, Sinauer Associates, 1980, p 77.
89. Weitzman ED. Biologic rhythms and hormone secretion patterns. *In* Krieger DT, Hughes JC (eds). Neuroendocrinology. Sunderland, MA, Sinauer Associates, 1980, p 85.
90. Moore-Ede MC, Czeisler CA, Richardson GS. Circadian timekeeping in health and disease. N Engl J Med 309:530, 1983.
91. Ishizuka B, Quigley ME, Yen SSC. Pituitary hormone release in response to food ingestion: Evidence for neuroendocrine signals from gut to brain. J Clin Endocrinol Metab 57:1111, 1983.
92. Yen SSC, Rebar RW. Endocrine rhythms in gonadotropins and ovarian steroids with reference to reproductive processes. *In* Krieger DT (ed). Endocrine Rhythms. New York, Raven Press, 1979, pp 259–298.
93. Matsuo H, Baba Y, Nair RM, et al. Structure of the porcine LH- and FSH-releasing hormone: I. The proposed amino acid sequence. Biochem Biophys Res Commun 43:1334, 1971.
94. Kakar SS, Musgrove LC, Devor DC, et al. Cloning, sequencing, and expression of human gonadotropin releasing hormone (GnRH) receptor. Biochem Biophys Res Commun 189:289, 1992.
95. Barry J, Barette B. Immunofluorescence study of LRF neurons in primates. Cell Tissue Res 164:163, 1975.
96. Silverman AJ, Jhamandas J, Renaud LP. Localization of luteinizing hormone–releasing hormone (LHRH) neurons that project to the median eminence. J Neurosci 7:2312, 1987.
97. Standish LJ, Adams LA, Vician L, et al. Neuroanatomical localization of cells containing gonadotropin-releasing hormone messenger ribonucleic acid in the primate brain by in situ hybridization histochemistry. Mol Endocrinol 1:371, 1987.
98. Anthony ELP, King JC, Stopa EG. Immunocytochemical localization of LHRH in the median eminence, infundibular stalk, and neurohypophysis: Evidence for multiple sites of releasing hormone secretion in humans and other mammals. Cell Tissue Res 236:5, 1984.
99. Jennes L, Eyigor O, Janovick JA, et al. Brain gonadotropin releasing hormone receptors: Localization and regulation. Recent Prog Horm Res 52:475, 1997.
100. Seeburg PH, Adelman JP. Characterization of cDNA for precursor of human luteinizing hormone releasing hormone. Nature 311:666, 1984.
101. Seeburg PH, Mason AJ, Stewart TA, et al. The mammalian GnRH gene and its pivotal role in reproduction. Recent Prog Horm Res 43:69, 1987.
102. Ackland JF, Nikolics K, Seeburg P, et al. Molecular forms of gonadotropin-releasing hormone associated peptide (GAP): Changes within the rat hypothalamus and release from hypothalamic cells in vitro. Neuroendocrinology 48:376, 1988.
103. Ronnekleiv OK, Naylor BR, Bond CT, et al. Combined immunohistochemistry for gonadotropin-releasing hormone (GnRH) and pro-GnRH, and in situ hybridization for GnRH messenger ribonucleic acid in rat brain. Mol Endocrinol 3:363, 1989.
104. Ronnekleiv OK, Adelman JP, Weber E, et al. Immunohistochemical demonstration of pro-GnRH and GnRH in the preoptic-basal hypothalamus of the primate. Neuroendocrinology 45:518, 1987.
105. Knobil E. Neuroendocrine control of the menstrual cycle. Recent Prog Horm Res 36:53, 1980.
106. Knobil E. The electrophysiology of the GnRH pulse generator. J Steroid Biochem 33:669, 1989.
107. Minami S, Frautschy SA, Plotsky PM, et al. Facilitatory role of neuropeptide on the onset of puberty: Effect of immunoneutralization of neuropeptide Y on the release of luteinizing hormone–releasing hormone. Neuroendocrinology 52:112, 1990.
108. Clarke IJ, Cummins JT. The temporal relationship between gonadotropin releasing hormone (GnRH) and luteinizing hormone (LH) secretion in ovariectomized ewes. Endocrinology 111:1737, 1982.
109. Rasmussen DD, Gambacciani M, Swartz W, et al. Pulsatile gonadotropin-releasing hormone release from the human mediobasal hypothalamus in vitro: Opiate receptor–mediated suppression. Neuroendocrinology 49:150, 1989.
110. Wetsel WC, Valenca MM, Merchenthaler I, et al. Intrinsic pulsatile secretory activity of immortalized LHRH secreting neurons. Proc Natl Acad Sci USA 89:4149, 1992.
111. Mellon PL, Windle JJ, Goldsmith P, et al. Immortalization of hypothalamic GnRH neurons by genetically targeted tumorigenesis. Neuron 5:1, 1990.
112. Wetsel WC, Liposits Z, Seidah NG, et al. Expression of candidate pro-LHRH processing enzymes in rat hypothalamus and in immortalized hypothalamic neuronal cell line. Neuroendocrinology 62:166, 1995.
113. Silverman AJ, Roberts JL, Dong KW, et al. Intrahypothalamic injection of a cell line secreting gonadotropin-releasing hormone results in cellular differentiation and reversal of hypogonadism in mutant mice. Proc Natl Acad Sci USA 89:10668, 1992.
114. Krsmanovic LZ, Stojilkovic SS, Catt KJ. Pulsatile gonadotropin-releasing hormone release and its regulation. Trends Endocrinol Metab 7:56, 1996.
115. Turgeon JL. Gonadotropin-releasing hormone neuron cell biology. Trends Endocrinol Metab 7:55, 1996.
116. Cesnjaj M, Krsmanovic LZ, Catt KJ, et al. Autocrine induction of *c-fos* expression in GT1 neuronal cells by gonadotropin-releasing hormone. Endocrinology 133:3042, 1993.
117. Padmanabhan V, Evans NP, Dahl GE, et al. Evidence for short or ultrashort loop negative feedback of gonadotropin-releasing hormone secretion. Neuroendocrinology 62:248, 1995.
118. Kalra SP, Kalra PS. Opioid-adrenergic-steroid connection in regulation of luteinizing hormone in the rat. Neuroendocrinology 38:418, 1984.
119. Grosser PM, O'Byrne KT, Williams CL, et al. Effects of naloxone on estrogen-induced changes in hypothalamic gonadotropin-releasing hormone pulse generator activity in the rhesus monkey. Neuroendocrinology 57:115, 1993.
120. Nazian SJ, Landon CS, Muffly KE, et al. Opioid inhibition of adrenergic and dopaminergic but not serotonergic stimulation of luteinizing hormone releasing hormone release from immortalized hypothalamic neurons. Mol Cell Neurosci 5:642, 1994.
121. Findell PR, Wong KH, Jackman JK, et al. β_1-Adrenergic and dopamine (D_1)–receptors coupled to adenylyl cyclase activation in GT1 gonadotropin-releasing hormone neurosecretory cells. Endocrinology 132:682, 1993.
122. Martinez de la Escalera G, Gallo F, Choi ALH, et al. Dopaminergic regulation of the GT_1 gonadotropin-releasing hormone (GnRH) neuronal cell lines: Stimulation of GnRH release via D_1-receptors positively coupled to adenylate cyclase. Endocrinology 131:2965, 1992.

123. Olson BR, Scott DC, Wetsel WC, et al. Effects of insulin-like growth factors I and II and insulin on the immortalized hypothalamic GT1–7 cell line. Neuroendocrinology 62:155, 1995.
124. Tsai PS, Werner S, Weiner RI. Basic fibroblast growth factor is a neurotropic factor in GT1 gonadotropin-releasing hormone neuronal cell lines. Endocrinology 136:3831, 1995.
125. Martinez-Hernandez A, Bell KP, Norenberg ND. Glutamine synthetase: Glial localization in brain. Science 195:1356, 1977.
126. Potashner SJ. Baclofen inhibits aspartate and glutamate release from slices. Eur J Pharmacol 240:325, 1979.
127. Weisskopf MG, Zalutsky RA, Nicoll RA. The opioid peptide dynorphin mediates heterosynaptic depression of hippocampal mossy fibre synapses and modulates long-term potentiation. Nature 362:423, 1993.
128. Stojilkovic S, Krsmanovic LZ, Spergel D, et al. Gonadotropin-releasing hormone neurons. Intrinsic pulsatility and receptor-mediated regulation. Trends Endocrinol Metab 5:201, 1994.
129. Evans RM. The steroid and thyroid hormone receptor superfamily. Science 240:889, 1988.
130. Mangelsdorf DJ, Thummel C, Beato M, et al. The nuclear receptor superfamily: The second decade. Cell 83:835, 1995.
131. Chandran UR, Attardi B, Friedman R, et al. Glucocorticoid repression of the mouse gonadotropin-releasing hormone gene is mediated by promoter elements that are recognized by heteromeric complexes containing glucocorticoid receptor. J Biol Chem 271:20412, 1996.
132. Attardi B, Tsujii T, Friedman R, et al. Glucocorticoid repression of gonadotropin-releasing hormone gene expression and secretion in morphologically distinct subpopulations of GT1–7 cells. Mol Cell Endocrinol 131:241, 1997.
133. Ahima RS, Harlan RE. Glucocorticoid receptors in LHRH neurons. Neuroendocrinology 56:845, 1992.
134. Morte B, Ĩniguez MA, Lorenzo PI, et al. Thyroid hormone–regulated expression of RC3/neurogranin in the immortalized hypothalamic cell line GT1–7. J Neurochem 69:902, 1997.
135. Jansen HT, Lubbers LS, Macchia E, et al. Thyroid hormone receptor (α) distribution in hamster and sheep brain: Colocalization in gonadotropin-releasing hormone and other identified neurons. Endocrinology 138:5039, 1997.
136. Scott REM, Wu-Peng XS, Yen PM, et al. Interactions of estrogen- and thyroid hormone receptors on a progesterone receptor estrogen response element (ERE) sequence: A comparison with the vitellogenin A2 consensus ERE. Mol Endocrinol 11:1581, 1997.
137. Kaufman J-M, Kesner JS, Wilson RC, et al. Electrophysiological manifestation of luteinizing hormone–releasing hormone pulse generator activity in the rhesus monkey: Influence of α-adrenergic and dopaminergic blocking agents. Endocrinology 116:1327, 1985.
138. Gearing M, Terasawa E. The α_1-adrenergic neuronal system is involved in the pulsatile release of luteinizing hormone–releasing hormone in the ovariectomized female rhesus monkey. Neuroendocrinology 53:373, 1991.
139. Leblanc H, Lachelin GCL, Abu-Fadil S, et al. Effects of dopamine infusion on pituitary hormone secretion in humans. J Clin Endocrinol Metab 43:668, 1976.
140. Lachelin GCL, Leblanc H, Yen SSC. The inhibitory effect of dopamine infusion on pituitary hormone secretion in humans. J Clin Endocrinol Metab 44:728, 1977.
141. Pehrson JJ, Jaffee WL, Vaitukaitis JL. Effect of dopamine on gonadotropin-releasing hormone induced gonadotropin secretion in postmenopausal women. J Clin Endocrinol Metab 56:889, 1983.
142. Williams CL, Nishihara M, Thalabard J-C, et al. Duration and frequency of the multiunit electrical activity associated with the hypothalamic gonadotropin releasing hormone (GnRH) pulse generator in the rhesus monkey: Differential effects of morphine. Neuroendocrinology 52:225, 1990.
143. Ferin M, Wehrenberg WB, Lam NY, et al. Effects and site of action of morphine on gonadotropin secretion in the female rhesus monkey. Endocrinology 111:1652, 1982.
144. Van Vugt DA, Webb MY, Reid RL. Comparison of the duration of action of nalmefene and naloxone on the hypothalamic-pituitary axis of the rhesus monkey. Neuroendocrinology 49:275, 1989.
145. Williams CL, Nishihara M, Thalabard J-C, et al. Corticotropin-releasing factor and gonadotropin-releasing hormone pulse generator activity in the rhesus monkey: Electrophysiological studies. Neuroendocrinology 52:133, 1990.
146. Fischer UG, Wood SH, Bruhn J, et al. Effect of human corticotropin-releasing hormone on gonadotropin secretion in cycling and postmenopausal women. Fertil Steril 58:1108, 1992.
147. Brann DW, Chorich LP, Mahesh VB. Effect of progesterone on galanin mRNA levels in the hypothalamus and the pituitary: Correlation with the gonadotropin surge. Neuroendocrinology 58:531, 1993.
148. Woller MJ, Terasawa E. Estradiol enhances the action of neuropeptide Y on in vivo luteinizing hormone–releasing hormone release in the ovariectomized rhesus monkey. Neuroendocrinology 56:921, 1992.
149. Schwanzel-Fukuda M, Pfaff DW. Origin of luteinizing hormone–releasing hormone neurons. Nature 338:161, 1989.
150. Ronnekleiv OK, Resko JA. Ontogeny of gonadotropin-releasing hormone–containing neurons in early fetal development of rhesus macaques. Endocrinology 126:498, 1990.
151. Schwanzel-Fukuda M, Jorgenson KL, Bergen HT, et al. Biology of normal luteinizing hormone–releasing hormone neurons during and after their migration from olfactory placode. Endocr Rev 13:623, 1992.
152. Schwanzel-Fukuda M, Bick D, Pfaff DW. Luteinizing hormone–releasing hormone (LHRH) expressing cells do not migrate normally in an inherited hypogonadal (Kallmann syndrome). Mol Brain Res 6:311, 1989.
153. Kaplan SL, Grumbach MM, Aubert ML. The ontogenesis of pituitary hormones and hypothalamic factors in the human fetus: Maturation of central nervous system regulation of anterior pituitary function. Recent Prog Horm Res 32:161, 1976.
154. Rossmanith WG, Swartz WH, Tueros VS, et al. Pulsatile GnRH-stimulated LH release from the human fetal pituitary in vitro: Sex associated differences. Clin Endocrinol (Oxf) 33:719, 1990.
155. Kaplan SL, Grumbach MM. Pituitary and placental gonadotropins and sex steroids in the human and subhuman primate fetus. J Clin Endocrinol Metab 7:487, 1978.
156. Reyes RI, Boroditsky RS, Winter JSD, et al. Studies on human sexual development: II. Fetal and maternal serum gonadotropin and sex steroid concentrations. J Clin Endocrinol Metab 38:612, 1974.
157. Rasmussen DD, Liu JH, Wolf PL, et al. Endogenous opioid regulation of gonadotropin-releasing hormone release from the human fetal hypothalamus in vitro. J Clin Endocrinol Metab 57:881, 1983.
158. Rasmussen DD, Liu JH, Swartz WH, et al. Human fetal hypothalamic GnRH neurosecretion: Dopaminergic regulation in vitro. Clin Endocrinol (Oxf) 25:127, 1986.
159. Ross JL, Loriaux DL, Cutler GB. Developmental changes in neuroendocrine regulation of gonadotropin secretion in gonadal dysgenesis. J Clin Endocrinol Metab 57:288, 1983.
160. Wildt L, Marshall GR, Knobil E. Experimental induction of puberty in the infantile female rhesus monkey. Science 207:1373, 1980.
161. Medhamurthy R, Gay VL, Plant TM. The prepubertal hiatus in gonadotropin secretion in the male rhesus monkey *(Macaca mulatta)* does not appear to involve endogenous opioid peptide restraint of hypothalamic gonadotropin-releasing hormone release. Endocrinology 126:1036, 1990.
162. Petraglia F, Bernasconi S, Iughetti L, et al. Naloxone induced luteinizing hormone secretion in normal, precocious, and delayed puberty. J Clin Endocrinol Metab 63:1112, 1986.
163. Wiemann JN, Clifton DK, Steiner RA. Pubertal changes in gonadotropin-releasing hormone and proopiomelanocortin gene expression in the brain of the male rat. Endocrinology 124:1760, 1989.
164. Donoso AO, Lopez FJ, Negro-Vilar A. Glutamate receptors of the non *N*-methyl-D-aspartic acid type mediate the increase in luteinizing hormone–releasing hormone release by excitatory amino acids in vitro. Endocrinology 126:414, 1990.
165. Plant TM, Gay VL, Marshall GR, et al. Puberty in monkeys is triggered by chemical stimulation of the hypothalamus. Proc Natl Acad Sci USA 86:2506, 1989.
166. Kapen S, Boyar RM, Finkelstein JW, et al. Effect of sleep-wake cycle reversal on luteinizing hormone secretory pattern in puberty. J Clin Endocrinol Metab 39:293, 1974.
167. Apter D, Viinikka L, Vihko R. Hormonal pattern of adolescent menstrual cycles. J Clin Endocrinol Metab 47:944, 1978.

168. Hazum E, Conn PM. Molecular mechanism of gonadotropin releasing hormone (GnRH) action: I. The GnRH receptor. Endocr Rev 9:379, 1988.
169. Karten MJ, Rivier JE. Gonadotropin-releasing hormone analog design. Structure function studies toward the development of agonists and antagonists: Rationale and perspective. Endocr Rev 7:44, 1986.
170. Handelsman DJ, Swerdloff RS. Pharmacokinetics of gonadotropin-releasing hormone and its analogs. Endocr Rev 7:95, 1986.
171. Lemay A, Maheux R, Faure N, et al. Reversible hypogonadism induced by a luteinizing hormone–releasing hormone (LHRH) agonist (buserelin) as a new therapeutic approach for endometriosis. Fertil Steril 41:863, 1984.
172. Cann CE, Martin MC, Genant HK, et al. Decreased spinal mineral content in amenorrheic women. JAMA 251:626, 1984.
173. Matta WH, Shaw RW, Hesp R, et al. Reversible trabecular bone density loss following induced hypo-oestrogenism with the GnRH analogue buserelin in premenopausal women. Clin Endocrinol (Oxf) 29:45, 1988.
174. Cetel NS, Rivier JE, Vale WW, et al. The dynamics of gonadotropin inhibition in women induced by an antagonistic analog of gonadotropin-releasing hormone. J Clin Endocrinol Metab 57:62, 1983.
175. Mais V, Kazer RR, Cetel NS, et al. The dependency of folliculogenesis and corpus luteum function on pulsatile gonadotropin secretion in cycling women using a gonadotropin-releasing hormone antagonist as a probe. J Clin Endocrinol Metab 62:1250, 1986.
176. Kessel B, Dahl KD, Kazer RR, et al. The dependency of bioactive FSH on gonadotropin releasing hormone in hypogonadal and cycling women. J Clin Endocrinol Metab 66:361, 1988.
177. Pavlou SN, DeBold CR, Island DP, et al. Single subcutaneous doses of a luteinizing hormone–releasing hormone antagonist suppress serum gonadotropin and testosterone levels in normal men [published erratum appears in J Clin Endocrinol Metab 63:940, 1986]. J Clin Endocrinol Metab 63:303, 1986.
178. Mortola JF, Sathanandan M, Pavlou S, et al. Suppression of bioactive and immunoreactive follicle-stimulating hormone and luteinizing hormone levels by a potent gonadotropin-releasing hormone antagonist: Pharmacodynamic studies. Fertil Steril 51:957, 1989.
179. Pavlou SN, Wakefield G, Schlechter NL, et al. Mode of suppression of pituitary and gonadal function after acute or prolonged administration of a luteinizing hormone–releasing hormone antagonist in normal men. J Clin Endocrinol Metab 68:446, 1989.
180. Eldelstein MC, Gordon K, Williams RF, et al. Single dose long-term suppression of testosterone secretion by a gonadotropin-releasing hormone antagonist (antide) in male monkeys. Contraception 42:209, 1990.
181. Behre HM, Bockers A, Schlingheider A, et al. Daily injections of the new GnRH antagonist cetrorelix effectively suppress serum gonadotropins and testosterone in normal men. Presented at the Symposium of Gonadotropins, GnRH, GnRH Analogs and Gonadal Peptides; May 20–24, 1992; Paris, France.
182. Behre HM, Kliesch S, Puhse G, et al. High loading and low maintenance doses of a gonadotropin-releasing hormone antagonist effectively suppress serum luteinizing hormone, follicle-stimulating hormone, and testosterone in normal men. J Clin Endocrinol Metab 82:1403, 1997.
183. Sharp SC, Farley GM, Lindner J, et al. Suppression of pituitary and gonadal function in normal men during chronic administration of a highly potent GnRH antagonist. Presented at the 74th annual meeting of the Endocrine Society; June 24–27, 1992; San Antonio, TX.
184. Fujimoto VY, Monroe SE, Nelson LR, et al. Dose-related suppression of serum luteinizing hormone in women by a potent new gonadotropin-releasing hormone antagonist (ganirelix) administered by intranasal spray. Fertil Steril 67:469, 1997.
185. Pavlou SN, Wakefield G, Island DP, et al. Suppression of pituitary-gonadal function by a potent new luteinizing hormone–releasing hormone antagonist in normal men. J Clin Endocrinol Metab 64:931, 1987.
186. Andreyko JL, Monroe SE, Marshall LA, et al. Concordant suppression of serum immunoreactive luteinizing hormone (LH), follicle-stimulating hormone, α subunit, bioactive LH, and testosterone in postmenopausal women by a potent gonadotropin releasing hormone antagonist (detirelix). J Clin Endocrinol Metab 74:399, 1992.
187. Crowley EF, McArthur JW. Stimulation of the normal menstrual cycle in Kallmann's syndrome by pulsatile administration of luteinizing hormone–releasing hormone (LHRH). J Clin Endocrinol Metab 51:173, 1980.
188. Miller DS, Reid R, Cetel N, et al. Pulsatile administration of low dose gonadotropin-releasing hormone (GnRH) for the induction of ovulation and pregnancy in patients with hypothalamic amenorrhea. JAMA 250:2937, 1983.
189. Leyendecker G, Wildt L, Hansmann M. Pregnancies following chronic intermittent (pulsatile) administration of GnRH by means of a portable pump (Zyklomat): A new approach in the treatment of infertility in hypothalamic amenorrhea. J Clin Endocrinol Metab 51:1214, 1980.
190. Schoemaker J, Simons AHM, von Osnabrugge GJC, et al. Pregnancy after prolonged pulsatile administration of luteinizing hormone–releasing hormone in a patient with clomiphene-resistant secondary amenorrhea. J Clin Endocrinol Metab 52:882, 1981.
191. Reid RL, Leopold GR, Yen SSC. Induction of ovulation and pregnancy with pulsatile luteinizing hormone releasing factor: Dosage and mode of delivery. Fertil Steril 36:553, 1981.
192. Skarin G, Nillius SJ, Wibell L, et al. Chronic pulsatile low dose GnRH therapy for induction of testosterone production and spermatogenesis in a man with secondary hypogonadotropic hypogonadism. J Clin Endocrinol Metab 55:723, 1982.
193. Hoffman AR, Crowley WF Jr. Induction of puberty in men by long-term pulsatile administration of low-dose gonadotropin-releasing hormone. N Engl J Med 307:1237, 1982.
194. Finkelstein JS, Spratt DI, O'Dea LSL, et al. Pulsatile gonadotropin secretion after discontinuation of long term gonadotropin-releasing hormone (GnRH) administration in a subset of GnRH deficient men. J Clin Endocrinol Metab 69:377, 1989.
195. West CP, Lumsden MA, Lawson S, et al. Shrinkage of uterine fibroids during therapy with goserelin (Zoladex): A luteinizing hormone–releasing hormone agonist administered as a monthly subcutaneous depot. Fertil Steril 48:45, 1987.
196. Kessel B, Liu JH, Mortola JF, et al. Treatment of uterine fibroids with agonist analogs of gonadotropin-releasing hormone. Fertil Steril 49:538, 1988.
197. Healy DL, Fraser HM, Lawson SL. Shrinkage of a uterine fibroid after subcutaneous infusion of an LHRH agonist. Br Med J 289:1267, 1984.
198. Andreyko JA, Blumenfeld Z, Marshall LA, et al. Use of an agonistic analog of gonadotropin-releasing hormone (nafarelin) to treat leiomyomas: Assessment of magnetic resonance imaging. Am J Obstet Gynecol 158:908, 1988.
199. Carr BR, Marshburn PB, Weatherall PT, et al. An evaluation of the effect of gonadotropin-releasing hormone analogs and medroxyprogesterone acetate on uterine leiomyomata volume by magnetic resonance imaging: A prospective, randomized, double blind, placebo-controlled, crossover trial. J Clin Endocrinol Metab 76:1217, 1993.
200. Manni A. Endocrine therapy of breast and prostate cancer. Endocrinol Metab Clin North Am 18:569, 1989.
201. Kuhn J-M, Billebaud T, Navratil H, et al. Prevention of the transient adverse effects of a gonadotropin-releasing hormone analogue (buserelin) in metastatic prostatic carcinoma by administration of an antiandrogen (nilutamide). N Engl J Med 321:413, 1989.
202. Crawford ED, Eisenberger MA, McLeod DG, et al. A controlled trial of leuprolide with and without flutamide in prostatic carcinoma. N Engl J Med 321:419, 1989.
203. Labrie F, Dupont A, Belanger A, et al. Treatment of prostate cancer with gonadotropin-releasing hormone agonists. Endocr Rev 7:67, 1986.
204. Vale WW, Speiss J, Rivier C, et al. Characterization of a 41–amino acid residue ovine hypothalamic peptide that stimulates the secretion of corticotropin and β-endorphin. Science 213:1394, 1981.
205. Thompson RC, Seasholtz AF, Douglass J, et al. The rat corticotropin-releasing hormone gene. Ann N Y Acad Sci 512:7, 1987.

206. Arbiser JL, Morton CC, Bruns GA, et al. Human corticotropin releasing hormone gene is located on the long arm of chromosome 8. Cytogenet Cell Genet 47:113, 1988.
207. Rivier C, Plotsky PM. Mediation by corticotropin-releasing factor (CRF) of adenohypophysial hormone secretion. Annu Rev Physiol 48:475, 1986.
208. DeSouza EB, Grigoriadis DE. Corticotropin-releasing factor. Physiology, pharmacology, and role in central nervous system and immune disorders. *In* Bloom FE, Kupfer DJ (eds). Psychopharmacology: The Fourth Generation of Progress. New York, Raven Press, 1995, pp 505–517.
209. Menzaghi F, Heinrichs SC, Pich EM, et al. The role of limbic corticotropin-releasing factor in behavioral responses to stress. Ann N Y Acad Sci 697:142, 1993.
210. Vamvakopoulos NC, Chrousos GP. Hormonal regulation of human corticotropin-releasing hormone gene expression: Implications for the stress response and immune/inflammatory reaction. Endocr Rev 15:409, 1994.
211. Palkovits M. Anatomy of neural pathways affecting CRH secretion. Ann N Y Acad Sci 512:139, 1987.
212. Swanson LW, Sawchenko PE, Rivier J, et al. Organization of ovine corticotropin-releasing factor immunoreactive cells and fibers in the rat brain: An immunohistochemical study. Neuroendocrinology 36:165, 1983.
213. Gibbs DM, Stewart RD, Liu JH, et al. Effects of synthetic corticotropin-releasing factor and dopamine on the release of immunoreactive β-endorphin/β-lipotropin and α-melanocyte–stimulating hormone from human fetal pituitaries in vitro. J Clin Endocrinol Metab 55:1149, 1982.
214. Plotsky PM, Cunningham ET Jr, Widmaier EP. Catecholaminergic modulation of corticotropin-releasing factor and adrenocorticotropin secretion. Endocr Rev 10:437, 1989.
215. Frim DM, Emanuel RL, Robinson BG, et al. Characterization and gestational regulation of corticotropin-releasing hormone messenger RNA in human placenta. J Clin Invest 82:287, 1988.
216. Usui T, Nakai Y, Tsukada T, et al. Expression of adrenocorticotropin-releasing hormone precursor gene in placenta and other non-hypothalamic tissues in man. Mol Endocrinol 2:871, 1988.
217. DiBlasio AM, Giraldi FP, Vigano P, et al. Expression of corticotropin-releasing hormone and its R1 receptor in human endometrial stromal cells. J Clin Endocrinol Metab 82:1594, 1997.
218. Mastorakos G, Scopa CD, Kao LC, et al. Presence of immunoreactive corticotropin-releasing hormone in human endometrium. J Clin Endocrinol Metab 81:1046, 1996.
219. Asakura H, Zwain IH, Yen SSC. Expression of genes encoding corticotropin-releasing factor, type 1 CRF receptor (CRF-R1), and CRF-binding protein (CRF-BP) and localization of the gene products in the human ovary. J Clin Endocrinol Metab 82:2720, 1997.
220. Erden HF, Zwain IH, Asakura H, et al. Corticotropin-releasing factor (CRF) inhibits LH-stimulated P450c17 gene expression and androgen production by isolated theca cells of human ovarian follicles. J Clin Endocrinol Metab 83:448, 1998.
221. Ekman R, Servenius B, Castro MG, et al. Biosynthesis of corticotropin-releasing hormone in human T-lymphocytes. J Neuroimmunol 44:7, 1993.
222. Bruhn TO, Engeland WC, Anthony ELP, et al. Corticotropin-releasing factor in adrenal medulla. Ann N Y Acad Sci 512:115, 1987.
223. Kasckow JW, Parkes DG, Owens MJ, et al. The BE(2)-M17 neuroblastoma cell line synthesizes and secretes corticotropin-releasing factor. Brain Res 654:159, 1994.
224. Robinson BG, Emanuel RL, Frim DM, et al. Glucocorticoid stimulates expression of corticotropin-releasing hormone gene in human placenta. Proc Natl Acad Sci USA 85:5244, 1988.
225. Linton EA, Lowry PJ. Corticotrophin releasing factor in man and its measurement: A review. Clin Endocrinol (Oxf) 31:225, 1989.
226. Sawchenko PE, Imaki T, Potter E, et al. The functional neuroanatomy of corticotropin-releasing factor. Ciba Found Symp 172:5, 1993.
227. Swanson LW, Simmons DM. Differential steroid hormone and neural influences on peptide mRNA levels in CRH cells of the paraventricular nucleus: A hybridization histochemical study in the rat. J Comp Neurol 285:413, 1989.
228. Spinedi E, Johnston CA, Chisari A, et al. Role of central epinephrine on the regulation of corticotropin-releasing factor and adrenocorticotropin secretion. Endocrinology 122:1977, 1988.
229. Suda T, Tozawa F, Yamada M, et al. Insulin-induced hypoglycemia increases corticotropin-releasing factor messenger ribonucleic acid levels in rat hypothalamus. Endocrinology 123:1371, 1988.
230. Tozawa F, Suda T, Yamada M, et al. Insulin-induced hypoglycemia increases proopiomelanocortin messenger ribonucleic acid levels in rat anterior pituitary gland. Endocrinology 122:1231, 1988.
231. Ellis MJ, Schmidli RS, Donald RA, et al. Plasma corticotrophin-releasing factor and vasopressin responses to hypoglycaemia in normal man. Clin Endocrinol 32:93, 1990.
232. Thorne N, Suda T, Nakagkami Y, et al. Adrenergic modulation of adrenocorticotropin responses to insulin-induced hypoglycemia and corticotropin-releasing hormone. J Clin Endocrinol Metab 68:87, 1989.
233. Tsagarakis S, Navara P, Rees LH, et al. Morphine directly modulates the release of stimulated corticotropin-releasing factor-41 from rat hypothalamus in vitro. Endocrinology 124:2330, 1989.
234. Tsagarakis S, Rees LH, Besser GM, et al. Neuropeptide Y stimulates CRF41 release from rat hypothalami in vitro. Brain Res 502:167, 1989.
235. Turnbull AV, Rivier C. Corticotropin-releasing factor (CRF) and endocrine responses to stress: CRF receptors, binding protein, and related peptides. Soc Exp Biol Med 215:1, 1997.
236. Chang C-P, Pearse RV II, O'Connell S, et al. Identification of a seven transmembrane helix receptor for corticotropin-releasing factor and sauvagine in mammalian brain. Neuron 11:1187, 1993.
237. Ross PC, Kostas CM, Ramabhadran TV. A variant of the human corticotropin-releasing factor (CRF) receptor: Cloning expression and pharmacology. Biochem Biophys Res Commun 205:1836, 1994.
238. Rivier C, Vale W. Involvement of corticotropin-releasing factor and somatostatin in stress-induced inhibition of growth hormone secretion in the rat. Endocrinology 117:2478, 1985.
239. Rivier C, Rivier J, Vale W. Stress-induced inhibition of reproductive functions: Role of endogenous corticotropin-releasing factor. Science 231:606, 1986.
240. DeSouza EB. Corticotropin-releasing factor receptors: Physiology, pharmacology, biochemistry and role in central nervous system and immune disorders. Psychoneuroendocrinology 20:789, 1995.
241. Schwartz J, Vale W. Dissociation of the adrenocorticotropin secretory responses to corticotropin-releasing factor (CRF) and vasopressin or oxytocin by using a specific cytotoxic analog of CRF. Endocrinology 122:1695, 1988.
242. Pozzoli G, Bilezikjian L, Perrin M, et al. Corticotropin-releasing factor (CRF) and glucocorticoids modulate the expression of type I CRF receptor messenger ribonucleic acid in rat anterior pituitary cell cultures. Endocrinology 137:65, 1995.
243. Luo X, Kiss A, Rabadan-Diehl C, et al. Regulation of hypothalamic and pituitary corticotropin-releasing hormone receptor messenger ribonucleic acid by adrenalectomy and glucocorticoids. Endocrinology 136:3877, 1995.
244. Makino S, Schulkin J, Smith MA, et al. Regulation of corticotropin-releasing hormone receptor messenger ribonucleic acid in the rat brain and pituitary by glucocorticoids and stress. Endocrinology 136:4517, 1995.
245. Aubry JM, Turnbull AV, Pozzoli G, et al. Endotoxin decreases corticotropin-releasing factor receptor 1 messenger ribonucleic acid levels in the rat pituitary. Endocrinology 138:1621, 1997.
246. Makino S, Takemura T, Asaba K, et al. Differential regulation of type-1 and type-2alpha corticotropin-releasing hormone receptor mRNA in the hypothalamic paraventricular nucleus of the rat. Brain Res Mol Brain Res 47:170, 1997.
247. Behan DP, DeSouza EB, Lowry PJ, et al. Corticotropin-releasing factor (CRF) binding protein: A novel regulator of CRF and related peptides. Front Neuroendocrinol 16:362, 1995.
248. Potter E, Behan DP, Fischer WH, et al. Cloning and characterization of the cDNAs for human and rat corticotropin-releasing factor–binding proteins. Nature 349:423, 1991.
249. McLean M, Bisits A, Davies J, et al. A placental clock controlling the length of human pregnancy. Nat Med 1:460, 1995.
250. Behan DP, Heinrichs SC, Troncoso JC, et al. Displacement of corticotropin-releasing factor from its binding protein as a possible treatment for Alzheimer's disease. Nature 378:284, 1995.

251. Vaughan J, Donaldson C, Bittencourt J, et al. Urocortin, a mammalian neuropeptide related to fish urotensin I and to corticotropin-releasing factor. Nature 378:287, 1995.
252. Spina M, Merlo-Pich E, Chan RK, et al. Appetite-suppressing effects of urocortin, a CRF-related neuropeptide. Science 273:1561, 1996.
253. Wong ML, al-Shekhlee A, Bongiorno PB, et al. Localization of urocortin messenger RNA in rat brain and pituitary. Mol Psychiatry 1:307, 1996.
254. Iino K, Sasano H, Oki Y, et al. Urocortin expression in human pituitary gland and pituitary adenoma. J Clin Endocrinol Metab 82:3842, 1997.
255. Petraglia F, Florio P, Gallo R, et al. Human placenta and fetal membranes express human urocortin mRNA and peptide. J Clin Endocrinol Metab 81:3807, 1996.
256. Behan DP, Khongsaly O, Ling N, et al. Urocortin interaction with corticotropin-releasing factor (CRF) binding protein (CRF-BP): A novel mechanism for elevating 'free' CRF levels in human brain. Brain Res 725:263, 1996.
257. Chrousos GP, Gold PW. The concepts of stress and stress system disorders: Overview of physical and behavioral homeostasis. JAMA 267:1244, 1992.
258. Saper CB, Lowey AD, Swanson LW, et al. Direct hypothalamo-autonomic connections. Brain Res 117:305, 1976.
259. Chrousos GP. The hypothalamic-pituitary-adrenal axis and immune-mediated inflammation. N Engl J Med 332:1351, 1995.
260. Gold PW, Gwirtsman H, Avgerinos PC, et al. Abnormal hypothalamic-pituitary-adrenal function in anorexia nervosa. Pathophysiologic mechanisms in underweight and weight-corrected patients. N Engl J Med 314:1335, 1986.
261. Linkowski P, Mendlewicz J, Leclercq R, et al. The 24-hour profile of adrenocorticotropin and cortisol in major depressive illness. J Clin Endocrinol Metab 61:429, 1985.
262. Suh BY, Liu JH, Berga S, et al. Hypercortisolism in patients with functional hypothalamic-amenorrhea. J Clin Endocrinol Metab 66:733, 1988.
263. Berga SL, Mortola JF, Girton L, et al. Neuroendocrine aberrations in women with functional hypothalamic amenorrhea. J Clin Endocrinol Metab 68:301, 1989.
264. Laughlin GA, Dominguez DE, Yen SSC. Nutritional and endocrine-metabolic aberrations in women with functional hypothalamic amenorrhea. J Clin Endocrinol Metab 83:25, 1998.
265. Biller BM, Federoff HJ, Koenig JI, et al. Abnormal cortisol secretion and responses to corticotropin-releasing hormone in women with hypothalamic amenorrhea. J Clin Endocrinol Metab 70:311, 1990.
266. Loucks AB, Mortola JF, Girton L, et al. Alterations in the hypothalamic-pituitary-ovarian and the hypothalamic-pituitary-adrenal axes in athletic women. J Clin Endocrinol Metab 68:402, 1989.
267. Laughlin GA, Yen SSC. Nutritional and endocrine-metabolic aberrations in amenorrheic athletes. J Clin Endocrinol Metab 81:4301, 1996.
268. Gold PW, Loriaux DL, Roy A, et al. Responses to corticotropin-releasing hormone in the hypercortisolism of depression and Cushing's disease. Pathophysiologic and diagnostic implications. N Engl J Med 314:1329, 1986.
269. Kaye WH, Gwirtsman H, George DT, et al. Elevated cerebrospinal fluid levels of immunoreactive corticotropin-releasing hormone in anorexia nervosa: Relation to state of nutrition, adrenal function, and intensity of depression. J Clin Endocrinol Metab 64:203, 1987.
270. Nemeroff CB. The role of corticotropin-releasing factor in the pathogenesis of major depression. Pharmacopsychiatry 21:76, 1988.
271. Xiao E, Luckhaus J, Niemann W, et al. Acute inhibition of gonadotropin secretion by corticotropin-releasing hormone in the primate: Are the adrenal glands involved? Endocrinology 124:1632, 1989.
272. Petraglia F, Sutton S, Vale W, et al. Corticotropin-releasing factor decreases plasma luteinizing hormone levels in female rats by inhibiting gonadotropin-releasing hormone release into hypophysial-portal circulation. Endocrinology 120:1083, 1987.
273. Gambacciani M, Yen SSC, Rasmussen DD. GnRH release from the mediobasal hypothalamus: In vitro inhibition by corticotropin releasing factor. Neuroendocrinology 43:533, 1986.
274. Blalock JE. A molecular basis for bidirectional communication between the immune and neuroendocrine systems. Physiol Rev 69:1, 1989.
275. Karalis K, Sano H, Redwine J, et al. Autocrine or paracrine inflammatory actions of corticotropin-releasing hormone in vivo. Science 254:421, 1991.
276. Aird F, Clevenger CV, Prystowsky MB, et al. Corticotropin-releasing factor mRNA in rat thymus and spleen. Proc Natl Acad Sci USA 90:7104, 1993.
277. Webster EL, Elenkov IJ, Chrousos GP. The role of corticotropin-releasing hormone in neuroendocrine-immune interactions. Mol Psychiatry 2:368, 1997.
278. Stephanou A, Jessop DS, Knight RA, et al. Corticotrophin-releasing factor–like immunoreactivity and mRNA in human leukocytes. Brain Behav Immun 4:67, 1990.
279. Woods RJ, Grossman A, Saphier P, et al. Association of human corticotropin-releasing hormone to its binding protein in blood may trigger clearance of the complex. J Clin Endocrinol Metab 78:73, 1994.
280. Mastorakos G, Weber JS, Magiakou MA, et al. Hypothalamic-pituitary-adrenal axis activation and stimulation of systemic vasopressin secretion by recombinant interleukin-6 in humans: Potential implications for the syndrome of inappropriate vasopressin secretion. J Clin Endocrinol Metab 79:934, 1994.
281. Farrar WL, Hill JM, Harel-Belland A, et al. The immune logical brain. Immunol Rev 100:361, 1987.
282. Breder CD, Binarello CA, Saper CB. Interleukin-1 immunoreactive innervation of the human hypothalamus. Science 240:321, 1988.
283. Martin JB. Interleukin-1 directly stimulates the release of corticotropin releasing factor from rat hypothalamus. *In* Martini L, Ganong WF (eds). Frontiers in Neuroendocrinology. New York, Raven Press, 1976, p 129.
284. Berkenbosch F, van Oers J, del Rey A, et al. Corticotropin releasing factor producing neurons in the rat activated by interleukin-1. Science 238:524, 1987.
285. Sapolsky RM, Rivier C, Yamamoto G, et al. Interleukin-1 stimulates the secretion of hypothalamic corticotropin releasing factor. Science 238:522, 1987.
286. Tsagarakis S, Gillies G, Rees LH, et al. Interleukin-1 directly stimulates the release of corticotropin releasing factor from rat hypothalamus. Neuroendocrinology 49:98, 1989.
287. Imura H, Fukata J, Mori T. Cytokines and endocrine function: An interaction between the immune and neuroendocrine systems. Clin Endocrinol (Oxf) 35:107, 1991.
288. Van Cauter E, Leproult R, Kupfer DJ. Effects of gender and age on the levels of circadian rhythmicity of plasma cortisol. J Clin Endocrinol Metab 81:2468, 1996.
289. Givalois L, Li S, Pelletier G. Age-related decrease in the hypothalamic CRH mRNA expression is reduced by dehydroepiandrosterone (DHEA) treatment in male and female rats. Mol Brain Res 48:107, 1997.
290. Khorram OA, Vu L, Yen SSC. Activation of immune function by dehydroepiandrosterone (DHEA) in age advanced men. J Gerontol 52A:M1, 1997.
291. Meany MJ, Aitken DH, Sharma S, et al. Basal ACTH, corticosterone and corticosterone binding globulin levels over diurnal cycle and hippocampal type I and type II corticosteroid receptors in young and old handled and nonhandled rats. Neuroendocrinology 55:204, 1992.
292. Finkelstein JW, Roffwarg HP, Boyar RM, et al. Age-related change in the twenty-four-hour spontaneous secretion of growth hormone. J Clin Endocrinol Metab 35:665, 1972.
293. Miller JD, Tannenbaum GS, Colle E, et al. Daytime pulsatile growth hormone secretion during childhood and adolescence. J Clin Endocrinol Metab 55:989, 1982.
294. Dawson-Hughes B, Stern D, Goldman J, et al. Regulation of growth hormone and somatomedin-C secretion in postmenopausal women: Effect of estrogen therapy. J Clin Endocrinol Metab 63:424, 1986.
295. Huseman CA, Hassing JM. Evidence for dopaminergic stimulation of growth velocity in some hypopituitary children. J Clin Endocrinol Metab 58:419, 1984.
296. Chikara K, Minamitani N, Kaji H, et al. Noradrenergic modulation of human pancreatic growth hormone releasing factor [hpGHRF(1–44)]–induced growth hormone release in conscious

male rabbits: Involvement of endogenous somatostatin. Endocrinology 114:1402, 1984.

297. Golstein J, Cauter EV, Desir D, et al. Effects of "jet lag" on hormonal patterns. IV. Time shifts increase growth hormone release. J Clin Endocrinol Metab 56:433, 1983.
298. Salomon F, Cuneo RC, Hesp R, et al. The effects of treatment with recombinant human growth hormone on body composition and metabolism in adults with growth hormone deficiency. N Engl J Med 321:1797, 1989.
299. Daughaday WH, Rotwein P. Insulin-like growth factor I and II: Peptide, messenger ribonucleic acid and gene structures, serum, and tissue concentrations. Endocr Rev 10:68, 1989.
300. Miller WL, Eberhardt NL. Structure and evaluation of growth hormone gene family. Endocr Rev 4:97, 1983.
301. Chen EY, Yu-Cheng L, Smith DH, et al. The human growth hormone locus: Nucleotide sequence, biology, and evolution. Genomics 4:479, 1989.
302. Smith RG, Van der Ploeg LHT, Howard AD, et al. Peptidomimetic regulation of growth hormone secretion. Endocr Rev 18:621, 1997.
303. Chapman IM, Bach MA, Van Cauter E, et al. Stimulation of the growth hormone (GH)–insulin-like growth factor I axis by daily oral administration of a GH secretogogue (MK-677) in healthy elderly subjects. J Clin Endocrinol Metab 81:4249, 1996.
304. Berelowitz M, Szabo M, Frohman LA, et al. Somatomedin-C mediates growth hormone negative feedback by effects on both the hypothalamus and the pituitary. Science 212:1279, 1981.
305. Tannenbaum GS, Guyda HJ, Posner BI. Insulin-like growth factors: A role in growth hormone negative feedback and body weight regulation via brain. Science 220:77, 1983.
306. Liposits Z, Merchenthaler I, Paull WK, et al. Synaptic communication between somatostatinergic axons and growth hormone–releasing factor (GRF) synthesizing neurons in the arcuate nucleus of the rat. Histochemistry 89:247, 1988.
307. Guillemin R, Brazeau P, Bohlen P. Somatocrinin, the growth hormone releasing factor. Recent Prog Horm Res 40:233, 1984.
308. Lin HD, Bollinger J, Ling N, et al. Immunoreactive growth hormone–releasing factor in human stalk median eminence. J Clin Endocrinol Metab 58:1197, 1984.
309. Wehrenberg WB, Ling N, Bohlen P, et al. Physiological roles of somatocrinin and somatostatin in the regulation of growth hormone secretion. Biochem Biophys Res Commun 109:562, 1982.
310. Martin JB. Functions of central nervous system neurotransmitters in regulation of growth hormone secretion. Fed Proc 39:2902, 1980.
311. Vance ML, Kaiser DL, Evans WS, et al. Pulsatile growth hormone secretion in normal man during a continuous 24-hour infusion of human growth hormone releasing factor (1–40). J Clin Invest 75:1584, 1985.
312. Brain CE, Hindmarsh PC, Brook CGD. Continuous subcutaneous GHRH(1–29)NH_2 promotes growth over 1 year in short, slowly growing children. Clin Endocrinol 32:153, 1990.
313. Thorner MO, Frohman DA, Leong J, et al. Extrahypothalamic growth-hormone releasing factor (GRF) secretion is a rare cause of acromegaly: Plasma GRF levels in 177 acromegalic patients. J Clin Endocrinol Metab 59:846, 1984.
314. Mayo KE, Cerelli GM, Lebo RV, et al. Gene encoding human growth hormone–releasing factor precursor: Structure, sequence, and chromosomal assignment. Proc Natl Acad Sci USA 82:63, 1985.
315. Patel YC. Growth hormone stimulates hypothalamic somatostatin. Life Sci 24:1589, 1979.
316. Chomczynski P, Downs TR, Frohman LA. Feedback regulation of growth hormone (GH)–releasing hormone gene expression by GH in rat hypothalamus. Mol Endocrinol 2:236, 1988.
317. Reichlin S. Somatostatin: Basic and Clinical Status. New York, Plenum Publishing, 1987.
318. Lamberts SWJ. The role of somatostatin in the regulation of anterior pituitary hormone secretion and the use of its analogs in the treatment of human pituitary tumors. Endocr Rev 9:417, 1988.
319. Vance ML, Kaiser DL, Martha PM Jr, et al. Lack of in vivo somatotroph desensitization or depletion after 14 days of continuous growth hormone (GH)–releasing hormone administration in normal men and a GH-deficient boy. J Clin Endocrinol Metab 68:22, 1989.
320. Brazeau P, Vale W, Burgur R, et al. Hypothalamic polypeptide that inhibits the secretion of immunoreactive growth hormone. Science 179:77, 1973.
321. Toni R, Jackson IMD, Lechan RM. Neuropeptide Y–immunoreactive innervation of thyrotropin-releasing hormone synthesizing neurons in the rat hypothalamic paraventricular nucleus. Endocrinology 126:2444, 1990.
322. Engel WK, Siddique T, Nicoloff JT. Effect on weakness and spasticity in amyotrophic lateral sclerosis of thyrotropin-releasing hormone. Lancet 2:73, 1983.
323. Metcalf G, Jackson IMD. Thyrotropin-releasing hormone: Biomedical significance. Ann N Y Acad Sci 553:1, 1989.
324. Yamada M, Wondisford FE, Radovick S, et al. Assignment of human preprothyrotropin releasing hormone (TRH) gene to chromosome 3. Somat Cell Mol Genet 17:97, 1991.
325. Lee SL, Sevarino K, Roos BA, et al. Characterization and expression of the gene-encoding rat thyrotropin-releasing hormone (TRH). Ann N Y Acad Sci 553:14, 1989.
326. Segerson TP, Kauer J, Wolfe HC, et al. Thyroid hormone regulates TRH biosynthesis in the paraventricular nucleus of the rat hypothalamus. Science 238:78, 1987.
327. Dyess EM, Sergerson TP, Liposits Z, et al. Triiodothyronine exerts direct cell-specific regulation of thyrotropin-releasing hormone gene expression in the hypothalamic paraventricular nucleus. Endocrinology 123:2291, 1988.
328. Gershengorn MC. Mechanism of signal transduction by TRH. Ann N Y Acad Sci 53:191, 1989.
329. Weintraub BD, Gesundheit N, Taylor T, et al. Effect of TRH on TSH glycosylation and biological action. Ann N Y Acad Sci 553:205, 1989.
330. du Vigneaud V. Hormones of the posterior pituitary gland: Oxytocin and vasopressin. Harvey Lect 50:1, 1956.
331. Brownstein MJ, Russell JT, Gainer H. Synthesis, transport, and release of posterior pituitary hormones. Science 207:373, 1980.
332. Land H, Schutz G, Schmale H, et al. Nucleotide sequence of cloned cDNA encoding bovine arginine vasopressin–neurophysin II precursor. Nature 295:299, 1982.
333. Verbalis JG, Robinson AG. Characterization of neurophysin-vasopressin prohormones in human posterior pituitary tissue. J Clin Endocrinol Metab 57:115, 1983.
334. Crowley WR, Armstrong WE. Neurochemical regulation of oxytocin secretion in lactation. Endocr Rev 13:33, 1992.
335. Scheffer JM, Liu J, Hsueh AJW, et al. The presence of neurohypophyseal hormones in human oviduct, ovary and follicular fluid. J Clin Endocrinol Metab 59:970, 1984.
336. Tan GJS, Tweedale R, Biggs JSG. Oxytocin may play a role in the control of human corpus luteum. Endocrinology 95:65, 1982.
337. Ivell R, Richter D. The gene for the hypothalamic peptide hormone oxytocin is highly expressed in the bovine corpus luteum: Biosynthesis, structure and sequence analysis. EMBO J 3:2351, 1984.
338. Adashi EY, Hsueh AJW. Direct inhibition of testicular androgen biosynthesis revealing antigonadal activity of neurohypophysial hormones. Nature 293:650, 1981.
339. Phillips HS, Hains J, Leung DW, et al. Vascular endothelial growth factor is expressed in rat corpus luteum. Endocrinology 127:965, 1990.
340. Poulain DA, Wakerley JB. Electrophysiology of hypothalamic magnocellular neurones secreting oxytocin and vasopressin. Neuroscience 7:773, 1982.
341. Husain MK, Frantz AG, Ciarochi F, et al. Nicotine-stimulated release of neurophysin and vasopressin in humans. J Clin Endocrinol Metab 41:1113, 1975.
342. Jijima K, Ogawa T. An HRP study on cell types and their regional topography within the locus coeruleus innervating the supraoptic nucleus of the rat. Acta Histochem 67:127, 1980.
343. Clarke G, Wood P, Merrick L, et al. Opiate inhibition of peptide release from the neurohumoral terminals of hypothalamic neurones. Nature 282:746, 1979.
344. Watson SJ, Akil H, Chazarossian VE, et al. Dynorphin immunocytochemical localization in brain and peripheral nervous system: Preliminary studies. Proc Natl Acad Sci USA 78:1260, 1981.
345. Bicknell RJ, Leng G. Endogenous opiates regulate oxytocin but not vasopressin secretion from the neurohypophysis. Nature 298:161, 1982.

346. Bondy CA, Gainer H, Russell JT. Dynorphin A inhibits and naloxone increases the electrically stimulated release of oxytocin but not vasopressin from the terminals of the neural lobe. Endocrinology 122:1321, 1988.
347. Zamir N, Zamir D, Eiden LE, et al. Methionine and leucine enkephalin in rat neurohypophysis: Different responses to osmotic stimuli and T2 toxin. Science 228:606, 1985.
348. Summy-Long JY, Rosella-Dampman LM, McLemore GL, et al. Kappa opiate receptors inhibit release of oxytocin from the magnocellular system during dehydration. Neuroendocrinology 51:376, 1990.
349. Sawchenko PE, Plotsky P, Pfeiffer SW, et al. Inhibin β in central neural pathways involved in the control of oxytocin secretion. Nature 334:615, 1988.
350. Johnson AE, Coirini H, Ball GF, et al. Anatomical localization of the effects of 17β-estradiol on oxytocin receptor binding in the ventromedial hypothalamic nucleus. Endocrinology 124:207, 1989.
351. Amico JA, Hempel J. An oxytocin precursor intermediate circulates in the plasma of humans and rhesus monkeys administered estrogen. Neuroendocrinology 51:437, 1990.
352. Shukovski L, Healy DL, Findlay JK. Circulating immunoreactive oxytocin during the human menstrual cycle comes from the pituitary and is estradiol dependent. J Clin Endocrinol Metab 68:455, 1989.
353. Shoji M, Share L, Crofton JT. Effect on vasopressin release of microinjection of angiotensin II into the paraventricular nucleus of conscious rats. Neuroendocrinology 50:327, 1989.
354. Miselis RR, Shapiro RE, Hand PJ. Subfornical organ efferents to neural systems for control of body water. Science 205:1022, 1979.
355. Ramsay DJ, Ganong WF. Regulation of salt and water intake. *In* Krieger DT, Hughes JC (eds). Neuroendocrinology. Sunderland, MA, Sinauer Associates, 1980, p 123.
356. Beinfeld MC, Meyer DK, Brownstein MJ. Cholecystokinin octapeptide in the rat hypothalamo-neurohypophysial system. Nature 288:376, 1980.
357. Rowe JW, Shelton RL, Helderman JH, et al. Influence of the emetic reflex on vasopressin release in man. Kidney Int 16:729, 1979.
358. Miaskiewicz SL, Stricker EM, Verbalis JG. Neurohypophyseal secretion in response to cholecystokinin but not meal-induced gastric distention in humans. J Clin Endocrinol Metab 68:837, 1989.
359. Weitzman RE, Firemark HM, Glatz TH, et al. Thyrotropin-releasing hormone stimulates release of arginine vasopressin and oxytocin in vivo. Endocrinology 104:904, 1979.
360. Thibonnier M, Bayer AL, Leng Z. Cytoplasmic and nuclear signaling pathways of V1–vascular vasopressin receptors. Regul Pept 45:79, 1993.
361. Thibonnier M, Preston JA, Dulin N, et al. The human V_3 pituitary vasopressin receptor: Ligand binding profile and density-dependent signaling pathways. Endocrinology 138:4109, 1997.
362. Miller M, Moses AM. Clinical states due to alteration of ADH release and action. *In* Moses AM, Share L (eds). Neurohypophysis. Basel, S Karger, 1977, p 153.
363. Dunn FL, Brennan TJ, Nelson AE, et al. The role of blood osmolality and volume in regulating vasopressin secretion in the rat. J Clin Invest 52:3212, 1973.
364. Jougasaki M, Wei CM, Aarhus LL, et al. Renal localization and actions of adrenomedullin: A natriuretic peptide. Am J Physiol 268:F657, 1995.
365. Clinkingbeard C, Sessions C, Shenker Y. The physiological role of atrial natriuretic hormone in the regulation of aldosterone and salt and water metabolism. J Clin Endocrinol Metab 70:582, 1990.
366. Liu JH, Muse K, Contreras P, et al. Augmentation of ACTH-releasing activity of synthetic corticotropin releasing factor (CRF) by vasopressin in women. J Clin Endocrinol Metab 57:1087, 1983.
367. Kimura T, Tanizawa O, Mori K, et al. Structure and expression of a human oxytocin receptor. Nature 356:526, 1992.
368. Fisher DA. Maternal-fetal neurohypophyseal system. Clin Perinatol 10:695, 1983.
369. Fuchs AR, Fuchs F, Husslein P, et al. Oxytocin receptors and human parturition: A dual role for oxytocin in the initiation of labor. Science 215:1396, 1983.
370. McNeilly AS, Robinson ICAF, Houston MJ, et al. Release of oxytocin and prolactin in response to suckling. Br Med J 286:257, 1983.
371. Murphy MR, Seckl JR, Burton S, et al. Changes in oxytocin and vasopressin secretion during sexual activity in men. J Clin Endocrinol Metab 65:738, 1987.
372. Carmichael MS, Humbert R, Dixen J, et al. Plasma oxytocin increases in the human sexual response. J Clin Endocrinol Metab 64:27, 1987.
373. de Wied D, Gaffori O, van Ree JM, et al. Central target for the behavioural effects of vasopressin neuropeptides. Nature 308:276, 1984.
374. Weingartner H, Gold P, Ballenger JC, et al. Effects of vasopressin on human memory functions. Science 211:601, 1981.
375. Ferrier BM, Kennett DJ, Devlin MC. Influence of oxytocin on human memory processes. Life Sci 27:2311, 1980.
376. Pedersen CA, Ascher JA, Monroe YL, et al. Oxytocin induces maternal behavior in virgin female rats. Science 216:648, 1982.
377. Moses AM. Diabetes insipidus and ADH regulation. *In* Krieger DT, Hughes JC (eds). Neuroendocrinology. Sunderland, MA, Sinauer Associates, 1980, p 149.
378. Roenneberg T, Aschoff J. Annual rhythm of human reproduction: I. Biology, sociology, or both. J Biol Rhythms 5:195, 1990.
379. Roenneberg T, Aschoff J. Annual rhythm of human reproduction: II. Environmental correlations. J Biol Rhythms 5:217, 1990.
380. Bronson FH. Seasonal variation in human reproduction: Environmental factors. Q Rev Biol 70:141, 1995.
381. Rojansky N, Brzezinski A, Schenker JG. Seasonality in human reproduction: An update. Hum Reprod 7:735, 1992.
382. Levine RJ. Male factors contributing to the seasonality of human reproduction. Ann N Y Acad Sci 709:29, 1994.
383. Wehr TA, Giesen HA, Moul DE, et al. Suppression of human responses to seasonal changes in day-length by modern artificial lighting. Am J Physiol 269:R173, 1995.
384. Gwinner E. Circannual Rhythms. New York, Springer-Verlag, 1986.
385. Wehr TA. Melatonin and seasonal rhythms. J Biol Rhythms 12:518, 1997.
386. Wurtman RJ, Axelrod J, Phillips LS. Melatonin synthesis in the pineal gland: Control by light. Science 142:1071, 1963.
387. Arendt J. Melatonin. Clin Endocrinol (Oxf) 29:205, 1988.
388. Cagnacci A. Melatonin in relation to physiology in adult humans. J Pineal Res 21:200, 1996.
389. Brzezinski A. Melatonin in humans. N Engl J Med 336:186, 1997.
390. Cagnacci A, Elliott JA, Yen SSC. Melatonin: A major regulator of the circadian rhythm of core temperature in humans. J Clin Endocrinol Metab 75:447, 1992.
391. Axelrod J. The pineal gland: A neurochemical transducer. Science 184:1341, 1974.
392. Tamarkin L, Baird CJ, Almeida OFX. Melatonin: A coordinating signal for mammalian reproduction? Science 227:714, 1985.
393. Pangerl B, Pangerl A, Reiter RJ. Circadian variations of adrenergic receptors in the mammalian pineal gland: A review. J Neural Transm 81:17, 1990.
394. Romero JA, Zatz M, Kebabian JW, et al. Circadian cycles in binding of ^{3}H-alprenolol receptor sites in rat pineal. Nature 258:435, 1975.
395. Gonzalez-Brito A, Jones DJ, Ademe RM, et al. Characterization and measurement of [125]iodopindolol binding in individual rat pineal glands: Existence of a 24-hour-rhythm in β-adrenergic receptor density. Brain Res 438:108, 1988.
396. Pangerl A, Pangerl B, Reiter RJ, et al. Twenty-four-hour variation of α_1-adrenergic receptors in the pineal gland of the male Syrian hamster. Brain Res 490:166, 1989.
397. Romero JA, Axelrod J. Pineal β-adrenergic receptor: Diurnal variations in sensitivity. Science 184:1091, 1974.
398. Klein DC, Sugden D, Weller JL. Postsynaptic α-adrenergic receptors potentiate the β-adrenergic stimulation of pineal serotonin *N*-acetyltransferase. Proc Natl Acad Sci USA 80:599, 1983.
399. Palazidou E, Franey C, Arendt J, et al. Evidence for a functional role of alpha-1 adrenoceptors in the regulation of melatonin secretion in man. Psychoneuroendocrinology 14:131, 1989.
400. Thompson C, Stinson D, Smith A. Seasonal affective disorder and season-dependent abnormalities of melatonin suppression by light. Lancet 336:703, 1990.
401. Tosini G, Menaker M. Circadian rhythms in cultured mammalian retina. Science 272:419, 1996.

402. Campbell SS, Murphy PJ. Extraocular circadian phototransduction in humans. Science 279:396, 1998.
403. Waldhauser F, Weiszenbacher G, Tatzer E, et al. Alterations in nocturnal serum melatonin levels in humans with growth and aging. J Clin Endocrinol Metab 66:648, 1988.
404. Kivelä A, Kauppila A, Leppäluoto J, et al. Melatonin in infants and mothers at delivery and in infants during the first week of life. Clin Endocrinol (Oxf) 32:593, 1990.
405. Wilson ME, Gordon TP. Nocturnal changes in serum melatonin during female puberty in rhesus monkeys: A longitudinal study. J Endocrinol 121:553, 1989.
406. Ehrenkranz JRL, Tamarkin L, Comite F, et al. Daily rhythm of plasma melatonin in normal and precocious puberty. J Clin Endocrinol Metab 55:307, 1982.
407. Berga SL, Jones KL, Kaufmann S, et al. Nocturnal melatonin levels are unaltered by ovarian suppression in girls with central precocious puberty. Fertil Steril 52:936, 1989.
408. Iguchi H, Kato K, Ibayashi H. Age dependent reduction in serum melatonin concentration in healthy human subjects. J Clin Endocrinol Metab 55:27, 1982.
409. Berga SL, Yen SSC. Circadian pattern of plasma melatonin concentrations during four phases of the human menstrual cycle. Neuroendocrinology 51:606, 1990.
410. Brzezinski A, Lynch HJ, Seibel MM, et al. The circadian rhythm of plasma melatonin during the normal menstrual cycle and in amenorrheic women. J Clin Endocrinol Metab 66:891, 1988.
411. Luboshitzky R, Dharan M, Goldman D, et al. Immunohistochemical localization of gonadotropin and gonadal steroid receptors in human pineal glands. J Clin Endocrinol Metab 82:977, 1997.
412. Brzezinski A, Seibel MM, Lynch HJ, et al. Melatonin in human preovulatory follicular fluid. J Clin Endocrinol Metab 64:865, 1987.
413. Rönnberg L, Kauppila A, Leppäluoto J, et al. Circadian and seasonal variation in human preovulatory follicular fluid melatonin concentration. J Clin Endocrinol Metab 71:493, 1990.
414. Kauppila A, Kivelä A, Pakarinen A, et al. Inverse seasonal relationship between melatonin and ovarian activity in humans in a region with a strong seasonal contrast in luminosity. J Clin Endocrinol Metab 65:823, 1987.
415. Webley GE, Luck MR. Melatonin directly stimulates the secretion of progesterone by human and bovine granulosa cells. J Reprod Fertil 78:711, 1986.
416. McIntyre IM, Norman TR, Burrows GD, et al. Human melatonin suppression by light is intensity dependent. J Pineal Res 6:149, 1989.
417. Cagnacci A, Soldani R, Yen SSC. The effect of light on core body temperature is mediated by melatonin in women. J Clin Endocrinol Metab 76:1036, 1993.
418. Arendt J, Skene DJ, Middleton B, et al. Efficacy of melatonin treatment in jet lag, shift work, and blindness. J Biol Rhythms 12:604, 1997.
419. Reppert SM. Melatonin receptors: Molecular biology of a new family of G protein–coupled receptors. J Biol Rhythms 12:528, 1997.
420. Cassone VM, Roberts MH, Moore RY. Melatonin inhibits metabolic activity in the rat suprachiasmatic nuclei. Neurosci Lett 81:29, 1987.
421. Bispink G, Zimmermann R, Weise HC, et al. Influence of melatonin on the sleep-independent component of prolactin secretion. J Pineal Res 8:97, 1990.
422. James SP, Mendelson WB, Sack DA, et al. The effect of melatonin on normal sleep. Neuropsychopharmacology 1:41, 1987.
423. Waldhauser F, Saletu B, Trinchard-Lugan I. Sleep laboratory investigations on hypnotic properties of melatonin. Psychopharmacology 100:222, 1990.
424. Arendt J, Aldhous M, Marks M, et al. Some effects of jetlag and its treatment by melatonin. Ergonomics 30:1379, 1987.
425. Lamberts SWJ, van den Beld AW, van der Lely A-J. The endocrinology of aging. Science 278:419, 1997.
426. Coevorden AV, Mockel J, Laurent E, et al. Neuroendocrine rhythms and sleep in aging men. Am Physiol Soc 260:E651, 1991.
427. Yen SSC. Estrogen withdrawal syndrome (Editorial). JAMA 255:1614, 1986.
428. Wise PH, Kashon ML, Krajnak KM, et al. Aging of the female reproductive systems: A window into brain aging. Recent Prog Horm Res 52:279, 1997.
429. Herman SM, Panayiotis D, Tsitouk AS, et al. Reproductive hormone in aging men. J Clin Endocrinol Metab 54:547, 1982.
430. Ravaglia G, Forti P, Maioli F, et al. The relationship of dehydroepiandrosterone sulfate (DHEAS) to endocrine-metabolic parameters and functional status in the oldest-old. Results from an Italian study on healthy free-living over-ninety-year-olds. J Clin Endocrinol Metab 81:1173, 1996.
431. Labrie F, Belanger A, Cusan L, et al. Marked decline in serum concentrations of adrenal C19 sex steroid precursors and conjugated androgen metabolites during aging. J Clin Endocrinol Metab 82:2396, 1997.
432. Parker CR Jr, Mixon RL, Brissie RM, et al. Aging alters zonation in the adrenal cortex of men. J Clin Endocrinol Metab 82:3898, 1997.
433. Wilkinson CW, Peskind ER, Raskind MA. Decreased hypothalamic-pituitary-adrenal axis sensitivity to cortisol feedback inhibition in human aging. Neuroendocrinology 65:79, 1997.
434. McEwen BS, Sapolsky RM. Stress and cognitive function. Curr Opin Neurobiol 5:205, 1995.
435. Seeman TE, McEwen BS, Singer BH, et al. Increase in urinary cortisol excretion and memory declines: MacArthur studies of successful aging. J Clin Endocrinol Metab 82:2458, 1997.
436. Guazzo EP, Kirkpatrick PJ, Goodyer IM, et al. Cortisol, dehydroepiandrosterone (DHEA), and DHEA sulfate in the cerebrospinal fluid of man: Relation to blood levels and the effects of age. J Clin Endocrinol Metab 81:3951, 1996.
437. Corpas E, Harman SM, Blackman MR. Human growth hormone and human aging. Endocr Rev 14:20, 1993.
438. Hesse V, Jahreis G, Schambach H, et al. Insulin-like growth factor-I correlation to changes of the hormonal status in puberty and age. Exp Clin Endocrinol 102:289, 1994.
439. Rudman D, Feller AG, Nagraj HS, et al. Effects of human growth hormone in men over 60 years old. N Engl J Med 323:1, 1990.
440. Holloway L, Butterfield G, Hintz RL, et al. Effects of recombinant human growth hormone on metabolic indices, body composition and bone turnover in healthy elderly women. J Clin Endocrinol Metab 79:470, 1994.
441. Thompson JL, Butterfield GE, Marcus R, et al. The effects of recombinant human insulin-like growth factor-I and growth hormone on body composition in elderly women. J Clin Endocrinol Metab 80:1845, 1995.
442. Cagnacci A, Soldani R, Yen SSC. Hypothermic effect of melatonin and nocturnal core body temperature decline are reduced in aged women. J Appl Physiol 78:314, 1995.

GONADOTROPIC HORMONES: Biosynthesis, Secretion, Receptors, and Action

Lisa M. Halvorson • William W. Chin

CHAPTER OUTLINE

KEY POINTS

- LH, acting initially on the theca cells, promotes androgen production to supply substrate for aromatization to estrogen; FSH is important for early granulosa cell maturation, including the development of LH/CG receptors.
- The anterior pituitary cell types responsible for the synthesis and secretion of LH and FSH are the gonadotropes.
- LH and FSH are composed of two different, noncovalently associated, carbohydrate-containing protein subunits called α and β.
- In the gonadotrope, the subunit genes are transcribed into mRNAs, which are in turn translated into the subunit precursors.
- The biosynthesis of the gonadotropin subunits proceeds by translation of the subunit mRNAs, post-translational modifications of the precursor subunits and subunit folding and combination, mature hormone packaging, and hormone secretion.
- Gonadotropin expression is modulated by hypothalamic factors (primarily GnRH), intrapituitary factors (primarily the peptides activin and follistatin), and gonadal feedback (both steroidal and peptide).
- The gonadotropin hormone receptors are members of the G protein–coupled receptor superfamily.
- Abnormal reproductive function due to alterations in gonadotropin expression and/or its action could be caused by activating or inactivating mutations of genes important in the hypothalamic-gonadotrope-gonadal axis.
- Abnormal synthesis and secretion of the gonadotropins occur in a variety of neoplasms.

The pituitary gonadotropins, luteinizing hormone (lutropin; LH) and follicle-stimulating hormone (follitropin; FSH), are critical for the regulation of gonadal function and reproduction in humans, subhuman primates, and other mammalian species. These hormones are released in a well-orchestrated manner, under the control of numerous factors including hypothalamic gonadotropin-releasing hormone (GnRH), and bind to specific, high-affinity receptors in the ovary and testis to regulate gametogenesis and sex steroid synthesis and secretion. LH acts on the Leydig cells of the testis and the theca cells of the ovary to regulate local and peripheral concentrations of the gonadal steroid hormones that are crucial for normal sexual development and reproductive function. In the ovary, LH is essential for ovulation by causing rupture of the preovulatory follicle and release of the ovum. FSH acts on the granulosa cells of the ovary and the Sertoli cells of the testis to promote germ cell development in these gonadal tissues.

PITUITARY GONADOTROPES

The anterior pituitary cell types responsible for the synthesis and secretion of LH and FSH are known as gonadotropes and first appear in the anterior pituitary gland during early fetal development. Other major anterior pituitary cell types include thyrotropes, corticotropes, somatotropes, and lactotropes that produce and secrete thyrotropin (TSH), adrenocorticotropin, growth hormone, and prolactin, respectively. Gonadotropes represent 7 to 15 percent of the total number of anterior pituitary cells.[3]

These pituitary cells, including gonadotropes, have been studied extensively by use of light and electron microscopy employing antisera specific for the intact hormones or their subunits. Gonadotropes are distinctive in structure and resemble the thyrotropes, the cell type that produces TSH. LH, FSH, and TSH are structurally related and belong to the family of glycoprotein hormones (Fig. 3–1). Inasmuch as LH and FSH contain carbohydrate moieties, the hormone-containing granules in gonadotropes can be stained by carbohydrate-sensitive chemicals such as alcian blue and the periodic acid–Schiff reagent.[1–3]

In most mammalian species, gonadotropes are composed of a heterogeneous population of cells. On the basis of morphologic features, at least two populations of gonadotropes may be discerned in the human pituitary gland—one containing large, ovoid cells and another with small, angular cells. In the rat, a major class of cells are large and round, contain two granule populations of 200 and 400 to 500 nm in diameter, and possess irregularly arranged and vesicular forms of rough endoplasmic reticulum. In the human pituitary, gonadotropes are sparsely dispersed throughout the pars distalis among acini composed predominantly of other anterior pituitary cell types. These gonadotropes react with antisera to both LH and FSH and the common α-subunit and contain granules from 275 to 375 nm in diameter (Fig. 3–1). They exhibit complex morphologic and cytologic properties, with differences between those of male and female animals, and are in varying states of secretory activity.[1, 4, 5]

Further, immunohistochemical studies using single- and double-labeling schemes demonstrated the presence of bihormonal and monohormonal groups of gonadotropes. In the rat pituitary, some gonadotropes contain both FSH and LH, whereas others contain only one of these hormones. The smaller gonadotropes are mainly monohormonal cells producing LH or FSH, whereas the larger cells store both LH and FSH or FSH alone. About 70 percent of the gonadotropes in the adult male rat pituitary contain both LH and FSH, 15 percent contain LH alone, and 15 percent contain FSH alone. However, the distribution of the two populations is not fixed. Instead, dynamic shifts in both the number and proportion of bihormonal and monohormonal gonadotropes are observed after castration, on GnRH administration, and during the estrous cycle in the rat. It is not clear whether such changes reflect the presence of a precursor pool of gonadotropes or plasticity in this pituitary cell type.[1, 4, 6]

The coexistence of LH and FSH in a major pituitary cell population in the human, the monkey, and the rat is consistent with the coupled secretion of LH and FSH at midcycle in the primate and with the simultaneous effects of GnRH on LH and FSH secretion. However, bihormonal or monohormonal populations of gonadotropes may underlie differential LH and FSH release under physiologic conditions. Another possible mechanism for such nonparallel release of LH and FSH may be revealed in the observation that gonadotrope secretory granules may selectively store either LH or FSH.[1–3]

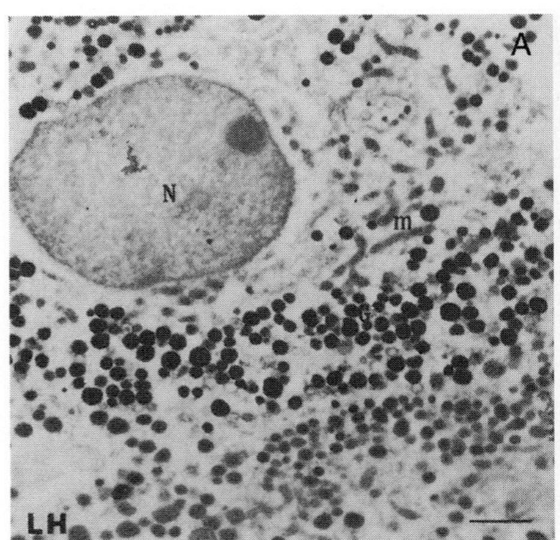

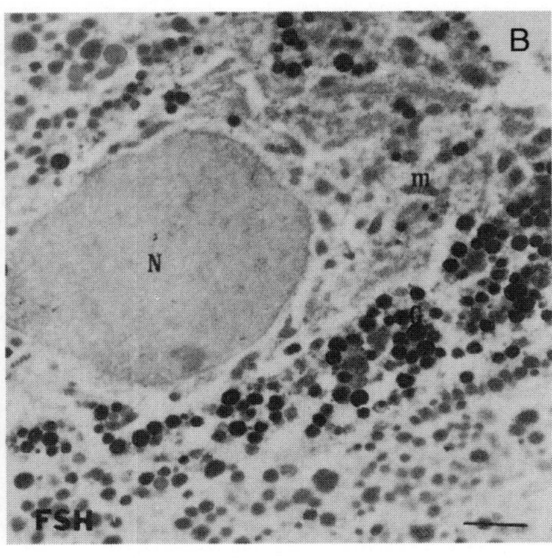

Figure 3–1 ■ A human gonadotrope containing secretory granules stained for LH *(A)* and FSH *(B)*. Serial sections of the cell were stained selectively for LH (with antiserum to hLH β-subunit) and FSH (with antiserum to hFSH β-subunit) by the avidin-biotin complex technique. Magnification × 5000; the bar is 1 μm. N, nucleus; m, mitochondria; G, cluster of stained granules. (Photographs courtesy of Dr. G. V. Childs, University of Texas Medical School, Galveston, TX.)

STRUCTURES OF LH AND FSH AND THEIR SUBUNITS

LH and FSH, together with thyroid-stimulating hormone (TSH), constitute one of the three major groups of anterior pituitary hormones. Growth hormone and prolactin form a second group of structurally related hormones; and corticotropin, together with its associated lipotropin, melanotropin, and the endorphins constitute the third group. LH, FSH, and TSH belong to the family of glycoprotein hormones that also includes the LH homologue expressed in human and equine placenta, chorionic gonadotropin (CG).

Subunit Structure of LH and FSH

LH and FSH share similar chemical and structural features. They are composed of two different, noncovalently associated, carbohydrate-containing protein subunits called α and β. Within a species, the α-subunit of LH, FSH, and TSH, along with that of human chorionic gonadotropin (hCG), possesses an identical polypeptide backbone or apoprotein. Hence, it is also called the "common" glycoprotein hormone subunit. In contrast, the β-subunit of each hormone is different, having unique protein sequence. The β-subunit confers specific activity on the αβ heterodimer because it is the β-subunit that dictates this effect in subunit recombination experiments. Importantly, only the dimer possesses biologic activity. In contrast, although the subunits can be found in the unassociated form in the pituitary gland and in circulation, these "free" subunits have little known activity. Of note, Thotakura and Blithe[7] have shown that the free α-subunit may stimulate prolactin release from human decidual cells. Each subunit is cysteine rich (α, 10; β, 12) and contains multiple disulfide linkages. Sugar moieties are attached to each subunit at specific sites and play key roles in the biologic activity and metabolic fate of the glycoprotein hormones.[8, 9]

LH and FSH have been isolated from anterior pituitaries of many species, including humans, rodents, cattle, swine, horses, amphibia, fish, and a variety of other vertebrates. They have been purified from pituitary glands by acid-ethanol extraction and ethanol precipitation, followed by ion exchange and size exclusion chromatography. There is relatively low abundance of LH and FSH compared with growth hormone, with roughly 70 mg LH, 20 mg FSH, and 5000 mg growth hormone isolated from 1000 human glands. At low pH, the intact hormones may be dissociated and then the α- and β-subunits isolated and purified by chromatographic techniques. The molecular sizes of LH and FSH are approximately 28,000 and 33,000 daltons, respectively; the molecular size of the common α-subunit is about 14,000 daltons. Heterogeneity of the attached carbohydrate groups and minor differences in the amino acid compositions probably account for the imprecise assessment of the apparent sizes of the hormones and their subunits.[8, 10]

The amino acid sequence of the α-subunit of human LH and FSH is shown in Figure 3–2. The 92–amino acid apoproteins of the human α-subunits are identical, being translated from a common α-subunit messenger ribonucleic acid (mRNA). Comparison of α-subunits among species shows sequence conservation at a level of 74 to 95 percent similarity. This finding is consistent with the observation that an α-subunit from one species can recombine with the β-subunits of other species. However, there are sufficient differences among α-subunits from different species to allow immunologic specificity.[10–13] The amino acid sequences of the human LH-β/FSH-β subunits in comparison with that of the related hCG-β are shown in Figure 3–3. Except for their extreme C-terminal ends, LH-β and CG-β are highly homologous, whereas FSH-β shows limited similarity at the level of 30 to 40 percent. All three gonadotropin β-subunits and the TSH β-subunit contain the same number and maintain positions of the 12 cysteine residues. They also contain an invariant Cys-Ala-Gly-Tyr or CAGY sequence that may be involved in subunit-subunit interaction. These features and the ability of the β-subunits to combine with the common α-subunit suggest that the genes that encode the β-subunits are derived from a common ancestral gene. However, it is still not known which domains among the β-subunit sequences are crucial for conferring LH versus FSH activity.[8, 10, 11, 14–16]

Carbohydrate Moieties and the LH/FSH Subunits

A special chemical feature of the LH and FSH subunits is the presence of carbohydrate moieties, with two oligosaccharide groups on the α-subunit (Asn 52 and Asn 78), one in human LH β-subunit (Asn 13), and two in human FSH β-subunit (Asn 13 and Asn 30), as indicated in Figures 3–2 and 3–3. The major sugar groups of the subunits of the pituitary gonadotropins are of the asparagine or *N*-linked type, that is, *N*-acetylglucosamine coupled to specific asparagine residues in the subunit apoprotein. The detailed structures of these oligosaccharide chains are shown in Figure 3–4. The carbohydrate structures of LH and FSH are similar; the sugar content of LH is about 16 percent by weight, and that of FSH is somewhat higher. The monosaccharide residues in both hormones include *N*-acetylglucosamine, mannose, galactose, fucose, glucosamine, *N*-acetylgalactosamine, and sialic (or neuraminic) acid. Each oligosaccharide is branched, either biantennary or triantennary, and is markedly heterogeneous at its peripheral branches, terminating largely with sialic acid and

```
                                10                                   20                                  30                                 40
ALA PRO ASP VAL GLN ASP CYS PRO GLU CYS THR LEU GLN GLU ASN PRO PHE PHE SER GLN PRO GLY ALA PRO ILE LEU GLN CYS MET GLY CYS CYS PHE SER ARG ALA TYR PRO THR PRO

                                50      ▼                            60                                  70                          ▼      80
LEU ARG SER LYS LYS THR MET LEU VAL GLN LYS ASN VAL THR SER GLU SER THR CYS CYS VAL ALA LYS SER TYR ASN ARG VAL THR VAL MET GLY GLY PHE LYS VAL GLU ASN HIS THR

                                90
ALA CYS HIS CYS SER THR CYS TYR TYR HIS LYS SER-COOH
```

Figure 3–2 ■ The amino acid sequence of the α-subunit of human glycoprotein hormones. The solid, inverted triangles indicate the sites of attachment of carbohydrate moieties, which are *N*-linked to asparagine residues 52 and 78.

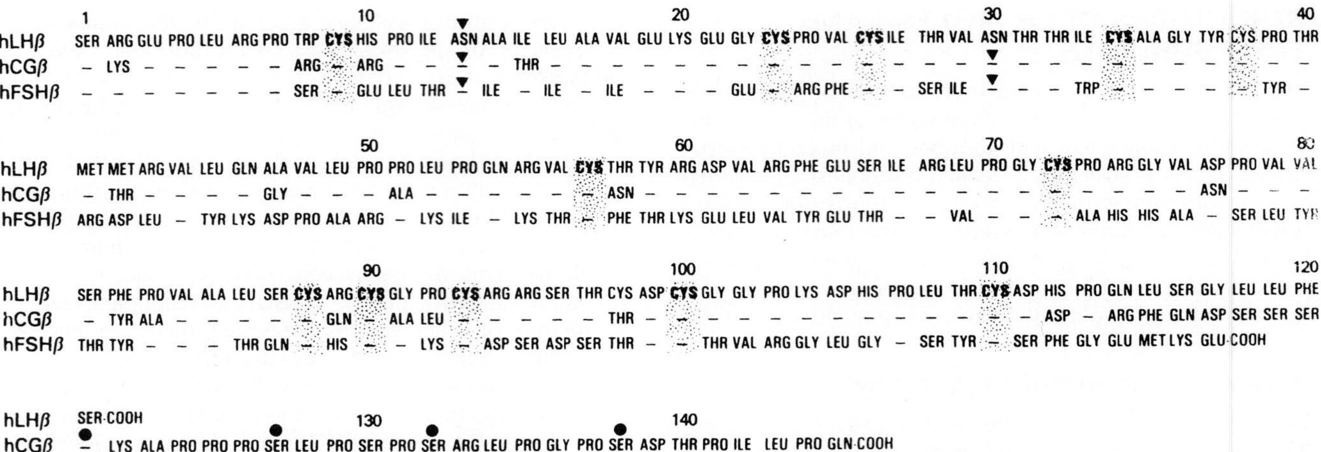

Figure 3–3 ■ Amino acid sequences of the hormone-specific human LH-β, CG-β, and FSH-β subunits. The dashes indicate identical amino acids between the LH-β and CG-β/FSH-β sequences. The conserved cysteine residues are shaded, and the *N*-linked and *O*-linked oligosaccharide moieties are shown as solid inverted triangles and circles, respectively.

fucose and occasionally galactose. In addition, many of the oligosaccharide branches in LH, but not FSH, terminate in sulfated *N*-acetylgalactosamine.[17] From an appreciation of the heterogeneity of the sugar groups on LH and FSH and the major synthesis of the two hormones in the same cell, it is apparent that there are both tissue- and hormone-specific patterns of glycosylation. In this light, recent work suggests that a series of tissue-specific glycosyltransferases reside in gonadotropes and thyrotropes to mediate the synthesis of these different sugar groups.[18–21]

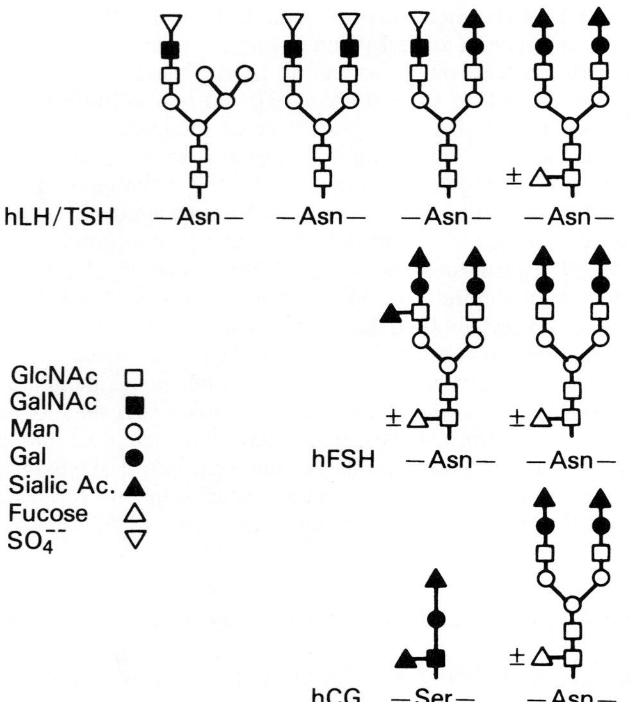

Figure 3–4 ■ Carbohydrate side chains of the pituitary glycoprotein hormones and human chorionic gonadotropin. (Modified from Sairam MR. Role of carbohydrates in glycoprotein hormone signal transduction. FASEB J 3:1915–1926, 1989.)

In addition to the *N*-linked oligosaccharides present in LH and FSH, the hCG β-subunit contains four *O*-linked oligosaccharides attached to serine residues in its unique C-terminal extension peptide, a region not present in the LH β-subunit. Further, the bovine pituitary and the human placenta have been shown to produce a free α-subunit with an additional *O*-linked oligosaccharide unit.[22] The presence of this *O*-linked sugar on the free α-subunit effectively prevents combination with the β-subunit; chemical removal of the sugar restores recombinational activity. The sialic acid content among the glycoprotein hormones is variable. There are 20, 5, and 1 to 2 sialic acid residues per molecule in human CG, FSH, and LH, respectively. The variations in isoelectric points (pIs) of the gonadotropins, ranging from 3 to 5 for hCG, 4.5 to 5 for FSH, and 6 to 10 for LH, are due largely to differences in this charged sugar residue. LH exhibits six isoforms, with a pI range of 8 to 10, that can be resolved by isoelectric focusing of rat pituitary extracts. A more heterogeneous profile is observed in human pituitary extracts and plasma, with a large proportion in the pI range from 6.5 to 10. In general, the most alkaline forms of LH have the highest biologic activity in vitro bioassays and are most rapidly cleared from the circulation. Conversely, the more acidic isoforms are less active in vitro but are present in higher concentrations in circulation because they are also more slowly metabolized and thus are more active in vivo.[10, 21, 23]

Enzymatic removal of the terminal sialic acid residues greatly shortens the circulating half-lives of these hormones with little effect on their abilities to act on their target cellular receptor. As a result, the biologic activities of desialylated human LH, hCG, and FSH are much reduced in vivo but are maintained in vitro on membrane receptors and isolated target cells. Further, removal of the *N*-linked carbohydrate groups strongly reduces the ability of the hormones to activate target cells in the testis and the ovary but exerts little effect on their binding to their receptor sites. For example, LH and FSH virtually lose their abilities to stimulate adenylate cyclase activity, yet retain high binding affinity for gonadal receptors after almost complete removal of their *N*-linked oligosaccharide moieties. As anticipated, such deglycosylated hormones can act in vitro as competitive antagonists of the actions of the intact glycoprotein hormones with respect to cyclic adenosine monophosphate (cAMP) and other second messenger production and, to a lesser extent, steroid hormone production.[10, 20, 21, 23, 24]

Other Structural Features of the Subunits

The three-dimensional structure of hCG has been determined by use of x-ray crystallographic analysis and gives important insights into the conformation of the hCG subunits in its heterodimer and that of LH and FSH[25] (Fig. 3–5). The structure shows that each subunit has several intramolecular disulfide linkages: five in the α-subunit and six in each β-subunit. These disulfide linkages form a motif called a "cystine knot" that is present in a number of growth factors such as nerve growth factor, platelet-derived growth factor-β, and transforming growth factor-β (TGF-β).[25] Thus, the glycoprotein hormones are members of a yet larger family of related proteins. In addition, the α- and β-subunits are apparently closely entwined through noncovalent forces between the subunits. Consistent with the presence of multiple intrachain disulfides and the high proline content, the main secondary structural feature of the subunits is β-sheet, rather than α-helix. Inasmuch as each β-subunit can combine with a common α-subunit (from the same or different species), three-dimensional structures of the β-subunits, from either direct crystal data or molecular modeling, reveal remarkable similarity.

Thus, by extrapolation, it might be conjectured that regions of the β-subunit with less well conserved sequences alone may be responsible for hormone binding and confer functional specificity to the intact heterodimer. Studies of deglycosylated (obtained enzymatically, chemically, or by in vitro mutagenesis) and recombined α- and β-subunits have, however, provided a surprising result. They show that the carbohydrate moieties of the α-subunit, but not the β-subunit, of a hormone are critical for activation of the cognate receptor and its associated G protein–coupled signaling systems. In particular, one of the two oligosaccharides in the α-subunit (linked to the Asn residue at position 52) is the most critical carbohydrate side chain in this activity. Finally, chemical and enzymatic modification studies suggest that regions of the common α-subunit, as well as those of the specific LH-β/FSH-β subunits, interact with the cognate gonadotropin receptor site.[10, 20, 21, 23, 24]

The reason that α combination is important for expression of hormonal activity is not clear. However, two roles can be postulated for the α-subunit in the active heterodimer. The first is that only the combined α-subunit possesses the requisite conformation, with or without appropriate post-translational modification, for effective interaction with the receptor. The second is that the β-subunit acquires an active conformation only after its combination with the α-subunit. Thus, it appears that a major role of the β-subunit among glycoprotein hormones may be to "force" the α-subunit into a conformation that allows the interaction of both subunits of the heterodimer with the cognate hormone receptor to activate the appropriate downstream signaling pathways.

GENE STRUCTURE/CHROMOSOMAL LOCALIZATION

The subunits of LH and FSH are encoded on separate genes located on different chromosomes. In the gonadotrope, the subunit genes are transcribed into mRNAs, which are in

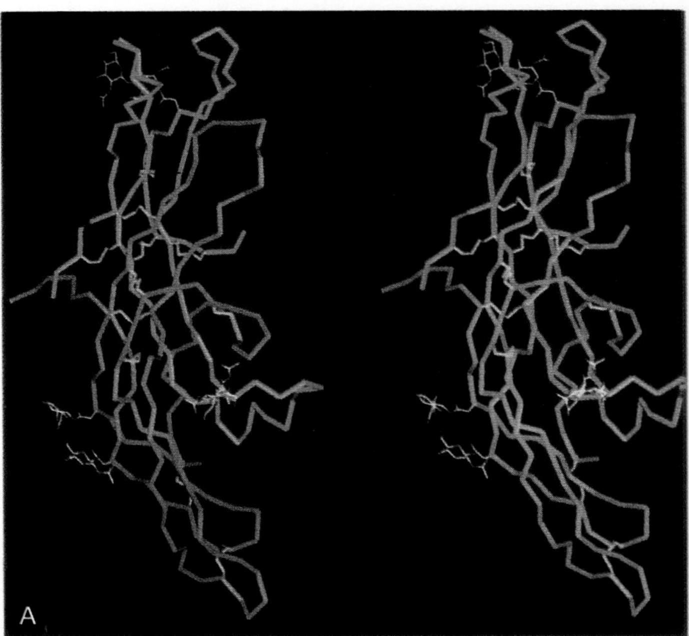

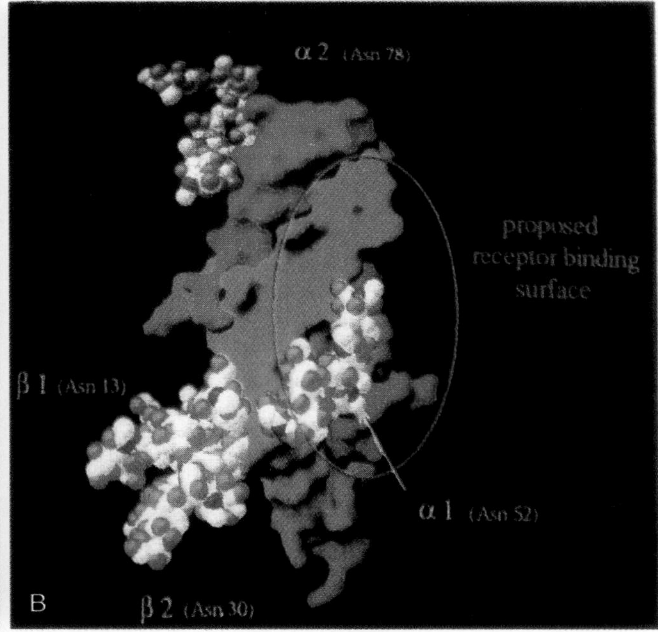

Figure 3–5 ■ Molecular models of hCG based on x-ray crystallographic studies. *A*, The structure of the α and CG-β heterodimer (α, blue; CG-β, green; carbohydrate moieties color-coded for atom type: red (O), white (C), and blue (N); and yellow, Cys-Cys bridges). *B*, A model of *N*-linked carbohydrate on hCG with the surfaces of the α and CG-β subunits denoted by blue and green surfaces, respectively, and a space-filling model of the carbohydrate moieties with atom type color coding as for *A*. (From Lapthorn AJ, Harris DC, Littlejohn A, et al. Crystal structure of human chorionic gonadotropin. Nature 369:455–461, 1994.)

turn translated into the subunit precursors. Typical of secretory proteins, the nascent subunit polypeptide includes a 20- to 24–amino acid leader or signal peptide, in addition to the subunit apoprotein. In a cotranslational process, this signal peptide is cleaved, and oligosaccharide moieties are attached to the appropriate asparagine residues. Then, the partially glycosylated α- and β-subunits combine in the endoplasmic reticulum, and the oligosaccharides undergo further processing in the Golgi complex. The mature glycoprotein hormones are packaged thereafter into secretory granules. Great progress has been achieved during past 20 years in the isolation and characterization of the genes and mRNAs encoding the α-subunit and LH-β/FSH-β. These extensive studies have confirmed the amino acid sequences of the subunits and provided new insights into their structure and evolution. In addition, other studies have given important details concerning the regulation of the transcription of the subunit genes by steroid hormones, GnRH, and other regulatory factors as well as the nature of the post-transcriptional events in the biosynthesis of the hormones.

α-Subunit Genes

The genes and complementary deoxyribonucleic acids (cDNAs) encoding the α-subunits in several species (human, cow, rat, and mouse) have been isolated and extensively characterized[9, 11, 12] (Fig. 3–6). The α-subunits are encoded by single loci of 8 to 16.5 kilobases (kb) in size and are composed of four exons, which encode the mRNA, and three introns. The α-subunit gene is located on human chromosome 6p21.1–23.[26] The marked difference in sizes among these genes is due largely to a wide variation in the sizes of the first intron. The mature α-subunit mRNAs are 730 to 800 nucleotides in length and show 70 to 90 percent similarity between species. Each subunit mRNA is translated to yield a precursor polypeptide that contains a 24–amino acid leader sequence and the 96– or 92 (human)–amino acid α-subunit apoprotein sequence. The promoter regions of the α-subunit genes have also been studied in detail. Of note, there is an 18–base pair (bp) sequence, just upstream of the transcription initiation site, that confers responsiveness to cAMP in itself and other genes, and it is termed a cAMP-regulatory element (CRE). Such regulatory elements are present in the 5′ flanking regions of many genes that are regulated by cAMP and have been found to interact with specific transcription factors, such as CRE-binding protein, that are in turn modulated by phosphorylation by the cAMP-regulated A kinase. The roles of such elements in the control of α-subunit expression and gonadotropin synthesis are discussed below.

β-Subunit Genes

Each β-subunit is encoded by a separate gene located on separate chromosomes. There is a single LH β-subunit gene in human, cow, rat, and mouse with a size (1.1 kb) smaller than the α-subunit genes and that contains three exons and two introns (Fig. 3–6). As noted later, the human LH β-subunit gene is present in a complex LH/CG-β gene cluster on human chromosome 19q13.3.[26] The LH β-subunit mRNA is 700 nucleotides in size and codes for a precursor protein with a 24–amino acid leader peptide and a 121–amino acid β-subunit polypeptide backbone. The human LH and CG β-subunits show about 82 percent similarity in their amino acid sequences and confer almost identical biologic properties when associated with the α-subunit. However, the hCG β-subunit contains an additional 24–amino acid extension at the C terminus and is more heavily glycosylated and, in particular, more sialylated than is hLH.[9, 11, 14–16]

In the human genome, the LH and CG β-subunit genes are encoded by two genes among a cluster of seven distinct LH-β/hCG-β–like genes (five are noncoding or pseudogenes), arranged in groups of tandem and inverted pairs

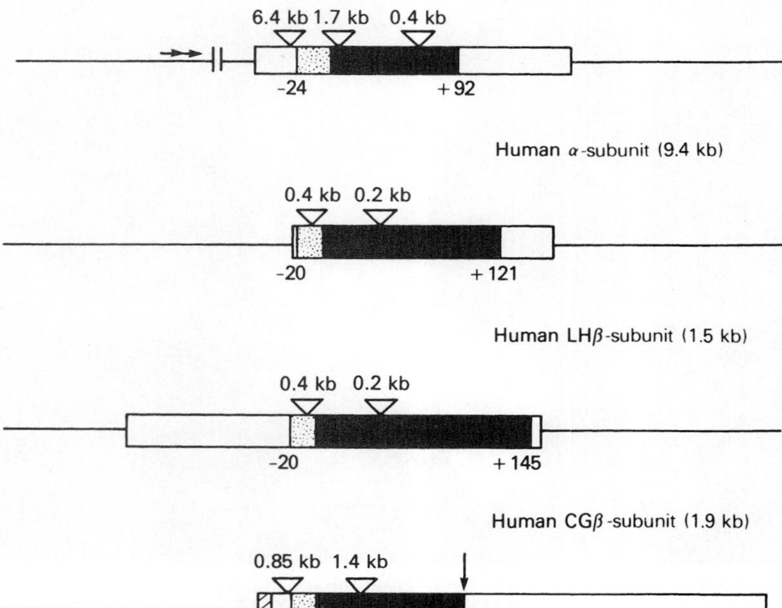

Figure 3–6 ■ Structures of the human α, LH-β, CG-β, and FSH-β subunit genes. Untranslated regions are shown as open bars, signal regions are stippled, and mature apoproteins are indicated in black. Inverted triangles indicate the position of introns, with sizes as labeled. Amino acid positions are numbered with respect to the first amino acid of the mature protein. The cyclic adenosine monophosphate regulatory element is shown by arrows. (Modified from Gharib SD, Wierman ME, Shupnik MA, Chin WW. Molecular biology of the pituitary gonadotropins. Endocr Rev 11:177–199, 1990.)

that probably have arisen by duplication of a LH-β–like ancestral gene[14] (Fig. 3–7). The genes encoding the β-subunits of other mammals have many structural features in common with the human LH-β and CG-β genes. Thus, the rat LH β-subunit gene contains three exons interrupted by two introns with strict conservation of the sites of intron-exon junctions between encoding genes. A high degree of similarity is also observed in the 200 base pairs of the 5′ flanking or promoter region, indicating that these sequences may be involved in the tissue-specific expression and hormonal regulation of the gene.

The protein coding regions of the LH and CG β-subunit genes differ only in the extreme C-terminal end, whereas the hCG-β gene apparently employs a different promoter and transcriptional start site than that used by the LH-β gene.[9, 14] Such an arrangement could result from pressure to maintain hCG-β gene expression and hCG production in the presence of high levels of estrogen to sustain the corpus luteum of pregnancy and to participate in the initiation of male sexual differentiation. The regulatory regions of the rat LH β-subunit gene promoter have recently been explored and are discussed later. Of note, it contains a 15-bp estrogen response element within 2 kb of the transcription start site.[27]

The FSH β-subunit is encoded by a single gene located on human chromosome 11p13 and contains three exons and two introns.[15, 28] The rat FSH-β mRNA is about 1.8 to 2.0 kb in size and encodes a precursor of the FSH β-subunit including a 20–amino acid signal peptide and a 110–amino acid residue apoprotein. There is a high level (approximately 80 percent) of nucleotide and amino acid similarity among species. Unlike the other glycoprotein subunit mRNAs, the FSH β-subunit mRNA possesses a relatively long 3′ untranslated (1 to 1.5 kb) region. The function of this unusual 3′ untranslated region is not known. The transcription of the human FSH β-subunit gene and subsequent post-transcriptional events lead to multiple mRNAs secondary to alternate splicing of the first exon and polyadenylation site choice.

Recombinant DNA technology has proved extremely valuable for the production of synthetic gonadotropins for clinical use in infertility and other conditions. cDNAs encoding α-subunit, LH-β, and FSH-β cDNAs, either as α, LH-β or α, or FSH cDNA pairs in suitable vectors, are introduced into mammalian cells by stable transfection. These recombinant cells are capable of synthesizing these complex glycoproteins because processing, including glycosylation and combination of the subunits, and secretion are achieved at high levels. Such recombinant hormones are also valuable for studies on the biosynthesis, conformation, and biologic properties of gonadotropins and the role of the carbohydrate residues in their biologic activities. They are also purer and potentially more active than those extracted from human pituitary tissue or postmenopausal urine and free of the risk of slow virus infection. Alternatively, synthesis of nonglycosylated hormones with antagonist activity, in appropriate expression systems, could provide information about the molecular conformation necessary to produce an effective antagonist for in vivo applications.

TRANSLATION, POST-TRANSLATIONAL PROCESSING, AND COMBINATION OF GONADOTROPIN SUBUNITS

The steps in the biosynthesis of the gonadotropin subunits proceed by the translation of the subunit mRNAs on the ribosome, followed by post-translational modifications of the precursor subunits and subunit folding and combination, mature hormone packaging, and hormone secretion. In paired cotranslational events, the nascent α- and β-subunit polypeptide precursors are subjected to proteolytic cleavage for removal of the signal peptides and to the attachment of sugar moieties. In the latter process, the gonadotropin subunit apoproteins undergo addition of high-mannose oligosaccharides that are transferred from a dolichol-bound precursor to form *N*-acetylglucosamine linkages with asparagine residues in the sequences Asn-X-Ser/

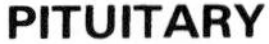

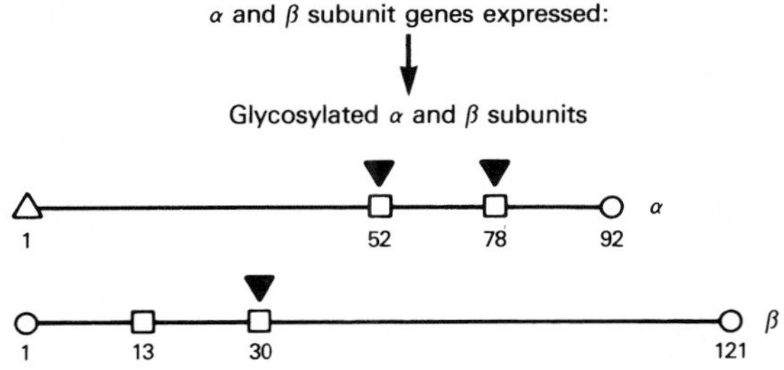

PLACENTA

Identical α and different β subunit genes expressed:
(Ancestral pituitary β gene with single base deletion
and incorporation of 3′-untranslated region)

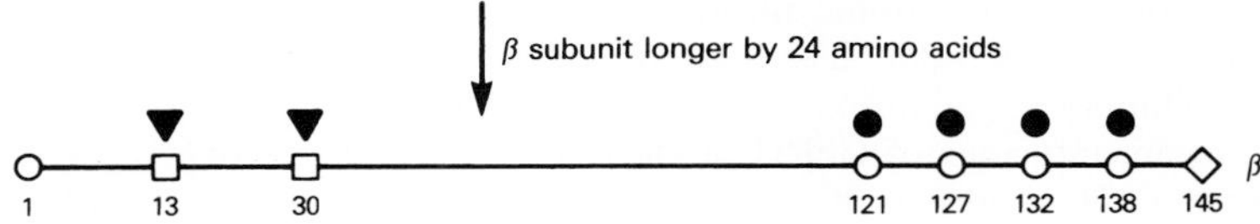

Figure 3–7 ■ Structures of human pituitary luteinizing hormone (LH) and placental chorionic gonadotropin (CG). The α-subunits of the two glycoprotein hormones are identical, but the CG β-subunit has several amino acid differences and an additional *N*-glycosylation site in the region homologous with hLH-β; it also has a 24–amino acid C-terminal extension containing four *O*-glycosylation sites, resulting from a single base deletion, apparent frame shift, and expression of part of the 3′ untranslated region of an ancestral β-subunit gene. Symbols: ○, serine; □, asparagine; Δ, alanine; ◇, glutamine. (Modified from Sairam MR. Role of carbohydrates in glycoprotein hormone signal transduction. FASEB J 3:1915–1926, 1989.)

Thr to the growing peptide chain and enter the lumen of the endoplasmic reticulum. Soon thereafter, subunit folding, formation of multiple intramolecular disulfide linkages, and subunit combination occur. The initial *N*-linked precursor oligosaccharides are remodeled by removal of their terminal glucose and several mannose residues by exoglycosidases in the endoplasmic reticulum and cis-Golgi apparatus and by the stepwise addition of outer sugars, including *N*-acetylglucosamine, galactose, sialic acid, and fucose, catalyzed by specific glycosyltransferases in the medial- and trans-Golgi apparatus. Another post-translational event is the addition of *O*-linked oligosaccharides to serine or threonine residues of the unassociated or free α-subunit and the C-terminal extension of the hCG β-subunit. Presumably, the α-subunit, in the absence of a combined β-subunit, appears conformationally "different" to permit the addition of the *O*-linked sugars.

Although the details of the formation and combination of the α- and β-subunits are not completely known, it is clear that the β-subunit is the rate-limiting factor in the biosynthesis of the glycoprotein hormones. The production of the β-subunit occurs more actively in both the pituitary and the placenta, and infusion of GnRH causes release of both LH and α-subunit in normal men. Conversely, the concentration of free β-subunit in the pituitary and the placenta is relatively low, and unassociated β-subunits are rarely found in plasma. At the mRNA level, there is always excess α-subunit versus β-subunit mRNA in both pituitary and placenta. In choriocarcinoma cells, the α-subunit of hCG is synthesized in molar excess (onefold to fivefold) over the β-subunit, and αβ dimers are rapidly formed from the α and β precursors before the trimming of their *N*-linked high-mannose oligosaccharides has occurred. Such rapid combination of α- and β-subunit precursors also occurs during LH and TSH synthesis and is followed by a rate-limiting step during the trimming of the high-mannose oligosaccharide in the endoplasmic reticulum. The final steps of glycosylation to form complex carbohydrate chains occur rapidly thereafter and are followed by secretion of mature hCG as it is formed in placental cells or by storage of mature LH and FSH in secretory granules in the pituitary gonadotropes.

LH AND FSH SYNTHESIS AND SECRETION

The content of LH and FSH in the human pituitary has generally been difficult to assess. However, analysis of pituitary LH content after sudden death in women at defined stages of the cycle showed a decrease during the early follicular phase, then a gradual rise up to the time of ovulation, followed by a sharp fall and a subsequent increase at the beginning of the cycle. Pituitary FSH content showed less marked fluctuations but also decreased during the early follicular phase and after ovulation. Such changes in pituitary hormone content are of interest but are not necessarily correlated with the secretory activity of the gonadotropes. Additional information about gonadotropin storage and secretion has been provided by analysis of the pituitary gonadotropin response to infusions of GnRH. Constant infusions of GnRH produce a biphasic profile of plasma LH, similar to the release of other hormones stored as granules; these findings suggest the existence of two pools of LH in the human pituitary. The biphasic release of LH is observed during GnRH infusion in both men and women and in hypogonadal patients and appears to be influenced by gonadal steroids. The initial release of LH peaks at 30 minutes, and the secondary rise begins after 90 minutes and continues for up to 4 hours. The size of the second response is augmented by estradiol, whereas progesterone increases both early and late responses after estrogen treatment. Such observations suggest the existence of a preformed LH pool that is rapidly released by GnRH and may be the source of LH released during the pulsatile pattern of plasma LH that occurs in normal men and women as well as in those with disorders of the hypothalamus, pituitary, or gonads. It is possible that the "early pool" that is observed during GnRH infusion represents recruitment of granules in proximity to the gonadotrope cell membrane and that episodic peaks of plasma LH represent the same response to endogenous pulses of GnRH from the hypothalamus. This finding would be consistent with in vitro observations that the initial LH release in response to GnRH does not require protein synthesis.

The second pool could represent the more coordinated release of the gonadotrope granule population together with stimulation of hormone biosynthesis. The size of the second, or reserve, pool increases markedly during the follicular phase, a change that can be reproduced by estradiol treatment. Such an increase in the quantity of LH released from the pituitary during GnRH infusion correlates well with the increasing content of pituitary LH observed up to the time of ovulation in the postmortem studies described earlier. Unlike the biphasic response of plasma LH, only a single progressive rise in plasma FSH occurs during infusion of GnRH. The absence of an early response in plasma FSH might reflect the lack of an acutely releasable FSH pool as a granule population in the gonadotropes or the need for stimulation by a more specific FSH-releasing factor to evoke release from an early pool. Favoring the latter possibility is the frequent occurrence of acute FSH release as "spikes" synchronous with those of LH and the more marked elevations of plasma FSH than LH in hypogonadal subjects.

In rat gonadotropes, GnRH stimulates LH release in seconds and secretory granule dissolution in minutes, with a corresponding rise in plasma LH measured in vivo. Immunocytochemical studies on the localization of biotin-labeled GnRH have shown specific binding of the ligand to about 15 percent of the cell population of the rat pituitary gland. Binding of GnRH to gonadotropes is followed rapidly by capping or aggregation of the receptor-bound peptide and the development of blebs into which gonadotropins become concentrated before their release from the cell. This regional sequestration of secretion granules can be so marked as to deplete the remainder of the cell of gonadotropin, suggesting that much of the stored hormone within individual gonadotropes can be released during the secretory response to GnRH.

In addition to the release of preformed gonadotropins from secretory granules, there is evidence for increased synthesis of α- and β-subunits during states of enhanced gonadotropin secretion. The amounts of both α and β mRNAs are regulated by gonadal steroids, and the pituitary content of β-subunit mRNAs is increased fourfold to eightfold during the preovulatory LH surge in the normal estrous cycle of the sheep. The stimulatory effect of estradiol on gonadotropin synthesis is complemented by the ability of pulsatile GnRH stimulation to enhance the rate of formation of LH-α and LH-β subunits in the gonadotrope, a combined action that is maximally effective around the time of the preovulatory LH surge. The regulation of gonadotropin synthesis and secretion by the interacting effects of gonadal steroids and GnRH is an intricate process that becomes especially complex during the control of the female reproductive cycle. An optimal frequency of GnRH pulsatile stimulation of the pituitary is essential to maintain appropriate plasma levels of LH and FSH, and circulating gonadotropins decline when the frequency of GnRH pulses is too low and also when GnRH stimulation is too frequent or continuous. The susceptibility of the human pituitary to desensitization by continued treatment with GnRH superagonist analogues has been of value for the suppression of gonadotropin secretion in the treatment of precocious puberty, prostatic and mammary cancer, endometriosis, fibroids, and other gonadal steroid–dependent disorders as well as in fertility regulation and in vitro fertilization.

LH AND FSH METABOLISM AND EXCRETION

The molecular properties of circulating glycoprotein hormones are generally similar to those of the hormones extracted from the pituitary. Pituitary and plasma gonadotropins show minor size differences, but there is no convincing evidence for larger prehormones or smaller active forms of LH and FSH. The gel filtration profile of postmenopausal plasma shows a single peak of biologically active plasma LH, coincident with the position of immunoreactive LH. Subtle changes in the properties of pituitary and circulating forms of LH and FSH have been observed in animals after changes in gonadal steroid–pituitary feedback. In the rat, androgen treatment increases the biologic activity of pituitary FSH relative to its immunoreactivity and reduces the rate of clearance of FSH from the circulation. In rhesus monkeys, ovariectomy is followed by changes in the properties of pituitary LH and FSH, which show a slight increase in molecular size and are less rapidly cleared from the circulation. The increased molecular size of pituitary LH and FSH is reversed by estrogen replacement in castrated animals and is reduced by digestion of pituitary extracts with neuraminidase to remove sialic acid residues. It is likely that these estrogen-regulated qualitative changes in pituitary gonadotropins depend on alterations in the carbohydrate composition of the hormone molecules and, specifically, on their degree of sialylation. The sialic acid content of gonadotropic hormones and other glycoproteins has a marked effect on their rate of clearance from the circulation and also influences their apparent molecular size as determined by gel filtration analysis. In addition to these minor variations in apparent size of gonadotropins, variations in oligosaccharide content and structure also cause charge microheterogeneity in both pituitary and circulating gonadotropic hormones, with serum isoforms separating over the pI range of 6.5 to 10 on electrofocusing.

RADIOIMMUNOASSAYS AND BIOASSAYS OF LH AND FSH

Radioimmunoassay and Bioassay

The circulating concentrations of immunoreactive LH and FSH have been extensively evaluated by specific radioimmunoassays employing antisera raised against the purified hormones. Antisera to hCG were previously employed in assays for LH, based on the close structural and immunologic similarities between the two hormones, but this practice has been superseded by the use of antisera to purified LH. Radioimmunoassays employing antisera against the hCG β-subunit or its unique C-terminal sequence are highly specific for the measurement of plasma or urinary hCG, even in the presence of significant levels of hLH. Subunit antisera are also valuable for the detection of circulating hormone subunits secreted by the pituitary and the placenta, or ectopically by certain neoplasms, and for heterologous assays in species for which homologous radioimmunoassays are not available.

The biologic activity of the low gonadotropin concentrations in plasma can be measured by radioligand-receptor binding assays and by in vitro bioassays employing gonadal target cells. Newer approaches use mammalian cells transfected with cDNAs encoding LH and FSH receptors and CRE-containing reporter gene constructs. Then the amount of reporter protein is proportional to the activation of the LH or FSH receptor. Radioligand-receptor assays for LH/hCG are sensitive to nanogram quantities of gonadotropin and readily measure hCG concentrations during pregnancy, even from the first few days after implantation of the blastocyst. Plasma LH and FSH levels measured by radioligand-receptor assays in postmenopausal women are commensurate with, or somewhat higher than, those measured by radioimmunoassay. A much more sensitive biologic assay for plasma LH and hCG employs dispersed interstitial cells from the rat or mouse testis that are highly sensitive to primate gonadotropins in vitro and respond with dose-dependent increments in testosterone production when incubated with low concentrations of LH and hCG.

Such in vitro bioassays permit accurate measurement of the biologic activity of circulating LH and hCG in human plasma under all physiologic circumstances. In addition, the combination of bioassay and radioimmunoassay permits calculation of bioactive/immunoreactive ratios, which provide a useful index of qualitative changes of the LH molecule. Biochemical changes in secreted LH, such as the degree of glycosylation and sulfation, often modify the bioactive/immunoreactive ratio and may reflect pathophysiologic changes in the hypothalamic-pituitary complex. In human and monkey sera, the immunoactive and bioactive LH profiles are in general well correlated during the menstrual cycle and other physiologic changes. However, significant discrepancies in the biologic and immunologic activities of serum LH occur under several circumstances (see later) and are of diagnostic value in certain disorders of gonadotropin secretion.

Plasma concentrations of LH and FSH are usually expressed in terms of standards calibrated in biologic units (e.g., the pituitary gonadotropin reference preparations distributed by the National Institutes of Health and the World Health Organization). Some laboratories still employ the urinary gonadotropin standard of human menopausal gonadotropin, formerly distributed as the Second International Reference Preparation (2nd IRP). The use of different standards has given a wide range of values for gonadotropins measured in individual laboratories, but all show identical profiles of plasma hormones during the menstrual cycle and other physiologic changes. In terms of purified hormone, the basal plasma levels of LH and FSH are equivalent to a few nanograms per milliliter, or approximately 10^{-11} mol/L.

Radioimmunoassay of Plasma LH and FSH Levels

Plasma gonadotropins undergo well-defined changes during the menstrual cycle, with frequent short-term elevations that reflect the pulsatile release of LH and FSH and long-term changes dominated by the midcycle peak of gonadotropin release. Plasma LH rises slightly in the late follicular phase, followed by a marked and sometimes biphasic preovulatory surge and a decline during the luteal phase. Plasma FSH shows a rise during the late luteal and early follicular phases, followed by a decline that is interrupted at midcycle by a small surge coinciding with the preovulatory LH peak. These profiles are well known and are constant in the normal cycle.

In abnormal cycles, marked changes in the patterns of gonadotropin secretion have been recognized. Thus, in the polycystic ovary syndrome, inappropriately elevated plasma LH levels are maintained by exaggerated pulses of LH, whereas FSH values are low and nonpulsatile. These changes reflect disordered secretion as a result of inappropriate estrogen feedback, derived from androgens formed by the chronically overstimulated ovaries, with increased pituitary sensitivity to GnRH and suppression of FSH secretion. In menstrual cycles characterized by a short luteal phase, FSH levels are low before ovulation and may lead to inadequate corpus luteum function after ovulation from an incompletely developed follicle. In perimenopausal women, the depletion of ovarian follicles leads to lower plasma estradiol and elevated plasma FSH with normal plasma LH levels. Such cycles often show a shortened follicular phase that is responsible for the progressive decrease in cycle length with increasing age. The importance of follicular function in regulating FSH secretion is indicated by the increase in plasma FSH that occurs when ovarian follicles are depleted or absent. The presence of increased FSH with normal LH indicates that differential regulation of gonadotropin secretion can occur and suggests the participation of ovarian inhibin (and possibly an additional hypothalamic factor) in the regulation of FSH secretion. Inhibin has recently been purified from bovine follicular fluid and cloned, and it has been shown to exert potent FSH-inhibitory actions in male and female animals.

In addition to the monthly fluctuations that characterize the menstrual cycle, short-term variations and episodic changes occur in the secretion of gonadotropins at various stages of development. At birth, plasma hCG and estrogen are elevated and FSH and LH are low. Within a week, hCG is no longer detectable in the circulation and plasma estrogens fall to the prepubertal range. In male infants, this is followed by a rapid but transient rise in serum FSH and LH levels with a secondary brief increase in plasma testosterone and estradiol. Serum FSH and LH rise rapidly during the first few weeks of life and then decline to prepubertal values at about 4 months of age. In girls, the postnatal FSH rise is more marked and more prolonged, and plasma values do not fall to the prepubertal level until 4 years of age.

The gonadotropin responses to GnRH show commensurate changes with age and sex. During the first year of life, the LH response is much more marked than the FSH response in boys, whereas the FSH response exceeds the LH response in girls. Thus, during infancy, there is higher FSH secretion and reserve in girls and a higher LH reserve in boys. At the onset of puberty, plasma FSH levels rise more rapidly than plasma LH in girls, and LH rises more sharply in boys. There is a marked rise in LH release after GnRH stimulation in both sexes, but the concomitant release of FSH is higher in girls at all stages of sexual maturation. The sex difference in sensitivity to GnRH and releasable FSH could be a factor in the higher incidence of precocious puberty in girls and delayed adolescence in boys. Another feature of puberty is the appearance of pulsatile release of gonadotropins, at first only during sleep. Augmentation of LH secretion during sleep is an early, central nervous system–mediated determinant of puberty that sometimes occurs before the onset of overt pubertal changes. Such nocturnal increases in LH secretion stimulate the testis to secrete androgen in pubertal boys and probably exert a similar but delayed action on estrogen production by the ovary in pubertal girls. As puberty progresses, the LH response to GnRH becomes greatly increased, and the pulsatile pattern of gonadotropin secretion becomes established during waking hours as well as during sleep. Although the mean plasma gonadotropin concentrations rise progressively during puberty, the absolute changes are not large and the overall increase is only about twofold in comparison with prepubertal values. However, the increase in gonadotropin secretion is much larger than suggested by the plasma levels, as indicated by the considerable rises in urinary gonadotropin excretion during puberty, with a 4-fold increase in FSH excretion and a 12-fold increase in LH excretion. In addition, there is a progressive rise in the bioactivity of circulating LH during puberty (see later).

The pulsatile nature of gonadotropin release in both men and women is well established by the end of puberty and is readily detected in blood samples taken at short intervals. The pulses are characterized by a rapid upsurge during 10 to 15 minutes followed by a fall with a half-time of 50 minutes for LH and somewhat more for FSH, reflecting the different clearance rates of the two gonadotropins. The pulses of FSH are much smaller than the LH pulses and are frequently, but not always, coincident with them. During the menstrual cycle, pulses occur at intervals of 1 to 2 hours in the follicular phase and about 4 hours in the luteal phase. At midcycle, there is an increase in pulse frequency and magnitude, the latter being consistent with the increase in sensitivity of the pituitary to GnRH near the time of ovulation. After menopause or castration, circulating gonadotropins are markedly elevated, FSH values rise to exceed LH levels, and episodic secretion continues with large pulses of both LH and FSH.

GONADOTROPIN-RELEASING HORMONE RECEPTOR

Hypophysial portal GnRH binds to the GnRH receptor (GnRH-R) on the cell surface of the gonadotrope with high affinity ($K_d \approx 0.3$ nM).[29, 30] There is considerable evidence in vivo and in vitro that the number of GnRH-Rs on the cell surface of the gonadotrope is regulated by varying GnRH pulse frequencies and other hormonal factors.[31] Changes in GnRH-R concentration on the surface of the gonadotrope are often correlated with alterations in gonadotrope response to GnRH. A major example is the increase in apparent sensitivity of the gonadotrope to GnRH that leads to the midcycle surge in LH and FSH that is probably mediated in part by increases in GnRH-R levels. As determined by GnRH binding, the concentration of GnRH-R in the pituitary gland is highest with a GnRH pulse frequency of 30 minutes. Lower concentrations are seen with a GnRH pulse frequency of 2 hours. Such changes in GnRH-R are correlated with optimal release and synthesis of LH and FSH, respectively. The relative amount of GnRH-R observed between high- and low-frequency GnRH pulses is twofold to threefold.[32–34] The variations in levels of GnRH-R during pituitary development, estrous cycle, pregnancy, lactation, and gonadectomy with and without estrogen replacement indicate that such changes are important in reproductive physiology.[35–37]

Recently, cDNAs for the mouse GnRH-R were obtained by screening cDNA libraries derived from a gonadotrope cell line, αT3–1, using frog oocyte expression.[38, 39] Soon thereafter, GnRH-R cDNAs from the human, rat, cow, pig, and sheep were isolated and characterized.[40–42] These data revealed a high level of similarity among the encoded receptors. The GnRH-R, approximately 320- to 330–amino acid residues in size, is a member of a large superfamily of seven membrane-spanning, G protein–coupled, cell surface receptors.[43] Special features include DRY to DRS consensus sequence in the second intracytoplasmic loop, interchange of conserved D and N residues in the second and seventh intramembrane domains, and absence of a COOH-terminal intracytoplasmic tail.[44, 45] In addition, the mouse, human, and ovine GnRH-R genes have recently been isolated and characterized.[46–49] The single-copy GnRH-R genes are more than 20 to 25 kb in size, contain three exons, and are localized to human chromosome 4q13.2–21.1 and sheep chromosome 6.[50–52] The promoter regions of the mouse and human genes have been examined, revealing complex organization with multiple transcriptional start-sites that are occasionally associated with TATA boxes.[46, 47] Further, there is evidence that alternative splicing of RNA transcripts results in multiple mouse GnRH-R mRNAs that code for truncated proteins (261 and 177 amino acids) in addition to the full-length receptor.[53]

Before the availability of GnRH-R cDNAs, the presence of GnRH binding sites in tissues other than the pituitary gland and pituitary cell lines was established. Studies show that multiple GnRH-R mRNAs with different sizes (5.0 to 5.5, 4.5, and 1.8 kb in the rat) are present in pituitary and extrapituitary tissues.[34, 54] Extrapituitary sites detected in rat and human include ovary, testes, brain (hippocampus, hypothalamus, and GT1–7 hypothalamic neuron cell line), prostate, breast, and placenta.[55, 56] The physiologic roles of the extrapituitary sites of GnRH-R expression are not known. The ontogeny of the GnRH-R in the anterior pituitary gland has been described. Binding and in situ hybridization approaches show that the protein and mRNA are expressed at mouse embryonic day 13.[57] Thus, GnRH-R appears after the α-subunit but several days before LH-β and FSH-β subunits during pituitary development.[58, 59]

By use of blot hybridization, ribonuclease protection, oocyte expression, and reverse transcription–polymerase chain reaction assays, studies on the regulation of pituitary GnRH-R gene expression at the mRNA level have been performed. GnRH-R mRNAs are increased by gonadectomy (twofold to fivefold) in rats and thereafter decreased by sex steroid replacement.[34] In perifused cultured rat pituitary cells, pulsatile GnRH for 16 hours increased GnRH-R mRNA levels by more than fivefold to sixfold, whereas continuous GnRH was not effective.[34] Other studies have confirmed the importance of pulsatile GnRH in the stimulation of GnRH-R mRNA in vivo.[37, 60, 61] Also, there is a threefold increase in pituitary GnRH-R mRNA on the afternoon of proestrus compared with the morning of metestrus in the rat estrous cycle.[62, 63] Recent work indicates that GnRH-R mRNA is stimulated by estradiol, progesterone, and inhibin in sheep[64, 65] and by estradiol and activin in rat.[36, 66] Lactation is associated with decreased pituitary GnRH-R mRNA.[67] In αT3–1 cells, GnRH has no effect on GnRH-R mRNA; however, forskolin decreases levels of GnRH-R mRNA but phorbol esters do not.[68] Finally, nuclear runoff and transfection studies establish the ability of activin A to stimulate GnRH-R gene expression at the transcriptional level.[66]

REGULATION OF GONADOTROPIN BIOSYNTHESIS AND SECRETION

The biosynthesis and secretion of the gonadotropins are tightly regulated across the reproductive cycle. Although this has been an area of active investigation for many years, the mechanisms by which this precise regulation is attained are still being elucidated. As seen in Figure 3–8, gonadotropin expression is modulated by hypothalamic factors (primarily GnRH), intrapituitary factors (primarily the peptides, activin and follistatin), and gonadal feedback (both steroidal and peptide). Gonadotropin expression can be modulated at many levels, including (1) alterations in transcription rates, (2) mRNA stabilization, (3) increased protein subunit synthesis, (4) post-translational modifications such as glycosylation, and (5) changes in gonadotrope cell number. The following sections discuss the roles of GnRH, the gonadal steroids, and the activin-inhibin-follistatin system on gonadotropin gene expression at both the biosynthetic and secretory levels.

Hypothalamic Control

Hypothalamic control of gonadotropin expression occurs primarily through the action of GnRH, a decapeptide encoded by a gene located on the short arm of chromosome 8.[69] Although GnRH was originally identified as the LH-releasing hormone (and therefore also called LHRH), it is now known that a single peptide stimulates release of both LH and FSH. During development, GnRH-secreting

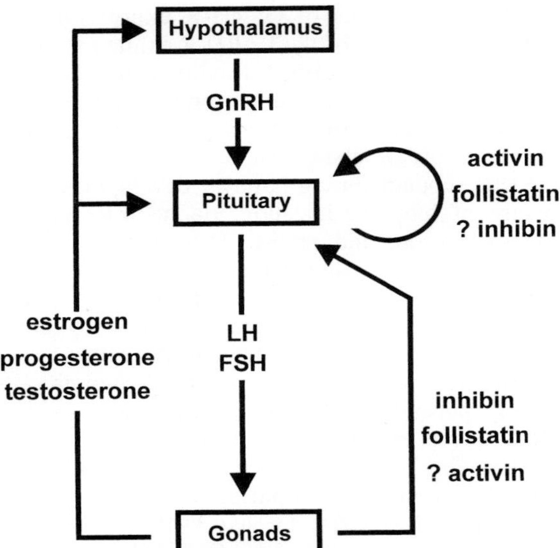

Figure 3–8 ■ Hypothalamus-pituitary-gonadal axis: schematic representation of peptide and steroidal factors that regulate gonadotropin biosynthesis and secretion.

neurons originate in the olfactory placode and migrate to the medial basal hypothalamus (MBH). In primates, the majority of the GnRH neuronal cell bodies are located within the arcuate nucleus of the MBH, with additional cells residing in the preoptic area of the anterior hypothalamus.[70] GnRH produced in these cells is transported down axons within the tuberoinfundibular tract to the median eminence where it is released into the hypophysial portal system that bathes the anterior pituitary (adenohypophysis). GnRH neurons also project to the limbic system as well as the amygdala, hippocampus, and periaqueductal gray matter.[71] These regions may participate in the control of reproductive behavior and may serve to modulate GnRH release; however, only lesions that prevent GnRH transport to the median eminence significantly affect gonadotropin secretion.

GnRH is normally released as a pulsatile rather than a continuous signal. Using a primate model, Knobil and colleagues[72] first demonstrated that this pulsatile pattern of GnRH release is required to increase gonadotropin expression (Fig. 3–9). This observation has been confirmed in humans by the restoration of gonadotropin secretion in GnRH-deficient males and females after exogenous pulsatile GnRH treatment.[73] Conversely, after a transient stimulatory period, continuous GnRH exposure suppresses gonadotrope function. Administration of an Nal-Glu GnRH antagonist to women in the follicular phase of the menstrual cycle reduced secretion of LH, FSH, and free α-subunit, with an overall greater sensitivity of LH to suppression.[74] The inhibitory effect of continuous GnRH has been exploited in the treatment of various gonadal steroid–dependent disorders including precocious puberty, endometriosis, prostate cancer, and breast cancer, as well as in control of the menstrual cycle for infertility treatment.[75]

Because of a short half-life of GnRH and the large dilutional effect, peripheral GnRH serum levels are too low for pulse characteristics to be determined in humans with reliability. Measurement of hypophysial portal GnRH levels is contraindicated for obvious technical reasons. Fortuitously, circulating levels of LH have been shown to correlate closely with GnRH release as determined by simultaneous measurement of both hypophysial portal and peripheral venous blood samples in a number of species.[76, 77] Therefore, frequent measurement of LH pulses can be used as an accurate indicator of GnRH secretion patterns. Whereas FSH secretion is also correlated with GnRH secretion, it is less useful as a marker because of its long half-life.

Episodic release of GnRH appears to be the result of a "pulse generator" within the MBH, because discrete pulses of GnRH can be measured from both fetal and adult human MBH tissue by use of a perifusion system.[78] Whether this intrinsic pulsatile pattern resides within the GnRH neurons themselves or is due to electrochemical communication within a local neural network remains to be proven. Of interest, immortalized GnRH neurons demonstrate pulsatile secretion in perifusion, suggesting that neither additional neuronal nor non-neuronal cell types are needed to produce the observed pattern of release.

GnRH pulse frequency differs across the normal female reproductive cycle. On the basis of LH measurements in the human, it has been estimated that GnRH pulses occur every 94 minutes in the early follicular phase, increasing to a frequency of every 71 minutes in the late follicular phase. Pulse frequency is lowest in the late luteal phase, with a pulse occurring every 216 minutes.[79] The relationship of gonadotropin secretion to GnRH pulse pattern has been studied in hypophysectomized animals receiving exogenous GnRH as well as in numerous in vitro systems. In general, more rapid pulse frequencies favor LH secretion, whereas slower pulse frequencies favor FSH.[80] Thus, variations in GnRH pulse frequency markedly influence both the absolute levels and the ratio of LH and FSH release.

The observed variations in GnRH pulsatility are believed to be achieved primarily through modulation of the "intrinsic" pulse pattern by gonadal steroid feedback. In ewes, estradiol causes an increase in GnRH pulse frequency and thereby an increase in LH release. Conversely, elevated progesterone levels, as occur during the luteal phase, are correlated with decreased LH pulsatility, presumably mediated by central modulation of GnRH pulse pattern.[81] Thus, increased luteal progesterone levels may cause a decrease in GnRH pulse frequency and, thereby, lead to the preferential biosynthesis and secretion of FSH that is observed in the late luteal phase of the menstrual cycle.[82]

Although less fully characterized, GnRH pulsatility is further fine-tuned by the action of locally released factors. Norepinephrine is believed to stimulate GnRH release; opioids exert inhibitory effects. Dopamine treatment can produce both stimulatory and inhibitory GnRH responses, depending on physiologic state. Because dopamine increases β-endorphin release, which in turn blunts dopaminergic release, it has been suggested that an intrahypothalamic neural network acts to regulate GnRH pulsatility.[83]

There are several lines of evidence to suggest that GnRH stimulates gonadotropin biosynthesis in addition to its effects on secretion. First, incorporation of radiolabeled precursor amino acids into LH and FSH is increased by the addition of GnRH to cultured pituitary cells.[84] Second,

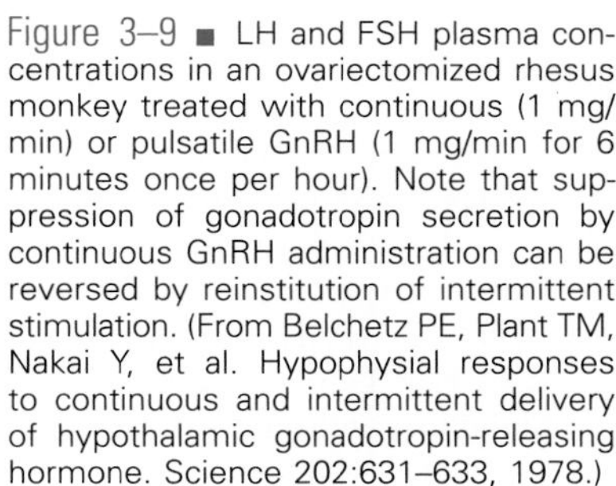

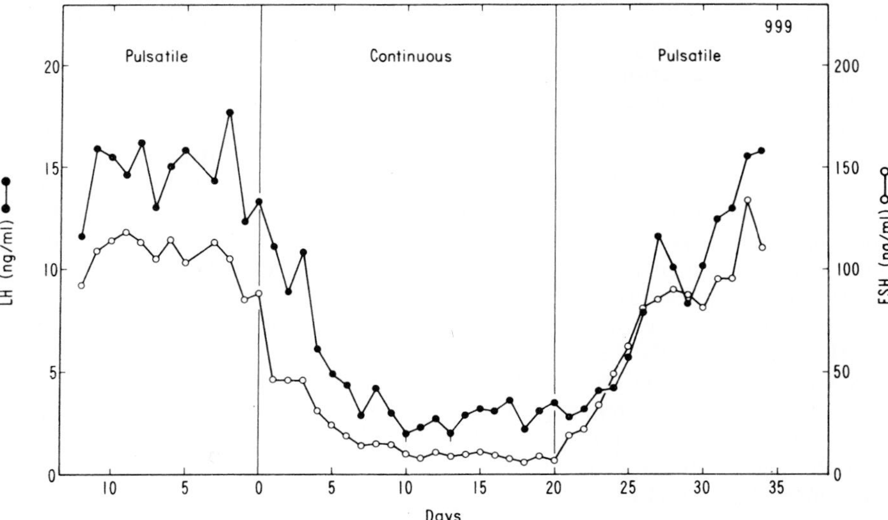

Figure 3–9 ■ LH and FSH plasma concentrations in an ovariectomized rhesus monkey treated with continuous (1 mg/min) or pulsatile GnRH (1 mg/min for 6 minutes once per hour). Note that suppression of gonadotropin secretion by continuous GnRH administration can be reversed by reinstitution of intermittent stimulation. (From Belchetz PE, Plant TM, Nakai Y, et al. Hypophysial responses to continuous and intermittent delivery of hypothalamic gonadotropin-releasing hormone. Science 202:631–633, 1978.)

blocking mRNA synthesis by actinomycin D inhibits GnRH-induced LH synthesis and release.[85] Third, a number of in vivo and in vitro models have demonstrated up-regulation of gonadotropin subunit mRNA expression by endogenous or exogenous GnRH. Treatment of male or female rats with a GnRH antagonist blunts the postcastration rise in all three gonadotropin subunit mRNAs.[86] In another model, the hypothalamic-pituitary disconnect sheep, α-subunit and LH β-subunit levels that had dropped to nearly undetectable levels were restored by pulsatile GnRH.[87] In castrated, testosterone-replaced male rats in which endogenous GnRH pulses are suppressed, treatment with pulsatile GnRH increased mRNA levels for all three gonadotropin subunits. Interestingly, short pulse intervals (every 8 to 30 minutes) stimulated α-subunit transcription rates, whereas longer pulse intervals of 120 minutes preferentially increased FSH-β mRNA synthesis. LH-β gene transcription rates increased maximally with 30-minute intervals between pulses.[82] Divergent regulation of gonadotropin subunit biosynthesis by variations in GnRH pulsatility has been confirmed in vitro.[88]

Although the mechanism by which GnRH pulse pattern is translated into differential regulation of gonadotropin gene expression (both biosynthesis and secretion) is currently unknown, alterations in gonadotrope GnRH-R number may contribute. It is well known that pulsatile GnRH up-regulates GnRH-R expression, with continuous GnRH exposure decreasing both receptor number and sensitivity. Furthermore, an increase in pituitary GnRH-Rs has been noted in the preovulatory period in rats, sheep, and monkeys.[89] In support of this theory, maximal stimulation of GnRH-R mRNA levels is attained with a GnRH pulse frequency (every 30 minutes) that results in preferential biosynthesis and secretion of LH relative to FSH.[90]

Increases in steady-state gonadotropin mRNA levels, as described before, can be achieved through mRNA stabilization as well as through increases in transcription rate. By nuclear runoff assay, pulsatile GnRH has been shown to increase the transcription rate of all three gonadotropin subunit mRNAs in perifused female rat pituitary fragments, with greater effects on the α-subunit and LH β-subunit mRNAs.[91] An increase in mRNA stabilization can be achieved through an increase in length of the polyadenylation "tail" located at the 3′ end of mRNA transcripts. Pulsatile GnRH treatment has been shown to increase the length of the 3′ end of both α-subunit and LH β-subunit mRNAs, but not of the FSH-β mRNAs, implying increased length of the polyadenylation tail and, therefore, increased mRNA stabilization.[92]

In addition to GnRH, a number of other neuropeptides are known to modulate gonadotropin gene expression. These factors may act indirectly, through regulation of GnRH pulsatility, or by exerting direct effects on gonadotroph function. Neuropeptide Y (NPY)–releasing nerve terminals impinge on both the MBH and the median eminence, locations well suited to regulation of GnRH neuronal function. In the presence of gonadal steroids, NPY increases GnRH release from the median eminence. At the level of the pituitary, NPY facilitates GnRH-induced LH release, possibly by altering GnRH-R affinity for GnRH. NPY may also have a paracrine effect on gonadotrope function, because it is produced in the thyrotropes and levels increase after ovariectomy.[93] The neuropeptides galanin and pituitary adenylate cyclase–activating polypeptide have also been implicated in the up-regulation of LH secretion.[94, 95]

Gonadal Steroid Feedback

Gonadotropin biosynthesis and secretion are modulated by two gonadal feedback systems—the gonadal steroid and activin-inhibin-follistatin systems. The actions of these two systems are superimposed on the pulsatile stimulatory action of GnRH. Because gonadectomy results in a prompt increase in serum gonadotropin levels, the overall effect of these systems can be seen to be inhibitory.

The gonadal steroids include the estrogens, progesterones, and androgens. Attempts to define the precise site of action of these hormones in gonadotropin regulation have produced contradictory results that have been attributed to interspecies variations, sexual dimorphism, or differences in model systems. Nevertheless, current data suggest that these steroids exert their effects at both the hypothalamus and the anterior pituitary.

Estrogen, progesterone, and androgen receptors have been identified in the gonadotrope cells of multiple species, including the monkey, consistent with the ability of the associated steroid to act directly on the anterior pituitary.[96, 97] Within the hypothalamus, receptors for the sex steroids have been identified in multiple neuronal cell types, including those that release dopamine and β-endorphin; however, receptors have not been detected in the GnRH-containing neurons of the arcuate nucleus.[98, 99] These data suggest that the gonadal steroids alter hypothalamic GnRH release indirectly through modulation of neural systems known to impinge on GnRH neurons. Interestingly, however, both positive and negative estrogen-responsive DNA-regulatory regions have been identified in the GnRH gene promoter with use of heterologous (non-GnRH) cell lines, implying a direct action that requires further investigation.[100]

Depending on the reproductive state, estrogen can either increase or decrease gonadotropin gene expression. Loss of estrogen feedback after ovariectomy is associated with marked increases in circulating levels of LH and FSH as well as elevated α-subunit, LH-β, and FSH-β mRNA levels.[101] Estradiol replacement reverses this postcastration increase in gonadotropin subunit mRNAs, most likely through decreases in transcription rate.[102]

The majority of estrogen's inhibitory effects are likely to be mediated through the pituitary gland. Hypothalamic-lesioned (i.e., GnRH-deficient) monkeys given hourly infusions of GnRH demonstrate decreased LH secretion in response to estradiol.[103] Furthermore, estrogen has been shown to decrease GnRH-mediated LH secretion but not unstimulated secretion in cultured pituitary cells.[104] Other investigations have indicated that estrogen may also exert negative effects at the level of the hypothalamic pulse generator. For example, estradiol administration in monkeys leads to a decrease in LH pulse frequency, known to reflect GnRH pulsatility.[105]

Estrogen exerts positive feedback effects on gonadotropin secretion at the time of the midcycle LH surge. This effect is estimated to require a sustained serum estradiol concentration of more than 200 pg/ml for approximately 50 hours in women.[106] In support of a pituitary site of action, Knobil[103] has demonstrated that the entire monkey menstrual cycle, including the gonadotropin surge, can be artificially induced by estradiol treatment in hypothalamic-lesioned animals. Hypothalamic actions may also contribute to the positive estrogen effects, however, because GnRH release pulse frequency is increased at the time of the LH surge.[107]

Progesterone effects have been even more difficult to define and may be dependent on estrogen priming. In a rat model system, estrogen treatment decreased α-subunit and LH β-subunit mRNA levels. Whereas progesterone treatment alone had no effect, administration of progesterone in the presence of estrogen resulted in synergistic suppression of the mRNA levels of these subunits. At least part of this effect may be achieved through a decrease in GnRH pulse frequency mediated through increases in the hypothalamic β-endorphin system.[108]

Androgens are also likely to exert effects at both the hypothalamus and pituitary, with differential effects on each of the gonadotropin subunit genes. As noted previously, estradiol replacement suppresses the postovariectomy rise in all three gonadotropin subunit mRNAs. In contrast, testosterone treatment after orchiectomy decreases α-subunit and LH β-subunit mRNA levels but fails to blunt FSH-β mRNA levels.[101] The differential expression of the gonadotropin genes may be attributed to opposing effects on FSH-β gene expression between the hypothalamus and the pituitary. In vivo and in vitro experiments in both sexes have suggested that, within the pituitary, androgens stimulate FSH-β mRNA levels and FSH secretion with minimal if any effects on α or LH-β gene expression.[109, 110] In contrast, within the hypothalamus, androgens most likely exert an inhibitory action, as demonstrated in men by an increase in LH pulsatility after androgen receptor blockade with flutamide.[111]

Activin-Inhibin-Follistatin System

Within the past decade, three polypeptide factors—inhibin, activin, and follistatin—have been isolated from follicular fluid on the basis of their selective effects on FSH gene expression. As suggested by their names, inhibin decreases and activin stimulates gonadotrope function. Follistatin also suppresses FSH-β gene expression, but at approximately one third the potency of inhibin. Whereas changes in LH-β gene expression have been detected in the presence of these peptides in some experimental situations, these effects have generally been of low magnitude and have been limited to interactive effects with GnRH. Therefore, although they may play a minor role in the modulation of LH expression, these three peptides are appropriately considered to be FSH-dominant in their effects.[112, 113]

Inhibin and activin are closely related peptides consisting of an α-subunit (relative molecular mass M_r = 18 kDa) linked by a disulfide bridge to one of two highly homologous β-subunits (approximate M_r = 14 kDa) to form either inhibin A ($\alpha\beta_A$) or inhibin B ($\alpha\beta_B$). Activin is composed of homodimers or heterodimers of the same β-subunits to form activin A ($\beta_A\beta_A$), activin AB ($\beta_A\beta_B$), or activin B ($\beta_B\beta_B$).[114, 115] More recently, a third β-subunit (β_C) has been identified.[116] On the basis of the β-subunit protein sequence, activin belongs to the TGF-β superfamily, a group of growth and differentiation factors that includes TGF-β, müllerian-inhibiting substance, and the bone morphogenic proteins.

It is currently unknown whether the different isoforms of inhibin and activin serve divergent functions. The preferential formation of αβ (inhibin) versus ββ (activin) dimers in cells that produce both subunits is also poorly understood. Differential expression of the two subunits probably serves as one regulatory mechanism, with an excess of α-subunits shifting production toward inhibin. Nevertheless, the biochemical relatedness of activin and inhibin provides a system in which cells may alternate relatively easily between the production of two factors with opposing actions.[112]

Follistatin (FS) is structurally unrelated to either inhibin or activin. A highly glycosylated polypeptide, follistatin is organized into three homologous domains. Alternative mRNA splicing produces a longer mRNA that encodes FS-

315 and a shorter mRNA form that encodes FS-288. The latter C-truncated form is believed to have increased biologic potency. The existence of two follistatin isoforms may provide a mechanism for the control of follistatin activity through alterations in post-transcriptional processing.[117–119]

Just as activin structurally resembles TGF-β, the activin receptor and signaling system demonstrates homology to the TGF-β receptor system. Activin receptors can be divided into two major classes: type I (Act-RI) and type II (Act-RII), each of which contains multiple isoforms.[120] As currently understood for the activin receptor B isoforms, it is believed that activin binds directly to Act-RIIB, a serine-threonine kinase, thereby increasing association with Act-RIB. Formation of this complex results in the hyperphosphorylation of Act-RIB, which in turn activates a member of the Mad transcription factor family. Activation of cytoplasmic Mad protein promotes translocation to the nucleus, where this protein, in conjunction with other coactivators, regulates gene transcription.[121, 122] As predicted by the well-described ability of activin to modulate gonadotrope function, the mRNAs that encode both the Act-RI and Act-RII receptors have been detected in whole pituitaries from a number of species as well as from a gonadotrope-derived mouse cell line.[123] Of note, studies have thus far failed to identify an inhibin-specific receptor. Because inhibin can bind to the Act-RII receptor, inhibin may act through competition with activin for activin receptor sites. The isolation of a follistatin receptor has also remained elusive. It has been demonstrated, however, that follistatin can bind to the common activin/inhibin β-subunit and that follistatin inhibits the interaction of activin A with the activin type II receptor. These results suggest that follistatin may act through modulation of activin or inhibin action.[124]

Of the three gonadal peptides, inhibin is currently believed to be the most important of the peptides for the feedback regulation of gonadotropin gene expression. In contrast, activin and follistatin effects on gonadotrope function most likely occur through the action of locally released peptides acting as autocrine/paracrine factors, as described later in this chapter.

Serum inhibin levels are widely regulated during the menstrual cycle as well as across stages of the reproductive life. Across the menstrual cycle, serum inhibin levels are estimated to range from 100 IU/L to more than 1500 IU/L.[125] Inhibin levels remain low in the follicular phase, correlating with a period of increasing FSH-β gene expression. During the luteal phase, circulating inhibin levels increase sharply, peaking in the midluteal phase and decreasing abruptly at the luteal-follicular transition, at which time FSH levels again begin to rise. This circulating inhibin is believed to be primarily gonadal in origin because serum levels drop abruptly after castration.[126] The correlation between circulating inhibin levels and FSH secretion is consistent with a role for inhibin in the modulation of pituitary function by a feedback mechanism.

Activin can also be detected in the serum; however, in contrast to inhibin, activin levels are relatively low and remain stable across the reproductive cycle.[126] The accurate measurement of dimeric activin and inhibin has been complicated by the high levels of binding proteins, both follistatin and α_2-macroglobulin, in serum and follicular fluid, as well as by difficulty in distinguishing dimeric proteins from free α-subunit.

Follistatin is also present in serum and may be produced by the ovary, with follicular levels exceeding circulating levels by as much as 150-fold. Nevertheless, follistatin levels have been found to be similar in eugonadal women, GnRH-deficient women, postmenopausal women, and women after oophorectomy, arguing against the ovary as the source of circulating follistatin. Furthermore, serum follistatin levels are stable across the menstrual cycle, suggesting that circulating follistatin may not play a significant role in the regulation of gonadotrope function.[127, 128]

Although they were originally isolated from the follicular fluid, it is now evident that these so-called gonadal peptides are expressed by a wide variety of reproductive and nonreproductive tissues and subserve diverse, tissue-specific functions beyond the control of FSH secretion.[129] Because these peptides are often present in low concentrations, most of the information regarding tissue distribution has been based on the detection of the corresponding mRNAs. Despite this caveat, the mRNAs that encode the inhibin/activin subunits, follistatin, and the activin receptor have been detected in the pituitary, ovary, testes, and placenta as well as in the brain, liver, kidney, adrenal, and bone marrow.

Within the pituitary, the gonadotropes as well as other cell subtypes have been shown to secrete follistatin and to produce the inhibin/activin α- and β-subunits.[129–131] Pituitary cells have been shown to contain dimeric activin β_B, which is functionally active, because treatment with an activin-blocking antibody decreases FSH secretion both in vivo and in vitro.[132, 133] Whereas inhibin α-subunit is present in gonadotropes, the production of αβ dimers (i.e., inhibin) has yet to be proven. Therefore, gonadotropin gene expression is modulated by members of the activin-inhibin-follistatin system that are produced both locally and in the gonads.

Pituitary-derived follistatin and inhibin/activin α- and β_B-subunit mRNAs are increased after ovariectomy in female rats. Treatment with exogenous estradiol prevents the increase in inhibin subunit expression while further augmenting the increase in follistatin gene expression.[130, 134] GnRH has also been demonstrated to increase follistatin mRNA and protein expression.[135] Pituitary follistatin mRNA levels have also been found to increase at the time of the periovulatory gonadotropin surge.[123] Therefore, GnRH and gonadal steroids may regulate gonadotropin gene expression directly as well as by altering intrapituitary levels of these three peptides, which in turn modulate FSH expression, allowing fine-tuning of pituitary function.

Within the ovary, activin acts to increase FSH-induced aromatase activity, FSH receptor expression, and LH receptor expression; follistatin appears to blunt many of these effects. Therefore, activin may act at the pituitary to increase FSH secretion while simultaneously increasing FSH sensitivity at the level of the ovary. These peptides may also modulate the process of spermatogenesis, for example, by activin-induced stimulation of spermatogonial proliferation.

The ability of activin, inhibin, and follistatin to regulate gonadotropin biosynthesis and secretion has been firmly established by use of a wide variety of in vitro and in vivo model systems. Injection of recombinant human inhibin preparations into both immature and adult-ovariectomized animals has been shown to suppress selectively both FSH-β mRNA and serum FSH levels. In the same system, injected recombinant activin increased FSH-β gene expression. Conversely, infusion with antiserum against the inhibin α-subunit produces marked hypersecretion of FSH in rats and monkeys.[136, 137] It is not yet known whether these increases in FSH-β mRNA levels are due to increased synthesis or stability of the mRNA; however, evidence is accumulating to suggest that both mechanisms are operative.[138]

Similar results have been detected with use of in vitro systems. Treatment of static pituitary cell cultures with purified porcine inhibin or follistatin significantly decreases FSH β-subunit mRNA levels with parallel decreases in FSH secretion. In contrast, exogenous recombinant human activin stimulates FSH-β gene expression[139] (Fig. 3–10). In a pituitary perifusion system, activin increases and inhibin decreases FSH-β mRNA levels when it is given alone or in the presence of pulsatile GnRH. This activin effect is blunted by cotreatment with inhibin, consistent with competition of activin and inhibin for the same receptors. In secretory studies, activin increases basal FSH secretion and augments GnRH-mediated FSH pulses.[133]

These peptides may also regulate gonadotropin biosynthesis by mechanisms beyond direct activation of the FSH-β gene. For example, activin A induces GnRH-R biosynthesis as well as increasing the proportion of immunoreactive FSH-containing cells in pituitary cell culture.[66, 140, 141]

DNA-Regulatory Elements in the Gonadotropin Genes

Studies have begun to elucidate the molecular mechanisms by which regulation of gonadotropin subunit gene expression is achieved. The activation or inhibition of gene transcription is attained through the interaction of nuclear transcription factors (proteins) with *cis*-acting DNA-regulatory sequences (*cis* elements) present in the promoter region of the gene located 5′ (upstream) of the transcriptional start site. These protein-DNA interactions provide basal, tissue-specific, and hormonally responsive gene expression. Of the gonadotropin genes, the transcriptional regulation of the α-subunit gene has been most thoroughly characterized, as seen in Figure 3–11.

The human glycoprotein α-subunit is expressed in the gonadotropes and thyrotropes of the anterior pituitary gland as well as in the placenta, contributing to the synthesis of the gonadotropins, TSH, and hCG, respectively. Pituitary-specific expression of the the α-subunit gene has been attributed to the presence of both a pituitary glycoprotein basal element that binds LH-2 and a gonadotrope-specific element (GSE) that binds the transcription factor steroidogenic factor 1 (SF-1).[142–144] The α-subunit gene promoter also contains an upstream regulatory element, a trophoblast-specific element, and tandem repeat CREs, all critical for placenta-specific expression.[145, 146]

Hormonally responsive *cis*-acting regulatory regions have also been identified in the human α-subunit gene promoter, including an activating GnRH response element and a repressor (inhibitory) androgen response element.[147, 148] It remains unclear whether the α-subunit gene promoter contains an estrogen response element. Whereas estrogen regulates expression of DNA constructs containing the α-subunit gene promoter, the promoter region lacks a high-affinity estrogen binding site.[149]

Only recently have investigators begun to identify the DNA-regulatory elements that are responsible for transcriptional regulation of the gonadotropin β-subunit genes. On the basis of studies in transgenic mice, gonadotrope-specific expression of the LH-β gene has been attributed to the proximal 776 base pairs of the 5′ flanking sequence.[150] A functional estrogen response element has also been detected in the rat LH-β gene promoter. Interestingly, LH-β gene expression was stimulated in the presence of this promoter sequence, perhaps providing a molecular explanation for the positive feedback effects of estrogen, at least in this species.[27]

In vivo and in vitro data have also implicated the orphan nuclear receptor SF-1 in regulation of LH-β gene promoter activity. SF-1 is expressed in the pituitary gland, the adrenal gland, and the gonads and has been shown to play a role in sexual differentiation and in the regulation of steroidogenic enzyme activity. SF-1 is also essential for the formation of the ventromedial hypothalamus, a region believed to be important for reproductive behavior. Within the pituitary, SF-1 expression is restricted to the gonadotrope subpopulation, consistent with a role in regulation of the gonadotropin subunits. Transgenic mice null for expression of SF-1 fail to express LH-β or FSH-β mRNAs and exhibit markedly reduced levels of α-subunit mRNA.[151, 152] In vitro studies have confirmed the ability of SF-1 to bind to and transactivate the rat LH-β promoter through action at two GSEs, and the mutation of the 5′ GSE site in the bovine LH-β promoter nearly eliminates promoter activity in a transgenic mouse model.[153, 154] Studies have also defined the presence of two functional DNA-binding sites for the immediate early gene product, Egr-1.[155] These Egr-1 regulatory elements may be important in mediating hormone responsiveness in this gene because Egr-1 expression can be increased by activation of the protein kinase C system, a major signaling pathway for GnRH. Investigations have also suggested a role for the transcription factor Sp1 in the mediation of GnRH responsiveness.

The FSH-β gene promoter is known to contain two AP-1 (jun/fos)–binding sites that provide protein kinase C responsiveness. By sequence analysis, the FSH-β gene promoter also contains nucleotide regions with homology to the GSE and the GnRH response elements found in the α-subunit; however, it is not yet known whether these sequences have functional significance.

GONADOTROPIN RECEPTORS

The receptors for the glycoprotein hormones are located in the plasma membrane where they interact with hormones present in the extracellular fluid. Whereas receptors are expressed at relatively low concentrations (thousands per cell), they exhibit high affinity and specificity.[156] The interaction between receptor and dimeric hormone leads to a conformational change in the receptor, which in turn activates a membrane-associated, G protein–coupled signaling system. Interestingly, receptor binding and receptor activa-

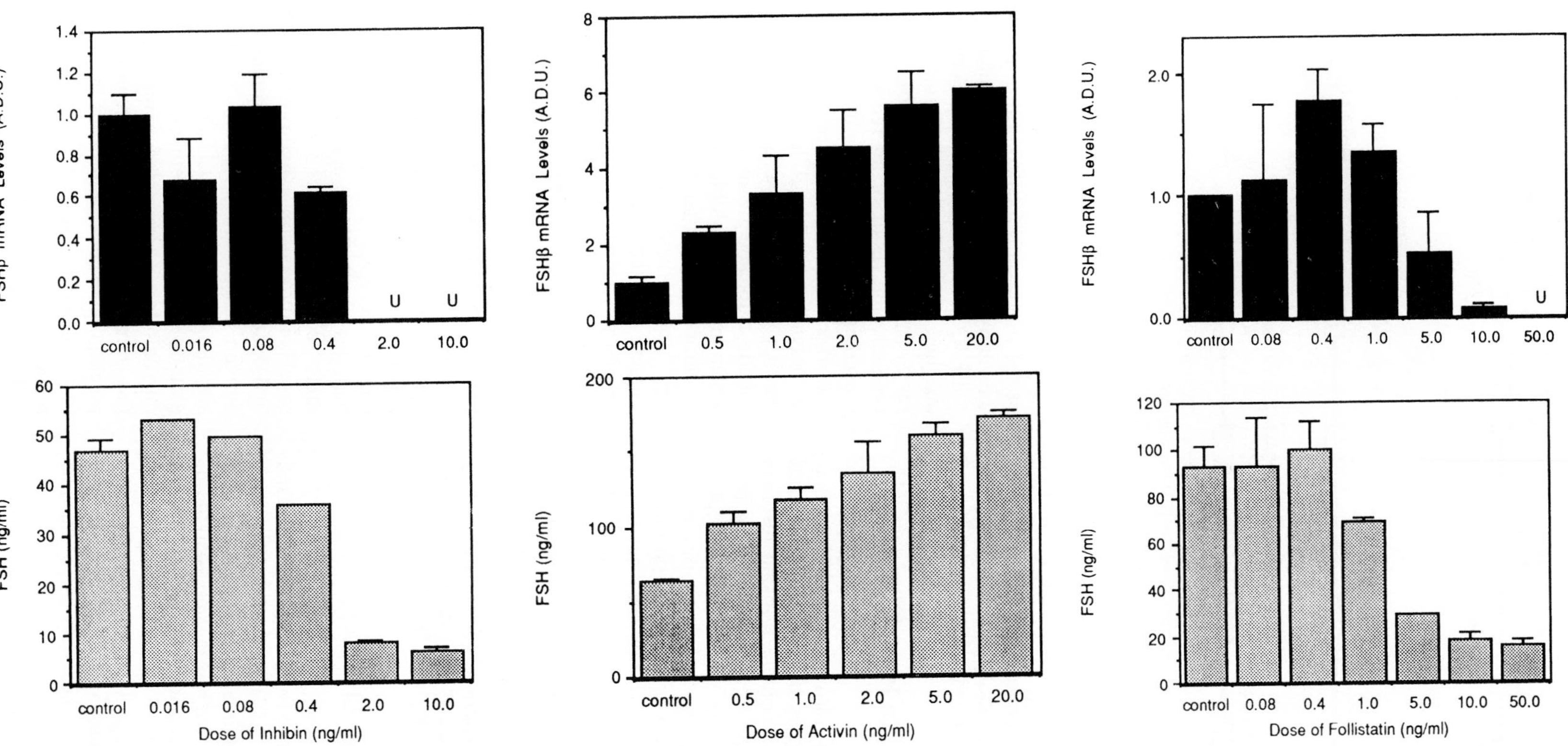

Figure 3–10 ■ Effects of recombinant human activin, purified porcine inhibin, and purified porcine follistatin on FSH β-subunit mRNA levels and FSH secretion by male rat primary pituitary cell cultures. (From Carroll RS, Corrigan AZ, Gharib SD, et al. Inhibin, activin, and follistatin: Regulation of follicle-stimulating hormone messenger ribonucleic acid levels. Mol Endocrinol 3:1969–1976, 1989.)

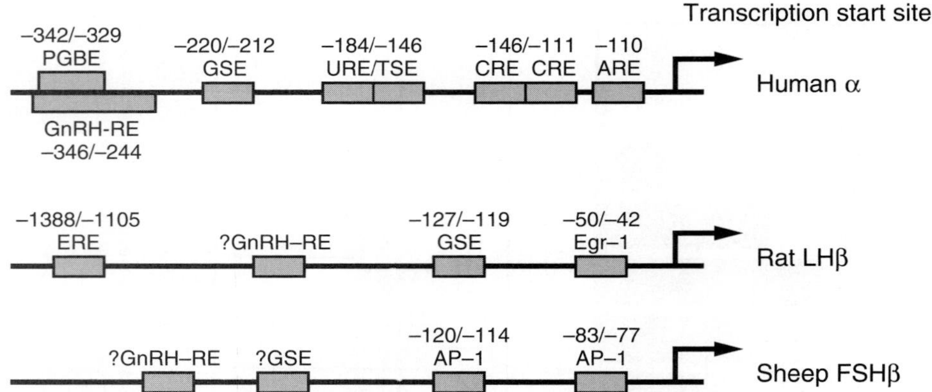

Figure 3–11 ■ Schematic representation of characterized and putative DNA-regulatory elements among the promoters of the gonadotropin subunit genes. PGBE, pituitary glycoprotein basal element; GSE, gonadotrope-specific element; URE, upstream regulatory element; TSE, trophoblast-specific element; CRE, AMP response element; ARE, androgen response element; ERE, estrogen response element; GnRH-RE, gonadotropin-releasing hormone response element; Egr-1, early growth response protein 1 regulatory element; AP-1, activating protein 1 regulatory element.

tion with intracellular signal generation are distinct events that can be separated experimentally and that may be differentially affected in pathologic states.

Characterization of Peptide Hormone Receptors

The ability of the glycoprotein hormones to bind to their receptors has been characterized by the use of radiolabeled ligands. Glycoprotein hormones contain tyrosine residues that can be radioiodinated with ^{125}I without altering biologic activity. The binding affinity of hormone receptors is determined by adding increasing concentrations of the radioactive hormone to a known quantity of purified or membrane-bound receptor and allowing the reaction to reach equilibrium. The amount of "free" hormone is then compared with the amount of "bound" hormone. The concentration of free hormone causing half-maximal saturation of the sites is equal to the molar dissociation constant, K_d.[157, 158] The K_d is the reciprocal of the association constant, K_a. The latter is often applied to hormone-binding data because its magnitude increases with increasing affinity as derived from the equation $K_a = [HR]/ [H][R]$.

Structural Features of the LH Receptor Gene and Protein

Of the LH and FSH receptors, the former has been studied most extensively. Because both LH and hCG bind to a single receptor, the LH receptor is also known as the LH/CG receptor. This receptor is a single-chain polypeptide of 674 (ovary) or 669 (testis) amino acids whose cDNAs have recently been cloned.[159–161] Because of the slightly higher affinity of hCG for this receptor as well as the availability of purified hCG preparations, many of the properties of the LH/CG receptor have been determined with use of hCG as the ligand.

The LH/CG receptor gene has been localized to chromosome 2 in humans.[162] Unlike most members of the G protein family, which are encoded by a single exon, the LH/CG receptor consists of 10 introns and 11 exons. All of the introns are located within the region coding for the unusually long extracellular domain.[163]

LH/CG receptor mRNA transcripts demonstrate marked size heterogeneity, with three major species detected in the rat ovary (5.8, 2.6, and 2.3 kb).[164] The size variations are probably the result of altered mRNA splicing in view of the complex intronic structure of this gene, although the use of alternative transcriptional start sites and variations in polyadenylation tail length may also contribute.[163] A number of lesser transcripts have also been identified that encode truncated forms of the LH/CG receptor, some of which are water soluble and therefore have been postulated to compete with membrane-bound forms for ligand binding.[165] Nevertheless, most of the currently available data suggest that these alternative forms do not participate in normal physiology.

In most systems studied, the various LH/CG receptor mRNA species are regulated in parallel, with the largest species being consistently the most abundant.[164] Furthermore, receptor protein levels are closely correlated to mRNA levels in states of both induction and homologous desensitization.

As indicated earlier, by sequence homology, the gonadotropin hormone receptors are members of the G protein–coupled receptor superfamily, a family of receptors that includes the GnRH, β-adrenergic, α-adrenergic, and dopamine receptors[43] (Fig. 3–12). Members of this receptor superfamily contain a hydrophilic extracellular domain, a hydrophobic transmembrane domain, and an intracellular domain. Characteristic of receptors that couple to G protein signaling systems, the LH/CG receptor transmembrane region spans the cell membrane seven times. Whereas the intracellular C-terminal domain is short for a member of this family, the LH/CG receptor exhibits a number of potential phosphorylation sites that have been demonstrated to be important for protein activation and deactivation in related receptors.[159]

The extracellular domain of the LH/CG receptor is large, comprising nearly half of the amino acids. The presence of this domain has been shown to be both necessary and sufficient for hormone binding. This extracellular region is

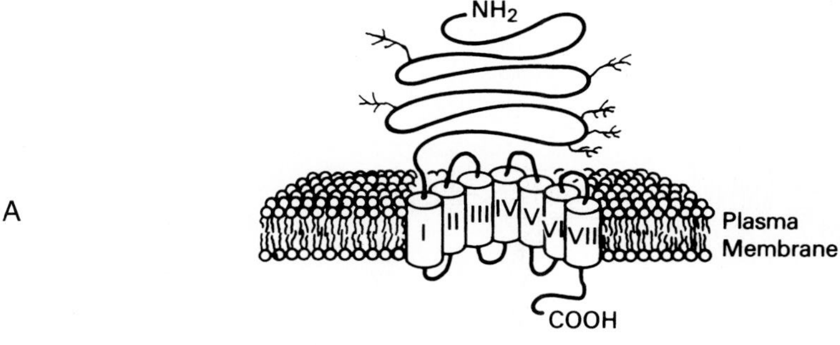

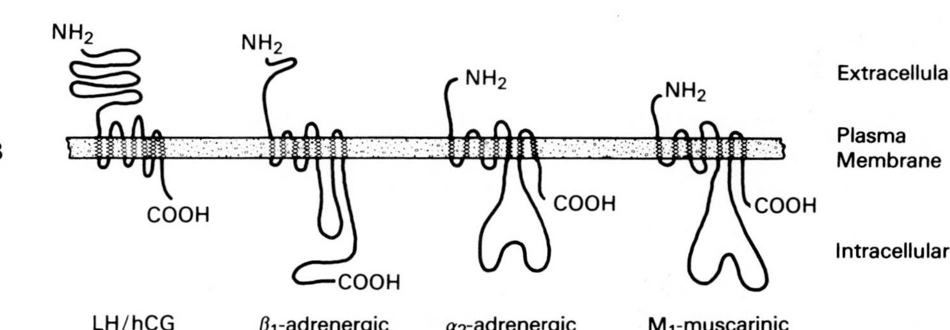

Figure 3–12 ■ Structure of the LH receptor. *A*, General structure of extracellular region and transmembrane domains. *B*, Comparison of LH receptor with other G protein–coupled receptors indicating the differences in extracellular regions and third intracellular loops.

also notable for containing 14 copies of a so-called leucine-rich repeat. This repeated motif may allow formation of amphipathic helices that would allow the hydrophilic surface of the extracellular domain to interact with the hydrophobic transmembrane domain, theoretically providing a mechanism for receptor activation after formation of the hormone-receptor complex.[166]

The extracellular domain also contains six potential *N*-linked glycosylation sites. Although it is presently unclear which of these sites are glycosylated in the native receptor, each of these sites is conserved across species, implying functional significance. Because molecular size is decreased after deglycosylation, it is clear that at least some of these sites are glycosylated in the intact state.[167] To determine the role of glycosylation in receptor function, investigators have either mutated the putative glycosylated amino acid residues to nonglycosylated residues or have treated receptor preparations with glycosidases. Because mutations in the receptor frequently impair receptor expression on the cell surface, these experiments have been somewhat difficult to interpret. Nevertheless, current data suggest that glycosylation does not significantly alter receptor binding affinity but may be a critical determinant of tertiary receptor function, which is in turn required for receptor activation.[168]

In an attempt to localize the exact site of the hormone-receptor interaction, hCG binding affinity has been compared between the native and either *N*-terminal truncated or internally deleted mutant receptors. As an alternative approach, artificially synthesized peptides containing regions of the extracellular domain or the extracellular connecting loops of the transmembrane domain have been tested for their ability to compete with the native receptor for binding radiolabeled hCG. These studies suggest that hCG contacts its receptor in the region of extracellular domain residues 21 to 38, 102 to 115, and 253 to 272 as well as in a portion of the third connecting loop.[169]

Gonadotropin Receptor Second Messenger Signaling Pathways

The LH and FSH receptors are coupled to a subset of guanosine triphosphate (GTP)–binding regulatory proteins, or G proteins, that activate the protein kinase A system (Fig. 3–13). G proteins are heterotrimers consisting of a stimulatory α-subunit ($G_{s\alpha}$) with GTP-ase activity linked to a complex consisting of one β and one γ chain. The interaction of gonadotropin with its receptor leads to activation of the receptor, presumably through the induction of conformational changes in receptor structure. Formation of the gonadotropin-receptor complex results in the replacement of α-subunit–bound guanosine diphosphate with GTP, leading to dissociation of the G protein α-subunit from the βγ complex. The free α-subunit then binds to adenylate cylase, which converts adenosine triphosphate to cAMP, increasing intracellular cAMP levels, which activate protein kinase A. Protein kinase A modulates the function of a wide variety of intracellular proteins through phosphorylation at specifically defined serine and threonine amino acid residues.[170]

Whereas the majority of data implicates cAMP as the principal mediator of LH and FSH receptor actions, additional evidence suggests that activation of the protein kinase C pathway may also occur. In this pathway, a different G protein, G_q, is linked to the gonadotropin receptor. Activation of this G complex activates phospholipase C, which cleaves membrane phospholipids to produce inositol 1,4,5-triphosphate ($InsP_3$) and 1,2-diacylglycerol (DAG). $InsP_3$

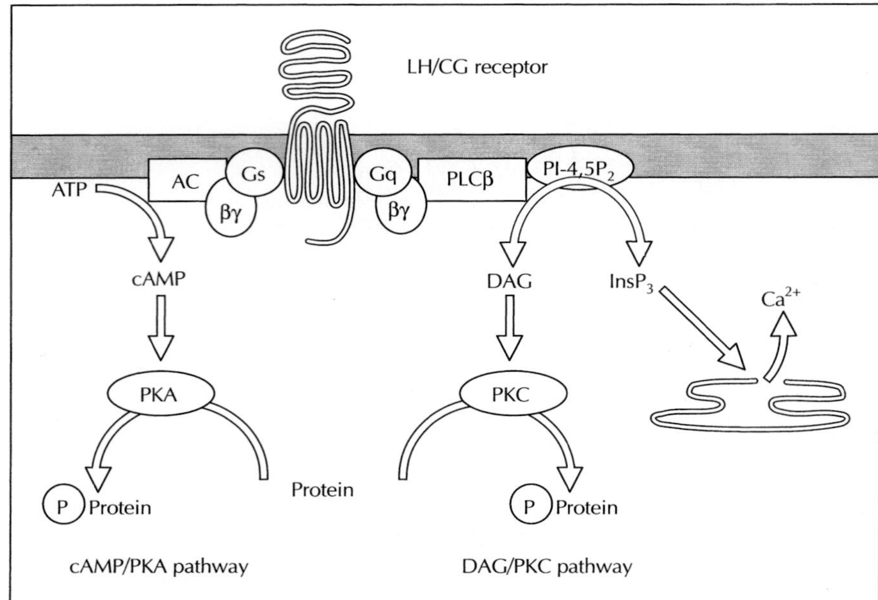

Figure 3–13 ■ Ligand interaction with the LH/CG receptor activates multiple signal transduction pathways. Inositol 1,4,5-triphosphate ($InsP_3$) mobilizes intracellular Ca^{2+} from the endoplasmic reticulum. The second messengers cAMP and diacylglycerol (DAG) activate families of serine-threonine protein kinases, protein kinase A (PKA) and protein kinase C (PKC), respectively, which phosphorylate specific intracellular proteins. (From Davis JS. Mechanisms of hormone action: Luteinizing hormone receptors and second-messenger pathways. Curr Opin Obstet Gynecol 6:254–261, 1994.)

causes the release of sequestered calcium into the intracellular space, increasing cytosolic calcium levels; DAG activates protein kinase C.

Thus, the gonadotropin receptors may stimulate both the protein kinase A and C signaling pathways. Activation of phospolipase C generally requires higher doses of LH/CG than are needed to achieve increases in cAMP levels, and the degree of phospholipase C activation is often lower than can be attained with other protein kinase C activators tested in the same system. Characterization of gonadotropin receptor–mediated signal transduction is further complicated by the existence of multiple adenylate cyclase and protein kinase C isoforms, each of which may be expressed in a cell-specific manner.[169, 171]

Desensitization

In addition to cell activation, the process of a hormone's binding to its receptor also initiates a process called desensitization, which reduces the cell's responsiveness to repetitive or ongoing stimulation. Homologous desensitization is attained through a fast mechanism, termed uncoupling, that occurs within minutes as well as through a slower process termed down-regulation.

In uncoupling, post-translational modifications in the receptor result in reduced receptor activity without changes in receptor number. Whereas the exact modifications involved have yet to be elucidated, uncoupling is known to require the presence of the C-terminal (intracellular) portion of the receptor.[172] Largely on the basis of studies of the β-adrenergic receptor, uncoupling may involve receptor autophosphorylation.[173] Although it has been shown that both ovarian and testicular LH/CG receptor can be phosphorylated after hCG treatment or by the catalytic subunit of protein kinase A, uncoupling of the receptor from the adenylate cyclase system has not been uniformly correlated with phosphorylation.[167, 174]

Down-regulation is achieved initially through an increase in the rate of receptor internalization and lysosomal accumulation, resulting in an increased degradation rate. In the second phase of down-regulation, which occurs after 3 to 4 hours, receptor biosynthesis is decreased as indicated by a decrease in steady-state receptor mRNA levels.[169, 175]

Tissue Distribution of the Gonadotropin Receptors

As implied by their names, gonadotropin receptor expression is classically thought to be restricted to gonadal cell populations. Whereas FSH receptor expression appears to be restricted to the granulosa cells of the ovary and Sertoli cells of the testes, studies have identified LH/CG receptors in the human endometrium, myometrium, fallopian tubes, and brain.[176, 177] These results clearly suggest extragonadal functions for the gonadotropins that remain to be elucidated.[178]

Within the ovary, the LH/CG receptor is expressed on differentiated granulosa, luteal, theca, and interstitial cells. Although levels of LH/CG receptor mRNA are nearly undetectable in the granulosa cells of preantral follicles, these levels are markedly increased with development to the preovulatory stage.[177] In ovarian theca cells, LH/CG receptor mRNA expression is detectable in preantral follicles. As observed for granulosa cells, theca LH/CG receptor mRNA levels are also induced during follicular maturation; however, the degree of induction is less pronounced than observed in granulosa cells.[177, 179] Corpus luteum cells express high levels of LH/CG receptor transcripts, with maintenance of expression dependent on prolactin or placental lactogen stimulation, at least in the rat.[180]

FSH Receptor Gene

The FSH receptor gene extends over 85 kilobases and contains 10 exons, 9 of which encode the extracellular domain. The human FSH receptor contains 678 amino acids and shows significant sequence similarity to the LH/CG receptor, with more than 80 percent homology in the transmembrane region.[181] As in the LH/CG receptor, the FSH receptor contains a large extracellular domain with a leucine-rich repeat region as well as multiple potential *N*-linked glycosylation sites (four rather than the six identified in the LH/CG receptor).[182] In common with the LH/CG receptor, the FSH receptor acts primarily through the cAMP signaling system.

REGULATION OF GONADAL FUNCTION BY GONADOTROPINS

LH and FSH exert their effects through activation of gonadotropin receptors present on the plasma membrane of granulosa and theca cells (in the ovary) and Sertoli and Leydig cells (in the testes). Activation of these receptors, in turn, stimulates the adenylate cyclase system to regulate both steroidogenesis and gametogenesis. Strong parallels exist between gonadotropin action in the ovary and the testes. In this section, we focus on ovarian effects; the role of gonadotropins in testicular function is discussed in Chapter 23.

Regulation of Follicular Maturation

A defined sequence of hormonal changes is required for normal follicular development and steroidogenesis. The concentration of gonadotropins and steroids in human follicular fluid has been determined across the menstrual cycle.[183] The concentrations of FSH, LH, estradiol, and progesterone in follicular fluid are generally highly correlated with circulating levels. During the midfollicular phase, however, the larger follicles (more than 8 mm) contain high levels of FSH despite falling levels of serum FSH, possibly reflecting retention of the hormone because FSH receptor levels are high in these follicles. Of note, even those granulosa cells that lack gonadotropin receptors may respond to gonadotropin stimuli owing to the presence of gap junctions between neighboring granulosa cells.[184]

The initiation of follicular growth can occur independently of gonadotropin stimulation, as demonstrated by early follicular maturation in gonadotropin-deficient mice.[185] Unless rescued by the early follicular rise in FSH, however, these early follicles will rapidly undergo atresia.[186] During the follicular phase of the menstrual cycle, FSH activates granulosa cell proliferation and steroidogenesis, inducing aromatase activity in the granulosa cells, which allows the conversion of thecally derived androgens to estrogens.[187, 188] FSH also regulates granulosa cell production of inhibin during the follicular phase; luteal inhibin synthesis is under the control of LH.[189, 190] Inhibin, in conjunction with a wide variety of locally produced growth factors and peptides, acts to modulate gonadotropin effects.

FSH regulates expression of its own receptor in a dose-dependent manner. As demonstrated in the rat, follicular levels of FSH lead to an increase in FSH receptor mRNA levels, whereas ovulatory surge concentrations decrease FSH receptor transcript number.[191] FSH also induces LH/CG receptor formation in granulosa cells, an effect that requires estradiol and is inhibited by androgens.[192, 193] FSH-stimulated increases in both FSH and LH/CG receptor expression are blunted by ovarian-derived epidermal growth factor and basic fibroblast growth factor as well as by GnRH.[191, 194]

LH/CG receptor number is further augmented by LH itself.[195] Consistent with observations for the FSH receptor, low levels of intracellular cAMP (as would be seen with low-dose FSH or LH) increase LH/CG receptor mRNA levels, whereas high concentrations produce a rapid decline in these transcripts.[179] Because receptor number and mRNA levels decrease abruptly after the midcycle gonadotropin surge, it has been postulated that an LH-induced increase in cAMP concentration is responsible for the decrease in receptor expression observed at this stage.

Whereas theca cells lack FSH receptors, LH/CG receptors are present in high numbers even in the early follicle. Although receptor number increases during follicular maturation, the change is less pronounced than observed in granulosa cells.[177, 179] Acting through its receptor, LH increases thecal expression of P450c17, the rate-limiting enzymatic step in the conversion of 21-carbon substrates into androgens. These androgens are a necessary precursor for the production of estrogens by granulosa cells, which lack the P450c17 enzyme.[196]

As antral formation progresses (in the periovulatory period), LH stimulates the expression of progesterone receptors on the granulosa cells of the dominant follicle,[197] promoting luteinization and early progesterone production, which slows granulosa cell proliferation.[198] Progesterone also enhances the positive feedback effects of estrogen, contributing to the development of the midcycle gonadotropin surge.[199]

Taken together, these observations suggest that LH and FSH play different but equally important roles in follicular development. FSH is important for early granulosa cell maturation, including the development of LH/CG receptors; LH, acting initially on the theca cells, promotes androgen production to supply substrate for aromatization to estrogen. As follicular maturation progresses, progesterone production begins in the granulosa cells under the influence of preovulatory LH secretion. This concept is supported by results obtained in gonadotropin-deficient women treated with recombinant human FSH. Whereas early follicular growth and low levels of estrogen production are observed in these women, the high estrogen levels required for induction of the LH surge and final follicular maturation are never attained. Thus, although only FSH is required for early folliculogenesis, full ovarian steroidogenesis is LH-dependent.[200, 201]

Midcycle Gonadotropin Surge

The midcycle LH surge leads to the resumption of meiosis, expansion of the cumulus oophorus, further luteinization of the granulosa cells, and synthesis of prostaglandins and plasminogen activator required for follicular rupture.[202] This elevation in LH serum levels normally lasts 48 to 50 hours, with ovulation occurring approximately 10 to 12 hours after peak levels are attained.[203, 204]

Many mechanisms have been proposed to explain the decline of the LH surge. The observed periovulatory decreases in pituitary GnRH-R number may lead to a decrease in the biosynthesis and secretion of LH.[33] Alternatively, decreased estrogen and increased circulating progesterone levels may contribute to the decrease in LH secretion through feedback at both the hypothalamus and pituitary. The existence of a gonadotropin surge-attenuating factor has also been postulated. Although the exact nature of this factor remains to be elucidated, it is believed to be an FSH-induced ovarian-derived peptide, distinct from inhibin, that acts at the pituitary to blunt the gonadotrope response to GnRH stimulation.[205]

Gonadotropin Action in the Luteal Phase

The luteal phase is characterized by increased progesterone production under the influence of LH.[190] On the basis of studies of human follicular development, normal luteal function requires the adequate induction of LH/CG receptors by FSH and estrogen during the follicular phase.[206] Decreased follicular-phase serum FSH levels are associated with depressed midluteal progesterone production as well as a decrease in luteal cell mass.[207] LH stimulates progesterone production through two major mechanisms: (1) induction of low-density lipoprotein (LDL) receptors, which allows increased uptake of LDL cholesterol, the substrate for progesterone production; and (2) increased expression of the mRNAs that encode P450scc and 3β-hydroxysteroid dehydrogenase, the steroidogenic enzymes required for progesterone synthesis.[208, 209] Whereas maintenance or a normal luteal phase is LH-dependent, demise of the corpus luteum approximately 14 days after ovulation does not appear to be due to changes in LH stimulation.[210] In contrast to nonprimate species, no luteolytic factor has been identified in the primate, although some studies suggest a role for estrogens, perhaps modulated by local prostaglandin levels.[211]

During the luteal-follicular transition, waning luteal cell biosynthetic capacity results in the loss of both inhibin and steroid (progesterone and estrogen) production.[212] Decreased circulating levels of inhibin allow an increase in FSH production, which in turn rescues the developing cohort of follicles from androgen-dominant atresia (primarily through induction of aromatase activity). Increased GnRH pulsatility secondary to the loss of inhibitory steroidal feedback also contributes to the rise in both FSH and LH serum levels.[213, 214]

GENETIC DISORDERS AFFECTING GONADOTROPIN EXPRESSION

Abnormal reproductive function due to alterations in gonadotropin expression could theoretically be caused by mutations in (1) the GnRH gene, (2) the GnRH-R gene, (3) the gonadotropin subunit genes, (4) the gonadotropin receptor genes, (5) G protein subunit genes required to transduce gonadotropin receptor signals, (6) genes that encode transcription factors that modulate gonadotropin biosynthesis, or (7) genes required for normal development of GnRH neurons or gonadotropes. These mutations could be either activating or inactivating and would be expected to present with predictable phenotypes. Mutations have now been described for a number of these categories, with the likelihood that more examples will be detected in the future.

Mutations Resulting in Abnormal GnRH Function

Although the GnRH gene has been sequenced in a number of patients with idiopathic hypogonadotropic hypogonadism (IHH), thus far no GnRH gene mutations have been identified.[215] In contrast, a family has been identified in which the presence of compound heterozygous mutations in the GnRH-R gene results in IHH. In this family, one of the mutant alleles contains a mutation in the first extracellular loop of the GnRH-R, resulting in decreased ligand binding. In the second mutant allele, mutation of the third intracellular loop decreases the ability of the bound receptor to activate phospholipase C.[216]

Interestingly, a subset of patients with the X-linked form of Kallmann's syndrome (IHH and anosmia) have been found to have mutations, not in the genes encoding GnRH or GnRH-R, but in the *KAL* gene, which encodes a neural cell adhesion–like molecule believed to be critical for normal migration of both olfactory and GnRH neurons from the olfactory placode.[215, 217] Mutation in the *KAL* gene causes GnRH deficiency, as confirmed by the pubertal development and fertility achieved in both males and females treated with exogenous GnRH.[73, 217]

Mutations in the Gonadotropin Genes

Inactivating mutations in both the LH-β and FSH-β genes have been described. A naturally occurring LH-β gene mutation (Arg for Gln at codon 54) produces hypogonadotropic hypogonadism in the homozygous state; heterozygous males have a high incidence of infertility. Interestingly, these patients have elevated immunoreactive LH levels with marked loss of bioactivity, which has been attributed to loss of receptor binding.[218] Additional LH-β sequence alterations have been detected, which occur in high frequency in the Finnish population (24 percent of alleles). These alterations are currently thought to represent polymorphisms, although ongoing studies suggest effects on bioactivity and hormonal half-life.[219, 220]

In the FSH-β gene, Matthews and colleagues[221] have identified a 2–base pair deletion at codon 61 that creates a premature termination codon, resulting in primary amenorrhea in the homozygous state. More recently, a female patient has been described who harbors both the codon 61 mutation and a missense mutation at codon 51. This patient, a compound heterozygote for FSH β-subunit mutations, presented with marked estrogen deficiency and delayed puberty due to inadequate ovarian aromatization.[222]

Mutations in the Gonadotropin Receptor Genes

Both activating and inactivating mutations have been identified in the genes that encode the gonadotropin receptors. Shenker and colleagues[223] reported an activating mutation in the LH receptor that produces familial male precocious puberty in heterozygotes. This mutation, an aspartate to glycine substitution at position 578, results in constitutive receptor activity as demonstrated by an increase in basal intracellular cAMP levels when this mutated receptor is expressed in an in vitro system. Females harboring this mutation are unaffected, because circulating estrogen levels are not altered in the presence of normal FSH receptor levels. It would be predicted, however, that these women may have elevations in ovarian androgen levels, a possibility that remains to be investigated. To date, 11 different LH receptor mutations have been described that produce a similar phenotype. Interestingly, the majority of these mutations are located in the sixth transmembrane segment and adjacent third intracellular loop, suggesting that this region of the receptor is critical for G protein coupling.

An inactivating missense mutation in the sixth transmembrane domain of LH receptor gene has also been described.[224] Although the mutant receptor binds hormone with normal affinity, it is unable to transduce a signal. Males homozygous for this mutation are unable to produce testosterone and therefore do not masculinize during development, resulting in male pseudohermaphroditism. Females with this mutation would be predicted to undergo normal female sexual differentiation; however, they would perhaps remain prepubertal owing to inadequate production of the androgen precursors required for pubertal levels of estrogen production.

An inactivating mutation has also been reported for the FSH receptor. This mutation, located in exon seven, adversely affects both hormone binding and signal transduction, producing hypergonadotropic ovarian failure in homozygous females. Homozygous males with the identical mutation were found to have variable degrees of spermatogenic failure, suggesting that FSH may be less important for male than for female fertility.[225, 226]

McCune-Albright Syndrome

In the McCune-Albright syndrome, a point mutation in the $G_{s\alpha}$ subunit produces ligand-independent activation of adenylate cyclase with an associated increase in cAMP accumulation. In the presence of this G protein mutation, the gonads function as if both the LH and FSH receptors are constitutively activated, resulting in gonadotropin-independent precocious puberty in both sexes. Because the $G_{s\alpha}$ subunit is expressed in a wide variety of tissues, this syndrome is associated with a large number of phenotypic abnormalities including polyostotic fibrous dysplasia (bony dysplasia), café au lait skin pigmentation changes, and other endocrine defects.[227]

Mutations Affecting Expression of DAX-1

Adrenal hypoplasia congenita is an X-linked disorder characterized by primary adrenal insufficiency and hypogonadotropic hypogonadism. This disorder has been linked to deletions and mutations in the gene that encodes for the transcription factor DAX-1.[228] Whereas the gonadotropin deficiency could be due to either a hypothalamic or pituitary defect, abnormal responses to exogenous GnRH in several patients suggest that at least part of the defect is at the level of the gonadotrope.[229] Studies have demonstrated that DAX-1 forms protein-protein interactions with the transcription factor SF-1. As described elsewhere in this chapter, SF-1 has been shown to regulate LH-β gene expression. Therefore, it has been postulated that DAX-1 may exert its effects indirectly by modulating SF-1 action.[230]

EUTOPIC AND ECTOPIC GONADOTROPIN SECRETION

The nature and significance of ectopic hormone secretion are considered in more detail elsewhere.

Abnormal synthesis and secretion of the gonadotropins occur in a variety of neoplasms. Hypersecretion of the glycoprotein hormone subunits by cells that normally express the gonadotropins (i.e., the pituitary gonadotropes and placental trophoblast) is termed eutopic production. Ectopic biosynthesis implies production of gonadotropins by a tumor whose cell of origin does not normally produce these peptides. Ectopic hormone production is generally attributed to the derepression or abnormal regulation of gene expression. Some investigators, however, have argued that nearly all normal tissues synthesize low levels of the peptide hormones (as detected by newly available, highly sensitive assays) and that all tumor production should therefore be deemed to be eutopic.[231]

Eutopic Production of Gonadotropins by Pituitary Neoplasms

Whereas the majority of patients with pituitary tumors demonstrate classical hypersecretory syndromes such as acromegaly or Cushing's disease, as many as one fourth of these patients have clinically nonfunctioning adenomas.[232] It has been determined by immunocytochemistry that the majority of these "nonfunctioning" tumors synthesize intact glycoprotein hormones or "free" (i.e., monomeric) glycoprotein hormone subunits. Although in vivo hormone production has proved more difficult to evaluate, increased levels of free α-subunit, the FSH β-subunit, and dimeric FSH are detected more commonly than intact LH. Interestingly, in contrast to the observed pattern in normal gonadotrophs, the FSH β-subunit is produced in excess of the α-subunit in FSH-secreting tumors.[233]

On the basis of their homogeneous pattern of X chromosome inactivation, pituitary adenomas are believed to be monoclonal in origin rather than the result of excessive stimulation of a polyclonal population.[234] Gonadotrope adenomas, often hormonally "silent," most commonly present as macroadenomas with symptoms and signs attributable to their size, such as visual changes, headache, and varying degrees of hypopituitarism. Reproductive abnormalities are usually in the form of hypogonadism secondary to destruction of the normal gonadotropes with inadequate gonadal stimulation by the aberrantly secreted, often monomeric gonadotropins. Mild hyperprolactinemia due to destruction of inhibitory dopamine pathways may also be present in these patients.[232] Rarely, eutopic secretion of LH or FSH may result in precocious puberty.[235]

Ectopic Production of Gonadotropins

Ectopic production of the gonadotropin subunits occurs in a wide variety of neoplasms. The most commonly detected subunits, the α-subunit and hCG β-subunit, may be produced by carcinomas of the lung, pancreas, liver, ovary, or cervix.[236, 237] As a result, elevations in serum gonadotropin subunit levels have proved to be a useful tumor marker during the management of these malignant neoplasms.[236, 238]

Comparisons of ectopically produced with pituitary-derived gonadotropin hormones have suggested differences primarily at the level of post-translational processing, although alterations in amino acid composition have also been observed. Despite chemical and immunologic similarity to the normal α-subunit, minimal functional activity is detected when a mixture of ectopic α-subunits and hCG β-subunits is tested in a rat testicular assay.[239] These results suggest that ectopic gonadotropin subunits may be relatively deficient either in their ability to form dimers or in their ability to activate the appropriate receptor once they are dimerized. As predicted by this observation, the majority of patients with gonadotropin-secreting tumors do not demonstrate reproductive abnormalities as the result of their malignant neoplasms. Nevertheless, a subset of patients may present with precocious puberty, a finding most commonly observed in males with tumors producing elevated serum hCG levels that stimulate testicular testosterone production.[240]

Acknowledgment

We acknowledge Dr. K. J. Catt and Dr. M. L. Dufau for the use of some of the materials in this chapter. Dr. Catt and Dr. Dufau were the authors of this chapter in the third edition.

References

1. Childs GV. Division of labor among gonadotropes. Vitamin Horm 50:215–286, 1995.
2. Childs GV. Functional ultrastructure of gonadotropes: A review. Curr Top Neuroendocrinol 7:49–97, 1986.
3. Childs GV, Hyde C, Naor Z, et al. Heterogeneous luteinizing hormone and follicle-stimulating hormone storage patterns in subtypes of gonadotropes separated by centrifugal elutriation. Endocrinology 113:2120–2128, 1983.
4. Childs GV, Naor Z, Hazum E, et al. Cytochemical characterization of pituitary target cells for biotinylated gonadotropin-releasing hormone. Peptides 4:549–555, 1983.
5. Pelletier G, Robert F, Hardy J. Identification of human anterior pituitary cells by immunoelectron microscopy. J Clin Endocrinol Metab 46: 534–542, 1978.
6. Wang CF, Lasley BL, Lein A, et al. The functional changes of the pituitary gonadotrophs during the menstrual cycle. J Clin Endocrinol Metab 42:718–728, 1976.
7. Thotakura NR, Blithe DL. Glycoprotein hormones: Glycobiology of gonadotrophins, thyrotrophin and free α subunit. Glycobiology 5:3–10, 1995.
8. Pierce JG, Parsons TF. Glycoprotein hormones: Structure and function. Annu Rev Biochem 50:465–495, 1981.
9. Chin WW. Glycoprotein hormone genes. *In* Habener JF (ed). Genes Encoding Hormones and Regulatory Peptides. Clifton, NJ, Humana Press, 1986, pp 137–172.
10. Ryan RJ, Charlesworth MC, McCormick DJ, et al. The glycoprotein hormones: Recent studies of structure-function relationships. FASEB J 2:2661–2669, 1988.
11. Gharib SD, Wierman ME, Shupnik MA, et al. Molecular biology of the pituitary gonadotropins. Endocr Rev 11:177–199, 1990.
12. Fiddes JC, Talmadge K. Structure, expression, and evolution of the genes for the human glycoprotein hormones. Recent Prog Horm Res 40:43–78, 1984.
13. Fiddes JC, Goodman HM. The gene encoding the common alpha subunit of the four human glycoprotein hormones. J Mol Appl Genet 1:3–18, 1981.
14. Talmadge K, Vamvakopoulos NC, Fiddes JC. Evolution of the genes for the beta subunits of human chorionic gonadotropin and luteinizing hormone. Nature 307:37–40, 1984.
15. Jameson JL, Becker CB, Lindell CM, et al. Human follicle-stimulating hormone β-subunit gene encodes multiple messenger ribonucleic acids. Mol Endocrinol 2:806–815, 1988.
16. Jameson JL, Chin WW, Hollenberg AN, et al. The gene encoding the β-subunit of rat luteinizing hormone. J Biol Chem 259:15474–15480, 1984.
17. Parsons TF, Pierce JG. Oligosaccharide moieties of glycoprotein hormones: Bovine lutropin resists enzymatic deglycosylation because of terminal *O*-sulfated *N*-acetylhexosamines. Proc Natl Acad Sci USA 77:7089–7093, 1980.
18. Baenziger JU. Regarding the glycoprotein hormones and their sulphated oligosaccharides (Letter). Glycobiology 5:459, 1995.
19. Baenziger JU. Glycosylation: To what end for the glycoprotein hormones? Endocrinology 137:1520–1522, 1996.
20. Chen H-C, Shimohigashi Y, Dufau ML, et al. Characterization and biological properties of chemically deglycosylated human chorionic gonadotropin. J Biol Chem 257:14446–14452, 1982.
21. Sairam MR. Role of carbohydrates in glycoprotein hormone signal transduction. FASEB J 3:1915–1926, 1989.
22. Parsons TF, Pierce JG. Free α-like material from bovine pituitaries: Removal of its *O*-linked oligosaccharide permits combination with lutropin-β. J Biol Chem 259:2662–2666, 1984.
23. Ulloa-Aguirre A, Midgley AR Jr, Beitins IZ, et al. Follicle-stimulating isohormones: Characterization and physiological relevance. Endocr Rev 16:765–787, 1995.
24. Matzuk MM, Boime I. Mutagenesis and gene transfer define site-specific roles of the gonadotropin oligosaccharides. Biol Reprod 40:48–53, 1989.
25. Lapthorn AJ, Harris DC, Littlejohn A, et al. Crystal structure of human chorionic gonadotropin. Nature 369:455–461, 1994.
26. Naylor SL, Chin WW, Goodman HM, et al. Chromosome assignments of genes encoding the alpha and beta subunits of glycoprotein hormones in man and mouse. Somat Cell Genet 9:757–770, 1983.
27. Shupnik WA, Weinmann CM, Notides AC, et al. An upstream region of the rat luteinizing hormone β gene binds estrogen receptor and confers estrogen responsiveness. J Biol Chem 264:80–86, 1989.
28. Gharib SD, Roy A, Wierman ME, et al. Isolation and characterization of the gene encoding the β-subunit of rat follicle-stimulating hormone. DNA 8:339–349, 1989.
29. Clayton RN. Gonadotropin-releasing hormone: Its actions and receptors. Endocr Rev 120:11–19, 1989.
30. Conn PM. The molecular basis of gonadotropin-releasing hormone action. Endocr Rev 7:3–10, 1986.
31. Marian J, Cooper RL, Conn PM. Regulation of the rat pituitary gonadotropin-releasing hormone receptor. Mol Pharmacol 19:399–405, 1981.
32. Loumaye E, Catt KJ. Homologous regulation of gonadotropin-releasing hormone receptors in cultured pituitary cells. Science 215:983–985, 1982.
33. Katt JA, Duncan JA, Herbon L, et al. The frequency of gonadotropin-releasing hormone stimulation determines the number of pituitary gonadotropin-releasing hormone receptors. Endocrinology 116:2113–2115, 1985.
34. Kaiser UB, Jakubowiak A, Steinberger A, et al. Regulation of rat pituitary gonadotropin-releasing hormone receptor mRNA levels in vivo and in vitro. Endocrinology 133:931–934, 1993.
35. Clayton RN, Catt KJ. Gonadotropin-releasing hormone receptors: Characterization, physiological regulation, and relationship to reproductive function. Endocr Rev 2:186–209, 1981.
36. Bauer-Dantoin AC, Weiss J, Jameson JL. Roles of estrogen, progesterone, and gonadotropin-releasing hormone (GnRH) in the control of pituitary GnRH receptor gene expression at the time of the preovulatory gonadotropin surges. Endocrinology 136:1014–1019, 1995.
37. Yasin M, Dalkin AC, Haisenleder DJ, et al. Gonadotropin-releasing hormone (GnRH) pulse pattern regulates GnRH receptor gene expression: Augmentation by estradiol. Endocrinology 136:1559–1564, 1995.
38. Reinhart J, Mertz LM, Catt KJ. Molecular cloning and expression of cDNA encoding the murine gonadotropin-releasing hormone receptor. J Biol Chem 267:21281–21284, 1992.
39. Tsutsumi M, Zhou W, Millar RP, et al. Cloning and functional expression of a mouse gonadotropin-releasing hormone receptor. Mol Endocrinol 6:1163–1169, 1992.

40. Eidne KA, Sellar RE, Couper G, et al. Molecular cloning and characterization of the rat pituitary gonadotropin-releasing hormone (GnRH) receptor. Mol Cell Endocrinol 90:R5–R9, 1992.
41. Kaiser UB, Zhao D, Cardona GR, et al. Isolation and characterization of cDNAs encoding the rat pituitary gonadotropin-releasing hormone receptor. Biochem Biophys Res Commun 189:1645–1652, 1992.
42. Kakar SS, Musgrove LC, Devor DC, et al. Cloning, sequencing, and expression of human gonadotropin-releasing hormone (GnRH) receptor. Biochem Biophys Res Commun 189:289–295, 1992.
43. Probst WC, Snyder LA, Schuster DI, et al. Sequence alignment of the G-protein coupled receptor superfamily. DNA Cell Biol 11:1–20, 1992.
44. Sealfon SC, Millar RP. Functional domains of the gonadotropin-releasing hormone receptor. Cell Mol Neurobiol 15:25–42, 1995.
45. Stojilkovic SS, Reinhart J, Catt KJ. Gonadotropin-releasing hormone receptors: Structure and signal transduction pathways. Endocr Rev 15:462–499, 1994.
46. Albarracin CT, Kaiser UB, Chin WW. Isolation and characterization of the 5′- flanking region of the mouse gonadotropin-releasing hormone receptor gene. Endocrinology 135:2300–2306, 1994.
47. Clay CM, Nelson SE, DiGregorio GB, et al. Cell-specific expression of the mouse gonadotropin-releasing hormone (GnRH) receptor gene is conferred by elements residing within 500 bp of proximal 5′ flanking region. Endocrine 3:615–622, 1995.
48. Fan NC, Peng C, Krisinger J, et al. The human gonadotropin-releasing hormone receptor gene: Complete structure including multiple promoters, transcription initiation sites and poly-adenylation signals. Mol Cell Endocrinol 107:R1–R8, 1995.
49. Zhou W, Flanagan C, Ballesteros JA, et al. A reciprocal mutation supports helix 2 and helix 7 proximity in the gonadotropin-releasing hormone receptor. Mol Pharmacol 45:165–170, 1994.
50. Fan NC, Jeung EB, Peng C, et al. The human gonadotropin-releasing hormone (GnRH) receptor gene: Cloning, genomic organization and chromosomal assignment. Mol Cell Endocrinol 103:R1–R6, 1994.
51. Montgomery GW, Penty JM, Lord EA, et al. The gonadotrophin-releasing hormone receptor gene maps to sheep chromosome 6 outside of the region of the FecB locus. Mamm Genome 6:436–438, 1995.
52. Kaiser UB, Dushkin H, Altherr MR, et al. Chromosomal localization of the gonadotropin-releasing hormone receptor gene to human chromosome 4q13.1–q21.1 and mouse chromosome 5. Genomics 20:506–508, 1994.
53. Zhou W, Sealfon SC. Structure of the mouse gonadotropin-releasing hormone receptor gene: Variant transcripts generated by alternative processing. DNA Cell Biol 13:605–614, 1994.
54. Alexander JM, Klibanski A. Gonadotropin-releasing hormone receptor mRNA expression by human pituitary tumors in vitro. J Clin Invest 93:2332–2339, 1994.
55. Jennes L, Conn PM. Gonadotropin-releasing hormone and its receptors in rat brain. Front Neuroendocrinol 15:51–77, 1994.
56. Minaretzis D, Jakubowski M, Mortola JF, et al. Gonadotropin-releasing hormone receptor gene expression in human ovary and granulosa-lutein cells. J Clin Endocrinol Metab 80:430–434, 1995.
57. Kartun KF, Mellon PL. The activin βB and activin type II receptor genes are expressed in gonadotrope cell lines (Abstract). 77th Annual Meeting of the Endocrine Society, Washington, DC, June 14–17, 1995.
58. Aubert ML, Begeot M, Winiger BP, et al. Ontogeny of hypothalamic luteinizing hormone–releasing hormone (GnRH) and pituitary GnRH receptors in fetal and neonatal rats. Endocrinology 116:1565–1576, 1985.
59. Japon MA, Rubenstein M, Low MJ. In situ hybridization analysis of anterior pituitary hormone gene expression during fetal mouse development. J Histochem Cytochem 42:1117–1125, 1994.
60. Lerrant Y, Kottler ML, Bergametti F, et al. Expression of gonadotropin-releasing hormone (GnRH) receptor gene is altered by GnRH agonist desensitization in a manner similar to that of gonadotropin β-subunit gene in normal and castrated rat pituitary. Endocrinology 136:2803–2808, 1995.
61. Turzillo AM, Campion CE, Clay CM, et al. Regulation of gonadotropin-releasing hormone (GnRH) receptor messenger ribonucleic acid and GnRH receptors during the early preovulatory period in the ewe. Endocrinology 135:1353–1358, 1994.
62. Bauer-Dantoin AC, Hollenberg AN, Jameson JL. Dynamic regulation of gonadotropin-releasing hormone mRNA levels in the anterior pituitary gland during the rat estrous cycle. Endocrinology 133:1911–1914, 1993.
63. Funabashi T, Brooks PJ, Weesner GD, et al. Luteinizing hormone–releasing hormone receptor messenger ribonucleic acid expression in the rat pituitary during lactation and the estrous cycle. J Neuroendocrinol 6:261–266, 1994.
64. Wu JC, Sealfon SC, Miller WL. Gonadal hormones and gonadotropin-releasing hormone (GnRH) alter messenger ribonucleic acid levels for GnRH receptors in sheep. Endocrinology 134:1846–1850, 1994.
65. Hamernik DL. Molecular biology of gonadotrophins. J Reprod Fertil Suppl 49:257–269, 1995.
66. Fernandez-Vazquez G, Kaiser UB, Albarracin CT, et al. Transcriptional activation of the gonadotropin-releasing hormone receptor gene by activin A. Mol Endocrinol 10:356–366, 1996.
67. Smith MS, Reinhart J. Changes in pituitary gonadotropin-releasing hormone receptor messenger ribonucleic acid content during lactation and after pup removal. Endocrinology 133:2080–2084, 1993.
68. Alarid ET, Mellon PL. Down-regulation of the gonadotropin-releasing hormone receptor messenger ribonucleic acid by activation of adenylyl cyclase in αT3–1 pituitary gonadotrope cells. Endocrinology 136:1361–1366, 1995.
69. Hayflick JS, Adelman JP, Seeburg PH. The complete nucleotide sequence of the human gonadotropin-releasing hormone gene. Nucleic Acids Res 17:6403–6404, 1989.
70. Schwanzel-Fukuda M, Pfaff DW. Origin of luteinizing hormone–releasing hormone neurons. Nature 338:161–164, 1989.
71. King JC, Anthony ELP. LHRH neurons and their projections in humans and other mammals: Species comparisons. Peptides 5:195–207, 1984.
72. Belchetz PE, Plant TM, Nakai Y, et al. Hypophysial responses to continuous and intermittent delivery of hypothalamic gonadotropin-releasing hormone. Science 202:631–633, 1978.
73. Crowley WF, McArthur JW. Simulation of the normal menstrual cycle in Kallmann's syndrome by pulsatile administration of luteinizing hormone–releasing hormone (LHRH). J Clin Endocrinol Metab 51:173–175, 1980.
74. Hall JE, Whitcomb RW, Rivier JE, et al. Differential regulation of luteinizing hormone, follicle-stimulating hormone, and free α-subunit secretion from the gonadotrope by gonadotropin-releasing hormone (GnRH): Evidence from the use of two GnRH antagonists. J Clin Endocrinol Metab 70:328–335, 1990.
75. Sandow J. Clinical applications of LHRH and its analogues. Clin Endocrinol (Oxf) 18:571–592, 1983.
76. Neill JD, Patton JM, Dailey RA, et al. Luteinizing hormone releasing hormone (LHRH) in pituitary portal blood of rhesus monkeys: Relationship to level of LH release. Endocrinology 101:430–434, 1977.
77. Levine JE, Ramirez VD. LHRH release during the rat estrous cycle and after ovariectomy, as estimated with push-pull cannulae. Endocrinology 111:1439–1448, 1982.
78. Rassmussen DD, Gambacciani M, Schwartz W, et al. Pulsatile gonadotropin-releasing hormone release from the human mediobasal hypothalamus in vitro: Opiate receptor–mediated suppression. Neuroendocrinology 49:150–156, 1989.
79. Filicori M, Santoro N, Merriam GR, et al. Characterization of the physiologic pattern of episodic gonadotropin secretion throughout the human menstrual cycle. J Clin Endocrinol Metab 62:1136–1144, 1986.
80. Wildt L, Hausler A, Marshall G, et al. Frequency and amplitude of gonadotropin-releasing hormone stimulation and gonadotropin secretion in the rhesus monkey. Endocrinology 109:376–385, 1981.
81. Wildt L, Hutchison JS, Marshall G, et al. On the site of action of progesterone in the blockade of the estradiol-induced gonadotropin discharge in the rhesus monkey. Endocrinology 109:1293–1294, 1981.
82. Haisenleder DJ, Dalkin AC, Ortolano GA, et al. A pulsatile gonadotropin-releasing hormone stimulus is required to increase transcription of the gonadotropin subunit genes: Evidence for differential regulation of transcription by pulse frequency in vivo. Endocrinology 128:509–517, 1991.
83. Yen SSC, Quigley ME, Reid RL, et al. Neuroendocrinology of

opioid peptides and their role in the control of gonadotropin and prolactin secretion. Am J Obstet Gynecol 152:485–493, 1985.
84. Khar A, Debeljuk L, Jutisz M. Biosynthesis of gonadotropins by rat pituitary cells in culture and pituitary homogenates: Effect of gonadotropin-releasing hormone. Mol Cell Endocrinol 12:53–65, 1978.
85. Liu TC, Jackson GL. Modifications of luteinizing hormone biosynthesis and release by gonadotropin-releasing hormone, cycloheximide, and actinomycin D. Endocrinology 103:1253–1263, 1978.
86. Wierman ME, Rivier J, Wang C. Gonadotropin-releasing hormone (GnRH)–dependent regulation of gonadotropin subunit mRNA levels in the rat. Endocrinology 124:272–278, 1989.
87. Hamernik DL, Nett TM. Gonadotropin-releasing hormone increases the amount of messenger ribonucleic acid for gonadotropins in ovariectomized ewes after hypothalamic-pituitary disconnection. Endocrinology 122:959–966, 1988.
88. Kaiser UB, Jakubowiak A, Steinberger A, et al. Differential effects of gonadotropin-releasing hormone (GnRH) pulse frequency on gonadotropin subunit and GnRH receptor messenger ribonucleic acid levels in vitro. Endocrinology 138:1224–1231, 1997.
89. Crowder ME, Nett TM. Pituitary content of gonadotropins and receptors for gonadotropin-releasing hormone (GnRH) and hypothalamic content of GnRH during the periovulatory period of the ewe. Endocrinology 114:234–239, 1984.
90. Kaiser UB, Sabbagh E, Katzenellenbogen RA, et al. A mechanism for the differential regulation of gonadotropin subunit gene expression by gonadotropin-releasing hormone. Proc Natl Acad Sci USA 92:12280–12284, 1995.
91. Shupnik MA. Effects of gonadotropin-releasing hormone on rat gonadotropin gene transcription in vitro: Requirement for pulsatile administration for luteinizing hormone-β gene stimulation. Mol Endocrinol 4:1444–1450, 1990.
92. Weiss J, Crowley WF, Jameson JL. Pulsatile gonadotropin-releasing hormone modifies polyadenylation of gonadotrophin subunit messenger ribonucleic acids. Endocrinology 130:415–420, 1992.
93. Kalra SP, Crowley WR. Neuropeptide Y: A novel neuroendocrine peptide in the control of pituitary hormone secretion, and its relation to luteinizing hormone. Front Neuroendocrinol 13:1–46, 1992.
94. Lopez FJ, Merchenthaler I, Ching M, et al. Galanin: A hypothalamic-hypophysiotropic hormone modulating reproductive functions. Proc Natl Acad Sci USA 88:4508–4512, 1991.
95. Rawlings SR, Hezareh M. Pituitary adenylate cyclase–activating polypeptide (PACAP) and PACAP/vasoactive intestinal polypeptide receptors: Actions on the anterior pituitary gland. Endocr Rev 17:4–29, 1996.
96. Huang X, Harlan RE. Absence of androgen receptors in LHRH immunoreactive neurons. Brain Res 624:309–311, 1993.
97. Sprangers SA, Brenner RM, Bethea CL. Estrogen and progestin receptor immunocytochemistry in lactotropes versus gonadotropes of monkey pituitary cell cultures. Endocrinology 124:1462–1470, 1989.
98. Sar M. Estradiol is concentrated in tyrosine hydroxylase containing neurons of the hypothalamus. Science 223:938–940, 1984.
99. Romano GJ, Krust A, Pfaff DW. Expression and estrogen regulation of progesterone receptor mRNA in neurons of the mediobasal hypothalamus: An in situ hybridization study. Mol Endocrinol 3:1295–1300, 1989.
100. Radovick S, Ticknor CM, Nakayama Y, et al. Evidence for direct estrogen regulation of the human gonadotropin-releasing hormone gene. J Clin Invest 88:1649–1655, 1991.
101. Gharib SD, Wierman ME, Badger TM, et al. Sex steroid hormone regulation of follicle-stimulating hormone subunit messenger ribonucleic acid (mRNA) levels in the rat. J Clin Invest 80:294–299, 1987.
102. Shupnik MA, Gharib SD, Chin WW. Estrogen suppresses rat gonadotropin gene transcription in vivo. Endocrinology 122:1842–1846, 1988.
103. Knobil E. The neuroendocrine control of the menstrual cycle. Recent Prog Horm Res 36:53–88, 1981.
104. Frawley S, Neill JD. Biphasic effects of estrogen on gonadotropin-releasing hormone–induced luteinizing hormone release in monolayer cultures of rat and monkey pituitary cells. Endocrinology 114:659–663, 1984.
105. Yamaji T, Dierschke DJ, Bhattacharya AN, et al. The negative feedback control by estradiol and progesterone of LH secretion in the ovariectomized rhesus monkey. Endocrinology 90:771–777, 1972.
106. Young JR, Jaffe RB. Strength-duration characteristics of estrogen effects on gonadotropin response to gonadotropin-releasing hormone in women. J Clin Endocrinol Metab 42:432–442, 1976.
107. Clarke IJ, Cummins JT. Increased gonadotropin-releasing hormone pulse frequency associated with estrogen-induced luteinizing hormone surges in ovariectomized ewes. Endocrinology 116:2376–2383, 1985.
108. Van Vugt DA, Lam NY, Ferin M. Reduced frequency of pulsatile luteinizing hormone secretion in the luteal phase of the rhesus monkey: Involvement of endogenous opiates. Endocrinology 315:1095–1101, 1984.
109. Wierman ME, Wang C. Androgen selectively stimulates follicle-stimulating hormone-β mRNA levels after gonadotropin-releasing hormone antagonist administration. Biol Reprod 42:563–571, 1990.
110. Gharib SD, Leung PCK, Carroll RS, et al. Androgens positively regulate follicle-stimulating hormone β-subunit mRNA levels in rat pituitary cells. Mol Endocrinol 4:1620–1626, 1990.
111. Urban RJ, Davis MR, Rogol AD, et al. Acute androgen receptor blockade increases luteinizing hormone secretory activity in men. J Clin Endocrinol Metab 67:1149–1155, 1988.
112. Dye RB, Rabinovici J, Jaffe RB. Inhibin and activin in reproductive biology. Obstet Gynecol Surv 47:173–185, 1992.
113. Weiss J, Crowley WF Jr, Halvorson LM, et al. Perifusion of rat pituitary cells with gonadotropin-releasing hormone, activin, and inhibin reveals distinct effects on gonadotropin gene expression and secretion. Endocrinology 132:2307–2311, 1993.
114. Vale W, Rivier J, Vaughan J, et al. Purification and characterization of an FSH release protein from porcine ovarian follicular fluid. Nature 321:776–779, 1986.
115. Mason AJ, Hayflick JS, Ling N. Complementary DNA sequences of ovarian follicular fluid inhibin show precursor structure and homology with transforming growth factor β. Nature 318:659–663, 1985.
116. Hotten G, Neidhardt H, Schneider C, et al. Cloning of a new member of the TGF-beta family: A putative new activin beta C chain. Biochem Biophys Res Commun 206:608–613, 1995.
117. Esch FS, Shimasaki S, Mercado M, et al. Structural characterization of follistatin: A novel follicle-stimulating hormone release–inhibiting polypeptide from the gonad. Mol Endocrinol 1:849–855, 1987.
118. Nakamura T, Takio K, Eto Y, et al. Activin-binding protein from rat ovary is follistatin. Science 247:836–838, 1990.
119. Inouye S, Guo Y, DePaolo L, et al. Recombinant expression of human follistatin with 315 and 288 amino acids: Chemical and biological comparison with native porcine follistatin. Endocrinology 129:815–822, 1991.
120. Matthews LS, Vale WW. Expression cloning of an activin receptor, a predicted transmembrane serine kinase. Cell 65:973–982, 1991.
121. Attisano L, Wrana JL, Montalvo E, et al. Activation of signalling by the activin receptor complex. Mol Cell Biol 16:1066–1073, 1996.
122. Baker JC, Harland RM. A novel mesoderm inducer, Madr2, functions in the activin signal transduction pathway. Genes Dev 10:1880–1889, 1996.
123. Halvorson LM, DeCherney AH. Inhibin, activin, and follistatin in reproductive medicine. Fertil Steril 65:459–469, 1996.
124. de Winter JP, ten Dijke P, de Vries CJ, et al. Follistatins neutralize activin bioactivity by inhibition of activin binding to its type II receptors. Mol Cell Endocrinol 116:105–114, 1996.
125. Lenton EA, de Kretser DM, Woodward AJ, et al. Inhibin concentrations throughout the menstrual cycles of normal, infertile, and older women compared with those during spontaneous conception cycles. J Clin Endocrinol Metab 73:1180–1190, 1991.
126. Demura R, Suzuki T, Tajima S, et al. Human plasma free activin and inhibin levels during the menstrual cycle. J Clin Endocrinol Metab 76:1080–1082, 1993.
127. Khoury RH, Wang QF, Crowley WF Jr, et al. Serum follistatin levels in women: Evidence against an endocrine function of ovarian follistatin. J Clin Endocrinol Metab 80:1361–1368, 1995.
128. Kettel LM, DePaolo LV, Morales AJ, et al. Circulating levels of follistatin from puberty to menopause. Fertil Steril 65:472–476, 1996.

129. Meunier H, Rivier C, Evans RM, et al. Gonadal and extragonadal expression of inhibin α, βA, and βB subunits in various tissues predicts diverse functions. Proc Natl Acad Sci USA 85:247–251, 1988.
130. Roberts V, Meunier H, Vaughan J, et al. Production and regulation of inhibin subunits in pituitary gonadotropes. Endocrinology 124:552–554, 1989.
131. Kaiser UB, Lee BL, Carroll RS, et al. Follistatin gene expression in the pituitary: Localization in gonadotrophs and folliculostellate cells in diestrous rats. Endocrinology 130:3048–3056, 1992.
132. Corrigan AZ, Bilezikjian LM, Carroll RS, et al. Evidence for an autocrine role of activin B within rat anterior pituitary cultures. Endocrinology 128:1682–1684, 1991.
133. DePaolo LV, Bald LN, Fendly BM. Passive immunoneutralization with a monoclonal antibody reveals a role for endogenous activin-B in mediating FSH hypersecretion during estrus and following ovariectomy of hypophysectomized pituitary-grafted rats. Endocrinology 130:1741–1743, 1992.
134. Kaiser UB, Chin WW. Regulation of follistatin messenger ribonucleic acid levels in the rat pituitary. J Clin Invest 91:2523–2531, 1993.
135. Besecke LM, Guendner MJ, Schneyer AL, et al. Gonadotropin-releasing hormone regulates follicle-stimulating hormone-beta gene expression through an activin/follistatin autocrine or paracrine loop. Endocrinology 137:3667–3673, 1996.
136. Dalkin AC, Knight CD, Shupnik MA, et al. Ovariectomy and inhibin immunoneutralization acutely increase follicle-stimulating hormone-β messenger ribonucleic acid concentrations: Evidence for a nontranscriptional mechanism. Endocrinology 132:1297–1304, 1993.
137. Medhamurthy R, Culler MD, Gay VL, et al. Evidence that inhibin plays a major role in the regulation of follicle-stimulating hormone secretion in the fully adult male rhesus monkey *(Macaca mulatta)*. Endocrinology 129:389–395, 1991.
138. Carroll RS, Kowash PM, Lofgren JA, et al. In vivo regulation of FSH synthesis by inhibin and activin. Endocrinology 129: 3299–3394, 1991.
139. Carroll RS, Corrigan AZ, Gharib SD, et al. Inhibin, activin, and follistatin: Regulation of follicle-stimulating hormone messenger ribonucleic acid levels. Mol Endocrinol 3:1969–1976, 1989.
140. Braden TD, Conn PM. Activin-A stimulates the synthesis of gonadotropin-releasing hormone receptors. Endocrinology 130:2101–2105, 1992.
141. Katayama T, Shiota K, Takahashi M. Activin A increases the number of follicle-stimulating hormone cells in anterior pituitary cultures. Mol Cell Endocrinol 69:179–185, 1990.
142. Schoderbek WE, Kim KE, Ridgway EC, et al. Analysis of DNA sequences required for pituitary-specific expression of the glycoprotein hormone α-subunit gene. Mol Endocrinol 6:893–903, 1992.
143. Roberson MS, Schoderbek WE, Tremml G, et al. Activation of the glycoprotein hormone α-subunit promoter by a LIM-homeodomain transcription factor. Mol Cell Biol 14:2985–2993, 1994.
144. Horn F, Windle JJ, Barnhart KM, et al. Tissue-specific gene expression in the pituitary: The glycoprotein hormone α-subunit gene is regulated by a gonadotrope-specific protein. Mol Cell Biol 12:2143–2153, 1992.
145. Jameson JL, Albanese C, Habener JF. Distinct adjacent protein-binding domains in the glycoprotein hormone alpha gene interact independently with a cAMP-responsive enhancer. J Biol Chem 264:16190–16196, 1989.
146. Delegeane AM, Ferland LH, Mellon PL. Tissue-specific enhancer of the human glycoprotein hormone alpha-subunit gene: Dependence on cyclic AMP-inducible elements. Mol Cell Biol 7:3994–4002, 1987.
147. Kay TWH, Jameson JL. Identification of a gonadotropin-releasing hormone–responsive region in the glycoprotein hormone α-subunit promoter. Mol Endocrinol 6:1767–1773, 1992.
148. Clay CM, Keri RA, Finicle AB, et al. Transcriptional repression of the glycoprotein hormone α subunit gene by androgen may involve direct binding of androgen receptor to the proximal promoter. J Biol Chem 268:13556–13564, 1993.
149. Keri RA, Anderson B, Kennedy GC, et al. Estradiol inhibits transcription of the human glycoprotein hormone α-subunit gene despite the absence of a high affinity binding site for the estrogen receptor. Mol Endocrinol 5:725–733, 1991.
150. Keri RA, Wolfe MW, Saunders TL, et al. The proximal promoter of the bovine luteinizing hormone beta-subunit gene confers gonadotrope-specific expression and regulation by gonadotropin-releasing hormone, testosterone, and 17 beta-estradiol in transgeneic mice. Mol Endocrinol 8:1807–1816, 1994.
151. Ingraham HA, Lala DS, Ikeda Y, et al. The nuclear receptor steroidogenic factor 1 acts at multiple levels of the reproductive axis. Genes Dev 8:2302–2312, 1994.
152. Ikeda Y, Luo X, Abbud R, et al. The nuclear receptor steroidogenic factor 1 is essential for the formation of the ventromedial hypothalamic nucleus. Mol Endocrinol 9:478–486, 1995.
153. Halvorson LM, Kaiser UB, Chin WW. Stimulation of luteinizing hormone β gene promoter activity by the orphan nuclear receptor, steroidogenic factor-1. J Biol Chem 271:6645–6650, 1996.
154. Keri RA, Nilson JH. A steroidogenic factor-1 binding site is required for activity of the luteinizing hormone beta subunit promoter in gonadotropes of transgenic mice. J Biol Chem 271:10782–10785, 1996.
155. Lee SL, Sadovsky Y, Swirnoff AH, et al. Luteinizing hormone deficiency and female infertility in mice lacking the transcription factor NGFI-A (Egr-1). Science 273:1219–1221, 1996.
156. Yamoto M, Shima K, Nakano R. Gonadotropin receptors in human ovarian follicles and corpora lutea throughout the menstrual cycle. Horm Res 37:5–11, 1992.
157. Catt KJ, Ketelslegers JM, Dufau ML. Receptors for gonadotropic hormone. *In* Blecher, M (ed). Methods in Receptor Research. New York, Marcel Dekker, 1976, p 175.
158. Rodbard D. Mathematics and statistics of ligand assays: An illustrated guide. *In* Langan J, Clapp J (eds). Ligand Assay: Analysis of International Developments on Isotopic and Nonisotopic Immunoassay. New York, Masson Publishing, 1981, p 45.
159. McFarland KC, Sprengel R, Phillips HS, et al. Lutropin-choriogonadotropin receptor: An unusual member of the G protein–coupled receptor family. Science 245:494–499, 1989.
160. Loosfelt H, Misrahi M, Atger M, et al. Cloning and sequencing of porcine LH-hCG receptor cDNA: Variants lacking transmembrane domain. Science 245:525–528, 1989.
161. Minegishi T, Nakamura K, Takakura Y, et al. Cloning and sequencing of human LH/hCG receptor cDNA. Biochem Biophys Res Commun 172:1049–1054, 1990.
162. Rousseau-Merck MF, Misrahi M, Atger M, et al. Localization of the human luteinizing hormone/choriogonadotropin receptor gene (LHCGR) to chromosome 2p21. Cytogenet Cell Genet 54:77–79, 1990.
163. Tsai-Morris CH, Buczko E, Wang W, et al. Structural organization of the rat luteinizing hormone (LH) receptor gene. J Biol Chem 266:11355–11359, 1991.
164. Hu ZZ, Tsai-Morris CH, Buczko E, et al. Hormonal regulation of LH receptor mRNA and expression in the rat ovary. FEBS Lett 274:181–184, 1990.
165. Tsai-Morris CH, Buczko E, Wang W, et al. Intronic nature of the rat LH receptor gene defines a soluble receptor subspecies with hormone binding activity. J Biol Chem 265:19385–19388, 1990.
166. Krantz DD, Zidovetzki R, Kagan BL, et al. Amphipathic beta structure of a leucine-rich repeat peptide. J Biol Chem 266:16801–16807, 1991.
167. Minegishi T, Delgado C, Dufau ML. Phosphorylation and glycosylation of the luteinizing hormone receptor. Proc Natl Acad Sci USA 86:1470–1474, 1989.
168. Liu X, Davis D, Segaloff DL. Disruption of potential sites for *N*-linked glycosylation does not impair hormone binding to the lutropin/choriogonadotropin receptor if Asn-173 is left intact. J Biol Chem 268:1513–1516, 1993.
169. Segaloff DB, Ascoli M. The lutropin/choriogonadotropin receptor . . . 4 years later. Endocr Rev 14:324–347, 1993.
170. Alberts B, Bray D, Lewis J, et al. Cell signaling. *In* The Molecular Biology of the Cell. New York, Garland Publishing, 1984, p 681.
171. Davis JS. Mechanisms of hormone action: Luteinizing hormone receptors and second-messenger pathways. Curr Sci 6:254–261, 1994.
172. Sanchez-Yague J, Rodriguez MC, Segaloff DL, et al. Truncation of the cytoplasmic tail of the lutropin choriogonadotropin receptor prevents agonist-induced uncoupling. J Biol Chem 267:7217–7220, 1992.

173. Lefkowitz RJ, Hausdorff WP, Caron MG. Role of phosphorylation in desensitization of the beta-adrenoreceptor. Trends Pharmacol Sci 11:190–194, 1990.
174. Zhu X, Gudermann T, Birnbaumer M, et al. A luteinizing hormone receptor with a severely truncated cytoplasmic tail (LHR-ct628) desensitizes to the same degree as the full-length receptor. J Biol Chem 268:1723–1728, 1993.
175. Ascoli M. Internalization and degradation of receptor-bound human choriogonadotropin in Leydig tumor cells. Fate of the hormone subunits. J Biol Chem 257:13306–13311, 1982.
176. Sprengel R, Braun T, Nikolics K, et al. The testicular receptor for follicle-stimulating hormone: Structure and functional expression of cloned cDNA. Mol Endocrinol 4:525–530, 1990.
177. Camp TA, Rahal JO, Mayo KE. Cellular localization and hormonal regulation of follicle-stimulating hormone and luteinizing hormone receptor messenger RNAs in the rat ovary. Mol Endocrinol 5:1405–1417, 1991.
178. Ziecik AJ, Derecka-Reszka K, Rzucidlo SJ. Extragonadal gonadotropin receptors, their distribution and function. J Physiol Pharmacol 43:33–49, 1992.
179. Segaloff DL, Wang H, Richards JS. Hormonal regulation of luteinizing hormone/chorionic gonadotropin receptor mRNA in rat ovarian cells during follicular development and luteinization. Mol Endocrinol 4:1856–1865, 1990.
180. Holt JA, Richards JS, Midgley AR Jr, et al. Effect of prolactin on LH receptor in rat luteal cells. Endocrinology 98:1005–1013, 1976.
181. Heckert LL, Daley I, Griswold MD. Structural organization of the follicle-stimulating hormone receptor gene. Mol Endocrinol 6:70–80, 1992.
182. Minegishi T, Nakamura K, Takakura Y, et al. Cloning and sequencing of human FSH receptor cDNA. Biochem Biophys Res Commun 175:1125–1130, 1991.
183. McNatty KP, Hunter WM, MacNeilly AS, et al. Changes in the concentration of pituitary and steroid hormones in the follicular fluid of human graafian follicles throughout the menstrual cycle. J Endocrinol 64:555–571, 1975.
184. Fletcher WH, Greenan JRT. Receptor mediated action without receptor occupancy. Endocrinology 116:1660, 1985.
185. Halpin DMG, Jones A, Fink G, et al. Postnatal ovarian follicle development in hypogonadal (hpg) and normal mice and associated changes in the hypothalamic-pituitary axis. J Reprod Fertil 77:287–296, 1986.
186. Vermesh M, Kletzky OA. Longitudinal evaluation of the luteal phase and its transition into the follicular phase. J Clin Endocrinol Metab 65:653–658, 1987.
187. Yong EL, Baird DT, Hillier SG. Mediation of gonadotropin-stimulated growth and differentiation of human granulosa cells by adenosine-3′,5′-monophosphate: One molecule, two messages. Clin Endocrinol (Oxf) 37:51–58, 1992.
188. McNatty KP, Makris A, DeGrazia C, et al. The production of progesterone, androgens, and estrogens by granulosa cells, thecal tissue, and stromal tissue from human ovaries in vitro. J Clin Endocrinol Metab 49:687–699, 1979.
189. Buckler HM, Healy DL, Burger HG. Purified FSH stimulates inhibin production from the human ovary. J Endocrinol 122:279–285, 1989.
190. McLachlan RI, Cohen NL, Vale WE, et al. The importance of luteinizing hormone in the control of inhibin and progesterone secretion by the human corpus luteum. J Clin Endocrinol Metab 68:1078–1085, 1989.
191. Tilly JL, LaPolt PS, Hsueh AJ. Hormonal regulation of follicle-stimulating hormone receptor messenger ribonucleic acid levels in cultured rat granulosa cells. Endocrinology 130:1296–1302, 1992.
192. Jia XC, Kessel B, Welsh TH Jr, et al. Androgen inhibition of follicle-stimulating hormone–stimulated luteinizing hormone receptor formation in cultured rat granulosa cells. Endocrinology 117:13–22, 1985.
193. Erickson GF, Wang C, Hsueh AJW. FSH induction of functional LH receptors in granulosa cells cultured in a chemically defined medium. Nature 270:336–338, 1979.
194. Piquette GN, LaPolt PS, Oikawa M, et al. Regulation of luteinizing hormone receptor messenger ribonucleic acid levels by gonadotropins, growth factors, and gonadotropin releasing hormone in cultured rat granulosa cells. Endocrinology 128:2449–2456, 1991.
195. Jia XC, Hsueh AJW. Homologous regulation of hormone receptors: Luteinizing hormone increases its own receptors in cultured rat granulosa cells. Endocrinology 115:2433–2439, 1984.
196. Mills TM. Effect of luteinizing hormone and cyclic adenosine 3′,5′-monophosphate on steroidogenesis in the ovarian follicle of the rabbit. Endocrinology 96:440–445, 1975.
197. Hild-Petito S, Stouffer RL, Brenner RM. Immunocytochemical localization of estradiol and progesterone receptors in the monkey ovary throughout the menstrual cycle. Endocrinology 123:2896–2905, 1988.
198. Chaffkin LM, Luciano AA, Peluso JJ. Progesterone as an autocrine/paracrine regulator of human granulosa cell proliferation. J Clin Endocrinol Metab 75:1404–1408, 1992.
199. Liu JH, Yen SSC. Induction of midcycle gonadotropin surge by ovarian steroids in women: A critical evaluation. J Clin Endocrinol Metab 57:797–802, 1983.
200. Shoham Z, Mannaerts B, Insler V, et al. Induction of follicular growth using recombinant human follicle-stimulating hormone in two volunteer women with hypogonadotropic hypogonadism. Fertil Steril 59:738–742, 1993.
201. Schoot DC, Coelingh-Bennink HJT, Mannaerts BM, et al. Human recombinant follicle-stimulating hormone induces growth of preovulatory follicles without concomitant increase in androgen and estrogen biosynthesis in a woman with isolated gonadotropin deficiency. J Clin Endocrinol Metab 74:1471–1473, 1992.
202. Peng X-R, Hsueh AJ, Ny T. Transient and cell-specific expression of tissue-type plasminogen activator and plasminogen-activator-inhibitor type 1 results in controlled and directed proteolysis during gonadotropin-induced ovulation. Eur J Biochem 214:147–156, 1993.
203. Hoff JD, Quigley ME, Yen SSC. Hormonal dynamics at midcycle: A reevaluation. J Clin Endocrinol Metab 57:792–796, 1983.
204. Investigators World Health Organization Task Force. Temporal relationships between ovulation and defined changes in the concentration of plasma estradiol-17β, luteinizing hormone, follicle stimulating hormone, and progesterone. Am J Obstet Gynecol 138:383–390, 1980.
205. Fowler PA, Templeton A. The nature and function of putative gonadotropin surge-attenuating/inhibiting factor (GnSAF/IF). Endocr Rev 17:103–120, 1996.
206. McNatty KP, Sawers RS. Relationship between the endocrine environment within the graafian follicle and the subsequent rate of progesterone secretion by human granulosa cells in culture. J Endocrinol 66:391–400, 1975.
207. Smith SK, Lenton EA, Cooke ID. Plasma gonadotrophin and ovarian steroid concentrations in women with menstrual cycles with a short luteal phase. J Reprod Fertil 75:363–368, 1985.
208. Brannian JD, Shiigi SM, Stouffer RL. Gonadotropin surge increases fluorescent-tagged low-density lipoprotein uptake by macaque granulosa cells from preovulatory follicles. Biol Reprod 47:355–360, 1992.
209. Ravindranath N, Little-Ihrig L, Benyo DF, et al. Role of luteinizing hormone in the expression of cholesterol side-chain cleavage cytochrome P450 and 3β-hydroxysteroid dehydrogenase Δ^{5-4} isomerase messenger ribonucleic acids in the primate corpus luteum. Endocrinology 131:2065–2070, 1992.
210. Zeleznik AJ, Little-Ihrig LL. Effect of reduced luteinizing hormone concentrations on corpus luteum function during the menstrual cycle of rhesus monkeys. Endocrinology 125:2237–2244, 1990.
211. Auletta FJ, Flint AP. Mechanisms controlling corpus luteum function in sheep, cows, nonhuman primates, and women especially in relation to the time of luteolysis. Endocr Rev 9:88–105, 1988.
212. Roseff SJ, Bangah ML, Kettel LM, et al. Dynamic changes in circulating inhibin levels during the luteal-follicular transition of the human menstrual cycle. J Clin Endocrinol Metab 69:1033–1039, 1989.
213. Hall JE, Schoenfeld DA, Martin KA, et al. Hypothalamic gonadotropin-releasing hormone secretion and follicle-stimulating hormone dynamics during the luteal-follicular transition. J Clin Endocrinol Metab 74:600–607, 1992.
214. Nippoldt TB, Reame NE, Kelch RP, et al. The roles of estradiol and progesterone in decreasing luteinizing hormone pulse frequency in the luteal phase of the menstrual cycle. J Clin Endocrinol Metab 69:67–76, 1989.

215. Weiss J, Adams E, Whitcomb RW, et al. Normal sequence of the gonadotropin-releasing hormone gene in patients with idiopathic hypogonadotropic hypogonadism. Biol Reprod 45:743–747, 1991.
216. de Roux N, Young J, Misrahi M, et al. A family with hypogonadotropic hypogonadism and mutations in the gonadotropin-releasing hormone receptor gene. N Engl J Med 337:1597–1602, 1997.
217. Franco B, Guioli S, Pragliola A, et al. A gene deleted in Kallmann's syndrome shares homology with neural cell adhesion and axonal path-finding molecules. Nature 353:529–536, 1991.
218. Weiss J, Axelrod L, Whitcomb RW, et al. Hypogonadism caused by a single amino acid substitution in the beta subunit of luteinizing hormone. N Engl J Med 326:179–183, 1992.
219. Haavisto AM, Pettersson K, Bergendahl M, et al. Occurrence and biological properties of a common genetic variant of luteinizing hormone. J Clin Endocrinol Metab 80:1257–1263, 1995.
220. Nilsson C, Pettersson K, Millar RP, et al. Worldwide frequency of a common genetic variant of luteinizing hormone: An international collaborative research. Fertil Steril 67:988–1004, 1997.
221. Matthews CH, Borgato S, Beck-Peccoz P, et al. Primary amenorrhoea and infertility due to a mutation in the beta-subunit of follicle-stimulating hormone. Nat Genet 5:83–86, 1993.
222. Layman LC, Lee E-J, Peak DB, et al. Delayed puberty and hypogonadism caused by mutations in the follicle-stimulating hormone β-subunit gene. N Engl J Med 337:607–611, 1997.
223. Shenker A, Laue L, Kosugi S, et al. A constitutively activating mutation of the luteinizing hormone receptor in familial male precocious puberty. Nature 365:652–654, 1993.
224. Kremer H, Kraaij R, Toledo SP, et al. Male pseudohermaphroditism due to a homozygous missense mutation of the luteinizing hormone receptor gene. Nat Genet 9:160–164, 1995.
225. Aittomaki K, Herva R, Stenman UH, et al. Clinical features of primary ovarian failure caused by a point mutation in the follicle-stimulating hormone receptor gene. J Clin Endocrinol Metab 81:3722–3726, 1996.
226. Tapanainen JL, Aittomaki K, Min J, et al. Men homozygous for an inactivating mutation of the follicle-stimulating hormone (FSH) receptor gene present variable suppression of spermatogenesis and fertility. Nat Genet 15:205–206, 1997.
227. Shenker A, Weinstein LS, Moran A, et al. Severe endocrine and nonendocrine manifestations of the McCune-Albright syndrome associated with activating mutations of stimulatory G protein G_S. J Pediatr 123:509–518, 1993.
228. Muscatelli F, Strom TM, Walker AP, et al. Mutations in the DAX-1 gene give rise to both X-linked adrenal hypoplasia congenita and hypogonadotropic hypogonadism. Nature 372:672–667, 1994.
229. Habiby RL, Boepple P, Nachtigall L, et al. Adrenal hypoplasia congenita with hypogonadotropic hypogonadism: Evidence that DAX-1 mutations lead to combined hypothalamic and pituitary defects in gonadotropin production. J Clin Invest 98:1055–1062, 1996.
230. Ito M, Yu R, Jameson JL. DAX-1 inhibits SF-1–mediated transactivation via a carboxy-terminal domain that is deleted in adrenal hypoplasia congenita. Mol Cell Biol 17:1476–1483, 1997.
231. Odell WD, Wolfsen AR. Humoral syndromes associated with cancer: Ectopic hormone production. Prog Clin Cancer 8:57–74, 1982.
232. Katznelson L, Alexander JM, Klibanski A. Clinically nonfunctioning pituitary adenomas. J Clin Endocrinol Metab 76:1089–1094, 1993.
233. Katznelson L, Alexander JM, Bikkal HA, et al. Imbalanced follicle-stimulating hormone beta-subunit hormone biosynthesis in human pituitary adenomas. J Clin Endocrinol Metab 74:1343–1351, 1992.
234. Alexander JM, Biller GMK, Bikkal H, et al. Clinically nonfunctioning pituitary tumors are monoclonal in origin. J Clin Invest 86:336–340, 1990.
235. Ambrosi B, Bassetti M, Ferrario R, et al. Precocious puberty in a boy with a PRL-, LH- and FSH-secreting pituitary tumour: Hormonal and immunocytochemical studies. Acta Endocrinol (Copenh) 122:569–576, 1990.
236. Rosen SW, Weintraub BD, Vaitukaitis JL, et al. Placental proteins and their subunits as tumor markers. Ann Intern Med 82:71–83, 1975.
237. Das S, Mukherjee K, Bhattacharya S, et al. Ectopic production of placental hormones (human chorionic gonadotropin and human placental lactogen) in carcinoma of the uterine cervix. Cancer 51:1854–1857, 1983.
238. Kourides IA, Schorr-Toshav NL. Alpha subunit of the glycoprotein hormones: Secretion by human malignancies. Clin Bull 11:106–109, 1981.
239. Weintraub BD, Krauth G, Rosen SW, et al. Differences between purified ectopic and normal alpha subunits of human glycoprotein hormones. J Clin Invest 56:1043–1052, 1975.
240. Arshad RR, Woo SY, Abbassi V, et al. Virilizing hepatoblastoma: Precocious sexual development and partial response of pulmonary metastases to cis-platinum. CA Cancer J Clin 32:293–300, 1982.

Chapter 4

STEROID HORMONES: Metabolism and Mechanism of Action

Bert W. O'Malley • Charles A. Strott

■ CHAPTER OUTLINE

KEY POINTS

- Steroid synthesis consists of two general pathways, a pregnenolone pathway and a progesterone pathway.
- Steroid hormones interact with serum binding proteins and undergo peripheral tissue transformations.
- Steroids enter peripheral target tissues, interact with specific intracellular receptors, and turn on select target genes that in turn mediate the biologic endpoint responses.
- Steroid-receptor complexes regulate gene expression.
- Sequence signals within genes allow regulated expression of steroid hormones.
- Key structural elements of steroid receptors allow interaction with DNA and the transcriptional machinery.
- Coregulator proteins (coactivators and corepressors) act as intermediaries in the mechanism by which the steroid-receptor complex recruits RNA polymerase to target genes.

Steroids are primordial molecules that evolved before eukaryotes approximately 2 billion years ago. They constitute one of the earliest forms of information transmitters, having been described as ancient bioregulators that exerted their message in their cell of origin.[1] Thus, the present-day hormonal role of steroids has emerged as a result of target organ specialization and not as a result of steroid evolution.[1] Steroids make up a subclass of lipids distinguished by a basic skeletal structure of four fused rings termed perhydrocyclopentanophenanthrene (Fig. 4–1). The steroid subcategory of molecules is part of an extraordinarily large and diverse family of chemical compounds that come under the rubric of terpenes or isoprenoids. This disparate group includes, in part, natural rubber, gutta-percha, numerous fragrant oils, turpentine hydrocarbons, the phytol side chain of chlorophyll, carotenoids, and the fat-soluble vitamins. What these substances have in common is that they are formed by the polymerization of a 5-carbon isoprene unit (Fig. 4–2). Hence, isopentenyl pyrophosphate, the activated isoprene unit, is the building block precursor of the various and sundry terpenes present in nature. In animals, isopentenyl pyrophosphate, derived from acetyl coenzyme A, is directed into four major prenyl derivatives (Fig. 4–3): (1) isopentenyl transfer ribonucleic acid (tRNA), which has a role in deoxyribonucleic acid (DNA) synthesis during the S-phase of the cell cycle; (2) ubiquinone, a component of the electron transfer chain; (3) dolichols, long-chain alcohols that function as glycosylated intermediates in the transfer of sugars to polypeptides; and (4) cholesterol, an important component of cell membranes and the parent compound of bile acids, vitamin D, and steroids.

Cholesterol (*chole,* bile, and *stereos,* solid) is produced by the condensation of two farnesyl pyrophosphates (6 isoprene units) to form squalene, a compound with 30 carbon atoms (see Fig. 4–3). The final stage in cholesterol biosynthesis involves cyclization and the eventual removal of three methyl groups to form cholesterol with its 27 carbon atoms. Cholesterol has the distinction of being the first isopentenoid isolated in pure form, and from it the generic term steroid is derived. The synthesis of cholesterol from squalene, as well as the conversion of cholesterol

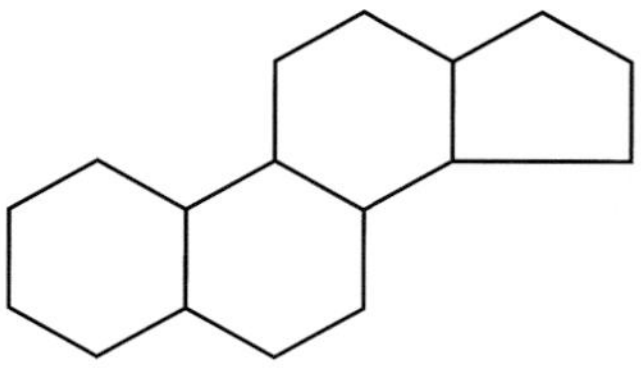

Figure 4–1 ■ Perhydrocyclopentanophenanthrene ring structure.

into steroid hormones, involves hydroxylation reactions requiring the reduced form of nicotinamide adenine dinucleotide phosphate (NADPH) and molecular oxygen, reactions carried out by specific cytochrome P450 monooxygenases or mixed function oxidases (half of the oxygen is reduced to H_2O). The initial stage in steroid biosynthesis is the conversion of cholesterol to the C_{21} compound, pregnenolone, with loss of a 6-carbon fragment (Fig. 4–4). This step involves two hydroxylations before cleavage, is mediated by a single cytochrome P450 named cholesterol side-chain cleavage or P450scc, and takes place within mitochondria of cells capable of initiating steroidogenesis.[2] In addition to the well-recognized capacity of cells in the adrenal cortex, ovary, testis, and placenta to perform cholesterol side-chain cleavage,[3–6] cells in specific areas of the brain can also perform this function.[7, 8] In the adrenal and gonad, the regulated step in the rapid steroidogenic response to an inducer (e.g., the trophic peptide hormones adrenocorticotropic hormone and luteinizing hormone) is the translocation of cholesterol from the outer mitochondria membrane to the inner membrane where the cholesterol side-chain cleavage enzyme system is located.[9–11] The intramitochondrial transfer of cholesterol requires a rapidly turning over protein,[12] recently identified as a 30-kDa phosphoprotein designated steroidogenic acute regulatory (StAR) protein.[13–15] Interestingly, however, expression of the StAR protein does not occur in either the placenta or the brain, the other tissues capable of cholesterol side-chain cleavage activity.[13] Three other proteins, that is, sterol carrier protein 2,[16–18] steroidogenesis activator polypeptide,[19, 20] and a protein homologous to endozepine or diazepam binding inhibitor,[21, 22] have been described and implicated in the acute steroidogenic response to trophic hormones in the adrenal and gonads; however, their precise involvement remains to be clearly determined.

The synthesis of steroid hormones involves up to five different hydroxylases, two dehydrogenases, a reductase, and an aromatase. The steroid hydroxylases and aromatase are members of the cytochrome P450 supergene family that has been given the designation of CYP as indicated in Table 4–1.[23] Steroid synthesis can be thought of as consisting of two general pathways, a pregnenolone (the embryonic precursor from which all biologically active steroid hormones are produced) pathway and a progesterone (produced from pregnenolone by the action of 3β-hydroxysteroid dehydrogenase) pathway. Synthesis of the primary C_{21} glucocorticoid cortisol and the primary C_{21} mineralocorticoid aldosterone is illustrated in Figure 4–5; synthesis of the C_{19} androgenic hormones testosterone and dihydrotestosterone and the C_{18} estrogenic steroids estrone and estradiol is depicted in Figure 4–6. The kinds of steroids produced and secreted will depend on the physiologic (or pathophysiologic) nature of the steroidogenic cell and the activity of inherent enzyme systems. The adrenal cortex can carry out, to all intents and purposes, the reactions shown in Figures 4–5 and 4–6, although it normally produces inconsequential amounts of estrogens and dihydrotestosterone; the testis and ovary carry out the reactions denoted in Figure 4–6. Whereas the production of estrogens and dihydrotestosterone is normally limited, the testis, nevertheless, is the principal source of circulating estrogens in men.[24] The production of dihydrotestosterone by the ovary probably does not occur. The placenta produces essentially only pregnenolone and progesterone from cholesterol; however, it does produce estrogens from C_{19} precursors derived from extraplacental sources.[25]

$$CH_2{=}C(CH_3){-}CH_2{-}CH_2$$

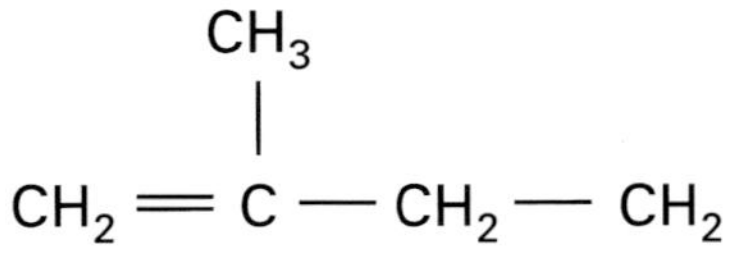

Figure 4–2 ■ Five-carbon isoprene unit.

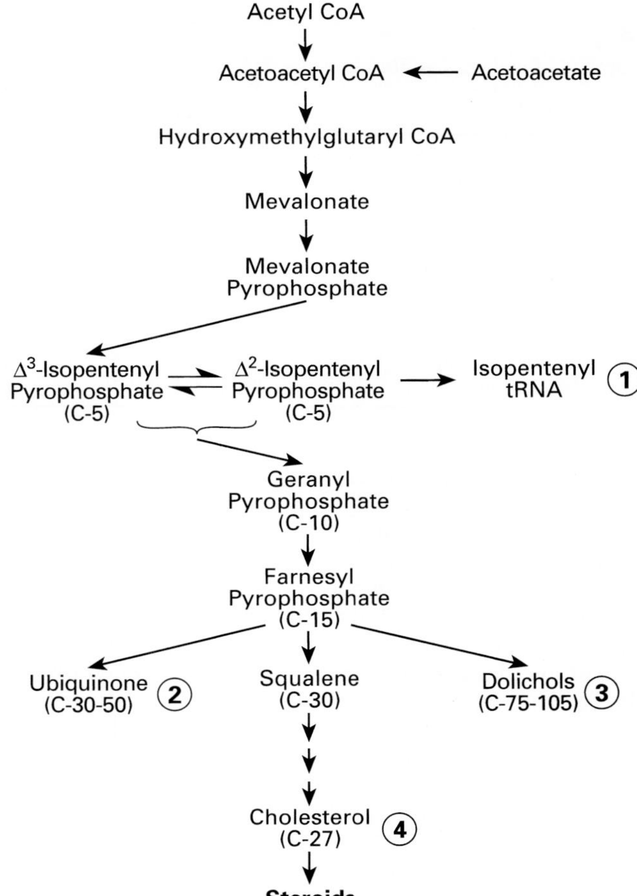

Figure 4–3 ■ Formation of activated isoprene and terpenoids from acetyl coenzyme A.

During the course of steroid synthesis (normal and abnormal), precursor or intermediate forms can leach out of cells and enter the circulation where they can be detected and quantified. In fact, in certain conditions of abnormal

■ TABLE 4–1
Enzymes Employed in Steroidogenesis

ENZYME	DESIGNATION
Cholesterol side-chain cleavage	CYP11A
17α-Hydroxylase	CYP17
17,20-Lyase	CYP17
21-Hydroxylase	CYP21
11β-Hydroxylase	CYP11B1
Aldosterone synthase	CYP11B2
Aromatase	CYP19
3β-Hydroxysteroid dehydrogenase	3βHSD
17β-Hydroxysteroid dehydrogenase	17βHSD
5α-Reductase	5αRed

steroid synthesis, the concentration of steroid intermediates in plasma can be markedly elevated. For instance, in all but one form of congenital adrenal hyperplasia, a group of disorders resulting from deficient steroidogenic enzymes, steroid intermediates in blood are strikingly elevated[26]; the exception is in the rare form called lipoid congenital adrenal hyperplasia, which is due to StAR protein deficiency.[27] Steroid intermediates in blood can also be elevated by the clinical and therapeutic use of agents that act to inhibit steroidogenic enzymes; an example would be the use of metyrapone, a drug used for testing the pituitary-adrenal axis.[28] In addition, steroids are metabolized within steroidogenic cells; the most prominent example is sulfoconjugation.[29–31]

Mechanisms of trophic peptide hormone regulation of steroidogenesis in gonadal tissue are discussed in Chapters 3, 6, and 7 and thus will not be dealt with here. This chapter, which is primarily concerned with steroids after they are released from their cell of origin, is composed of two major sections; the first encompasses steroid metabolism, and the second pertains to molecular mechanisms apropos steroids at their site of action.

STEROID METABOLISM

Nomenclature and Configuration of Steroids

Steroid carbon atoms are numbered, and the perhydrocyclopentanophenanthrene rings are indicated by letters as illustrated in Figure 4–7. The spatial orientation of atoms or groups about asymmetric centers is depicted in Figure 4–8, in which the perhydrocyclopentanophenanthrene ring is depicted as a projection onto the plane of the paper; bonds to atoms or groups lying below the plane of the paper are shown as broken lines and termed α; bonds to atoms or groups lying above the plane of the paper are shown as solid lines and termed β. Unless stated to the contrary, use of a steroid name implies that atoms or groups attached at ring junctions 8, 9, 10, 13, and 14 are oriented as shown, that is, a hydrogen atom is α-oriented at carbons 9 and 14 and β-oriented at carbon 8, and the methyl groups attached at carbons 10 and 13 are β-oriented; furthermore, a carbon chain attached at position 17 is assumed to be β-oriented. When steroids have saturated rings A and B, the conformation of the hydrogen atom at position 5 must always be indicated. This is illustrated in Figure 4–9 for two pregnane compounds; also, as illustrated in Figure 4–9, the conformation of substituents at position 20 of pregnane compounds is denoted by either α (for a substituent shown to the right of the side chain) or β (for a substituent shown to the left of the side chain).

The natural steroids are named after the saturated hydrocarbons, and when all rings are saturated, the parent name ends in -ane (Fig. 4–10). Note that for the compounds in Figure 4–10, the orientation of the hydrogen at position 5, although not denoted, could be in either the α or β conformation. The names for unsaturated or aromatic steroids are derived from the saturated compounds by changing the terminal -ane to -ene, -diene, or -triene, preceded by the number of the lowest carbon atom involved (Fig. 4–11). The terminal -e of saturated and unsaturated compounds is omitted if it precedes a vowel (see examples in Table 4–2).

Most substituents can be designated as either prefixes or suffixes. A few can be named only as prefixes: halogens, alkyl groups, or nitro groups. When possible, one type of substituent must be designated as a suffix. When more than one type is present that could be designated as a suffix, one type only may be so expressed and the other types must be designated as prefixes. Choice of suffix is made according to an order of decreasing preference: onium salt, acid, lactone, ester, aldehyde, ketone (prefix oxo-, suffix -one), alcohol (prefix hydroxy-, suffix -ol), amine, ether. Suffixes are added to the name of the saturated or unsatu-

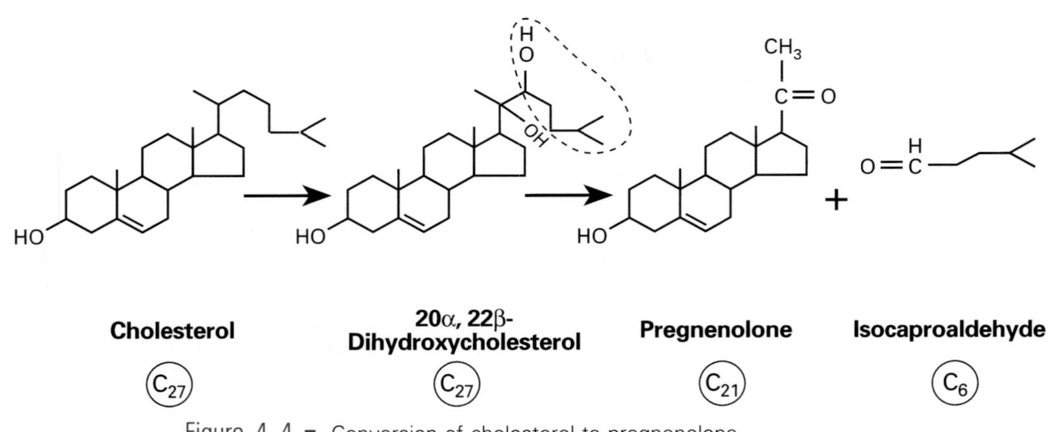

Figure 4–4 ■ Conversion of cholesterol to pregnenolone.

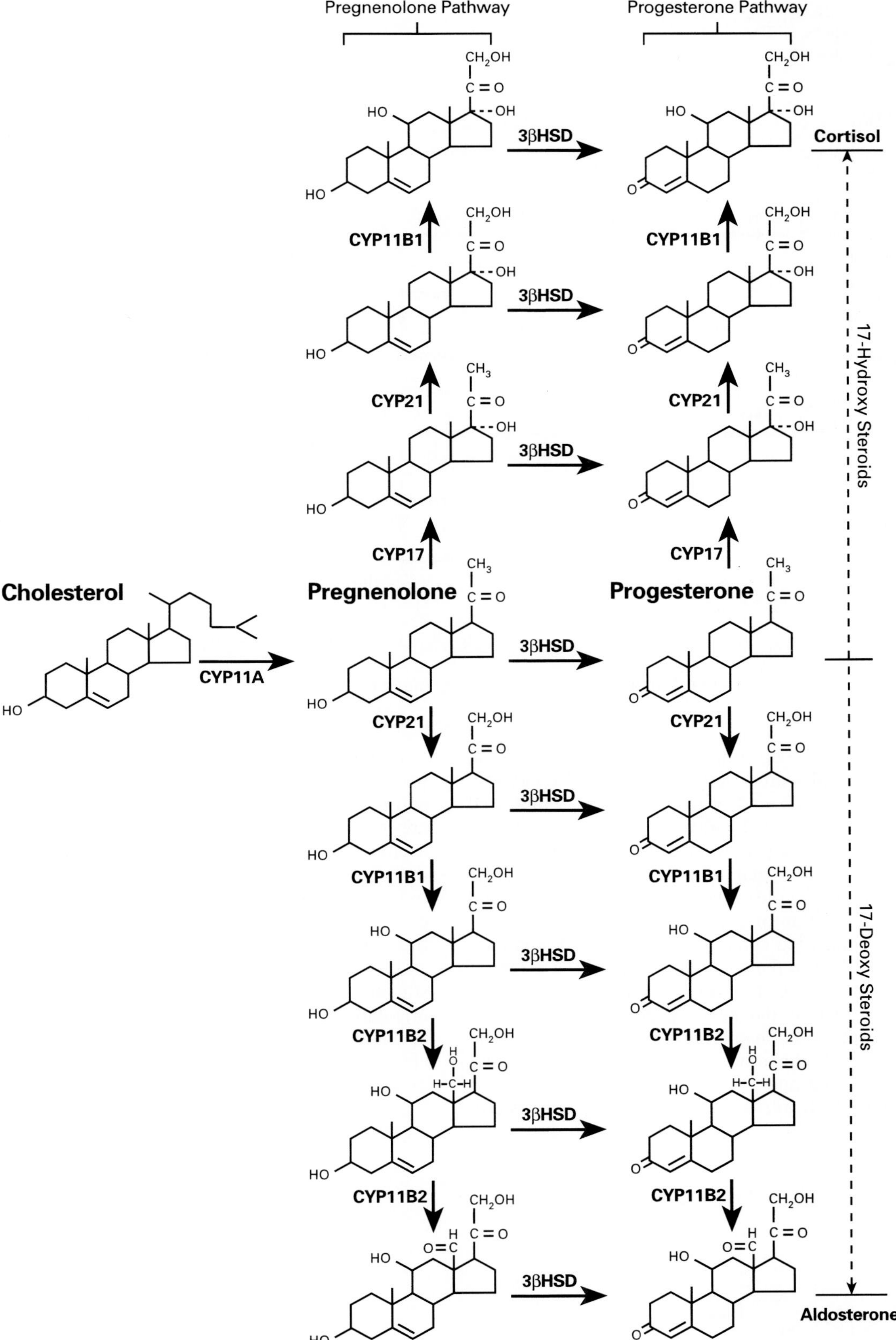

Figure 4–5 ■ General scheme for synthesis of cortisol and aldosterone.

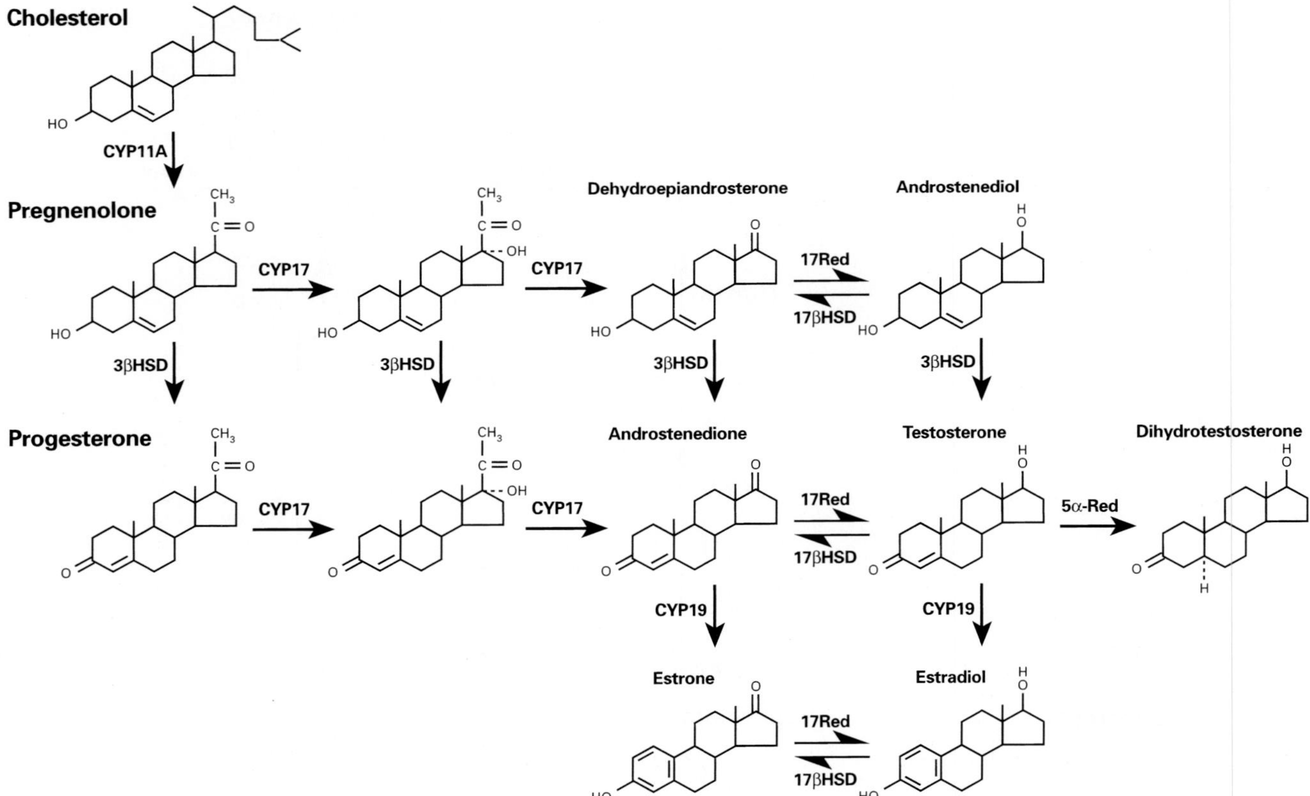

Figure 4–6 ■ General scheme for synthesis of estrogens and androgens.

rated parent system. Many important steroids have trivial names; some examples are listed in Table 4–2. In addition, prefixes can be used to modify trivial names as indicated in Table 4–3. The prefixes dihydro-, tetrahydro-, dehydro-, hydroxy-, deoxy-, and others refer to the addition or deletion of hydrogen and oxygen atoms from the parent molecule; the prefix epi- denotes inversion of a substituent, and nor- denotes elimination of a methyl group.

Steroid conjugates are commonly encountered, and they are named according to the following system. For esters of monohydric steroids, the steroid hydrocarbon radical name is followed by that of the acyloxy group in its anionic form. The steroid radical name is formed by replacing the terminal -e of the hydrocarbon name by -yl and inserting before this the locant and Greek letter; an example would be 5-cholesten-3β-yl sulfonate (trivial name, cholesterol sulfonate).

Figure 4–12 depicts a C_{19} steroid with the perhydrocyclopentanophenanthrene nucleus in its planar configuration and the conformation or spatial orientation of atoms that are free to rotate with respect to each other about an asymmetric carbon. That is, orientations can assume two distinguishable positions: equatorial (e), when they lie close to the plane of the ring, and axial (a), when they are more or less perpendicular to the plane of the ring. Several biochemical generalizations based on the spatial orientation of substituents have been put forth.[32] For example, a substituent is more stable in the equatorial than in the axial orientation; an equatorial hydroxyl group is more easily acylated than is an axial group at the same position (rule also applies to the hydrolysis of esters). Stereoconfiguration of the perhydrocyclopentanophenanthrene nucleus is al-

Figure 4–7 ■ Steroid configuration. Steroid carbon atoms are numbered, and ring structures are designated by letters.

Figure 4–8 ■ Orientation of atoms or groups about steroid asymmetric centers.

CH_3 | H—C—OH CH_3 | HO—C—H

5α-Pregnan-20α-ol   **5β-Pregnan-20β-ol**

Figure 4–9 ■ Configuration of hydrogen at steroid carbon 5; substituents at position 20 of a pregnane derivative.

■ TABLE 4–2
Trivial Names of Steroids

TRIVIAL NAME	SYSTEMATIC NAME
Cholesterol	5-Cholesten-3-β-ol
Cholestanol	5α-Cholestan-3-β-ol
Coprostanol	5β-Cholestan-3-β-ol
Androstenedione	4-Androstene-3,17-dione
Testosterone	17β-Hydroxy-4-androsten-3-one
Androsterone	3α-Hydroxy-5α-androstan-17-one
Etiocholanolone	3α-Hydroxy-5β-androstan-17-one
Estrone	3-Hydroxy-1,3,5(10)-estratrien-17-one
Estradiol	1,3,5(10)-Estratriene-3,17β-diol
Estriol	1,3,5(10)-Estratriene-3,16α,17β-triol
Pregnenolone	3β-Hydroxy-5-pregnen-20-one
Progesterone	4-Pregnene-3,20-dione
Pregnanolone	3α-Hydroxy-5β-pregnan-20-one
Pregnanediol	5β-Pregnane-3α,20α-diol
Cortisone	17α,21-Dihydroxy-4-pregnene-3,11,20-trione
Cortisol	11β,17α,21-Trihydroxy-4-pregnene-3,20-dione
Cortol	5β-Pregnane-3α,11β,17α,20α,21-pentol
Cortolone	3α,17α,20α,21-Tetrahydroxy-5β-pregnane-11-one
Aldosterone	11β,21-Dihydroxy-3,20-dioxo-4-pregnen-18-al

ways *trans* at the junctions of rings B and C and essentially always at the C and D rings but can be either *cis* or *trans* at rings A and B. For example, the 5α-reduced metabolite of testosterone, 5α-dihydrotestosterone, is A/B *trans* and takes the shape of a planar molecule (Fig. 4–13*B*). In contrast, the 5β-reduced metabolite of testosterone, 5β-dihydrotestosterone, is A/B *cis* and forms a nonplanar molecule with an almost right-angle bend (Fig. 4–13*C*). The presence of a double bond involving carbon 5, either a 4 to 5 double bond in ring A or a 5 to 6 double bond in ring B, also creates a planar molecule as demonstrated by the structure of testosterone (Fig. 4–13*A*). In fact, the shapes of testosterone and 5α-dihydrotestosterone are similar as illustrated by the top and side views for each steroid presented in Figure 4–13*A* and *B*, respectively. These structural similarities and distinctions have significant functional implications. For instance, 5α-dihydrotestosterone and testosterone both bind to the human prostatic androgen receptor and demonstrate biologic activity, whereas 5β-dihydrotestosterone binds weakly and is essentially devoid of biologic activity.[33, 34] Similarly, the 5α-reduced metabolite of progesterone (5α-dihydroprogesterone) in the chicken oviduct is biologically as active as progesterone, in contrast to the 5β-reduced metabolite (5β-dihydroprogesterone), which demonstrates limited activity.[35] Furthermore, the biologic activity of 5α-dihydroprogesterone presumably relates to its ability to bind to the progesterone receptor; 5β-dihydroprogesterone, in contrast, binds poorly to the progesterone receptor and has little biologic activity.[36]

Clinical Evaluation

Investigation of the physiology or pathophysiology of a steroid hormone–producing endocrine gland necessitates consideration of the amount of particular steroids being produced. Initially, this commonly involves the determination of steroid concentrations in blood and in some instances the measurement of unconjugated steroids or steroid metabolites excreted in urine. In analyzing plasma

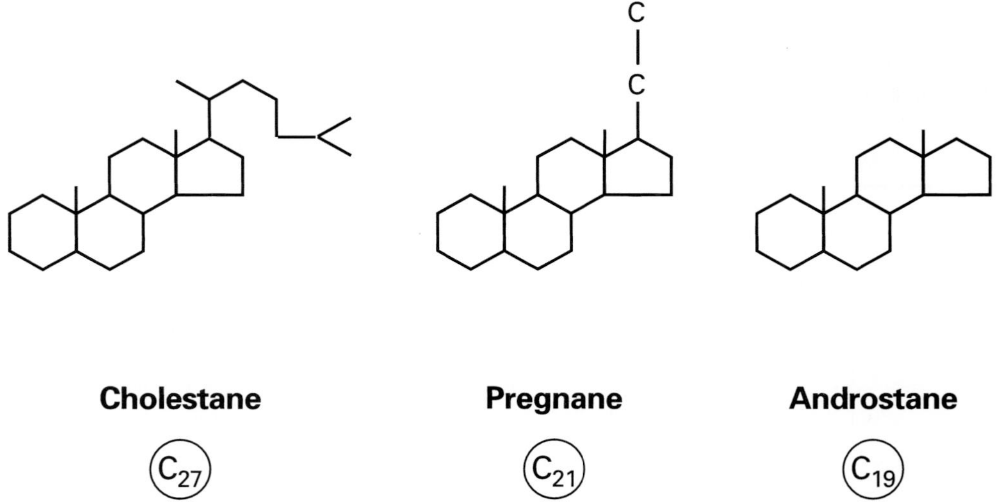

Figure 4–10 ■ Parent compounds when all steroid rings are saturated.

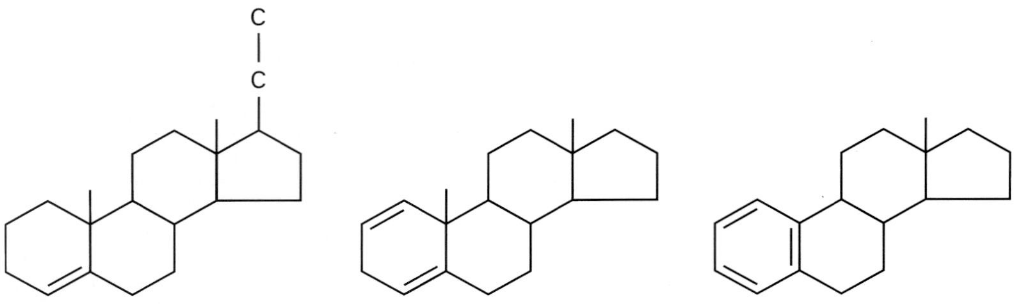

C
C

4-Pregnene **1,4-Androstadiene** **1,3,5(10)-Estratriene**

Figure 4–11 ■ Steroid ring unsaturation.

steroid levels, certain considerations could come into play, for instance, the age and sex of the patient, diurnal—episodic—and cyclic steroid secretion, and the peripheral interconversion of steroids.

Steroid concentrations in blood have traditionally been expressed in units such as micrograms per deciliter, picograms per milliliter, and so forth. The Commission on Quantities and Units (International Union of Pure and Applied Chemistry) has recommended that SI units (Système International d'Unités), which express a substance concentration as moles per liter, be used. In fact, the employment of SI units is more helpful in understanding physiologic mechanisms. For example, steroid receptors are generally measured in moles, and the measurement of steroid blood concentrations in moles per liter facilitates comparison of a circulating steroid level with receptor availability. Reference ranges for selected steroids in blood, determined for the most part by a single laboratory, are listed in Table 4–4. It is important that each laboratory develop its own norms, and the clinician or investigator should ascertain that such norms have been established and are in use.

The measurement of steroid concentrations in urine is of little value because urinary volume is highly variable relative to steroid clearance. The amount of a steroid excreted in the urine is usually expressed as micrograms or milligrams per 24 hours. The accepted way to express urinary steroid values has been in terms of unit mass of creatinine, because creatinine is commonly thought to be excreted at a constant rate; thus, determining a steroid:creatinine ratio allows for variation in the urine volume. It turns out, however, that this is not strictly the case because significant variability in urinary creatinine excretion can occur.[37] Nonetheless, in the clinical evaluation of adrenocortical function, measurement of urinary corticoids or metabolites is still commonly used. In reproductive endocrinology,

■ TABLE 4–3

Modified Trivial Names of Steroids

MODIFIED TRIVIAL NAME	SYSTEMATIC NAME
25-Hydroxycholesterol	5-Cholesten-3β,25-diol
Dihydrotestosterone	17β-Hydroxy-5α-androstan-3-one
19-Nortestosterone	17β-Hydroxy-4-estren-3-one
Dehydroepiandrosterone	3β-Hydroxy-5-androsten-17-one
17-Hydroxyprogesterone	17α-Hydroxy-4-pregnene-3,20-dione
20α-Dihydroprogesterone	20α-Hydroxy-4-pregnen-3-one
11-Deoxycortisol	17α,21-Dihydroxy-4-pregnene-3,20-dione
Tetrahydrocortisone	3α,17α,21-Trihydroxy-5β-pregnane-11,20-dione
Tetrahydrocortisol	3α,11β,17α,21-Tetrahydroxy-5β-pregnan-20-one
Allocortol	5α-Pregnane-3α,11β,17α,20α,21-pentol
Allocortolone	3α,17α,20α,21-Tetrahydroxy-5α-pregnane-11-one

■ TABLE 4–4

Reference Ranges for Selected Reproductive Steroids in Adult Human Serum

STEROID	SUBJECTS	REFERENCE VALUES
Androstenedione	Men	2.8–7.3 nmol/L
	Women	3.1–12.2 nmol/L
Testosterone	Men	6.9–34.7 nmol/L
	Women	0.7–2.8 nmol/L
Dihydrotestosterone	Men	1.03–3.10 nmol/L
	Women	0.07–0.86 nmol/L
Dehydroepiandrosterone	Men/women	5.5–24.3 nmol/L
Dehydroepiandrosterone sulfonate	Men/women	2.5–10.4 μmol/L
Progesterone	Men	<0.3–1.3 nmol/L
	Women	
	Follicular	0.3–3.0 nmol/L
	Luteal	19.0–45.0 nmol/L
Estradiol	Men	<37–210 pmol/L
	Women	
	Follicular	<37–360 pmol/L
	Midcycle	625–2830 pmol/L
	Luteal	699–1250 pmol/L
	Postmenopausal	<37–140 pmol/L
Estrone	Men	37–250 pmol/L
	Women	
	Follicular	110–400 pmol/L
	Luteal	310–660 pmol/L
	Postmenopausal	22–230 pmol/L
Estrone sulfonate	Men	600–2500 pmol/L
	Women	
	Follicular	700–3600 pmol/L
	Luteal	1100–7300 pmol/L
	Postmenopausal	130–1200 pmol/L

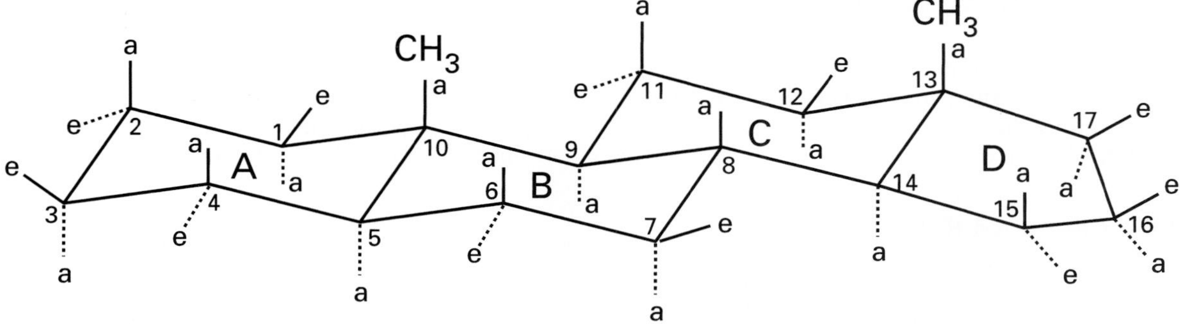

Figure 4–12 ■ Planar configuration of a C_{19} steroid showing confirmation or spatial orientation of atoms free to rotate with respect to each other about an asymmetric carbon.

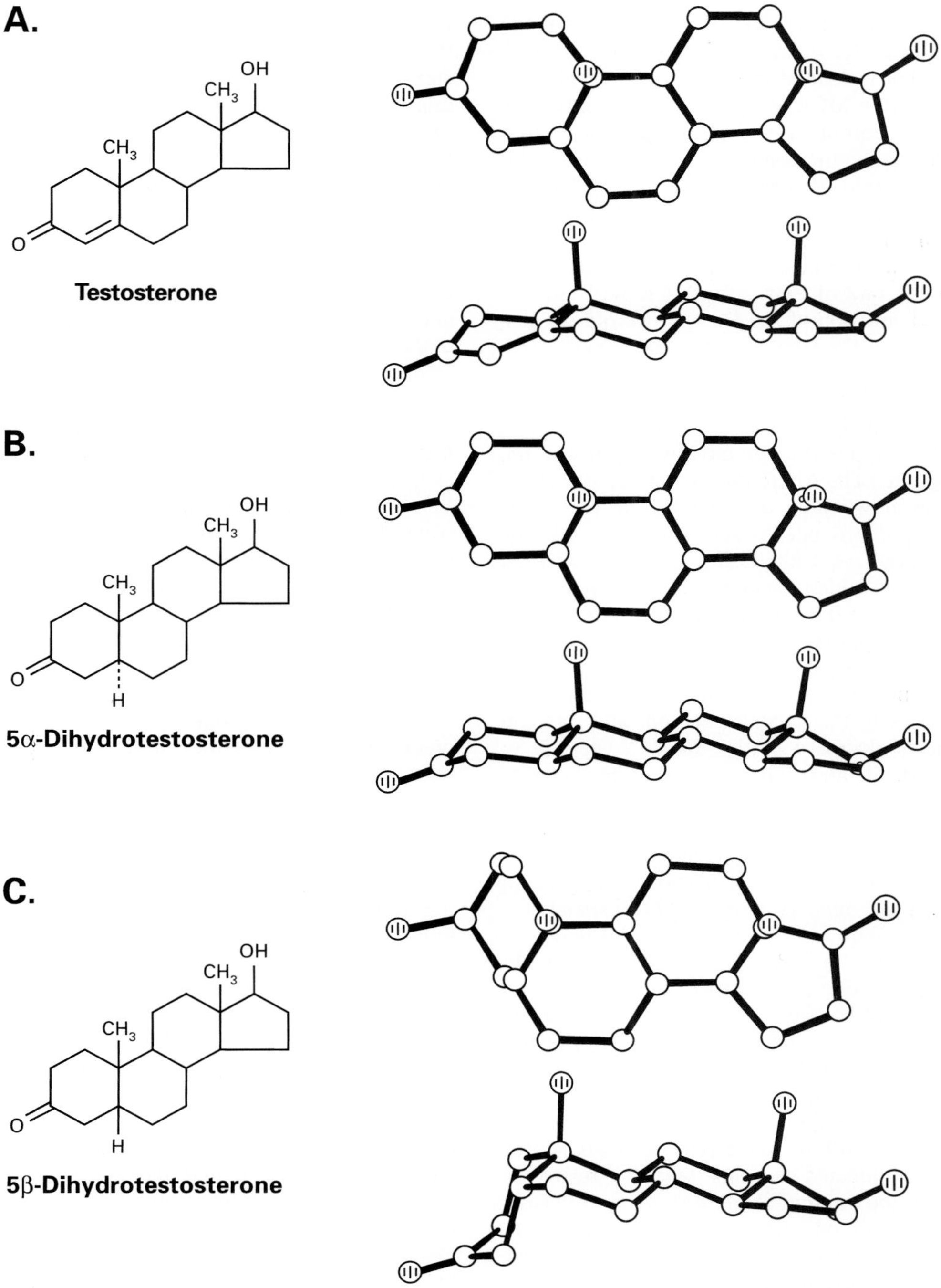

A.

OH

CH_3

CH_3

O

Testosterone

B.

OH

CH_3

CH_3

O

H

5α-Dihydrotestosterone

C.

OH

CH_3

CH_3

O

H

5β-Dihydrotestosterone

Figure 4–13 ■ Configuration of testosterone *(A),* 5α-dihydrotestosterone *(B),* and 5β-dihydrotestosterone *(C)* with top and side structural views.

though, it is the analysis of plasma steroids and not urinary metabolites that forms the common approach. A detailed discussion regarding the evaluation of the hormonal status is presented in Chapter 26.

Metabolic Clearance Rate

A steroid is secreted and enters the blood compartment, and as the blood flows through each tissue in the body, a certain amount of the steroid will be removed or extracted. The metabolic clearance rate (MCR) is defined as the volume of blood that has been completely cleared of a substance per unit time (L/day).[38] The rate of clearance of a steroid from the blood of the whole body is the sum of steroid clearance rates for each tissue or organ, and it is the overall value that is termed the MCR. The usual technique for measuring the MCR is to continuously infuse an isotopically labeled steroid at a constant rate and, after sufficient time, determine the concentration of the unconjugated radioactive steroid in peripheral venous blood to verify the presence of a steady state. At equilibrium, the concentration of the isotopic steroid in blood will be constant, and the rate of clearance of the steroid from blood will be equal to the rate of entry; the MCR will then be equal to the rate of infusion of the isotopic steroid divided by the concentration of the labeled steroid in blood:

$$\text{cpm/min} \div \text{cpm/ml} = \text{ml/day or L/day}$$

The liver is the principal tissue for removing steroids from blood, and it is possible to directly determine the hepatic clearance rate. The MCR minus the hepatic clearance rate indicates how much of the total clearance has occurred in extrahepatic tissue. Because hepatic blood flow is in the neighborhood of 1500 L/day, a steroid with an MCR in excess of this value indicates that tissue other than the liver is extracting the steroid. For example, androstenedione has an MCR of approximately 2000 L/day, indicating that a substantial extrahepatic clearance is present. The MCR can also be influenced by posture, because hepatic blood flow decreases in the upright position, and this can lead to a significant decrease in the MCR.[39] The fall in MCR, when one goes from a lying to a standing position, can result in an increase in the plasma steroid concentration without a change in the secretion rate for the steroid (although a change in the secretion rate could also occur).

The binding of steroids to explicit plasma proteins such as testosterone-estradiol–binding globulin (TEBG) and corticosteroid-binding globulin (CBG or transcortin) will suppress peripheral metabolism.[40] This is reflected in relatively low MCRs for testosterone and cortisol. Furthermore, an increase in the level of a discrete steroid-binding plasma protein can further suppress the MCR of the specifically bound steroid. Many unconjugated steroids bind to albumin, but unlike specific steroid binding to TEBG and CBG, the binding of unconjugated steroids to albumin is nonspecific and of low affinity. This results in MCRs for albumin-bound unconjugated steroids that are relatively high, indicating that the binding of these steroids to plasma albumin has little effect on metabolism.[40] In contrast to the situation with unconjugated steroids, however, steroid sulfoconjugates bind avidly to plasma albumin[41] and as a result are cleared slowly from the blood compartment.[42, 43] The low MCR for steroid sulfonates is reflected in an increase in their plasma concentration; steroid sulfonates circulate at concentrations several-fold higher than their unconjugated form[44, 45] (see Table 4–4).

Secretion and Production Rates

Biologically active steroids, for the most part, are secreted by a primary steroid endocrine gland such as the gonad or adrenal cortex. Steroid precursors and intermediates (see Figs. 4–5 and 4–6), however, can leach out of the steroid-producing tissue, and it is possible for them to be converted to a biologically active form in peripheral tissue such as the skin or adipose tissue. Thus, the secreted inactive steroid acts as a *prehormone*, in that it is converted peripherally to an active hormone.[46] For instance, androstenedione (prehormone) can be converted in peripheral tissue to testosterone (hormone). In addition, testosterone, the major androgen secreted by the testis and the primary circulating androgen in males, also functions as a prehormone in that it is converted to two other potent hormones, namely, dihydrotestosterone and estradiol. In fact, it is the former compound that serves as the principal androgenic mediator and is the major androgen bound to the androgen receptor in tissues such as accessory sexual glands, genital skin, sebaceous glands, hair follicles, and the anterior pituitary.[47]

To speak of a *secretion rate* refers to the total secretion from endocrine glands. To speak of a *production rate* refers to the entry of a steroid into the blood compartment from all possible sources, endocrine glands and peripheral sites. In a steady state, the amount of a steroid being cleared from the blood will be equal to the amount of steroid entering the circulation, and the blood production rate will equal the MCR multiplied by the plasma steroid concentration ($PR = MCR \times [S]$). When the peripheral conversion of a precursor does not contribute significantly to the amount of hormone entering the blood compartment, the blood production rate will be equal to the secretion rate. For example, aldosterone, a steroid that has no peripheral precursor and enters the circulation only as a result of secretion by the adrenal cortex, has a secretion rate that is equivalent to the blood production rate. When the peripheral conversion of a precursor does contribute significantly to the total amount of steroid hormone entering the blood compartment, the blood production rate will be greater than the secretion rate. The additional amount of steroid hormone is derived from the endocrine secretion of an inactive precursor that undergoes conversion in the periphery to the active form and then re-enters the circulation to mix with the endocrine-secreted steroid hormone. The fraction of secreted steroid precursor that is converted to the steroid hormone product is referred to as the rho (ρ) value. As a means of determining the ρ value, a radioactive form of the precursor is infused at a constant rate until equilibrium is reached, and the plasma concentrations of unconjugated radioactive precursor and radioactive product are determined. The ratio of the radioactivity in the product to the precursor determines the percentage of conversion of the precursor to the product. The conversion ratio multiplied by the ratio of the MCRs of the product and precursor determines the ρ value:

$$\frac{cpm^{product}}{cpm^{precursor}} \times \frac{MCR^{product}}{MCR^{precursor}} = \rho^{pre\text{-}pro}$$

If the blood production rate of the precursor is known, then the $\rho^{pre\text{-}pro}$ multiplied by the production rate of the precursor will yield the amount of the product entering the circulation that is derived from the precursor. In steroid endocrinology, precursor-product peripheral conversions can significantly influence the physiologic or pathophysiologic status. More specifically, in reproductive endocrinology, important precursor-product conversions are androstenedione to estrone, estrone to estradiol, androstenedione to testosterone, testosterone to estradiol, and testosterone to dihydrotestosterone. Figure 4–14 depicts ρ values for four sex steroid interconversions obtained from the excellent in-depth review of the concepts of MCR, production rate, and steroid interconversion presented by Baird and associates.[48]

The secretion of a steroid by an endocrine gland can be determined by selective catheterization. The concentration of the steroid is measured simultaneously in the effluent venous blood and in the peripheral circulation; if a steroid gradient can be established by subtracting the peripheral venous concentration, glandular secretion is confirmed. With the additional measurement of the effluent blood flow, a reasonable estimate of the glandular secretion rate for the steroid can be made. Whereas this is a valuable technique for examining glandular steroid secretion, there are certain caveats to bear in mind: blood removed from the effluent vein can be diluted by inadvertent mixture with peripheral blood, and the stress of the procedure may alter the effluent blood flow.

On the basis of considerations of MCRs, secretion and production rates, and ρ values, the following particulars have been determined. In normal menstruating women, approximately 60 percent of circulating testosterone and essentially 100 percent of circulating dihydrotestosterone are derived from the peripheral conversion of androstenedione; 30 to 40 percent of testosterone is directly secreted. On the other hand, greater than 95 percent of circulating estradiol is directly secreted, the rest being derived from the peripheral conversion of estrone; approximately two thirds of circulating estrone is secreted, with the remaining derived from the peripheral conversion of estradiol and androstenedione. In normal men, greater than 95 percent of plasma testosterone is directly secreted, with a small amount derived peripherally from androstenedione. Two thirds or more of circulating estradiol in men results from direct testicular secretion, with the remainder derived from the peripheral conversion of testosterone and estrone.[24, 49] Likewise, the majority of circulating estrone in men is secreted (about 60 to 70 percent from the testis; 10 percent from the adrenal), with the rest coming from the peripheral conversion of estradiol and androstenedione.[24, 48] Similar to that in women, circulating dihydrotestosterone in men is mostly derived from peripheral conversion (60 percent from testosterone; 15 percent from androstenedione), with only 25 percent being secreted. Blood production rates, secretion rates, and MCRs for reproductive steroid hormones are listed in Table 4–5.

Plasma Protein Binding

The fact that steroid hormones bind to circulating plasma proteins presents them in two forms in the circulation: bound and unbound.[40, 50, 51] Greater than 97 percent of testosterone and estradiol is bound to plasma proteins,

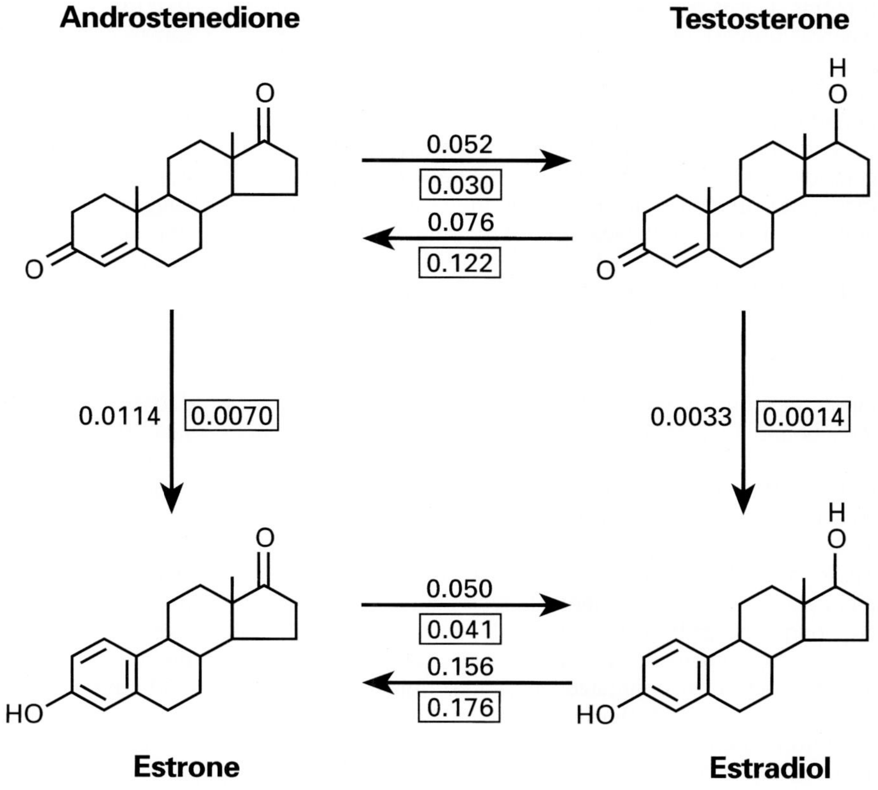

Androstenedione → Testosterone: 0.052 [0.030]; Testosterone → Androstenedione: 0.076 [0.122]

Androstenedione → Estrone: 0.0114 [0.0070]; Testosterone → Estradiol: 0.0033 [0.0014]

Estrone → Estradiol: 0.050 [0.041]; Estradiol → Estrone: 0.156 [0.176]

Figure 4–14 ■ Mean rho (ρ) values for androgens and estrogens. Values for women are boxed. (From Baird DT, Horton R, Longcope C, Tait JF. Steroid dynamics under steady-state conditions. Recent Prog Horm Res 25:611–664, 1969.)

■ TABLE 4–5

Blood Production Rate, Secretion Rate, and Metabolic Clearance Rate for Reproductive Steroid Hormones

STEROID		MCR (L/day)	PR (mg/day)	SR (mg/day)
Men				
Androstenedione		2200	2.8	1.6
Testosterone		950	6.5	6.2
Estrone		2050	0.15	0.11
Estradiol		1600	0.06	0.05
Estrone sulfonate		167	0.08	Insig
Women				
Androstenedione		2000	3.2	2.8
Testosterone		500	0.19	0.06
Estrone	F	2200	0.11	0.08
	L	2200	0.26	0.15
	PM	1610	0.04	Insig
Estradiol	F	1200	0.09	0.08
	L	1200	0.25	0.24
	PM	910	0.006	Insig
Estrone sulfonate	F	146	0.10	Insig
	L	146	0.18	Insig
Progesterone	F	2100	2.0	1.7
	L	2100	25.0	24.0

MCR, metabolic clearance rate; PR, production rate; SR, secretion rate; F, follicular phase of menstrual cycle; L, luteal phase of menstrual cycle; PM, postmenopausal; Insig, insignificant.

specifically to TEBG and nonspecifically to albumin. Testosterone is bound more to TEBG (men, 65 percent; women, 78 percent) than to albumin (men, 33 percent; women, 20 percent). Because estradiol has a somewhat weaker binding affinity than does testosterone for TEBG, binding to albumin (men, 68 percent; women, 40 percent) is increased relative to TEBG (men, 30 percent; women, 58 percent). The same situation exists for cortisol and progesterone; more than 97 percent is also bound to plasma proteins. Cortisol is bound primarily to CBG (90 percent), whereas progesterone, because CBG has a somewhat lower affinity for progesterone than for cortisol and the cortisol concentration usually far exceeds that of progesterone, is bound mainly to albumin (80 percent). The specific binding of testosterone (and dihydrotestosterone) to TEBG and of cortisol to CBG is reflected in relatively low MCRs for these steroids. In contrast, other unconjugated steroids bound primarily (but weakly) to albumin have relatively high MCRs.

The MCRs for unconjugated steroids can be thought of as forming a continuum from a relatively low to high level, covering essentially an order of magnitude (as an approximation, about 200 to 2000 L/day). Where a particular steroid falls on this continuum is dictated by the degree it is bound to a specific plasma-binding protein. For instance, cortisol, in both men and women, is highly bound to CBG (90 percent) and has an MCR of around 200 L/day; testosterone is bound to a somewhat lower degree by TEBG (women, 78 percent; men, 65 percent) and has an MCR of about 500 L/day for women and 950 L/day for men. On the other hand, androstenedione and progesterone are bound primarily by albumin and have MCRs of roughly 2000 L/day; however, in contrast to the rather weak albumin binding of unconjugated steroids, sulfonate conjugates of steroids (e.g., testosterone sulfonate and dehydroepiandrosterone sulfonate) are strongly bound by albumin and as a consequence have extremely low MCRs, in the neighborhood of 20 L/day.[42, 43] Steroid sulfonates are cleared from the circulation more slowly than are steroids conjugated as glucuronates.[52] This reflects a major difference in the protein binding of sulfonate conjugates (strong) versus glucuronate conjugates (weak).[53]

Steroids are ordinarily measured in blood as the total concentration, although an analysis of the bound and unbound fractions is possible. It has been accepted for some time that the unbound fraction is the biologically important fraction because it can freely diffuse into tissue during transit of the capillary bed.[54] On the other hand, the protein-bound fraction is thought to act primarily as a reservoir for steroid hormones. Unconjugated steroids bound to albumin, because of low binding affinities and rapid dissociation rates, are generally treated as being free and biologically available.[55, 56] Interestingly, there is immunologic evidence suggesting that TEBG and CBG may themselves have important functions in target tissues.[56] In addition, it has been demonstrated that cell membranes have specific binding sites for TEBG[57] and CBG.[58, 59] Whereas some cell types appear to actively internalize CBG and TEBG, the biologic impact of these interactions is not well understood.[60] There is no definitive evidence that steroid-binding plasma proteins facilitate entry of steroids into cells.[61] In fact, the hepatic uptake of cortisol from serum can be entirely accounted for by the pool of free cortisol.[62] It thus appears that the action of steroid hormones in target tissue does not require the extracellular presence of TEBG and CBG; however, it has been proposed that these specific steroid-binding proteins might function to modulate hormonal responsivity by controlling the availability of the free steroid molecule.[63, 64] Regardless, at this juncture, a precise biologic function for extracellular, high-affinity steroid-binding proteins remains to be elucidated.[64]

Because the clinical evaluation of a steroid hormone routinely involves an interpretation of the steroid's total circulating concentration, it is important to take into ac-

■ TABLE 4–6

Factors and Endocrine Status that Influence the Binding Capacity of Testosterone-Estradiol–Binding Globulin and Cortisol-Binding Globulin

FACTORS AND ENDOCRINE STATUS	BINDING CAPACITY	
	TEBG	**CBG**
Exogenous estrogen	↑	↑
Pregnancy	↑	↑
Exogenous androgen	↓	↓
Anabolic steroids	↓	n.c.
Danazol (androgenic properties)	↓	n.c.
Progestins (androgenic properties)	↓	n.c.
Thyroid hormones (severe hyperthyroidism)	↑	↓
Prolactin (hyperprolactinemia)	↓	n.c.
Growth hormone (acromegaly)	↓	n.c.
Old age (men)	↑	—
Postmenopausal	↓	—
Obesity	↓	n.c.

TEBG, testosterone-estradiol–binding globulin; CBG, cortisol-binding globulin; n.c., no change.

count the influence of specific steroid-binding proteins on the total plasma steroid hormone level. There are conditions associated with either a significant increase or decrease in TEBG and CBG levels in blood that are reflected in a relative increase or decrease in respective steroid concentrations[65] (Table 4–6); and, as noted previously, a change in the plasma level of TEBG or CBG will affect the MCR of steroid hormones bound to them.[40] For example, estrogen treatment increases TEBG and CBG levels in blood along with the total concentration of testosterone and cortisol; concomitantly, the MCRs for testosterone and cortisol are reduced as a result of reduced tissue extraction and metabolism. Nonetheless, in such cases, when a state of equilibrium is re-established, the free steroid level will be essentially normal, indicating that the free steroid level is a better index of the hormonal status.[66]

Steroid Transformation and Conjugation

Circulating steroids are transformed primarily in the liver by a series of reactions, and the altered metabolites are conjugated and excreted in the urine mostly as glucuronides (glucosiduronates) but also to some extent as sulfonate esters[67, 68] (Fig. 4–15). The steroid glucuronides are formed by the action of glucuronosyltransferase, present in liver microsomes, and uridine diphosphoglucuronic acid. Steroid sulfonates are formed by the action of soluble steroid sulfotransferases and the universal sulfonate donor, 3′-phosphoadenosine 5′-phosphosulfate. Major reactions in the transmutation of neutral steroids are

1. reduction of the double bond between carbons 4 and 5 of ring A;
2. reduction of the 3-keto group in ring A;
3. oxidation of the 11β-hydroxyl group of cortisol;
4. oxidation of the 17β-hydroxyl group in C_{19} steroids;
5. reduction of the 20-keto group of progesterone and corticoids;
6. cleavage of the side chain of C_{21} steroids, thereby producing 17-ketosteroids;
7. esterification to either glucuronic acid or sulfuric acid.

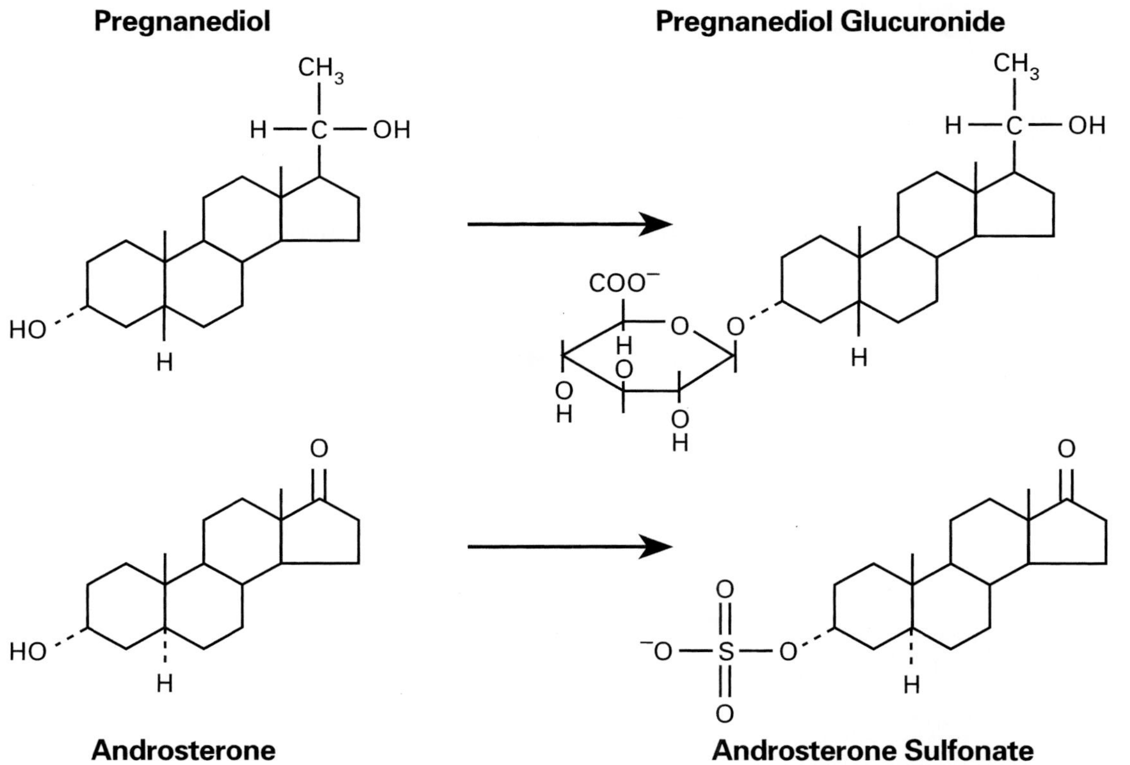

Pregnanediol → Pregnanediol Glucuronide

Androsterone → Androsterone Sulfonate

Figure 4–15 ■ Steroid conjugates.

An important biotransformation for cortisol involves the 11β-hydroxyl group and interconversion with cortisone (Fig. 4–16*A*). The reversible oxidation-reduction enzyme system (11βHSD1) uses both nicotinamide adenine dinucleotide and nicotinamide adenine dinucleotide phosphate, with the latter being more effective, and is widely distributed but predominant in the liver. Under normal conditions, the reaction is somewhat in favor of the oxidized (cortisone) form, which has reduced biologic activity. 11βHSD1 is a principal determinant of the level of circulating cortisol and is strongly influenced by thyroid hormone, which accelerates the oxidative reaction. The liver irreversibly reduces the ring A double bond of cortisol and cortisone (Fig. 4–16*A*), progesterone (Fig. 4–16*B*), and testosterone and androstenedione (Fig. 4–17*A*); reduction of the ring A double bond is followed by reduction of the 3-keto group. The two reduction steps are commonly combined and referred to as ring A reduction. In the reduction of ring A, the hydrogen at C-5 can be introduced in either the α or the β position (see Fig. 4–9); the reductases of liver require NADPH and are located in either microsomes (5α-reductase) or the cell sap (5β-reductase). β-Reduction at C-5 of cortisol, cortisone, and progesterone is predominant in humans, whereas reduction of the 3-keto group usually results in formation of a 3α-hydroxyl group (see Figs. 4–16 and 4–17*A*). Cortisol, cortisone, and progesterone also undergo reduction of the 20-keto group, principally as indicated in Figure 4–16. The tetrahydro-derivatives of cortisol and cortisone are found in urine largely as glucuronides with trace amounts as sulfonates.

Testosterone and androstenedione undergo ring A reduction in a similar manner (about half 5α and half 5β), and the 17β-hydroxyl group of testosterone is oxidized to 17-ketone (see Fig. 4–17*A*); these compounds are then excreted as glucuronides or sulfonates. Estrogens are largely excreted in the urine as glucuronides and sulfonates of estrone, estradiol, and estriol along with 2-hydroxyestrone; the last compound can be further metabolized by methylation at C-2 (see Fig. 4–17*B*). Estrone and 2-hydroxyestrone are the major metabolites in normal subjects.

Steroids can be transferred from blood to urine without being changed, but in amounts that are quite small in comparison to reduced and conjugated metabolites. Although steroids and their metabolites can be quantified in urine, it is customary in the field of reproductive endocrinology to determine the concentrations of biologically active steroid hormones in plasma or serum and forgo urinary measurements.

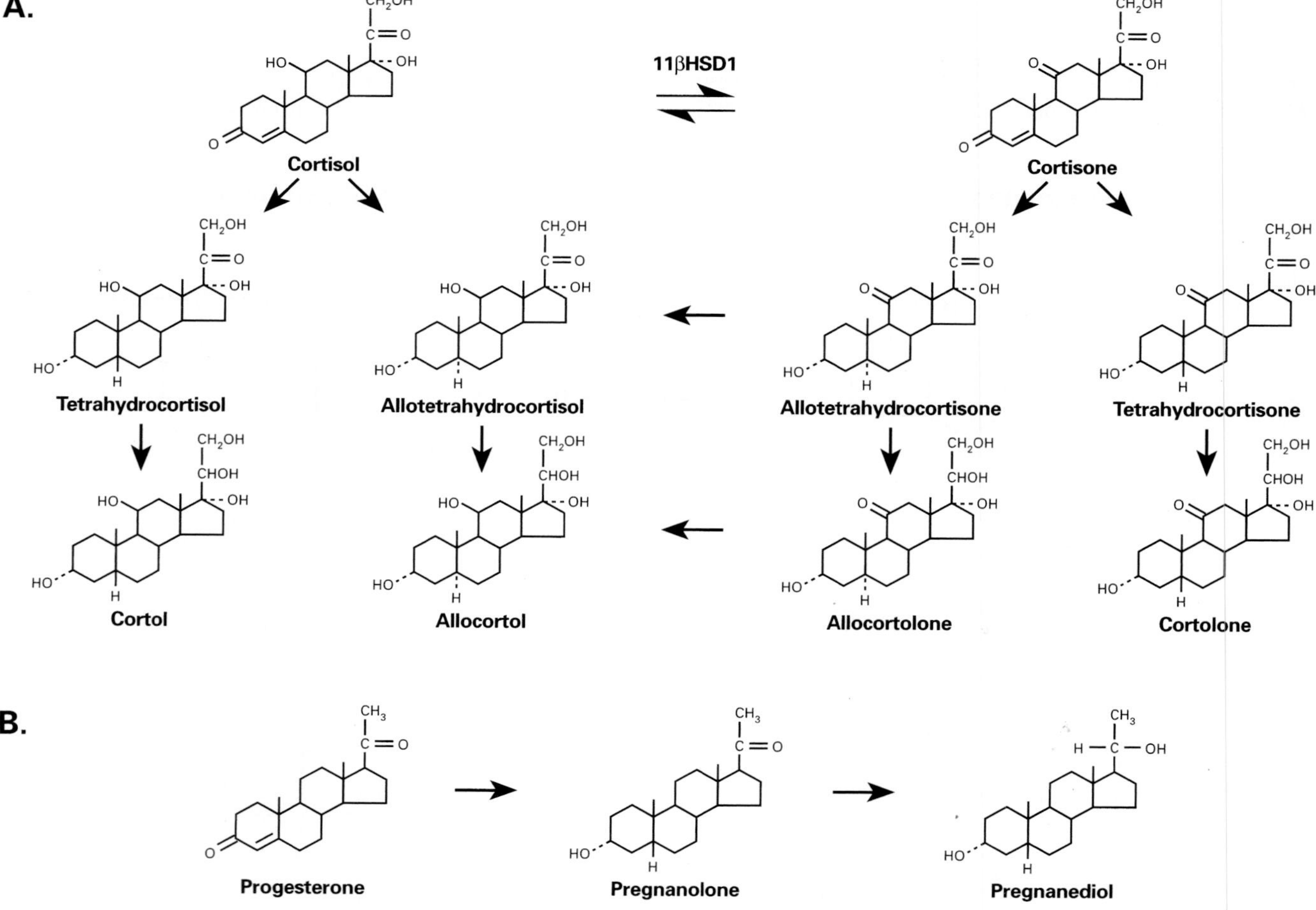

Figure 4–16 ■ Cortisol *(A)* and progesterone *(B)* metabolism.

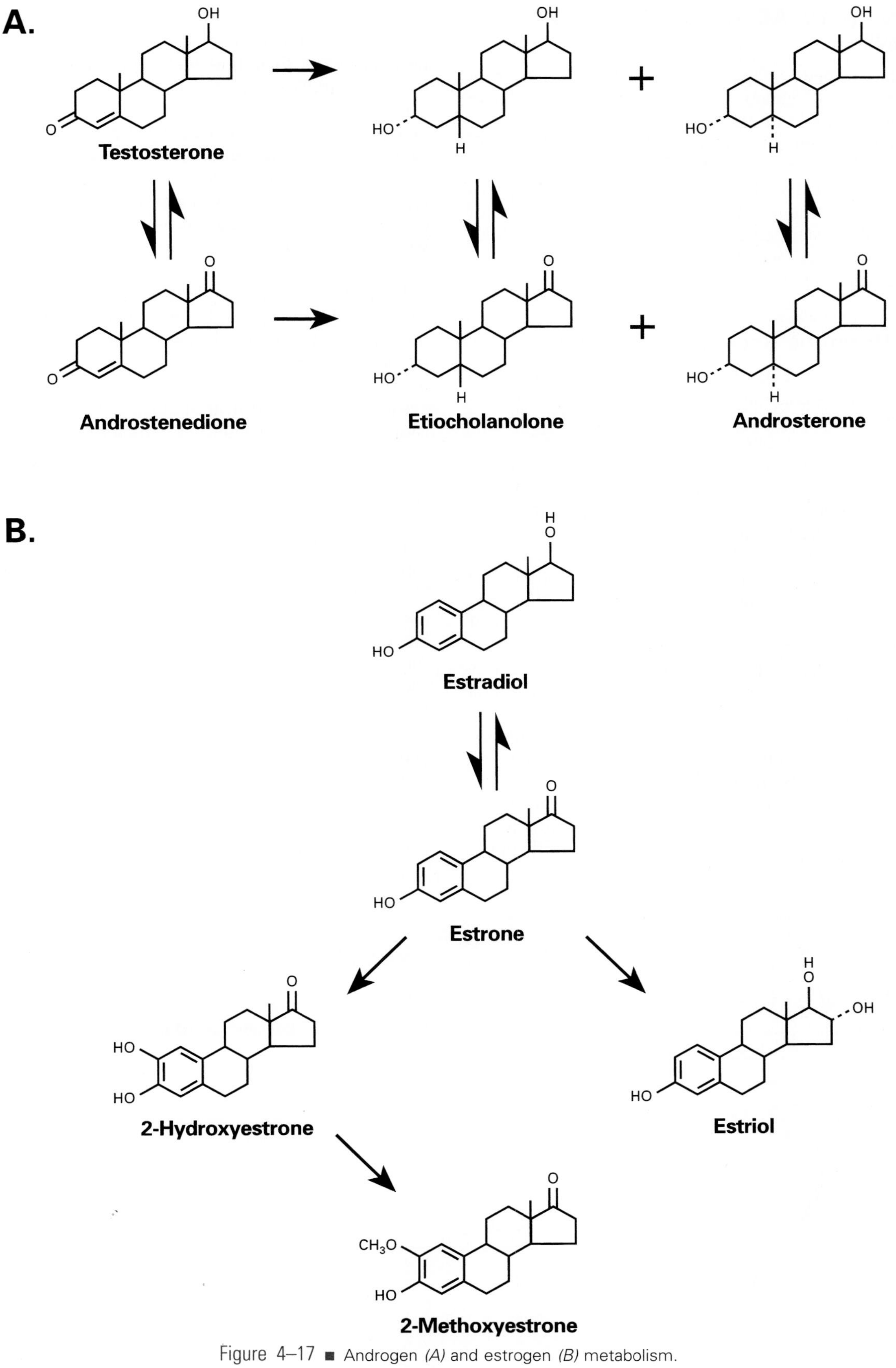

A.

Testosterone ⇌ Androstenedione

Testosterone → Etiocholanolone (17-OH) + Androsterone (17-OH)

Androstenedione → Etiocholanolone + Androsterone

B.

Estradiol ⇌ Estrone

Estrone → 2-Hydroxyestrone → 2-Methoxyestrone

Estrone → Estriol

Figure 4–17 ■ Androgen *(A)* and estrogen *(B)* metabolism.

MECHANISM OF ACTION OF STEROID HORMONES

All functions in cells of species as diverse as plants, fish, birds, animals, and humans are controlled by genes. There are between 80,000 and 100,000 functional genes in humans, and these genes are contained in the DNA of all human cells. In each cell type, approximately 2000 to 15,000 genes are active. These genes code for the proteins that compose the structural scaffold of cells, the enzymes of cells that control intermediary metabolism, and the cellular regulatory molecules, which in turn exert feedback influences on the genes themselves.

Steroid Hormone Receptors: Overview

Of the class of proteins that regulate gene function in human, animal, avian, and amphibian cells, the receptors for steroid hormones are a prime example. The classic steroidal hormones are estrogens, progesterone, androgens, glucocorticoids, mineralocorticoids, and vitamin D. These are potent hormones that regulate the developmental and physiologic functions of female phenotype (estrogen), pregnancy (progesterone), male phenotype (androgen), metabolism and stress responses (glucocorticoid), salt and water balance (mineralocorticoid), and calcium metabolism and skeletal growth (vitamin D). To accomplish this task, the steroid hormones must bind and activate a group of specific gene-regulatory molecules called receptors. These receptors are proteins that are present in cells in low amounts but that bind steroid hormones specifically and tightly.

Our current understanding of the biochemical pathway of steroid hormone action in cells can be summarized briefly as follows. The hormones are secreted from their respective endocrine glands into the blood stream, where they circulate, mostly bound (95 percent) to plasma transport proteins, which provide a reservoir for steroid supply to cells. The free steroids diffuse into cells and combine with specific receptors present in the target cells in which they will exert their functions. The receptor for estrogens (e.g., estradiol) exists primarily in female-specific target cells such as uterus, vagina, breast, and brain. In contrast, glucocorticoids (e.g., cortisol) have receptors in all cells because they must regulate metabolism and the stress response in all cells. After binding tightly to their specific receptors, the steroid hormones cause the receptors to undergo a conformational (allosteric) change in structure, which converts the receptors from an inactive to an active conformation. At this point, the receptors have the capacity to bind to the regulatory elements of genes and activate (or suppress) their function. If a gene is activated, for example, the enzyme RNA polymerase transcribes the information in the gene into messenger ribonucleic acid (mRNA), an intermediate molecule that carries the information to the cytoplasmic compartment of cells. There the information is again decoded (translated) on structures termed ribosomes, which produce the appropriate protein product specified by the gene in question. This pathway of steroid hormone action has been described in the past two decades[69–78] and is detailed in Figure 4–18.

Free steroid enters the cell and binds to inactive receptors in either the cytoplasmic or nuclear compartment. On complexing with hormone, the receptor undergoes an allosteric conformational change into an active form capable of affecting nuclear gene transcription. For efficient function directly, the receptor must dimerize, interact with specific DNA sequences, and then couple to other transcription factors to form a stable multimeric complex, which entices RNA polymerase to initiate transcription at that gene. A large pre-mRNA that includes all exons and introns of the gene is synthesized. The pre-mRNA is processed by a "splicing complex" that edits out all introns and assembles the exons into a contiguous sequence that codes for the respective protein product of the gene.

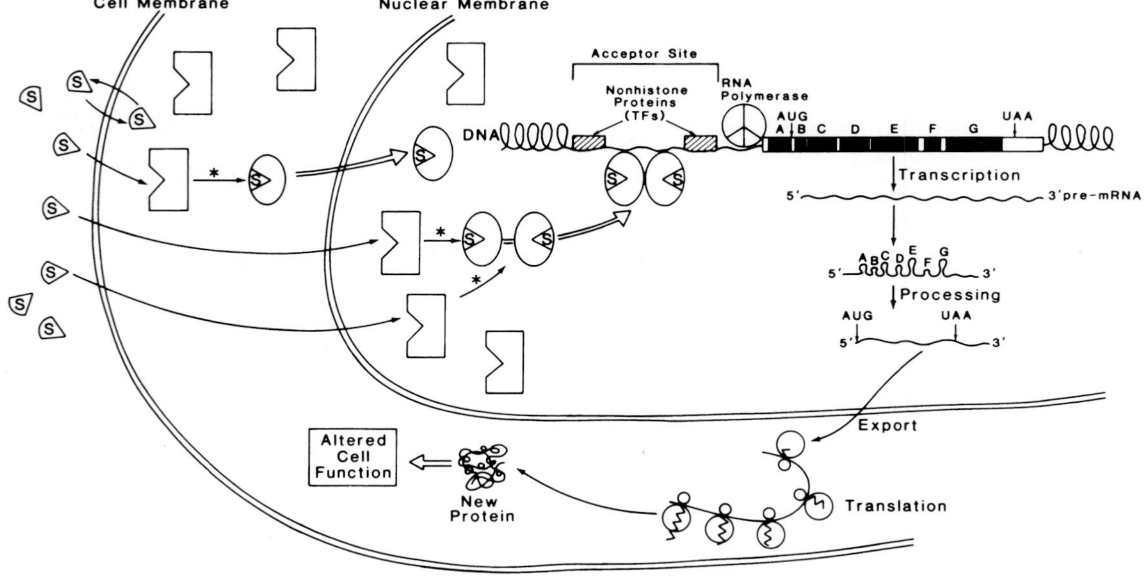

Figure 4–18 ■ Molecular pathway of steroid hormone action. TFs, transcription factors.

Receptor Gene Structure

To understand how steroid receptors might regulate gene function, we must first review the structure of genes in more detail.[79–81] A typical array of regulatory components for a steroid hormone–regulated gene is shown at the top of Figure 4–19. The structural gene contains the information transcribed into mRNA and later into the protein product of the gene. The mRNA is not synthesized, however, unless the regulatory elements of the gene are intact and "activated." These elements are linked to the gene and located near the beginning (5′ end) of the gene; they are termed *cis* elements because they are linked to the same strand of DNA (gene unit). The *cis* elements, which regulate expression of steroid-controlled genes, are classified into four main groups: (1) promoters, (2) steroid-responsive enhancers, (3) silencers, and (4) hormone-independent enhancers.

Receptor Gene Function

Promoters

The promoter is required absolutely for the gene to be transcribed and for mRNA to be produced. The promoter sets the basal rate of transcription and also controls accuracy of transcriptional initiation. Only one promoter is required, and it is usually located within 100 bases (deoxyribonucleotides) of the beginning of the gene (see Fig. 4–19).

The promoter is often composed of two distinct subelements. The TATA box is a 7–base pair (bp) adenine-thymine–rich sequence located approximately 30 bp from the start site of transcription for a gene. It is required absolutely for gene expression. The requirement for an upstream promoter (see Fig. 4–19) is more variable; when present, it increases promoter function and is usually located slightly farther upstream (~90 bp) from the first nucleotide (+1) of the transcript. Both of these subelements are activated to function when protein complexes bind specifically to these sites.

Steroid-Responsive Enhancers

Located farther upstream from the 5′ end of the gene, and not constrained to any particular site, is one or more copies of the steroid-responsive enhancer. Enhancers are short DNA sequences (~15 bp) that are potent stimulators of transcription and may be located close to or at a distance from their cognate genes. The enhancers, which respond to signals from steroid hormones, serve as DNA binding sites for the activated steroid-receptor complexes and are termed steroid response elements (SREs).[82] Such SRE sites have been shown to contain copies of a particularly important set of deoxyribonucleotides whose fundamental sequence composition contains binding sites for specific receptors.

Silencers

In contrast, silencers are *cis* elements that work in an opposite manner from enhancers. They act to decrease or silence transcription of genes. A particular gene may have one or more silencers. If a silencer is present, the adjacent

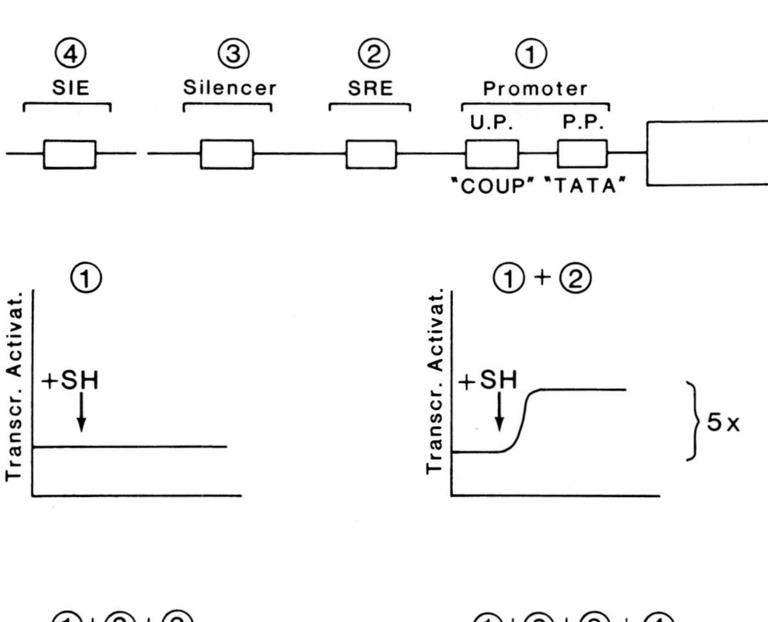

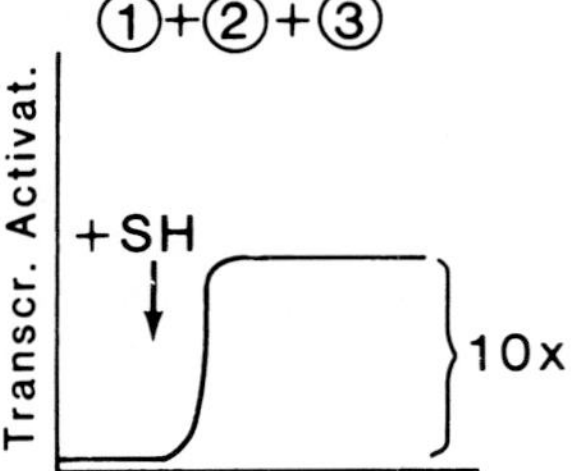

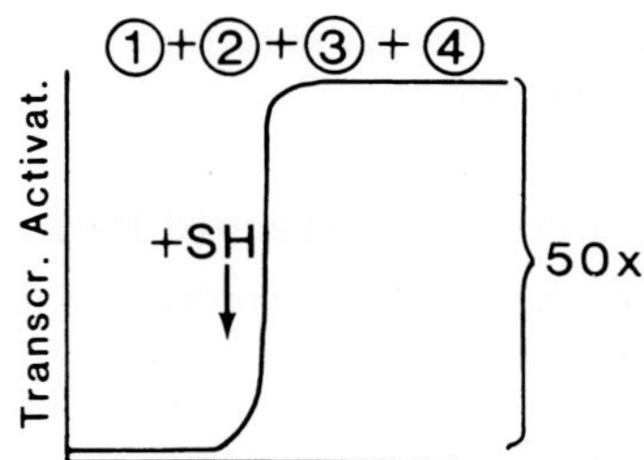

Figure 4–19 ■ Evolution of a tightly controlled gene with a marked inductive response to steroid hormone. SIE, steroid-independent enhancer; SRE, steroid response element; UP, upstream promoter; SH, steroid hormone.

gene has no basal rate of transcription in the absence of steroid hormone stimulation. Activation of the SRE will override the silencer effect, however, and turn on expression of the gene.

Hormone-Independent Enhancers

Finally, steroid-independent enhancers, one or more, may be located within the regulatory region of the gene. These *cis* elements tend to augment SRE function by further raising the maximal rate of inducible gene expression.

The manner by which these four types of *cis* elements cooperate to achieve precise regulation of expression of a gene is summarized schematically in Figure 4–19. In the absence of a promoter, a gene is not transcribed at a constant (constitutive) rate (see Fig. 4–19, panel 1). If the promoter is a "strong" one, the rate of transcription is high; if the promoter is "weak," it is expressed at a lower rate. In this case, the transcription of the gene is not subject to stimulation (or suppression) by steroid hormones. In contrast, the existence of a nearby SRE (enhancer) allows the gene to be placed under control of steroid hormones (see Fig. 4–19, panel 2). For example, hormone stimulation might increase the rate of transcription another fivefold above the basal level. If a silencer element is then added to the regulatory cassette, the basal level is decreased to near zero, but the maximal attainable level after hormone stimulation remains unaltered. This combination, however, now permits a 10-fold level of stimulation by hormone (see Fig. 4–19, panel 3). Finally, the addition of one or more steroid-independent enhancers leads to synergistic increases in the maximal level of expression in response to hormone (see Fig. 4–19, panel 4) but does not influence the basal level of transcription in the absence of hormone.

Such combinations of regulatory *cis* elements have been assembled around genes during thousands of millions of years of evolution. The process of evolution allows each gene to gather and retain the particular combination of *cis* elements that suits its own cellular needs. Assembly of these elements occurs by random DNA recombination, and retention occurs by positive evolutionary selection; that is to say, when a *cis* element "jumps" into the vicinity of a gene, it is retained in the gene's regulatory cassette if it provides a selective advantage for the cell's function and survival. There is no particular reason that a given gene may not have multiple similar or identical copies of each type of *cis* element. Such a case would simply magnify the quantitative effect of each type of response. We find that the ovalbumin gene of the chicken is an example of the type of gene portrayed in panel 4 of Figure 4–19. It has a strong promoter, is totally silent in the absence of hormone, and is induced to an extremely high rate of expression by steroid hormones as a result of the presence of a particularly efficient combination of SREs and steroid-independent enhancers.

Structure of Steroid Response Elements

The SREs are noteworthy in their structure. For example, this *cis* element is composed of two half-sites for glucocorticoid receptor binding, each with the composition similar to TGTTCT. Consequently, a prototypic SRE, such as that which promotes glucocorticoid or progesterone response, has a composition of GGTACANNNTGTTCT (N = any base). The SRE half-sites are usually located on complementary strands of DNA and point in the opposite direction to form a twofold axis of symmetry (palindrome). Their sequence varies only slightly for different hormone responsiveness, indicating a reaction of great specificity. For example, GGTCANNNTGACC causes the estrogen receptor to bind and activate this cognate SRE sequence, and a slightly different SRE is required for thyroid hormone or vitamin D response, and so forth. Although the precise mechanisms of receptor binding to the SRE are not known at present, recent evidence suggests that one molecule of activated steroid-receptor complex binds to each of the two half-sites to form a dimer.

The receptor proteins are tightly controlled molecules in cells that, because of their obvious importance and potency, are nurtured from their initial synthesis to their end-stage degradation. The genes that code for the receptors are themselves under hormonal control. For example, the gene that directs synthesis of the receptor for the pregnancy hormone progesterone is a complex gene of greater than 40,000 bp in length composed of eight exons (coding regions) that, when processed into the final mRNA product, will direct the cell to synthesize receptor. In turn, the progesterone receptor gene appears to be stimulated to produce its product by estrogenic hormones. This experimental observation demonstrates the cooperation that occurs among hormones in the endocrine system and fits with the clinical observation that for progesterone to act on the female uterus and allow implantation and growth of a fertilized egg, the woman (or animal) must have had prior exposure to endogenous estradiol or exogenous estrogenic drugs.

The cooperation between estrogenic and progestational hormones at the receptor gene level is illustrated in Figure 4–20. To prevent dangerous chronic stimulation of cellular target genes responsive to the hormone-activated receptors, the receptors exert a feedback regulatory effect on transcription of their own parent genes. In other words, the progesterone-receptor complex causes a "down-regulation" of the synthesis of its own receptor through a poorly understood inhibition of production or increase in turnover of progesterone receptor mRNA. In this manner, potential overstimulation with progesterone is minimized and the cell is protected from resultant damage. In fact, most receptor genes are down-regulated by their activated receptor products, no doubt reflecting a more general mechanism by which the homeostatic milieu of hormonal regulation is maintained within the endocrine system.

After mRNA is generated by transcription of receptor genes, the receptor mRNA migrates to the cytoplasm of cells, where it is translated on ribosomes. Certain of the nascent receptor molecules, such as those for glucocorticoid, progesterone, estrogen, and androgen, are then released into their cells complexed with "heat shock" proteins. These heat shock proteins are thought to help the receptor fold into an appropriate conformation that permits subsequent biologic activity and tends to protect them from degradation by cellular proteases. The heat shock proteins are named because their activities are stimulated in all cells by the "shock" of severe stress, such as elevated

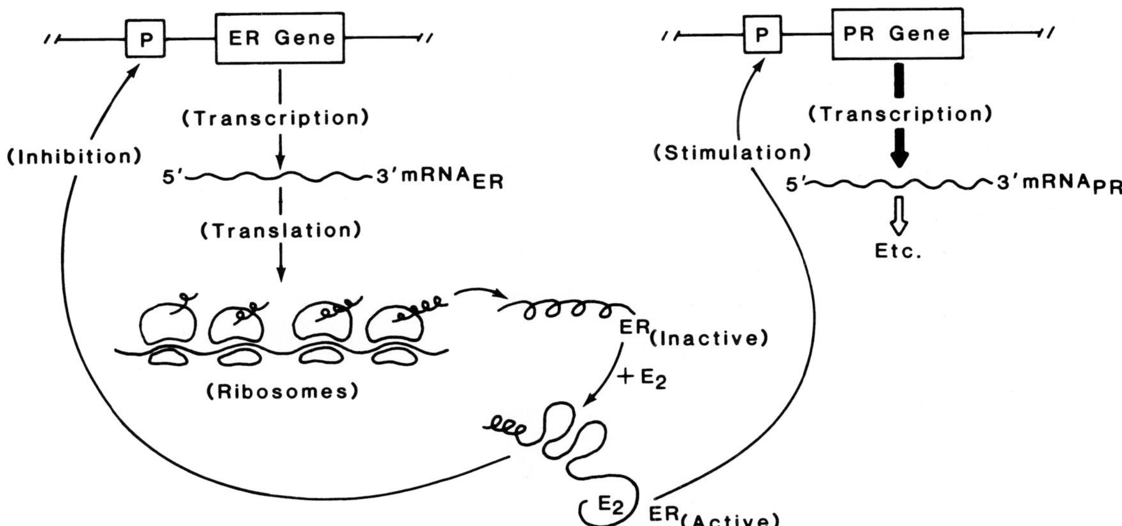

Figure 4–20 ■ Feedback control within endocrine network of steroid receptor genes. mRNA, messenger ribonucleic acid; E_2, estradiol; ER, estrogen receptor; P, progesterone; PR, progesterone receptor.

temperature or chemicals. They are thought to aid in the synthesis, folding, and transport of a number of complex eukaryotic proteins. While complexed to heat shock protein, steroid receptors cannot bind well to DNA. On binding of the steroid hormones to receptors, the heat shock proteins are released, and their native capacity to bind specifically to their cognate SRE is unleashed. No evidence for such an association with heat shock proteins exists for thyroid hormone or vitamin D receptors.

Functions of Steroid Receptors

Biochemical studies of steroid receptors in a large number of laboratories during the past 20 years have led to the conclusion that these important regulatory molecules have at least three major functions. They were known (1) to bind their respective hormone, (2) to bind to DNA, and (3) to regulate gene transcription. Thus, it was predicted that they would have three types of structural domains, a DNA binding domain, a transcription modulation domain, and a steroid hormone binding domain that regulated the functional activation of the receptor molecule. These conclusions were supported by a number of studies using proteolytic enzymes, which have the capacity to chip the receptor apart into separate fragments that could be tested for their individual functional characteristics.

Molecular cloning of the complementary DNA (cDNA) for receptors during the past several years has confirmed the suspected structure, because separate binding domains were observed for steroid hormone and DNA binding.[79–81] The glucocorticoid receptor was cloned first. In close temporal fashion, the estrogen receptor and the progesterone receptor were cloned. Next, the mineralocorticoid receptor was cloned, followed by the vitamin D receptor. Finally, the cloning of the thyroid hormone receptor, the vitamin A (retinoic acid) receptor, and the androgen receptor were reported and the structures deduced. These receptors all showed a marked similarity in structure, which indicated that they were members of a superfamily of genes (Fig. 4–21). This family of gene products shares an overall similarity in structure of 40 to 50 percent in the DNA binding region (I), with closely related molecules sharing a homology of up to 94 percent. Two regions of lesser homology (II, III) are found in the C-terminal half of the molecules. The most primitive of these genes appeared to be the vitamin D, thyroid hormone, and retinoic acid receptors, which have major effects on early development of animals and humans. Theoretically, the expansion of this gene family occurred through evolutionary duplication and divergence of the more primitive receptor genes to form the more recent family members (e.g., glucocorticoid, progesterone), which regulate acute reactions in differentiated cells. The relative structures and domain sizes of the members of this receptor family are represented schematically in Figure 4–21. The most highly conserved (homologous) domain is the DNA binding domain (domain I), which is conserved to a level of approximately 45 to 50 percent among all of the molecules and establishes each as a member of this superfamily of genes. Moderate similarities ($\sim$22 percent) among family members are noted in domains II and III, located in the steroid binding (regulatory) domain of the receptors; these homologies are more evident when closely related receptors, such as glucocorticoid and progesterone or thyroid hormone and vitamin D receptors, are compared.

The tremendous effort given to cloning and determination of the amino acid structure of these receptors led to only a few surprises. Among the most novel observations were the following. There was more than one form of the thyroid and retinoic acid receptors, and the existence of tissue-specific forms was evident. That is, instead of one form of the thyroid receptor being present in all cells in which thyroid hormone is to act, different cells have a different form of the receptor, presumably specialized to carry out slightly different gene-regulatory function. This is the case also for the estrogen receptor, which has two isoforms (ERλ and ERβ) that are produced from two distinct genes. There are also isoforms of the progesterone

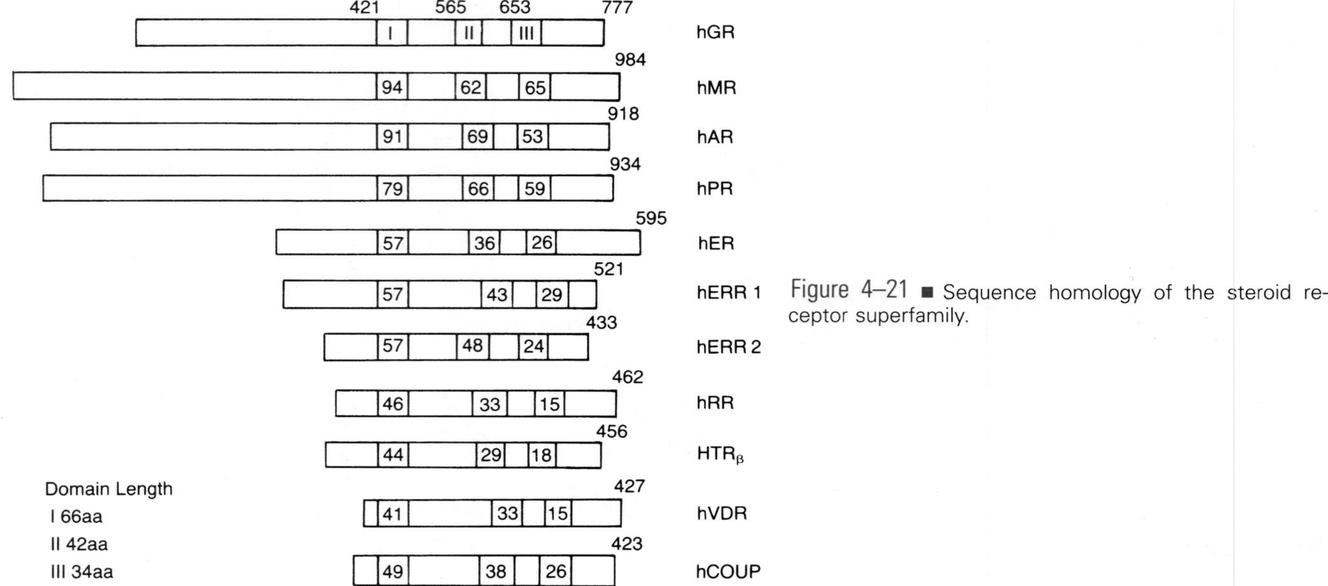

Figure 4–21 ■ Sequence homology of the steroid receptor superfamily.

receptor (PR_A and PR_B), but these are produced from the same gene.

A series of new genes coding for "receptors" with no known function or activating ligand have been observed. There are as many as 40 to 50 of these molecules, many of which still have not been published because of the lack of a defined function. Two of the first of these molecules, ERR1 and ERR2, were reported by the Evans laboratory[83] (see Fig. 4–21). Another of the first described "orphan receptors" has been shown to be a promoter transcription factor for a series of genes.[84, 85] It was defined originally as a binding protein for the chicken ovalbumin upstream promoter and was termed COUP transcription factor.[85] It also serves to regulate the insulin, apolipoprotein (very low density lipoprotein), and pro-opiomelanocortin gene promoters. The results now define the receptor gene family to include many novel transcription factors and raise the question as to the possible ligands for orphan receptors. The shear number of members in this steroid receptor superfamily predicts it to be the largest family of eukaryotic transcription factors and promises to generate a wealth of new biology in the next decade. These observations show that the superfamily of receptor genes is much larger than it was thought to be previously and that many new regulatory hormones for these orphan receptors could be discovered in the near future.

A question of great interest to scientists in this field relates to how the receptors function to turn on genes. The suspected domain structure of these receptors is conserved among family members and is illustrated for the estrogen receptor and the progesterone receptor in Figure 4–22. The C-terminal region of the protein contains the ligand (hormone) binding domain. Deletions and mutations of amino acids over a broad range in this domain lead to loss of some transcriptional activity and loss of all hormone binding. Consequently, such receptor deletions lose the capacity to be activated by hormone. At present, it is impossible to determine the exact amino acids involved in steroid interaction in this domain, although studies have implicated cysteine as an important contact amino acid for molecular interactions in this region. A series of studies of different receptors show that the hormone (agonist) and antihormone (antagonist) interact with different residues in distinct regions of the C-terminal domain.

A nuclear localization signal (see Fig. 4–22) is located just C-terminal to the DNA binding domain. The nuclear localization signal is responsible for sending the molecule into the nucleus after its synthesis on cytoplasmic ribosomes. The DNA binding domain contains the eight cysteine residues that complex two zinc atoms to form the two well-known zinc fingers (type II) comprising the region of the receptors responsible for specific and high-affinity binding to nuclear DNA elements (SREs; hormone response elements) located usually in the 5′ flanking regions

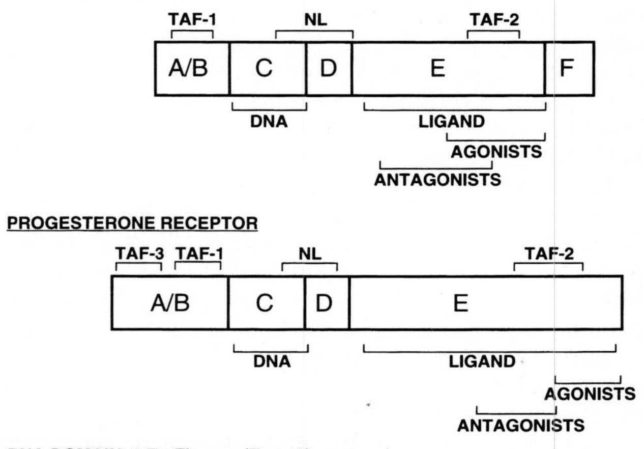

Figure 4–22 ■ Structure-function domains of the estrogen receptor to progesterone receptor. NL, nuclear localization signal.

of target genes. Also contained in the receptor molecules are two or more activation functions, usually one in the C terminus of the molecules and one or more in the N-terminal region. These activation functions are domains that, when mutated, destroy the capacity of receptors to activate transcription. They are thought to bind additional transcription factors that serve as intermediates between the receptors and the general transcription factors bound to the promoter (TATA box) of target genes. As shown in Figure 4–22, the estrogen receptor has two activation function regions, whereas the progesterone receptor has three. The activation functions participate synergistically to stimulate transcription.

Domain II could be considered the "active site" of the molecule, because it seems to be the region responsible for specific binding to DNA at its target SRE. Domain II contains nine perfectly conserved cysteine residues, eight of which are complexed into two zinc fingers. Each zinc finger contains one zinc ion bound to four cysteine residues, holding the intervening amino acids into a finger-like projection. A deletion of this domain destroys all receptor activity. In addition, many single amino acid changes in domain II are deleterious to function, especially changes in any of the cysteine amino acids. In some receptors (e.g., glucocorticoid and progesterone), domain II alone can have some stimulatory effect on transcription, albeit smaller and less specific than that of the intact molecule. In any event, this domain appears to be the heart of the molecule as far as specific DNA binding.

Domain I is more enigmatic as far as its precise function. Domain I exerts an important influence on transcriptional modulation. If domain I is deleted, we find that the receptor's effect on transcriptional regulation is diminished. Recent experiments have shown that domain I in the estrogen and progesterone receptor may be involved in selective activation of different hormone-regulatable genes.

The domain structure of steroid receptors is not as simple and defined as we might expect. For instance, a series of studies showed that domain III not only binds hormone but also contains protein sequences that must have a powerful effect on transcriptional activation as well. Also, mutational studies have shown that one can switch the order of domains (e.g., place domain III at the N terminus) or duplicate domains and the molecule remains functional and regulatable on reintroduction into cells.

After synthesis, there are post-translational modifications that are required to produce a fully functional receptor molecule and perhaps to signal changes in the receptor that are coincident with inactivation. Although other modifications may yet be discovered, it is clear that phosphorylation of the receptor does occur. In fact, present evidence from a number of laboratories indicates that some steroid receptors may undergo as many as 5 to 10 independent phosphorylations. These multiple phosphorylations are complex and difficult to relate to specific functions. Our best guess is that they enhance or retard some or all of the following processes: (1) specific hormone binding; (2) dimerization of receptors and stable interaction with DNA; (3) interactions with other transcription factors and RNA polymerase; and (4) inactivation and degradation of receptor. This is a topic of great interest at present, and more precise information on the physiologic consequences of phosphorylation should be forthcoming in the near future.

To understand how proteins bind to DNA and activate regulatory *cis* elements located near genes, we must first consider *trans*-acting factors as a whole. It is perhaps most simple to think of them as proteins that are produced by a distinct gene and that diffuse and bind to their new site of action, that is, to regulatory *cis* elements located at the gene on which they are to exert their effect. In this sense, steroid receptors are *trans* factors because they are produced from genes located elsewhere and must diffuse to their cognate SRE elements, which are located usually in the 5′ regulatory regions of their target genes. SRE elements are *cis* elements that appear to function only when one or more *trans* factors are bound to them. In fact, gene function in animals and humans appears to occur only when a group of *trans* factors touch each other in a precise and complex manner so that RNA polymerase is recruited to the gene and stimulated to act. RNA polymerase is a nuclear enzyme whose job is to transcribe or express the inherited information in genes. There is not a great excess of RNA polymerase in cells, and active genes are in competition for it. To compete effectively, the gene must have assembled an appropriate set of *cis* elements that provide strong transcription capacities. To be activated to function, these *cis* elements in turn must bind *trans* factors. These factors are sequence-specific DNA-binding proteins that establish a structural network near the beginning (5′ end) of genes that attract RNA polymerase. Many of these factors have been purified and studied, but a detailed discussion of their properties is beyond the scope of this chapter.

The steroid receptors have a natural predilection for their SRE sequences, which could be more than 100 times greater than their affinity for nonspecific DNA sequences. The receptor-SRE complex is strengthened further by protein-protein interactions with other transcription factors at adjacent DNA sites. Although when hormone binds to receptors its affinity for DNA may be increased a bit more, it appears that the receptor's native affinity for an SRE is a dominant force in its ability to sift through the 3 billion base pairs in the human genome and to find this small 15-bp SRE-regulatory sequence. Obviously, this reaction is of prime importance for selective regulation of genes by steroid hormones.

We have learned only recently how the steroid-activated receptor molecule binds to its enhancer element (SRE). The SRE is composed of two half-sites, each of which binds one molecule of steroid receptor. This dimer of receptor is now bound tightly and stably and has a significant ability to stimulate gene transcription. Stability is important in this instance because the length of receptor residence time on the SRE should relate to the potency for stimulation of transcription. In fact, optimal stability seems to be provided when a second dimer binds to another nearby enhancer and the two dimers touch each other. It is well known that two SREs have a much greater functional effect (greater than 10-fold) on gene expression than does one; in this case, 1 + 1 = 10, not 2. If the two SREs are located at a distance from one another, it is thought that the DNA can bend in such a way that the receptor dimers can come into proximity with each other and couple.[78, 86, 87]

In turn, the receptor multimer is thought to exert a further stabilizing force on the promoter complex. For example, the TATA box of the promoter must be occupied by a specific binding protein called TATA-binding protein as a protein complex (transcription factor IID) for RNA polymerase to initiate gene transcription. It is an unstable association that is functionally stabilized by protein-protein interactions with a large complex (>30) of protein factors that are common to most genes. This complex of factors is referred to as the general transcription factor complex. It functions to promote initiation of transcription. The promoter complex can be stabilized by receptor interactions at nearby enhancer elements. This stable complex will now draw RNA polymerase to this gene repeatedly for transcriptional initiations. These types of protein-protein interactions seem to be a general mechanism whereby *trans* factors are stabilized at the respective *cis* elements of many genes and transcription is thereby stimulated. Further positive enhancement occurs when nearby enhancer elements (SREs) are occupied by receptor dimers. This "action at a distance" is thought to occur by some type of DNA looping that allows the receptors to fold back and exert a further stabilization effect on the promoter complex. By this means, steroid hormones can drive transcription of such target genes to high levels.

Coregulator Proteins for Receptors

A series of receptor-associated proteins have been discovered that act as intermediaries in receptor stimulation or inhibition of transcription. These coregulator proteins fall into two main functional classes: coactivators, which enhance receptor capacity to stimulate gene transcription; and corepressors, which aid receptors in turning off transcription of target genes. In a manner not well understood, these coregulators help "bridge" the DNA-bound receptors to the core promoter complex (general transcription factors) and provide the majority of the potency of receptors to regulate gene expression.

Coactivators are represented by the subgroup of coregulator proteins that enhance the capacity of receptors to activate target genes. The first of such molecules to be shown to have a coactivator activity in animal cells was SRC-1 (steroid receptor coactivator 1).[88] This coactivator has two forms (160 kDa and 125 kDa) and is present in all cells, but in varying concentrations. A typical effect of SRC-1 on progesterone receptor activity in cultured cells is shown in Figure 4–23. In the absence of progestin ligand, the transfection of an expression vector containing SRC-1 into the cells has no effect on basal transcription. In the presence of a strong progestin (R5020), however, the SRC-1 enhances receptor capacity to activate its target gene more than 10-fold. Such coactivators bind at the activation function regions (see Fig. 4–22) of receptors and contain their own "activation domains" that influence the growth hormone–releasing factor (GRF) complex at the promoter to recruit RNA polymerase to the target gene. SRC-1 has broad activity on most members of the steroid receptor superfamily and appears to play a prominent role in receptor activation of genes; it is only one of a complex of proteins that appear to act together. Another prominent player in this complex is CBP (CREB [cAMP response element–binding protein]—binding protein),[89] a coregulator initially thought only to mediate cyclic adenosine monophosphate (cAMP) signaling to target genes but now known to enhance effects of most transcription factors. Its broad effect on many signaling pathways for transcription has led to its being considered an "integrator."[89] Other proteins within this complex are beyond the scope of this discussion but are nonetheless important (Fig. 4–24).

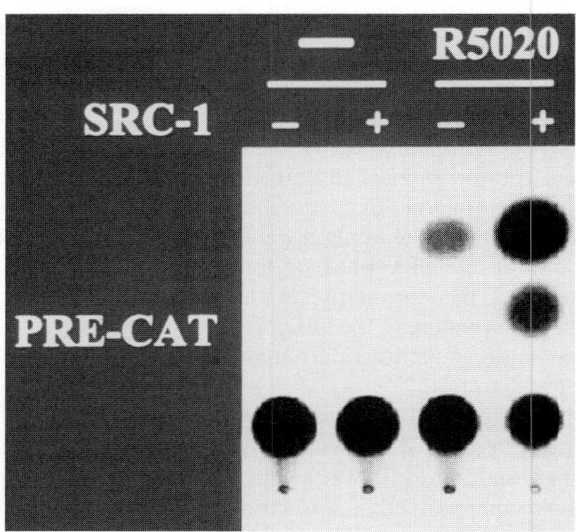

Figure 4–23 ■ Effect of SRC-1 on progesterone receptor activity in cultured cells. Lanes 1 and 2, no hormone. Lanes 3 and 4 have progestin (R5020) added.

Unoccupied receptors (e.g., thyroid hormone receptor, retinoic acid receptor) are often found bound to target DNA elements and, in most cases, suppress basal gene transcription. In certain instances, ligand-bound receptors repress nuclear transcription of target genes. These functions of receptors are mediated by corepressors, proteins that function in an opposite manner to coactivators (see Fig. 4–24). Two homologous corepressors have been identified to date and have been termed N-CoR (nuclear factor corepressor) and SMRT (silencing mediator for retinoid and thyroid hormone receptors). These molecules have two major functional roles, to bind to receptors (primarily in

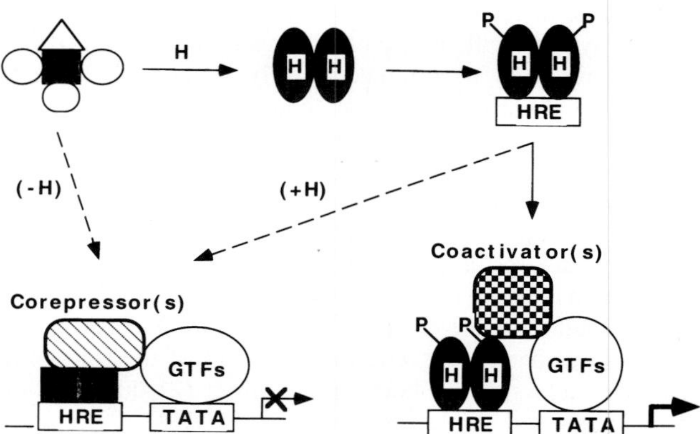

Figure 4–24 ■ Functions of steroid receptors are mediated by coactivators and corepressors. GTFs, general transcription factors; HRE, hormone response element.

the C-terminal domains of receptors) and to touch the GRFs in such a way that GRF function is inhibited. Corepressors are present in all cells also, but their concentrations vary in different cell types. The active conformations of receptors have a higher affinity for coactivators, whereas the inactive receptor conformations have a higher affinity for corepressors.[90, 91]

Much of the pharmacology and physiology of steroid hormone action can be explained by biochemical studies of steroid receptors. For instance, steroid hormone potency correlates with (1) the affinity of receptor for the hormone (or drug) and (2) the efficiency of the activated hormone-receptor complex to regulate transcription. High affinities lead to prolonged occupancy of the SRE and sustained transcriptional stimulation. The mechanism of action of certain drugs that are antihormones can be understood on this basis. For instance, the drug tamoxifen, an antiestrogen used in the therapy of breast cancer, binds to the normal estrogen receptor in a nonproductive manner. Although it has a high affinity for its target SRE, the nonproductive receptor-tamoxifen complex cannot couple efficiently to *trans* factors and RNA polymerase in a way that stimulates target gene transcription. The limited concentration of receptor (approximately 20,000 molecules per cell) is then tied up in an inactive complex with the antihormone tamoxifen. Finally, as described before for estrogen and progesterone, interactions among hormones can alter the net levels of a receptor within a cell and can alter its potential for function in a direct correlative manner. When estrogen induces the level of progesterone receptor in a target cell, that cell displays a greatly increased ability to respond to progesterone.

There appears to be a functional interplay in animal cells between various coregulators. In terms of gene activation by nuclear receptors, a high level of coactivator promotes efficient gene activation, whereas a high concentration of corepressor acts to retard gene activation by receptors. Such coregulator proteins are important in determining the kinetics of gene induction by steroid hormones. In some instances, they may even determine the tissue-specific effects of mixed antagonist/agonist molecules such as tamoxifen. Tamoxifen is a good antagonist in breast cells but is an agonist in the uterus and bone. Such tissue-specific effects may result from the following reasoning (Fig. 4–25). Tamoxifen induces a receptor conformation intermediate to that induced by a pure agonist (estradiol) or pure antagonist. This conformation has an intermediate affinity for both coactivators and corepressors. Consequently, if the cellular concentration of corepressors is high, tamoxifen could act as an antagonist. Conversely, if the cellular concentration of corepressors is high, tamoxifen could act as an agonist. Because the discovery of receptor coregulator proteins is rather recent, it seems certain that much of ligand cell physiology will be shown to be determined by the relative intracellular concentrations of coactivators and corepressors.

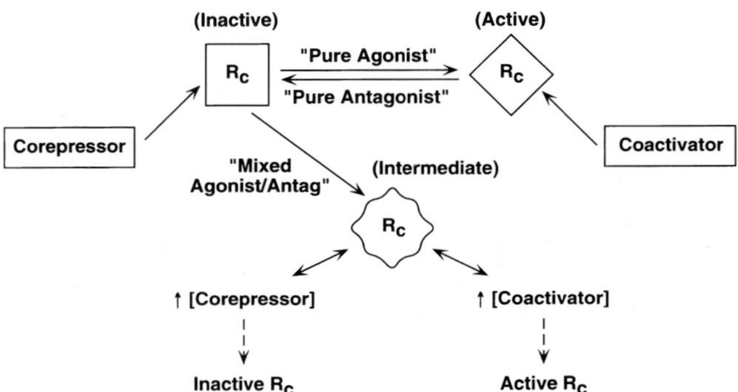

Figure 4–25 ■ Tissue specificity of a mixed antagonist/agonist may result from divergent cell levels of corepressor and coactivator.

Inherited defects in receptors can serve as a basis for certain genetic diseases.[92] For example, in vitamin D–resistant rickets (type II), patients suffer low calcium, retarded bone growth, hair loss, and other clinical symptoms inherent to this deficiency. This syndrome results from a recessive inherited defect in the receptor for vitamin D that prevents its normal gene-regulatory function. The nuclear gene coding for the vitamin D receptor was one of the first analyzed in a number of patients and shown to produce a human disease when mutated.[93] Initial results revealed that a substitution of a single amino acid in the tip of either one of the DNA-binding zinc fingers (in domain II) of the receptor led to defective function and concomitantly to a resistant state in which the patient is unresponsive to treatment with vitamin D in any amounts. Other forms of the disease are caused by inherited stop codons for translation of the receptor mRNA, which does not result in the production of a functional vitamin D receptor or mutations in other regions of the receptor that interfere with its transcriptional activation function. Similar alterations in the gene coding for the androgen receptor have been uncovered in certain patients born with subtypes of the genetic disease called testicular feminization (see Chapter 14). In this disease, a genetic male presents with a female phenotype and is clearly resistant to endogenous circulating testosterone or exogenous treatment with androgens. In many cases, a defect in the androgen receptor has been suspected, and experimental studies show this to be true. The cloned cDNA and nuclear genes for all steroid receptors that are now available for this type of screening of DNA from patients should provide many important new insights into the causes of clinical syndromes of steroid hormone "unresponsiveness." This includes syndromes as diverse as unexplained long bone growth (estrogen receptor), vitamin deficiencies (retinoic acid receptor), infertility (progesterone receptor), unexplained salt and water loss (mineralocorticoid receptor), and inability to cope with stress and uncontrolled emotional responses (glucocorticoid receptor).[92]

References

1. Sandor T, Mehdi AZ. Steroids and evolution. *In* Barrington EJW (ed). Hormones and Evolution. New York, Academic Press, 1979, pp 1–72.
2. Simpson ER. Cholesterol side-chain cleavage, cytochrome P_{450}, and the control of steroidogenesis. Mol Cell Endocrinol 13:213, 1979.
3. Kimura T. ACTH stimulation on cholesterol side chain cleavage activity of adrenocortical mitochondria. Mol Cell Biochem 36:105, 1981.
4. Kashiwagi K, Defeldecker WP, Salhanick HA. Purification and characterization of mitochondrial cytochrome P-450 associated with cholesterol side chain cleavage from bovine corpus luteum. J Biol Chem 255:2606, 1980.

5. Hall PF. Cellular organization for steroidogenesis. Int Rev Cytol 86:53, 1984.
6. Goldring NB, Farkash Y, Goldschmit D, Orly J. Immunofluorescent probing of the mitochondrial cholesterol side-chain cleavage P450 expressed in differentiating granulosa cells in culture. Endocrinology 119:2821, 1986.
7. Le Goascogne C, Robel P, Gouezou M, et al. Neurosteroids: Cytochrome P-450scc in rat brain. Science 237:1212, 1987.
8. Hu ZY, Bourreau E, Jung-Testas I, et al. Neurosteroids: Oligodendrocyte mitochondria convert cholesterol to pregnenolone. Proc Natl Acad Sci USA 84:8215, 1987.
9. Privalle CT, Crivello JF, Jefcoate CR. Regulation of intramitochondrial cholesterol transfer to side-chain cleavage cytochrome P-450 in rat adrenal gland. Proc Natl Acad Sci USA 80:702, 1983.
10. Jefcoate CR, McNamara BC, DiBartolemeis MJ. Control of steroid synthesis in adrenal fasciculata cells. Endocr Res 12:315, 1986.
11. Privalle CT, McNamara BC, Dhariwal MS, Jefcoate CR. ACTH control of cholesterol side-chain cleavage at adrenal mitochondrial cytochrome P-450_{scc}. Regulation of intramitochondrial cholesterol transfer. Mol Cell Endocrinol 53:87, 1987.
12. Strott CA. The search for the elusive adrenal steroidogenic "regulatory" protein. Trends Endocrinol Metab 1:312, 1990.
13. Sugawara T, Holt JA, Driscoll D, et al. Human steroidogenic acute regulatory protein: Functional activity in COS-1 cells, tissue-specific expression, and mapping of the structural gene to 8p11.2 and a pseudogene to chromosome 13. Proc Natl Acad Sci USA 92:4778, 1995.
14. Clark BJ, Soo S-C, Caron KM, et al. Hormonal and developmental regulation of the steroidogenic acute regulatory protein. Mol Endocrinol 9:1346, 1995.
15. King SR, Ronen-Fuhrmann T, Timberg R, et al. Steroid production after in vitro transcription, translation, and mitochondrial processing of protein products of complementary deoxyribonucleic acid for steroidogenic acute regulatory protein. Endocrinology 136:5165, 1995.
16. Chanderbhan R, Noland BJ, Scallen TJ, Vahouny GV. Sterol carrier $protein_2$: Delivery of cholesterol from adrenal lipid droplets to mitochondria for pregnenolone synthesis. J Biol Chem 257:8928, 1982.
17. Vahouny GV, Chanderbhan R, Noland BJ, et al. Sterol carrier $protein_2$: Identification of adrenal sterol carrier $prtoein_2$ and site of action for mitochondrial cholesterol utilization. J Biol Chem 258:11731, 1983.
18. Vahouny GV, Dennis P, Chanderbhan R, et al. Sterol carrier $protein_2$ (SCP_2)–mediated transfer of cholesterol to mitochondrial inner membranes. Biochem Biophys Res Commun 122:509, 1984.
19. Pedersen RC, Brownie AC. Steroidogenesis-activator polypeptide isolated from a rat Leydig cell tumor. Science 236:188, 1987.
20. Mertz LM, Pedersen RC. Steroidogenesis activator polypeptide may be a product of glucose regulated protein 78 (GRP 78). Endocr Res 15:101, 1989.
21. Yanagibashi K, Ohno Y, Kawamura M, Hall PF. The regulation of intracellular transport of cholesterol in bovine adrenal cells: Purification of a novel protein. Endocrinology 123:2075, 1988.
22. Besman MJ, Yanagibashi K, Lee TD, et al. Identification of des-(gly-ile)-endozepine as an effector of corticotropin-dependent adrenal steroidogenesis: Stimulation of cholesterol delivery is mediated by the peripheral benzodiazepine receptor. Proc Natl Acad Sci USA 86:4897, 1989.
23. Nelson DR, Kamataki T, Waxman DJ, et al. The P450 superfamily: Update on new sequences, gene mapping, accession numbers, early trivial names of enzymes, and nomenclature. DNA Cell Biol 12:1, 1993.
24. Baird DT, Galbraith A, Fraser IS, Newsam JE. The concentration of oestrone and oestradiol-17 in spermatic venous blood in man. J Endocrinol 57:285, 1973.
25. Simpson ER, MacDonald PC. Endocrine physiology of the placenta. Annu Rev Physiol 43:163, 1981.
26. Donohoue PA, Parker K, Migeon CJ. Congenital adrenal hyperplasia. *In* Scriver CR, Beaudet AL, Sly WS, Valle D (eds). The Metabolic and Molecular Basis of Inherited Disease. New York, McGraw-Hill, 1995, pp 2929–2966.
27. Lin D, Sugawara T, Strauss JF III, et al. Role of steroidogenic acute regulatory protein in adrenal and gonadal steroidogenesis. Science 267:1828, 1995.
28. Liddle GW, Estep HL, Kendall JW, et al. Clinical application of a new test of pituitary reserve. J Clin Endocrinol Metab 19:875, 1959.
29. Payne AH, Singer SS. The role of steroid sulfatase and sulfotransferase enzymes in the metabolism of C_{21} and C_{19} steroids. *In* Hobkirk R (ed). Steroid Biochemistry, Vol 1. Boca Raton, FL, CRC Press, 1979, pp 111–145.
30. Roy AB. Sulfotransferases. *In* Mulder GJ (ed). Sulfation of Drugs and Related Compounds. Boca Raton, FL, CRC Press, 1981, pp 83–130.
31. Hobkirk R. Steroid sulfotransferases and steroid sulfate sulfatases: Characteristics and biological roles. Can J Biochem Cell Biol 63:1127, 1985.
32. Fieser LF, Fieser M. Steroids. New York, Reinhold Publishing, 1959, p 14.
33. Mainwaring WIP, Milroy EJG. Characterization of the specific androgen receptors in the human prostate gland. J Endocrinol 57:371, 1973.
34. Baulieu E-E, Lasnitzki I, Robel P. Metabolism of testosterone and action of metabolites on prostate glands grown in organ culture. Nature 219:1155, 1968.
35. Strott CA. Metabolism of progesterone in the chick oviduct: Relation to the progesterone receptor and biological activity. Endocrinology 95:826, 1974.
36. Smith HE, Smith RG, Toft DO, et al. Binding of steroids to progesterone receptor proteins in chick oviduct and human uterus. J Biol Chem 249:5924, 1974.
37. Greenblatt DJ, Ransil BJ, Harmatz JS, et al. Variability of 24-hour urinary creatinine excretion by normal subjects. J Clin Pharmacol 16:321, 1976.
38. Tait JF. Review: The use of isotopic steroids for the measurement of production rates in vivo. J Clin Endocrinol Metab 23:1285, 1963.
39. Flood C, Hunter AS, Lloyd CA, Longcope C. The effects of posture on the metabolism of androstenedione and estrone in males. J Clin Endocrinol Metab 36:1180, 1973.
40. Siiteri PK, Murai JT, Hammond GL, et al. The serum transport of steroid hormones. Recent Prog Horm Res 38:457, 1982.
41. Puche RC, Nes WR. Binding of dehydroepiandrosterone sulfate to serum albumin. Endocrinology 70:857, 1962.
42. Wang DY, Bulbrook RD. The metabolic clearance rates of dehydroepiandrosterone, testosterone and their sulphate esters in man, rat and rabbit. J Endocrinol 38:307, 1967.
43. Wang DY, Bulbrook RD, Coombs MM. Metabolic clearance rates of pregnenolone, 17-acetoxypregnenolone and their sulphate esters in man, rat and rabbit. J Endocrinol 39:395, 1967.
44. Nieschlag E, Loriaux DL, Ruder HJ, et al. The secretion of dehydroepiandrosterone and dehydroepiandrosterone sulphate in man. J Endocrinol 57:123, 1973.
45. Nishikawa T, Strott CA. Unconjugated and sulfoconjugated steroids in plasma and zones of the adrenal cortex of the guinea pig. Steroids 41:105, 1983.
46. Baird DT, Horton R, Longcope C, Tait J. Steroid prehormones. Perspect Biol Med 3:384, 1968.
47. Wilson JD. Disorders of androgen action. Clin Res 35:1, 1987.
48. Baird DT, Horton R, Longcope C, Tait JF. Steroid dynamics under steady-state conditions. Recent Prog Horm Res 25:611, 1969.
49. Fishman LM, Sarfaty GA, Wilson H, Lipsett MB. The role of the testis in oestrogen production. *In* Wolstenholme GEW, O'Connor M (eds). Ciba Foundation Colloquia on Endocrinology, Vol 16. Endocrinology of the Testis. London, J & A Churchill, 1967, pp 156–166.
50. Westphal U. Steroid-Protein Interactions, Vol II. New York, Springer-Verlag, 1986.
51. Dunn JF, Nisula BC, Rodbard D. Transport of steroid hormones: Binding of 21 endogenous steroids to both testosterone-binding globulin and corticosteroid-binding globulin in human plasma. J Clin Endocrinol Metab 53:58, 1981.
52. Vande Wiele RL, MacDonald PC, Gurpide E, Lieberman S. Studies on secretion and interconversion of the androgens. Recent Prog Horm Res 19:275, 1963.
53. Mulder GJ, Jakoby WB. Sulfation. *In* Mulder GJ (ed). Conjugation Reactions in Drug Metabolism: An Integrated Approach. New York, Taylor & Francis, 1990, pp 107–161.
54. Giorgi E. The transport of steroid hormones into animal cells. Int Rev Cytol 65:49, 1980.
55. Manni A, Pardridge WM, Cefalu W, et al. Bioavailability of albumin-bound testosterone. J Clin Endocrinol Metab 61:705, 1985.

56. Englebienne P. The serum steroid transport proteins: Biochemistry and clinical significance. Mol Aspects Med 7:313, 1984.
57. Hryb DJ, Kahn MS, Rosner W. Testosterone-estradiol–binding globulin binds to prostatic cell membranes. Biochem Biophys Res Commun 128:432, 1985.
58. Hryb DJ, Kahn MS, Romas NA, Rosner, W. Specific binding of human corticosteroid-binding globulin to cell membranes. Proc Natl Acad Sci USA 83:3253, 1986.
59. Hsu BR-S, Siiteri PK, Kuhn RW. Interactions between corticosteroid-binding globulin (CBG)a and target tissue. *In* Forest MG, Pugeat M (eds). Binding Proteins of Steroid Hormones. London, John Libbey Eurotext, 1986, pp 577–591.
60. Hammond GL. Potential functions of plasma steroid-binding proteins. Trends Endocrinol Metab 6:298, 1995.
61. Rosner W. The functions of corticosteroid-binding globulin and sex hormone-binding globulin: Recent advances. Endocr Rev 11:80, 1990.
62. Mendel CM, Kuhn RW, Weisiger RA, et al. Uptake of cortisol by the perfused rat liver: Validity of the free hormone hypothesis applied to cortisol. Endocrinology 124:468, 1989.
63. Baulieu E-E. Steroid hormone binding plasma proteins and their intra- and extra-cellular congeners. *In* Forest MG, Pugeat M (eds). Binding Proteins of Steroid Hormones. London, John Libbey Eurotext, 1986, pp 1–11.
64. Joseph DR. Structure, function, and regulation of androgen-binding protein/sex hormone–binding globulin. Vitam Horm 49:197, 1994.
65. Vermeulen A. TEBG and CBG as an index of endocrine function. *In* Forest MG, Pugeat M (eds). Binding Proteins of Steroid Hormones. London, John Libbey Eurotext, 1986, pp 383–395.
66. Vermeulen A, Storia T, Verdonck L. The apparent free testosterone concentration: An index of androgenicity. J Clin Endocrinol Metab 33:759, 1971.
67. McKerns KW. Steroid Hormones and Metabolism. New York, Appleton-Century-Crofts, 1969.
68. Briggs MH, Brotherton J. Steroid Biochemistry and Pharmacology. New York, Academic Press, 1970.
69. Jensen EV, Jacobson HI, Flesher JW, et al. Estrogen receptors in target tissues. *In* Pincus G, Nakao T, Tait JF (eds). Steroid Dynamics. New York, Academic Press, 1966, pp 133–156.
70. O'Malley BW, McGuire WL, Kohler PO, Korenman S. Studies on the mechanism of steroid hormone regulation of synthesis of specific proteins. Recent Prog Horm Res 25:105, 1969.
71. Gorski J, Gannon F. Current models of steroid hormone action: A critique. Annu Rev Biochem 28:425, 1976.
72. Katzenellenbogan BS. Dynamics of steroid hormone receptor action. Annu Rev Physiol 42:17, 1980.
73. O'Malley BW. Steroid hormone action in eukaryotic cells. J Clin Invest 74:207, 1984.
74. Yamamoto K. Steroid receptor regulated transcription of specific genes and gene networks. Annu Rev Genet 19:209, 1985.
75. Ringold G. Steroid hormone regulation of gene expression. Annu Rev Pharmacol Toxicol 25:529, 1985.
76. Walters MR. Steroid hormone receptors and the nucleus. Endocr Rev 6:512, 1985.
77. Haussler MR. Vitamin D receptors: Nature and function. Annu Rev Nutr 6:527, 1986.
78. Tsai MJ, O'Malley BW. Molecular mechanisms of action of steroid/thyroid receptor superfamily members. Annu Rev Biochem 673:451, 1994.
79. Evans RM. The steroid and thyroid hormone receptor superfamily. Science 240:889, 1988.
80. Beato M. Gene regulation by steroid hormones. Cell 56:335, 1989.
81. Green S, Chambon P. Oestradiol induction of a glucocorticoid-responsive gene by a chimeric receptor. Nature 325:75, 1987.
82. Berg JM. Binding specificity of steroid receptors. Cell 57:1065, 1989.
83. Giguere V, Yang N, Segui P, Evans R. Identification of a new class of steroid hormone receptors. Nature 331:91, 1988.
84. Wang LH, Tsai SY, Sagami I, O'Malley BW. Purification and characterization of COUP transcription factor from HELA cells. J Biol Chem 262:16080, 1987.
85. Wang L-H, Tsai SY, Cook RG, et al. COUP transcription factor is a member of the steroid receptor superfamily. Nature 340:163, 1989.
86. Charron J, Drouin J. Glucocorticoid inhibition of transcription from episomal proopiomelanocortin gene promoter. Proc Natl Acad Sci USA 83:8903, 1986.
87. Akerblom I, Slater E, Beato M, et al. Negative regulation by glucocorticoids with a cAMP responsive enhancer. Science 241:350, 1988.
88. Õnate SA, Tsai SY, Tsai MJ, O'Malley BW. Sequence and characterization of a coactivator for the steroid hormone receptor superfamily. Science 270:1354, 1996.
89. Lin SC, Heyman RA, Rose DW, et al. A CBP integrator complex mediates transcriptional activation and AP-1 inhibition by nuclear receptors. Cell 85:403, 1996.
90. Kurokawa R, Soderstrom M, Horlein A, et al. Polarity-specific activities of retinoic acid receptors determined by a co-repressor. Nature 377:451, 1995.
91. Chen JD, Evans RM. A transcriptional co-repressor that interacts with nuclear hormone receptors. Nature 377:454, 1995.
92. Tsai SY, Tsai MJ, O'Malley BW. The steroid receptor superfamily: Transactivators of gene expression. *In* Parker MG (ed). Nuclear Hormone Receptors: Molecular Mechanisms, Cellular Functions, and Clinical Abnormalities. San Diego, Academic Press, 1991, pp 103–124.
93. Hughes MR, Malloy PJ, Kieback DG, et al. Point mutations in the human vitamin D receptor gene associated with hypocalcemic rickets. Science 242:1702, 1988.

Chapter 5

PROSTAGLANDINS AND PROSTAGLANDIN-LIKE PRODUCTS IN REPRODUCTION: Eicosanoids, Peroxides, and Oxygen Radicals

Aydin Arici • Harold R. Behrman • David L. Keefe

■ CHAPTER OUTLINE

KEY POINTS

- Prostaglandins are derived from essential fatty acids by enzyme-catalyzed oxidation.
- Prostaglandins are short-lived paracrine agents whose actions are mediated by specific plasma membrane receptors.
- The commonly known steroidal and nonsteroidal anti-inflammatory agents block the synthesis of prostaglandins.
- Prostaglandins are mediators of GnRH secretion, ovulation, luteal regression, cervical ripening, and parturition, and they maintain a patent ductus arteriosus.
- Prostaglandins are pathophysiologic mediators of inflammation and dysmenorrhea.

Prostaglandins, thromboxanes, and leukotrienes derived enzymatically from essential fatty acids constitute a unique class of polyunsaturated, hydroxylated, 20-carbon fatty acids categorized as eicosanoids. Eicosanoids evoke a variety of biologic actions in diverse tissues at extremely low concentrations. They are produced ubiquitously, and some, but not exclusive, tissue specificity may exist for the selective production and response to particular eicosanoids within this broad classification.

Supported by NIH-HD-01041 (A. A.), NIH-HD-10718 (H. B.), and NIH-HD-01099 (D. K.).

Interaction of polyunsaturated fatty acids with oxygen radicals results in peroxidation and the formation of other hydroxylated fatty acids by nonenzymatic mechanisms. The generation of reactive oxygen species is in many instances a regulated process, occurs widely, and has profound and often deleterious effects on cell function.

In many cases, eicosanoids and other products of oxygen radical attack serve as paracrine and autocrine modulators of cellular function; they are metabolized rapidly, which leads to loss of biologic activity. This chapter deals with salient features of eicosanoid and oxygen radical synthesis and metabolism and delineates actions that may be of particular significance for the reproductive system.

BIOSYNTHESIS OF EICOSANOIDS

Interrelationships with Essential Fatty Acids

Eicosanoids are derived from essential fatty acids, long known to be required nutrients. Indeed, essential fatty acids deficiency leads to impaired fertility, skin lesions, failure of growth, and eventual death. However, the addition of small amounts of linoleic, linolenic, or arachidonic acid (but not saturated fatty acids) reverses the effects of essential fatty acid deficiency. Monoenoic fatty acids, such as oleic acid, are not essential nutrients, whereas long-chain fatty acids with two or more bonds (e.g., linoleic and arachidonic acid) are essential for cell structure and function. Conversion of linoleic acid to the 20-carbon fatty acids that serve as substrates for eicosanoid synthesis occurs readily. Dietary replacement with prostaglandins has not resulted in complete amelioration of essential fatty acids deficiency symptoms, not surprising in view of the variety of biologically active compounds within the eicosanoid family. Much of the current information on the synthesis and metabolism of eicosanoids is limited to products of arachidonic acid metabolism, the most abundant of the prostaglandin precursors (Fig. 5–1).

Storage and Release of Arachidonic Acid

In addition to enzymatic synthesis of arachidonic acid by chain elongation and desaturation, a major source of arachidonic acid is the diet (Fig. 5–2). Little unesterified or "free" arachidonic acid is present in the intracellular milieu. Esterified arachidonic acid is not a substrate for eicosanoid synthesis. The predominant esterified source of arachidonic acid that serves as a prosubstrate for eicosanoid synthesis is the phospholipids, although substantial amounts are also extant in triglycerides and as esters of cholesterol.

The enzymes that catalyze the formation of eicosanoids exist in a substrate-limiting environment. Consequently, liberation of arachidonic acid from esterified stores results in the prompt formation of these products. Release of arachidonic acid is facilitated by the hydrolytic action of

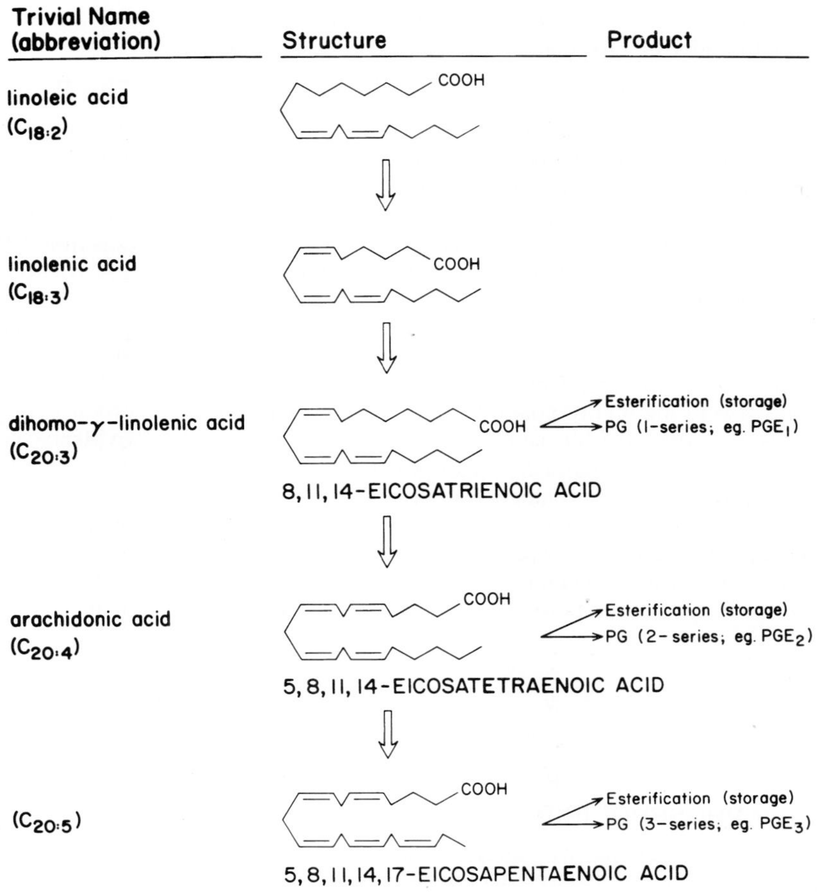

Trivial Name (abbreviation)	Structure	Product
linoleic acid ($C_{18:2}$)	COOH	
linolenic acid ($C_{18:3}$)	COOH	
dihomo-γ-linolenic acid ($C_{20:3}$)	COOH 8,11,14-EICOSATRIENOIC ACID	Esterification (storage) PG (1-series; eg. PGE_1)
arachidonic acid ($C_{20:4}$)	COOH 5,8,11,14-EICOSATETRAENOIC ACID	Esterification (storage) PG (2-series; eg. PGE_2)
($C_{20:5}$)	COOH 5,8,11,14,17-EICOSAPENTAENOIC ACID	Esterification (storage) PG (3-series; eg. PGE_3)

Figure 5–1 ■ Interrelationships of prostaglandins with essential fatty acids. Fatty acids with two or more double bonds (18-carbon fatty acids are the most common) may undergo desaturation and chain elongation to form substrates for prostaglandin biosynthesis.

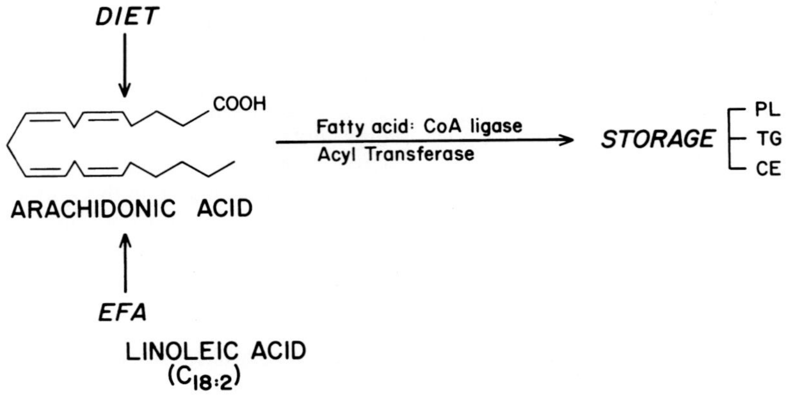

DIET

COOH

Fatty acid: CoA ligase

Acyl Transferase

STORAGE [PL TG CE]

ARACHIDONIC ACID

EFA

LINOLEIC ACID ($C_{18:2}$)

Figure 5–2 ■ Origins of arachidonic acid. Both diet and biosynthesis from essential fatty acids (EFA) are sources of arachidonic acid. Little "free" arachidonic acid is present in cells, because most is esterified in phospholipids (PL), triglycerides (TG), and cholesterol esters (CE).

phospholipases (Fig. 5–3). Phospholipase A_2, in particular a cytosolic form of the enzyme that shows selectivity for arachidonyl-containing phospholipids,[1] releases arachidonic acid and appears to be under tonic inhibition by phospholipid binding and sequestering proteins termed annexins.[2] There is considerable interest in the pharmacologic control of phospholipase activity, because regulation of these enzymes appears to be intimately related to the availability of arachidonic acid for conversion to eicosanoids.

Pathways of Arachidonic Acid Metabolism

The liberation of intracellular free arachidonic acid is followed rapidly by enzymatic oxidation in at least two separate pathways (Fig. 5–4). One pathway is catalyzed by an enzyme complex referred to as prostaglandin (PG) synthase, or cyclooxygenase, which leads to production of prostaglandins and thromboxane. The initial dihydroperoxy fatty acid formed in this reaction is PGG_2. The peroxide moiety at the 15-carbon position is rapidly reduced to form PGH_2 as a result of the inherent peroxidase activity of cyclooxygenase.[3] Both PGG_2 and PGH_2 are short-lived.

Other pathways of arachidonic acid oxidation are catalyzed by lipoxygenases, enzymes that catalyze the formation of hydroxylated, but noncyclized, fatty acids. The 5-hydroxylated product, 5-hydroperoxyeicosatetraenoic acid, gives rise to the highly potent leukotrienes.[4] Other lipoxygenases catalyze the formation of 12- and 15-hydroxylated fatty acids. In the adrenal, a 15-lipoxygenase metabolite appears to mediate steroidogenesis in response to low levels of adrenocorticotropic hormone.[5] Production of hydroperoxy fatty acids also occurs nonenzymatically by lipid peroxidation from oxygen radical attack followed by reduction with glutathione peroxidase. Indeed, bioactive prostaglandin-like products are formed by such nonenzymatic oxidative processes that are referred to as isoprostanes.[6]

The Leukotrienes

Lipoxygenase-catalyzed oxidation of arachidonic acid leads to noncyclized, hydroxylated derivatives at the 5-carbon position, and these compounds show potent biologic activities (Fig. 5–5). These include leukotrienes C_4, D_4, and E_4, which represent the long-known, slow-reacting substance of anaphylaxis.[7] The hydroxylated product, 5-hydroxyeicosatetraenoic acid (5-HETE), shows chemotactic activity for human neutrophils and eosinophils, but the most potent chemotactic and leukocyte-activating agent is leukotriene B_4.[8]

The Prostaglandins and Thromboxanes

Cyclooxygenase- or PGH synthase–catalyzed oxidation of arachidonic acid results in production of prostaglandins and thromboxane (Fig. 5–6). At present, two PGH synthases are known, which are encoded by separate genes. One is a constitutive enzyme that is found in virtually all tissues and referred to as PGH synthase-1 or cyclooxygenase-1. The second enzyme, called PGH synthase-2 or cyclooxygenase-2, is inducible and is often markedly up-regulated during cellular differentiation by cytokines or hormones.[9, 10]

Since the early discovery of $PGF_{2\alpha}$ and PGE_2, four major products of endoperoxide metabolism have been described. Evidence points to tissue specificity in the nature of the prostaglandin formed. Thus, platelets appear to synthesize a relative abundance of thromboxane A_2 (TXA_2), a potent platelet-aggregating substance and vasoconstrictor. TXA_2 has a short life (seconds) and is rapidly degraded in water to TXB_2. Prostacyclin, or PGI_2, is produced in considerable quantities by endothelial cells.[11] PGI_2 is a potent vasodilator

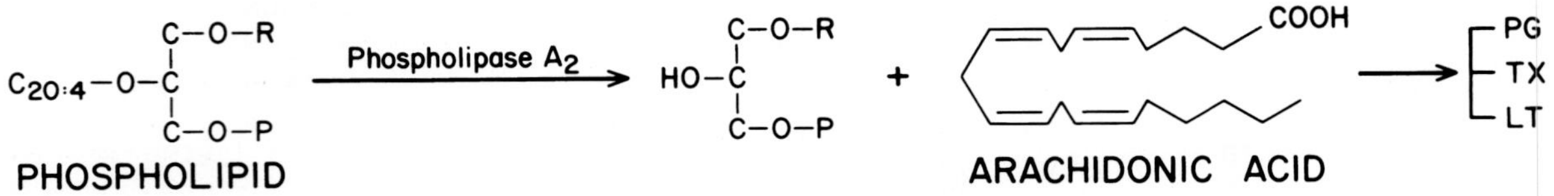

C—O—R | $C_{20:4}$—O—C | C—O—P

PHOSPHOLIPID

Phospholipase A_2

C—O—R | HO—C | C—O—P

+

COOH

ARACHIDONIC ACID

[PG TX LT]

Figure 5–3 ■ Mobilization of arachidonic acid from esterified pools. Phospholipids are a prominent pool of arachidonic acid that is released by phospholipase A_2. Free arachidonic acid is available for conversion to prostaglandins (PG), thromboxane (TX), or leukotrienes (LT).

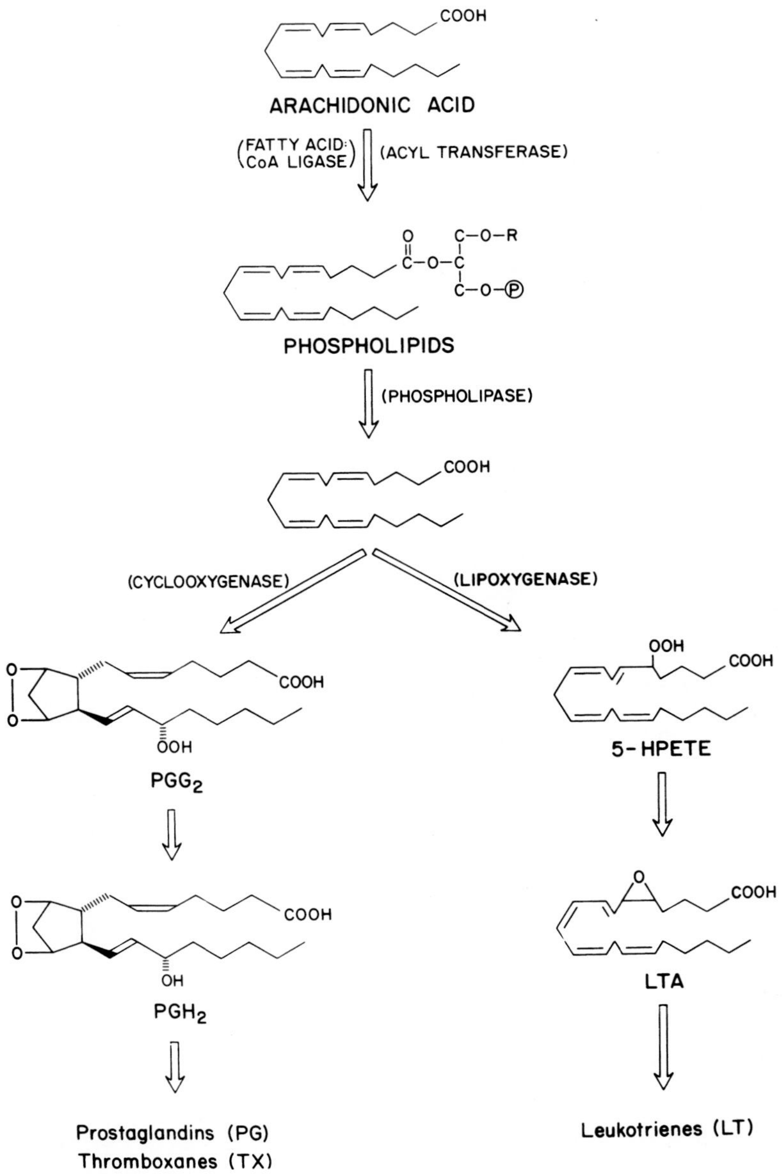

Figure 5–4 ■ Pathways of arachidonic acid metabolism. In addition to catabolism by beta oxidation, arachidonic acid is metabolized by the cyclooxygenase or lipoxygenase pathway. 5-HPETE, 5-hydroperoxyeicosatetraenoic acid.

and inhibitor of platelet aggregation. These properties, which are directly antagonistic to those of TXA_2, permit PGI_2 and TXA_2 to modulate platelet aggregation and vessel wall repair.[12] Separate enzymes catalyze the production of TXA_2 and PGI_2.

PGE_2 and $PGF_{2\alpha}$ are produced by virtually every tissue, and substantial amounts are seen in the follicle, uterus, and brain. Whether enzyme-catalyzed production of PGE_2 is necessary is questioned because PGE_2 is readily formed by simple nonoxidative rearrangement,[10] whereas $PGF_{2\alpha}$ is formed by reduction of PGH_2 by a unique enzyme.[10] Both are potent stimulators of smooth muscle. A wide variety of other cells also respond directly to PGE_2 and $PGF_{2\alpha}$, and the nature of the response to all prostaglandins is dictated by the nature of the receptor with which the tissue is endowed.

PGD_2 is formed from PGH_2 by 11-ketoisomerase; but like that of PGE_2, the formation of PGD_2 may occur by simple nonenzymatic rearrangement. PGD_2 is abundant in brain and platelets. Hydroxyheptadecatrienoic acid and malondialdehyde have no known biologic functions.

Little is known of the products of PGH_1 metabolism, although PGF_1, $PGF_{1\alpha}$, PGD_1, and TXB_1 have been described.[13] However, PGG_1 and PGH_1 were not found to be substrates for prostacyclin synthase, but PGG_3 and PGH_3 were.[14] Although the cyclooxygenase and lipoxygenase pathways result in the formation of PGG_3 (see Fig. 5–1), little information is available on this series of eicosanoids. Interestingly, some populations ingest high levels of fatty acid precursors for the 3-series of prostaglandins (n-3 or omega-3 fatty acids), which may be relevant to the low incidence of myocardial infarction in these people.[15] Cyclooxygenase shows a preference for arachidonic acid,[13] and other omega-3 fatty acids may inhibit prostaglandin synthesis by acting as competitive substrates.

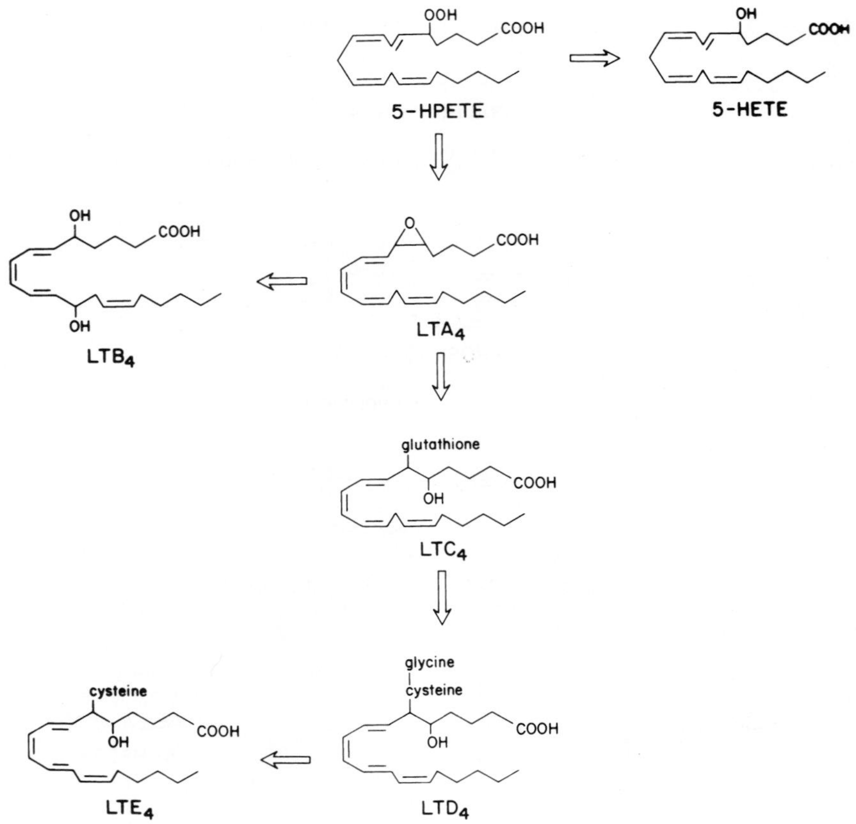

Figure 5–5 ■ Biosynthesis of leukotrienes. 5-HPETE, 5-hydroperoxyeicosatetraenoic acid; 5-HETE, 5-hydroxyeicosatetraenoic acid.

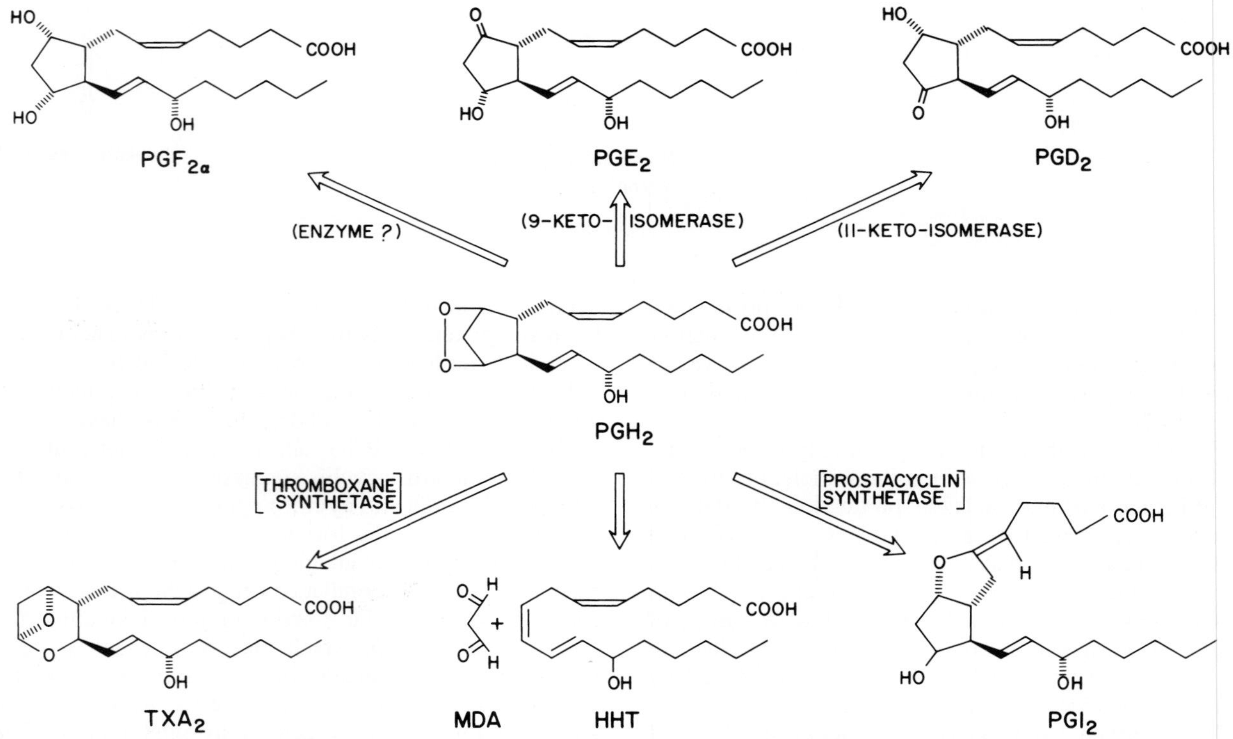

Figure 5–6 ■ Biosynthesis of prostaglandins and thromboxane. HHT, hydroxyheptadecatrienoic acid; MDA, malondialdehyde.

Nomenclature

Structurally, all prostaglandins have a "hairpin" configuration and contain a cyclopentanone nucleus with a carboxyl and an aliphatic side chain. They are named from the archetypal (but hypothetical) structure prostanoic acid (Fig. 5–7). Primary prostaglandins contain a 15-hydroxyl group with a double bond at carbon 13, which is essential for bioactivity. Each group of prostaglandins is allocated a letter (A, B, C, D, E, F, G, H, or I), which denotes particular functional groups in the cylopentanone ring. The degree of unsaturation of the side chains is indicated by the subscript numeral after the letter; thus PGE_1, PGE_2, and PGE_3 have one, two, and three double bonds, respectively (see Fig. 5–7). A description of the stereochemistry at position 9 in the cyclopentanone ring is denoted by the subscript α or β; thus, the configuration of $PGF_{2\alpha}$ has the orientation of the 9-hydroxyl moiety oriented below the plane of the ring. $PGF_{2\beta}$ (the inactive isomer of $PGF_{2\alpha}$) has the 9-hydroxyl group oriented above the plane of the ring.

A similar system is used for nomenclature of thromboxane that is based on a hypothetical structure—thrombanoic acid. The thromboxanes, too, are composed of 20 carbons with a hairpin configuration. For leukotrienes (see Fig. 5–5), the abbreviation used for the trivial name denotes the presence of three conjugated double bonds in the molecule, and the subscript number describes the total number of double bonds in the structure.[4]

Metabolism

A characteristic feature of eicosanoids is the transient nature of their existence. In some instances, the mere presence of water produces an immediate "facile" hydrolysis into inactive products (e.g., TXA_2, PGI_2, PGG_2, PGH_2). In other instances, a plethora of degrading enzymes in the lung, the liver, the kidney, and other tissues results in a virtually complete loss of the biologic activity within one circulation of blood. It is not surprising, therefore, that few instances of eicosanoids acting as "hormones" occur, except when a specialized vascular organization is present to permit local delivery (e.g., countercurrent diffusion, blood portal system).

The first and most important catabolic step from the standpoint of biologic inactivation of prostaglandin is conversion of the 15-hydroxyl group to a 15-keto moiety (Fig. 5–8), a reaction catalyzed by 15-hydroxyprostaglandin dehydrogenase (15-OH-PGDH).[16] In general, highest concentrations of 15-OH-PGDH are found in the lungs, the placenta, the spleen, and the kidney cortex. The brain has relatively low levels of 15-OH-PGDH activity, as do the ovary and the testis. Substrates for 15-OH-PGDH include PGE, PGF, and PGI, but the last prostaglandin is degraded rapidly by facile hydrolysis.

The second step in the sequential degradation of prostaglandins is reduction of the double bond at position 13 (see Fig. 5–8) by 13,14-prostaglandin reductase, which is highly specific for 15-keto prostaglandins[17]; this enzyme has a tissue distribution similar to that of 15-OH-PGDH. The metabolites then undergo both beta (i.e., carboxyl chain) and omega oxidation, resulting in urinary excretion of the final products. Although Figure 5–8 depicts the series of catabolic steps of PGE_2, a sequence of virtually identical events occurs with $PGF_{2\alpha}$.

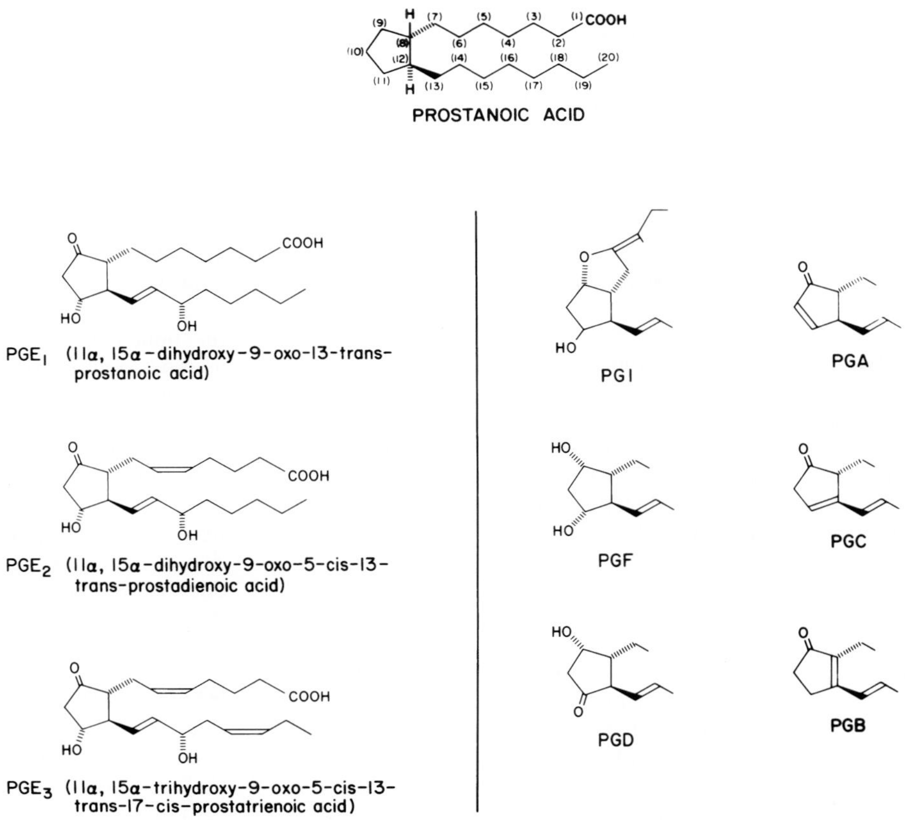

PROSTANOIC ACID

PGE_1 (11α, 15α-dihydroxy-9-oxo-13-trans-prostanoic acid)

PGE_2 (11α, 15α-dihydroxy-9-oxo-5-cis-13-trans-prostadienoic acid)

PGE_3 (11α, 15α-trihydroxy-9-oxo-5-cis-13-trans-17-cis-prostatrienoic acid)

PGI PGA PGF PGC PGD PGB

Figure 5–7 ■ Nomenclature and structure of the prostaglandins.

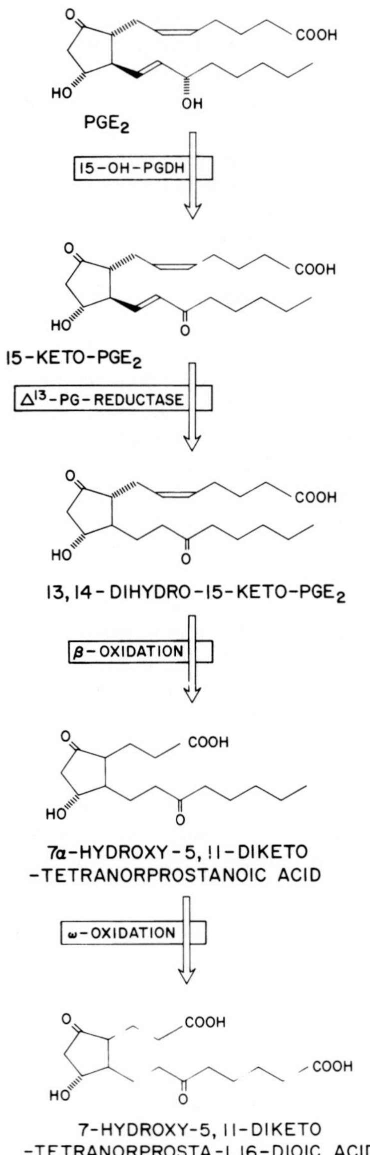

Figure 5–8 ■ Metabolism of prostaglandin E_2.

PGI_2 is unstable in aqueous solutions, particularly at neutral to acid pH, in which it rapidly undergoes hydrolysis to form 6-keto $PGF_{1\alpha}$, a major but inactive metabolite.[18] PGI_2 is also metabolized by 15-OH-PGDH in vascular endothelium[18] (Fig. 5–9). TXA_2 rapidly undergoes facile hydrolysis to form the inactive metabolite TXB_2 followed by beta oxidation[19] (Fig. 5–9).

PHARMACOLOGY OF THE ARACHIDONIC ACID CASCADE

The discovery of eicosanoids and their diverse biologic activities allows a greater understanding of the pharmacology of familiar and established drugs and provides a foundation for development of novel compounds with more selective therapeutic modalities. Aspirin, the oldest and most common drug in our pharmacopeia, produces analgesic and antipyretic effects by inhibition of prostaglandin synthesis.[20] A variety of drugs are now known to influence the arachidonic acid cascade, and these are summarized in Figure 5–10.

Phospholipase

Availability of unesterified arachidonic acid plays a pivotal role in eicosanoid synthesis, and phospholipases serve a fundamental role in this process (see Fig. 5–4). Dogma states that phospholipase A_2 serves a fundamental role in the release of free arachidonic acid from esterified stores and at least five separate phospholipases have been identified,[21] but a cytosolic form appears to result in hormone-dependent release. Phospholipases C and D may also increase arachidonic acid release from esterified stores.[10]

Glucocorticoids are potent anti-inflammatory agents, and it was once believed that their anti-inflammatory activity resided solely in their ability to inhibit phospholipase A_2 activity, thereby decreasing the availability of arachidonic acid. The mechanism of the inhibitory action of glucocorticoids on eicosanoid synthesis was thought to occur by the induction of proteins termed lipocortins.[22] Lipocortins belong to the general class of proteins termed annexins, which sequester phospholipids[2] and thereby prevent phospholipase A_2 action. Although this remains one action of glucocorticoids, recent evidence indicates that glucocorticoids also rapidly inhibit phospholipase activation by blocking enzyme phosphorylation.[23] More recent evidence favors the inhibitory action of glucocorticoids on prostaglandin synthesis by blockade of prostaglandin synthase-2 induction (see later).

Lipoxygenase

No drugs now available selectively inhibit lipoxygenase activity and preferentially inhibit production of leukotrienes (see Fig. 5–5). An older chemical often used experimentally to inhibit lipoxygenase is nordihydroguaiaretic acid, but it is best known for its antioxidant properties. On the other hand, there are drugs that inhibit both the lipoxygenase and the cyclooxygenase pathways. These include the competitive inhibitor analogues of arachidonic acid, such as eicosatetraynoic acid. This synthetic compound has triple bonds at each of the positions in which arachidonic acid has double bonds (see Fig. 5–1). The potent chemotactic activity of leukotriene B_4 and the deleterious effects of leukotrienes C_4, D_4, and E_4 (slow-reacting substances of anaphylaxis) have spurred interest in the search for selective inhibitors of lipoxygenase activity. The common nonsteroidal anti-inflammatory drugs (NSAIDs) do not inhibit lipoxygenase activity at therapeutic levels. Indeed, inhibition of cyclooxygenase activity may lead to enhanced production of lipoxygenase products, probably by increasing the availability of arachidonic acid to the latter pathway.[24]

Cyclooxygenase

There is now strong evidence that glucocorticoids block cytokine induction of PGH synthase-2, and this may be the major basis for their ability to inhibit eicosanoid synthesis.[2, 10] Virtually all of the aspirin-like drugs of

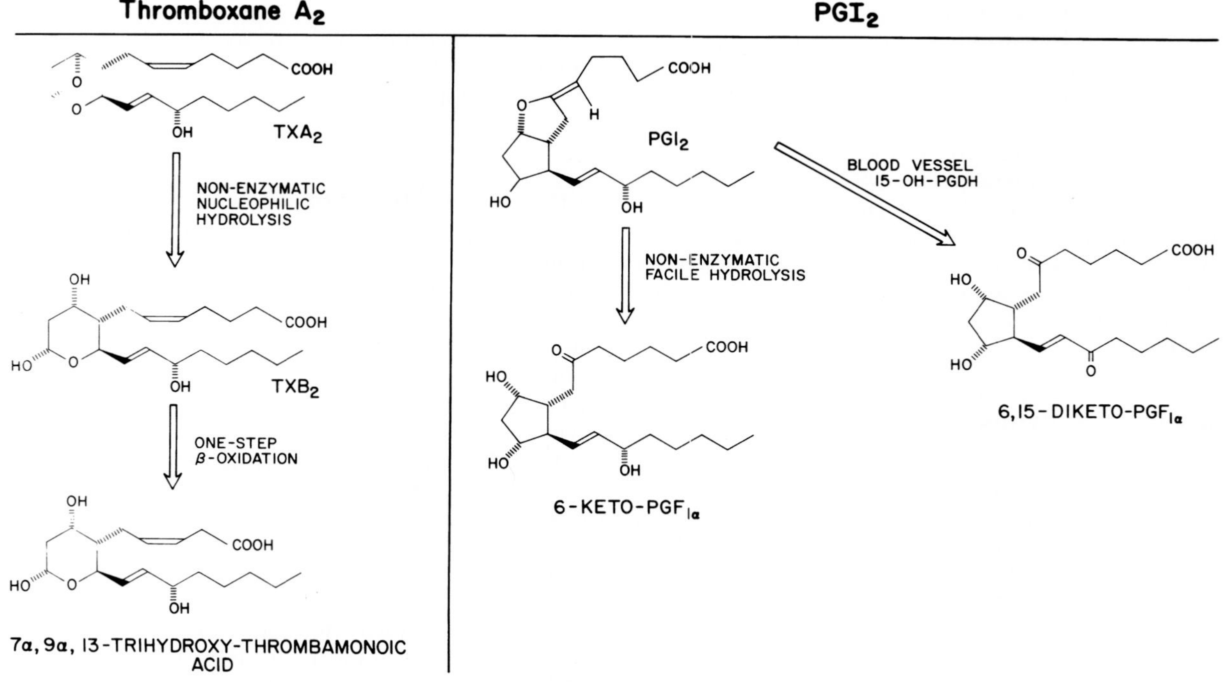

Figure 5–9 ■ Deactivation of thromboxane A_2 and PGI_2 by nonenzymatic facile hydrolysis.

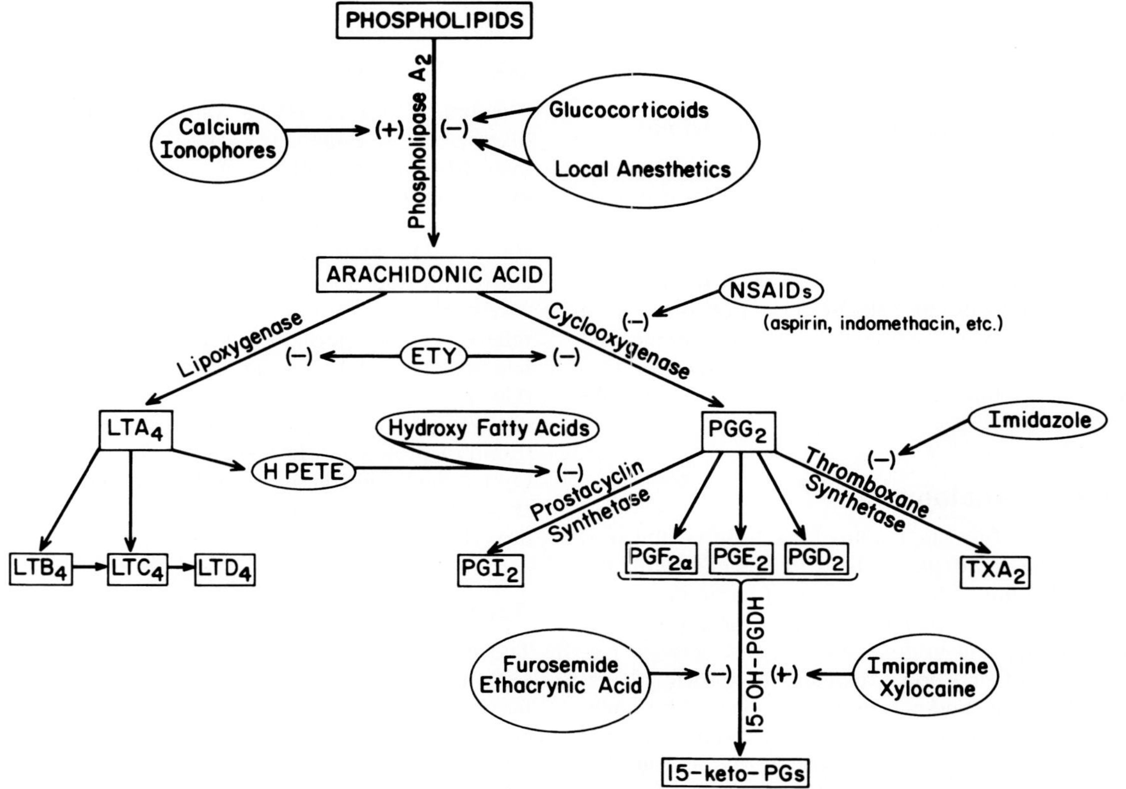

Figure 5–10 ■ Pharmacology of the arachidonic acid cascade. NSAIDs, nonsteroidal anti-inflammatory drugs; ETY, eicosatetraynoic acid; HPETE, hydroperoxyeicosatetraenoic acid.

NSAIDs are inhibitors of prostaglandin production (see Fig. 5–10) and act by direct inhibition of cyclooxygenase.[20] Although lipoxygenase inhibition occurs with some NSAIDs, high drug concentrations are necessary, and probably no inhibition of lipoxygenase activity occurs at therapeutic concentrations. Indeed, leukotriene production may be increased, as described earlier. NSAIDs are about 100 times more potent as inhibitors of prostaglandin synthase-1 than of prostaglandin synthase-2.[9, 10] This may be the basis for high levels of NSAIDs that are required to block prostaglandin synthesis when prostaglandin synthase-2 has been up-regulated, such as in the ovulatory follicle or arthritic joint.

Prostacyclin Synthase

The enzyme prostacyclin synthase catalyzes the transformation of PGG_2 to PGI_2 (see Fig. 5–10). No selective inhibitors of this enzyme are available commercially, but hydroperoxy fatty acids inhibit formation of PGI_2 in vitro.[12] PGI_2 production in cardiac tissue is inhibited by nicotine, but nicotine has no effect on platelet TXA_2 production.[25] It is not known if this is a direct effect of nicotine on prostacyclin synthase.

Thromboxane Synthase

Formation of TXA_2 in the platelet is inhibited by a variety of agents that block cyclooxygenase activity, such as NSAIDs, but few inhibitors of conversion of PGG_2 to TXA_2 are known. Imidazole and its derivatives may selectively inhibit thromboxane synthase,[26] although this same drug also inhibits prostacyclin synthase, albeit at higher concentrations.

15-Hydroxyprostaglandin Dehydrogenase

There is considerable evidence that inhibition of prostaglandin catabolism may lead to increased levels of prostaglandins. In this regard, lidocaine and the antidiuretic drugs furosemide and ethacrynic acid inhibit 15-OH-PGDH activity.[27] This may explain the diuretic action of these drugs, because PGE_2 produces diuresis by an action directly in the kidney. The tricyclic antidepressants imipramine and desipramine activate swine kidney 15-OH-PGDH activity.[27] A review of drugs that affect this enzyme has been published.[16]

Prostaglandin Analogues

Several analogues of prostaglandins have been synthesized to circumvent the rapid metabolism that occurs with the natural prostaglandins. The clinical use of natural and synthetic analogues of prostaglandins includes those for induction of luteal regression in domestic animals, cervical ripening, induction of abortion, treatment of gastric ulcers, erectile dysfunction, and vascular disorders. The early promise of these potent drugs led to disappointment, primarily because of the inability to separate smooth muscle–stimulating activity from other desired actions. As a consequence, side effects such as nausea, vomiting, diarrhea, headache, and other disturbing occurrences have led to some disenchantment with this avenue of drug development. The recent discovery of specific receptors that mediate different responses to prostaglandins may permit the synthesis of analogues with more selective action and clinical usefulness.

Prostaglandin Receptors

Prostaglandin receptors are classified on the basis of functional activities of natural and synthetic agonists and a few antagonists into the categories of DP, EP, FP, IP, and TP in which the first letter denotes the prostaglandin type and the letter P denotes "prostanoid."[28] Subsequent studies by binding analysis and most recently by molecular cloning techniques have confirmed the presence of distinct receptor types and the presence of three or four subtypes of EP (EP_{1-4}). Plasma membrane prostaglandin receptors belong to the superfamily of G protein–coupled receptors with characteristic seven transmembrane spanning regions.[29] Intracellular second messengers of prostaglandin receptors include cyclic adenosine monophosphate (cAMP), protein kinase C, and calcium.[28, 29] The various receptors show remarkable specificity for the eicosanoid with at least a 100-fold preference for the ligand. At high concentrations, PGE_2 and $PGF_{2\alpha}$ interact with the DP receptor; similarly, $PGF_{2\alpha}$ will activate the EP receptor, whereas PGD_2 and PGE_2 will interact with the FP receptor at high concentrations. Most tissues contain a mixture of receptors, which appears to be the basis for often opposite effects of a particular prostaglandin at different doses. A brief summary of the ligands and their receptor types is shown in Table 5–1.[28, 29]

OXYGEN RADICALS AND PEROXIDES

The importance of oxygen radicals in aging, health, and disease is now established. The reproductive system, however, has until recently been ignored with regard to these endogenous, highly reactive products. Reactive oxygen species include singlet oxygen ($^1O_2$), superoxide anion ($O_2^-\cdot$), $HO_2\cdot$, hydrogen peroxide (H_2O_2), the hydroxyl radical ($OH\cdot$), and lipid hydroperoxides.[30, 31] Cells are readily permeable to H_2O_2 in contrast to $O_2^-\cdot$, and H_2O_2, although relatively nontoxic alone, is rapidly converted to $OH\cdot$ in the presence of $O_2^-\cdot$ and ferrous iron (Fe^{2+}) or copper (Cu^+). The hydroxyl radical is extremely reactive, and cell injury produced by this species is believed to occur at the origin of production in a site-specific manner.[32] Thus, both $O_2^-\cdot$ (which can directly produce damage) and H_2O_2 derived from $O_2^-\cdot$ participate in the production of the hydroxyl radical.

Actions of Reactive Oxygen Species

The cell membrane is a major site of action of oxygen radicals, and nonezymatic peroxidation of polyunsaturated fatty acids within membrane phospholipids is particularly notable.[33, 34] Lipoperoxides have profound effects on membrane function, which include increased membrane rigidity, loss of elasticity, alteration in membrane permeability, impaired anchoring of the cytoskeleton, and others.[35] Membrane peroxidation increases phospholipase A_2 activity,[36]

■ TABLE 5–1
A Summary of Prostanoid Receptors, Their Ligands, and Second Messengers

LIGAND	RECEPTOR	MEDIATOR	TISSUE
PGI_2	IP	↑ cAMP	Platelets, vasculature, monocytes, T cells
PGD_2	DP	↑ cAMP; ↑ NO	Nervous tissue, uterus, platelets, coronary arteries
PGE_2	EP_1	↑ Ca^{2+}; ↑ PKC	Uterus, ileum
	EP_2	↑ cAMP	Ovary, uterus, mast cells, basophils
	EP_3	↓ cAMP	Uterus, adipocytes, vasculature, gastrointestinal tract
	EP_4	↑ cAMP	Vasculature
$PGF_{2\alpha}$	FP	↑ Ca^{2+}; ↑ PKC	Corpus luteum, theca, vasculature
TXA_2	TP	↑ Ca^{2+}; ↑ PKC	Platelets, vasculature, uterus

cAMP, cyclic adenosine monophosphate; NO, nitric oxide; PKC, protein kinase C.

thereby increasing synthesis of eicosanoids. Lysophosphatides produced by phospholipase activation also contribute to membrane damage, activation of leukocytes, and cell lysis.

Deoxyribonucleic acid (DNA) strand scission is a notable response to oxygen radicals, a phenomenon associated with the mutagenic actions of these reactive species. In fact, depletion of cell levels of adenosine triphosphate (ATP) by oxygen radicals is linked to DNA damage because DNA repair mechanisms deplete cellular nicotinamide adenine dinucleotide.[36]

Proteins are attacked directly by the hydroxyl radical, causing cross-linking and a consequent loss of function. Decomposition of lipid peroxides results in the formation of malondialdehyde, a highly reactive substance on primary amino groups of proteins. Oxygen radicals also directly oxidize amino acids within proteins; histidine, arginine, lysine, and proline are particularly sensitive to this effect.[37]

Origins of Reactive Oxygen Species

There is direct evidence for the generation of oxygen radicals in the reproductive system, and a predominant source is leukocytes. Infiltration of leukocytes is a hallmark of luteolysis,[38] as is the infiltration of leukocytes in the preovulatory follicle after exposure to luteinizing hormone (LH).[39] Human sperm produce oxygen radicals,[40] and oxygen radicals are used in lower animals in formation of the cross-linked fertilization envelope.[41] Interestingly, mammalian predictyate oocytes do not have functional DNA repair mechanisms,[42] which makes them highly susceptible to radical attack. Uterine and amniotic sepsis are known to induce leukocytic infiltration, and uterine contractions are induced by peroxide in a prostaglandin-dependent mechanism[43] that may cause premature delivery.

Phagocytic leukocytes have a unique membrane-associated oxidase that on activation produces a violent release of oxygen radicals.[44] The respiratory burst is triggered by some cytokines and by phagocytosis. Activated or primed macrophages produce tumor necrosis factor-α (TNF-α) and interleukin (IL)-1, which trigger the release of oxygen radicals from neutrophils.[45] Oxygen radicals stimulate further TNF-α production, which sets in motion a chain reaction of oxygen radical production through leukocytic interactions.[46] Activation of the membrane-associated NADPH oxidase is under complex regulation by unsaturated fatty acid, G proteins, and cytosolic peptides.[47–49] Eicosanoids and other cytokines are involved in the chemotaxis, adherence, extravasation, and activation of neutrophils. Provocatively, in the corpus luteum, interferon (IFN)-γ induces antigens, macrophages produce TNF-α, macrophages are resident, and phagocytosis is extensively documented.[38, 50, 51] Thus, all the elements for immune cell–derived release of oxygen radicals are present in the ovary and the reproductive tract.

Endothelial cells are another source of oxygen radicals. These cells not only are phagocytic but also evoke release of oxygen radicals.[52] The cytokines IL-1 and IFN-γ and activators of protein kinase C stimulate oxygen radical production by endothelial cells.[53] Other major stimuli for production of oxygen radicals in endothelium are ischemia and reperfusion.[54]

Ovarian parenchymal cells are another source of oxygen radicals. Steroidogenic enzymes produce oxygen radicals in hydroxylation and side-chain cleavage reactions, and superoxide and hydrogen peroxide are generated in the corpus luteum.[55, 56] These effects are the probable basis for depletion of ascorbic acid produced by LH and $PGF_{2\alpha}$.[57]

It has been estimated that each mitochondrion generates about 10^7 oxygen radicals per day. NADH dehydrogenase and the ubiquinone–cytochrome *b* complex produce much of the superoxide, and hydrogen peroxide arises from dismutation of superoxide.[58] Mitochondria play an important role in the pathophysiology of oxygen radicals, not only because they generate oxygen radicals but also because they are especially sensitive to oxygen radical attack. Deterioration of mitochondrial function from accumulated exposure to oxygen radicals is one of the leading theories of senescence[59, 60] because mitochondrial DNA (mtDNA) accumulates mutations in postmitotic tissues with age.[61–63] This susceptibility to oxygen radical–induced mutations occurs because mtDNA is close to radical-generating enzymes on the mitochondrial inner membrane; lacks histones, which protect nuclear DNA; assumes a small superhelical structure, which readily intercalates environmental mutagens; lacks introns, so mtDNA contains more densely packed coding information than does nuclear DNA; contains only a single known DNA polymerase, with minimal repair capacity; and contains multiple repeated sequences, which predisposes mtDNA to deletions through slippage-replication.[64]

Defenses Against Oxygen Radicals

The reproductive system with its vital role in propagation of the species must, from necessity, be uniquely protected from these extremely toxic but ubiquitous oxygen byproducts. One defensive mechanism is to provide a low oxygen environment such as that seen with developing germ cells within their barrier of protective nurse cells and in the fallopian tube. Beyond structural mechanisms, inhibition of production, detoxification, and repair of damaged cell products are the remaining avenues of defense against oxygen radicals.

Recent evidence shows that production of oxygen radicals by leukocytes is inhibited by growth factors and other cytokines. Provocatively, transforming growth factor-β (TGF-β) and IFN-α prevent activation of macrophages,[65, 66] and adenosine prevents activation of neutrophils.[33, 34] Both adenosine and TGF-β are produced by the ovary, and IFN-α–like trophoblast proteins rescue the corpus luteum of pregnancy in domestic animals.[67] Thus, the cellular and chemical elements for regulation of both production and inhibition of oxygen radicals are present in the ovary. These processes may be extant in rescue, maintenance, and regression of the corpus luteum; in follicle rescue and atresia; and in ovulation.

A major line of defense is detoxification of oxygen radicals, catalyzed by superoxide dismutase, catalase, and glutathione peroxidase.[30, 31] Both mitochondria and cytosol contain unique enzymes that catalyze the dismutation of superoxide into hydrogen peroxide and oxygen. Cytosolic superoxide dismutase is a copper-zinc metalloenzyme (also found in the extracellular fluid), and the mitochondrial form is a manganese metalloenzyme.[30] Hydrogen peroxide is detoxified by two major enzymes: catalase and glutathione peroxidase. Catalase is found in virtually every cell, primarily within peroxisomes and cytosol. Glutathione peroxidase, in contrast to catalase, detoxifies lipid peroxides as well as hydrogen peroxide. Glutathione peroxidase is a selenium metalloenzyme located in the cytosol and mitochondria.

Another major defensive strategy against radicals is through antioxidant vitamins, with E serving such a role in lipid-enriched membranes and C in aqueous compartments. Membranes are major sites of damage by radicals, and the protective role of vitamin E is of paramount importance in terminating peroxidation chain reactions of unsaturated lipids. Vitamin C recycles oxidized E back to the reduced state, and oxidized C is either reduced by transhydrogenases or replaced from extracellular sources. Thus, depletion of vitamin C is directly related to the production of oxygen radicals; and such depletion, seen in response to LH and $PGF_{2\alpha}$ in the corpus luteum, may occur by such a process. The cellular accumulation of ascorbic acid occurs by an active transport system that is endocrine regulated in the ovary.[57, 68]

Repair processes invoked to remove damaged cellular components are the final avenue of defense against radicals. Removal of peroxidized fatty acids in membrane phospholipids by activation of phospholipase A_2 is one example. Another is the activation of poly(adenosine diphosphate–ribose)polymerase produced by damage of DNA described earlier. There appears to be less information on the role of proteases in removal, or repair, of proteins subjected to oxidative damage, but such phenomena would be expected.

Oxygen Radicals and the Reproductive System

Oxygen radicals may be important mediators of luteolysis. Plasma membranes from regressing rat corpora lutea produce superoxide and hydrogen peroxide[55, 56] and show an increase in lipid peroxidation.[69, 70] In luteal cells, oxygen radicals abruptly abrogate LH-sensitive adenylate cyclase activity, inhibit progesterone synthesis, and deplete ATP.[71] Provocatively, these antigonadotropic actions of oxygen radicals are similar to those produced by $PGF_{2\alpha}$, but they are of much greater magnitude. Whereas $PGF_{2\alpha}$ does not mediate the actions of hydrogen peroxide,[71] reactive oxygen species are generated by $PGF_{2\alpha}$ in the corpus luteum.[55, 56]

Reactive oxygen species may also serve a role in follicular atresia, in ovulation, and in oocyte function. Interestingly, ascorbic acid deficiency causes marked follicular atresia and oocyte destruction,[72] and ascorbic acid blocks apoptosis in granulosa cells of cultured follicles.[73] Evidence points to the production of oxygen radicals at ovulation and in the oocyte.[41, 72, 74] Oxygen radicals are used in lower animals in the formation of the cross-linked fertilization envelope,[41] and vitamin E deficiency is known to impair gamete survival. Production of oxygen radicals at ovulation, in response to LH, may signal differentiation of the oocyte. However, radical overproduction may cause injury, such as that seen in atresia, characterized by the presence of lipofuscin and "glassy membranes," histologic landmarks of radical production.

Oocytes are postmitotic, long-lived cells, and their developmental capacity deteriorates with age. Mitochondrial DNA deletions were identified first in ovaries from older women[75] and more recently in individual oocytes that failed to fertilize after attempted in vitro fertilization.[76, 77] There is considerable evidence that oxygen radicals influence sperm function. Lipid peroxidation directly parallels loss of sperm motility, yet human sperm produce oxygen radicals on stimulation,[78] and exposure of human zona to oxygen radicals markedly enhances sperm attachment.[40]

Oxygen is toxic to embryos, most likely because it promotes formation of oxygen radicals. Embryos develop under low oxygen concentrations, especially during the peri-implantation period. A number of experimental conditions that reduce oxygen radical levels in vitro have been shown to positively influence embryo developmental potential. A rise in hydrogen peroxide levels coincides with the time of the two-cell block in mice,[79] and addition of reduced glutathione to the culture medium improves the development of mouse zygotes through the two-cell block.[80] Alteration of media to eliminate inorganic metals or to add antioxidants also improves embryo development.[81–83] Interestingly, an extramitochondrial NADPH-dependent oxidase activity, capable of generating superoxide and hydrogen peroxide, resides in the trophoblast layer of the blastocyst.[84] The function of such a radical generator is unknown, but it may be involved in implantation.

Uterine contractions are induced by oxygen radicals coincident with the production of prostaglandins.[43] These

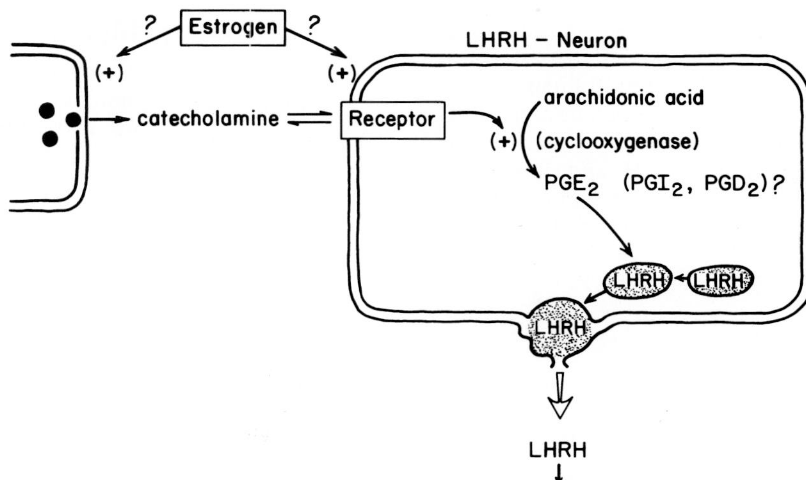

Figure 5–11 ■ Role of prostaglandins in hypothalamic gonadotropin-releasing hormone (GnRH or luteinizing hormone–releasing hormone [LHRH]) secretion. Question marks indicate a lack of information concerning whether estrogen directly or indirectly stimulates prostaglandin production in GnRH neurons. The endogenous and active prostaglandin in the GnRH neuron has not been established. Plus signs indicate stimulation.

findings may be related to the fact that uterine and amniotic sepsis results in premature delivery.[85] However, it is also possible that generation of oxygen radicals may serve a role in the induction of parturition.[85]

EICOSANOIDS AND GONADOTROPIN SECRETION

Since the finding that aspirin and indomethacin block ovulation,[86] evidence implicates prostaglandins, particularly PGE_2, as regulators of gonadotropin-releasing hormone (GnRH) secretion.[87] Prostaglandins have little direct effect on pituitary secretion of gonadotropins, but either peripheral or third-ventricle injection of PGE_2 stimulates gonadotropin secretion. PGE_2 stimulates the release of GnRH from the hypothalamus,[88] and pretreatment of animals with antisera to neutralize endogenous GnRH prevents release of LH produced by PGE_2 administration.[89] Catecholaminergic stimuli increase PGE and GnRH release from medial basal hypothalamic tissue in vitro, PGE_2 directly stimulates GnRH release from such tissue, and indomethacin blocks stimulation of GnRH induced by catecholamine.[90] Thus, GnRH release may be regulated directly by intraneuronal PGE_2 production and serve as a mediator of catecholamine on GnRH secretion (Fig. 5–11). Estrogen is known to stimulate LH secretion, and this effect of estrogen may also be mediated by prostaglandin, because indomethacin inhibits estrogen-stimulated LH secretion.[91]

EICOSANOIDS IN THE OVARY

The Preovulatory Follicle

Prostaglandins play a pivotal role in follicular rupture in a variety of species. Inhibitors of prostaglandin synthesis block ovulation, neutralization of endogenous $PGF_{2\alpha}$ with antiserum inhibits ovulation, and elevated levels of prostaglandins occur in preovulatory follicles.[87] Both PGE_2 and $PGF_{2\alpha}$ levels are increased in follicular fluid, but it has not been established completely whether PGE_2, $PGF_{2\alpha}$, or both are the physiologic inducers of the follicular rupture process. Cyclooxygenase-2 is induced by LH in the preovulatory follicle.[92] No FP receptors are present in granulosa cells of the preovulatory follicle, but they are present in the theca.[93] Thus, if $PGF_{2\alpha}$ is essential for ovulation, its action must be restricted to the thecal layer. Lipoxygenase-derived products have also been implicated as mediators of the ovulatory process.[94]

The surge of gonadotropins stimulates follicular eicosanoid biosynthesis by a cAMP-mediated process that is dependent on gene activation but is independent of steroidogenesis. The mechanisms by which eicosanoids induce the rupture process is not clear, although protease activation seems to be involved (Fig. 5–12). A marked preovulatory increase in neutrophil density has been observed in the theca concomitant with the LH surge,[95] and

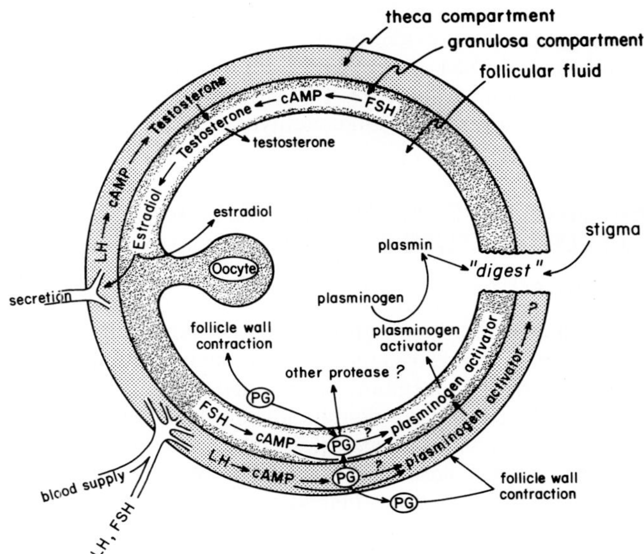

Figure 5–12 ■ Role of prostaglandins in follicular rupture. Follicular production of prostaglandins is induced by both luteinizing hormone (LH) and follicle-stimulating hormone (FSH) that is mediated by cAMP but is not dependent on steroidogenesis. Prostaglandins (PG) may induce follicular rupture by an action in follicular fluid (e.g., protease), by an action on the follicle wall (e.g., contraction, collagen breakdown), or by both.

leukocytes may play a role in timely follicular rupture by secreting proteolytic enzymes, oxygen radicals, and prostaglandins. Intrafollicular concentration of IL-8, a neutrophil chemoattractant/activating factor, rises markedly around the time of ovulation and was found to be up-regulated by LH and human chorionic gonadotropin (hCG).[96] Thus, IL-8 seems to be responsible for the timely recruitment of neutrophils in and around the periovulatory follicles.

The Corpus Luteum

The role of eicosanoids in human luteal regression is enigmatic; in nonprimate mammalian species, $PGF_{2\alpha}$ is a physiologic luteolysin.[87] $PGF_{2\alpha}$ induces functional regression of the corpus luteum by a receptor-mediated process, independent initially of changes in ovarian or luteal blood flow.[97] Within minutes, $PGF_{2\alpha}$ depletes ascorbic acid,[57] uncouples the occupied LH receptor from adenylate cyclase, and decreases transport of gonadotropin from capillaries to the luteal cell.

Whereas $PGF_{2\alpha}$ may serve a role as a luteolysin in the human, this conclusion must be tempered by the relative insensitivity of the human corpus luteum in vivo to the luteolytic action of exogenous $PGF_{2\alpha}$. Unlike in animals, the human uterus plays no role in the luteolytic process. However, $PGF_{2\alpha}$ is produced by the human corpus luteum, and specific receptors for $PGF_{2\alpha}$ are located in human luteal tissue.[98] In the human, $PGF_{2\alpha}$ inhibits gonadotropin-stimulated progesterone production by luteinized cells in vitro.[99] Conversely, PGE_2 stimulates progesterone secretion in human luteal cells,[99] but the decrease in progesterone secretion produced by $PGF_{2\alpha}$ is transient.[100]

Estrogens induce premature luteal regression in the human.[101] On the basis of studies in the monkey, this action of estrogen appears to be at the level of the ovary.[102] In the monkey, there is evidence that the luteolytic action of estrogen is linked to prostaglandin production, because estrogen treatment increases $PGF_{2\alpha}$ levels in ovarian blood and indomethacin blocks the luteolytic effect of estrogen.[103]

EICOSANOIDS IN THE UTERUS AND FALLOPIAN TUBES

Endometrium

The endometrium is not only a site of synthesis but also a site of action of prostaglandin. The main prostaglandins produced by nonpregnant endometrium are $PGF_{2\alpha}$ and PGE_2, although other eicosanoids are also evident and production is greater during the secretory phase than during the proliferative phase of the cycle. The synthesis of prostaglandins is greater in the glandular epithelium than in the stroma of the endometrium.[104, 105] Mechanisms for steroid hormone regulation of prostaglandin synthesis are difficult to interpret because estrogens increase and progestins decrease the endometrial production of prostaglandins in vitro, findings that do not correspond to those seen in vivo. This discrepancy may be due to leukocyte interactions, which can occur only in vivo, that are known to increase prostaglandin production.

Myometrium

The myometrium produces predominantly PGI_2, unlike the amnion, chorion, and decidua. PGI_2 is a powerful vasodilator and smooth muscle relaxer and has been shown to inhibit the increase in uterine tone produced by $PGF_{2\alpha}$ in vitro.[106] Although the myometrium is not a major producer of eicosanoids, it is one of the main target tissues of prostaglandins. $PGF_{2\alpha}$ and PGE_2 are known to stimulate myometrial contractility, because they increase intracellular calcium by the interaction with specific receptors. Neither the density nor the affinity of the receptor seems to change during parturition.[107] The increased contractile activity during labor is directly related to the rise of $PGF_{2\alpha}$ and PGE_2 and to the production of other eicosanoids by the fetoplacental unit.

Cervix

The strength of the cervix as a connective tissue organ is related to the absolute collagen content and the degree of intermolecular cross-links. During pregnancy, the cervical collagen content decreases, and close to term the cervix has greater water retention and a soft, swollen appearance. These changes are associated with increases in the activity of two extracellular enzymes capable of degrading collagen: collagenase and leukocyte elastase. The duration of the dilatation phase of labor is directly related to the cervical collagen concentration and collagen extractibility.[108]

Various prostaglandins are produced in the uterine cervix, and their increased production is associated with cervical ripening.[109] Receptor sites for PGE and PGF are present in the cervix.[110] The local administration of prostaglandins to the cervix in pregnant women results in clinical, histologic, and biochemical changes that are consistent with those observed during physiologic cervical ripening; PGE_2 is 10 times more potent than $PGF_{2\alpha}$. The mechanism of action of prostaglandins in cervical ripening is not known. A frequent problem is the need to achieve delivery in patients with an unripe cervix, and the administration of prostaglandins to induce cervical ripening before induction has had great appeal. Local application of PGE_2 is accomplished by vaginal or intracervical administration, and both routes are equally effective.[111]

Dysmenorrhea

Dysmenorrhea is the occurrence of pain associated with menstruation. This disorder is classified into primary and secondary types. Primary dysmenorrhea is common, typically occurs in adolescence in the absence of recognizable pelvic disease, and usually begins shortly after menarche with severe spasmodic cramps superimposed on a constant background pain. In more severe cases, nausea, diarrhea, and headache also occur. Secondary dysmenorrhea is less common and typically occurs in women in their 30s and 40s; it is usually attributable to a pelvic disease such as endometriosis, adenomyosis, or pelvic inflammatory disease. The current thinking is that primary dysmenorrhea results from uterine hypercontractility, hypertonus, and resulting ischemia. Solid evidence implicates prostaglandins in the pathophysiology of primary dysmenorrhea. Elevated levels of $PGF_{2\alpha}$ and PGE_2 occur in the endometrium and menstrual fluid of women with dysmenorrhea with an elevated ratio of $PGF_{2\alpha}$ to PGE_2. Intrauterine administration of $PGF_{2\alpha}$ induces uterine contractility and dysmenorrhea-like pain, and the administration of antiprostaglandin agents results in a marked improvement of pain in nearly 80 percent of dysmenorrheic women.

The mechanisms responsible for an alteration in eicosanoid bioavailability in dysmenorrhea have not been established. It has been known for some years that plasma concentrations of vasopressin are elevated at the time of menstruation and are higher in women with dysmenorrhea. The administration of vasopressin stimulates uterine contractility, decreases uterine blood flow, and causes dysmenorrhea-like pain.[112] Vasopressin infusion results in an elevation of the plasma concentration of $PGF_{2\alpha}$; interestingly, the effect of vasopressin on uterine activity is not blocked by antiprostaglandin agents. Finally, plasma vasopressin levels are elevated in women whose dysmenorrhea is successfully treated with prostaglandin inhibitors, suggesting that vasopressin may have an etiologic role that is mediated through some pathway other than uterine prostaglandin synthesis.[113]

These results suggest a direct effect of vasopressin on myometrium or an alternative mechanism for vasopressin to stimulate uterine contractility. Studies in rats indicate that vasopressin-induced uterine contractions are inhibited by nordihydroguaiaretic acid (a lipoxygenase inhibitor and antioxidant) but not by prostaglandin synthase inhibitors.[114] Thus, arachidonate lipoxygenase metabolites may modulate or mediate the effect of vasopressin-induced uterine contractility.

Patients with primary dysmenorrhea who wish to take contraceptives can be given the oral contraceptive pill, which produces almost complete relief of dysmenorrhea in up to 50 percent of women; a further 30 to 40 percent experience marked relief.[115] Combination birth control pills have been shown to decrease the menstrual fluid content of $PGF_{2\alpha}$. Patients who do not wish to take oral contraceptives may be given antiprostaglandin agents.

Fallopian Tubes and the Treatment of Ectopic Pregnancy

Prostaglandins have been implicated in the regulation of ovum transport in the fallopian tubes. $PGF_{2\alpha}$, when administered subcutaneously to rabbits soon after ovulation, accelerates ovum transport.[116] In vitro studies evaluating the response of fallopian tube smooth muscle layers in the human suggest that $PGF_{2\alpha}$ has a stimulatory effect, whereas PGE_2 is inhibitory on spontaneous contractions.[117] Whether endogenous prostaglandins are responsible for the spontaneous motility of the human fallopian tube remains controversial. However, indomethacin inhibits the contractions of the fallopian tube, suggesting that prostaglandins may be involved in the spontaneous motility of the human fallopian tube.[118]

The finding that $PGF_{2\alpha}$ causes strong contractions together with vasoconstriction and the fact that $PGF_{2\alpha}$ is luteolytic led to the use of prostaglandins in the treatment of unruptured tubal pregnancy. Unruptured tubal pregnancy has been successfully treated with $PGF_{2\alpha}$ injected locally into the affected tube and corpus luteum.[119] Thus, local $PGF_{2\alpha}$ injection seems to provide good clinical results, provided that the initial serum hCG concentration is below 2500 mIU/ml. Injections into the corpus luteum should be avoided because of increased side effects such as cardiac arrhythmia and lung edema that can sometimes be life threatening.[120]

EICOSANOIDS IN PREGNANCY

Implantation

In rodents, the levels of $PGF_{2\alpha}$ and PGE_2 are elevated at the site of implantation.[121] Indomethacin, an inhibitor of prostaglandin synthesis, alters the local increase in vascular permeability and blocks or delays implantation in animals and is reversed by injection of prostaglandins. Platelet-activating factor (PAF) may be another signal for implantation with its unique vasodilating properties.[122] It is not clear, however, whether PAF acts alone or by triggering the local production of prostaglandins by endometrial gland cells.[123] PAF is produced not only by human embryos during early pregnancy[124] but also by endometrial stromal cells, where the level is increased by progesterone and PGE_2.[125] On the other hand, PAF induces a dose-dependent increase in the synthesis of PGE_2 from secretory-phase endometrial glands in culture.[105] Local vascular changes induced by PAF and PGE_2 play an important role in the penetration phase of the implantation process, causing stromal edema, which offers a loose interstitium for trophoblast invasion and also allows the volume expansion of the decidual cells.

Termination of Pregnancy

Prostaglandins stimulate uterine contractility and induce cervical ripening at any stage of pregnancy and can be employed as abortifacients in the first or second trimester. The high incidence of side effects of PGE_2 and $PGF_{2\alpha}$ precludes their widespread clinical application, which has led to the use of prostaglandin analogue. The E analogues are superior in efficacy to and have a lower incidence of side effects than the F analogues.[126] In randomized clinical trials, vacuum aspiration and the use of PGE analogues were equally efficacious in pregnancy termination.[127] Women treated with PGE analogues showed more gastrointestinal disturbances and a longer mean duration of bleeding than did those treated with vacuum aspiration. However, mean blood loss and hemoglobin concentrations were not significantly different between the two groups. Overall, patients receiving prostaglandins required more analgesia. The use of prostaglandins in first-trimester termination of pregnancy is becoming more popular worldwide with the introduction of progesterone antagonists such as RU 486. When used alone, RU 486 has an unacceptable rate of incomplete abortion.[128] The combined use of the orally active methyl ester of PGE_1 with RU 486 overcomes many of these problems and has proved to be a safe and effective method of early termination of pregnancy.[129, 130]

Termination of pregnancy in the second trimester may be accomplished either by dilatation and evacuation or by prostaglandins. Dilatation and evacuation is an effective, rapid, convenient, and safe method for pregnancy termination. However, concerns about the potential consequences of surgical dilatation of the cervix and uterine perforation, coupled with personal preference, have precluded dilatation and evacuation from becoming the method of choice for midtrimester termination of pregnancy in the United States. Comparisons between intra-amniotic $PGF_{2\alpha}$ and hypertonic saline show that procedures performed with $PGF_{2\alpha}$ are shorter but are associated with a higher rate of gastrointestinal side effects, heavy bleeding, requirement for transfusions, and surgical re-evacuation.[131] The rate of live-born fetuses after $PGF_{2\alpha}$ administration is 5 to 40 times higher than with hypertonic saline. Other routes of prostaglandin administration for midtrimester abortion are in the extra-ovular space, intracervically, and vaginally. The requirement of an invasive procedure for administration and the availability of alternative methods for midtrimester abortion have decreased the popularity of intra-amniotic $PGF_{2\alpha}$. The two most widely used prostaglandin regimens are vaginal suppositories of PGE_2 and intramuscular administration of prostaglandin analogues. The most common side effects include fever, chills, nausea, vomiting, and diarrhea. Abortion is generally complete in 14 hours; patients may require narcotic analgesia, antiemetics, and antipyretics during the procedure. An acceptable alternative to intravaginal PGE_2 administration is the intramuscular injection of 15-methyl-$PGF_{2\alpha}$. Because cervical fistulas and lacerations have been observed after midtrimester abortion with prostaglandin, it has been recommended that laminaria tents be placed before the procedure to allow cervical ripening.[132]

Management of the third-trimester pregnancy complicated by an intrauterine fetal death is accomplished by either expectant management or use of prostaglandin followed by induction with oxytocin. Expectant management is associated with an increased risk of disseminated intravascular coagulopathy and emotional distress. Oxytocin alone is often ineffective in the induction of labor. A frequently used regimen is vaginal administration of PGE_2 in combination with oxytocin infusion, which seems to reduce the incidence of undesirable side effects.[133, 134]

Preterm and Term Parturition

Prostaglandins are widely accepted to be involved in the onset of labor.[135] They play a major role in the two essential physiologic components of normal parturition: myometrial contractility and cervical dilatation and effacement. There is extensive evidence to support this conclusion. First, administration of PGE_2 and $PGF_{2\alpha}$ to women during pregnancy will result in myometrial contractility and may lead to first- and second-trimester abortion and induction of labor.[136, 137] Second, the administration of PGH_2 synthase inhibitors delays the progress of midtrimester abortion and the onset of labor at term[138]; these agents can also arrest preterm labor.[139] Third, the concentrations of prostaglandins in amniotic fluid,[140] maternal plasma, and urine[141] and amniotic fluid concentrations of arachidonic acid, which is the precursor of prostaglandins, are increased during spontaneous labor at term. Fourth, intra-amniotic injection of arachidonic acid leads to the onset of labor, an effect blocked by aspirin administration.[142] Finally, prostaglandins cause the contraction of smooth muscle tissues in vitro.

Lipoxygenase-derived metabolites of arachidonic acid may also play a role in parturition. Spontaneous labor in women at term is associated with increased amniotic fluid concentrations of HETEs and leukotrienes.[143] Amniotic fluid concentrations of 5-HETE and leukotriene C_4 increase 1 week before the onset of labor in the rhesus monkey, an effect associated with the appearance of a nocturnal pattern of uterine contractility. A further increase in the concentrations of these metabolites occurs during active labor.[144, 145] Finally, intravenous administration of arachidonic acid increases myometrial tone after antigen challenge and indomethacin treatment in the guinea pig, but this effect is prevented by the administration of a selective leukotriene antagonist.[146]

Although the evidence implicating prostaglandins in the onset of spontaneous labor at term is compelling, their participation in and contribution to the onset of preterm labor are less clear. Amniotic fluid concentrations of PGE_2 and $PGF_{2\alpha}$ and their respective metabolites are elevated in the amniotic fluid of women with intra-amniotic infection and preterm labor. However, in women with preterm labor and without intra-amniotic infection, amniotic fluid concentrations of prostaglandins and their metabolites are either not elevated or elevated only to a small extent.[147, 148]

Fetal membranes (amnion and chorion), decidua, myometrium, and placenta are established sources of eicosanoids. Studies of the rate of PGF and PGE production by dispersed cells (from amnion, chorion, decidua, and placenta) indicate that the production rate by amnion and decidua is higher after spontaneous labor than after elective delivery by cesarean section in women without labor. In contrast, chorion cells obtained after spontaneous labor have an increased output of prostaglandin F metabolite (PGFM), which is not reflected in changed production of PGE and PGF. This observation led to the proposition that the function of chorion in prostaglandin metabolism is mainly catabolic. Indeed, the chorion has considerable PGDH activity and, thus, could act as a metabolic barrier, preventing prostaglandin in the amnion from reaching the myometrium.[107] Transport experiments to study this possibility have yielded contradictory results.

Intrauterine tissues also produce HETEs and leukotrienes. Indeed, this may be the main metabolic pathway during pregnancy, and spontaneous labor may be due to a relative shift in favor of the cyclooxygenase pathway.[149] PGE_2 is several times more potent than $PGF_{2\alpha}$ in stimulating myometrial contractility.[150] Despite this, the prevalent view is that $PGF_{2\alpha}$ is more important than PGE_2 in the context of parturition. The evidence to support this view is that amniotic fluid concentrations of $PGF_{2\alpha}$ are higher than those of PGE_2 in women in active labor at term,[151] and plasma concentrations of the metabolite of $PGF_{2\alpha}$, but not those of PGE_2, are increased during parturition.

On the other hand, the elevated prostaglandin concentration in amniotic fluid in labor is much higher in the compartment formed below the head in the amniotic sac (the forebag).[152] Because this fluid is more likely to be collected at membrane rupture, a disproportionately high concentration of prostaglandin has been reported in earlier studies. The increase in prostaglandins may be a consequence of the inflammatory changes associated with the trauma of labor and partly produced in response to the interaction of cytokines and prostaglandins present in cervical and vaginal fluids with the parietal decidua, which becomes exposed as the cervix softens, is effaced, and dilates. Thus, prostaglandins during labor may not be initiating signals but rather reflect the process of labor.

Potential signals for increased synthesis of prostaglandins by intrauterine tissues include several growth factors and PAF. PAF, secreted by the fetal lung and kidney, is capable of stimulating prostaglandin production by human amnion and inducing myometrial contractions directly. PAF is absent in the amniotic fluid of nonlaboring women, but it appears and increases significantly after the onset of labor.[153] Regulation of PAF availability probably depends on acetylhydrolase in human decidua, the activity of which decreases in peripheral blood as pregnancy progresses in the rabbit.[154]

Fetus

Prostaglandins play a major role in fetal circulation and breathing. Throughout intrauterine life, the oxygen tension of the fetal blood is low and the ductus arteriosus remains open. After birth, the ductus arteriosus closes following the increase in the blood oxygen tension that occurs after spontaneous breathing. The effect of the changing oxygen tension on the ductus arteriosus is believed to be mediated by the actions of prostaglandins on the ductus. PGE_2 appears to be the major stimulator for dilatation of the ductus arteriosus and is involved in maintaining normal patency in utero. Inhibitors of prostaglandin synthase, when given to the mother, may lead to premature closure of the ductus arteriosus[155] but can be used pharmacologically to close a symptomatic patent ductus arteriosus postnatally.[156]

Placental PGE_2 is believed to suppress fetal breathing by acting in the fetal brain. Occlusion of the umbilical cord followed by the rapid clearance of PGE_2 stimulates strong breathings by the newborn.[157] Fetal renal circulation is also sensitive to prostaglandins, and this allowed indomethacin to be used therapeutically to reduce amniotic fluid volume in cases of polyhydramnios.[158, 159]

References

1. Lin LL, Lin AY, Knopf JL. Cytosolic phospholipase A_2 is coupled to hormonally regulated release of arachidonic acid. Proc Natl Acad Sci USA 89:6147, 1992.
2. Mitchell MD, Trautman MS. Molecular mechanisms regulating prostaglandin action. Mol Cell Endocrinol 93:C7, 1993.
3. Lands WEM. The biosynthesis and metabolism of prostaglandins. Rev Physiol 41:633, 1979.
4. Samuelsson B, Borgeat P, Hammarstrom S, et al. Introduction of a nomenclature: Leukotrienes. Prostaglandins 17:785, 1979.
5. Yamazaki T, Higuchi K, Kominami S, Takemori S. 15-Lipoxygenase metabolite(s) of arachidonic acid mediates adrenocorticotropin action in bovine adrenal steroidogenesis. Endocrinology 137:2670, 1996.
6. Morrow JD, Roberts LJ II. The isoprostanes. Current knowledge and directions for future research. Biochem Pharmacol 51:1, 1995.
7. Morris HR, Taylor GW, Piper PJ, et al. Structure of slow-reacting substance of anaphylaxis from guinea pig lung. Nature 286:264, 1980.
8. Ford-Hutchinson AW, Bray MA, Dorg MW, et al. Leukotriene B, a potent chemokinetic and aggregation substance released from polymorphonuclear leukocytes. Nature 286:264, 1980.
9. Wu KK. Inducible cyclooxygenase and nitric oxide synthase. Adv Pharmacol 33:179, 1995.
10. Smith WL. Prostanoid biosynthesis and mechanisms of action. Am J Physiol 263:F181, 1992.
11. Bunting S, Moncada A, Vane JR. Antithrombotic properties of vascular endothelium. Lancet 11:1075, 1977.
12. Gryglewski RJ, Bunting S, Moncada S, et al. Arterial walls are protected against deposition of thrombi by a substance which they make from prostaglandin endoperoxides. Prostaglandins 12:685, 1976.
13. Falardeau P, Hamberg M, Samuelsson B. Metabolism of 8, 11, 14-eicosatrienoic acid in human platelets. Biochim Biophys Acta 411:193, 1976.
14. Vane JR, Bergstrom S. Prostacyclin. New York, Raven Press, 1979, p 11.
15. Dyerberg J, Bang HO, Stoffersen E, et al. Eicosapentaenoic acid and prevention of thrombosis and arteriosclerosis. Lancet 2:117, 1978.
16. Hansen HS. 15-Hydroxyprostaglandin dehydrogenase: A review. Prostaglandins 12:647, 1976.
17. Lee SC, Levine L. Purification and properties of chicken heart prostaglandin 13-reductase. Biochem Biophys Res Commun 61:14, 1974.
18. Wong PYK, Sun FF, McGiff JC. Metabolism of prostacyclin in blood vessels. J Biol Chem 253:5555, 1978.
19. Jackson-Roberts L, Sweetman BJ, Oates JA. Metabolism of thromboxane B_2 in the monkey. J Biol Chem 253:5305, 1978.
20. Vane JR. Inhibition of prostaglandin synthesis as a mechanism of action for aspirin-like drugs. Nature New Biol 321:232, 1971.
21. Dennis EA. Diversity of group, types, regulation, and function of phospholipase A_2. J Biol Chem 269:13057, 1994.
22. Rothhut B, Russo-Marie F. Lipocortins. Adv Exp Med Biol 245:209, 1988.
23. Croxtall JD, Choudhury Q, Newman S, et al. Lipocortin 1 and the control of $cPLA_2$ phosphorylation. Biochem Pharmacol 52:351, 1996.
24. Jackschik BA, Falkenhein S, Parker CW. Precursor role of arachidonic acid in slow reacting substance release from rat basophilic leukemia cells. Proc Natl Acad Sci USA 74:4577, 1977.
25. Wennmole A. Effects of nicotine on cardiac prostaglandin and platelet thromboxane synthesis. Br J Pharmacol 64:559, 1978.
26. Moncada S, Bunting S, Mullane K, et al. Imidazole: A selective potent antagonist of thromboxane synthesis. Prostaglandins 13:611, 1977.
27. Tai H-H, Hollander CS. Kinetic evidence of a distinct regulatory site on 15-hydroxyprostaglandin dehydrogenase. *In* Samuelsson B, Paoletti R (eds). Advances in Prostaglandin and Thromboxane Research, Vol 1. New York, Raven Press, 1976, p 171.
28. Coleman RA, Smith WL, Narumiya S. International Union of Pharmacology classification of prostanoid receptors: Properties, distribution, and structure of the receptors and their subtypes. Pharmacol Rev 46:205, 1994.
29. Thierauch K-H, Dinter H, Stock G. Prostaglandins and their receptors: I. Pharmacologic receptor description, metabolism and drug use. J Hyperten 11:1315, 1993.
30. Fridovich I. The biology of oxygen radicals: General concepts. *In* Halliwell B (ed). Oxygen Radicals and Tissue Injury. Proceedings of a Brook Lodge Symposium, Augusta, Michigan, April 27–29, 1987. Bethesda, MD, Federation of American Societies of Experimental Biology, 1988, p 1.
31. Chance B, Sies H, Boveris A. Hydroperoxide metabolism in mammalian organs. Physiol Rev 59:527, 1979.
32. Fridovich I. Biological effects of the superoxide radical. Arch Biochem Biophys 247:1, 1986.
33. Roberts P, Newby A, Hallett M, et al. Inhibition by adenosine of reactive oxygen metabolite production by human polymorphonuclear leukocytes. Biochem J 227:669, 1985.
34. Cronstein B, Kubersky S, Weissmann G. Engagement of adenosine receptors inhibits hydrogen peroxide (H_2O_2) release by activated human neutrophils. Clin Immunol Immunopathol 42:76, 1987.
35. Lippman R. Free radical–induced lipoperoxidation and aging. *In* Miquel J, Quintanilha AT, Weber H (eds). Handbook of Free Radicals and Antioxidants in Biomedicine. Boca Raton, FL, CRC Press, 1989, p 187.
36. Schraufstatter I, Hyslop P, Hinshaw D, et al. Hydrogen peroxide–induced injury of cells and its prevention by inhibitors of poly(ADP-ribose)polymerase. Proc Natl Acad Sci USA 83:4908, 1986.

37. Amici A, Levine R, Tsai L, et al. Conversion of amino acid residues in proteins and amino acid homopolymers to carbonyl derivatives by metal-catalyzed oxidation reaction. J Biol Chem 264:3341, 1989.
38. Adams E, Hertig A. Studies on the human corpus luteum: I. Observations on the ultrastructure of development and regression of luteal cells during the menstrual cycle. J Cell Biol 41:696, 1969.
39. Cavender J, Murdoch W. Morphological studies of the microcirculatory system of periovulatory ovine follicles. Biol Reprod 39:459, 1988.
40. Aitken R, Clarkson J. Cellular basis of defective sperm function and its association with the genesis of reactive oxygen species by human spermatozoa. J Reprod Fertil 81:459, 1987.
41. Somers C, Battaglia D, Shapiro B. Localization and developmental fate of ovoperoxidase and proteoliaisin, two proteins involved in fertilization envelope assembly. Dev Biol 131:226, 1989.
42. Guli C, Smyth D. UV-induced DNA repair is not detectable in predictyate oocytes of the mouse. Mutat Res 208:115, 1988.
43. Cherouny P, Ghodgaonkar R, Niebyl J, et al. Effect of peroxide on prostaglandin production and contractions of the pregnant rat uterus. Am J Obstet Gynecol 159:1390, 1988.
44. Gabig T, Kipnes R, Baboir B. Solubilization of the O_2-forming activity responsible for the respiratory burst in human neutrophils. J Biol Chem 253:6663, 1978.
45. Ward P, Johnson K, Warren J, et al. Immune complexes, oxygen radicals, and lung injury. *In* Halliwell B (ed). Oxygen Radicals and Tissue Injury: Proceedings of a Brook Lodge Symposium, Augusta, Michigan, April 27–29, 1987. Bethesda, MD, Federation of American Societies of Experimental Biology, 1988, p 107.
46. Clark I, Thumwood C, Chaudri G, et al. Tumor necrosis factor and reactive oxygen species: Implications for free radical–induced tissue injury. *In* Halliwell B (ed). Oxygen Radicals and Tissue Injury: Proceedings of a Brook Lodge Symposium, Augusta, Michigan, April 27–29, 1987. Bethesda, MD, Federation of American Societies of Experimental Biology, 1988, p 122.
47. Badwey JA, Curnutte JT, Karnovsky ML. *cis*-Polyunsaturated fatty acids induce high levels of superoxide production by human neutrophils. J Biol Chem 256:12640, 1981.
48. Lu DJ, Grinstein S. ATP and guanine nucleotide dependence of neutrophil activation. J Biol Chem 265:13721, 1990.
49. Fujimoto S, Smith RM, Curnutte JT, et al. Evidence that activation of the respiratory burst oxidase in a cell-free system from human neutrophils is accomplished in part through an alteration of the oxidase-related 67-kDa cytosolic protein. J Biol Chem 264:21629, 1989.
50. Fairchild D, Pate J. Interferon-gamma induction of major histocompatibility complex antigens on cultured bovine luteal cells. Biol Reprod 40:453, 1989.
51. Bagavandoss P, Kunkel S, Wiggins R, et al. Tumor necrosis factor-α (TNF-α) production and localization of macrophages and T lymphocytes in the rabbit corpus luteum. Endocrinology 122:1185, 1988.
52. Ryan U. Endothelial Cells. Boca Raton, FL, CRC Press, 1988.
53. Matsubara T, Ziff M. Increased superoxide anion release from human endothelial cells in response to cytokines. J Immunol 137:3295, 1986.
54. Halliwell B. Oxidants and human disease: Some new concepts. FASEB J 1:358, 1987.
55. Sawada M, Carlson J. Superoxide radical production in plasma membrane samples from regressing corpora lutea. Can J Physiol Pharmacol 67:465, 1989.
56. Riley JCM, Behrman HR. In vivo generation of hydrogen peroxide in the rat corpus luteum during luteolysis. Endocrinology 128:1749, 1991.
57. Musicki B, Kodaman PH, Aten RF, et al. Endocrine regulation of ascorbic acid transport and secretion in luteal cells. Biol Reprod 54:399, 1996.
58. Turrens JP, Boveris A. Generation of superoxide anion by NADPH dehydrogenase of bovine heart mitochondria. Biochem J 191:421, 1980.
59. Harmon D. The biologic clock: The mitochondria? J Am Geriatr Soc 4:145, 1972.
60. Miguel J, Economos AC, Fleming J, et al. Mitochondrial role in aging. Exp Gerontol 15:575, 1980.
61. Cortopassi GA, Arnheim N. Detection of a specific mitochondrial DNA deletion in tissue of older humans. Nucleic Acids Res 18:6927, 1990.
62. Wallace JL. Prostaglandins, NSAIDs and cytoprotection. Gastroenterol Clin North Am 21:631, 1992.
63. Linnane AW, Ozawa T, Marzuki S, et al. Mitochondrial DNA mutations as an important contributor to ageing and degenerative disease. Lancet 1:642, 1989.
64. Wallace DC. Mitochondrial DNA variation in human evolution, degenerative disease and aging. Am J Hum Genet 57:201, 1994.
65. Tsunawaki S, Sporn M, Ding A, et al. Deactivation of macrophages by transforming growth factor-β. Nature 334:260, 1988.
66. Yoshida R, Murray H, Nathan C. Agonist and antagonist effects of interferon α and β on activation of human macrophages. J Exp Med 167:1171, 1988.
67. Roberts R. Conceptus interferons and maternal recognition of pregnancy. Biol Reprod 40:449, 1989.
68. Behrman HR, Preston SL, Aten RF, et al. Hormone induction of ascorbic acid transport in immature granulosa cells. Endocrinology 137:4316, 1996.
69. Sawada M, Carlson J. Association of lipid peroxidation during luteal regression in the rat and natural aging in the rotifer. Exp Gerontol 20:179, 1985.
70. Aten RF, Duarte KM, Behrman HR. Regulation of ovarian antioxidant vitamins, reduced glutathione, and lipid peroxidation by luteinizing hormone and prostaglandin $F_{2\alpha}$. Biol Reprod 46:401, 1992.
71. Behrman H, Preston S. Luteolytic actions of peroxide in rat ovarian cells. Endocrinology 124:2895, 1989.
72. Kramer MM, Harman MT, Brill AK. Disturbances of reproduction and ovarian changes in the guinea-pig in relation to vitamin C deficiency. Am J Physiol 106:611, 1933.
73. Tilly JL, Tilly KI. Inhibitors of oxidative stress mimic the ability of follicle-stimulating hormone to suppress apoptosis in cultured rat ovarian follicles. Endocrinology 136:242, 1995.
74. Turner E, Hager L, Shapiro B. Ovothiol replaces glutathione peroxidase as a hydrogen peroxide scavenger in sea urchin eggs. Science 242:939, 1988.
75. Kitagawa T, Suganuma N, Nawa A, et al. Rapid accumulation of deleted mitochondrial deoxyribonucleic acid in postmenopausal ovaries. Biol Reprod 49:730, 1993.
76. Keefe DL, Niven-Fairchild T, Powell S, et al. Mitochondrial deoxyribonucleic acid deletions in oocytes and reproductive aging in women. Fertil Steril 64:577, 1995.
77. Chen X, Prosser R, Simonetti S, et al. Rearranged mitochondrial genomes are present in human oocytes. Am J Hum Genet 57:239, 1995.
78. Alvarez J, Touchstone J, Blasco L. Spontaneous lipid peroxidation and production of hydrogen peroxide and superoxide in human spermatozoa. J Androl 8:338, 1987.
79. Nasr-Esfahani MM, Aitken JR, Johnson MH. Hydrogen peroxide levels in mouse oocytes and early cleavage stage embryos developed in vitro or in vivo. Development 109:501, 1990.
80. Legge M, Sellens MH. Free radical scavengers ameliorate the two-cell block in mouse embryo culture. Hum Reprod 6:867, 1991.
81. Umaoka Y, Noda Y, Narimoto K, et al. Developmental potentiality of embryos cultured under low oxygen tension with superoxide dismutase. J In Vitro Fert Embryo Transf 8:245, 1991.
82. Takahashi M, Nagai T, Hamano S, et al. Effect of thiol compounds on in vitro development and intracellular glutathione content of bovine embryos. Biol Reprod 49:228, 1993.
83. Nonogaki T, Noda Y, Narimoto K, et al. Protection from oxidative stress on mouse embryo development in vitro. Hum Reprod 6:1305, 1991.
84. Manes C. Cyanide-resistant reduction of nitroblue tetrazolium and hydrogen peroxide production by the rabbit blastocyst. Mol Reprod Dev 31:114, 1992.
85. Minkoff H. Prematurity: Infection as an etiologic factor. Obstet Gynecol 62:137, 1983.
86. Orczyk GP, Behrman HR. Ovulation blockade by aspirin and indomethacin: In vivo evidence for a role of prostaglandin in gonadotropin secretion. Prostaglandins 1:3, 1972.
87. Behrman HR. Prostaglandins in hypothalamopituitary and ovarian function. Annu Rev Physiol 41:685, 1979.

88. Ojeda SR, Wheaton JE, McCann SM. Prostaglandin E_2–induced release of luteinizing hormone releasing factor (LRF). Neuroendocrinology 17:283, 1975.
89. Chobsieng P, Naor Z, Koch Y, et al. Stimulatory effect of PGE_2 on LH release in the rat: Evidence for hypothalamic site of action. Neuroendocrinology 17:12, 1975.
90. Ojeda SR, Negro-Vilar A, McCann S. Release of prostaglandin E by hypothalamic tissue: Evidence for their involvement in catecholamine-induced luteinizing hormone release. Endocrinology 104:617, 1979.
91. Ojeda SR, Harms PG, McCann SM. Effect of inhibitors of prostaglandin synthesis on gonadotropin release in the rat. Endocrinology 97:843, 1975.
92. Sirois J, Richards JAS. Purification and characterization of a novel distinct isoform of prostaglandin endoperoxide synthase induced by human chorionic gonadotropin in granulosa cells of rat preovulatory follicles. J Biol Chem 267:6382, 1992.
93. Orlicky DJ, Fisher L, Dunscomb N, et al. Immunohistochemical localization of $PGF_{2\alpha}$ receptor in the rat ovary. Prostaglandins Leukot Essent Fatty Acids 46:223, 1992.
94. Reich R, Kohen F, Slager R, et al. Ovarian lipoxygenase activity and its regulation by gonadotropin in the rat. Prostaglandins 30:581, 1985.
95. Brannstrom M, Pascoe V, Norman RJ, McClure N. Localization of leukocyte subsets in the follicle wall and in the corpus luteum throughout the human menstrual cycle. Fertil Steril 61:488, 1994.
96. Arici A, Oral E, Bukulmez O, et al. Interleukin-8 expression and modulation in human preovulatory follicles and ovarian cells. Endocrinology 137:3762, 1996.
97. Pang C, Behrman H. Acute effects of $PGF_{2\alpha}$ on ovarian and luteal blood flow, luteal gonadotropin uptake in vivo and gonadotropin binding in vitro. Endocrinology 108:2239, 1981.
98. Powell WS, Hammarstrom S, Samuelsson B, et al. Prostaglandin $F_{2\alpha}$ receptor in human corpora lutea. Lancet 1:1120, 1974.
99. McNatty KP, Henerson KM, Sawers RS. Effects of $PGF_{2\alpha}$ and E_2 on the production of progesterone in human granulosa cells in tissue culture. J Endocrinol 67:231, 1975.
100. McDougall AN, Walker FM, Watson J. The effect of cloprostenol on human luteal steroid and prostaglandin secretion in vitro. Br J Pharmacol 60:425, 1977.
101. Johansson EDB, Gemzell C. Plasma levels of progesterone during the luteal phase in normal women with synthetic estrogens. Acta Endocrinol (Copenh) 68:551, 1971.
102. Karsch FJ, Sutton GP. An intraovarian site for the luteolytic action of estrogen in the rhesus monkey. Endocrinology 98:553, 1976.
103. Auletta FJ, Caldwell BV, Speroff L. Estrogen-induced luteolysis in the rhesus monkey: Reversal with indomethacin. Prostaglandins 11:745, 1976.
104. Rees MCP, Anderson ABM, Demers LM, et al. Endometrial and myometrial prostaglandin release during the menstrual cycle in relation to menstrual blood loss. J Clin Endocrinol Metab 58:813, 1984.
105. Smith SK, Kelly RW. Effect of platelet-activating factor on the release of $PGF_{2\alpha}$ and PGE_2 by separated cells of human endometrium. J Reprod Fertil 82:271, 1988.
106. Omini C, Folco GC, Pasargiklian R, et al. Prostacyclin (PGI_2) in pregnant human uterus. Prostaglandins 17:113, 1979.
107. Okazaki T, Casey ML, Okita JR, et al. Initiation of human parturition: XII. Biosynthesis and metabolism of prostaglandins in human fetal membranes and uterine decidua. Am J Obstet Gynecol 139:373, 1981.
108. Ekman G, Malmstrom A, Uldbjerg N, et al. Cervical collagen: An important regulator of cervical function in term labor. Obstet Gynecol 67:633, 1986.
109. Ellwood DA, Mitchell MD, Anderson ABM. The in vitro production of prostanoids by the human cervix during pregnancy: Preliminary observations. Br J Obstet Gynaecol 87:210, 1980.
110. Bauknecht T, Krahe B, Rechenbach U, et al. Distribution of prostaglandin E_2 and prostaglandin $F_{2\alpha}$ receptors in human myometrium. Acta Endocrinol (Copenh) 98:446, 1981.
111. Rix P, Ladehoff P, Moller AM, et al. Cervical ripening and induction of delivery by local administration of prostaglandin E_2 gel or vaginal tablets is equally effective. Acta Obstet Gynecol Scand 75:45, 1996.
112. Akerlund M, Kostrzewska A, Melin T, et al. Vasopressin effects on isolated non-pregnant myometrium and uterine arteries and their inhibition by deamino-ethyl-lysine-vasopressin and deamino-ethyl-oxytocin. Br J Obstet Gynaecol 90:732, 1983.
113. Stromberg P, Forsling ML, Akerlund M. Effects of prostaglandin inhibition on vasopressin levels in women with primary dysmenorrhea. Obstet Gynecol 58:206, 1981.
114. Demers LM, Hahn DW, McGuire JL. Newer concepts in dysmenorrhea research. *In* Dawood MY, McGuire JL, Demers LM (eds). Premenstrual Syndrome and Dysmenorrhea. Baltimore, Urban & Schwarzenburg, 1984, p 205.
115. Kremser E, Mitchell GM. Treatment of primary dysmenorrhea with combined-type oral contraceptive: A double blind study. J Am Coll Health Assoc 19:195, 1971.
116. Chang MD, Hunt DM. Effect of prostaglandin $E_{2\alpha}$ on the early pregnancy of rabbits. Nature 236:120, 1972.
117. Hahlin M, Bokstrom H, Lindblom B. Ectopic pregnancy: In vitro effects of prostaglandins on the oviduct and corpus luteum. Fert Steril 47:935, 1987.
118. Lindblom B, Wilhelmsson M, Wikland M, et al. Prostaglandins and oviductal function. Acta Obstet Gynecol Scand 113:43, 1983.
119. Lindblom B, Kallfelt B, Hahlin M, et al. Local prostaglandin $F_{2\alpha}$ injection for termination of ectopic pregnancy. Lancet 1:776, 1987.
120. Egarter C, Husslein P. Prostaglandins in the treatment of tubal pregnancy. Eicosanoids Fatty Acids 5:44, 1988.
121. Kennedy TG, Zamecnik J. The concentration of 6-keto-prostaglandin $F_{1\alpha}$ is markedly elevated at the site of blastocyst implantation in the rat. Prostaglandins 61:599, 1978.
122. Alecozay AA, Casslen BG, Riehl RM, et al. Platelet activating factor in human luteal phase endometrium. Biol Reprod 41:578, 1989.
123. Kennedy TG. Embryonic signals and the initiation of blastocyst implantation. Aust J Biol Sci 36:531, 1983.
124. Roberts TK, Adamson LM, Smart YC, et al. An evaluation of peripheral blood platelet enumeration as a monitor of fertilization and early pregnancy. Fert Steril 47:848, 1987.
125. Alecozay AA, Harper MJK, Schenken RS, et al. Paracrine interaction between and prostaglandins in hormonally-treated human luteal phase endometrium in vitro. J Reprod Fertil 91:301, 1991.
126. Bieniarz J, Hunter G, Scommegna A, et al. Efficacy and acceptability of 15(*S*)-methyl-prostaglandin E_2 methyl ester for midtrimester pregnancy termination. Am J Obstet Gynecol 120:840, 1974.
127. World Health Organization Task Force on Post-ovulatory Methods for Fertility Regulation. Menstrual regulation by intramuscular injections of 16-phenoxy-tetranor-PGE_2 methyl sulfonylamide or vacuum aspiration. Br J Obstet Gynaecol 94:949, 1987.
128. Cameron IT, Baird DT. Early pregnancy termination: A comparison between vacuum aspiration and medical abortion using prostaglandin (16, 16 dimethyl-trans-delta2-PGE_1 methyl ester) or the antiprogestogen RU 486. Br J Obstet Gynaecol 95:271, 1988.
129. Norman JE, Thong KJ, Baird DT. Uterine contractility and induction of abortion in early pregnancy by misoprostol and mifeprostone. Lancet 338:1233, 1991.
130. Peyron R, Aubeny E, Targosz V, et al. Early termination of pregnancy with mifeprostone (RU 486) and the orally active prostaglandin misoprostol. N Engl J Med 328:1509, 1993.
131. Grimes DA, Cates W. The comparative efficacy and safety of intraamniotic prostaglandin $F_{2\alpha}$ and hypertonic saline for second-trimester abortion: A review and critique. J Reprod Med 22:248, 1979.
132. Stubblefield PG, Naftolin F, Frigoletto FD, et al. Pretreatment with laminaria tents before midtrimester abortion with intra-amniotic prostaglandin $F_{2\alpha}$. Am J Obstet Gynecol 118:284, 1974.
133. MacKenzie IZ, Davies AJ, Embrey MP. Fetal death in utero managed with vaginal prostaglandin E_2 gel. Br Med J 1:764, 1979.
134. Hill NCW, Selinger M, Ferguson J, et al. Management of intra-uterine fetal death with vaginal administration of gemeprost or prostaglandin E_2: A random allocation controlled trial. J Obstet Gynecol 11:422, 1991.
135. Liggins GC, Fairclough RJ, Grieves SA, et al. The mechanism of initiation of parturition in the ewe. Recent Prog Horm Res 29:111, 1973.
136. Thiery M. Induction of labor with prostaglandins. *In* Keirse MJNC, Anderson A, Gravenhorst JB (eds). Human Parturition:

New Concepts and Developments. Leiden, The Netherlands, Leiden University Press, 1979, p 155.

137. Novy MJ, Liggins GC. Role of prostaglandins, prostacyclin, and thromboxanes in the physiologic control of the uterus and in parturition. Semin Perinatol 4:45, 1980.
138. Novy MJ, Cook MJ, Manaugh L. Indomethacin block of normal onset of parturition in primates. Am J Obstet Gynecol 118:142, 1974.
139. Besinger RE, Niebyl JR. The safety and efficacy of tocolytic agents for the treatment of preterm labor. Obstet Gynecol Surv 45:415, 1990.
140. Dray F, Frydman R. Primary prostaglandins in amniotic fluid in pregnancy and spontaneous labor. Am J Obstet Gynecol 126:13, 1976.
141. Hamberg M. Quantitative studies on prostaglandin synthesis in man: III. Excretion of the major urinary metabolite of prostaglandins $F_{1\alpha}$ and $F_{2\alpha}$ during pregnancy. Life Sci 14:247, 1974.
142. MacDonald PC, Schultz FM, Duenhoelter JH, et al. Initiation of human parturition. Obstet Gynecol 44:629, 1974.
143. Romero R, Wu YK, Mazor M, et al. Increased amniotic fluid leukotriene C_4 concentration in term human parturition. Am J Obstet Gynecol 159:655, 1988.
144. Walsh SW. 5-Hydroxyeicosatetraenoic acid, leukotriene-C_4 and $PGF_{2\alpha}$ in amniotic fluid before and during term and preterm labor. Am J Obstet Gynecol 161:1352, 1989.
145. Bennett PR, Elder MG, Myatt L. The effects of lipoxygenase metabolites of arachidonic acid on human myometrial contractility. Prostaglandins 33:837, 1987.
146. Carraher R, Hahn DW, Ritchie DM, et al. Involvement of lipoxygenase products in myometrial contractions. Prostaglandins 26:23, 1983.
147. Romero R, Emamian M, Wan M, et al. Prostaglandin concentrations in amniotic fluid of women with intra-amniotic infection and preterm labor. Am J Obstet Gynecol 157:1461, 1987.
148. Romero R, Wu YK, Mazor M, et al. Amniotic fluid prostaglandin E_2 in preterm labor. Prostaglandins Leukot Essent Fatty Acids 34:141, 1988.
149. Myatt L, Rose MP, Elder MG. Lipoxygenase products of arachidonic acid in human fetal membranes. 32nd Annual Meeting of the Society for Gynecologic Investigation; March 21–25, 1985; Phoenix, AZ.
150. Embrey MP. The effect of prostaglandins on human pregnant uterus. J Obstet Gynaecol Br Commonw 76:783, 1969.
151. Keirse MJNC, Turnbull AC. E prostaglandins in amniotic fluid during late pregnancy and labour. J Obstet Gynaecol Br Commonw 80:970, 1973.
152. MacDonald PC, Casey ML. The accumulation of prostaglandins (PG) in amniotic fluid is an after-effect of labor and not indicative of a role for PGE_2 or $PGF_{2\alpha}$ in the initiation of human parturition. J Clin Endocrinol Metab 76:1332, 1993.
153. Billah MM, Johnston JM. Identification of phospholipid platelet-activator factor (1-0-alkyl-2-acetyl-sn-glycero-3-phosphocholine) in human amniotic fluid and urine. Biochem Biophys Res Commun 113:51, 1983.
154. Maki N, Hoffman DR, Johnston JM. Platelet-activating factor acetylhydrolase activity in maternal, fetal and newborn rabbit plasma during pregnancy and lactation. Proc Natl Acad Sci USA 85:1, 1988.
155. Eronen M, Personen E, Kurki T, et al. The effects of indomethacin and a β-sympathomimetic agent on the fetal ductus arteriosus during treatment of premature labor: A randomized double-blind study. Am J Obstet Gynecol 164:141, 1991.
156. Brash AR, Hickey DE, Graham TP, et al. Pharmacokinetics of indomethacin in the neonate: Relation of plasma indomethacin levels to response of the ductus arteriosus. N Engl J Med 305:67, 1981.
157. Thorburn GD. The placenta, PGE_2 and parturition. Early Hum Dev 29:63, 1992.
158. Cabrol D, Landesman R, Muller J, et al. Treatment of polyhydramnios with prostaglandin synthetase inhibitor (indomethacin). Am J Obstet Gynecol 157:422, 1987.
159. Kirshon B, Cotton DB. Polyhydramnios associated with a ring chromosome managed with indomethacin. Am J Obstet Gynecol 158:1063, 1988.

Chapter 6

THE OVARIAN LIFE CYCLE

John Yeh • Eli Y. Adashi

■ CHAPTER OUTLINE

KEY POINTS

- The ovary is a dynamic organ that is crucial for the survival of the species.
- The ovarian follicular compartments interact in a highly integrated manner to secrete sex steroids and produce a fertilizable ovum.
- Primordial follicular units develop into the highly differentiated preovulatory stage of antral follicles.
- Regulation of follicular atresia involves peptide growth factors.
- Steroidogenesis and protein biosynthesis are operational characteristics of the ovary.
- Putative intraovarian regulators may modulate growth and function of the ovarian cell compartments.
- The ovary is active in initiation and maintenance of reproductive cyclicity.
- Dynamic events governing follicular maturation lead to ovulation and to formation and function of the corpus luteum.
- The menopausal ovary is capable of producing androgens.

The underpinning of ovarian function draws on the fundamental need to preserve the species. Accordingly, the ovary is designed to subserve a single central objective, the generation of a fertilizable ovum. In this respect, the ovary may be viewed as the "master gland," with its function facilitated by the contribution of the various other components of the hypothalamic-pituitary-ovarian axis. This view differs from the more traditional outlook ascribing the role of a master gland to the pituitary, an organ that is highly dependent on hypothalamic principles. However, current information suggests that the ovary plays an active role in the initiation and maintenance of reproductive cyclicity. The hypothalamus and pituitary are viewed as playing a permissive tonic role in this connection. Indeed, it is the changing tide of ovarian signals that appears to help determine the activities of the hypothalamic-pituitary unit. It is for these reasons that the ovary has often been likened to a pelvic clock, dictating the comings and goings of the reproductive process. Stated differently, it might be considered that the ovary does in effect possess a "mind" of its own. This is attested to by a multitude of putative intraovarian regulators that act in ways previously viewed as the domain of the central nervous system.

It is the objective of this chapter to provide a contemporary view of the ovarian life cycle, a dramatic process schematically illustrated in Figure 6–1.

ONTOGENY

The ovary, an ever-changing tissue, is a multicompartmental structure with different and variable biologic properties. Responding to cyclic pituitary gonadotropin secretion, the various follicular compartments interact in a highly integrated manner to secrete sex steroids and to produce a fertilizable ovum. The following section attempts to delineate the key events in the ontogeny of the ovary and the central players in this complex equation.

The Oocyte: Depletion of a Finite Endowment

The primordial germ cells are known to originate from the endoderm of the yolk sac (near the caudal end of the embryo). At this site, they can be identified as early as the end of the third week of gestation by alkaline phosphatase staining.[1] Migration of germ cells toward the genital ridge

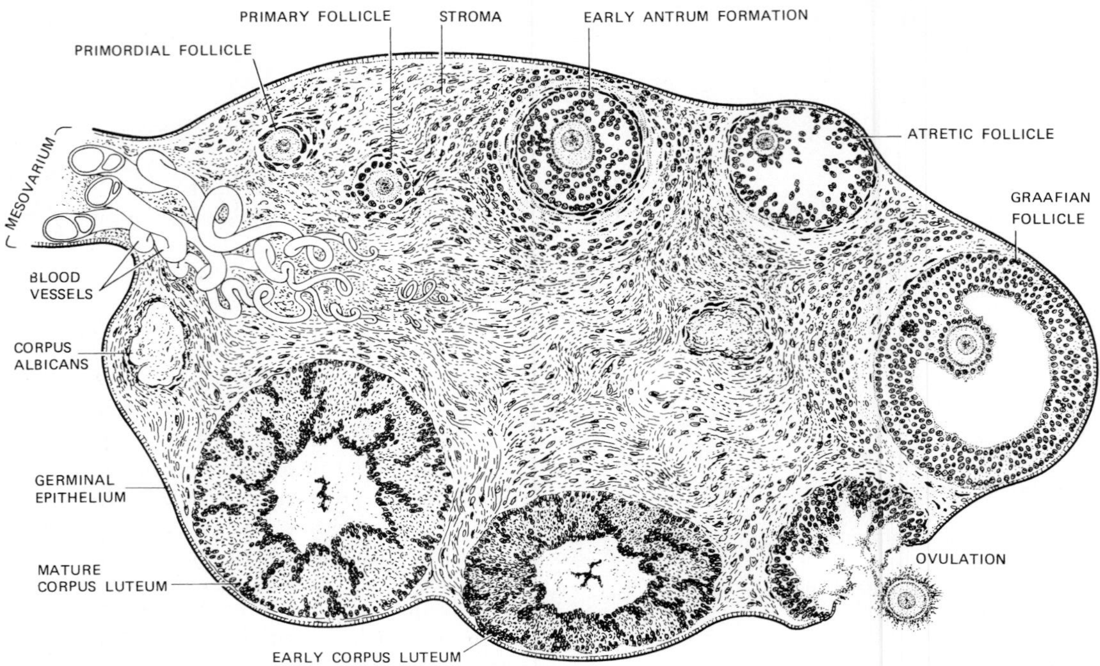

Figure 6–1 ■ The life cycle of the human ovary. (Modified from Ham AW, Leeson TS. Histology, 4th ed. Philadelphia, JB Lippincott, 1961.)

occurs by ameboid movements, with the aid of pseudopodia.[2] The route of migration along the dorsal mesentery of the hindgut is interrupted only by the required lateral crossing of the coelomic angle at the level of the genital ridge. Whereas some chemotaxis is clearly operational, the precise cellular mechanisms underlying the guidance of germ cells to the genital ridge remain uncertain. Importantly, germ cells appear unable to persist outside the genital ridge, which may thus be viewed as the only region competent to sustain gonadal development. By the same token, germ cells play an indispensable role in the induction of gonadal development. In fact, no functional gonad is to be expected in the absence of germ cells.

On arrival at the genital ridge by the fifth week of gestation, the premeiotic germ cells are referred to as oogonia.[3] During the subsequent 2 weeks of intrauterine life (weeks 5 to 7 of gestation), the "indifferent stage," the primordial gonadal structure constitutes no more than a bulge on the medial aspect of the urogenital ridge. This protuberance is created by proliferation of surface (coelomic) germinal epithelium, by growth of the underlying mesenchyme, and by oogonial multiplication. The oogonia total 10,000 by around 6 to 7 weeks of intrauterine life. Because meiosis and oogonial atresia are not operational, the actual number of germ cells is dictated by mitotic division at this time.

It is during this indifferent phase that the gonadal cortex and medulla are first delineated. However, short of cytogenetic evidence, the precise sexual identity of the gonadal ridge cannot be ascertained at this point. Nevertheless, the absence of testicular development beyond 7 weeks of gestation is generally considered presumptive evidence of ovarian formation. Additional clues to the sexual identity of the gonad can be derived from the detection of oogonial meiosis at about 8 weeks of gestation because no comparable process will be observed in the testis until puberty. The sexual identity of the gonadal ridge is clear by 16 weeks of gestation, when the first primordial follicles can be visualized.

By about 8 weeks of intrauterine life, persistent mitosis increases the total number of oogonia to 600,000.[4] From this point on, the oogonial endowment is subject to three simultaneous ongoing processes: mitosis, meiosis, and oogonial atresia. Stated differently, the onset of oogonial meiosis and oogonial atresia is now superimposed on oogonial mitosis. As a result of the combined impact of these processes, that is, mitosis counterbalanced by meiosis and oogonial atresia, the number of germ cells peaks at 6 to 7 $\times$ 10^6 by 20 weeks of gestation. At this time, two thirds of the total germ cells are intrameiotic primary oocytes; the remaining third can still be viewed as oogonial. The midgestational peak (and the post peak decline) are accounted for, if only in part, by the progressively decreasing rate of oogonial mitosis, a process destined to end entirely by about 7 months of intrauterine life. Equally relevant is the increasing rate of oogonial atresia, which peaks at about month 5 of gestation. During this period, regulation of the ovarian developmental process could be hypothesized to be complex, including the involvement of peptide growth factors[5–8] (Fig. 6–2).

From midgestation onward, relentless and irreversible attrition progressively diminishes the germ cell endowment of the gonad.[9] Ultimately, some 50 years later, this is finally exhausted. For the most part, this is accomplished through follicular atresia, rather than oogonial atresia, and begins around month 6 of gestation and continues throughout life. In contrast, oogonial atresia (see later) is destined to end at 7 months of intrauterine life as follicular atresia sets in. As expected, follicular atresia does not and cannot start until follicles have formed. However, once follicular atresia

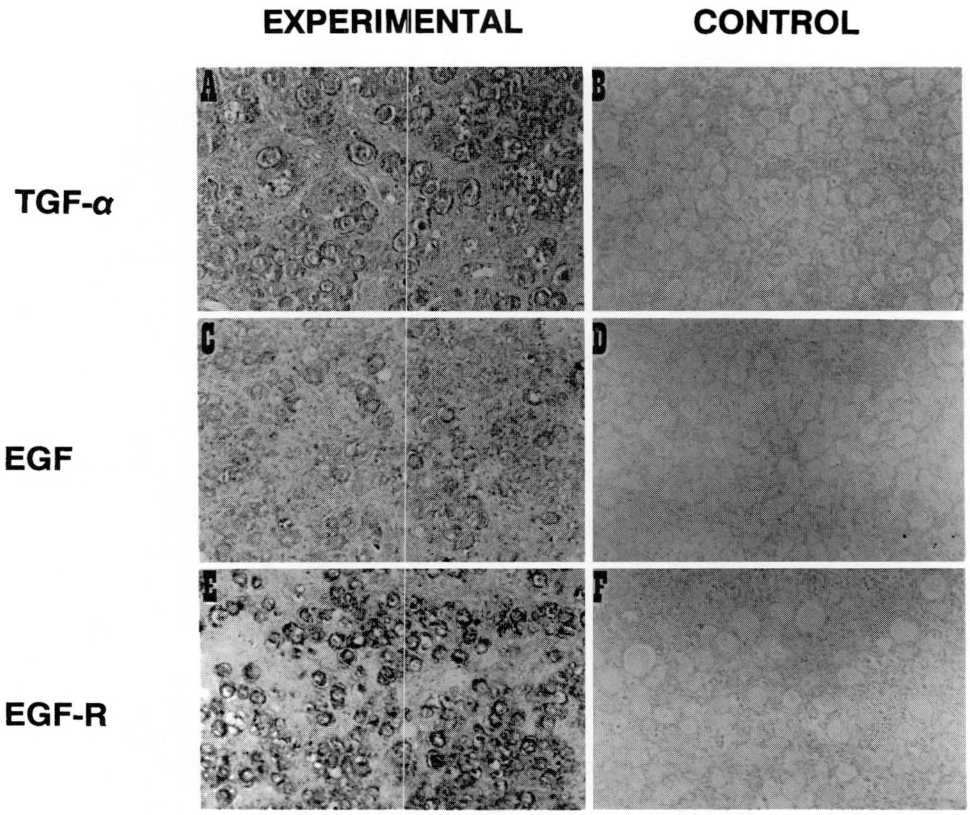

EXPERIMENTAL CONTROL

TGF-α

EGF

EGF-R

A B C D E F

Figure 6–2 ■ Immunohistochemical localization of transforming growth factor-α (TGF-α), epidermal growth factor (EGF), and EGF receptor (EGF-R) in 22-week-old human fetal ovaries. Note the intense staining of the oocytes for each antigen. (From Bennett RA, Osathanondh R, Yeh J. Immunohistochemical localization of transforming growth factor-α, epidermal growth factor (EGF), and EGF receptor in the human fetal ovary. J Clin Endocrinol Metab 81:3073–3076, 1996. The Endocrine Society.)

is in motion, there is little question that it has a profound effect on germ cell endowment, given that only 1 to 2 × 10^6 germ cells are present at birth.[10] Remarkably, this dramatic depletion of the germ cell mass occurs during a period as short as 20 weeks. No similar rate of depletion will be seen again. Consequently, newborn females enter life still far from realizing reproductive potential, having lost as much as 80 percent of their germ cell endowment. This decreases further to approximately 300,000 by the onset of puberty. Of these follicles, only 400 to 500 (i.e., less than 1 percent of the total) will ovulate in the course of a reproductive life span.[11]

Between weeks 8 and 13 of fetal life, some of the oogonia depart from the mitotic cycle to enter the prophase of the first meiotic division. It is this change that marks the conversion of these cells to primary oocytes well before actual follicle formation. Meiosis (beginning at about 8 weeks of gestation) provides temporary protection from oogonial atresia, thereby allowing the germ cells to invest themselves with granulosa cells and to form primordial follicles. Accordingly, oogonia that persist beyond the seventh month of gestation and have not entered meiosis will be subject to oogonial atresia. Consequently, no oogonia are usually present at birth.

Once formed, the primary oocyte persists in prophase of the first meiotic division until the time of ovulation, when meiosis is resumed and the first polar body is formed and extruded. Although the exact cellular mechanisms responsible for this meiotic arrest remain uncertain, it is generally presumed that a granulosa cell–derived putative meiosis inhibitor is in play. This hypothesis is based on the observation that denuded (granulosa-free) oocytes are capable of spontaneously completing meiotic maturation in vitro.

The primary oocyte is converted into a secondary oocyte by completion of the first meiotic metaphase and formation of the first polar body, before actual ovulation but after the luteinizing hormone (LH) surge. At ovulation, the secondary oocyte and the surrounding granulosa cells (cumulus oophorus) are extruded and enter the fallopian tube. If sperm penetration occurs, the secondary oocyte undergoes a second meiotic division, after which the second polar body is eliminated.

The Granulosa Cell Compartment

The oocyte and the granulosa cells are separated from the surrounding stroma by a membrane referred to as the basal lamina.[12] The granulosa cells do not have a direct vascular supply.

It is the avascular nature of the granulosa cell compartment that necessitates intercellular contact between neighboring cells. Thus, the granulosa cells are interconnected by extensive intercellular gap junctions, which result in their coupling to yield an expanded integrated and functional syncytium[13–15] (Fig. 6–3). Gap junctions are composed of proteins called connexins. Connexin-37 is present in gap junctions in follicles, and connexin-37–deficient mice lack graafian follicles, fail to ovulate, and develop inappropriate corpora lutea.[16] It is generally presumed that the specialized cell junctions may be important in metabolic exchange and in the transport of small molecules between neighboring granulosa cells. Moreover, the granulosa cells (presumed to originate from either germinal epithelium or the rete ovarii) extend cytoplasmic processes to form gap junctions with the plasma membrane of the oocyte (Fig. 6–4). In the connexin-37–deficient mice, the authors also found that oocyte development is arrested before meiotic competence.[16] Thus, gap junctions represent a crucial communication system that is responsible in large measure for the tight control exerted by the cumulus granulosa cells on the resumption of meiosis by the enclosed primary oocyte.

Follicular granulosa cells are heterogeneous in nature, and their level of differentiation is not uniform. A large body of information suggests that the follicular granulosa cells are stratified in a manner allowing the distinction of at least three populations of cells, the mural, antral, and cumulus granulosa cells. The mural granulosa cells (i.e., cells abutting the basement membrane) may well be the most active, as judged by various functional parameters. For example, mural granulosa cells have been considered the most active steroidogenically, with high intracellular levels of 3β-hydroxysteroid dehydrogenase, glucose-6-phosphate dehydrogenase, and cytochrome P450.[17, 18] In addition, the mural granulosa cells appear to possess a generous level of LH receptors.

These observations markedly differ from those made for the antral granulosa cells (i.e., those cells closest to the antral cavity) or the cumulus cells (i.e., those surrounding the oocyte). At ovulation, the granulosa cell constituents of the cumulus oophorus are extruded with the oocyte, whereas the remaining granulosa cells become incorporated into the corpus luteum. Moreover, the absence of cytochrome P450 activity in cumulus cells suggests the absence of aromatase activity. Likewise, the overall LH receptor content and level of LH responsiveness appear substantially diminished in cumulus granulosa cells relative to that of their mural counterparts.[19–22] These observations suggest that the cumulus granulosa cells may function in a stem cell capacity. According to this view, cumulus granulosa

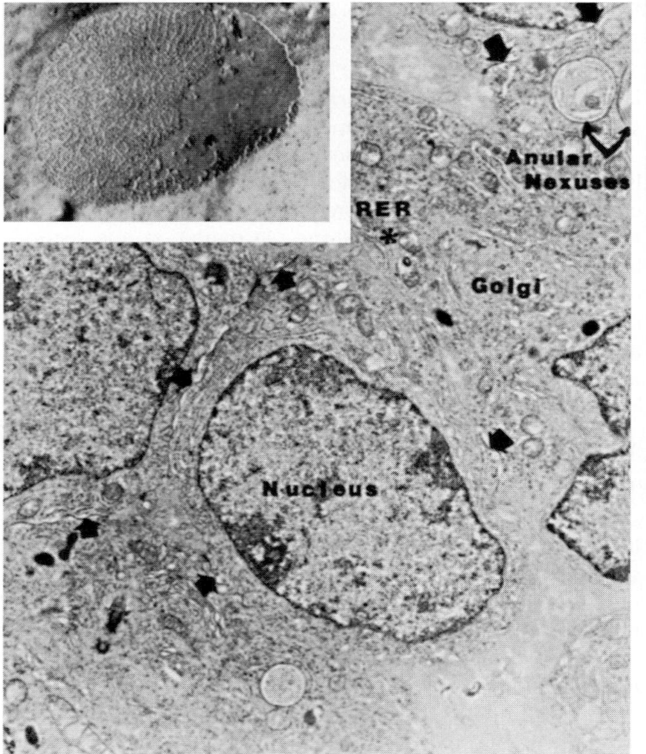

Figure 6–3 ■ Numerous gap junctions *(arrows)* are noted between FSH-stimulated granulosa cells of a dominant graafian follicle. RER, rough endoplasmic reticulum. *Inset:* Replica of granulosa cell membrane fracture demonstrating the hexagonally ordered protein particles of the gap junctions. (From Erickson GF. An analysis of follicle development and ovum maturation. Semin Reprod Endocrinol 4:233, 1986. Thieme Medical Publishers, New York. Reproduced by permission.)

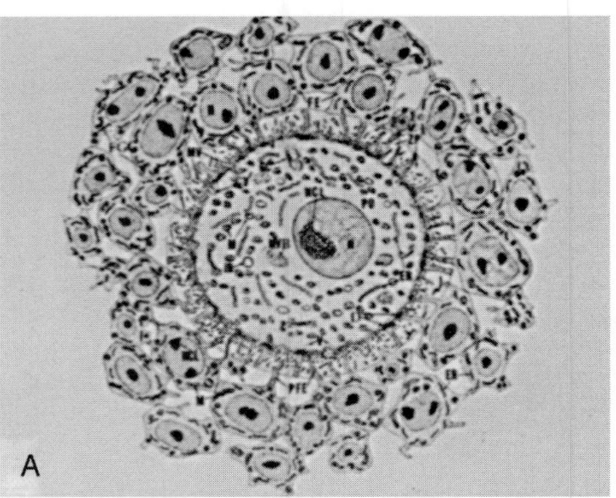

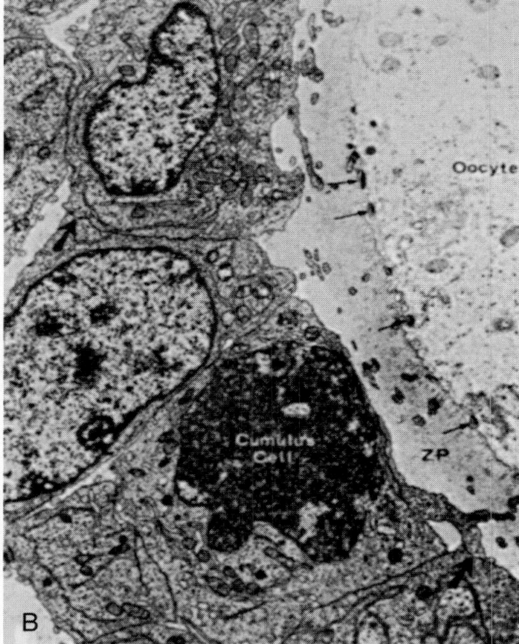

Figure 6–4 ■ Structural relationship between the granulosa cell and the oocyte. *A,* Microvilli of an oocyte interdigitate with cytoplasmic extensions of granulosa cells, penetrating the zona pellucida (ZP). *B,* Note the penetration of the zona pellucida by cytoplasmic processes of granulosa cells. Small gap junctions *(thin arrows)* are observed between processes of the granulosa cell and the oocyte membrane. The thick arrow indicates a gap junction between granulosa cells. (*A* and *B* from Erickson GF. An analysis of follicle development and ovum maturation. Semin Reprod Endocrinol 4:233, 1986. Thieme Medical Publishers, New York. Reproduced by permission.)

cells may be likened to a "feeder" layer engaged in active multiplication contributing to and thereby forming the membrana granulosa. This view arose from observations revealing multiplication of cumulus granulosa cells in the face of a relatively undifferentiated state. In this respect, these observations are consistent with the notion that the processes of granulosa cellular proliferation and differentiation may be mutually exclusive.

Although the granulosa cell population is highly heterogeneous, little information is available about the significance of this stratification. Accordingly, a more detailed understanding of the nature of the heterogeneity in question constitutes a major goal of contemporary ovarian physiology.

The Interstitial (Interfollicular) Compartment

Theca-Interstitial Cells

The demonstration that the theca-interstitial cells are the androgen-producing unit was made by Ryan and Petro.[23] Rice and Savard[24, 25] noted the ability of the theca interna and interstitial tissue to undertake de novo synthesis of androgens. The androgen-producing cells are located in the loose connective tissue of both the cortex and the medulla,[26] arising in all likelihood from a population of unspecialized mesenchymal cells in the stromal compartment.

The cells making up the theca-interstitial compartment are heterogeneous in nature. One contemporary view of the dynamic alterations characteristic of this ovarian compartment is by Erickson.[27] Four classes of interstitial cells have been identified.

Primary Interstitial Cells. Primary interstitial cells constitute a transient population of androgen-producing cells located in the medullary compartment of the fetal ovary.[28] Although apparent at about 12 weeks of gestation, these cells disappear by 20 weeks. Their function remains a mystery. Morphologically resembling fetal testicular Leydig cells, primary interstitial cells are functionally limited in terms of their steroidogenic capacity. Specifically, these cells appear to be incapable of de novo steroidogenesis, presumably owing to the lack of cholesterol side-chain cleavage activity. These cells are unresponsive to gonadotropic stimulation and could conceivably be employing circulating steroidogenic precursors to yield androgens.

Theca-Interstitial Cells. Theca-interstitial cells are the constant feature of all developing follicles (secondary or later follicles). They are the main mature androgen-producing component concerned with the sustenance and atresia of the follicle.

Secondary Interstitial Cells. Secondary interstitial cells represent hypertrophied theca interna remnants surviving follicular atresia. These cells settle in the region of the old follicle but otherwise remain functionally and structurally unchanged. The secondary interstitial cells (unlike theca-interstitial cells) are the target of noradrenergic innervation (see later).

Hilar Interstitial Cells. Hilar interstitial cells are constituents of the ovarian hilum. They are large steroidogenic lutein-like cells with structural and functional characteristics indistinguishable from those of differentiated testicular Leydig cells. Both types of cells contain a unique hexagonal array of crystal lattice named after Reinke. Hilar cells are intimately associated with nonmyelinated sympathetic nerve fibers. The secretory function (i.e., androgen biosynthesis) of these cells is strongly suggested by their prominence at the time of puberty, during pregnancy, and around the menopause.

Resident Ovarian White Blood Cells

Unlike the testicular seminiferous tubule, the ovary does not constitute an immunologically privileged site. Thus, resident ovarian mononuclear phagocytes (macrophages), lymphocytes, and polymorphonuclear granulocytes can be observed at various stages of the ovarian life cycle. For example, macrophages, but not other white blood cells, are known to constitute a major cellular component of the interstitial (i.e., interfollicular) ovarian compartment.[29] In part, these macrophages are present within the ovarian stroma near perifollicular capillaries (Fig. 6–5). Unfortu-

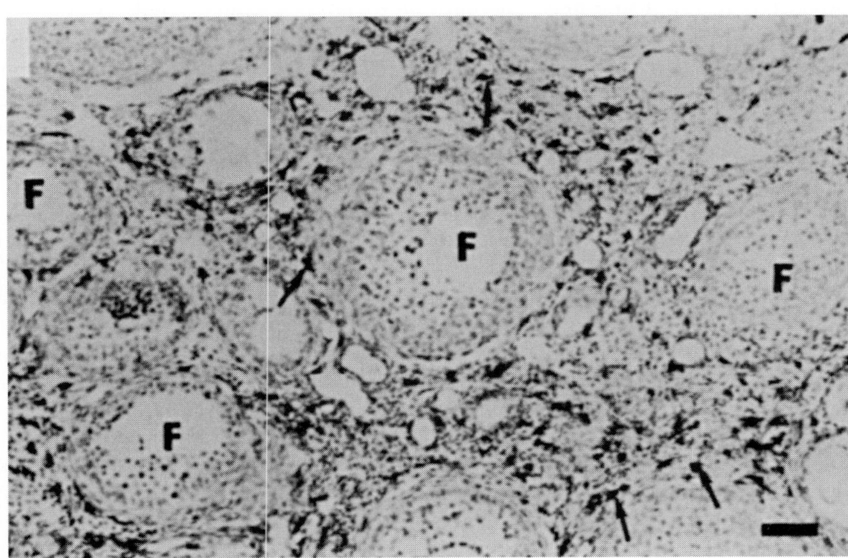

Figure 6–5 ■ Resident ovarian macrophages constitute a major cellular component of the interstitial (i.e., interfollicular) ovarian compartment. F, follicles. (From Hume DA, Halpin D, Charlton H, Gordon S. The mononuclear phagocyte system of the mouse defined by immunohistochemical localization of antigen F4/80: Macrophages of endocrine organs. Proc Natl Acad Sci USA 81:4174–4177, 1984.)

nately, little is known about this apparently permanent, noncyclic presence.

With the exception of macrophages, few other white blood cells have been observed in the early phases of follicular development. However, this is altered as preovulatory events or atresia prompts massive ovarian infiltration by several different types of white blood cells.[30] Paving the way are mast cells,[31–33] which increase progressively during the latter portion of the follicular phase. This invasion culminates with their degranulation in response to the proestrus LH surge.[34] The resultant follicular hyperemia,[35–39] coupled with chemotactic signaling,[40, 41] appears to play a crucial role in subsequent luteal function[42] and heralds a sequence of events reminiscent of an acute inflammatory response.[43] The follicular hyperemia observed is initiated by histamine and propagated by prostaglandin E_2.[43] Both agents cause vasodilatation and enhanced capillary/venule permeability by relaxing vascular smooth muscle.[43] The released histamine may also affect gonadal steroidogenesis.

Next to arrive are eosinophils and T lymphocytes, which migrate into the corpus luteum.[44] Ovine corpora lutea have been shown to secrete a specific chemoattractant for eosinophils.[45] Infiltration and subsequent degranulation of these cells have been reported to occur before evidence of either functional or structural luteal regression.

Activated T cells are known to produce lymphokines that attract and activate macrophages. Accordingly, T lymphocytes are followed in short sequence by phagocytic monocytes with features similar to those observed in other body sites.[46] Macrophages within the pericapillary spaces represent, in all likelihood, the dark stellate K cells that have been seen scattered among the granulosa cells in light micrographs.[47] In this connection, cocultures of ovarian macrophages and luteal cells were seen to make discrete cell-cell contacts.[46] As the corpus luteum matures, these macrophages are characterized by the presence of many electron-dense lysosomal granules and phagocytotic granules of variable configuration and structure throughout their cytoplasm.[48]

The invasion of macrophages and T lymphocytes into the corpus luteum is delayed by pregnancy and thus is not strictly a function of the age of the corpus luteum. Indeed, only a few macrophages and T lymphocytes were observed in rabbit corpora lutea of day 19 pregnancy, whereas the numbers of these cells were sixfold to eightfold higher in corpora lutea of day 19 pseudopregnancy. By the day of parturition, however, macrophages do begin to infiltrate the corpora lutea of pregnancy.[49]

The significance of the preceding observations may be that resident ovarian representatives of the white blood cell series constitute potential in situ modulators of ovarian function, acting through the local secretion of regulatory cytokines.[50] Because the flow of information is probably multidirectional, the same cells are probably targeted for steroidal and peptidergic input. Moreover, immune cells are endowed with steroidogenic capabilities that could, in their own right, affect steroid economy.[51, 52]

The potential relevance of macrophages becomes more evident if consideration is given to their ability to elaborate growth factors previously implicated as putative intraovarian regulators.[50, 53] Indeed, noncytokine secretory products of the macrophage, such as growth factors, have been shown to exert modulatory effects on the growth and functional development of the ovarian granulosa-luteal cells.

Follicular Development

The transformation of ovarian follicles into a corpus luteum was first described in 1672 by Regnier de Graaf.[54] Since that time, ovarian follicles have clearly been shown to constitute the fundamental functional unit of the ovary. These traverse a developmental track that propels primordial follicular units into the highly differentiated preovulatory stage of antral (graafian) follicles.[55, 56]

In infant human ovaries, several preantral follicular classes were noted by Lintern-Moore:[57]

1. Primordial follicles (30 to 60 μm in diameter) were found to be composed of a late diplotene primary oocyte (9 to 25 μm in diameter) surrounded by a single layer of flattened (noncuboidal) pregranulosa cells.
2. Primary follicles (>60 μm in diameter) were characterized by a primary oocyte surrounded by a single layer of cuboidal granulosa cells.
3. Secondary follicles (≤120 μm) consisted of a primary oocyte surrounded by several layers of cuboidal granulosa cells (≤600).

According to Gougeon,[58] the various follicular classes, defined in large measure by the number of follicular granulosa cells observed, represent the stages of development that a follicle would have to traverse on its way to complete maturity. Although this scheme of follicular development is subject to individual variation, it is nevertheless based on morphometric data, which provide a solid working model for further conceptual developments[58, 59] (Fig. 6–6).

Primordial Follicle Formation

The first primordial follicle, a complex consisting of an oocyte and spindle-shaped pregranulosa cells enclosed by the basal lamina, is found by around 16 weeks of intrauterine life (Fig. 6–7). It is generally accepted that primordial follicle formation ends no later than 6 months post partum. Indeed, although oogonial divisions and oogonial meiosis have ceased by the seventh month of gestation, primary oocytes continue to invest themselves with granulosa cells as primordial follicles are being generated. This stage of follicular development is entirely gonadotropin independent. Little information exists about the morphogenic agents responsible for follicular organization.

Preantral Growth Phase

In this follicular development phase, primordial follicles (30 μm in diameter) are converted to mature secondary follicles (120 μm in diameter). The process is continuously operational throughout the reproductive life span, remaining uninterrupted until menopause (Fig. 6–8). Initiated during the fifth to sixth month of gestation, the process becomes evident when the spindle-shaped granulosa cell precursors of some primordial follicles differentiate into a single layer of cuboidal cells, thereby yielding primary follicles. Concurrently, the granulosa cells synthesize and

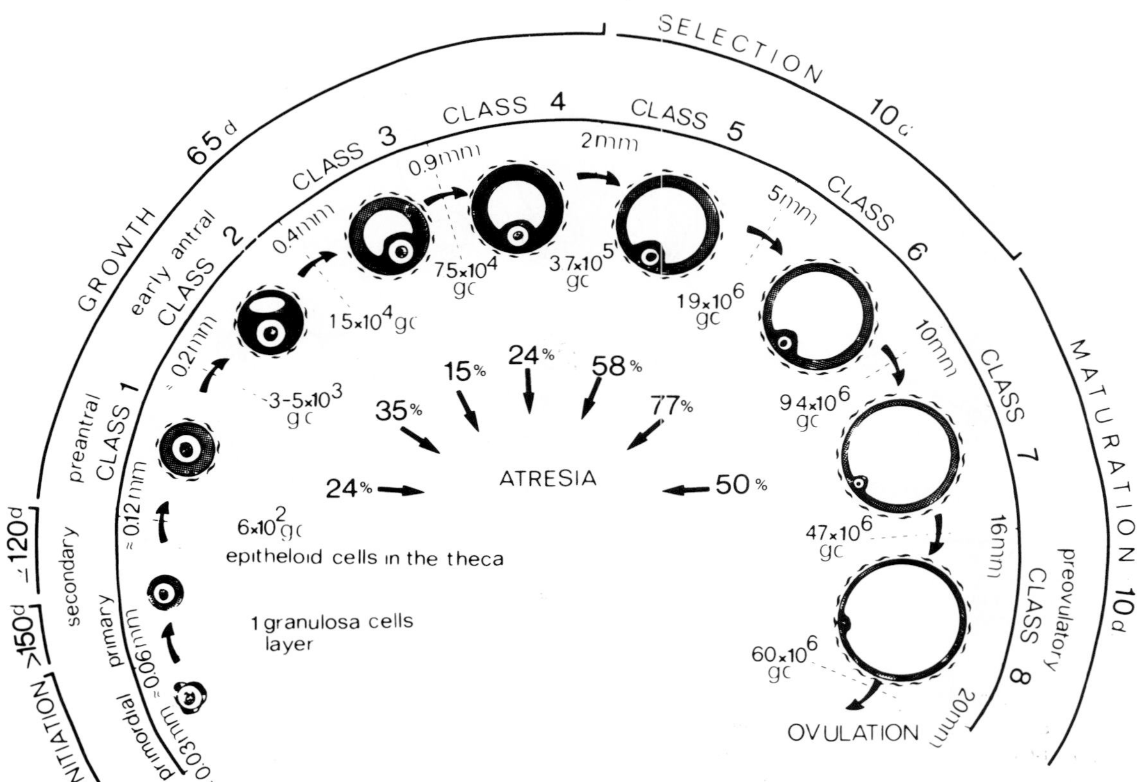

Figure 6–6 ■ Stages of follicular genesis in the adult human ovary and level of atresia in the eight classes of growing follicles. The classes under study are defined by the granulosa cell (gc) numbers and the corresponding estimated follicular diameter (mm). (From Gougeon A. Dynamics of follicular growth in the human: A model from preliminary results. Hum Reprod 1:81–87, 1986.)

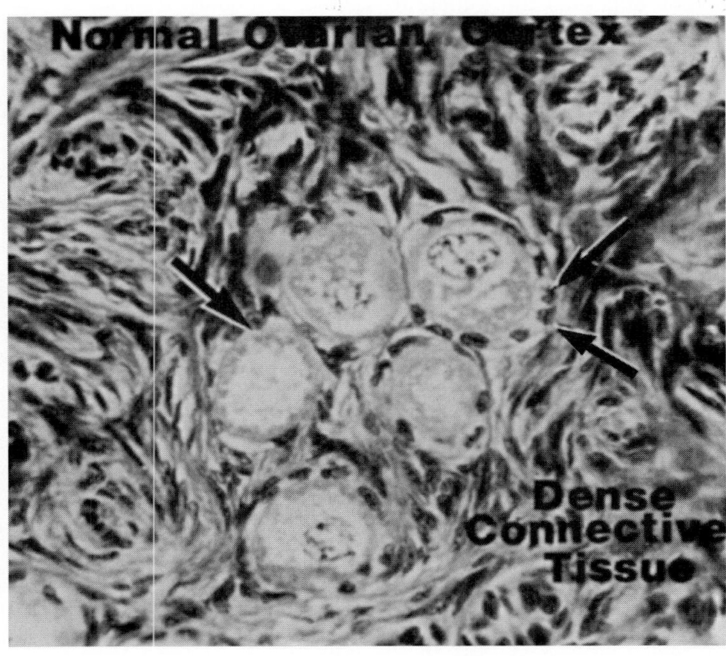

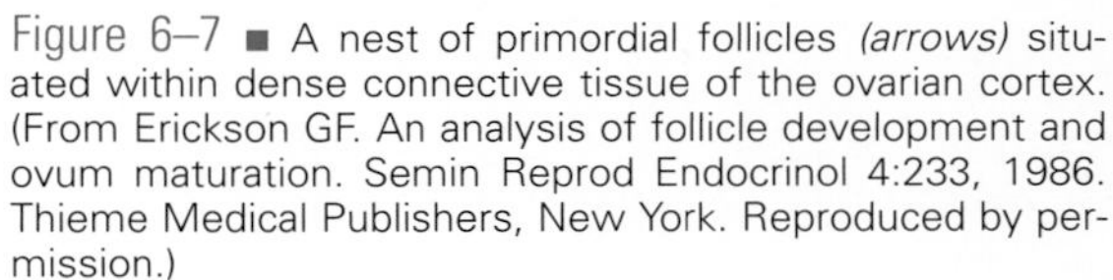
Figure 6–7 ■ A nest of primordial follicles *(arrows)* situated within dense connective tissue of the ovarian cortex. (From Erickson GF. An analysis of follicle development and ovum maturation. Semin Reprod Endocrinol 4:233, 1986. Thieme Medical Publishers, New York. Reproduced by permission.)

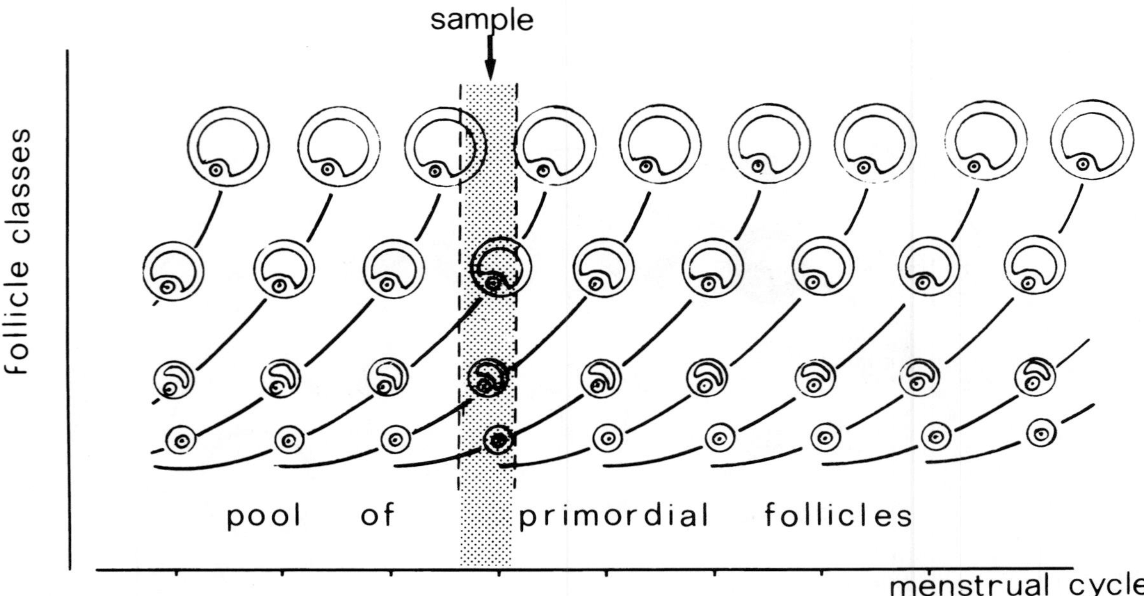

Figure 6–8 ■ Follicular growth waves underlie the nonsynchronous heterogeneous state of development of ovarian follicles at any given point in time. (From Gougeon A. Dynamics of follicular growth in the human: A model from preliminary results. Hum Reprod 1:81–87, 1986.)

secrete mucopolysaccharides, giving rise to a translucent halo surrounding the oocyte known as the zona pellucida.[60] The cytoplasmic processes of granulosa cells traverse the zona pellucida to maintain intimate gap junctional contact with the plasma membrane of the oocyte.[12] These cytoplasmic contacts provide an avenue for the transfer of information and nutrients to the oocyte. Accordingly, granulosa cells maintaining contact with the oocyte have distinctive properties. Ultimately, proliferation of primary follicular granulosa cells gives rise to multiple layers of cells, thereby enlarging the follicle to yield a secondary follicle (Fig. 6–9). The combination of granulosa cell proliferation and differentiation, hypertrophy of theca cells, and growth of the oocyte all work to increase the diameter of maturing follicles. A significant component of this growth phase is dedicated to oocyte differentiation and growth. This includes the acquisition of the zona pellucida, which is a pathognomonic feature of the preantral primary follicle. At the same time, however, the total granulosa cell endowment of secondary follicles will increase to 600, concurrent with the progression of thecal differentiation. The mature secondary follicles constitute the pool of preantral follicles from which tonic (probably follicle-stimulating hormone [FSH] dependent) recruitment of follicles takes place.

The limited growth and premature atresia of follicles in fetal and premenarchal ovaries were attributed, until recently, to absent pituitary gonadotropin secretion. However, the human fetal pituitary gland is now known to secrete gonadotropins.[61] In fact, circulating immunoreactive FSH levels in fetal serum collected from the fifth to the seventh month of gestation are comparable to those in postmenopausal women. The apparent importance of gonadotropins in the primate fetus was further illustrated by the observation that hypophysectomy of the fetal rhesus monkey results in oocyte depletion[62] (Fig. 6–10).

Thus, this early phase of follicular development is likely to be dependent on gonadotropins.[62] This aspect of early human follicular growth is highlighted by studies of the "resistant ovary" syndrome. In this syndrome, the cardinal manifestations include sexual immaturity, primary amenorrhea, hypoestrogenism, and compensatory hypergonadotropinism.[63] The ovaries of these patients are small and contain many primordial follicles that show no evidence of maturation despite high concentrations of endogenous gonadotropins. The lack of response in these patients to high doses of exogenous menopausal gonadotropins indi-

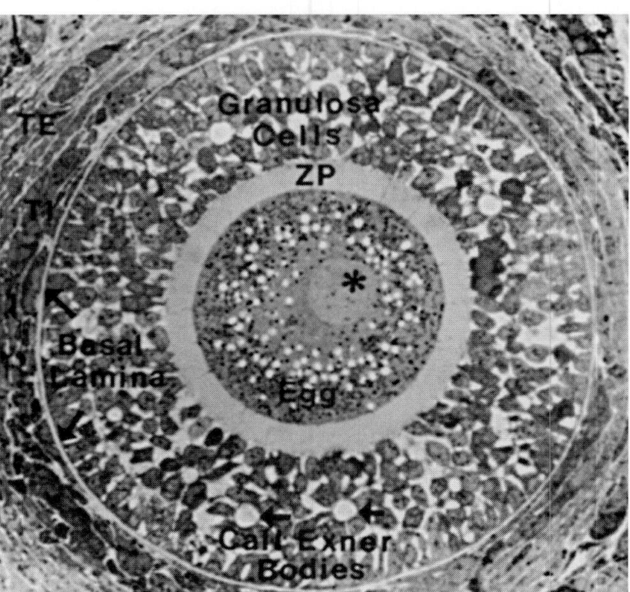

Figure 6–9 ■ Photomicrograph of a section through a preantral follicle. The dictyate oocyte contains a large germinal vesicle (*) and a zona pellucida (ZP). TI, theca interna; TE, theca externa. (From Erickson GF, Magoffin DA, Dyer CA, Hofeditz C. The ovarian androgen producing cells: A review of structure/function relationships. Endocr Rev 6:371–399, 1985. © The Endocrine Society.)

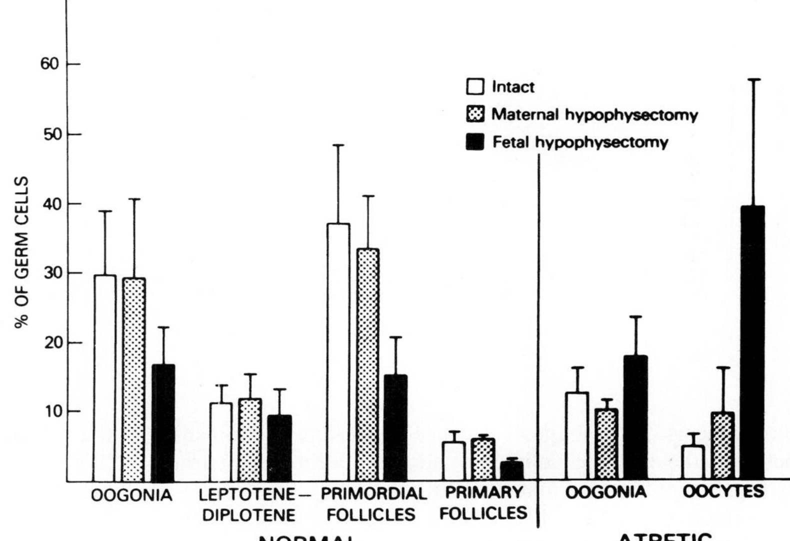

Figure 6–10 ■ Effect of fetal hypophysectomy on follicular development in newborn rhesus monkeys. (From Gulyas BJ, Hodgen GD, Tullner WW, Ross GT. Effects of fetal or maternal hypophysectomy on endocrine organs and body weight in infant rhesus monkeys *[Macaca mulatta]* with particular emphasis on oogenesis. Biol Reprod 16:216–227, 1977.)

cates that the disease is a primary ovarian disorder. As such, this model demonstrates the absolute gonadotropin dependence of follicular growth beyond the primordial follicle stage.

The role of ovarian steroids is more clearly evident in patients afflicted with 17α-hydroxylase deficiency.[64–66] This congenital enzyme deficiency results in decreased ovarian biosynthesis of estrogens and, hence, sexual immaturity and primary amenorrhea. Laboratory studies reveal elevated levels of progesterone, low estrogen levels, and high levels of gonadotropins. Serial sections of ovarian tissue from these women reveal a failure of normal follicular growth. Antral formation is commonly observed, a phenomenon leading to clinically significant follicular cyst formation. These observations suggest that the high circulating levels of FSH are capable of promoting antrum formation. On the other hand, the lack of synergistic interactions between gonadotropins and estrogens dooms the follicles to abnormal and premature demise. Although estrogen replacement has not been shown to normalize follicular growth in these women, administration of 17α-hydroxyprogesterone has been shown to stimulate estrogen

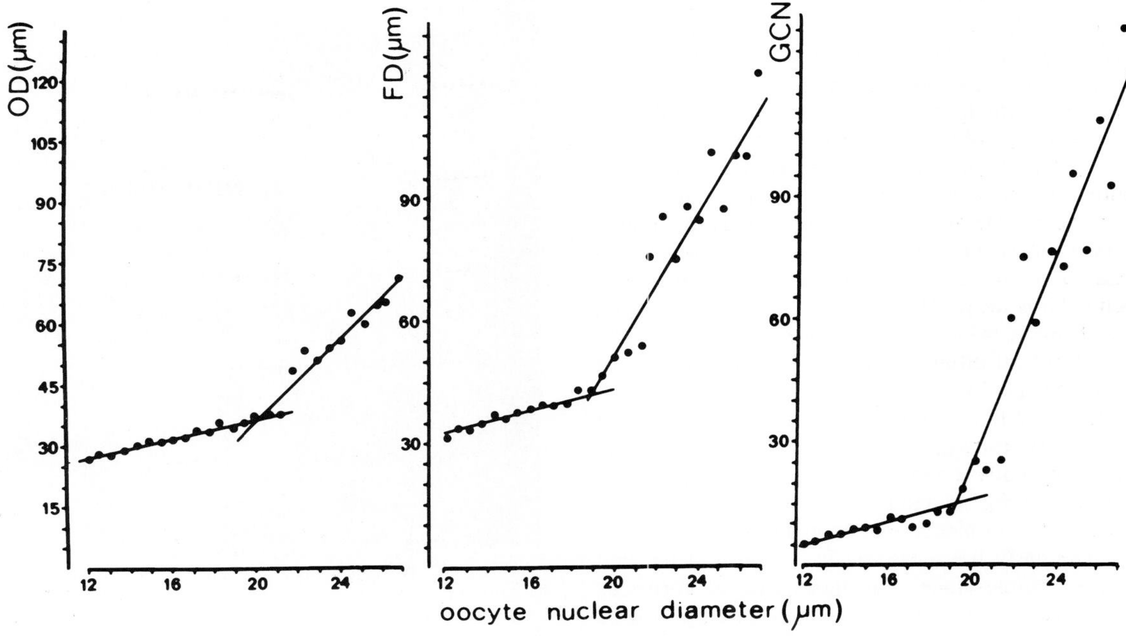

Figure 6–11 ■ Biphasic preantral growth phase: oocyte diameter (OD), follicular diameter (FD), and follicular granulosa cell number (GDN) as a function of oocyte nuclear diameter. (From Gougeon A. Dynamics of follicular growth in the human: A model from preliminary results. Hum Reprod 1:81–87, 1986.)

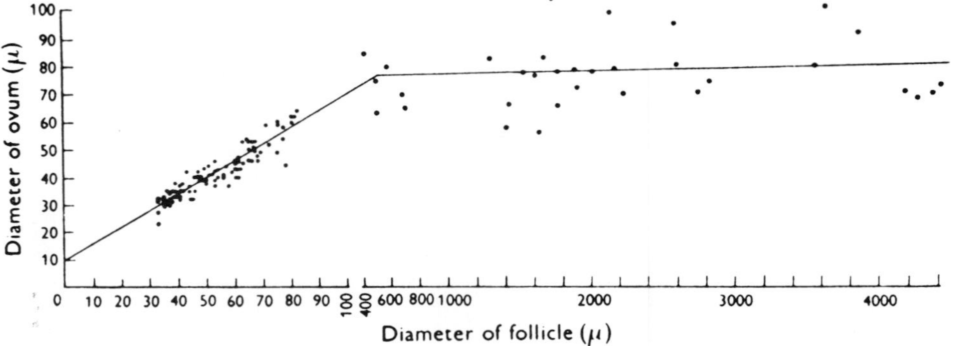

Figure 6–12 ■ Regression lines constructed by plotting oocyte diameter as a function of follicle size in human ovaries. (From Erickson GF. An analysis of follicle development and ovum maturation. Semin Reprod Endocrinol 4:233, 1986. Thieme Medical Publishers, New York. Reproduced by permission.)

biosynthesis. This suggests a cause and effect relationship between the enzyme deficiency and the failure of ovarian estrogen secretion by maturing follicles.

Collectively, these observations suggest that both early and late follicular maturation in the human ovary depends on adequate pituitary gonadotropin secretion and also on ovarian sex steroid hormone secretion in response to gonadotropic stimulation.

The conversion of a primordial follicle into a primary follicle is marked by little if any real follicular growth until the germinal vesicle reaches a diameter of 20 μm. This corresponds to a mean primordial follicular diameter of 40 μm and a total of about 15 granulosa cells. Up to this point, little change can be documented in primary oocyte diameter, follicular diameter, or the number of granulosa cells (Fig. 6–11). It may be concluded that follicles enter the "real" growth phase when the diameter of the germinal vesicle exceeds 20 μm. Thereafter, follicular growth is characterized by progressive increments of all parameters evaluated, including follicular diameter and granulosa cell number.

When a primordial follicle begins to grow (germinal vesicle >20 μm), the dictyate primary oocyte embarks on a series of ultrastructural and biochemical changes. This culminates in the formation of a fully grown (mean diameter, 75 to 80 μm) and physiologically differentiated ovum, surrounded by the zona pellucida and a single layer of cuboidal granulosa cells (i.e., a primary follicle). Increases in oocyte and follicular diameters are positively correlated until well into the secondary follicle stage when oocytes reach a mean diameter of 80 μm. This stage corresponds to a follicular diameter of 110 to 120 μm and a granulosa endowment of about 600 cells (Figs. 6–12 and 6–13). The germinal vesicle itself attains a mean maximal diameter of 26 to 27 μm at this follicular size.

As a secondary follicle is being formed, the granulosa cells develop FSH, estrogen, and androgen receptors and become physiologically coupled by gap junctions. Moreover, the differentiating secondary follicle migrates into the medulla where it completes the acquisition of a thecal component. The early theca interna is acquired at the end of the primary follicle stage. The theca externa forms as the follicle expands and compresses surrounding stroma (see Fig. 6–9).

The emergence of the thecal layer of the follicle is associated with the acquisition of follicular blood supply. Indeed, simultaneously with the development of the theca, the follicle acquires arterioles that terminate in a wreath-like network of capillaries adjacent to the basement membrane. Lymphatics are added on as well. As the capillaries form, the theca-interstitial cells appear to embark on a differentiation pathway with acquisition of LH receptors and steroidogenic biosynthetic capacity. Once the pretheca stromal cells reach the basement membrane, they engage in concentric layering. They become aligned parallel to one another and form a radial arrangement of highly elongated fibroblast-like cells around the entire follicle. Moreover, increasing proportions of the spindle-shaped theca cells proximal to the basal lamina accumulate cytoplasm, become epithelioid in appearance, and acquire organelles characteristic of steroid hormone–secreting cells. They are known as theca interna cells. More peripheral layers of these cells retain their spindle-shaped configuration and merge with stromal cells. These are known as the theca externa cells (see Fig. 6–9).

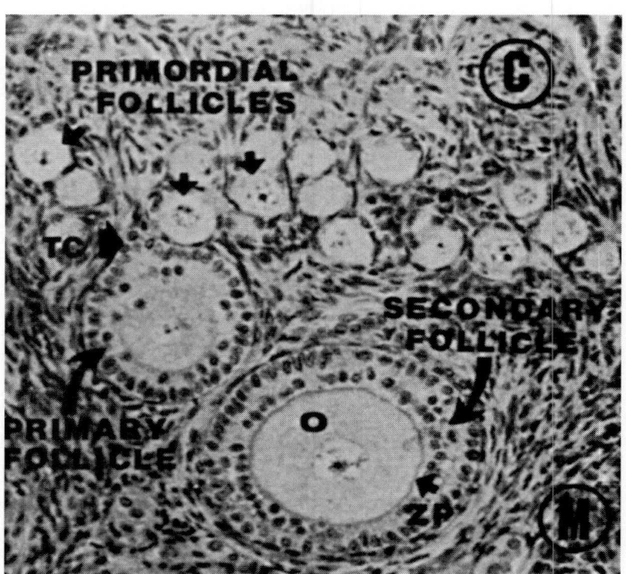

Figure 6–13 ■ Progressive follicular development from primordial to primary to secondary follicles is accompanied by a dramatic increase in the oocyte size and differentiation. Note that during oocyte growth, the recruited follicles migrate out of the cortex (C) into the medulla (M) by actions presumed to involve the theca cone (TC). (From Erickson GF. An analysis of follicle development and ovum maturation. Semin Reprod Endocrinol 4:233, 1986. Thieme Medical Publishers, New York. Reproduced by permission.)

The stromal transformation is initiated by an unknown signal capable of triggering surrounding unspecialized mesenchymal cells to migrate to the outer surface of the follicle. Although the nature of the signal remains uncertain, it could be of circulatory or intraovarian origin.

Tonic Growth Phase

This phase of follicular development corresponds to the conversion of class 1 (still preantral) follicles (0.12 to 0.2 mm in diameter) to class 4 (antral) follicles with a diameter of up to 2 mm (Fig. 6–14). Growth is characterized by a 600-fold increase in granulosa cell numbers, concurrent with a greater than 15-fold increase in overall follicular diameter. This overall increase in follicular size is accomplished by both granulosa cell proliferation and enlargement of the antrum. The term tonic growth is used here to distinguish this phase of follicular development from the exponential growth phase characteristic of follicular classes 5 to 8. Thus, tonic follicular growth is not gonadotropin independent. In fact, gonadotropin support is necessary if a follicle is to progress past early preantral development. However, progress is slow with low circulating levels of gonadotropins. It is during this phase of follicular development that atresia does not appear to be directly related to the cyclic changes characteristic of circulating gonadotropins. In this respect, this phase of follicular growth contrasts with later stages of follicular development when atresia appears to be closely related to the cyclic changes in the circulating levels of FSH.

The limited ability of follicles to grow with relatively low circulating levels of pituitary gonadotropins is amply documented. For example, antral follicles have been documented in the ovaries of prepubertal females. Similar morphologic observations were made in hypogonadotropic conditions such as anorexia nervosa. Also, graafian follicles have rarely been observed in patients with Kallmann's syndrome.[67–71] Limited follicular development is also found in users of oral contraceptives or in pregnant women.[72, 73] Thus, low levels of gonadotropins are probably required and sufficient for follicles to grow.

On the acquisition of a theca interna, class 1 follicles are presumed to become responsive to gonadotropic stimulation. Indeed, it is presumed that the presence of thecal LH and granulosa FSH receptors[74] and the establishment of a granulosa–theca-interstitial cell interrelationship result in the formation of a functional follicular unit. Accordingly, the entry of secondary follicles into the class 1 variety (still preantral) is thought to occur in the early part of the luteal phase. This is several days after ovulation, days 15 to 19 of the cycle. This arbitrary ovulatory cycle is designated cycle 1. About 25 days later (i.e., between days 11 and 15 of the subsequent ovulatory cycle, cycle 2), conversion of the class 1 follicle into a class 2 follicle (early antral) can be observed. Still 20 days later, during the tail end of the luteal phase of this same cycle (cycle 2), class 2 follicles become class 3 follicles. Fifteen days later, during the late follicular phase of the next cycle (cycle 3), the class 3 follicles are converted to class 4 follicles. The transition into class 5 is presumed to occur 10 days later during the

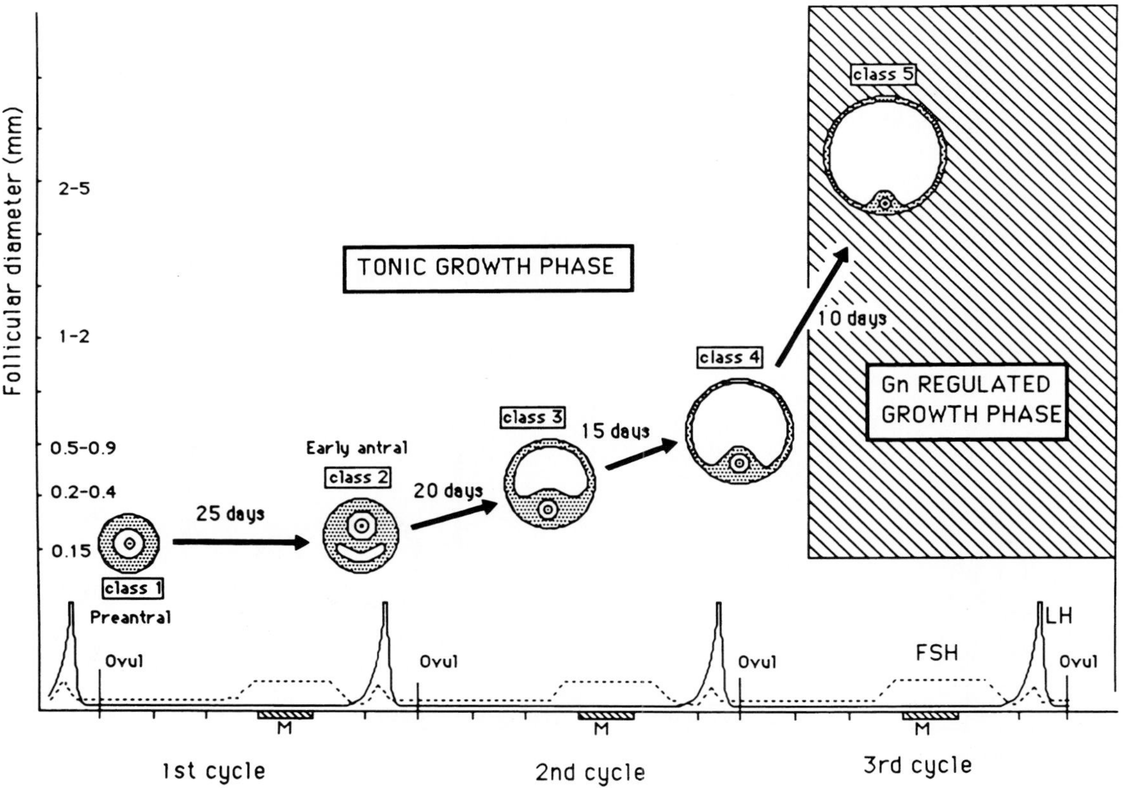

Figure 6–14 ■ Tonic (periantral) follicular growth: conversion of a class 1 into a class 5 follicle. M, menses; Gn, gonadotropin; LH, luteinizing hormone; FSH, follicle-stimulating hormone. (Courtesy of A. Gougeon.)

late luteal phase, days 25 to 28 of cycle 3, and is a key step in follicular growth preceding final maturation.

When follicular diameters reach 200 to 400 μm, localized accumulation of fluid appears among the granulosa cells. These so-called Call-Exner bodies are areas of liquefaction or of granulosa cell secretion. These accumulations increase in size, become confluent, and give rise to a central fluid-filled cavity referred to as the antrum. The appearance of the antrum transforms the follicle into a graafian follicle in which the oocyte occupies an eccentric position and is surrounded by two to three layers of granulosa cells. They are collectively referred to as the cumulus oophorus. Cells in the cumulus oophorus are contiguous with mural granulosa cells, which constitute the membrana granulosa that surrounds the central antrum.

Antral fluid contains steroid hormones, proteins, proteoglycans, and electrolytes.[75] Plasma proteins, gonadotropins, and prolactin reach the antral fluid, an ultrafiltrate, by diffusion from vascular spaces outside the basal lamina. In contrast, proteoglycans are FSH-dependent secretory products of granulosa cells.[76–81] Although the role of intraovarian proteoglycans remains speculative, it is presumed that they may enhance antrum formation and maintenance through increased viscosity. The origin of antral fluid steroids is less clear. Some of the steroids are secreted by theca and interstitial cells and diffuse across the basal lamina into the antral fluid. Although some antral fluid steroids (e.g., estrogens) are secreted by granulosa cells, the interfollicular variations in antral fluid hormone concentration suggest that regulation is more complicated than can be ascribed to diffusion alone.

Gonadotropin-Dependent (Exponential) Growth Phase

Although earlier stages of follicular development are likely to be gonadotropin dependent, the final stages of follicular development are the ones heavily dependent on gonadotropins. Indeed, larger follicles need gonadotropic support if they are to reach ovulatory size. According to this view, late luteal–phase class 5 follicles constitute the cohort from which the follicles destined to ovulate in the next cycle will be recruited. The residual growth to be accomplished will take place during the follicular phase of ovulatory cycle 4. This growth is gonadotropin dependent, is exponential with a 160-fold increase in granulosa cell endowment, and results in an increase in follicular size from 5 to 20 mm in diameter. Thus, a follicle is projected to spend around 5 days in each of the remaining follicular classes (6 to 8) before ovulation. It is during this time that follicular selection and dominance are accomplished (Figs. 6–15 and 6–16).

In the early follicular phase, FSH stimulates granulosa cell aromatase activity, resulting in increased follicular concentrations of estrogen. The rising estrogen increases the follicular uptake of FSH and thereby increases the

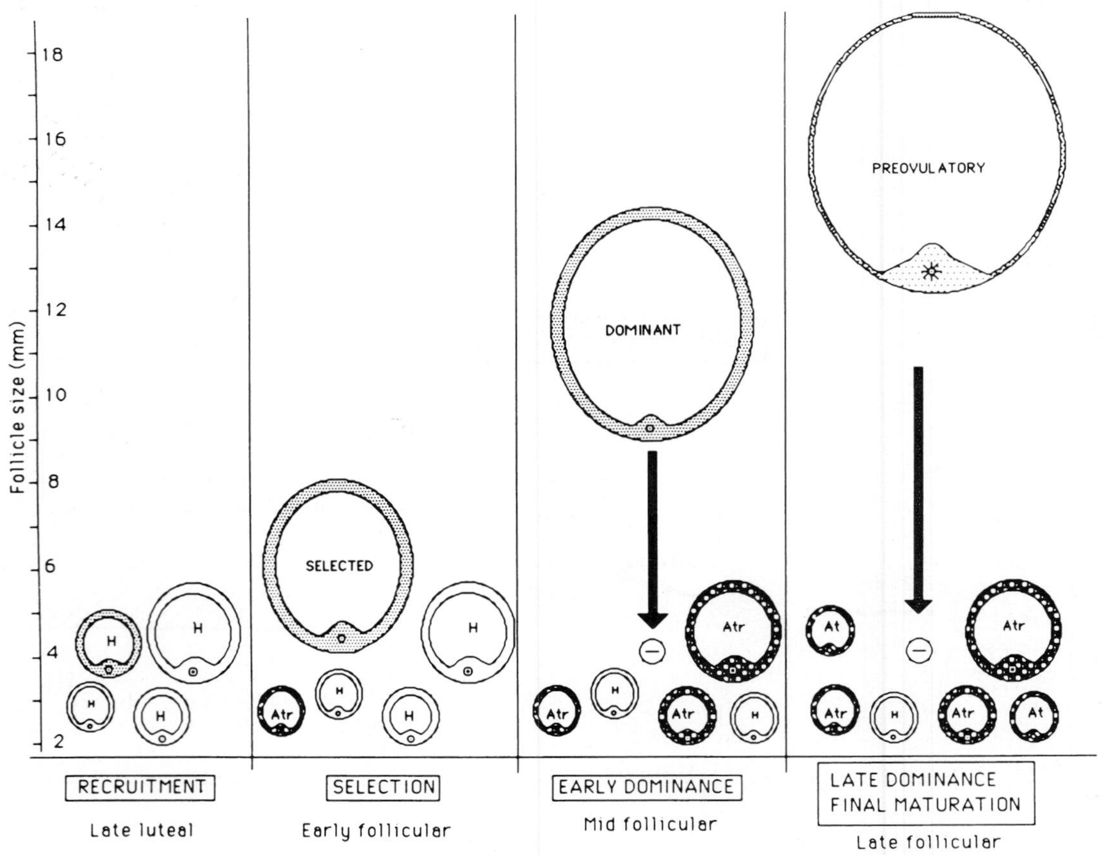

Figure 6–15 ■ Gonadotropin-dependent (exponential) follicular growth phase: recruitment, selection, and the attainment of dominance. H, healthy follicle; At and Atr, atretic follicle. (Courtesy of A. Gougeon.)

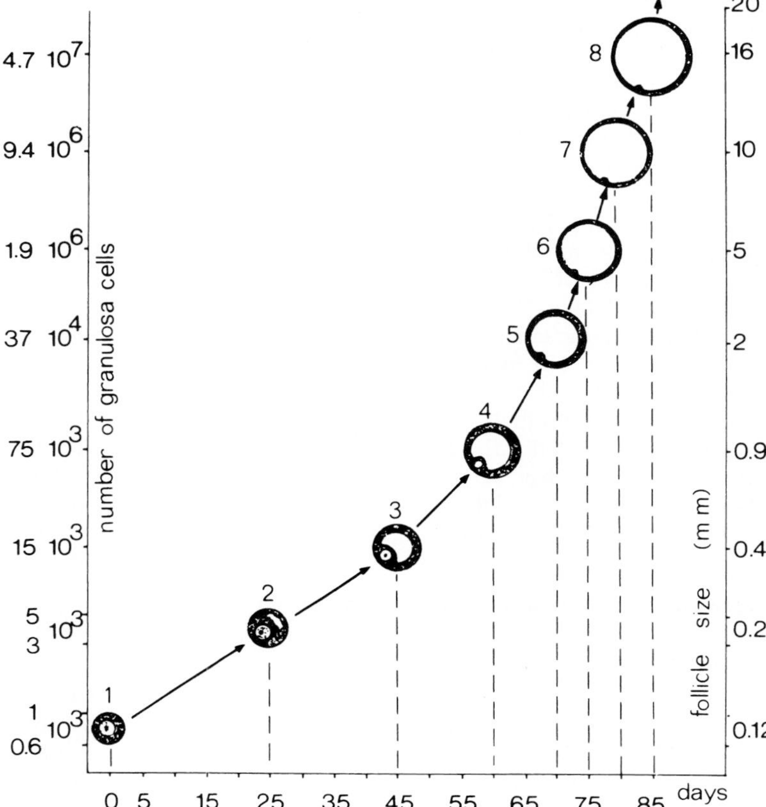

Figure 6–16 ■ Rate of follicular growth (classes 1 to 8) in the human ovary. (From Gougeon A. Dynamics of follicular growth in the human: A model from preliminary results. Hum Reprod 1:81–87, 1986.)

sensitivity of the follicle to FSH hormonal action. By the midfollicular phase, one follicle (probably by chance) has produced relatively more estrogen than the other follicles in its cohort. Estrogen production by this dominant follicle is responsible for the asymmetry in estrogen concentrations seen in the ovarian vein effluent by days 5 through 7 of the follicular phase. Enhanced antrum formation and LH receptor acquisition are to be anticipated. The dominant follicle thus enjoys an orderly sequence of events in which FSH and estrogen stimulate growth, antrum formation, and the appearance of LH receptors.

The dramatic increase in estrogen production by the dominant follicle during the second half of the follicular phase is accompanied by falling circulating levels of FSH.[82] As a result, the nondominant follicles of the same cohort fail to thrive. These follicles are marked by diminished estrogen biosynthesis as well as elevated intrafollicular androgen levels and diminished sensitivity to FSH. Whereas local factors may be at play, the intrafollicular concentrations of gonadotropins and of steroids are undoubtedly central to the self-amplification process.

There are thecal changes associated with the development of the dominant follicle. Indeed, by the seventh day of the cycle, the follicle destined to ovulate is surrounded by theca that selectively takes up more LH than the theca of other members of the developing cohort.[83, 84] By day 9 of the follicular phase, the vascularity of the theca of the dominant follicle is twice that of other follicles. This increased vascularity leads to increased delivery of LH and low-density lipoprotein (LDL) to the theca and of FSH to the granulosa cells.

It has been suggested that the dominant follicle secretes a protein capable of inhibiting aromatase activity of adjacent ipsilateral smaller follicles, with those in the contralateral ovary being similarly affected. The dominant follicle then takes an active role in ensuring its preferred status. Others think that the emergence of the dominant follicle is a consequence of growth arrest of smaller members of the follicular cohort. According to this view, the relative inability of nondominant members of the cohort to thrive does not reflect an active action on the part of the dominant follicle but rather reflects a deteriorating endocrine environment where only the dominant follicle survives. This differential effect may reflect the relative inability of smaller follicles to survive the fall in the circulating levels of FSH occurring in the midfollicular phase, which presumably results as a response to increasing negative ovarian feedback. Importantly, enhanced FSH responsiveness appears to be coupled to a marked increase in the mitotic index of the developing granulosa cells. Such conclusions are in keeping with the observations whereby the granulosa cells of the largest follicles were shown to be significantly more sensitive to FSH, in terms of aromatase activity, compared with smaller follicles.

Postnatal Follicular Development

From the fifth month of fetal life until the menopause, follicular maturation is continuous. Thus, all stages of follicular development (with the exception of ovulation) can be observed in the infant ovary.[85–88] Indeed, progression to the level of an antral follicle (and in many cases follicular cyst) may be relatively common during the first year of postnatal life, consistent with the observed hypergonadotropinism.[89, 90] In fact, by the fourth to sixth month of postnatal life, follicular development has been found to progress to the point of antrum formation in virtually all ovaries examined.[91] Beyond that point, however, the number of maturing antral follicles is strikingly lower, even though the cycles of follicular growth and atresia continue throughout childhood.[92] Thus, growth ceases and atresia begins before any graafian follicle achieves the characteristic preovulatory size seen in ovulatory women. The follicular size achieved is clearly age related in that the diameter of the largest atretic follicle is generally observed in ovaries of older premenarchal girls. Furthermore, this increase in follicular diameter has been shown to parallel an age-related increase in the weight of premenarchal ovaries from less than 1 gm at birth to 5 to 10 gm at menarche.

Maternal (Gestational) Follicular Growth

It is assumed that maternal follicular maturation is suspended during the early period of gestation and that the ovaries are resistant to gonadotropin stimulation. However, it has been demonstrated that exogenous gonadotropins can readily promote gestational follicular maturation. Moreover, after 8 to 10 weeks of gestation, follicular growth and atresia continue until term. Although progressive maturation beyond antrum formation can be observed, the process commonly terminates in atresia, well before the achievement of ovulatory size.[93] The morphologic appearance of such preantral follicles[94, 95] remains unaffected by the high concentrations of human chorionic gonadotropin (hCG). However, hCG stimulates hypertrophy and "luteinization" of the thecal component of both normal and atretic antral follicles in a manner far more intensely than that found in comparable follicles examined during the cycle.[26] These changes, coupled with the luteinization of granulosa cells in some atretic follicles, give rise to numerous corpora lutea atretica.[74] Virtually no immunoreactive FSH is detectable in the maternal circulation throughout pregnancy.

Follicular Atresia

In ovarian physiology, atresia is the process whereby oocytes and follicles are eliminated from the ovary. Apoptosis, programmed cell death, may be the method by which the ovary eliminates the follicles.[96, 97] Apoptosis is a nontoxic mode of cell death that eliminates single cells in tissues without eliciting an inflammatory response. This process requires protein synthesis and, usually, has a typical pattern of internucleosomal deoxyribonucleic acid (DNA) fragmentation that requires a calcium- and magnesium-dependent endonuclease. Specific genes and proteins regulate this process.

The fact that estrogens are secreted by the ovaries of premenarchal girls indicates that follicles destined to undergo atresia may secrete hormones that are active in stimulating the development of secondary sexual characteristics.

Gonadotropin-independent atresia refers to the process that begins in utero and continues relentlessly thereafter. The frequency with which this subtype of atresia is encountered is strongly correlated with follicular size, approaching 100 percent in follicles that exceed 1 mm in diameter, that is, follicles in the early antral stage.

Gonadotropin-dependent atresia represents a cyclic process involving follicles of different sizes, including those with a diameter of less than 1 mm (Fig. 6–17). This point was elegantly illustrated by means of a systematic evaluation of the morphologic correlates of ovarian cyclicity.[98] Specifically, reciprocal relationships were noted between the numbers of normal and atretic antral (≥1 mm in diameter) follicles. In fact, the number of normal follicles peaked twice during the cycle, just before the midcycle preovulatory gonadotropin surge and in the midluteal phase. Each of these peaks coincided with a reduction in the proportion of such follicles undergoing atresia.

Using animal models, several studies have demonstrated

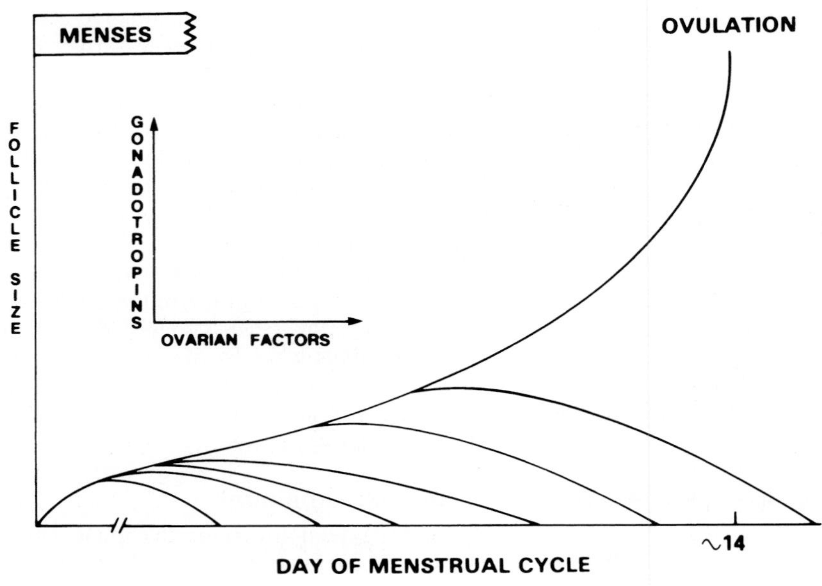

Figure 6–17 ■ Trajectory of follicular growth. Follicular maturation and atresia are determined by the interaction between gonadotropins and putative intraovarian regulators. (From Goodman AL, Hodgen GD. The ovarian triad of the primate menstrual cycle. Recent Prog Horm Res 39:1–73, 1983.)

an association between apoptosis and follicular atresia. In atretic follicles from avian and porcine ovaries, DNA fragmentation patterns typical of apoptosis have been found.[99] In addition, using a histologic technique in which DNA fragmentation can be detected in situ, Palumbo and Yeh[100] have found that it is the atretic follicles that have evidence of apoptosis, not healthy follicles (Fig. 6–18). In in vitro studies, granulosa cells are affected differently by different growth factors; epidermal growth factor (EGF), transforming growth factor-α (TGF-α), and basic fibroblast growth factor (bFGF) have protective effects on granulosa cell apoptosis.[101] Thus, the regulation of atresia in follicles involves peptide growth factors in addition to other agents like FSH and steroids.

There is little doubt that the structural and functional integrity of the follicular complex hinges on the intactness of the oocyte. As the oocyte degenerates, other follicular components follow suit, with the process being irreversible in nature. Whereas death and degeneration of the oocyte are an inevitable consequence of atresia, resumption of meiosis and extrusion of at least the first polar body may be among the earlier manifestations of atresia in some follicles. In either case, the oocyte ultimately displays pyknosis followed by necrosis and complete resorption (most likely involving phagocytosis). Changes in the other follicular components differ with the stage of follicular maturation at the time that atresia occurs.

As noted earlier, granulosa cells in the cumulus oophorus and the membrana granulosa possess different characteristics. Some of these differences are highly apparent in follicles undergoing atresia. Indeed, reduction in mitotic index and cytolysis, which is preceded by nuclear pyknosis, karyorrhexis, and karyolysis, are first observed in granulosa cells farthest from the oocyte. In contrast, these same changes are observed much later (i.e., only after atresia is far advanced) in cells adjacent to the oocyte or in the cumulus.

Significantly, the preceding sequence of events, terminating in cytolysis, is not always the initial response of granulosa cells in follicles undergoing atresia. In some instances, granulosa cells from the membrana granulosa are exfoliated and float free in antral fluid. In other cases, granulosa cells undergo luteinization,[102] resulting in the formation of corpora lutea atretica containing oocytes in various stages of degeneration. The frequency with which this phenomenon is observed in the ovaries of pregnant women indicates that it may well be related to the unique ovarian hormonal milieu characteristic of gestation. Regardless of the initial changes, granulosa cells are ultimately replaced by fibroblasts in follicles undergoing atresia. The antrum is invaded by capillaries and fibroblasts and ultimately collapses, with the zona pellucida frequently being the last of the follicular components to disappear. All components inside the basal lamina of follicles are ultimately replaced by avascular scars (corpora albicantia), thereby completing the process of absorption and obliteration.

Theca cells hypertrophy outside the basal lamina of follicles undergoing atresia, which is sometimes referred to as theca cell luteinization. Ultimately, these theca cells are thought to become part of the interstitial cell pool and thus are morphologically indistinguishable from other stromal cells. These secondary interstitial cells retain the capacity to hypertrophy in response to stimulation with LH/hCG, particularly during pregnancy.

Although the precise cellular mechanisms underlying atresia remain unknown,[103] a large body of information appears to implicate theca-interstitial cell–derived androgens in this connection.[104] According to this view, LH-supported theca-interstitial cell androgen biosynthesis may produce adverse androgen receptor–mediated effects in the adjacent granulosa cells.[105] That androgens may promote atresia has been suggested by experiments in which treatment with antisera to either LH[106] or androstenedione[107] resulted in increased ovulation rates, which is presumed to involve diminished atresia in graafian follicles. Moreover, systemic (or perhaps intraovarian) hyperandrogenism, resulting from small doses of hCG or testosterone, inhibits granulosa cell proliferation and increases atresia in preantral follicles of estrogen-primed immature female rats. In vitro, Billig and colleagues[108] have shown that treatment of granulosa cells with testosterone results in increased DNA ladder formation, consistent with the notion that androgens

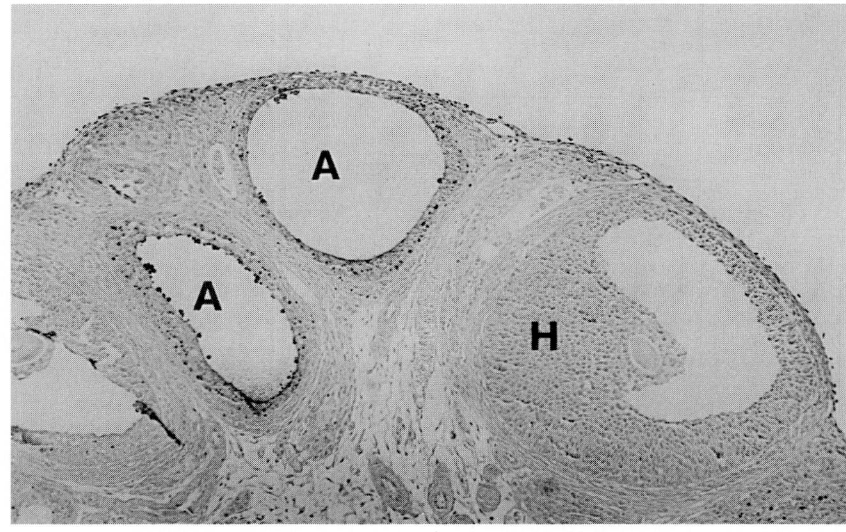

Figure 6–18 ■ Photomicrograph of a section of a rat ovary during atresia. The histologic technique stains nuclei that are undergoing apoptosis. Note staining of nuclear fragments in the atretic follicles. H, healthy follicle; A, atretic follicle. (From Palumbo A. and Yeh J. In situ localization of apoptosis in the rat ovary during follicular atresia. Biol Reprod 51:888–895, 1994.)

are promoters of apoptosis in the process of follicular atresia. Thus, in the absence of gonadotropic support, the primary effect of androgens on estrogen-stimulated preantral follicles is follicular atresia. This antiestrogenic effect of androgens is expected, because androgens reduce the ovarian concentration of estrogen receptors. Follicular atresia can also be induced by the withdrawal of estrogenic support from immature hypophysectomized rats.

OPERATIONAL CHARACTERISTICS

Steroidogenesis

The human fetal ovary is not steroidogenically quiescent.[109–112] It has been shown that the fetal human ovary possesses not only cholesterol side-chain cleavage activity but also 17α-hydroxylase as well as 17,20-desmolase activities.[113–115] Limited information is available on the steroidogenic function of the fetal ovary.[116] However, the operational characteristics of the adult ovary have been the subject of intense investigation. In the following section, we describe some characteristics of adult ovarian steroidogenesis.

The steroid hormone content of ovarian vein effluents and peripheral venous blood were compared to distinguish steroids secreted by the ovary from those secreted by the adrenal and from those produced by peripheral conversion of precursors.[117] These studies revealed that the ovaries secrete pregnenolone, progesterone, 17α-hydroxyprogesterone, dehydroepiandrosterone, androstenedione, testosterone, estrone, and estradiol-17β.[118, 119] Although such measurements provide insights to the steroidogenic pathways under study, they do not identify the specific ovarian cells involved. To make these distinctions, steroid hormones have been identified and quantified from whole (sliced or minced) ovaries, microdissected follicles, or ovarian cell suspensions. It is this combined body of knowledge that underlies our current understanding of adult ovarian steroidogenesis.

Studies using microdissected follicles identified estrone and estradiol as the major steroid products. Progesterone and 17α-hydroxyprogesterone proved to be the major products of the corpus luteum. Studies using steroid precursors revealed that the isolated granulosa cell is capable of producing mostly progesterone and estrogens, along with 17α-hydroxyprogesterone.[120–122] In contrast, isolated theca cells produced progesterone, 17α-hydroxyprogesterone, and androstenedione.[121, 123]

Estrogen Biosynthesis

Granulosa cells are the source of the two most important ovarian steroids, estradiol and progesterone. Although granulosa cells are capable of producing progesterone independently, the biosynthesis of estrogens requires cooperation between the granulosa cells and their thecal neighbors. The participation of these two cell types and of the two gonadotropins (FSH and LH) in ovarian estrogen biosynthesis underlies the concept of the two-cell/two-gonadotropin hypothesis, that an integrative process is required for ovarian estrogen biosynthesis (Fig. 6–19). According to this view, theca-derived, LH-dependent androgens are aromatized by FSH-inducible granulosa cells. Indeed, ovarian estrone and estradiol derive from the aromatization of their androgen precursors, androstenedione and testosterone, respectively. A broader view of this concept could include intercellular exchanges of other steroidogenic substrates.

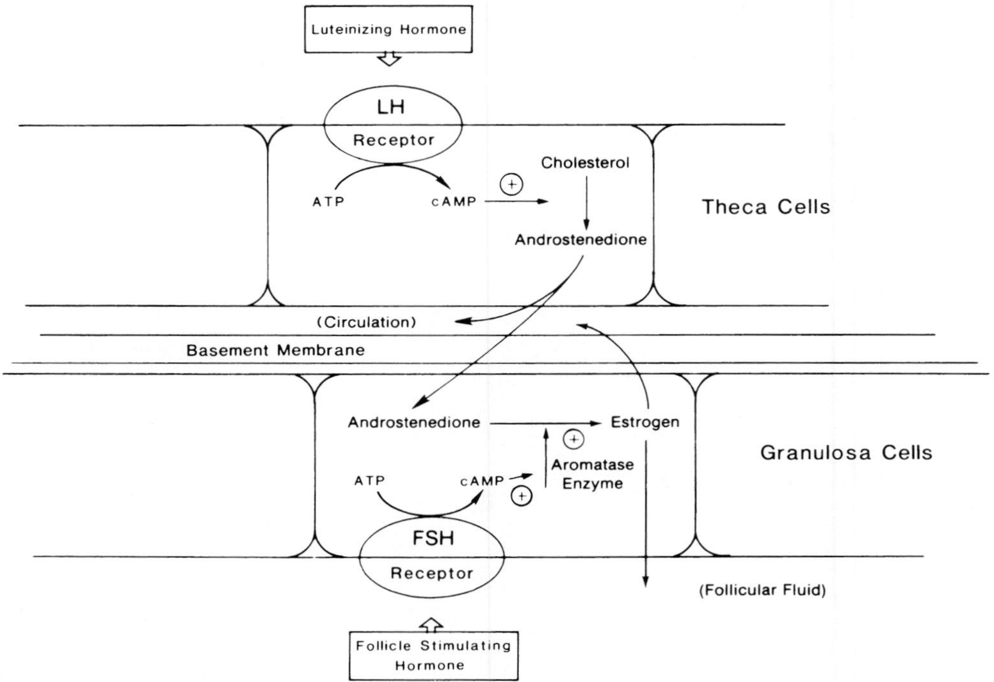

Figure 6–19 ■ The two-cell/two-gonadotropin hypothesis of follicular estrogen production. FSH, follicle-stimulating hormone; ATP, adenosine triphosphate; cAMP, cyclic adenosine monophosphate.

Indeed, some studies suggest that intercellular exchanges of steroids occur at multiple levels.

That follicular estrogen biosynthesis requires both the granulosa and theca-interstitial cells was first discovered by Falck.[124] The biochemical basis of this two-cell/two-gonadotropin theory was provided by Ryan and Petro,[23] whose findings revealed that the theca-interstitial cells are the producers of C_{19} androgens. The granulosa cells are the primary cellular site of aromatization. Moreover, Ryan and colleagues[125] found that the conversion of acetate to estrogen is substantially enhanced by the coincubation of granulosa and theca cells. Bjersing[126] summarized the process as "C_{19} precursor steroids are elaborated by theca-interstitial cells and are transferred across the basement membrane of the follicle to the granulosa cells where they are aromatized to estrogens."

In keeping with these conclusions, studies of isolated granulosa cells revealed that FSH, but not LH, stimulates estrogen production when the cells are provided with aromatizable androgenic substrate. In contrast, isolated theca did not produce significant amounts of estrogens under any experimental circumstances. Indeed, aromatase activity of granulosa cells was estimated to be at least 700 times greater in large preovulatory follicles than in theca cells.[127] These results are consistent with the hypothesis that granulosa cells are the principal site of estrogen biosynthesis in the dominant preovulatory follicle. These observations suggest that androgen, mainly androstenedione, produced by LH-stimulated theca cells is the main substrate for estrogen biosynthesis by FSH-stimulated granulosa cells (see Fig. 6–19). Although estrone is produced from androstenedione, it is readily converted to estradiol by the granulosa cell–based steroidogenic enzyme 17β-hydroxysteroid dehydrogenase.[128] Aromatization involves the loss of the C-19 methyl group and the stereospecific elimination of the 1β and 2β hydrogens of the A ring of the androgen precursor. A total of three hydroxylation reactions are required per estrogen formed.

As illustrated in Figure 6–19, both LH and FSH hormonal action appears to require the membrane-associated enzyme adenylate cyclase.[129] Indeed, gonadotropin-mediated stimulation of adenylate cyclase results in the conversion of intracellular adenosine triphosphate to cyclic adenosine monophosphate (cAMP). In turn, cAMP is thought to bind to the regulatory subunit of a protein kinase (commonly referred to as kinase A); the catalytic subunit of the enzyme is activated and dissociated, which in turn phosphorylates key intracellular proteins central to signal transduction.

Progestin Biosynthesis

The granulosa cell, like the theca-interstitial cell, is amply endowed for progestin biosynthesis. Central to this process is the availability of abundant supplies of cholesterol, which serves as the starting material for steroidogenic biosynthesis. Studies have shown that cholesterol used for membrane synthesis and steroid hormone production is derived primarily from circulating serum lipoproteins[130] rather than from de novo cellular synthesis from acetate[131] (Fig. 6–20). LDL is known to bind to specific membrane receptors, with the LDL-receptor complexes entering the cell by endocytosis.[132, 133] Thereafter, the endocytotic vesicles are known to fuse to lysosomes, where LDL cholesterol esters are hydrolyzed to yield free cholesterol.[134] The free cholesterol, in turn, is re-esterified and is stored in the cytoplasm in lipid droplets. When needed, the cholesterol ester is hydrolyzed and the free cholesterol transported to mitochondria for steroidogenic synthesis.

The importance of LDL cholesterol for ovarian progesterone secretion is demonstrated by the observation that LDL is required for maximal progesterone secretion by cultured cells.[135] High-density lipoprotein does not support human ovarian progesterone biosynthesis. Thus, the availability of LDL to various ovarian compartments could influence steroid hormone production. For example, human follicular fluid contains little or no LDL, thereby limiting the ability of preovulatory granulosa cells to produce progesterone.[136] However, after ovulation, vascularization of the corpus luteum provides the means by which LDL is

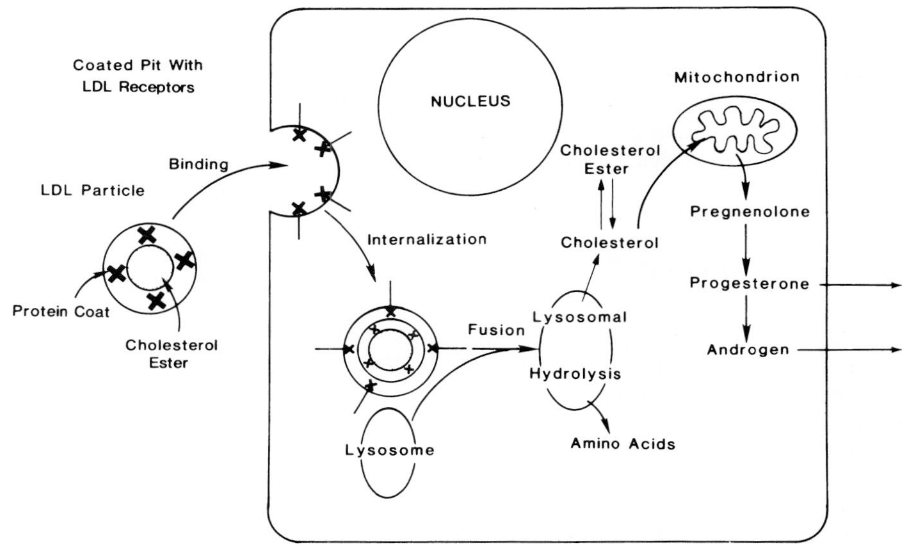

Figure 6–20 ■ Circulating low-density lipoprotein (LDL) constitutes the major source of cellular cholesterol substrate for steroidogenesis. Circulating LDL particles, containing a cholesterol ester core surrounded by a protein coat, bind to specific cell membrane receptors. The LDL-receptor complex is internalized and fuses to lysosomes. The cholesterol ester is hydrolyzed to cholesterol and the protein coat to amino acids.

delivered to the luteinized granulosa cells, thereby allowing progesterone biosynthesis.

Although lipoproteins constitute the most abundant source, endogenously produced cholesterol may also be employed in steroid biosynthesis.[137, 138] Cholesterol is converted to pregnenolone through the rate-limiting step of cholesterol side-chain cleavage in the mitochondria.[139] The subsequent conversion of pregnenolone to progesterone occurs readily by the relatively abundant cytoplasmic enzymes 3β-hydroxysteroid dehydrogenase/Δ^4,Δ^5-isomerase.[140] Although the human granulosa cell has been reported to contain low levels of 17α-hydroxylase activity and thus have ability to convert progesterone to 17α-hydroxyprogesterone, the significance of this finding remains uncertain. Little is known with respect to the functional role, if any, of the steroidogenic enzymes 20α-hydroxysteroid dehydrogenase and 5α-reductase in human granulosa cells.

Androgen Biosynthesis

Studies of isolated human theca reveal that the thecal layer is the major cellular source of follicular androgen. In addition, it is LH rather than FSH that stimulates thecal androgen production.[141] In contrast, androgen production by isolated cultured human granulosa cells is negligible, with or without added gonadotropins.

The biosynthesis of C_{19} androgens is the domain of the theca-interstitial cell. Accordingly, this cell type is amply endowed with the machinery to produce the progestin precursors. More important, however, the theca-interstitial cell is amply endowed with 17α-hydroxylase/17,20-desmolase activity,[142] which is capable of converting the precursors pregnenolone and progesterone to the C_{19} steroids dehydroepiandrosterone and androstenedione, respectively. Consequently, the presence of 17α-hydroxylase/17,20-desmolase activity can be viewed as an exclusive feature of the ovarian theca-interstitial cell.

Protein Biosynthesis

There is little doubt that the granulosa and theca-interstitial cells are capable of elaborating a large number of proteins. The identity of most of the proteins remains a mystery. On the other hand, a measurable number of identifiable proteins have been studied and are addressed in this chapter. Many, such as steroidogenic enzymes and cell surface receptors, are self-evident. Others receive mention in the appropriate context.

Established Ovarian Regulators

Improved understanding of regulatory phenomena in humans poses formidable experimental challenges. Although studies of subhuman primates constitute a highly satisfactory alternative, they are costly and technically difficult. Accordingly, reliance has been placed on nonprimate animal models that can more easily be acquired, maintained, and manipulated.[143, 144] In recognizing the utility of such an approach, one must also recognize the dangers inherent in extrapolating data from one species to another.

Signaling Systems

Steroid receptor profiles have been accurately determined for granulosa cells isolated from preantral follicles of immature hypophysectomized female rats.[145, 146] The cells contain proteins that specifically bind estrogens, androgens, and progestins.[147–155] These proteins possess characteristics similar to those of receptors found in the cells of other steroid-responsive tissues.[156] Moreover, in common with steroid-responsive cells in other tissues, estrogens and androgens accumulate in the nuclei of granulosa cells. As is the case for the granulosa cell, the actions of estrogens at the level of theca-interstitial cells are most likely receptor mediated. Stumpf[157] has demonstrated [^{3}H]estradiol uptake in nuclei of theca-interstitial and secondary interstitial cells. The role of receptors for other steroids in the theca-interstitial cells remains unknown.

Preantral granulosa cells are targeted primarily by FSH.[158] Negligible LH binding is observed in preantral granulosa cells.[159] The binding of LH and hCG is confined to thecal and interstitial cells.[160] Antral granulosa cells appear capable of binding both LH and FSH.[159] Thus, FSH receptors are found in granulosa cells from follicles of all sizes,[161] but LH receptors are found only in granulosa cells of large preovulatory follicles.[162–166] These observations are consistent with the notion that the acquisition of LH receptors is under the influence of FSH.[167, 168]

The complementary DNA sequence of the human FSH receptor has been determined, and it has been shown that this transmembrane protein is a G-protein–coupled receptor.[169, 170] It has been localized to the p21 region of chromosome 2.[171] The LH/hCG receptor has been cloned and has been determined to contain 701 amino acids. Sequence analysis demonstrated that this protein has a 341-residue extracellular domain and a 333-residue region containing seven transmembrane segments. This membrane-spanning region displays significant similarity with all members of the G protein receptor family. Analysis of the chromosomal structure of this protein demonstrates that this gene encompasses 70 kilobases and has 11 exons.[172]

Given the preceding, granulosa cells would be expected to respond, at the minimum, to estrogens, androgens, progestogens, FSH, and LH.[173] Similarly, the theca-interstitial cell can be expected to respond to LH and estrogens. In addition, ovarian cells are endowed with other receptor systems, which receive mention in the following.

Role of Follicle-Stimulating Hormone

As indicated by its name, FSH is the main promoter of follicular maturation. Given that FSH receptors have been exclusively localized to granulosa cells, it is generally presumed that FSH action in the ovary involves the granulosa cells. The ability of FSH to orchestrate follicular growth and differentiation depends on its ability to exert multiple actions concurrently.

In vivo rodent studies suggest that FSH is capable of increasing the number of its own receptors in the granulosa cell. Whereas estradiol by itself may be without effect on the distribution, number, or affinity of granulosa cell FSH receptors, estrogens have been shown to synergize with FSH to enhance the overall number of granulosa cell FSH receptors.[174] Consequently, changes in the production of estradiol by preantral follicles could increase their response to FSH through the regulation of the cell surface receptors.

There is little doubt that one of the major actions of FSH is the induction of granulosa cell aromatase activity.[175] Thus, little or no estrogen can be produced by FSH-unprimed granulosa cells even if they are supplied with aromatizable androgen precursors. On the other hand, treatment with FSH enhances the aromatization capability of granulosa cells, an effect due to an enhancement of the granulosa cell aromatase content.[176–178]

Treatment with FSH has also been shown to induce LH receptors in granulosa cells.[179] The ability of FSH to induce LH receptors is augmented by the concomitant presence of estrogens.[180] Furthermore, progestins, androgens, and LH itself may also induce LH receptors. Once induced, the granulosa cell LH receptor requires the continued presence of FSH for its maintenance.

Although estrogens are the most important mitogen for granulosa cells,[181] FSH may also promote granulosa cell division.[182] Treatment with FSH also increases the number of gap junctions as well as the amount of junctional membrane between granulosa cells.

Role of Luteinizing Hormone

LH plays a major role in the sustenance of corpus luteum function. In addition, a follicular role other than the induction of follicular rupture is also possible.[183] First, it is likely that LH plays a major role in the promotion of theca-interstitial cell androgen production. In addition, LH may well synergize with FSH in the more advanced phases of follicular development. Last, small and sustained increments in the circulating levels of LH are both necessary and sufficient to cause small antral follicles to grow and develop to the preovulatory stage.[184, 185] It is presumed that LH is acting on theca-interstitial cells of small follicles where it promotes androgen biosynthesis.[186] The consequent increase in estrogen production is presumed to contribute to the growth and development of the follicles. Treatment with small doses of LH also presumably results in an increase in the LH receptor content[187] as well as in the induction of the key steroidogenic enzyme 17α-hydroxylase/17,20-desmolase.

Role of Estrogens

In addition to their multiple systemic effects, estrogens exert a variety of critical actions at the level of the ovary.[188–197] Both granulosa and theca-interstitial cells appear to be sites of estrogen action. In the granulosa cell, estrogens promote cellular division[198–201] and exert an antiatretic effect.[202–204] In addition, estrogens play important roles in the promotion of intercellular gap junction formation,[205, 206] in the enhancement of antrum formation,[184] and in the increase in the estrogen receptor content.[207] Importantly, estrogens synergize with gonadotropins at several levels,[208] including the promotion of ovarian growth,[209–211] LH and FSH receptor formation, and enhancement of aromatase activity.[212] The ability of estrogens to increase the enzyme responsible for their own formation accounts for the exponential preovulatory rise in the circulating levels of estradiol. This form of self-amplification may also play a central role in the process of follicular selection as well as in the establishment of follicular dominance. However, in keeping with the complexity of intraovarian control mechanisms, estrogens can also inhibit ovarian androgen production directly by blocking the conversion of C_{21} progestins to C_{19} androgens.[213–217]

Role of Androgens

Aside from serving as substrates for estrogen production, androgens exert a variety of receptor-mediated effects in the granulosa cell.[218–221] Androgens possess the capacity to promote gonadotropin-stimulated granulosa cell aromatase activity.[222, 223] Thus, androgens augment FSH-stimulated aromatase activity by acting as a substrate and also by exerting a direct paracrine effect, which results in the up-regulation of this steroidogenic enzyme.[224] Androgens have also been shown to promote progestin biosynthesis.[225, 226] On the other hand, high follicular concentrations of 5α-reduced androgens such as dihydrotestosterone may act as competitive inhibitors of granulosa cell aromatase activity.[227]

In the absence of gonadotropins, androgens promote follicular atresia and antagonize estrogen-associated ovarian weight increases in hypophysectomized immature rats.[228] Similarly, treatment with dihydrotestosterone abolishes the ability of granulosa cells to have LH receptors induced by FSH.[229] It has been postulated that these and other androgenic effects may be due to an androgen receptor–mediated decrease in the ovarian estrogen receptor content. As such, these findings are in keeping with the observation that an increased androgen to estrogen ratio is associated with the morphologic features of atresia. Although androgens undoubtedly play regulatory roles in the theca-interstitial cells, no experimental information is available with respect to this.

Putative Intraovarian Regulators

The cyclic process of ovarian folliculogenesis is marked by dramatic proliferation and differentiation of the developing components of the maturing follicle. Although the central role of gonadotropins and of gonadal steroids is well accepted, the different fates of follicles suggest the existence of additional intraovarian modulatory systems.[230] Stated differently, it may be presumed that gonadotropin action may be "fine-tuned" in situ. This accounts for the observed differences in the rate and extent of development of ovarian follicles (e.g., not all follicles mature to the same extent before becoming atretic). Other phenomena such as initiation and arrest of meiosis or dominant follicle selection cannot be accounted for solely by altered gonadotropin release. Similarly, it is likely that the stages of follicular growth generally considered to be gonadotropin independent may involve intraovarian signaling.

The concept of local gonadal regulators dates to the time when the embryology of the ovary was the subject of intense scrutiny. Although other contributors must be acknowledged, the notion of intraovarian regulators was promoted with vigor by the late Cornelia Post Channing, whose pioneering experiments ushered in contemporary molecular endocrinology as it is applied to ovarian physiology.

Among potential intraovarian regulators, growth factors, cytokines, and neuropeptides have been the subject of intense investigation. Most of these agents are not expected to act in the traditional endocrine manner, given their local intraovarian production. Thus, current speculation favors the notion that a host of putative intraovarian regulators may, in fact, engage in subtle in situ modulation of the growth and function of the ovarian cell compartments. In this capacity, a given putative intraovarian regulator may modulate the proliferation or differentiation of a developing ovarian cell, acting either in its own right or as an amplifier or attenuator of gonadotropin action. Such putative intraovarian regulators may also be concerned with intercompartmental communication, allowing a tighter linking of different ovarian cell populations. For example, a growing body of evidence now suggests that granulosa cell–derived modulators may, in fact, regulate the adjacent theca-interstitial cell compartment to coordinate follicular development. In doing so, the granulosa cell may exert some control over its own destiny, in that it may regulate the inflow of androgen substrates from the neighboring theca.

According to contemporary views, potential intraovarian intercellular communication may take on one of the following configurations:

1. Paracrine communication, which involves diffusion of regulators from producer cells to distinct local target cells. This is a phenomenon involving more than one cell type.
2. Autocrine communication, which involves the action of a regulator on surface receptors at its cell of origin. This is a self-stimulatory phenomenon by which a single cell type serves as the site of regulator production, reception, and action.

To qualify as an intraovarian regulator, the putative regulatory agent needs to meet the minimal criteria of (1) local production, (2) local reception, and (3) local action. In addition, evidence of indispensability to in vivo ovarian function needs to be provided.

For the most part, few of the putative intraovarian regulators currently under study have satisfactorily met these criteria. Indeed, much remains to be learned about local intraovarian regulation. Accordingly, the information provided here can be viewed merely as a prelude to what the future holds. It is certain that novel factors will be added to this preliminary list, requiring modification of current views. The following is a brief listing of a select group of putative intraovarian regulators.

Insulin-like Growth Factor Family

Insulin-like growth factors (IGFs) constitute a family of essentially two homologous, low-molecular-weight, single-chain polypeptide growth factors named for their remarkable structural and functional similarity to insulin. IGF-I is a member of the so-called basic IGFs, peptides whose isoelectric point is anywhere between 8.1 and 8.5. A 70–amino acid polypeptide, IGF-I plays a variety of metabolic roles, not the least of which is the promotion of linear skeletal growth. IGF-I, now known to be ubiquitous, has been found to subserve a variety of tissue-specific functions in keeping with the needs dictated by the tissue in question. IGF-II is a 67–amino acid polypeptide that has 62 percent homology with IGF-I. IGF-II is expressed in both fetal and adult human tissues.

A large body of information now suggests that the ovary is a site of IGF production, reception, and action.[231] In the human, by use of in situ hybridization and immunohistochemistry, IGF-I has been described in preantral follicles; IGF-II has been localized to both preantral and dominant follicles.[232–234] For the IGF-I receptor, in situ studies demonstrated that it is present in the granulosa cells of dominant follicles. The IGF-II receptor is found in theca and granulosa cells. In follicular fluid, both IGF-I and IGF-II have been identified. The conclusions are that IGF-II is the principal IGF in humans[235] and that in small antral follicles, IGF-II is an autocrine agent in theca cells whereas it serves as a paracrine agent in granulosa cells.[232, 233] In the dominant follicles, IGF-II serves as a paracrine regulator. These observations suggest that IGFs may engage in intercompartmental communication in the interest of coordinated follicular development. Although multiple ovarian actions have been ascribed to the IGFs, their main projected role in humans is the amplification of gonadotropin hormonal action.

IGF hormonal action appears subject to further modulation through the local elaboration of low-molecular-weight binding proteins. Six IGF-binding proteins (IGFBPs) have been described and may regulate the effects of IGFs on ovarian function by their binding to the polypeptides or by direct effects on ovarian steroidogenesis. In humans, IGFBP-1 through IGFBP-5 have been identified either in follicular fluid or by analysis of messenger ribonucleic acid (mRNA) from granulosa cells.[236–239] The regulation of IGFBP expression is by both FSH and IGFs.[239] Thus, the IGF system in the human is complex and is subject to multiple sites of modulation.

In a patient with Laron dwarfism, which is characterized by low levels of IGF-I secondary to growth hormone receptor deficiency, ovulation induction with human menopausal gonadotropins after administration of a gonadotropin-releasing hormone (GnRH) analogue resulted in development of mature, fertilizable oocytes.[240] This case suggests that in the human, IGF-I is not an essential agent for normal follicular development.

At the clinical level, IGF-I may have a bearing on the puberty-promoting effect of growth hormone. An association appears to exist between isolated growth hormone deficiency and delayed puberty in both rodents and human subjects, a process reversed by systemic hormone replacement therapy.

Epidermal Growth Factor Family

Purified on the basis of its ability to stimulate precocious eyelid opening and tooth eruption in newborn mice, EGF was initially found in male mouse submaxillary glands and later in human urine as urogastrone. Mature EGF comprises a single polypeptide chain of 53 amino acids displaying three internal disulfide bonds. EGF was originally thought to have a limited range of tissue expression, but recent in situ hybridization analysis of sections of whole newborn mice indicates that RNA complementary to cloned EGF probes may be present in a large variety of tissues.

TGF-α, a structural analogue of EGF, is a single-chain, 50–amino acid polypeptide capable of binding to an apparently common EGF/TGF-α receptor.[241] Not only do EGF and TGF-α both recognize the same cellular receptor, they are apparently equally potent in most systems studied. TGF-α is a member of a family of polypeptides best known for their ability to produce an acute albeit reversible phenotypic transformation of normal mammalian cells. TGF-α can thus be defined operationally by its ability to stimulate anchorage-independent growth in soft agar of cells that are otherwise anchorage dependent.

At the level of the ovary, EGF has been observed to exert potent regulatory effects on granulosa cell proliferation and differentiation.[242–245] These effects of EGF are presumably mediated by specific cell membrane receptors, the existence of which has been demonstrated on bovine, ovine, and murine granulosa cells.[246, 247] TGF-α, like EGF, proved a potent inhibitor of gonadotropin-supported granulosa cell differentiation.

In humans, analyses of follicular fluid have demonstrated that TGF-α is present while EGF is present in low levels.[248] By immunohistochemistry, TGF-α and EGF have been found to be present in oocytes.[249, 250] TGF-α has been described in granulosa and theca cells of antral follicles and in the luteal cells of corpora lutea.[251] Their common receptor, the EGF receptor, has been found in granulosa cells, theca cells, and corpora lutea.[249] By in situ hybridization, EGF mRNA has not been detected in human ovaries; TGF-α has been found in theca and luteinized theca cells, and the EGF receptor has been localized to both follicles and corpora lutea.[252]

Transforming Growth Factor Family

Transforming growth factors are a family of 25-kDa polypeptides composed of two homodimeric chains. Three mammalian isoforms (TGF-β1, TGF-β2, and TGF-β3) have been identified, and they have up to 80 percent homology between them. They are now recognized as polyfunctional regulatory molecules.[253] Originally identified by its ability to elicit a reversible phenotypic transformation of normal mammalian cells, TGF-β has now been shown to exert numerous regulatory actions in a wide variety of both normal and neoplastic cells.[253] TGF-β uses two receptors for signal transduction, the type 1 and type 2 receptors. At the level of the ovary, TGF-β1 has been shown to profoundly alter the proliferation and differentiation of rat granulosa cells.[254–264] In addition, an increasing body of evidence now suggests that the ovarian theca-interstitial[265] as well as granulosa cells may be sites of TGF-β production and action.

In humans, TGF-β has been found in follicular fluids.[266] TGF-β1 and TGF-β2 mRNA has been demonstrated in granulosa cells. By immunohistochemistry, TGF-β1 has been demonstrated in oocytes, granulosa cells, and theca cells.[250, 267] The levels appear to increase with increasing follicular development. TGF-β2 has been localized to theca cells and small luteal cells of corpora lutea. In vitro, TGF-β1 and TGF-β2 appear to modulate inhibin and activin production in human granulosa-luteal cells.[268]

Inhibin and activin, two other members of the TGF-β protein superfamily, and the activin-binding protein follistatin are discussed briefly.

INHIBIN

Inhibin is a 32-kDa glycoprotein composed of two subunits, named α (18 kDa) and β (12 kDa), linked by disulfide bonds.[269] Structurally, inhibin is a heterodimer composed of a common α-subunit but different β-subunits, denoted β_A and β_B. The forms of inhibin, $\alpha\beta_A$ and $\alpha\beta_B$, are named A and B, respectively. Although inhibin is produced by a number of tissues in the body, the majority is derived from the gonads. In the ovary, the source of inhibin is granulosa cells. The main role for inhibin, for which it was discovered and named, is to suppress FSH production in the pituitary.

Although both isoforms of inhibin seem to have similar biologic properties, their synthesis is regulated differently during the follicular and luteal phases. Inhibin B is secreted mainly during the early follicular phase, with levels decreasing in midfollicular phase and becoming undetectable after the LH surge.[270] Inhibin A levels are low during the first half of the follicular phase but increase gradually during midfollicular phase with a peak during the luteal phase. By immunohistochemistry and in situ hybridization, all three subunits are expressed in small antral follicles.[271–273] In the dominant follicle and in the corpus luteum, the α and β_A subunits are found. The three subunits are found to be expressed in response to gonadotropins or factors that increase intracellular cAMP.[274, 275] The mechanisms underlying the differential synthesis of inhibin A and B during the different parts of the menstrual cycle need further study for a fuller understanding.

ACTIVIN

Activin, unlike inhibin, is composed of dimers of the β-subunits of inhibin ($\beta_A\beta_B$, $\beta_A\beta_A$, or $\beta_B\beta_B$).[276, 277] Activin was found in follicular fluid during the process of purification of inhibin and was named because of its stimulatory effects on FSH secretion in cultured pituitary cells. Unlike inhibin, activin may not play an endocrine role in the pituitary-gonadal axis in that almost all immunoreactive activin in human serum is bound to proteins (particularly follistatin). Bound activin is, therefore, unable to bind target cells. Variation in activin A during the normal menstrual cycle is less than that observed for inhibin. It has been reported that levels are highest during midcycle and the late luteal phase–early follicular phase.[278, 279] In addition, serum activin levels are significantly higher in pregnancy.[280] Granulosa cell–derived activin has also been shown to enhance the FSH-supported induction of granulosa cell LH receptors and, in theca cells, suppresses LH-stimulated androgen synthesis. In human granulosa cells, activin suppresses basal and gonadotropin-stimulated progesterone and estrogen production.[281]

FOLLISTATIN

Another protein is follistatin, a single-chain polypeptide (315 amino acids) originally isolated from porcine follicular fluid on the basis of its FSH-suppressing activity.[276, 282] Although structurally distinct from both inhibin and activin, this FSH-inducible granulosa cell–derived polypeptide appears to suppress the release of pituitary FSH, but not LH, in a manner reminiscent of inhibin. The interest in follistatin derives from the finding that it is an activin-binding protein that neutralizes activin bioactivity. In human granulosa cells, follistatin stimulates progesterone production, although it is not clear whether this is a direct effect of follistatin or a consequence of its binding of activin.[281] Serum concentrations of follistatin show that it is relatively constant through the menstrual cycle.[283, 284] Histologic studies show that follistatin is expressed in small antral and preovulatory follicles.[272]

Fibroblast Growth Factor Family

Basic FGF, a 146–amino acid polypeptide, is a mitogen for a wide variety of mesoderm-derived and neuroectoderm-derived cells. It belongs to the FGF family of at least five homologous polypeptides. For bFGF, an amino terminal truncated form lacking the first 15 residues has been identified in the ovarian corpus luteum.[285] Although the physiologic relevance of bFGF to ovarian function remains under investigation, several lines of evidence suggest that bFGF may play a central role in supporting the growth and development of the granulosa-luteal cell. Indeed, bFGF constitutes the main mitogenic factor isolated from crude luteal extract and has previously been shown to stimulate the replicative life span of cultured granulosa cells of bovine, porcine, rabbit, guinea pig, and human origin.[286–288]

In humans, bFGF is mitogenic for granulosa-luteal cells.[289] Messenger RNA for bFGF and the FGF receptor has been demonstrated in human granulosa cells.[290, 291] Functionally, it has been hypothesized that this polypeptide may modulate angiogenesis, proliferation, progesterone synthesis, and apoptosis in the ovary.[289, 292, 293]

Interleukins

Interleukin (IL)–1, a polypeptide cytokine predominantly produced and secreted by activated macrophages, has been shown to possess a wide range of biologic functions.[294–296] In the ovary, IL-1 has been observed to suppress the functional and morphologic luteinization of cultured murine and porcine granulosa cells.[297–301] Exerted at "physiologic" (10^{-9} M) concentrations, IL-1 action could not be attributed to altered cell viability. Rather, the antigonadotropic activity of IL-1 appeared to involve sites of action both proximal and distal to cAMP generation. Later work by Kasson and Gorospe[302] shed additional light on the ovarian relevance of interleukins. Both IL-1α and IL-1β augmented the FSH-stimulated accumulation of 20α-dihydroprogesterone. In all cases, less IL-1β than IL-1α was required to produce a comparable affect. IL-2 slightly, but significantly, enhanced both FSH-stimulated progesterone and 20α-dihydroprogesterone production but had no effect on FSH-stimulated estrogen production or LH/hCG receptor induction. IL-3 potentiated the 20α-dihydroprogesterone response to FSH by up to 65 percent but had no effect on FSH-stimulated progesterone or estrogen production or LH/hCG receptor induction. More recent studies suggest that the theca-interstitial cell may also be a site of IL-1 (but not IL-2) reception and action.

The circulating levels of IL-1 have been observed to be elevated during the luteal (but not preovulatory) phase of normally cycling women.[303] The possible role of progesterone in this regard is supported by the observation that IL-1 activity in human pelvic macrophages is subject to hormonal regulation by gonadal steroids.[304] Specifically, low concentrations of progesterone appear to up-regulate macrophage expression of the gene encoding IL-1.[305] In contrast, higher concentrations of progesterone significantly inhibit IL-1 activity.[305]

Although the relevance of IL-1 to ovarian physiology remains a matter of study, it is tempting to speculate that IL-1 could be the elusive intraovarian luteinization inhibitor, the putative suppressor of premature follicular luteinization. Such speculation is intriguing in light of the apparent progesterone dependence of IL-1 gene expression.[303] Regarding the intraovarian cellular origin of IL-1, resident interstitial ovarian macrophages could well be a site of hormonally regulated expression of the gene encoding IL-1 given the reported gonadotropin dependence of their testicular counterparts.[306–308]

In humans, significant amounts of IL-1–like activity have been detected in follicular fluid.[309, 310] Moreover, Kokia and Adashi[311] have demonstrated the existence of a highly compartmentalized, hormonally dependent intraovarian IL-1 system with ligands, receptor, and receptor antagonist. This suggests that the cytokine system is a potential actor in follicular function.

Tumor Necrosis Factor-α

The potential ovarian relevance of another macrophage product, tumor necrosis factor-α (TNF-α), has recently been explored.[49, 312–315] TNF-α, a 157–amino acid polypeptide, was originally named for its oncolytic activity as displayed in the serum of bacille Calmette-Guérin–immunized, endotoxin-challenged mice.[316, 317] Indeed, TNF-α proved capable of inducing tumor necrosis in vivo and of exerting nonspecies-specific cytolytic or cytostatic effects on a broad range of transformed cell lines in vitro. Although TNF-α was initially thought to be tumor selective, it has become clear that certain nontumor cells possess TNF-α receptors and that TNF-α may be a regulatory monokine with pleiotropic noncytotoxic activities in addition to its antitumor properties. Most important, TNF-α has been shown to engage in the differentiation of a variety of cell types.

At the level of the ovary, TNF-α was found capable of attenuating the differentiation of cultured granulosa cells from immature rats through virtual neutralization of FSH hormonal action at sites proximal but not distal to cAMP generation.[310, 314] In other studies, TNF-α has been found to effect complex dose-dependent alterations in the elaboration of progesterone and androstenedione but not of estrogen by explanted preovulatory follicles of murine origin.[313]

TNF-α may be locally derived from activated resident ovarian macrophages, as has been shown for regressing (but not young) corpora lutea. Although basal TNF-α activity was undetectable in corpora lutea of both pregnancy and pseudopregnancy, TNF-α activity was markedly stimulated in the presence of lipopolysaccharide.[49] However, the detection of TNF-α activity in some luteal tissue on day 5 and the scarcity of macrophages at this stage raise the possibility that cells other than macrophages may also produce TNF-α in the corpus luteum.

In humans, TNF-α has been demonstrated in the antral layer of granulosa cells and in follicular fluid.[318] Atretic follicles also contained TNF-α, as did corpora lutea. In vitro, human granulosa-lutein cells have been shown to produce TNF-α in response to FSH.

Catecholaminergic Input

Evidence suggests that ovarian theca-interstitial cells may be the recipients of direct sympathetic innervation by noradrenergic nerve terminals.[319–330] Electrical stimulation of the ovarian plexus of hypophysectomized rats has been shown to morphologically transform theca-interstitial cells to assume ultrastructural features typical of active steroid-secreting cells.[331] In contrast, ovarian denervation has been shown to result in a decrease in the activity of 3β-hydroxysteroid dehydrogenase in the pregnant rat.[332] Moreover, murine theca-interstitial cells can produce androgens under catecholaminergic stimulation.[333] Perhaps most significant is that electrical stimulation of the hypothalamus in hypophysectomized and adrenalectomized rats results in the alteration of ovarian steroid biosynthesis, independent of changes in ovarian blood flow.[334] These findings suggest the existence of an independent central nervous system–ovarian neural axis distinct from and parallel to the hypothalamic-pituitary-ovarian hormonal axis.

In the granulosa cell, catecholamines activate the cAMP transduction sequence, resulting in the promotion of progesterone, but not estrogen, synthesis.[335–343] It is difficult to envision how the follicle-enclosed granulosa cells could be subjected to catecholaminergic modulation. Although diffusion across the basement membrane cannot be excluded, it appears more likely that the adrenergic innervation of the ovary targets the theca-interstitial rather than the nonluteinized granulosa cell.

The potential role of catecholamines in ovarian androgen biosynthesis has received relatively limited attention. This is perplexing given the large body of evidence documenting direct sympathetic innervation of the theca-interstitial compartment. In the rat, the noradrenergic nerve supply to the ovary constitutes an outflow of the sympathetic nervous system originating from the lower thoracic region of the spinal cord. Reaching the ovary by the superior ovarian nerve and the ovarian plexus along the ovarian artery, noradrenergic nerve fibers invest the ovarian blood vessels and exhibit a network of varicosities around secondary interstitial and theca-interstitial cells. The nonvascular innervation of the ovary is provided by the superior ovarian nerve, whereas the plexus nerve originates mainly perivascular fibers.

The theca-interstitial cell is a site of catecholamine reception and action.[332, 333] Specifically, it appears that catecholamines, acting through β_2-selective adrenergic recognition sites, possess the ability to synergize with gonadotropins in the promotion of ovarian androgen production. It is likely that adrenergically supported androgen production may play a role in the regulation of granulosa cell estrogen production, thereby participating in the process of follicular recruitment and selection. In addition, it is conceivable that excessive activation of thecal adrenergic receptors may play a role in the pathogenesis of conditions associated with ovarian hyperandrogenism. Indeed, histochemical evaluation of ovarian tissue obtained from patients with the polycystic ovary syndrome revealed markedly enhanced innervation of the theca-interstitial cell compartment.[344] Thus, although the theca-interstitial cells are structurally and functionally intact, the genesis and maintenance of the polycystic ovary syndrome may be explained by enhanced adrenergic exposure of the ovarian androgen-producing cell. This is in keeping with the observation that psychologic stress may be more prevalent in women with the polycystic ovary syndrome and that direct central nervous system input may be at work.[345]

Other Peptides

THE OVARIAN RENIN-ANGIOTENSIN SYSTEM

Renin is a protease capable of cleaving its substrate angiotensinogen to form angiotensin I. Angiotensin I, in turn, is converted to angiotensin II by angiotensin-converting enzymes. Angiotensin II is viewed as the main active peptide of the renin-angiotensin system. Evidence suggests the existence of an intrinsic ovarian renin-angiotensin system.[346] The activity of the ovarian renin-angiotensin system fluctuates in the course of the normal cycle, reaching a peak at around midcycle. Similarly, angiotensin II receptors display cyclic variation. It has been suggested that the high preovulatory levels of angiotensin II in follicular fluid may be involved in the maturation of the oocyte and in ovulation either directly or through other ovarian regulators. It has also been suggested that angiotensin II may play a role in the formation of the corpus luteum as well as in the regulation of steroid secretion by luteal cells.

CORTICOTROPIN-RELEASING FACTOR

Corticotropin-releasing factor (CRF) mRNA and protein have been localized in the thecal and stromal cells of human ovaries.[347] Granulosa cells appear to be negative for this protein. In addition, the receptor for CRF was detected in the theca cells but not in stroma or granulosa cells. Finally, CRF-binding protein immunostaining, but not mRNA, was detected in thecal and stromal cells. Thus, CRF may serve as an autocrine or paracrine regulator in the thecal-stromal compartment of the human ovary.

LUTEINIZATION INHIBITOR

The existence of luteinization inhibitor, still a speculative entity, has been strongly suggested by the ability of granulosa cells from large preovulatory (but not small) follicles to undergo spontaneous luteinization in vitro.[348] Presumably, then, luteinization inhibitor may be provided by granulosa cells from small follicles, larger preovulatory follicles being inactive in this regard.

OOCYTE MATURATION INHIBITOR

Although the exact biochemical nature of oocyte maturation inhibitor remains a mystery, its existence has been proposed in an effort to address the otherwise enigmatic process of meiotic arrest. Indeed, little is known with respect to the mechanisms responsible for holding the mammalian oocyte in abeyance in the late diplotene stage. That an inhibitor is involved is suggested by the fact that the removal of an oocyte from its intrafollicular environment will result in the spontaneous resumption of meiosis once it is in culture.[349–351] Because oocyte maturation inhibitor inhibits the resumption of meiosis only when it is applied to cumulus-oocyte complexes, it appears likely that oocyte inhibition requires the intermediacy of the surrounding granulosa cumulus cells.

GONADOTROPIN SURGE-INHIBITING FACTOR

Gonadotropin surge-inhibiting factor refers to a nonsteroidal substance that inhibits the surge of LH and FSH secretion induced by either estradiol or GnRH. The activity of gonadotropin surge-inhibiting factor is distinct from that of inhibin, which selectively suppresses pituitary release of FSH but not of LH. That the substance under study is short-lived and of ovarian origin was shown by the return of normal pituitary responsiveness within 30 minutes after bilateral oophorectomy.

CYCLICITY

Follicular Growth and Development: Recruitment, Selection, and Dominance

Recruitment is the term used to indicate that a follicle has entered the so-called growth trajectory, that is, the process by which the follicle departs from the resting pool to begin a well-characterized pattern of growth and development. It is recognized that growing follicles are vulnerable to atresia and thus may depart from the trajectory at any point. Consequently, recruitment, although obligatory, does not guarantee ovulation. Stated differently, recruitment is a necessary but not a sufficient condition for ovulation to occur.

Selection refers to the process by which the maturing follicular cohort is decreased to a size equal to the species-specific ovulatory quota. Accordingly, selection is complete when the number of healthy follicles, those with ovulatory potential, in the cohort equals the size of the ovulatory quota. Like recruitment, selection does not guarantee ovulation. However, given its greater temporal proximity to ovulation, selection may, with high probability, be expected to be followed by ovulation in a typical cycle.

During the late luteal phase, the largest healthy follicle may not be the one selected because smaller follicles may harbor granulosa cells with a mitotic index greater than that of the presumptive leading follicle. Consequently, the apparent growth delay of nonleading follicles could well be compensated for in a matter of days, with the final selection occurring in the early part of the subsequent follicular phase. However, even in the early follicular phase, no morphologic differences exist between the selected follicle and other healthy members of the cohort. This notwithstanding, the leading follicle can be distinguished from other members of the cohort by its sheer size and the high mitotic index of its granulosa cells. Moreover, only the leading follicle can at this point boast detectable levels of FSH in its follicular fluid. This same follicle also displays significant follicular levels of estradiol. Indeed, it is generally agreed that the capacity to aromatize androgens efficiently is an important determinant of the chosen follicle. Most important, the follicle destined to ovulate displays a granulosa cell mitotic index that is high enough to ensure that smaller albeit healthy follicles are unlikely to catch up.

Dominance refers to the status of the follicle destined to ovulate given its presumed key role in regulating the size of the ovulatory quota. The selected follicle becomes dominant about a week before ovulation. Consequently, it must maintain its dominance during the week before ovulation. Stated differently, the follicle selected for ovulation is functionally (not merely morphologically) dominant in that it is presumed to inhibit the development of other competing follicles on both ovaries. Inevitably, the dominant follicle (i.e., the sole follicle destined to ovulate) continues to thrive under circumstances it has made inhospitable for others.[352–354]

The preceding and related concepts were formulated in large measure by the seminal work of Hodgen.[355] There is little doubt that this work affected the thinking of ovarian physiologists grappling with the difficult issues of ovarian cyclicity. A crucial series of experiments were made by Goodman and Hodgen[356] in which it was observed that cauterization of the largest visible follicle on days 8 to 12 in the primate delayed the expected time of the next preovulatory surge of pituitary gonadotropins (Fig. 6–21). In contrast, luteectomy during the midluteal phase (days 16 to 19) advanced the expected time of the next preovulatory gonadotropin surge.[357] Similar observations were made in women when the interval from ablation of the dominant follicle or corpus luteum to the next ovulation proved to be 14 days.[358] As such, these findings are consistent with the hypothesis that the ovary itself may play a "time giver" role during the menstrual cycle and that this time-keeping function is subserved by the activities of the cyclic structures of the dominant ovary. The 28-day menstrual cycle is thus the result of the intrinsic life span of the cyclic ovarian dominant structures and not the result of timed changes dictated by the brain or pituitary. The dominant follicle therefore determines the length of the follicular phase, with the corpus luteum determining the length of the luteal phase.[358] Similar conclusions might be extended to the human.

The preceding finding also suggested that the selection of the follicle destined to ovulate had already occurred by the time of cautery (i.e., by day 8 of the cycle). Indeed, it would appear that no other member of the follicular cohort was competent to serve as a surrogate for the cauterized follicle to achieve a timely, midcycle ovulation. Thus, the dominant follicle may play a key role in regulating the size of the ovulatory quota by inhibiting the development of any competing follicles in either ovary. A similar function is served by the corpus luteum. Thus, the ovulatory follicle, once selected in midfollicular phase, and the corpus luteum are the dominant ovarian structures. Accordingly, the next round of follicular growth occurs only after the interference by the cyclic structure is removed either naturally after the demise of the corpus luteum or artificially by experimental intervention. Further insight was gained from studies in which progesterone-replaced luteectomized primates were evaluated. These studies revealed progesterone to be the principal luteal hormone responsible for the inhibition of

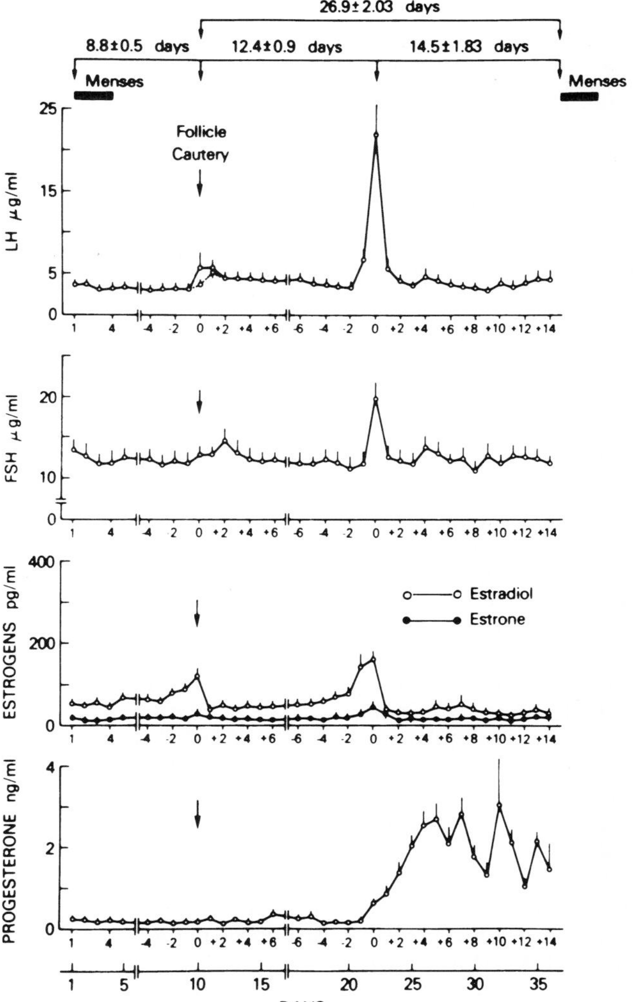

Figure 6–21 ■ Hormonal patterns before and after cautery of the largest visible follicle in rhesus monkeys. (From Goodman AL, Nixon WE, Johnson DK, Hodgen GD. Regulation of folliculogenesis in the cycling rhesus monkey: Selection of the dominant follicle. Endocrinology 100:155–161, 1977. © The Endocrine Society.)

luteal follicular growth. Circulating gonadotropin levels were apparently maintained after follicular or luteal ablation, and follicle recruitment occurred without an attendant increase in circulating gonadotropins. Thus, the inhibition of follicular growth by the cyclic structures of the ovary was not due to a decrease in the circulating levels of gonadotropins. Rather, it appeared to be due to local intraovarian influences.

Further insight was derived from experiments revealing that the follicle destined to ovulate attains dominance 5 to 7 days after the demise of the corpus luteum. This conclusion was based on the observation that the levels of estradiol in ovarian veins were significantly different between ovaries by days 5 to 7 of the cycle. This difference in estrogen levels between ovaries provides the earliest hormonal index attesting to the emergence of the dominant follicle.

Follicles with a diameter of less than 8 mm show a relatively low intrafollicular estrogen to androgen ratio. However, from the midfollicular phase onward, this ratio is reversed. With its increased capacity to aromatize androstenedione, the chosen follicle is able to synthesize estradiol in sufficient quantities to result in appreciable passage of this hormone into the general circulation, thereby resulting in asymmetry of ovarian function as early as days 5 to 7 of the cycle.[359] In the late follicular phase, the intrafollicular concentrations of estradiol are maximal at a time when the circulating estradiol levels surge to a peak. With the ovulatory LH surge, the intrafollicular concentrations of estradiol decrease along with a parallel decrease in the intrafollicular concentrations of androstenedione. Concurrently, progressive increases have been noted for the intrafollicular content of both progesterone and 17α-hydroxyprogesterone, reflecting early granulosa cell luteinization.[360]

Antral fluid concentrations of estrone, estradiol, androstenedione, testosterone, and progesterone have been measured in specimens collected from ovarian follicles of women undergoing surgery.[361–364] Results of such studies have been reasonably consistent; data from one laboratory have been adapted for graphic display in Figure 6–22. Despite large differences, the mean antral concentrations of steroid hormones tended to vary with the time in the cycle and with the size of the follicle. Throughout the cycle, antral fluid levels of androgens and estrogens vary, with higher ratios of androgens to estrogens in smaller follicles than in larger follicles. The concentration of progesterone is elevated in large follicles sampled late in the follicular phase. Thus, higher antral concentrations of estrogens and progestogens and lower concentrations of androgens constitute a characteristic steroid hormone profile of preovulatory follicles.[365] In contrast, hormone profiles of smaller follicles sampled late in the follicular phase have been characterized by higher concentrations of androgens and lower concentrations of estrogens and progesterone. Although the data do not establish whether antral fluid steroid hormone profiles determine the ovulatory follicle, they do establish that the profiles of individual follicles are distinctive. In other words, mechanisms exist for regulating the antral fluid steroid hormone milieu in individual human ovarian follicles.

Because steroid secretion depends on gonadotropin stimulation, the antral fluid levels of gonadotropin were also evaluated.[366] In one study in which antral fluid FSH, LH, and prolactin levels were determined, evidence for follicle size- and cycle time–associated differences was noted. LH was detected in the antral fluid of only 16 percent of smaller follicles but in 70 percent of larger follicles around midcycle. FSH levels were measurable in antral fluid from both small and large follicles. However, in relation to serum FSH levels, antral FSH concentrations tended to be higher in larger follicles. It was also observed that estradiol levels were higher in antral fluids marked by measurable levels of FSH. Thus, antral fluid levels of FSH and estradiol are positively correlated. Moreover, incubation with FSH induces aromatase activity in granulosa cells recovered from follicles with low antral fluid estradiol levels, usually follicles less than 8 to 10 mm in diameter. It was therefore postulated that the presence or absence of measurable FSH was responsible for differences observed in antral fluid ratios of androgen to estrogen.

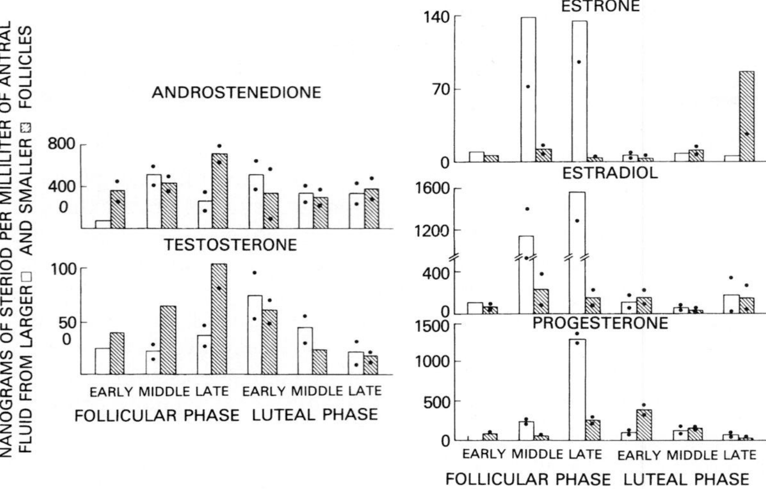

Figure 6–22 ■ Steroidal content of follicular fluid recovered from larger *(clear bars)* and smaller *(hatched bars)* antral follicles sampled at the indicated time during the menstrual cycle. (Adapted from McNatty KP, Hunter WM, McNeilley AS, Sawers PS. Changes in the concentration of pituitary and steroid hormones in the follicular fluid of human graafian follicles throughout the menstrual cycle. J Endocrinol 64:1, 1975. © The Endocrine Society.)

Taken together, these data are consistent with the concept that hormone concentrations are regulated in the microenvironment of individual follicles. Moreover, a functional role was assigned to the hormonal composition of the microenvironment when it was shown that it affected progesterone synthesis by isolated granulosa cells in vitro. Thus, granulosa cells exposed to antral fluid containing FSH, LH, and estradiol in vivo secreted more progesterone than did cells isolated from follicles devoid of and thus unexposed to these hormones.[367]

Ovulation

As midcycle approaches, there is a dramatic rise in estrogen, followed by an LH and to a lesser extent an FSH surge. This triggers the dominant follicle to ovulate. For reasons not well understood, but possibly because of unique microenvironmental circumstances, one follicle ovulates and gives rise to a corpus luteum during each menstrual cycle. In the human, both LH and hCG have been shown to stimulate rupture of mature follicles. However, in hypophysectomized rats, highly purified FSH can serve as the "ovulatory hormone" after follicular maturation has been stimulated by the administration of FSH and LH. Inhibitors of prostaglandin synthesis (introduced systemically or locally into the antrum) have been shown to inhibit ovulation in rats and rabbits. Because LH has been shown to stimulate prostaglandin biosynthesis by ovarian follicles,[368–376] increased prostaglandin synthesis might mediate the ovulatory stimulus of LH.

Mechanically, ovulation consists of rapid follicular enlargement followed by protrusion of the follicle from the surface of the ovarian cortex. Ultimately, rupture of the follicle results in the extrusion of an oocyte-cumulus complex. In the human ovary, this sequence may well begin 5 to 6 days before the onset of the preovulatory LH surge. However, it is the latter event that marks the end of the follicular phase of the cycle and precedes actual rupture by as much as 36 hours.

Fortuitous endoscopic visualization of the ovary around the time of ovulation reveals that elevation of a conical "stigma" on the surface of the protruding follicle precedes rupture[377] (Fig. 6–23). Rupture of this stigma is accompanied by gentle rather than explosive expulsion of the oocyte and antral fluid, which suggests that the fluid is not under high pressure.[378, 379] Indeed, direct measurements have demonstrated that intrafollicular pressure is low in preovulatory follicles.[380]

Several hypotheses have been advanced to account for the rapid increase in size and rupture of the follicle. Consideration has to be given to changes in the composition of the antral fluid during the period of rapid preovulatory follicular enlargement. In addition, an increase in colloid osmotic pressure has been noted. Although the granulosa cell–derived proteoglycans play a role in regulating the colloid osmotic pressure, little information is available about their involvement.[381–384] Thus, a cause and effect relationship between the altered composition of antral fluid

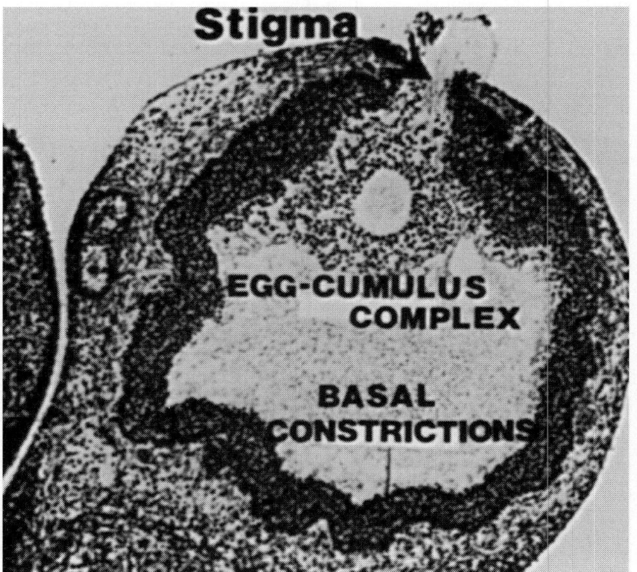

Figure 6–23 ■ Ovulation of the cumulus-oocyte complex through the stigma. (From Erickson GF. An analysis of follicle development and ovum maturation. Semin Reprod Endocrinol 4:233, 1986. Thieme Medical Publishers, New York. Reproduced by permission.)

and the enlargement and rupture of the follicle remains to be established. Alternatively, stigma formation and rupture may reflect the effects of enzymes acting locally on protein substrates in the basal lamina.[385, 386] In keeping with this theory, instillation of protease inhibitors into the antral fluid inhibits ovulation. One such proteolytic enzyme, plasminogen activator, has been localized in increasing concentrations in the walls of rat ovarian follicle just before ovulation.[387] Plasminogen activator, a serine protease, stimulates the conversion of plasminogen, a follicular fluid constituent, into the proteolytically active enzyme plasmin. This is known to activate collagenase, presumptively obligatory in the dissolution of the basal membrane and the perifollicular stroma in ovulation. Thus, plasminogen activator–mediated conversion of plasminogen to plasmin may contribute to the proteolytic digestion of the follicular wall, which is a prerequisite of follicular rupture. Consideration is also given that plasminogen activator may be involved in gap junction disruption and thereby disrupt the communication between the oocyte and the surrounding cumulus cells. Although the physiologic significance of plasminogen activator remains a matter of study, there is little doubt that ovarian cells produce this protease in measurable amounts in a manner subject to tight hormonal regulation. The FSH-dependent production of plasminogen activators by granulosa cells is particularly well documented.

Corpus Luteum Formation and Demise

After ovulation, the dominant follicle reorganizes to become the corpus luteum. After rupture of the follicle, capillaries and fibroblasts from the surrounding stroma proliferate and penetrate the basal lamina. This rapid vascularization of the corpus luteum may be guided by angiogenic factors, some of which are detected in the follicular fluid.[388] Vascular endothelial growth factor has been isolated from corpora lutea and has been postulated, along with bFGF, to be a potential angiogenic agent in corpora lutea.[389, 390] Concurrently, the mural granulosa cells undergo morphologic changes collectively referred to as luteinization. These cells, along with the surrounding theca-interstitial cells and the invading vasculature, intermingle to give rise to a corpus luteum. These cells have gap junctions to serve as part of the machinery that facilitates communication between the luteal cells, and connexin-43 has been identified as a protein in these luteal gap junctions.[391]

It is this endocrine gland that is the major source of sex steroid hormones secreted by the ovary during the postovulatory phase of the cycle. An important aspect of this phenomenon is the penetration of the follicle basement membrane by blood vessels, which provides the granulosa-luteal cells with LDL.[387] As stated earlier, LDL cholesterol serves as the substrate for corpus luteum progesterone production. A key regulator of the steroidogenesis is LH. Duncan and colleagues[392] showed that in humans the LH receptor is maintained throughout the functional life span of corpora lutea and not down-regulated during the maternal recognition of pregnancy. In addition to LH, another potential regulator of corpora luteal function is IGF-I, which has been shown to promote estrogen and progesterone production in human luteal cells.[393] Estrogen receptors and progesterone receptors have also been localized to human corpora lutea, and it has been hypothesized that estrogen and progesterone may also regulate luteal function.[394]

The functional life span of the corpus luteum is normally 14 ± 2 days. Thereafter, the corpus luteum spontaneously regresses. It is replaced, unless pregnancy occurs, by an avascular scar referred to as the corpus albicans.

The mechanisms underlying luteal life span remain unclear. Factors that may regulate this process include hormones such as hCG, maintenance of luteal vascularization, and immune cells.[395] There is little doubt about the central role of LH in the maintenance of corpus luteum function. Withdrawal of LH support in a variety of experimental circumstances has almost invariably resulted in luteal regression.[396] However, in pregnancy, hCG secreted by the gestational trophoblast maintains the ability of the corpus luteum to elaborate progesterone, which helps to maintain the early gestation until the luteoplacental shift.[397] Accordingly, the corpus luteum doubles its size (compared with the pre-pregnancy size) during the first 6 weeks of gestation.[398] This increase is due to proliferation of connective tissues and blood vessels, along with hypertrophy of the luteinized granulosa and theca cells. This early hypertrophy is later followed by regression. The corpus luteum at term is only half the size of that during the menstrual cycle. Furthermore, hormones such as estrogens[399] and prostaglandins[400] have been suggested as important factors in the promotion of luteal demise. In terms of the hypothesis regarding angiogenic maintenance of luteal function, as mentioned before, several angiogenic peptide growth factors have been described in the corpus luteum. For the immunologic regulation of luteal life span, it has been demonstrated that corpus luteal regression is associated with a progressive infiltration of lymphocytes and macrophages.[395]

For the actual mechanism for luteal regression, apoptosis may be the means by which human corpora lutea are deleted. Shikone and colleagues[401] have shown that early corpora lutea have no evidence of apoptotic DNA fragmentation. Midluteal and late luteal corpora have evidence of the DNA fragmentation. In corpora of early pregnancy, they found no evidence of apoptotic DNA fragmentation. Rodger and associates[402] localized BCL2, an apoptosis-related protein, in granulosa-lutein cells, theca-lutein cells, endothelial cells, and blood vessels. However, they found no evidence of changes in the BCL2 level during the normal luteal phase or after hCG administration. These studies represent first steps in understanding the actual mechanisms for deletion of cells during human luteolysis.

DECLINE

The Climacteric Ovary: Hormone-Dependent Androgen Production

The postmenopausal ovary is an atrophic, yellowish, lusterless structure with a wrinkled surface weighing less than 10 gm.[403–405] This is despite exposure to high circulating levels of gonadotropins. On microscopic examination, the cortex is thin and usually devoid of follicles. A few primordial follicles and follicles undergoing maturation and atresia may be found for up to 5 years after the last menses.

Linear extrapolation in women with regular menses predicts that by the mean age of the menopause (50 years of age), each ovary would still contain 2500 to 4000 primordial follicles. However, the fact that the menopausal ovary is largely devoid of follicles strongly suggests that follicular depletion accelerates in the last decade of menstrual life.

The postmenopausal ovarian stroma of the human ovary is capable of producing androgens.[25] In support of this, incubation of postmenopausal ovarian stromal slices with pregnenolone yielded progesterone, dehydroepiandrosterone, and testosterone. Consistent with this, it has been histochemically established that the cortical stroma of the postmenopausal ovary is endowed with steroidogenic enzymes. Moreover, the postmenopausal cortical stroma has been shown to produce measurable amounts of androstenedione (and progesterone) in vitro.[406] In fact, the addition of hCG to postmenopausal stromal strips elicited a significant increase in cAMP formation, which indicates preserved responsiveness to gonadotropins.

The postmenopausal ovarian cortex occasionally shows evidence of stromal hyperplasia. When stromal hyperplasia is florid, the ovary may be enlarged, consisting almost entirely of hyperplastic stromal nodules. In such cases, the lipid-rich luteinized cells of the hyperplastic stroma resemble the theca interna cells of the follicle. Such specimens have been shown to produce larger amounts of androstenedione than normal stroma does.[407] Thus, ovaries with stromal hyperthecosis may produce enough androgens to result in circulating testosterone within the male range, hirsutism, and virilization.[408]

The medulla of the postmenopausal ovary is large in relation to the cortex and is traversed by sclerosed blood vessels. Functionally, the most important medullary component may well be the hilar cells. Groups of large epithelioid cells closely connected to bundles of nonmyelinated nerve fibers and small vessels are the prominent cellular component of the hilum. These hilar cells are presumed to have the same embryonic origin as testicular Leydig cells. Histochemically similar to the interstitial cells of the testes, hilar cells are generally assumed to display considerable steroidogenic potential. Indeed, hilar cells have been reported to show morphologic and histochemical changes in response to treatment with hCG.

Incubation of strips of ovarian hilar tissue from postmenopausal women revealed a steroidogenic pattern similar to that of the postmenopausal ovarian stroma. However, the overall amount of steroids produced was substantially increased compared with stroma. These findings imply that the hilar cells may be of greater importance than the stromal cells in the overall steroidogenic potential of the postmenopausal ovary. Addition of hCG to hilar cells results in increased cAMP formation and steroid biosynthesis, indicating preserved responsiveness to gonadotropins.

Hilar cells can give rise to functional neoplasms (i.e., hilar cell tumors).[409–413] These usually produce excess amounts of androgens leading to signs and symptoms of virilism. However, signs and symptoms of estrogen excess may also be evident in circumstances of significant peripheral aromatization.

Although devoid of follicles, the menopausal ovary is not a defunct endocrine organ. Indeed, analysis of peripheral and ovarian vein blood from menopausal women indicates that the menopausal ovary secretes predominantly androstenedione and testosterone. In fact, the concentrations of testosterone and androstenedione in ovarian veins of menopausal women are 15 and 4 times higher, respectively, than their peripheral levels (Fig. 6–24).

It is estimated that the postmenopausal ovary contributes no more than 20 percent of the daily production of androstenedione. This conclusion is supported by the following observations:

1. Serum androstenedione is minimally (≤30 percent) reduced after oophorectomy (Fig. 6–25).
2. The circulating level of androstenedione has a diurnal rhythm, suggesting a substantial adrenal contribution.
3. Serum androstenedione is markedly reduced after treatment with dexamethasone.
4. The circulating levels of androstenedione increase after the systemic administration of adrenocorticotropic hormone (ACTH) but not of hCG.
5. The increase of androstenedione levels found in the ovarian veins of menopausal women is of a lesser magnitude than that found in premenopausal women.

The ovarian secretion of testosterone is greater in menopausal than in premenopausal women. The circulating level of testosterone is only slightly lower than that observed in premenopausal women. Most of the menopausal testosterone production reflects direct ovarian secretion, a contribution greater than that made by the premenopausal ovary (see Fig. 6–24). That a significant proportion of circulating

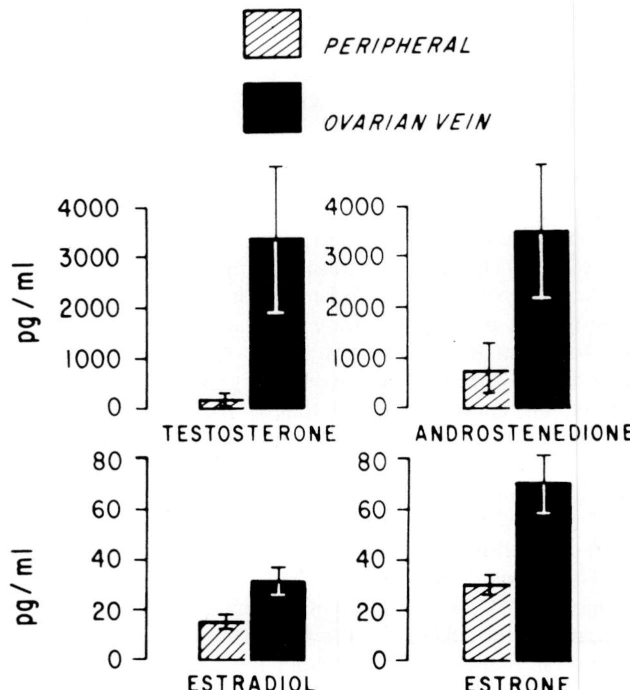

Figure 6–24 ■ Circulating levels of key androgens and estrogens in peripheral and ovarian vein blood of postmenopausal women. (From Judd HL, Judd GE, Lucas WE, Yen SSC. Endocrine function of the postmenopausal ovary: Concentration of androgens and estrogens in ovarian and peripheral vein blood. J Clin Endocrinol Metab 39:1020–1024, 1974. © The Endocrine Society.)

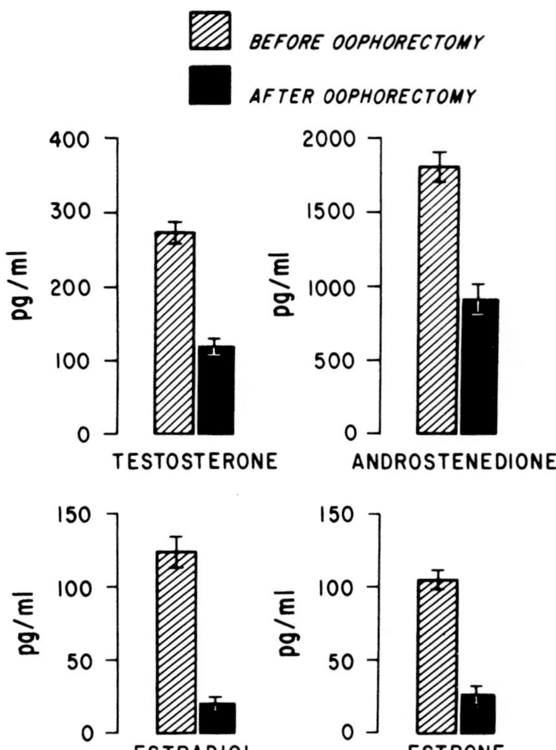

Figure 6–25 ■ Effect of oophorectomy on the circulating levels of key androgens and estrogens in postmenopausal women. (From Judd HL, Judd GE, Lucas WE, Yen SSC. Endocrine function of the postmenopausal ovary: Concentration of androgens and estrogens in ovarian and peripheral vein blood. J Clin Endocrinol Metab 39:1020–1024, 1974. © The Endocrine Society.)

testosterone appears to be derived from the postmenopausal ovary is suggested by the following:

1. Serum testosterone decreases 50 percent after oophorectomy.
2. The marked step-up of testosterone found in the ovarian vein of postmenopausal women is greater than that observed in premenopausal women.

Estrogen production in postmenopausal women is almost exclusively due to extraglandular aromatization of androstenedione. Thus, estrone, the major estrogen in the blood of postmenopausal women, derives predominantly from peripheral aromatization of adrenal androstenedione. Oophorectomy results in no significant reduction in urinary estrogen excretion by postmenopausal women. However, adrenalectomy after oophorectomy virtually eliminates measurable estrogens from the urine. The daily production rate of estrogen by this mechanism is related at least in part to body weight and perhaps also to age.

Whereas little doubt remains about the dominant role of peripheral aromatization, controversy still exists with respect to the possibility of direct ovarian contribution to the circulating estrogen pool. Longcope[414] was unable to document a concentration gradient across the ovary for estradiol. Mattingly and Huang's[415] in vitro studies suggested that the postmenopausal ovarian stroma is unable to aromatize androgens to estrogens. These observations are in keeping with those of Grodin and colleagues[416] indicating that the main steroid produced by the ovary is androstenedione, from which testosterone and estradiol are peripherally converted. On the other hand, Judd and coworkers[417] have suggested that the postmenopausal ovary may synthesize limited amounts of estrogens. This was based on the observation that the concentrations of estradiol and estrone are two times higher in ovarian vein blood than in peripheral blood of postmenopausal women. Denefors[406, 407] found measurable in vitro formation of estradiol by postmenopausal cortical stroma and hilar cells, indicating aromatization capability.

Ovarian androgen production in postmenopausal women might be gonadotropin dependent. Indeed, Judd and coworkers[418] proposed that gonadotropin stimulation may be the cause of the apparently increased ovarian production of testosterone in postmenopausal women. In this connection, Vermeulen[419] showed that the administration of hCG to postmenopausal women results in a small increase in the circulating levels of testosterone. Similarly, Poliak and colleagues[420] observed that the daily injection of hCG gave rise to marked hyperplasia of the ovarian hilar cell and to histochemical evidence suggesting active steroidogenesis. These results support the view that the postmenopausal hilar cells may respond to exogenous hCG with an increase in steroid biosynthesis. In related studies, Greenblatt and associates[421] demonstrated that hCG administration, but not ACTH, resulted in increased androgen (but not estrogen) production by the ovaries. Dowsett and colleagues[422] showed that treatment of postmenopausal women with a long-acting GnRH agonist results in a significant decrease in the circulating levels of total testosterone, an effect associated with a 22 percent decrease in the levels of estradiol. The fall in serum estradiol levels was presumed to be the consequence of the reduction in serum testosterone levels. Taken together, the observations suggest that ovarian androgen biosynthesis is at least partially gonadotropin dependent.

Given that the menopausal ovary may be a site of gonadotropin action, it would be reasonable to hypothesize the existence of ovarian gonadotropin receptors.[423] Such binding sites were localized by autoradiography after incubation of postmenopausal ovarian sections with labeled gonadotropins. Binding sites for both LH and FSH were identified in the cortical stroma and in hilar cells.[424] Because the hilar cells appear to contain steroidogenic enzymes, it is likely that steroidogenesis in these cells is controlled by circulating gonadotropins.

References

1. Baker TG. A quantitative and cytological study of germ cells in human ovaries. Proc R Soc Biol 158:417, 1963.
2. Witschi E. Migration of the germ cells of human embryos from the yolk sac to the primitive gonadal folds. Contrib Embryol 32:67, 1948.
3. Baker TG, Franchi LL. The fine structure of oogonia and oocytes in human ovaries. J Cell Sci 2:213, 1967.
4. Ohno S, Klinger H, Atkin N. Human oogenesis. Cytogenetics 1:42, 1962.
5. Yeh J, Osathanondh R, Villa-Komaroff L. Expression of messenger ribonucleic acid for epidermal growth factor receptor and its ligands, epidermal growth factor and transforming growth factor-α, in human first- and second-trimester fetal ovary and uterus. Am J Obstet Gynecol 168:1569, 1993.

6. Yeh J, Osathanondh R. Expression of messenger ribonucleic acids encoding for basic fibroblast growth factor (FGF) and alternatively spliced FGF receptor in human fetal ovary and uterus. J Clin Endocrinol Metab 77:1367, 1993.
7. Shifren J, Osathanondh R, Yeh J. Human fetal ovaries and uteri: Developmental expression of genes encoding the insulin, insulin-like growth factor-I, and insulin-like growth factor II receptors. Fertil Steril 59:1036, 1993.
8. Bennett RA, Osathanondh R, Yeh J. Immunohistochemical localization of transforming growth factor-α (TGFα), epidermal growth factor (EGF), and EGF-receptor (EGF-R) in the human fetal ovary. J Clin Endocrinol Metab 81:3073, 1996.
9. Peters H. Intrauterine gonadal development. Fertil Steril 27:493, 1976.
10. Himelstein-Braw R, Byskov AG, Peters H, Faber M. Follicular atresia in the infant human ovary. J Reprod Fertil 46:55, 1976.
11. Franchi LL, Mandl AM, Zuckerman S. The development of the ovary and the process of oogenesis. *In* Zuckerman S, Mandl AM, Eckstein P (eds). The Ovary. London, Academic Press, 1962, pp 1–88.
12. Weakly BS. Electron microscopy of the oocyte and granulosa cells in the developing ovarian follicles of the golden hamster. J Anat 100:503, 1966.
13. Albertini DF, Anderson E. The appearance and structure of intercellular connections during the ontogeny of the rabbit ovarian follicle with particular reference to gap junctions. J Cell Biol 63:234, 1974.
14. Amsterdam A, Joseph SR, Lieberman ME, Lindner HR. Organization of intramembrane particles in freeze-cleaved gap junctions of rat graafian follicles: Optical diffraction analysis. J Cell Sci 21:93, 1976.
15. Amsterdam A, Knecht M, Catt KJ. Hormonal regulation of cytodifferentiation and intercellular communication in cultured granulosa cells. Proc Natl Acad Sci USA 78:300, 1981.
16. Simon AM, Goodenough DA, Li E, Paul DL. Female infertility in mice lacking connexin 37. Nature 385:525, 1997.
17. Zoller LC, Weisz J. A quantitative cytochemical study of glucose-6-phosphate dehydrogenase and Δ^5-3β-hydroxysteroid dehydrogenase activity in the membrana granulosa of the ovulable type of follicle of the rat. Histochemistry 62:125, 1979.
18. Zoller LC, Weisz J. Identification of cytochrome P-450, and its distribution in the membrana granulosa of the preovulatory follicle using quantitative cytochemistry. Endocrinology 103:310, 1979.
19. Channing CP, Bae I-H, Stone SL, et al. Porcine granulosa and cumulus cell properties. LH/hCG receptors, ability to secrete progesterone and ability to respond to LH. Mol Cell Endocrinol 22:359, 1981.
20. Hillensjo T, Magnusson C, Svensson U, Thelander H. Effect of LH and FSH on progesterone synthesis in cultured rat cumulus cells. Endocrinology 108:1920, 1981.
21. Lawrence TS, Dekel M, Beers WH. Binding of human chorionic gonadotropin by rat cumuli, oophori and granulosa cells: A comparative study. Endocrinology 106:1114, 1980.
22. Magnusson C, Billig H, Aneroth P, et al. Comparison between the progestin secretion responsiveness to gonadotropins of rat cumulus and mural granulosa cells in vitro. Acta Endocrinol 101:611, 1982.
23. Ryan KJ, Petro Z. Steroid biosynthesis by human ovarian granulosa and thecal cells. J Clin Endocrinol Metab 26:46, 1966.
24. Rice BF, Savard K. Steroid hormone formation in the human ovary. IV. Ovarian stromal compartment; formation of radioactive steroids from acetate-1-^{14}C and action of gonadotropins. J Clin Endocrinol Metab 26:593, 1966.
25. Savard K, Marsh JM, Rice BF. Gonadotropins and ovarian steroidogenesis. Recent Prog Horm Res 21:285, 1965.
26. Mossman HW, Koering MJ, Ferry D. Cyclic changes of interstitial gland tissue of the human ovary. Am J Anat 115:235, 1964.
27. Erickson GF, Magoffin DA, Dyer CA, Hofeditz C. The ovarian androgen producing cells: A review of structure/function relationships. Endocr Rev 6:371, 1985.
28. Gondos B, Hobel CJ. Interstitial cells in the human fetal ovary. Endocrinology 93:736, 1973.
29. Hume DA, Halpin D, Charlton H, Gordon S. The mononuclear phagocyte system of the mouse defined by immunohistochemical localization of antigen F4/80: Macrophages of endocrine organs. Proc Natl Acad Sci USA 81:4174, 1984.
30. Parr EL. Histological examination of the rat ovarian follicle wall prior to ovulation. Biol Reprod 11:483, 1974.
31. Jones RE, Duvall D, Guillette LJ. Rat ovarian mast cells: Distribution and cyclic changes. Anat Rec 197:489, 1980.
32. Shinohara H, Nakatani T, Morisawa S, et al. Mast cells in the ovarian bursa of the golden hamster. Biol Reprod 36:445, 1987.
33. Nakamura Y, Smith M, Krishna A, Terranova PF. Increased number of mast cells in the dominant follicle of the cow: Relationships among luteal, stromal, and hilar regions. Biol Reprod 37:546, 1987.
34. Krishna A, Terranova PF. Alterations in mast cell degranulation and ovarian histamine in the proestrous hamster. Biol Reprod 32:1211, 1985.
35. Szego CM, Gitin ES. Ovarian histamine depletion during acute hyperaemic response to luteinizing hormone. Nature 201:682, 1964.
36. Wurtman RJ. An effect of luteinizing hormone on the fractional perfusion of the rat ovary. Endocrinology 75:927, 1964.
37. Morikawa H, Okamura H, Okazaki T, Nishimura T. Changes in histamine in rabbit ovary during ovulation. Acta Obstet Gynecol 28:504, 1976.
38. Murdoch WJ, Nix KJ, Dunn TG. Dynamics of ovarian blood supply to periovulatory follicles of the ewe. Biol Reprod 28:1001, 1983.
39. Krishna A, Terranova PF, Matteri RL, Papkoff H. Histamine and increased ovarian blood flow mediate LH-induced superovulation in the cyclic hamster. J Reprod Fertil 76:23, 1986.
40. Halterman SD, Murdoch WJ. Ovarian function in ewes treated with antihistamines. Endocrinology 119:2417, 1986.
41. Seow WK, Thong YH, Waters M, et al. Isolation of a chemotactic protein for neutrophils from human ovarian follicular fluid. Int Arch Allergy Appl Immunol 86:331, 1988.
42. Cavender JL, Murdoch WJ. Morphological studies of the microcirculatory system of periovulatory ovine follicles. Biol Reprod 39:989, 1988.
43. Espey L. Ovulation and an inflammatory reaction—a hypothesis. Biol Reprod 22:73, 1980.
44. Murdoch WJ, Steadman LE, Belden EL. Immunoregulation of luteolysis. Med Hypotheses 27:197, 1988.
45. Murdoch WJ. Treatment of sheep with prostaglandin $F_{2\alpha}$ enhances production of a luteal chemoattractant for eosinophils. Am J Reprod Immunol Microbiol 15:52, 1987.
46. Kirsch TM, Friedman AC, Vogel RL, Flickinger GL. Macrophages in corpora lutea of mice: Characterization and effects on steroid secretion. Biol Reprod 25:629, 1981.
47. Gillim SW, Christensen AK, McLennan CE. Fine structure of the human menstrual corpus luteum at its stage of maximum secretory activity. Am J Anat 126:409, 1969.
48. Lobel B, Rosenbaum R, Deane H. Enzymic correlates of physiological regression of follicles and corpora lutea in ovaries of normal rats. Endocrinology 68:232, 1961.
49. Bagavandoss P, Wiggins RC, Kunkel SL, Keyes PL. Localization of macrophages and T lymphocytes and induction of tumor necrosis factor-α (TNF-α) in corpora lutea of pregnant and pseudo-pregnant rabbits. Biol Reprod 38:56, 1988.
50. Takemura R, Werb Z. Secretory products of macrophages and their physiological functions. Am J Physiol 246:C1, 1984.
51. Reynolds H, Nathan P, Srivastava L, Hess E. Release of estradiol from fetal bovine serum by rat thymus, spleen, kidney, lung and lung macrophage cultures. Endocrinology 110:2213, 1982.
52. Milewich L, Chen G, Lyons C, et al. Metabolism of androstenedione by guinea-pig peritoneal macrophages: Synthesis of testosterone and 5α-reduced metabolites. J Steroid Biochem 17:61, 1982.
53. Rapolee DA, Mark D, Banda MJ, Werb Z. Wound macrophages express TGF-α and other growth factors in vivo: Analysis by mRNA phenotyping. Science 241:708, 1988.
54. Jocelyn HD, Setchell BP. Regnier de Graaf on the human reproductive organs. Chapter XII, "Concerning the 'testicles' of women, or rather their ovaries." J Reprod Fertil Suppl 17:131, 1972.
55. Hisaw FL. Development of the graafian follicle and ovulation. Physiol Rev 27:95, 1947.
56. Peters H, Byskov AG, Himelstein-Braw R, Faber M. Follicular growth: The basic event of the mouse and human ovary. J Reprod Fertil 45:559, 1975.

57. Lintern-Moore S, Peters H, Moore GPM, Faber M. Follicular development in the infant human ovary. J Reprod Fertil 39:53, 1974.
58. Gougeon A. Dynamics of follicular growth in the human: A model from preliminary results. Hum Reprod 1:81, 1986.
59. Gougeon A, Chainy GBN. Morphometric studies of small follicles in ovaries of women at different stages. J Reprod Fertil 81:433, 1987.
60. Chiquoine HD. The development of the zona pellucida of the mammalian ovum. Am J Anat 106:149, 1960.
61. Kaplan SL, Grumbach MM, Aubert ML. The ontogenesis of pituitary hormones and hypothalamic factors in the human fetus: Maturation of central nervous system regulation of anterior pituitary function. Recent Prog Horm Res 32:161, 1976.
62. Gulyas BJ, Hodgen GD, Tullner WW, Ross GT. Effects of fetal or maternal hypophysectomy on endocrine organs and body weight in infant rhesus monkeys *(Macaca mulatta)* with particular emphasis on oogenesis. Biol Reprod 16:216, 1977.
63. Seegar-Jones G, de Moraes-Ruehsen M. A new syndrome of amenorrhea in association with hypergonadotropism and apparently normal ovarian follicular apparatus. Am J Obstet Gynecol 104:597, 1969.
64. Goldsmith O, Solomon DH, Horton R. Hypogonadism and mineralocorticoid excess. The 17-hydroxylase deficiency syndrome. N Engl J Med 277:673, 1967.
65. Biglieri EG, Herron MA, Brust N. 17-Hydroxylation deficiency in man. J Clin Invest 45:1946, 1966.
66. Mallin SR. Congenital adrenal hyperplasia secondary to 17-hydroxylase deficiency. Ann Intern Med 70:69, 1969.
67. Kallmann F, Shonfeld WA, Barrera SE. The genetic aspects of primary eunuchoidism. Am J Ment Defic 48:203, 1944.
68. Gauthier G. Olfacto-genital dysplasia (agenesis of the olfactory lobes with absence of gonadal development) at puberty [in French]. Acta Neuroveg (Wien) 21:345, 1960.
69. Goldenberg RL, Powell RD, Rosen SW, et al. Ovarian morphology in women with anosmia and hypogonadotropic hypogonadism. Am J Obstet Gynecol 126:91, 1976.
70. Mroueh A, Kase N. Olfactory-genital dysplasia. Am J Obstet Gynecol 100:525, 1968.
71. Tagatz G, Fialkow PJ, Smith D, Spadoni L. Hypogonadotropic hypogonadism associated with anosmia in the female. N Engl J Med 283:1326, 1970.
72. Starup J, Visfeldt J. Ovarian morphology and pituitary gonadotropins in serum during and after long-term treatment with oral contraceptives. Acta Obstet Gynecol Scand 53:161, 1974.
73. Starup J, Visfeldt J. Ovarian morphology in early and late human pregnancy. Acta Obstet Gynecol Scand 53:211, 1974.
74. Huhtaniemi I, Yamamoto M, Ranta T, et al. Follicle-stimulating hormone receptors appear earlier in the primate fetal testis than in the ovary. J Clin Endocrinol Metab 65:1210, 1987.
75. Edwards RG. Follicular fluid. J Reprod Fertil 37:189, 1974.
76. Jensen CE, Zacharie F. Studies on the mechanism of ovulation. II. Isolation and analysis of acid mucopolysaccharides in bovine follicular fluid. Acta Endocrinol (Copenh) 27:356, 1958.
77. Mueller PL, Schreiber JR, Lucky AW, et al. Follicle-stimulating hormone stimulates ovarian synthesis of proteoglycans in the estrogen-stimulated hypophysectomized immature female rat. Endocrinology 102:824, 1978.
78. Schweitzer M, Jackson JC, Ryan RJ. The porcine ovarian follicle. VII. FSH stimulation of in vitro [^{3}H]-glucosamine incorporation into mucopolysaccharides. Biol Reprod 24:332, 1981.
79. Yanagashita M, Hascall VC. Biosynthesis of proteoglycans by rat granulosa cells cultured in vitro: Modulation by gonadotropins, steroid hormones, prostaglandins, and a cyclic nucleotide. Endocrinology 109:1641, 1979.
80. Yanagashita M, Rodbard D, Hascall VC. Isolation and characterization of proteoglycans from porcine ovarian follicular fluid. J Biol Chem 254:911, 1979.
81. Zachariae F. Acid mucopolysaccharides in the ovary and their role in the mechanism of ovulation. Acta Endocrinol Suppl 47:33, 1959.
82. Fritz MA, Speroff L. The endocrinology of the menstrual cycle, the interaction of folliculogenesis and neuroendocrine mechanisms. Fertil Steril 38:509, 1982.
83. DiZerega GS, Richardson CM, Davis TF, et al. Fluorescence localization of LH/hCG uptake in the primate ovary: Characterization of the preovulatory ovary. Fertil Steril 34:379, 1980.
84. Zeleznik AJ, Schuler HM, Reichert LE. Gonadotropin-binding sites in the rhesus monkey ovary: Role of the vasculature in the selective distribution of hCG to the preovulatory follicle. Endocrinology 109:356, 1981.
85. Forest MG. Function of the ovary in the neonate and infant. Eur J Obstet Gynaecol Reprod Biol 9:145, 1979.
86. Valdes-Dapena MA. The normal ovary of childhood. Ann N Y Acad Sci 142:597, 1967.
87. Peters H. The human ovary in childhood and early maturity. Eur J Obstet Gynaecol Reprod Biol 9:137, 1979.
88. Peters H, Himelstein-Braw R, Faber M. The normal development of the ovary in childhood. Acta Endocrinol (Copenh) 82:617, 1976.
89. Kulin HE, Reiter EO. Gonadotropins during childhood and adolescence: A review. Pediatrics 51:260, 1973.
90. Winter JS, Faiman C. Pituitary-gonadal relations in female children and adolescents. Pediatr Res 7:948, 1973.
91. Polhemus DW. Ovarian maturation and cyst formation in children. Pediatrics 1:588, 1953.
92. Winter JSD, Faiman C, Reyes FI, Hobson WC. Gonadotropins and steroid hormones in the blood and urine of prepubertal girls or other primates. Clin Endocrinol Metab 7:512, 1978.
93. Nelson WW, Greene RR. Some observations on the histology of the human ovary during pregnancy. Am J Obstet Gynecol 76:66, 1958.
94. Lynch MJG, Kyle PR, Bruce-Lockhart P. Unusual ovarian changes (hyperthecosis) in pregnancy. Am J Obstet Gynecol 77:335, 1959.
95. Ryan KJ. Granulosa–thecal cell interaction in ovarian steroidogenesis. J Steroid Biochem 11:799, 1979.
96. Palumbo A, Yeh J. Apoptosis as a basic mechanism in the ovarian cycle: Follicular atresia and luteal regression. J Soc Gynecol Invest 2:565, 1995.
97. Yeh J, Kim HH. Polycystic ovarian syndrome (PCOS): The possible roles of apoptosis in human granulosa cells. *In* Chang RJ (ed). Polycystic Ovarian Syndrome. New York, Springer-Verlag, 1996, p 51.
98. Block E. Quantitative morphological investigations of the follicular system in women. Acta Endocrinol (Copenh) 8:33, 1951.
99. Tilly JL, Kowalski KI, Johnson AL, Hsueh AJW. Involvement of apoptosis in ovarian follicular atresia and postovulatory regression. Endocrinology 129:2799, 1991.
100. Palumbo A, Yeh J. In situ localization of apoptosis in the rat ovary: A role for apoptosis in follicular atresia. Biol Reprod 51:888, 1994.
101. Tilly JL, Billig H, Kowalski KI, Hsueh AJW. Epidermal growth factor and basic fibroblast growth factor suppress the spontaneous onset of apoptosis in cultured rat ovarian granulosa cells and follicles by a tyrosine kinase–dependent mechanism. Mol Endocrinol 6:1642, 1992.
102. Terranova PF. Steroidogenesis in experimentally induced atretic follicles of the hamster: A shift from estradiol to progesterone synthesis. Endocrinology 108:1885, 1981.
103. Braw RH, Tsafriri A. Follicles explanted from pentobarbitone-treated rats provide a model for atresia. J Reprod Fertil 59:259, 1980.
104. Uilenbroek JTJ, Woutersen PJA, Van der Schoot P. Atresia in preovulatory follicles: Gonadotropin binding in steroidogenic activity. Biol Reprod 23:219, 1980.
105. Ross GT. Gonadotropins and preantral follicular maturation in women. Fertil Steril 25:522, 1974.
106. Terranova PF, Greenwald GS. Increased ovulation rate in the cyclic guinea pig after a single injection of an antiserum to LH. J Reprod Fertil 61:37, 1981.
107. Scaramuzzi RJ, Davidson WG, Van Look PFA. Increasing ovulation rate in sheep by active immunization against an ovarian steroid androstenedione. Nature 269:817, 1977.
108. Billig H, Furuta I, Hsueh AJW. Estrogens inhibit and androgens enhance ovarian granulosa cell apoptosis. Endocrinology 133:2204, 1993.
109. Goldman A, Yakovac W, Bongiovanni A. Development of activity of 3β-hydroxysteroid dehydrogenase in human fetal tissues and in two anencephalic newborns. J Clin Endocrinol 26:14, 1966.

110. Jungmann R, Schweppe J. Biosynthesis of sterols and steroids from acetate-C by human fetal ovaries. J Clin Endocrinol 28:1599, 1968.
111. Roberts JD, Warren JC. Steroid biosynthesis in the fetal ovary. Endocrinology 74:846, 1964.
112. Schindler AE, Friedrich E. Steroid metabolism of foetal tissues. I. Metabolism of pregnenolone-4-^{14}C by human foetal ovaries. Endokrinologie 65:72, 1975.
113. Block E. Metabolism of [4-^{14}C]-progesterone by human fetal testis and ovaries. Endocrinology 74:833, 1964.
114. Payne AH, Jaffe RB. Androgen formation from pregnenolone sulfate by the human fetal ovary. J Clin Endocrinol Metab 39:300, 1974.
115. Voutilainen R, Miller W. Developmental expression of genes for the steroidogenic enzymes P450scc (20,22-desmolase), P450c17 (17α-hydroxylase/17,20-lyase), and P450c21 (21-hydroxylase) in the human fetus. J Clin Endocrinol Metab 63:1145, 1986.
116. Wilson EA, Jawad MJ. The effects of trophic agents on fetal ovarian steroidogenesis in organ culture. Fertil Steril 32:73, 1979.
117. Barlow J, Emerson K, Saxena B. Estradiol production after ovariectomy for carcinoma of the breast. N Engl J Med 28:633, 1969.
118. Baird DT, Burger P, Heavon-Jones GD, Scaramuzzi RJ. The site of secretion of androstenedione in non-pregnant women. J Endocrinol 63:201, 1974.
119. Baird DT, Fraser IJ. Concentration of estrone and estradiol-17β in follicular fluid and ovarian venous blood of women. Clin Endocrinol (Oxf) 4:171, 1969.
120. Fowler RE, Fox NL, Edwards RG, et al. Steroidogenesis by cultured granulosa cells aspirated from human follicles using pregnenolone and androgens as precursors. J Endocrinol 77:171, 1978.
121. Channing CP. Steroidogenesis and morphology of human ovarian cell types in tissue culture. J Endocrinol 45:297, 1969.
122. Tsang BK, Armstrong DT, Whitfield JF. Steroid biosynthesis by isolated human ovarian follicular cells in vitro. J Clin Endocrinol Metab 51:1407, 1980.
123. McNatty KP, Makris A, DeGrazia C, et al. The production of progesterone, androgens, and estrogens by granulosa cells, thecal tissue, and stromal tissue from human ovaries in vitro. J Clin Endocrinol Metab 49:687, 1979.
124. Falck B. Site of production of oestrogen in rat ovary as studied by micro-transplants. Acta Physiol Scand Suppl 47:1, 1959.
125. Ryan KJ, Petro Z, Kaiser J. Steroid formation by isolated and recombined granulosa and thecal cells. J Clin Endocrinol Metab 28:355, 1968.
126. Bjersing L. On the morphology and endocrine function of granulosa cells of ovarian follicles and corpora lutea. Acta Endocrinol Suppl (Copenh) 125:5, 1967.
127. Hillier SG, Reichert LE, van Hall EV. Control of preovulatory follicular estrogen biosynthesis in the human ovary. J Clin Endocrinol Metab 52:847, 1981.
128. Bjersing L. Histochemical demonstration of Δ^5-3β- and 17β-hydroxysteroid dehydrogenase activities in porcine ovary. Histochemie 10:295, 1967.
129. Knecht M, Nanta T, Katz MS, Catt KJ. Regulation of adenyl cyclase activity by follicle-stimulating hormone and a gonadotropin-releasing hormone agonist in cultured rat granulosa cells. Endocrinology 112:1247, 1983.
130. Brown MS, Goldstein JL. Receptor-mediated control of cholesterol metabolism. Science 191:150, 1976.
131. Andersen JM, Dietschy JM. Relative importance of high and low density lipoproteins in the regulation of cholesterol synthesis in the adrenal gland, ovary, and testis in the rat. J Biol Chem 253:9024, 1978.
132. Goldstein JL, Anderson RG, Brown MS. Coated pits, coated vesicles, and receptor mediated endocytosis. Nature 279:679, 1979.
133. Anderson RG, Brown MS, Goldstein JL. Role of the coated endocytotic vesicle in the uptake of receptor-bound low density lipoprotein in human fibroblasts. Cell 10:351, 1977.
134. Brown MS, Dana SE, Goldstein JL. Receptor-dependent hydrolysis of cholesterol esters contained in plasma low density lipoprotein. Proc Natl Acad Sci USA 72:2925, 1975.
135. Schreiber JR, Hsueh AJW, Weinstein DB, Erickson GF. Plasma lipoproteins stimulate progestin production by rat ovarian granulosa cells cultured in serum free medium. J Steroid Biochem 13:1009, 1980.
136. Simpson ER, Rochelle DB, Carr BR, MacDonald PC. Plasma lipoproteins in follicular fluid of human ovaries. J Clin Endocrinol Metab 51:1469, 1980.
137. Schuler LA, Scavo L, Kirsch TM, et al. Regulation of de novo biosynthesis of cholesterol and progestins, and formation of cholesteryl ester in rat corpus luteum by exogenous sterol. J Biol Chem 254:8662, 1979.
138. Tureck RW, Strauss JF III. Progesterone synthesis by luteinized human granulosa cells in culture: The role of de novo sterol synthesis and lipoprotein-carried sterol. J Clin Endocrinol Metab 54:367, 1982.
139. Dimino MJ, Campbell MD. Progesterone synthesis by luteal mitochondria in vitro. Proc Soc Exp Biol Med 152:54, 1976.
140. Sulimovici S, Boyd GS. The Δ^5-3β-hydroxysteroid dehydrogenase of rat ovarian tissue. Eur J Biochem 7:549, 1969.
141. Tsang BK, Moon YS, Simpson CW, Armstrong DT. Androgen biosynthesis in human ovarian follicles: Cellular source, gonadotropic control, and adenosine 3′5′ monophosphate mediation. J Clin Endocrinol Metab 48:153, 1979.
142. Sasano H, Okamoto M, Mason JI, et al. Immunolocalization of aromatase, 17α-hydroxylase and side-chain-cleavage cytochromes P-450 in the human ovary. J Reprod Fertil 85:163, 1989.
143. Hsueh AJW, Adashi EY, Jones PBC, Welsh TH. Hormonal regulation of the differentiation of cultured ovarian granulosa cells. Endocr Rev 5:76, 1984.
144. Richards JS. Hormonal control of ovarian follicular development: A 1978 perspective. Recent Prog Horm Res 35:343, 1979.
145. Richards J. Estradiol receptor content in rat granulosa cells during follicle development: Modification by estradiol and gonadotropins. Endocrinology 97:1174, 1975.
146. Milwidsky A, Younes M, Besch N, et al. Receptor-like binding proteins for testosterone and progesterone in the human ovary. Am J Obstet Gynecol 138:93, 1980.
147. Saiduddin S, Zassenhaus HP. Effect of testosterone and progesterone on the estradiol receptor in the immature rat ovary. Endocrinology 102:1069, 1978.
148. Saiduddin S, Zassenhaus HP. Estradiol-17β receptors in the immature rat ovary. Steroids 29:197, 1977.
149. Saiduddin S, Milo GE Jr. Effect of hypophysectomy and pretreatment on uptake and retention of estradiol by the ovary. Proc Soc Exp Biol Med 146:513, 1974.
150. Saiduddin S. ^{3}H-estradiol uptake by the rat ovary. Proc Soc Exp Biol Med 138:651, 1971.
151. Schreiber JR, Reid R, Ross GT. A receptor-like testosterone binding protein in ovaries from estrogen stimulated hypophysectomized immature female rats. Endocrinology 98:1206, 1976.
152. Schreiber JR, Ross GT. Further characterization of a rat ovarian testosterone receptor with evidence for nuclear translocation. Endocrinology 99:590, 1976.
153. Schreiber JR, Erickson GF. Progesterone receptor in the rat ovary. Further characterization and localization in the granulosa cell. Steroids 34:459, 1979.
154. Schreiber JR, Hsueh AJ. Progesterone “receptor” in rat ovary. Endocrinology 105:915, 1979.
155. Tjalve H, Appelgren LE. Chromosomal accumulation of ^{3}H-estradiol in the ovarian granulosa cells and ovarian squash preparations. Experientia 29:1143, 1973.
156. Ullberg S, Bengtsson G. Autoradiographic distribution studies with natural oestrogens. Acta Endocrinol (Copenh) 43:75, 1963.
157. Stumpf WE. Nuclear concentration of ^{3}H-estradiol in target tissues. Dry-mount autoradiography of vagina, oviduct, ovary, testes, mammary tumor, liver and adrenal. Endocrinology 85:31, 1969.
158. Midgley AR Jr. Autoradiographic analysis of gonadotropin binding to rat ovarian tissue sections. Adv Exp Med Biol 36:365, 1973.
159. Amsterdam A, Koch Y, Lieberman ME, Lindner HR. Distribution of binding sites for human chorionic gonadotropin in the preovulatory follicle of the rat. J Cell Biol 67:894, 1975.
160. Bortolussi M, Marini G, Dal Lago A. Autoradiographic studies of the distribution of LH (hCG) receptors in the ovary of untreated and gonadotropin-primed immature rats. Cell Tissue Res 183:329, 1977.
161. Nimrod A, Erickson GF, Ryan KJ. A specific FSH receptor in rat

granulosa cells: Properties of binding in vitro. Endocrinology 98:56, 1976.
162. Nimrod A, Bedrak E, Lamprecht SA. Appearance of LH-receptors and LH-stimulatable cyclic AMP accumulation in granulosa cells during follicular maturation in the rat ovary. Biochem Biophys Res Commun 78:977, 1977.
163. Kammerman S, Canfield RE, Kolena J, Channing CP. The binding of iodinated hCG to porcine granulosa cells. Endocrinology 91:65, 1972.
164. Kammerman S, Ross J. Increase in numbers of gonadotropin receptors on granulosa cells during follicular maturation. J Clin Endocrinol Metab 41:546, 1975.
165. Channing CP, Kammerman S. Binding of gonadotropins to ovarian cells. Biol Reprod 10:179, 1974.
166. Jaaskelainen K, Markkanen S, Rajaniemi H. Internalization of receptor-bound human chorionic gonadotropin in preovulatory rat granulosa cells in vivo. Acta Endocrinol (Copenh) 103:406, 1983.
167. Uilenbroek JTJ, Richards JS. Ovarian follicular development during the rat estrous cycle: Gonadotropin receptors and follicular responsiveness. Biol Reprod 20:1159, 1979.
168. Zeleznik AJ, Midgley AR, Reichert LE. Granulosa cell maturation in the rat; increased binding of human chorionic gonadotropin following treatment with follicle-stimulating hormone in vivo. Endocrinology 95:818, 1974.
169. Minegishi T, Nakamura K, Takakura Y, et al. Cloning and sequencing of human FSH receptor cDNA. Biochem Biophys Res Commun 175:1125, 1991.
170. Kelton CA, Cheng SV, Nugent NP, et al. The cloning of the human follicle stimulating hormone receptor and its expression in COS-7, CHO, and Y-1 cells. Mol Cell Endocrinol 89:141, 1992.
171. Rousseau-Mereck MF, Atger M, Loosfelt H, et al. The chromosomal localization of the human follicle-stimulating hormone receptor gene (FSHR) on 2p21–p16 is similiar to that of the luteinizing hormone receptor gene. Genomics 15:222, 1993.
172. Atger M, Misrahi M, Sar S, et al. Structure of the human luteinizing hormone–choriogonadotropin receptor gene: Unusual promoter and 5′ non-coding regions. Mol Cell Endocrinol 111:113, 1995.
173. Zeleznik AJ, Keyes PL, Menon MJ, et al. Development-dependent responses of ovarian follicles to FSH and hCG. Am J Physiol 233:E229, 1977.
174. Richards JS, Ireland JJ, Rao MC, et al. Ovarian follicular development in the rat: Hormone receptor regulation by estradiol, follicle-stimulating hormone and luteinizing hormone. Endocrinology 99:1562, 1976.
175. Dorrington JH, Moon YS, Armstrong DT. Estradiol-17β biosynthesis in cultured granulosa cells from hypophysectomized immature rats: Stimulation by follicle-stimulating hormone. Endocrinology 97:1328, 1975.
176. Armstrong DT, Papkoff H. Stimulation of aromatization of exogenous and endogenous androgens in ovaries of hypophysectomized rat in vivo by follicle-stimulating hormone. Endocrinology 99:1144, 1976.
177. Moon YS, Tsang BK, Simpson CW, Armstrong DT. Estradiol-17β biosynthesis in cultured granulosa and theca cells of human ovarian follicles: Stimulation by follicle-stimulating hormone. J Clin Endocrinol Metab 47:263, 1978.
178. Moon YS, Dorrington JH, Armstrong DT. Stimulatory action of follicle-stimulating hormone on estradiol-17β secretion by hypophysectomized rat ovaries in organ culture. Endocrinology 97:244, 1975.
179. Erickson GF, Wang C, Hsueh AJW. FSH induction of functional LH receptors in granulosa cells cultured in a chemically defined medium. Nature 279:336, 1979.
180. Rani CSS, Salhanick AR, Armstrong DT. Follicle-stimulating hormone induction of luteinizing hormone receptor in cultured rat granulosa cells: An examination of the need for steroids in the induction process. Endocrinology 108:1379, 1981.
181. Penchartz RI. Effect of estrogens and androgens alone and in combination with chorionic gonadotropin on the ovary of the hypophysectomized rat. Science 91:554, 1940.
182. Peluso JJ, Steger RW. Role of FSH in regulating granulosa cell division and follicular atresia in rats. J Reprod Fertil 54:275, 1978.
183. Louvet JP, Harman SM, Ross GT. Effects of human chorionic gonadotropin, human interstitial cell–stimulating hormone, and human follicle-stimulating hormone on ovarian weights in estrogen-primed hypophysectomized immature female rats. Endocrinology 96:1179, 1975.
184. Richards JS, Jongssen JA, Kersey KA. Evidence that changes in tonic luteinizing hormone secretion determine the growth of preovulatory follicles in the rat. Endocrinology 107:641, 1980.
185. Richards JS, Bogvich K. Effects of human chorionic gonadotropin and progesterone on follicular development in the immature rat. Endocrinology 111:1429, 1982.
186. Bogvich K, Richards JS. Androgen biosynthesis in developing ovarian follicle: Evidence that luteinizing hormone regulates theca 17α-hydroxylase and C17-20 lyase activity. Endocrinology 111:1201, 1982.
187. Ireland JJ, Richards JS. A previously undescribed role for luteinizing hormone (LH:hCG) on follicular cell differentiation. Endocrinology 102:1458, 1978.
188. Goldenberg RL, Vaitukaitis JL, Ross GT. Estrogen and follicle-stimulating hormone interactions on follicle growth in rats. Endocrinology 90:1492, 1972.
189. Goldenberg RL, Reiter EO, Ross GT. Follicle response to exogenous gonadotropins: An estrogen-mediated phenomenon. Fertil Steril 24:121, 1973.
190. Croes-Buth S, Paesi JA, deJongh SE. Stimulation of ovarian follicles in hypophysectomized rats by low dosages of oestradiol benzoate. Acta Endocrinol (Copenh) 32:399, 1959.
191. Johnson DC, Cheng HC. Effect of diethylstilbestrol on ovarian responses to pregnant mare's serum gonadotropin in hypophysectomized immature rats. Endocrinology 102:1563, 1978.
192. Meyer JE, Bradbury JT. Influence of stilbestrol on the immature rat ovary and its response to gonadotrophin. Endocrinology 66:121, 1960.
193. Smith BD. The effect of diethylstilbestrol on the immature rat ovary. Endocrinology 69:238, 1961.
194. Smith BD, Bradbury JT. Ovarian weight response to varying doses of estrogens in intact and hypophysectomized rats. Proc Soc Exp Biol Med 107:946, 1961.
195. Williams PC. Effect of stilboestrol on the ovaries of hypophysectomized rats. Nature 145:388, 1940.
196. Williams PC. Ovarian stimulation by oestrogens: Effect in immature hypophysectomized rats. Proc R Soc Lond Biol 132:189, 1944.
197. Williams PC. Ovarian stimulation by oestrogens: 2. Stimulation in the absence of hypophysis, uterus, and adrenal glands. J Endocrinol 4:125, 1945.
198. Bradbury JT. Direct action of estrogen on the ovary of the immature rat. Endocrinology 68:115, 1961.
199. De Wit JC. The effect of oestradiol monobenzoate on follicles of various sizes in the ovary of the hypophysectomized rat. Acta Endocrinol (Copenh) 12:123, 1953.
200. Payne RW, Hellbaum AA. The effect of estrogens on the ovary of the hypophysectomized rat. Endocrinology 57:193, 1955.
201. Rao MC, Midgley AR Jr, Richards JS. Hormonal regulation of ovarian cellular proliferation. Cell 14:71, 1978.
202. Harman SM, Louvet JP, Ross GT. Interaction of estrogen and gonadotropins on follicular atresia. Endocrinology 96:1145, 1975.
203. Ingraham DL. The effect of oestrogen on the atresia of ovarian follicles. J Endocrinol 19:123, 1959.
204. Ingraham DL. The effect of gonadotrophins and oestrogen on ovarian atresia in the immature rat. J Endocrinol 19:117, 1959.
205. Burghardt RC, Matheson RL. Gap junction amplification in rat ovarian granulosa cells. Dev Biol 94:206, 1982.
206. Merk FB, Botticelli CR, Albright JT. An intercellular response to estrogen by granulosa cells in the rat ovary; an electron microscope study. Endocrinology 90:992, 1972.
207. Richards JS. Maturation of ovarian follicles, actions and interactions of pituitary and ovarian hormones on follicular cell differentiation. Physiol Rev 60:51, 1980.
208. Simpson ME, Evans HM, Fraenkel-Conrat HL, Li CH. Synergism of estrogens with pituitary gonadotropins in hypophysectomized rats. Endocrinology 28:37, 1941.
209. Payne RW, Runser RH. The influence of estrogen and androgen on the ovarian response of hypophysectomized immature rats to gonadotropins. Endocrinology 62:313, 1958.
210. Reiter EO, Goldenberg RL, Vaitukaitis JL, et al. Evidence for a role of estrogen in the ovarian augmentation reaction. Endocrinology 91:1518, 1972.

211. Reiter EO, Goldenberg RL, Vaitukaitis JL, Ross GT. A role for endogenous estrogen in normal ovarian development in the neonatal rat. Endocrinology 91:1537, 1972.
212. Adashi EY, Hsueh AJW. Estrogens augment the stimulation of ovarian aromatase activity by follicle-stimulating hormone in cultured rat granulosa cells. J Biol Chem 257:6077, 1982.
213. Leung PCK, Goff AK, Kennedy TG, Armstrong DT. An intraovarian inhibitory action of estrogen on androgen production in vivo. Biol Reprod 19:641, 1978.
214. Leung PCK, Armstrong DT. Estrogen treatment of immature rats inhibits ovarian androgen production in vitro. Endocrinology 104:1411, 1979.
215. Leung P, Armstrong DT. A mechanism for the intraovarian inhibitory action of estrogen on androgen production. Biol Reprod 21:1035, 1979.
216. Magoffin DA, Erickson GF. Mechanism by which estradiol inhibits ovarian androgen production in the rat. Endocrinology 108:962, 1981.
217. Magoffin DA, Erickson GF. Direct inhibitory effect of estrogen on LH-stimulated androgen synthesis by ovarian cells cultured in defined medium. Mol Cell Endocrinol 28:81, 1982.
218. Hillier SG, Knazek R, Ross GT. Androgenic stimulation of progesterone production by granulosa cells from preantral ovarian follicles: Further in vitro studies using replicate cell cultures. Endocrinology 100:1539, 1977.
219. Hillier SG, Ross GT. Effects of exogenous testosterone on ovarian weight, follicular morphology and intraovarian progesterone concentration in estrogen-primed hypophysectomized immature female rats. Biol Reprod 20:261, 1979.
220. Louvet JP, Harman SM, Schreiber JR, Ross GT. Evidence for a role of androgens in follicular maturation. Endocrinology 97:366, 1975.
221. Moon YS, Duleba AJ, Leung PCK. Androgenic alteration in pathways of C_{19}-steroid metabolism by cultured rat granulosa cells. Biochem Biophys Res Commun 113:948, 1983.
222. Daniel SAJ, Armstrong DT. Enhancement of follicle-stimulating hormone–induced aromatase activity by androgens in cultured rat granulosa cells. Endocrinology 107:1027, 1980.
223. Hillier SG, DeZwart FA. Evidence that granulosa cell aromatase induction/activation by follicle-stimulating hormone is an androgen receptor–regulated process in vitro. Endocrinology 109:1303, 1981.
224. Armstrong DT, Dorrington JH. Androgens augment FSH-induced progesterone secretion by cultured rat granulosa cells. Endocrinology 99:1411, 1976.
225. Lucky AW, Schreiber JR, Hillier SG, et al. Progesterone production by cultured preantral rat granulosa cells; stimulation by androgens. Endocrinology 100:128, 1977.
226. Nimrod A, Lindner HT. The synergistic effect of androgen on the stimulation of progesterone secretion by FSH in cultured rat granulosa cells. Mol Cell Endocrinol 5:315, 1976.
227. Hillier SG, van den Boogard AJM, Reichart LE Jr, van Hall EV. Alterations in granulosa cell aromatase activity accompanying preovulatory follicular development in the rat ovary with evidence that 5α-reduced C_{19} steroids inhibit the aromatase reaction in vitro. J Endocrinol 84:409, 1980.
228. Payne RW, Hellbaum AA, Owens JN Jr. The effect of androgens on the ovaries and uterus of the estrogen-treated hypophysectomized immature rat. Endocrinology 59:306, 1956.
229. Farookhi R. Effects of androgen on induction of gonadotropin receptors and gonadotropin-stimulated adenosine 3′,5′-monophosphate production in rat ovarian granulosa cells. Endocrinology 106:1216, 1980.
230. Franchimont P, Channing CP (eds). Intragonadal Regulation of Reproduction. London, Academic Press, 1981.
231. Adashi EY. The intraovarian insulin-like growth factor system. *In* Adashi EY, Leung PCK (eds). The Ovary. New York, Raven Press, 1993, p 319.
232. el-Roeiy A, Chen X, Roberts VJ, et al. Expression of insulin-like growth factor-I (IGF-I) and IGF-II and the IGF-I, IGF-II, and insulin receptor genes and localization of the gene products in the human ovary. J Clin Endocrinol Metab 77:1411, 1993.
233. el-Roeiy A, Chen X, Roberts VJ, et al. Expression of the genes encoding the insulin-like growth factors (IGF-I and II), the IGF and insulin receptors, and IGF-binding proteins 1–6 and the localization of their gene products in normal and polycystic ovary syndrome ovaries. J Clin Endocrinol Metab 78:1488, 1994.
234. Zhou J, Bondy C. Anatomy of the human insulin-like growth factor system. Biol Reprod 48:467, 1993.
235. Geisthovel F, Moretti-Rojas I, Asch RH, Rojas FJ. Expression of insulin-like growth factor-II (IGF-II) messenger ribonucleic acid (mRNA), but not IGF-I mRNA, in human preovulatory granulosa cells. Hum Reprod 4:899, 1989.
236. Giudice LC, Milki AA, Milkowski DA, el Danasouri I. Human granulosa contain messenger ribonucleic acids encoding insulin-like growth factor–binding proteins (IGFBPs) and secrete IGFBPs in culture. Fertil Steril 56:475, 1991.
237. San Roman GA, Magoffin DA. Insulin-like growth factor binding proteins in ovarian follicles from women with polycystic ovarian disease: Cellular source and levels in follicular fluid. J Clin Endocrinol Metab 75:1010, 1992.
238. Grimes RW, Barber JA, Shimasaki S, et al. Porcine ovarian granulosa cells secrete insulin-like growth factor–binding proteins-4 and -5 and express their messenger ribonucleic acids: Regulation by follicle-stimulating hormone and insulin-like growth factor-1. Biol Reprod 50:695, 1994.
239. Iwashita M, Kudo Y, Yoshimura Y, et al. Physiological role of insulin-like-growth-factor-binding protein-4 in human folliculogenesis. Horm Res 46(suppl)1:31, 1996.
240. Dor J, Ben-Sclomo I, Lunenfeld B, et al. Insulin-like growth factor-I (IGF-I) may not be essential for ovarian follicular development: Evidence from IGF-I deficiency. J Clin Endocrinol Metab 74:539, 1992.
241. Yeh J, Yeh YC. Transforming growth factor-alpha and human cancer. Biomed Pharmacother 43:651, 1989.
242. Vlodavsky I, Brown KD, Gospodarowicz D. A comparison of the binding of epidermal growth factor to cultured granulosa and luteal cells. J Biol Chem 253:3744, 1978.
243. Knecht M, Catt KJ. Modulation of cAMP-mediated differentiation in ovarian granulosa cells by epidermal growth factor and platelet-derived growth factor. J Biol Chem 258:2789, 1983.
244. Schomberg DW, May JV, Mondschein JS. Interactions between hormones and growth factors in the regulation of granulosa cell differentiation in vitro. J Steroid Biochem 19:291, 1983.
245. Yeh J, Lee GY, Anderson E. Presence of transforming growth factor-alpha messenger ribonucleic acid (mRNA) and absence of epidermal growth factor mRNA in rat ovarian granulosa cells and the effects of these factors on steroidogenesis in vitro. Biol Reprod 48:1071, 1993.
246. Mock EJ, Niswender GD. Differences in the rates of internalization of ^{125}I-labeled human chorionic gonadotropin, luteinizing hormone, and epidermal growth factor by ovine luteal cells. Endocrinology 113:259, 1983.
247. St-Arnaud R, Walker P, Kelly PA, Labrie F. Rat ovarian epidermal growth factor receptors: Characterization and hormonal regulation. Mol Cell Endocrinol 31:43, 1983.
248. Mason HD, Carr L, Leake R, Franks S. Production of transforming growth factor-alpha by normal and polycystic ovaries. J Clin Endocrinol Metab 80:2053, 1995.
249. Maruo T, Ladines-Llave CA, Samoto T, et al. Expression of epidermal growth factor and its receptor in the human ovary during follicular growth and regression. Endocrinology 132:924, 1993.
250. Chegini N, Williams RS. Immunocytochemical localization of transforming growth factors (TGFs) TGF-alpha and TGF-beta in human ovarian tissues. J Clin Endocrinol Metab 74:973, 1992.
251. Li S, Maruo T, Ladines-Llave CA, et al. Expression of transforming growth factor-alpha in the human ovary during follicular growth, regression and atresia. Endocr J 41:693, 1994.
252. Tamura M, Sasano H, Suzuki T, et al. Expression of epidermal growth factors and epidermal growth factor receptor in normal cycling human ovaries. Hum Reprod 10:1891, 1995.
253. Sporn MB, Roberts AB, Wakefield LM, Assoian RK. Transforming growth factor-β: Biological function and chemical structure. Science 233:532, 1986.
254. Dorrington J, Chuma AV, Bendell JJ. Transforming growth factor β and follicle-stimulating hormone promote rat granulosa cell proliferation. Endocrinology 123:353, 1988.
255. Adashi EY, Resnick CE. Antagonistic interactions of transforming growth factors in the regulation of granulosa cell differentiation. Endocrinology 119:1243, 1986.
256. Feng P, Catt KJ, Knecht M. Transforming growth factor β

regulates the inhibitory actions of epidermal growth factor during granulosa cell differentiation. J Biol Chem 261:14167, 1986.
257. Knecht M, Feng P, Catt KJ. Transforming growth factor-beta regulates the expression of luteinizing hormone receptors in ovarian granulosa cells. Biochem Biophys Res Commun 139:800, 1986.
258. Dodson WC, Schomberg DW. The effect of transforming growth factor-β on follicle-stimulating hormone–induced differentiation of cultured rat granulosa cells. Endocrinology 120:512, 1987.
259. Hutchinson LA, Findlay JK, de Vos FL, Robertson DM. Effects of bovine inhibin, transforming growth factor-β and bovine activin-A on granulosa cell differentiation. Biochem Biophys Res Commun 146:1405, 1987.
260. Blair EI, Kim I-C, Estes JE, et al. Human platelet-derived growth factor preparations contain a separate activity which potentiates follicle stimulating hormone mediated induction of luteinizing hormone receptor in cultured rat granulosa cells: Evidence for transforming growth factor β. Endocrinology 123:2003, 1988.
261. Zhiwen Z, Findlay JK, Carson RD, et al. Transforming growth factor β enhances basal and FSH-stimulated inhibin production by rat granulosa cells in vitro. Mol Cell Endocrinol 58:161, 1988.
262. Adashi EY, Resnick CE, Hernandez ER, et al. Ovarian transforming growth factor-β (TGF-β): Cellular site(s), and mechanism(s) of action. Mol Cell Endocrinol 61:247, 1989.
263. Knecht M, Feng P, Catt K. Bifunctional role of transforming growth factor-β during granulosa cell development. Endocrinology 120:1243, 1987.
264. Ying SY, Becker A, Ling N, et al. Inhibin and β type transforming growth factor (TGFβ) have opposite modulating effects on the follicle stimulating hormone (FSH)–induced aromatase activity of cultured rat granulosa cell. Biochem Biophys Res Commun 136:969, 1986.
265. Magoffin DA, Gancedo B, Erickson GF. Transforming growth factor-β promotes differentiation of ovarian thecal-interstitial cells but inhibits androgen production. Endocrinology 125:1951, 1989.
266. McWilliam R, Leake RE, Coutts JR. Growth factors in human ovarian follicle fluid and growth factor receptors in granulosa-luteal cells. Int J Biol Markers 10:216, 1995.
267. Chegini N, Flanders KC. Presence of transforming growth factor-beta and their selective cellular localization in human ovarian tissue of various reproductive stages. Endocrinology 130:1707, 1992.
268. Eramaa M, Ritvos O. Transforming growth factor-beta 1 and -beta 2 induce inhibin and activin beta B-subunit messenger ribonucleic acid levels in cultured human granulosa-luteal cells. Fertil Steril 65:954, 1996.
269. Burger HG, Farnworth PG, Findlay JK, et al. Aspects of current and future inhibin research. Reprod Fertil Dev 7:992, 1995.
270. Groome NP, Illingworth PJ, O'Brien M, et al. Measurement of dimeric inhibin B throughout the human menstrual cycle. J Clin Endocrinol Metab 81:1401, 1996.
271. Jaatinen TA, Penttila TL, Kaipia A, et al. Expression of inhibin alpha, beta A and beta B messenger ribonucleic acids in the normal human ovary and in polycystic ovarian syndrome. J Endocrinol 143:127, 1994.
272. Roberts VJ, Barth S, el-Roeiy A, Yen SSC. Expression of inhibin/activin subunits and follistatin messenger ribonucleic acids and proteins in ovarian follicles and the corpus luteum during the human menstrual cycle. J Clin Endocrinol Metab 77:1402, 1993.
273. Roberts VJ, Barth S, el-Roeiy A, Yen SSC. Expression of inhibin/activin system messenger ribonucleic acids and proteins in ovarian follicles from women with polycystic ovarian syndrome. J Clin Endocrinol Metab 79:1434, 1994.
274. Aloi JA, Dalkin AC, Schwartz NB, et al. Ovarian inhibin subunit gene expression: Regulation by gonadotropins and estradiol. Endocrinology 136:1227, 1995.
275. Eramaa M, Tuuri T, Hilden K, Ritvos O. Regulation of inhibin alpha- and beta A-subunit messenger ribonucleic acid levels by chorionic gonadotropin and recombinant follicle-stimulating hormone in cultured human granulosa-luteal cells. J Clin Endocrinol Metab 79:1670, 1994.
276. Peng C, Ohno T, Khorasheh S, Leung PC. Activin and follistatin as local regulators in the human ovary. Biol Signals 5:81, 1996.
277. Li R, Phillips DM, Mather JP. Activin promotes ovarian follicle development in vitro. Endocrinology 136:849, 1995.
278. Knight PG, Muttukrishna S, Groome NP. Development and application of a two-site enzyme immunoassay for the determination of 'total' activin-A concentrations in serum and follicular fluid. J Endocrinol 148:267, 1996.
279. Muttukrishna S, Fowler PA, George L, et al. Changes in peripheral serum levels of total activin A during the human menstrual cycle and pregnancy. J Clin Endocrinol Metab 81:3328, 1996.
280. Harada K, Shintani Y, Sakamoto Y, et al. Serum immunoreactive activin levels in normal subjects and patients with various diseases. J Clin Endocrinol Metab 81:2125, 1996.
281. Cataldo NA, Rabinovici J, Fujimoto VY, Jaffe RB. Follistatin antagonizes the effects of activin-A on steroidogenesis in human luteinizing granulosa cells. J Clin Endocrinol Metab 79:272, 1994.
282. Erickson GF, Chung DG, Sit A, et al. Follistatin concentrations in follicular fluid of normal and polycystic ovaries. Hum Reprod 10:2120, 1995.
283. Khoury RH, Wang QF, Crowley WF Jr, et al. Serum follistatin levels in women: Evidence against an endocrine function of ovarian follistatin. J Clin Endocrinol Metab 80:1361, 1995.
284. Kettel LM, DePaolo LV, Morales AJ, et al. Circulating levels of follistatin from puberty to menopause. Fertil Steril 65:472, 1996.
285. Gospodarowicz D, Cheng J, Lui G-M, et al. Corpus luteum angiogenic factor is related to fibroblast growth factor. Endocrinology 117:2283, 1985.
286. Gospodarowicz D, Ill CR, Birdwell CR. Effects of fibroblast and epidermal growth factors on ovarian cell proliferation in vitro: I. Characterization of the response of granulosa cells to FGF and EFG. Endocrinology 100:1108, 1977.
287. Gospodarowicz D, Bialecki H. The effect of epidermal and fibroblast growth factor on the replicative lifespan of bovine granulosa cells in culture. Endocrinology 103:854, 1978.
288. Gospodarowicz D, Bialecki H. Fibroblast and epidermal growth factors are mitogenic agents for cultured granulosa cells of rodent, porcine, and human origin. Endocrinology 104:757, 1979.
289. Tapanainen J, Leinonen PJ, Tapanainen P, et al. Regulation of human granulosa-luteal progesterone production and proliferation by gonadotropins and growth factors. Fertil Steril 48:576, 1987.
290. Watson R, Anthony F, Pickett M, et al. Reverse transcription with nested polymerase chain reaction shows expression of basic fibroblast growth factor transcripts in human granulosa and cumulus cells from in vitro fertilisation patients. Biochem Biophys Res Commun 187:1227, 1992.
291. Di Blasio AM, Vigano P, Cremonesi L, et al. Expression of the genes encoding basic fibroblast growth factor and its receptor in human granulosa cells. Mol Cell Endocrinol 96:R7, 1993.
292. Reynolds LP, Killilea SD, Redmer DA. Angiogenesis in the female reproductive system. FASEB J 6:886, 1992.
293. Chun SY, Eisenhauer KM, Minami S, et al. Hormonal regulation of apoptosis in early antral follicles: Follicle-stimulating hormone as a major survival factor. Endocrinology 137:1447, 1996.
294. Dinarello CA. Interleukin-1 and the pathogenesis of the acute-phase response. N Engl J Med 311:1413, 1984.
295. Duff G. Many roles for interleukin-1. Nature 313:352, 1985.
296. Dinarello CA. Biology of interleukin-1. FASEB J 21:108, 1988.
297. Fukuoka M, Mori T, Taii S, Yasuda K. Interleukin-1 inhibits luteinization of porcine granulosa cells in culture. Endocrinology 122:367, 1987.
298. Gottschall PE, Katsuura G, Hoffman ST, Arimura A. Interleukin-1: An inhibitor of luteinizing hormone receptor formation in cultured rat granulosa cells. Endocrinology 117:2313, 1988.
299. Gottschall PE, Katsuura G, Dahl RR, et al. Discordance in the effects of interleukin-1 on rat granulosa cell differentiation induced by follicle-stimulating hormone or activators of adenylate cyclase. Biol Reprod 39:1074, 1988.
300. Gottschall PE, Katsuura G, Hoffmann ST, Arimura A. Interleukin 1: An inhibitor of luteinizing hormone receptor formation in cultured rat granulosa cells. FASEB J 2:2492, 1988.
301. Fukuoka M, Yasuda K, Taii S, et al. Interleukin-1 stimulates growth and inhibits progesterone secretion in the cultures of porcine granulosa cells. Endocrinology 124:884, 1989.
302. Kasson B, Gorospe W. Effects of interleukins 1, 2 and 3 on follicle-stimulating hormone–induced differentiation of rat granulosa cells. Mol Cell Endocrinol 62:103, 1989.
303. Cannon JG, Dinarello CA. Increased plasma interleukin-1 activity in women after ovulation. Science 227:1247, 1985.

304. Pacifici R, Rifas L, McCracken R, et al. Ovarian steroid treatment blocks a postmenopausal increase in blood monocyte interleukin 1 release. Proc Natl Acad Sci USA 86:2398, 1989.
305. Polan ML, Carding S, Louides J. Progesterone modulates interleukin-1β (IL-1β) mRNA production by human pelvic macrophages. Fertil Steril 50:S4, 1988.
306. Yee JB, Hutson JC. Testicular macrophages: Isolation, characterization and hormone responsiveness. Biol Reprod 29:1319, 1983.
307. Yee J, Hutson J. In vitro effects of follicle-stimulating hormone on testicular macrophages. Biol Reprod 32:880, 1985.
308. Yee J, Hutson J. Biochemical consequences of follicle-stimulating hormone binding to testicular macrophages in culture (Abstract). Biol Reprod 32:872, 1985.
309. Khan SA, Schmidt K, Hallin P, et al. Human testis cytosol and ovarian follicular fluid contain high amounts of interleukin-1–like factor(s). Mol Cell Endocrinol 58:221, 1988.
310. Takakura K, Taii S, Fukuoka M, et al. Interleukin-2 receptor/p55(Tac)–inducing activity in porcine follicular fluid. Endocrinology 125:618, 1989.
311. Kokia E, Adashi EY. Potential role of cytokines in ovarian physiology: The case for interleukin-1. *In* Adashi EY, Leung PCK (eds). The Ovary. New York, Raven Press, 1993, p 383.
312. Bagavandoss P, Kunkel SL, Wiggins RC, Keys PL. Tumor necrosis factor-α (TNF-α) production and localization of macrophages and T lymphocytes in the rabbit corpus luteum. Endocrinology 122:1185, 1987.
313. Emoto N, Baird A. The effect of tumor necrosis factor/cachectin on follicle-stimulating hormone–induced aromatase-activity in cultured rat granulosa cells. Biochem Biophys Res Commun 153:792, 1988.
314. Roby KF, Terranova PF. Tumor necrosis factor alpha alters follicular steroidogenesis in vitro. Endocrinology 123:2952, 1988.
315. Adashi E, Resnick C, Croft C, Payne D. Tumor necrosis factor α inhibits gonadotropin hormonal action in non-transformed ovarian granulosa cells. J Biol Chem 264:1, 1989.
316. Unanue E, Allen P. The basis for the immunoregulatory role of macrophages and other accessory cells. Science 236:551, 1987.
317. Harrison L, Campbell I. Cytokines: An expanding network of immuno-inflammatory hormones. Mol Endocrinol 2:1151, 1988.
318. Terranova PF, Sancho-Tello M, Hunter VJ. Tumor necrosis factor-alpha and ovarian function. *In* Adashi EY, Leung PCK (eds). The Ovary. New York, Raven Press, 1993, p 395.
319. Owman CH, Rosengren E, Sjoberg NO. Adrenergic innervation of the human female reproductive organs: A histochemical and chemical investigation. Obstet Gynecol 30:763, 1967.
320. Jacobowitz D, Wallach EE. Histochemical and chemical studies of the autonomic innervation of the ovary. Endocrinology 81:1132, 1967.
321. Neilson D, Jones GS, Woodruff JD, Goldberg B. The innervation of the ovary. Obstet Gynecol Surv 25:889, 1970.
322. Walles B, Groschel-Stuart U, Owman CH, et al. Fluorescence histochemical demonstration of a relationship between adrenergic nerves and cells containing actin and myosin in the rat ovary with special reference to the follicle wall. J Reprod Fertil 52:175, 1978.
323. Burden HW. Adrenergic innervation in ovaries of the interstitial gland in the guinea pig ovary. Neuroendocrinology 17:40, 1972.
324. Svensson KG, Owman CH, Sjoberg NO, et al. Ultrastructural evidence for adrenergic innervation of the interstitial gland in the guinea pig ovary. Neuroendocrinology 17:40, 1975.
325. Lawrence IE, Burden HW. The origin of the extrinsic adrenergic innervation to the rat ovary. Anat Rec 196:51, 1980.
326. Gilbert AB. Innervation of the ovarian follicle of the domestic hen. Q J Exp Physiol 1:437, 1965.
327. Dahl E. Studies of the fine structure of ovarian interstitial tissue. III. The innervation of the thecal gland of the domestic fowl. Z Zellforsch Mikrosk Anat 109:212, 1970.
328. Moshin S, Pennefather JN. The sympathetic innervation of the mammalian ovary, a review of pharmacological and histological studies. Clin Exp Pharmacol Physiol 6:335, 1979.
329. Marshall JM. Adrenergic innervation of the female reproductive tract: Anatomy, physiology and pharmacology. Ergeb Physiol 62:6, 1970.
330. Stefenson A, Owman CH, Sjoberg NO, et al. Comparative study of the autonomic innervation of the mammalian ovary, with particular regard to the follicular system. Cell Tissue Res 215:47, 1981.
331. Capps ML, Lawrence IE, Burden HW. Ultrastructure of the cells of the ovarian interstitial gland in hypophysectomized rats. The effects of stimulation of the ovarian plexus and of denervation. Cell Tissue Res 193:433, 1978.
332. Burden HW, Lawrence LE. The effect of denervation on the localization of Δ^5-3β-hydroxysteroid dehydrogenase activity in the rat ovary during pregnancy. Acta Anat 97:286, 1977.
333. Dyer CA, Erickson GF. Norepinephrine amplifies human chorionic gonadotropin-stimulated androgen biosynthesis by ovarian theca-interstitial cells. Endocrinology 116:1645, 1985.
334. Kawakami M, Kubo K, Vemuira T, et al. Involvement of ovarian innervation in steroid secretion. Endocrinology 109:136, 1981.
335. Condon WA, Black DL. Catecholamine-induced stimulation of progesterone by the bovine corpus luteum in vitro. Biol Reprod 15:573, 1976.
336. Godkin JD, Black DL, Duby RT. Stimulation of cyclic AMP and progesterone synthesis by LH, PGE_2 and isoproterenol in the bovine CL in vitro. Biol Reprod 17:514, 1977.
337. Jordan AW III, Caffrey JL, Niswender GD. Catecholamine-induced stimulation of progesterone and adenosine 3′,5′-monophosphate production by dispersed ovine luteal cells. Endocrinology 103:385, 1978.
338. Ratner A, Sanborn CR, Weiss GK. β-Adrenergic stimulation of cAMP and progesterone in rat ovarian tissue. Am J Physiol 239:E139, 1980.
339. Veldhuis JD, Harrison TS, Hammond JM. β_2-Adrenergic stimulation of ornithine decarboxylase activity in porcine granulosa cells in vitro. Biochim Biophys Acta 627:123, 1980.
340. Kliachko S, Zor U. Increase in catecholamine-stimulated cyclic AMP and progesterone synthesis in rat granulosa cells during culture. Mol Cell Endocrinol 23:23, 1981.
341. Adashi EY, Hsueh AJW. Stimulation of β_2-adrenergic responsiveness by follicle-stimulating hormone in rat granulosa cells in vitro and in vivo. Endocrinology 108:2170, 1981.
342. Aguado LI, Ojeda SR. Prepubertal ovarian function is finely regulated by direct adrenergic influences. Role of noradrenergic innervation. Endocrinology 114:1845, 1984.
343. Aguado LI, Ojeda SR. Ovarian adrenergic nerves play a role in maintaining preovulatory steroid secretion. Endocrinology 114:1944, 1984.
344. Semenova II. Adrenergic innervation of ovaries in Stein-Leventhal syndrome. Vestn Akad Med Nauk SSSR 24:58, 1969.
345. Erickson GF, Yen SSC. New data on follicle cells in polycystic ovaries: A proposed mechanism for the genesis of cystic follicles. Semin Reprod Endocrinol 2:231, 1984.
346. Pepperell JR, Nemeth G, Palumbo A, Naftolin F. The intraovarian renin-angiotensin system. *In* Adashi EY, Leung PCK (eds). The Ovary. New York, Raven Press, 1993, p 363.
347. Asakura H, Zwain IH, Yen SSC. Expression of genes encoding corticotropin-releasing factor (CRF), type 1 CRF receptor, and CRF-binding protein and localization of the gene products in the human ovary. J Clin Endocrinol Metab 82:2720, 1997.
348. Ledwitz-Rigby F, Rigby BW, Gay VL, et al. Inhibitory action of porcine follicular fluid upon granulosa cell luteinization in vitro. J Endocrinol 74:175, 1977.
349. Stone SL, Pomerantz SH, Schwartz-Kripner A, Channing CP. Inhibition of oocyte maturation from porcine follicular fluid. Further purification and evidence for reversible action. Biol Reprod 19:585, 1978.
350. Tsafriri A, Channing CP. An inhibitory influence of granulosa cells and follicular fluid upon porcine oocyte meiosis in vitro. Endocrinology 96:922, 1975.
351. Edwards RG. Maturation in vitro of mouse, sheep, cow, pig, rhesus monkey, and human oocytes. Nature 208:349, 1965.
352. DiZerega GS, Marrs RP, Roche PL, et al. Identification of proteins in pooled human follicular fluid which suppress follicular response to gonadotropins. J Clin Endocrinol Metab 56:35, 1983.
353. DiZerega GS, Goebelsmann U, Nakamura RM. Identification of protein(s) secreted by the preovulatory ovary which suppresses the follicle response to gonadotropins. J Clin Endocrinol Metab 54:1091, 1982.
354. DiZerega GS, Hodgen GD. The primate ovarian cycle: Suppression of human menopausal gonadotropin-induced follicular growth in presence of the dominant follicle. J Clin Endocrinol Metab 50:819, 1980.

355. Hodgen GD. The dominant ovarian follicle. Fertil Steril 38:281, 1982.
356. Goodman AL, Hodgen GD. Between ovary interaction in the regulation of follicle growth, corpus luteum function, and gonadotropin secretion in the primate ovarian cycle. I. Effects of follicle cautery and hemiovariectomy during the follicular phase in cynomolgus monkeys. Endocrinology 104:1304, 1979.
357. Goodman AL, Hodgen GD. Between ovary interaction in the regulation of follicle growth, corpus luteum function, and gonadotropin in the primate ovarian cycle. II. Effects of luteectomy and hemiovariectomy during the luteal phase in cynomolgus monkeys. Endocrinology 104:1310, 1979.
358. Nilsson L, Wikland M, Hamberger L. Recruitment of an ovulatory follicle in the human following follicle-ectomy and luteectomy. Fertil Steril 37:30, 1982.
359. DiZerega GS, Marut EL, Turner CK, Hodgen GD. Asymmetrical ovarian function during recruitment and selection of the dominant follicle in the menstrual cycle of the rhesus monkey. J Clin Endocrinol Metab 51:698, 1980.
360. Brailly S, Gougeon A, Milgram E, et al. Androgens and progestins in the human ovarian follicle: Differences in the evolution of preovulatory, healthy nonovulatory, and atretic follicles. J Clin Endocrinol Metab 53:128, 1981.
361. McNatty KP. Hormonal correlates of follicular development in the human ovary. Aust J Biol Sci 34:249, 1981.
362. McNatty KP, Baird DT, Bolton A, et al. Concentration of oestrogens and androgens in human ovarian venous plasma and follicular fluid throughout the menstrual cycle. J Endocrinol 71:77, 1976.
363. McNatty KP. Cyclic changes in antral fluid hormone concentrations in humans. Clin Endocrinol Metab 7:577, 1978.
364. McNatty KP, Moore-Smith D, Makris A, et al. The microenvironment of the human antral follicle: Interrelationships among the steroid levels in antral fluids, the population of granulosa cells, and the status of the oocyte in vivo and in vitro. J Clin Endocrinol Metab 49:851, 1979.
365. Sanyal MK, Berger MJ, Thompson IE, et al. Development of graafian follicles in adult human ovary. I. Correlation of estrogen and progesterone concentration in antral fluid with growth of follicles. J Clin Endocrinol Metab 38:828, 1974.
366. McNatty KP, Hunter WM, McNeilley AS, Sawers PS. Changes in the concentration of pituitary and steroid hormones in the follicular fluid of human graafian follicles throughout the menstrual cycle. J Endocrinol 64:555, 1975.
367. McNatty KP, Sawers RS. Relationship between the endocrine environment within graafian follicle and the subsequent rate of progesterone secretion by human granulosa cells in vitro. J Endocrinol 66:391, 1975.
368. Bauminger S, Lindner HR. Periovulatory changes in ovarian prostaglandin formation and their hormonal control in the rat. Prostaglandins 9:737, 1975.
369. Armstrong DT. Role of prostaglandins in follicular responses to luteinizing hormone. Ann Biol Anim Biochim Biophys 15:181, 1975.
370. Armstrong DT, Grinwich DL. Blockage of spontaneous and Lh-induced ovulation in rats by indomethacin, an inhibitor of prostaglandin synthesis. Prostaglandins 1:21, 1972.
371. Armstrong DT, Zamecnik J. Pre-ovulatory elevation of rat ovarian prostaglandin F, and its blockade by indomethacin. Mol Cell Endocrinol 2:125, 1975.
372. Armstrong D, Grinwich D, Moon Y, Zamecnik J. Inhibition of ovulation in rabbits by intrafollicular injection of indomethacin and prostaglandin F antiserum. Life Sci 14:129, 1974.
373. Erickson GF, Challis JRG, Ryan KJ. Production of prostaglandin F by rabbit granulosa cells and thecal tissue. J Reprod Fertil 49:133, 1977.
374. Marsh JM, Yang NST, LeMaire WJ. Prostaglandin synthesis in rabbit graafian follicles in vitro. Effect of luteinizing hormone and cyclic AMP. Prostaglandins 7:269, 1974.
375. Triebwasser WF, Clark MR, LeMaire WJ, Marsh JM. Localization and in vitro synthesis of prostaglandins in components of rabbit preovulatory graafian follicles. Prostaglandins 16:621, 1978.
376. Tsafriri A, Lindner HR, Zor U, Lamprecht SA. Physiological role of prostaglandins in the induction of ovulation. Prostaglandins 2:1, 1972.
377. Doyle JB. Exploratory culdotomy for observation of tubo-ovarian physiology at ovulation time. Fertil Steril 2:475, 1951.
378. Espey LL, Lipner H. Measurements of intrafollicular pressures in the rabbit ovary. Am J Physiol 205:1067, 1963.
379. Blandau R, Rumery R. Measurements of intrafollicular pressure in ovulatory and preovulatory follicles in the rat. Fertil Steril 14:330, 1963.
380. Blandau RJ. Anatomy of ovulation. Clin Obstet Gynecol 10:347, 1969.
381. Gebauer H, Lindner HR, Amsterdam A. Synthesis of heparin-like glycosaminoglycans in rat ovarian slices. Biol Reprod 18:350, 1978.
382. Bellin ME, Lenz RW, Steadman LE, Ax RL. Proteoglycan production by bovine granulosa cells in vitro occurs in response to FSH. Mol Cell Endocrinol 29:51, 1983.
383. Ax RL, Ryan RJ. The porcine ovarian follicle. IV. Mucopolysaccharides at different stages of development. Biol Reprod 20:1123, 1979.
384. Ax RL, Ryan RJ. FSH stimulation of ^{3}H-glucosamine-incorporation into proteoglycans by porcine granulosa cells in vitro. J Clin Endocrinol Metab 49:696, 1979.
385. Espey LL. Ovarian proteolytic enzymes and ovulation. Biol Reprod 10:216, 1974.
386. Bjersing L, Cajander S. Ovulation and the mechanism of follicle rupture. IV: Ultrastructure of membrana granulosa of rabbit graafian follicles prior to induced ovulation. Cell Tissue Res 153:1, 1974.
387. Beers WH, Strickland S, Reich E. Ovarian plasminogen activator: Relationship to ovulation and hormonal regulation. Cell 6:387, 1975.
388. Frederick JL, Shimanuki T, DiZerega GS. Initiation of angiogenesis by human follicular fluid. Science 224:389, 1984.
389. Kamat BR, Brown LF, Manseau EJ, et al. Expression of vascular permeability factor/vascular endothelial growth factor by human granulosa and theca lutein cells. Role in corpus luteum development. Am J Pathol 146:157, 1995.
390. Redmer DA, Dai Y, Li J, et al. Characterization and expression of vascular endothelial growth factor (VEGF) in the ovine corpus luteum. J Reprod Fertil 108:157, 1996.
391. Khan-Dawood FS, Yang J, Dawood MY. Expression of gap junction protein connexin-43 in the human and baboon *(Papio anubis)* corpus luteum. J Clin Endocrinol Metab 81:835, 1996.
392. Duncan WC, McNeilly AS, Fraser HM, Illingworth PJ. Luteinizing hormone receptor in the human corpus luteum: Lack of down-regulation during maternal recognition of pregnancy. Hum Reprod 11:2291, 1996.
393. Johnson MC, Devoto L, Retamales I, et al. Localization of insulin-like growth factor (IGF-I) and IGF-I receptor expression in human corpora lutea: Role on estradiol secretion. Fertil Steril 65:489, 1996.
394. Revelli A, Pacchioni D, Cassoni P, et al. In situ hybridization study of messenger RNA for estrogen receptor and immunohistochemical detection of estrogen and progesterone receptors in the human ovary. Gynecol Endocrinol 10:177, 1996.
395. Bukovsky A, Caudle MR, Keenan JA, et al. Is corpus luteum an immune-mediated event? Localization of immune system components and luteinizing hormone receptor in human corpora lutea. Biol Reprod 53:1373, 1995.
396. Casper R, Yen SSC. Induction of luteolysis in the human with a long acting analog of luteinizing hormone–releasing factor. Science 205:408, 1979.
397. Yoshimi T, Strott C, Marshall J, Lipsett M. Corpus luteum function in early pregnancy. J Clin Endocrinol Metab 29:225, 1969.
398. Gillman J, Stein H. The human corpus luteum of pregnancy. Surg Gynecol Obstet 72:129, 1941.
399. Schoonmaker JN, Victery W, Karsch FJ. A receptive period for estradiol-induced luteolysis in the rhesus monkey. Endocrinology 108:1874, 1981.
400. O'Gray JP, Kohorn EI, Glass RH, et al. Inhibition of progesterone synthesis in vitro by prostaglandin $F_{2\alpha}$. J Reprod Fertil 30:153, 1972.
401. Shikone T, Yamoto M, Kokawa K, et al. Apoptosis of human corpora lutea during cyclic luteal regression and early pregnancy. J Clin Endocrinol Metab 81:2376, 1996.

402. Rodger FE, Fraser HM, Duncan WC, Illingworth PJ. Immunolocalization of bcl-2 in the human corpus luteum. Hum Reprod 10:1566, 1995.
403. Hertig AT. The aging ovary, a preliminary note. J Clin Endocrinol Metab 4:581, 1944.
404. Woll E, Hertig AT, Smith GVS, et al. The ovary in endometrial carcinoma with notes on the morphological history of the aging ovary. Am J Obstet Gynecol 56:617, 1948.
405. Bigelow B. Comparison of ovarian and endometrial morphology spanning the menopause. Obstet Gynecol 11:487, 1958.
406. Dennefors BL, Janson PO, Knutson F, Hamberger L. Steroid production and responsiveness to gonadotropin in isolated stromal tissue of human postmenopausal ovaries. Am J Obstet Gynecol 136:997, 1980.
407. Dennefors BL, Janson PO, Hamberger FK. Hilus cells from human postmenopausal ovaries: Gonadotrophin sensitivity, steroid and cyclic AMP production. Acta Obstet Gynecol Scand 61:413, 1982.
408. Braithwaite SS, Erkman-Balis B, Avila TD. Postmenopausal virilization due to ovarian stromal hyperthecosis. J Clin Endocrinol Metab 46:295, 1978.
409. Mandel FP, Voet RL, Weiland AJ, Judd HL. Steroid secretion by masculinizing and "feminizing" hilus cell tumors. J Clin Endocrinol Metab 52:779, 1981.
410. Merkow LP, Slifkin M, Acevedo HF, Greenberg WV. Ultrastructure of an interstitial (hilar) cell tumor of the ovary. Obstet Gynecol 37:845, 1971.
411. Carson RS, Findlay JK, Burger HG, Trounson AO. Gonadotropin receptors of the ovine ovarian follicle during follicular growth and atresia. Biol Reprod 21:75, 1979.
412. Schnoy N. Ultrastucture of a virilizing ovarian Leydig cell-tumor. Virchows Arch Pathol Anat 397:17, 1982.
413. Sternberg WH. The morphology, androgenic function, hyperplasia, and tumors of the human ovarian hilus cèlls. Am J Pathol 25:493, 1947.
414. Longcope C. Metabolic clearance and blood production of estrogens in postmenopausal women. Am J Obstet Gynecol 111:778, 1971.
415. Mattingly RF, Huang WY. Steroidogenesis of the menopausal and postmenopausal ovary. Am J Obstet Gynecol 103:679, 1969.
416. Grodin JM, Siiteri PK, MacDonald PC. Source of estrogen production in postmenopausal women. J Clin Endocrinol Metab 36:207, 1973.
417. Judd HL, Judd GE, Lucas WE, Yen SSC. Endocrine function of the postmenopausal ovary: Concentration of androgens and estrogens in ovarian and peripheral vein blood. J Clin Endocrinol Metab 39:1020, 1974.
418. Judd HL, Lucas WE, Yen SSC. Effect of oophorectomy on circulating testosterone and androstenedione levels in patients with endometrial cancer. Am J Obstet Gynecol 118:793, 1974.
419. Vermeulen A. The hormonal activity of the postmenopausal ovary. J Clin Endocrinol Metab 42:247, 1976.
420. Poliak A, Jones GES, Goldberg B, et al. Effect of human chorionic gonadotropin on postmenopausal women. Am J Obstet Gynecol 101:731 1968.
421. Greenblatt RB, Colle ML, Mahesh VB. Ovarian and adrenal steroid production in the postmenopausal woman. Obstet Gynecol 47:383, 1976.
422. Dowsett M, Cantwell B, Anshumala LAL, et al. Suppression of postmenopausal ovarian steroidogenesis with the luteinizing hormone–releasing hormone agonist goserelin. J Clin Endocrinol Metab 66:672, 1988.
423. Peluso JJ, Steger RW, Jaszczak S, Hafez ESE. Gonadotropin binding sites in human postmenopausal ovaries. Fertil Steril 27:789, 1976.
424. Nakano R, Shima K, Yamoto M, et al. Binding sites for gonadotrophins in human postmenopausal ovaries. Obstet Gynecol 73:196, 1989.

Chapter 7

THE HUMAN MENSTRUAL CYCLE: Neuroendocrine Regulation

S. S. C. Yen

CHAPTER OUTLINE

KEY POINTS

- Menarche, a dynamic neuroendocrine-metabolic process, reflects the establishment of nutritional microenvironments and the functional activity of hypothalamic GnRH pulse generator—the seat in activation of the gonadotropin-ovarian axis and inauguration of menstrual cyclicity.
- The neuroendocrine system that controls the human menstrual cycle is the pulsatile nature of gonadotropin secretion, which is a direct result of episodic release of GnRH from the neuronal terminals at the arcuate nucleus–median eminence region and delivery to the gonadotroph through the portal vessels.
- The origin of the GnRH pulse generator may reside within the GnRH neuron itself, and the pulsatile frequency and amplitude are dictated by central (i.e., opioidergic system) and peripheral (i.e., ovarian steroids) feedback signals.
- The follicular phase of the cycle is regulated by high frequency and low amplitude of GnRH/LH pulses. Increasing frequency in the late follicular phase occurs as a consequence of feedback action of increasing levels of estradiol by the preovulatory follicle.
- The menstrual cycle is interrupted, when estradiol attains a crucial level, by the onset of the midcycle gonadotropin surge, the duration of which is amplified by the feedback action of progesterone. This event is pivotal in the process of ovulation—a dynamic phase of follicular-luteal transition.
- The luteal phase of the cycle is dominated by LH pulses of slow frequency but high amplitude. The production of progesterone and its feedback action on the opioidergic neuronal system exert an inhibitory influence on frequency modulation. Progesterone, together with estradiol and inhibin A, also provides a negative feedback action on FSH secretion whereby folliculogenesis is prevented.
- The initiation of follicular growth of the ensuing cycle depends on the regression of the antecedent corpus luteum. The key event is the inverse dynamic between the fall of inhibin A, progesterone, and estradiol and the rise of FSH. These events, together with the emerging of high-frequency LH pulses that occur 2 days before the onset of menses, initiate a new round of folliculogenesis—a dynamic process of luteal-follicular transition.

THE MENSTRUAL CYCLE: CHARACTERISTICS

Menarche

The initiation of puberty depends on a complex series of events that occur within the brain and appears to require interactive participation of neuronal circuitries and glial networks as well as peripheral endocrine-metabolic signals. The progression of pubertal development and maturation in girls is marked by the onset of the menstrual period (the menarche). During the first few months and up to a year, the hypothalamic-pituitary-ovarian axis is not completely synchronized, resulting in anovulatory cycles with irregular lengths.[1]

There has been a trend in the last century toward an earlier onset of puberty and menarche in affluent societies, attributed primarily to the improvement of nutritional status and general health of younger generations of women.[2, 3] The onset of menarche is closely related to the attainment of a crucial percentage of body fat.[2, 4, 5] The increased percentage of body fat is governed by the availability of metabolic substrates. Thus, nutrition is the crucial factor in the timing of sexual maturation, which is expressed in the establishment of hypothalamic pulsatile release of gonadotropin-releasing hormone (GnRH)—the seat in the activation of the gonadotropin-ovarian axis and the inauguration of menstrual cyclicity.

The age at which girls develop menarche varies between 9 and 16 years with a mean of 12.5 years. Peripherally originated metabolic signals that can act centrally to modify neuronal function have recently been identified. Insulin-like growth factor I (IGF-I) and leptin possess attributes as candidates to convey messages to inform the hypothalamus of the adequacy of nutritional microenvironments for reproduction.

IGF-I serum levels increase during childhood, with highest values attained at puberty, and thereafter IGF-I levels decline with advancing age.[6, 7] Girls older than 8 years have measurable free IGF-I levels that account for approximately 1 percent of the total IGF-I concentration (Fig. 7–1). The more than 10-fold increase in IGF-I parallels the rapid increase in serum levels of dehydroepiandrosterone sulfate (DHEA-S), a marker of adrenarche. Thus, IGF-I and DHEA-S may jointly participate in the events of adrenarche and puberty.[8] The presence of IGF-I receptors on GnRH neurons and the median eminence and the dose-dependent IGF-I–induced increase in GnRH messenger ribonucleic acid (mRNA) and secretion from GT-1–7 cells[9, 10] are consistent with a feedback effect of IGF-I on GnRH neurons. Furthermore, the temporal pattern of binding of IGF-I to its receptor in the hypothalamus was found to peak during the period of increasing GnRH gene expression in vivo,[11–13] and IGF-I knockout mice do not undergo reproductive development. IGF-I may also enhance basal and GnRH-stimulated luteinizing hormone (LH) release by pituitary cells.[14] These attributes, together with experiments showing that IGF-I administered intraventricularly to immature rats induces LH secretion and advances puberty,[15] raise the possibility that the acute elevation of IGF-I during human puberty may serve as a metabolic signal for the maturation of the neuroendocrine axis and the onset of menarche.

Leptin, the hormone product of the *ob* gene, acts through functional receptors in the arcuate nucleus of the hypothalamus and serves as an afferent satiety signal regulating appetite, body weight, and energy expenditure as well as sexual maturation.[16–18] Neuropeptide Y (NPY) in the arcuate nucleus appears to be the mediator of food intake and reproductive function.[18] Rising leptin levels inhibit NPY in the arcuate nucleus and, thus, the inhibitory effect of NPY on GnRH neuronal activity is removed, allowing sexual maturation and reproductive function to proceed.[19] A large body of evidence now supports the existence of a negative feedback loop regulating food intake, leptin secretion, and hypothalamic NPY expression,[20, 21] and leptin may represent a metabolic gate for the onset of puberty in female rats.[22]

In a prospective study, body composition and serum leptin levels were measured and the timing of menarche was recorded in 393 pubertal girls during 4 years.[23] The rise of serum leptin concentrations up to 12.2 ng/ml was associated with a decline in age at menarche (Fig. 7–2). A serum leptin level of 12.2 ng/ml corresponded to a relative percentage body fat of 29.7 percent, a body mass index of 22.3, and body fat of 16.0 kg. A gain in body fat of 1 kg

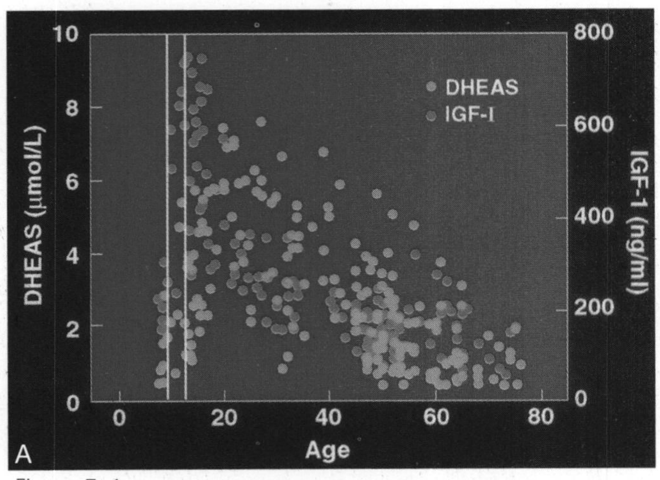

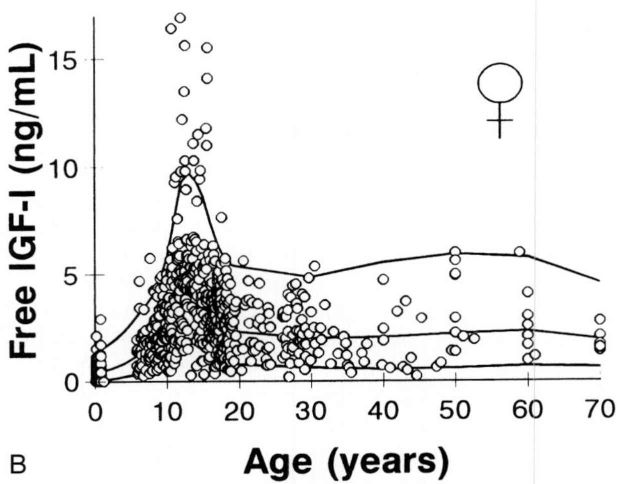

Figure 7–1 ■ Acute elevations of IGF-I levels *during the window* of initiation and maturation of puberty and the onset of menarche. *A*, Serum concentrations of total IGF-I and DHEA-S as related to age in females. (From Laughlin and Yen, unpublished data.) *B*, Serum concentrations of free IGF-I as related to age in females. The lines represent the mean (± SE) value and upper and lower limits. (From Juul A, Holm K, Kastrup KW, et al. Free insulin-like growth factor I serum levels in 1430 healthy children and adults, and its diagnostic value in patients suspected of growth hormone deficiency. J Clin Endocrinol Metab 82:2497–2502, 1997. © The Endocrine Society.)

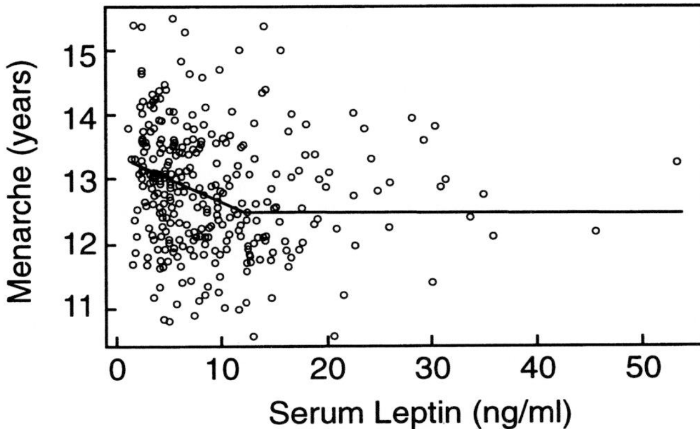

Figure 7–2 ■ Relationship between serum leptin concentrations before menarche and age at menarche in 311 young girls. The scatter plot is shown with the linear-plateau least squares fit model. The 95 percent confidence interval at the change point (serum leptin levels) between two regression lines showing the inverse relation between menarche and leptin is −0.12 to −0.05 years. The 95 percent confidence interval for the change point (serum leptin: × 0) is 7.6 to 16.7 ng/ml. (From Matkovic V, Ilich JZ, Skugor M, et al. Leptin is inversely related to age at menarche in human females. J Clin Endocrinol Metab 82:3239–3245, 1997. © The Endocrine Society.)

lowered the time of menarche by 13 days. An increase of 1 ng/ml in serum leptin lowered the age at menarche by 1 month. These findings are consistent with the postulated critical body fat hypothesis in the onset of menarche[5] and demonstrate that a critical blood leptin level is necessary to initiate menarche. Leptin may be viewed as a mediator between adipose tissue and reproductive ability.[23] Thus, leptin and IGF-I are important players in subserving peripheral signals for the maturation of the reproductive axis and the onset of menarche. It is anticipated that other peripheral signals, such as thyroid hormone, may also be important in this process.

Hormonal Dynamics

Clinical Characteristics

Studies of the periodicity of the human menstrual cycle have demonstrated that the median interval between menstrual periods is 28 days during the active reproductive years, but an increase in the intermenstrual intervals occurs at the two ends of the reproductive life of the individual[24] (Fig. 7–3). These prolonged menstrual intervals are associated with the *frequent* occurrence of anovulatory cycles during adolescence[25–28] and the menopausal transition.[29] At these times, the aberrant secretion of estradiol and gonadotropin results in asynchrony of the various elements of the system and is manifested as luteal-phase defects or anovulatory cycles.[27, 29]

The menstrual cycle is a repetitive expression of the interaction of the hypothalamic-pituitary-ovarian system with associated structural and functional changes in the target tissues—uterus, oviducts, endometrium, and vagina—of the reproductive tract. Each cycle culminates in menstrual bleeding, the first day of which is accepted as a clinical reference point marking the beginning of a menstrual cycle.

Pituitary gonadotropins follicle-stimulating hormone (FSH) and LH serve as links between the hypothalamus and the ovary. An overview of changing patterns of gonadotropin secretion in the human female before, during, and after the reproductive years is shown in Figure 7–4. In the absence of appropriate ovarian function, as found in the prepubertal and menopausal phases of the life cycle, the levels of circulating FSH are greater than those of LH. A marked reduction in the *FSH to LH ratio* is typical of the reproductive years. The low gonadotropin secretion during the prepubertal phase is causally related to insufficient hypothalamic GnRH stimulation.[27] As girls enter puberty, the appearance of pulsatile LH secretion and sleep-entrained LH increments occur, reflecting activation of GnRH neuronal activities. The disappearance of the sleep-related amplification of LH pulses after puberty[30, 31] serves as a marker of maturational processes of the GnRH neuronal system. The elevation of FSH levels associated with the menopausal years is due primarily to a decline in negative feedback because of reduced ovarian estradiol and inhibin levels.[32]

Hormonal Dynamics

The human menstrual cycle can be divided into four functional phases on the basis of structural, morphologic, and sex steroid production by the ovary[33] (Table 7–1):

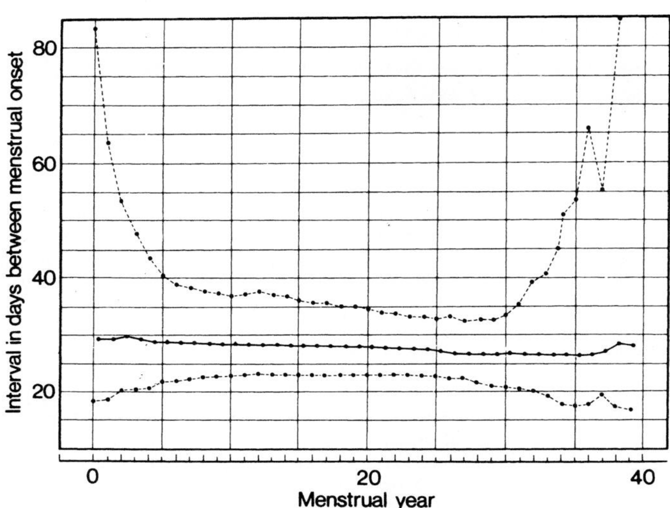

Figure 7–3 ■ Median menstrual cycle lengths throughout the reproductive life of women from menarche (year 0) to menopause (year 40). Ninety percent of all cycles fall within the upper and lower broken lines. (From Treloar AE, Boynton RE, Behn BG, Brown BW. Variation of the human menstrual cycle through reproductive life. Int J Fertil 12:77–126, 1970.)

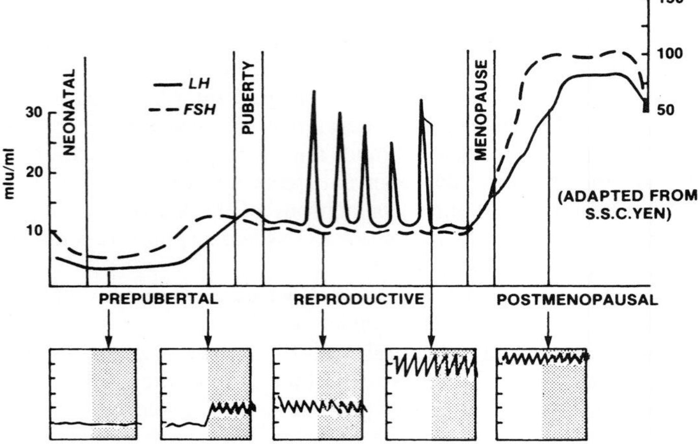

Figure 7–4 ■ The changing pattern and ratio of LH to FSH before, during, and after the reproductive phase of the human female's life cycle. The lower boxes illustrate the amplitude of pulsatile LH release through which circulating concentrations are maintained. The shaded areas represent periods of nocturnal sleep. Note that sleep-induced LH rise is uniquely found during pubertal sexual maturation. (From Yen SSC, et al. Neuroendocrine rhythms of gonadotropin secretion in women. *In* Ferin M, et al [eds]. Biorhythms and Human Reproduction. New York, John Wiley & Sons, 1974, pp 219–238.)

- a *follicular* phase (subdivided into early, mid, and late);
- an *ovulatory* phase (follicular-luteal transition);
- a *luteal* phase (subdivided into early, mid, and late); and
- a *menstrual* phase (luteal-follicular transition).

The circulating levels of gonadotropins, estrogens, progesterone, and inhibins during the normal ovulatory cycle in women exhibit well-defined cyclic patterns. The time course of and relative changes in these hormonal levels, as measured daily, are illustrated in Figure 7–5*A*.

THE FOLLICULAR PHASE

The first half of the cycle is referred to as the follicular phase and is characterized by a progressive increase in circulating levels of estradiol and inhibin B by the developing graafian follicle. However, folliculogenesis begins in the *late luteal* phase of the preceding cycle and continues during the luteal-follicular transition. At this time, the demise of the corpus luteum and the associated rapid decline of levels of inhibin A, as well as of estradiol and progesterone, permit a rise in FSH secretion about 2 days before the onset of menstruation (Fig. 7–5*B*).

The rise of dimeric inhibin B (follicular phase) and inhibin A (luteal phase) noted before has been determined by recently developed enzyme-linked immunosorbent assays.[34, 35] The inhibin levels shown in Figure 7–5 were measured by immunoassay and appear to closely resemble the pattern of dimeric inhibin A (Fig. 7–6). The increase in FSH levels, together with the return from low to high LH pulse frequency, initiates follicle recruitment during the first 4 to 5 days of the follicular phase. This is followed by selection of a single follicle from a cohort of follicles (days 5 to 7), the maturation of the dominant follicle (days 8 to 12), and ultimately ovulation (days 13 to 15).[36] This process constitutes the follicular phase of the cycle, lasts approximately 13 days, and is directed to the genesis of one preovulatory follicle while the others undergo atresia.

The selection of a single follicle destined to ovulate is associated with a high capacity for androgen, estrogen, progesterone, and inhibin B biosynthesis and secretion.[37–40] The integrity of the production of these hormones is dependent on the interaction between theca and granulosa cells; the activities of each are modulated by changes in cytochrome P450 steroidogenic enzymes[41] and by a variety of growth factors that operate through paracrine and autocrine mechanisms.[42, 43] As trophic hormones, LH and FSH have an inherent ability to modify the rate of follicular growth and maturation and the associated microenvironments within the ovarian follicle.

Because both estradiol and inhibin are potent suppressors of FSH secretion, the time course of FSH decline during the mid to late follicular phase may be causally related to feedback suppression by ovarian estradiol and inhibin.[38, 44, 45] In contrast, corresponding circulating LH levels exhibit a progressive increasing trend (see Fig. 7–5*A*).

■ TABLE 7–1

Production Rate of Sex Steroids in Women at Different Stages of the Menstrual Cycle

	DAILY PRODUCTION RATE		
SEX STEROIDS*	Early Follicular	Preovulatory	Midluteal
Progesterone (mg)	1	4	25
17-Hydroxyprogesterone (mg)	0.5	4	4
Dehydroepiandrosterone (mg)	7	7	7
Androstenedione (mg)	2.6	4.7	3.4
Testosterone (μg)	144	171	126
Estrone (μg)	50	350	250
Estradiol (μg)	36	380	250

From Baird DT, Fraser IS. Blood production and ovarian secretion rates of estradiol-17β and estrone in women throughout the menstrual cycle. J Clin Endocrinol Metab 38:1009–1017, 1974. © The Endocrine Society.

*Values are expressed in milligrams or micrograms per 24 hours.

THE OVULATORY PHASE (FOLLICULAR-LUTEAL TRANSITION)

Because the peak of the midcycle LH surge cannot be accurately defined, the *onset* of the LH surge is employed to provide a relatively precise reference point for timing hormonal and intrafollicular dynamics at midcycle[46] (Fig. 7–7). During the last 2 to 3 days before the onset of the midcycle surge, the increment in circulating estradiol levels (doubling time, 61.3 hours) parallels that in inhibin, progesterone, and 17α-hydroxyprogesterone levels (see Fig. 7–7). This increase in progestin concentrations reflects the pro-

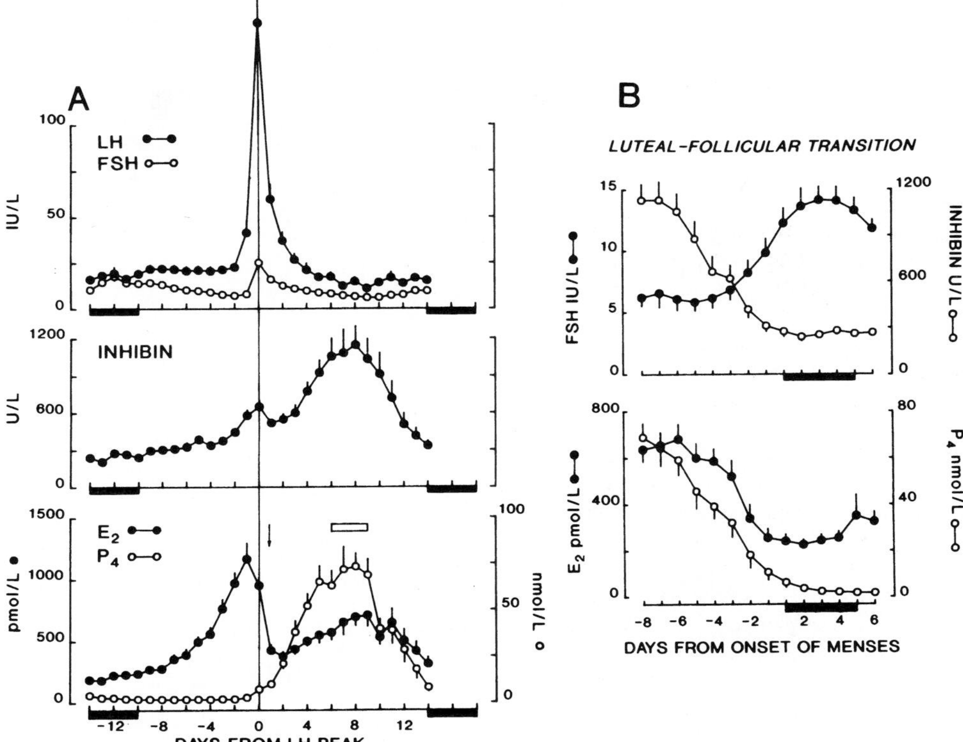

Figure 7–5 ■ *A,* The hormonal pattern in the human menstrual cycle. The data (mean ± SE) are centered on the day of midcycle peak of LH and FSH. Ovarian estradiol (E_2), progesterone (P_4), and inhibin levels are shown in the lower two panels. The arrow indicates the estimated time of ovulation, and the open box depicts the time of implantation during the midluteal phase. The closed boxes represent menstrual periods.

B, The relationship of FSH, inhibin, and ovarian steroids during corpus luteum regression, the onset of menses, and the initiation of folliculogenesis for the next cycle. These are key changes in hormonal levels during the luteal-follicular transition. (Data from Roseff SJ, Bangah ML, Kettel LM, et al. Dynamic changes in circulating inhibin levels during the luteal-follicular transition of the human menstrual cycle. J Clin Endocrinol Metab 69:1033–1039, 1989. © The Endocrine Society.)

cess of luteinization of the granulosa cells after acquisition of LH receptors and the resulting ability of LH to initiate biosynthesis of 17α-hydroxyprogesterone and progesterone.[47, 48]

The LH and FSH surges begin abruptly (LH levels double within 2 hours) and are temporally associated with the attainment of peak estradiol levels and the initiation of a rapid rise of progesterone 12 hours earlier. The mean duration of the *LH surge is 48 hours*, with a rapidly ascending limb (doubling time, 5.2 hours) lasting 14 hours and accompanied by a rapid decline in circulating estradiol, 17α-hydroxyprogesterone, and inhibin B concentrations but a rise in serum inhibin A levels (see Fig. 7–6). The longer descending limb (half-time, 9.6 hours), lasting 20 hours, is associated with a second rapid rise in progesterone and inhibin A and a further decline in circulating 17α-hydroxyprogesterone, estradiol, and inhibin B levels, beginning 36 hours after surge onset or 12 hours before termination of the surge. Inhibin secretion during the periovulatory interval is not coupled with that of either estradiol or progesterone. Changing inhibin levels at this time may represent the sum contributions by the preovulatory follicle and the emerging corpus luteum.[38] The cellular mechanisms responsible for the acute shift in steroidogenesis to favor progesterone production are probably due to the increasing P450 17α-hydroxylase activity in the preovulatory follicle.[41] The relative role of inhibin A and inhibin B in the regulation of FSH secretion during this phase of the cycle remains to be determined.

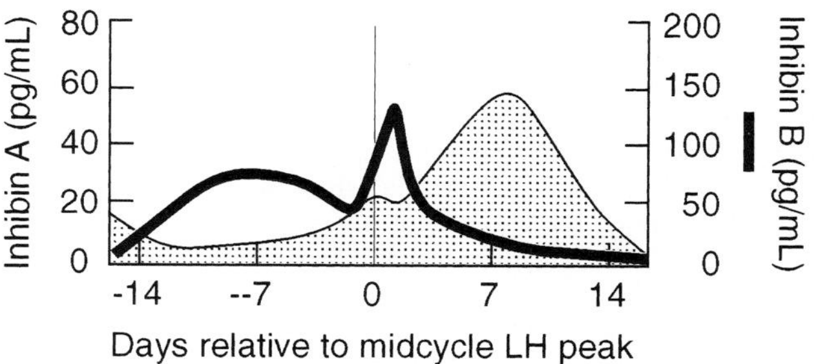

Figure 7–6 ■ Major elevations of mean circulating concentrations of inhibin B (follicular phase) and inhibin A (luteal phase) during the menstrual cycle. Time zero represents midcycle LH surge. (Drawing based on data from Groome NP, Illingworth PJ, O'Brien M, et al. Measurement of dimeric inhibin B throughout the human menstrual cycle. J Clin Endocrinol Metab 81:1401–1405, 1996.)

The precise time interval between the onset of the LH surge and ovulation in women appears to be 1 to 2 hours before the final phase of the progesterone rise or *35 to 44 hours after the onset* of the LH surge.[38, 46]

THE LUTEAL PHASE

The hallmark of the luteal phase of the menstrual cycle is the shift from the estrogen-dominated follicular phase to progesterone dominance. The luteinization of the theca-granulosa cells after ovulation is associated with an abundance of all P450 steroidogenic enzymes in luteal cells[41] and an increasing ability to synthesize large amounts of progesterone and, to a lesser extent, estradiol. The peak concentrations of progesterone and estradiol attained at the midluteal phase constitute the *3-day window* in which the secretory endometrium is conducive to implantation (see Fig. 7–5*A*). Although inhibin A also reaches a peak level at this time, it does not play a role in implantation. Unless

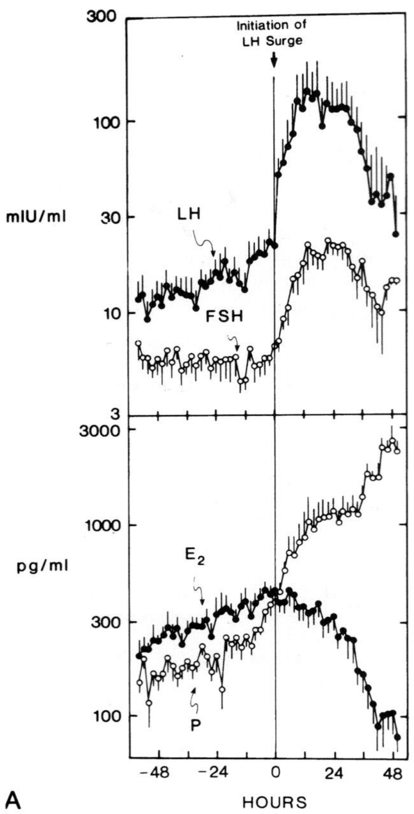

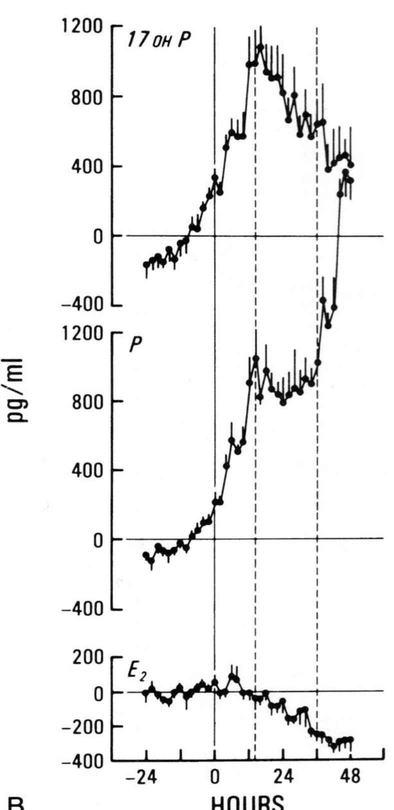

Figure 7–7 ■ Midcycle hormone dynamics.

A, Mean (± SE) levels of serum LH, FSH, estradiol (E_2), and progesterone (P) measured every 2 hours for 5 days at midcycle in seven studies. The initiation of the gonadotropin surge provides the reference point (time zero) around which the data are presented. Note that the hormone concentrations are plotted on a logarithmic scale.

B, The temporal relationship of 17-hydroxyprogesterone (17OHP), progesterone (P), and estradiol (E_2) before and during the LH surge is shown. Time zero is referenced at the onset of the surge. (*A* and *B* from Hoff JD, Quigley ME, Yen SSC. Hormonal dynamics at midcycle: A reevaluation. J Clin Endocrinol Metab 57:792–796, 1983. © The Endocrine Society.)

implantation occurs, luteolysis ensues, with a prompt linear decline in circulating progesterone, estradiol, and inhibin A levels during the last 4 to 5 days of the functional life of the corpus luteum.[38, 49]

The secretory activity of the corpus luteum and its functional life span are dependent on appropriate LH support.[50–52] Interruption of LH pulsatility by means of GnRH antagonist administration during various stages of the luteal phase induces rapid reduction of progesterone, estradiol, and inhibin levels, followed by luteolysis and the onset of menses.[49, 51] Levels of FSH are suppressed during the luteal phase to reach the lowest levels during the entire cycle; FSH is not required for the maintenance of the corpus luteum. The combination of inhibin with estrogen and progesterone synergistically suppresses FSH secretion and thus prevents the initiation of folliculogenesis during the luteal phase of the cycle.

THE MENSTRUAL PHASE (LUTEAL-FOLLICULAR TRANSITION)

The initiation of follicular growth of the ensuing cycle is dependent on the regression of the antecedent corpus luteum. The key event is the inverse relationship between the fall of inhibin A levels and the rise in FSH levels that occurs 2 days before the onset of menses, thereby initiating follicular recruitment for the ensuing cycle[49, 53] (see Fig. 7–5*B*). Thus, the luteal-follicular transition represents a sequence of dynamic changes involving the termination of luteal function and a shift from low-frequency and high-amplitude LH pulses to high-frequency and low-amplitude LH pulses. This is accompanied by a rise in FSH, which in turn stimulates inhibin B production by the developing follicles.[49, 53, 54] These dynamic changes are consequences of withdrawal of the inhibitory effects of the corpus luteum steroids, inhibin, and hypothalamic opioid peptides.[38, 49–51, 55]

Animal Models of the Reproductive Cycle

In the past, much of the understanding of the regulation of the menstrual cycle in humans was deduced from experimental findings in laboratory animals, the best known of which involved the rat. The most dynamic segment of the cycle in the rat occurs just before ovulation, when the estrogen level is high and the animal exhibits mating behavior. This time is known as the period of "heat" or "estrus" and is the interval during which the male is accepted by a female. Although endometrial development is necessary for implantation in all viviparous animals, regression of the endometrium in the form of menstrual bleeding occurs only in primates; most mammals do not undergo significant endometrial sloughing, although at estrus there may be slight vaginal spotting in addition to swelling of the external genitalia and willingness to mate. The neuroendocrine clocks that determine the timing of ovulation in the rat are (1) the ovarian estradiol signal, which establishes the day, and (2) the surges of GnRH and gonadotropin, which occur at fixed hours for the initiation of ovulation.[56]

Although most mammals, including women, are spontaneous and cyclic ovulators, the rabbit and the cat are outstanding examples of so-called reflex ovulators. These animals have long periods of estrus with the presence of multiple mature follicles, and multiple ovulation is achieved by a neurogenic reflex in which coitus is the stimulus that triggers an acute discharge of ovulating hormone (LH), thereby maximizing the reproductive capacity.[57]

Reproductive cycles in seasonal breeders, such as sheep, represent still another type of cyclicity. Ewes have regular 16-day estrous cycles that start in the autumn and cease in the spring. The principal stimulus controlling the seasonal reproductive rhythm in the ewe is the environmental daylight length. During the reproductive season, the ewe shows estrous behavior for only 1 day of 16, and ovulation occurs about 24 hours after the onset of estrus.[57]

NEUROENDOCRINE CONTROL OF THE MENSTRUAL CYCLE

Pulsatile Secretion of Gonadotropins

Follicular Phase

An essential feature in the gonadotropic control of ovarian function is the pulsatile nature of LH and FSH release by the pituitary gland. Pulse frequency and amplitude of gonadotropin release are profoundly modulated by ovarian steroids. In the absence of such gonadal feedback, as in postmenopausal or ovariectomized women, the elevated gonadotropin levels are maintained by increased amplitude and frequency of their pulsatile release.[58–61]

Whereas hypogonadal subjects exhibit pulses of high amplitude and high frequency (approximately one pulse per 60 minutes), normally cycling women provide a changing pattern of high-frequency and low-amplitude pulses during the follicular phase and low-frequency and high-amplitude pulses uniquely found during the luteal phase of the cycle.[58, 60, 62–65] Although the pattern of LH pulsatility during the menstrual cycle was described nearly three decades ago, reliable analytic tools for accurate appraisal of pulse dynamics were only recently devised. Conventional pulse analysis of serum LH concentrations does not provide direct information regarding the nature of underlying secretory events because circulating LH concentrations reflect the combined contributions of secretion and metabolic clearance. By use of a multiple-variable deconvolution technique, quantitative assessments of simultaneous LH secretion and clearance during different phases of the menstrual cycle have been made.[66] As displayed in Figure 7–8 and tabulated in Table 7–2, changes in LH secretory dynamics related to the pulse frequency, the pulse amplitude, the secretory half-life, and the cumulative secretion in a 24-hour day occur in different steroid environments. A periodicity of 80 minutes is seen during the early follicular phase, with an increase in frequency and amplitude in the late follicular phase. A remarkable reduction in pulse frequency with varying amplitudes occurs during the midluteal phase. Ovarian estradiol appears to be most effective in modulating the amplitude, whereas progesterone acts to lower the LH pulse frequency.[44, 67]

Midcycle Surge

The frequency of LH pulses does not appear to change during the preovulatory surge in women and in rhesus monkeys.[63, 68, 69] As depicted in Figure 7–9, the onset of LH surge is acute, with an unequivocal progressive increase in pulse amplitude, the excursions of which are comparable with those seen in hypogonadal postmenopausal women. As noted before, the duration of the midcycle surge lasts 48 hours, and ovulation occurs at approximately 36 hours after initiation of the surge[46] (see Fig. 7–7).

Luteal Phase

During the midluteal phase, pulsatile cosecretion of estradiol, progesterone, and LH has been observed (Fig. 7–10), suggesting a coordinated signal for synchronizing pulses of pituitary LH and corpus luteum steroids.[52, 70, 71] Resumption of high-frequency LH pulses becomes evident 1 day before the onset of menses or near the completion of luteolysis. A concordance in the LH and FSH pulses has been identified through the use of time-series analysis,[64] which has overcome the blurring effect of the long circulating half-life of FSH.[72] Levels of the biologically active form of LH during a secretory episode are consistently higher than those of immunoreactive LH for both spontaneous and exogenous GnRH-stimulated pulses.[73, 74] The dependency of both bioactive LH and FSH secretion by the gonadotroph on appropriate GnRH stimulation has been

■ TABLE 7–2

Mean (±SEM) Luteinizing Hormone Secretory Burst Characteristics During Phases of the Menstrual Cycle*

NUMBER (24 hr)	PERIODICITY (min)	AMPLITUDE† (mIU/ml/min)	HALF-DURATION† (min)	LH HALF-LIFE (min)	TOTAL DAILY SECRETION (mIU/ml/24 hr)
Early follicular 175 ± 1.4a	80 ± 3a	0.43 ± 0.02a	6.5 ± 1.0a	131 ± 13a	49 ± 6a
Late folicular 26.9 ± 1.6b	53 ± 1b	0.70 ± 0.03b	3.5 ± 0.9b	128 ± 12a	56 ± 8a
Midluteal 10.1 ± 1.0c	177 ± 15c‡	0.26 ± 0.02c‡	11.0 ± 1.1c	103 ± 7a	52 ± 4a
	395 ± 37d‡	0.95 ± 0.05d‡			

*Entries in each column identified by a, b, c, d differ significantly (Duncan's multiple-range test, $P < .05$). Periodicity is intersecretory burst interval. LH, Luteinizing hormone.

†Duration of the deconvolution-resolved LH secretory burst at half-maximal amplitude.

‡Maximal rate of LH secretion attained with the deconvolution-resolved LH secretory burst. The midluteal phase has been divided into small (less than 0.65 mIU/ml/min) and large (greater than 0.65 mIU/ml/min) secretory burst amplitudes.

Data from Sollenberger MJ, Carlsen EC, Johnson ML, et al. Specific physiological regulation of LH secretory events throughout the human menstrual cycle. New insights into the pulsatile mode of gonadotropin release. J Neuroendocrinol 2:845, 1990.

Early Follicular

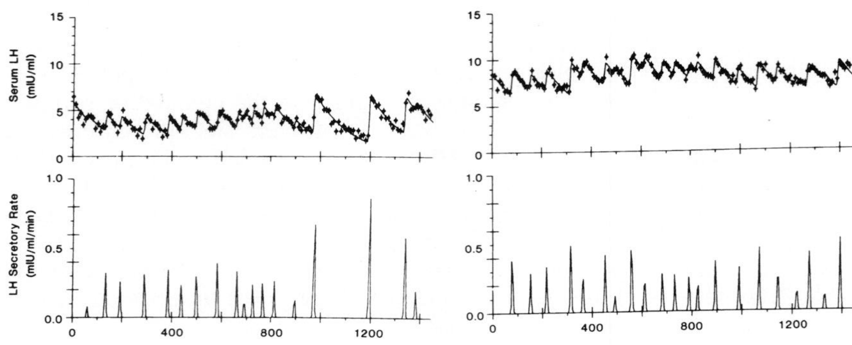

Late Follicular

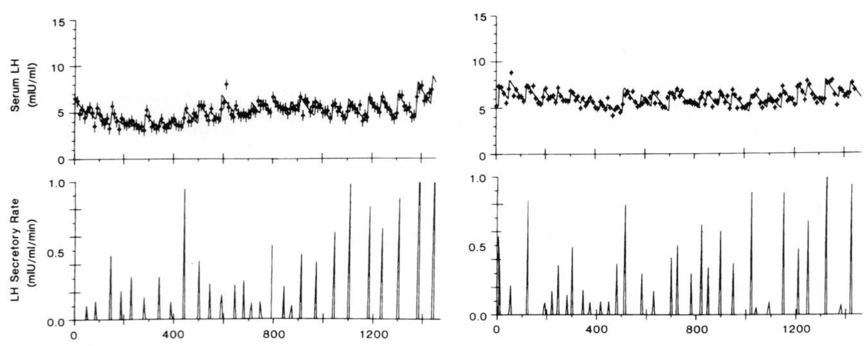

Mid Luteal

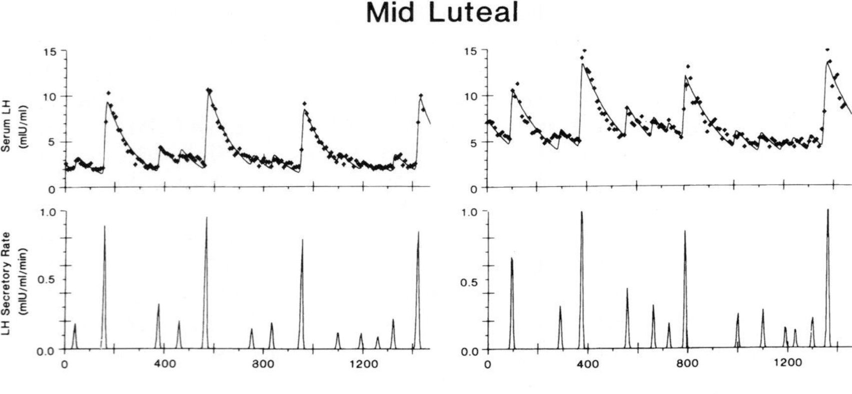

Time (min)

Figure 7–8 ■ Variations of LH pulsatile activity and pituitary LH secretory rates as measured by LH pulse pattern in serum (deconvolution analysis) during three phases of the human menstrual cycle. Note the cessation of pituitary secretion between acute, short-lasting pulsatile releases. (From Sollenberger MJ, Carlsen EC, Johnson ML, et al. Specific physiological regulation of LH secretory events throughout the human menstrual cycle. New insights into the pulsatile mode of gonadotropin release. J Neuroendocrinol 2:845, 1990. Courtesy of S. Karger AG, Basel.)

demonstrated by blockade of GnRH action through the use of GnRH antagonists.[75, 76]

Hypothalamic GnRH Pulse Generator

The biosynthetic and secretory activities of the GnRH neuronal system are detailed in Chapter 2. Evidence for the existence of the hypothalamic pulse generator that governs the episodic release of GnRH is established. Experiments conducted in the rhesus monkey revealed that the rhythmic acute and short-lasting secretory activity of GnRH occurs at approximately hourly intervals and has its origin in the vicinity of the arcuate nucleus within the medial basal hypothalamus (MBH).[77] A remarkable synchrony can be observed among pulses of GnRH in the portal blood, electrophysiologic multiunit activity of the MBH, and LH pulses in the peripheral blood.[77, 78] Thus, an ultradian rhythm within the MBH governs the pulsatile discharge of GnRH from the nerve terminals at the median eminence and represents the key controller of pituitary pulsatile gonadotropin secretion.

Measurements of GnRH concentrations in the hypophysial portal blood of intact rhesus monkeys and ovariectomized ewes have revealed a distinct pulsatile pattern of

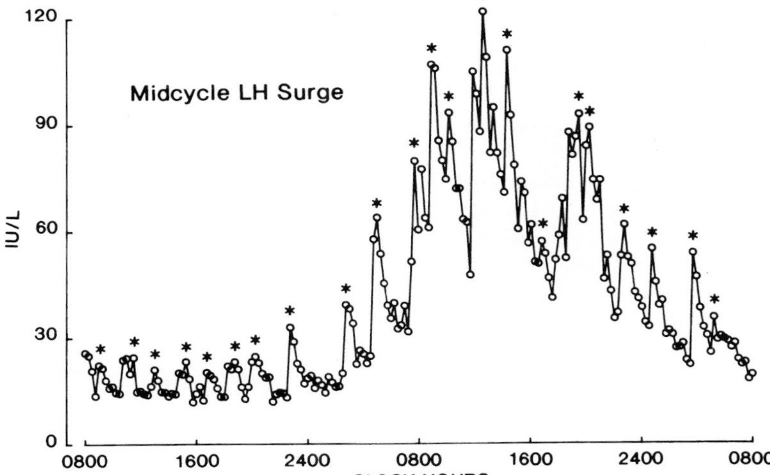

Figure 7–9 ■ Pulsatile LH secretion measured at 15-minute intervals *(open circles)* for a 24-hour period during the midcycle surge in an ovulatory woman. Asterisks indicate a significant pulse of LH.

release. During the midcycle surge, the peaks and valleys of GnRH pulses varied from 400 to 0 pg/ml, respectively.[79–81] Similar pulsatile patterns of GnRH release in response to estradiol-induced gonadotropin surge were seen in the cerebrospinal fluid of the third ventricle.[82, 83] The secretion of GnRH into the third ventricle resembles that of other hypothalamic releasing factors, such as corticotropin-releasing factor.

The relative changes in the GnRH pulse generator activity during different phases of the menstrual cycle, monitored continuously in a rhesus monkey, revealed changes of high-frequency to low-frequency GnRH pulses from the follicular to the luteal phase similar to those observed in the human menstrual cycle.[77] The pulse frequency of the GnRH pulse generator activity is markedly reduced at night during the follicular phase of the cycle, an observation that affirms a GnRH-mediated slowing of LH pulses during sleep in the early follicular phase of the human menstrual cycle.[84–86] When estrogen and progesterone concentrations begin to fall during the late luteal phase, a temporal increase in the GnRH pulse generator activity becomes apparent and continues to increase through the first few days of the follicular phase, when maximal frequencies are attained.

In humans, hypothalamic pulsatile GnRH secretion and the site of the putative GnRH pulse generator have been indirectly investigated. In nonhuman primates, all of the neural elements composing the GnRH pulse generator reside within the MBH and are capable of functioning as an intrinsic pacemaker independently of neural innervation from the remainder of the brain. This self-contained functional capacity of MBH has been used to explore the pulse generator in isolated human MBHs. Discrete pulsatile GnRH release from the isolated MBH of the human fetus (20 to 30 weeks of gestation) and the adult has been observed in an in vitro perfusion system (see Chapter 2).[87] The periodicity of GnRH pulses is approximately 60 minutes for the fetal MBH and 60 to 100 minutes for the adult MBH. These findings confirm that in humans, as in monkeys, the hypothalamic GnRH pulse-generating system appears to be located entirely within the MBH. However, it remains to be determined whether the pulse generator is an intrinsic property of the GnRH neuron itself or is influenced by coupling with other neurons within the MBH. This crucial question appeared to be resolved by the observations of spontaneous pulsatile GnRH release by the GT-1 neuronal cells in culture. Thus, *GnRH neurons per se* may constitute the GnRH pulse generator, a proposition that requires additional study.[88]

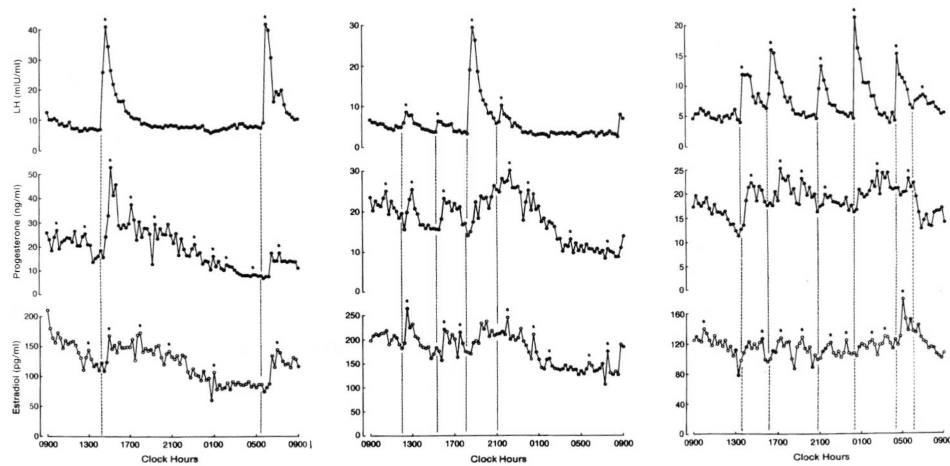

Figure 7–10 ■ Representative 24-hour pulsatile profiles of LH, estradiol, and progesterone in three women during midluteal phase of the cycle. Coordinated temporal copulsatile release is apparent. (From Rossmanith WG, Laughlin GA, Mortola JF, et al. Pulsatile cosecretion of estradiol and progesterone by the midluteal phase corpus luteum: Temporal link to luteinizing hormone pulses. J Clin Endocrinol Metab 70:990–995, 1990. © The Endocrine Society.)

Pulsatile GnRH on the Gonadotroph

There is abundant evidence both in vivo and in vitro that the frequency and the amplitude of GnRH pulses are critical in determining gonadotropin subunit biosynthesis, coupling, and glycosylation by the gonadotroph as well as GnRH receptor density.

In patients with endogenous GnRH deficiency (e.g., Kallmann syndrome) and hypogonadotropic amenorrhea, activation of pulsatile release of FSH and LH can be achieved by pulsed GnRH administration programmed at physiological frequency (i.e., 60–90 minutes) and dosage (i.e., 5–10 μg per pulse).[89] Increasing the frequency beyond the physiologic range (i.e., three pulses per hour) causes down-regulation of pituitary responsiveness and markedly reduces the secretion of LH and FSH. Lower frequency (i.e., once every 3 hours) induces preferential secretion of FSH.[90, 91]

Subunits of gonadotropin mRNA are also regulated by the frequency and the amplitude of GnRH pulses. Higher frequency of GnRH pulses induces an increase in α-subunit mRNA but with a greater increase for LH-β than FSH-β. Physiologic frequency (approximately two pulses per hour in the rat) of GnRH pulses increases the mRNA levels for all three gonadotropin subunits, whereas lower frequency (one pulse every 2 hours) selectively increases FSH-β mRNA.[88, 92, 93]

Functional disruption of gonadotropin response to GnRH signals can also be achieved by the use of GnRH antagonists or GnRH antisera. Under these experimental conditions, the postcastration rise of the mRNA levels of all three subunits is prevented.[94, 95] In humans, there is a significantly greater reduction in bioactive than in immunoreactive LH and FSH after blockade of GnRH receptors by GnRH antagonists, suggesting that impairment of gonadotropin processing occurs as a result of GnRH deprivation.[75, 76]

In summary, high-frequency GnRH pulses favor increases in LH-β but not FSH-β mRNAs. Low-frequency pulses selectively induce FSH-β mRNA, whereas physiologic frequency of GnRH promotes mRNA of all three subunits of gonadotropins. In addition, appropriate GnRH input is required for glycosylation and coupling of subunits, thereby generating biologically active LH and FSH molecules.[96] It follows that in women with hypogonadotropism due to endogenous GnRH deficiencies, administration of pulses of GnRH at a frequency of 90 minutes initiates a normal sequence of follicular development, ovulation, and corpus luteum formation (see Chapters 2 and 19 for details).

GnRH Receptors

The gonadotroph response to binding of GnRH by its receptor includes synthesis and release of gonadotropins and regulation of GnRH receptor density. Changes in the number of steady-state GnRH receptors induced by GnRH appear to reflect a complex series of events involving the rate of generation of receptors (synthesis, unmasking, and recycling) and loss of functional receptors (degradation, internalization, and inactivation). Studies on the rat pituitary[97] demonstrated that GnRH causes a significant *increase in the rate of synthesis of GnRH receptors* on gonadotrophs independently of Ca^{2+}.[97] This is analogous to other ligand-receptor systems in which ligands up-regulate their own receptors (i.e., estrogen and androgen).[98, 99] GnRH-stimulated synthesis of GnRH receptors is independent of the GnRH dose, and a discernible up-regulation can be observed in 20 minutes. About 13 to 15 hours are required for generating half the population of receptors.

Priming and Releasing Actions

Studies in humans have shown that the priming function and the releasing action of GnRH are dissociable; large doses tend to stimulate release, whereas small doses induce the priming effect preferentially.[100] When infusion of small amounts of GnRH (0.005 μg/m^2/min) is continued for 20 hours, the self-priming effect of GnRH on LH release not observed during the first 4 hours becomes evident thereafter and induces an increased amplitude of LH pulses throughout the remaining infusion period. The priming effect of minute doses of GnRH is unaccompanied by LH release initially but is manifested by an enhanced LH pulse amplitude after 4 hours, indicating an enhanced endogenous GnRH action, in all probability reflecting a progressive increase in levels of GnRH receptor number.[100] These observations are consistent with the in vitro data cited earlier that generation of increasing numbers of GnRH receptors requires at least 4 hours and that the priming and releasing actions of GnRH may operate in separate pathways. In addition, factors such as estradiol play an important role in augmenting the GnRH receptor number induced by GnRH.[101] The demonstration of GnRH receptor on GnRH GT-1 neuronal cells raises the possibility of an autoregulation of GnRH receptor by GnRH in vivo (see Chapter 2 for details).

Modulation of Hypothalamic-Pituitary Function

From the foregoing, it is evident that the basic tenet of hypothalamic control of the menstrual cycle is the rhythmic discharge of GnRH into the hypothalamic portal circulation by the GnRH neuronal system within the arcuate nucleus of the MBH. It is also apparent that the observed changes in GnRH/LH pulsatile activity during the menstrual cycle, particularly its frequency, must be dictated by modulating factors from central and peripheral neuroendocrine signals.

The role of catecholamines, neuropeptides, and ovarian steroids and inhibins in the functional activities of GnRH neurons and secretion has been studied extensively in the rat and nonhuman primates. In humans, relevant information, albeit indirect, is also rapidly expanding. An account of the complex factors modulating the GnRH-gonadotroph system is given in the following with emphasis on physiologic relevance, pharmacologically demonstrated effects, experimental conditions, ovarian steroid milieu, and species differences.

Central Modulation

α-ADRENERGIC SYSTEM

Considerable evidence suggests that norepinephrine is an important neurotransmitter that exerts a stimulatory effect on hypothalamic GnRH neurons. An increased norepinephrine turnover occurs during the proestrous period, and blockade of α-adrenergic receptors abolishes pulsatile LH release in the rat.[102] The ascending pathways of two major norepinephrine systems from the brain stem are projected to hypothalamic areas, where GnRH neurons are found (Fig. 7–11): the locus ceruleus norepinephrine system and the medullary norepinephrine system. Direct synaptic links between the norepinephrine terminals and GnRH neurons have not yet been unequivocally demonstrated. Instead, there is good evidence that the ascending noradrenergic fibers make synaptic contact with the *γ-aminobutyric acid (GABA)–ergic interneurons.* Evidence from several studies suggests that norepinephrine stimulation of GnRH neurons is mediated by inhibiting the tonic release of GABA-ergic interneurons through α- but not β-adrenergic receptors.[103, 104]

In nonhuman primates, a stimulatory effect of the α-adrenergic system on GnRH secretion has also been established. The activity of the GnRH pulse generator is markedly suppressed by α-adrenergic blockers in ovariectomized monkeys.[105] However, the involvement of the α-adrenergic system in the regulation of GnRH/LH secretion during the menstrual cycle, particularly in the preovulatory surge, has not been demonstrated in monkeys or humans. Primates may differ from rats in that spontaneous and estradiol-induced LH surges persist after total deafferentation of the MBH in the rhesus monkey,[106] indicating that the neural (i.e., noradrenergic) signal arising outside the MBH is not essential for the control of GnRH secretion. On the other hand, whether the influence of the α-adrenergic system on GnRH-gonadotropin secretion may be activated during stressful conditions remains to be delineated. The role of norepinephrine in the regulation of gonadotropin secretion in humans has not yet been defined.

DOPAMINERGIC INPUT

Despite extensive investigation, the role of dopamine in the regulation of GnRH secretion remains controversial. Depending on the experimental conditions, both a stimulatory and inhibitory influence has been observed. Demonstrations of a stimulatory action of dopamine on GnRH secretion include the perifused MBH isolated from human hypothalami in vitro[107] and the electrophysiologically monitored GnRH pulse generator in ovariectomized monkeys.[105] These findings are in opposition to those noting the inhibitory action of dopamine in cycling and postmenopausal women[108] and under a variety of experimental conditions in the rat.[102] These conflicting results are further complicated by the demonstration in human MBH of dopaminergic stimulation of endogenous opioid release, which in turn inhibits GnRH secretion.[109] Considering that dopamine can stimulate hypothalamic β-endorphin release and that β-endorphin inhibits hypothalamic dopaminergic turnover and release,[110] an interacting neural system of dopamine and β-endorphin in the control of GnRH secretion within the arcuate nucleus has been proposed[109] (see Fig. 7–11). In this regard, administration of a dopamine agonist (bromocriptine) to postmenopausal women was found to restore LH responses to naloxone infusion, suggesting that an increased endogenous opioid activity had occurred.[111]

Immunocytochemical and electron microscopic studies demonstrated synaptic contacts between dopamine neurons and GnRH neurons.[103, 112] Further, dopamine receptor D_1 subtype has been identified in GnRH neuronal cells, and activation of D_1 receptor by dopamine stimulated GnRH release.[113, 114] Thus, the modulation of GnRH neuronal activity by dopamine may be conducted by several pathways.

ENDOGENOUS OPIOIDS

Compelling evidence indicates that, in humans as in experimental animals, endogenous opioid peptides play a pivotal role in the neural control of gonadotropin secretion by way of an inhibitory effect on hypothalamic GnRH secretion.[55, 83] A single injection of morphine to ovariectomized monkeys can bring about immediate cessation of GnRH pulse generator activity.[77] Administration of β-endorphin to women in vivo and to isolated human MBH perifused

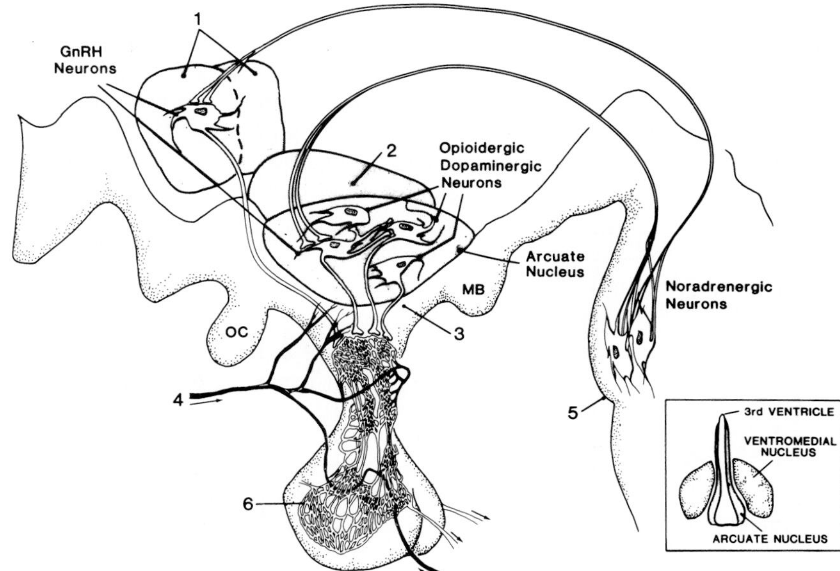

Figure 7–11 ■ Neuroanatomic relationship of noradrenergic, dopaminergic, opioidergic, and GnRH neurons within the arcuate nucleus–median eminence region and within the preoptic anterior hypothalamic area. Note GnRH opioid peptides and dopamine axons terminating onto the portal capillaries. 1, preoptic anterior hypothalamic area; 2, ventromedial nucleus; 3, median eminence (MB); 4, superior hypophysial artery; 5, brain stem (locus ceruleus); 6, hypophysial portal loops; 7, inferior hypophysial artery; OC, optic chiasm.

Inset, Relationship of arcuate nucleus, third ventricle, and ventromedial nucleus is illustrated.

in vitro induces a prompt suppression of GnRH/LH pulses.[87, 115]

The hypothalamic opioidergic system is a well-defined neuronal network within the arcuate nucleus of the MBH, and it is in close contact with the GnRH neuronal system (see Fig. 7–11). This anatomic and functional relationship between opioidergic activity and GnRH secretion becomes more apparent in high-estrogen and particularly high-estrogen and high-progesterone environments[111] (Fig. 7–12). The opioid influence is shown by the observation that the opioid receptor antagonist naloxone induces an increase in the frequency and the amplitude of pulsatile GnRH/LH secretion.[83, 116, 117] Further evidence of ovarian steroid mediation is the failure of opioid receptor blockade by naloxone to modify gonadotropin secretion in postmenopausal women, suggesting uncoupling of the opioidergic influence on GnRH release in the absence of adequate ovarian steroids.[118] This phenomenon may explain the high frequency and amplitude of LH pulses and the unrestrained gonadotropin secretion in postmenopausal women. Sequential administration of estrogen and progesterone to hypogonadal and agonadal women and ovariectomized monkeys readily restores the opioidergic inhibition on GnRH/LH pulsatile activity, which resembles that found during the late follicular and midluteal phases of the cycle.[83, 119–121] Thus, the negative feedback effect of estrogen, and especially the synergistic action of estrogen and progesterone, on gonadotropin secretion may, in part, be functionally linked to an increase in the opioidergic inhibition of GnRH secretion.

The endogenous opioid peptides may also play a role in the regulation of sleep-entrained slowing of GnRH pulses in the early follicular phase and the initiation of midcycle gonadotropin surge. Infusion of naloxone (30 μg/kg/hr) for 24 hours at a constant rate completely reversed the sleep-associated slowing of LH pulses, whereas the daytime LH pulse characteristics were unaltered in the early follicular phase in women.[86] This observation suggests that a nocturnal increase in opioidergic inhibition may be responsible for the slowing of LH pulses. A diurnal variation of hypothalamic opiate-binding site, as observed in prepubertal rats, may be deduced to account for this neuroendocrine event.[122]

The midcycle gonadotropin surge in women, as in other mammalian species, is initiated by the feedback action of increasing levels of serum estradiol on the hypothalamic-pituitary unit, inducing an augmentation of the self-priming action of GnRH on gonadotrophs and modulating the neuronal activity that governs GnRH secretion. Among the many pathways that may regulate GnRH neuronal activity at the time of gonadotropin surge is the hypothalamic opioidergic system, as alluded to before. The sex steroid milieu at this time may be critically important. When opioid receptors are blocked by constant infusion of naloxone (30 μg/kg/hr) for 24 hours in the late follicular–phase woman, a robust increase in pulsatile release of LH and FSH, with a progressive increase in pulse amplitude, is elicited, indistinguishable from that observed during the onset of spontaneous midcycle surge. The responsiveness to naloxone in this regard is conditioned by the presence of preovulatory levels of estradiol.[123] It is proposed that a change of opioidergic activity occurs near the midcycle, which may be a component of neuroendocrine events for the initiation of the gonadotropin surge. It is not clear, however, whether this change is attributable to a decreased opioid receptor sensitivity or density or to a reduced opioid concentration at the neuronal regulatory sites.[124]

The Ovarian Clock

FOLLICULAR-PHASE ESTRADIOL AS A CRITICAL SIGNAL

Negative Feedback. The tonic secretion of LH and FSH appears to be controlled by the classic negative feedback loop. Interrupting this negative feedback loop in normally cycling women by ovariectomy leads to a prompt increase in gonadotropin levels. The rise in LH and FSH levels continues until a plateau is reached after about 3 weeks to levels 10 times the preovariectomy value.[125] Reversal of this hypersecretion of gonadotropin in the open-loop feedback system can be readily achieved in hypogonadal women by the administration of estradiol.[126] Identical results have been observed in rhesus monkeys under similar experimental conditions.[127]

In the absence of ovarian feedback, the elevated gonadotropin levels are reflections of marked increase in the amplitude of pulses of LH and FSH without significant changes in pulse frequency compared with that observed during the follicular phase of the cycle. Conversely, estradiol administration reduces the amplitude of LH pulses.[126–128]

The negative feedback action of estradiol, however, is not stationary but exhibits a time-dependent change from the initial inhibitory effect followed in a few days by an increase in gonadotropin secretion.[126–129] This biphasic

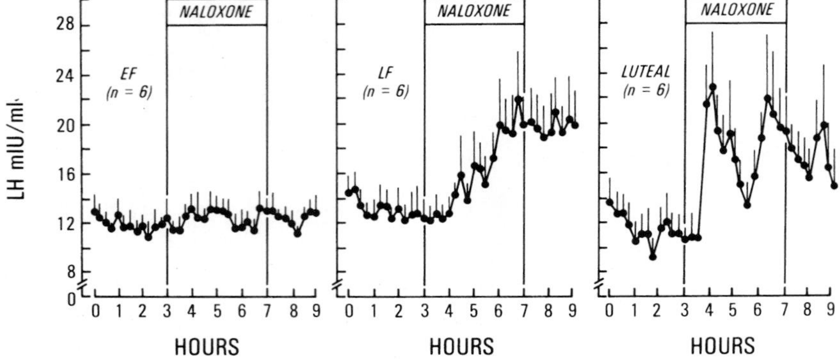

Figure 7–12 ■ Infusion of naloxone, an opiate receptor antagonist, elicits an incremental change of LH in subjects during the late follicular (LF) and midluteal phases of the cycle (but not in the early follicular [EF] phase), indicating a progressive increase in endogenous opioid inhibition of GnRH secretion, especially during the luteal phase. (From Quigley ME, Yen SSC. The role of endogenous opiates in LH secretion during the menstrual cycle. J Clin Endocrinol Metab 51:179–181, 1980. © The Endocrine Society.)

feedback action of estradiol (discussed later) involves the development of a *positive*, or stimulatory, feedback effect on gonadotropin secretion.

Progesterone administered in pharmacologic dosages to hypogonadal women and ovariectomized monkeys has little effect in reducing the elevated gonadotropin levels.[126, 127] However, during the luteal phase of the menstrual cycle or after estrogen priming, progesterone induces a decreased LH pulse frequency with an increased amplitude. As already noted, this effect of progesterone is mediated by its action on hypothalamic β-endorphin, which is known to decrease the frequency of the GnRH pulse generator. In the context of the negative feedback action of ovarian steroids, therefore, estradiol and progesterone represent the principal signals and possess synergistic effects.[127, 128]

Positive Feedback. The initiation of the preovulatory surge of gonadotropin is the consequence of a positive feedback action of estradiol. When the rising circulating estradiol concentration seen in the late follicular phase is experimentally simulated by exogenous administration of estradiol in hypogonadal states to approximately 300 pg/ml for a period of 2 to 3 days, a gonadotropin surge is elicited in women[130, 131] and monkeys.[127] A fourfold increase in progesterone levels secreted by the preovulatory follicle amplifies the duration of the surge and augments the positive feedback action of estradiol.[46, 130] Although the preovulatory progesterone secretion may be required for the full expression of the gonadotropin surge in women, this effect of progesterone is not demonstrable in rhesus monkeys.[127] Thus, the timing of the LH surge is not instigated by the hypothalamus but is governed by signals from the preovulatory follicle—hence, the concept of *an ovarian clock* in the control of GnRH-gonadotropin–mediated menstrual cyclicity in humans and primates.

The Midcycle Surge (the Switch from Negative to Positive Feedback Actions). Although the ability of ovarian estradiol to exert both negative and positive feedback may seem paradoxical, the development of positive feedback is known to require prior negative feedback.[132–134] The pituitary is unquestionably the major site of estradiol action[127, 128] as evidenced by the remarkable increase in pituitary sensitivity and capacity of gonadotropin release in response to a small dose of GnRH infusion (4 hours) during the course of increasing estrogen levels (Fig. 7–13). This more than 20-fold increase in sensitivity and capacity of pituitary gonadotropin release from early follicular phase to midcycle surge in parallel with the rise of estradiol levels could be implicated as the primary event in the initiation of midcycle surge. However, recent evidence indicates a hypothalamic site of action as well. In the brain, receptors for estradiol and progesterone are present in discrete neuronal populations in the MBH (see Chapter 2). As in other target tissues, estradiol is capable of inducing progesterone-receptor mRNA levels in neurons of the MBH.[135] By use of combined immunocytochemistry, autoradiography, and in situ hybridization studies, specific cells that expressed nuclear estrogen and progesterone receptors have been identified[135–138]:

- Dopamine neurons (tyrosine hydroxylase immunoreactive neurons) in the arcuate nucleus possess both estrogen (approximately 30 percent) and progesterone (approximately 90 percent) receptors.

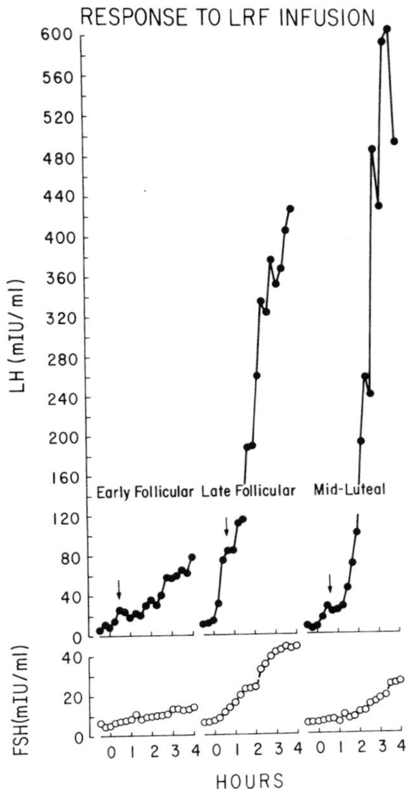

Figure 7–13 ■ The dramatic increase in pituitary gonadotroph sensitivity and capacity on LH and FSH release in response to a small dose of GnRH infusion (0.2 μg/min•4 hr) during early to late follicular phase and during the midluteal phase of the cycle. (From Yen SSC, Lasley BL, Wang CF, et al. The operating characteristics of the hypothalamic-pituitary system during the menstrual cycle and observations of biological action of somatostatin. Recent Prog Horm Res 31:321–363, 1975.)

- β-Endorphin neurons contain receptors for both estrogen (approximately 20 percent) and progesterone (approximately 30 percent).
- GnRH neurons of GT-1 cells express receptors for both estrogen and progesterone (unpublished observation).
- The induction of c-*fos* (a proto-oncogene and marker of early gene expression) in GnRH neurons by estrogen indicates cellular activation.

These findings, together with the evidence of marked augmentation of pituitary sensitivity and capacity as noted before, suggest that the positive feedback action of estradiol involves both the hypothalamic neuronal systems and pituitary gonadotroph in the generation of midcycle surge.

Although ovarian steroids can act directly on GnRH neurons, the presence of both estrogen and progesterone receptors in dopaminergic and β-endorphinergic neurons provides a functional and anatomic basis for the role of these neuronal systems as mediators. As noted before, both β-endorphin and dopamine have axoaxonal synapses with GnRH neurons and have the ability to influence the GnRH pulse generator, GnRH secretion, and response to estrogen and progesterone feedback action. However, direct evidence to implicate the requirement of GnRH surge to trigger the onset of midcycle gonadotropin discharge in humans and in monkeys remains to be established. As indicated earlier, orderly follicular maturation and ovulation can be readily achieved in the absence of hypothalamic GnRH function in humans (i.e., Kallmann's syndrome) and in rhesus monkeys (i.e., hypothalamic clamp model) by the administration of pulsatile GnRH at a fixed dose and frequency.[128, 139] If proven to occur, they are not obligatory for the initiation of the surge in humans and primates.

THE LUTEAL PHASE

It is clear that the most dramatic event of the menstrual cycle is the generation of midcycle gonadotropin surge that causes the ovulatory process by the graafian follicle. Thereafter, the formation and maintenance of the corpus luteum and its production of progesterone in concert with estradiol constitute the feedback signals to convert the high-frequency LH pulses to low-frequency and high-amplitude LH pulses. Further, these two ovarian steroids transform the endometrium from a proliferative phase to a secretory phase that is essential for implantation.

During the luteal phase of the cycle, the development of new follicles is inhibited. This phenomenon is probably attributable to a reduction in FSH secretion by the combined negative feedback action of estrogens and progesterone.[140] The rise in circulating FSH at the end of the luteal phase (see Fig. 7–5) cannot be the consequence of waning concentrations of progesterone because it cannot be prevented by extended progesterone treatment in monkeys or in women[140]; neither can the luteal-follicular transitional increase in LH pulse frequency be inhibited unless luteal-phase levels of both progesterone and estradiol are maintained.[140] The importance of the role of estradiol in this regard is supported by the finding in women that estradiol antagonists (clomiphene citrate or tamoxifen) in the luteal phase of the cycle cause an increase in LH pulse frequency and a rise in circulating FSH levels.[141, 142] The fall in circulating levels of inhibin A that occurs at the end of the luteal phase by itself cannot account for the perimenstrual rise in FSH because neutralization of α-subunit by antiserum in the midluteal phase does not elicit a premature rise in FSH.[143] Thus, the rapid decline of progesterone, estradiol, and inhibin, in combination, may be required to disinhibit the hypothalamic-pituitary unit and to initiate the rise of FSH levels and the increased LH pulse frequency occurring during luteal-follicular transition.

OVARIAN STEROIDOGENESIS (HIGH-DENSITY LIPOPROTEIN CHOLESTEROL AS SUBSTRATE)

Cholesterol and cholesterol esters, hydrophobic molecules, are carried through the hydrophilic environment of the blood stream in lipoproteins. Perhaps the most familiar, low-density lipoprotein (LDL) delivers cholesterol and its metabolites to cells by binding to specific receptors on the cell surface. In this process of "holoparticle uptake," *the entire LDL particle is bound, endocytosed, and ultimately delivered to lysosomes where degradation of both protein and lipid occurs.* Although uptake of high-density lipoprotein (HDL) into most tissues can probably occur by a similar mechanism, HDL also uses a more selective means of delivering its cargo. In certain cells, HDL attaches ("docks"), delivers some of its cholesterol esters (and perhaps other lipids), and then dissociates from the cell surface and continues to circulate in the blood, now as a partially lipid-depleted particle[144] (Fig. 7–14). *A receptor for HDL that mediates this "selective cholesterol ester uptake" has been identified by Acton and colleagues[145] and is reported to be SR-BI, a previously reported cell surface molecule.*

Once internalized, the cholesterol esters are either hydrolyzed and directly used for steroidogenesis or stored in the cell as cholesterol esters until needed. The utilization of stored cholesterol esters is a hormone-regulated event because it does not occur until the cells are further stimulated to increase progesterone secretion. In human granulosa cells, Azhar and coworkers[146] have demonstrated the internalization processes and utilization of HDL cholesterol esters by the cells (see Fig. 7–14). Thus, HDL-derived cholesterol is an important substrate for steroidogenesis, in addition to LDL cholesterol, by the ovarian cells.

In summary, the first half of the ovarian cycle is directed by pulsatile gonadotropin secretion, which eventuates in a preovulatory gonadotropin surge when estradiol produced by the developing graafian follicle surpasses threshold levels in the circulation. The second half of the cycle is dominated by progesterone secreted in response to the luteotropic action of LH released at a reduced pulse frequency. Follicular development is inhibited. The ovarian cycle is terminated by luteolysis, allowing resumption of follicular development in response to gonadotropic stimulation with an increased frequency. The graafian follicle and the corpus luteum provide elements of the *ovarian clock* that times the menstrual cycle. The functional activities of the ovarian clock, in turn, are dependent on the coordinated behavior of the GnRH pulse generator.

Inhibins, Activins, and Follistatin

A family of inhibin proteins with diverse functions has been identified; inhibin is composed of α- and β-subunits that are derived from separate genes.[147] Although the αβ heterodimer of inhibin suppresses FSH secretion, the ββ homodimer stimulates FSH release.[148] The inhibins, heterodimers composed of an α-subunit and one of at least two β-subunits forming inhibin A and inhibin B, have now been isolated from follicular fluid and characterized on the basis of their ability to inhibit FSH secretion selectively from pituitary cells.[148] A changing pattern of inhibin subunit mRNA expression has been determined to occur in ovarian granulosa, theca, and lutein cells across reproductive cycles in a variety of animal species,[148] including the human.[149–151] *These studies indicate that* β_A *subunit expression* is highest in the corpus luteum and the dominant follicle, that β_B *subunit expression is highest in the granulosa cells of antral follicles*[151, 152] that are present at the time of the luteal-follicular transition, and that α-subunit expression appears relatively constant throughout follicular development after the antral stage.[151] In general, the secretion of inhibin A and inhibin B across the menstrual cycle mirrors these changes in mRNA levels.[39, 49, 153] Declining inhibin A estrogen and progesterone from the corpus luteum may collectively contribute to the luteal-follicular rise in FSH.[49] The pattern of secretion of inhibin B from

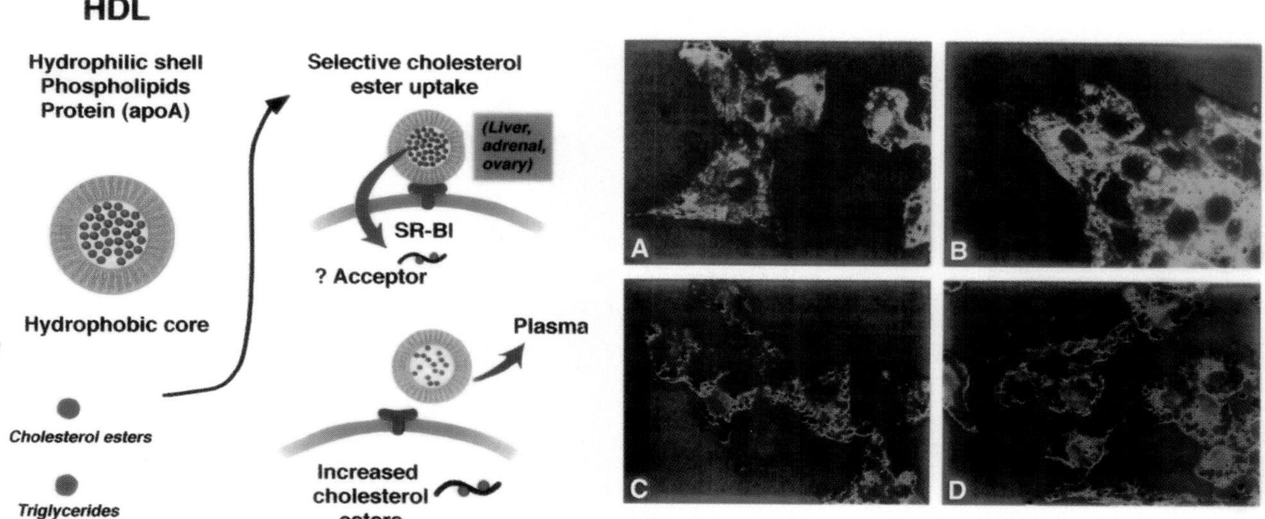

Figure 7–14 ■ The left side of the illustration depicts cholesterol esters and triglycerides released from the hydrophobic core *(left box)*. Cholesterol ester uptake by the steroidogenic cells occurs through interaction with the specific receptor (SR-BI). Once internalized, it is stored in the cell for steroidogenesis when needed *(right circle)*. (From Steinberg D. A docking receptor for HDL cholesterol esters. Science 271:460–461, 1996.)

The right side of the figure shows uptake and intracellular transport of rec-HDL–cholesterol ester to lipid droplets of a preparation of human granulosa cells. All granulosa cells in the preparation show a reticular pattern of low-level *(greenish yellow)* fluorescence. *A*, Granulosa cells were incubated with rec-HDL for 15 minutes. The cells accumulated a small number of yellow (medium fluorescent) and red (highly fluorescent) droplets. *B* to *D*, Granulosa cells were incubated with rec-HDL for 1, 3, and 6 hours, respectively. The cells increasingly took in and stored cholesterol esters as incubation time increased. By 6 hours, most of the non-Golgi cytoplasmic areas were bright *red*, indicating the presence of closely packed lipid droplets containing cholesterol esters. Perinuclear (putative Golgi) areas contained medium-level *(yellow)* fluorescence throughout the 1- to 3-hour experimental period. (From Azhar S, Tsai L, Medicheria S, et al. Human granulosa cells use high density lipoprotein cholesterol for steroidogenesis. J Clin Endocrinol Metab 83:983–991, 1998. © The Endocrine Society.)

developing follicles suggests that its release from granulosa cells may, in turn, be stimulated by FSH[39] (see Fig. 7–6).

Follistatin protein has no structural similarity to inhibins or activins.[154, 155] It is now known that follistatin functions as a binding protein for activin.[156] One follistatin monomer binds to one β-subunit.[157] Although follistatin may circulate with activins bound to it, follistatin has also been shown to bind to heparan sulfate proteoglycan on the cell surface.[156] In this way, follistatin may directly regulate the action of activins at the cell surface by acting as either a reservoir for activins or by directly presenting activins to bind to the type II activin receptor (Fig. 7–15). Activin type II receptors then interact with either free or follistatin-bound activins. Although type II activin receptors can bind activins, they alone cannot elicit a signal transduction event. A type II activin receptor is required for formation of type II receptor–activin type I receptor complex[158] for signal transduction.

Circulating levels of immunoreactive follistatin in men and in women during the menstrual cycle are relatively constant.[159–161] A two-site chemoluminescent assay revealed that virtually all circulating follistatin is bound to activin with little if any free circulating follistatin in men and women independent of hormonal status.[160] These observations indicate that the biologic role of circulating follistatin is to restrict activin bioavailability. In contrast, a substantial amount of free follistatin has been detected in the ovary (i.e., follicular fluid) and pituitary with an average value of 250 ng/ml.[160] These high concentrations (~100 times) may contribute to circulating follistatin and its inhibitory effect on bioavailability of activins. This proposition is consistent with the relatively low concentrations of circulating total activin A of 100 to 200 pg/ml during the human menstrual cycle with approximately fivefold greater concentrations seen in postmenopausal women.[162] In view of the heparan sulfate proteoglycan–binding property of follistatin, the delivery of activins to the cell surface and its subsequent coupling with activin receptors may be important to the target cell action[163] (see Fig. 7–15).

ACTIONS ON THE ANTERIOR PITUITARY

Inhibins are potent inhibitors of basal FSH release by cultured pituitary cells, confirming the earlier observation of an inhibin-like substance from cultured granulosa cells that selectively suppresses FSH release.[164] The effect of inhibins on FSH release requires a latent period of several hours, and maximal suppression is not reached until 8 to 24 hours after exposure to inhibins either in vitro or in vivo.[148] Inhibins also suppress GnRH-induced up-regulation of GnRH receptors in cultured rat pituitary cells. This action of inhibin occurs at the intracellular level beyond the stage of Ca^{2+} mobilization.[165]

Activin A ($\beta_A\beta_A$) is a potent and selective FSH secretagogue in vitro. Like that of inhibins, the effect of activins on FSH release is independent of GnRH and requires a long latency.[166] Activins and inhibins appear functionally to antagonize one another: inhibin decreases the spontaneous production of FSH and obscures the effects of low concentrations of activin, whereas higher concentrations of activin overcome the effect of inhibin, resulting in a net stimula-

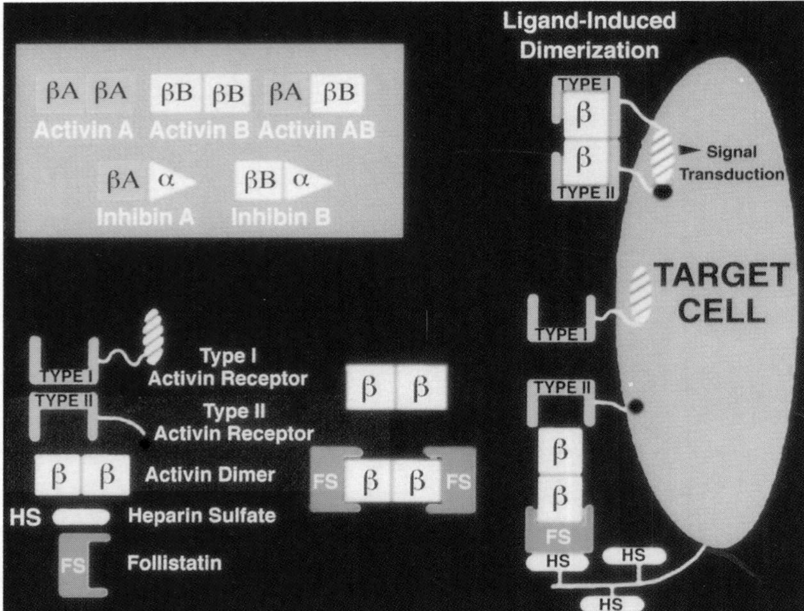

Figure 7–15 ■ Interactions of activins, activin receptors, and follistatin at the cell surface and in the circulation. In the upper lefthand corner are the structures of the inhibins and activins. The α-subunit is unique to the inhibins and the β_A and β_B subunits are shared between the inhibins and activins. Follistatin (FS) has been shown to bind the β-subunits of activins (β:β) in vitro (1 FS:1 β-subunit). In vivo, follistatin may be bound to activins in the circulation or to heparan sulfate proteoglycans (HS) on the cell surface. Type II activin receptors can bind activins but cannot transduce the activin signal in the absence of type I activin receptors. Type I receptors do not bind activins in the absence of a type II receptor. (From Matzuk MM, Kumar TR, Shou W, et al. Transgenic models to study the roles of inhibins and activins in reproduction, oncogenesis, and development. Recent Prog Horm Res 51:123–154, 1996.)

tion of FSH secretion. The highest concentrations of activin completely abolish the effects of inhibin. These opposing actions are further demonstrated by showing that inhibin decreases FSH mRNA to undetectable levels in 72 hours, with a parallel change in FSH secretion, in rat pituitary cell cultures. Addition of activin induced a marked increase in FSH mRNA levels, with concomitant increases in FSH secretion. *Follistatin* at doses of 10 to 50 ng/ml in cell cultures also results in a significant reduction in FSH mRNA. In no experiments have changes in LH-β mRNA been observed.[96, 148] The physiologic significance of the functional interaction between inhibins and activins on the pituitary release of FSH remains to be defined because the gonadotroph itself produces inhibins, activins, and follistatin.[167, 168]

OVARIAN PRODUCTION OF INHIBIN

Bioassay, immunocytochemistry, and in situ hybridization methods have established that inhibin and its subunits are produced by the granulosa cells of the ovary.[169] However, inhibin α-subunit mRNA and immunoreactivity have been found in theca interna cells.[170] The ability of both theca interna and granulosa cells to produce α-subunits of inhibin is consistent with the observation that levels of α-subunit mRNA in the ovary are always much higher than β-subunit mRNA.[171, 172] Ovarian follicular fluids contain relatively more αβ than ββ dimers, and this explains the net inhibitory effect of follicular fluids on FSH secretion.[148]

The inhibin production by the granulosa cell is regulated by FSH. In addition to FSH, a number of hormones and growth factors play a role in modulating inhibin production by the granulosa cells. LH augments the inhibin production in granulosa cells after acquisition of LH receptors. IGF-I and vasoactive intestinal peptide, both present in the ovary, are capable of stimulating inhibin production by the granulosa cell. Further, estradiol may exert a positive intraovarian effect on inhibin production, because it stimulates the secretion of immunoreactive inhibin in hypophysectomized rats.[169, 173, 174]

In human ovaries, in situ hybridization/immunohistochemistry studies revealed that both theca and granulosa cells in human ovarian follicles are endowed with the ability to synthesize inhibin, activin, and follistatin.[175] Human theca cells pretreated with LH/IGF-I display *augmentation* of androgen synthesis in response to inhibin A, whereas activin inhibits androgen production.[176, 177] The stimulatory action of inhibin was achieved at lower concentrations than the inhibitory effects of activin. The relative preponderance of C_{19} steroids compared with progesterone in the inhibin-treated cell culture was considered to indicate stimulation of 17α-hydroxylase activity.[178] Furthermore, androgens and inhibin seem to have a reciprocal interaction with a significant enhancement of FSH-stimulated inhibin production in human granulosa cells in vitro by testosterone and dihydrotestosterone but not estrogen.[178] The mechanisms of inhibin and activin action have yet to be defined because receptors for these peptides in the human ovary remain to be characterized.

INTEGRATED CONTROL (FUNCTIONAL INTERACTION OF THE HYPOTHALAMIC-PITUITARY-OVARIAN AXIS)

On the basis of the foregoing, the operation of the neuroendocrine system that controls the human menstrual cycle may be formulated (Fig. 7–16). The current rapid flow of new knowledge will undoubtedly refine or modify the construction of the present understanding of control of the menstrual cycle.

The pulsatile nature of gonadotropin secretion by the pituitary is a direct result of episodic release of GnRH from the neuronal terminals at the arcuate nucleus–median eminence region with delivery to the gonadotroph through hypothalamic-hypophysial portal vessels. The origin of this

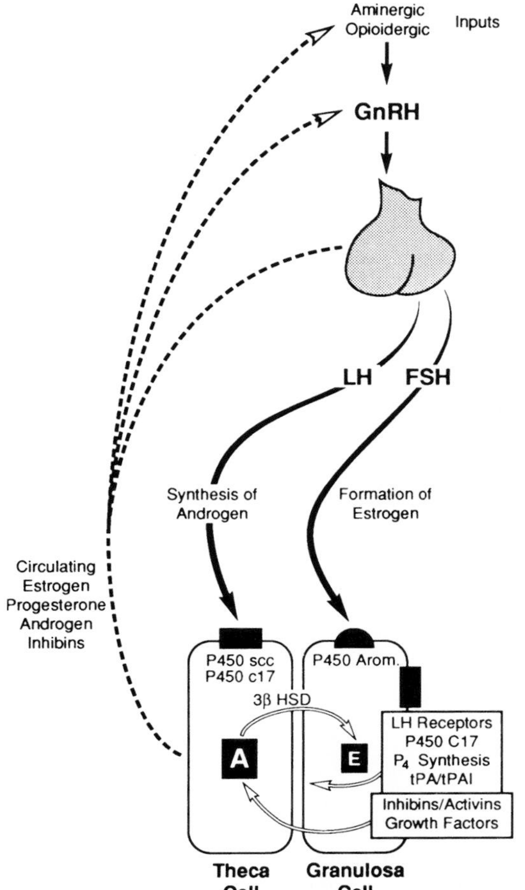

Figure 7–16 ■ Diagrammatic representations of the hypothalamic-pituitary-ovarian interaction in the control of the human menstrual cycle. The pulsatile release of LH and FSH, mediated by the hypothalamic GnRH, functions to induce ovarian theca and granulosa cell steroidogenesis and follicular maturation. The theca cell is endowed with LH receptors, which mediate LH-induced P450 steroidogenic enzymes and the synthesis of androgens as well as function as targets of modulators from the granulosa cells (paracrine). The multifunctional granulosa cell has the capacity to generate FSH-mediated LH receptors. P450c17 enzyme, and progesterone synthesis (P_4). In addition, it has the ability to produce locally a variety of autocrine/paracrine regulators (such as growth factors and tissue plasminogen activator and inhibitors [tPA and tPAI]).

intermittent delivery of GnRH appears to be the behavior of the GnRH neuron itself as judged by the observations of GT-1 neuronal cells. The pulsatile GnRH activity appears to be modulated by the neighboring neurons and astrocytes, the degree of which is ovarian steroid dependent: the inhibitory effect of the opioidergic system is most evident in the late follicular and midluteal phase of the cycle. Ovarian steroid withdrawal during luteolysis results in an increased GnRH-gonadotropin pulse frequency due to disinhibition of this opioidergic modulation of GnRH neuronal activity.

The rapid decline of ovarian steroid and inhibin A levels after luteolysis initiates the rise of pituitary FSH release that occurs 2 days before the onset of menses, thereby inaugurating a new round of folliculogenesis. The frequency and the amplitude of GnRH pulses are crucial for determining the synthesis and the secretion of gonadotropic hormones by the pituitary. A positive autoregulation of GnRH receptors by GnRH (self-priming) and prevailing estradiol concentrations augment GnRH-receptive gonadotrophs in conjunction with marked increases in synthesis and gene expression of α-subunit, LH-β, and FSH-β.[179] In combination, they induce a remarkable increase in pituitary capacity and sensitivity. When estradiol levels exceed a threshold for a period of 2 to 3 days, a change in the functional capacity of the gonadotroph occurs, as manifested by the marked increase in sensitivity to small pulses of exogenous GnRH (Fig. 7–17) and by a rapid shift of gonadotropins from the large reserve pool to the acute releasable pool, from which a midcycle surge may be initiated. Whereas estradiol serves as a trigger in the onset of the surge, the rise in progesterone secreted by the preovulatory follicle appears to amplify the duration of the surge.

Although the site of feedback action is principally at the level of the pituitary, there is cogent evidence of a hypothalamic site of estradiol action on GnRH neurons. Progesterone can also exert its feedback effect directly on GnRH neurons. The requirement of GnRH surge during the midcycle in humans and nonhuman primates remains unclear.[180] That the onset of the LH surge and ovulation occur in response to an intermittent delivery of fixed amounts of exogenous GnRH in monkeys with lesions of the arcuate nucleus[127] and in women with endogenous GnRH deficiency[139] provides presumptive evidence that an increment of GnRH release may not be required in humans and primates.

PHYSIOLOGIC AND BEHAVIORAL VARIABLES

Many myths, superstitions, and fears have surrounded the menstrual cycle to the extent that in folklore it frequently becomes incorporated into unrelated symptoms and even religious rituals in a negative way. For example, women in some primitive societies were isolated from the rest of the tribe during the time of menstruation. The advances in the biologic and behavioral sciences during the past decades have dispelled most of the myths by providing explanations of some of the manifestations associated with the hormonal changes during the menstrual cycle.

It has been recognized for some time that hormonal modifications in the menstrual cycle are correlated with several discernible changes in other functional systems. Lately, more interest has been taken in the subject because these variations lead to alterations of responsiveness, tolerance, and performance, as has been shown in states with desynchronization of circadian rhythms.[181] The following accounts are historical or descriptive, and the underlying mechanisms remain to be defined in most instances.

Seasonality of the Human Menstrual Cycle

Seasonal reproduction in mammals is a crucial strategy of adaptation to environmental changes. For maximal survival, the times of conception and birth of the young must occur in harmony with food availability, ambient temperature, light-dark cycles, and a variety of social cues.

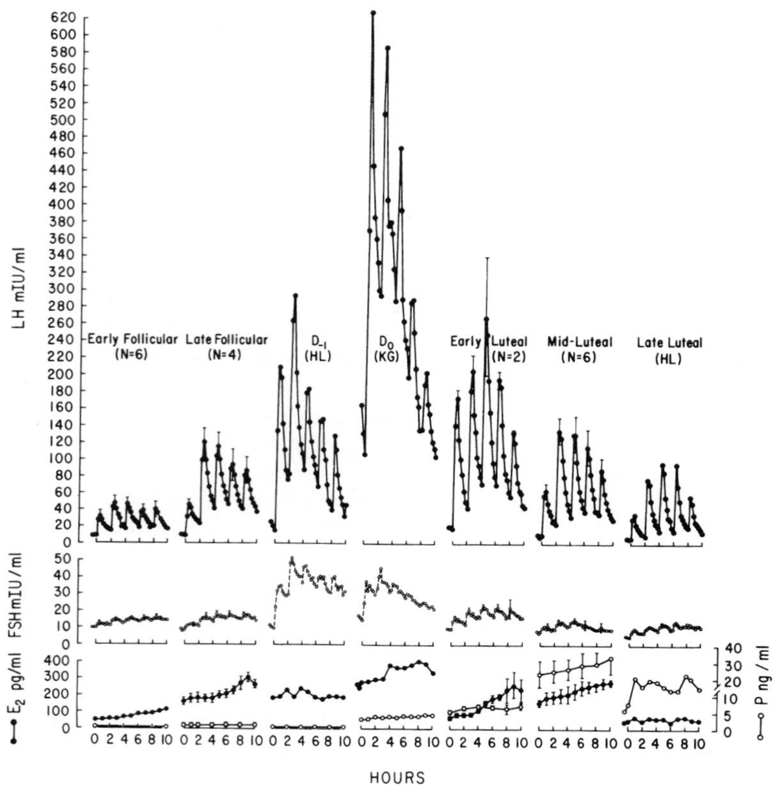

Figure 7–17 ■ Functional capacity and sensitivity of gonadotrophs to five pulses of exogenous GnRH (10 μg at 2-hour intervals) exhibit a remarkable cyclic change. The sensitivity is defined as the acute release of LH and FSH in response to the first dose of GnRH, and the capacity is estimated from the sum of gonadotropin release during the subsequent four pulses of GnRH stimulation. The self-priming action of GnRH (i.e., the response to the second dose is significantly greater than that to the first dose of GnRH) can be seen during the late follicular and midluteal phases of the cycle. Basal levels of estradiol (E_2) and progesterone (P) and their resposes to GnRH-induced gonadotropin rise are also shown. D_{-1}, day before onset of midcycle surge; D_0, day of midcycle surge. (From Wang CF, Lasley BL, Lein A, Yen SSC. The functional changes of the pituitary gonadotrophs during the menstrual cycle. J Clin Endocrinol Metab 42:718–728, 1976. © The Endocrine Society.)

Natural selection has provided mammals with a number of signaling systems that couple environmental cues to appropriate neuroendocrine responses.[182] The most spectacular model of an environmental cue related to the phenomenon of seasonal breeding is the sheep. The breeding season begins in early autumn when the photoperiod is decreasing. After 5 months of gestation, lambs are born in the spring when chances for survival are maximal. The breeding season ends in the late winter, when the photoperiod is increasing, and is followed by a 7-month anestrous period. This annual recurrence of switches between reproductive activity and quiescence, a natural process of reversible fertility, is associated with *activation and suppression*, respectively, of *GnRH pulse generator activity*.[183] The link between the seasonal switch to reproductive activity and neuroendocrine control of GnRH secretion is the daily rhythm of melatonin secretion by the pineal gland in all mammalian species, including humans. Melatonin secretion is stimulated by darkness and is inhibited by light. This signal reflects the changing environmental light-dark cycle.[184] Thus, in seasonal breeders, temporal signals to the reproductive system are synchronized by the duration of melatonin secretion (see Chapter 2 for details).[184–186]

Primates also exhibit seasonal variation in menstrual cyclicity and fertility, with the breeding season extending from autumn to spring. This period is accompanied by regular ovulatory cycles of relatively constant duration. With lengthening of daylight, the cycles become anovulatory, or luteal phase deficient, with reduced circulating levels of LH, FSH, estradiol, and progesterone.[187–191] With onset of the breeding season, resumption of normal gonadotropin secretion and ovulatory cycles becomes evident.[189] Melatonin measurements were not made in these studies. In rhesus monkeys kept under laboratory conditions in which environmental variables are constant, seasonal manifestation of the reproductive cycle does not occur.[192]

In humans, seasonality in reproductive activity is also discernible.[182] Cumulative data show that birth rates are lowest around April and May, indicating that conception rate is low during the summer months.[193] Environmental cues, particularly the light-dark cycle, may influence seasonal reproductive capacity in humans, notably in regions with strong contrast in seasonal luminosity, such as the Arctic, Sweden, and Finland.[194, 195] In these northern regions, the amount of daylight is 20 to 22 hours in May and June and about 3 hours in November to January. Under these extreme light-dark cycle changes, the activity of the pituitary-ovarian axis and the conception rate are decreased in the dark months of the year.[195–197] In addition, an inverse relationship between levels of melatonin and gonadotropin–ovarian hormones during the dark season has been observed, suggesting that an elevated melatonin secretion may be linked to low reproductive capacity.[195] Because the circadian pattern of plasma melatonin concentrations is unaltered by fluctuation of ovarian steroids and by phases of the menstrual cycle in women,[198] the increased melatonin secretion observed during the dark season is induced by the environmental cue. In warm climates, there is a reduced birth rate in spring. This effect appears to be related to *deterioration in quality and quantity of semen* during the summer months and may account for low fertility rates in high-temperature environments.[199]

Although melatonin is implicated as a timekeeping seasonal reproductive pacemaker, how it does so is unclear.

Further, underlying mechanisms of melatonin action on seasonal reproductive activity and quiescence may differ from species to species, depending on various modes of *adaptation* to their environmental cues. Thus, the evidence that environmental cues influence reproductive activity in humans must be viewed within the context of the ability of humans to modify their environment and social *adjustment* to account for the attenuation of the seasonal pattern of reproduction (see Chapter 2).

Core Body Temperature

The elevation of basal body temperature after ovulation and during the second half of the menstrual cycle begins at the time of the characteristic temperature dip preceding the rise; these temperature excursions were recognized long before the discovery of progesterone.[200] Although the thermogenic effect of progesterone is now well known, the site and mechanisms of its action remain unclear. Owing to many confounding factors, the reliability of oral measurements of basal body temperature is poor, and these measurements are frequently not reproducible. Assessment of *core body temperature* by either rectal or vaginal probes provides a reproducible recording of temperature, which conforms to a well-defined circadian rhythm. As shown in Figure 7–18, the elevation of core temperature by 0.4 to 0.6°C during the luteal phase is accompanied by a phase delay in nocturnal melatonin secretion with a 40 percent attenuation in circadian amplitude of the nocturnal temperature nadir compared with the follicular phase.[201] A similar recording has been reported by the use of a rectal thermistor probe.[202] The increased core body temperature during the luteal phase of the cycle may serve an important biologic purpose in human reproduction by providing a relatively stable intrauterine environment conducive for implantation.

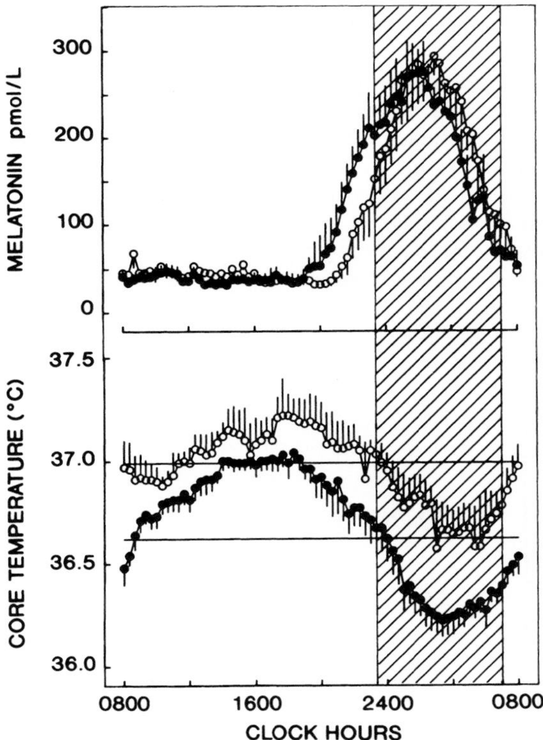

Figure 7–18 ■ Mean ± SE circadian rhythms of melatonin *(top)* and core body temperature *(bottom)* in seven women during the early follicular phase (days 3 to 6, ●) and luteal phase (days 20 to 23, ○) of the menstrual cycle. Hatched area indicates sleep time. The horizontal lines represent the 24-hour mean temperature. (From Cagnacci A, Soldani R, Laughlin GA, Yen SSC. Modification of circadian body temperature rhythm during the luteal menstrual phase: Role of melatonin. J Appl Physiol 80:25–29, 1996.)

Sensory Acuity

Several studies reported that sensory detection for taste, smell, hearing, touch, and two-point discrimination is relatively more acute during the follicular phase than during the luteal phase of the cycle. Among these sensory modalities, variation in *olfactory acuity* was most apparent.[203, 204] These changes were relative to the phases of the cycle and were generally within normal limits for each sensory modality.

The increase in olfactory sensitivity during the high-estrogen phase of the cycle in women resembles that of the lower species, in which the olfactory system functions as an active component in the processing of information, particularly in matters related to sexual activities.[205, 206] Studies provide some clues concerning the neuroendocrine integration of olfaction and sex steroids:

- During exposure to receptive female rats, there is a threefold increase in norepinephrine release by the olfactory bulbs from the male rats in vivo.[206]
- Corticotropin-releasing hormone is localized and expressed in olfactory bulbs, and it may subserve the gamut of odor-mediated responses.[207]
- Estrogen can activate neuropeptide gene expression in the olfactory pathway.[208]

The enhanced sensitivity of reproductive neural systems brought about by estrogen would therefore be an important mechanism by which sex hormones control the access of specific sensory cues to neural circuits mediating various aspects of reproductive function. These findings may be relevant to the *menstrual synchronization* observed among young women in college dormitories.[209] Of related interest is the nasal pit origin of the GnRH neuronal system in several species studied, including humans.[210] The recently described olfactory marker protein gene[211] and a G_s protein within sensory neurons of the olfactory epithelium (termed G_{olf})[212] and in situ biosynthesis of Δ^5-steroids in the olfactory bulbs[213] may permit future identification of selective expression in these cells for the transmission of olfactory information relevant to reproduction.

Sexual Activity

Assessments of sexual activity patterns as related to the phases of the menstrual cycle are limited. Confounding factors, such as social customs, adaptations, religious practices, and many others, preclude accurate quantitation. On theoretical grounds, one might expect an increase in human female sexual behavior around midcycle, because mammals, including nonhuman primates, exhibit heightened sexual receptivity at estrus in response to central action of estrogen and progesterone.[214] Earlier studies showed premenstrual and postmenstrual rises in coital frequency.[215, 216] In a study designed to test the hypothesis of midcycle peaks of sexual activity, a significant increase was found at the time of ovulation in female-initiated sexual activity, including both autosexual and heterosexual modes, but it was not apparent in male-initiated sexual behavior.[216] The increased sexual arousability in late follicular phase was confirmed in two studies.[217, 218] The neuroendocrine mediation of sexual response during the arousal and orgasmic phases of coitus is discussed in Chapter 2.

Eating Behavior and Body Weight

Fluctuations in food intake and body weight during the human menstrual cycle have been known for centuries. Results of earlier studies are conflicting. By controlling for confounding factors and refining measurement, several reports showed that food intake is significantly greater during the luteal phase than during the follicular phase of the cycle.[219–221] The increased food intake during the luteal phase has no discernible effect on body weight because this pattern of food intake is balanced by an increase in basal metabolic rate[222] and daily energy expenditure.[223] Similar findings have been reported for nonhuman primates.[224] This increase in appetite and eating behavior during the luteal phase is often associated with low serotonin activity.[225]

The Breast

The human breast is known to respond to fluctuations of hormone levels during the menstrual cycle with cyclic changes in breast volume and cellular morphologic features. Measurements of mitotic activity and of deoxyribonucleic acid synthesis ([^{3}H]thymidine incorporation) display a substantial increase in the latter part of the luteal phase, indicating that maximal epithelial proliferation occurs after peaks of estrogen and progesterone levels.[226–228] In contrast to its influence on the endometrium, progesterone does not have a decisive inhibitory effect on estrogen-mediated proliferation in the breast and may even potentiate the action of estrogen[226] (Fig. 7–19). Thus, the general view that progesterone counteracts estrogen effects may not be applicable to mammary tissue. The mechanism by which progestins affect cellular proliferation in the breast in vivo is not clear. In vitro studies suggest that progestins may induce transcription of specific genes involved directly or indirectly in the control of the cell cycle.[229] IGF-I exerts a decisive stimulatory effect on the production of mammary progesterone receptors independently of estrogen. Because mammary cells are known to be sites of IGF-I and IGF-I–binding protein production, reception, and action, they may act in paracrine and autocrine pathways in the stimulation of progesterone receptor production. The production of IGF-I, and IGF-I–binding proteins in turn, is regulated by estrogen. Thus, progesterone receptors and the action of progesterone in the mammary cells are modulated by hormones and growth factors.[230]

Significant numbers of women experience breast discomfort characterized by heaviness, tenderness, or pain during the luteal phase of the cycle. Cyclical mastalgia is a relatively common complaint in women of reproductive age and it is not associated with psychologic abnormality.[231] The hormonal basis of this syndrome is strongly suggested because spontaneous resolution occurs with the onset of menopause and after ovariectomy. Although ovarian steroid fluctuations are linked to mastalgia, the mechanisms to account for the fact that some but not all women suffer from mastalgia are not clear. Mastalgia occurs predominantly during the premenstrual phase, coinciding with the maximal epithelial proliferation of the mammary gland. It seems plausible that progesterone and estrogen withdrawal at this time of the cycle induces production of increasing numbers of prolactin receptors, thereby enhancing the stimulatory action of prolactin on the mammary gland[232] and the consequent sensation of breast volume increase. Suppression of prolactin secretion by the use of dopamine agonists, such as bromocriptine, has been effective in reducing symptoms. Further, improvement of symptoms is maintained for at least 6 months after completion of the 6-month treatment.[233]

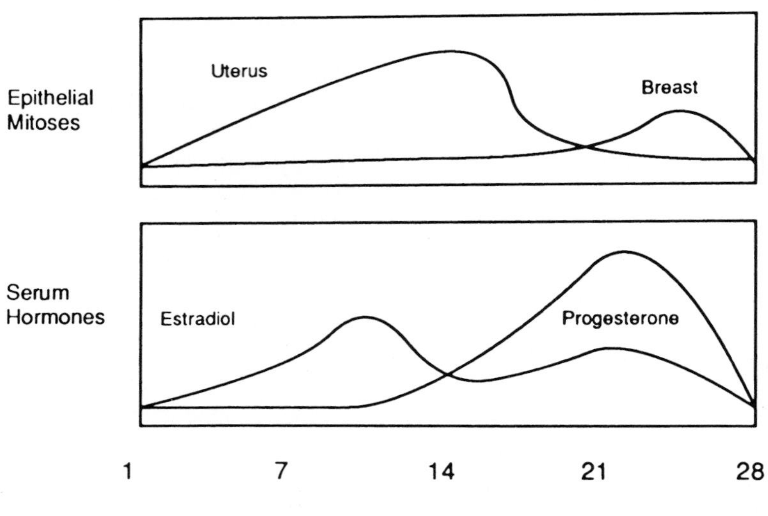

Figure 7–19 ■ Changes in epithelial mitosis of breast and endometrium and serum estradiol and progesterone levels during the human menstrual cycle. (Adapted from Clarke CL, Southerland RL. Progestin regulation of cellular proliferation. Endocr Rev 11:266–301, 1990; based on original data from Longacre TA, Bartow SA. A correlative morphologic study of human breast and endometrium in the menstrual cycle. Am J Surg Pathol 10:382–393, 1986.)

Mood and Behavior

A variety of emotional and physical changes have been linked to hormonal fluctuation during the menstrual cycle. The luteal phase and particularly the premenstrual period in many women appear to be associated with psychologic symptoms, such as depression, irritability, and tension, and with physical symptoms, such as breast tenderness, abdominal bloating, headache, and fatigue.[234] Further, psychoneuroendocrine responses to stress exhibit a greater epinephrine and norepinephrine excretion and negative mood states during the luteal phase than during the follicular phase.[235] Similarly, enhanced performance on tests of articulation and fine-motor skills was observed during the late follicular phase of the cycle.[236]

Several studies, although confirming the relationship between physical symptoms and increased food intake during the late luteal phase, failed to establish the association of hormonal fluctuation and affective changes during the premenstrual period.[237–239] Several explanations may account for this discrepancy. First, because most of these studies were conducted in college student volunteers of younger age, and because behavior of volunteer college students may vary from that of a random population sampling because of the restricted educational level and the lack of occupational status, experiments that report perceptual, cognitive, or physiologic responses may be biased in systematic fashion by sampling error. Second, studies of mood-cycle relationship were significantly influenced by expectancies.[238] Finally, the cycle phases studied were not defined by hormonal characteristics, resulting in inconsistent designations of stages of the menstrual cycle.

In sum, mood and behavioral fluctuations related to the menstrual cycle may not exist in most normal women. Premenstrual physical symptoms are present in most women but with varying degrees of perceptions.

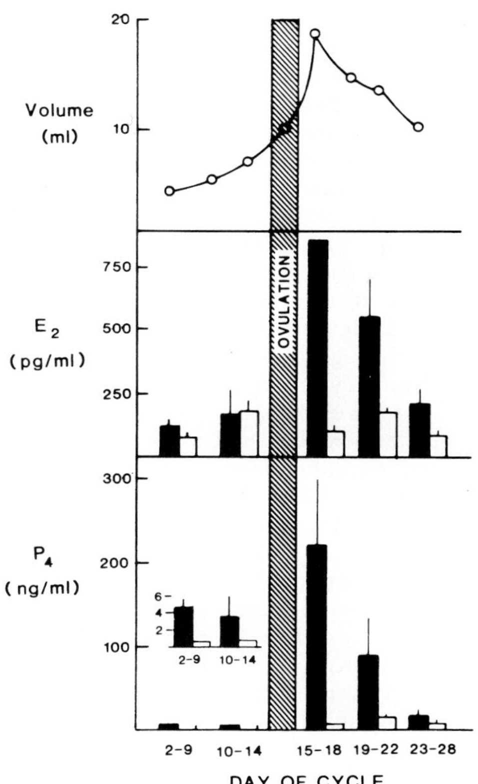

Figure 7–20 ■ Changes in the volume and concentrations (mean ± SE) of estradiol (E_2) and progesterone (P_4) in the peritoneal fluid *(closed bars)* and plasma *(open bars)* during the course of the menstrual cycle. (Modified from Konickx PR, Heyns W, Verhoeven G, et al. Biochemical characterization of peritoneal fluid in women during the menstrual cycle. J Clin Endocrinol Metab 51:1239–1244, 1980; and Konickx PR, Renaer M, Brosens IA. Origin of peritoneal fluid in women: An ovarian exudation product. Br J Obstet Gynaecol 87:177–183, 1980.)

Luteinized Unruptured Follicle Syndrome

In recent years, a condition characterized by the presence of regular menses and presumptive ovulation but without release of the ovum or the ovulation stigma has been described.[240, 241] This condition is known as the luteinized unruptured follicle (LUF) syndrome. Studies have revealed a cyclic hormonal profile similar to that seen in normal ovulatory women. Ovulation failures are documented by

- the absence of stigma at laparoscopy;
- the lack of ultrasonic signs of ovulation;
- the histologic evidence of a persistent luteinized cyst.[242, 243]

This condition, in which the follicle becomes luteinized but without release of the ovum, cannot be diagnosed by the usual methods of ovulation assessments. One source of peritoneal fluid seems to be through exudation from the ovary bearing the dominant follicle and by direct discharge of follicular fluid during and after ovulation.[244] When LUF occurs, a smaller volume of peritoneal fluid with lower estradiol and progesterone concentrations is found, in marked contrast to the findings in normal ovulatory cycles (Fig. 7–20), when the volume of peritoneal fluid increases progressively during the follicular phase, with an abrupt elevation at ovulation, and then slowly declines thereafter.[241] Concentrations of both estradiol and progesterone are consistently higher in peritoneal fluid than in plasma in normal cycling women, with a 5- to 10-fold difference after ovulation.[244] However, there are conflicting data on the value of peritoneal fluid steroid levels in establishing the diagnosis of LUF syndrome.[245]

Although LUF syndrome has been implicated as a factor in women with unexplained infertility, the causal relationship remains to be established. Furthermore, in a prospective study by Kerin and colleagues,[243] in which 66 normally cycling women were monitored by daily ultrasonography for a total of 183 cycles, the incidence of LUF was found to be 4.5 percent. Thus, the so-called LUF syndrome appears to be a sporadic and infrequent phenomenon; it is an uncommon cause of infertility and should be considered to represent a biologic variable rather than a syndrome.[243] The mechanism for this occasional failure of follicle rupture is presumably inadequate follicular development and reduced blood flow to these follicles.[246]

Functional Decline with Age

The fertility rate declines after age 35 years in women with regular menstrual cycles.[247, 248] Assessments of the functional integrity have been made by several investigators to discern the underlying causes for the subfertility status in the presence of regular cyclicity. A few years before the onset of menopause, the *perimenopausal phase* of reproductive life, ovarian dysfunctions are evident. Circulating FSH levels are elevated, and inhibin concentrations are reduced. This is accompanied by irregular menstrual cycles with intermittent anovulation.[249, 250] These findings are reflections of impaired folliculogenesis as age progresses in concert with an accelerated decline in the number of primordial follicles in the ovary as menopause approaches.[248] Studies in different age groups have revealed that between the age of 40 and 45 years, women with regular ovulatory cycles manifest accelerated follicle recruitments and development of dominant follicles in the presence of elevated FSH and a shorter follicular phase with elevated estradiol levels compared with those in younger woman.[251–253] That these follicles are not atretic is indicated by the high ratio of estradiol to androstenedione in the follicle fluid.

A large cohort cross-sectional study in 380 cycling women (age 45 to 56 years) divided according to the degree of menstrual irregularities revealed that there was an age-related increase in FSH levels, accompanied by decreases in estradiol and inhibin levels.[32] After adjustment for age and body mass index, the most striking hormone change was elevated FSH levels with concentrations two to five times greater in women who had not experienced menses for 3 months. The decline of inhibin and estradiol reflects the paucity of follicle numbers, which decline at a rapid rate after age 37 years.[254] These findings have important clinical implications; for example, serum FSH may be in the postmenopausal range during the follicular phase in women with regular cycles who are older than 45 years. In fact, studies have suggested that serum FSH levels increase slowly, but significantly, as a function of increasing age starting at age 27 years.[255] In addition, enhancement of LH pulse frequency and elevated mean LH levels were found in cycling women older than 40 years.[256]

These data are consistent with progressive aging of the ovary and reduced negative feedback action of estradiol and inhibin. They are also compatible with aging processes in general that are evident after age 25 years. In this context, the decline of ovarian function appears to parallel that of adrenal DHEA and the growth hormone–IGF-I systems (see Fig. 7–1*A*). GnRH gene expression in the MBH is increased in postmenopausal women,[257] a finding arguing against the proposal that hypothalamic aging plays a key role in the initiation of reproductive decline as indicated in rodents.[258]

References

1. Venturoli S, Porcu E, Fabbri R, et al. Longitudinal evaluation of the different gonadotropin pulsatile patterns in anovulatory cycles of young girls. J Clin Endocrinol Metab 74:836, 1992.
2. Zacharias L, Wurtman RJ. Age at menarche. N Engl J Med 280:868, 1969.
3. Wyshak G, Frisch RE. Evidence for a secular trend in age of menarche. N Engl J Med 306:1033, 1982.
4. Maclure M, Travis LB, Willett W, et al. A prospective cohort study of nutrient intake and age at menarche. Am J Clin Nutr 54:649, 1991.
5. Frisch RE, McArthur JW. Menstrual cycles: Fatness as a determinant of minimum weight for height necessary for their maintenance or onset. Science 185:949, 1974.
6. Laughlin GA, Yen SSC. Dynamic changes in serum IGF-I concentrations from prepubertal girls to aging women. Unpublished work, 1998.
7. Juul A, Holm K, Kastrup KW, et al. Free insulin-like growth factor I serum levels in 1430 healthy children and adults, and its diagnostic value in patients suspected of growth hormone deficiency. J Clin Endocrinol Metab 82:2497, 1997.
8. Hesse V, Jahreis G, Schambach H, et al. Insulin-like growth factor I correlations to changes of the hormonal status in puberty and age. Exp Clin Endocrinol 102:289, 1994.
9. Olson BR, Scott DC, Wetsel WC, et al. Effects of insulin-like growth factors I and II and insulin on the immortalized hypothalamic GT1-7 cell line. Neuroendocrinology 62:155, 1995.
10. Longo KM, Sun Y, Gore AC. Insulin-like growth factor-I effects on gonadotropin-releasing hormone biosynthesis in GT1-7 cells. Endocrinology 139:1125, 1998.
11. Wolfe AM, Wray S, Westphal H, et al. Cell-specific expression of the human gonadotropin-releasing hormone gene in transgenic animals. J Biol Chem 271:20018, 1996.
12. DueZas M, Luquin S, Chowen JA, et al. Gonadal hormone regulation of insulin-like growth factor-I–like immunoreactivity in hypothalamic astroglia of developing and adult rats. Neuroendocrinology 59:528, 1994.
13. Gore AC, Roberts JL. Regulation of gonadotropin-releasing hormone gene expression in vivo and in vitro. Front Neuroendocrinol 18:209, 1997.
14. Soldani R, Cagnacci A, Yen SSC. Insulin, insulin-like growth factor-I (IGF-I), and IGF-II enhance basal and GnRH-stimulated LH release from rat anterior pituitary cells in vitro. Acta Endocrinol (Copenh) 131:641, 1994.
15. Hiney JK, Srivastava V, Nyberg CL, et al. Insulin-like growth factor 1 of peripheral origin acts centrally to accelerate the initiation of female puberty. Endocrinology 137:3717, 1996.
16. Steiner RA. Lords and ladies leapin' on leptin. Endocrinology 137:4533, 1996.
17. Rogol AD. Leptin and puberty (Editorial). J Clin Endocrinol Metab 83:1089, 1998.
18. Kiess W, Blum WF, Aubert ML. Leptin, puberty and reproductive function: Lessons from animal studies and observations in humans. Eur J Endocrinol 138:26, 1998.
19. Catzeflis C, Pierroz DD, Rohner-Jeanrenaud F, et al. Neuropeptide Y administered chronically into the lateral ventricle profoundly inhibits both the gonadotropic and the somatotropic axis in intact adult female rats. Endocrinology 132:224, 1993.
20. Campfield LA, Smith FJ, Guisez Y, et al. Recombinant mouse OB protein: Evidence for a peripheral signal linking adiposity and central neural networks. Science 269:546, 1995.
21. Schwartz MW, Seeley RJ. The new biology of body weight regulation. J Am Diet Assoc 97:54, 1997.
22. Cheung CC, Thornton JE, Kuijper JL, et al. Leptin is a metabolic gate for the onset of puberty in the female rat. Endocrinology 138:855, 1997.
23. Matkovic V, Ilich JZ, Skugor M, et al. Leptin is inversely related to age at menarche in human females. J Clin Endocrinol Metab 82:3239, 1997.
24. Treloar AE, Boynton RE, Benn BG, et al. Variation of human menstrual cycle through reproductive life. Int J Fertil 12:77, 1967.
25. Fraser IS, Michie EA, Wide L, et al. Pituitary gonadotropins and ovarian function in adolescent dysfunctional uterine bleeding. J Clin Endocrinol Metab 37:407, 1973.
26. Venturoli S, Porcu E, Fabbri R, et al. Longitudinal evaluation of the different gonadotropin pulsatile patterns in anovulatory cycles of young girls. J Clin Endocrinol Metab 74:836, 1992.
27. Lemarchand-Beraud T, Zufferey MM, Reymond M, et al. Maturation of the hypothalamo-pituitary-ovarian axis in adolescent girls. J Clin Endocrinol Metab 54:241, 1982.
28. Apter D, Viinikka L, Vihko R. Hormonal pattern of adolescent menstrual cycles. J Clin Endocrinol Metab 47:944, 1978.
29. Sherman BM, West JH, Korenman SG. The menopausal transition: Analysis of LH, FSH, estradiol, and progesterone concentrations during menstrual cycles of older women. J Clin Endocrinol Metab 42:629, 1976.
30. Boyar RM, Finkelstein JW, David R, et al. Twenty-four hour

patterns of plasma luteinizing hormone and follicle-stimulating hormone in sexual precocity. N Engl J Med 289:282, 1973.
31. Boyar RM, Finkelstein JW, Roffwarg H, et al. Twenty-four-hour luteinizing hormone and follicle-stimulating hormone secretory patterns in gonadal dysgenesis. J Clin Endocrinol Metab 37:521, 1973.
32. Burger HG, Dudley EC, Hopper JL, et al. The endocrinology of the menopausal transition: A cross-sectional study of a population-based sample. J Clin Endocrinol Metab 80:3537, 1995.
33. Baird DT, Fraser IS. Blood production and ovarian secretion rates of estradiol-17β and estrone in women throughout the menstrual cycle. J Clin Endocrinol Metab 38:1009, 1974.
34. Groome NP, Illingworth PJ, O'Brien M, et al. Measurement of dimeric inhibin B throughout the human menstrual cycle. J Clin Endocrinol Metab 81:1401, 1996.
35. Robertson DM, Cahir N, Findlay JK, et al. The biological and immunological characterization of inhibin A and B forms in human follicular fluid and plasma. J Clin Endocrinol Metab 82:889, 1997.
36. Goodman AL, Hodgen GD. The ovarian triad of the primate menstrual cycle. Recent Prog Horm Res 39:1, 1983.
37. Hillier SG, Reichert LEJ, Van Hall EV. Control of preovulatory follicular estrogen biosynthesis in the human ovary. J Clin Endocrinol Metab 52:847, 1981.
38. McLachlan RI, Cohen NL, Dahl KD, et al. Serum inhibin levels during the periovulatory interval in normal women: Relationships with sex steroid and gonadotrophin levels. Clin Endocrinol (Oxf) 32:39, 1990.
39. Groome NP, Illingworth PJ, O'Brien M, et al. Measurement of dimeric inhibin B throughout the human menstrual cycle. J Clin Endocrinol Metab 81:1401, 1996.
40. Judd HL, Yen SS. Serum androstenedione and testosterone levels during the menstrual cycle. J Clin Endocrinol Metab 36:475, 1973.
41. Sano Y, Suzuki K, Arai K, et al. Changes in enzyme activities related to steroidogenesis in human ovaries during the menstrual cycle. J Clin Endocrinol Metab 52:994, 1981.
42. Erickson GF. Follicular maturation and atresia. *In* Flamigni C, Givens JR. The Gonadotropins: Basic Science and Clinical Aspects in Females. New York, Academic Press, 1982, p 171.
43. Hsueh AJ, Jones PB, Adashi EY, et al. Intraovarian mechanisms in the hormonal control of granulosa cell differentiation in rats. J Reprod Fertil 69:325, 1983.
44. Yen SS, Vandenberg G, Siler TM. Modulation of pituitary responsiveness to LRF by estrogen. J Clin Endocrinol Metab 39:170, 1974.
45. Marshall JC, Case GD, Valk TW, et al. Selective inhibition of follicle-stimulating hormone secretion by estradiol. Mechanism for modulation of gonadotropin responses to low dose pulses of gonadotropin-releasing hormone. J Clin Invest 71:248, 1983.
46. Hoff JD, Quigley ME, Yen SS. Hormonal dynamics at midcycle: A reevaluation. J Clin Endocrinol Metab 57:792, 1983.
47. McNatty KP, Makris A, DeGrazia C, et al. The production of progesterone, androgens, and estrogens by granulosa cells, thecal tissue, and stromal tissue from human ovaries in vitro. J Clin Endocrinol Metab 49:687, 1979.
48. McNatty KP, Smith DM, Makris A, et al. The microenvironment of the human antral follicle: Interrelationships among the steroid levels in antral fluid, the population of granulosa cells, and the status of the oocyte in vivo and in vitro. J Clin Endocrinol Metab 49:851, 1979.
49. Roseff SJ, Bangah ML, Kettel LM, et al. Dynamic changes in circulating inhibin levels during the luteal-follicular transition of the human menstrual cycle. J Clin Endocrinol Metab 69:1033, 1989.
50. McLachlan RI, Cohen NL, Vale WW, et al. The importance of luteinizing hormone in the control of inhibin and progesterone secretion by the human corpus luteum. J Clin Endocrinol Metab 68:1078, 1989.
51. Mais V, Cetel NS, Muse KN, et al. Hormonal dynamics during luteal-follicular transition. J Clin Endocrinol Metab 64:1109, 1987.
52. Filicori M, Butler JP, Crowley WFJ. Neuroendocrine regulation of the corpus luteum in the human. Evidence for pulsatile progesterone secretion. J Clin Invest 73:1638, 1984.
53. Welt CK, Martin KA, Taylor AE, et al. Frequency modulation of follicle-stimulating hormone (FSH) during the luteal-follicular transition: Evidence for FSH control of inhibin B in normal women. J Clin Endocrinol Metab 82:2645, 1997.
54. Hall JE, Schoenfeld DA, Martin KA, et al. Hypothalamic gonadotropin-releasing hormone secretion and follicle-stimulating hormone dynamics during the luteal-follicular transition. J Clin Endocrinol Metab 74:600, 1992.
55. Yen SS, Quigley ME, Reid RL, et al. Neuroendocrinology of opioid peptides and their role in the control of gonadotropin and prolactin secretion. Am J Obstet Gynecol 152:485, 1985.
56. Bogdanove EM. Hypothalamic-hypophyseal interrelationships: Basic aspects. *In* Balin H, Glasser S. Reproductive Biology. Amsterdam, Excerpta Medica, 1972, pp 5–70.
57. Short RV. Reproduction. Annu Rev Physiol 29:373, 1967.
58. Yen SS, Tsai CC, Naftolin F, et al. Pulsatile patterns of gonadotropin release in subjects with and without ovarian function. J Clin Endocrinol Metab 34:671, 1972.
59. Santen RJ, Bardin CW. Episodic luteinizing hormone secretion in man. Pulse analysis, clinical interpretation, physiologic mechanisms. J Clin Invest 52:2617, 1973.
60. Yen SSC, Vandenberg G, Tsai CC, et al. Ultradian fluctuations of gonadotropins. In Ferin M, Halberg F, Richart RM, VandeWiele RL. Biorhythms and Human Reproduction. New York, John Wiley & Sons, 1974, pp 203–218.
61. Filicori M, Marseguerra M, Mimmi P, et al. The pattern of LH and FSH pulsatile release: Physiological and clinical significance. *In* Flamigni C, Givens JR. The Gonadotropins: Basic Science and Clinical Aspects in Females. New York, Academic Press, 1982, pp 365–375.
62. Santen RJ, Bardin CW. Episodic luteinizing hormone secretion in man. Pulse analysis, clinical interpretation, physiologic mechanisms. J Clin Invest 52:2617, 1973.
63. Reame N, Sauder SE, Kelch RP, et al. Pulsatile gonadotropin secretion during the human menstrual cycle: Evidence for altered frequency of gonadotropin-releasing hormone secretion. J Clin Endocrinol Metab 59:328, 1984.
64. Filicori M, Santoro N, Merriam GR, et al. Characterization of the physiological pattern of episodic gonadotropin secretion throughout the human menstrual cycle. J Clin Endocrinol Metab 62:1136, 1986.
65. Backstrom CT, McNeilly AS, Leask RM, et al. Pulsatile secretion of LH, FSH, prolactin, oestradiol and progesterone during the human menstrual cycle. Clin Endocrinol (Oxf) 17:29, 1982.
66. Sollenberger MJ, Carlsen EC, Johnson ML, et al. Specific physiological regulation of LH secretory events throughout the human menstrual cycle: New insights into the pulsatile mode of gonadotropin release. J Neuroendocrinol 2:845, 1990.
67. Soules MR, Steiner RA, Clifton DK, et al. Progesterone modulation of pulsatile luteinizing hormone secretion in normal women. J Clin Endocrinol Metab 58:378, 1984.
68. Rossmanith WG, Liu CH, Laughlin GA, et al. Relative changes in LH pulsatility during the menstrual cycle: Using data from hypogonadal women as a reference point. Clin Endocrinol (Oxf) 32:647, 1990.
69. Djahanbakhch O, Warner P, McNeilly AS, et al. Pulsatile release of LH and oestradiol during the periovulatory period in women. Clin Endocrinol (Oxf) 20:579, 1984.
70. Rossmanith WG, Laughlin GA, Mortola JF, et al. Pulsatile cosecretion of estradiol and progesterone by the midluteal phase corpus luteum: Temporal link to luteinizing hormone pulses. J Clin Endocrinol Metab 70:990, 1990.
71. Veldhuis JD, Christiansen E, Evans WS, et al. Physiological profiles of episodic progesterone release during the midluteal phase of the human menstrual cycle: Analysis of circadian and ultradian rhythms, discrete pulse properties, and correlations with simultaneous luteinizing hormone release. J Clin Endocrinol Metab 66:414, 1988.
72. Yen SC, Llerena LA, Pearson OH, et al. Disappearance rates of endogenous follicle-stimulating hormone in serum following surgical hypophysectomy in man. J Clin Endocrinol Metab 30:325, 1970.
73. Sawyer-Steffan JE, Lasley BL, Hoff JD, et al. Comparison of in-vitro bioactivity and immunoreactivity of serum LH in normal cyclic and hypogonadal women treated with low doses of LH-RH. J Reprod Fertil 65:45, 1982.
74. Veldhuis JD, Johnson ML, Dufau ML. Preferential release of

bioactive luteinizing hormone in response to endogenous and low dose exogenous gonadotropin-releasing hormone pulses in man. J Clin Endocrinol Metab 64:1275, 1987.
75. Kessel B, Dahl KD, Kazer RR, et al. The dependency of bioactive follicle-stimulating hormone secretion on gonadotropin-releasing hormone in hypogonadal and cycling women. J Clin Endocrinol Metab 66:361, 1988.
76. Mortola JF, Sathanandan M, Pavlou S, et al. Suppression of bioactive and immunoreactive follicle-stimulating hormone and luteinizing hormone levels by a potent gonadotropin-releasing hormone antagonist: Pharmacodynamic studies. Fertil Steril 51:957, 1989.
77. Knobil E. Electrophysiological approaches to the hypothalamic GnRH pulse generator. *In* Yen SSC, Vale W. Neuroendocrine Regulation of Reproduction. Norwell, MA, Serono Symposia, USA, 1990, pp 3–9.
78. Neill JD, Patton JM, Dailey RA, et al. Luteinizing hormone releasing hormone (LHRH) in pituitary stalk blood of rhesus monkeys: Relationship to level of LH release. Endocrinology 101:430, 1977.
79. Carmel PW, Araki S, Ferin M. Pituitary stalk portal blood collection in rhesus monkeys: Evidence for pulsatile release of gonadotropin-releasing hormone (GnRH). Endocrinology 99:243, 1976.
80. Pau KY, Berria M, Hess DL, et al. Preovulatory gonadotropin-releasing hormone surge in ovarian-intact rhesus macaques. Endocrinology 133:1650, 1993.
81. Clarke IJ, Cummins JT. The temporal relationship between gonadotropin releasing hormone (GnRH) and luteinizing hormone (LH) secretion in ovariectomized ewes. Endocrinology 111:1737, 1982.
82. Xia L, Van Vugt D, Alston EJ, et al. A surge of gonadotropin-releasing hormone accompanies the estradiol-induced gonadotropin surge in the rhesus monkey. Endocrinology 131:2812, 1992.
83. Ferin M, Van Vugt D, Wardlaw S. The hypothalamic control of the menstrual cycle and the role of endogenous opioid peptides. Recent Prog Horm Res 40:441, 1984.
84. Kapen S, Boyar R, Hellman L, et al. The relationship of luteinizing hormone secretion to sleep in women during the early follicular phase: Effects of sleep reversal and a prolonged three-hour sleep-wake schedule. J Clin Endocrinol Metab 42:1031, 1976.
85. Soules MR, Steiner RA, Cohen NL, et al. Nocturnal slowing of pulsatile luteinizing hormone secretion in women during the follicular phase of the menstrual cycle. J Clin Endocrinol Metab 61:43, 1985.
86. Rossmanith WG, Yen SS. Sleep-associated decrease in luteinizing hormone pulse frequency during the early follicular phase of the menstrual cycle: Evidence for an opioidergic mechanism. J Clin Endocrinol Metab 65:715, 1987.
87. Rasmussen DD, Gambacciani M, Swartz W, et al. Pulsatile gonadotropin-releasing hormone release from the human mediobasal hypothalamus in vitro: Opiate receptor–mediated suppression. Neuroendocrinology 49:150, 1989.
88. Wetsel WC, Valenca MM, Merchenthaler I, et al. Intrinsic pulsatile secretory activity of immortalized LHRH secreting neurons. Proc Natl Acad Sci USA 89:4149, 1992.
89. Marshall JC, Kelch RP. Gonadotropin-releasing hormone: Role of pulsatile secretion in the regulation of reproduction. N Engl J Med 315:1459, 1986.
90. Wildt L, Hausler A, Marshall G, et al. Frequency and amplitude of gonadotropin-releasing hormone stimulation and gonadotropin secretion in the rhesus monkey. Endocrinology 109:376, 1981.
91. Belchetz PE, Plant TM, Nakai Y, et al. Hypophysial responses to continuous and intermittent delivery of hypothalamic gonadotropin releasing hormone. Science 202:631, 1978.
92. Kaiser UB, Sabbagh E, Katzenellenbogen RA, et al. A mechanism for the differential regulation of gonadotropin subunit gene expression by gonadotropin-releasing hormone. Proc Natl Acad Sci USA 92:12280, 1995.
93. Dalkin AC, Haisenleder DJ, Ortolano GA, et al. The frequency of gonadotropin-releasing-hormone stimulation differentially regulates gonadotropin subunit messenger ribonucleic acid expression. Endocrinology 125:917, 1989.
94. Wierman ME, Rivier JE, Wang C. Gonadotropin-releasing hormone–dependent regulation of gonadotropin subunit messenger ribonucleic acid levels in the rat. Endocrinology 124:272, 1989.
95. Lalloz MR, Detta A, Clayton RN. Gonadotropin-releasing hormone is required for enhanced luteinizing hormone subunit gene expression in vivo. Endocrinology 122:1681, 1988.
96. Gharib SD, Wierman ME, Shupnik MA, et al. Molecular biology of the pituitary gonadotropins. Endocr Rev 11:177, 1990.
97. Braden TD, Conn PM. Altered rate of synthesis of gonadotropin-releasing hormone receptors: Effects of homologous hormone appear independent of extracellular calcium. Endocrinology 126:2577, 1990.
98. Eckert RL, Mullick A, Rorke EA, et al. Estrogen receptor synthesis and turnover in MCF-7 breast cancer cells measured by a density shift technique. Endocrinology 114:629, 1984.
99. Syms AJ, Norris JS, Panko WB, et al. Mechanism of androgen-receptor augmentation. Analysis of receptor synthesis and degradation by the density-shift technique. J Biol Chem 260:455, 1985.
100. Hoff JD, Lasley BL, Yen SS. The functional relationship between priming and releasing actions of luteinizing hormone–releasing hormone. J Clin Endocrinol Metab 49:8, 1979.
101. Davis M-T, Preston JF III. Gonadotropin-releasing hormone receptor binding and pituitary responsiveness in estradiol-primed monkeys. Science 213:1388, 1981.
102. Ramirez VD, Feder HH, Sawyer CH. The role of brain catecholamines in the regulation of LH secretion: A critical inquiry. In Martini L, Ganong WF. Frontiers in Neuroendocrinology. New York, Raven Press, 1984, p 27.
103. Leranth C, MacLusky NJ, Shanabrough M, et al. Catecholaminergic innervation of luteinizing hormone–releasing hormone and glutamic acid decarboxylase immunopositive neurons in the rat medial preoptic area. An electron-microscopic double immunostaining and degeneration study. Neuroendocrinology 48:591, 1988.
104. Gitler MS, Barraclough CA. Stimulation of the medullary A1 noradrenergic system augments luteinizing hormone release induced by medial preoptic nucleus stimulation. Evaluation of A1 projections to the hypothalamus and of drugs which affect norepinephrine synthesis and adrenoceptors. Neuroendocrinology 48:351, 1988.
105. Kaufman JM, Kesner JS, Wilson RC, et al. Electrophysiological manifestation of luteinizing hormone–releasing hormone pulse generator activity in the rhesus monkey: Influence of alpha-adrenergic and dopaminergic blocking agents. Endocrinology 116:1327, 1985.
106. Pohl CR, Knobil E. The role of the central nervous system in the control of ovarian function in higher primates. Annu Rev Physiol 44:583, 1982.
107. Rasmussen DD, Liu JH, Swartz WH, et al. Human fetal hypothalamic GnRH neurosecretion: Dopaminergic regulation in vitro. Clin Endocrinol (Oxf) 25:127, 1986.
108. Yen SSC. Studies of the role of dopamine in the control of prolactin and gonadotropin secretion in humans. *In* Fuxe K, Hokfelt T, Luft R. Central Regulation of the Endocrine System. New York, Plenum Publishing, 1979, p 387.
109. Rasmussen DD, Liu JH, Wolf PL, et al. Neurosecretion of human hypothalamic immunoreactive beta-endorphin: In vitro regulation by dopamine. Neuroendocrinology 45:197, 1987.
110. Wilkes MM, Yen SS. Reduction by beta-endorphin of efflux of dopamine and DOPAC from superfused medial basal hypothalamus. Life Sci 27:1387, 1980.
111. Melis GB, Cagnacci A, Gambacciani M, et al. Chronic bromocriptine administration restores luteinizing hormone response to naloxone in postmenopausal women. Neuroendocrinology 47:159, 1988.
112. Kuljis RO, Advis JP. Immunocytochemical and physiological evidence of a synapse between dopamine- and luteinizing hormone releasing hormone–containing neurons in the ewe median eminence. Endocrinology 124:1579, 1989.
113. Findell PR, Wong KH, Jackman JK, et al. $Beta_1$-adrenergic and dopamine (D_1)–receptors coupled to adenylyl cyclase activation in GT1 gonadotropin-releasing hormone neurosecretory cells. Endocrinology 132:682, 1993.
114. Martinez de la Escalera, Gallo F, Choi AL, et al. Dopaminergic regulation of the GT1 gonadotropin-releasing hormone (GnRH) neuronal cell lines: Stimulation of GnRH release via D_1-receptors positively coupled to adenylate cyclase. Endocrinology 131:2965, 1992.

115. Reid RL, Hoff JD, Yen SS, et al. Effects of exogenous beta h-endorphin on pituitary hormone secretion and its disappearance rate in normal human subjects. J Clin Endocrinol Metab 52:1179, 1981.
116. Quigley ME, Yen SS. The role of endogenous opiates in LH secretion during the menstrual cycle. J Clin Endocrinol Metab 51:179, 1980.
117. Ropert JF, Quigley ME, Yen SS. Endogenous opiates modulate pulsatile luteinizing hormone release in humans. J Clin Endocrinol Metab 52:583, 1981.
118. Reid RL, Quigley ME, Yen SS. The disappearance of opioidergic regulation of gonadotropin secretion in postmenopausal women. J Clin Endocrinol Metab 57:1107, 1983.
119. Melis GB, Paoletti AM, Gambacciani M, et al. Evidence that estrogens inhibit LH secretion through opioids in postmenopausal women using naloxone. Neuroendocrinology 39:60, 1984.
120. Shoupe D, Montz FJ, Lobo RA. The effects of estrogen and progestin on endogenous opioid activity in oophorectomized women. J Clin Endocrinol Metab 60:178, 1985.
121. Cagnacci A, Melis GB, Paoletti AM, et al. Influence of oestradiol and progesterone on pulsatile LH secretion in postmenopausal women. Clin Endocrinol (Oxf) 31:541, 1989.
122. Jacobson W, Wilkinson M. Association of diurnal variations in hypothalamic but not cortical opiate ([^{3}H]-naloxone)-binding sites with the ability of naloxone to induce LH release in the prepubertal female rat. Neuroendocrinology 44:132, 1986.
123. Rossmanith WG, Mortola JF, Yen SS. Role of endogenous opioid peptides in the initiation of the midcycle luteinizing hormone surge in normal cycling women. J Clin Endocrinol Metab 67:695, 1988.
124. Jacobson W, Kalra SP. Decreases in mediobasal hypothalamic and preoptic area opioid ([^{3}H]naloxone) binding are associated with the progesterone-induced luteinizing hormone surge. Endocrinology 124:199, 1989.
125. Yen SS, Tsai CC. The effect of ovariectomy on gonadotropin release. J Clin Invest 50:1149, 1971.
126. Yen SS, Tsai CC, Vandenberg G, et al. Gonadotropin dynamics in patients with gonadal dysgenesis: A model for the study of gonadotropin regulation. J Clin Endocrinol Metab 35:897, 1972.
127. Knobil E. The neuroendocrine control of the menstrual cycle. Recent Prog Horm Res 36:53, 1980.
128. Yen SS, Lasley BL, Wang CF, et al. The operating characteristics of the hypothalamic-pituitary system during the menstrual cycle and observations of biological action of somatostatin. Recent Prog Horm Res 31:321, 1975.
129. Yen SS, Tsai CC. The biphasic pattern in the feedback action of ethinyl estradiol on the release of pituitary FSH and LH. J Clin Endocrinol Metab 33:882, 1971.
130. Liu JH, Yen SS. Induction of midcycle gonadotropin surge by ovarian steroids in women: A critical evaluation. J Clin Endocrinol Metab 57:797, 1983.
131. Keye WRJ, Jaffe RB. Strength-duration characteristics of estrogen effects on gonadotropin response to gonadotropin-releasing hormone in women. I. Effects of varying duration of estradiol administration. J Clin Endocrinol Metab 41:1003, 1975.
132. Yen SS, Lein A. The apparent paradox of the negative and positive feedback control system on gonadotropin secretion. Am J Obstet Gynecol 126:942, 1976.
133. Yen SS, Tsai CC. Acute gonadotropin release induced by exogenous estradiol during the mid-follicular phase of the menstrual cycle. J Clin Endocrinol Metab 34:298, 1972.
134. Nillius SJ, Wide L. Induction of a midcycle-like peak of luteinizing hormone in young women by exogenous oestradiol-17. J Obstet Gynaecol Br Commonw 78:822, 1971.
135. Romano GJ, Krust A, Pfaff DW. Expression and estrogen regulation of progesterone receptor mRNA in neurons of the mediobasal hypothalamus: An in situ hybridization study [published erratum appears in Mol Endocrinol 3:1860, 1989]. Mol Endocrinol 3:1295, 1989.
136. Fox SR, Harlan RE, Shivers BD, et al. Chemical characterization of neuroendocrine targets for progesterone in the female rat brain and pituitary. Neuroendocrinology 51:276, 1990.
137. Sar M. Estradiol is concentrated in tyrosine hydroxylase–containing neurons of the hypothalamus. Science 223:938, 1984.
138. Hoffman GE, Lee WS, Attardi B, et al. Luteinizing hormone–releasing hormone neurons express c-*fos* antigen after steroid activation. Endocrinology 126:1736, 1990.
139. Crowley WFJ, McArthur JW. Simulation of the normal menstrual cycle in Kallman's syndrome by pulsatile administration of luteinizing hormone–releasing hormone (LHRH). J Clin Endocrinol Metab 51:173, 1980.
140. Nippoldt TB, Reame NE, Kelch RP, et al. The roles of estradiol and progesterone in decreasing luteinizing hormone pulse frequency in the luteal phase of the menstrual cycle. J Clin Endocrinol Metab 69:67, 1989.
141. Maruncic M, Casper RF. The effect of luteal phase estrogen antagonism on luteinizing hormone pulsatility and luteal function in women. J Clin Endocrinol Metab 64:148, 1987.
142. Lumsden MA, West CP, Baird DT. Tamoxifen prolongs luteal phase in premenopausal women but has no effect on the size of uterine fibroids. Clin Endocrinol 31:335, 1989.
143. Fraser HM, Smith KB, Lunn SF, et al. Immunoneutralization and immunocytochemical localization of inhibin alpha subunit during the midluteal phase in the stump-tailed macaque. J Endocrinol 133:341, 1992.
144. Steinberg D. A docking receptor for HDL cholesterol esters. Science 271:460, 1996.
145. Acton S, Rigotti A, Landschulz KT, et al. Identification of scavenger receptor SR-BI as a high density lipoprotein receptor. Science 271:518, 1996.
146. Azhar S, Tsai L, Medicherla S, et al. Human granulosa cells use high density lipoprotein cholesterol for steroidogenesis. J Clin Endocrinol Metab 83:983, 1998.
147. Mason AJ, Niall HD, Seeburg PH. Structure of two human ovarian inhibins. Biochem Biophys Res Commun 135:957, 1986.
148. Vale W, Hsueh AJ, Rivier C, et al. The inhibin/activin family of hormones and growth factors. *In* Sporn MB, Roberts AB. Peptide Growth Factors and Their Receptors II. New York, Springer-Verlag, 1990, pp 211–248.
149. Davis SR, Krozowski Z, McLachlan RI, et al. Inhibin gene expression in the human corpus luteum. J Endocrinol 115:R21, 1987.
150. Yamoto M, Minami S, Nakano R, et al. Immunohistochemical localization of inhibin/activin subunits in human ovarian follicles during the menstrual cycle. J Clin Endocrinol Metab 74:989, 1992.
151. Roberts VJ, Barth S, el-Roeiy A, et al. Expression of inhibin/activin subunits and follistatin messenger ribonucleic acids and proteins in ovarian follicles and the corpus luteum during the human menstrual cycle. J Clin Endocrinol Metab 77:1402, 1993.
152. Schwall RH, Mason AJ, Wilcox JN, et al. Localization of inhibin/activin subunit mRNAs within the primate ovary. Mol Endocrinol 4:75, 1990.
153. Lambert-Messerlian GM, Hall JE, Sluss PM, et al. Relatively low levels of dimeric inhibin circulate in men and women with polycystic ovarian syndrome using a specific two-site enzyme-linked immunosorbent assay. J Clin Endocrinol Metab 79:45, 1994.
154. Ueno N, Ling N, Ying SY, et al. Isolation and partial characterization of follistatin: A single-chain Mr 35,000 monomeric protein that inhibits the release of follicle-stimulating hormone. Proc Natl Acad Sci USA 84:8282, 1987.
155. Robertson DM, Klein R, de Vos FL, et al. The isolation of polypeptides with FSH suppressing activity from bovine follicular fluid which are structurally different to inhibin. Biochem Biophys Res Commun 149:744, 1987.
156. Nakamura T, Takio K, Eto Y, et al. Activin-binding protein from rat ovary is follistatin. Science 247:836, 1990.
157. Shimonaka M, Inoye S, Shimasaki S, et al. Follistatin binds both activin and inhibin through the common β subunit. Endocrinology 128:3313, 1991.
158. Mathews LS. Activin receptors and cellular signaling by the receptor serine kinase family. Endocr Rev 15:310, 1994.
159. Khoury RH, Wang QF, Crowley WF Jr, et al. Serum follistatin levels in women: Evidence against an endocrine function of ovarian follistatin. J Clin Endocrinol Metab 80:1361, 1995.
160. McConnell DS, Wang Q, Sluss PM, et al. A two-site chemiluminescent assay for activin-free follistatin reveals that most follistatin circulating in men and normal cycling women is in an activin-bound state. J Clin Endocrinol Metab 83:858, 1998.
161. Kettel LM, DePaolo LV, Morales AJ, et al. Circulating levels of follistatin from puberty to menopause. Fertil Steril 65:472, 1996.
162. Knight PG, Muttukrishna S, Groome NP. Development and application of a two-site enzyme immunoassay for the

determination of "total" activin-A concentrations in serum and follicular fluid. J Endocrinol 148:267, 1996.
163. Matzuk MM, Kumar TR, Shou W, et al. Transgenic models to study the roles of inhibins and activins in reproduction, oncogenesis, and development. Recent Prog Horm Res 51:123, 1996.
164. Erickson GF, Hsueh AJ. Secretion of "inhibin" by rat granulosa cells in vitro. Endocrinology 103:1960, 1978.
165. Wang QF, Farnworth PG, Findlay JK, et al. Inhibitory effect of pure 31-kilodalton bovine inhibin on gonadotropin-releasing hormone (GnRH)–induced up-regulation of GnRH binding sites in cultured rat anterior pituitary cells. Endocrinology 124:363, 1989.
166. Vale W, Rivier J, Vaughan J, et al. Purification and characterization of an FSH releasing protein from porcine ovarian follicular fluid. Nature 321:776, 1986.
167. Roberts V, Meunier H, Vaughan J, et al. Production and regulation of inhibin subunits in pituitary gonadotropes. Endocrinology 124:552, 1989.
168. Kaiser UB, Lee BL, Carroll RS, et al. Follistatin gene expression in the pituitary: Localization in gonadotropes and folliculostellate cells in diestrous rats. Endocrinology 130:3048, 1992.
169. Bicsak TA, Tucker EM, Cappel S, et al. Hormonal regulation of granulosa cell inhibin biosynthesis. Endocrinology 119:2711, 1986.
170. Meunier H, Cajander SB, Roberts VJ, et al. Rapid changes in the expression of inhibin alpha-, beta A–, and beta B–subunits in ovarian cell types during the rat estrous cycle. Mol Endocrinol 2:1352, 1988.
171. Davis SR, Dench F, Nikolaidis I, et al. Inhibin A-subunit gene expression in the ovaries of immature female rats is stimulated by pregnant mare serum gonadotrophin. Biochem Biophys Res Commun 138:1191, 1986.
172. Mason AJ, Hayflick JS, Ling N, et al. Complementary DNA sequences of ovarian follicular fluid inhibin show precursor structure and homology with transforming growth factor-beta. Nature 318:659, 1985.
173. Zhang Z, Lee VW, Carson RS, et al. Selective control of rat granulosa cell inhibin production by FSH and LH in vitro. Mol Cell Endocrinol 56:35, 1988.
174. Rivier C, Vale W. Immunoreactive inhibin secretion by the hypophysectomized female rat: Demonstration of the modulating effect of gonadotropin-releasing hormone and estrogen through a direct ovarian site of action. Endocrinology 124:195, 1989.
175. Roberts VJ, Barth S, el-Roeiy A, et al. Expression of inhibin/activin system messenger ribonucleic acids and proteins in ovarian follicles from women with polycystic ovarian syndrome. J Clin Endocrinol Metab 79:1434, 1994.
176. Hillier SG, Yong EL, Illingworth PJ, et al. Effect of recombinant activin on androgen synthesis in cultured human thecal cells. J Clin Endocrinol Metab 72:1206, 1991.
177. Hillier SG, Yong EL, Illingworth PJ, et al. Effect of recombinant inhibin on androgen synthesis in cultured human thecal cells. Mol Cell Endocrinol 75:R1, 1991.
178. Hillier SG. Regulatory functions for inhibin and activin in human ovaries. J Endocrinol 131:171, 1991.
179. Lloyd JM, Childs GV. Changes in the number of GnRH-receptive cells during the rat estrous cycle: Biphasic effects of estradiol. Neuroendocrinology 48:138, 1988.
180. Norman RL, Gliessman P, Lindstrom SA, et al. Reinitiation of ovulatory cycles in pituitary stalk–sectioned rhesus monkeys: Evidence for a specific hypothalamic message for the preovulatory release of luteinizing hormone. Endocrinology 111:1874, 1982.
181. Czeisler CA, Johnson MP, Duffy JF, et al. Exposure to bright light and darkness to treat physiologic maladaptation to night work [see comments]. N Engl J Med 322:1253, 1990.
182. Bronson FH. Mammalian reproduction: An ecological perspective. Biol Reprod 32:1, 1985.
183. Karsch FJ, Woodfill CJ. I. Neuroendocrinology of seasonal breeding: Mode of action of melatonin. *In* Yen SSC, Vale W. Neuroendocrine Regulation of Reproduction. Norwell, MA, Serono Symposia, USA, 1990, pp 9–18.
184. Arendt J. Melatonin. Clin Endocrinol (Oxf) 29:205, 1988.
185. Kaynard AH, Malpaux B, Robinson JE, et al. Importance of pituitary and neural actions of estradiol in induction of the luteinizing hormone surge in the ewe. Neuroendocrinology 48:296, 1988.
186. Tamarkin L, Baird CJ, Almeida OF. Melatonin: A coordinating signal for mammalian reproduction? Science 227:714, 1985.
187. Dailey RA, Neill JD. Seasonal variation in reproductive hormones of rhesus monkeys: Anovulatory and short luteal phase menstrual cycles. Biol Reprod 25:560, 1981.
188. Keverne EB, Michael RP. Annual changes in the menstruation of rhesus monkeys. J Endocrinol 48:669, 1970.
189. Walker ML, Wilson ME, Gordon TP. Endocrine control of the seasonal occurrence of ovulation in rhesus monkeys housed outdoors. Endocrinology 114:1074, 1984.
190. Wehrenberg WB, Dyrenfurth I. Photoperiod and ovulatory menstrual cycles in female macaque monkeys. J Reprod Fertil 68:119, 1983.
191. Hutz RJ, Dierschke DJ, Wolf RC. Seasonal effects on ovarian folliculogenesis in rhesus monkeys. Biol Reprod 33:653, 1985.
192. Valerio DA, Pallotta AJ, Courtney KD. Experiences in large-scale breeding of simians for medical experimentation. Ann N Y Acad Sci 162:282, 1969.
193. Natality Statistics Analysis, United States—1962. Washington, DC, National Center for Health Statistics, U.S. Department of Health, Education, and Welfare, Vital and Health Statistics, 1964. Public Health Service publication Series 21, No. 1.
194. Ehrenkranz JR. Seasonal breeding in humans: Birth records of the Labrador Eskimo. Fertil Steril 40:485, 1983.
195. Kauppila A, Kivela A, Pakarinen A, et al. Inverse seasonal relationship between melatonin and ovarian activity in humans in a region with a strong seasonal contrast in luminosity. J Clin Endocrinol Metab 65:823, 1987.
196. Ronkainen H, Pakarinen A, Kirkinen P, et al. Physical exercise–induced changes and season-associated differences in the pituitary-ovarian function of runners and joggers. J Clin Endocrinol Metab 60:416, 1985.
197. Sandahl B. Seasonal birth pattern in Sweden in relation to birth order and maternal age. Acta Obstet Gynecol Scand 57:393, 1978.
198. Berga SL, Yen SS. Circadian pattern of plasma melatonin concentrations during four phases of the human menstrual cycle. Neuroendocrinology 51:606, 1990.
199. Levine RJ, Mathew RM, Chenault CB, et al. Differences in the quality of semen in outdoor workers during summer and winter [see comments]. N Engl J Med 323:12, 1990.
200. Tompkins P. The use of basal temperature graphs in determining the date of ovulation. JAMA 124:698, 1944.
201. Cagnacci A, Soldani R, Laughlin GA, et al. Modification of circadian body temperature rhythm during the luteal menstrual phase: The role of melatonin. J Appl Physiol 80:25, 1996.
202. Lee KA. Circadian temperature rhythms in relation to menstrual cycle phase. J Biol Rhythms 3:255, 1988.
203. Henkin RI. Sensory changes during the menstrual cycle. *In* Ferin M, Halberg F, Richart RM, vande Wiele RL. Biorhythms and Human Reproduction. New York, John Wiley & Sons, 1974, pp 277–285.
204. Vierling JS, Rock J. Variations in olfactory sensitivity to exaltolide during the menstrual cycle. J Appl Physiol 22:311, 1967.
205. Keverne EB, de la Riva C. Pheromones in mice: Reciprocal interaction between the nose and brain. Nature 296:148, 1982.
206. Dluzen DE, Ramirez VD. Receptive female rats stimulate norepinephrine release from olfactory bulbs of freely behaving male rats. Neuroendocrinology 49:28, 1989.
207. Imaki T, Nahon JL, Sawchenko PE, et al. Widespread expression of corticotropin-releasing factor messenger RNA and immunoreactivity in the rat olfactory bulb. Brain Res 496:35, 1989.
208. Simerly RB, Young BJ, Capozza MA, et al. Estrogen differentially regulates neuropeptide gene expression in a sexually dimorphic olfactory pathway. Proc Natl Acad Sci USA 86:4766, 1989.
209. McClintock MK. Menstrual synchrony and suppression. Nature 229:244, 1971.
210. Schwanzel-Fukuda M, Bick D, Pfaff DW. Luteinizing hormone–releasing hormone (LHRH)–expressing cells do not migrate normally in an inherited hypogonadal (Kallmann) syndrome. Brain Res Mol Brain Res 6:311, 1989.
211. Danciger E, Mettling C, Vidal M, et al. Olfactory marker protein gene: Its structure and olfactory neuron-specific expression in transgenic mice. Proc Natl Acad Sci USA 86:8565, 1989.
212. Jones DT, Reed RR. Golf: An olfactory neuron specific–G protein involved in odorant signal transduction. Science 244:790, 1989.

213. Le Goascogne C, Robel P, Gouezou M, et al. Neurosteroids: Cytochrome P-450scc in rat brain. Science 237:1212, 1987.
214. Pfaff D. Molecular consequences of sex steroid actions on hypothalamic nerve cells. In Yen SSC, Vale W. Neuroendocrine Regulation of Reproduction. Norwell, MA, Serono Symposia, USA, 1990, pp 71–94.
215. Hart RD. Monthly rhythm of libido in married women. Br Med J 1:1023, 1960.
216. Adams DB, Gold AR, Burt AD. Rise in female-initiated sexual activity at ovulation and its suppression by oral contraceptives. N Engl J Med 299:1145, 1978.
217. Slob AK, Bax CM, Hop WC, et al. Sexual arousability and the menstrual cycle. Psychoneuroendocrinology 21:545, 1996.
218. Burleson MH, Gregory WL, Trevathan WR. Heterosexual activity: Relationship with ovarian function. Psychoneuroendocrinology 20:405, 1995.
219. Gong EJ, Garrel D, Calloway DH. Menstrual cycle and voluntary food intake. Am J Clin Nutr 49:252, 1989.
220. Dalvit SP. The effect of the menstrual cycle on patterns of food intake. Am J Clin Nutr 34:1811, 1981.
221. Pliner P, Fleming AS. Food intake, body weight, and sweetness preferences over the menstrual cycle in humans. Physiol Behav 30:663, 1983.
222. Solomon SJ, Kurzer MS, Calloway DH. Menstrual cycle and basal metabolic rate in women. Am J Clin Nutr 36:611, 1982.
223. Webb P. 24-hour energy expenditure and the menstrual cycle. Am J Clin Nutr 44:614, 1986.
224. Rosenblatt H, Dyrenfurth I, Ferin M, et al. Food intake and the menstrual cycle in rhesus monkeys. Physiol Behav 24:447, 1980.
225. Dye L, Blundell JE. Menstrual cycle and appetite control: Implications for weight regulation. Hum Reprod 12:1142, 1997.
226. Longacre TA, Bartow SA. A correlative morphologic study of human breast and endometrium in the menstrual cycle. Am J Surg Pathol 10:382, 1986.
227. Going JJ, Anderson TJ, Battersby S, et al. Proliferative and secretory activity in human breast during natural and artificial menstrual cycles. Am J Pathol 130:193, 1988.
228. Anderson TJ, Battersby S, King RJ, et al. Oral contraceptive use influences resting breast proliferation. Hum Pathol 20:1139, 1989.
229. Clarke CL, Southerland RL. Progestin regulation of cellular proliferation. Endocr Rev 11:266, 1990.
230. Katzenellenbogen BS, Norman MJ. Multihormonal regulation of the progesterone receptor in MCF-7 human breast cancer cells: Interrelationships among insulin/insulin-like growth factor-I, serum, and estrogen [published erratum appears in Endocrinology 126:3217, 1990]. Endocrinology 126:891, 1990.
231. Preece PE, Mansel RE, Hughes LE. Mastalgia: Psychoneurosis or organic disease? Br Med J 1:29, 1978.
232. Djiane J, Durand P. Prolactin-progesterone antagonism in self regulation of prolactin receptors in the mammary gland. Nature 266:641, 1977.
233. Mansel RE, Dogliotti L. European multicentre trial of bromocriptine in cyclical mastalgia. Lancet 335:190, 1990.
234. Dennerstein L, Abraham SF. Affective changes and the menstrual cycle. *In* Beaumont PJV, Burrows GD. Handbook of Psychiatry and Endocrinology. Amsterdam, Elsevier, 1982, pp 367–400.
235. Collins A, Eneroth P, Landgren BM. Psychoneuroendocrine stress responses and mood as related to the menstrual cycle. Psychosom Med 47:512, 1985.
236. Hampson E. Estrogen-related variations in human spatial and articulatory-motor skills. Psychoneuroendocrinology 15:97, 1990.
237. Laessle RG, Tuschl RJ, Schweiger U, et al. Mood changes and physical complaints during the normal menstrual cycle in healthy young women. Psychoneuroendocrinology 15:131, 1990.
238. Olasov B, Jackson J. Effects of expectancies on women's reports of moods during the menstrual cycle. Psychosom Med 49:65, 1987.
239. Sommer B. How does menstruation affect cognitive competence and psychophysiological response? *In* Gotub S. Lifting the Curse of Menstruation. New York, Hayworth Press, 1983, pp 53–90.
240. Marik J, Hulka JF. Luteinized unruptured follicle syndrome: A subtle cause of infertility. Fertil Steril 29:270, 1978.
241. Koninckx PR, DeMoor P, Brosens IA. Diagnosis of the luteinized unruptured follicle syndrome by steroid hormone assays on peritoneal fluid. Br J Obstet Gynaecol 87:929, 1980.
242. Coulam CB, Hill LM, Breckle R. Ultrasonic evidence for luteinization of unruptured preovulatory follicles. Fertil Steril 37:524, 1982.
243. Kerin JF, Kirby C, Morris D, et al. Incidence of the luteinized unruptured follicle phenomenon in cycling women. Fertil Steril 40:620, 1983.
244. Koninckx PR, Heyns W, Verhoeven G, et al. Biochemical characterization of peritoneal fluid in women during the menstrual cycle. J Clin Endocrinol Metab 51:1239, 1980.
245. Janssen-Caspers HA, Kruitwagen RF, Wladimiroff JW, et al. Diagnosis of luteinized unruptured follicle by ultrasound and steroid hormone assays in peritoneal fluid: A comparative study. Fertil Steril 46:823, 1986.
246. Zaidi J, Jurkovic D, Campbell S, et al. Luteinized unruptured follicle: Morphology, endocrine function and blood flow changes during the menstrual cycle. Hum Reprod 10:44, 1995.
247. Menken J, Trussell J, Larsen U. Age and infertility [published erratum appears in Science 234:413, 1986]. Science 233:1389, 1986.
248. Erickson GF. Dissociation of endocrine and gametogenic ovarian function. *In* Lobo RA. Perimenopause. Norwell, MA, Serono Symposia, USA, 1997, pp 101–118.
249. Sherman BM, West JH, Korenman SG. The menopausal transition: Analysis of LH, FSH, estradiol, and progesterone concentrations during menstrual cycles of older women. J Clin Endocrinol Metab 42:629, 1976.
250. MacNaughton J, Banah M, McCloud P, et al. Age related changes in follicle stimulating hormone, luteinizing hormone, oestradiol and immunoreactive inhibin in women of reproductive age. Clin Endocrinol (Oxf) 36:339, 1992.
251. Klein NA, Battaglia DE, Fujimoto VY, et al. Reproductive aging: Accelerated ovarian follicular development associated with a monotropic follicle-stimulating hormone rise in normal older women. J Clin Endocrinol Metab 81:1038, 1996.
252. Klein NA, Battaglia DE, Miller PB, et al. Ovarian follicular development and the follicular fluid hormones and growth factors in normal women of advanced reproductive age. J Clin Endocrinol Metab 81:1946, 1996.
253. Santoro N, Brown JR, Adel T, et al. Characterization of reproductive hormonal dynamics in the perimenopause. J Clin Endocrinol Metab 81:1495, 1996.
254. Richardson SJ, Senikas V, Nelson JF. Follicular depletion during the menopausal transition: Evidence for accelerated loss and ultimate exhaustion. J Clin Endocrinol Metab 65:1231, 1987.
255. Ahmed E, Lenton EA, Cooke ID. Hypothalamic-pituitary ageing: Progressive increase in FSH and LH concentrations throughout the reproductive life in regularly menstruating women. Clin Endocrinol (Oxf) 41:199, 1994.
256. Reame NE, Kelch RP, Beitins IZ, et al. Age effects of follicle-stimulating hormone and pulsatile luteinizing hormone secretion across the menstrual cycle of premenopausal women. J Clin Endocrinol Metab 81:1512, 1996.
257. Rance NE, Uswandi SV. Gonadotropin-releasing hormone gene expression is increased in the medial basal hypothalamus of postmenopausal women. J Clin Endocrinol Metab 81:3540, 1996.
258. Wise PM, Kashon ML, Krajnak KM, et al. Aging of the female reproductive system: A window into brain aging. Recent Prog Horm Res 52:279, 1997.

Chapter 8

THE ENDOMETRIUM AND MYOMETRIUM: Regulation and Dysfunction

Jerome Strauss III • Christos Coutifaris

■ CHAPTER OUTLINE

KEY POINTS

- The endometrium and myometrium function in concert to receive the embryo, support its growth, and ultimately assist in its timely expulsion.
- The preparation of a receptive uterine environment is programmed by ovarian steroid hormones that act directly on the endometrium and myometrium and indirectly through the intermediacy of various growth factors and cytokines.
- The endometrium is populated by unique immune cells that produce regulatory cytokines and allow the fetal semiallograft to be accepted by the maternal host.
- The components of a receptive endometrium include the luminal epithelium, which must express cell adhesion molecules and extracellular matrix proteins that permit the blastocyst to adhere to the uterine lining; glandular epithelial cells, which secrete substances that support blastocyst development and trophoblast invasion; a stroma composed of an extracellular matrix that facilitates trophoblast invasion; and decidual cells and large granular lymphocytes that modulate trophoblast function through the secretion of growth factors, growth factor–binding proteins, and cytokines.
- A vascular system nourishes the endometrium in the initial receptive phase and is remodeled by invading trophoblasts to establish the placental blood supply.
- The coordinated contractile activity of the myometrium promotes sperm migration, followed by hormone-imposed hyperplasia and quiescence that accommodate embryo growth and development.
- In the absence of conception, the endometrium is shed through an orchestrated remodeling process involving matrix metalloproteinases, the production of vasoactive substances, and uterine contractions that promote hemostasis and the expulsion of the shed endometrial lining.
- Endometrial dysfunction includes abnormalities in the preparation of a receptive state, neoplasia of epithelial cells, and intrinsic endometrial defects or host abnormalities that permit the attachment and proliferation of endometrial glands and stroma at ectopic sites.
- Abnormalities in programmed cell death permit hormone-facilitated clonal expansion of myometrial smooth muscle cells.

The two main compartments of the uterus, the endometrium and the myometrium, are regulated in a coordinated manner to receive the embryo, to accommodate its growth and development, and ultimately to ensure the timely expulsion of the mature fetus. This chapter describes the structural and functional changes in the human endometrium and myometrium during the normal menstrual cycle and pregnancy, providing a basis for the consideration of clinical methods to assess endometrial function and the pathophysiology of abnormalities of the endometrium and myometrium.

STRUCTURE AND MORPHOLOGY

Morphogenesis of the Uterus

The female reproductive tract arises from the paired müllerian (paramesonephric) ducts, which are derived from longitudinal invaginations of the coelomic epithelium of the mesonephros during week 6 of gestation.[1–3] Directed by a combinatorial code of homeobox (HOX9-13) genes controlling the transcription of morphogenetic regulators that undoubtedly include growth factors (e.g., epidermal growth factor, basic fibroblast growth factor, and later insulin-like growth factors), their receptors, and cell adhesion molecules, the paramesonephric ducts form the fallopian tubes, fusing by week 10 of gestation to produce the primordial uterus and upper portion of the vagina. Dysregulated expression or absence of expression of the homeobox genes or their downstream target genes leads to malformations of the reproductive tract and, in some instances, abnormal function of the adult tissues.[4, 5] This program of morphogenesis can be played out only in the absence of müllerian-inhibiting substance. Although it is independent of the ovaries and estrogen, the normal program of differentiation can be disrupted by exogenous estrogens, probably acting on the estrogen receptors that are present in mesenchymal cells.[6]

The primordial uterus is initially lined by a simple cuboidal epithelium that subsequently becomes columnar and pseudostratified. Beneath this epithelium lies a condensed mesenchyme that gives rise to the endometrial stroma and the myometrium. By week 22 of gestation, the uterus has taken on the structure of the adult organ. Glandular secretory activity, glycogen accumulation, and stromal edema are evident by week 32 under the influence of placentally derived estrogens. After delivery and the precipitous fall in estrogens, the endometrium regresses to an atrophic state, containing a few small-caliber glands and a poorly vascularized stroma.

Mesenchymal-epithelial interactions are crucial to the formation of the reproductive tract.[7] In isolation, the epithelial and mesenchymal components of the reproductive tract will not undergo morphogenesis. The mesenchyme is the major target for factors that govern organ formation; it also mediates responses to sex steroid hormones.[7a] Thus, estrogen receptors are detected in the embryonic mesenchyme of the female reproductive tract well before the receptors appear in epithelial cells. The mesenchyme communicates with the epithelium through paracrine effectors

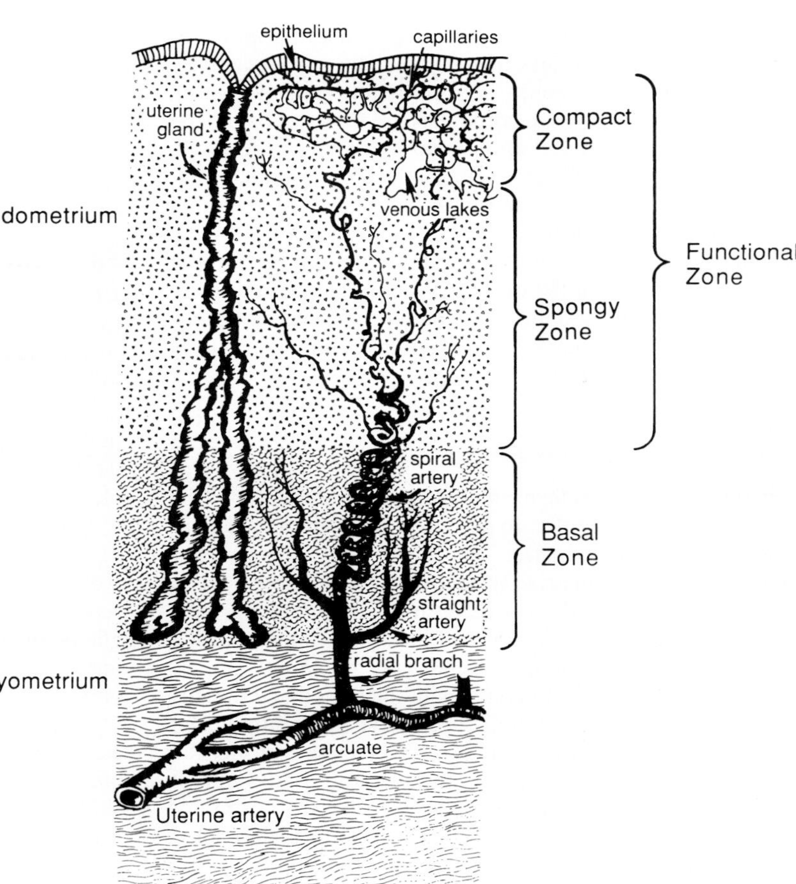

Figure 8–1 ■ Diagram of the histologic organization of secretory-phase human endometrium. (Modified from Blandau RJ. Weiss-Greep Histology, 4th ed. New York, McGraw-Hill, 1977, p 911. © Williams & Wilkins Company, Baltimore.)

that encompass local growth regulators, differentiation factors, and extracellular matrix components that signal the epithelial cells through integrins and other cell adhesion molecules.

Structure of the Adult Endometrium and Dynamic Changes During the Menstrual Cycle

The primate endometrium can be divided into two major layers on the basis of morphology and functional inferences[8] (Fig. 8–1). The transient functional layer, or functionalis, contains a compact zone including the stroma subjacent to the luminal epithelium and an intermediate spongy zone that contains more densely packed tortuous glands, giving it a lacy appearance on histologic examination. The basal layer, or basalis, lies underneath the spongy zone and adjacent to the myometrium. It contains the gland fundi and supporting vasculature. Although these layers are histologically definable during the secretory phase, the distinctions between them should more properly be considered the reflection of polarized gradients of cells with different phenotypes. Thus, moving from functionalis to basalis, the proliferative activity of cells declines. The functionalis undergoes a striking progression of histologic changes during the menstrual cycle, whereas the basalis shows only modest alterations. Patterns of gene expression also show gradients across the layers as described later.

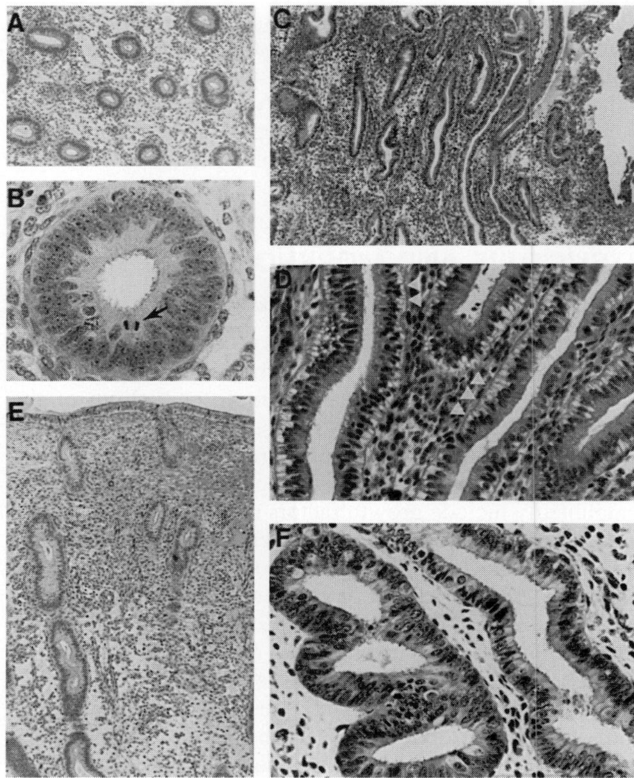

Figure 8–2 ■ Histology of the endometrium during the menstrual cycle.

A and *B*, Proliferative endometrium. Mitoses are present *(arrow)*. Nuclei in the glandular epithelium are pseudostratified.

C and *D*, Secretory endometrium, day 18. Subnuclear glycogen vacuoles are uniformly present in glandular epithelium *(arrowheads)*.

E and *F*, Midsecretory endometrium. Glandular secretory activity is present, and the stroma is edematous. The stromal cells in the more superficial layers as well as around vessels *(E)* have become pseudodecidualized and exhibit a flattened, polygonal configuration with distinct cell borders.

The Early Proliferative Phase

During the early proliferative phase, the endometrium usually has a thickness of less than 2 mm. The mitotic activity of cells in the basal zones and epithelial cells persisting in the lower uterine and cornual segments results in the restoration of the luminal epithelium by day 5 of the cycle. During the early proliferative phase, the glands are straight, narrow, and tubular and lined with low columnar cells that have round nuclei located near the cell base (Fig. 8–2*A*). Mitotic activity in both the glandular epithelium and stroma is evident by day 5 of the cycle. At the ultrastructural level, the epithelial cell cytoplasm contains numerous polyribosomes, but the endoplasmic reticulum and Golgi complexes of these cells are not well developed.

The Late Proliferative Phase

The endometrium thickens in the late proliferative phase as a result of glandular hyperplasia and an increase in stromal extracellular matrix. The glands are widely separated near the endometrial surface and more crowded and tortuous deeper into the endometrium. The glandular epithelial cells increase in height and become pseudostratified as the time of ovulation approaches (Fig. 8–2*B*).

The luminal epithelium contains both ciliated and nonciliated cells that differ in their secretory capabilities. The ratio of nonciliated to ciliated cells changes during the menstrual cycle, decreasing in the late proliferative phase and increasing in the secretory phase. In general, estradiol levels correlate directly with the presence of ciliated cells, and withdrawal of estrogen is associated with loss of cilia.

Early Secretory Phase

After ovulation, the zonation of the endometrium referred to earlier is most evident. Mitotic activity in epithelial and stromal cells is rare in the secretory phase, being restricted to the first 3 days after ovulation. The nuclei of glandular epithelial cells and stromal cells develop heterochromatin in the early secretory phase (Fig. 8–2*C* and *D*). The glandular epithelial cells begin to accumulate glycogen-rich vacuoles at their base, displacing the nuclei to the midregions of the columnar cells. Evidence for modest secretory activity is seen in histologic preparations as a light eosinophilic collection in the gland lumina. Although it is named the secretory phase of the cycle, the endometrial luminal and glandular epithelial cells also display secretory activity during the proliferative phase. A reticular network of argyrophilic fibers containing fibrillar collagens (type III and type I collagen fibers) is established in the stroma by the early secretory phase. Stromal edema contributes to the thickening of the endometrium at this time.

Ultrastructural studies of the endometrial epithelial cells reveal progressive accumulation of glycogen throughout the proliferative and early secretory phases. The endoplasmic reticulum of the cells is abundant, and the mitochondria become unusually large with prominent cristae. An ordered spherical stack of interdigitating tubules, the nucleolar channel system, appears in the nucleoli of the secretory-phase epithelial cells[8] (Fig. 8–3). There is an invagination of the cytoplasm into the nucleus near the nucleolar channel system that might provide a direct connection to the perinuclear space for transport of messenger ribonucleic acid (mRNA) to the cytoplasm. The nucleolar channel system forms in response to progesterone and is an ultrastructural hallmark of the early secretory phase.

The Midsecretory and Late Secretory Phases

The endometrium in the midsecretory and late secretory phases is 5 to 6 mm thick and well vascularized. A characteristic feature of this phase of the cycle is the development of the spiral arteries. These vessels become increasingly coiled as they lengthen more rapidly than the endometrium thickens.

The endometrial luminal epithelium undergoes cycle-dependent changes that potentially facilitate initial events in embryo implantation. Scanning electron microscopy reveals that on the second day after ovulation, the luminal cells are oval[9] (Fig. 8–4). Long, thick microvilli are prominent, and numerous small droplets 0.3 to 0.6 μm in diameter cover their surfaces. Large cytoplasmic projections appear on cycle days 20 to 22, which coincides with the expected time of implantation. These projections, termed pinopods, also appear on rat endometrial luminal cells during the window of implantation. Thus, it has been proposed that the appearance of pinopods is a morphologic marker of the receptive phase of the human endometrium. The formation of pinopods appears to be dependent on progesterone. Estrogen causes regression of pinopods. Functional studies on pinopods in rats suggest that they mediate epithelial uptake of fluid (pinocytosis) and macromolecules (endocytosis), which may be involved in signal transmission between the blastocyst and epithelial cells. However, the true significance of pinopods with respect to implantation remains obscure.

The endometrial glands are tortuous in the midsecretory

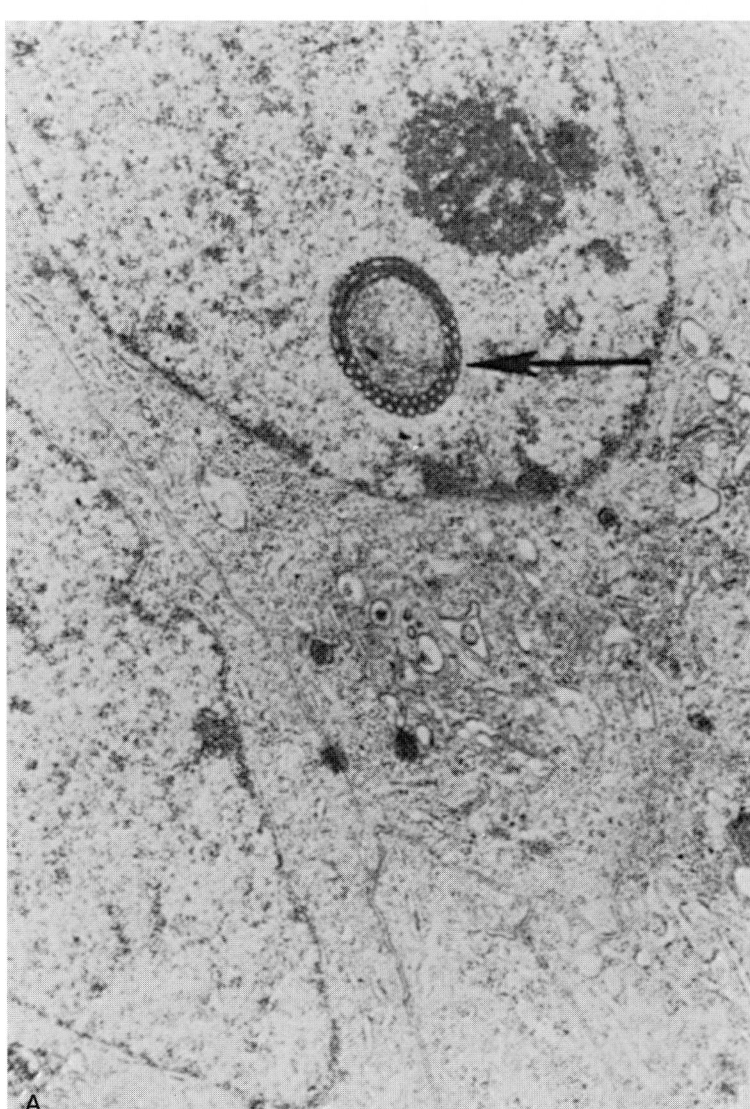

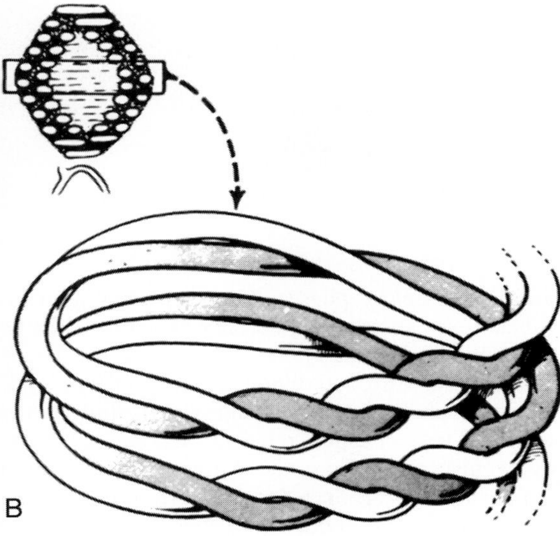

Figure 8–3 ■ Postovulatory secretory endometrium (cycle day 17).

A, Transmission electron microscopy of a glandular epithelial cell with a nucleolar channel system (*arrow*).

B, Schematic representation of nucleolar channel system. (*A* and *B* from Wynn RM. The Human Endometrium. Cyclic and Gestational Changes. *In* Wynn RM, Jollie WP: Biology of the Uterus. New York, Plenum Publishing, 1989, pp 289–331.)

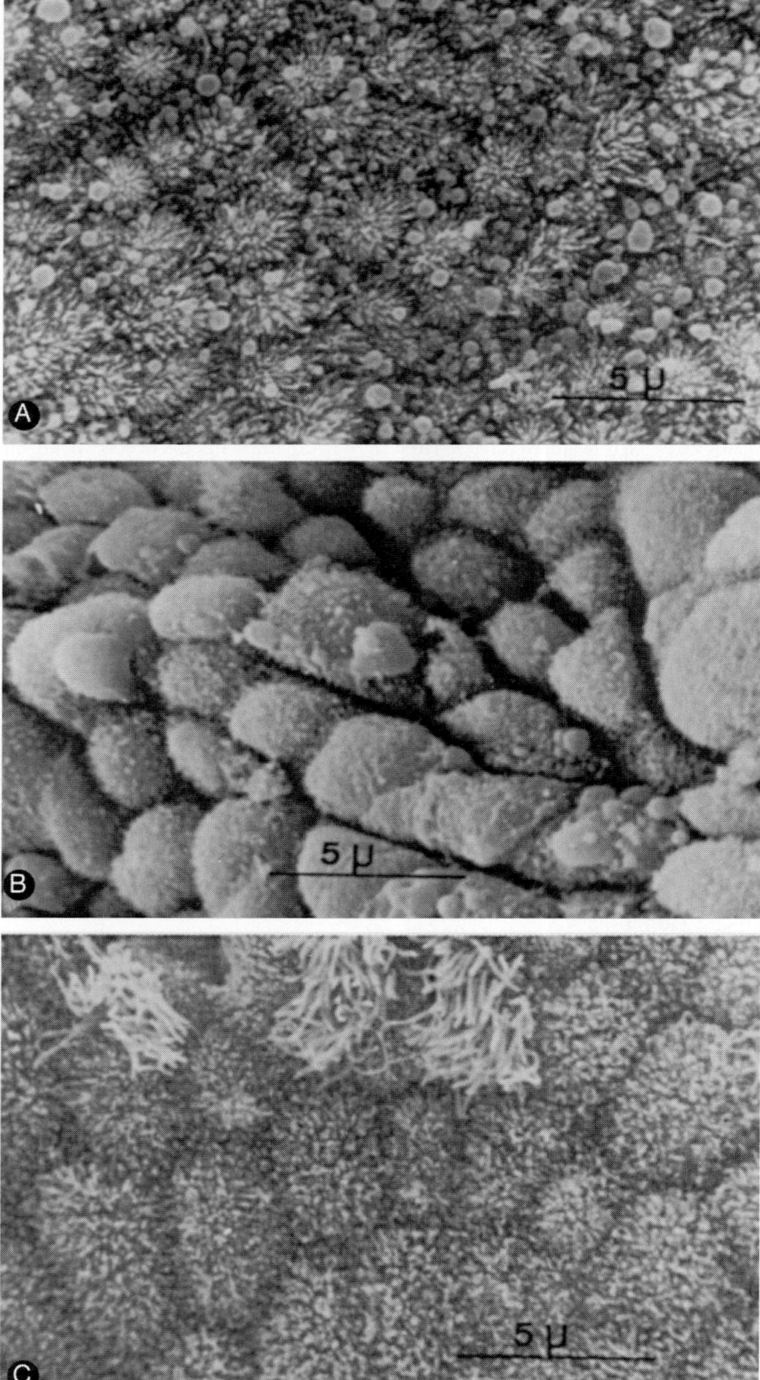

Figure 8–4 ■ Scanning electron microscopy of the uterine lumen.

A, Luminal epithelium, 2 days after ovulation during a spontaneous menstrual cycle.

B, Luminal epithelium on day 6 after ovulation during a spontaneous menstrual cycle.

C, Luminal epithelium on day 9 after ovulation during a spontaneous menstrual cycle. (*A* to *C* from Martel D, Frydman R, Sarantis L, et al. Scanning electron microscopy of the uterine luminal epithelium as a marker of the implantation window. *In* Yoshinaga K [ed]. Blastocyst Implantation. Boston, Adams Publishing Group, 1989, p 179.)

and late secretory phases. Their secretory activity reaches a maximum about 6 days after ovulation, when few vacuoles are found in the epithelial cells (see Fig. 8–2*E* and *F*). Stromal cells around blood vessels enlarge and acquire an eosinophilic cytoplasm and a pericellular extracellular matrix. These changes, referred to as predecidualization to distinguish them from the further transformation of the stroma that occurs in a fertile cycle, subsequently spread, accentuating the demarcation between the subepithelial compact zone and the spongy zone. The fact that the predecidual changes occur first near blood vessels suggests that humoral factors provoke them. At the ultrastructural level, the predecidual stromal cells display well-developed Golgi complexes and parallel lamellae of endoplasmic reticulum. Their surrounding matrix consists of laminin, fibronectin, heparan sulfate, and type IV collagen.[10, 11]

The stromal cells of the midsecretory and late secretory phase express a repertoire of proteins that promote hemostasis, including tissue factor, a membrane-associated protein that initiates coagulation when it contacts blood, and plasminogen activator inhibitor type 1 (PAI-1), which restrains fibrinolysis.[12, 13] This pattern of gene expression prevents focal hemorrhage that might result from trophoblast invasion during implantation.

The Premenstrual Phase and Menstruation

With the decline in the secretion of progesterone and estradiol by the corpus luteum, a program of endometrial remodeling is initiated; alterations in the extracellular matrix and infiltration of leukocytes lead to hypoxia/reperfusion injury and sloughing of the functionalis, followed by activation of hemostatic and regenerative processes. The main histologic features of the premenstrual phase are degradation of the stromal reticular network; stromal infiltration by polymorphonuclear and mononuclear leukocytes; and "secretory exhaustion" of the endometrial glands, whose epithelial cells now have basal nuclei. The nucleolar channel system and giant mitochondria characteristic of the early and midsecretory phases vanish. The endometrium shrinks preceding menstruation, in part as a result of the diminished secretory activity and the catabolism of extracellular matrix.

Menstruation is the final consequence of progesterone and estrogen withdrawal. The classic studies of Markee[14] suggest that an ischemic phase caused by vasoconstriction of the arterioles and coiled arteries precedes the onset of menstrual bleeding by 4 to 24 hours. Bleeding occurs after the arterioles and arteries relax, leading to hypoxia/reperfusion injury. The superficial endometrial layers are distended by the formation of hematomas, and fissures subsequently develop, leading to the detachment of tissue fragments. Autophagy and heterophagy are evident, as is apoptosis.[15] There is debate about the amount of endometrium lost during menstruation. Examination of hysterectomy specimens suggests that the functionalis is shed and subsequently regenerated from the basalis layer. In contrast, examination of endometrial biopsy specimens indicates that shedding is less extensive with regeneration from the spongy zone.

The menstrual effluent consists of fragments of tissue mixed with blood, liquefied by the fibrinolytic activity of the endometrium that is expressed with the withdrawal of progesterone. Clots of varying size may be present if blood flow is excessive. The duration of menses in ovulatory cycles is variable, generally 4 to 6 days and usually similar from cycle to cycle in any individual ovulatory woman. The amount of blood lost in a normal menses ranges from 25 to 60 ml, being greater when coagulation and platelet disorders are present.

The Biochemical Events Associated with Menstruation

The biochemical basis for the dramatic structural changes in the endometrium in the perimenstrual period is only partially understood. Lysosomes as well as specific matrix-degrading proteases, the matrix metalloproteinases (MMPs), appear to be involved, although the evidence implicating the latter is much stronger than for the former.[16–18] Lysosomal involvement was proposed because of the high specific activity of certain lysosomal hydrolases in endometrial tissue in the menstrual phase, an increase in the abundance of lysosomes in the endometrium during the late secretory phase, and the cytochemical demonstration of acid phosphatase in the perimenstrual endometrium. A decline in progesterone was postulated to increase lysosomal membrane fragility. However, these associations do not establish a direct link between lysosomal activation and menstruation.

The MMPs are members of a family of enzymes that have overlapping substrate specificities for collagens and other matrix components. The genes encoding MMPs are under the transcriptional control of various cytokines and growth factors; their products are secreted as latent enzymes that must be activated to display their proteolytic activities. Endogenous inhibitors, the tissue inhibitors of matrix metalloproteinases (TIMPs), bind to and inactivate the MMPs. In the primate endometrium, MMPs and TIMPs are expressed in cell- and menstrual cycle–specific patterns.

The expression of interstitial collagenase (MMP-1), stromelysin 2 (MMP-10), and gelatinase B (MMP-9) in the stroma is essentially restricted to the perimenstrual period, with MMP-1 and MMP-9 localized to the functionalis layer (Fig. 8–5). Matrilysin (MMP-7) is expressed in epithelial cells during the proliferative phase before ovulation and is then lost from the epithelium during the secretory phase, returning in the premenstrual period, when it is also detected in the stroma. Stromelysin 1 (MMP-3) and stromelysin 3 (MMP-11) are present in the stroma during the proliferative phase, suppressed during the secretory period, and up-regulated with menstruation. Gelatinase A (MMP-2) expression is reduced by progesterone; it is increased in stromal cells as a consequence of progesterone withdrawal at the end of the luteal phase. The fibrinolytic system, urokinase and tissue plasminogen activator, also increases in the endometrium around menstruation as progesterone is withdrawn. Moreover, PAI-1 expression is reduced, allowing the plasminogen activators to activate plasmin, which can proteolytically cleave and activate the PRO-MMPs.[19] TIMP-1 is markedly up-regulated in the epithelium and stroma in the premenstrual and menstrual phases of the cycle, providing a restraint to the MMP-mediated extracellular matrix proteolysis. Organ culture studies employing enzyme inhibitors have documented that MMPs are directly involved in the catabolism of the collagenous matrix and that the induction of the MMPs is triggered by a decline in progesterone and estrogen levels.

The endothelins are a family of potent vasoconstrictors produced by endothelial cells that act on two types of receptors present on vascular smooth muscle. Endothelin 1, produced by endometrial epithelial or stromal cells, may act on spiral artery smooth muscle cells to promote vasoconstriction. The enzyme that degrades endothelin 1 and other vasoactive peptides, enkephalinase, a membrane-bound metalloendopeptidase, is present in highest levels in the midsecretory endometrium.[20] Expression of the gene encoding enkephalinase is up-regulated by progesterone. The decline in progesterone levels at the end of the luteal phase results in a subsequent fall in enkephalinase, which prolongs the biological life of endothelin 1. Vasopressin

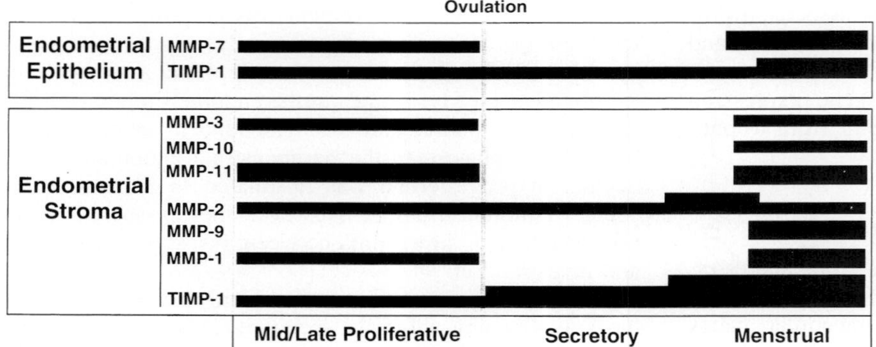

Figure 8–5 ■ Schematic of matrix metalloproteinase expression in the human endometrium during the menstrual cycle. (Modified from Rodgers WH, Matrisian LM, Giudice LC, et al. Patterns of matrix metalloproteinase expression in cycling endometrium imply differential functions and regulation by steroid hormones. J Clin Invest 94:946–953, 1994.)

may also function as a vasoconstrictor in the endometrium during the menstrual phase of the cycle.[21]

The production of endometrial prostaglandins, particularly $PGF_{2\alpha}$ and other eicosanoids, is enhanced by lysosomal phospholipases that liberate arachidonic acid, which in turn is metabolized into prostanoids.[22] The premenstrual fall in progesterone is followed by a decline in endometrial 15-hydroxyprostaglandin dehydrogenase activity, which inactivates $PGF_{2\alpha}$, resulting in increased availability of prostaglandins, which trigger myometrial contractions that compress the endometrial vasculature and promote hemostasis.[23]

Endometrial Perfusion

A number of methods have been used to assess uterine and specifically endometrial blood flow. By measuring the clearance of radioactive xenon gas, highest endometrial perfusion was reported between days 10 and 12 and days 21 and 26 of the cycle.[24] Transvaginal color Doppler studies suggest that endometrial perfusion is increased around the presumed time of ovulation.[25] Microvascular perfusion has been assessed more recently by laser Doppler fluximetry, a technique that monitors red blood cell flux, with transvaginal placement of a fiberoptic probe into the uterine cavity.[26] With use of this technique, endometrial perfusion demonstrated the short-term temporal changes expected during the cardiac cycle. Mean endometrial perfusion was highest during the proliferative phase and the early secretory phase, not too dissimilar from the finding based on ^{133}Xe clearance. Interestingly, no episodes of transient ischemia were noted in women studied during the menstrual phase of the cycle. This observation contradicts the dogma of ischemia and reperfusion injury, but the apparent discrepancy may be explained by the fact that the fluximetry method measures perfusion in a small tissue volume. Thus, significant changes in tissue perfusion may have gone undetected.

The Endometrium in the Cycle of Conception and Pregnancy

The examination of hysterectomy specimens revealed that the first consistent structural changes in the endometrium of pregnancy are recrudescence or accentuation of glandular secretory activity, edema, and the predecidual reaction.[27] The increased prominence of the vasculature is considered to be a manifestation of increased blood flow, which may account for the associated edema. Endometrial biopsies in the cycle of conception suggest that stromal edema and vascular congestion are the earliest persistent morphologic features of the endometrium of pregnancy, whereas secretory changes are more subtle and not routinely detectable.[28] The discrepancies between the reports based on examination of hysterectomy specimens and those of endometrial biopsy specimens may reflect the more limited sampling achieved in the biopsy procedure.

Within the first weeks of gestation, the endometrium undergoes characteristic changes in which the epithelium folds and the epithelial cells become distended with a clear cytoplasm (Fig. 8–6). Many of the epithelial cells develop enlarged and hyperchromatic nuclei. The enlarged nuclei are polyploid. These changes are commonly referred to as the Arias-Stella reaction.[29, 30] The ultrastructural characteristics of the endometrium are consistent with a hypersecretory state. Parallel channels of endoplasmic reticulum and large mitochondria are abundant in the epithelial cells, and the Golgi complexes have numerous stacked saccules. The Arias-Stella reaction has an irregular distribution in the uterus and is present in about 50 percent of the uteri of women with ectopic pregnancies.

As pregnancy continues, the endometrium exhibits significant changes in cellular composition that are reflected in the marked alterations in the synthesis and secretion of endometrial proteins (discussed later). As gestation advances, endometrial glands atrophy and are scarce at term. The decidua develops with continued exposure of the uterus to progesterone, secreted initially by the corpus luteum and later by the trophoblast of the placenta. The plump, polygonal decidual cells are arranged in a cobblestone configuration with distinct cell borders resulting from the accumulation of a pericellular matrix[10, 11] (Fig. 8–7). The abundant decidual cell prolyl hydroxylase, an enzyme involved in collagen synthesis, indicates the important role of these cells in extracellular matrix production. The ultrastructural features of the decidual cells, including prominent Golgi complexes, dilated rough endoplasmic reticulum, and dense membrane-bound secretory granules, are characteristic of secretory cells. The secretory products of the decidual cells, particularly insulin-like growth factor–binding protein 1 (IGFBP-1) and transforming growth factor-β (TGF-β), may restrain the invasion of trophoblast cells.[31]

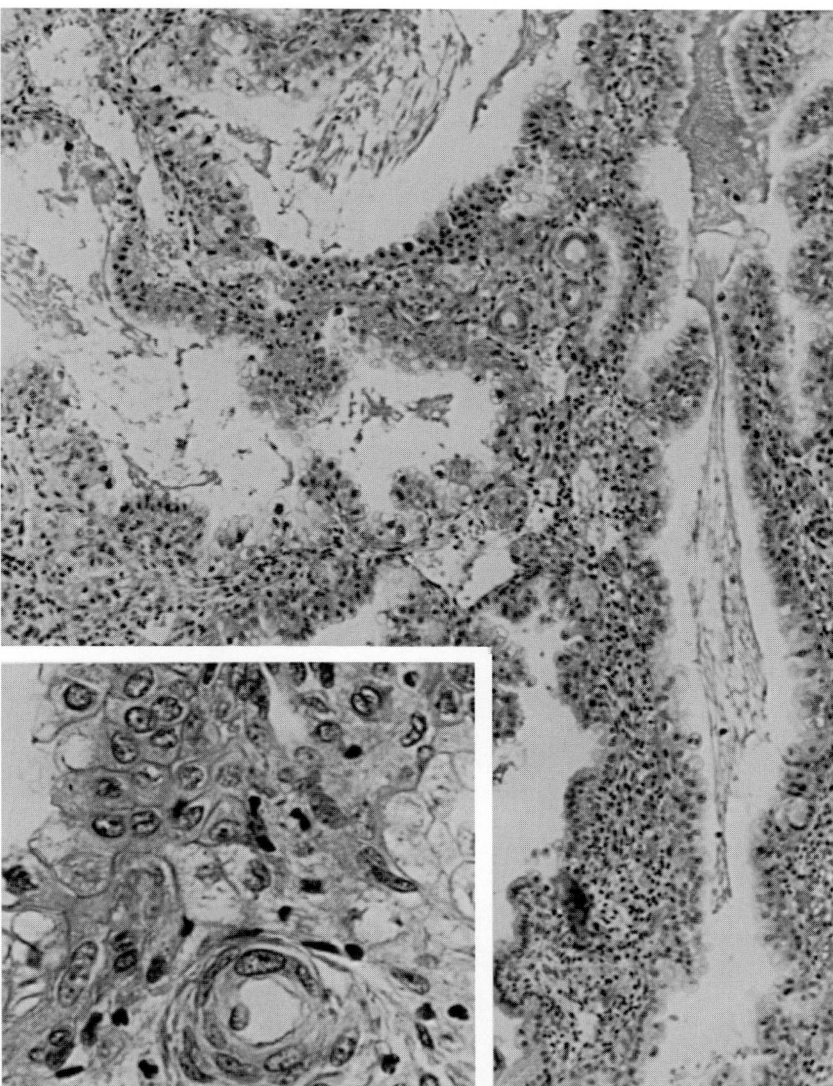

Figure 8–6 ■ Arias-Stella reaction. Hypersecretory glands with enlarged hyperchromatic nuclei are present. The glands have scalloped borders. *Inset:* High-power view.

The decidualized stroma represents the field that allows trophoblast invasion and placentation; its remodeling is crucial to the morphogenesis of the placenta and the establishment of the uteroplacental circulation. Moreover, the decidualized stroma represents the arena where the fetal allograft is exposed to maternal immunologically competent cells.

Transformation of the endometrial stroma begins to take place on day 21. The stroma becomes looser owing to the accumulation of amorphous components, including high-molecular-weight proteins with voluminous saccharide moieties, as well as partial breakdown and reorganization of the fibrillar collagens. Type V collagen epitopes are unmasked; collagen type VI, "stiff" short collagen fibers that bridge other fibrillar collagens, disappears from most of the stroma, persisting only in association with vessels and the basement membrane of the glands. The deposition of a basement membrane–type matrix containing laminin and type II collagens around the decidual cells that contributes to the formation of a looser stroma serves as a substrate for the invading trophoblasts. Entactin, a component of this basement membrane–like matrix, promotes trophoblast cell adhesion and migration. The decidual matrix is also a rich source of cytokines, protease inhibitors, protease precursors, and other factors that modulate cell behavior.

The Endometrium in Advancing Age

The basal endometrium interdigitates with the myometrium with advancing age, resulting in a degree of superficial adenomyosis that is a normal finding in the uterus in the fifth decade of life. This infiltrating endometrium does not undergo normal cyclic changes. After menopause, endometrial atrophy is apparent and mitotic activity ceases. Epithelial cells shrink in size, and the stroma becomes fibrotic. A compact eosinophilic material is found in the lumina of the endometrial glands, occasionally engorging them and giving rise to the histologic pattern referred to as cystic atrophy (Fig. 8–8).

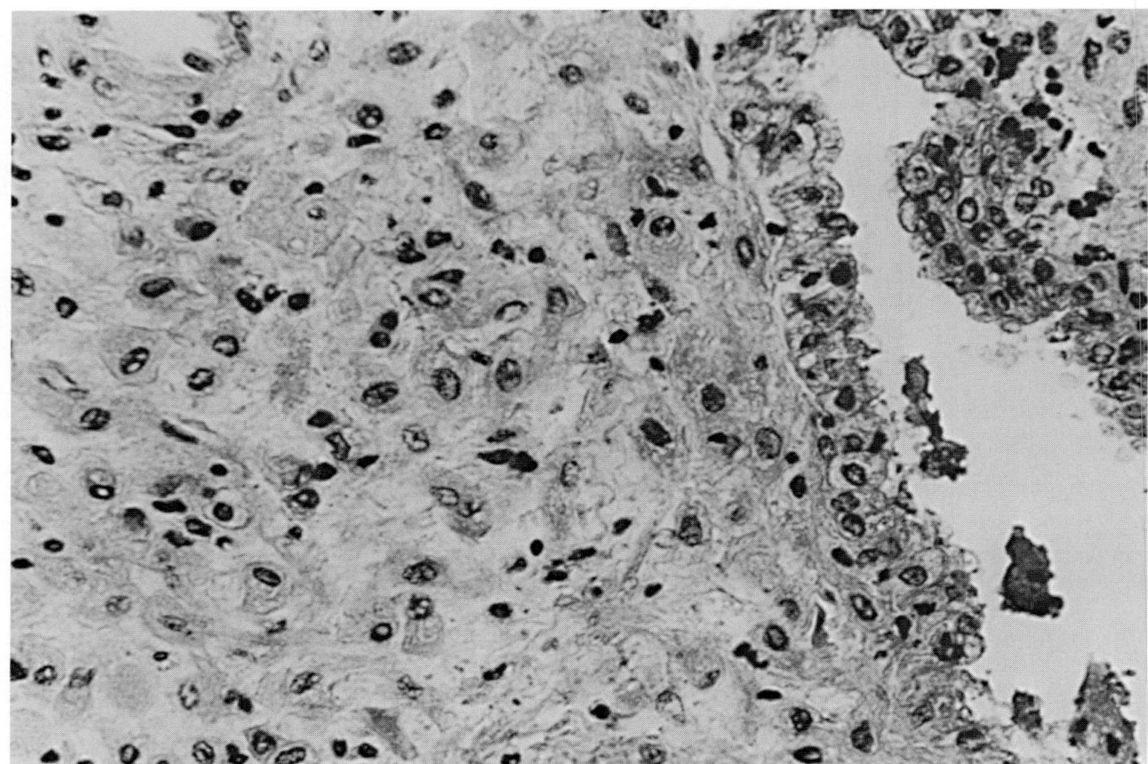

Figure 8–7 ■ Decidua of pregnancy. Decidualized stromal cells are plump and have distinct cell borders. Glands are atrophic.

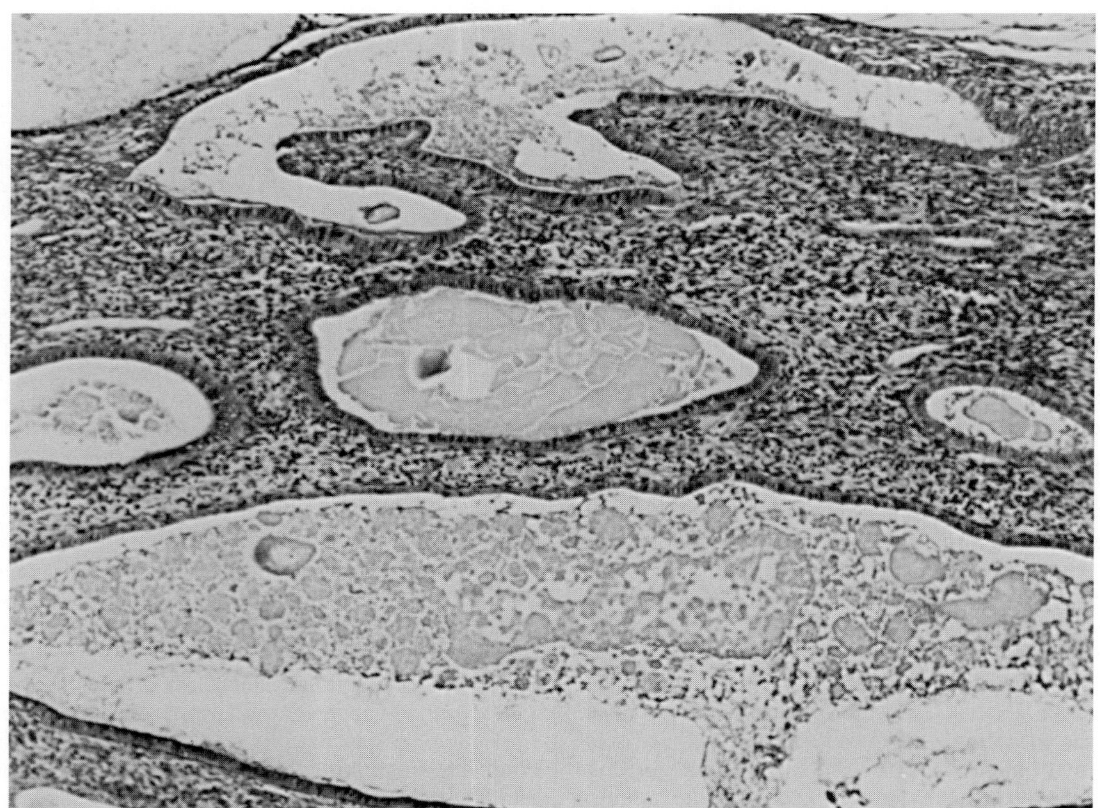

Figure 8–8 ■ Postmenopausal endometrium. Epithelial cells are flat. Stroma is fibrotic and compact. Eosinophilic material has accumulated in gland lumina.

The Immune Cell Population of the Uterus

The human endometrial stroma is enriched with lymphoid and myeloid cells; at any time during the menstrual cycle, 10 to 15 percent of the endometrial cells are leukocytes.[32–35] These cells are distributed singly or as aggregates, with the aggregates being primarily localized in the basalis. Suppressor T cells predominate, but helper T cells are also present. This pattern distinguishes the endometrial lymphoid system because of its large population of suppressor-cytotoxic cells and few B cells and plasma cells.

A unique member of the lymphoid lineage is found in the endometrium. Granulated lymphocytes are round cells that characteristically have bilobed or indented nuclei and a pale cytoplasm containing acidophilic granules. Granulated lymphocytes appear to be a specialized subset of natural killer cells on the basis of their expression of cell surface antigens ($CD3^-$, $CD16^+$, and $CD56^+$). When activated by interleukin (IL)–2 in vitro, the granulated lymphocytes become competent to kill malignant and some normal cells through the release of cytotoxic proteins including perforin and serine esterases. Granulated lymphocytes accumulate in the endometrium during the luteal phase and persist in the decidua during the first trimester, when they compose 70 percent of the decidual leukocyte population. In a nonfertile cycle, the granulated lymphocytes that amass during the secretory phase undergo programmed cell death.

The granulated lymphocytes have been proposed to play a role in modulating trophoblast invasion during implantation and placentation because of the abundance of these cells in the decidua during the first trimester. Although in vitro studies document the killing activity of cytokine-activated granulated lymphocytes, there is little evidence for destruction of trophoblast cells in vivo. Thus, any restraining activity that granulated lymphocytes exert on invading trophoblast cells appears to be through a noncytotoxic mechanism that may involve secreted cytokines including colony-stimulating factor 1 (CSF-1), IL-1, leukemia inhibitory factor (LIF), and interferon-γ. The apparent resistance of trophoblast cells to killing both in vitro and in vivo may be explained by the fact that trophoblast cells express a nonclassical and nonpolymorphic major histocompatibility complex (MHC) class I antigen, HLA-G, and the suppression of killing activity by endometrial stromal cells. The most convincing evidence for an important role for granulated lymphocytes in pregnancy comes from mouse models lacking these cells. In the transgenic mouse line TgE26, abnormal implantation sites are found, followed by fetal demise in association with changes in uterine arterioles suggestive of arteriosclerosis and hypertension.[36] These histopathologic changes are reminiscent of preeclampsia in humans.

The relatively large population of T lymphocytes in the endometrium may also have an important influence on stromal and epithelial cell function through the release of cytokines for which the stromal and epithelial cells have receptors. Cytokines are produced by activated T cells, and there is good reason to believe that endometrial T cells are activated in situ as judged by their expression of antigens that are characteristic of the activated state, including the MHC class II molecules HLA-DR, HLA-DP, and HLA-DQ and very late antigen 1.

The Myometrium During the Menstrual Cycle

The myometrium is organized into three strata, an external hood-like layer covering the fundus beneath which lies a dense network of fibers. Sphere-like fibers composing the innermost layer surround the internal os and tubal ostia. The myometrium undergoes functional changes during the menstrual cycle. During the follicular phase, there is an increasing frequency and intensity of subendometrial and myometrial peristaltic waves. As the time of ovulation approaches, the number of waves with a fundocervical direction decreases in favor of waves with a cervicofundal direction.[37, 38] These peristaltic waves may aid in sperm transport. The endometrial wave-like activity is reported to correlate with fecundability; cycles in which conception occurs show less activity than in nonconception cycles.[39] During menstruation, contractions move from the fundus toward the cervix with irregular frequency varying from one to three per minute, facilitating expulsion of the shed functionalis.

Uterine contractility can be influenced by pharmacologic agents. Instillation of $PGF_{2\alpha}$ into the uterine cavity increases uterine contractions. Administration of RU 486 in the postovulatory period also increases uterine contractions.

The myometrial compartment changes dramatically during pregnancy primarily as a result of muscle hypertrophy, the elaboration of extracellular matrix, and an increase in lymphatics and blood vessels. These changes are promoted by estrogen and progesterone acting in part through growth factors including the insulin-like growth factors (IGFs).

Clinical Evaluation of the Endometrium

The Endometrial Biopsy

The endometrial biopsy has been used as the gold standard in assessing endometrial maturation. The histologic evaluation of postovulatory endometrial development was summarized in the classic paper by Noyes and colleagues.[40] These authors compared the histologic characteristics of the endometrium with changes in the basal body temperature and developed standardized criteria for "dating" the endometrium that remain in use today. The major changes in endometrial histology described by Noyes and colleagues are presented in Figure 8–9. The morphologic changes occurring in the first week after ovulation are primarily seen in the glandular components of the endometrium, including mitoses, basal vacuolation, and secretion. Stromal changes predominate in the second week and consist of edema, the predecidual reaction, and leukocyte infiltration. Noyes and colleagues found that the day of the secretory phase as assessed by morphologic criteria agreed well with the corresponding day of the cycle as determined by basal body temperature and not necessarily with the date of the next menstrual flow.

METHOD AND INTERPRETATION

Normal endometrial development is assumed when the histologic and chronologic endometrial dates agree within 2 days. When they differ by more than 2 days, the endometrium is considered to be out of phase. Understanding the limitations of this test is important if treatments are based

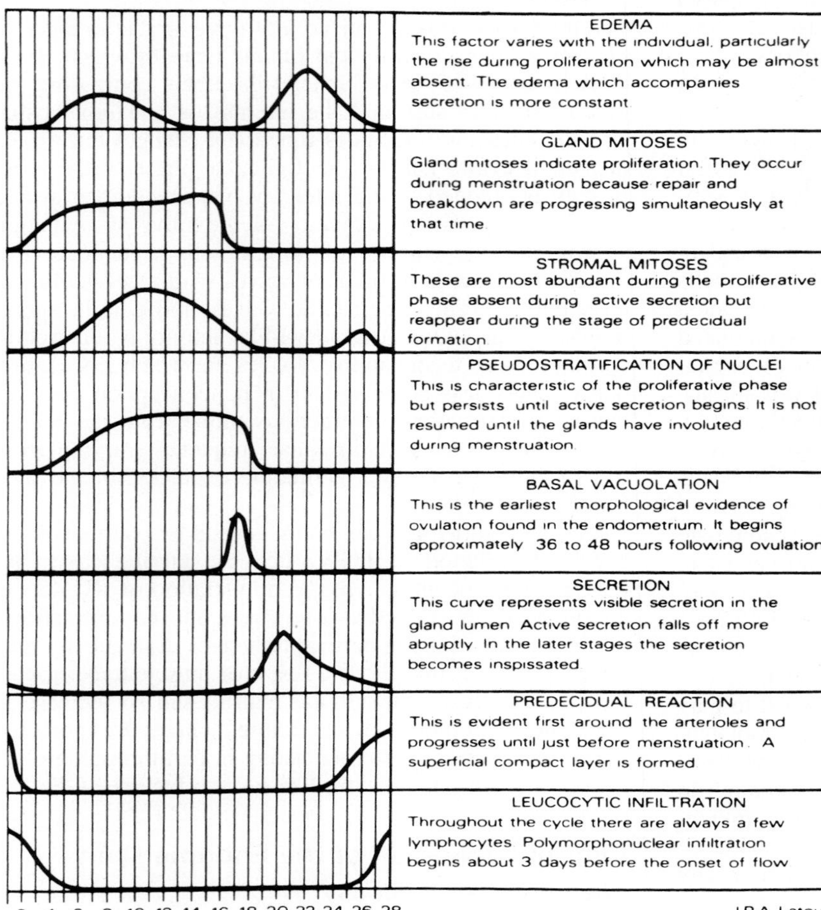

Figure 8–9 ■ Events occurring in various components of the endometrium during the menstrual cycle. (From Noyes RW, Hertig AT, Rock J. Dating the endometrial biopsy. Fertil Steril 1:3, 1950. Reproduced with permission of the publisher, The American Fertility Society. Redrawn by Dr. J. P. A. Latour, Royal Victoria Hospital, Montreal, Canada.)

on biopsy results, because the true sensitivity and specificity of the endometrial biopsy for the diagnosis of infertility are unknown. Issues that should be considered include

- Technique and timing of the biopsy
- Interobserver variation in biopsy interpretation
- Variance in the histologic interpretation of "early" versus "late" biopsies
- Stromal-epithelial dyssynchrony
- Chronic endometritis

TECHNIQUE AND TIMING OF THE BIOPSY

The endometrial sampling usually encompasses a small fragment from the anterior fundal area of the uterus. However, observations suggest that human embryo implantation occurs in the posterior endometrium, possibly as the result of three-dimensional relationships between the ostium of the fallopian tube, the anatomic position of the uterus, and gravitational forces. Alternatively, this selectivity in the site of implantation may indicate the existence of regional differences in the endometrium. Therefore, the functional significance of morphologic and molecular findings derived from endometrial biopsies may not be perfectly linked to uterine receptivity.

Sampling from the lower uterine segment may yield misleading results because of differences in the morphologic responses of the lower segment to steroid hormones compared with the fundus.

Experimental work with laboratory animals has revealed that there is a temporal window during which the endometrium is permissive to embryo attachment and invasion.[41] As described later, experience with the assisted reproductive technologies indicates that such a temporal window permissive to implantation also exists in humans. The work of Bergh and Navot[42] suggests that the window of initial interaction between the embryo and the endometrium spans days 20 to 24 of the normalized menstrual cycle. Presumably, the establishment of the receptive state of the human endometrium depends on the exposure of the tissue to appropriate levels of steroid hormones. It can be hypothesized that because of either deficient plasma concentrations of these steroid hormones or decreased responsiveness of the endometrium to appropriate levels of hormones, there may be a delay in the establishment of the receptive state, and thus implantation will fail even though a potentially normal embryo is present in the endometrial cavity. These considerations are of importance in selecting the optimal time to perform biopsy of the endometrium. It has been argued that the late luteal–phase biopsy is most appropriate because it reflects the cumulative effects of steroids on the endometrium, which thus makes it a better predictor of the "adequacy" of the luteal phase.[43, 44] Nevertheless, a biopsy performed during the window of implantation (days 20 to 24) that exhibits delay in maturation may have greater clinical significance, even though that endometrium may "catch up" at the later stages of the luteal phase (days 26 to 28). Indeed, recent findings indicate that an endometrial biopsy performed in the midluteal phase may detect a greater number of women with delayed endometrial maturation during the temporal window of implantation.[45] Most of the women with out-of-phase midluteal-phase biopsy results in this study had normal late luteal endometrium.

PRECISION OF ENDOMETRIAL DATING BY HISTOLOGIC CRITERIA

The dating of endometrial biopsies is most consistent when a single observer interprets the specimens. Interobserver variation is estimated to be 0.96 ± 0.08 days.[46] Even with one observer, there may be considerable variability in dating that is related to the time in the luteal phase at which the biopsy specimen is obtained. The estimate of "false-positive" readings of an out-of-phase endometrium as high as 18 percent may account, in part, for the high frequency of out-of-phase endometrial biopsy results reported by some investigators (see later).[47–49] Detection of the luteinizing hormone (LH) surge by semiquantitative urinary LH immunoassays or timing ovulation by ultrasonographic monitoring of ovarian structure provides the most reliable endometrial dating.[50, 51]

Improvements in the precision of histologic dating may also be gained by the application of morphometric techniques, although these have not gained wide acceptance in clinical practice.[52] Dockery and associates[53] employed a quantitative electron microscopic analysis and demonstrated that the structural variation in biopsy specimens collected in the luteal phase of normal fertile women is small. However, it is not certain whether this conclusion can be extended to infertile women. Moreover, this analysis is expensive and laborious and cannot be employed as a routine diagnostic tool.

STROMAL-EPITHELIAL DYSSYNCHRONY

Glandular-stromal dyssynchrony has been noted in many endometrial biopsy studies but its clinical significance is uncertain.[54–56] It has been considered to be an indication that the biopsy specimen was obtained from the lower uterine segment. Nevertheless, the consistency of this finding in hormone replacement cycles invites re-examination of its significance. The observation described in most of these studies was that even though there may have been dyssynchrony in the early biopsy during the presumed window of implantation, the late luteal–phase biopsy indicated catch-up of the histologic features of both endometrial compartments. The successful establishment of pregnancy in a subsequent cycle indicated that the dyssynchrony may have been of no clinical significance. Thus, the dogma that there should be synchrony of development between the stromal and glandular endometrial components needs to be re-evaluated.

CHRONIC ENDOMETRITIS

A chronic inflammatory process in the endometrium may adversely affect the establishment of pregnancy. Nevertheless, it has been hypothesized that an acute inflammatory reaction may actually enhance implantation.

OUT-OF-PHASE BIOPSIES IN FERTILE WOMEN

The incidence of out-of-phase biopsies in ovulatory, fertile women has not been clearly defined.[57–59] Four studies of limited statistical power of parous, ovulatory women indicated incidences ranging from 0 to 20 percent for an out-of-phase biopsy in the first study cycle.[60–63] In addition, there are two other studies of ovulating women who were not necessarily fertile in which the incidence of an out-of-phase biopsy on the first study cycle was 0 percent[50] and 20 percent.[64] In Balasch's study,[60] the criterion was delayed histologic endometrial maturation of greater than 2 days. This approach yielded an incidence of luteal-phase defect of 12.9 percent in 359 infertile women compared with only 4 percent in 25 fertile women. In another widely quoted study by Davis and colleagues,[61] repeated endometrial biopsies were carried out in the same women. Five women underwent 35 biopsies, and on 18 occasions (51 percent), the biopsy results were out of phase by use of the criterion of more than a 2-day lag; 31 percent were out of phase if more than a 3-day lag was used as a criterion. When two consecutive cycles were evaluated in 30 biopsy pairs, eight (27 percent) showed out-of-phase endometrial morphologic changes by 2 days, two (7 percent) when the 3-day or more criterion was applied. The studies described are difficult to compare because the approaches used were different. The denominator was the patient for the Balasch study, whereas it was the cycle or cycle pair for the Davis study. Davis compared endometrial dating with the onset of the next menstrual period, and the reference point for the Balasch study is uncertain.

These and other studies point out the significant variation in endometrial development in fertile as well as in infertile women that must be considered when a diagnosis of luteal-phase deficiency is entertained. Therefore, most authorities suggest that the diagnosis of abnormal endometrial development be based on two consecutive out-of-phase biopsy results, a practice that reduces the theoretical false-positive rate. However, uncertainty arises in patients who have one in-phase and one out-of-phase biopsy result. Furthermore, it is difficult to rigorously assess response to treatment when multiple samplings are needed to establish the diagnosis. Unfortunately, the literature on luteal-phase deficiencies has been clouded by the lack of attention to these issues, which bear heavily on the accuracy of diagnosis and the evaluation of treatment efficacy.[57, 58, 62, 65]

Ultrasonography

Growth of the endometrium can be monitored by ultrasonography (Fig. 8–10). Sequential monitoring of endometrial thickness in women treated with human menopausal gonadotropins reveals rapid daily growth of 0.5 mm from day −3 to day +2 (day 0 being the day of human chorionic gonadotropin [hCG] administration), followed by a slower growth rate of 0.1 mm/day. For the purpose of this

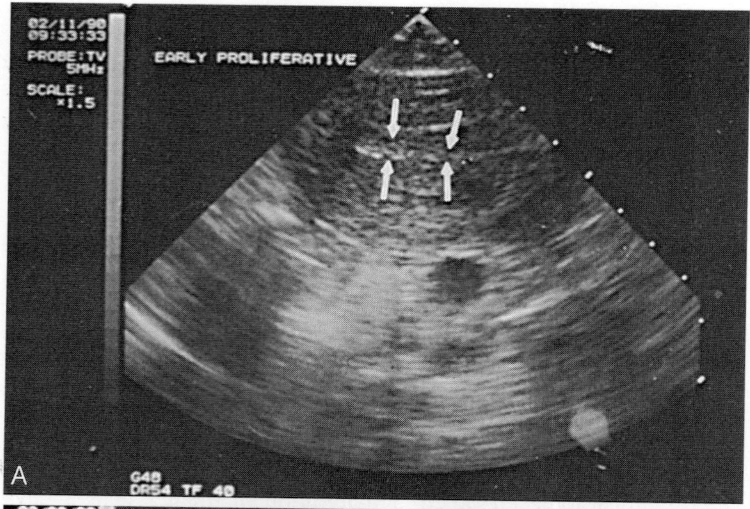

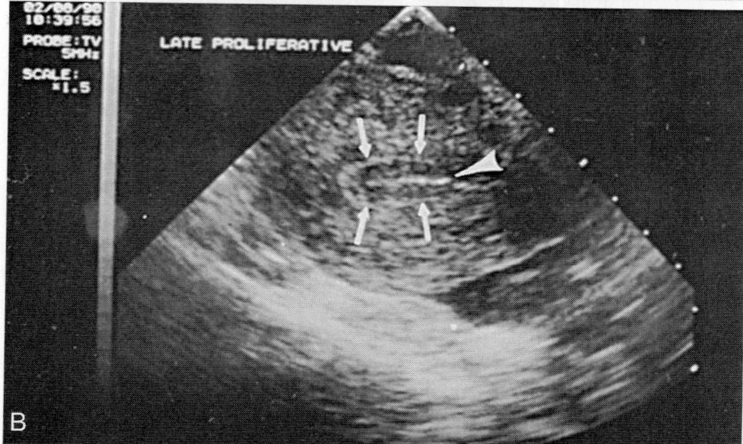

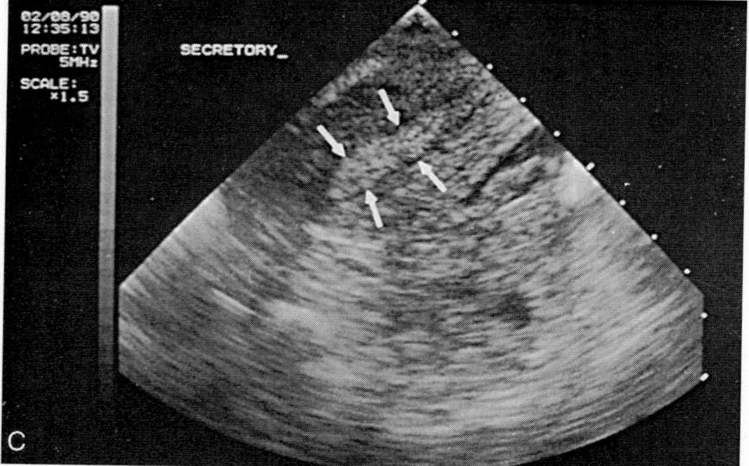

Figure 8–10 ■ Ultrasonographic appearance of the endometrium during phases of the menstrual cycle.
A, Early proliferative phase: 2- to 3-mm echo-dense endometrial stripe *(arrows).*
B, Late proliferative phase: thickened endometrial stripe (8 to 12 mm; *arrows*) with an echo-dense area in the endometrial-myometrial junction, then a relatively echo-lucent area and a bright echo-dense stripe in the region of the endometrial cavity *(arrowhead).*
C, Secretory phase. The endometrial stripe remains thickened (8 to 12 mm) but assumes an echo-dense, uniform appearance *(arrows).*

imaging technique, thickness is defined as the total distance between the basal layers of the two apposing surfaces of anterior and posterior endometrium. Most authors report that endometrial growth does not correlate with serum estradiol or progesterone levels and suggest that a thickness of 8 mm or more in the late proliferative phase with a trilaminar ultrasonographic pattern may be a prerequisite for success in in vitro fertilization and embryo transfer (IVF-ET) cycles.[66]

Sonohysterography

Instillation of sterile saline into the endometrial cavity during ultrasonographic evaluation of the uterus has enhanced the capability of the examiner to identify space-occupying lesions such as polyps or submucous myomas (Fig. 8–11). The capacity of this diagnostic test to evaluate specific uterine anomalies (i.e., septa) is less certain. Although this technique appears promising in the evaluation of the endometrial cavity, the specificity and sensitivity

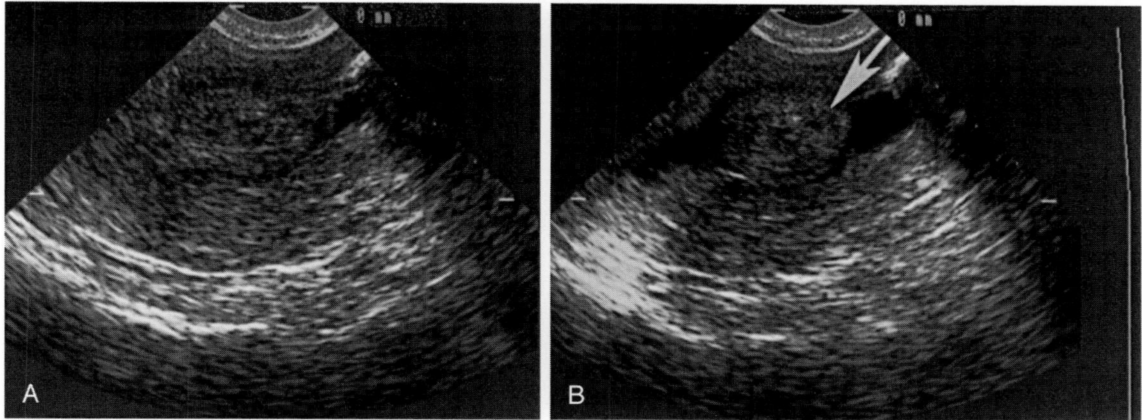

Figure 8–11 ■ Sonohysterography. Instillation of sterile saline within the endometrial cavity results in delineation of intracavitary abnormalities. An indistinct mass *(A)* becomes well defined after instillation of the echo-lucent liquid *(B, arrow)*. (Courtesy of Dr. Samantha Pfeifer, University of Pennsylvania, Philadelphia, PA.)

of sonohysterography in identifying the various lesions encountered within the uterus have not been clearly defined at this writing.[67]

Magnetic Resonance Imaging

Magnetic resonance imaging reveals a pattern of endometrial growth similar to that detected by ultrasonography, with the exception that a junctional zone in the endometrium, which may represent the arcuate vessels, is also demonstrated.[68] Magnetic resonance imaging has been shown to provide useful information in cases of congenital uterine anomalies, especially in the distinction between bicornuate and septate uterus.

Hysteroscopy

Direct visualization of the endometrial cavity by hysteroscopy has proved useful in the assessment of abnormal uterine bleeding, intrauterine foreign bodies, infertility, and recurrent pregnancy loss.[69] In the infertile patient, hysteroscopic evaluation of the endometrial cavity after an abnormal hysterosalpingogram can be informative. The diagnosis of some müllerian fusion defects and intrauterine adhesions as well as their therapy is possible by hysteroscopy.

BIOCHEMISTRY AND MOLECULAR BIOLOGY OF UTERINE GROWTH AND DIFFERENTIATION

Steroid Hormone and Growth Factor Regulation of Endometrial Cell Proliferation and Differentiation

Steroid Hormone Metabolism in the Uterus

The level of bioactive hormone in the uterus is determined by the concentration of hormone presented in plasma as well as the activities of uterine enzymes that form active molecules from prohormones and degrade these hormones.[70] The enzymes that carry out transformations of steroid hormones are subject to regulation during the menstrual cycle. Estradiol taken up from the plasma can be converted into estrone by the action of 17β-hydroxysteroid dehydrogenases or converted to sulfated conjugates by estrogen sulfotransferase[71, 72] (Fig. 8–12). Two different 17β-hydroxysteroid dehydrogenases capable of oxidizing estradiol to estrone, the type II and type IV enzymes, have been found in endometrium.[73, 74] The type II enzyme is associated with microsomes; type IV enzyme appears to be

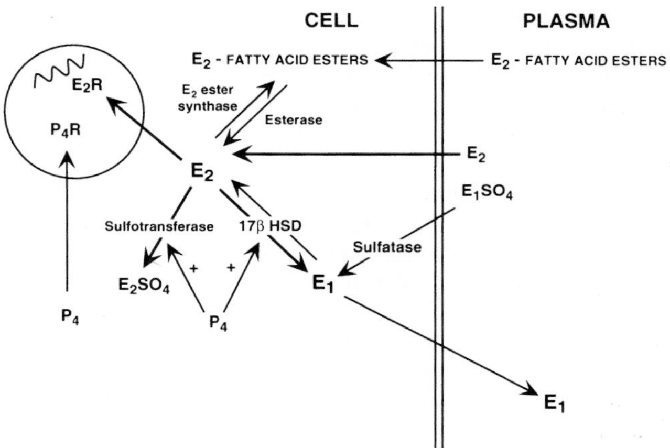

Figure 8–12 ■ Scheme indicating metabolic processes leading to the synthesis and removal of estradiol from epithelial cells of human endometrium. Progesterone increases the activities of estradiol 17β-hydroxysteroid dehydrogenases (17βHSD) and sulfotransferase. In addition, progesterone lowers estrogen receptor concentrations. These hormonal effects influence estradiol levels and actions during the luteal phase. E_1, estrone; E_2, estradiol; E_1SO_4, estrone sulfate; E_2SO_4, estradiol sulfate; P_4, progesterone; R, steroid hormone receptor. (Based on data from Satyaswaroop PG, Wartell DJ, Mortel R. Distribution of progesterone receptor, estradiol dehydrogenase, and 20α-dihydroprogesterone dehydrogenase activities in human endometrial glands and stroma. Endocrinology 111:743–749, 1982; King RJ, Townsend PT, Whitehead MI, et al. Biochemical analyses of separated epithelium and stroma from endometria of premenopausal and postmenopausal women receiving estrogen and progestins. J Steroid Biochem 14:979–987, 1981; Tseng L, Liu HC. Stimulation of arylsulfotransferase activity by progestins in human endometrium in vitro. J Clin Endocrinol Metab 53:418–421, 1981; and Clarke CL, Adams JB, Wren BG. Induction of estrogen sulfotransferase in the human endometrium by progesterone in organ culture. J Clin Endocrinol Metab 55:70–75, 1982.)

in peroxisomes. Both enzymes use the oxidized form of nicotinamide adenine dinucleotide as a cofactor and are predominantly localized to glandular epithelium in the secretory phase. Progesterone enhances the conversion of estradiol to estrone in endometrial cells by increasing expression of the type II and type IV enzymes and estradiol sulfation by increasing expression of estrogen sulfotransferase.

The normal endometrium does not appear to express aromatase, whereas eutopic and ectopic endometrial tissue from subjects with endometriosis does, allowing the conversion of circulating androgens into bioactive estrogens.[75] This biochemical distinction between normal endometrium and endometrium from subjects with endometriosis may be related to aromatase induction by cytokines (IL-6 and IL-11) in women with endometriosis.

Progesterone is also subject to catabolism in the endometrium. The type II 17β-hydroxysteroid dehydrogenase is a 20α-hydroxysteroid dehydrogenase.[73, 74] Thus, in the secretory phase, there is an increased level of an enzyme capable of inactivating both estradiol and progesterone in the glandular epithelium.

Steroid Hormone Receptors in the Uterus

There are striking spatial and temporal changes in steroid hormone receptor expression during the primate menstrual cycle[76, 77] (Figs. 8–13 and 8–14). Estrogen receptor concentrations are highest during the proliferative phase, declining after ovulation as a result of the suppressive effects of progesterone. Endometrial progesterone receptors peak at the time of ovulation, a pattern reflecting the ability of estradiol to induce progesterone receptor expression and the down-regulatory actions of progesterone on its own receptor.

Immunohistochemical studies reveal that estrogen receptors are localized to the nuclei of epithelial, stromal, and myometrial cells during the proliferative phase. The epithelial cell staining is most prominent. After progesterone levels rise, estrogen receptor staining is restricted to the deep basal glands and vascular smooth muscle.

Progesterone receptors are also localized to nuclei but are most prominent in epithelial cells during the proliferative phase and postovulatory days 1 to 3.[76–78] By day 4 after ovulation, progesterone receptor staining of the epithelial cells declines markedly and remains weak or absent during the secretory phase. In contrast, staining of stromal cells remains moderate to strong throughout the secretory phase. Progesterone receptors have not been detected in vascular smooth muscle.

Two forms of the progesterone receptor, A and B, have been identified. These isoforms are derived from a single gene through use of alternative transcription sites so that the A form lacks a 164 amino acid N-terminal sequence present in the B form. The A and B forms of the progesterone receptor have different functions, and the differential expression of the two isoforms determines tissue responses.[79] The A form of the progesterone receptor can function as a transcriptional activator or repressor, depending on the context. The expression pattern of the two forms of the progesterone receptor has not been comprehensively mapped in the human endometrium.

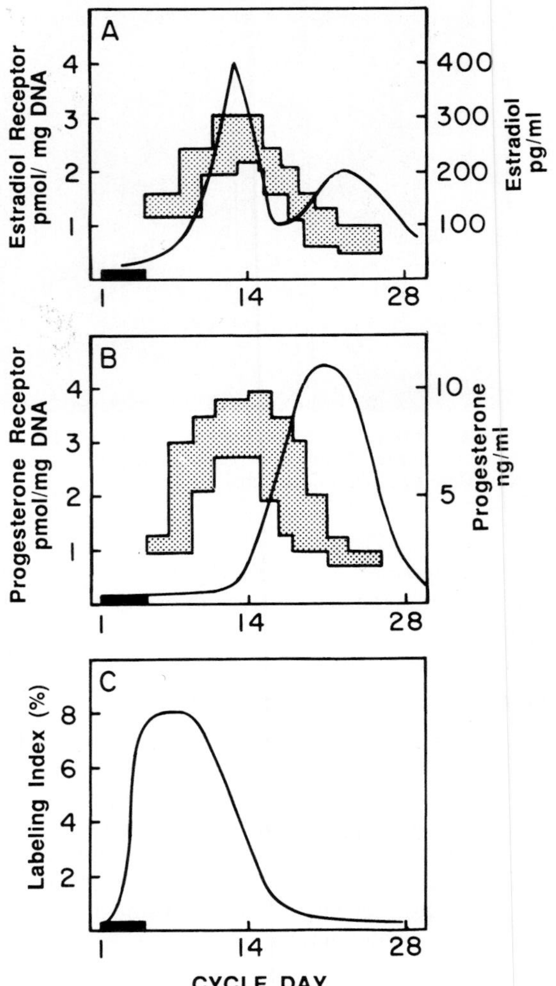

Figure 8–13 ■ Estradiol and progesterone receptors in endometrial cells during the normal menstrual cycle. The concentrations of estradiol receptor *(A)* and progesterone receptor *(B)*, mean values of plasma estradiol and progesterone, and endometrial proliferation as assessed by incorporation of [^{3}H]thymidine in vitro (labeling index, *C*). (Modified from Frolich M, Brand EC, van Hall EV. Serum levels of unconjugated aetiocholanolone, androstenedione, testosterone, dehydroepiandrosterone, aldosterone, progesterone, and oestrogens during the normal menstrual cycle. Acta Endocrinol [Copenh] 81:548–562, 1976.)

Steroid Hormone Regulation of Uterine Growth

The proliferation of the epithelial and stromal cells that results in the regeneration of the functionalis is under the influence of estradiol and various growth factors. The potent effects of estrogens on endometrial growth are evident from the well-documented dose-dependent development of endometrial hyperplasia in postmenopausal women receiving estrogen preparations as hormone replacement therapy. Conversely, targeted mutation of the estrogen receptor-α in the mouse results in a normally formed but hypoplastic uterus in females homozygous for the targeted allele.[80]

Estradiol exerts transcriptional control over a variety of genes through the intermediacy of the estradiol receptor, including IGF-1, TGF-α, and epidermal growth factor

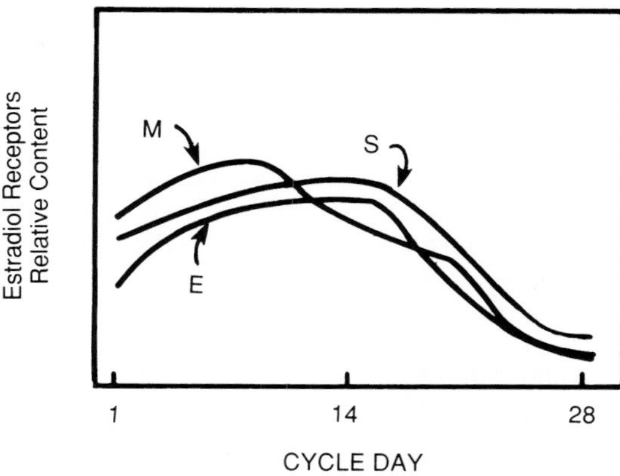

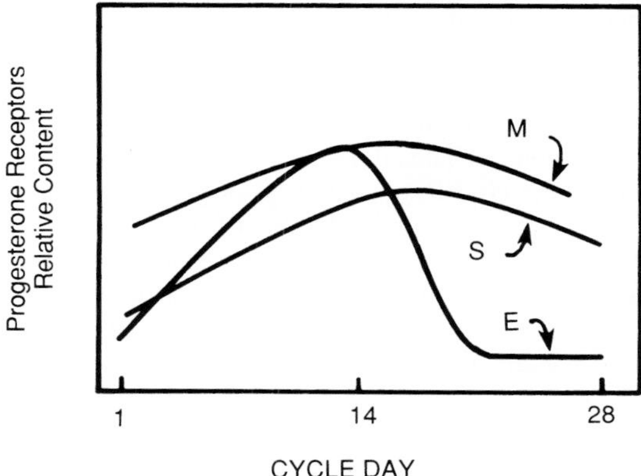

Figure 8–14 ■ Relative levels of uterine estrogen and progesterone receptor immunostaining intensity throughout the menstrual cycle in glandular epithelium (E), stroma (S), and myometrium (M). (Modified from Lessey BA, Killam AP, Metzger DA, et al. Immunohistochemical analysis of human uterine estrogen and progesterone receptors throughout the menstrual cycle. J Clin Endocrinol Metab 67:334–340, 1988. © The Endocrine Society.)

(EGF).[81, 82] Estradiol may also enhance expression of proto-oncogenes involved in stimulating cell proliferation, including *MYC, FOS, JUN,* and *RAS.*[83] The correlation of *MYC,* endometrial deoxyribonucleic acid (DNA) polymerase, and estrogen is consistent with this notion. The mitogenic effects of estrogen on epithelial cells appear to result from paracrine actions, with estradiol affecting the release of factors from mesenchymal cells.[7a] Stromal cells produce IL-6, which inhibits epithelial replication. Estradiol reduces IL-6 production, removing the restraint on epithelial cell proliferation.

The effects of progesterone on endometrial growth are complex, encompassing zone-specific inhibitory as well as stimulatory effects on endometrial cell proliferation. Mice lacking a progesterone receptor develop uterine hyperplasia and uterine inflammation, reflecting an inability to counteract the proliferative actions of estrogens.[84] The inflammatory changes suggest that progesterone normally exerts anti-inflammatory actions in the uterus through the progesterone receptor.

DNA synthesis assessed by [^{3}H]thymidine incorporation into cells of the endometrium of the rhesus monkey in vivo or into explants of human endometrium in vitro is greatest in the epithelial cells of the functionalis and low in the deep zona basalis during the proliferative phase.[85] Labeling indices fall dramatically in the luteal phase with the exception of the basalis, where thymidine incorporation increases as progesterone levels rise, suggesting that progestins stimulate the formation of precursor cells in preparation for the next cycle. In vitro studies using animal stromal cells have shown progesterone-stimulated cell proliferation in the presence of a variety of growth factors.

Growth Factors and Receptors Expressed in the Endometrium

A variety of growth factors have been implicated in the dramatic morphologic changes that occur in the endometrium during the menstrual cycle and pregnancy (Fig. 8–15). Among the growth factors whose expression has been demonstrated in the human endometrium and decidua are EGF and TGF-α; acidic and basic fibroblast growth factor (FGF); IGF-I and IGF-II; IL-1 and IL-6; LIF; macrophage colony-stimulating factor (M-CSF); granulocyte-macrophage colony-stimulating factor (GM-CSF); TGF-β; platelet-derived growth factor (PDGF); tumor necrosis factor-α (TNF-α); and endothelins 1, 2, and 3. Several of these factors have been proposed to play crucial roles in endometrial function and during pregnancy.[86–88] The endometrium and decidua have also been shown to express receptors for many of these factors, including the EGF/TGF-α, IGF-I and IGF-II, IL-1, M-CSF, GM-CSF, PDGF, and endothelin receptors. With such a wide array of growth factors, it has become difficult to determine with clarity the role of each factor in endometrial growth and differentiation as well as in processes involving maternal embryonic interaction and placental development.[89, 90] A number of growth factors have been shown to exert regulatory effects on the expres-

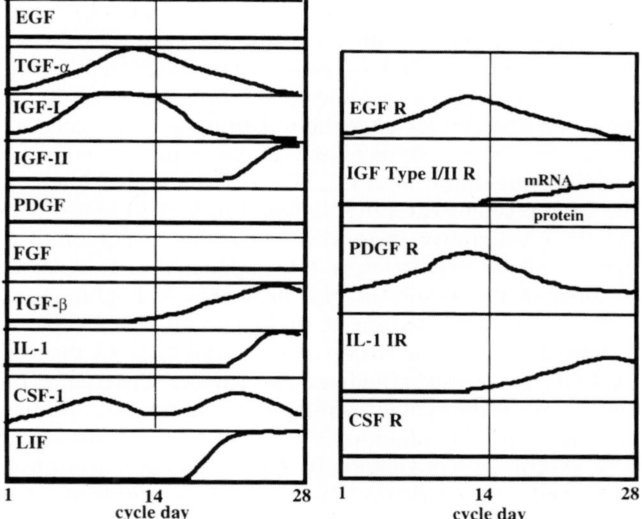

Figure 8–15 ■ Growth factors and their receptors in human endometrium during the menstrual cycle. Schematic represents tissue levels relative to the proliferative phase of the cycle. (From Giudice LC, Saleh W. Growth factors in reproduction. Trends Endocrinol Metab 6:60, 1995. Reproduced with permission of Elsevier Science Inc.)

sion of extracellular matrix proteins and their cellular receptors (integrins), which also influence cell growth and differentiation.[91–95]

TRANSFORMING GROWTH FACTOR-β FAMILY

The TGF-β family, multifunctional proteins that regulate cell growth and differentiation, includes five dimeric polypeptides encoded by related genes.[96–98] They bind to three cell surface proteins designated type I, II, and III receptors. The type I and type II receptors are thought to mediate the actions of TGF-β. In the human endometrium, the highest level of expression of TGF-β mRNA and protein in the epithelial and stromal cells is seen in the late proliferative and early secretory to midsecretory phases.[99] The type II receptor parallels the expression of the TGFs-β. In vitro, TGFs-β inhibit endometrial cell proliferation, and it has been postulated that TGFs-β participate in the transition of the endometrium from the proliferative to the secretory phase. TGF-β is even more abundant in the decidua in the first trimester of pregnancy, where it is thought to restrain trophoblast invasion by promoting trophoblast differentiation away from the invasive phenotype. TGFs-β up-regulate the expression of cellular fibronectin by trophoblast cells[100–102] and induce TIMPs and PAI-1. TGF-β1 is also angiogenic in vivo, and it regulates extracellular matrix organization during angiogenesis. Thus, TGF-β1 may have roles in neovascularization during the regeneration of the endometrium as well as during implantation and placentation. Finally, TGF-β1 is a potent immunosuppressant that may prevent the maternal immune rejection of the fetal allograft.

EPIDERMAL GROWTH FACTOR AND RELATED MOLECULES

EGF and TGF-α stimulate the proliferation of endometrial stromal cells.[103–105] These growth factors also enhance the morphologic and functional differentiation of decidual cells in vitro. EGF is present in the endometrium, and its cellular distribution changes with the phase of the cycle. In the proliferative phase, EGF is predominantly localized in stromal cells; during the secretory phase, it is increased in the glandular and surface epithelium. During the late secretory phase, expression is increased in the stromal cells surrounding the spiral arteries. TGF-α, which also binds to the EGF receptor (EGF-R), is found in highest levels during the proliferative phase, declining after ovulation. The primary site of expression is in the epithelial cells. Another member of this family of growth factors is amphiregulin, which is also detected in the endometrium. The synthesis of fibronectin and vitronectin by epithelial cells is enhanced by EGF. EGF also stimulates stromal cell differentiation and enhances the synthesis of laminin and fibronectin. This contrasts with the inhibitory effect of EGF on laminin and type IV collagen production by human uterine adenocarcinoma cells. EGF has recently been shown to influence the expression of integrins by human endometrial cells.

EGF has not been identified in the circulation of cycling or menopausal women, but it has been detected in the serum of pregnant women with peak concentrations in early pregnancy. Binding studies indicate that EGF-R peaks at the time of ovulation or shortly thereafter and declines during the secretory phase to a nadir immediately before menses. The binding sites are present on both stromal and epithelial cells as well as in decidua of pregnancy. Immunohistochemical studies suggest that decidualization is associated with an increase in EGF-R. Abnormal EGF and EGF-R activity has been reported in cases of intrauterine growth retardation. Although its role in embryo implantation is still unknown, it has been hypothesized that EGF and related molecules play a role in the induction of trophoblast differentiation.

INSULIN-LIKE GROWTH FACTORS

IGF-I and IGF-II are polypeptides of approximately 7 kDa that have structural homology to insulin.[104] They bind to specific (type I and type II) IGF receptors on the membranes of a variety of cells to promote mitosis and differentiation. Both IGFs stimulate the proliferation of human endometrial stromal cells via the type I receptor. IGF-I expression is greatest in the late proliferative and early secretory phase, whereas IGF-II is most abundant in the midsecretory endometrium and decidua of the first trimester of pregnancy. The IGFs are bound by a family of binding protein (IGFBPs) that are thought to modulate their activities in target tissues.[106–108] One of the binding proteins, IGFBP-1, is a major secretory product of decidualized stromal cells, and it has been hypothesized to play a role in modulating trophoblast invasion. Both IGFBP-1 and IGFBP-2 contain the Arg-Gly-Asp (RGD) amino acid sequence that is recognized by a number of integrins. IGFBP-1 has been demonstrated to bind to the $\alpha_5\beta_1$ integrin through this motif.

IGF-I and IGF-II are produced by the human placenta; IGF-I mRNA is localized by in situ hybridization primarily in the syncytial trophoblast. IGF-II mRNA has been demonstrated in mesenchymal fibroblasts of the villous core but has also been shown to be expressed in first-trimester and term cytotrophoblasts. The expression of IGFs in the placenta seems to be under the regulatory control of hormones (insulin, human placental lactogen, and estrogens) as well as growth factors, including PDGF. Type IGF-I receptors have been detected in the placenta during the earliest periods of gestation, and it has been hypothesized that IGFs promote trophoblast proliferation.

PLATELET-DERIVED GROWTH FACTOR

PDGF is produced by endometrial stromal cells and also released in the endometrium by activated platelets.[104] PDGF is a potent mitogen that acts on endometrial receptors that are most abundant in the proliferative phase of the cycle.

FIBROBLAST GROWTH FACTORS

FGFs encompass a family of growth factors that can stimulate growth of endometrial cells and smooth muscle cells.[109, 110] Acidic and basic FGFs bind to proteoglycans. Because these proteins do not contain secretory signal sequences, they may be most important in the endometrium during menstruation when they could be released from dying cells. Basic FGF is angiogenic but also stimulates stromal cell proliferation in the presence of progesterone. FGF-7, also known as keratinocyte growth factor, stimulates epithelial cell proliferation. FGF-7 mRNA is expressed at highest level in the late secretory–phase endometrium in the stroma; its receptor is most abundant in the glandular epithelium in the late proliferative phase. These findings suggest that FGF-7 is progesterone dependent, whereas its receptor is estrogen sensitive. FGF-8 is a uterine growth factor isolated from bovine uterus.

VASCULAR ENDOTHELIAL GROWTH FACTOR

Vascular endothelial growth factor (VEGF) exists in multiple forms as a consequence of alternative splicing.[111, 112] VEGF stimulates angiogenesis as well as vascular permeability. Four different VEGF transcripts have been detected in the human endometrium. Although it is present in the proliferative phase, the greatest level of expression of VEGF appears to be in the glandular epithelial cells in the menstrual phase of the cycle, when it may participate in the vascular events associated with the sloughing of the functional layer and the subsequent regeneration and neovascularization of the endometrium.

TUMOR NECROSIS FACTOR-α

TNF-α is a pleiotropic factor that exerts inflammatory, mitogenic, mitostatic, angiogenic, and immunomodulatory effects in a variety of tissues.[113] It is a membrane-bound 14-kDa polypeptide that is derived by proteolytic cleavage from the 26-kDa precursor. Expression of TNF-α mRNA and protein has been demonstrated in human endometrium, decidua, and trophoblasts. Its receptors have also been found in all these tissues. TNF-α in the human endometrium seems to be subject to regulation by steroid hormones, namely, estrogens and progesterone.

TNF-α and its receptors (TNF-R) are expressed by trophoblasts, during both early and late gestation.[114] There is differential expression of the two genes encoding TNF-R, thus allowing some regulation of TNF-α activity. In cultured human chorionic cells, TNF-α affects cellular fibronectin secretion. It has been hypothesized that along with other endometrial and trophoblast factors, TNF-α controls trophoblast adhesion and invasion.[115]

COLONY-STIMULATING FACTORS

Colony-stimulating factors are a group of cytokines that were initially identified by their characteristic stimulation of hematopoietic stem cells, prompting them to form colonies in semisolid culture media.[116] The first of these factors to be purified was macrophage-colony stimulating factor (M-CSF), also known as CSF-1, which, in the hematopoietic system, regulates the proliferation and maturation of monocytes and enhances mature macrophage cell function.[117, 118] There is widespread distribution of both M-CSF and its receptor in the endometrium, decidua, and placenta,[119–121] suggesting that it plays a role in local events during pregnancy. The receptor (CSF1R encoded by FMS) is highly expressed by extravillous trophoblasts in the cell columns that anchor the placenta to the uterus[122]; the endometrial cells, both of local and of bone marrow origin, that are in proximity to the anchoring trophoblasts appear to be the major source of the M-CSF found at the placental-uterine interface.[123, 124] During pregnancy, accumulation of M-CSF in amniotic fluid has been demonstrated.[125] Although M-CSF has been proposed to regulate trophoblast morphogenesis and differentiation,[126] the exact functions of this cytokine at these sites in the reproductive tract are yet to be determined.

LEUKEMIA INHIBITORY FACTOR

LIF, a cytokine of the IL-6 family, acquired its name by its capacity to inhibit the proliferation of a mouse leukemic cell line.[127, 128] LIF is expressed by both the mouse and the human endometrium. Observations in the mouse have clearly demonstrated that LIF of endometrial origin is crucial in the process of blastocyst implantation. Stewart and colleagues[129] showed that homozygous LIF-deficient females failed to become pregnant, whereas transfer of their embryos to pseudopregnant, wild-type females resulted in viable pregnancies. The role of LIF in human endometrial function and embryo implantation is less clear at present. Nevertheless, LIF mRNA and protein are present in human endometrium and peak in the secretory phase of the cycle.[130] LIF receptor is present in endometrial cells throughout the cycle.[130] Of interest is that secretion of LIF from cultured endometrium in patients with repeated implantation failures or unexplained infertility has been shown to be decreased.[131, 132] This observation, coupled with the presence of LIF receptor on human blastocysts and placenta,[133] is suggestive but certainly not conclusive of a role of LIF in human implantation, trophoblast differentiation, or placentation.[134, 135] The cycle-dependent expression of LIF in human endometrium may be a function of other growth factors (i.e., TGF-β) rather than a direct effect of steroid hormones.

Myometrial Growth

The wet weight of the human uterus increases 10-fold during pregnancy, and its carrying capacity increases from 300 ml to 4.5 L largely owing to hypertrophy and hyperplasia of the myometrium. The myometrial hyperplasia is steroid hormone dependent and probably mediated by growth factors, particularly the IGFs.[106] The primate myometrium expresses all components of the IGF signaling system, including IGF-I and IGF-II and the type I growth factor receptor as well as IGFBPs 2, 3, 4, and 5. IGF-I and IGFBPs 2, 4, and 5 are up-regulated by estrogen, whereas IGFBP-3 is suppressed by estrogen. Progesterone enhances expression of IGF-I and IGFBP-2 mRNA stimulated by estrogen. The stimulation of IGF-I expression by estrogen is accompanied by an increased number of Ki-67–positive myometrial cells, indicating myometrial cell proliferation.

Secretory Products of the Uterus

The endometrium and myometrium secrete a number of proteins that probably have important autocrine and paracrine functions. Some of these proteins also enter into the general circulation. A remarkable increase in secretory activity is associated with the luteal phase and early pregnancy, with increased activity of the epithelial cells of the glands and decidualization of the stroma.[136–140] Several secretory proteins produced by the endometrium deserve special attention because of their potential physiologic relevance to endometrial and trophoblast function or their utility as markers of endometrial function (Fig. 8–16).

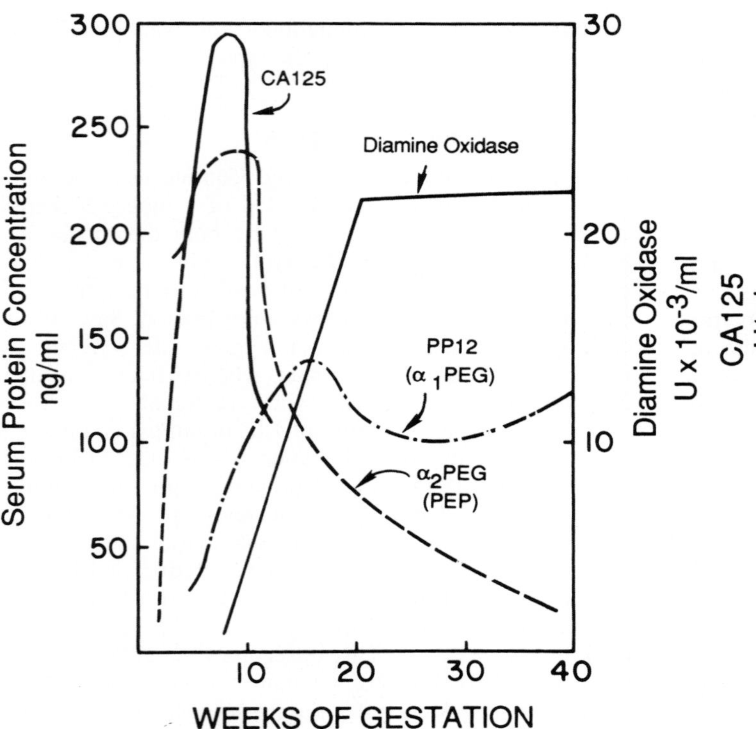

Figure 8–16 ■ Levels of CA-125, diamine oxidase, progesterone-associated endometrial protein (PEP), and pregnancy-associated endometrial α1-globulin (α_1-PEG) in the sera of pregnant women. (Modified from Bell SC. Secretory endometrial and decidual proteins: Studies and clinical significance of a maternally derived group of pregnancy-associated serum proteins. Hum Reprod 1:129–143, 1986.)

Progesterone-Associated Endometrial Protein (Glycodelin)

Progesterone-associated endometrial protein (PEP) is also known by a number of other names including placental protein 14 (an erroneous name because it is a decidual product), and glycodelin α_2-microglobulin, α-uterine protein, and pregnancy-associated α_2-globulin.[141–143] PEP is a dimeric glycoprotein produced mainly by the glandular epithelium but also by decidual tissue. The mature form of the protein contains 162 amino acid residues and is 17.5 percent by weight carbohydrate. It has extensive structural homology with the β-lactoglobulins and retinol-binding proteins. PEP has been postulated to play a role as an immunosuppressant, but this hypothesis remains to be convincingly established. PEP appears in peripheral serum in the late secretory phase when progesterone levels are declining. During pregnancy, maternal PEP levels increase several-fold during the first trimester.

The discordant pattern of PEP and progesterone in serum may reflect the slower turnover of the protein. Levels of PEP in serum fail to rise in women using combination-type oral contraceptives and in some patients with luteal-phase defects, presumably because of an inadequate luteal steroidal impact on the endometrium. There is a good but not perfect correlation between the progestational activity of steroids and their ability to stimulate PEP synthesis.

Insulin-like Growth Factor–Binding Protein 1

IGFBP-1, also known as pregnancy-associated α_1-protein and placental protein 12, is a major secretory product of decidual cells.[144, 145] The protein undergoes post-translational modification by phosphorylation. IGFBP-1 is one of a number of proteins that bind IGF-I and IGF-II, affecting the ability of these growth factors to interact with the IGF receptors. Consequently, the binding proteins can have significant roles in modulating IGF effects. IGFBP-1 derived from the decidua has been proposed to control the invasion and proliferation of trophoblast cells during implantation and placentation by sequestering IGFs.[108] Because IGFBP-1 contains the Arg-Gly-Asp (RGD) motif recognized by cell surface integrins that bind fibronectin, its actions may be more complex than simple IGF sequestration when it is presented to cells that express the RGD-binding integrins.

Stromal cell IGFBP-1 mRNA levels are regulated by progesterone as well as by IGFs and other growth factors. Serum levels of IGFBP-1 do not change across the menstrual cycle but rise markedly during the first trimester in parallel with the decidual response, reaching peak concentrations at 15 to 20 weeks of gestation. They then decline but rise again in late pregnancy. Pregnancy termination with RU 486 causes a marked decline in IGFBP-1 levels before a fall in hCG levels, confirming the progesterone dependence of IGFBP-1 production by decidual cells. IGFBP-1 also accumulates in amniotic fluid.

Prolactin

Prolactin is produced by both the endometrium and the myometrium.[146–152] Human leiomyomas secrete prolactin and express prolactin mRNA. Progesterone inhibits prolactin secretion, whereas estrogen tends to increase it. The function of prolactin in the uterus is not known, although prolactin receptors have been found in animal endometrium and myometrium, raising the possibility that prolactin may have some paracrine or autocrine functions in this organ, possibly as a modulator of cells of the immune system. During pregnancy, prolactin produced by the decidua accumulates in the amniotic fluid, where it has been postulated to have effects on osmoregulation and fetal lung development.[153]

CA-125

CA-125 is a high-molecular-weight glycoprotein of 200,000 to 400,000 daltons containing 24 percent by weight carbohydrate that is recognized by a monoclonal antibody, OC-125, generated against an ovarian carcinoma cell line.[154] The CA-125 antigen is detectable in decidualized endometrium. CA-125 appears in the serum during early pregnancy in a pattern that parallels that of PEP. It also accumulates in amniotic fluid during the first trimester. CA-125 levels are elevated in certain women with endometriosis, and the degree of elevation is generally correlated with the severity of the disease. However, the sensitivity of serum CA-125 determinations for the diagnosis of endometriosis is low, which precludes serum measurements as a screening test. There is, however, a reasonably good correlation between serum CA-125 levels and the course of endometriosis, including regression in response to treatment.

Cell Adhesion Molecules

The cyclic regeneration of the functionalis layer during the menstrual cycle and the process of embryo implantation involve events of cell adhesion and migration. These dynamic processes encompass homotypic and heterotypic cell-cell encounters as well as cell–extracellular matrix interactions.[155]

There are four main classes of cell adhesion molecules: the integrins, the cadherins, the selectins, and molecules belonging to the immunoglobulin superfamily. Mucins have recently attracted attention because of their possible involvement in nonspecific cell-cell and cell-substratum interactions. All of these classes of molecules and several of their matrix ligands are expressed by the endometrium and have been implicated in endometrial regeneration and embryo implantation.[155]

Integrins are heterodimeric transmembrane glycoproteins, each composed of an α and β subunit.[156–158] A wide repertoire of integrins are expressed by the endometrium and by human trophoblasts.[159, 160] It is interesting that although certain integrins are constitutively expressed, others appear to be spatially and temporally regulated, suggesting that the latter molecules serve specific functions during the different stages of the endometrial cycle.

Unlike other epithelia, the endometrium undergoes cycles of regeneration and maturation that are under tight hormonal control. The endometrial epithelium appears to express the α_2, α_3, α_6, and β_4 subunits constitutively. These integrins are common in many epithelia and may play a role in the organization of a polarized continuous epithelial layer. Subunits α_2 (laminin and collagen type IV receptor) and α_3 (laminin, collagen type IV, and fibronectin receptor) display a pericellular distribution. The distribution of α_6 (laminin receptor) is mostly basal and lateral, indicating a close relationship with the basement membrane. Integrin subunit β_4 is confined to the lateral cell surfaces.[161, 162]

Conflicting data are arising on integrin expression owing to the availability of multiple antibodies (many of which may identify different moieties of the integrin molecules), the molecular complexity and versatility of the integrin molecules, and the variability of endometrial maturation between subjects or between cycles in the same individuals.[160, 163, 164]

After estrogen priming, progesterone induces profound modifications of the endometrial epithelium. Integrin α_1 subunit, a receptor for collagen type IV and laminin, is expressed in vivo throughout the entire secretory phase but not in the proliferative phase.[161] In addition, the α_4 integrin subunit (a fibronectin receptor recognizing the IIICS region of fibronectin, distant from the RGD domain) is expressed in the early luteal phase.[165] This molecule was observed throughout the midsecretory phase and declined by day 24 of the cycle. Another integrin subunit that is not typical to epithelial cells, the α_v integrin subunit, is immunohistochemically detected in the endometrial epithelium slightly before ovulation and continues its expression during the secretory phase.[161, 165] Multiple β integrin subunits may pair with α_v. For example, $\alpha_v\beta_1$ integrin is an RGD-recognizing receptor that binds fibronectin and vitronectin; $\alpha_v\beta_5$ is an RGD-recognizing receptor for vitronectin, fibronectin, and osteopontin; $\alpha_v\beta_6$ binds fibronectin; and $\alpha_v\beta_3$ is an RGD-recognizing receptor that binds multiple ligands including vitronectin, fibronectin, fibrinogen, von Willebrand's factor, osteopontin, and thrombospondin, as well as, indirectly, laminin and collagen.

Another integrin subunit, also atypical for epithelial cells, displays an interesting pattern of regulation in the human endometrium; β_3 integrin is expressed in endometrial epithelial cells after day 19 of the menstrual cycle.[161] Expression of $\alpha_v\beta_3$ integrin by polarized epithelial cells is a novel finding in cell biology, and it has its counterpart in the trophectoderm covering the preimplantation embryo as well as the villous syncytiotrophoblast.[166] A plausible function of this molecule may be to provide support for adhesion of extracellular matrix molecules on the endometrial lumen, possibly offering adhesion sites for the blastocyst. The appearance of β_3 integrin subunit on the endometrial surface coincides temporally with the decline of progesterone receptors in the endometrial epithelium,[167, 168] suggesting complex regulatory mechanisms underlying the onset of its expression.[169] Although it is speculative as it relates to the endometrium, extracellular matrix signaling through integrin receptors is a well-recognized phenomenon that contributes to cell differentiation and tissue morphogenesis.[170]

THE ENDOMETRIUM AND IMPLANTATION

The Endometrium in the Peri-implantation Period and the Concept of Endometrial Receptivity

Embryos enter the uterine cavity at the morula stage, approximately 2 to 3 days after fertilization. Implantation begins several days later, around the sixth to seventh day after fertilization. Studies in experimental and domestic animals have demonstrated that there must be synchronous development of the embryo and endometrium for normal implantation and development to occur.[171] In laboratory animals, there is a discrete window for implantation, which in some species lasts only a matter of hours. Because the human blastocyst can implant at ectopic sites, it may not have rigorous requirements for nidation.

The concept of a window of implantation has been advanced in animal models and in the human,[9, 40, 172–174] but the molecular basis for alterations in uterine receptivity remains unclear. Uterine receptivity, in the strictest sense, is defined as the temporal window of endometrial maturation during which the trophectoderm of the blastocyst can attach to the endometrial epithelial cells and subsequently can proceed to invade the endometrial stroma. The transition from the nonreceptive to the receptive endometrial state is presumably determined by the regulated expression of membrane-bound, soluble or secretory factors that are permissive to trophoblast attachment and subsequent migration. In the study of *human* endometrial receptivity, a key question is the determination of the temporal window of implantation. Only factors expressed during this temporal window can be considered either markers or functional mediators of the receptive state.

Even though embryos from various species, including the human, are capable of attachment and spreading on various extracellular matrix components or other cells, it is evident that there is a defined period of time during which such a process can occur in vivo and within the uterus.

The Window of Embryo Transfer

The temporal window of uterine receptivity can be inferred from what has been learned from transfer of embryos to uteri of women primed with exogenous estrogen and progesterone preparations. There is a distinct window for *embryo transfer* leading to implantation which spans endometrial cycle days 16 to 20. Presumably, the actual window of *implantation* follows this window of transfer because embryos need to further develop from the 4- to 8-cell stage to the blastocyst stage before initiation of attachment and frank invasion.

Rogers and Murphy[174] summarized data on 52 pregnancies achieved with donor oocytes and, on the basis of the chronologic age of the endometrium relative to the embryo, concluded that the human implantation window must be at least 3½ days. Formigli and associates[175] flushed embryos from donors at 5 days after ovulation and reported pregnancies after transfer to recipients anywhere from 4 days in front to 3 days behind the donor at the time of ovulation, suggesting a period of uterine receptivity of up to 7 days. However, the possibility of spontaneous pregnancy in the recipients was not ruled out. Using serum hCG as a marker of initial embryonic-maternal interaction, Bergh and Navot[42] defined the window of implantation in the human as being from day 20 through day 24 of the cycle (Fig. 8–17). Thus, it appears that the window of implantation in the human is wide (approximately 4 days). These recent observations agree with the earlier morphologic data from Hertig and colleagues,[176] which suggested that the onset of uterine receptivity to human trophoblast implantation occurs at approximately days 19 to 20. Therefore, in attempting to define molecular mediators of uterine receptivity in the human, the expression of the "factor" should span days 19 to 20 through 24 of the endometrial cycle.

Regulation of the Endometrium with Exogenous Steroid Hormones

Oocyte donation and assisted reproductive technologies have been used in the treatment of women with ovarian failure.[177] The clinical indications for use of donated oocytes have broadened to include premenopausal women younger than 40 years or who have shown poor ovarian reserve, normally cycling women in whom IVF has failed previously, or women who have genetic disorders. In addition, replacement cycles driven by exogenously administered hormones after gonadotropin-releasing hormone (GnRH) agonist down-regulation are routinely used for transfer of cryopreserved embryos. These clinical applications have provided unique opportunities to examine the hormonal requirements for endometrial maturation. A number of hormone replacement protocols have been proposed, and many pregnancies have resulted from donor oocytes in women with and without ovarian failure. The success of these procedures has ranged between 35 and 50 percent per transfer.

The adequacy of hormone replacement regimens has been assessed by histologic analysis of endometrial biopsy specimens. Biopsies on day 20 to day 22 typically reveal dyssynchrony between glands and stroma. The glandular components at this time are more characteristic of day 17 to day 18 endometrium, whereas the stroma appears more consistent with days 21 to 23. However, biopsies in the late phase reveal day 25 to day 26 stroma and glands. Therefore, the glandular elements exhibit delayed maturation early during progesterone administration on days 20 to 22, the time of expected implantation, but catch up by day 26. Despite this apparent dyssynchrony, the pregnancy rate in these patients with donor oocytes is higher than in conventional IVF.[55, 56, 175, 177, 178]

Davis and Rosenwaks[179] treated 15 patients with 21 transfers of donor oocytes and reported higher pregnancy rates when the endometrium was judged to be in phase on a day 21 biopsy during a "mock" replacement cycle. Those whose biopsy results were more than 2 days out of phase yielded no pregnancies. Navot and coworkers,[55] in an attempt to define the dose and length of exogenous hormone administration, explored the histologic characteristics of replacement cycles of varying "follicular phase" lengths in four protocols: (1) standard 28-day cycle, (2) short follicular phase (6 mg/day estradiol for 6 days), (3) long follicular phase with stepwise increases in estradiol during 3 to 5 weeks, and (4) accelerated secretory transformation with 150 mg progesterone administered intramuscularly in the luteal phase. This study revealed that the length of estrogen priming is not critical for achieving the appropriate endometrial conditions for embryo transfer. This observation has been confirmed in a more recent study by Michalas and colleagues.[180]

At present, the most common protocols use a step-up administration of oral micronized estradiol in 2-, 4-, and 6-mg daily doses followed by 4 to 6 mg of estradiol com-

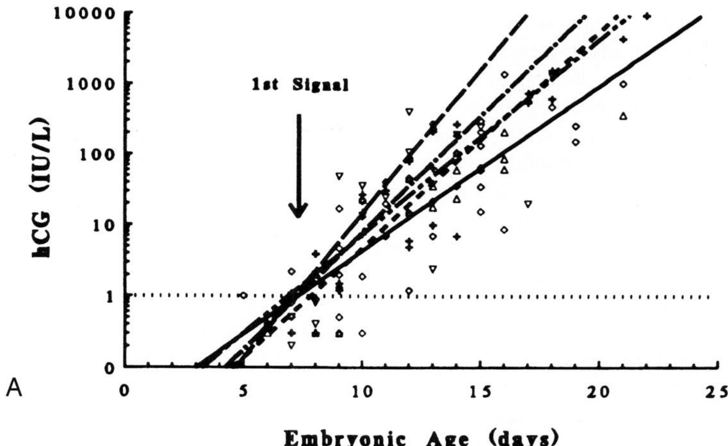

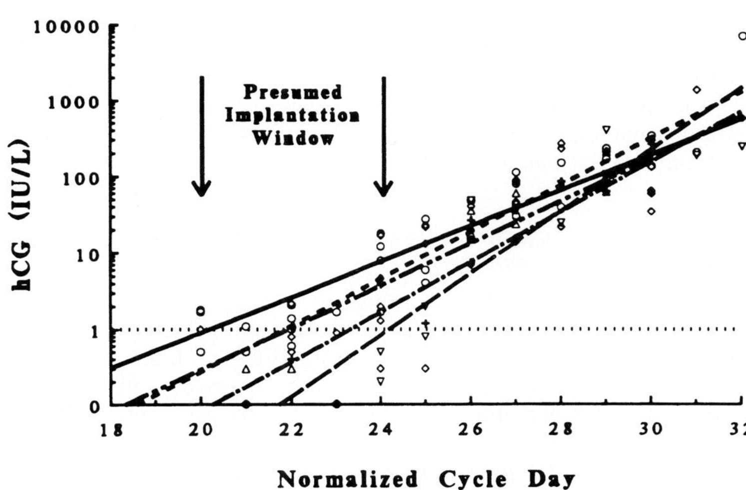

Figure 8–17 ■ Definition of the "window of implantation" in the human as assessed by the first detection of hCG in the maternal circulation by use of an ultrasensitive assay. When the hCG concentration from individual pregnancies was plotted against endometrial dating *(B)*, the window spans days 20 to 24. When the individual pregnancy hCG concentrations were plotted against embryonic age *(A)*, it appears that it is the day 7 embryo that initiates the implantation process. (From Bergh PA, Navot D. The impact of embryonic development and endometrial maturity on the timing of implantation. Fertil Steril 58:537–542, 1992. Reproduced with permission of the American Society for Reproductive Medicine.)

bined with daily parenteral progesterone (50 mg) to promote the secretory transformation. Serum estradiol levels in these subjects during the replacement "follicular" phase reach preovulatory peak levels of 800 to 1000 pg/ml. Intramuscular injection of 50 mg of progesterone usually generates serum levels of more than 10 ng/ml. More recently, oral, micronized progesterone has been employed, but the pharmacokinetics of this preparation requires dosing four times a day to achieve adequate serum levels. The length of exposure to progesterone, but not absolute plasma progesterone concentrations achieved after an adequate priming of the endometrium with estrogens, is a key factor for the development of uterine receptivity.

Early Implantation in the Human

Before any type of interaction between the trophoblast layer of the blastocyst and the maternal cells, whether these are located in the uterus or at an ectopic site, the zona pellucida has to be either completely or partially degraded. Gradual zona thinning as well as complete hatching of embryos can be observed in vitro. The existence of ectopic implantation suggests that the endometrium is not obligatory for this process to be successfully completed. Nevertheless, there may be more subtle regulation of hatching within the endometrial cavity. Although the process of the degradation of the zona pellucida is driven by the embryo, the presence of inhibitors or agents that induce "zona hardening" may affect the timing of the process. These factors may play a role in the establishment of the window of implantation.

Work on subhuman primates demonstrates that mononuclear cytotrophoblasts of the trophectoderm of the blastocyst have fused into syncytia before the attachment of these cells to the endometrial epithelium.[181] Careful histologic examination of very early human implantation sites such as those studied by Hertig and colleagues[176] and by Hamilton and Boyd[182] indicate that it is the syncytial trophoblast layer of the human embryo that comprises the invading front during the first few days of implantation. Thus, the consensus appears to be that it is a syncytial trophoblast cell that initially interacts with and adheres to the endometrial epithelium, and it is only after the human embryo is completely embedded in the endometrium that cytotrophoblast cell columns start to stream out of the trophoblastic shell and further invade the uterus.[183, 184] This process starts approximately 1 week after the initiation of implantation and continues well into the second trimester of pregnancy. The early human implantation sites that have been examined histologically demonstrate that by day 12 after ovulation, the embryo is almost completely covered by endometrium. The endometrial stroma around the implantation site displays the predecidual reaction and is edematous. By the classic histologic criteria of Noyes and associates,[40] the endometrium of the implantation site is not different from the nonpregnant midsecretory-phase endometrium. The glands adjacent to the embryo are themselves deflected by invading trophoblasts but still have the tortuosity and secretion-filled appearance typical for this stage of the menstrual cycle. In vitro observations using human embryos or human trophoblasts have attempted to characterize some morphologic features of the early events of trophoblast-endometrial interactions.[185, 186]

The Window of Implantation and Markers of Endometrial Receptivity

Several attempts have been made to correlate biochemical markers as well as histochemical or ultrastructural features with uterine receptivity (Fig. 8–18). Morphologic studies initially related the disappearance of surface microvilli and of the ciliated cells, the flattening of cell surface with smoothening of their contour, and the development of apical protrusions as features of endometrial maturation supporting implantation.[9] The development of pinopods on the apical surface of endometrial epithelial cells has been considered an important morphologic feature of peri-implantation endometrium that is progestin dependent.[9] Together with organelle formation, a profound modification of the composition of the surface glycocalyx has been documented, reflecting changes in surface saccharide moieties and glycoproteins.[187] Mucin MUC-1 and keratan sulfate are two transmembrane glycoproteins that have been shown to significantly increase in the glandular cell surface during the peri-implantation period. The expression of MUC-1 on the endometrial surface appears to be down-regulated at the time of the opening of the window of implantation.[188, 189] This observation has led investigators to propose that such down-regulation of a relatively large cell surface molecule allows the "unmasking" of smaller molecules such as integrins or cadherins, which may mediate the specific adhesion of the trophectoderm to the endometrial epithelial cell during the receptive phase of the cycle.

Experiments conducted in laboratory animals suggest that the period of uterine receptivity to the blastocyst is signaled by a decrease in the negative surface charge of the endometrial epithelium.[190] This has been revealed by various histochemical techniques, including binding of cationic ferritin and alcian blue staining. The significance of minimal negative charge on the endometrial epithelium is that adhesive events such as the attachment of the blastocyst will be enhanced by the reduction in repulsive charges. The human secretory endometrium appears to have little negative surface charge as assessed by these techniques.[28]

A novel cell surface molecule, trophinin, has been identified and has been shown to mediate trophoblast-endometrial adhesion in vitro.[191] Its menstrual cycle expression and its function, in vitro, need further characterization. Nevertheless, the in vitro observations are promising as to a functional role of this molecule in trophoblast-endometrial interactions.

The observation that endometrial epithelium expresses integrins on the luminal surface and that several of these molecules are regulated in an on-off pattern has led to the search for markers of the window of implantation among this superfamily of molecules.[159] Moreover, the observation that the trophectoderm of the preimplantation blastocyst expresses integrins as well as their ligands has fostered the attractive concept that these molecules may take part in the mechanisms underlying early events in implantation.[155] The subunit β_3, for instance, is expressed after day 19 of the cycle (day 5 after ovulation), suggesting that the functional dimer $\alpha_v\beta_3$ appears on the endometrial surface at the time of the "opening" of the window of implantation. This integrin is almost never encountered in epithelial cells, and the fact that it is also expressed by the human trophectoderm[166] makes it even more interesting. A possible ligand for α_v integrins is osteopontin, a phosphorylated secretory glycoprotein of 42 to 58 kDa.[192–194] Osteopontin, which is expressed by secretory endometrial epithelium, may provide a substratum for the attachment of the trophoblast. Therefore, a possible role of the α_v family of integrins can be envisioned in human implantation. However, patients with Glanzmann's thrombasthenia who have an inherited absence of β_3 have not been described to be infertile. Thus, the β_3 integrin may be participatory but not obligatory in the process of implantation. Redundancy in integrin subunits (i.e., β_1, β_3, or β_5 pairing with α_v) may explain this observation. Alternatively, the regulated expression of integrins in human endometrium and trophoblasts may influence other processes, as yet uncharacterized, that may have little to do with implantation.

To date, no single integrin molecule can be claimed as *the* molecule identifying the window of implantation. Adaptation of the data to fit in the concept of the window of implantation requires the presumption that either a yet unidentified adhesion or other molecule defines uterine receptivity or, alternatively, a set of coexpressed integrins (and possibly their ligands) represent the molecular basis for this process. The observation that α_4 integrin subunit is turned off in endometrial epithelial cells by day 24 of the cycle has led to the hypothesis that the coexpressed $\alpha_v\beta_3$ and $\alpha_4\beta_1$ integrins are more reliable markers of the window of endometrial receptivity.[162, 169] However, a functional role for these molecules has not been demonstrated. Although their usefulness in clinical medicine is unclear at present, further investigation into their roles as either markers or functional mediators of cellular processes in endometrial development, regulation, and embryo implantation is warranted.

Molecular epidemiologic studies have been initiated in an effort to characterize normal and abnormal patterns of expression of integrins in the human endometrium. Expres-

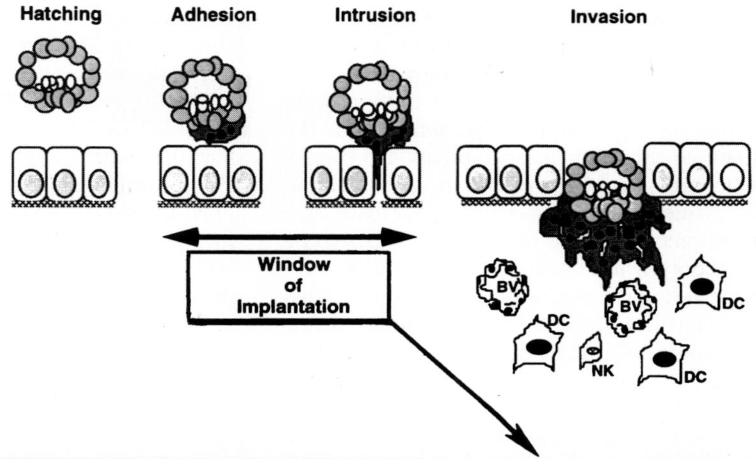

Some Factors with Potential Roles in the Establishment of a Receptive Endometrium		Early Secretory	Mid Secretory	Late Secretory
Morphologic	Pinopodes	-	+	-
Cell-associated	MUC-1	+	-	-
	α1	+	+	+
	α4	+	+	-
	αv	+	+	+
	β1	+	+	+
	β3	-	+	+
	β5	+	+	+
	Trophinin	+	?	?
Secretory	LIF	-	+	+
	M-CSF	+	++	+
	IL-1	+	++	++
	IGFBP-1	+	+	+
	OPN	+	++	++
	C3	+	+	+

Figure 8–18 ■ Schematic representation of the early phases of human implantation *(top)* and a listing of some of the morphologic, cell-associated, and secretory endometrial factors with potential roles in the establishment of the receptive endometrium. Note that with the exception of LIF (and only in the mouse), no other factor has been conclusively shown to have a functional role in implantation. Nevertheless, some of these factors may be markers of appropriate endometrial maturation during the period of endometrial receptivity. LIF, leukemia inhibitory factor; IGFBP-1, insulin-like growth factor–binding protein 1; M-CSF, macrophage colony-stimulating factor; OPN, osteopontin; α1, α4, αv, β1, β3, and β5, integrin subunits; MUC-1, mucin 1.

sion of β_3 has been shown to be absent from the endometrium of patients identified as having infertility secondary to maturational delay. A significant number of patients with so-called unexplained infertility by standard criteria were found to have aberrant expression of β_3 integrin in the endometrial epithelium. Some of these subjects had biopsy results that were actually out of phase by histologic criteria, whereas another group was found to display histologic maturity of the endometrium but lacked β_3.[169] Klentzeris and coworkers[195] reported the absence of α_4 integrin subunit from secretory endometrial epithelium among patients with unexplained infertility. Interestingly, in a few patients with a luteal-phase defect defined by histologic criteria in biopsies performed between days 20 and 24 of the cycle, treatment with clomiphene citrate and progesterone vaginal suppositories corrected the maturational delay and restored expression of the β_3 integrin in a subsequent cycle.[162, 169] In this study, patients with unexplained infertility did not display significant differences in the expression of α_4 integrin subunit. In contrast to these studies, expression of $\alpha_1\beta_1$ and $\alpha_v\beta_3$ integrins in the luteal phase is not affected by high-dose estrogen and progesterone administered for emergency contraception, which raises some questions about the functional significance of the immunohistochemical findings.[196]

Integrin research on the endometrium may change the way we approach the diagnostic work-up of endometrial maturation. In fact, if crucial molecular events occur between days 20 and 24, biopsies of the endometrium to assess appropriate maturation may need to be performed during that window.[45]

Trophoblast Invasion

During nidation and placentation, trophoblasts adhere and migrate within the endometrial stroma and finally invade the maternal vessels and establish the hemochorial placenta (Fig. 8–19). This process includes cell-cell and cell-substratum interactions involving degradation of the matrix to allow migration of the cells as well as matrix remodeling.[197–201] Cell adhesion has been shown to directly modulate the expression of extracellular matrix components.[202] Present knowledge suggests that a number of proteinases play important roles in the degradation of the basement membrane and extracellular matrix during the process of human trophoblast invasion.[203–208] Specifically, MMP-9 appears to be one of the major determinants of the capability of human trophoblasts to degrade laminin/type IV collagen–rich basement membranes. Regulation of MMP-9 activity is achieved, at least in part, through TIMPs, specifically TIMP-3, which appears to be unique in its expression by human trophoblasts. In vitro studies using mouse blastocysts have contributed significantly to our understanding of the role of extracellular matrix ligands and their integrin receptors in embryo attachment, outgrowth, and signaling.[209–214] Urokinase-type plasminogen activator is another proteinase that either directly or indirectly through activation of pro-MMPs may increase the capacity of human trophoblast to degrade extracellular matrix.[215, 216] This proteinase may be kept in check by trophoblast or endometrial plasminogen activator inhibitors, particularly PAI-1.[217] Recent work suggests that the low-density lipoprotein receptor–related protein may also play a crucial role in regulating the activity of urokinase in human trophoblasts.[218–220] The factors that promote the elaboration of these proteinases may include cytokines such as IL-1β.

The binding of specific extracellular matrix proteins to their integrin receptors on the cell membrane can also regulate cellular migratory activity. The process of trophoblast migration and invasion is associated with predictable switching of specific integrins on the trophoblast mem-

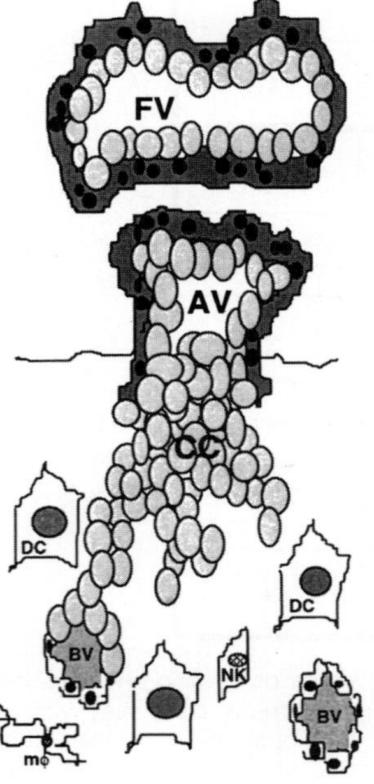

Villous Trophoblasts:

	E-cad	OPN	αv	β3	β5	PECAM-1
Cytotrophoblasts	+	+	-	-	-	-
Syncytiotrophoblasts	-	-	+	+	+	-/+

Extravillous Trophoblasts:

Cytotrophoblast cell column	E-cad	α6	β4	α1	β1	α5	Cellular FN	β3	β5	PECAM-1
Proximal	+	+	+	-	-	-	-	-	-	-
Distal	-	-	-	+	+	+	+	+	-	?+

	PECAM-1	VCAM-1	E-cad	VE-cad	α1	αv	α4	β1	β3	β6
Endovascular trophoblasts	+	+	-	+	+	?	+	+	+	-

Figure 8–19 ■ Schematic of a floating (FV) and an anchoring (AV) chorionic villus and some of the cell adhesion molecules expressed by human villous trophoblasts, trophoblasts of cell columns (CC), and endovascular trophoblasts. E-cad, E-cadherin; VE-cad, vascular endothelial cadherin; PECAM-1, platelet-endothelial cell adhesion molecule 1; VCAM-1, vascular cell adhesion molecule 1; FN, fibronectin; OPN, osteopontin; α1, α4, α5, α6, αv, β1, β3, β5, and β6, integrin subunits; DC, decidual cell; BV, blood vessel; mφ: macrophage; NK, other nonresident cells (e.g., natural killer cells).

branes. Immunohistochemical examination of cytotrophoblast cell columns in human implantation sites demonstrated that the proximal cells of the anchoring villus express $\alpha_6\beta_4$ (laminin receptor).[200, 221] As the trophoblast cells invade, they up-regulate the $\alpha_1\beta_1$ integrin (a collagen/laminin receptor). In vitro studies suggest that this integrin and its binding to type IV collagen or laminin may contribute significantly to the establishment of the invasive phenotype of these cells.[221] In addition, trophoblast cells within the proximal cytotrophoblast cell column also express the α_v integrin subunit. Several β-subunits have been shown to combine with the α_v subunit to form heterodimers with differing effects on cell function in response to adhesion to the same matrix ligand. For example, in vitro functional experiments indicate that binding of $\alpha_v\beta_3$ by some of its several ligands (i.e., vitronectin) mediates the adhesion of the cell to the substratum and up-regulates the expression and activity of type IV collagenases.[222] In addition, the β_3 integrin subunit has been associated with tumor progression and metastasis.[223, 224] A matrix binding to the α_v heterodimers not only mediates the adhesion of the cell to the substratum but also promotes cell migration.[225] These observations make it attractive to hypothesize that in addition to $\alpha_6\beta_4$ and $\alpha_1\beta_1$, α_v integrins may participate in conferring the migratory, invasive phenotype to trophoblast cells.

In contrast to the integrins expressed by the cells of the proximal cytotrophoblast cell column, which have been associated with promotion of the migratory invasive phenotype, cells of the mid and distal column of the anchoring villus have turned off their expression of $\alpha_6\beta_4$ and have up-regulated their expression of the $\alpha_5\beta_1$ integrin[200, 221] and of its specific ligand, fibronectin.[226] In vitro studies have suggested that attachment of human trophoblast cells to fibronectin by the $\alpha_5\beta_1$ integrin inhibits invasion, which has led to the hypothesis that expression of $\alpha_5\beta_1$ and its ligation by fibronectin confer the stationary or noninvasive phenotype to the cells.[221] Abnormal integrin expression has been linked to conditions of pregnancy thought to have their pathogenesis associated with abnormal implantation.[227]

At present, the endometrial factors that contribute to the regulation of the adhesive, migratory, and invasive properties of human trophoblasts are not completely understood. Several proteins capable of binding to integrins known to be expressed by trophoblasts are present in the endometrial milieu. Specifically, laminin and type IV collagen (which bind to $\alpha_6\beta_4$ and $\alpha_1\beta_1$) are integral components of basement membranes, and osteopontin (which binds to α_v integrins) and IGFBP-1 (which can bind to $\alpha_5\beta_1$) are both expressed by secretory endometrium and by the decidua of pregnancy.[107, 192, 213, 228] In addition, several endometrial factors have been shown to regulate the expression of integrins and their ligands by trophoblasts. TGF-β up-regulates cellular fibronectin and M-CSF regulates both fibronectin[91] and its α_5 integrin receptor in these cells.[229] Both of these growth factors are abundantly expressed by the human endometrium. Other factors such as LIF may modulate trophoblast behavior during implantation by as yet uncharacterized molecular mechanisms.[230–232]

Other cell adhesion molecules, such as vascular endothelial cadherin and platelet-endothelial cell adhesion molecule 1 in combination with several integrins, have been proposed to be involved in the invasion of maternal vessels by trophoblasts.[155, 233] A functional role for some of these molecules is suggested by their altered expression in preeclampsia, a condition of abnormal implantation.[234]

EFFECTS OF CONTRACEPTIVE AGENTS AND DEVICES ON THE ENDOMETRIUM

Contraceptive Steroid Hormones

Oral contraceptives produce characteristic atrophic changes in the endometrium.[235] The histologic appearance depends on the length of exposure, the regimen, the steroid content, and to a lesser extent the specific steroidal compounds themselves. In women using combination-type pills, the endometrial glands are narrow, widely spaced, and lined with an atrophic cuboidal epithelium. The thickness of the endometrium is diminished, and mitotic figures are rarely observed. The nuclear channel system and giant mitochondria, which are characteristic of glandular epithelial cells in the secretory phase, are absent. The number of ciliated cells in the luminal epithelium is reduced, as is the number of microvilli on epithelial cell surfaces, which are short and clubbed when present. The stroma shows predecidual changes that depend on the dose of progestin in the pills. Sporadic areas of edema may be present in the stroma. Pills containing steroids with a high progestational potency may cause the stroma to appear "pseudosarcomatous" because of the presence of spindle-shaped stromal cells. Spiral arteries fail to develop. Thrombosis and capillary distention lead to focal stromal hemorrhagic necrosis, resulting in spotting. Multiphasic preparations produce changes in the endometrium similar to those produced by monophasic preparations with the exception that spiral artery development is not inhibited.

Low-dose progestin-only pills initially produce a secretory pattern in the endometrium in approximately 50 percent of users. With prolonged administration, many of the changes seen in the endometrium of combination pill users are found. Irregular bleeding is associated with distended capillary networks and incomplete spiral arteriole development. After 6 months, an atrophic endometrium is present in most users. Progestins administered in a depot injection (medroxyprogesterone 17-acetate) or in implants (levonorgestrel) produce similar changes in the endometrium.

Intrauterine Devices

The endometrium initially responds to foreign bodies with infiltration of polymorphonuclear leukocytes.[236, 237] Microabscesses are occasionally formed. The uterine stroma is compressed by the presence of the device, leading to subsequent fibrosis and plasma cell infiltration. In some instances, chronic inflammatory changes can be intense and extend throughout the endometrium. The inflammatory reaction, although confined in many instances to the area surrounding the device, appears to widely influence the reproductive tract to discourage gamete viability, embryo development, and implantation.

Copper-containing intrauterine devices (IUDs) generally produce the same effects on the endometrium as those of inert devices, although leukocyte infiltration is less with the copper-containing IUDs. The copper leaches from the device and accumulates in the adjacent superficial endometrial layers, where it may affect the function of proteins including enzymes and steroid hormone receptors, contributing to the contraceptive action of the IUD.

Progestagen-containing devices produce atrophic changes surrounding the device, including a reduced number of glands, reduced height of the glandular epithelium during the proliferative phase, and stromal predecidual changes. The normal histologic changes during the cycle near the device are disrupted. The steroids and their metabolites accumulate in the superficial layers of the endometrium adjacent to the device, but little steroid penetrates into the deeper endometrial layers.[238] A reduced number of capillary vessels is found in the endometrium and there is less epithelial surface erosion and microthrombosis of stromal capillaries in women wearing a progestagen-containing IUD compared with inert and copper-containing devices. This may account for the reduced incidence of spotting and menorrhagia associated with progestagen-containing IUDs.

PATHOPHYSIOLOGY OF ENDOMETRIAL AND MYOMETRIAL DYSFUNCTION

Luteal-Phase Defects

Inadequate secretory transformation of the endometrium resulting from deficient ovarian progesterone secretion or possibly an intrinsic uterine defect was first described in 1949 by Jones as a cause of infertility and recurrent abortion.[239–240] In the literature, luteal-phase defects are diagnosed in 3 to 20 percent of infertile patients and 25 to 60 percent of patients with recurrent abortion. They are reported to occur in 20 to 50 percent of anovulatory women treated with clomiphene citrate.[241–249] However, the true incidence of bona fide luteal-phase defects is difficult to assess because of the variation in diagnostic criteria, the relative lack of precision of endometrial dating, and the lack of a clear understanding of the normal variation of endometrial histology and function in fertile women.[250, 251] With the exception of recurrent abortion, luteal-phase defects are not associated with any characteristic symptoms.[252]

Several types of luteal-phase defects have been described: (1) endometrium chronologically out of phase with a luteal phase of normal length; (2) dyssynchronous development of the endometrial glands and stroma; and (3) in-phase endometrium with a curtailed luteal phase (less than 10 days). It is assumed that a lag in chronologic development in the endometrium and glandular-stromal dyssynchrony impair fertility by discouraging implantation.[241] In women with short luteal phases (assessed by basal body temperature), there appears to be a higher incidence of "subclinical abortions" detected by transient appearance of hCG in the blood or urine.

The pathophysiology of luteal-phase defects has been postulated to encompass several different mechanisms, including (1) abnormal follicular development, leading to ovulation failure (luteinized unruptured follicle syndrome); (2) inadequate luteinization and subsequent deficient progesterone secretion; (3) hypocholesterolemia (hypobetalipoproteinemia), causing reduced progesterone secretion as a result of diminished supplies of steroid precursors; and (4) uterine abnormalities disrupting endometrial function, including submucous myomas that may compromise endometrial vascularization, endometritis, and defects in steroid hormone receptors (e.g., variant estrogen receptor).

Abnormal follicular development occurs in the extremes of reproductive life (postmenarchal and premenopausal stages). Hyperprolactinemia, in some cases transient, is thought to be a rare cause of luteal-phase defects as a result of reduced gonadotropin secretion as well as direct inhibitory effects of prolactin on granulosa cell function. Stress and calorie restriction may cause abnormal follicle-stimulating hormone (FSH) and LH release, leading to abnormal follicular growth and luteinization. Tubal ligation and endometriosis have also been implicated in the genesis of luteal-phase defects. However, it is now generally accepted that tubal ligation does not cause luteal-phase abnormalities. The relationships, if any, between luteal-phase defects and endometriosis are a topic of current debate.

Pharmacologic manipulation of ovarian function (e.g., induction of ovulation with GnRH, menopausal gonadotropins, and clomiphene citrate) is associated with luteal-phase deficiency.[253] An incidence of luteal-phase defects, ranging from 25 to 50 percent of cycles, has been claimed in patients treated with clomiphene citrate. This abnormal endometrial maturation is postulated to be a major factor causing the relatively low conception to ovulation ratio and the increased spontaneous abortion rate associated with clomiphene therapy. Suboptimal FSH secretion or an inadequate LH surge in clomiphene-treated women can result in a corpus luteum with deficient secretory function. A direct antiestrogenic effect of clomiphene on the endometrium could also theoretically contribute to altered maturation. However, endometrial steroid hormone receptor levels are not necessarily distorted in clomiphene-treated women.[254] There appears to be no relationship between the dose of clomiphene citrate used and the incidence of out-of-phase endometrium. Thus, the occurrence of luteal-phase defects in clomiphene-treated women may reflect abnormalities in the anovulatory patient rather than intrinsic actions of the drug.

Women with luteal-phase defects are reported to have low FSH levels and low FSH to LH ratios in the early and midfollicular phase. Low serum levels of progesterone and estrogen in the midluteal phase have been found in several studies.[255–257] Analyses of endometrial steroid hormone receptors in women diagnosed with luteal-phase defects have yielded inconsistent results.[258, 259] In a study of sequential biopsies, patients with luteal-phase defects had significantly lower nuclear progesterone receptors in the proliferative phase than did women with normal endometrial maturation, a finding suggestive of diminished estrogenic stimulation of the endometrium. Elevated cytosolic progesterone receptors in secretory endometrium of patients diagnosed with luteal-phase defects have also been reported, a finding consistent with diminished luteal-phase progesterone levels. However, some authors find no significant alterations in endometrial steroid receptors in luteal-phase defects. These divergent results probably reflect the heterogeneity in the populations of patients studied and differences in diagnostic criteria.

On the basis of the assumption that histologic features

accurately reflect tissue function (i.e., the ability to support pregnancy), the primary tool for the diagnosis of luteal-phase defects is the endometrial biopsy taken close to the expected time of menses. As discussed earlier, the precision of endometrial dating by use of the criteria of Noyes and coauthors is such that it is generally accepted that subjects should demonstrate an out-of-phase biopsy result or abnormal luteal-phase length in two consecutive cycles to establish the diagnosis of luteal-phase defect. In view of the occurrence of out-of-phase biopsy results in women of proven fertility, one might conclude that the condition is not necessarily a cause of infertility. Alternatively, one may argue that it is a generalized phenomenon and that it accounts for the failure to conceive in most women; this seems unlikely, given the experience with IVF-ET in which pregnancies occur despite appreciable histologic variation in the endometrium.[260] Thus, the incidence of physiologically significant luteal-phase defects has probably been overstated, particularly when relaxed diagnostic criteria have been employed.

Basal body temperature monitoring can be used to detect short luteal phases, but it cannot diagnose other forms of luteal-phase deficiency. Although reduced progesterone levels have been documented in some patients with luteal-phase defects, random progesterone determinations do not offer sufficient sensitivity and specificity for the diagnosis of the condition. The pulsatile secretion of progesterone in the luteal phase is one factor that diminishes the usefulness of serum progestin assays, causing significant overlap between normal and abnormal values. Multiple sampling (three values between days 4 and 11 before expected menses), which increases the specificity of the approach, is an inconvenient and relatively expensive diagnostic option.[261]

A failure of PEP to rise in serum has been reported in patients with luteal-phase defects. However, this has not achieved wide use as a laboratory test. The application of various immunologic probes for the examination of endometrial biopsy specimens also remains a research tool yet to be proven effective in the diagnosis of luteal-phase defects.

Treatment of luteal-phase defects has been designed to address the suspected cause of the disorder. However, there have been no randomized double-blind controlled studies of sufficient statistical power from which to draw conclusions regarding the efficacy of various protocols.[262] Although numerous studies describe a beneficial response to supplemental progesterone, the small number of patients studied and the varied diagnostic criteria make critical evaluation of the benefits of this treatment impossible. Bromocriptine has been employed to treat hyperprolactinemia associated with luteal-phase defects. Clomiphene is reported to correct spontaneous luteal-phase defects. Treatment with menotropins and addition of hCG to clomiphene therapy are also advocated; the reported success of the latter treatments may be related more to superovulation than to correction of a hormonal imbalance.

Endometriosis

Endometriosis is a common disorder characterized by the presence and proliferation of endometrial tissue outside of the uterine cavity.[263, 264] The glands and stroma of endometriosis are usually responsive to gonadal hormones, although steroid receptor levels are somewhat lower than those in normal endometrium. The biochemical changes in the ectopic endometrium mimic those of the uterine cavity in response to the late luteal–phase decline in progesterone, including increased production of prostanoids, which promote inflammation, fibrosis, and adhesion formation.

The incidence of endometriosis is difficult to assess because lesions exist in many patients without causing symptoms. As a result of increased awareness of the disease, there is a rising reported occurrence. It is estimated that endometriosis affects 10 to 15 percent of all women of reproductive age. In infertile women, the incidence of endometriosis may be as high as 40 to 50 percent. Endometriosis is common in adolescent girls.[265] Asymptomatic as well as symptomatic endometriosis has also been reported in postmenopausal women.[266] Symptoms of abdominal pain, bleeding, and intestinal and urinary tract obstruction may bring the postmenopausal woman to the physician. Because of the relative rarity of this condition, the diagnosis is usually not considered and may occasion radical operative procedures for suspected malignant disease. There appears to be a correlation between postmenopausal endometriosis and relatively high levels of estrogen. Development of symptomatic lesions has been associated with hormone replacement therapy.

The most common site of endometriosis is the pelvis; the ovaries, posterior broad ligament, anterior cul-de-sac, posterior cul-de-sac, and uterosacral ligaments are the structures most often involved. The rectovaginal septum, uterine serosa, cervix, vagina, ileum, appendix, cecum, bladder, and ureters are less frequently affected. Widespread disease enmeshes pelvic organs, peritoneal surfaces, and bowel. Unusual sites of involvement include the umbilicus, laparotomy and episiotomy scars, pleura, lungs, diaphragm, kidney, and spinal canal.

Location, size, and age of the lesions determine the gross appearance of endometriosis. Small fluid-containing vesicles are seen on the surface of the peritoneum early in the disease process. The vesicular fluid turns brown after bleeding has occurred, producing the "powder burn," a puckered black lesion, usually surrounded by a stellate scar. Endometriomas, cysts filled with dark-colored old blood, are characteristic of ovarian involvement. Fibrotic reactions are variable but are prominent when endometriosis involves smooth muscle. Lesions involving large bowel can cause thickening of the muscularis, leading to strictures. Several classifications of endometriosis have been proposed, but the most widely accepted is that endorsed by the American Society for Reproductive Medicine, which was recently revised.[267] Notably, an analysis of pregnancy rates revealed that there is not significant difference in pregnancy rates among the four classifications, indicating that the classification does not adequately assess the anatomic features of endometriosis that have an impact on fertility or that biochemical factors not evaluated in the classification are more important determinants of fertility and fecundity.[268] Levels of CA-125 and PEP, which are frequently found to be elevated in the sera of women with significant disease, can be used to monitor the progress of disease and response to treatment in some patients.

Three main theories have been advanced to explain the

etiology of endometriosis: transplantation of exfoliated endometrial cells, metaplasia of coelomic epithelium, and generation from embryonic rests.[264, 269] Evidence supporting the origin of endometriosis from transplanted exfoliated cells from retrograde menstruation, iatrogenic causes, or vascular and lymphatic spread is most compelling. Dissemination by these routes can account for the occurrence of endometriosis in the most common and rare sites. The evidence supporting this hypothesis includes the common occurrence of retrograde menstruation in ovulatory women; the existence of viable endometrial cells in menstrual fluid; the presence of endometrial cells in fallopian tubes and the peritoneal cavity; and the observation that endometrial tissue can implant and grow within the peritoneal cavity and the abdominal wall.

Regurgitation of menstrual flow through the fallopian tubes is suggested by the appearance of bloody peritoneal dialysates at the time of menses and detection of blood in the peritoneal cavity at laparotomy or laparoscopy performed in the perimenstrual period. Relative hypotonia of the uterotubal junction may permit retrograde flow and thus predispose certain women to the development of endometriosis. Egress of endometrial tissue through the fallopian tubes and the effects of gravity can account for the frequency of lesions in the vicinity of the tubal ostia (i.e., the ovary, uterosacral ligaments, and base of the broad ligaments).

Several other observations are consistent with the origin of endometriosis by transplantation through retrograde flow. Women with endometriosis have shorter cycles and longer duration of menses. Dysmenorrhea, which is produced by increased uterine smooth muscle tone, is associated with endometriosis. Finally, in women with outflow obstruction of the reproductive tract, endometriosis is more likely to develop.

Hematogenous and lymphatic spread can explain the rare occurrence of endometriosis at sites other than the pelvic viscera and peritoneum. Vascular seeding (e.g., during surgery) can account for endometriosis in tissues like lungs, skin, and muscle. The potential for lymphatic spread has been documented by the detection of microscopic endometrial tissue in lymph nodes at autopsy and in lymphadenectomy specimens.

Endometriosis has also been suggested to arise from metaplasia of peritoneal mesothelium. This mechanism may explain the occurrence of endometriosis in women with müllerian agenesis, in postmenopausal subjects, and in women years after hysterectomy. However, there is scant experimental evidence supporting the concept of coelomic metaplasia. Moreover, the distribution of lesions and the preponderance of disease in women of reproductive age are not easily explained by the metaplasia hypothesis.

The development of endometriosis from embryonic rests may account for prostatic endometriosis in men receiving high-dose estrogen therapy. This may arise from the prostatic utricle, which corresponds developmentally to the uterus. However, if this is a general mechanism by which endometriosis is derived, the disease might be expected to occur most frequently along the distribution of müllerian duct precursors, including the urogenital ridges. This clearly is not the case, which argues against genesis from embryonic rests as a primary mechanism.

A role for environmental toxins, including dioxin and dioxin-like compounds, in the pathogenesis of human endometriosis is a topic of current interest.[270] Compounds acting through the aryl hydrocarbon receptor, have been linked to the development of endometriosis in subhuman primates.

Because retrograde menstruation is relatively common, one must search for reasons why endometriosis progresses in some women. There may be a genetic predisposition to endometriosis that is inherited maternally,[271, 272] although more recent reports indicate that the risk for disease susceptibility is polygenic. Immunologic factors, programmed by genetic differences, may cause women to be susceptible to endometriosis.[273–276] Indeed, some investigators have queried whether endometriosis is an immunologic disorder. This has led to the postulation that the development of endometriosis hinges on the balance of retrograde menstruation and cell-mediated cytotoxicity. Infertile women with moderate to severe endometriosis suffer significant depression in cytotoxic lymphocyte response but do not differ from age-matched fertile control subjects in terms of nonspecific immune function. High frequencies of autoantibodies in the peripheral blood and body fluids have also been demonstrated in women with endometriosis. Finally, increased numbers of activated macrophages in the peritoneal cavity are characteristic of endometriosis. The activated monocytes and macrophages produce growth factors that may promote proliferation of the ectopic endometrium and angiogenesis. Once ectopic implants are established, the secretory products of the inflammatory cells may promote disease progression as part of a reinforcing cycle. However, with the exception of the apparent deficiency in cytotoxic T-cell function, the other reported alterations in the immune system may be a result rather than a cause of endometriosis. Nonetheless, the idea of an immunological component to endometriosis is attractive and has been supported by findings in a subhuman primate model. In addition, the immune suppressive action of danazol, an effective treatment for endometriosis, is consistent with this hypothesis. Alternatively, the endometrial tissue may be biochemically distinct in aggressive endometriosis.[277, 278] Evidence for this notion includes the finding that endometrial tissue from patients with endometriosis expresses aromatase, whereas normal endometrium does not. The pattern of integrin expression is also reported to be altered on the endometrium in subjects with endometriosis in that $\alpha_v\beta_3$ integrin is reduced.[279] The patterns of secretory proteins produced and MHC class II antigen expression also differ, suggestive of an intrinsic endometrial abnormality.[280, 281]

The invasive features of aggressive endometriosis suggest parallels with neoplasia. Studies of allelic loss in endometriosis lesions have revealed a significant loss of heterozygosity at candidate loci for tumor suppressor genes including 9p, 11q, and 22q.[282] Moreover, invasive endometriosis tissue has been found to have lost expression of E-cadherin. This is a feature of metastatic cancers.[283] These findings suggest that inactivation of a tumor suppressor gene may play a role in the development of endometriosis.

The relationship between endometriosis and infertility is complex and controversial.[284–287] Although there is no doubt that extensive disease impairs fertility and that infertile women are more likely to have endometriosis than are fertile women, the role of minimal to moderate disease in the etiology of infertility is less clear. A critical review of existing literature reveals that experimental evidence supporting a causal relationship between minimal to moderate endometriosis and infertility is sparse. The lack of clear temporal and dose-response relationships between onset and extent of disease and infertility call into question claims based on retrospective analyses that less extensive disease is a major cause of infertility. Indeed, conclusions from poorly controlled studies have not been confirmed on more rigorous evaluation. Work of Guzick and coworkers has attempted to address some of these issues in a more comprehensive and scientific manner.[268]

Prostanoids, thought to be produced by the ectopic endometrial tissue and activated macrophages, figure prominently in the theories of how endometriosis might disrupt normal reproductive processes. Significantly elevated levels of prostanoids, including PGE_2 and metabolites of prostacyclin (6-keto-$PGF_{1\alpha}$) and thromboxane B_2, are found in peritoneal fluid of women with endometriosis.[288] In addition, endometriotic tissue produces complement component 3, which can yield chemotactic peptides as well as play a role in macrophage activation, promoting release of monokines and lymphokines that may also disrupt crucial events in conception.

Luteinized unruptured follicles and luteal-phase defects have been reported to be prevalent in women with endometriosis. It has been suggested that failure of follicular rupture results from a deficiency of LH receptors caused perhaps by the action of prostaglandins in the peritoneal fluid and in endometriosis implants around the tubes. However, there is no direct evidence that eicosanoids at the concentrations reported have any significant effect on human ovarian or tubal physiology.

Peritoneal fluids of patients with endometriosis reduce survival of sperm and are embryotoxic in the mouse embryo bioassay system. Substances released by endometrium and inflammatory cells, including monokines and cytokines such as TNF-α, IL-1, IL-6, and IL-8 are believed to be responsible for these observations. Factors released from macrophages also inhibit sperm penetration of zona-free hamster ova. Although these data suggest mechanisms for impaired infertility, they are derived from in vitro studies and rely heavily on animal models, which may not be relevant to human reproductive processes.

Endometrial Neoplasia

Endometrial Hyperplasia and Carcinoma

HYPERPLASIA

There is a substantial literature indicating that endometrial hyperplasia is a precursor to endometrial malignant neoplasia, particularly when changes such as nuclear atypia and complex glandular crowding are present.[289, 290] The prevailing notion has been that endometrial hyperplasias represent a histologic and biologic continuum extending from exaggerated proliferation of normal endometrium to carcinoma in situ. This concept is consonant with the coexistence of adenocarcinoma and hyperplasia. Unfortunately, the literature on endometrial hyperplasia has suffered from a profusion of classifications and definitions that have made comparisons between study populations difficult. The International Society of Gynecologic Pathologists has proposed a classification based on the architecture of glands and cytologic features of the cells. The hyperplasias are described as either simple or complex, depending on the extent of proliferation and crowding of the glands. The cytologic evaluation is based on nuclear features. Cytologic atypia is characterized by large round nuclei with prominent nucleoli. Simple hyperplasia is characterized by proliferation of glands and stroma where the glands are round and regular or focally dilated (cystic hyperplasia). Complex hyperplasia, or adenomatous hyperplasia without atypia, is defined as glandular crowding without cytologic atypia. Nuclear atypia is often found in association with stratification of glandular cells and loss of polarity. Other features of this seemingly more aggressive type of hyperplasia include abundant and eosinophilic cytoplasm and ultrastructural modifications, such as irregular cytoplasmic membranes, distended nuclear membranes, and reduced cilia and microvilli.

Reports have demonstrated an impressive rate of progression of endometrial hyperplasia with cytologic atypia to carcinoma (24 to 57 percent of patients). In contrast, there is a relatively low likelihood of progression of simple or complex hyperplasia without atypia to cancer. In one large study, less than 2 percent of women who had been diagnosed with endometrial hyperplasia without atypia subsequently developed cancer more than 1 year after the diagnosis of hyperplasia was made, whereas 23 percent of the subjects with hyperplasia and cellular atypia developed cancer. This has led some investigators to consider hyperplasia with cellular atypia as a separate biologic lesion distinguished from other histologic forms with lower potential for malignant change. The existing data on the effects of estrogens on endometrial neoplasia (see later) are best interpreted in the context of lesions having differing biologic potential for malignant behavior.

Endometrial epithelial metaplasias, defined as the replacement of endometrial epithelium by another type not normally found in the endometrium (i.e., squamous, tubal, papillary, eosinophilic, and clear cell types), bear superficial resemblance to endometrial hyperplasia with cellular atypia. Endometrial metaplasia and hyperplasia may coexist, and the microscopic differentiation between the two is based on histologic patterns and cytologic alterations (e.g., nuclear pleomorphism, nuclear polarity, mitoses). Endometrial metaplasias are identified most frequently in postmenopausal or perimenopausal women taking exogenous estrogen. They can also be found in young, often infertile women with unopposed estrogen (e.g., polycystic ovary syndrome). Although opinions vary as to the biologic meaning of the endometrial metaplasias, these lesions do not appear to have great clinical significance.

CARCINOMA

Adenocarcinoma is the most common form of uterine cancer. These tumors frequently have foci of squamous metaplasia; less frequently, both components are malignant (adenosquamous carcinoma). Tumor grade, which is assessed in the glandular component only, is a significant prognostic factor. The presence of squamous metaplasia has no prognostic significance. Risk factors identified in existing literature for the development of endometrial cancer include nulliparity, late menopause, radiation to the pelvis, obesity, diabetes, and exogenous estrogen use. The correlation between endometrial cancer and obesity may relate to the twofold to threefold greater production of estrogens in obese women as a result of extraglandular aromatization of adrenal androgens by adipose stromal tissue; the storage of estrogen esters in adipose tissue; and the association of obesity with reduced sex hormone–binding globulin levels, permitting increased metabolism of circulating androgens and greater bioavailability of generated estrogens. Use of combination-type oral contraceptives may reduce the risk of endometrial cancer.

The histologic diagnosis of early adenocarcinoma of the endometrium is difficult in the absence of frank invasion of the stroma. Intraglandular bridges lacking stromal support and cribriforming of the epithelial cells are associated with stromal invasion. Assessment of nuclear DNA content by flow cytometry has been of limited value in distinguishing malignant lesions, because many endometrial cancers have diploid or nearly diploid DNA contents, in contrast to other nonhematologic cancers, which are associated with a far greater incidence of aneuploidy.

Genetic abnormalities are found in many endometrial cancers that in some cases correlate with tumor progression.[291–293] An inactivating mutation in the *KRAS* gene has been found in 10 to 20 percent of premalignant endometrial hyperplasias and invasive cancers. Mutations that inactivate the tumor suppressor gene *P53* are found in 10 to 20 percent of advanced tumors, and the *ERBB2* oncogene is overexpressed in 10 percent of tumors. In addition, allelic deletions in a number of chromosomes have been reported (10q and 14q), with loss of heterozygosity at 14q being strongly correlated with poor outcome. The tumor suppressor gene located on 10q23-q26 may be the PTEN1 gene, a gene that is mutated in a variety of cancers including primary endometrial cancer.

Steroid hormone receptors have been quantified in endometrial cancers. Progesterone receptors are frequently found in primary endometrial tumors, with the presence and level of receptors being correlated with the tumor grade. The majority of well-differentiated tumors (approximately 50 percent) contain receptors, whereas the undifferentiated tumors express receptors less frequently (33 percent). There has been a survival advantage in women whose tumors were progesterone receptor–positive. Although there are relatively few studies that examine the predictive value of steroid receptor analyses with respect to response to hormone therapy, there appears to be a relationship. The overall response rate to hormone therapy is about 34 percent.

Estrogens and Endometrial Hyperplasia and Carcinoma

The dose- and duration-dependent development of endometrial hyperplasia in women receiving estrogen has been well documented.[293, 294] A significant percentage of women with granulosa theca cell ovarian tumors have cystic and adenomatous hyperplasia, and 9 percent are diagnosed with endometrial carcinoma. Endometrial hyperplasia is also more prevalent in anovulatory women with polycystic ovary syndrome whose endometrium is chronically exposed to unopposed estrogens. In the 1970s, case-control and cohort epidemiologic studies pointed out a relationship between endometrial cancer and exogenous estrogens. Cramer and Knapp[294] concluded that the cumulative risk of endometrial cancer in postmenopausal women older than 50 years is 7 percent after 15 years of estrogen treatment, whereas it is less than 1 percent among those not exposed to estrogens. Meta-analyses of published studies confirm an increased risk of endometrial cancer with long duration of unopposed estrogen use.[295] However, tumors that have occurred in women receiving exogenous estrogens have usually been stage I, grade I lesions and have been associated infrequently with myometrial invasion. Thus, survival with endometrial cancer is greater in women diagnosed with endometrial cancers who are estrogen users compared with those who are nonusers.

Early investigators suggested that estrone was more likely than estradiol or estriol to promote endometrial carcinoma on the basis of first retrospective epidemiologic studies suggesting an association between exogenous estrogens and endometrial malignant neoplasia in which most women had received conjugated estrogens, which are approximately 65 percent estrone sulfate. However, it is evident that equivalent doses of conjugated estrogens and estradiol produce the same degree of endometrial stimulation and the same incidence of hyperplasia.[296] The administration of estriol to women in regimens that take into account its rapid absorption and metabolic clearance has been associated with the development of endometrial hyperplasia as well. Moreover, no significant differences in the effects of estradiol on the endometrium are found when it is administered with or without estriol, dispelling the notion that estriol protects against estradiol-induced endometrial stimulation. Although natural estrogens do not appear to have selective actions on the endometrium, some pharmacological agents do show tissue selectivity. Raloxifene exerts estrogenic effects on bone and lipid profiles but is an estrogen antagonist in the uterus. Conversely, the antiestrogen tamoxifen, used in the treatment of estrogen-dependent breast cancer, promotes endometrial hyperplasia.

THE IMPACT OF PROGESTAGENS

Progestins reduce endometrial estrogen receptor content and induce 17β-hydroxysteroid dehydrogenases, which convert estradiol to estrone, and sulfotransferase, which converts estrogens to inactive sulfates. The impact of progestagens on the endometrial response to exogenous estrogens has been documented in several clinical studies. Whitehead and Fraser[296] found that the incidence of endometrial hyperplasia ranges from 16 to 32 percent in women treated with cyclic estrogens but that progestagen treatment for 7 days each month reduces the incidence of hyperplasia to 3 to 4 percent. Studd and Thom[297] found that extending progestagen treatment to 10 days reduces the incidence even further (2 percent), and treatment for 13 days per month reduces the incidence to zero. A 9-year prospective study indicated that women treated with combinations of estrogen and progestin have a significantly lower incidence of endometrial cancer than do estrogen users and untreated women.

PREDICTION OF RISK AND MONITORING RESPONSE TO REPLACEMENT THERAPY

Several strategies have been suggested to identify women at risk for development of endometrial cancer who are receiving exogenous hormone therapy and to monitor endometrial changes during replacement. Endometrial biopsy remains the standard tool. Various methods for obtaining endometrial samples for cytologic analysis have been developed, including saline lavage, brush cytology, vacuum aspiration, and jet washing. However, the reliability of these methods has been questioned (high incidence of unsatisfactory specimens and false-negative results), raising sufficient concern to preclude their use in lieu of traditional endometrial biopsy. Pretreatment biopsy specimens reveal a low incidence of premalignant lesions, and one can question the cost-effectiveness of biopsy as a screening test before replacement therapy. Sonohysterography and hysteroscopy also have a place in the evaluation of women receiving hormone replacement therapy who develop unscheduled bleeding.

Dysmenorrhea

Primary dysmenorrhea, menstrual pain not associated with recognizable pelvic disease, is due to intrinsic uterine dysfunction. Occurring only in ovulatory cycles, the symptoms of dysmenorrhea usually commence a few hours before the onset of the menstrual flow. Pain is greatest when the endometrium is shedding rapidly, approximately 12 hours after flow begins. The diagnosis of primary dysmenorrhea is based on medical history and normal findings on pelvic and rectovaginal examination.

The painful cramps of dysmenorrhea are associated with uterine contractions; in women with dysmenorrhea, uterine contractile activity is heightened during menses, and basal myometrial tone and amplitude of contractions are increased. During intense contractions, there is a reduction in blood flow to the endometrium, suggesting that ischemia, in part, causes the pain of dysmenorrhea.

The uterine contractions are prompted by prostaglandins, which are potent uterotonic agents both in vitro and in vivo acting through cell surface prostaglandin receptors.[21] Prostanoids may also directly sensitize uterine pain fibers. The notion that prostanoids are central to the pathogenesis of dysmenorrhea is supported by the observations that eicosanoids, most prominently $PGF_{2\alpha}$, are found in high concentrations in menstrual fluid and that $PGF_{2\alpha}$ levels are higher in the endometrium and menstrual fluid of women complaining of dysmenorrhea than in women with pain-free menses.[22] All drugs effective in inhibiting prostaglandin synthesis, including the potent nonsteroidal anti-inflammatory drugs ibuprofen, naproxen, and mefenamic acid, alleviate symptoms of dysmenorrhea.[298] Calcium antagonists, such as nifedipine, are also effective because they prevent uterine contraction. Combination-type oral contraceptives, which reduce endometrial mass and thus total endometrial prostaglandin synthesis, prevent dysmenorrhea in 90 percent of cases.

In addition to prostanoids, other uterotonic substances including lipoxygenase products, vasopressin, and oxytocin may have a role in dysmenorrhea. Thus, antagonists of the V_1 receptor and oxytocin receptor have a therapeutic effect in dysmenorrheic subjects. Reductions in nitric oxide (NO), which relaxes uterine smooth muscle, may also contribute to the intensified contractions associated with dysmenorrhea.[299]

Uterine Leiomyomas

Leiomyomas are monoclonal tumors that occur in up to 30 percent of women of reproductive age. The pathogenesis of these growths appears to be rooted in the actions of steroid hormones, genetic alterations in the leiomyoma cells, and possibly abnormal cell–extracellular matrix interactions.[300]

Leiomyomas are responsive to both estrogens and progestins; they shrink in volume after menopause or with suppression of ovarian function through use of desensitizing GnRH agonist therapy. Evidence for estrogen regulation of leiomyoma growth beyond the clinical observations includes the finding that leiomyomas have an increased concentration of estrogen receptors compared with normal myometrium isolated from the same uterus.

The action of progestins on leiomyomas has been debated in the literature. Published clinical observations and in vitro studies collectively favor the view that progestins increase leiomyoma growth. Progesterone receptors appear to be more abundant in leiomyomas than in adjacent myometrium. The A form of the progesterone receptor predominates. In support of this view, the peak mitotic activity in the normal myometrium and leiomyomas is detected during the luteal phase. A number of clinical studies suggest that progestins increase leiomyoma growth and that the antiprogestin RU 486 causes a significant reduction in tumor volume.[301]

The actions of steroid hormones on leiomyoma growth may be either direct or mediated through the action of locally produced growth factors. Leiomyoma cells express EGF, TGF-β, PDGF, IGF-I, and IGF-II and their receptors. The density of IGF-I receptors is greater in leiomyomas than in normal myometrium. GnRH agonist treatment reduces the EGF receptor, TGF-β and TGF-β receptor contents of leiomyomas, and their production of IGF-I and IGF-II. These observations are consistent with the idea that local growth factors produced in response to steroid hormones contribute to leiomyoma growth. A novel leiomyoma-derived growth factor with homology to cysteine-rich protein has been extracted from human myomas. In contrast, in vitro studies of cultured normal myometrial cells and leiomyoma cells reveal that the normal cells are more responsive to exogenous growth factors.

Although GnRH agonists cause a hypoestrogenemic state through the suppression of pituitary gonadotropin secretion that is associated with shrinkage of myomas, the GnRH analogues may also have a direct effect on the tumors. Leiomyomas express the genes encoding both GnRH and the GnRH receptor, and GnRH treatment reportedly reduces thymidine incorporation into myometrial cells in culture and blocks the effects of estrogen and progestins on myometrial cell proliferation.

Expression of the cell survival gene *BCL2* is significantly increased in leiomyomas.[302] The increased levels of *BCL2* may inhibit the normal programmed cell death cycles, extending the life span of the leiomyoma cells. Progesterone treatment up-regulates *BCL2* expression in cultured leiomyoma cells.

The abnormal growth of leiomyoma cells has a genetic component, which may be acquired as a consequence of increased proliferative activity of leiomyoma precursor cells. Distinct cytogenetic abnormalities are frequently observed in leiomyomas, mostly involving chromosomes 7 (7q21–32), 12 (12q14–15), and 14 (14q21–24).[303] The chromosomal rearrangements in bands 12q14–15 are of particular interest because these are also found in other mesenchymal tumors (e.g., lipomas). A member of the high-mobility group family of DNA-binding proteins, HMGI-C, encoded by a gene located on 12q14–15, appears to be involved in growth regulation. Rearrangements at 12q14–15 affecting the gene encoding HMGI-C where the HMGI-C DNA binding domain fuses to a *trans*-activation domain, producing a transcription factor that promotes benign neoplastic growth.[304] Another related protein, HMG(Y), may also be involved in leiomyoma formation.[305]

Leiomyomas contain an abundant collagenous extracellular matrix accounting for their designation as fibroid tumors. The change in tumor volume after induction of hypoestrogenemia with GnRH agonists is due mostly to a shrinkage in the leiomyoma cells, not the extracellular matrix. Leiomyomas contain 50 percent more collagen, mostly type I collagen, than does normal myometrial tissue. Mutations in the paired COL4A5 and COL4A6 collagen genes, which reside on the X chromosome, are also associated with diffuse leiomyomatosis, demonstrating that the extracellular matrix can exert important regulatory control on uterine smooth muscle growth.[306]

Adenomyosis

The presence of endometrial glands and stroma deep within the myometrium is not an infrequent finding on histologic examination of hysterectomy specimens.[307] However, the histologic criteria for diagnosis of adenomyosis vary; some pathologists hold that ectopic glands and stroma should be located 2 to 3 mm below the endometrial surface, and others define adenomyosis as glands and stroma invading the myometrium to the depth of at least one third of the thickness of the uterine wall. The glands of adenomyosis are derived from the basal layer. With extensive adenomyosis, the uterus is moderately enlarged, boggy, or nodular in consistency.

Adenomyosis is most common in parous women in the fourth or fifth decade, with an incidence variably reported from 5 to 70 percent. The substantial difference in incidence probably reflects different diagnostic criteria. The most widely accepted idea is that obstetric trauma or postpartum endomyometritis causes a breakdown of the endometrium-myometrium border, allowing penetration of glands into the myometrium. An estrogenic milieu may also be permissive to the development of adenomyosis, and medical therapy that produces a hypoestrogenemic state or antagonizes estrogen action may be effective in some cases (e.g., danazol and GnRH analogues).

References

1. O'Rahilly R. Prenatal human development. *In* Wynn RA, Jollie PA. Biology of the Uterus. New York, Plenum Publishing, 1989, p 35.
2. Szamborski J, Laskowska H. Some observations on the developmental histology of the human foetal uterus. Biol Neonate 13:298, 1968.
3. Yeh J, Thiet M-P, Laohaprasitiporn C, et al. Growth factors in the fetal uterus. Semin Reprod Endocrinol 13:102, 1995.
4. Taylor HS, Vandem GB, Igarashi P. A conserved Hox axis in the mouse and human female reproductive system: Late establishment and persistent adult expression of the Hoxa cluster genes. Biol Reprod 57:1338, 1997.
5. Hsieh-Li HM, Witte DP, Weinstein M, et al. Hoxa 11 structure, extensive antisense transcription, and function in male and female fertility. Development 121:1373, 1995.
6. Greco TL, Duello TM, Gorski J. Estrogen receptors, estradiol, and diethylstilbestrol in early development: The mouse as a model for the study of estrogen receptors and estrogen sensitivity in embryonic development of male and female reproductive tracts. Endocr Rev 14:59, 1993.
7. Cunha GR, Chung LQK, Shannon JM, et al. Hormone-induced morphogenesis and growth: Role of mesenchymal-epithelial interactions. Recent Prog Horm Res 39:559, 1983.

7a. Cooke PS, Buchanan DL, Young P, et al. Stromal estrogen receptors mediate mitogenic effects of estradiol on uterine epithelium. Proc Natl Acad Sci USA 94:6535, 1997.

8. Wynn RM. Histology and ultrastructure of the human endometrium. *In* Wynn RM. Biology of the Uterus. New York, Plenum Publishing, 1977, pp 341–376.
9. Martel D, Frydman R, Sarantis L, et al. Scanning electron microscopy of the uterine luminal epithelium as a marker of the implantation window. *In* Yoshinaga K. Blastocyst Implantation. Boston, Adams Publishing Group, 1989, p 225.
10. Aplin JD, Charlton AK, Ayad S. An immunohistochemical study of human endometrial extracellular matrix during the menstrual cycle and first trimester of pregnancy. Cell Tissue Res 253:231, 1988.
11. Iwahashi M, Muragaki Y, Ooshima A, et al. Alterations in distribution and composition of the extracellular matrix during decidualization of the human endometrium. J Reprod Fertil 108:147, 1996.
12. Schatz F, Aigner S, Papp C, et al. Plasminogen activator activity during decidualization of human endometrial stromal cells is regulated by plasminogen activator inhibitor 1. J Clin Endocrinol Metab 80:2504, 1995.
13. Lockwood CH, Nemerson Y, Krikun G, et al. Steroid-modulated stromal cell tissue factor expression: A model for the regulation of endometrial hemostasis and menstruation. J Clin Endocrinol Metab 77:1014, 1993.
14. Markee JE. Menstruation in intraocular endometrial transplants in the rhesus monkey. Contrib Embryol 28:219, 1940.
15. Kokawa K, Shikone T, Nakano R. Apoptosis in the human uterine endometrium during the menstrual cycle. J Clin Endocrinol Metab 81:4144, 1996.
16. Marbaix E, Kokorine I, Moulin P, et al. Menstrual breakdown of human endometrium can be mimicked in vitro and is selectively and reversibly blocked by inhibitors of matrix metalloproteinases. Proc Natl Acad Sci USA 93:9120, 1996.
17. Rodgers WH, Matrisian LM, Giudice LC, et al. Patterns of matrix metalloproteinase expression in cycling endometrium imply differential functions and regulation by steroid hormones. J Clin Invest 94:946, 1994.
18. Irwin JC, Kirk D, Gwatkin RB, et al. Human endometrial matrix metalloproteinase-2, a putative menstrual proteinase. Hormonal regulation in cultured stromal cells and messenger RNA expression during the menstrual cycle. J Clin Invest 97:438, 1996.
19. Casslen B, Andersson A, Milsson IM, et al. Hormonal regulation of the release of plasminogen activators and of a specific activator inhibitor from endometrial tissue in culture. Proc Soc Exp Biol Med 182:419, 1986.
20. Head JR, MacDonald PC, Casey ML. Cellular localization of membrane metalloendopeptidase (enkephalinase) in human endometrium during the ovarian cycle. J Clin Endocrinol Metab 76:769, 1993.
21. Akerlund A. Vascularization of human endometrium. Uterine blood flow in healthy condition and in primary dysmenorrhoea. Ann N Y Acad Sci 734:47, 1994.
22. Bieglmayer C, Hofer G, Kainz C, et al. Concentrations of various

arachidonic acid metabolites in menstrual fluid are associated with menstrual pain and are influenced by hormonal contraceptives. Gynecol Endocrinol 9:307, 1995.
23. Casey ML, Hemsell DL, MacDonald PC, et al. NAD$^+$ dependent 15-hydroxy prostaglandin dehydrogenase activity in human endometrium. Prostaglandins 19:115, 1980.
24. Fraser IS, McCarron G, Hutton B, et al. Endometrial blood flow measured by xenon 133 clearance in women with normal menstrual cycles and dysfunctional uterine bleeding. Am J Obstet Gynecol 156:158, 1987.
25. Kapesic S, Kurjak A. Uterine and ovarian perfusion during the periovulatory period assessed by transvaginal color Doppler. Fertil Steril 60:439, 1993.
26. Gannon BJ, Corati CJ, Vecco CJ. Endometrial perfusion across the normal human menstrual cycle assessed by laser Doppler fluximetry. Hum Reprod 12:132, 1997.
27. Hertig AT. Gestational hyperplasia of endometrium: A morphologic correlation of ova, endometrium, and corpora lutea during early pregnancy. Lab Invest 31:1153, 1964.
28. Mazur MT, Duncan DA, Younger JB. Endometrial biopsy in the cycle of conception: Histologic and lectin histochemical evaluation. Fertil Steril 51:764, 1989.
29. Thrasher TV, Richart TM. Ultrastructure of the Arias-Stella reaction. Am J Obstet Gynecol 112:113, 1972.
30. Arias-Stella J. Atypical endometrial changes associated with presence of chorionic tissue. Arch Pathol 58:112, 1954.
31. Fazleabas AT, Hild-Petito S, Verhage HG. The primate endometrium. Morphological and secretory changes during early pregnancy—implications of the insulin-like growth factor axis. Semin Reprod Endocrinol 13:120, 1995.
32. Kamat BR, Isaacson PG. The immunocytochemical distribution of leukocytic subpopulations in human endometrium. Am J Pathol 127:66, 1987.
33. Whitelaw PF, Croy BA. Granulated lymphocytes of pregnancy. Placenta 17:533, 1996.
34. Tabibzadeh S. Cytokines and endometrial microenvironments. Semin Reprod Endocrinol 13:133, 1995.
35. Hunt JS. Immunologically relevant cells in the uterus. Biol Reprod 50:461, 1994.
36. Guimond M-J, Luross JA, Wang B, et al. Absence of natural killer cells during murine pregnancy is associated with reproductive compromise in TgE26 mice. Biol Reprod 56:169, 1997.
37. Kunz G, Beil D, Deininger H, et al. The dynamics of rapid sperm transport through the female genital tract: Evidence from vaginal sonography of uterine peristalsis and hysterosalpingoscintigraphy. Hum Reprod 11:627, 1996.
38. Chalubinski K, Deutinger J, Bernaschek G. Vaginosonography for recording of cycle-related myometrial contractions. Fertil Steril 59:225, 1993.
39. Itland MM, Evers JLH, Dengelman GAJ, et al. Relation between endometrial wavelike activity and fecundability in spontaneous cycles. Fertil Steril 67:492, 1997.
40. Noyes RW, Hertig AT, Rock J. Dating the endometrial biopsy. Fertil Steril 1:3, 1950.
41. Psychoyos A. Hormonal control of ovoimplantation. Vitam Horm 31:201, 1973.
42. Bergh PA, Navot D. The impact of embryonic development and endometrial maturity on the timing of implantation. Fertil Steril 58:537, 1992.
43. Wentz AC, Jones GS. Endometrial biopsy in the evaluation of infertility. Fertil Steril 33:121, 1980.
44. Wentz AC, Kossoy LR, Parker RA. The impact of luteal phase inadequacy in an infertile population. Am J Obstet Gynecol 162:937, 1990.
45. Castelbaum AJ, Wheeler J, Coutifaris C, et al. Timing of the endometrial biopsy may be critical for the accurate diagnosis of luteal phase deficiency. Fertil Steril 61:443, 1994.
46. Scott RT, Snyder RR, Strickland DM, et al. The effect of interobserver variation in dating endometrial histology on the diagnosis of luteal phase defects. Fertil Steril 50:888, 1988.
47. Li T-C, Dockery P, Rogers AW, et al. How precise is histologic dating of endometrium using the standard dating criteria? Fertil Steril 51:759, 1989.
48. Dockery P, Li T-C, Rogers AW, et al. An examination of the variation in timed endometrial biopsies. Hum Reprod 3:715, 1988.
49. Gibson M, Badger GJ, Byrn F, et al. Error in histologic dating of secretory endometrium: Variance component analysis. Fertil Steril 56:242, 1991.
50. Shoupe D, Mishell DR Jr, Lacarra M, et al. Correlation of endometrial maturation with four methods of estimating day of ovulation. Obstet Gynecol 73:88, 1989.
51. Li T-C, Rogers AW, Lenton EA, et al. A comparison between two methods of chronological dating of human endometrial biopsies during the luteal phase, and their correlation with histologic dating. Fertil Steril 48:928, 1987.
52. Li T-C, Rogers AW, Dockery P, et al. A new method of histologic dating of human endometrium in the luteal phase. Fertil Steril 50:52, 1988.
53. Dockery P, Warren MA, Li T-C, et al. A morphometric study of the human endometrial stroma during the peri-implantation period. Hum Reprod 5:112, 1990.
54. Andoh K, Mizunuma H, Nakazato Y, et al. Endometrial dating in the conception cycle. Fertil Steril 58:1127, 1992.
55. Navot D, Anderson TL, Droesch K, et al. Hormonal manipulation of endometrial maturation. J Clin Endocrinol Metab 68:801, 1989.
56. Navot D, Laufer N, Kopolovic J, et al. Artificially induced endometrial cycles and establishment of pregnancies in the absence of ovaries. N Engl J Med 314:806, 1986.
57. Askel S. Sporadic and recurrent luteal phase defects in cyclic women: Comparison with normal cycles. Fertil Steril 33:372, 1980.
58. Balasch J, Vanrell JA. Corpus luteum insufficiency in fertility: A matter of controversy. Hum Reprod 2:557, 1987.
59. Li T-C, Cooke ID. Evaluation of the luteal phase. Hum Reprod 6:484, 1991.
60. Balasch J, Creus M, Marquez M, et al. The significance of luteal phase deficiency on infertility: A diagnostic and therapeutic approach. Hum Reprod 1:145, 1986.
61. Davis OK, Berkeley AS, Naus GJ, et al. The incidence of luteal phase defect in normal, fertile women, determined by serial endometrial biopsies. Fertil Steril 51:582, 1989.
62. Hecht BR, Bardawil WA, Khan-Dawood FS, et al. Luteal insufficiency: Correlation between endometrial dating and integrated progesterone output in clomiphene citrate–induced cycles. Am J Obstet Gynecol 163:1986, 1990.
63. Li T-C, Dockery P, Rogers AW, et al. A quantitative study of endometrial development in the luteal phase: Comparison between women with unexplained infertility and normal fertility. Br J Obstet Gynaecol 97:576, 1990.
64. Grunfeld L, Sandler B, Fox J, et al. Luteal phase deficiency after completely normal follicular and periovulatory phases. Fertil Steril 52:919, 1989.
65. Batista MC, Cartledge TP, Merino MJ, et al. Midluteal phase endometrial biopsy does not accurately predict luteal function. Fertil Steril 59:294, 1993.
66. Glissant A, de Mouzon J, Frydman R. Ultrasound study of the endometrium during in vitro fertilization cycles. Fertil Steril 44:786, 1985.
67. Graham D, Chung SN. Office sonohysterography. *In* Rock JA, Faro S, Gant NF, et al. Advances in Obstetrics and Gynecology, Vol 4. St. Louis, CV Mosby, 1997, p 137.
68. Wiczyk HP, Janus CL, Richards CJ, et al. Comparison of magnetic resonance imaging and ultrasound in evaluating follicular and endometrial development throughout the normal cycle. Fertil Steril 49:969, 1988.
69. Hysteroscopy. Obstet Gynecol Clin North Am 22:1, 1995.
70. Gurpide E. Enzyme modulation of hormonal action at the target tissue. J Toxicol Environ Health 4:249, 1978.
71. Tseng L, Mazella J. Cyclic changes of estradiol metabolic enzymes in human endometrium during the menstrual cycle. *In* Kimball FA. The Endometrium. New York, SP Medical and Scientific Books, 1980, pp 211–226.
72. Strott CA. Steroid sulfotransferases. Endocr Rev 17:670, 1996.
73. Andersson S. 17β-Hydroxysteroid dehydrogenase: Isozymes and mutations. J Endocrinol 146:197, 1995.
74. Luu-The V, Zhang Y, Poirier D, et al. Characteristics of human types 1, 2 and 3 17β-hydroxysteroid dehydrogenase activities: Oxidation/reduction and inhibition. J Steroid Biochem Mol Biol 55:581, 1995.
75. Noble LS, Simpson ER, Johns A, Bulun SE. Aromatase expression in endometriosis. J Clin Endocrinol Metab 81:174, 1996.

76. Lessey BA, Killam AP, Metzger DA, et al. Immunohistochemical analysis of human uterine estrogen and progesterone receptors throughout the menstrual cycle. J Clin Endocrinol Metab 67:334, 1988.
77. Levy C, Robel P, Gautray JP, et al. Estradiol and progesterone receptors in human endometrium: Normal and abnormal cycles and early pregnancy. Am J Obstet Gynecol 136:646, 1980.
78. Press MF, Udove JA, Greene GL. Progesterone receptor distribution in the human endometrium. Am J Pathol 131:112, 1988.
79. Viville B, Charnock-Jones DS, Sharkey AM, et al. Distribution of the A and B forms of the progesterone receptor messenger ribonucleic acid and protein in uterine leiomyomata and adjacent myometrium. Hum Reprod 12:815, 1997.
80. Lubahn DB, Moyer JS, Golding TS, et al. Alteration of reproduction function but not prenatal sexual development after insertional disruption of the mouse estrogen receptor gene. Proc Natl Acad Sci USA 90:11162, 1993.
81. Dichson RB, Lippman ME. Estrogenic regulation of growth and polypeptide growth factor secretion in human breast carcinoma. Endocr Rev 8:29, 1989.
82. Beato M. Gene regulation by steroid hormones. Cell 56:335, 1989.
83. Odom LD, Varrett JM, Pantazis CG, et al. Immunocytochemical study of *ras* and *myc* proto-oncogene polypeptide expression in the human menstrual cycle. Am J Obstet Gynecol 161:1663, 1989.
84. Lydon JP, DeMayo FJ, Funk CR, et al. Mice lacking progesterone receptor exhibit pleiotropic reproductive abnormalities. Genes Dev 9:2266, 1995.
85. Ferenczy A, Bertrand G, Gelfand MM. Proliferation kinetics of human endometrium during the normal menstrual cycle. Am J Obstet Gynecol 133:859, 1979.
86. Hill JA. Cytokines considered critical in pregnancy. Am J Reprod Immunol 28:123, 1992.
87. Rutanen EM. Cytokines in reproduction. Ann Med 25:343, 1993.
88. Giudice LC, Saleh W. Growth factors in reproduction. Trends Endocrinol Metab 6:60, 1995.
89. Ohlsson R. Growth factors, protooncogenes and human placental development. Cell Differ Dev 28:1, 1989.
90. Sharkey AM, Dellow K, Blayney M, et al. Stage-specific expression of cytokine and receptor messenger ribonucleic acids in human preimplantation embryos. Biol Reprod 53:974, 1995.
91. Adams JC, Watt FM. Regulation of development and differentiation by the extracellular matrix. Development 117:1183, 1993.
92. Adamson ED. Activities of growth factors in preimplantation embryos. J Cell Biochem 53:280, 1993.
93. Santala P, Heino J. Regulation of integrin-type cell adhesion receptors by cytokines. J Biol Chem 266:23505, 1991.
94. Wahl SM, Allen JB, Weeks BS, et al. Transforming growth factor beta enhances integrin expression and type IV collagenase secretion in human monocytes. Proc Natl Acad Sci USA 90:4577, 1993.
95. Zambruno G, Marchisio PC, Marconi A, et al. Transforming growth factor-β1 modulates β_1 and β_5 integrin receptors and induces the de novo expression of the $\alpha_v\beta_6$ heterodimer in normal human keratinocytes: Implications for wound healing. J Cell Biol 129:853, 1995.
96. Roberts AB, Sporn MB. Differential expression of TGF-beta isoforms in embryogenesis suggests specific roles in developing and adult tissues. Mol Reprod Dev 32:91, 1992.
97. Sporn MB, Roberts AB, Wakefield LM, et al. Transforming growth factor-β: Biological function and chemical structure. Science 233:532, 1986.
98. Sporn MB, Roberts AB. The transforming growth factor-betas: Past, present and future. Ann N Y Acad Sci 593:1, 1990.
99. Kauma S, Matt D, Strom S, et al. Interleukin-1β, human leukocyte antigen HLA-DRα, and transforming growth factor-β expression in endometrium, placenta and placental membranes. Am J Obstet Gynecol 163:1430, 1990.
100. Feinberg RF, Kliman HJ, Wang C-L. Transforming growth factor-β stimulates trophoblast oncofetal fibronectin synthesis in vitro: Implications for trophoblast implantation in vivo. J Clin Endocrinol Metab 78:1241, 1994.
101. Ignotz RA, Massagué J. Transforming growth factor-β stimulates the expression of fibronectin and collagen and their incorporation into the extracellular matrix. J Biol Chem 261:4337, 1986.
102. Jackson GM, Edwin SS, Varner MW, et al. Regulation of fetal fibronectin production in human chorion cells. Am J Obstet Gynecol 169:1431, 1993.
103. Irwin JC, Utian WH, Eckert RL. Sex steroids and growth factors regulate the growth and differentiation of cultured human endometrial stromal cells. Endocrinology 129:2385, 1991.
104. Giudice LC. Growth factors and growth modulators in human uterine endometrium: Their potential relevance to reproductive medicine. Fertil Steril 61:1, 1994.
105. Carpenter G. Receptors for epidermal growth factor and other polypeptide mitogens. Annu Rev Biochem 56:881, 1987.
106. Adesanya OO, Zhou J, Bondy CA. Cellular localization of sex steroid regulation of insulin-like growth factor binding protein messenger ribonucleic acids in the primate myometrium. J Clin Endocrinol Metab 81:2495, 1996.
107. Julkunen M, Koistinen R, Suikkari A-M, et al. Identification by hybridization histochemistry of human endometrial cells expressing mRNAs encoding a uterine β-lactoglobulin homologue and insulin-like growth factor–binding protein-1. Mol Endorinol 4:700, 1990.
108. Ritvos O, Ranta T, Jalkanen J, et al. Insulin like growth factor (IGF) binding protein from human decidua inhibits the binding and biological action of IGF-1 in cultured choriocarcinoma cells. Endocrinology 122:150, 1988.
109. Fujimoto J, Hori M, Ichigo S, et al. Expression of basic fibroblast growth factor and its mRNA in uterine endometrium during the menstrual cycle. Gynecol Endocrinol 10:193, 1996.
110. Rusnati M, Casarotti G, Pecorelli S, et al. Basic fibroblast growth factor in ovulatory cycle and postmenopausal human endometrium. Growth Factors 3:299, 1990.
111. Li HF, Gregory J, Ahmed A. Immunolocalisation of vascular endothelial growth factor in human endometrium. Growth Factors 11:277, 1994.
112. Shifren JL, Tseng JF, Zaloudek CJ, et al. Ovarian steroid regulation of vascular endothelial growth factor in the human endometrium: Implications for angiogenesis during the menstrual cycle and in the pathogenesis of endometriosis. J Clin Endocrinol Metab 81:3112, 1996.
113. Hunt JS. Expression and regulation of the tumor-necrosis factor alpha gene in the female reproductive tract. Reprod Fertil Dev 5:141, 1993.
114. Hampson J, McLaughlin PJ, Johnson PM. Low affinity receptors for tumour necrosis factor-alpha, interferon gamma, and granulocyte-macrophage colony-stimulating factor are expressed on human placental syncytiotrophoblasts. Immunology 79:485, 1993.
115. Todt JC, Yang Y, Lei J, et al. Effects of tumor necrosis factor-alpha on human trophoblast cell adhesion and motility. Am J Reprod Immunol 36:65, 1996.
116. Das SK, Stanley ER, Guilbert LJ, et al. Discrimination of a colony stimulating factor by a specific receptor on a macrophage cell line. J Cell Physiol 104:359, 1980.
117. Tushinski RJ, Oliver IT, Guilbert LJ, et al. Survival of mononuclear phagocytes depends on a lineage. Cell 28:71, 1982.
118. De Nichilo MO, Burns GF. Granulocyte-macrophage and macrophage colony-stimulating factors differentially regulate α_v integrin expression on cultured human macrophages. Proc Natl Acad Sci USA 90:2517, 1993.
119. Daiter E, Pollard JW. Colony stimulating factor-1 (CSF-1) in pregnancy. Reprod Med Rev 1:83, 1992.
120. Daiter E, Pampfer S, Yeung YG, et al. Expression of colony-stimulating factor-1 in the human uterus and placenta. J Clin Endocrinol Metab 74:850, 1992.
121. Pampfer S, Daiter E, Barad D, et al. Expression of the colony-stimulating factor-1 receptor (c-*fms* proto-oncogene product) in the human uterus and placenta. Biol Reprod 46:48, 1992.
122. Jokhi PP, Chumbley G, King A, et al. Expression of the colony stimulating factor-1 receptor (*cfms* product) by cells at the uteroplacental interface. Lab Invest 68:308, 1993.
123. Kauma SW, Aukerman SL, Eierman D, Turner T. Colony-stimulating factor-1 and *c-fms* expression in human endometrial tissues and placenta during the menstrual cycle and early pregnancy. J Clin Endocrinol Metab 73:746, 1991.
124. Jokhi PP, King A, Boocock C, Loke YW. Secretion of colony stimulating factor-1 by human first trimester placental and decidual cell populations and the effect of this cytokine on trophoblast thymidine uptake in vitro. Hum Reprod 10:2800, 1995.

125. Ringler GE, Coutifaris C, Strauss JF III, et al. Accumulation of colony-stimulating factor 1 in amniotic fluid during human pregnancy. Am J Obstet Gynecol 160:655, 1989.
126. Saito S, Saito M, Enomoto M, et al. Human macrophage-colony-stimulating factor induces the differentiation of trophoblast. Growth Factors 9:11, 1993.
127. Hilton DJ, Nicola NA, Gough NM, et al. Resolution and purification of three distinct factors produced by Kregs ascites cells which have differentiation-inducing activity on murine myeloid leukemic cell lines. J Biol Chem 263:9238, 1988.
128. Hilton DJ, Gough NM. Leukemia inhibitory factor: A biological perspective. J Cell Biochem 46:21, 1991.
129. Stewart CL, Kaspar P, Brunet LJ, et al. Blastocyst implantation depends on maternal expression of leukaemia inhibitory factor. Nature 359:76, 1992.
130. Cullinan EB, Abbondanzo SJ, Anderson PS, et al. Leukemia inhibitory factor (LIF) and LIF receptor expression in human endometrium suggests a potential autocrine/paracrine function in regulating embryo implantation. Proc Natl Acad Sci USA 93:3115, 1996.
131. Delage G, Moreau JF, Taupin JL, et al. In vitro modulation of the production of the cytokine HILDA/LIF, secreted by human endometrial explants: Preliminary results [in French]. Contracept Fertil Sex 23:622, 1995.
132. Chaouat G, Menu E, Delage G, et al. Immuno-endocrine interactions in early pregnancy. Hum Reprod 10:55, 1995.
133. Sharkey AM, Dellow K, Flayney M, et al. Stage-specific expression of cytokine and receptor messenger ribonucleic acids in human preimplantation embryos. Biol Reprod 53:974, 1995.
134. Stewart CL. Leukaemia inhibitory factor and the regulation of pre-implantation development of the mammalian embryo. Mol Reprod Dev 39:233, 1994.
135. Nachtigall MJ, Kliman HJ, Feinberg RF, et al. The effect of leukemia inhibitory factor (LIF) on trophoblast differentiation: A potential role in human implantation. J Clin Endocrinol Metab 81:801, 1996.
136. Bell SC. Secretory endometrial and decidual proteins: Studies and clinical significance of a maternally derived group of pregnancy-associated serum proteins. Hum Reprod 1:129, 1986.
137. Isaacson KB, Coutifaris C, Garcia CR, et al. Production and secretion of complement component C3 by endometriotic implants and ovarian endometriomas. J Clin Endocrinol Metab 69:1003, 1989.
138. Isaacson KB, Galman M, Coutifaris C, et al. Endometrial synthesis and secretion of complement component 3 (C3) by patients with and without endometriosis. Fertil Steril 53:836, 1990.
139. Bell SC, Patel SR, Kirwan PH, et al. Protein synthesis and secretion by the human endometrium during the menstrual cycle and the effect of progesterone in vitro. J Reprod Fertil 77:221, 1986.
140. Hasty LA, Lambris JD, Lessey BA, et al. Hormonal regulation of complement components and receptors throughout the menstrual cycle. Am J Obstet Gynecol 170:168, 1994.
141. Joshi SG. A progestagen-associated protein of the human endometrium: Basic studies and potential clinical applications. J Steroid Biochem 19:751, 1983.
142. Seppälä M, Koistinen H, Koistinen R, et al. Glycodelins as regulators of early events of reproduction. Clin Endocrinol (Oxf) 46:381, 1997.
143. McRae MA, Galle PC, Joshi SG. The role of measurement of progestagen-associated endometrial protein in predicting adequate endometrial differentiation. Hum Reprod 6:761, 1991.
144. Bell SC. Decidualization and insulin-like growth factor (IGF) binding protein: Implications for its role in stromal cell differentiation and the decidual cell in haemochorial placentation. Hum Reprod 4:125, 1989.
145. Giudice LC. Endometrial growth factors and proteins. Semin Reprod Endocrinol 13:93, 1995.
146. Maslar IA. The progestational endometrium. Semin Reprod Biol 6:115, 1988.
147. Maslar IA, Riddick DH. Prolactin production by human endometrium during the normal menstrual cycle. Am J Obstet Gynecol 135:751, 1979.
148. Kauma S, Shapiro SS. Immunoperoxidase localization of prolactin in endometrium during normal menstrual, luteal phase defect, and corrected luteal phase defect cycles. Fertil Steril 46:37, 1986.
149. Heffner LJ, Iddenden DA, Lyttle CR. Electrophoretic analyses of secreted human endometrial proteins: Identification and characterization of luteal phase prolactin. J Clin Endocrinol Metab 62:1288, 1986.
150. Maier DB, Kuslis ST. Human uterine luminal fluid volumes and prolactin levels in normal menstrual cycles. Am J Obstet Gynecol 159:434, 1988.
151. McRae MA, Newman GR, Walker SM, et al. Immunohistochemical identification of prolactin and 24K protein in secretory endometrium. Fertil Steril 45:643, 1986.
152. Ying Y-K, Walters CA, Kuslis S, et al. Prolactin production by explants of normal, luteal phase defective, and corrected luteal phase defective late secretory endometrium. Am J Obstet Gynecol 151:801, 1985.
153. Tyson JE, Hwang P, Guyda H, et al. Studies of prolactin secretion in human pregnancy. Am J Obstet Gynecol 113:12, 1972.
154. Jacobs I, Bast RC Jr. The CA 125 tumor-associated antigen: A review of the literature. Hum Reprod 4:1, 1989.
155. Coutifaris C, Dardik R, Omigbodun A. Cell adhesion molecules and embryo implantation. *In* Rock JA, Faro S, Gant NF, et al. Advances in Obstetrics and Gynecology, Vol 4. St. Louis, CV Mosby, 1997, p 163.
156. Albelda S, Buck C. Integrins and other cell adhesion molecules. FASEB J 4:2868, 1991.
157. Ruoslahti E, Noble NA, Kagami S, et al. Integrins. Kidney Int 45(Suppl):S17, 1994.
158. Ruoslahti E, Pierschbacher MD. New perspectives in cell adhesion: RGD and integrins. Science 238:491, 1987.
159. Sueoka K, Shiokawa S, Miyazaki T, et al. Integrins and reproductive physiology: Expression and modulation in fertilization, embryogenesis, and implantation. Fertil Steril 67:799, 1997.
160. Bronson RA, Fusi FM. Integrins and human reproduction. Mol Hum Reprod 2:153, 1996.
161. Lessey BA, Damjanovich L, Coutifaris C, et al. Integrin adhesion molecules in the human endometrium: Correlation with normal and abnormal menstrual cycle. J Clin Invest 90:188, 1992.
162. Lessey BA. Endometrial integrins. Endocrinologist 5:214, 1995.
163. Vinatier D. Integrins and reproduction. Eur J Obstet Gynecol Reprod Biol 59:71, 1995.
164. Tabibzadeh S. Patterns of expression of integrin molecules in human endometrium throughout the menstrual cycle. Hum Reprod 7:876, 1992.
165. Lessey BA. The use of integrins for the assessment of uterine receptivity. Fertil Steril 61:850, 1994.
166. Campbell S, Swann HR, Seif MW, et al. Cell adhesion molecules on the oocyte and preimplantation human embryo. Hum Reprod 10:1571, 1995.
167. Garcia E, Bouchard P, DeBrux J, et al. Use of immunocytochemistry of progesterone and estrogen receptors for endometrial dating. J Clin Endocrinol Metab 64:80, 1988.
168. Lessey BA, Killam AP, Metzger DA, et al. Immunohistochemical analysis of human uterine estrogen and progesterone receptors throughout the menstrual cycle. J Clin Endocrinol Metab 647:334, 1988.
169. Lessey BA, Yet IJ, Castelbaum AJ, et al. Endometrial progesterone receptors and markers of uterine receptivity in the window of implantation. Fertil Steril 65:427, 1996.
170. Juliano RL, Haskill S. Signal transduction from the extracellular matrix. J Cell Biol 120:577, 1993.
171. Pope WF. Uterine asynchrony: A cause of embryonic loss. Biol Reprod 39:999, 1988.
172. Finn CA. The implantation reaction. *In* Wynn RM. Biology of the Uterus. New York, Plenum Publishing, 1977, pp 245–303.
173. Psychoyos A. Uterine receptivity for nidation. Ann N Y Acad Sci 476:36, 1986.
174. Rogers PAW, Murphy CR. Uterine receptivity for implantation: Human studies in blastocyst implantation. *In* Yoshinaga K. Blastocyst Implantation. Boston, Adams Publishing Group, 1989, p 231.
175. Formigli L, Formigli G, Roccio C. Donation of fertilized uterine ova to infertile women. Fertil Steril 47:162, 1988.
176. Hertig AJ, Rock J, Adams EC. A description of 34 human ova within the first 17 days of development. Am J Anat 98:435, 1956.
177. Rosenwaks Z. Donor eggs: Their application in modern reproductive technologies. Fertil Steril 47:895, 1987.

178. Sauer MV, Paulson RJ. Oocyte and embryo donation. Curr Opin Obstet Gynecol 7:193, 1995.
179. Davis OK, Rosenwaks Z. Preparation of the endometrium for oocyte donation. J Assist Reprod Genet 10:457, 1993.
180. Michalas S, Loutradis D, Drakakis P, et al. A flexible protocol for the induction of recipient endometrial cycles in an oocyte donation programme. Hum Reprod 11:1063, 1996.
181. Enders AC. Current topic: Structural responses of the primate endometrium to implantation. Placenta 12:309, 1991.
182. Hamilton WJ, Boyd JD. Development of the human placenta. *In* Philipp EE, Barnes J, Newton M. Scientific Foundations of Obstetrics and Gynecology. London, William Heinemann, 1970, pp 185–254.
183. Benirschke K, Kaufmann P. Early development of the human placenta. *In* Benirschke K, Kaufmann P. Pathology of the Human Placenta. New York, Springer-Verlag, 1991, pp 13–21.
184. Larsen JF. Electron microscopy of nidation in the rabbit and observations on the human trophoblastic invasion. *In* Hubinont PO, Leroy F, Robyn C, Leleux P. Ovo-Implantation, Human Gonadotrophins and Prolactin. Basel, S Karger, 1970, pp 38–51.
185. Lindenberg S, Pedersen B, Hamberger L, et al. Models for human implantation derived from implantation in vitro. Reprod Fertil Dev 4:653, 1992.
186. Coutifaris C, Babalola GO, Feinberg RF, et al. Purified human cytotrophoblasts: Surrogates for the blastocysts in in vitro models of implantation. *In* Mashiach S, Ben-Rafael A, Laufer N, Schenker JG. Advances in Assisted Reproductive Technologies. New York, Plenum Publishing, 1990, pp 687–695.
187. Aoki D, Kawakami H, Nozawa S, et al. Differences in lectin binding patterns of normal human endometrium between proliferative and secretory phases. Histochemistry 92:177, 1989.
188. Hey NA, Graham RA, Seif MW, et al. The polymorphic epithelial mucin MUC1 in human endometrium is regulated with maximal expression in the implantation phase. J Clin Endocrinol Metab 78:337, 1994.
189. Aplin JD, Seif MW, Graham RA, et al. The endometrial cell surface and implantation. Expression of the polymorphic mucin MUC-1 and adhesion molecules during the endometrial cycle. Ann N Y Acad Sci 734:103, 1994.
190. Christensen S, Verhage HG, Nowak G, et al. Smooth muscle myosin II and alpha smooth muscle actin expression in the baboon *(Papop anubis)* uterus is associated with glandular secretory activity and stromal cell transformation. Biol Reprod 53:598, 1995.
191. Fukuda MN, Sato T, Nakayama J, et al. Trophinin and tastin, a novel cell adhesion molecule complex with potential involvement in embryo implantation. Genes Dev 9:1199, 1995.
192. Young MF, Kerr JM, Termine JD, et al. cDNA cloning, mRNA distribution and heterogeneity, chromosomal location, and RFLP analysis of human osteopontin (OPN). Genomics 7:491, 1990.
193. Kiefer MC, Bauer DM, Barr PJ. The cDNA and derived amino acid sequence for human osteopontin. Nucleic Acids Res 17:3306, 1989.
194. Miyauchi A, Alvarez J, Greenfield EM, et al. Recognition of osteopontin and related peptides by an $\alpha_v\beta_3$ integrin stimulates immediate cell signals in osteoclasts. J Biol Chem 266:2369, 1991.
195. Klentzeris LD, Bulmer JN, Trejdosiewicz LK, et al. β1 integrin cell adhesion molecules in endometrium of fertile and infertile women. Hum Reprod 8:1223, 1993.
196. Taskin O, Brown RW, Young DC, et al. High doses of oral contraceptives do not alter endometrial α_1 and $\alpha_v\beta_3$ integrins in the late implantation window. Fertil Steril 61:850, 1994.
197. Aplin JD. Implantation, trophoblast differentiation and hemochorial placentation: Mechanistic evidence in vivo and in vitro. J Cell Sci 99:681, 1991.
198. Aplin JD. The cell biology of human implantation. Placenta 17:269, 1996.
199. Damsky C, Sutherland A, Fisher S. Extracellular matrix 5: Adhesive interactions in early mammalian embryogenesis, implantation and placentation. FASEB J 7:1320, 1993.
200. Damsky CH, Fitzgerald ML, Fisher SJ. Distribution patterns of extracellular matrix components and adhesion receptors are intricately modulated during first trimester differentiation along the invasive pathway, in vivo. J Clin Invest 89:210, 1992.
201. Graham CH, Lala PK. Mechanisms of placental invasion of the uterus and their control. Biochem Cell Biol 70:867, 1992.
202. Dhawan J, Lichtler AC, Rowe DW, et al. Cell adhesion regulates pro-alpha 1(I) collagen mRNA stability and transcription in mouse fibroblasts. J Biol Chem 266:8470, 1991.
203. Bischof P, Friedelli E, Martelli M, et al. Expression of extracellular matrix–degrading metalloproteinases by cultured human trophoblast cells. Effect of cell adhesion and purification. Am J Obstet Gynecol 165:1791, 1991.
204. Burrows TD, King A, Loke YW. Expression of integrins by human trophoblast and differential adhesion to laminin or fibronectin. Hum Reprod 8:475, 1993.
205. Fisher SJ, Cui T-Y, Zhang L, et al. Adhesive and degradative properties of human placental cytotrophoblast cells in vitro. J Cell Biol 109:891, 1989.
206. Lala PK, Graham CH. Mechanisms of trophoblast invasiveness and their control: The role of proteases and proteinase inhibitors. Cancer Metastasis Rev 9:369, 1990.
207. Librach CL, Werb Z, Fitzgerald ML, et al. 92-kD type IV collagenase mediates invasion of human cytotrophoblasts. J Cell Biol 113:437, 1991.
208. Moll UM, Lane BL. Proteolytic activity of first trimester human placenta: Localization of interstitial collagenase in villous and extravillous trophoblast. Histochemistry 94:555, 1990.
209. Armant DR, Kaplan HA, Lennarz WJ. Fibronectin and laminin promote in vitro attachment and outgrowth of mouse blastocysts. Dev Biol 116:519, 1986.
210. Schultz JF, Armant DR. β_1- and β_3-class integrins mediate fibronectin binding activity at the surface of developing mouse peri-implantation blastocysts. J Biol Chem 270:11522, 1995.
211. Yelian FD, Yang Y, Hirata JD, et al. Molecular interactions between fibronectin and integrins during mouse blastocyst outgrowth. Mol Reprod Dev 41:435, 1995.
212. Carson DD, Tang JP, Gay S. Collagens support embryo attachment and outgrowth in vitro: Effects of the Arg-Gly-Asp sequence. Dev Biol 127:368, 1988.
213. Fay TN, Grudzinskas JG. Human endometrial peptides: A review of their potential role in implantation and placentation. Hum Reprod 6:1311, 1991.
214. Haimovici F, Anderson DJ. Effects of growth factors and growth factor–extracellular matrix interactions on mouse trophoblast outgrowth in vitro. Biol Reprod 49:124, 1993.
215. Queenan JT Jr, Kao LC, Arboleda A, et al. Regulation of urokinase-type plasminogen activator production by cultured human cytotrophoblasts. J Biol Chem 262:10903, 1987.
216. Zini JM, Murray SC, Graham CH, et al. Characterization of urokinase receptor expression by human placental trophoblasts. Blood 79:2917, 1992.
217. Feinberg RF, Kao L-C, Haimowitz JE, et al. Plasminogen activator inhibitor types 1 and 2 in human trophoblasts: PAI-1 is an immunocytochemical marker of invading trophoblasts. Lab Invest 61:20, 1989.
218. Coukos G, Gafvels ME, Wisel S, et al. Expression of α_2-macroglobulin receptor/low density lipoprotein receptor–related protein and the 39 kd receptor–associated protein in human trophoblasts. Am J Pathol 144:383, 1994.
219. Gafvels ME, Coukos G, Sayegh R, et al. Regulated expression of the trophoblast α_2-macroglobulin receptor/low density lipoprotein receptor protein: Differentiation and cAMP modulate protein and mRNA levels. J Biol Chem 267:21230, 1992.
220. Strickland S, Richards WG. Invasion of the trophoblasts. Cell 71:355, 1992.
221. Damsky CH, Librach C, Lim K-H, et al. Integrin switching regulates normal trophoblast invasion. Development 120:3657, 1994.
222. Seftor REB, Seftor EA, Gehlsen KR, et al. Role of the $\alpha_v\beta_3$ integrin in human melanoma cell invasion. Proc Natl Acad Sci USA 89:1557, 1992.
223. Albelda SM. Role of integrins and other cell adhesion molecules in tumor progression and metastasis. Lab Invest 68:4, 1993.
224. Albelda SM, Mette SA, Elder DE, et al. Integrin distribution in malignant melanoma: Association of the β3 subunit with tumor progression. Cancer Res 50:6757, 1990.
225. Cheresh DA, Smith JW, Cooper HM, Quaranta V. A novel vitronectin receptor integrin ($\alpha_v\beta_x$) is responsible for distinct adhesive properties of carcinoma cells. Cell 57:59, 1989.
226. Feinberg RF, Kliman HJ, Lockwood CJ. Is oncofetal fibronectin a

trophoblast glue for human implantation? Am J Pathol 138:537, 1991.
227. Zhou Y, Damsky CH, Chiu K, et al. Preeclampsia is associated with abnormal expression of adhesion molecules by invasive cytotrophoblasts. J Clin Invest 91:950, 1993.
228. Brown LF, Berse B, Van de Water L, et al. Expression and distribution of osteopontin in human tissues: Widespread association with luminal epithelial surfaces. Mol Biol Cell 3:1169, 1992.
229. Omigbodun A, Ziolkiewicz P, Coukos G, et al. Macrophage-colony stimulating factor (M-CSF) regulates the expression of fibronectin and its $\alpha5$ integrin receptor. Endocrinology (in press).
230. Bischof P, Haenggeli L, Campana A. Effect of leukemia inhibitory factor on human cytotrophoblast differentiation along the invasive pathway. Am J Reprod Immunol 34:225, 1995.
231. Haimovici F, Anderson DJ. Cytokines and growth factors in implantation. Microsc Res Tech 25:201, 1993.
232. Defilippi P, Silengo L, Tarone G. Alpha 6.beta 1 integrin (laminin receptor) is down-regulated by tumor necrosis factor-alpha and interleukin-1 beta in human endothelial cells. J Biol Chem 267:18303, 1992.
233. Zhou Y, Fisher SJ, Janatpour M, et al. Human cytotrophoblasts adopt a vascular phenotype as they differentiate: A strategy for successful endovascular invasion? J Clin Invest 99:2139, 1997.
234. Zhou Y, Damsky CH, Fisher SJ. Preeclampsia is associated with failure of human cytotrophoblasts to mimic a vascular adhesion phenotype: One cause of defective endovascular invasion in this syndrome? J Clin Invest 99:2152, 1997.
235. Hesla JS, Kurman RJ, Rock JA. Histologic effects of oral contraceptives on the uterine corpus and cervix. Semin Reprod Endocrinol 7:213, 1989.
236. Sheppard BL. Endometrial morphological changes in IUD users: A review. Contraception 36:1, 1987.
237. Shaw ST Jr, Macaulay LR, Hohman WR. Morphologic studies on IUD-induced metrorrhagia. I. Endometrial changes and clinical correlations. Contraception 19:47, 1979.
238. Ermini M, Carpino F, Petrozza V, Benagiano G. Distribution and effect on the endometrium of progesterone released from a Progestasert device. Hum Reprod 3:221, 1989.
239. Jones GES. Some newer aspects of the management of infertility. JAMA 141:1123, 1949.
240. Jones GS. The luteal phase defect. Fertil Steril 27:351, 1976.
241. Peters AJ, Wentz AC. Luteal phase inadequacy. Diagnosis, management and cost concerns. Semin Reprod Endocrinol 13:162, 1995.
242. McNeely MJ, Soules MR. The diagnosis of luteal phase deficiency: A critical review. Fertil Steril 50:l, 1988.
243. Doody KJ, Carr BR. Diagnosis and treatment of luteal dysfunction. *In* Hillier SG. Ovarian Endocrinology. London, Blackwell Scientific Publications, 1991, pp 260–318.
244. Seppala M, Julkunen M, Koskimies A, et al. Proteins of the human endometrium. Basic and clinical studies toward a blood test for endometrial function. Ann N Y Acad Sci 54:432, 1988.
245. Brodie BL, Wentz AC. An update of the clinical relevance of luteal phase inadequacy. Semin Reprod Endocrinol 7:138, 1989.
246. Davidson BJ, Thrasher TV, Seraj JM. An analysis of endometrial biopsies performed for infertility. Fertil Steril 48:770, 1987.
247. Dor J, Homburg R, Rabau E. An evaluation of etiologic factors and therapy in 665 infertile couples. Fertil Steril 28:74, 1977.
248. Gibson M. Clinical evaluation of luteal function. Semin Reprod Endocrinol 8:130, 1990.
249. Tabibzadeh S. Immunoreactivity of human endometrium: Correlation with endometrial dating. Fertil Steril 54:624, 1990.
250. Soules MR, McLachlar RI, Ek M, et al. Luteal phase deficiency: Characterization of reproductive hormones over the menstrual cycle. J Clin Endocrinol Metab 69:804, 1989.
251. Thatcher SS, Breuel K. Infertility and the luteal phase. Assist Reprod Rev 3:203, 1993.
252. Vanrell JA, Balasch J. Luteal phase defects in repeated abortion. Int J Gynecol Obstet 24:111, 1986.
253. Manners CV. Endometrial assessment in a group of infertile women on stimulated cycles for IVF: Immunohistochemical findings. Hum Reprod 5:128, 1990.
254. Hecht B, Khan-Dawood FS, Dawood MY. Peri-implantation phase endometrial estrogen and progesterone receptors: Effect of ovulation induction with clomiphene citrate. Am J Obstet Gynecol 161:1688, 1989.
255. Miller MM, Hoffman DI, Creinin M, et al. Comparison of endometrial biopsy and urinary pregnanediol glucuronide concentration in the diagnosis of luteal phase defect. Fertil Steril 54:1008, 1990.
256. Rosenfeld DL, García C-R. A comparison of endometrial histology with simultaneous plasma progesterone determinations in infertile women. Fertil Steril 27:1256, 1976.
257. Rosenfeld DL, García C-R. Endometrial biopsy in the cycle of conception. Fertil Steril 26:1088, 1975.
258. Jacobs MH, Balash J, Gonzalez-Merlow JN, et al. Endometrial cytosolic and nuclear progesterone receptors in the luteal phase defect. J Clin Endocrinol Metab 64:472, 1987.
259. McRae MA, Blasco L, Lyttle CR. Serum hormones and their receptors in women with normal and inadequate corpus luteum function. Fertil Steril 42:58, 1984.
260. Graf MJ, Reyniak JV, Battle-Muher P, et al. Histologic evaluation of the luteal phase in women following follicle aspiration for oocyte retrieval. Fertil Steril 49:616, 1988.
261. Jordan J, Craig K, Clifton DK, et al. Luteal phase defect: The sensitivity and specificity of diagnostic methods in common clinical use. Fertil Steril 62:54, 1994.
262. Karamardian LM, Grimes DA. Luteal phase deficiency: Effect of treatment on pregnancy rates. Am J Obstet Gynecol 167:1391, 1992.
263. Gerbie AB, Merill JA. Pathology of endometriosis. Clin Obstet Gynecol 31:779, 1988.
264. Olive DL, Schwartz LB. Endometriosis. N Engl J Med 328:1759, 1993.
265. Chatman DL, Ward AB. Endometriosis in adolescents. J Reprod Med 27:156, 1982.
266. Kempers RD, Dockerty MB, Hunt AB, et al. Significant postmenopausal endometriosis. Surg Gynecol Obstet 111:348, 1960.
267. Revised American Society for Reproductive Medicine classification of endometriosis: 1996. Fertil Steril 67:817, 1997.
268. Guzick DS, Silliman NP, Adamson GD, et al. Prediction of pregnancy in infertile women based on the American Society for Reproductive Medicine's revised classification of endometriosis. Fertil Steril 67:822, 1997.
269. Metzger D, Haney AF. Etiology of endometriosis. Obstet Gynecol Clin North Am 16:1, 1989.
270. Zegneloglu HB, Arici A, Olive DL. Environmental toxins and endometriosis. Obstet Gynecol Clin North Am 24:307, 1997.
271. Ranney B. Endometriosis IV. Hereditary tendency. Obstet Gynecol 37:734, 1991.
272. Mahmood TA, Templeton A. Prevalence and genesis of endometriosis. Hum Reprod 6:5344, 1991.
273. Dmowski WP. Immunological aspects of endometriosis. Int J Gynaecol Obstet 50(suppl 1):S3, 1995.
274. Vinatier D, Dufour P, Oosterlynck D. Immunological aspects of endometriosis. Hum Reprod Update 2:371, 1996.
275. Grosskinsky CM, Halme J. Endometriosis: The host response. Baillieres Clin Obstet Gynaecol 7:701, 1993.
276. Dmowski WP, Gebel HM, Braun DP. The role of cell-mediated immunity in pathogenesis of endometriosis. Acta Obstet Gynecol Scand Suppl 159:7, 1994.
277. Oral E, Arici A. Peritoneal growth factors and endometriosis. Semin Reprod Endocrinol 14:257, 1996.
278. Osteen KG, Bruner KL, Sharpe-Timms KL. Steroid and growth factor regulation of matrix metalloproteinase expression and endometriosis. Semin Reprod Endocrinol 14:247, 1996.
279. Lessey BA, Castelbaum AJ, Sawin SW, et al. Aberrant integrin expression in the endometrium of women with endometriosis. J Clin Endocrinol Metab 79:643, 1994.
280. Sharpe KL, Zimmer LR, Griffin WT, et al. Polypeptides synthesized and released by human endometriosis differ from those of uterine endometrium in cell and tissue explant culture. Fertil Steril 60:839, 1993.
281. Ota H, Igarashi S. Expression of major histocompatibility complex class II antigen in endometriotic tissue in patients with endometriosis and adenomyosis. Fertil Steril 60:854, 1993.
282. Jiang X, Hitchcock A, Bryan EJ, et al. Microsatellite analysis of endometriosis reveals loss of heterozygosity at candidate tumor suppressor gene loci. Cancer Res 56:3534, 1996.

283. Gaetje R, Kotzian S, Herrmann G, et al. Non-malignant epithelial cells, potentially invasive in human endometriosis, lack the tumor suppressor molecule E-cadherin. Am J Pathol 150:461, 1997.
284. Evers JL. Endometriosis does not exist; all women have endometriosis. Hum Reprod 9:2206, 1994.
285. Koninckx PR. Is mild endometriosis a condition occurring intermittently in all women? Hum Reprod 9:2202, 1994.
286. Pellicer A, Oliveira N, Ruiz A, et al. Exploring the mechanism(s) of endometriosis related infertility: An analysis of embryo development and implantation in assisted reproduction. Hum Reprod 10(suppl 2):91, 1995.
287. Brosens IA. Is mild endometriosis a progressive disease? Hum Reprod 9:2209, 1994.
288. Oral E, Olive DL, Arici A. The peritoneal environment in endometriosis. Hum Reprod Update 2:385, 1996.
289. Silverberg SG. Hyperplasia and carcinoma of the endometrium. Semin Diagn Pathol 5:135, 1988.
290. Kurman RJ, Kaminski PF, Norris HJ. The behavior of endometrial hyperplasia: A long-term study of "untreated" hyperplasia in 170 patients. Cancer 56:403, 1985.
291. Enomoto T, Inoue M, Peratoni AO, et al. K-*ras* activation in premalignant and malignant lesions of the human uterus. Cancer Res 51:5308, 1991.
292. Kohler MF, Berchuck A, Davidoff AM, et al. Overexpression and mutation of p53 in endometrial carcinoma. Cancer Res 52:1622, 1992.
293. Bandera CA, Boyd J. The molecular genetics of endometrial carcinoma. Prog Clin Biol Res 396:185, 1997.
294. Cramer DW, Knapp RC. Review of epidemiologic studies of endometrial cancer and exogenous estrogen. Obstet Gynecol 54:521, 1979.
295. Grady D, Gebretsadik T, Kerlikowske K, et al. Hormone replacement therapy and endometrial cancer risk—a metaanalysis. Obstet Gynecol 85:304, 1995.
296. Whitehead MI, Fraser D. The effects of estrogens and progestogens on the endometrium: Modern approach to treatment. Obset Gynecol Clin North Am 14:299, 1987.
297. Studd JWW, Thom JH. Oestrogens and endometrial cancer. *In* Studd JWW. Progress in Obstetrics and Gynecology, Vol 1. Edinburgh, Churchill Livingstone, 1981, pp 182–198.
298. Russell PT, Owens OM. Dysmenorrhoea and other menstrual disorders. *In* Bygdeman M, Berger GS, Keith LG. Prostaglandins and Their Inhibitors in Clinical Obstetrics and Gynaecology. Norwell, MA, Kluwer Academic Publishers, 1986, p 315.
299. Norman J. Nitric oxide and the myometrium. Pharm Therap 70:91, 1996.
300. Rein MS, Nowak RA. Biology of uterine myomas and myometrium in vitro. Semin Reprod Endocrinol 10:310, 1992.
301. Yen SSC. Use of antiprogestin in the management of endometriosis and leiomyoma. *In* Donalson MS, Dorflinger L, Brown SS, Benet LZ (eds). Clinical Application of Mifepristone (RU 486) and Other Antiprogestins. Washington, DC, National Academy Press, 1993, p 189.
302. Matsuo H, Maruo T, Samoto T. Increased expression of Bcl-2 protein in human uterine leiomyoma and its up regulation by progesterone. J Clin Endocrinol Metab 82:293, 1997.
303. Barbieri RL, Andersen J. Uterine leiomyomas. The somatic mutation theory. Semin Reprod Endocrinol 10:301, 1992.
304. Ashar HR, Fejzo MS, Tkachenko A, et al. Disruption of the architectural factor HMGI-C: DNA-binding AT hook motifs fused in lipomas to distinct transcriptional regulatory domains. Cell 82:57, 1995.
305. Williams AJ, Powell WL, Collins T, et al. HMG(Y) expression in human uterine leiomyomata. Involvement of another high motility group architectural factor in a benign neoplasm. Am J Pathol 150:911, 1997.
306. Zhou J, Mochizuki T, Smeets H, et al. Deletion of the paired alpha 5(IV) and alpha 6(IV) collagen genes in inherited smooth muscle tumors. Science 261:1167, 1997.
307. Siegler AM, Camilien L. Adenomyosis. J Reprod Med 39:841, 1994.

Chapter 9

PROLACTIN IN HUMAN REPRODUCTION

S. S. C. Yen • Robert B. Jaffe

■ CHAPTER OUTLINE

KEY POINTS

- Prolactin and its receptor have been conserved across species.
- Prolactin subsumes different roles in different species, including maintenance of the corpus luteum and regulation of fluid and electrolyte flux. In the human and many other species, prolactin regulates casein and α-lactalbumin synthesis necessary for milk production, its major known function in adult women postpartum.
- Prolactin may play a role in tissue differentiation and development in the human fetus.
- Prolactin is closely related to growth hormone, with which it shares common ancestry and structural similarities. Differentiation of the lactotroph and somatotroph are under transcriptional regulation by Pit-1; point mutations of Pit 1 gene results in hypopituitarism.
- Prolactin is under tonic inhibitory control, primarily by hypothalamic dopamine produced by tuberoinfundibular neurons.
- Prolactin is not regulated in a classic endocrine manner by feedback from target tissue hormones; a variety of autocrine/paracrine factors, neurotransmitters, and peripheral hormones participate in its regulation.
- Prolactin secretion is episodic, sleep- and food-entrained, and responsive to stress and other psychologic secretagogues.
- Prolactin-secreting pituitary tumors can cause galactorrhea and interfere with menstrual function in women, cause impotence in men and cause visual field changes and headaches in both sexes. Pituitary stalk damage and primary hypothyroidism, as well as pituitary tumors, can be associated with hyperprolactinemia.
- Prolactin, like growth hormone, plays a role in immune function, exerting endocrine control on the immune system and also acting as a cytokine released by immune cells that can regulate the lymphocyte response by paracrine and autocrine mechanisms.

When viewed from an evolutionary perspective, prolactin (PRL)—a lactogenic hormone—has been and is indispensable for the preservation of the species. Survival of the young is dependent on a unique biologic system that shifts the source of metabolic fuel from the uterus to the mammary gland and thus enables the mother to continue providing nutrients after the birth of the child. Failure of this system would obviously mean extinction of all mammalian species, including humans. The existence of a pituitary lactogenic hormone, distinct from pituitary growth hormone (hGH), was demonstrated in humans in 1970,[1] and a radioimmunoassay was developed soon thereafter.[2]

The PRL molecule is a single polypeptide containing 198 amino acid residues with a molecular weight (MW) of

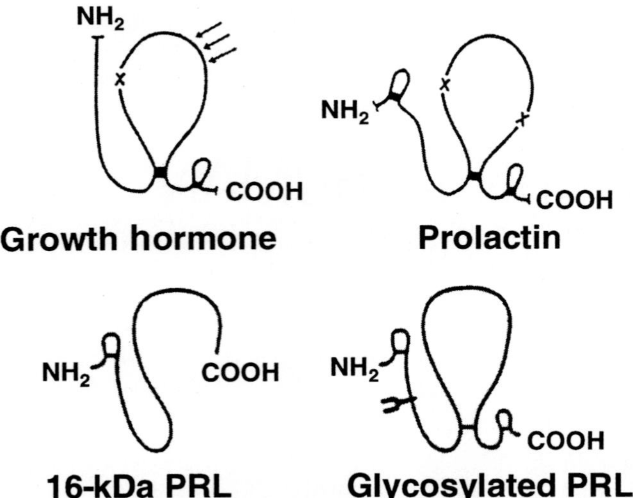

Figure 9–1 ■ Diagrammatic representation of the high degree of similarity between the structures of pituitary growth hormone (PGH) and prolactin. Connecting solid blocks represent the disulfide bridges; X indicates position of tryptophan residues; arrows indicate site of enzymatic cleavage of hGH to yield forms with enhanced biologic activity. Also illustrated are the 16-kDa fragment of prolactin and a glycosylated form of prolactin. (Modified from Niall HD. The chemistry of prolactin. *In* Jaffe RB [ed]. Prolactin. New York, Elsevier North-Holland, 1981.)

22,000. Its structure is remarkably similar to hGH[3] (Fig. 9–1). The structure is folded into a globular shape, and the folds are connected by three disulfide bonds. The degree of homology of the amino acid sequence among PRL, hGH, and human placental lactogen (hPL) is striking (Fig. 9–2).

PROLACTIN GENE STRUCTURE AND ITS KINSHIP

The hPRL gene, which was cloned in 1981, is on human chromosome 6,[4] which is also the locus of human leukocyte antigen. The significance of this association, if any, is currently unknown. Extensive sequence homology between hGH and hPL[5, 6] has been observed. Additional members of the PRL gene family have been described; the human decidual PRL complementary deoxyribonucleic acid (cDNA) has been cloned, and the sequence is almost identical with that of the pituitary cDNA, confirming that there is only a single copy of the hPRL gene per haploid genome.[7] The hPRL gene appears to have been derived from a common somatomammotropic (hGH-hPRL-hPL) precursor some 400 million years ago, the period when fish and quadrupeds started to diverge.[8] By use of transgenic mice, it was established that there is a common precursor stem cell of both hGH- and hPRL-producing cells; the progenitor is a growth hormone–expressing stem-somatotroph, with the capacity of differentiating into lactotrophs through postmitotic events.[9] These stem-somatotrophs are still present in adult pituitaries and are capable of repopulating mature growth hormone– and PRL-producing cells. Somatomammotrophs have been found in both human fetal[10] and normal and neoplastic adult pituitaries.[11]

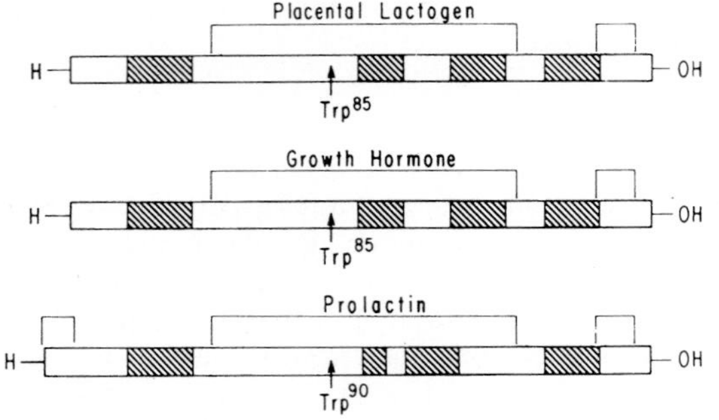

Figure 9–2 ■ Structural similarities of the somatomammotropin family of hormones. The bars represent the peptide chains, with the amino terminal to the left and the carboxyl terminal to the right. The hatched areas represent the recognizable portions of replicating sequences. The line above each bar represents the position of disulfide bridges. Trp, tryptophan. (From Niall HD, Hogan ML, Sauer R, et al. Sequences of pituitary and placental lactogenic and growth hormones: Evolution from a primordial peptide by gene reduplication. Proc Natl Acad Sci USA 68:866–870, 1971.)

THE PITUITARY LACTOTROPH

The lactotroph of the adenohypophysis is the cell that synthesizes and secretes PRL. In human pituitaries, lactotrophs constitute 40 to 50 percent of the total pituitary cell population[11] and are aggregated mainly in the posterior lateral wings of the adenohypophysis. The hPRL content in the pituitary is relatively low (approximately 135 μg per gland), about 1 percent of the content of hGH. The disparity between pituitary content of hPRL and lactotroph population is probably because hPRL has a considerably higher turnover rate than does hGH and thus is stored in smaller quantity. Rapid accumulation and depletion of PRL stores have been observed in the absence of and in response to mammary nerve stimulation, respectively.[12] However, corresponding PRL release, as measured by radioimmunoassay, does not reflect the rapid turnover of PRL within the adenohypophysis. This is due to the release of a PRL molecule with relatively low immunoreactivity in response to suckling.[12, 13]

Lactotroph During Pregnancy

The pituitary of late pregnancy enlarges to twice its normal size, principally because of an increase in the size and number of lactotrophs. These so-called pregnancy cells, previously called chromophobes, are clearly hypertrophic and hyperplastic lactotrophs with high secretory activity.[14]

Isoforms of hPRL

Heterogeneity of the hPRL molecule has been described in both human plasma and the pituitary.[15–17] Serum PRL levels, as measured by radioimmunoassay, do not always correlate with clinical findings. For example, some patients with very high radioimmunoassayable serum PRL levels have normal menstrual cycles and no galactorrhea, and the converse is also observed. These discrepancies are due to the heterogeneity of molecular forms, with varying ratios of immunoactivity to bioactivity (glycosylated versus nonglycosylated) of circulating PRL.[15–17] The following distinct forms of circulating PRL have been described:

1. "Little" PRL (MW ~ 23,000), corresponding to the nonglycosylated monomeric hormone with high receptor binding, bioactivity, and full immunoactivity;
2. Two glycosylated forms of hPRL (MW ~ 25,000), differing in the carbohydrate units: G^1-hPRL and G^2-hPRL, both with reduced immunoreactivity; G^1-hPRL has only one fourth the bioactivity of G^2-hPRL;
3. "Big" PRL (MW ~50,000), consisting of a mixture of dimeric and trimeric forms of glycosylated PRL (G-PRL); and
4. "Big-big" PRL (MW ~100,000), possibly representing G-PRL coupled covalently with immunoglobulin.[18]

These heterogeneous forms of PRL have been found in both normal and hyperprolactinemic states, and the big and big-big forms apparently have lower receptor-binding properties.[15] Normal fertility is maintained in patients with hyperprolactinemia due mainly to big-big PRL. However, circulating big PRL in human plasma can be converted to little PRL by reduction of its disulfide bonds.[19] Glycosylated forms of hPRL are less immunoreactive than little PRL and are the predominant forms present in most human plasma.[20] Differential release of glycosylated and nonglycosylated isoforms of PRL under physiologic conditions and in response to stimulation has been described.[21] Until a more sensitive and reliable bioassay becomes available, the relationship between the various forms of hPRL and their apparently discrepant clinical effects will remain unresolved.

The 16-kDa Fragment of Prolactin

Interestingly, Clapp and associates[22] have found that a 16-kDa fragment of PRL (16K-PRL) has potent inhibitory effects on angiogenesis, the formation of new capillaries from an established microvasculature. This has important clinical implications for such diverse processes as wound healing, inhibition of tumor growth, diabetic retinopathy, and rheumatoid arthritis, in all of which neovascularization is involved. A number of investigators are studying antiangiogenic factors as potential agents for inhibiting tumor growth, because solid tumors cannot grow beyond 1 to 3 mm in the absence of an adequate blood supply.

PRL can be cleaved enzymatically both in the pituitary gland and in PRL-responsive tissues. One of these cleavage products is 16K-PRL. Clapp and associates found that recombinant human 16K-PRL is a potent inhibitor of human vascular endothelial cells that had been stimulated by two angiogenic factors, vascular endothelial growth factor and basic fibroblast growth factor. This inhibition occurred with nanomolar concentrations of 16K-PRL, suggesting that it is potent at biologically meaningful concentrations. They also found that 16K-PRL is biologically active at PRL receptors. The antimitogenic activity of 16K-PRL appears to be specific for vascular endothelial cells. Intact PRL, however, does not appear to have antiangiogenic activity. Cleaved forms of PRL are present in the circulation of humans. The 16K-PRL appears to be mediated by a novel receptor that is being characterized at the time of this writing.

Prolactin Receptors and Signaling Mechanisms

The PRL receptor was cloned initially in the rat and subsequently in the human.[23] Like the growth hormone receptor, it is a single-pass transmembrane receptor member of the hematopoietic receptor superfamily. Human PRL does not bind to the human growth hormone (hGH) receptor, but hGH binds to both the hGH receptor and hPRL receptor. The crystal structure of a complex of hGH bound to the extracellular domain of the hPRL receptor has been described.[24] There are both long and short forms of the receptor, both of which can bind PRL with high affinity. Both the short and long forms can induce PRL responsive cells to grow.[25]

Interestingly, the PRL receptor is widely distributed, in some instances in the same tissue in which the ligand, PRL, is also expressed. The receptor has been found in the hypothalamus,[26] pituitary gland (both normal and neoplastic),[27] gastrointestinal tract,[28] prostate,[29] bone,[30] decidua,[31] fetal membranes,[31] and Leydig cells[32] as well as in normal and neoplastic breast tissue.[33, 34]

That both PRL and its receptor are expressed in such diverse tissues (pituitary gland, gastrointestinal tract, prostate, decidua, and breast) suggests the presence of an autocrine/paracrine loop in these tissues. Because a classic endocrine feedback loop between pituitary PRL and its target tissues has not been described, this potential autocrine/paracrine action suggests another possible mode of action for this hormone. PRL has been conserved across species and subsumes different functions in different species. For example, it controls fluid and electrolyte flux in fish, maintains the corpus luteum in rodents and sheep, and stimulates casein synthesis for milk production in the breasts of many species. This may explain its wide tissue distribution.

In the human fetus, there is intense PRL receptor immunoreactivity in tissues derived from embryonic mesoderm, including the periadrenal and perinephric mesenchyme; the pulmonary and duodenal mesenchyme; the cardiac and skeletal myocytes; and the mesenchymal precartilage and maturing chondrocytes of the endochondral craniofacial and long bones, vertebrae, and ribs.[35] Marked changes in the cellular distribution and extent of PRL receptor expression were seen in many tissues during fetal development. In the fetal adrenal gland, the initial PRL receptor expression in periadrenal mesenchyme was followed by immunoreactivity in deeper fetal cortical cell layers. In the fetal kidney and lung, invagination of cortical mesenchyme was accompanied by progressive PRL receptor immunoreactivity in bronchial and renal tubular epithelial cells. In addition, in the pancreas, the PRL receptor was expressed primarily in acinar cells and ducts in early gestation, whereas in late gestation and in the postnatal period, the receptor was expressed primarily in pancreatic islets where it colocalized with insulin and glucagon.[35] These observations suggest that PRL may play a role in tissue differentiation and organ development during human fetal intrauterine life.

Information has emerged in recent years concerning the signaling mechanisms involved after PRL binding to its receptor. One of the earliest responses to PRL binding, at least in an experimental cell line and in mouse mammary gland explants, is an increase in tyrosine phosphorylation of cellular proteins. The tyrosine kinase Jak_2 may serve as an early, and perhaps initial, signaling molecule for PRL, as may tyrosine kinases of the Src family.

In addition to the Janus kinase (Jak) and Src families, PRL induces activation of Ras, an oncogenic protein that supports an alternative route from the membrane to the nucleus.[36] This route provides a possible molecular bridge between activation of the PRL receptor–associated tyrosine kinases and subsequent stimulation of the serine/threonine kinase Raf-1, a Ras target that is activated by PRL.

Further, the gene for whey acidic protein in the rat contains a mammary gland–specific and hormonally regulated DNase I–hypersensitive site.[37] Nuclear factor I binding is the major DNA-protein interaction within this tissue-specific nuclease hypersensitive region. Interestingly, a recognition site for mammary gland factor (signal transducer and activator of transcription [STAT-5]), which mediates PRL induction of milk protein gene expression, is immediately proximal to the nuclear factor I binding sites.

Functional Heterogeneity

Functional heterogeneity within the population of lactotrophs also exists. By use of the reverse hemolytic plaque assay for measurement of PRL secretion by individual lactotrophs, two subpopulations of cells were found, one secreting small amounts and the other secreting 150-fold more PRL.[38] The latter group of cells is preferentially responsive to the inhibitory effects of dopamine (DA). Similarly, on the basis of electrophysiologic responses, two functional types of lactotrophs were characterized: one with high resting potential that is thyrotropin-releasing hormone (TRH) sensitive/DA insensitive, and the other with low resting potential that is TRH insensitive/DA sensitive.[39] These functional differences may be related to the intrinsic cell cycle of secretory activities.

CONTROL OF LACTOTROPH DEVELOPMENT AND PROLACTIN SECRETION

The pituitary-specific transcriptional factor Pit-1, a member of the POU domain family, activates and regulates the transcription of both growth hormone and PRL promoters.[40] Although Pit-1 messenger ribonucleic acid (mRNA) was detected in all five types of pituitary cells in rodents, Pit-1 protein was limited to three cell types: lactotrophs, somatotrophs, and thyrotrophs.[41] In humans, point mutations in the gene encoding Pit-1 have been reported in cases of combined deficiencies of growth hormone, PRL, and thyrotropin (thyroid-stimulating hormone [TSH]).[42]

Specific DNA-dependent interactions have been found between Pit-1 and the nuclear receptors, thyroid hormone receptor, glucocorticoid receptor, and estrogen receptor (ER).[43] In human pituitary glands and pituitary adenomas, ERs have been found,[44] and Pit-1 mRNA and ER mRNA were colocalized with PRL immunoreactivity in pituitary adenoma cells.[45] This raises the possibility of interactions between Pit-1 and the ER in the functional differentiation and development of PRL-secreting adenomas, discussed subsequently.

In contrast to the role of Pit-1 in pituitary PRL expression, transcriptional regulation of PRL gene expression in certain nonpituitary sites, including decidua and lymphocytes, as well as in a uterine sarcoma cell line, is independent of Pit-1.[46] There is a decidual/lymphoid promoter located approximately 6 kilobases upstream of the pituitary-specific start site regulating PRL expression,[46] and Pit-1 is not involved. Activation of this promoter can be induced by cyclic adenosine monophosphate (cAMP), suggesting that a signal transduced through the cAMP signaling pathway is a primary inducer of decidual PRL gene expression. In a uterine sarcoma cell line, the decidual upstream promoter is not used, but transcription of the PRL gene is effected by a downstream pituitary-type transcription start site. This uterine sarcoma line lacks Pit-1.

The synthesis and release of pituitary PRL, like those of growth hormone, are under a complex hypothalamic dual regulatory system that involves both inhibitory PRL-inhibiting factors (PIFs) and stimulatory PRL-releasing factors (PRFs). At the pituitary level, PRL is regulated by autocrine and paracrine mechanisms discussed before and subsequently. Peripheral hormones, including estrogens, thyroid hormones, vitamin D, and glucocorticoids, are potent modulators of PRL synthesis and release and of PRL gene expression (Fig. 9–3). Thus, lactotrophs possess numerous membrane and nuclear receptors, each of which transduces a particular functional signal. The minute-to-minute regulation of PRL secretion by the lactotroph appears to be largely controlled by the balance of inhibitory (PIF) and stimulatory (PRF) inputs transmitted to the pituitary from the hypothalamus as well as modulated by peripheral hormones.

Prolactin Synthesis and Release

As in other protein hormone–secreting cells, PRL synthesis and release follow a processing scheme that includes receptor activation, generation of second messengers, and gene transcription. After hormone synthesis and packaging into secretory granules, PRL is stored in the cytoplasm before release. On exposure to secretagogues, lactotrophs release PRL from a readily releasable pool, and newly synthesized PRL goes to replenish the releasable pool as well as to a storage pool.[47]

In addition to Pit-1 discussed before, PRL gene expression is regulated by a number of different hormones acting through diverse intracellular mechanisms. DA, TRH, and estradiol have all been shown to alter transcription of the PRL gene.[48–50]

In addition, the neuropeptide galanin is distributed widely in the central and peripheral nervous systems, anterior pituitary gland, and adrenal medulla. In the anterior pituitary, galanin colocalizes with corticotropin (adrenocorticotropic hormone) in the corticotroph in the human pituitary and, at least in the rodent, in the lactotroph. Pituitary galanin expression is sensitive to estrogen status; a marked elevation occurs during pregnancy and lactation, and exogenous 17β-estradiol can induce a marked (4000-fold) in-

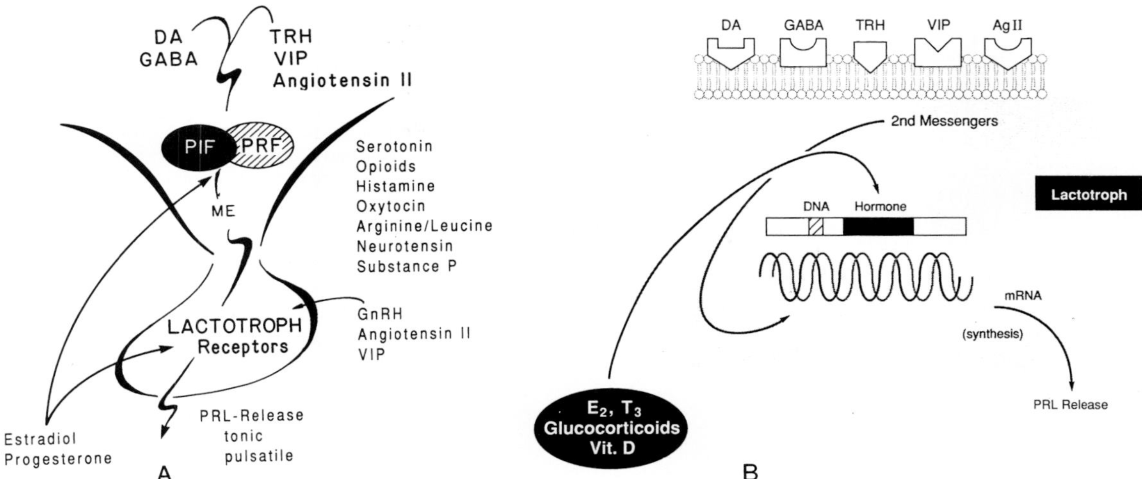

Figure 9–3 ■ Diagrammatic representation of neuroendocrine regulation of lactotroph function and prolactin secretion.

A, A variety of hypothalamic prolactin-inhibiting factors (PIFs) and prolactin-releasing factors (PRFs) as well as central and peripheral modulators are depicted. Several peptides regulate prolactin (PRL) secretion within the pituitary gland by means of autocrine and paracrine mechanisms. Peripheral hormones, particularly estradiol and progesterone, exert their influence through both hypothalamic and pituitary sites.

B, Lactotrophs possess multiple membrane receptors for a variety of regulatory factors, and their functional inhibition (dopamine, γ-aminobutyric acid) and activation (thyrotropin-releasing hormone, vasoactive intestinal peptide, angiotensin II) of PRL synthesis and release are mediated by induction of second messengers after binding to their specific receptors. A number of peripheral hormones (E_2, T_3, glucocorticoids, and vitamin D) targeted at the specific nuclear binding sites in the regulation of lactotroph function are also shown.

crease in mRNA levels of galanin. In rats, galanin is secreted by a minority of lactotrophs and is essential for the regulation of basal and vasoactive intestinal peptide (VIP)–stimulated PRL release.[51] Increased concentrations of estrogen increase the number of galanin-secreting cells, and the resulting increase in basal PRL release is completely abolished by treatment with galanin antiserum. Further, galanin is a potent lactotroph growth factor, and galanin immunoneutralization inhibits the mitogenic effects on the lactotroph.[51] Thus, in the rodent, there appear to be paracrine effects of galanin on lactotroph function. In addition, the effect of estrogen on lactotroph proliferation and PRL release appears to be mediated by locally secreted galanin.

Galanin also stimulates basal and growth hormone–releasing hormone (GHRH)–stimulated growth hormone in humans. However, the role of galanin in regulating PRL secretion in humans is not clear. In healthy men, whereas intravenous galanin caused a significant increase in growth hormone levels and enhanced the growth hormone response to GHRH, baseline and TRH-stimulated PRL levels were not altered by galanin.[52] In another study, the intravenous infusion of porcine galanin to normal women alone and in combination with TRH caused an increase in serum growth hormone but did not modify spontaneous PRL secretion.[53] Furthermore, intravenous infusion of human galanin to normal men resulted in an increase in circulating growth hormone but not in PRL.[54] Thus, it appears possible that if galanin does affect PRL secretion in humans, its effect may be a local autocrine/paracrine effect, perhaps modulated by the endogenous estrogen environment.

Prolactin-Inhibiting Factors

Dopamine

The role of hypothalamic DA as a major PIF is firmly established.[55] DA is secreted into the portal vessels by the tuberoinfundibular DA (TIDA) system, the cell bodies of which are located in the arcuate nucleus, with axons terminating in the external layer of the median eminence (ME). The biosynthesis and release of DA occur in the axonic terminals, which abut the portal capillaries. DA is bound to DA receptors on the lactotroph with resultant inhibition of PRL secretion.[56] The concentration of DA in the central portal vessels is twice as high as that in the lateral vessels.[57] This topographic difference in the concentration of portal DA may have implications for the frequent occurrence of adenoma formation in the lateral wings of the adenohypophysis.

Dopamine Synthesis and Release by the Tuberoinfundibular Dopamine System

The pathway for synthesis of DA is covered in Chapter 2 and is outlined here in brief. The pathway for biosynthesis and release of DA is illustrated in Figure 9–4*A*. Tyrosine, an essential amino acid and the precursor for biosynthesis of all catecholamines, is transported actively into the brain. As a substrate, tyrosine is taken up by catecholaminergic neurons, such as TIDA. Within the neurons, tyrosine is converted to L-dihydroxyphenylalanine (DOPA) by the rate-limiting enzyme tyrosine hydroxylase. This enzyme is regulated, in part, by end-product inhibition, so that increases of intraneuronal DA concentration result in decreased DA synthesis, and vice versa. DOPA is rapidly decarboxylated to DA by L-amino acid decarboxylase. The newly synthesized DA can then be released or stored in nerve terminals. The DA released at the outer layer of the ME enters the portal circulation and binds to DA receptors on the lactotroph. DA at the nerve terminals is subject to oxidative deamination by monoamine oxidase to form an inactive metabolite, dihydroxyphenylacetic acid. Unlike other catecholamine neurons, DA released by TIDA neu-

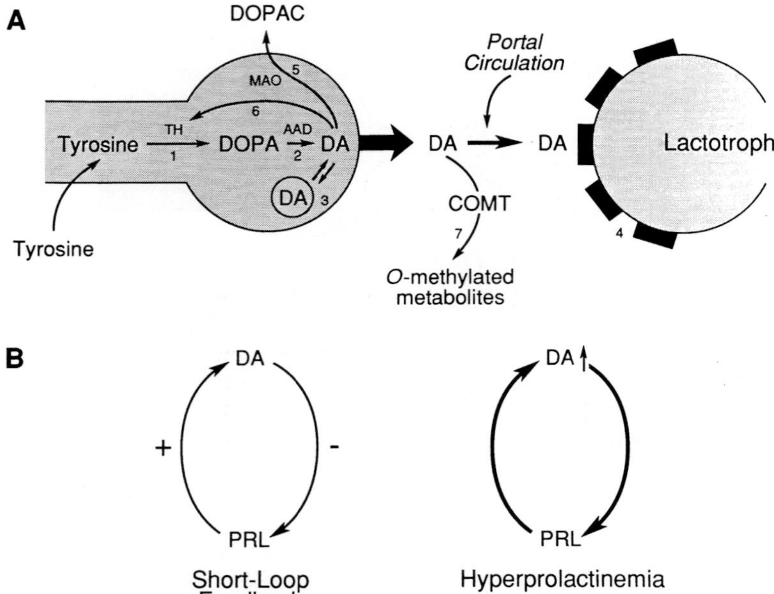

Figure 9–4 ■ Prolactin and dopamine turnover.

A, Schematic representation of dopaminergic nerve terminals and dopamine (DA) receptors on the lactotroph. Tyrosine is transported into the neurons and converted to L-dihydroxyphenylalanine (DOPA) by the rate-limiting enzyme tyrosine hydroxylase (TH, step 1). This enzyme is regulated in part by end-product inhibition, so that decreases of intraneural DA concentration result in increased DA synthesis and vice versa. DOPA is rapidly decarboxylated to DA by L-aromatic amino acid decarboxylase (AAD, step 2). The newly synthesized DA can be released or stored (step 3). The DA released at the outer layer of the median eminence enters the portal circulation, where binding to DA receptors on the lactotroph takes place (step 4). DA in the nerve terminals is oxidatively deaminated by monoamine oxidase (MAO) to form an inactive metabolite (dihydroxyphenylacetic acid, step 5). Two unique features of the tuberoinfundibular dopamine system are (1) the possibility that further metabolism of DA by catechol *O*-methyltransferase (COMT) will not occur and (2) the absence of autoreceptors for local negative feedback regulation.

B, Short-loop feedback system of prolactin (PRL) and dopamine (DA) regulation.

rons may not be further metabolized by catechol *O*-methyltransferase, and local negative feedback is absent because of the lack of autoreceptors of the TIDA system.

Prolactin, through short-loop feedback, increases DA turnover (Fig. 9–4*B*); accordingly, an increase in PRL secretion by the lactotroph induces enhanced DA release, thereby inhibiting PRL secretion. Evidence for such an autoregulatory system has been demonstrated both in vitro and in vivo.[58] The autoregulation by PRL of PRL release is mediated by the PRL receptors in the ME that stimulate DA release.[59] Central administration of α-melanocyte–stimulating hormone, a product of pro-opiomelanocortin, activates TIDA neurons, thereby decreasing the secretion of PRL by the lactotrophs.[59] An unidentified PIF from the posterior lobe may play a role in the regulation of PRL secretion.[60]

The principal site of inactivation of DA after release into the portal system is the DA membrane receptor on the target lactotroph. Thus, TIDA in the control of PRL secretion serves as a neurohormone rather than as a neurotransmitter.

Dopamine Control of Prolactin Secretion

The inhibitory effect of DA on PRL release can be shown by the administration of L-dopa, a metabolic precursor of DA; L-dopa readily crosses the blood-brain barrier and increases the rate of formation of DA beyond the rate-limiting step, tyrosine hydroxylase. As a consequence, PRL levels decline to a nadir 2½ hours after L-dopa administration (0.5 gm), and the recovery includes a rebound above basal level (Fig. 9–5). L-Dopa suppresses PRL levels even when conversion to norepinephrine is blocked by diethyldithiocarbonate, a DA β-hydroxylase inhibitor,[55] demonstrating that norepinephrine is not required in the regulation of PRL secretion and that hypothalamic DA acts directly as a potent PIF.

DA infusion at a variety of rates (from 0.02 to 8 μg/kg/min) for 3 to 4 hours produces a dose-related suppression of PRL levels in normal men and women as well as in patients with hyperprolactinemia.[61–63] Although DA does not cross the blood-brain barrier, both the ME and the adenohypophysis are outside the blood-brain barrier, and DA infused into the general circulation can therefore be effectively delivered to the lactotroph. Significant suppression of PRL levels can be achieved by as little as 0.02 μg/kg/min, and maximal suppression occurs at 4 μg/kg/min. This inhibition is followed by a marked rebound in PRL secretion on cessation of DA infusion, suggesting that PRL synthesis is not disrupted by the DA inhibition of PRL release[61] (Fig. 9–6).

DA receptors located in the plasma membrane on the lactotroph are classified as D_2 subtypes, and the cDNA of the D_2 DA receptor has been cloned.[64] Lactotroph D_2 receptors are coupled to signal transduction mechanisms. A model depicting DA action on the lactotroph is shown in Figure 9–7. After binding of DA, the DA-receptor complex activates a membrane inhibitory G_i protein, which is negatively coupled to adenylate cyclase and phospholipase C

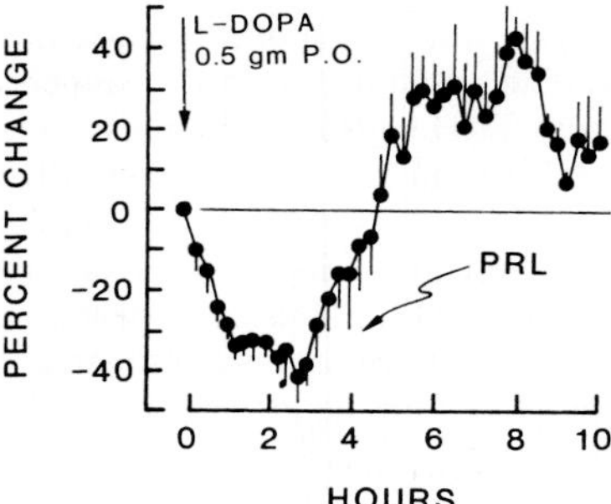

Figure 9–5 ■ The effect of L-dopa showing an acute inhibition of prolactin (PRL) secretion by the pituitary. (From Leblanc H, Yen SSC. The effect of L-dopa and chlorpromazine on prolactin and growth hormone secretion in normal women. Am J Obstet Gynecol 126:162–164, 1976.)

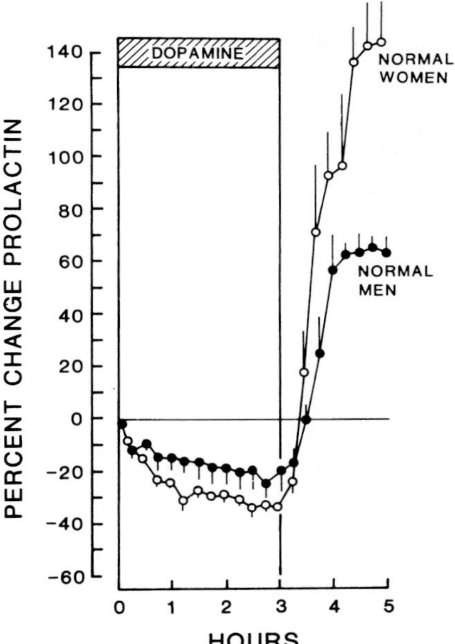

Figure 9–6 ■ Plasma prolactin concentration during and after dopamine infusion (0.4 μg/kg/min) in normal male and female subjects. Prolactin release is inhibited in all subjects and rebounds on discontinuation of the infusion. (From Leblanc H, Lachelin GC, Abu-Fadil S, Yen SSC. Effects of dopamine infusion on pituitary hormone secretion in humans. J Clin Endocrinol Metab 43:668–674, 1976. © The Endocrine Society.)

systems,[64, 65] thereby reducing PRL release and mRNA transcription.[66, 67] The transmembrane signal evoked by DA withdrawal elicits rapid release of PRL. This event involves effector pathways of adenylate cyclase with the formation of the second messenger cAMP and the phospholipase C enzyme, resulting in the hydrolysis of intramembrane phosphatidylinositol bisphosphate to generate inositol triphosphate and diacylglycerol. Inositol triphosphate functions as a second messenger to mobilize Ca^{2+} from the intracellular Ca^{2+} store in the endoplasmic reticulum, which initiates PRL release. In additional, diacylglycerol serves to activate the protein kinase C system and to trigger a Ca^{2+}-dependent PRL release. The protein kinase C pathway regulating PRL release may also be activated when receptors for secretagogues, such as TRH, are activated. In the DA withdrawal model, the effect of TRH on protein kinase C activation appears to be prolonged, thereby potentiating the PRL-releasing activity of TRH.[68]

Apomorphine and ergots (e.g., bromocriptine) are agonists with high affinity for D_2 receptors and are potent inhibitors of PRL release. Haloperidol, metoclopramide, and domperidone are examples of D_2 receptor antagonists, and they induce PRL release by antagonizing endogenous DA binding in vivo and in vitro (Table 9–1). These agonistic and antagonistic actions in corresponding reduction and augmentation of PRL secretion are well established in humans.

Paradoxically, although it is well established that DA, through D_2 DA receptors, inhibits PRL production, it can actually increase PRL release under appropriate experimental conditions. The D_1 and D_5 DA receptors can activate adenylate cyclase. In a cell type that secretes PRL but does not express DA receptors (GH_4Cl) that was transfected with D_1 and D_5 receptors, DA increased PRL release. Thus, D_1 and D_5 receptors are capable of mediating the stimulatory effects of DA on PRL release. The mRNA for D_5 DA receptors is present in rat anterior pituitary glands.[69]

γ-Aminobutyric Acid

Several lines of evidence, both in vivo and in vitro, suggest that γ-aminobutyric acid (GABA), in addition to DA, may function as a PIF:

1. GABA nerve terminals are present in the internal and external layers of the ME.[70]
2. GABA is secreted into the portal blood, and specific GABA receptors are present on the pituitary lactotroph.[71] Concentrations of GABA in portal blood are inversely related to PRL secretion.[72]

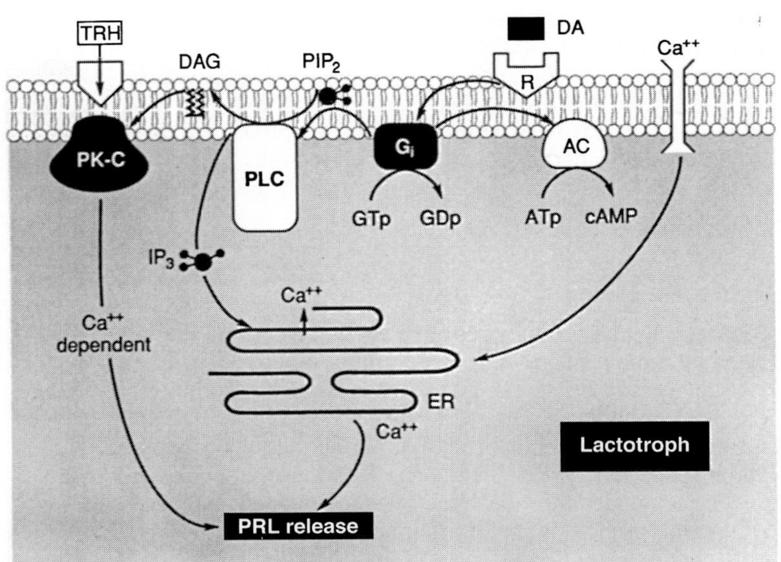

Figure 9–7 ■ Schematic illustration of mechanisms of inhibitory action of dopamine (DA) and stimulatory action of thyrotropin-releasing hormone (TRH) on prolactin (PRL) release by the lactotroph. The model depicts the negatively coupled DA receptor and the G_i protein, which functions to inhibit the adenylate cyclase (AC)/cyclic adenosine monophosphate (cAMP) system as well as phospholipase C (PLC). Dopamine withdrawal would activate these systems to generate intracellular messengers, cAMP, inositol triphosphate (IP_3), and diacylglycerol (DAG), thereby inducing Ca^{2+}-dependent cellular events of PRL release. When coupled to its receptors, TRH induces a similar pathway resulting in protein kinase C (PK-C) activation and generates Ca^{2+}-dependent PRL release. ER, endoplasmic reticulum.

■ TABLE 9–1

Conditions Associated with Inappropriate Prolactin Secretion

PHARMACOLOGIC CAUSES	PATHOLOGIC CAUSES
Estrogen therapy	Hypothalamic lesions
Anesthesia	Craniopharyngioma
DA receptor blocking agents	Glioma
Phenothiazines	Granulomas
Haloperidol	Histiocytosis X
Metoclopramide	Sarcoid
Domperidone	Tuberculosis
Pimozide	Stalk transection
Sulpiride	Postsurgical or head injury
DA reuptake blocker	Irradiation damage of the hypothalamus
Nomifensine	Pseudocyesis (functional)
CNS DA-depleting agents	Pituitary tumors
Reserpine	Cushing's disease
Methyldopa	Acromegaly
Monoamine oxidase inhibitor	Prolactinoma
Inhibition of DA turnover	Mixed GH or ACTH- and PRL-secreting adenomas
Opiates	"Nonfunctional" adenomas
Stimulation of serotoninergic system	Reflex causes
Amphetamines	Chest wall injury and herpes zoster neuritis
Hallucinogens	Upper abdominal surgery
Histamine H_2 receptor antagonists	Hypothyroidism
Cimetidine	Renal failure
	Ectopic production
	Bronchogenic carcinoma
	Hypernephroma

DA, dopamine; CNS, central nervous system; GH, growth hormone, ACTH, adenocorticotropic hormone; PRL, prolactin.

3. Enhancement of endogenous GABA-ergic tone induced by sodium valproate (an inhibitor of GABA transaminase that degrades GABA at central and peripheral sites) reduces basal and breast-stimulated PRL release in women.[73]

The inhibitory activity of DA is far greater than that of GABA. The marked rebound in PRL release, seen both in vitro and in vivo after the cessation of DA infusion, does not occur with GABA, suggesting different mechanisms of action for DA and GABA. DA, but not GABA, permits the lactotroph to accumulate newly synthesized PRL, which appears to be rapidly released after withdrawal of DA inhibition.[74] It has been proposed that, unlike DA, GABA as a PIF may function episodically in response to certain stimuli rather than being constantly secreted into the portal blood.

Prolactin-Releasing Factors

Although hypothalamic control of PRL secretion is dominated by a tonic inhibitory mechanism, a functional role of PRF appears to be necessary for acute secretory activities. For example, under certain conditions, incremental PRL secretion is not accompanied by a measurable decrease in portal blood DA levels,[75] and acute PRL release can occur under maximal inhibition by DA. Experimental evidence in several species, including humans, suggests that TRH, VIP, angiotensin II (AII), and several other substances may be involved in the control of PRL secretion. Thus, neuroregulation of PRL secretion appears to be multifactorial (see Fig. 9–3).

Thyrotropin-Releasing Hormone

Hypothalamic TRH is a potent stimulator of the release of pituitary PRL both in vivo and in vitro.[76] The TRH concentration required to elicit an in vitro PRL release (10^{-9} M) is within the range found in the portal plasma (200 to 500 pg/ml). Specific receptors for TRH are present on the lactotroph, and TRH stimulates PRL gene transcription within minutes. The result is an increase in mRNA accumulation in the cytoplasm as well as acute release of PRL. The effect of TRH is thought to involve phospholipase C–mediated hydrolysis of inositol phospholipids, resulting in Ca^{2+} release from an intracellular pool and activation of calcium-lipid–dependent protein kinase C–mediated PRL release[77] (see Fig. 9–7).

Further evidence that TRH plays a role in the regulation of PRL release is provided by the reduction of PRL as well as TSH secretion in rats after the administration of TRH antiserum.[78] Although the PRL- and TSH-releasing actions of TRH are separate and distinct, circulating levels of thyroxine (T_4) and triiodothyronine (T_3) do influence the PRL release in response to TRH stimulation; subnormal serum levels of T_3 and T_4, as in primary hypothyroidism, increase TRH-induced PRL release, whereas higher than normal serum levels of T_3 and T_4 inhibit PRL mRNA accumulation and release.[79] Although thyroid hormone and estradiol receptors are members of a superfamily of genes, they have opposing actions on PRL synthesis and release by lactotrophs. Estradiol, in contrast to T_3, induces preferential augmentation of basal and TRH-stimulated PRL release (Fig. 9–8). Thus, TRH-mediated PRL release can be modulated by circulating thyroid hormones, estradiol, and antithyroid medication in patients with hyperthyroidism.

Vasoactive Intestinal Peptide and Oxytocin

The presence of VIP and oxytocin in high concentrations in hypophyseal portal blood and the presence of specific receptors in the anterior pituitary suggest that these neuropeptides are involved in regulating anterior pituitary function.[80] Indeed, VIP and oxytocin are established PRFs.

VIP stimulates the secretion of PRL in the rat by acting at both the hypothalamic and the pituitary levels. The PRL-releasing action of VIP is mediated by stimulation of oxytocin release.[81] At the pituitary level, VIP appears to interfere with the inhibitory action of DA on the adenylate cyclase–cAMP system. In addition, VIP is produced locally within the lactotroph and has been shown to stimulate PRL release. This autocrine action of VIP may explain the high rate of "spontaneous" PRL secretion attributed to lactotrophs deprived of hypothalamic influences.[82] In humans, infusion of VIP induces a prompt rise in PRL levels.[83]

Angiotensin II

AII is a potent secretagogue for the release of PRL both in vivo and in vitro.[84] It acts on a specific receptor on the

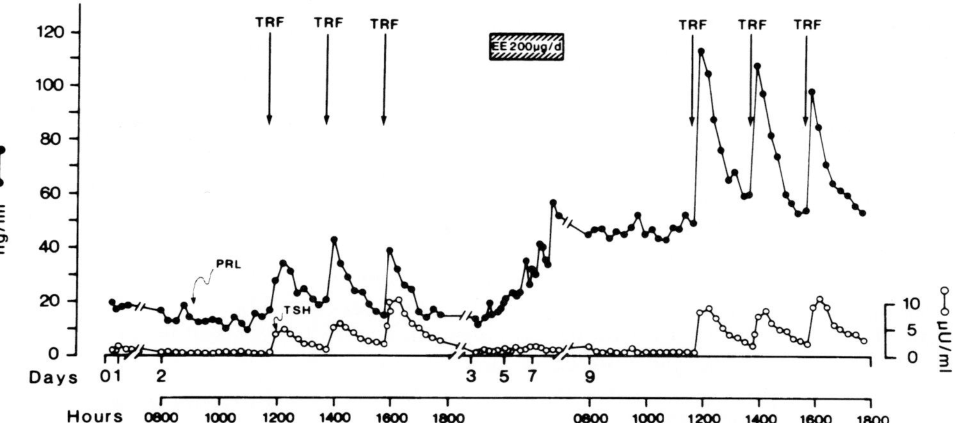

Figure 9–8 ■ Marked augmentation of basal and thyrotropin-releasing hormone (TRH, 200 μg intravenous bolus)–stimulated prolactin (PRL) release in a hypogonadal woman treated with large doses of ethinyl estradiol (EE, 200 μg/day) for 1 week (days 3 to 9) compared with pretreatment values (days 1 and 2). Note that thyroid-stimulating hormone (TSH) levels and responses to TRH were unaltered by estrogen administration. TRF, thyrotropin-releasing factor.

lactotroph, and its PRL-releasing action can be blocked by an AII antagonist (saralasin).[85] The PRL-releasing activity of AII is more potent than that of TRH, and the action is fast (peak at 10 minutes) but brief.

AII, an octapeptide, has been identified in the brains of several species, including humans. The immunoreactivity for AII is concentrated in the hypothalamus and ME and possibly is released into the portal circulation to serve as a PRF in the regulation of PRL release. Pituitary AII receptors are also exposed to peripherally circulating AII; thus, peripheral changes in activity of the renin-angiotensin system may influence PRL secretion.[84] Moreover, all of the components of the renin-angiotensin system have been colocalized within the human pituitary lactotroph, but not in other pituitary cells. Thus, an autocrine action of AII on PRL release has been proposed.[86] However, the relative effectiveness of central, peripheral, and autocrine modes of AII regulation of PRL secretion by the lactotroph is unclear.

Neurotransmitter Mediation of Prolactin Release

Several neurotransmitters and neuromodulators appear to be involved in the control of PRL release by the hypothalamus. Interactions among and between these neurotransmitters, PIFs and PRFs, may provide integrated control of PRL secretion under a variety of physiologic and stressful conditions.

Serotonin

A serotoninergic pathway appears to be involved in the control of PRL secretion. Because serotonin (5-hydroxytryptamine) does not cross the blood-brain barrier, a variety of pharmacologic agents have been used to test the serotonin effect; the results indicate that enhanced serotonin activity causes PRL release, whereas lowered serotonin activity reduces PRL secretion. The effects of serotonin on PRL secretion are independent of DA. The experimental findings include the following:

1. Administration of 5-hydroxytryptophan to rats pretreated with fluoxetine, a serotonin uptake inhibitor, causes a significant increase in PRL levels.[87] Activation of serotonin receptors in the medial basal hypothalamus by intracerebral injection of serotonin induces a dose-related rise in plasma PRL concentrations.[88]
2. Quipazine, a serotonin receptor agonist, stimulates PRL secretion.[87]
3. Acute PRL release occurs in men after infusion or ingestion of 5 to 10 gm of L-tryptophan, the substrate for biosynthesis of serotonin.[89, 90]
4. Administration of cyproheptadine, a serotonin antagonist, blocks the PRL-releasing effect of oral administration of 5-hydroxytryptophan in men.[91]
5. Methysergide, a drug with serotonin-blocking properties, significantly depresses resting PRL levels.[92]
6. In postpartum women, methysergide blocks both basal and acute PRL release induced by mechanical stimulation of the nipples and suckling.[93]

These results suggest that in humans, as in rats, activation of the serotoninergic pathway causes PRL release. The signal that triggers serotoninergic input appears to originate at the dorsal raphe nucleus, with the ultimate release of serotonin at the terminal of the medial basal hypothalamus.

Endogenous Opioids

Experimental evidence indicates that the opioidergic control of PRL secretion in the rat is mediated through its inhibition of DA turnover by the tuberoinfundibular neurons.[94, 95] If this functional relationship operates in vivo, assuming that the naloxone-sensitive opiate receptor is involved, a decrement in PRL release should occur after opiate receptor blockade by naloxone. Such a relationship has been demonstrated in rats and monkeys.[96, 97]

In humans, PRL release occurs in response to exogenous administration of opiates and opioid peptides.[98] Naloxone infusion at different dose regimens, however, does not appear to affect basal PRL release or PRL release induced by exercise, hypoglycemia, or stress.[99] In addition, high doses of naloxone do not suppress puerperal hyperprolactinemia,[100] suckling-stimulated PRL release, or hyperprolactinemia due to pituitary microadenomas.[101] Thus, whereas exogenous opioids do induce PRL release in humans, the role of *endogenous* opioids in regulating PRL secretion under physiologic and pathologic conditions remains unclear.

Histamine

Histamine is a putative hypothalamic transmitter found in highest concentrations in the ME; it binds to two types of receptors, H_1 and H_2.[102] In the rat, intracerebroventricular administration of histamine induces prompt PRL release, whereas cimetidine or ranitidine, each an H_2 receptor blocking agent, abolishes histamine-stimulated or stress-induced PRL release.[103] Cimetidine has been shown to induce PRL release and galactorrhea in humans.[104] Histamine-stimulated PRL release appears, in part, to be mediated by serotoninergic pathways.[105]

Neurotensin and Substance P

Both neurotensin and substance P, isolated from bovine hypothalamus, have been shown to stimulate the release of PRL in the rat.[106] Intracerebroventricular administration of substance P in rhesus monkeys induces a rapid increase in serum PRL levels.[107] The effect of neurotensin and substance P on PRL release in humans is not known.

Short-Loop Feedback Control (Autoregulation)

Because release of PRL is not regulated by negative feedback signals from peripheral target sites, short-loop feedback, operating by way of hypothalamic regulation (through retrograde PRL flow), assumes particular physiologic significance (see Fig. 9–4). Such an autoregulatory mechanism is supported by a variety of experimental evidence, including:

1. PRL binding sites are localized in the ME;
2. Intracerebroventricular injection of PRL results in an increase both in DA turnover in the ME and in DA concentration in the portal blood[108];
3. The high turnover rate of DA in the ME, found during lactation and pregnancy, is reduced by hypophysectomy or by reducing PRL secretion through a direct pituitary inhibition by bromocriptine administration[109, 110]; and
4. Hyperprolactinemia, induced by pituitary transplants, decreases VIP release (PRF) and increases DA secretion, resulting in reduced PRL output.[111]

Thus, PRL controls its own secretion rate through feedback regulation of hypothalamic releasing (VIP) and inhibiting (DA) factors. In addition, as noted previously, PRL receptors are present in both the hypothalamus and pituitary gland.

Paracrine and Autocrine Control of Prolactin Release

The autocrine control of PRL secretion by VIP and AII has been described earlier in this chapter. The ability of exogenous gonadotropin-releasing hormone (GnRH) and GnRH agonists to elicit PRL release by the pituitary in humans has been demonstrated.[112] Moreover, synchronized pulsatile release of PRL and luteinizing hormone (LH) has been observed in postmenopausal women[113] and in midluteal-phase women in response to naloxone.[114] These observations suggest that endogenous pulsatile release of GnRH may induce the secretion of both LH and PRL. The most likely explanation for the PRL-releasing action of GnRH involves an intrapituitary mechanism wherein gonadotrophs interact with the lactotrophs by means of a paracrine factor. This concept, supported by experimental data,[115] is consistent with the close anatomic association between lactotrophs and gonadotrophs within the pituitary.

Peripheral Hormones

Several peripheral hormones exert influence on biosynthesis and secretion of PRL. These hormones have in common the ability to bind to members of the steroid receptor superfamily gene products.

Glucocorticoids

Dexamethasone inhibits PRL gene transcription. The negative regulation of PRL secretion by glucocorticoids appears to be exerted by interference with the DNA-binding region of the glucocorticoid receptor, thereby reducing gene transcription.[116] This effect of glucocorticoids may, in part, explain the association of hypoprolactinemia in functional states associated with hypercortisolism.

Vitamin D

A direct inhibitory action of $1,25(OH)_2D_3$ (vitamin D_3) on PRL mRNA accumulation and release has been demonstrated in a rat pituitary cell line.[117] Hyperprolactinemia in chronic renal failure can be reversed by vitamin D_3 treatment.[118] Limited information precludes the assignment of a regulatory role of vitamin D_3 on PRL secretion at this time.

Estrogen

Estrogen significantly promotes both the synthesis and release of PRL by the pituitary. This effect appears to be dose and duration dependent. Administration of pharmacologic doses of estrogen induces a rapid and profound rise in PRL release within 2 days in postmenopausal women[119] (Fig. 9–9) and in men,[120] with a corresponding suppression of serum LH and follicle-stimulating hormone (FSH) levels. The increasing levels of PRL during estrogen treatment appear to be maintained by an increase in the amplitude but not frequency of episodic PRL release throughout the 24-hour period.[121]

In reproductive-age women, administration of estradiol in amounts that produce circulating levels normally seen in the preovulatory period results in a rise in nocturnal PRL secretion with little change in daytime secretion.[122]

This positive influence of estrogen on PRL turnover in the pituitary can be accounted for by several mechanisms:

1. Binding of estrogen to its nuclear receptor on the lactotroph[123] leads to the activation of gene transcription and accumulation of PRL mRNA.[124, 125]

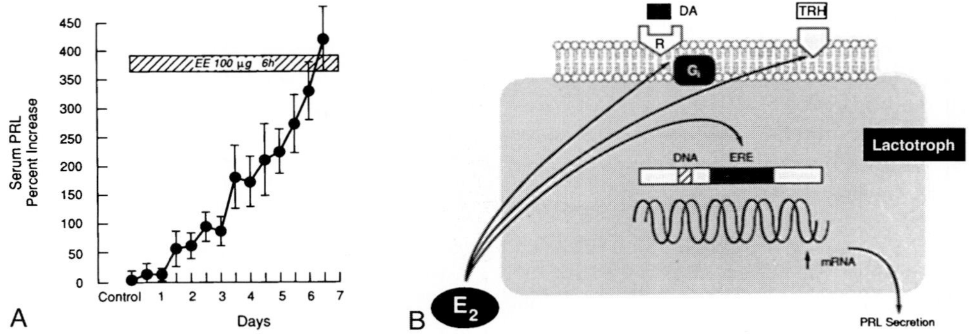

Figure 9–9 ■ Circulating levels of prolactin (PRL) in response to estrogen treatment in hypogonadal women.

A, The data are expressed as percentage change from pretreatment values. *Note:* A 400 percent increase of PRL concentration was attained after 7 days of ethinyl estradiol (EE) administration.

B, The positive effect of estradiol (E_2) on PRL dynamics is exerted at multiple sites; E_2 inhibits the coupling of DA receptor to G_i protein; up-regulation of TRH receptors and binding of the E_2-receptor complex to the intracellular E_2 response element (ERE) lead to gene activation, accumulation of mRNA, and PRL synthesis.

2. An antidopaminergic effect of estrogen at the pituitary level markedly decreases the ability of DA to inhibit PRL secretion.[126] This effect of estrogen appears to be exerted by preventing the D_2 receptor from activating the G_1 protein, thereby interrupting the inhibitory signal of DA and resulting in increased PRL synthesis and release.[127] However, this antidopaminergic effect of estrogen demonstrated in the rat has not been observed in humans.[128]
3. Estrogen up-regulates the TRH receptor on the lactotroph, permitting an increased sensitivity to the PRL-releasing action of TRH[129] (see Fig. 9–9).

Thus, the up-regulating action of estrogen on PRL synthesis and release is exerted by multiple mechanisms: increased PRL DNA synthesis, increased TRH receptors, and reduced DA action. The last remains to be demonstrated in humans. Estradiol appears to exert less effect on PRL secretion in humans than in rodents.

Progesterone

Progesterone administration after estrogen priming causes an acute release of PRL as well as of LH in ovariectomized women[130] and in monkeys.[131] Although the lactotroph is richly endowed with receptors for estrogen but not for progesterone, this is markedly different from the gonadotroph, in which both estrogen and progesterone receptors are present.[123] Thus, the progesterone effect on PRL secretion, as described before, probably does not involve a direct effect on the lactotroph. The precise mechanism is unknown, but a hypothalamic site of progesterone action is possible. Progesterone may induce GnRH release, thereby providing a paracrine effect from gonadotroph to lactotroph. This proposed mode of action is consistent with the ability of estrogen to induce progesterone receptors in the hypothalamus and in GnRH receptors on the gonadotroph as demonstrated in primates.[132, 133]

PROLACTIN AND THE IMMUNE SYSTEM

Interactions between the neuroendocrine and immune systems have been recognized for more than two decades. Indeed, as indicated in a review,[134] the nervous, endocrine, and immune systems must be integrated at all levels to maintain homeostasis. The concept is evolving that the anabolic hormones (growth hormone, PRL, and the insulin-like growth factors) not only regulate body growth, metabolism, tissue repair, and cell survival but also serve to integrate the growth, maintenance, repair, and function of the immune system.[134] The immune response is regulated by locally produced cytokines. That PRL can influence immune function was shown by its ability to reverse the involution of the thymus and normalize the defective immune system of dwarf mice.[135] PRL, in addition to being secreted by the pituitary gland and exerting endocrine control on the immune system, can also act as a cytokine, because it is released within immune cells, particularly by T cells and thymocytes, and can regulate the lymphocyte response by paracrine and autocrine mechanisms. PRL, like growth hormone and somatostatin, can stimulate thymic cell development as well as mature immunocompetent cells. Pituitary PRL and lymphocyte PRL both can be regulated by immune factors: human PRL synthesis by lymphocytes can be induced by T-cell stimuli,[136] and increased release of PRL by the pituitary can be observed in vivo after immune challenge. Both hyperprolactinemia and hypoprolactinemia appear to be immunosuppressive in rats.[137] Therefore, physiologic levels of circulating PRL are probably necessary to maintain immunocompetence. As a generalization, low levels of PRL inhibit immune function whereas elevated levels enhance immunity, at least in rodents.

In humans, thymocytes can produce a 23- to 24-kDa form of PRL,[138] and peripheral blood lymphocytes produce a 27-kDa form.[139] Thymocytes and peripheral lymphocytes can also synthesize an 11-kDa PRL that is released together with the larger form. Whereas both the 24- and 11-kDa forms have biologic activity in vitro (Nb_2 node lymphoma bioassay), their function in vivo, if any, remains to be determined.

Interestingly, 8 human malignant neoplasms of a variety of types, of 32 studied, expressed but did not secrete PRL[140]; and in another study,[141] serum PRL was elevated in 16 of 28 acute myeloblastic leukemia patients.[141] The PRL-like mRNA detected in extrapituitary sites has a sequence identical to that of pituitary PRL in the protein-coding region. Therefore, the existence of different isoforms that have been found in many of these sites suggests post-transcriptional modifications. A 60-kDa form of PRL, which has been found in human peripheral circulating mononuclear cells,[142] differs from the dimeric form in serum. The form of PRL used as a signaling molecule by lymphocytes remains to be determined. In clones of T cells, the 24-kDa form mediated interleukin (IL)-2–stimulated progression to the S phase in the cell cycle.[143] In the aggregate, the data suggest that different PRL isoforms participate in different functions in the immune system. PRL can act as an autocrine/paracrine factor to regulate proliferation of previously stimulated immunocompetent cells.

Hyperprolactinemia can increase IL-4 and IL-6 mRNA expression by murine splenocytes[144] and decrease the serum levels of IL-2 in patients with PRL-secreting adenomas.[145] After bromocriptine treatment of the tumors, IL-2 serum levels are restored. High circulating PRL levels inhibit suppressor (CD8t) T cells, thereby activating autoantibody-producing B-cell clones.[146] PRL may be considered a permissive factor in the development of a pre-existing abnormal response.[137]

PRL may also participate in lymphocyte maturation and activation. The proliferative response of human T cells in response to mitogens (phytohemagglutinin and concanavalin A) is inhibited by PRL antiserum.[142]

Among the cells on which PRL receptors are found are the lymph node Nb_2 cell line,[147] B and T lymphocytes,[148] NK cells,[149] and lymphoid/myeloid leukemia cell lines.[149] The binding affinity at these sites suggests that they can respond to physiologic circulating PRL levels. Furthermore, PRL receptors are strongly expressed in the thymus and bone marrow.[150] Finally, the PRL receptor is a member of the hematopoietic receptor superfamily, which includes receptors for IL-2, IL-3, IL-4, IL-6, IL-7, granulocyte-macrophage colony-stimulating factor, granulocyte colony-stimulating factor, growth hormone, and erythropoietin.[151] (For a discussion of postreceptor signaling events, particularly involving the Jak family of tyrosine kinases, see the reviews of this entire subject by Matera[137] and Weigent.[152])

PROLACTIN SECRETION UNDER PHYSIOLOGIC CONDITIONS

Physiologic conditions associated with increased PRL release are summarized in Table 9–2.

■ TABLE 9–2

Physiologic Conditions Associated with Increased Prolactin Release

CONDITIONS	FEATURES
Sleep	Entrained neuroendocrine rhythm
Feeding	High-protein meal, especially at noon
Exercise	Mechanism unknown
Stress	Both physical and emotional stress
Coitus	Marked elevation in association with orgasm
Menstrual cycle	Late follicular and luteal phases
Pregnancy	Tenfold increase near term
Amniotic fluid	Peak at second trimester, with extraordinarily high levels secreted by the decidua
Puerperium	First 3 to 4 weeks
Nursing	Acute short-lasting release
Fetus	Higher than in mother near term
Neonate	First 2 to 3 weeks after birth

Episodic Secretion and Clearance

PRL is released in pulses of varying amplitude superimposed on continuous basal secretion.[153] The metabolic clearance rate of PRL in humans is correlated with body surface area.[154] The mean metabolic clearance rate for PRL is 40 to 45 ml/min/m^2 with no gender difference.[155, 156] The calculated daily secretion of PRL is approximately 350 μg.[156] If the nocturnal sleep-entrained rise in circulating PRL were taken into account, the true production rate would be higher.

The disappearance of ^{125}I-labeled human PRL from plasma is multiexponential, with an initial half-life ($t_{1/2}$) of 50 to 60 minutes,[157] which is two to three times that of previous estimates. Because of the heterogeneity of circulating PRL, further studies are needed to firmly establish the disappearance rates of the various forms of plasma PRL in humans.

Sleep-Entrained and Food-Entrained Prolactin Release

The highest plasma PRL concentration occurs during nocturnal sleep[156, 157] (Fig. 9–10). This nocturnal augmentation of PRL release is sleep entrained, but it also has an intrinsic circadian rhythm[158] (see later). PRL release begins to increase shortly (10 to 60 minutes) after the onset of sleep; this increase involves a series of secretory pulses (three to eight spikes), resulting in an elevated plasma concentration that persists during the remaining hours of sleep.[158] During the first hour after waking, plasma PRL concentration falls rapidly, with the lowest concentration beginning in the late morning (between 9:00 AM and 11:00 AM). This diurnal sleep-entrained pituitary PRL cycle is present in prepubertal and pubertal boys and girls as well as in adults.[159] There is an increased ratio of bioactive PRL (MW 23,000) to the glycosylated form of PRL released during sleep.[21] The physiologic significance of a diurnal rhythm of PRL secretion remains to be defined. As noted, estradiol augments the nocturnal PRL rise in reproductive-age women.[122]

An acute release of PRL concomitant with a cortisol rise

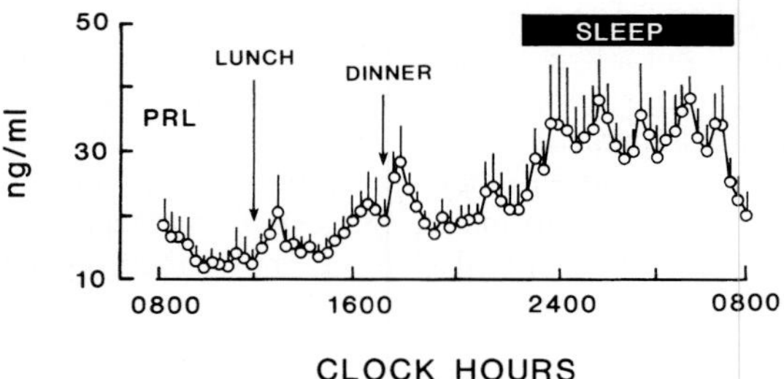

Figure 9–10 ■ Around-the-clock prolactin (PRL) concentrations in eight normal women. Acute elevation of PRL level occurs shortly after the onset of sleep and begins to decline shortly before awakening. Note the increase of PRL levels during lunch.

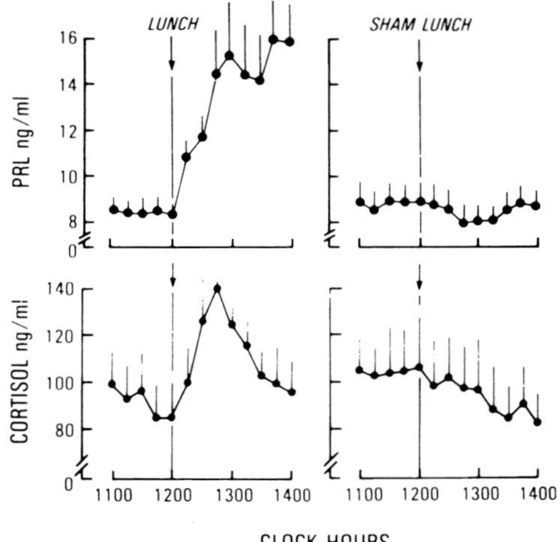

Figure 9–11 ■ Mean (±SE) serum prolactin (PRL) and cortisol levels in seven normal fasting volunteers before and after the ingestion of a regular mixed meal or "sham" meal (seeing and chewing only) at 1200 hours. (From Ishizuka B, Quigley ME, Yen SSC. Pituitary hormone release in response to food ingestion: Evidence for neuroendocrine signals from gut to brain. J Clin Endocrinol Metab 57:1111–1116, 1983. © The Endocrine Society.)

occurs after ingestion of a standardized mixed meal given at noon[160] (Fig. 9–11). No consistent increments occur in either of these hormones after breakfast (8:00 AM) or dinner (6:00 PM).[90] The magnitude of the PRL and cortisol release in response to lunch is not significantly influenced by a preceding breakfast. On the other hand, the composition of the midday meal has a clear effect. Whereas carbohydrate meals induce no discernible effects, high-protein meals cause a large increment in both serum PRL and cortisol, and high-fat meals stimulate a selective release of PRL.[90] Ingestion of the neurotransmitter substrates L-tyrosine, L-tryptophan, and 5-hydroxytryptophan induces remarkable increments in serum concentrations of both PRL and cortisol, suggesting that these essential amino acids may be active components of the high-protein meal[90] (Fig. 9–12). Infusion of L-arginine also elicits a rapid rise of PRL levels.[161] The meal-mediated PRL and cortisol release is unaffected by prior receptor blockade of the opioidergic and cholinergic systems with naloxone or atropine, respectively.[90] The cephalic-vagal pathway appears not to be required, as suggested by the lack of effect of "sham" meals. Thus, the protein component of the noon meal may represent the stimulus for surges of PRL and cortisol.[90]

The high-protein noon meal may serve to link the gut and brain by providing neurotransmitter substrates, thus modifying central catecholamine and serotonin biosynthesis. These may then influence hypothalamic factors that control pituitary PRL and adrenocorticotropic hormone secretion.[90, 91, 162] The possibility that the release of gastrointestinal hormones, such as cholecystokinin, after meals may also serve to influence the hypothalamic-pituitary system remains to be explored.

A sleep-independent circadian rhythm of PRL was recently described in both men and women.[158] The amplitude of this rhythm was significantly greater in women than in men and, in women, was present in the follicular and luteal phases of the cycle. It was speculated that this sleep-independent PRL circadian rhythm, like other endogenous endocrine rhythms, is driven by the human circadian pacemaker in the hypothalamic suprachiasmatic nucleus.

Prolactin Rhythm After "Jet Lag"

Experiments have been conducted to determine the effects of 7-hour jet lag between Chicago and Brussels on sleep-related PRL secretion. One day after the westward flight, a brief elevation of serum PRL concentration was observed during wakefulness, at the time of anticipated sleep-associated increase according to Brussels time, and the nocturnal PRL peak occurred earlier in sleep with declining levels throughout the rest of the night. Normalization of the PRL

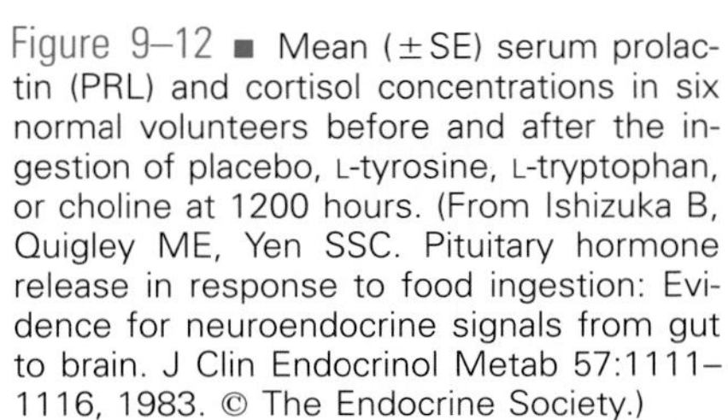

Figure 9–12 ■ Mean (±SE) serum prolactin (PRL) and cortisol concentrations in six normal volunteers before and after the ingestion of placebo, L-tyrosine, L-tryptophan, or choline at 1200 hours. (From Ishizuka B, Quigley ME, Yen SSC. Pituitary hormone release in response to food ingestion: Evidence for neuroendocrine signals from gut to brain. J Clin Endocrinol Metab 57:1111–1116, 1983. © The Endocrine Society.)

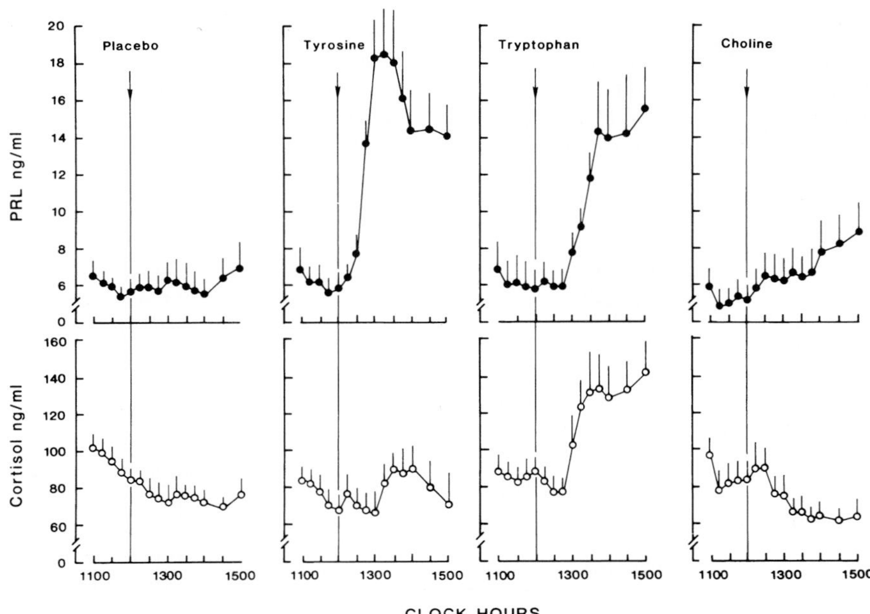

secretory pattern occurred 11 to 21 days after arrival in Chicago.[163]

One day after eastward travel, the sleep-related increase in PRL level was gradual, reaching its peak only at the anticipated onset of sleep according to Chicago time, and PRL levels declined less abruptly after awakening. Full return to a normal pattern took 11 to 21 days after arrival in Brussels. Sleep deprivation experiments showed PRL patterns similar to those observed immediately after the eastward flight. These observations strongly suggest that the nighttime rise in PRL is not solely sleep dependent but also has an intrinsic circadian rhythm.

Stress and Other Stimuli

An elevated rate of PRL secretion is induced by a number of stress stimuli, including venipuncture, physical exercise, surgery, hypoglycemia, and general or conduction anesthesia in both men and women[120] (Fig. 9–13). Sexual intercourse is a potent stimulus for PRL release, and a greater rise (10-fold) in serum PRL has been found in women experiencing orgasm. Limited studies indicate that coitus does not induce a PRL rise in men.[120] Thus, PRL release is found in many types of stress that may be either physical or emotional or both.

Puberty and the Menstrual Cycle

At the time of puberty in girls, mean serum PRL levels increase significantly to reach the adult female range.[164] No such change in mean serum PRL concentrations occurs in boys as they approach pubertal age, and the average PRL level in adult men thus remains lower than that of adult women.[157] PRL concentrations generally decrease after menopause.

Some investigators have found that PRL levels reach a peak at midcycle and remain high during the luteal phase, with the overall pattern of circulating PRL concentration during the menstrual cycle resembling that of estradiol.[157, 165] The increased PRL concentration during high estrogen phases of the cycle is temporally related to amplified episodic PRL pulsatility.[157] Other investigators have not found definite menstrual cycle changes. PRL release in response to TRH appears to be greater during the luteal phase than during the midfollicular phase of the cycle.[166]

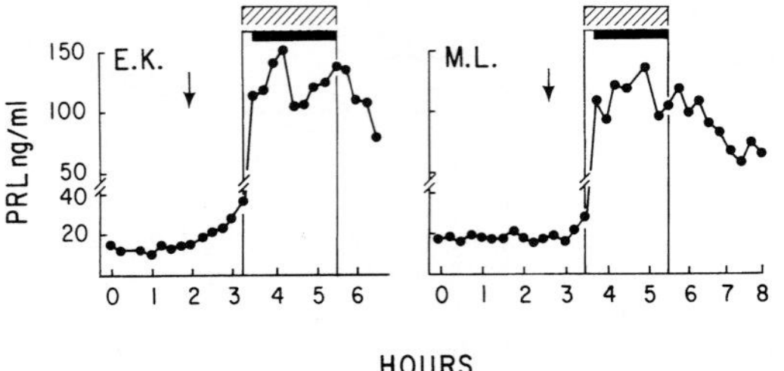

Figure 9–13 ■ The acute release of prolactin (PRL) in response to anesthesia and surgical stress in women undergoing pelvic laparotomy. Arrows indicate the time of premedication. The hatched and black bars represent the duration of anesthesia and surgical procedures, respectively.

Pregnancy, Parturition, and Lactation

The Mother

Maternal serum immunoreactive PRL begins to rise in the first trimester of pregnancy and increases in an approximately linear pattern to 10 times the concentration of nonpregnant women at term[167, 168] (Fig. 9–14). This rise is probably related causally to supramaximal estrogen stimulation and is a functional reflection of hypertrophy and hyperplasia of the pituitary lactotrophs. The isoforms of PRL during the course of pregnancy exhibit a shift from glycosylated (G-PRL, MW 25,000) to the more bioactive form of nonglycosylated PRL (MW 23,000); G-PRL is the predominant molecular species during the first trimester of pregnancy, and the 23,000 MW PRL represents the major component of immunoactive PRL near term.[169, 170] Thus, in response to the changing hormonal milieu of pregnancy, the isoforms of PRL shift in favor of the more biologically active form—23 kDa.

The episodic and sleep-entrained patterns of PRL release observed in nonpregnant women are maintained during pregnancy.[171] The midday surge of PRL (and cortisol) secretion in response to lunch also persists in pregnant women but with a greater magnitude.[172] In contrast to PRL levels in nonpregnant women, the levels in women at late pregnancy do not appear to be influenced by surgical stress or by anesthesia.[173]

The physiologic significance of pregnancy-induced hyperprolactinemia and of the concomitant release of PRL and cortisol in response to lunch is unclear. Experimental data suggest that PRL may play a role in the regulation of storage and mobilization of fat[174] and that cortisol can synergize with PRL influence on fat metabolism.[175] In hyperprolactinemic patients, insulin secretion in response to glucose is exaggerated, as is the suppression of glucagon by glucose. This finding resembles that of normal pregnancy.[176] The metabolic effects of PRL, together with the well-recognized anti-insulin and catabolic actions of cortisol, ultimately may be shown to serve as components of the integrated endocrine control of metabolic homeostasis in pregnancy.

The Fetus

The synthesis, storage, and secretion of PRL in the pituitary gland of the human fetus are found after the 12th week of gestation and occur at an accelerated rate during the last few weeks of intrauterine life.[177] These findings are consistent with the first detection of pituitary lactotrophs at 18 weeks of gestation and a sharp increase in numbers after 22 weeks of gestation[178] (see also Chapter 27). At term, the mean umbilical vein concentration of PRL is higher than that in the maternal plasma (see Fig. 9–14). This high PRL level then declines progressively to the normal range of children by the end of the first week of postnatal life. Serum PRL levels and the PRL content of the lactotrophs in anencephalic infants are essentially the same as those in normal infants.[178] The normal pattern of PRL levels in anencephalic fetuses is probably due to the anatomic isolation of lactotrophs from the hypothalamus as well as to direct estrogen stimulation of lactotrophs in the fetal pituitary.

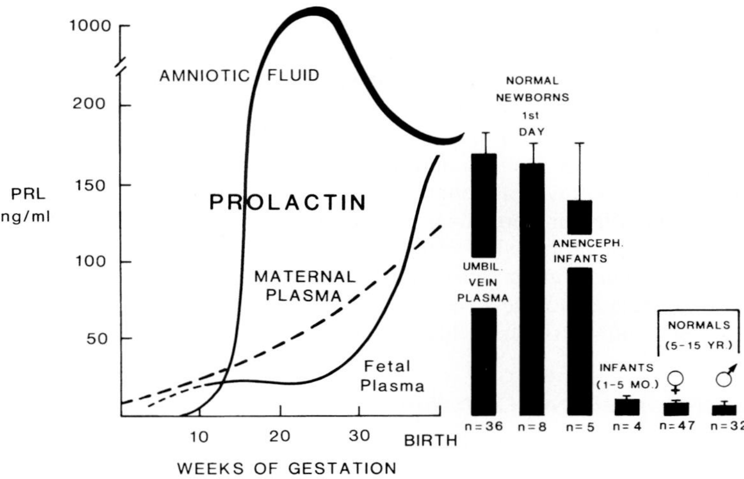

Figure 9–14 ■ Comparison of patterns of maternal, fetal, and amniotic fluid prolactin (PRL) levels during the course of human pregnancy. On the right, plasma levels of prolactin in normal and anencephalic newborns are compared with those of normal infants and adults. (From Aubert ML, Grumbach MM, Kaplan SL. The ontogenesis of human fetal hormones. III. Prolactin. J Clin Invest 56:155–164, 1975, © by permission of the American Society of Clinical Investigation; and Schenker JG, Ben-David M, Polishuk WZ. Prolactin in normal pregnancy: Relationship of maternal, fetal, and amniotic fluid levels. Am J Obstet Gynecol 123:834–838, 1975.)

The physiologic roles of fetal PRL are not completely clear. The changing patterns of PRL receptor expression in the human fetus discussed previously suggest that PRL may play a role in intrauterine tissue differentiation and organ development. In addition, experimental evidence suggests that fetal PRL may participate in osmoregulation by the kidney and in lung maturation. In rats, experimentally imposed hyperprolactinemia results in a decrease in water, sodium, and potassium excretion by the kidney.[179] In the human fetus, indirect evidence also supports a role of PRL in the regulation of water and salt balance[180] (see also previous discussion of PRL receptor localization in the human fetus in the section on PRL receptors and signaling mechanisms).

Amniotic Fluid Compartment

The highest PRL concentration is found in the amniotic fluid, where it is 5- to 10-fold greater than in maternal serum.[181] Of special interest is the observation that this high PRL concentration in amniotic fluid peaks during the second trimester of pregnancy, when both the fetal and maternal PRL concentrations are relatively low (see Fig. 9–14). The human chorion-decidua is capable of de novo biosynthesis of PRL, which is identical to that derived from the pituitary,[182] and, as indicated previously, PRL receptors are found in the decidua and fetal membranes. The secretion of PRL by human decidual tissue in vitro is not under dopaminergic control, which is known to inhibit both fetal and maternal pituitary PRL release. Amniotic fluid PRL is mainly in the glycosylated form (G-PRL) and is covalently bound to immunoglobulin.[18] It has been proposed that the G-PRL–immunoglobulin complex serves as a shuttle for transferring PRL from amniotic fluid to the fetus by placental passage of immunoglobulin, thus providing local immune function within the uterus. If proven, this mode of delivery of PRL may exert a stimulatory function on fetal thymic hormone production during the period in which fetal pituitary PRL secretion is relatively low.[183]

PRL-binding sites have been demonstrated in human amnion[184] and in the lung, adrenal gland, and liver of the fetal rhesus monkey.[185] A 50 percent decrease in amniotic fluid volume can be induced in rhesus monkeys by intra-amniotic injection of ovine PRL, an effect that persists for about 24 hours.[186] Thus, PRL produced locally may participate in the osmotic regulation and immune function of the amniotic fluid and fetal compartments.

Multiphasic Prolactin Release During Parturition

PRL secretion in the periparturitional period follows a remarkable multiphasic pattern not found in patients who undergo elective cesarean section[173] (Fig. 9–15). PRL concentration, which rises continuously throughout pregnancy, declines precipitously during active labor, reaching a nadir

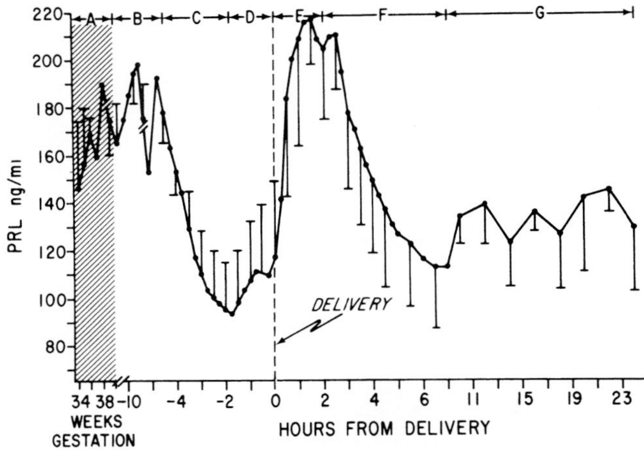

Figure 9–15 ■ The multiphasic pattern of prolactin (PRL) levels (mean ± SE) during the periparturitional periods. During the last few weeks of pregnancy (phase A), PRL levels show frequent fluctuations. These levels are maintained during early hours of labor (phase B). However, during the ensuing hours of active labor, a remarkable decline in PRL levels occurs, reaching a nadir about 2 hours before delivery (phase C). There is some recovery during the last 2 hours before delivery (phase D), leading to a dramatic upward surge of PRL during the first 2 hours after delivery (phase E). PRL levels fall progressively during the subsequent 5 hours (phase F) and reach a relatively constant level with random fluctuation during the next 16 hours (phase G). (From Rigg LA, Yen SSC. Multiphasic prolactin [PRL] secretion during parturition in humans. Am J Obstet Gynecol 128:215–218, 1977.)

approximately 2 hours before delivery. Just before and immediately after delivery, a surge of PRL release occurs, reaching a peak within 2 hours post partum. This multiphasic PRL release is not correlated with changes in steroid hormone concentration, including cortisol. The neuroendocrine mechanism that accounts for this pattern of PRL release is unknown, although a transient rise and fall in tuberoinfundibular dopaminergic activity during active labor has been proposed.[173] Alternatively, the rapid decline of PRL levels during active labor and delivery may be causally related to the central release of oxytocin, which has been shown to inhibit PRL secretion in the rat.[187]

Lactogenesis and Lactation

PRL is the key hormone controlling milk production. The entire process of lactogenesis, however, requires a cascade of events that involve multiple hormonal interactions on the mammary gland[188] (Fig. 9–16). The initial growth of the ductal system is dependent on estrogen, with which growth hormone (hGH) and cortisol synergize. The development of the lobuloalveolar system requires both estrogen and progesterone in the presence of PRL. The synthesis of milk protein (casein and α-lactalbumin) and fat is regulated principally by PRL and facilitated by hGH, insulin, and cortisol.[189] It has been shown that hGH induces lactogenesis in a variety of test systems, and binding of hGH to the PRL receptor may account for the intrinsic PRL-like activity of hGH.[190] The binding affinity of hGH for the extracellular binding domain of the hPRL receptor is enhanced 8000-fold in the presence of zinc. This hormone-receptor "zinc sandwich" offers a molecular link to the lactogenic properties of hGH.[191]

During pregnancy, the increasing levels of PRL, cortisol, placental lactogen, estrogens, and progesterone combine to stimulate the development of the secretory apparatus of the breast, but lactogenesis is minimal and lactation absent. This phenomenon may be attributed to the inhibitory effect of progesterone on lactogenesis by two interdependent mechanisms: progesterone reduces the ability of PRL to up-regulate its own receptor,[192] and progesterone inhibits the number of estrogen receptors. In addition, progesterone inhibition of cortisol binding to its receptor has been suggested as one of the mechanisms by which progesterone antagonizes cortisol-induced stimulation of casein mRNA accumulation in the mammary cell.[193] After delivery, estrogen and progesterone levels fall rapidly; this results in an unopposed PRL autoregulatory mechanism with a prompt increase in PRL receptors. When PRL receptors in the glandular mammary tissue become abundant soon after delivery, lactogenesis and milk secretion are established.

During lactation, basal levels of PRL are not substantially elevated. In fact, PRL levels decline to the upper normal range by the third week post partum. Lactation is maintained by periodic surges of bioactive (MW 23,000) PRL release stimulated by suckling,[194] and this acts to prime the breast for the next feeding.

Transfected cells expressing the human PRL receptor gene treated with hGH or PRL activate two milk protein genes, β-lactoglobulin and β-casein, in a dose-dependent manner. Glycosylated and nonglycosylated hPRL were equally effective in activating the β-casein promoter.[195] There does not appear to be a relationship between the concentration of PRL in plasma of lactating women and the rate of milk synthesis in either the short term (between breast feedings) or long term (from 1 to 6 months of lactation).[196] Optimal lactation is dependent on the frequency but not on the duration of suckling.

A role for insulin and insulin-like growth factors (IGF-I and IGF-II) in the support of lactogenesis and lactation has been proposed. Receptors for insulin, IGF-I, and IGF-II are present in mammary tissue, and lactation is associated with a preferential up-regulation of IGF-I receptors.[197] The type I IGF receptor has a high affinity for IGF-I and a lower affinity for IGF-II and insulin. Both IGF-I and insulin stimulate casein synthesis, but IGF-I is 10 to 20 times more potent than insulin.[198] At physiologic concentrations, IGF-I (approximately 100 ng/ml) exerts a significant augmentation of PRL-induced lactogenesis.[199] Although growth hormone receptors are not found in the mammary gland, growth hormone does increase milk production in the cow. Further, growth hormone treatment induces eleva-

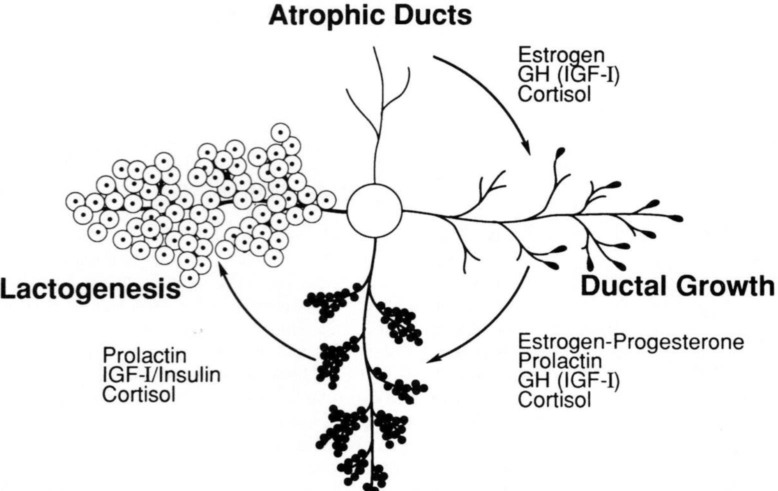

Figure 9–16 ■ The multihormonal interaction regulating the growth of the mammary gland and in the initiation of lactogenesis and lactation, delineated in the hypophysectomized-ovariectomized-adrenalectomized rat. GH, growth hormone; IGF-I, insulin-like growth factor type I. (From Lyons WP. Hormonal synergism in mammary growth. Proc R Soc Lond B 149:303, 1958.)

tion of IGF-I levels, which also could account for the observed increase in milk production.[200]

Neuroendocrinology of the Suckling Reflex

The maintenance of lactation in the puerperium is dependent on mechanical stimulation of the nipple by suckling, as indicated earlier. Sensory signals originating in the nipple during suckling and conveyed by an afferent pathway in the spinal cord ultimately reach the hypothalamus and induce an acute release of oxytocin and PRL. Elevated PRL secretion during lactation may act centrally to induce mother-infant bonding—the "fostering" behavior. Denervation of the nipple or lesions of the spinal cord and brain stem abolish the normal response to suckling.[201]

Three interrelated consequences of suckling are remarkable examples of neuroendocrine networks in the control of reproductive function: (1) facilitation of milk flow, (2) induction of lactogenesis, and (3) amenorrhea and a state of reproductive quiescence through inhibition of GnRH secretion.

Oxytocin release without concomitant release of vasopressin is induced by afferent signals from the nerve endings in the nipple transmitted to both paraventricular and supraoptic nuclei.[202] Activin-containing neurons are localized in the nucleus solitarius tract, which is a major recipient of visceral sensory information and includes projections to the paraventricular nuclei. Activin has been shown to convey signals for oxytocin release during suckling.[203] Oxytocin brings about contraction of the myoepithelial cells of the mammary alveoli and ducts to induce the ejection of milk. An increase in episodic oxytocin release occurs when the mother plays with the infant or in anticipation of nursing even before actual suckling. Milk "let-down" can then be observed[204] (Fig. 9–17). This phenomenon clearly illustrates the involvement of "higher centers" in the neuroendocrine control of oxytocin secretion. Most interesting is the finding of expression of c-*fos*, a transcription factor, activated by the suckling stimulus; strong signals of c-*fos* are found in catecholaminergic neurons in the locus caeruleus, in the nucleus solitarius tract of the lower brain stem, and in the paraventricular and supraoptic nuclei of the hypothalamus of lactating rats.[205] This observation indicates that the suckling stimulus activates multiple neuronal systems.

When nursing is initiated, there is a prompt and large release of PRL that is temporally associated with, but independent of, episodic oxytocin release[205] (see Fig. 9–17). This transient increase in PRL secretion, composed mostly of the bioactive form (MW 23,000), is sufficient to maintain lactogenesis and an adequate milk supply for the next feeding. The maintenance of milk production by the suckling reflex can be attenuated by both ethanol and nicotine through inhibitory effects of ethanol on oxytocin release[203] and of nicotine on PRL secretion.[206]

The suckling stimulus activates multiple inhibitory inputs on the GnRH pulse generator and is thereby instrumental in maintaining lactational amenorrhea. Postpartum amenorrhea is due entirely to GnRH suppression, as evidenced by the failure to respond to the positive feedback action of estradiol in primates (Fig. 9–18) and by the reactivation of the gonadotropin-ovarian axis and ovulation in women during the first few days post partum through the administration of pulsatile GnRH.[207] The mechanism responsible for suckling-induced suppression of GnRH may involve the activation of a series of inhibitors: (1) increased DA turnover in the arcuate nucleus, (2) serotoninergic activation, (3) GABA-ergic activation,[208] and (4) corticotropin-releasing factor–opioidergic activation.[209, 210]

Suckling-induced blockade of ovulation is of major biologic and social significance because it is the most important mechanism for spacing pregnancies in populations with no other means of birth control. Weiner and colleagues[211] demonstrated the presence of PRL receptors on GnRH neurons derived from transgenic mice. Thus, PRL may act directly, in a receptor-mediated manner, to suppress GnRH and therefore gonadotropin production.

INAPPROPRIATE PROLACTIN SECRETION

Causes

Hyperprolactinemia resulting from inappropriate PRL secretion is a common clinical entity. There are many causes for this condition; some reflect serious pathologic processes, and others are consequences of reversible functional disorders (see Table 9–1).

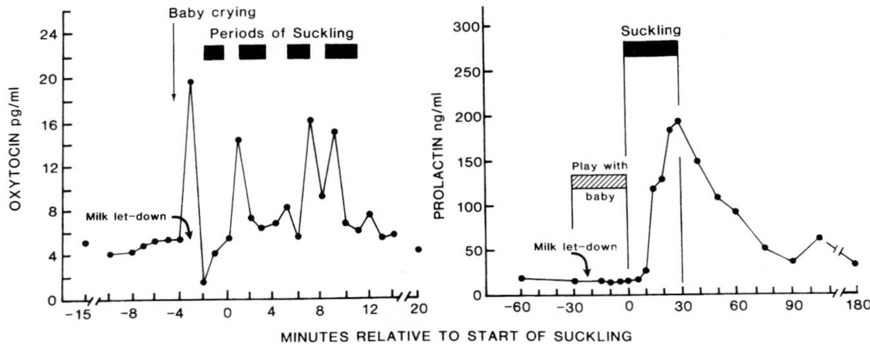

Figure 9–17 ■ Plasma oxytocin *(left)* and prolactin *(right)* concentrations in response to the anticipation of nursing and suckling in lactating women. Milk "let-down" occurred in association with acute release of oxytocin but not of prolactin. (Modified from Noel GL, Suh HK, Frantz AG. Prolactin release during nursing and breast stimulation in postpartum and nonpostpartum subjects. J Clin Endocrinol Metab 38:413–423, 1974. © The Endocrine Society; and McNeilly AS, Robinson CAF, Houston MJ, Howie PW. Release of oxytocin and prolactin in response to suckling. Br Med J 286:257–259, 1983.)

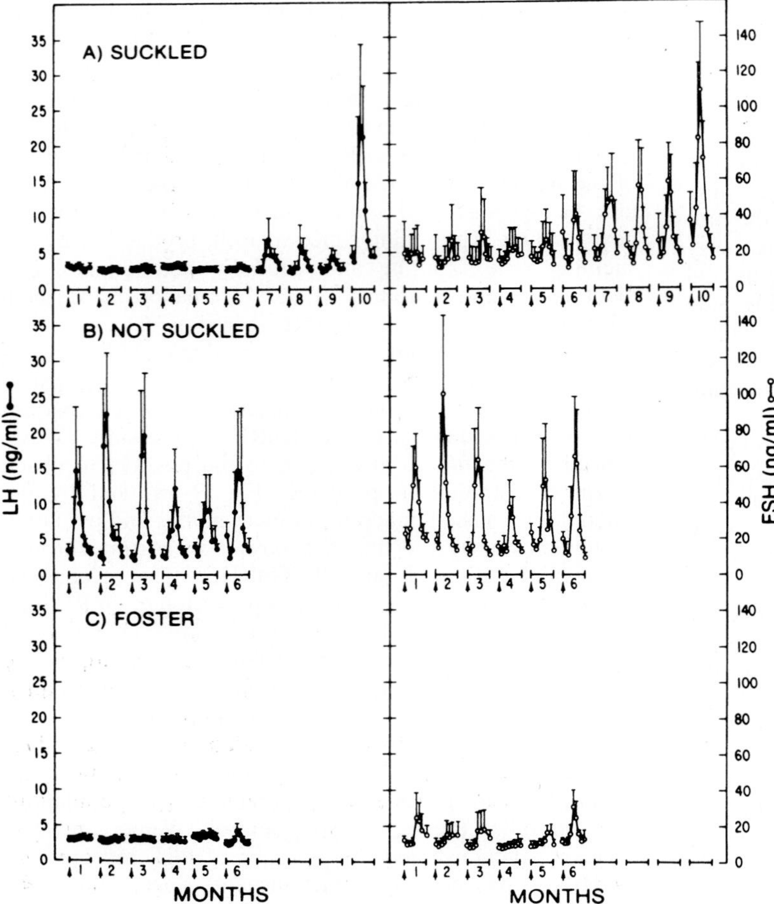

Figure 9–18 ■ Suckling-induced inhibition of the positive feedback effect of estradiol on luteinizing hormone (LH) and follicle-stimulating hormone (FSH) release in the rhesus monkey. Estradiol benzoate was injected subcutaneously *(arrows)* each month post partum into mothers suckled by their own infants *(A)*, into mothers whose infants were weaned on the day of parturition *(B)*, and into mothers suckled by foster infants from group B *(C)*. Note the absence of gonadotropin responses during the initial months of nursing in both natural and foster mothers but not in mothers weaned at the time of parturition. (From Plant TM, Schallenberger E, Hess DL, et al. Influence of suckling on gonadotropin secretion in the female rhesus monkey [*Macaca mulatta*]. Biol Reprod 23:760–766, 1980.)

Hypothalamic Hyperprolactinemia

This includes, among many other causes, the interruption of DA delivery to the portal system by stalk transection or expanding intrasellar tumors with impingement on the pituitary stalk. Under these circumstances, PRL hypersensitivity to DA suppression occurs,[62] probably as a result of the prolonged deprivation of DA; this has been shown experimentally in the rat.[212]

Pituitary Hyperprolactinemia

Although this condition is most commonly due to the presence of PRL-secreting adenomas, other types of pituitary tumors can also secrete PRL (see Table 9–1). PRL-secreting adenoma cells possess DA receptors that are functionally similar to those of the normal lactotrophs.[213] When DA is infused at the maximal effective dose (4 μg/kg/min) in normal women and in patients with hyperprolactinemia caused by microadenoma, PRL suppression is prompt.[63, 214] The resulting decline in serum PRL levels follows a multiexponential curve with a $t_{1/2}$ in the initial phase of approximately 55 minutes for both normal women and prolactinoma patients.

In contrast to DA infusion that delivers DA directly to the adenoma lactotroph, central dopaminergic augmentation by pharmacologic means has little or no effect on serum PRL levels.[215, 216] Administration of the DA antagonists metoclopramide[215] and sulpiride[217] also has no discernible effect on PRL levels in adenoma patients but does block the PRL inhibition induced by DA infusion. These observations suggest a relative deficiency of DA at the adenoma site. The relative deficiency of DA at the site at which an adenoma develops may also be the result of an altered blood supply to that area of the pituitary gland with peripheral blood with its lower DA concentration, rather than portal blood supplying the area where the adenoma develops.[218]

Prolactin-Secreting Adenomas and Their Management

PRL-secreting adenomas are the most common pituitary tumors in women. Signs and symptoms include hyperprolactinemia, galactorrhea, amenorrhea, headache, and bitemporal hemianopia. Although much more common in women than in men, they also do occur in men, in whom they usually attain large size before being diagnosed. In men, the most usual symptoms are headache, visual field changes, and impotence. Mean testosterone concentrations in these men are often slightly lower than normal.

Tumors are somewhat arbitrarily classified by size into microadenomas (<1 cm) and macroadenomas (>1 cm), the latter being associated with greater elevations of PRL concentrations (usually >100 ng/ml). PRL-secreting adenomas, although usually benign and often indolent, on occasion may undergo malignant change. The diagnosis of these tumors is made by PRL measurements and radiologic imaging. The preferred method of imaging currently is magnetic resonance imaging because of its sensitivity and relatively low radiation exposure. The tumors are usually in the lateral wings of the anterior pituitary gland.

The most usual form of treatment currently is with a DA agonist. Bromocriptine has been the most widely used of these, and tumors decrease in size in most patients; patients often become euprolactinemic, which in women is associated with resumption of menses and disappearance of galactorrhea and headaches. Treatment must usually be continued indefinitely to maintain the euprolactinemic state. Treatment should be administered to amenorrheic women even if pregnancy is not the goal, because osteopenia often occurs within 6 months of the amenorrhea either because of the associated hypoestrogenemia or as a direct effect of PRL on bone.[219] There does not appear to be a deleterious effect of continuing bromocriptine during pregnancy. Side effects of bromocriptine are not uncommon and include syncope, nausea, and vomiting. A long-acting form is available that decreases the incidence of side effects. More recently, more specific D_2 DA receptor agonists have become available, including cabergoline[220–222] and quinagolide.[223, 224] The latter has been shown to be useful in the treatment of bromocriptine-resistant tumors, in which there is decreased expression of the two D_2 DA receptor isoforms.[225] Previously, transsphenoidal resection of PRL-secreting adenomas was used more frequently in the treatment of these tumors. However, there is frequently a recurrence of hyperprolactinemia after about 5 to 7 years.[226, 227] On occasion, radiation or gamma knife therapy is helpful as a secondary form of therapy, particularly in cases in which the tumor abuts the cavernous sinus, making complete removal unlikely.

During pregnancy, enlargement of the tumors of clinical significance is relatively uncommon, particularly in microadenomas (~6 percent for microadenomas and 24 to 36 percent for macroadenomas).[228, 229] When this enlargement causes symptoms of chiasmal compression and headache, reinstitution of the DA agonist is often successful. Transsphenoidal resection during pregnancy is occasionally required. Pituitary apoplexy is an uncommon but serious complication.

Drugs

In humans, an increasing number of drugs that affect dopaminergic mechanisms or the putative PRL-releasing factors have been found to induce PRL secretion. Drugs that interfere with synthesis, metabolism, reuptake, or receptor binding of DA would reduce DA availability and consequently would result in hypersecretion of PRL (see Table 9–1). On the other hand, drugs with DA agonist activity, operating either by promoting synthesis of DA or by interacting with DA receptor sites, suppress PRL release. Thus, galactorrhea has been recognized as a relatively common complication in the treatment of patients with phenothiazine, metoclopramide, reserpine, methyldopa, and similar agents.[230, 231] Menstrual irregularities or amenorrhea often develop in these patients, thus reflecting the importance of neurotransmitters and hyperprolactinemia in the inhibition of GnRH secretion and impairment of ovarian function.

Thyroid Dysfunction

Elevated PRL levels are seen in some patients with thyroid disease, particularly primary hypothyroidism. The metabolic clearance rate of PRL is significantly higher than normal in hyperthyroidism and tends to be lower than normal in hypothyroidism.[154] Thus, in hyperthyroidism, an increase in the production rate of PRL may not result in an elevation of basal PRL levels. Enlargement of the pituitary gland is frequently seen in primary hypothyroidism but not in hyperthyroidism. Further, pituitary cells from hypothyroid rats show a striking increase in VIP, which also may contribute, together with the increased TRH, to the increased PRL release.[232] Elevated levels of total and free estradiol are found in patients with thyroid disorders and may play a part in the increased production rate of PRL, but this cannot explain the changes in the metabolic clearance rate. T_3 exerts an inhibitory effect on PRL mRNA as well as on the TRH receptor. Thus, a decrease in T_3 feedback on the lactotroph may induce an increase in the number of TRH receptors as well as VIP, thereby enhancing PRL-releasing actions of TRH and VIP.

Chronic Renal Failure

In chronic renal failure, 20 to 30 percent of patients have hyperprolactinemia; this increases to 80 percent in patients requiring hemodialysis.[233] The development of hyperprolactinemia in chronic renal failure is not related to retention of immunoreactive fragments or degradation products of endogenous PRL; it is the result of both a reduced metabolic clearance rate and an increased production rate of PRL. An impaired ability of DA to suppress PRL release has been observed; this defect may be related either to the presence in uremic patients of serum factors that interfere with the binding of DA to its receptor on the lactotroph or to the development of DA receptor abnormalities. Reversal to normoprolactinemia occurs after renal transplantation or treatment with vitamin D_3.[233]

Effects of Hyperprolactinemia on Endocrine-Metabolic Functions

Most of the experimental data on the biologic action of PRL are derived from in vivo and in vitro studies using ovine PRL; the use of this PRL in different species limits the conclusions that can be drawn regarding the physiology of PRL in humans. In addition, the majority of the observed actions of PRL may be secondary or indirect. However, observations made in human hyperprolactinemic individuals have enhanced, albeit indirectly, our understanding of the endocrine-metabolic effects of human PRL. A variety of changes in cells and systems have been described in hyperprolactinemic states, and these are summarized in Figure 9–19.

Osmoregulation

Among the extramammary actions of PRL in some species, osmoregulatory function is an important feature. Although

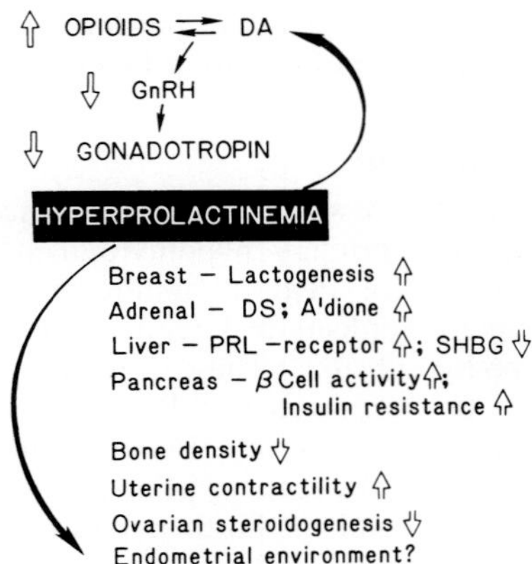

Figure 9–19 ■ Diagrammatic representation of neuroendocrine-metabolic effects of hyperprolactinemia; at the hypothalamic-pituitary level, high prolactin (PRL) levels induce increased dopamine (DA) and opioid peptide in the hypothalamus. These inhibitors in turn reduce pulsatile gonadotropin-releasing hormone (GnRH) secretion, resulting in hypogonadotropinism. An additional mechanism in the inhibition of gonadotropin secretion may involve binding of PRL to GnRH receptors (see text); at the peripheral level, prolactin may exert functional changes in many target tissues. DS, dehydroepiandrosterone sulfate; A'dione, androstenedione; SHBG, sex hormone–binding globulin.

conflicting data have been reported, PRL *does not* appear to play a role in osmoregulation in humans. Endogenous PRL elevation induced by TRH has no apparent effect on water and salt excretion.[234] On the other hand, the high concentration of PRL in amniotic fluid suggests that PRL may play an osmoregulatory role during the "aquatic" phase of human ontogenesis (see earlier).

Androgenic Effects

Hirsutism and elevated urinary 17-ketosteroids were observed in half of the patients in the original description of the Forbes-Albright syndrome more than 40 years ago.[235] In recent years, abnormal androgen secretion and metabolism in nearly 40 percent of the patients with hyperprolactinemia and pituitary adenoma have been reported.[236–238] When the polycystic ovary syndrome is excluded, the balance of the data shows that levels of adrenal androgens—dehydroepiandrosterone sulfate (DHEA-S) or both DHEA-S and dehydroepiandrosterone—are elevated, and normalization can be achieved after bromocriptine treatment. Studies by Lobo and Kletzky[238] have revealed that levels of DHEA-S and androstenedione are elevated, whereas testosterone, dihydrotestosterone, androstenediol, and estradiol levels are decreased. Plasma sex hormone–binding globulin is also reduced. Reversal of these changes occurs after lowering the PRL levels. Furthermore, the elevated androgen levels are suppressed by dexamethasone, suggesting that hyperprolactinemia may exert a stimulatory action on adrenal androgen secretion.

Although substantial numbers of patients with hyperprolactinemia have androgenic abnormalities, only a small number of them have overt androgenic manifestations such as hirsutism and acne. This disparity can be explained by the observation that the elevated total androgens are of relatively low biologic activity and that the increase in unbound testosterone and androstenediol due to the reduced sex hormone–binding globulin is only half of that found in hirsute women. Furthermore, unbound dihydrotestosterone is not increased because there is a relative decrease in 5α-reductase activity attributable to a PRL effect.[239] Because dihydrotestosterone is necessary for the expression of androgenic action in the hair follicle, this decreased 5α-reductase activity is consistent with the relatively uncommon occurrence of hirsutism in hyperprolactinemic patients. The mechanism by which inappropriate elevation of PRL stimulates adrenal androgen secretion and inhibits 5α-reductase activity, either directly or indirectly, remains unclear. The expression of the PRL receptor has been demonstrated in human adrenal glands.[240]

Bone Density

Decreased bone density has been observed in hyperprolactinemic women.[219, 241, 242] Although prolonged hypoestrogenic states can account for the reduced bone mineral content, some patients with normal estrogen levels are also found to have reduced bone density. Measurements of serum calcium, phosphorus, parathyroid hormone, and $1,25(OH)_2D_3$ have not revealed significant changes in hyperprolactinemic women. However, the role of calcitonin has not been evaluated. A striking decrease in circulating PRL levels occurs after calcitonin administration,[243] and the possibility exists that inappropriate PRL levels may suppress calcitonin and thus account for the demineralization of bone.

A direct action of PRL on calcium mobilization should also be considered. PRL has been shown to stimulate calcium mobilization from the bone independently of vitamin D and parathyroid hormone in the rat.[244] In addition, as indicated previously, PRL receptors have been found in a bone tumor cell line. Regardless of the mechanism, hyperprolactinemic patients are at risk for development of osteoporosis, and assessment of estrogen and bone mineral status is indicated. Early intervention to correct the hyperprolactinemic state is important clinically.

Hyperinsulinemia and Insulin Resistance

Exogenous PRL administered to the rat induces an exaggerated insulin response to an intravenous glucose challenge, and when their islets are perfused in vitro with glucose, more insulin is released than from islets of control rats.[245] In women, hyperprolactinemia, with or without pituitary adenomas, is associated with basal hyperinsulinemia but normoglycemia.[246] In addition, these patients exhibit an exaggerated incremental insulin release and glucagon suppression in response to a glucose tolerance test.[247] These features, observed in both animals and humans, resemble those seen in late pregnancy and suggest that PRL may directly stimulate pancreatic beta cells and increase peripheral or hepatic resistance to insulin action. The finding that immunoreactive PRL is selectively localized in the cytoplasm of the beta cells supports a link between PRL and insulin secretion.[248]

Hypothalamic-Pituitary Dysfunction

Hyperprolactinemic states are frequently associated with hypogonadism with or without galactorrhea, the best

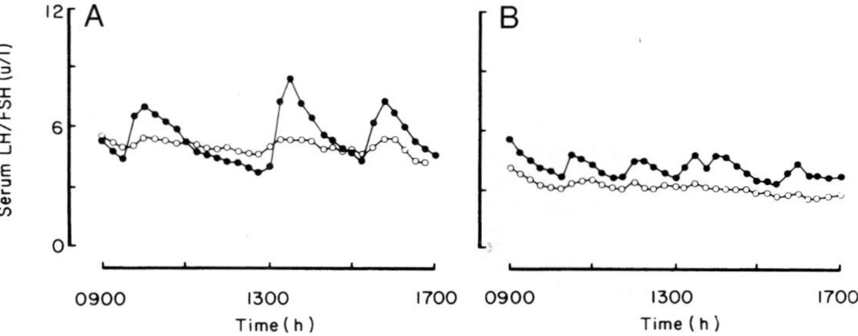

Figure 9–20 ■ In patients with hyperprolactinemia, either pulsatile luteinizing hormone (LH) activities are absent or the frequency is reduced with larger amplitude *(closed circles),* as shown in *A*. The return to normal follicular pulsatile LH secretory pattern occurs 1 week after prolactin suppression by bromocriptine treatment (*B*). Serum follicle-stimulating hormone (FSH) levels (*open circles*) showed no discernible changes. (Redrawn from Moult PA, Rees LH, Besser GM. Pulsatile gonadotrophin secretion in hyperprolactinaemic amenorrhoea and the response to bromocriptine therapy. Clin Endocrinol (Oxf) 16:153–162, 1982. Courtesy of Blackwell Scientific Publications Ltd.)

known of which are postpartum lactational amenorrhea and the galactorrhea-amenorrhea syndrome. Various studies have suggested that supraphysiologic concentrations of PRL exert an inhibitory effect on the hypothalamic-pituitary-ovarian axis. In addition, as indicated previously, there are PRL receptors on GnRH neurons.[211]

The observation that hypoestrogenism in association with hyperprolactinemia is not associated with hot flushes suggests alterations of central neurotransmission. Both hypothalamic DA and opioid peptides appear to serve as neuromodulators for the pulsatile secretion of GnRH. Available evidence suggests that hyperprolactinemia inhibits GnRH activity by interacting with the hypothalamic DA and opioidergic systems through the short-loop feedback mechanism or by a direct effect on GnRH neurons[211] (see Fig. 9–19). The following observations support this concept:

1. In hyperprolactinemic patients, LH pulses are either absent or reduced in frequency and amplitude.[249, 250] Normal LH pulsatility can be restored after PRL suppression with bromocriptine[251] (Fig. 9–20).
2. Estrogen fails to induce a positive feedback response of gonadotropin secretion in hyperprolactinemic women. Restitution of a normal response follows PRL suppression or surgical removal of a prolactinoma.[252, 253]
3. Increased dopaminergic inhibition of hypothalamic GnRH activity may exist in hyperprolactinemic women. After the administration of a DA receptor antagonist, metoclopramide, circulating LH rises in hyperprolactinemic patients but not in normal cycling women during the early follicular phase of the menstrual cycle (Fig. 9–21).
4. Increased endogenous opioid inhibition of the GnRH-gonadotropin system, as assessed by naloxone infusion, has been observed in some but not all patients with hyperprolactinemia. The decreased pulsatile LH secretion in these patients can be restored within hours, after naloxone infusion.[254]
5. Hyperprolactinemia, induced experimentally in the rat, is associated with reduced numbers of GnRH receptors in the pituitary.[255]
6. The loss of the sleep-entrained rise in serum PRL and the failure of PRL release in response to arginine infusion and to chlorpromazine challenge further suggest central nervous system–hypothalamic dysfunction.[249, 256]
7. PRL receptors have been demonstrated in a GnRH neuronal cell line derived from a GnRH-producing tumor.[211]

Ovarian Steroidogenesis

In contrast to some lower species, the role of PRL in the regulation of ovarian function in humans is poorly understood. In rats, PRL may inhibit FSH-mediated estrogen production and LH-mediated androgen secretion.[257, 258] In women, PRL may participate in the regulation of ovarian steroidogenesis, and hyperprolactinemia may also interfere with normal ovarian function. McNatty and associates[259] found that the PRL concentration in the follicular fluid of human ovaries varies markedly with follicle size in the absence of changes in circulating PRL levels; highest follicular concentrations of PRL occur in the fluid of small follicles, reaching levels fivefold to sixfold those in serum. Samples of follicular fluid obtained from mature follicles contain lower PRL concentrations approximating those found in serum. McNatty and Sawers[260] then demonstrated that progesterone secretion by cultured granulosa cells obtained from human ovarian follicles is almost completely inhibited by PRL at concentrations equivalent to those in follicular fluid (100 ng/ml) but not by lower concentrations (10 to 20 ng/ml). These observations suggest that the high PRL concentrations found in the early phase of follicular growth inhibit progesterone secretion and lower PRL levels in the mature follicle act permissively to allow enhanced progesterone secretion. In hyperprolactinemic models, impaired follicular development and luteal-phase defects have been observed. The cellular mechanism of PRL action in the human ovary remains to be elucidated.

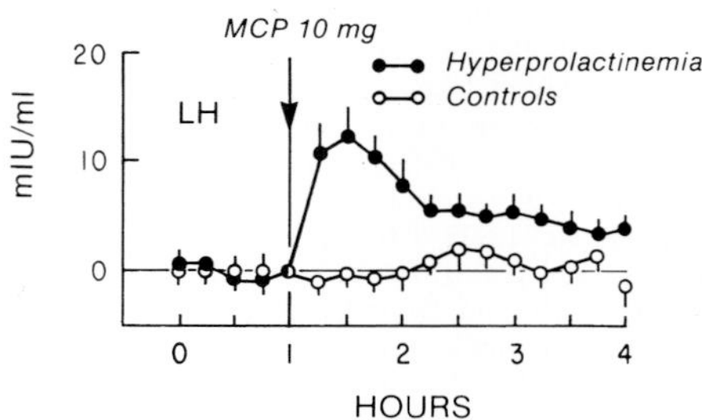

Figure 9–21 ■ Mean (±SE) net change in serum luteinizing hormone (LH) after administration of a dopamine receptor antagonist, metoclopramide (MCP, 10 mg intravenous bolus), to six patients with hyperprolactinemia with later surgical documentation of prolactinoma and six normal control women studied during the early follicular phase of the menstrual cycle. (From Quigley ME, Judd SJ, Gilliland GB, Yen SSC. Effects of a dopamine antagonist on the release of gonadotropin and prolactin in normal women and women with hyperprolactinemic anovulation. J Clin Endocrinol Metab 48:718–720, 1979. © The Endocrine Society.)

References

1. Lewis UJ, Singh NP, Seavey BK. Human prolactin: Isolation and some properties. Biochem Biophys Res Commun 44:1169, 1971.
2. Hwang P, Guyda H, Friesen H. A radioimmunoassay for human prolactin. Proc Natl Acad Sci USA 68:1902, 1971.
3. Niall HD. The chemistry of prolactin. *In* Jaffe RB (ed). Prolactin. New York, Elsevier North-Holland, 1981, p 1.
4. Owerbach D, Rutter WJ, Cooke NE, et al. The prolactin gene is located on chromosome 6 in humans. Science 212:815, 1981.
5. Miller WL, Eberhardt NL. Structure and evolution of the growth hormone gene family. Endoc Rev 4:97, 1983.
6. Truong AT, Duez C, Belayew A, et al. Isolation and characterization of the human prolactin gene. EMBO J 3:429, 1984.
7. Takahashi H, Nabeshima Y, Nabeshima Y-I, et al. Molecular cloning and nucleotide sequence of DNA complementary to human decidual prolactin mRNA. J Biochem 95:1491, 1984.
8. Cooke NE, Coit D, Shine J, et al. Human prolactin: cDNA structural analysis and evolutionary comparisons. J Biol Chem 256:4007, 1981.
9. Borrelli E, Heyman RA, Arias C, et al. Transgenic mice with inducible dwarfism. Nature 339:538, 1989.
10. Mulchahey JJ, Jaffe RB. Detection of a potential progenitor cell in the human fetal pituitary that secretes both growth hormone and prolactin. J Clin Endocrinol Metab 66:24, 1988.
11. Lloyd RV, Anagnostou D, Cano M, et al. Analysis of mammosomatotropic cells in normal and neoplastic human pituitary tissues by the reverse hemolytic plaque assay and immunocytochemistry. J Clin Endocrinol Metab 66:1103, 1988.
12. Mena F, Pacheco P, Grosvenor CE. Effect of electrical stimulation of mammary nerve upon pituitary and plasma prolactin concentrations in anesthetized lactating rats. Endocrinology 106:458, 1980.
13. Sinha YN, Gilligan TA. Identification of a less immunoreactive form of prolactin in the rat pituitary. Endocrinology 108:1091, 1981.
14. Goluboff LG, Ezrin C. Effect of pregnancy on the somatotroph and the prolactin cell of the human adenohypophysis. J Clin Endocrinol Metab 29:1533, 1969.
15. Farkouh NH, Packer MG, Frantz AG. Large molecular PRL with reduced receptor activity in human serum: High proportion in basal state and reduced after TRH. J Clin Endocrinol Metab 48:1026, 1979.
16. Lewis UJ, Singh RNP, Lewis LJ. Two forms of glycosylated human prolactin have different pigeon crop sac-stimulation activities. Endocrinology 124:1558, 1989.
17. Markoff E, Sigel MB, Lacour N, et al. Glycosylation selectively alters the biological activity of prolactin. Endocrinology 123:1303, 1988.
18. Heffner LJ, Gramates LS, Yuan RW. A glycosylated prolactin species is covalently bound to immunoglobulin in human amniotic fluid. Biochem Biophys Res Commun 165:299, 1989.
19. Benveniste R, Helman JD, Orth DN, et al. Circulating big hPRL: Conversion to small hPRL by reduction of disulfide bonds. J Clin Endocrinol Metab 48:883, 1979.
20. Markoff E, Lee DW. Glycosylated prolactin is a major circulating variant in human serum. J Clin Endocrinol Metab 65:1102, 1987.
21. Liu JH, Lee DW, Markoff E. Differential release of prolactin variants in postpartum and early follicular phase women. J Clin Endocrinol Metab 71:605, 1990.
22. Clapp C, Martial JA, Guzman RC, et al. The 16-kilodalton N-terminal fragment of human prolactin is a potent inhibitor of angiogenesis. Endocrinology 133:1292, 1993.
23. Boutin J-M, Edery M, Shirota M, et al. Identification of a cDNA encoding a long form of prolactin receptor in human hepatoma and breast cancer cells. Mol Endocrinol 3:1455, 1989.
24. Somers W, Ultsch M, De Vas AM, Kossiakoff A-A. The x-ray structure of a growth hormone–prolactin receptor complex. Nature 372:409, 1994.
25. Das R, Vonderhaar BK. Transduction of prolactin's (PRL) growth signal through both long and short forms of the PRL receptor. Mol Endocrinol 9:1750, 1995.
26. Crumeyrolle-Arias M, Latouche J, Jammes H, et al. Prolactin receptors in the rat hypothalamus: Autoradiographic localization and characterization. Neuroendocrinology 57:457, 1993.
27. Jin L, Quian X, Kulig E, et al. Prolactin receptor messenger ribonucleic acid in normal and neoplastic human pituitary tissues. J Clin Endocrinol Metab 82:963, 1997.
28. Nagano M, Chastre E, Choquet A, et al. Expression of prolactin and growth hormone receptor genes and their isoforms in the gastrointestinal tract. Am J Physiol 268:G431, 1995.
29. Nevalainen MT, Valve EM, Ingleton PM, et al. Prolactin and prolactin receptors are expressed and functioning in human prostate. J Clin Invest 99:618, 1997.
30. Bataille-Simoneau N, Gerland K, Chappard D, et al. Expression of prolactin receptors in human osteosarcoma cells. Biochem Biophys Res Commun 229:323, 1996.
31. Maaskant RA, Bogic LV, Gilger S, et al. The human prolactin receptor in the fetal membranes, decidua, and placenta. J Clin Endocrinol Metab 81:396, 1996.
32. Weiss-Messer E, Ber R, Barkey RJ. Prolactin and MA-10 Leydig cell steroidogenesis: Biphasic effects of prolactin and signal transduction. Endocrinology 137:5509, 1996.
33. Clevenger CV, Chang WP, Ngo W, et al. Expression of prolactin and prolactin receptor in human breast carcinoma. Evidence for an autocrine/paracrine loop. Am J Pathol 146:695, 1995.
34. Fuh G, Wells JA. Prolactin receptor antagonists that inhibit the growth of breast cancer cell lines. J Biol Chem 270:13133, 1995.
35. Freemark M, Driscoll P, Maaskant R, et al. Ontogenesis of prolactin receptors in the human fetus in early gestation. Implications for tissue differentiation and development. J Clin Invest 99:1107, 1997.
36. Erwin RA, Kirken RA, Malabarba MG, et al. Prolactin activates Ras via signaling proteins SHC, growth factor receptor bound 2, and son of sevenless. Endocrinology 136:3512, 1995.
37. Li S, Rosen JM. Nuclear factor I and mammary gland factor (STAT 5) play a critical role in regulating whey acidic gene expression in transgenic mice. Mol Cell Biol 15:2063, 1995.
38. Neill JD, Smith PF, Lugne EH, et al. Detection and measurement of hormone secretion from individual pituitary cells. Recent Prog Horm Res 43:175, 1987.
39. Israel JM, Kukstas LA, Vincent J-D. Plateau potentials recorded from lactating rat enriched lactotroph cells are triggered by thyrotropin releasing hormone and shortened by dopamine. Neuroendocrinology 51:113, 1990.
40. Mangalam HJ, Albert VR, Ingraham HA, et al. A pituitary POU domain protein, Pit-1, activates both growth hormone and prolactin promoters transcriptionally. Genes Dev 3:946, 1989.
41. Simmons DW, Voss JW, Ingraham HA, et al. Pituitary cell phenotypes involve cell-specific Pit-1 mRNA translation and synergistic interactions with other transcription factors. Genes Dev 4:695, 1990.
42. Phaffle RW, Di Mattia GE, Parks JS, et al. Mutation of the POU-specific domain of Pit-1 and hypopituitarism without pituitary hypoplasia. Science 257:1118, 1992.
43. Day RN, Koike S, Sakai M, et al. Both Pit-1 and the estrogen receptor are required for estrogen responsiveness of the rat prolactin gene. Mol Endocrinol 4:1964, 1990.
44. Stefaneanu L, Kovacs K, Horvath E, et al. In situ hybridization study of estrogen receptor messenger RNA in human adenohypophysial cells and pituitary adenomas. J Clin Endocrinol Metab 78:83, 1994.
45. Sanno N, Teramoto A, Matsuno A, et al. Expression of Pit-1 and estrogen receptor messenger RNA in prolactin-producing pituitary adenomas. Mod Pathol 9:526, 1996.
46. Gellersen B, Kempf R, Telgmann R, Di Mattia GE. Neopituitary human prolactin gene transcription is independent of Pit-1 and differentially controlled in lymphocytes and in endometrial stroma. Mol Endocrinol 8:356, 1994.
47. Stachura ME, Tyler JM, Kent PG. Pituitary immediate release pools of growth hormone and prolactin are preferentially refilled by new rather than stored hormone. Endocrinology 125:444, 1989.
48. Day RN, Mauer RA. The distal enhancer region of the rat prolactin gene contains elements conferring response to multiple hormones. Mol Endocrinol 3:3, 1989.
49. Murdoch GH, Waterman M, Evans RM, Rosenfeld MG. Molecular mechanisms of phorbol ester, thyrotropin-releasing hormone and growth factor stimulation of prolactin gene transcription. J Biol Chem 260:11852, 1985.
50. Waterman ML, Adler S, Nelson C, et al. A single domain of the

estrogen receptor confers deoxyribonucleic acid binding and transcriptional activation of the prolactin gene. Mol Endocrinol 2:14, 1988.
51. Wynick D, Hammond PJ, Akinsanya KO, Bloom SR. Galanin regulates basal and oestrogen-stimulated lactotroph function. Nature 364:529, 1993.
52. Giustine A, Licini M, Schettino M, et al. Physiological role of galanin in the regulation of anterior pituitary function in humans. Am J Physiol 266:E57, 1994.
53. Arvat E, Gianotti L, Ramunni J, et al. Effect of galanin on basal and stimulated secretion of prolactin, gonadotropins, thyrotropin, adrenocorticotropin and cortisol in humans. Eur J Endocrinol 133:300, 1995.
54. Murakami Y, Ohshina K, Mochizuki T, Yanaihara N. Effect of human galanin on growth hormone, prolactin, and antidiuretic hormone secretion in normal men. J Clin Endocrinol Metab 77:1436, 1993.
55. MacLeod RM, Kimura H, Login I. Inhibition of prolactin secretion by dopamine and piribedil (ET-495). *In* Pecile A, Muller EE (eds). Growth Hormone and Related Peptides. New York, Elsevier North-Holland, 1976, p 443.
56. Gibbs DM, Neill JD. Dopamine levels in hypophysial stalk blood in the rat are sufficient to inhibit prolactin secretion in vivo. Endocrinology 102:1895, 1978.
57. Reymond MJ, Speciale SG, Porter JC. Dopamine in plasma of lateral and medial hypophysial portal vessels: Evidence for regional variation in the release of hypothalamic dopamine into hypophysial portal blood. Endocrinology 112:1958, 1983.
58. Gregerson KA, Selmanoff M. Selection effects of hyperprolactinemia on in vitro dopamine release from median eminence synaptosomes. J Neurosci 8:2477, 1988.
59. Lindley SE, Lookingland KJ, Moore KE. Activation of tuberoinfundibular but not tuberohypophysial dopaminergic neurons following intracerebroventricular administration of alpha-melanocyte-stimulating hormone. Neuroendocrinology 51:394, 1990.
60. Murai I, Garris PA, Ben-Jonathan N. Time-dependent increase in plasma prolactin after pituitary stalk section: Role of posterior pituitary dopamine. Endocrinology 124:2343, 1989.
61. Leblanc H, Lachelin GC, Abu-Fadil S, Yen SSC. Effects of dopamine infusion on pituitary hormone secretion in humans. J Clin Endocrinol Metab 43:668, 1976.
62. Serri O, Kuchel O, Buu NT, Somma M. Differential effects of a low-dose dopamine infusion on prolactin secretion in normal and hyperprolactinemic subjects. J Clin Endocrinol Metab 56:225, 1983.
63. Martin MC, Weiner RI, Monroe SE, et al. Prolactin-secreting adenomas in women. VII. Dopamine regulation of prolactin secretion. J Clin Endocrinol Metab 59:485, 1984.
64. Bunzow JR, Van Tol HHM, Grandy DK, et al. Cloning and expression of a rat D_2 dopamine receptor cDNA. Nature 336:783, 1988.
65. Enjalbert A, Musset F, Chonard C, et al. Dopamine inhibits prolactin secretion stimulated by the calcium channel agonist Bay-K-8644 through a pertussis toxin–sensitive G protein in anterior pituitary cells. Endocrinology 123:406, 1988.
66. Maurer RA. Dopaminergic inhibition of prolactin synthesis and prolactin messenger RNA accumulation in cultured pituitary cells. J Biol Chem 255:8092, 1980.
67. Murdoch GH, Rosenfeld MG, Evans RM. Eukaryotic transcriptional regulation and chromatin-associated protein phosphorylation by cyclic AMP. Science 218:1315, 1982.
68. De la Escalera GM, Porter BW, Martin TFJ, Weiner RI. Dopamine withdrawal and addition of thyrotropin-releasing hormone stimulate membrane translocation of protein kinase-C and phosphorylation of an endogenous 80K substrate in enriched lactotrophs. Endocrinology 125:1168, 1989.
69. Porter TE, Grandy D, Bunzow J, et al. Evidence that stimulatory dopamine receptors may be involved in the regulation of prolactin secretion. Endocrinology 134:1263, 1994.
70. Vincent S, Hokfelt T, Wu JY. GABA neuron systems in the hypothalamus and the pituitary gland. Neuroendocrinology 34:117, 1982.
71. Grossman A, Delitala G, Yeo T, Besser GM. GABA and muscimol inhibit the release of prolactin from dispersed rat anterior pituitary cells. Neuroendocrinology 32:145, 1981.
72. Gudelsky GA, Apud JA, Masotto C, et al. Ethanolamine-*O*-sulfate enhances γ-aminobutyric acid secretion into hypophysial portal blood and lowers serum prolactin concentrations. Neuroendocrinology 37:397, 1983.
73. Melis GM, Fruzetti F, Paoletti AM, et al. Pharmacological activation of γ-aminobutyric acid–system blunts prolactin response to mechanical breast stimulation in puerperal women. J Clin Endocrinol Metab 58:201, 1984.
74. Lamberts SWJ, MacLeod RM. Studies on the mechanism of the GABA-mediated inhibition of prolactin secretion. Proc Soc Exp Biol Med 158:10, 1978.
75. Neill JD, Frawley LS, Plotsky PM, Tindall GT. Dopamine in hypophysial stalk blood of the rhesus monkey and its role in regulating prolactin secretion. Endocrinology 108:489, 1981.
76. Jacobs LS, Snyder PJ, Wilbur JF, et al. Increased serum prolactin after administration of synthetic thyrotropin releasing hormone (TRH) in man. J Clin Endocrinol Metab 33:996, 1971.
77. Gershengorn MC, Geras E, Spina Purello V, Rebecchi MJ. Inositol triphosphate mediates thyrotropin-releasing hormone mobilization of nonmitochondrial calcium in rat mammotropic pituitary cells. J Biol Chem 259:10675, 1984.
78. Koch Y, Goldhaber G, Fireman I, et al. Suppression of prolactin and thyrotropin secretion in the rat by antiserum to thyrotropin-releasing hormone. Endocrinology 100:1476, 1977.
79. Snyder PJ, Jacobs LS, Utiger RD, Daughaday WH. Thyroid hormone inhibition of the prolactin response to thyrotropin-releasing hormone. J Clin Invest 52:2324, 1973.
80. Abe H, Engler D, Molitch ME, et al. Vasoactive intestinal peptide is a physiological mediator of prolactin release in the rat. Endocrinology 116:1383, 1985.
81. Samson WK, Bianchi R, Mogg RJ, et al. Oxytocin mediates the hypothalamic action of vasoactive intestinal peptide to stimulate prolactin secretion. Endocrinology 124:812, 1989.
82. Nagy G, Mulchahey JJ, Neill JD. Autocrine control of prolactin secretion by vasoactive intestinal peptide. Endocrinology 122:364, 1988.
83. Yiangou Y, Gill JS, Chrysanthou BJ, et al. Infusion of prepro-VIP derived peptides in man: Effect on secretion of prolactin. Neuroendocrinology 48:615, 1988.
84. Dufy-Barbe L, Rodriguez F, Arsaut J, et al. Angiotensin II stimulates prolactin release in the rhesus monkey. Neuroendocrinology 35:242, 1982.
85. Aguilera G, Hyde CL, Catt KJ. Angiotensin II receptors and prolactin release in pituitary lactotrophs. Endocrinology 111:1045, 1982.
86. Saint-Andre J-P, Rohmer V, Alhenc-Gelas F, et al. Presence of renin, angiotensinogen, and converting enzyme in human pituitary lactotroph cells and prolactin adenomas. J Clin Endocrinol Metab 63:231, 1986.
87. Clemens JA, Sawyer BD, Cerimele B. Further evidence that serotonin is a neurotransmitter involved in the control of prolactin secretion. Endocrinology 100:692, 1977.
88. Willoughby JO, Menadue MF, Liebelt HJ. Activation of 5-HT 1 serotonin receptors in the medial basal hypothalamus stimulates prolactin secretion in the unanesthetized rat. Neuroendocrinology 47:83, 1988.
89. MacIndoe JH, Turkington RW. Stimulation of human prolactin secretion by intravenous infusion of L-tryptophan. J Clin Invest 52:1972, 1973.
90. Ishizuka B, Quigley ME, Yen SSC. Pituitary hormone release in response to food ingestion: Evidence for neuroendocrine signals from gut to brain. J Clin Endocrinol Metab 57:1111, 1983.
91. Kato Y, Nakai Y, Imura H, et al. Effect of 5-hydroxytryptophan (5-HTP) on plasma prolactin levels in man. J Clin Endocrinol Metab 38:695, 1974.
92. Del Pozo E, Lancranjan I. Clinical use of drugs modifying the release of anterior pituitary hormones. *In* Ganong W, Martini L (eds). Frontiers in Neuroendocrinology, Vol 5. New York, Raven Press, 1978, p 207.
93. Delitala G, Lodica G, Masala A, et al. Action of metergoline in suppressing prolactin release induced by mechanical breast emptying. J Clin Endocrinol Metab 44:763, 1977.
94. Van Loon GR, Ho D, Kim C. β-Endorphin–induced decrease in hypothalamic dopamine turnover. Endocrinology 106:76, 1980.
95. Wilkes MM, Yen SSC. Reduction by β-endorphin of efflux of

dopamine and DOPAC from superfused medial basal hypothalamus. Life Sci 27:1387, 1980.
96. Van Vugt DA, Meites J. Influence of endogenous opiates on anterior pituitary function. Fed Proc 39:2533, 1980.
97. Gold MS, Redmond DE, Donabedian RK. The effects of opiate agonist and antagonists on serum prolactin in primates: Possible role for endorphins in prolactin regulation. Endocrinology 105:284, 1979.
98. Von Graffenried B, Del Pozo E, Roubicek J, et al. Effects of the synthetic enkephalin analogue FK 33-824 in man. Nature 272:729, 1978.
99. Grossman A, Rees LH. The neuroendocrinology of opioid peptides. Br Med Bull 39:83, 1983.
100. Grossman A, Stubbs WA, Gaillard RC, et al. Studies of the opiate control of prolactin, GH and TSH. Clin Endocrinol (Oxf) 14:381, 1971.
101. Blankstein J, Reyes F, Winter J, Faiman C. Failure of naloxone to alter growth hormone and prolactin levels in acromegalic and hyperprolactinemic patients. Clin Endocrinol (Oxf) 11:475, 1979.
102. Knigge U, Dejgaard A, Wollesen F, et al. Histamine regulation of prolactin secretion through H_1- and H_2-receptors. J Clin Endocrinol Metab 55:118, 1982.
103. Knigge U, Matzen S, Warberg J. Histaminergic mediation of the stress-induced release of prolactin in male rats. Neuroendocrinology 47:68, 1988.
104. Carlson HE, Ippoliti AF. Cimetidine, an H_2-antihistamine, stimulates prolactin secretion in man. J Clin Endocrinol Metab 45:367, 1977.
105. Knigge U, Sleimann I, Matzen S, Warberg J. Histaminergic regulation of prolactin secretion: Involvement of serotoninergic neurons. Neuroendocrinology 48:527, 1988.
106. Rivier C, Brown M, Vale W. Effect of neurotensin, substance P and morphine sulfate on the secretion of prolactin and growth hormone in the rat. Endocrinology 100:751, 1977.
107. Eckstein N, Wehrenberg WB, Louis K, et al. Effects of substance P on anterior pituitary secretion in the female rhesus monkey. Neuroendocrinology 31:338, 1980.
108. Gudelsky GA, Porter JC. Release of dopamine from tuberoinfundibular neurons into pituitary stalk blood after prolactin or haloperidol administration. Endocrinology 106:526, 1980.
109. Hokfelt T, Fuxe K. Effects of PRL and ergot alkaloids on the tuberoinfundibular dopamine (DA) neurons. Neuroendocrinology 9:100, 1972.
110. Bybee DE, Nakawatase C, Szabo M, Frohman LA. Inhibitory feedback effects of prolactin on its secretion involve central nervous system dopaminergic mediation. Neuroendocrinology 36:27, 1983.
111. Sarkar DK. Evidence for prolactin feedback actions on hypothalamic oxytocin, vasoactive intestinal peptide and dopamine secretion. Neuroendocrinology 49:520, 1989.
112. Yen SSC, Hoff JD, Lasley BL, et al. Induction of prolactin release by LRF and LRF-agonist. Life Sci 26:1963, 1980.
113. Cetel NS, Yen SSC. Concomitant pulsatile release of prolactin and luteinizing hormone in hypogonadal women. J Clin Endocrinol Metab 56:1313, 1983.
114. Cetel NS, Quigley ME, Yen SSC. Naloxone-induced prolactin secretion in women: Evidence against a direct prolactin stimulatory effect of endogenous opioids. J Clin Endocrinol Metab 60:191, 1985.
115. Denef C, Andries M. Evidence for paracrine interaction between gonadotrophs and lactotrophs in pituitary cell aggregates. Endocrinology 112:813, 1983.
116. Schule R, Muller M, Otsuka-Murakami H, Renkawitz R. Cooperativity of the glucocorticoid receptor and the CACCC-box binding factor. Nature 332:87, 1988.
117. Murdoch GH, Rosenfield MG. Regulation of pituitary function and prolactin production in the GH_4 cell line by vitamin D. J Biol Chem 256:4050, 1981.
118. Verbeelen D, Vanhaelst L, Van Steirtegham AC, Sennesael J. Effect of 1,25-dihydroxyvitamin D_3 on plasma prolactin in patients with renal failure on regular dialysis treatment. J Endocrinol Invest 6:359, 1983.
119. Yen SSC, Ehara Y, Siler TM. Augmentation of prolactin secretion by estrogen in hypogonadal women. J Clin Invest 53:652, 1974.
120. Frantz AG, Kleinberg DL, Noel GL. Studies on prolactin in man. Recent Prog Horm Res 28:527, 1972.
121. Veldhuis JD, Evans WS, Johnson MD, Stumpf PG. Mechanisms that subserve estradiol's induction of increased prolactin concentrations: Evidence of amplitude modulation of spontaneous prolactin secretory bursts. Am J Obstet Gynecol 161:1149, 1989.
122. Marshall LA, Martin MC, Leong S, Jaffe RB. Influence of preovulatory estradiol concentrations on diurnal and pulsatile prolactin secretion patterns. Am J Obstet Gynecol 159:1558, 1988.
123. Sprangers SA, Brenner RM, Bethea CL. Estrogen and progestin receptor immunocytochemistry in lactotropes versus gonadotropes of monkey pituitary cell cultures. Endocrinology 124:1462, 1989.
124. Maurer RA. Estrogen regulates the transcription of the prolactin gene. J Biol Chem 257:2133, 1982.
125. Waterman ML, Adler S, Nelson C, et al. A single domain of the estrogen receptor confers deoxyribonucleic acid binding and transcriptional activation of the rat prolactin gene. Mol Endocrinol 2:14, 1988.
126. Raymond V, Beaulieu M, Labrie F, Boissier J. Potent antidopaminergic activity of estradiol at the pituitary level on prolactin release. Science 200:1173, 1978.
127. Munemura M, Agui T, Sibley DR. Chronic estrogen treatment promotes a functional uncoupling of the D_2 dopamine receptor in rat anterior pituitary gland. Endocrinology 124:346, 1989.
128. Judd SJ, Rigg LA, Yen SSC. The effects of ovariectomy and estrogen treatment on the dopamine inhibition of gonadotropin and prolactin release. J Clin Endocrinol Metab 49:182, 1979.
129. DeLean A, Garon M, Kelly PA, Labrie F. Changes in pituitary thyrotropin releasing hormone (TRH) receptor level and prolactin response to TRH during the rat estrous cycle. Endocrinology 100:105, 1977.
130. Rakoff JS, Yen SSC. The simultaneous release of prolactin and gonadotropins in response to progesterone administration in estrogen-primed ovariectomized women. J Clin Endocrinol Metab 47:918, 1978.
131. Williams RF, Gianfortoni JG, Hodgen GD. Hyperprolactinemia induced by an estrogen-progesterone synergy: Quantitative and temporal effects of estrogen priming in monkeys. J Clin Endocrinol Metab 60:126, 1985.
132. MacLusky NJ, Lieberburg I, Kerey LC, McEwen BS. Progestin receptors in the brain and pituitary of the Bonnet monkey (*Macaca radiata*): Differences between the monkey and the rat in the distribution of progestin receptors. Endocrinology 106:185, 1980.
133. Adams TE, Norman RL, Spies HG. Gonadotropin-releasing hormone receptor binding and pituitary responsiveness in estradiol-primed monkeys. Science 213:1388, 1981.
134. Clark R. The somatogenic hormones and insulin-like growth factor-1: Stimulators of lymphopoiesis and immune function. Endocr Rev 18:157, 1997.
135. Chen HW, Meier H, Heiniger H, Huebner RJ. Tumorigenesis in strain DW-J mice and induction by prolactin of the group-specific antigen of endogenous C-type RNA tumor virus. J Natl Cancer Inst 49:1145, 1972.
136. Hiestand PC, Mekler P, Nordmann R, et al. Prolactin as a modulator of lymphocyte responsiveness provides a possible mechanism for cyclosporine. Proc Natl Acad Sci USA 83:2599, 1986.
137. Matera L. Endocrine, paracrine and autocrine actions of prolactin on immune cells. Life Sci 59:599, 1996.
138. Montgomery DW, Shen GK, Ulrich ED, et al. Human thymocytes express a prolactin-like messenger ribonucleic acid and synthesize bioactive prolactin-like proteins. Endocrinology 131:3019, 1992.
139. Montgomery DW, Zukoski CF, Shah GN, et al. Concanavalin A–stimulated murine splenocytes produce a factor with prolactin-like bioactivity and immunoreactivity. Biochem Biophys Res Commun 145:692, 1987.
140. Rosen SW, Weintraub BD, Aaronson SA. Nonrandom ectopic protein production by malignant cells: Direct evidence in vitro. J Clin Endocrinol Metab 50:834, 1980.
141. Hatfill S, Kirby R, Hanley M, et al. Hyperprolactinemia in acute myeloid leukemia and indication of ectopic expression of human prolactin in blast cells of a patient of subtype M4. Leuk Res 14:57, 1990.
142. Sabharwal P, Glaser R, Lafuse W, et al. Prolactin synthesized and secreted by human peripheral blood mononuclear cells: An autocrine growth factor for lymphoproliferation. Proc Natl Acad Sci USA 89:7713, 1992.

143. Clevenger CV, Russell DH, Appasamy PM, Prystowsky M. Regulation of interleukin 2–driven T-lymphocyte proliferation by prolactin. Proc Natl Acad Sci USA 87:6460, 1990.
144. Lavalle C, Loyo E, Paniagua R, et al. Correlation study between prolactin and androgens in male patients with systemic lupus erythematosus. J Rheumatol 14:268, 1987.
145. Vidaller A, Llorente L, Larrea F, et al. T-cell dysregulation in patients with hyperprolactinemia: Effect of bromocriptine treatment. Clin Immunol Immunopathol 38:337, 1986.
146. Blank M, Krause I, Buskila D, et al. Bromocriptine immunomodulation of experimental SLE and primary antiphospholipid syndrome via induction of nonspecific T suppressor cells. Cell Immunol 162:114, 1995.
147. Shen GH, Montgomery DW, Ulrich ED, et al. Up-regulation of prolactin gene expression and feedback modulation of lymphocyte proliferation during acute allograft rejection. Surgery 112:387, 1992.
148. Russell DH, Kibler R, Matrisian L, et al. Prolactin receptors on human T and B lymphocytes: Antagonism of prolactin binding by cyclosporine. J Immunol 134:3027, 1985.
149. Matera L, Muccioli G, Cesano A, et al. Prolactin receptors on large granular lymphocytes: Dual regulation by cyclosporine A. Brain Behav Immunol 2:1, 1988.
150. Dardenne M, De Moraes MCL, Kelly PA, Gagnerault MC. Prolactin receptor expression in human hematopoietic tissues analyzed by flow cytofluorometry. Endocrinology 134:2108, 1994.
151. Bazan JF. A novel family of growth factor receptors: A common binding domain in the growth hormone, prolactin, erythropoietin and IL-6 receptors, and the p75 IL-2 receptor β-chain. Biochem Biophys Res Commun 164:788, 1989.
152. Weigent DA. Immunoregulatory properties of growth hormone and prolactin. Pharmacol Ther 69:237, 1996.
153. Leighton PC, McNeilly AS, Chard T. Short-term variation in blood levels of prolactin in women. J Endocrinol 68:177, 1976.
154. Cooper DS, Ridgway EC, Kliman B, et al. Metabolic clearance and production rates of prolactin in man. J Clin Invest 64:1669, 1979.
155. Sievertsen GD, Lim VS, Nakawatase C, Frohman LA. Metabolic clearance and secretion rates of human prolactin in normal subjects and in patients with chronic renal failure. J Clin Endocrinol Metab 50:846, 1980.
156. Ehara Y, Siler T, Vandenberg G, et al. Circulating prolactin levels during the menstrual cycle: Episodic release and diurnal variation. Am J Obstet Gynecol 117:962, 1973.
157. Sassin JF, Frantz AG, Weitzman ED, Kapen S. Human prolactin: 24-hour pattern with increased release during sleep. Science 177:1205, 1972.
158. Waldstein J, Duffy JF, Bronson EN, et al. Gender differences in the temporal organization of prolactin (PRL) secretion: Evidence for a sleep-independent circadian rhythm of circulating PRL levels—a clinical research center study. J Clin Endocrinol Metab 81:1483, 1996.
159. Weitzman ED, Boyar RM, Kapen S, Hellman L. The relationship of sleep stages to neuroendocrine secretion and biological rhythm in man. Recent Prog Horm Res 31:399, 1975.
160. Quigley ME, Ropert JF, Yen SSC. Acute prolactin release triggered by feeding. J Clin Endocrinol Metab 52:231, 1981.
161. Rakoff JS, Siler TM, Sinha YN, Yen SSC. Prolactin and growth hormone release in response to sequential stimulation by arginine and synthetic TRF. J Clin Endocrinol Metab 37:641, 1973.
162. Rasmussen DD, Ishizuka B, Quigley ME, Yen SSC. Effects of tyrosine and tryptophan ingestion on plasma catecholamine and 3,4-dihydroxyphenylacetic acid concentrations. J Clin Endocrinol Metab 57:760, 1983.
163. Desir D, Van Cauter E, L'Hermite M, et al. Effects of "jet lag" on hormonal patterns: III. Demonstration of an intrinsic circadian rhythmicity in plasma prolactin. J Clin Endocrinol Metab 55:849, 1982.
164. Lee PA, Xenakis T, Winer J, Matsenbaugh S. Puberty in girls: Correlation of serum levels of gonadotropins, prolactin, androgens, estrogens, and progestins with physical changes. J Clin Endocrinol Metab 43:775, 1976.
165. Vekeman M, Delvoye P, L'Hermite M, Robyn C. Serum prolactin levels during the menstrual cycle. J Clin Endocrinol Metab 44:989, 1977.
166. Boyd AE III, Sanchez-Frano F. Changes in the prolactin response to thyrotropin-releasing hormone (TRH) during the menstrual cycle. J Clin Endocrinol Metab 44:985, 1977.
167. Jaffe RB, Yuen BH, Keye WR Jr, Midgley AR Jr. Physiologic and pathologic profiles of circulating human prolactin. Am J Obstet Gynecol 117:757, 1973.
168. Rigg LA, Yen SSC. The pattern of increase in circulating prolactin levels during human gestation. Am J Obstet Gynecol 129:454, 1977.
169. Markoff E, Lee DW, Hollingsworth DR. Glycosylated and nonglycosylated prolactin in serum during pregnancy. J Clin Endocrinol Metab 67:519, 1988.
170. Larrea F, Escorza A, Valero A, et al. Heterogeneity of serum prolactin throughout the menstrual cycle and pregnancy in hyperprolactinemic women with normal ovarian function. J Clin Endocrinol Metab 68:982, 1989.
171. Boyar RM, Finkelstein JW, Kapen S, Hellman L. Twenty-four prolactin secretory pattern during pregnancy. J Clin Endocrinol Metab 40:117, 1975.
172. Quigley ME, Ishizuka B, Ropert JF, Yen SSC. The food-entrained prolactin and cortisol release in late pregnancy and prolactinoma patients. J Clin Endocrinol Metab 54:1109, 1982.
173. Rigg LA, Yen SSC. Multiphasic prolactin (PRL) secretion during parturition in humans. Am J Obstet Gynecol 128:215, 1977.
174. Nicoll CS. "Spinoff" from comparative studies on prolactin physiology of significance to the clinical endocrinologist. *In* Pasteels JL (ed). Human Prolactin. Amsterdam, Excerpta Medica, 1973, p 119.
175. Meier AH, Troliec TN, Joseph MM, John TM. Temporal synergism of prolactin and adrenal steroids in the regulation of fat stores. Proc Soc Exp Biol Med 137:408, 1971.
176. Gustafson AB, Banasiak MF, Kalkhoff RK, et al. Correlation of hyperprolactinemia with altered plasma insulin and glucagon: Similarity to effects of late human pregnancy. J Clin Endocrinol Metab 51:242, 1980.
177. Aubert ML, Grumbach MM, Kaplan SL. The ontogenesis of human fetal hormones. III. Prolactin. J Clin Invest 56:155, 1975.
178. Begeot M, Dubois MP, Dubois PM. Evolution of lactotropes in normal and anencephalic human fetuses. J Clin Endocrinol Metab 58:726, 1984.
179. Stier CT Jr, Cowden EA, Friesen HG, Allison MEM. Prolactin and the rat kidney: A clearance and micropuncture study. Endocrinology 115:362, 1984.
180. Pullano JG, Cohen-Addad N, Apuzzio JJ, et al. Water and salt conservation in the human fetus and newborn. I. Evidence for role of fetal prolactin. J Clin Endocrinol Metab 69:1180, 1989.
181. Schenker JG, Ben-David M, Polishuk WZ. Prolactin in normal pregnancy: Relationship of maternal, fetal, and amniotic fluid levels. Am J Obstet Gynecol 123:834, 1975.
182. Riddick DH, Kusmik WF. Decidua: A possible source of amniotic fluid PRL. Am J Obstet Gynecol 127:187, 1977.
183. Dardenne M, Savino W, Gagnerault M-C, et al. Neuroendocrine control of thymic hormonal production. I. Prolactin stimulates in vivo and in vitro the production of thymulin by human and murine thymic epithelial cells. Endocrinology 125:3, 1989.
184. McCoshen JA, Tomita K, Fernandez C, Tyson JE. Specific cells of human amnion selectively localize prolactin. J Clin Endocrinol Metab 55:166, 1982.
185. Josimovich JB, Merisko K, Boccella L, Tobon H. Binding of prolactin by fetal rhesus cell membrane fractions. Endocrinology 100:557, 1977.
186. Josimovich JB, Merisko K, Boccella L. Amniotic prolactin control over amniotic and fetal extracellular fluid water and electrolytes in the rhesus monkey. Endocrinology 100:564, 1977.
187. Lumpsin MD, Samson WK, McCann SM. Hypothalamic and pituitary sites of action of oxytocin to alter prolactin secretion in the rat. Endocrinology 112:1711, 1983.
188. Lyons WR. Hormonal synergism in mammary growth. Proc R Soc Lond B 149:303, 1958.
189. Topper YJ, Freeman CS. Multiple hormone interactions in the developmental biology of the mammary gland. Physiol Rev 60:1049, 1980.
190. Forsyth IA. Variation among species in the endocrine control of mammary growth and function. The role of prolactin, growth hormone, and placental lactogen. J Dairy Sci 69:886, 1986.

191. Cunningham BC, Bass S, Fuh G, Wells JA. Zinc mediation of binding of human growth hormone to the human prolactin receptor. Science 250:1709, 1990.
192. Djiane J, Durand P. Prolactin-progesterone antagonism in self-regulation of prolactin receptors in the mammary gland. Nature 266:614, 1977.
193. Ganguly R, Majumder PK, Ganguly N, Ganerfee ML. The mechanism of progesterone-glucocorticoid interaction in the regulation of casein gene expression. J Biol Chem 257:2182, 1982.
194. Konner M, Worthman C. Nursing frequency, gonadal function, and birth spacing among !Kung hunter-gatherers. Science 207:788, 1980.
195. Lochnan HA, Buteau H, Richards S, et al. Functional activity of the human prolactin receptor and its ligands. Mol Cell Endocrinol 114:91, 1995.
196. Cox DB, Owens RA, Hartmann PE. Blood and milk prolactin and the rate of milk synthesis in women. Exp Physiol 81:1007, 1996.
197. Dehoff MH, Elgin RG, Collier RJ, Clemmons DR. Both type I and II insulin-like growth factor receptor binding increase during lactogenesis in bovine mammary tissue. Endocrinology 122:2412, 1988.
198. Prosser CG, Sankaran L, Hinnighausen L, Topper YJ. Comparison of the roles of insulin and insulin-like growth factor I in casein gene expression and in the development of alpha-lactalbumin and glucose transport activities in the mouse mammary epithelial cell. Endocrinology 120:1411, 1987.
199. Duclos M, Houdebine L-M, Djiane J. Comparison of insulin-like growth factor I and insulin effects on prolactin-induced lactogenesis in the rabbit mammary gland in vitro. Mol Cell Endocrinol 65:129, 1989.
200. Hadsell DL, Campbell PG, Baumrucker CR. Characterization of the change in type I and II insulin-like growth factor receptor of bovine mammary tissue during the pre- and postpartum periods. Endocrinology 126:637, 1990.
201. Voloschin LM, Dottaviano EJ. The channeling of natural stimuli that evoke the ejection of milk in the rat: Effect of transections in the midbrain and hypothalamus. Endocrinology 99:49, 1976.
202. Cobo E. Neuroendocrine control of milk ejection in women. *In* Josimovich JB, Reynolds M, Cobo E (eds). Lactogenic Hormones, Fetal Nutrition, and Lactation. New York, John Wiley & Sons, 1974, p 433.
203. Sawchenko PE, Plotsky PM, Pfeiffer SW, et al. Inhibin β in central neural pathways involved in the control of oxytocin secretion. Nature 334:615, 1988.
204. McNeilly AS, Robinson CAF, Houston MJ, Howie PW. Release of oxytocin and PRL in response to suckling. Br Med J 286:257, 1983.
205. Smith MS, Lee L-R, Pohl CR, et al. Inhibitory effects of the suckling stimulus on hypothalamic GnRH release and pulsatile LH secretion. *In* Yen SSC, Vale W (eds). Symposium on Neuroendocrine Regulation of Reproduction. Norwell, MA, Serono Symposia, USA, 1990, pp 39–46.
206. Blake CA, Sawyer CH. Nicotine blocks the suckling-induced rise in circulating prolactin in lactating rats. Science 177:619, 1972.
207. Liu JH, Yen SSC. Endocrinology of the postpartum state. *In* Brody SA, Ueland K (eds). Endocrine Disorders in Pregnancy. East Norwalk, CT, Appleton & Lange, 1989, p 111.
208. Racagni G, Apud JA, Cocchi D, et al. Regulation of prolactin secretion during suckling: Involvement of the hypothalamo-pituitary GABAergic system. J Endocrinol Invest 7:481, 1984.
209. Ishizuka B, Quigley ME, Yen SSC. Postpartum hypogonadotropinism: Evidence for increased opioid inhibition. Clin Endocrinol 20:573, 1984.
210. Kooy A, deGreef WJ, Vreeburg JTM, et al. Evidence for the involvement of corticotropin-releasing factor in the inhibition of gonadotropin release induced by hyperprolactinemia. Neuroendocrinology 51:261, 1990.
211. Milenkov L, D' Angelo D, Kelly PA, Weiner RI. Inhibition of gonadotropin hormone–releasing hormone release by prolactin from GT1 neuronal cell lines through prolactin receptors. Proc Natl Acad Sci USA 91:1244, 1994.
212. Cheung CY, Weiner RI. In vitro supersensitivity of the anterior pituitary to dopamine inhibition of prolactin secretion. Endocrinology 102:1614, 1978.
213. Bethea CL, Ramsdell JS, Jaffe RB, et al. Characterization of the dopaminergic regulation of the human prolactin-secreting cells cultured on extracellular matrix. J Clin Endocrinol Metab 54:893, 1982.
214. Quigley ME, Judd SJ, Gilliland GB, Yen SSC. Functional studies of dopamine control of prolactin secretion in normal women and women with hyperprolactinemic pituitary microadenoma. J Clin Endocrinol Metab 50:994, 1980.
215. Fine SA, Frohman LA. Loss of central nervous system component of dopaminergic inhibition of prolactin secretion in patients with prolactin-secreting pituitary tumors. J Clin Invest 61:973, 1978.
216. Crosignani PG, Ferrari C, Malinverni A. Effect of central nervous system dopaminergic activation on prolactin secretion in man: Evidence for a common central defect in hyperprolactinemic patients with and without radiological signs of pituitary tumors. J Clin Endocrinol Metab 51:1068, 1980.
217. Crosignani PG, Reschini E, Peracchi M, et al. Failure of dopamine infusion to suppress the plasma prolactin response to sulpiride in normal and hyperprolactinemic subjects. J Clin Endocrinol Metab 45:841, 1977.
218. Schechter J, Goldsmith P, Wilson C, Weiner R. Morphological evidence for the presence of arteries in human prolactinomas. J Clin Endocrinol Metab 67:713, 1988.
219. Schlechte JA, Sherman B, Martin R. Bone density in amenorrheic women with and without hyperprolactinemia. J Clin Endocrinol Metab 56:1120, 1983.
220. Ciccarelli E, Giusti M, Miola C, et al. Effectiveness and tolerability of long term treatment with cabergoline, a new long-lasting ergoline derivative, in hyperprolactinemic patients. J Clin Endocrinol Metab 69:725, 1989.
221. Webster J, Piscitelli G, Polli A, et al for the Cabergoline Study Group. A comparison of cabergoline and bromocriptine in the treatment of hyperprolactinemic amenorrhea. N Engl J Med 331:904, 1994.
222. Andreotti AC, Pianezolla E, Persiani S, et al. Pharmacokinetics, pharmacodynamics, and tolerability of cabergoline, a prolactin-lowering drug, after administration of increasing oral doses (0.5, 1.0, and 1.5 milligrams) in healthy male volunteers. J Clin Endocrinol Metab 80:841, 1995.
223. Rasmussen C, Bergh T, Wide L, Brownell J. Long term treatment with a new non-ergot–long-acting dopamine agonist CV 205-502, in women with hyperprolactinemia. Clin Endocrinol (Oxf) 29:271, 1988.
224. Morange I, Barlier A, Pellegrini I, et al. Prolactinomas resistant to bromocriptine: Long-term efficacy of quinagolide and outcome of pregnancy. Eur J Endocrinol 135:413, 1996.
225. Caccavelli L, Feron F, Morange I, et al. Decreased expression of the two D_2 dopamine receptor isoforms in bromocriptine-resistant prolactinomas. Neuroendocrinology 60:314, 1994.
226. Serri O, Rasio E, Beauregard H, et al. Recurrence of hyperprolactinemia after selective transsphenoidal adenomectomy in women with prolactinoma. N Engl J Med 309:280, 1983.
227. Feigenbaum SL, Downey DE, Wilson CB, Jaffe RB. Transsphenoidal pituitary resection for preoperative diagnosis of prolactin-secreting pituitary adenoma in women: Long term follow-up. J Clin Endocrinol Metab 81:1711, 1996.
228. Molitch ME. Pregnancy and the hyperprolactinemic woman. N Engl J Med 312:1364, 1985.
229. Gemzell C, Wang CF. Outcome of pregnancy in women with pituitary adenoma. Fertil Steril 31:363, 1979.
230. Healy DL, Burger HG. Sustained elevation of serum prolactin by metoclopramide: A clinical model of idiopathic hyperprolactinemia. J Clin Endocrinol 46:709, 1978.
231. Kauppila A, Leinonen P, Vikho R, Ylostalo P. Metoclopramide-induced hyperprolactinemia impairs ovarian follicle maturation and corpus luteum function in women. J Clin Endocrinol Metab 54:955, 1982.
232. Lam KSL, Reichlin S. Pituitary vasoactive intestinal peptide regulates prolactin secretion in the hypothyroid rat. Neuroendocrinology 50:524, 1989.
233. Lim VS, Kathpalia S, Frohman LA. Hyperprolactinemia and impaired pituitary response to suppression and stimulation in chronic renal failure: Reversal after transplantation. J Clin Endocrinol Metab 48:101, 1979.
234. Baumann G, Loriaux DL. Failure of endogenous prolactin to alter renal salt and water retention and adrenal function in man. J Clin Endocrinol Metab 43:643, 1976.

235. Forbes A, Hanneman PH, Griswold GF, Albright F. Syndrome characterized by galactorrhea, amenorrhea, and low urinary FSH: Comparison with acromegaly and normal lactation. J Clin Endocrinol Metab 14:265, 1954.
236. Vermeulen A, Ando S. Prolactin and adrenal androgen secretion. Clin Endocrinol (Oxf) 8:295, 1978.
237. Glickman SP, Rosenfield RL, Bergenstal RM, Helke J. Multiple androgenic abnormalities, including elevated free testosterone, in hyperprolactinemic women. J Clin Endocrinol Metab 55:251, 1982.
238. Lobo RA, Kletzky OA. Normalization of androgen and sex hormone–binding globulin levels after treatment of hyperprolactinemic women. J Clin Endocrinol Metab 55:251, 1982.
239. Magrini G, Ebiner JR, Burchkardt P, Felber JP. Study on the relationship between plasma prolactin levels and androgen metabolism in man. J Clin Endocrinol Metab 43:944, 1976.
240. Glasow A, Breidert M, Haidan A, et al. Functional aspects of the effect of prolactin (PRL) on adrenal steroidogenesis and distribution of the PRL receptor in the human adrenal gland. J Clin Endocrinol Metab 81:3103, 1996.
241. Klibanski A, Neer R, Beitins I, et al. Decreased bone density in hyperprolactinemic women. N Engl J Med 303:1511, 1981.
242. Koppelmann MC, Kurtz DW, Morrish A, et al. Vertebral body bone mineral content in hyperprolactinemic women. J Clin Endocrinol Metab 59:1059, 1984.
243. Carman JS, Wyatt RJ. Reduction of serum-prolactin after subcutaneous salmon calcitonin. Lancet 1:1267, 1977.
244. Pahuja D, DeLuca H. Stimulation of intestinal calcium transport and bone calcium mobilization by prolactin in vitamin D–deficient rats. Science 214:1038, 1981.
245. Gustafson A, Banasiak M, Kalkhoff R, et al. Prolactin-induced hyperinsulinemia (abstract). Clin Res 26:720, 1978.
246. Tourniaire J, Pallo D, Pausset G, et al. Diminution de la tolerance glucidique et hyperinsulinisme dans l'adenome a prolactine. Nouv Presse Med 3:1705, 1974.
247. Gustafson AB, Banasiak MF, Kalkhoff RK, et al. Correlation of hyperprolactinemia with altered plasma insulin and glucagon: Similarity to effects of late human pregnancy. J Clin Endocrinol Metab 51:242, 1980.
248. Meuris S, Verloes A, Robyn C. Immunocytochemical localization of prolactin-like immunoreactivity in rat pancreatic islets. Endocrinology 112:2221, 1983.
249. Boyar RM, Kapen S, Finkelstein JW, et al. Hypothalamic-pituitary function in diverse hyperprolactinemic states. J Clin Invest 53:1588, 1974.
250. Bohnet HG, Dahlen HG, Wuttke W, Schneider HPG. Hyperprolactinaemic anovulatory syndrome. J Clin Endocrinol Metab 42:132, 1976.
251. Moult PJA, Rees LH, Besser GM. Pulsatile gonadotrophin secretion in hyperprolactinaemic amenorrhoea and the response to bromocriptine therapy. Clin Endocrinol 16:153, 1982.
252. Travaglini P, Ambrosi B, Beck-Pecoz P, et al. Hypothalamic-pituitary-ovarian function in hyperprolactinemic women. J Clin Invest 1:39, 1978.
253. Koike K, Aono T, Tsutsumi H, et al. Restoration of oestrogen-positive feedback effect on LH release in women with prolactinoma by transsphenoidal surgery. Acta Endocrinol 100:492, 1982.
254. Quigley ME, Sheehan KL, Casper RF, Yen SSC. Evidence for an increased opioid inhibition of luteinizing hormone secretion in hyperprolactinemic patients with pituitary microadenoma. J Clin Endocrinol Metab 50:427, 1980.
255. Marshetti B, Labrie F. Prolactin inhibits pituitary luteinizing hormone–releasing hormone receptors in the rat. Endocrinology 111:1208, 1982.
256. Zarate A, Jacobs S, Canales ES, et al. Functional evaluation of pituitary reserve in patients with the amenorrhea-galactorrhea syndrome utilizing luteinizing hormone–releasing hormone (LH-RH), L-dopa and chlorpromazine. J Clin Endocrinol Metab 37:855, 1973.
257. Dorrington J, Gore-Langton RE. Prolactin inhibits oestrogen synthesis in the ovary. Nature 290:600, 1981.
258. Magoffin DA, Erickson GF. Prolactin inhibition of luteinizing hormone–stimulated androgen synthesis in ovarian interstitial cells cultured in defined medium: Mechanism of action. Endocrinology 111:2001, 1982.
259. McNatty KP, Hunter WN, McNeilly AS, Sawers RS. Changes in the concentration of pituitary and steroid hormones in the follicular fluid of human graafian follicles throughout the menstrual cycle. J Endocrinol 64:555, 1975.
260. McNatty KP, Sawers RS. Relationship between the endocrine environment within the graafian follicle and the subsequent secretion of progesterone by human granulosa cells in culture. J Endocrinol 66:391, 1975.

Chapter 10

THE BREAST

Robert L. Barbieri

CHAPTER OUTLINE

KEY POINTS

- The main role of the breast is the secretion of milk. Breast milk consists of milk proteins including casein and lactalbumin, free fatty acids, and the milk sugar lactose. Prolactin and steroid hormones regulate the production of milk by altering the rate of transcription of key genes such as the β-casein and whey acidic protein genes.
- In lactating women, contraceptives containing both estrogen and progestin significantly decrease the daily milk production volume and alter the chemical composition of breast milk. Contraceptives containing only progestins tend to have a lesser impact on milk production volume.
- Bromocriptine, a dopamine agonist, suppresses prolactin secretion and suppresses milk production. In the peripartum period, bromocriptine has been reported to be associated with cases of hypertension and seizure.
- Approximately 75 percent of women with both galactorrhea and amenorrhea have hyperprolactinemia.
- Breast cancer is caused by both predisposing genetic traits and environmental exposures.
- Numerous epidemiologic and laboratory observations suggest that breast cancer is an endocrine disease.
- Estrogen antagonists are the mainstay of endocrine treatment of breast cancer.
- New, organ-selective estrogen antagonists are in active development.
- Oophorectomy is an effective hormonal treatment of breast cancer.
- The number of breast cancer survivors is increasing rapidly. For breast cancer survivors, issues such as the risk of pregnancy and estrogen replacement therapy are complex and require more data from clinical trials.

The breast overlies the second to the sixth ribs. The medial border of the breast is the sternum, and the lateral border is the latissimus dorsi. The superior and inferior borders are the clavicle and the costal margin and upper rectus sheath. The breast consists of glandular, adipose, and connective tissues. The glandular tissue of the breast is arranged in approximately 15 to 20 lobes (Fig. 10–1). Each lobe consists of a branching structure made up of lobules and finally acini (also referred to as alveoli). The acini are lined by a single layer of milk-secreting epithelial cells. Each acinus is encased in an interwoven pattern of contractile myoepithelial cells. The lumens of the acini connect to collecting intralobular ducts, which empty into the main 15 to 20 lobar collecting ducts. In turn, each lobe drains into the nipple. The nipple is surrounded by a pigmented areola. The sebaceous glands located on the perimeter of the areola are referred to as the glands of Montgomery. The glandular tissue is embedded in fat, which accounts for most of the mass of the breast. The lobules are separated by connective tissue septa, Cooper's ligaments, which run from the subcutaneous tissue to the chest wall.

The breast is sensitive to the sex steroids estradiol, progesterone, and testosterone and to numerous protein hormones, including prolactin and oxytocin.[1] During puberty and pregnancy, the breast is stimulated to grow.

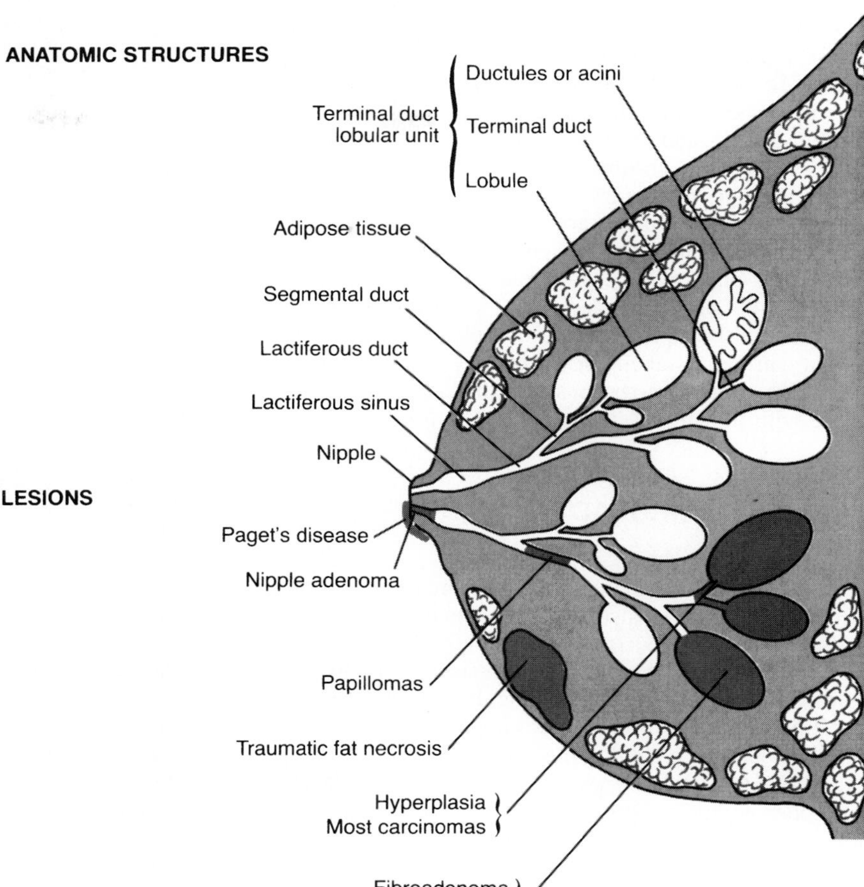

Figure 10–1 ■ Anatomy of the breast and major lesions at each site within the breast. (From Cotran RS, Kumar V, Robbins SL [eds]. Pathologic Basis of Disease, 5th ed. Philadelphia, WB Saunders, 1994, p 1090.)

In many mammals, estradiol is especially important in stimulating the growth of the ductal system, and progesterone is important in stimulating the growth of the acini and stromal elements. During pregnancy, estradiol, progesterone, and prolactin are important factors stimulating breast growth. Androgens tend to inhibit breast growth, an effect that can be characterized as antiestrogenic.

A genetic experiment of nature, androgen insensitivity syndrome, provides an example of the important interplay between estrogens and androgens in the regulation of breast growth.[2] In androgen insensitivity due to mutations in the androgen receptor, genetic males (46,XY) do not have a functional androgen receptor. Testosterone is produced by the testis, but target tissues are not capable of responding to the high levels of circulating androgens. In this syndrome, estradiol levels are in the range of 50 pg/ml, an estradiol concentration comparable to early follicular-phase levels.[3] Breast volume in individuals with androgen insensitivity is typically above average. This suggests that in the complete absence of androgen inhibition, modest levels of estradiol are capable of stimulating significant breast growth. Progesterone levels are low in individuals with loss of the androgen receptor. This suggests that breast volume is not absolutely dependent on progesterone stimulation. The antiestrogenic effect of androgen on breast growth can be used in the treatment of fibrocystic disease.

DEVELOPMENT OF THE BREAST

The development of the breast occurs in three major phases: in utero, at puberty, and during pregnancy. This process has been best studied in the rodent. During in utero development of the breast, the growth of epithelial elements into the underlying mesenchyme results in the development of a rudimentary ductal system. In the mouse, the majority of mammary morphogenesis occurs in the postnatal period. Immediately after birth, the mammary ducts are quiescent. At sexual maturity, the distal ends of the ducts proliferate and develop into the end buds, a structure similar to the human acinus. With the onset of pregnancy, a second round of proliferation occurs. Numerous hormones including estradiol, progesterone, androgens, prolactin, other lactogenic factors, thyroxine, glucocorticoid, insulin, growth hormone, transforming growth factor-β, and epidermal growth factor (EGF) play roles in this process.[4, 5]

During the normal menstrual cycle, the breast undergoes cycles of growth and quiescence. In the early follicular phase, the ductal cells proliferate and continue to develop throughout the remainder of the cycle. In the luteal phase of the cycle, progesterone stimulates the proliferation of the terminal duct structure, basal epithelial cells, and stromal cells. Accompanying these proliferative changes are an increase in stromal edema and vacuolization of epithelial cells. These effects may account, in part, for the sense of breast fullness women experience during the late luteal phase. At menses, the decrease in estradiol and progesterone is associated with a decrease in cell proliferation, stromal edema, and the size of the ducts and acini.[6]

The two most common congenital anomalies of the breast are supernumerary nipples and accessory axillary breast tissue. Supernumerary nipples are the result of the persistence of epidermal thickenings along the embryologic milk line. Supernumerary nipples can extend from the axilla to the suprapubic area. On occasion, breast tissue extends into the axillary fossa. Ectopic breast tissue in this region can be mistaken for an axillary mass or may cause pain after pregnancy because of the engorgement of the tissue with milk.[4, 6]

LACTATION, PROLACTIN, AND OXYTOCIN

In reproduction, the main role of the breast is secretion of milk. Breast milk consists of milk proteins including casein and lactalbumin, free fatty acids, and the milk sugar lactose. Lactose is a disaccharide consisting of glucose and galactose. During pregnancy, the breast is prepared for lactation by the actions of estradiol, progesterone, prolactin, and other factors including placental lactogen. During pregnancy, the breast is exposed to high levels of lactogenic hormones including prolactin, human placental lactogen, and placental growth hormone. In the nonpregnant woman, prolactin levels are typically below 25 ng/ml. During the third trimester of pregnancy, prolactin levels are typically 15-fold higher, in the range of 200 to 450 ng/ml.[7] Human placental lactogen reaches concentrations in the range of 6000 ng/ml during the third trimester. These lactogenic stimuli cause the breast to grow and prepare the alveoli for lactation. During pregnancy, the high concentration of progesterone blocks lactogenesis. After delivery, the decrease in circulating estradiol and progesterone concentrations and the continued elevated prolactin concentration result in an increase in the production of all of the components of milk.[8] The molecular mechanisms subserving these effects are discussed later. After the decrease in estradiol and progesterone, milk production requires 2 to 5 days to become established. In the postpartum interval, milk production can be suppressed by replacing estradiol and progesterone or by suppressing prolactin secretion.[9] Milk production also requires the synergistic action of growth hormone, insulin, thyroxine, and cortisol.

During suckling, sensory signals originating in the nipple travel through thoracic nerves 4, 5, and 6 to the central nervous system. When the suckling-induced signals reach the paraventricular and supraoptic nuclei, they stimulate the release of oxytocin from the posterior pituitary. Suckling-induced signals also cause the hypothalamus to induce an acute release of prolactin, in part by suppressing dopamine secretion.[10] Prolactin maintains lactogenesis by stimulating the transcription of the casein and lactalbumin genes and other genes needed for the synthesis of free fatty acids and lactose. Oxytocin release during suckling causes the contraction of the myoepithelial cells of the mammary acini and ducts to induce the flow of milk. In addition to suckling, oxytocin can be released from the posterior pituitary by visual and auditory stimuli.

The Effect of Prolactin on β-Casein Gene Function

The cellular mechanisms that control milk protein production have been best elucidated for the β-casein and whey acidic protein genes. For the β-casein gene, prolactin, progesterone, estradiol, insulin, glucocorticoids, thyroxine, cell substratum proteins, and growth factors such as EGF regulate gene function. In the mammary epithelial cell line HC11, expression of the β-casein milk protein gene is largely regulated at the transcriptional level.

Prolactin is the key endocrine regulator of β-casein gene transcription. The prolactin receptor appears to be a member of the cytokine receptor family.[11] These receptors are characterized by extracellular cysteine motifs, a single transmembrane-spanning domain, and the absence of an intrinsic receptor-associated tyrosine kinase in the intracellular domain. The prolactin receptor may be capable of activating an intracellular tyrosine kinase, which then phosphorylates substrates that act to regulate gene transcription.

The addition of prolactin to cultures of mammary epithelial cells results in casein gene transcription within 30 minutes. This effect requires the presence of both insulin and glucocorticoid. Deletion and point mutagenesis studies have demonstrated that in HC11 cells transfected with the rat β-casein promoter, a region of approximately 340 bases immediately upstream of the transcription start site is a major site for gene regulation.[12, 13] The 340 bases 5′ of the transcription start site contain the bases that confer gene inducibility by insulin, glucocorticoids, and prolactin.

Mammary gland–specific nuclear factor (MGF) is an 89-kDa transcription-regulatory factor that binds at bases −80 to −100, 5′ of the transcription start site, and activates β-casein gene transcription. MGF is a latent cytoplasmic factor that can be activated by lactogenic hormones such as prolactin or growth hormone. After activation, MGF translocates to the nucleus where it stimulates β-casein transcription.[14] The concentration of MGF is increased by lactogenic hormones and decreased by milk stasis.[13]

Deletion of bases −110 to −150 from the transcription start site results in constitutive β-casein expression in the absence of prolactin. The transcription-regulatory factor that interacts with a portion of this deoxyribonucleic acid (DNA) segment (−110 to −120) appears to be Ying-Yang 1.[15] Ying-Yang 1 is a 68-kDa zinc finger protein. Binding of Ying-Yang 1 to the promoter region of the β-casein gene results in inhibition of transcription. Conceptually, the activator effects of MGF and the repressor effects of Ying-Yang 1 may be a simple on-off system to regulate β-casein gene transcription[16] (Fig. 10–2).

In the promoter for the β-casein gene, there are multiple half-sites for glucocorticoid receptors between −250 and −79.[17] EGF decreases β-casein gene expression. No AP-1 sites have been identified in the β-casein promoter region, suggesting that the effect of EGF may be regulated through indirect mechanisms.[18] EGF also inhibits the transcription of the prolactin receptor messenger ribonucleic acid (mRNA).[19] Progesterone decreases both β-casein and pro-

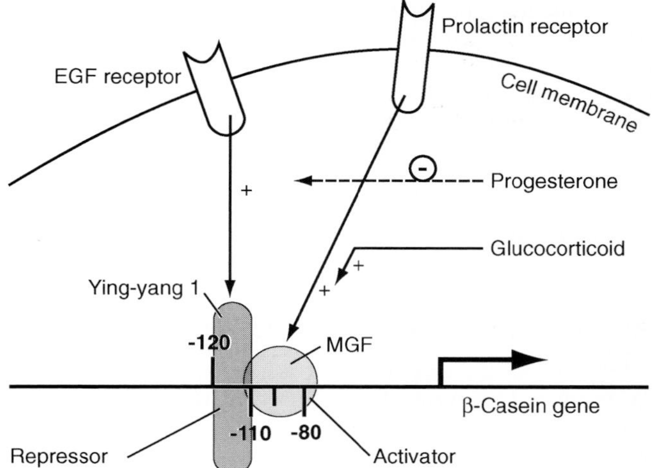

Figure 10–2 ■ Regulation of the β-casein gene, a major milk protein. β-Casein protein production is largely under transcriptional regulation. Transcription of the β-casein gene is regulated by many hormones including prolactin, progesterone, glucocorticoids, estradiol, insulin, thyroxine, and growth factors. Two proteins, mammary gland–specific nuclear factor (MGF), an activator of transcription, and Ying-Yang 1, a repressor of transcription, are major regulators of β-casein gene transcription. Prolactin acts through the prolactin receptor that activates MGF, which increases β-casein gene transcription. Glucocorticoids enhance this effect. Progesterone blocks the prolactin-induced activation of MGF and gene transcription. Epidermal growth factor (EGF) is one of many stimuli that increase Ying-Yang 1 activity and repress β-casein gene transcription.

lactin receptor gene transcription. Both EGF and progesterone are important negative regulators of lactogenesis.[19]

Lactation and Amenorrhea

Suckling activates multiple systems that inhibit gonadotropin-releasing hormone (GnRH) secretion. The inhibitory systems activated during suckling include dopamine, serotonin, γ-aminobutyric acid, and corticotropin-releasing factor-opioid.[20] The degree to which breast feeding suppresses GnRH secretion is modulated by the nutritional status of the mother, the body mass of the mother, and the intensity of the breast feeding. During exclusive breast feeding, approximately 40 percent of women will remain amenorrheic at 6 months post partum.[21] Women who remain amenorrheic during breast feeding may have higher prolactin levels than do women who become ovulatory while breast feeding.[22]

Women who are breast feeding and are amenorrheic have circulating estradiol levels in the range of 20 to 40 pg/ml. In contrast, normally cycling women have a preovulatory estradiol concentration in the range of 250 to 300 pg/ml. The hypoestrogenic state that is associated with breast feeding and amenorrhea can produce symptoms such as vaginal dryness. Many gynecologic diseases, such as endometriosis and uterine leiomyomas, are dependent on estradiol. The hypoestrogenic effect associated with amenorrhea and breast feeding may have a beneficial effect on these estrogen-dependent disease processes and may account for the laboratory and epidemiologic observation that the risk of estrogen-dependent disease is reduced.[23, 24]

Lactation and Steroid Contraceptives

In the puerperium, the episodic release of prolactin that is induced by suckling is important in maintaining the production of breast milk. High doses of estrogen, progestins, and androgens suppress lactation.[25] Steroid contraceptives, especially those containing both estrogen and progestin, significantly alter the daily production volume and composition of breast milk. In one study of more than 170 lactating women, the combination of 30 μg of ethinyl estradiol and 150 μg of levonorgestrel reduced daily milk volume by 42 percent. In contrast, a progestin-only minipill containing 75 μg of norgestrel reduced daily milk volume by only 12 percent.[26] Combination estrogen-progestin contraceptives also decrease the concentration of nitrogen, lactalbumin, lactoferrin, and lactose in breast milk. These changes in the composition of breast milk are modest and within the normal range of physiologic variation observed in lactating women who are not taking contraceptive steroids.[27]

The development of the newborn does not appear to be significantly affected by the changes in milk composition and volume associated with the use of combination estrogen-progestin oral contraceptives. In one study, both weight and neurologic development were similar in newborns of lactating mothers who did and did not take oral contraceptives.[26, 28] If a steroid contraceptive is to be recommended for a lactating woman, it is probably best to use a progestin-only regimen such as a minipill or depot medroxyprogesterone acetate.

Lactation Suppression

Prolactin secretion is crucial to the maintenance of lactation. Suppression of prolactin secretion with dopamine agonists such as bromocriptine will suppress lactation.[29] The frequency of adverse effects associated with bromocriptine use in the puerperium is low.[29] However, there are a few case reports of severe hypertension and seizures that occurred in postpartum women who used bromocriptine.[30] Owing to these adverse outcomes, many authorities do not recommend bromocriptine as a first-line agent to suppress lactation. There may be a few clinical situations, such as mothers assigning their newborn for adoption, in which bromocriptine could be considered for the suppression of lactation. In most mothers, lactation suppression can be achieved with minimization of the mechanical stimulation of the breast and nipple, ice packs, and antiprostaglandin treatment. Milk stasis appears to decrease the production of MGF, the main intracellular activator of milk protein production.[12, 13]

Induction of Lactation

Induced lactation is defined as breast feeding in the absence of a recent pregnancy. On occasion, adoptive mothers desire to breast feed. In countries in which access to formula is limited, induced lactation in a surrogate may be important if the biologic mother cannot continue to breast feed. The key hormone involved in lactation is prolactin. Medications that raise prolactin levels can be used to help induce lactation. For example, chlorpromazine, 25 mg three times daily, will cause an increase in prolactin secretion.[31] When it is coupled with nipple stimulation every few hours, lactation can be established in the majority of women.

Lactation and the Transmission of Human Immunodeficiency Virus

Many authorities state that breast feeding is the preferred method of infant feeding. On the basis of more than a dozen case reports, it appears that the human immunodeficiency virus (HIV) can be transmitted from mother to child by breast milk.[32] In some of these case reports, women who were HIV-negative during pregnancy became HIV-positive in the postpartum period. Their breast feeding children then became HIV-positive. The HIV virus was detected in breast milk. The Centers for Disease Control and Prevention have recommended that HIV-positive women should not breast feed HIV-negative infants.[33] In contrast, the World Health Organization has recommended that breast feeding of babies should be promoted and supported in all populations, regardless of the HIV status of the mother.[34]

Galactorrhea

Galactorrhea is the secretion of breast milk at a time remote from nursing. In contrast to other breast secretions, the unique feature of galactorrhea is that the secretion contains milk. This can be demonstrated by drying the secretion on a glass slide and staining for the presence of fat.

Galactorrhea is usually due to hyperprolactinemia or excessive sensitivity of the breast to normal circulating levels of prolactin. If the galactorrhea is associated with normal ovulatory menses, the most likely cause of the galactorrhea is excessive sensitivity of the breast to normal circulating levels of prolactin. If the galactorrhea is associated with amenorrhea, it is likely that the circulating prolactin level is elevated. Approximately 75 percent of women with galactorrhea and amenorrhea have hyperprolactinemia. The causes of hyperprolactinemia are reviewed in detail in Chapter 9. Briefly, the most common causes of hyperprolactinemia are a prolactin-secreting pituitary tumor, the use of dopamine antagonist medications (such as phenothiazines), and primary hypothyroidism. Galactorrhea of any cause can be suppressed by the use of dopamine agonist medications such as bromocriptine. In women with galactorrhea, normal ovulatory menses, and normal prolactin concentration, low doses of bromocriptine (1.25 to 2.5 mg) are often effective in the suppression of galactorrhea.

BENIGN BREAST DISEASE

Fibrocystic change is the most common benign breast abnormality. It is characterized histologically by hyperplastic changes of the lobular epithelium, ductal epithelium, or connective tissue.[6] The disorder is characterized clinically by breast tenderness that is particularly severe in the premenstrual phase of the menstrual cycle. Fibrocystic changes in the breast occur in a high percentage of women. Some authorities contend that fibrocystic change is a variant of normal breast physiology, not a disease state.

The medical management of fibrocystic disease continues to evolve. Danazol is an attenuated androgen that is effective in reducing symptoms associated with fibrocystic disease in 80 percent of patients.[35] Danazol is effective in the treatment of fibrocystic disease probably because of its antiestrogenic effects. The recommended dosage is between 100 and 400 mg daily. Danazol is a teratogen, and doses less than 400 mg daily do not reliably suppress ovulation. Women taking danazol should use a barrier contraceptive.

BREAST CANCER: AN ENDOCRINE DISEASE

In developed countries, breast cancer is the most common cancer of women. In the next millennium, breast cancer will cause more than 500,000 deaths annually.[36] In developed countries, the lifetime risk of developing breast cancer is approximately 10 percent. Approximately 20 percent of cases will be diagnosed before the age of 50 years, and 80 percent will be diagnosed after the age of 50 years. Numerous factors including genetics, hormones, diet, lifestyle, and other environmental exposures probably contribute to the risk of developing breast cancer.

Genetic factors are major contributors to breast cancer risk. In women with one affected first-degree relative, the risk of breast cancer is increased twofold to threefold.[37] If two first-degree relatives are affected, or if the disease was diagnosed in a family member before age 45 years, the risk is further increased.[37, 38] Overall, approximately 15 percent of breast cancer is related to family history, and about half this risk is attributed to cancer susceptibility genes.[38] Germ line mutations in at least four different genes are associated with an increased risk of breast cancer. These genes include *BRCA1, BRCA2,* the gene encoding ataxia-telangiectasia, and *P53* (Table 10–1).

BRCA1 is a tumor suppressor gene on chromosome 17 that is mutated in the germ line in about 5 percent of women with breast cancer.[39] The *BRCA1* gene is composed of 22 coding exons distributed over 100 kilobases of genomic DNA. The gene encodes a protein of 1863 amino acids.[40] The BRCA1 protein contains a zinc finger motif and is probably a nucleic acid–binding protein that acts as a tumor suppressor. Approximately 0.1 to 0.2 percent of all women have a germ line allele of a *BRCA1* gene that contains an inactivating mutation.[41] If the second allele of

■ TABLE 10–1

Calculated Risk of Breast Cancer by Age 70 Years in Women with a Mutated Allele in a Gene Causing a Cancer Syndrome

GENE	CHROMOSOME	CALCULATED RISK (%) OF BREAST CANCER BY AGE 70 YEARS
BRCA1	17q21	87
BRCA2	13q12–13	60
Ataxia-telangiectasia	11q22–23	17
P53	17q13	>50

From Ford D, Easton DF. The genetics of breast and ovarian cancer. Br J Cancer 72:805–812, 1995.

BRCA1 undergoes an inactivating somatic mutation, the affected woman has a high risk of developing breast cancer. Women who have a germ line mutation of one *BRCA1* allele have an 85 percent chance of developing breast cancer by the age of 70 years.[42] More than half of *BRCA1*-associated breast cancers will occur before age 50 years.

In families at high risk for breast cancer, more than 40 different mutations in *BRCA1* have been reported.[39] Most of the mutations are inactivating, which is consistent with *BRCA1* being a tumor suppressor gene. Most of the mutations are frameshift or nonsense mutations that prematurely truncate the protein and result in loss of protein function.

Women with a critical *BRCA1* mutation are at high risk for developing ovarian cancer. It is estimated that approximately 30 percent of women with a critical *BRCA1* mutation will develop ovarian cancer by age 60 years.[42] Among women of Ashkenazi Jewish origin, a frameshift mutation of the *BRCA1* gene, 185delAG, occurs with a carrier frequency of 1 percent. In a study of 31 Jewish women with ovarian cancer, 6 women had the 185delAG mutation (19 percent). In contrast, none of the control Jewish women without ovarian cancer had the mutation. For the Jewish women with ovarian cancer diagnosed before age 50 years, 38 percent had the 185delAG mutation.[43]

BRCA2 is a breast cancer susceptibility gene on chromosome 13q12–13.[44] *BRCA2* mutations are associated with a higher risk of male breast cancer and a lower risk of ovarian cancer than are *BRCA1* mutations.[45] Ataxia-telangiectasia is an autosomal recessive disorder with a phenotype of cerebellar ataxia and oculocutaneous telangiectasias.[46] Approximately 1 percent of the population carries one copy of a mutated gene for ataxia-telangiectasia. Female relatives of patients with ataxia-telangiectasia are at a twofold to threefold increased risk for breast cancer.[47] The Li-Fraumeni syndrome is associated with premenopausal breast cancers, brain tumors, adrenocortical cancers, and other tumors.[48] Germline mutations in *P53* have been identified in more than 50 percent of Li-Fraumeni families.[49] The risk of breast cancer in mutation carriers is approximately 50 percent.

In addition to genetic factors, many lifestyle factors and other environmental exposures modulate the risk of developing breast cancer. Physical activity appears to reduce the risk of breast cancer.[50] Consumption of 15 gm or more of alcohol per day increases the risk of breast cancer by about 50 percent relative to that of nondrinkers.[51] Fruit and vegetable consumption appears to decrease the risk of breast cancer.[52]

Hormones clearly play a role in the development of breast cancer. In men, the lifetime risk of breast cancer is low. In women who have had bilateral oophorectomy early in life, the risk of breast cancer is low. Although these observations strongly suggest a causative relationship between estrogen and breast cancer, the precise relationship between endogenous and exogenous hormones and breast cancer remains controversial.

On the basis of indirect epidemiologic evidence, endogenous estrogen production appears to be associated with breast cancer.[53, 54] Early age at menarche (before age 12 years) and late age at menopause (after age 55 years) are associated with an increased risk of breast cancer. Obesity increases risk of breast cancer, possibly by increasing the peripheral conversion of androgens to estrogens.[55] Breast feeding, a natural hypoestrogenic state, is associated with a reduced risk of breast cancer.[56]

Although indirect epidemiologic evidence suggests a relationship between estrogen and breast cancer, it has been difficult to demonstrate a relationship between circulating estrogen and breast cancer. A few case-control studies suggested that there is a relationship between increased circulating concentration of estrone and an increased risk of breast cancer.[57] Other investigators have reported that low sex hormone–binding globulin concentration, a state that would result in increased free estrogen and androgen concentrations, is associated with an increased risk of breast cancer.[58]

The relationship between exogenous hormones and breast cancer is controversial. To date, no consistent pattern of findings has emerged. This controversy is reviewed in greater detail in the following.

Oral Contraceptives and the Risk of Breast Cancer

The relationship between oral contraceptive use and breast cancer is unclear. A number of studies suggested that the use of oral contraceptives for more than 10 years is associated with a twofold increase in the risk of early breast cancer.[59] The Cancer and Steroid Hormone Study, one of the largest studies to examine this issue, found no relationship between the use of oral contraceptives and breast cancer.[60]

Hormone Replacement Therapy and the Risk of Breast Cancer

Scientific discourse often suffers by being drawn into controversial issues before the availability of objective and conclusive experimental data. At present, no information is available from controlled prospective randomized clinical trials to demonstrate a causal link between estrogen replacement therapy and the risk of developing breast cancer. The Women's Health Initiative clinical trial of estrogen replacement therapy is designed to examine the potential relationship between hormone replacement therapy and breast cancer. Data from this study will not be available until 2001. Pending the results from this study, scientists are limited to data from case-control and prospective cohort studies. Both case-control and prospective cohort studies are subject to bias because clinicians may be prescribing estrogen on the basis of clinical characteristics of the patients, which are independent determinants of breast cancer risk. For example, estrogen may be prescribed more often to women with high levels of physical activity, a clinical characteristic that is linked to a reduced risk of breast cancer.

In most epidemiologic studies, ever-use of hormone replacement therapy is not associated with an increased risk of breast cancer[61–65] (Fig. 10–3). In a few studies, hormone replacement therapy, including both current use and prolonged use (more than 10 years), is associated with a 30 percent increase in the risk of breast cancer.[63–65] One of the largest prospective studies in which this association was

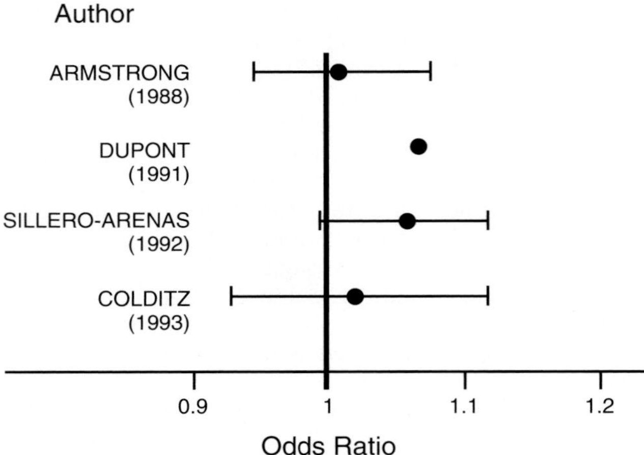

Figure 10–3 ■ Relative risk of breast cancer in ever users versus never users of hormone replacement therapy.

examined is the Nurses' Health Study.[65] A major strength of this study is that a large number of nurses, healthy at entry into the study, have been observed every 2 years for more than 15 years. Nurses are sophisticated clinicians and can accurately report the onset of new diseases. During 725,550 person-years of follow-up, the study documented 1935 new cases of breast cancer. The risk of breast cancer was significantly increased among women who were currently using estrogen alone (relative risk, 1.32; 95 percent confidence interval, 1.14 to 1.54) or estrogen plus progestin (relative risk, 1.41; 95 percent confidence interval, 1.15 to 1.74) compared with menopausal women who had never used hormones. For women who had used estrogen for 5 to 9 years, the risk of breast cancer was 1.46 (95 percent confidence interval, 1.22 to 1.74). For women who had used estrogen for 10 years or more, the relative risk of breast cancer was 1.46 (95 percent confidence interval, 1.20 to 1.76). The relative risk of death from breast cancer was 1.45 (95 percent confidence interval, 1.01 to 2.09) among women who had taken estrogen for 5 years or more. These data suggest that there is an association between the current use of estrogen replacement therapy and breast cancer but that the magnitude of the association is small.

The purpose of epidemiologic studies is to discover important associations between exposures and disease. Epidemiologic studies cannot demonstrate a cause-effect relationship between an exposure and a disease. Cause-effect relationships must be established in clinical trials or demonstrated in laboratory models. Until data are available from the Women's Health Initiative clinical trial, it is likely that the controversy surrounding the link between estrogen replacement therapy and breast cancer will remain unresolved. Clinicians and patients are challenged with the difficult task of balancing the beneficial effects of estrogen replacement on bone disease with the potential adverse effects on the breast. Quantitative analyses of the benefits and risks of hormone replacement therapy generally indicate that the benefits of therapy outweigh the risks in most populations of patients.

Alcohol Use, Hormone Replacement Therapy, and Breast Cancer Risk

Alcohol use by women appears to be associated with a decreased risk of heart disease and an increased risk of breast cancer.

Fuchs and colleagues[66] reported on the association between alcohol use and mortality from heart disease and breast cancer in the Nurses' Health Study. During 12 years of follow-up of 85,709 nurses (for a total of 1,010,209 person-years of follow-up), 2658 women died. A total of 503 women died of cardiovascular disease; 1495 died of cancer, including 350 of breast cancer. Accidents and suicides resulted in 203 deaths, and 52 deaths occurred because of cirrhosis of the liver.

Alcohol at doses of 1.5 to 29.9 gm/day reduced the risk of death. (Note: a 4-ounce glass of wine contains approximately 10.8 gm of alcohol; a standard drink of spirits contains 15.1 gm of alcohol; 12 ounces of beer contains 13.2 gm of alcohol.) At low doses (1.5 to 4.9 gm), alcohol consumption reduced risk of death from cardiovascular disease (relative risk, 0.57). At high doses (more than 30 gm daily), alcohol consumption increased the risk of death from breast cancer (relative risk, 1.67) and liver cirrhosis (relative risk, 2.55). These data suggest that alcohol consumption is an independent risk factor for breast cancer. Alcohol may increase the risk for breast cancer by increasing the bioavailability of estrogen.[67]

Recent data suggest that alcohol consumption may alter estrogen metabolism in women using estrogen replacement therapy. Ginsburg and colleagues[68] studied the effects of alcohol consumption on the half-life of estradiol in menopausal women using transdermal estradiol. In women using transdermal estradiol who consumed a carbohydrate beverage, the apparent half-life of estradiol was 245 minutes. After consumption of a large dose of ethanol (approximately 0.7 gm/kg), the apparent half-life of estradiol was 378 minutes. This suggests that alcohol decreases the clearance rate of estradiol. In a follow-up study, Ginsburg and colleagues[69] demonstrated that in women taking oral micronized estradiol, the acute consumption of alcohol resulted in an approximately 300 percent increase in circulating estradiol levels (Fig. 10–4). This suggests that alcohol may also increase the efficiency of absorption of estrogen from the gastrointestinal tract. These studies were performed with use of high doses of alcohol.

Additional studies are needed to determine whether alcohol consumed with meals or as cocktails can also produce a rise in circulating estradiol. If these studies demonstrate an effect of dietary alcohol intake on estradiol in women taking oral estradiol hormone replacement, it may be reasonable to adjust the estrogen replacement dose in a downward direction.

BREAST CANCER TREATMENT

Treatment of breast cancer has three main goals: (1) control of the primary tumor site, (2) minimization of the risk of developing metastatic disease, and (3) maintenance of the woman's quality of life. Surgical treatment, including lumpectomy or mastectomy combined with radiotherapy, is the

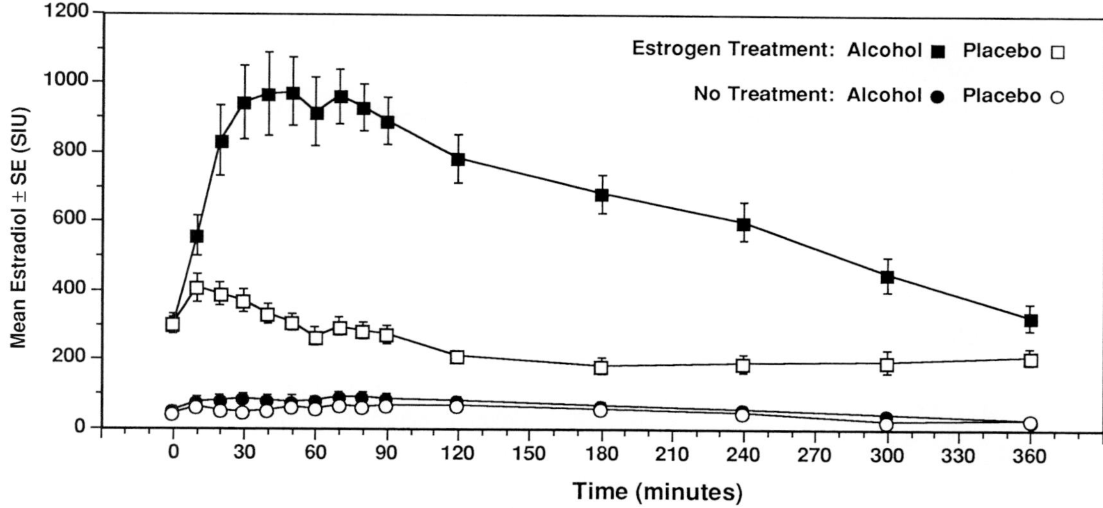

Figure 10–4 ■ Serum estradiol levels after alcohol or carbohydrate drink in postmenopausal women. Alcohol administration (0.7 gm/kg) is represented in the closed symbols. Carbohydrate drink (Polycose) administration is represented in the open symbols. After administration of alcohol or carbohydrate drink, blood samples were obtained for 6 hours. Estradiol levels for women who were receiving micronized estradiol, 1 mg daily, are shown as open and closed squares. Estradiol levels for women not receiving hormone replacement therapy are shown as open and closed circles. Mean SEM; N = 12; SIU = pmol/L. In menopausal women receiving micronized estradiol, serum estradiol significantly increased after administration of alcohol ($P < .001$). (From Ginsburg ES, Mello NK, Mendelson JH, et al. Effects of alcohol ingestion on estrogens in postmenopausal women. JAMA 276:1747–1751, 1996. Copyright 1997, American Medical Association.)

main method for controlling tumor recurrence at the site of the primary tumor. Hormonal treatment and chemotherapy are the main approaches to reduce the risk of developing metastatic tumors and to treat existing metastatic disease.

The Early Breast Cancer Trialists' Collaborative Group[70] reviewed the efficacy of various treatment regimens for breast cancer. Data were available from 133 trials that involved 75,000 women with early breast cancer, of whom 32 percent died during treatment and follow-up and 10 percent had new recurrences. The women participated in clinical trials that evaluated the efficacy of tamoxifen (30,000 women), oophorectomy (3000 women), polychemotherapy (11,000 women), single-agent chemotherapy (15,000 women), and immunotherapy (6000 women). Tamoxifen, oophorectomy in women younger than 50 years, and polychemotherapy all reduced recurrence of disease and mortality. Recurrence rates were reduced by 25 percent, 26 percent, and 25 percent by tamoxifen, oophorectomy in women younger than 50 years, and polychemotherapy, respectively. Mortality was reduced by 17 percent, 25 percent, and 16 percent by tamoxifen, oophorectomy in women younger than 50 years, and polychemotherapy. Oophorectomy after age 50 years and immunotherapy were not effective. Long courses of tamoxifen (2 to 5 years) were more effective than short courses. Short courses of polychemotherapy were as effective as long courses.

In general, adjuvant treatment is offered to women with greater than a 20 percent risk of recurrent disease. Clinical characteristics of this population of patients include positive lymph nodes, large primary tumor (greater than 2 cm), and invasion of lymphatic or vascular channels in the breast.

For women in this high-risk group who are younger than 50 years, chemotherapy with doxorubicin and cyclophosphamide every 3 weeks for four doses or therapy with cyclophosphamide, methotrexate, and fluorouracil for 6 months is often recommended. Oophorectomy may be as effective as polychemotherapy in this group of premenopausal women. For women older than 65 years, many authorities recommend tamoxifen regardless of the estrogen receptor status of the tumor. For women who are between the ages of 50 and 65 years, tamoxifen is recommended if the tumor is positive for estrogen receptors, and polychemotherapy is recommended if the tumor is negative for estrogen receptors.[71–73] For women with far-advanced disease, such as chest wall involvement, multimodal treatment including surgery, radiation, polychemotherapy, and hormone treatment may be warranted.

The Role of Tamoxifen

Tamoxifen is a triphenylethylene derivative structurally related to clomiphene (Fig. 10–5). At the standard dose of 20 mg daily, steady-state plasma concentrations are reached after approximately 4 weeks of therapy.[74, 75] One of tamoxifen's main bioactive metabolites, *N*-desmethyltamoxifen, reaches steady-state concentrations after 8 weeks of therapy.[74] Tamoxifen undergoes extensive hepatic metabolism, mainly by hydroxylation and conjugation pathways. The principal metabolite of tamoxifen, *N*-desmethyltamoxifen, has affinity for the estrogen receptor comparable to that of tamoxifen.[76]

A metabolite that is present at low concentrations, 4-hydroxytamoxifen, has affinity for the estradiol receptor similar to that of estradiol.[77, 78] Some authorities believe that 4-hydroxytamoxifen may account for a substantial portion of tamoxifen's antiestrogenic properties.

Tamoxifen, like most steroid analogues, is both an estrogen agonist and an estrogen antagonist. The observed effects of tamoxifen are dependent on endogenous estradiol concentration and the specific organ or cell type being studied. For example, in hypoestrogenic states, tamoxifen

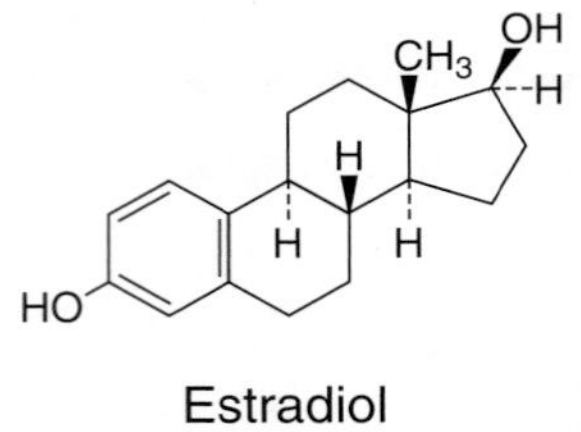

Figure 10–5 ■ Chemical structures of estradiol, clomiphene citrate, and tamoxifen citrate. Note the similarity in the structure of clomiphene, an agent used to induce ovulation, and tamoxifen, an antiestrogen used in the treatment of breast cancer.

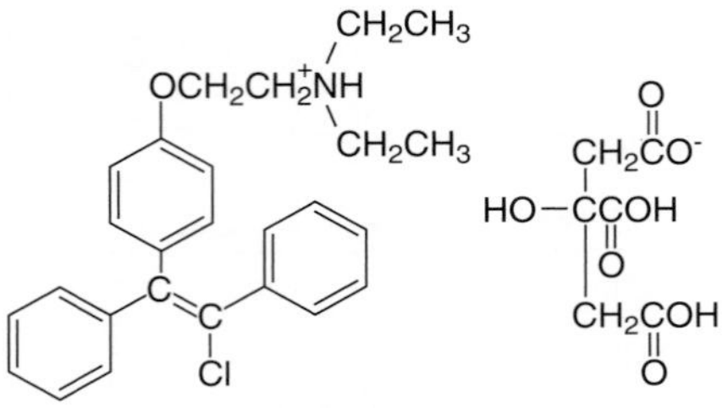

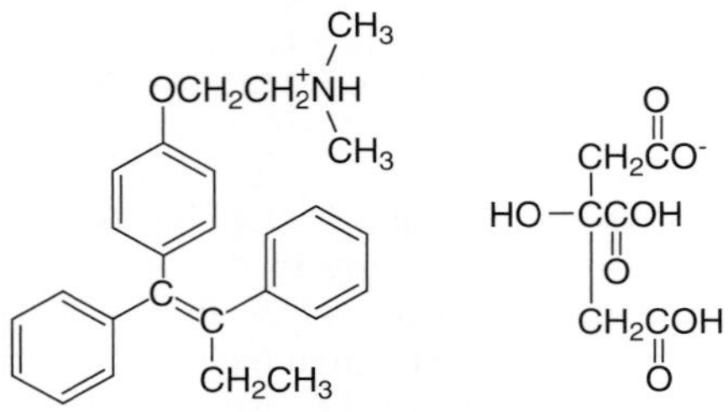

can be demonstrated to have estrogen agonist properties in the liver as demonstrated by increases in circulating high-density lipoprotein cholesterol and sex hormone–binding globulin.[79, 80] In hypoestrogenic states, tamoxifen can be demonstrated to increase progesterone receptors in the endometrium[81] and increase vaginal cornification,[82] both estrogen agonist effects. Finally, tamoxifen has been demonstrated to increase bone density in menopausal women.[83]

In contrast to these estrogen agonistic effects on the liver, bone, endometrium, and vaginal epithelium, tamoxifen has estrogen antagonist effects in breast tumor cells. Tamoxifen blocks human breast tumor growth in immunodeficient mice.[84, 85] Tamoxifen also blocks estradiol-stimulated DNA synthesis and transforming growth factor-β and EGF synthesis in breast cancer cells in vitro.[86, 87]

As noted before, tamoxifen delays the time to first relapse and significantly increases overall survival in both premenopausal and postmenopausal women with breast cancer. An important clinical issue is the optimal number of years that tamoxifen should be prescribed to women with breast cancer. The current recommendation is that tamoxifen therapy be prescribed for approximately 5 years. This recommendation is the result of more than 20 years of investigations. Initially, investigators demonstrated that 2 years of tamoxifen therapy was clearly better than placebo at extending disease-free and overall survival.[70] Comparative trials of 2 years versus 5 years demonstrated that 5 years of treatment resulted in longer disease-free and overall survival than did treatment for 2 years. In addition, second primary breast tumors were reduced by 50 percent in women treated for 5 years.[88] Studies have compared the effects of 5 years versus 10 years of tamoxifen treatment. Two studies suggested that 10 years of tamoxifen treatment is not associated with shorter disease-free intervals than is 5 years of treatment.[89] Consequently, the National Cancer Institute has recommended no more than 5 years of tamoxifen treatment.[89] Some experts have interpreted these findings to indicate that the estrogen antagonist tamoxifen may develop agonistic properties in breast tumors with long-term use.[90]

A major advantage of tamoxifen therapy is that it has no major life-threatening effects and has a beneficial effect on the quality of life. It is important to contrast this record of safety and acceptability with that of polychemotherapy. The most common side effects of tamoxifen are nausea and vomiting, which occur in up to 20 percent of women. Vaginal bleeding, irregular menses, and rash are reported by less than 10 percent of women. Tamoxifen clearly increases the risk of developing endometrial polyps and endometrial cancer. In one study of 4914 women participating in tamoxifen clinical trials, there was a sixfold increase in endometrial cancer and a threefold increase in gastrointestinal tract cancer in the women receiving tamoxifen.[91] In another study, there was an eightfold increase in the risk of developing endometrial cancer.[92] In this study, the rate of new endometrial cancer was 1.6 per 1000 woman-years in patients treated with tamoxifen versus 0.2 per 1000 woman-years in the placebo group.[92] In addition, tamoxifen therapy is associated with a 1.9-fold increase in the risk of developing colon cancer and a threefold increase in the risk of developing stomach cancer. These studies suggest that the endometrium and gastrointestinal tract may be targets for tamoxifen-induced carcinogenesis. An international consensus conference concluded that tamoxifen should be labeled a potential carcinogenic agent.

Endometrial disease reported in women receiving tamoxifen includes endometrial hyperplasia, polyps, endometrial cancer, clear cell cancer, and leiomyosarcoma.[93] These findings suggest that women receiving tamoxifen need to be carefully monitored by a gynecologist. One clinical strategy is to perform office hysteroscopy and directed endometrial biopsy on a yearly basis for women receiving tamoxifen. This strategy is expensive but provides high sensitivity and specificity in detecting endometrial abnormalities. Two less aggressive strategies are yearly sonography and hysterosonography with biopsies as indicated.

Clinicians should exercise caution when prescribing tamoxifen to premenopausal women. Tamoxifen is an antiestrogen in the central nervous and pituitary systems that control GnRH and gonadotropin secretion. In normal ovulatory premenopausal women treated with tamoxifen, elevations in gonadotropin levels result in multifollicular development, multiple follicular ovulation, and elevated concentrations of estradiol and progesterone[94–96] (Fig. 10–6). In premenopausal women, chronic tamoxifen therapy

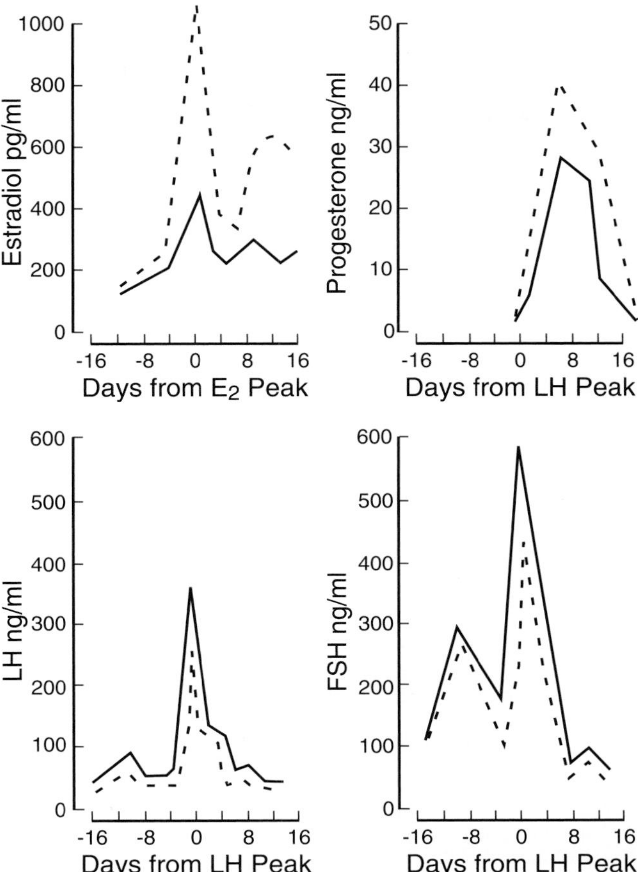

Figure 10–6 ■ The effects of tamoxifen treatment on luteinizing hormone (LH), follicle-stimulating hormone (FSH), estradiol (E_2), and progesterone levels in five normal premenopausal women during one baseline cycle (upper limit of response, *solid line*) and two tamoxifen treatment cycles (average response, *dashed lines*). Treatment of premenopausal women with tamoxifen resulted in an increase in circulating estradiol and progesterone. No significant changes in circulating LH or FSH were detected in this small study. In premenopausal women, tamoxifen treatment probably results in multifollicular development. (Adapted from Sherman BM, Chapler FK, Crickard K. Endocrine consequences of continuous antiestrogen therapy with tamoxifen in premenopausal women. J Clin Invest 64:398–404, 1979. Reproduced by copyright permission of The American Society for Clinical Investigation.)

can be associated with enlargement of the ovary due to multifollicular development and ovarian torsion.

Advances in the Development of Estrogen Agonist/Antagonists

Estrogen works by binding to intracellular estrogen receptors and regulating the transcription of specific genes. Estrogen diffuses into the nucleus of a cell and binds to the estrogen receptor. The estrogen–estrogen receptor complex then interacts with other transcription-regulatory factors and binds to the DNA. The binding of the activated estrogen-receptor complex to DNA can lead to an increase/decrease in the production of mRNA, which leads to an increase/decrease in the production of the protein product of the gene.

Recent information suggests that the estrogen receptor contains at least two important amino acid sequences that might control the agonist/antagonist properties of ligand analogues.[97–99] In the N-terminal portion of the receptor is an amino acid sequence named the AF-1 site. The AF-1 site may be able to bind to DNA and initiate estrogen agonist effects independent of estradiol binding to the receptor. Some of the estrogen agonist actions of antiestrogens may be mediated by the AF-1 site. The AF-2 site is an amino acid sequence in the C-terminal portion of the estradiol receptor that mediates ligand-dependent estrogen agonist effects. In addition, many coactivators interact with the estradiol–estrogen receptor complex. The functional state of these coactivators may mediate the estrogen agonist effects of the estradiol–estrogen receptor complex in various tissues.

Preliminary findings suggest that estrogen ligand analogues may be able to dissect out organ-specific properties of the estrogen receptor.[100–102] For example, some estrogen agonist/antagonists appear to be agonists in bone and liver and antagonists in the breast and endometrium. Other estrogen ligand analogues appear to be estrogen antagonists in all organs and tissues. New antisteroid compounds are in development that take advantage of these organ-specific effects. For example, droloxifene and idoxifene are effective in the treatment of breast cancer and appear to have much less estrogenic action on the uterus than does tamoxifen. It is hoped that droloxifene (3-hydroxytamoxifen) and idoxifene will not cause the increase in risk for uterine cancer observed with tamoxifen. Raloxifene is an estrogen receptor ligand that appears to act as an estrogen agonist in bone and liver and as an antagonist in the breast and uterus[103] (Fig. 10–7). An intriguing property of this agent is that it might be useful in the treatment of bone and lipid changes associated with the menopause without stimulating mitotic activity in breast tissue or the endometrium.

Antiprogestins also appear to be effective in the treatment of breast cancer. The antiprogestin onapristone appears to be effective in the treatment of breast cancer and appears to have increased efficacy when it is combined with an antiestrogen.[102]

Oophorectomy: An Effective Treatment of Breast Cancer

Polychemotherapy for breast cancer is associated with many adverse effects including nausea, vomiting, alopecia, myelosuppression, thrombophlebitis, and mucositis. For premenopausal women with estrogen receptor–positive breast cancer, oophorectomy has efficacy similar to polychemotherapy in the reduction of recurrences and mortality (Fig. 10–8). In one trial, 332 premenopausal women with node-positive breast cancer were randomized to receive either bilateral oophorectomy or cyclophosphamide, methotrexate, 5-fluorouracil polychemotherapy. After a maximum of 12 years of follow-up, there was no significant difference in disease-free survival or recurrences in the two groups. Actuarial survival at 8 years was 60 percent. Oophorectomy was associated with better survival than polychemotherapy in women with tumor estrogen receptor concentrations greater than 20 fmol/mg protein ("estrogen receptor–positive"). Polychemotherapy was more effective

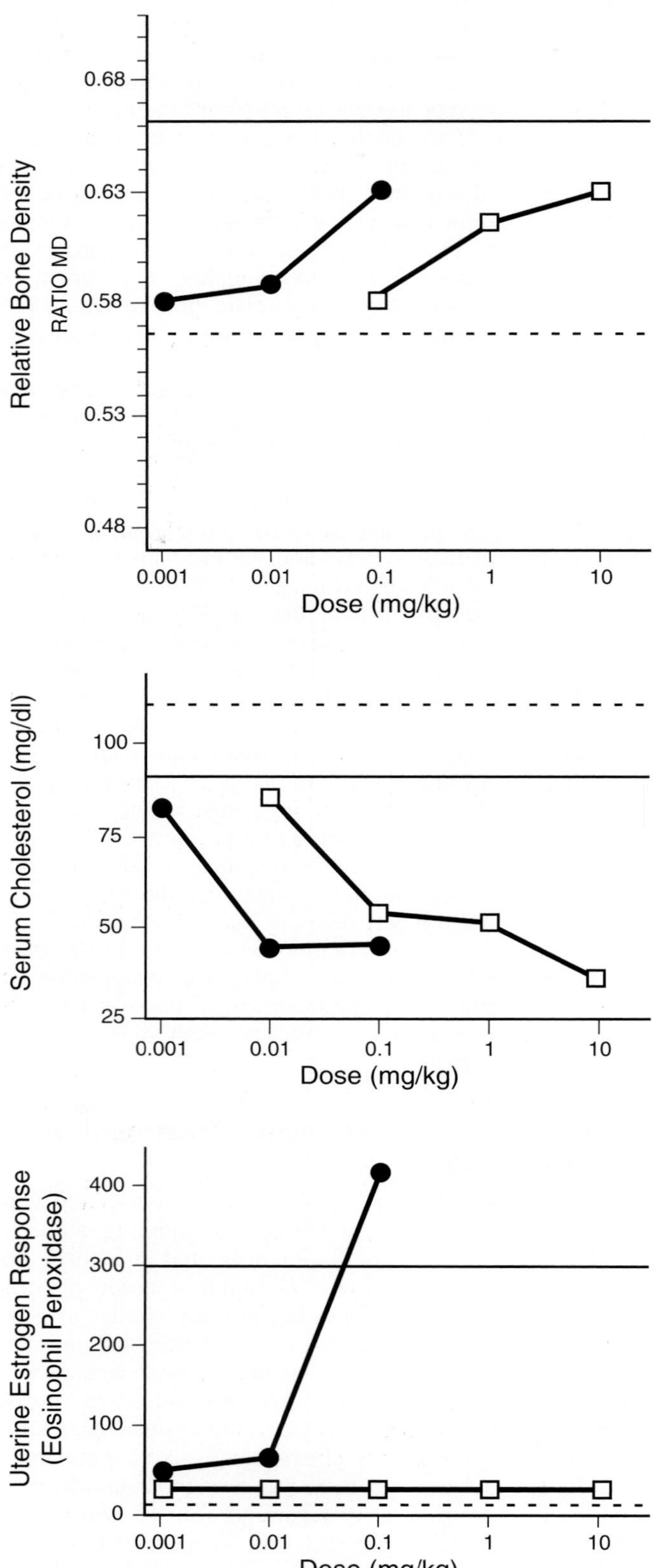

Figure 10–7 ■ The effects of sham oophorectomy *(solid line),* oophorectomy *(dashed line),* and replacement therapy after oophorectomy with ethinyl estradiol *(solid circles)* or raloxifene *(open squares)* on bone density, serum cholesterol, and uterine estrogen response (eosinophil peroxidase activity) in the rat. Ethinyl estradiol, a classic estrogen agonist, increases bone density, decreases serum cholesterol, and increases uterine eosinophil peroxidase activity. Raloxifene increases bone density and decreases cholesterol but has no significant effect on uterine eosinophil peroxidase activity. This suggests that the effects of different synthetic estrogens may be organ specific. Tamoxifen (results not shown), a mixed estrogen agonist/antagonist, increases bone density and has modest estrogen agonist effects on rat uterine eosinophil peroxidase activity (a biomarker of estrogen action in the uterus). (Adapted from Sato M, Rippy MK, Bryant HU. Raloxifene, tamoxifen, nafoxidene, or estrogen effects on reproductive and nonreproductive tissues in ovariectomized rats. FASEB J 10:905–912, 1996.)

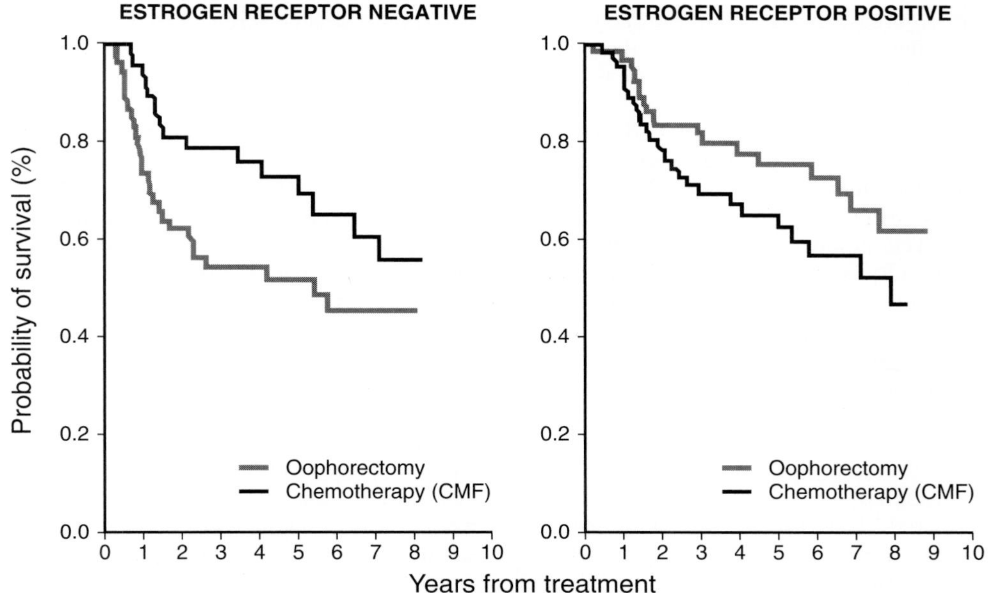

Figure 10–8 ■ The effects of oophorectomy versus polychemotherapy (cyclophosphamide, methotrexate, 5-fluorouracil [CMF]) on survival of premenopausal women with breast cancer. In premenopausal women with breast cancer, when the tumor was negative for estrogen receptors (<20 fmol/mg protein), polychemotherapy with CMF resulted in a trend to better survival than did oophorectomy. In premenopausal women with breast cancer, when the tumor was positive for estrogen receptors, oophorectomy resulted in a trend to better survival than did polychemotherapy with CMF. (Adapted from Scottish Cancer Trials Breast Group and ICRF Breast Unit. Adjuvant ovarian ablation versus CMF chemotherapy in premenopausal women with pathological stage II breast carcinoma: The Scottish trial. Lancet 341:1293–1298, 1993. © by The Lancet Ltd.)

than oophorectomy for women with tumors that were estrogen receptor–negative.[104]

This study suggested that premenopausal women with node-positive breast cancer can be given the option to choose bilateral oophorectomy if their tumor is estrogen receptor–positive. Advances in laparoscopic surgery make ambulatory bilateral oophorectomy a realistic choice in most medical centers. Laparoscopic bilateral oophorectomy is a cost-effective option compared with multiple courses of polychemotherapy. Gynecologists need to inform medical oncologists of the availability and benefits of laparoscopic oophorectomy.

Chemotherapy-Related Amenorrhea

The definition of chemotherapy-related amenorrhea varies by investigator from 3 to 12 months of amenorrhea in women undergoing chemotherapy who had menses within the 12 months preceding the initiation of chemotherapy.[105] A review of approximately 3000 premenopausal women receiving adjuvant chemotherapy for breast cancer demonstrated a 70 percent rate of chemotherapy-related amenorrhea.[105] The interval between initiation of chemotherapy and the cessation of menses was dependent on the age of the women treated. For women younger than 40 years, the onset of cessation of menses ranged from 6 to 16 months after initiation of chemotherapy. For women older than 40 years, the cessation of menses occurred 2 to 4 months after initiation of chemotherapy. In adjuvant chemotherapy for breast cancer, alkylating agents such as cyclophosphamide, L-PAM, and thiotepa are the agents most likely to cause ovarian dysfunction and depletion of the oocyte pool. The antimetabolites such as methotrexate and fluorouracil are less likely to cause ovarian dysfunction. There is a relationship between the dose of cyclophosphamide and the rate of chemotherapy-related amenorrhea. For women who received a cumulative dose of cyclophosphamide in the range of 400 mg/m^2, the rate of chemotherapy-related amenorrhea was between 10 and 30 percent, depending on the age of the woman. At cumulative cyclophosphamide doses in the range of 8000 mg/m^2, the rate of amenorrhea was 60 percent and 95 percent in younger and older age groups, respectively.[106]

Many women with chemotherapy-related amenorrhea have elevated follicle-stimulating hormone levels. Curiously, a significant number of women with breast cancer and chemotherapy-related amenorrhea will resume menses 6 to 24 months after completing chemotherapy.[107] Approximately 50 percent of women younger than 40 years will resume menses. Approximately 10 percent of women older than 40 years will resume menses. Interestingly, recurrence of breast cancer appears to be somewhat more common in women who resume menses after adjuvant chemotherapy.[107]

HORMONE REPLACEMENT THERAPY IN SURVIVORS OF BREAST CANCER

Many breast cancers are endocrine-dependent neoplasms. Some authorities believe that a goal of breast cancer treatment is to minimize the exposure of these tumors to estrogen. However, the hypoestrogenic state is associated with an increased risk of cardiovascular and bone disease as well as significant dyspareunia. Consequently, the decision to treat a survivor of breast cancer with estrogen is an exceedingly complex one. It involves weighing the risk of tumor recurrence and progression against the benefits of protection from cardiovascular and bone disease.

Three trends will increase the number of patients who ask clinicians for advice concerning estrogen replacement after breast cancer. One trend is that cancers are being diagnosed at an early stage owing to widespread cancer detection programs. The number of survivors of breast cancer will increase rapidly because of both early detection and the availability of more effective treatments. A second trend is that owing to the aging of the population, more women will be at risk for developing breast cancer. Finally, adjuvant polychemotherapy can induce premature menopause in young women with breast cancer. This effect will increase the number of young hypoestrogenic survivors of breast cancer, a group that might benefit substantially from estrogen replacement therapy.

DiSaia and coworkers[108] reported a series of 77 women with breast cancer who received estrogen replacement therapy (Table 10–2). The mean interval between primary therapy of the breast cancer and the initiation of estrogen replacement therapy was 24 months. The mean duration of therapy was 27 months. The majority of the women received standard doses of conjugated equine estrogens. During the follow-up period, seven women had recurrences of their breast cancer. Two women had discontinued estrogen before the detection of the recurrence. Five women were taking estrogen at the time the recurrence was detected. Of these five, four discontinued the estrogen. One died and three were alive, two with active disease. One woman continued the estrogen, and she was alive without detectable disease. The majority of the recurrences were in women with stage I disease.

Women who have a recurrence of breast cancer while they are receiving hormone replacement therapy should consider discontinuing the hormones. Dhodapkar and associates[109] discontinued estrogen replacement in four women with breast cancer who suffered a recurrence during estrogen replacement therapy. Discontinuation of the estrogen was associated with regression in the detectable metastatic disease in all four women.

■ TABLE 10–2

Hormone Replacement Therapy in Survivors of Breast Cancer: Effect by Stage and Node Status*

	PATIENTS TREATED	NUMBER OF RECURRENCES
Effect by Stage		
0	6	0
I	43	4
II	17	3
III	5	0
IV	0	0
Unknown	6	0
Total	77	7
Effect by Lymph Node Status		
Negative	58	5
Positive	13	2
Unknown	6	0

* Median interval between diagnosis of breast cancer and initiation of hormone replacement therapy was 2 years.

From DiSaia PJ, Odicino F, Grosen EA, et al. Hormone replacement therapy in breast cancer (Letter). Lancet 342:1232, 1993. © by the Lancet Ltd.

One innovative approach to hormone replacement in women with breast cancer is to combine tamoxifen and conjugated equine estrogen therapy. Powles and colleagues[110] described 35 women treated with this combination. Twenty-four women had relief of menopausal symptoms. Two women relapsed during the 43 months of mean follow-up time. An alternative approach is to use an agent such as raloxifene, which appears to be an estrogen agonist in the bone and liver but an estrogen antagonist in the breast and uterus.

The decision to use estrogen replacement in menopausal survivors of breast cancer ultimately rests on a quantitative analysis of the risks and benefits of such an approach. With the limited data available, Goodwin[111] reported that for women with node-negative breast cancer who have substantial menopausal symptoms, the benefits of estrogen outweigh the risks. Other experts have reached similar conclusions.

Ongoing clinical trials will help to further refine the risks and benefits of estrogen replacement therapy. In one trial, the criteria for entry include (1) stage I or stage II breast cancer and (2) a 24-month disease-free interval if the tumor was estrogen receptor–negative or a 10-year disease-free interval if the tumor was estrogen receptor–positive.[112] The decision to prescribe estrogen to survivors of breast cancer is likely to be one of the most challenging of all clinical problems for reproductive endocrinologists in the next millennium.

PREGNANCY IN SURVIVORS OF BREAST CANCER

No randomized clinical trials are available concerning the effects of pregnancy on breast cancer. A limited number of case reports have been published.[113–116] These studies suggested that pregnancy does not have an adverse effect on women who have survived breast cancer. For example, von Schoultz and associates[113] observed 50 women who became pregnant after treatment for breast cancer. Eight percent of the women who became pregnant after breast cancer treatment developed metastatic disease. In a cohort of comparable women who did not become pregnant, 24 percent developed metastatic disease. In most reports, women with breast cancer were advised to wait 2 to 3 years before becoming pregnant. This advice will avoid pregnancy in women who are destined to have recurrences shortly after primary treatment. Women with the most rapid recurrences after primary treatment are at the highest risk for death from breast cancer.

BREAST CANCER PREVENTION STRATEGIES

Breast cancer prevention is a novel concept that continues to evolve. The lack of a comprehensive physiologic model for the etiology of breast cancer makes it difficult to construct a detailed, rational approach to prevention. Clinicians should continue to emphasize screening and early detection as the primary method of reducing the impact of the disease. Current approaches to breast cancer prevention include pharmacologic interventions and lifestyle changes, such as (1) retinoids, (2) antiestrogens including tamoxifen, (3) GnRH agonist oophorectomy, (4) dietary changes, (5) prolonged lactation, and (6) avoidance of alcohol.

Many laboratory studies indicate that retinoids are antiproliferative and antiestrogenic in breast tissue.[117, 118] Recent laboratory findings suggest that the retinoic acid receptors RAR and RXR can compete with the estrogen receptor for two transcription-regulatory elements, estrogen receptor–associated proteins ERAP140 and ERAP160.[119] High retinoid levels in the breast may inhibit the ability of the estrogen–estrogen receptor complex to interact with genomic DNA and stimulate cell division. Investigators are currently evaluating the efficacy of a retinoid, 4-hydroxyphenyl retinamide,[120] to prevent the development of new primary breast cancer lesions in women previously treated for breast cancer. The major forms of toxicity associated with retinoids are hepatic and cutaneous toxicity and teratogenicity. If retinoids are demonstrated to reduce the risk of breast cancer, it is likely that the risk reduction will be modest.

Tamoxifen is currently being evaluated in large primary prevention trials in at least three countries.[121] As an estrogen agonist/antagonist, tamoxifen is clearly effective in reducing the rate of recurrence in women with breast cancer. Numerous studies suggest that in women with breast cancer, tamoxifen reduces the incidence of new primary malignant neoplasms in the contralateral breast.[122] It is likely that tamoxifen will prove effective in the prevention of breast cancer. As noted before, tamoxifen is associated with significant side effects, including endometrial cancer. New synthetic antiestrogens, such as raloxifene, with less agonistic activity in the uterus may reduce this risk.

Pharmacologic suppression of ovarian estrogen production is an alternative prevention strategy to antiestrogen treatment.[123] Ablation of ovarian estrogen production can be accomplished surgically with oophorectomy or by prolonged use of a GnRH agonist analogue, such as leuprolide acetate. An alternative approach to the inhibition of estrogen secretion is to use inhibitors of the estrogen synthase enzyme aromatase.[124] Suppression of ovarian estrogen production is associated with numerous adverse effects, such as vasomotor flushes, bone loss, and atrophy of the vagina.

The pharmacologic approaches reviewed have the disadvantages of unwanted side effects and the cost of the medication. Three lifestyle interventions that are low cost and have minimal side effects include dietary manipulations, encouraging lactation, and reducing alcohol intake.

In a large Canadian trial, the efficacy of a low-fat diet in the prevention of breast cancer is being evaluated. Controversy persists as to the potential role of dietary fat in the etiology of breast cancer. Worldwide comparison of fat intake and breast cancer prevalence indicates a high positive correlation ($r = 0.8$).[125] However, epidemiologic studies that directly assess diet composition do not consistently demonstrate a relationship between fat intake and breast cancer risk.[126] A competing hypothesis is that total calorie intake is a better predictor of breast cancer risk than is fat intake alone. This hypothesis suggests that it is not the fat content of the diet but total calorie consumption that is the link between diet and breast cancer. Studies in monkeys support the concept that high levels of calorie intake, regardless of the composition of the calories, may be a risk factor for cancer. Soy products may have estrogen antagonist properties that reduce the risk of breast cancer.[127]

Numerous epidemiologic studies indicate that prolonged lactation is associated with a low risk of developing breast cancer.[128] Encouraging women to lactate and providing more support for breast feeding are interventions with low cost and risk that deserve additional study. Many epidemiologic studies suggest that chronic alcohol intake, especially above 30 gm daily, increases the risk of breast cancer. Reducing alcohol consumption may reduce the risk of breast cancer and cirrhosis, but it may increase the risk of atherosclerotic heart disease.[66]

For women, one of the most feared diseases is breast cancer. A popular perception is that women would rather die 10 times from heart disease than once from breast cancer. Genetic predisposition and endocrine exposures are dominant factors in the etiology of breast cancer. Both the geneticist and the reproductive endocrinologist will play major roles in developing strategies to cure this devastating disease.

References

1. Mauvais-Jarvis P, Kutten F, Gompel A. Estradiol-progesterone interaction in normal and pathologic breast cells. Ann N Y Acad Sci 464:152–167, 1986.
2. Andler W, Zachmann M. Spontaneous breast development in an adolescent girl with testicular feminization after castration in early childhood. J Pediatr 94:304–305, 1979.
3. Naftolin F, Pujol-Amat P, Corker CS, et al. Gonadotropins and gonadal steroids in androgen insensitivity syndrome: Effects of castration and sex steroid administration. Am J Obstet Gynecol 147:491–496, 1983.
4. Rosen JM, Humphreys R, Krnacik S, et al. The regulation of mammary gland development by hormones, growth factors and oncogenes. Prog Clin Biol Res 387:95–111, 1994.
5. Dixon JM, Mansel RE. Congenital problems and aberrations of normal breast development and involution. Br Med J 309:797–780, 1994.
6. Cotran RS, Kumar V, Robbins SL. Pathologic Basis of Disease, 5th ed. Philadelphia, WB Saunders, 1994, pp 1089–1111.
7. Rigg LA, Yen SSC. The pattern of increase in circulating prolactin levels during human gestation. Am J Obstet Gynecol 129:454–458, 1977.
8. Neville MC, Casey C, Hay WW Jr. Endocrine regulation of nutrient flux in the lactating woman. Do the mechanisms differ from pregnancy? Adv Exp Med Biol 352:85–98, 1994.
9. Brun del Re R, Del Pozo E, De Grandi P, et al. Prolactin inhibition and suppression of puerperal lactation by CB 154. A comparison with estrogen. Obstet Gynecol 41:884–890, 1973.
10. McNeilly AS, Robinson CAF, Houston MJ, Howie PW. Release of oxytocin and prolactin in response to suckling. Br Med J 286:257–259, 1983.
11. Cosman D. A new cytokine receptor superfamily. Trends Biochem Sci 15:265–269, 1990.
12. Schmitt-Ney M, Doppler W, Ball RK, Groner B. β-Casein gene promoter activity is regulated by the hormone mediated relief of transcriptional repression and a mammary-gland–specific nuclear factor. Mol Cell Biol 11:3745–3755, 1991.
13. Schmitt-Ney M, Happ B, Hofer P. Mammary gland–specific nuclear factor activity is positively regulated by lactogenic hormones and negatively by milk stasis. Mol Endocrinol 6:1988–1997, 1992.
14. Tourkine N, Schindler C, Larose M, Houdebine LM. Activation of STAT factors by prolactin, interferon-gamma, growth hormones and a tyrosine phosphatase inhibitor in rabbit primary mammary epithelial cells. J Biol Chem 270:20925–20961, 1995.

15. Shi Y, Seto E, Chang LS, Shenk T. Transcriptional repression by YY1, a human GLI-Kruppel–related protein and relief of repression by adenovirus E1A protein. Cell 67:377–388, 1991.
16. Meier VS, Groner B. The nuclear factor YY-1 participates in repression of the β-casein gene promoter in mammary epithelial cells and is counteracted by mammary gland factor during lactogenic hormone induction. Mol Cell Biol 14:128–137, 1994.
17. Welte T, Philipp S, Cairns C, et al. Glucocorticoid receptor binding sites in the promoter region of milk protein genes. J Steroid Biochem Mol Biol 47:75–81, 1993.
18. Hynes NE, Taverna D, Harweth IM. Epidermal growth factor receptor, but not c-*erbB-2* activation, prevents lactogenic hormone induction of the β casein gene in mouse mammary epithelial cells. Mol Cell Biol 10:4027–4034, 1990.
19. Nishikawa S, Moore RC, Nonomura N, Oka T. Progesterone and EGF inhibit mouse mammary gland prolactin receptor and β-casein gene expression. Am J Physiol 267:C1467–C1472, 1994.
20. Yen SSC, Jaffe RB. Prolactin in human reproduction. *In* Yen SSC, Jaffe RB, Barbieri RL (eds). Reproductive Endocrinology, 4th ed. Philadelphia, WB Saunders, 1998.
21. Campbell OMR, Gray RH. Characteristics and determinants of postpartum ovarian function in women in the United States. Am J Obstet Gynecol 169:55–60, 1993.
22. Campino C, Ampuero S, Diaz S, Seron-Ferre M. Prolactin bioactivity and the duration of lactational amenorrhea. J Clin Endocrinol Metab 79:970–974, 1994.
23. Barragan JC, Brotons J, Ruiz JA, Acien P. Experimentally induced endometriosis in rats: Effect on fertility and the effects of pregnancy and lactation on the ectopic endometrial tissue. Fertil Steril 58:1215–1219, 1992.
24. London SJ, Colditz GA, Stampfer MJ, et al. Lactation and risk of breast cancer in a cohort of US women. Am J Epidemiol 132:17–26, 1990.
25. Kochenour NK. Lactation suppression. Clin Obstet Gynecol 23:1045–1059, 1980.
26. Taneykoon M, Dusitsin N, Chalapati S, et al. Effects of hormonal contraceptives on milk volume and infant growth. Contraception 30:505–522, 1984.
27. Lonnerdal B, Forsum E, Hambraeus L. Effect of oral contraceptives on composition and volume of breast milk. Am J Clin Nutr 33:816–824, 1980.
28. Nilsson S, Mellbin T, Hofvander Y, et al. Long term follow up of children breast fed by mothers using oral contraceptives. Contraception 34:443–457, 1986.
29. Morgans D. Bromocriptine and postpartum lactation suppression. Br J Obstet Gynecol 102:851–853, 1995.
30. Comabella M, Alvarez-Sabin J, Rovira A, Codina A. Bromocriptine and postpartum cerebral angiopathy: A causal relationship? Neurology 46:1754–1756, 1996.
31. Auerbach KG, Avery JL. Induced lactation. Am J Dis Child 135:340–342, 1981.
32. Ziegler JB, Cooper DA, Johnson RO, Gold J. Postnatal transmission of AIDS-associated retrovirus from mother to infant. Lancet 1:896–898, 1985.
33. Centers for Disease Control. Recommendations for assisting in the prevention of perinatal transmission of human T-lymphotropic virus type III/lymphadenopathy-associated virus and acquired immunodeficiency syndrome. MMWR Morb Mortal Wkly Rep 34:721–732, 1985.
34. World Health Organization Global Program on AIDS. Consensus statements from the WHO/UNICEF consultation on HIV transmission and breast feeding. Wkly Epidemiol Rec 67:177, 1992.
35. Vorherr H. Fibrocystic breast disease: Pathophysiology, pathomorphology, clinical picture and management. Am J Obstet Gynecol 154:161–179, 1986.
36. Pisani P, Parkin DM, Ferlay J. Estimates of the worldwide mortality from eighteen major cancers in 1985: Implications for prevention and projections of future burden. Int J Cancer 55:891–903, 1993.
37. Slattery ML, Kerber RA. A comprehensive evaluation of family history and breast cancer risk, the Utah population database. JAMA 270:1563–1568, 1993.
38. Weber BL, Garber JE. Family history and breast cancer, probabilities and possibilities. JAMA 270:1602–1603, 1993.
39. Shattuck-Eidens D, McClure MC, Simard J, et al. A collaborative survey of 80 mutations in the *BRCA1* breast and ovarian cancer susceptibility gene. JAMA 273:535–541, 1995.
40. Miki Y, Swensen J, Shattuck-Eidens D, et al. Isolation of *BRCA1,* the 17q-linked breast and ovarian cancer susceptibility gene. Science 266:66–71, 1994.
41. Ford D, Easton DF. The genetics of breast and ovarian cancer. Br J Cancer 72:805–812, 1995.
42. Easton DF, Ford D, Bishop DT. Breast and ovarian cancer incidence in *BRCA1* mutation carriers. Am J Hum Genet 56:265–271, 1995.
43. Muto MG, Cramer DW, Tangir J, et al. Frequency of the *BRCA1* 185 del AG mutation among Jewish women with ovarian cancer and matched population controls. Cancer Res 56:1250–1252, 1996.
44. Wooster R, Neuhausen S, Manigion J, et al. Localization of a breast cancer susceptibility gene *(BRCA2)* to chromosome 13q by genetic linkage analysis. Science 265:2088–2090, 1994.
45. Bishop DT, Cannon-Albright L, McLellan T, et al. Segregation and linkage analysis of 9 Utah breast cancer pedigrees. Genet Epidemiol 5:151–169, 1988.
46. Zakian VA. ATM related genes: What do they tell us about functions of the human gene? Cell 82:685–687, 1995.
47. Easton DF. Cancer risks in A-T heterozygotes. Int J Radiat Biol 66:s177–s182, 1994.
48. Li FP, Fraumeni JF, Mulvihill JJ, et al. A cancer family syndrome in twenty-four kindreds. Cancer Res 48:5358–5362, 1988.
49. Malkin D, Li FP, Strong LC, et al. Germline p53 mutations in a familial syndrome of breast cancer, sarcomas and other neoplasms. Science 250:1233–1238, 1990.
50. Freidenreich CM, Rohan TE. A review of physical activity and breast cancer. Epidemiology 6:311–317, 1995.
51. Longnecker MP. Alcoholic beverage consumption in relation to the risk of breast cancer: Meta-analysis and review. Cancer Causes Control 5:73–82, 1994.
52. Tichopoulou A, Katsouyanni K, Stuver S. Consumption of olive oil and specific food groups in relation to breast cancer risk in Greece. J Natl Cancer Inst 87:110–116, 1995.
53. Kelsey JL, Gammon MD, John EM. Reproductive factors and breast cancer. Epidemiol Rev 15:36–47, 1993.
54. Rosner B, Colditz G, Willet W. Reproductive risk factors in a prospective study of breast cancer: The Nurses' Health Study. Am J Epidemiol 139:819–835, 1994.
55. Sellers T, Kushi L, Potter DJ. Effect of family history, body fat distribution and reproductive factors on the risk of postmenopausal breast cancer. N Engl J Med 326:1323–1329, 1992.
56. Yoo KY, Tajima K, Kuroishi T. Independent protective effect of lactation against breast cancer: A case control study in Japan. Am J Epidemiol 135:726–733, 1992.
57. Cauley JA, Gutal JP, Kuller LH, et al. The epidemiology of serum sex hormones in postmenopausal women. Am J Epidemiol 132:1120–1131, 1989.
58. Toniolo PG, Levitz M, Zeleniuch-Jacquotte A, et al. A prospective study of endogenous estrogens and breast cancer in postmenopausal women. J Natl Cancer Inst 87:190–197, 1995.
59. Romieu I, Berlin JA, Colditz G. Oral contraceptives and breast cancer: Review and meta-analysis. Cancer 66:2253–2263, 1990.
60. Cancer and Steroid Hormone Study of the Centers for Disease Control and the National Institute of Child Health and Human Development. Oral contraceptive use and the risk of breast cancer. N Engl J Med 315:405–411, 1986.
61. Armstrong BK. Oestrogen therapy after the menopause—boon or bane? Med J Aust 148:213–214, 1988.
62. Dupont WD, Page DL. Menopausal estrogen replacement therapy and breast cancer. Arch Intern Med 151:67–72, 1991.
63. Steinberg KK, Thacker SB, Smith SJ. A meta-analysis of the effect of estrogen replacement therapy on the risk of breast cancer. JAMA 265:1985–1990, 1991.
64. Sillero-Arenas M, Delgado-Rodriguez M, Rodriguez-Canteras R. Menopausal hormone replacement therapy and breast cancer: A meta-analysis. Obstet Gynecol 79:286–294, 1992.
65. Colditz GA, Egan KM, Stampfer MJ. Hormone replacement therapy and the risk of breast cancer. Results from epidemiologic studies. Am J Obstet Gynecol 168:1473–1480, 1993.
66. Fuchs CS, Stampfer MJ, Colditz GA, et al. Alcohol consumption and mortality among women. N Engl J Med 332:1245–1250, 1995.

67. Reichman ME, Judd JT, Longcope C. Effects of alcohol consumption on plasma and urinary hormone concentration in premenopausal women. J Natl Cancer Inst 85:722–727, 1993.
68. Ginsburg ES, Walsh BW, Shea BF, et al. The effects of ethanol on the clearance of estradiol in postmenopausal women. Fertil Steril 63:1227–1230, 1995.
69. Ginsburg ES, Mello NK, Mendelson JH, et al. Effects of alcohol ingestion on estrogens in postmenopausal women. JAMA 276:1747–1751, 1996.
70. Early Breast Cancer Trialists' Collaborative Group. Systemic treatment of early breast cancer by hormonal, cytotoxic or immunotherapy: 133 randomized trials involving 31,000 recurrences and 24,000 deaths among 75,000 women. Lancet 339:1–15, 71–85, 1992.
71. Olivotto IA, Bajdik CD, Plenderleith IH. Adjuvant systemic therapy and survival after breast cancer. N Engl J Med 330:805–810, 1994.
72. Neville AM, Bettelheim R, Gelber RD. Factors predicting treatment responsiveness and prognosis in node-negative breast cancer. J Clin Oncol 10:696–705, 1992.
73. Bonadonna G, Valagussa P, Rossi A. Ten-year experience with CMF-based adjuvant chemotherapy in resectable breast cancer. Breast Cancer Res Treat 5:95–115, 1985.
74. Adams HK, Patterson JS, Kemp JV. Studies on the metabolism and pharmacokinetics of tamoxifen in normal volunteers. Cancer Treat Rep 64:761–764, 1980.
75. Jordan VC, Fritz NF, Tormey DC. Endocrine effects of adjuvant chemotherapy and long-term tamoxifen administration on node-positive patients with breast cancer. Cancer Res 47:624–630, 1987.
76. Kemp JV, Adam HK, Wakeling AE. Identification and biological activity of tamoxifen metabolites in human serum. Biochem Pharmacol 32:2045–2052, 1983.
77. Fabian C, Tilzer L, Sternson L. Comparative binding affinities of tamoxifen, 4-hydroxytamoxifen and desmethyltamoxifen for estrogen receptors isolated from human breast carcinoma: Correlation with blood levels in patients with metastatic breast cancer. Biopharm Drug Dispos 2:381–390, 1981.
78. Wakeling AE, Slater SR. Estrogen-receptor binding and biological activity of tamoxifen and its metabolites. Cancer Treat Rep 64:741–744, 1980.
79. Saki F, Cheix F, Clavel M. Increases in steroid binding globulins induced by tamoxifen in patients with carcinoma of the breast. J Endocrinol 76:219–226, 1978.
80. Love RR, Wiebe DP, Newcombe PA. Effects of tamoxifen on cardiovascular risk factors in postmenopausal women. Ann Intern Med 115:860–864, 1991.
81. Luciani L, Oriana S, Spatti G. Hormonal and receptor status in postmenopausal women with endometrial carcinoma before and after treatment with tamoxifen. Tumori 70:189–192, 1984.
82. Boccardo F, Bruzzi P, Rubagotti A. Estrogen-like action of tamoxifen on vaginal epithelium in breast cancer patients. Oncology 38:281–285, 1981.
83. Love RR, Mazess RB, Barden HS. Effects of tamoxifen on bone mineral density in postmenopausal women with breast cancer. N Engl J Med 326:852–856, 1992.
84. Gottardis MM, Jiang SY, Jeng MH, Jordan VC. Inhibition of tamoxifen stimulated growth of an MCF-7 tumor variant in athymic mice by novel steroid antiestrogens. Cancer Res 49:4090–4093, 1989.
85. Gottardis MM, Robinson SP, Satyaswaroop PG, Jordan VC. Contrasting actions of tamoxifen on endometrial and breast tumor growth in the athymic mouse. Cancer Res 48:812–814, 1988.
86. Coezy E, Borgna JL, Rochefort H. Tamoxifen and metabolites in MCF-7 cells. Correlation between binding to estrogen receptor and inhibition of cell growth. Cancer Res 42:317–323, 1982.
87. Imai Y, Leung CKH, Friesen HG. Epidermal growth factor receptors and effect of epidermal growth factor on growth of human breast cancer cells in long term tissue culture. Cancer Res 42:4394–4398, 1982.
88. Fisher B, Redmond C. New perspective on cancer of the contralateral breast: A marker for assessing tamoxifen as a preventive agent. J Natl Cancer Inst 83:1278–1280, 1991.
89. National Cancer Institute. Adjuvant therapy of breast cancer—tamoxifen update. US Department of Health and Human Services, National Institutes of Health, Public Health Service. Bethesda, MD, National Cancer Institute clinical announcement, November 30, 1995.
90. Santen RJ. Long term tamoxifen therapy: Can an antagonist become an agonist? (Editorial). J Clin Endocrinol Metab 81:2027–2029, 1996.
91. Rutqvist LE, Johansson H, Signomklao T, et al. Adjuvant tamoxifen therapy for early stage breast cancer and second primary malignancies. J Natl Cancer Inst 87:645–651, 1995.
92. Fisher JB, Costantino JP, Redmond CK. Endometrial cancer in tamoxifen treated breast cancer patients: Findings from the National Surgical Adjuvant Breast and Bowel Project. J Natl Cancer Inst 86:527–537, 1994.
93. Daniel Y, Inbar M, Bar-Am A, et al. The effects of tamoxifen treatment on the endometrium. Fertil Steril 65:1083–1089, 1996.
94. Jordan VC, Fritz NF, Langan-Fahey S. Alteration of endocrine parameters in premenopausal women with breast cancer with long term adjuvant therapy with tamoxifen as the single agent. J Natl Cancer Inst 83:1488–1491, 1991.
95. Groom GV, Griffiths K. Effects of the anti-estrogen tamoxifen on plasma levels of luteinizing hormone, follicle stimulating hormone, prolactin, estradiol and progesterone in normal pre-menopausal women. J Endocrinol 70:421–428, 1976.
96. Sherman BM, Chapler FK, Crickard K. Endocrine consequences of continuous antiestrogen therapy with tamoxifen in premenopausal women. J Clin Invest 64:398–404, 1979.
97. Mangelsdorf DJ, Thummel C, Beato M. The nuclear receptor superfamily: The second decade. Cell 83:835–839, 1995.
98. Mahfoudi A, Roulet E, Dauvois S, et al. Specific mutations in the estrogen receptor change the properties of antiestrogens to full agonists. Proc Natl Acad Sci USA 92:4206–4210, 1995.
99. Webb P, Lopez GN, Uht RMJ, Kushners PJ. Tamoxifen activation of the estrogen receptor/AP-1 pathway; potential origin for the cell-specific estrogen like effects of antiestrogen. Mol Endocrinol 9:443–456, 1995.
100. Geisler J, Haarstad H, Gundersen S, et al. Influence of treatment with the anti-estrogen 3-hydroxytamoxifen (droloxifene) on plasma sex hormone levels in postmenopausal patients with breast cancer. J Endocrinol 146:359–363, 1995.
101. Coombes RC, Haynes BP, Dowsett M, et al. Idoxifene: A report of a phase I study in patients with metastatic breast cancer. Cancer Res 55:1070–1074, 1995.
102. Black LJ, Sato M, Rowley ER, et al. Raloxifene prevents bone loss and reduces serum cholesterol without causing uterine hypertrophy in ovariectomized rats. J Clin Invest 93:63–69, 1994.
103. Sato M, Rippy MK, Bryant HU. Raloxifene, tamoxifen, nafoxidene or estrogen effects on reproductive and nonreproductive tissues in ovariectomized rats. FASEB J 10:905–912, 1996.
104. Scottish Cancer Trials Breast Group and ICRF Breast Unit. Adjuvant ovarian ablation versus CMF chemotherapy in premenopausal women with pathological stage II breast carcinoma: The Scottish trial. Lancet 341:1293–1298, 1993.
105. Bines J, Oleske DM, Cobleigh MA. Ovarian function in premenopausal women treated with adjuvant chemotherapy for breast cancer. J Clin Oncol 14:1718–1729, 1996.
106. Goldhirsch A, Gelber RD, Castiglione M. The magnitude of endocrine effects of adjuvant chemotherapy for premenopausal breast cancer patients. Ann Oncol 1:183–188, 1990.
107. Bianco AR, Del Mastro L, Gallo C. Prognostic role of amenorrhea induced by adjuvant chemotherapy in premenopausal patients with early breast cancer. Br J Cancer 63:799–803, 1991.
108. DiSaia PJ, Odicino F, Grosen EA, et al. Hormone replacement therapy in breast cancer (Letter). Lancet 342:1232, 1993.
109. Dhodapkar MV, Ingle JN, Ahman DL. Estrogen replacement therapy withdrawal and regression of metastatic breast cancer. Cancer 75:43–46, 1995.
110. Powles TJ, Hickish T, Casey S. Hormone replacement after breast cancer. Lancet 342:60–61, 1993.
111. Goodwin PJ. Decision analysis of estrogen replacement therapy in women made prematurely menopausal during adjuvant chemotherapy for breast cancer. Breast Cancer Res Treat 14:147–152, 1989.
112. Vassilopoulou-Sellin R, Theriault R. Randomized prospective trial of estrogen replacement therapy in women with a history of breast cancer. Monogr Natl Cancer Inst 16:153–159, 1994.
113. Von Schoultz E, Johannsson H, Wilking N, Rutqvist LE. Influence

of prior and subsequent pregnancy on breast cancer prognosis. J Clin Oncol 13:430–434, 1995.
114. Sutton R, Buzdar AU, Hortobagyi GN. Pregnancy and offspring after adjuvant chemotherapy in breast cancer patients. Cancer 65:847–850, 1990.
115. Ariel IM, Kempner R. The prognosis of patients who become pregnant after mastectomy for breast cancer. Int Surg 74:185–187, 1989.
116. Harvey JC, Rosen PP, Ashikari R, et al. The effect of pregnancy on the prognosis of carcinoma of the breast following mastectomy. Surg Gynecol Obstet 153:723–725, 1981.
117. Anzano MA, Byers SW, Smith JM. The prevention of breast cancer in the rat with 9-cis retinoic acid as a single agent and in combination with tamoxifen. Cancer Res 54:4610–4614, 1994.
118. DePalo G, Veronesi U, Camerini T. Can fenretinide protect women against ovarian cancer? J Natl Cancer Inst 87:146–147, 1995.
119. Halachmi S, Marden E, Martin G, et al. Estrogen receptor associated proteins: Possible mediators of hormone induced transcription. Science 264:1455–1458, 1994.
120. Abou-Issa H, Curley RW, Panigot MJ, et al. In vivo use of N-(4-hydroxyphenyl retinamide)-*O*-glucuronide as a breast cancer chemopreventive agent. Anticancer Res 13:1431–1436, 1993.
121. Nease RF Jr, Ross JM. The decision to enter a randomized trial of tamoxifen for the prevention of breast cancer in healthy women: An analysis of the tradeoffs. Am J Med 99:180–189, 1995.
122. Fisher B, Costantino J, Redmond C. A randomized clinical trial evaluating tamoxifen in the treatment of patients with node-negative breast cancer who have estrogen receptor positive tumors. N Engl J Med 320:479–484, 1989.
123. Pike MC, Spicer DV. The chemoprevention of breast cancer by reducing sex steroid exposure. J Cell Biochem Suppl 17G:26–36, 1993.
124. Brodie AM, Dowsett M, Coombes RC. Aromatase inhibitors as new endocrine therapy for breast cancer. Cancer Treat Res 39:51–65, 1988.
125. Prentice RL, Sheppard L. Dietary fat and cancer: Consistency of the epidemiologic data and disease prevention that may follow from a practical reduction in fat consumption. Cancer Causes Control 1:81–97, 1990.
126. Giovannucci E, Stampfer MJ, Colditz GA. A comparison of prospective and retrospective assessment of diet in the study of breast cancer. Am J Epidemiol 137:502–511, 1993.
127. Messina MJ, Pensky V, Setchell KD. Soy intake and cancer risk: A review of the in vitro and in vivo data. Nutr Cancer 21:113–131, 1994.
128. Mittendorf F, Greenberg ER, Clapp RW, et al. Lactation and reduced risk of premenopausal breast cancer. N Engl J Med 330:81–87, 1994.

Chapter 11

MENOPAUSE AND AGING

Robert B. Jaffe

■ CHAPTER OUTLINE

KEY POINTS

- There is an interval between reproductive age and the menopause, the "menopausal transition," characterized by menstrual irregularities, hormonal changes, and waning of fertility.
- By the year 2020, it is anticipated that there will be almost 46 million postmenopausal women in the United States alone.
- After the menopause, there is a marked increase in gonadotropins and a marked decrease in ovarian inhibin and sex steroids.
- There are profound effects on the cardiovascular, musculoskeletal, and central nervous systems, many of which are a result of the cessation of ovarian production of 17β-estradiol.
- Increased risks of coronary artery disease (the leading cause of death in women) and osteoporosis accompany the decrease in 17β-estradiol.
- Hormone replacement therapy for postmenopausal women obviates some of the consequences of cessation of ovarian 17β-estradiol secretion. However, there are also potential risks of prolonged hormone replacement therapy.
- The menopausal transition and menopause are integral components of the aging process, which affects most if not all organ and metabolic systems.

With many women in the developed countries now living out at least one third of their lives after the menopause (average age of menopause in the United States is 51 years), it is small wonder that so much media attention has been focused on health aspects of this crucial period. Topics such as osteoporosis, cardiovascular disease, and the benefits and risks of hormone replacement therapy have received markedly increased attention in both the lay and medical literature in the last few years.

THE MENOPAUSE AND PERIMENOPAUSAL PERIOD

The Menopausal Transition

Whereas the menopause, the final cessation of menses, represents a single event, there is a series of clinical changes beginning approximately 4 years before the menopause on the basis of menstrual irregularities,[1] approximately 8 years before the menopause when hormonal changes are considered, and about 10 years biologically when waning of fertility is considered, which constitute the menopausal transition. This transition is marked by increased variability in menstrual cycle length; a gradual rise in pituitary gonadotropins; a decline in the glycoprotein inhibin and mean ovarian secretion of sex steroids but with erratic, striking increases in estradiol shortly before the onset of the menopause (Fig. 11–1); and decreased fertility.

After about age 40 years, the number of regular ovulatory cycles begins to decline. Initially, there is little change in median cycle length as both long and short cycles increase in frequency. However, as ovarian function declines further, there is usually a reduction in cycle length because of a reduction in the length of the follicular phase.[2]

As the menopausal transition is initiated, there is an increase in circulating levels of follicle-stimulating hormone (FSH) and a decrease in estradiol, inhibin, and progesterone.[3, 4] Mean luteinizing hormone (LH) concentrations are similar to those in younger women.[5] These changes in circulating hormone levels frequently occur in the presence of ovulatory menstrual cycles. Thus, the ovary gradually becomes less responsive to gonadotropins several years before menses cease.

Factors responsible for the increase in FSH levels before the menopause without a concomitant increase in LH remain to be completely elucidated. Ovarian inhibin is secreted in decreasing amounts with advancing age. This heterodimeric glycoprotein preferentially inhibits the production of FSH. First described in the male, inhibin has

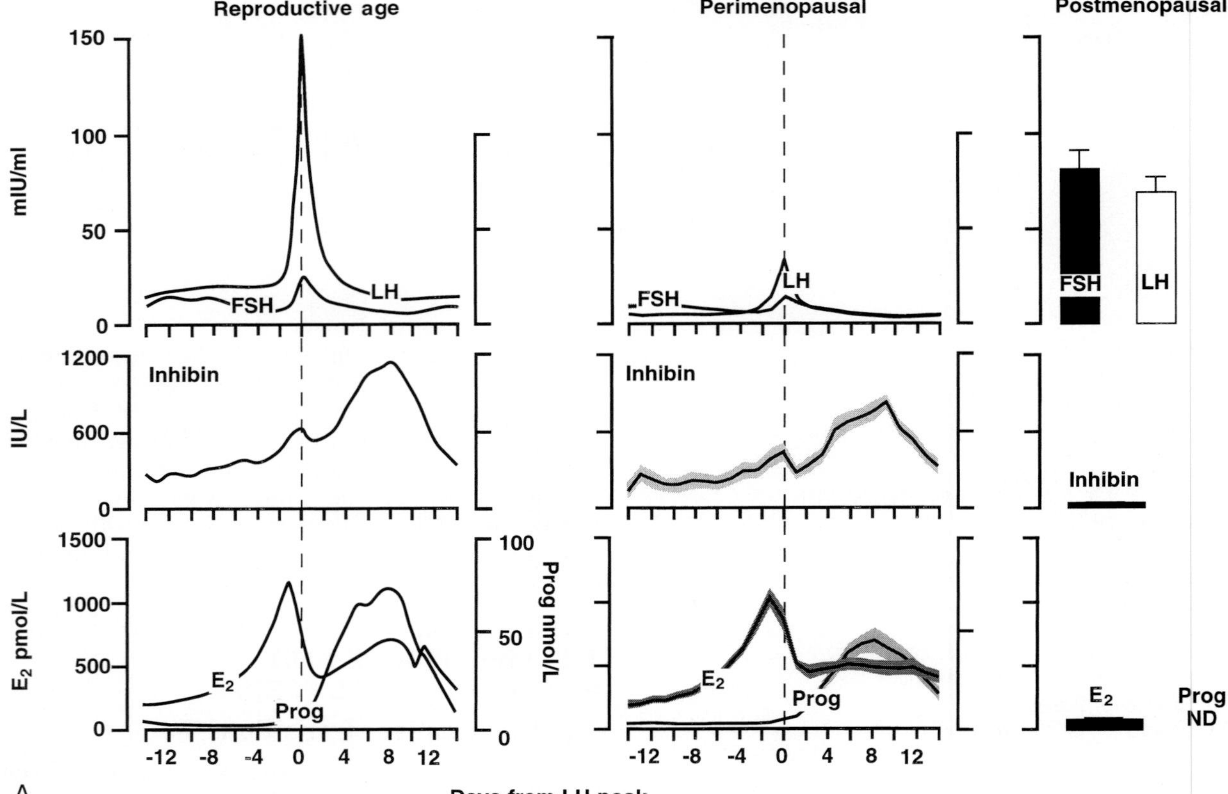

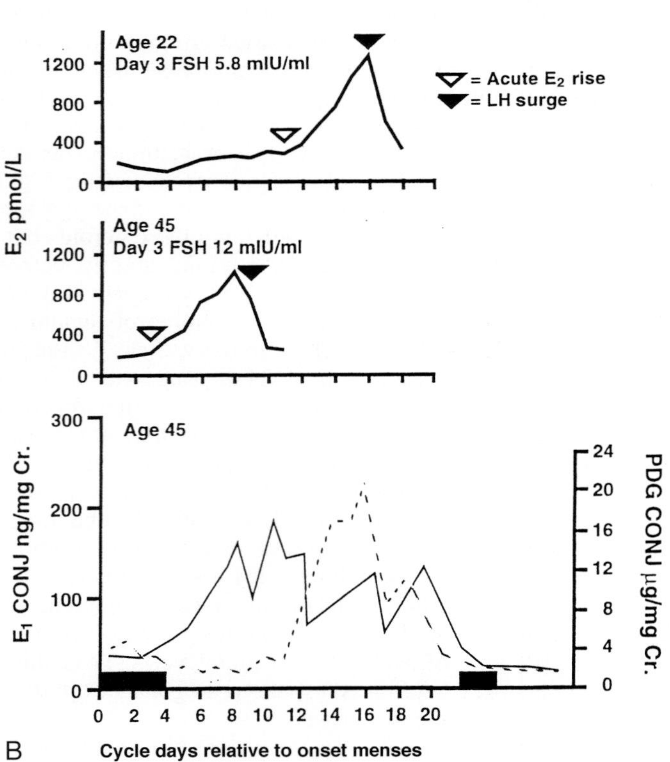

Figure 11–1 ■ *A*, Schematic illustration of follicle-stimulating hormone (FSH), luteinizing hormone (LH), inhibin, estradiol (E_2), and progesterone (Prog) in reproductive age women centered on day of LH surge, day 0 *(left panel)*; mean values of these hormones in perimenopausal women (shaded areas represent SEM, *(center panel)* and postmenopausal women *(right panel)*. ND, not detectable. (Reproductive age hormone profiles adapted from Roseff SJ, Bangah MZ, Kettel C, et al. Dynamic changes in circulating inhibin levels during the luteal-follicular transition of the human menstrual cycle. J Clin Endocrinol Metab 69:1033–1039, 1989. Perimenopausal data adapted from Klein NA, Battaglia DE, Fujimoto VY, et al. Reproductive aging: Accelerated ovarian follicular development associated with a monotropic follicle-stimulating hormone rise in normal older women. J Clin Endocrinol Metab 81:1038–1045, 1996. Postmenopausal inhibin value from Burger HG, Dudley EC, Hopper JC, et al. The endocrinology of the menopausal transition: A cross-sectional study of a population-based sample. J Clin Endocrinol Metab 80:3537–3545, 1995.)

B, Circulating estradiol (E_2) in a 22-year-old woman *(upper panel)* and a 45-year-old woman *(middle panel)*. Open inverted triangle illustrates day of acute E_2 rise, and filled inverted triangle represents day of LH surge. Note earlier onset of acute E_2 rise and LH surge in older women. In lower panel, concentrations of urinary conjugated estrogen (E_1 CONJ) and conjugated urinary metabolite of progesterone (pregnanediol glucuronide, PDG CONJ) in another 45-year-old woman. Filled horizontal bars represent days of menses. Note large, erratic rises in estrogen levels and shortness of cycle. (Adapted from Klein NA, Battaglia DE, Fujimoto VY, et al. Reproductive aging: Accelerated ovarian follicular development associated with a monotropic follicle-stimulating hormone rise in normal older women. J Clin Endocrinol Metab 81:1038–1045, 1996; and Shideler SE, DeVane GW, Kalra PS, et al. Ovarian-pituitary hormone interactions during the perimenopause. Maturitas 11:331–339, 1989.)

been demonstrated in follicular fluid, in the pituitary gland, and in the circulation.[6, 7] It is likely that the production of inhibin diminishes with ovarian age pari passu with a decreasing number of follicles.

Waning ovarian follicular activity and its eventual cessation, but with striking episodic increased secretion of estradiol, are key events in the endocrinologic changes occurring in the menopausal transition. Decreasing production of estradiol and inhibin by the ovary removes the negative feedback inhibition on the hypothalamic-pituitary system. This results in a gradual rise of gonadotropins, with FSH rising earlier and to higher levels than does LH. When ovaries are removed from women during their reproductive life, the length of time during which gonadotropins rise varies, but it often takes more than 1 month to reach final menopausal levels[8] (Fig. 11–2).

Endocrinologic Changes

Gonadotropins

With the cessation of menstrual function, gonadotropin levels rise markedly; concentrations of FSH rise earlier, and to higher levels, than those of LH. A hallmark of the menopause is further increases in gonadotropins as a result of increased amplitude rather than frequency.[9] Because metabolic clearance rates of FSH and LH in postmenopausal women are not appreciably different from those of women during reproductive life,[10] the increased circulating levels of these gonadotropins in menopausal women are a reflection of the increased pituitary production rate. Plasma concentrations of FSH and LH are consistently elevated in postmenopausal women compared with those observed throughout the normal menstrual cycle.[11] Concentrations of FSH are more consistently elevated in random samples from postmenopausal women than are LH levels. The ratio of FSH to LH levels is almost always greater than 1. A similar increase in pituitary content of FSH and LH in

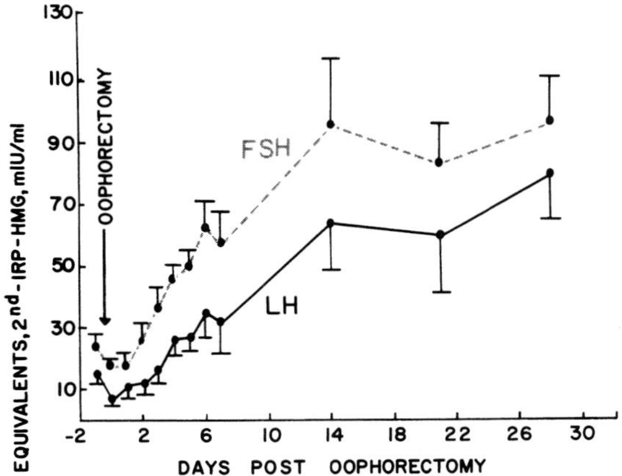

Figure 11–2 ■ Mean LH and FSH concentrations in six menstruating women before and after bilateral oophorectomy and total hysterectomy. The mean serum LH and FSH concentrations for the first 12 hours after oophorectomy depicted by the second set of data points represent 14 different observations of these patients. (From Monroe SE, Jaffe RB, Midgley AR Jr. Regulation of human gonadotropins. XIII. Changes in serum gonadotropins in menstruating women in response to oophorectomy. J Clin Endocrinol Metab 34:420–422, 1972. © The Endocrine Society.)

postmenopausal women occurs[12] independent of age.[11] In 72 postmenopausal women, LH concentration was 93.8 ± 5.4 and FSH concentration was 132.4 ± 5.6 mIU/ml.

There is a periodic pulsatile pattern of LH and FSH in postmenopausal women. The pulses of FSH are more pronounced in postmenopausal women than in women during the menstrual cycle. Pulses of gonadotropins occur at approximately 60- to 90-minute intervals.[9]

The pulsatile release of gonadotropins reflects the pulsatile release of gonadotropin-releasing hormone (GnRH) from the arcuate nucleus of the hypothalamus, the principal site of endogenous pulsatile GnRH discharge[13] (see Chapter 2 for detailed discussion). Administration of GnRH to postmenopausal women induces a marked rise in LH concentrations (4.1 × baseline) and a lesser rise (1.6 × baseline) in FSH.[11] In autopsy brain specimens, there was decreased hypothalamic GnRH content in ovariectomized and postmenopausal women compared with younger women.[14]

Steroids

Estrogen production by the postmenopausal ovary is minimal, and ovarian removal is not accompanied by any significant further decrease in levels of estrogens.[15, 16] However, in measurements of steroids in ovarian and peripheral venous blood from postmenopausal women, increased amounts of testosterone and androstenedione in the ovarian blood compared with those in the peripheral circulation were found.[16] Thus, the postmenopausal ovary continues to produce these androgens in significant amounts. In fact, the difference between ovarian and peripheral venous concentrations of testosterone in postmenopausal women is significantly higher than that found in premenopausal women, although the reverse is true in the case of androstenedione.[16] Presumably, the androgens are produced by the ovarian stromal and hilar (hilus) cells, which are capable of androgen production. Interestingly, approximately one third of testosterone production by the postmenopausal ovary is gonadotropin dependent, because administration of GnRH antagonists to postmenopausal women resulted in a decrease in circulating testosterone; circulating levels of the predominantly adrenal androgen dehydroepiandrosterone sulfate (DHEA-S) did not fall.[17, 18] Concentrations of androstenedione in the peripheral circulation after the menopause are reduced to a mean of approximately 800 to 900 pg/ml[19–22] from a mean value during the menstrual cycle of approximately 1500 pg/ml.[23] The concentrations of androstenedione in postmenopausal women are similar to those in premenopausal women after oophorectomy.[20] A further reflection of the predominantly adrenal source of androstenedione is its diurnal variation in older women, with a peak concentration between 8 AM and 12 noon and a nadir between 3 PM and 4 AM.[21] (Levels of the adrenal androgen DHEA-S progressively decrease in both sexes with advancing gestational age; see section on aging later in this chapter.)

Androstenedione is bound only minimally to sex hormone–binding globulin (SHBG)[24] and loosely to albumin. Because of this minimal binding, the metabolic clearance rate of androstenedione is rapid (1800 L/24 hr)[25, 26] in both premenopausal and postmenopausal women. The average production rate of androstenedione (the metabolic clearance rate times the plasma concentration) is 1.6 mg/24 hr in postmenopausal women.

As indicated earlier, the postmenopausal ovary contributes more significantly to the levels of circulating testosterone than to those of androstenedione. The mean concentration of testosterone in postmenopausal women (approximately 250 pg/ml) is only slightly less than that in premenopausal women.[17, 19, 27, 28]

In contrast to androstenedione, testosterone binds strongly to SHBG and therefore has a slower clearance rate (600 L/24 hr). Thus, the production rate is approximately 150 μg/24 hr. Although there is a slight increase in the concentrations of ovarian venous estrone and estradiol in contrast with those in the peripheral circulation, this is not enough to account for significant estrogen secretion by the postmenopausal ovary (Fig. 11–3).

Extragonadal Aromatization

If the ovary is not the source of estrogens in postmenopausal women, the question arises as to the origin of the estrogens often found in the circulation and the urine. The answer lies in an intriguing concept developed by Siiteri and MacDonald and their associates, extragonadal aromatization.[29, 30] According to this concept, androgens—particularly androstenedione produced principally in the adrenal gland—are converted (aromatized) to estrogen at extraglandular sites (i.e., outside of either the ovary or the adrenal gland). These sites have not been identified definitively, but the reaction has been shown to occur in fat, liver, kidney, and specific nuclei of the hypothalamus. It may be a ubiquitous process. This extraglandular estrogen formation mainly involves the conversion of androstenedione to estrone. The extent of extragonadal aromatization is influenced by age, sex, and weight. Heavy women have higher conversion rates and circulating estrogen concentrations than do slender women.[16, 21, 29, 30] The production rate of estrone derived from androstenedione is the product of the production rate of androstenedione multiplied by the percentage of conversion of androstenedione to estrone. This route can account for virtually all of the estrone produced by postmenopausal women. The average percentage of conversion (2.8 percent) is double that found in premenopausal women. The amount of estrone formed by this route is also increased in women with postmenopausal bleeding (Fig. 11–4), including many of those who develop endometrial carcinoma.

Although the adrenal gland is probably the major source of the androstenedione used in peripheral aromatization, it does not secrete appreciable amounts of estrogens, contrary to earlier belief. In fact, the normal adrenal gland secretes relatively little estrogen at any stage of adult life.[31]

Circulating concentrations of estradiol are low in postmenopausal women (approximately 13 pg/ml),[16, 19, 21, 22, 32] as are those in premenopausal women after oophorectomy. This estradiol is probably derived principally from conversion of precursors in peripheral tissues.

The circulating concentration of estrone is higher than that of estradiol after the menopause. The mean concentration approximates 35 pg/ml.[16, 19, 21, 22, 33] It is loosely bound to albumin and does not bind to SHBG. Therefore, it has a more rapid clearance rate (approximately 1600 L/24 hr) than does estradiol.[34] The estrone production rate, therefore, is approximately 55 μg/24 hr.

Causes of Menopausal Syndrome

The mechanism responsible for the appearance of the menopausal syndrome is not known, but it is likely that neuroendocrinologic factors related to changes in catecholamines, perhaps resulting from decreased estrogen levels, may be involved. Catecholamines, particularly those involved in dopamine and norepinephrine formation and metabolism, act as neurotransmitters. They play a significant role in modulating mood, behavior, and motor activities as well as hypothalamic-pituitary function.[35] In an excellent and provocative review of the regulation of the aging process, Finch[36] noted that in old mice there is a decrease in striatal dopamine and reduced conversion of L-tyrosine to L-dopa and to catecholamines in several areas of the brain, including the hypothalamus. In addition, the metabolism of total norepinephrine in the hypothalamus and total dopamine in the striatum is decreased. These findings suggest that aging may be associated with decreased activity of dopamine hydroxylase, increased activity of monoamine

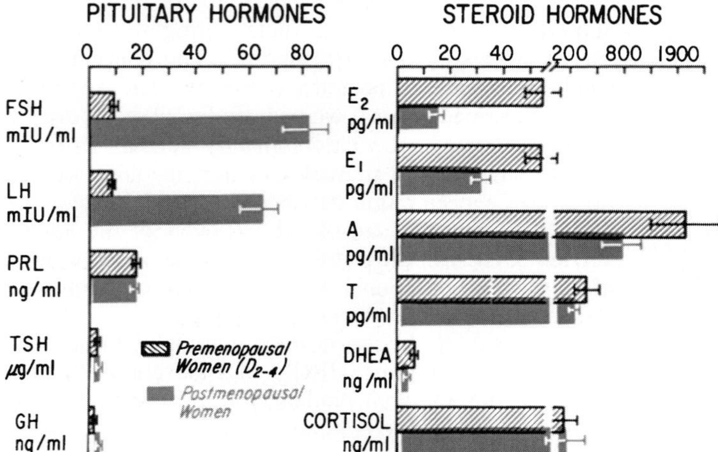

Figure 11–3 ■ Circulating levels of pituitary and steroid hormones in postmenopausal women compared with premenopausal women studied during the first week (days 2 to 4) of the menstrual cycle. FSH, follicle-stimulating hormone; LH, luteinizing hormone; PRL, prolactin; TSH, thyroid-stimulating hormone; GH, growth hormone; E_2, estradiol; E_1, estrone; A, androstenedione; T, testosterone; DHEA, dehydroepiandrosterone. (From Yen SSC. The biology of menopause. J Reprod Med 18:287–296, 1977.)

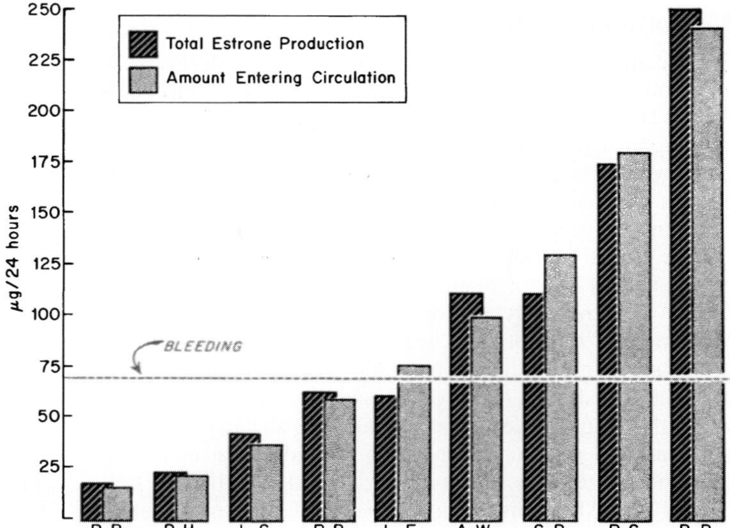

Figure 11–4 ■ Estrone production and the amount entering the circulation in postmenopausal women. (From MacDonald PC, Grodin JM, Siiteri PK. *In* Progress in Endocrinology: Proceedings of the Third International Congress of Endocrinology. Amsterdam, Excerpta Medica, 1969, p 775.)

oxidase or catechol *O*-methyltransferase, and reduced neuronal reuptake of catecholamines.[37]

Further, long-term administration of L-dopa significantly prolongs the life span of old male mice.[38] In addition, L-dopa can reinitiate a regular estrous cycle in old rats that are in constant estrus.[39] These observations suggest that a deficiency or an alteration of metabolism of catecholamines is associated with aging. Further evidence in humans is the development of fine tremors in older people that often respond to L-dopa administration.

Ovarian hormones may affect catecholamines in the central nervous system (CNS). Concentrations of dopamine decrease and those of norepinephrine increase in the hypothalamus after gonadectomy,[40, 41] and both the activity of tyrosine hydroxylase (the rate-limiting enzyme in catecholamine synthesis) and the turnover rate of norepinephrine in the hypothalamus increase after gonadectomy.[42, 43] Taken together, these observations suggest that estrogen withdrawal may cause an increase in the ratio of norepinephrine to dopamine levels that is independent of the aging process.[37] All of the consequences of gonadectomy noted previously can be reversed with estrogen administration.

Prostaglandins may play an intermediary role in the integration of neuroendocrine function.[44] Prostaglandins have been found in the rat brain,[45] including the hypothalamus. Vascular smooth muscle is a major site of action of prostaglandin F_2 (see Chapter 5). Thus, sympathetic stimulation may cause release of prostaglandins, which may have a vasodilatory action.[41] Further, prostaglandins are involved in the hypothalamic regulation of gonadotropin release.[46] These effects of prostaglandins can be obviated by the prostaglandin inhibitors aspirin and indomethacin. That estrogens play a role in prostaglandin synthesis and release in the brain is suggested by the observation that estrogen infusion in oophorectomized sheep attenuates the pulsatile pattern of CNS prostaglandin release.[47]

Estrogen deficiency in the CNS, a target tissue, may induce changes in both prostaglandins and catecholamines and may promote their interactions in the neurons located in the cervical region of the spinal cord, thereby reproducing regional vasodilatation.[37] Vasodilatation occurring in the brain may explain the signs and symptoms of menopausal hot flashes.

A group of symptoms, including nervousness, anxiety, irritability, and depression, has also been associated with the menopause. Whether these symptoms are related to changes in the CNS as a result of decreased estrogen levels or whether they have a different cause has not been ascertained.

CLINICAL CHANGES, EVALUATION, AND MANAGEMENT

Since the last edition of this textbook was written, there has been a plethora of articles and books written on various aspects of the perimenopause and postmenopausal period. This is not surprising because there are more than 30 million women older than 55 years in the United States alone, with an average life expectancy of approximately 30 years after the menopause. It is estimated that there will be 37.9 million by the year 2010 and 45.9 million by 2020.[48] About one half of all women reach menopause between 45 and 50 years, about one fourth before age 45 years, and one fourth after age 50 years. The mean age of menopause in one study was 51.4 years.[49]

Most signs and symptoms of the menopause result from diminution in circulating estrogen levels. These include vasomotor instability, vaginal dryness and irritation, loss of skin elasticity, and decreased size of the uterus and breasts. The vasomotor instability results in the characteristic hot flashes—a flushing of the skin accompanied by a feeling of warmth and profuse sweating. Interestingly, individuals who have never been exposed to normal female levels of endogenous circulating estrogens (e.g., patients with gonadal dysgenesis) do not experience symptoms of vasomotor instability. Although the majority of women evidence symptoms of estrogen deficiency (vasomotor symptoms and vaginal atrophy), not all do. This may be the result of extragonadal aromatization of sufficient magnitude to provide a continuing source of estrogen.

Menopausal Hot Flash

Several investigators have undertaken studies designed to elucidate the mechanisms involved in the hot flash (hot flush). Hot flashes have been observed in 65 to 76 percent of women who have spontaneous menopause or who have undergone bilateral oophorectomy.[50–52] More than 80 percent of women who have hot flashes experience them for more than 1 year.[51]

One of the earlier detailed clinical descriptions of the hot flash was that of Hannan,[50] subsequently reviewed by Judd.[53] The majority of the women noted that the first indication of the hot flash was a sensation of pressure in the head, akin to a headache. This progressed in intensity until the actual flush occurred. Occasional heart palpitations were also experienced. The actual flush usually began in the head and neck areas and then passed, often in waves, over the entire body. It was described as a feeling of heat or burning. After this, an immediate outbreak of sweating was described, involving the entire body but particularly marked in the head, neck, upper chest, and back. The entire episode varied from transient to as long as 30 minutes.[50]

There are profound physiologic changes associated with these flashes, both in the course of the day and during sleep at night.[54–58] Many investigators have measured the temperature of women with hot flashes.[54–61] Skin temperature measurements were performed on the fingers, the toes, and the forehead, and core body temperature was measured on the tympanic membrane and in the rectum. These investigators defined a prodromal period between the initiation of the subjective feeling of the flush and the first change in physiologic function that can be recorded (Fig. 11–5).

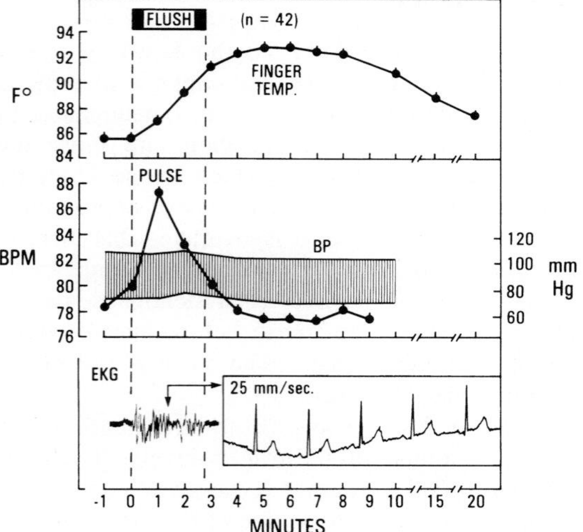

Figure 11–5 ■ Physical changes during 42 flushes monitored in six subjects. The mean (±SEM) duration of the subjective feeling of warmth (2.7 ± 0.1 minute) is indicated by the solid bar (FLUSH). A mean increase in finger temperature is seen at 6 minutes and persists after the subjective feeling of warmth. Pulse rate increases 9.1 beats per minute (BPM) with no associated change in blood pressure (BP). A dramatic electrocardiographic (EKG) fluctuation during the flush is shown at a paper speed of 1 mm/sec; but at the normal paper speed of 25 mm/sec in the inset, it is apparent that the rhythm and components of the electrocardiogram are normal. (From Casper R, Yen SSC: Menopausal flushes: A neuroendocrine link with pulsatile luteinizing hormone secretion. Science 205:823, 1979.)

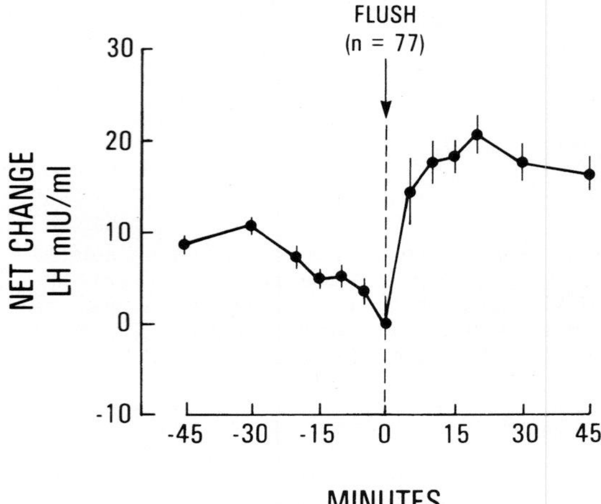

Figure 11–6 ■ Mean (±SEM) serum LH concentration during 77 flush episodes expressed as net change in milli-international units per milliliter from the onset of the flush at 0 on the X axis. This graph incorporates 5-minute sampling from 20 minutes before to 20 minutes after each flush episode. It can be seen that the flush onset is coincident with a rise in serum LH. (From Casper R, Yen SSC: Menopausal flushes: A neuroendocrine link with pulsatile luteinizing hormone secretion. Science 205:823, 1979.)

The hiatus between the prodrome and the first quantifiable episode of the flush may last up to 4 minutes. Skin conductance, a reflection of perspiration, is the first quantifiable sign of the flush.[56, 58, 61] An increase in skin temperature, reflecting cutaneous vasodilatation, occurs next. As a result of heat loss from the body by sweating and evaporation, a drop in core temperature occurs. The average decrease in core temperature is 0.2°C.[58, 61] In addition, increase in pulse rate accompanies flushing. The physiologic changes, which begin after the subjective sensation of the flush, persist for minutes after subjective symptoms are no longer present.

Circulating levels of estrone and estradiol do not fluctuate before or after flushes.[59] In contrast, there does appear to be a correlation between pulsatile LH release and the occurrence of hot flashes[60, 61] (Fig. 11–6). There is disagreement concerning a correlation with pulsatile FSH release; one study demonstrates such a correlation[61] and another does not.[60] The adrenal steroids cortisol, dehydroepiandrosterone (DHEA), and androstenedione have also been found to increase significantly in association with the hot flash.[59] So, too, have the pro-opiomelanocortin–derived peptides adrenocorticotropic hormone (ACTH), β-lipotropin, and β-endorphin.[62]

Although the mechanisms involved in the genesis of the hot flash have not been elucidated definitively, it appears that the flash represents an alteration in central thermoregulatory function. It has been suggested that it is effected by a sudden lowering of the central thermoregulating mechanism, and that this gives rise to the prodromal sensation of an impending flush. Subsequently, mechanisms promoting heat loss are activated to make the core temperature consonant with the new set-point, resulting in a decrease in the core temperature. Central factors, such as catecholamines, that govern both temperature regulation and GnRH production may be involved.

Of great practical importance is the loss of sleep associated with hot flashes. Nocturnal hot flashes are often associated with frequent episodes of waking, and this may produce significant sleep deprivation and fatigue.

Bone

Of the various changes associated with the menopause, changes in the bony skeleton and cardiovascular abnormalities (Table 11–1) have the most profound health implications. Recent data suggest that CNS function may also be affected. In osteoporosis, there is a reduction in the quantity of bone without alterations in its chemical composition.[63] In essence, osteoporosis is characterized by a decrease in bone mineral density resulting from an imbalance in the processes of bone formation and resorption. The decrease in bone mineral density leads to an increased risk of fracture. The most striking initial changes are in trabecular bone, in which there may be a loss of 50 percent with aging. Loss of cortical bone tends to develop later than that of trabecular bone, with a loss of approximately 5 percent per year. There is a loss of mineral mass in both men and women with age, men lose bone mass after 45 to 50 years of age and women after 30 years. After premenopausal oophorectomy or in untreated gonadal dysgenesis, there is an accentuation of the process.

An increase in the rate of bone destruction in relation to the rate of bone formation probably also contributes to postmenopausal osteoporosis. Estrogen replacement therapy may be the best available treatment for postmenopausal osteoporosis, but slowing down the already low rate of bone catabolism in elderly individuals by the administration of estrogen or other therapeutic means requires long periods of treatment before pronounced increases in the total mass of bone take place. Prophylactic administration of estrogen may produce better results.

Bone loss is most rapid during the first 3 or 4 years after the menopause; the annual rate of loss approximates 2.5 percent. Thereafter, the rate decreases to approximately 0.75 percent per year for the remainder of the individual's life.[74] Smoking augments the development of osteoporosis.[75] Slender women are more likely to develop osteoporosis than are heavier women.[75]

■ TABLE 11–1

Purported Benefits and Risks of Estrogen Therapy in Postmenopausal Women

ORGAN/SYSTEM	BENEFITS
Cardiovascular	Decreased incidence of coronary artery disease; reduction of cerebrovascular accidents
Bone	Decreased bone resorption; reduction of osteoarthritis
Central nervous system	Decreased risk and prolongation of age at onset of Alzheimer's disease; alleviation of hot flashes
Skin	Preservation of elasticity; maintenance of collagen matrix
Dental	Reduction of dental caries and tooth loss
Gastrointestinal	Reduced risk of colon cancer
Vagina	Reduces or eliminates vaginal dryness, atrophy, and infection
ORGAN/SYSTEM	**RISKS**
Breast	Possible increase in incidence of breast cancer
Liver	Increase in liver adenomas
Vascular	Thrombosis, thrombophlebitis, pulmonary embolus
Uterus	Increased risk of endometrial carcinoma if progestin not given concomitantly

The vertebral body is the most common site of fracture in postmenopausal women. However, the incidence of fractures of other bones, including the upper femur, the humerus, the ribs, and the distal forearm, is also increased. Approximately one in four white women in northern Europe has vertebral fractures by age 65 years and one in two by age 75 years.[76] The incidence of hip fracture, a major cause of morbidity and mortality in postmenopausal women, increases from 0.3 per 1000 at age 45 years to 20 per 1000 at age 85 years.[76]

The bulk of currently available data suggests a pivotal role of ovarian estrogen loss in the development of postmenopausal osteoporosis (see below). There is decreased calcium loss from bone in women treated with estrogen.[77] Further, there is an inverse correlation between estrone and estradiol levels and urinary calcium excretion, the latter a reflection of bone resorption.[78] There is also an inverse correlation between body weight or excess fat and calcium excretion, reflecting the increased incidence of osteoporosis in slender women. The increase in extragonadal aromatization with increasing weight thus may play a role in the lower incidence of osteoporosis in heavier women.

Estrogen Effects on Bone

Estrogens seem to act primarily to inhibit bone resorption rather than to stimulate its formation.[64] Estrogen receptors have been found in cultured bone cell lines.[65, 66] There have been suggestions that estrogens exert their effects by stimulating growth factors, such as fibroblast growth factor,[67] in bone. Estrogens have an effect on the blood-bone balance antagonistic to that of parathyroid hormone. A decrease in estrogenic activity leads to a slight elevation in plasma calcium levels, which results in hypercalciuria and a negative calcium balance. Increased plasma and urine concentrations of calcium, phosphorus, and hydroxyproline and collagen cross-links, thought to reflect collagen turnover in general and bone resorption in particular (Table 11–2), occur in women after the menopause, particularly when the menopause has been induced artificially. These changes are reversed after treatment with estrogens.

Other factors play a role in the development of osteoporosis. The disorder is found less frequently in blacks than in whites. Its incidence is lower in areas in which the fluoride content of the water is high. Sodium fluoride is concentrated in the bone and produces decreased osteoclastic activity and calcium retention. Thyrocalcitonin, which is involved in bone metabolism, inhibits resorption.

Bone mineral mass of the radius throughout adult life is greater in men than in women.[68] In men, it decreases after age 60 years; in women, it decreases earlier, at approximately 50 years, and the loss is greater. At the average age of 67 years, half of the normal white female population has less than the normal amount of bone in the radius. Premenopausal women older than 50 years do not show any decline of bone mineral mass, whereas in postmeno-

■ TABLE 11–2
Assessment of Bone Mineral Content and Turnover

RADIOLOGIC

Type	Bone Type Assessed
Dual-energy x-ray absorptiometry	Trabecular and cortical
Single-photon absorptiometry	Cortical (no longer used in the United States)
Dual-photon absorptiometry	Trabecular and cortical (rarely used currently)
Computed tomography	Trabecular

BIOCHEMICAL MARKERS

Resorption
Deoxypyridinoline
Pyridinoline
Cross-linked *N*-telopeptide
Hydroxyproline

Formation
Osteocalcin
Bone-specific alkaline phosphatase
Procollagen type 1 C-terminal peptide

■ TABLE 11–3
Agents Used in Treatment and Prevention of Bone Loss

Estrogens
Bisphosphonates
  Etidronate (Didronil)
  Alendronate (Fosamax)
Calcitonin
Estrogen "antagonists"
  Raloxifene
  Droloxifene
Fluoride
Intermittent parathyroid hormone

pausal women, regardless of age, there is a loss of bone mass related to the number of years after menopause; women who have had an oophorectomy have significantly less bone mass than do premenopausal women of the same average age. There is a decrease in the cortical thickness of the radius in women who have had an oophorectomy. This has been treated with a variety of preparations and dosages of estrogens after oophorectomy (Fig. 11–7; Tables 11–3 and 11–4). In a long-term follow-up study, untreated

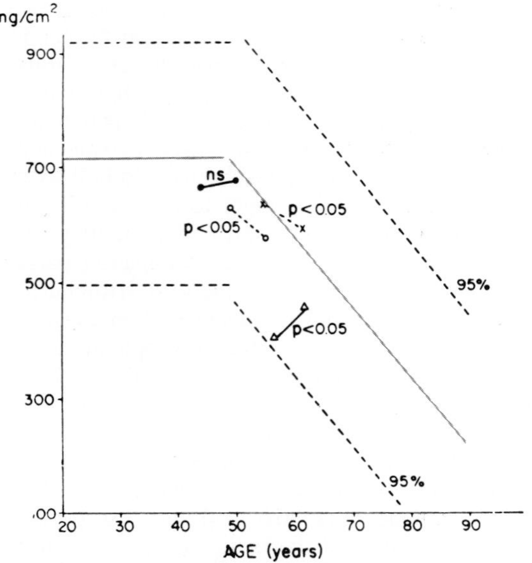

Figure 11–7 ■ Changes in bone mineral mass of the radius in two groups of untreated and two groups of estrogen-treated postmenopausal women in relation to the mean *(solid line)* and 95 percent confidence limits *(broken lines)* of normal women. x - - - x, natural menopause (untreated); ○ - - - ○, castrates (untreated); ■ - - - ■, natural menopause (estrogen treated); ● - - - ●, castrates (estrogen-treated); ns, not significant. (From Meema S, Meema HE. Isr J Med Sci 12:601–606, 1976.)

postmenopausal women (after a natural or an artificial menopause) demonstrated a significant loss of bone mass, whereas estrogen-treated postmenopausal women showed no such loss.[68]

In another report, prospective studies of bone mass in women after oophorectomy for benign conditions were performed,[69] and skeletal response to treatment with ethinyl estradiol 3-methyl ether (mestranol) was assessed by photon absorption densitometry. Untreated patients lost bone mass rapidly during the first 2 years after oophorectomy. When estrogen replacement was started within 2 months after oophorectomy, it prevented subsequent bone loss. Three years after oophorectomy, untreated women who had already lost bone tissue and then began to receive estrogen replacement showed a significant increase in their bone mass. The women in whom this treatment was delayed for 6 years did not respond.

In studies of women with postmenopausal osteoporosis before and after estrogen therapy,[70] increased bone resorption, normal bone formation, and decreased serum immunoreactive parathyroid hormone levels before treatment were found. In patients treated with replacement doses of estrogen, bone resorption decreased to normal levels and parathyroid hormone concentrations increased after short-term therapy; bone formation decreased to low levels after long-term therapy. Thus, both an intrinsic abnormality of bone cell function and a disruption of the normal regulation of bone turnover by parathyroid hormone and sex hormones, as a result of the menopause, are important in the pathogenesis of the menopause. However, the menopause alone does not adequately explain the higher than normal values for bone resorption in osteoporosis, because the degree of postmenopausal reduction in sex hormone production is similar in women with and without osteoporosis. It is possible that the biologic effect of serum estrogens is less marked in osteoporotic women, although the serum estrogen concentration is similar in menopausal women with and without osteoporosis. It is possible that a defect in the binding of sex steroids to specific receptors in target tissues, including bone, is one of the fundamental abnormalities in postmenopausal osteoporosis.

Calcitonin

Several studies have suggested that a deficiency of calcitonin may cause bone loss, and immunoreactive serum calcitonin concentrations are much lower in women than in men. This observation may be related to the increased

■ TABLE 11–4
Types of Estrogens, Usual Doses, and Routes of Administration

AGENT	BRAND NAME	USUAL DOSAGE	ROUTE OF ADMINISTRATION
Conjugated equine estrogens	Premarin	0.625 mg	Oral (available in 0.3, 0.625, 0.9, 1.2, 2.5 mg tablets)
	Prempro	1 tablet	Oral (contains 0.625 mg conjugated estrogen, 1.25 mg medroxyprogesterone acetate)
17β-estradiol	Estrace	1.2 mg (micronized)	Oral 1.2 mg
	Estrace	0.01% (micronized)	Vaginal cream (1 gm = 6.1 mg estradiol)
	Estraderm	0.05, 1.0 mg	Transdermal
	Climera		Transdermal
	Estring	2 mg (micronized)	Vaginal ring
Estrone sulfate (piperazine salt)	Ogen	0.625 mg	Oral (contains 0.75 mg estropipate)
Ethinyl estradiol	Estinyl	0.02, 0.05 mg	Oral (also available in 0.5 mg tablet)
Diethylstilbestrol	Diethylstilbestrol	1.5 mg	Oral
Quinestrol	Estrovis	100 μg	Oral
Estrone sulfate/equine estrogens	Estratab	0.625, 1.25 mg	Oral
Estrone sulfate/equine estrogens/testosterone	Estratest H.S.	1 tablet	Oral (contains 0.625 mg esterified estrogen, 1.25 mg methyltestosterone)
Estrone sulfate/equine	Estratest	1 tablet	Oral (contains 1.25 mg esterified estrogen, 2.5 mg methyltestosterone)

prevalence of symptomatic bone loss in women compared with men. Other investigators found normal values of circulating calcitonin in women with postmenopausal osteoporosis[71] but a reduced increment of calcitonin after calcium infusion.[72] Using improved techniques for quantifying calcitonin, one group concluded that postmenopausal osteoporosis is not associated with and does not result from calcitonin deficiency.[73] On the contrary, excessive skeletal calcium release may stimulate calcitonin secretion in patients with the disorder.

Collagen

Age-induced changes in the collagenous matrix, the main constituent of the organic portion of bone, are at least partially responsible for age-induced physiologic osteoporotic changes in the skeleton.[74] In particular, there seems to be a labile function of recently synthesized collagen in bone that loses its metabolic activity rapidly with advancing age.

Assessment of Bone Loss

It is important to have reliable means of accurately assessing bone loss quantitatively. Such quantitative bone mineral analysis is useful in assessing the efficacy of pharmacologic preparations used in the treatment or the prevention of osteoporosis. Such assessment might also potentially permit predictions as to which women are at greater risk for development of osteoporosis and thus permit selective therapeutic intervention. Both radiologic and biochemical assessments have been developed (see Table 11–2). Standard bone x-ray films are not too useful, because more than 30 percent of the bone must be lost before the loss is apparent. Previously, most clinical investigators used methods such as radiogrammetry and linear photon absorptiometry for mineral measurement in the peripheral skeleton. Subsequently, efforts were directed toward the development of techniques to measure either trabecular mineral in the peripheral skeleton by computed tomography[79] or total mineral in the axial skeleton by dual-photon absorptiometry[80] and neutron activation analysis. Methods of making serial vertebral measurements by quantitative computed tomography have also been described.[81] With use of quantitative computed tomography, vertebral cancellous bone loss in premenopausal women who have undergone oophorectomy could be detected by 12 months, whereas peripheral measurements showed no change. This method offers high precision and sensitivity and thus allows early detection of vertebral cancellous bone loss; however, it is expensive and requires considerable expertise. Single-photon absorptiometry was widely used but is not as sensitive or precise as dual-photon absorptiometry, quantitative computed tomography, or dual-energy x-ray absorptiometry and is rarely used currently. Dual-energy x-ray absorptiometry has been employed more recently, and it is currently the method of choice for assessing bone density in many institutions (see Table 11–2).

Whereas bone densitometry can detect established osteoporosis, it has limited value for early follow-up treatment of osteoporotic patients because densitometry cannot detect subtle differences in bone density. For this, biochemical markers of bone resorption and formation are useful. A variety of biochemical markers for diagnosis and monitoring treatment of osteoporosis have been described (see Table 11–2). Those markers that assess resorption include deoxypyridinoline, pyridinoline, cross-linked *N*-telopeptide, and hydroxyproline. The markers of bone formation include osteocalcin, bone-specific alkaline phosphatase, and procollagen type 1 C-terminal peptide.

Bone is not static; rather, it is in an active process of remodeling, which is a reflection of bone resorption and formation. The processes are mediated by osteoclasts (resorption) and osteoblasts (formation). The processes are coupled so that no net bone is lost. During the process of resorption, the bone matrix, or scaffolding, composed of mineralized deposits and proteins, is solubilized and digested by acids and enzymes produced by the osteoclasts.

The development of postmenopausal osteoporosis and the possibility of its prevention by estrogen therapy constitute one of the two most compelling reasons for the prophylactic use of estrogen in postmenopausal women, the other being reduction in cardiovascular disease (see following).

Cardiovascular System

Effects of Estrogen

Epidemiologic evidence of the beneficial effects of estrogen on coronary artery disease continues to mount.[82] Most epidemiologic studies indicate a decrease in the incidence of coronary artery disease of about 40 to 50 percent in postmenopausal women taking estrogen compared with those who do not. In contrast to these observational studies, recently a randomized blinded placebo-controlled secondary prevention trial of combined conjugated estrogen plus medroxyprogesterone acetate daily for ~ 4 years was performed in postmenopausal women with established coronary heart disease.[82a] The rate of thromboembolic events was increased early in the treatment course. Overall there were no significant differences between hormone-treated and placebo-treated groups in later occurrence of nonfatal or fatal coronary heart disease. However, a favorable pattern in coronary heart disease events existed after several years of treatment. Whether similar patterns would occur in women without preexisting coronary heart disease remains to be seen. The study emphasizes the need for controlled prospective clinical trials. However, the exact role of estrogens in the pathogenesis of atherosclerosis and myocardial infarction remains to be ascertained completely. Estrogen increases high-density lipoprotein cholesterol and decreases low-density lipoprotein cholesterol. Alterations in high-density and low-density lipoprotein cholesterol, however, probably do not account for more than 45 percent of the beneficial effects of estrogen on coronary artery disease. Estrogen receptors have been found on blood vessels, including the coronary arteries, and estrogen increases blood flow and decreases vascular resistance.[83] In addition, estrogen decreases concentrations of endothelin,[84] the most powerful endogenous vasoconstrictor described. A relation between decreased estrogen production and increased incidence of atherosclerosis in women during the sixth decade has been noted by a number of authors, and bilateral oophorectomy increases the severity of atherosclerosis. Further, oophorectomy before the natural menopause is associated with an increased frequency of coronary artery disease. Elevation of serum cholesterol levels and β-lipoprotein to α-lipoprotein ratios appear to be associated with the development of coronary atherosclerosis. However, the cholesterol to phospholipid ratio has been an unreliable atherogenic index.

The myocardial infarction rate in women lags 10 to 15 years behind that of men. This sex difference is virtually absent in Japanese, Bantus, and African-Americans[85] for reasons that have not been completely elucidated. The absence of a sex difference may be related in part to nutritional factors, because atherosclerosis is relatively uncommon in these groups.

A survey in Edinburgh, Scotland, dealing with the incidence of heart attacks in that city as a whole showed that although acute heart attacks were more common in men at all ages up to 69 years (the maximal age in the study), the rate of change was appreciably greater in women[86] (Fig. 11–8). This rise is probably related to the occurrence of the menopause.

The surgical removal of both ovaries from premenopausal women is followed by the premature development of the clinical features of coronary heart disease. However, the surgical removal of one ovary from women of comparable age does not influence the incidence of coronary heart disease 20 years later. After bilateral oophorectomy, the

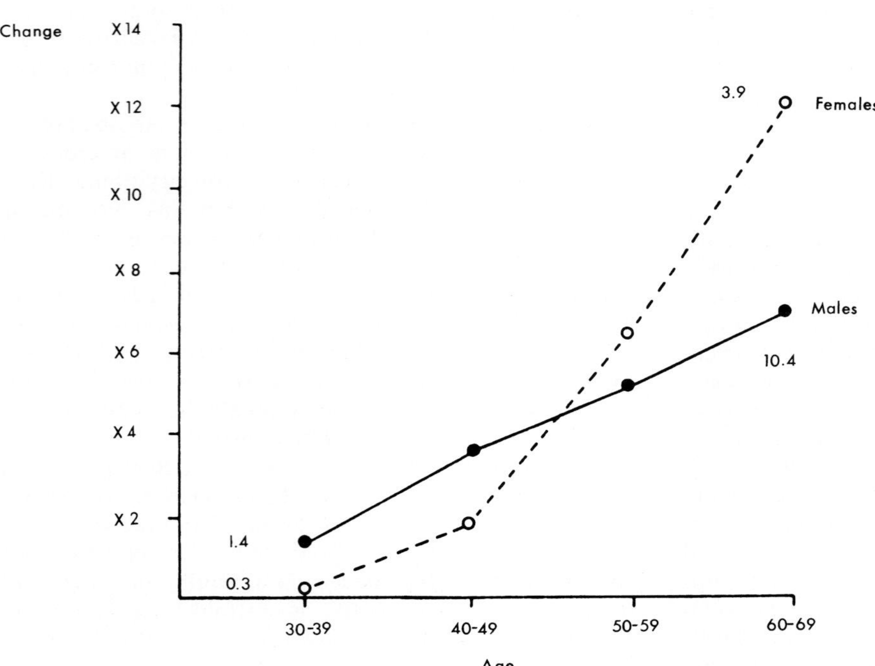

Figure 11–8 ■ Acute heart attacks: incidence rates per 1000 and change by age and sex in a study in Edinburgh, Scotland. (From Armstrong A, Duncan B, Oliver MF, et al. Natural history of acute coronary heart attacks: A community study. Br Heart J 34:67–80, 1972.)

serum lipid levels are higher than after unilateral oophorectomy.[87]

A significant increase in the incidence of coronary heart disease in women observed for 10 to 20 years after menstruation had ceased prematurely (before the age of 40 years) was reported.[88] Serum cholesterol and triglyceride levels in these women were significantly higher than those in women who continued to menstruate until they underwent a normal menopause. The serum lipid levels were found to increase with the length of time after the menopause.

There is no change in systolic or diastolic blood pressure around the menopause. However, hypertension is an important risk factor in the premature development of coronary heart disease, and the high male to female ratio is eliminated in its presence. This may explain the almost equal male and female incidence of coronary heart disease among African-Americans in the southern United States, where hypertension is common in women.

Other Organ Systems (see Table 11–1)

Central Nervous System

A recent study indicates that estrogen use by postmenopausal women may delay the onset and decrease the risk of Alzheimer's disease.[89] This study was performed in part because studies in rats indicated that estrogen promotes the growth of cholinergic neurons,[90] stimulates the secretase metabolism of the amyloid precursor protein,[91] and may interact with apolipoprotein E. All of these factors could affect the risk of Alzheimer's disease.

Gastrointestinal Tract

Two studies indicate that postmenopausal estrogen use decreases the risk of colon cancer.[92, 93] These studies are consistent with others suggesting a protective role of hormone therapy in the development of colon cancer. Because adenocarcinoma of the colon is one of the most common cancers and is associated with significant morbidity and mortality, these studies have important health implications.

Dental

In addition to its well-known effects on trabecular and cortical bone in postmenopausal women, estrogen has been reported to have beneficial effects on oral health, particularly tooth loss and alveolar residual ridge resorption.[94] There have been several studies demonstrating a relationship between severe osteoporosis and residual ridge resorption, and women with severe osteoporosis are three times more likely to experience edentia than are healthy age-matched control subjects.[94] Thus, it is not surprising that tooth loss and rates of edentia are significantly lower in estrogen users than in nonusers. The proportion of women with edentia decreases with increasing duration of estrogen use.

Osteoarthritis

A study indicates that estrogen therapy decreases the risk of osteoarthritis in elderly white women.[95] This might not be immediately apparent because estrogen therapy inhibits bone resorption, and increased bone mass tends to increase osteoarthritis of the hip in postmenopausal women. However, if this observation is replicated, it would be a significant benefit of estrogen therapy because osteoarthritis, the most common form of arthritis in elderly women, afflicts millions of women annually.

Vagina

Vaginal dryness, atrophy, and vaginal infections respond readily to local or systemic estrogen therapy.

HORMONE REPLACEMENT THERAPY

There have been several studies demonstrating an increased risk of carcinoma of the endometrium[96–98] in women receiving estrogen-only treatment. Whether there is an increased risk of carcinoma of the breast, probably the most troubling aspect of hormone replacement therapy to many women,[99, 100] also needs to be determined definitively.

Nevertheless, given all of the uncertainties, there does appear to be a consensus that estrogen should be used at least in the treatment of selected patients.[96] If it is borne in mind that endogenous sources of estrogen in some women are sufficient to obviate symptoms of vasomotor instability and vaginal dryness, the current thinking of some clinicians is that there should always be a clear indication for estrogen treatment. For this group of clinicians, whether treatment is indicated is dependent on the patient's symptoms, the physical findings, and the manner in which the patient reacts. Atrophic changes of the vulva, the vagina, the urethra, and the bladder or signs of beginning osteoporosis are indications for estrogen therapy. A case has been made for prophylactic treatment, and this has gained wide acceptance by gynecologists because there is a rationale for preventing symptoms of the deficiency syndrome rather than treating them after they occur. It is my practice to frequently use estrogen prophylactically because of the risk of osteoporosis and because of the salutary effect on the cardiovascular system. In many epidemiologic studies, use of estrogen treatment in postmenopausal women is associated with a decrease in the incidence of coronary artery disease of approximately 40 to 50 percent.[101] Studies also suggest a decreased incidence and longer time to development of Alzheimer's disease[89] and decreased incidence of colon cancer,[102] osteoarthritis,[95] and dental disease[94] (see Table 11–1).

The minimal dose of conjugated estrogen necessary to prevent osteoporosis is 0.5 mg.[103] This should be given with a synthetic progestin added for at least 10 days. One group found that the dose of conjugated estrogens could be reduced to 0.3 mg if adequate calcium was administered concomitantly.[104] A commonly employed regimen for the administration of estrogens and progestin is estrogens on the first 25 days of each month, with progestins added on the 14th or 16th through 25th days (Table 11–5). Some clinicians now administer estrogen continuously and punctuate the regimen with monthly administration of a progestin for 10 to 14 days. An increasingly common regimen is to use both estrogen (e.g., 0.625 mg conjugated estrogen) and progestin (e.g., medroxyprogesterone acetate 2.5 mg)

■ TABLE 11–5
Estrogen-Progestin Replacement Regimens

TYPE	AVERAGE DOSAGE REGIMENS
Intermittent estrogen and progestin	
Estrogen days 1–25	Conjugated estrogens, 0.625 mg or equivalent
Progestin days 14–25	Medroxyprogesterone acetate, 10 mg
Continuous estrogen and intermittent progestin	
Estrogen daily	Conjugated estrogens, 0.625 mg or equivalent
Progestin days 1–16	Medroxyprogesterone acetate, 10 mg
Continuous estrogen and progestin	Conjugated estrogens, 0.625 mg or equivalent Medroxyprogesterone acetate, 2.5 mg

daily without interruption. Although there may be irregular vaginal spotting and bleeding for the initial 4 to 6 months of this continuous therapy, most women become amenorrheic thereafter. A report from the Postmenopausal Estrogen/Progestin Intervention trial indicated that this continuous regimen was associated with a greater increase in bone density than intermittent regimens.[105] At present, there are no objective criteria for determining which patients should receive preventive therapy. However, the patient who has had oophorectomy early, the patient with premature ovarian failure or beginning osteoporosis, and the patient with an atrophic vaginal smear and climacteric symptoms probably should be treated.

There is some controversy as to the duration of estrogen therapy. Some clinicians believe that only severe symptoms should be treated, and then only with the lowest possible dosages for the shortest possible time. The contrary view is that treatment should be long term and that it should be continued as long as is reasonable in each individual case, even up to old age. Several studies indicate that to prevent hip fractures in older postmenopausal women, continued estrogen therapy is necessary,[106] even if the patient has received estrogen for 10 years after the menopause.

Because of studies strongly suggesting that combined estrogen-progestin therapy reduces or eliminates the risk of endometrial hyperplasia and cancer,[107–111] Weinstein and Schiff[112] evaluated the costs, risks, and benefits of estrogen-progestin and estrogen-only therapy in postmenopausal women. They concluded that estrogen-progestin therapy, in that it eliminates the excess risk of endometrial carcinoma, is estimated to offer increased life expectancy relative to estrogen-only therapy. Moreover, this treatment was estimated to increase life expectancy by up to 1 month, relative to no treatment, if continued on a long-term basis, owing to the reduction in hip fractures. They concluded that overall, on the basis of then available evidence, estrogen-progestin therapy appeared to be cost-effective, except in women who consider the adverse effects of continued withdrawal bleeding to offset the relief of menopausal symptoms. They cautioned that their conclusions must be viewed as tentative until the roles of estrogens and progestins in cardiovascular disease and breast cancer are clarified definitively. Because observational epidemiologic studies have indicated a strong association between estrogen use and decreased risk of coronary artery disease, cardiovascular benefit appears highly likely. The Postmenopausal Estrogen/Progestin Intervention study[105] and others have shown an improvement in lipid profiles in postmenopausal women receiving estrogen.

The dosage of estrogen used should be the lowest amount that is effective in obviating the signs and symptoms of estrogen deprivation. The paradox, of course, is that one of the most compelling reasons for the use of estrogens is the prevention of osteoporosis. Because there is no way at present to predict which women are most likely to develop osteoporosis (although the group of patients at highest risk are thin, sedentary whites who smoke), many believe that prophylactic estrogen therapy is indicated in all postmenopausal women other than those with specific contraindications (see later). Currently, oral estrogens are the most widely used. Whether attempts should be made to use naturally occurring estrogens, such as micropulverized 17β-estradiol[113] (see Table 11–4), and whether these have benefits over synthetic preparations have not been established. Daily doses of 1 to 2 mg of micronized estradiol are sufficient to control menopausal symptoms. In addition, other routes of administration of estradiol, including vaginal,[114] transdermal, and topical skin administration,[115] have been used (see Table 11–4). The transdermal delivery system for estradiol ("the patch") is now widely used. This is said to have the advantage of avoiding the "first pass" through the liver, thereby obviating potentially deleterious effects of estrogen on the liver. However, this may potentially decrease the effects of estrogen on lipoprotein cholesterol.

Progesterone inhibits the replenishment of estradiol receptors, thereby reducing the uptake and unopposed stimulation of target cells by estrogen.[116] For this reason, women who have not had a hysterectomy probably should receive progestins when estrogen therapy is employed. Concerns about decreased cardiovascular benefits when progestins are added to the estrogen regimen have not been borne out clinically; epidemiologic studies indicate as great a protective effect of estrogen and progestin as of estrogen alone, even though adding progestin decreases somewhat the beneficial effects on circulating lipids.[107]

Treatment of Osteoporosis

For the treatment of osteoporosis, bisphosphonates (see Table 11–3) can be used in women who cannot or do not wish to take estrogen. Several bisphosphonates have been studied.[117–121] Most recently, alendronate[121] was approved by the Food and Drug Administration in the United States. Side effects, particularly of the gastrointestinal tract, are frequent, and the medication must be taken in the morning, while vertical, with a great deal of water. Use of bisphosphonates will not have a beneficial effect on the cardiovascular system, however. Recently a lower dose of alendronate for prevention of osteoporosis has become available clinically. Calcitonin, recently made available in oral form, is also being evaluated for osteoporosis treatment. A nasal insufflation delivery system for calcitonin administration has recently been introduced for clinical use.

Breast Cancer and Estrogen Treatment

Probably the most frequent concern of women contemplating the use of estrogens in the postmenopausal period is the risk of breast cancer. In spite of numerous individual studies and several meta-analyses, no definitive, unequivocal answer has yet emerged.

Estrogen can stimulate mitogenesis in breast cancer cell lines in vitro.[122] In addition, it is thought that estrogen accelerates the growth of pre-existing breast cancer in vivo.

Prominent epidemiologists have derived data indicating that early menopause, both natural and surgically induced, reduces breast cancer risk; early menarche increases breast cancer risk; and postmenopausal estrogen replacement therapy increases breast cancer risk to a relatively small extent. They point out that the incidence of common, non–estrogen-dependent cancers rises continuously and rapidly with age, following a straight line when incidence is plotted on a log-log scale versus age; whereas the rate of breast cancer incidence, which also continues to rise with age, slows distinctly at about age 50 years, the age of menopause, and continues at this reduced rate for the remainder of a woman's life. They note that women whose natural menopause occurred before age 45 years had only half the breast cancer risk of those whose menopause occurred after age 55 years.[123] Bilateral oophorectomy and pelvic irradiation also reduced breast cancer risk. Thus, they argue that the hormonal pattern of premenopausal women causes a greater rate of increase in risk of breast cancer than does the hormonal pattern of postmenopausal women.[124] They also note that later menarche also decreases the risk of breast cancer and that the earlier regular menstruation is established, the greater the subsequent risk of breast cancer.[125, 126]

Further, epidemiologists note that population-based epidemiologic (as contrasted with hospital-based) studies usually show a positive association between estrogen treatment and breast cancer risk,[127] and they estimate that the effects of conjugated estrogen use show an increase in breast cancer risk of about 2.2% per year of estrogen use.

Some studies[127] support the contention that estrogens alone or estrogen and progestins increase the risk of breast cancer, whereas others[128] do not. It is apparent that a clear-cut, definitive answer to this clinically important question is currently not available. Until it is, clinicians should share available information with their postmenopausal patients and should help them balance the benefits of estrogen therapy on bone, the cardiovascular system, other forms of cancer, and other disease processes against the possible risks of breast cancer. A study indicates that except for women at no risk for coronary heart disease who have two first-degree relatives with breast cancer, hormone replacement therapy should increase the average life expectancy of most postmenopausal women.[129] However, another study indicates that whereas hormone replacement therapy decreases mortality in postmenopausal women for the first 10 years of use, the increased risk of breast cancer after 10 years obviates this benefit in the minority of patients with no cardiovascular risk factors (diabetes, hypercholesterolemia, hypertension, obesity, smoking), although the benefit persists in those women (the majority) who have cardiovascular risk factors.[130] It is possible that mixed estrogen agonistic/antagonistic preparations will be developed that will have beneficial (agonistic) effects on bone and the cardiovascular system and estrogen antagonistic effects on the breast and uterus. One such preparation recently was approved for clinical use in the United States (raloxifene), and others are being developed and undergoing testing.

Thromboembolic Disease

Three studies, appearing in the same issue of one journal, point to an increased risk of thromboembolic disease and pulmonary emboli.[131–133] Although the overall incidence is still low, it is threefold to fourfold higher in menopausal women receiving estrogen replacement than in those who are not.

PREMATURE AND PRIMARY OVARIAN FAILURE

There is a group of individuals, categorized as having premature ovarian failure, whose menstrual cycles terminate before the age of 40 years and who may have few or no menses and often no obvious demonstrable genetic abnormality. These individuals usually have the symptom complex of amenorrhea, elevated gonadotropin levels, and decreased estrogen concentrations. Mutations in genes for gonadotropin receptors have recently been identified in women presenting with premature ovarian failure.[134]

It has been suggested that the ovaries of patients with premature ovarian failure are depleted of ova early, resulting in an unduly early menopause. The rate of depletion of oocytes increases normally in the menopausal transition.[135] Those patients with premature ovarian failure grow normally during adolescence because they have normally functioning ovaries during that period. Thus, they are usually of normal stature because the condition usually develops after epiphyseal closure. The cause of the condition has not been elucidated, although both a deficient number of ova initially and excessive gonadotropic stimulation of the processes of follicular growth and atresia have been suggested. Not uncommonly, there is associated autoimmune disease, most commonly autoimmune thyroiditis. There may also be autoimmune adrenal and parathyroid disease as well as associated pernicious anemia. Premature ovarian failure can also be found in patients with myasthenia gravis and polyendocrinopathies. There may also be mucocutaneous candidiasis, hypoadrenalism, and hypoparathyroidism.[139, 140] It is possible that there are altered (i.e., biologically inactive) forms of gonadotropins in some of these patients. Antibodies have been found in many of these patients by use of an enzyme-linked immunosorbent assay.[136, 137] It is also possible that these individuals have developed antibodies to gonadotropins or gonadotropin receptors; these have been described,[138] as have genetic mutations in the FSH receptor.[134] As is true with menopause occurring at the usual time, the lack of adequate ovarian estrogen production and inhibin results in increased concentrations of FSH and LH.

Rebar and colleagues[138] detailed the clinical and endocrinologic characteristics of premature ovarian failure. They noted, as had been suggested in previous isolated cases, that ovarian failure is not always permanent, as indicated by reinitiation of menstrual cycles and even occasional pregnancy in some of these patients. All of the patients with premature ovarian failure reported by Rebar and colleagues had ovarian activity for less than half of the average reproductive life span. In many of these patients, menses were always irregular. In some patients, menarche was delayed, and incomplete sexual development was noted in some of these women.

In the study conducted by Rebar and Connolly,[141] patients were divided into three groups. One group was composed of women who failed to undergo complete sexual maturation and frequently had either primary amenorrhea or only a single spontaneous period; a second group included patients with complete maturation and regular menses for several years before the onset of amenorrhea or sporadic menses; and a third group had evidence of ovulation during or after the study period. Pregnancy occurred in several individuals in the last two groups. Many of the patients had typical hot flashes and accompanying changes in pulse rate and finger temperature that occurred concomitantly with LH pulses. Some of the patients had altered arm span to height measurements compatible with hypogonadism. There was little or no histologic evidence of follicular activity, even when viable oocytes were present. Beneath the cuboidal epithelium covering the ovary, there were thick layers of dense connective tissue. No evidence of developing follicles or corpora lutea was seen, nor were differentiated steroid-secreting cells observed.

Another histologic picture observed in ovaries of some of these patients is extensive lymphocytic infiltration surrounding the follicles, probably part of the immune process. Corticosteroid therapy has been tried in some of these patients, and at least two pregnancies have been reported.

Varying profiles of gonadotropins and steroid hormones are found in these patients. In many, typical postmenopausal gonadotropin levels are observed, with FSH levels greater than those of LH in most samples and low but fluctuating levels of estrogens and androgens. In other women, LH concentrations are frequently greater than those of FSH, and decreasing gonadotropin concentrations are observed in association with rising levels of estradiol and estrone, occasionally to levels observed before normal preovulatory LH surges. On occasion, cycles are, in fact, ovulatory.

On the basis of these observations, Rebar and colleagues concluded that elevated FSH levels cannot be considered absolute evidence of permanent premature ovarian failure. They suggested that the syndrome manifested in the three clinical groups they described may represent a continuum in which individuals may be affected at any stage before the expected age of menopause. They noted that "in some patients all follicles undergo atresia before final sexual maturation at puberty. In others, the final depletion of oocytes occurs during the pubertal years. In still others, ovarian failure occurs postpubertally. In some, the signs and symptoms of ovarian 'failure' may simply be transient." They found a surprisingly high frequency (23 of 97 patients with secondary amenorrhea) of subsequent evidence of follicular activity and even pregnancies. They correctly pointed out that "the presence of elevated circulating concentrations of FSH no longer can be termed indicative of irreversible ovarian failure."

Evaluation of affected patients, in addition to a careful history and physical examination, should include chromosome analysis (although usually this will not alter the patient's therapy); measurement of serum calcium, phosphate, and protein concentrations for evidence of hypoparathyroidism; and thyroid function studies, including evaluation of antibodies. Some form of assessment of adrenal reserve by administration of corticotropin (ACTH) should also be carried out.

A group of patients also has been described with primary amenorrhea in whom there is evidence of ovarian "resistance" to gonadotropins. These patients have small hypoplastic ovaries with unstimulated follicles and increased levels of gonadotropins. This disorder, which may represent a part of the spectrum of premature ovarian failure, has been termed the resistant ovary syndrome. More recent studies suggest that these patients have mutations in genes for the LH or FSH receptors.[134]

AGING

The effects of aging on reproductive processes are in many respects inextricably linked with the advent of the menopause. In some respects, the menopause can be viewed as a natural phase of the aging process. However, some endocrinologic changes, including those of the somatotrophic axis and those of adrenal androgen production, appear to reflect age-related phenomena, although even some of these are influenced by declining ovarian steroid production (Table 11–6).

■ TABLE 11–6
Endocrine-Metabolic Changes with Aging

Luteinizing hormone	↑
Follicle-stimulating hormone	↑
Growth hormone	↓
Adrenocorticotropic hormone	→*
Prolactin	↓
Thyroid-stimulating hormone	→*
Estradiol	↓
Estrone	↓
Progesterone	↓
Triiodothyronine	→
Thyroxine	→*
Cortisol	↓*
Dehydroepiandrosterone	↓
Dehydroepiandrosterone sulfate	↓
Testosterone	↑
Androstenedione (Δ^4)	↓
Inhibin	↓
Melatonin	↓
Insulin-like growth factor I	↓
Dopamine	↓
Norepinephrine	↑

*May be slight decrease or decrease in response to specific secretagogue (e.g., corticotropin-releasing hormone, thyrotropin-releasing hormone, somatostatin, growth hormone–releasing hormone, adrenocorticotropin) with age.

The Somatotrophic Axis

The growth hormone (GH) axis declines with advancing age, and there has been considerable controversy concerning the benefits and risks of administration of GH, its intermediaries, or its secretagogues to older individuals.

As detailed in Chapter 2, GH secretion by the anterior pituitary gland, which is pulsatile in nature, is regulated by growth hormone–releasing hormone (GHRH) and somatostatin. GHRH stimulates GH synthesis and secretion; somatostatin release–inhibiting factor inhibits GH release without altering GH synthesis.[142] In addition, insulin-like growth factor I (IGF-I), formerly called somatomedin, which is synthesized in response to GH in the liver and other tissues, acts as an intermediary in GH regulation of some metabolic phenomena.[143] IGF-I, in turn, can inhibit GH release from the pituitary gland rapidly.[144] In both men and women, GH secretion decreases with advancing age.[145] This decline with aging may be related to the changes in body composition that occur with age. These changes include a decrease in muscle mass of 20 to 50 percent, a decrease in bone mass of approximately 20 percent, and an increased proportion of body fat of approximately 100 percent. Further, there is a redistribution of fat from peripheral subcutaneous tissue to intra-abdominal adipose tissue depots.

The decline in GH secretion in both sexes occurs primarily before age 40 years.[146, 147] The reasons for this decline are not clear but may be related to increased somatostatin or decreasing GHRH; the administration of GHRH or a GHRH analogue to older men results in increased circulating concentrations of GH and IGF-I.[147, 148] The decline in ovarian steroid concentrations may also contribute to the decline in circulating GH levels in women. In one study, serum estradiol concentrations correlated with the differences in 24-hour integrated GH concentrations,[149] and estrogen replacement therapy increased 24-hour spontaneous and GHRH-stimulated GH release in postmenopausal women.[150, 151]

Several GH-releasing peptides, in addition to GHRH, have been synthesized.[152–154] At least one of them stimulates pulsatile GH secretion in humans, probably acting on both the hypothalamus and pituitary[151, 152] through a novel receptor.[155] Because GH is anabolic when it is administered in physiologic concentrations, stimulating muscle development and strength and causing loss of fat tissue while increasing bone density,[156] investigators have explored the effects of GH-releasing peptide administration.[148, 157] This is discussed in detail in Chapter 2.

Adrenal Steroids

A striking feature of advancing age is the decline in the adrenal androgens DHEA and DHEA-S (Fig. 11–9). A variety of putative benefits have been attributed to the administration of DHEA or DHEA-S, including inhibition of atherosclerosis, decrease in obesity, protection against viral infection, and inhibition of cancer. Whereas reduced atherosclerosis, improved immune function, tumor suppression, and improved memory are suggested by data in rodents (which do not have circulating DHEA-S), these effects have not been demonstrated definitively in humans.

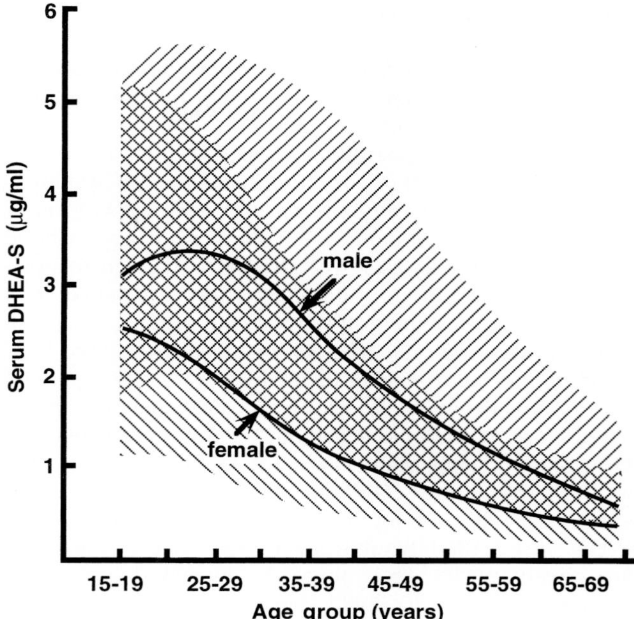

Figure 11–9 ■ Serum dehydroepiandrosterone sulfate (DHEA-S) concentrations throughout life in men *(upper curve, solid line)* and women *(lower curve, solid line)*. Shaded areas depict normal ranges for men (//////) and women (\\\\\\\\). (Adapted from Orentreich N, Brind JL, Rizer RL, Vogelman JH. Age changes and sex differences in serum dehydroepiandrosterone sulfate concentrations throughout adulthood. J Clin Endocrinol Metab 59:551–555, 1984.)

Earlier attempts to administer markedly supraphysiologic quantities of DHEA or DHEA-S were not associated with consistent beneficial effects. More recently, Yen and associates[159] administered nightly oral doses of DHEA to older men and women in a randomized, placebo-controlled crossover trial that produced circulating levels of this steroid and DHEA-S within the normal range for young adults. They described an increased sense of well-being, increased energy, and an increase in circulating IGF-I concentrations and a concomitant decrease in IGF-binding protein-1 (IGFBP-1). There was no significant increase in libido. In a more recent study,[160] the possible correlation between endogenous concentrations of DHEA-S and functional, psychologic, and mental status was assessed in a group of 620 men and women older than 65 years. Significantly lower concentrations of DHEA-S were found in women with functional limitations, as measured by the Activities of Daily Living scale. In addition, lower baseline DHEA-S levels were correlated with depressive symptoms, poor subjective perception of health, and lack of satisfaction with their lives. Thus, there appears to be some correlation between decreased DHEA-S levels and depression; a suggestion has been made that administration of DHEA improves older individuals' sense of well-being, also studied in a group of chronically depressed patients.[161]

In addition to the influence of changes in adrenal DHEA and DHEA-S secretion on aspects of mood, behavior, and mentation, it is possible that DHEA and DHEA-S produced locally in the brain influence CNS function. The formation of this novel class of steroids,[162–164] neurosteroids, which are synthesized de novo in the brain, may have significant effects on learning, memory, and behavior, at least in rodents.[165–167] Whether decreased formation of locally produced DHEA and DHEA-S in rodents or humans occurs with aging and whether this affects CNS function in older individuals remain to be ascertained.

There are several possible reasons, not mutually exclusive, for the beneficial effects observed after DHEA administration. It is possible that there was a rapid conversion of the DHEA to potent androgens that may exert anabolic effects. Much higher doses of oral DHEA given to postmenopausal women in a previous study[168] resulted in a significant increase in testosterone, androstenedione, and 5α-dihydrotestosterone. The estrogens estrone and 17β-estradiol also increase with this markedly supraphysiologic dose.[169] Another possible reason for the beneficial effects of the more physiologic doses of DHEA is the increase in IGF-I and corresponding decrease in IGFBP-1. As pointed out in the preceding section on the somatotrophic axis and aging, IGF-I is a major intermediary in GH action. The decline in IGFBP-1 would render even more of the IGF-I biologically active. Over time, the increased activity of the somatotrophic axis could lead to glucose-lowering and protein-sparing effects.

It is also possible that the DHEA was having a direct central effect. Both DHEA and DHEA-S bind to the γ-aminobutyric acid–receptor complex, resulting in neuronal excitability, at least in vitro.[170] There also appears to be memory enhancement and inhibition of aggressive behavior in rodents brought about by DHEA. Similar effects may occur in humans, and preliminary data suggest that DHEA has antidepressant and cognition-enhancing effects in middle-aged and elderly individuals with major depression (see Chapter 2).[169, 171, 172]

Cortisol

A comprehensive study by van Cauter and colleagues[173] demonstrated that cortisol levels are higher in older, postmenopausal women than in premenopausal women, although the qualitative characteristics of the circadian wave shape are preserved. There appears to be a progressive decline in the endogenous inhibition of nocturnal cortisol secretion during aging, reflected by a delay in the onset of the quiescent period and higher nocturnal cortisol levels. Van Cauter and colleagues suggest that this loss of resiliency is consistent with the "wear and tear" of lifelong exposure to stress, and may reflect neuronal loss in the hippocampal area. These hippocampal effects may underlie some of the memory deficits that occur in many adults. Further, the loss of resiliency may be related to the sleep disorders that affect many older individuals.

References

1. McKinlay SM, Brambella DJ, Posner NG. The normal menopausal transition. Maturitas 14:102, 1992.
2. Treolar AR, Bounton RE, Behn BG, Brown BW. Variation of the human menstrual cycle through reproductive life. Int J Infertil 12:77, 1967.
3. Sherman BW, West JH, Korenman SG. The menopausal transition: Analysis of LH, FSH, estradiol, and progesterone concentrations during menstrual cycles of older women. J Clin Endocrinol Metab 42:629, 1976.
4. Baird DT, Smith KB. Inhibin and related peptides in the regulation of reproduction. Oxf Rev Reprod Biol 15:191, 1993.
5. Van Look PF, Lothian H, Hunter WM, et al. Hypothalamic-pituitary ovarian function in perimenopausal women. Clin Endocrinol (Oxf) 7:13, 1977.
6. Groome NP, Illingworth PJ, O'Brien M, et al. Measurement of dimeric inhibin β throughout the human menstrual cycle. J Clin Endocrinol Metab 81:1401, 1996.
7. McLashlan RI, Robertson DM, Burger HG, deKretser DM. The radioimmunoassay of bovine and human follicular fluid and serum inhibin. Mol Cell Endocrinol 46:175, 1986.
8. Monroe SE, Jaffe RB, Midgley AR Jr. Regulation of human gonadotropins in menstruating women in response to oophorectomy. J Clin Endocrinol Metab 34:420, 1972.
9. Yen SSC, Tsai CC, Naftolin F, et al. Pulsatile patterns of gonadotropin release in subjects with and without ovarian function. J Clin Endocrinol Metab 34:671, 1972.
10. Kohler PO, Ross GT, Odell WD. Metabolic clearance and production rates of human luteinizing hormone in pre- and postmenopausal women. J Clin Invest 43:381, 1968.
11. Scaglin H, Medina M, Pinto-Ferreira AL, et al. Pituitary LH and FSH secretion and responsiveness in women of old age. Acta Endocrinol (Copenh) 81:673, 1976.
12. Verzar F. Anterior pituitary function in age. *In* Harris GW, Donovan BT (eds). The Pituitary Gland, Vol 2. London, Butterworth, 1966, p 444.
13. Plant TM, Krey LC, Moossy J, et al. The arcuate nucleus and the control of gonadotropin and prolactin secretion in the female rhesus monkey. Endocrinology 102:52, 1978.
14. Parker CR, Porter JC. LHRH and TRH in the hypothalamus of women: Effects of age and reproductive status. J Clin Endocrinol Metab 58:488, 1984.
15. Judd HL, Lucas WE, Yen SSC. Serum 17β-estradiol and estrone levels in post-menopausal women with and without endometrial cancer. J Clin Endocrinol Metab 43:272, 1976.
16. Judd HL, Judd GE, Lucas WE, Yen SSC. Endocrine function of the postmenopausal ovary: Concentrations of androgens and estrogens in ovarian and peripheral vein blood. J Clin Endocrinol Metab 39:1020, 1974.
17. Andreyko JL, Monroe SE, Marshall LA, et al. Concordant suppression of serum immunoreactive LH, FSH alpha subunit, bioactive LH and testosterone in postmenopausal women by a potent gonadotropin releasing hormone antagonist (detirelix). J Clin Endocrinol Metab 74:399, 1992.
18. Rabinovici J, Rothman P, Monroe SE, et al. Endocrine effects and pharmacokinetic characteristics of a potent new GnRH antagonist (ganirelix) with minimal histamine-releasing properties. J Clin Endocrinol Metab 75:1220, 1992.
19. Greenblatt RB, Colle ML, Mahesh VB. Ovarian and adrenal steroid production in the postmenopausal woman. Obstet Gynecol 47:383, 1976.
20. Judd HL, Lucas WE, Yen SSC. Effect of oophorectomy on circulating testosterone and androstenedione levels in patients with endometrial cancer. Am J Obstet Gynecol 118:793, 1974.
21. Vermeulen A. The hormonal activity of the postmenopausal ovary. J Clin Endocrinol Metab 42:247, 1976.
22. Vermeulen A, Verdonck L. Sex hormone concentrations in postmenopausal women. Clin Endocrinol (Oxf) 9:59, 1978.
23. Abraham GE. Ovarian and adrenal contribution to peripheral androgens during the menstrual cycle. J Clin Endocrinol Metab 39:340, 1974.
24. Rosner W. Interaction of adrenal and gonadal steroids with proteins in human plasma. N Engl J Med 281:658, 1969.
25. Bardin CW, Lipsett MB. Testosterone and androstenedione blood production rates in normal women and women with idiopathic hirsutism or polycystic ovaries. J Clin Invest 46:981, 1967.
26. Horton R, Tait JF. Androstenedione production and interconversion rates measured in peripheral blood and studies on the possible site of its conversion to testosterone. J Clin Invest 45:301, 1966.
27. Calanog A, Sall S, Gordon GG, et al. Testosterone metabolism in endometrial cancer. Am J Obstet Gynecol 124:60, 1976.
28. Lloyd CW, Lobotsky J, Baird DT, et al. Concentration of unconjugated estrogens, androgens and gestagens in ovarian and peripheral venous plasma of women: The normal menstrual cycle. J Clin Endocrinol Metab 32:155, 1971.

29. Grodin JM, Siiteri PK, MacDonald PC. Source of estrogen production in post-menopausal women. J Clin Endocrinol Metab 36:207, 1973.
30. Siiteri PK, MacDonald PC. Role of extraglandular estrogen in human endocrinology. *In* Greep RO, Astwood E (eds). Handbook of Physiology: Endocrinology, Vol 2. Washington, DC, American Physiological Society, 1973, p 615.
31. Ho Yuen B, Kelch RP, Jaffe RB. Adrenal contribution to plasma estrogens in adrenal disorders. Acta Endocrinol (Copenh) 76:117, 1974.
32. Baird DT, Guevara A. Concentration of unconjugated estrone and estradiol in peripheral plasma in nonpregnant women through the menstrual cycle, castrate and postmenopausal women and in men. J Clin Endocrinol Metab 29:149, 1969.
33. Radar MD, Flickinger GL, De Villa GO Jr, et al. Plasma estrogens in postmenopausal women. Am J Obstet Gynecol 116:1069, 1973.
34. Longcope C. Metabolic clearance and blood production rates of estrogens in postmenopausal women. Am J Obstet Gynecol 111:778, 1971.
35. Axelrod J. Relationship between catecholamines and other hormones. Recent Prog Horm Res 31:1, 1975.
36. Finch CE. The regulation of physiologic changes during mammalian aging. Q Rev Biol 51:49, 1976.
37. Yen SSC. The biology of menopause. J Reprod Med 18:287, 1977.
38. Catzias GC, Miller ST, Nicholson AR Jr, et al. Prolongation of the life span in mice adapted to large amounts of L-dopa. Proc Natl Acad Sci USA 71:2466, 1974.
39. Huang HH, Meites J. Reproductive capacity of aging female rats. Neuroendocrinology 17:289, 1975.
40. Donoso AI, Stefano IJE, Biscardi AM, Cukier J. Effects of castration on hypothalamic catecholamines. Am J Physiol 212:727, 1967.
41. Fuxe K, Hockfelt T, Nilsson O. Castration, sex hormones and tuberoinfundibular dopamine neurons. Neuroendocrinology 5:107, 1969.
42. Anton-Toy F, Wurtman RJ. Norepinephrine turnover in the rat brain after gonadectomy. Science 159:1245, 1968.
43. Bapna J, Neff H, Costa EA. A method for studying norepinephrine and serotonin metabolism in small regions of the rat brain; effect of ovariectomy on amine metabolism in anterior and posterior hypothalamus. Endocrinology 89:1345, 1971.
44. Brody MJ, Kadowitz PJ. Prostaglandins as modulators of the autonomic nervous system. Fed Proc 33:48, 1974.
45. Holmes SW, Horton EW. Prostaglandins and the central nervous system. *In* Ramwell P, Shaw J (eds). Prostaglandin Symposium of the Worcester Experimental Foundation for Biology. New York, Wiley-Interscience, 1968, p 21.
46. Harms PG, Ojeda SR, McCann SM. Prostaglandin involvement in hypothalamic control of gonadotropin and prolactin release. Science 181:760, 1973.
47. Roberts JS, McCracken JA. Prostaglandin F_2 production by the brain during estrogen-induced secretion of luteinizing hormone. Science 190:894, 1975.
48. US Bureau of the Census. Projection of the population of the United States: 1977 to 2050. Current Population Report Series P-25, No. 704.
49. Jaszmann LJB. Epidemiology of the climacteric syndrome. *In* Campbell S (ed). The Management of the Menopause and Postmenopausal Years. Baltimore, University Park Press, 1976, p 12.
50. Hannan JH. The flushings of the menopause. London, Baillière, Tindall and Cox, 1927, p 1.
51. Jaszmann LJB, Van Lith ND, Zaat JCA. The perimenopausal symptoms. Med Gynecol Sociol 4:268, 1969.
52. Thompson B, Hart SA, Durno D. Menopausal age and symptomatology in general practice. J Biol Sci 5:71, 1973.
53. Judd HL. Menopause and postmenopause. *In* Benson R (ed). Current Obstetric and Gynecologic Diagnosis and Treatment. Los Altos, CA, Lange Medical Publications, 1980, p 510.
54. Molnar GW. Body temperatures during menopausal hot flashes. J Appl Physiol 38:499, 1975.
55. Meldrum DR, Shamonki IM, Frumar AM, et al. Elevations in skin temperature of the finger as an objective index of postmenopausal hot flashes: Standardization of the technique. Am J Obstet Gynecol 135:713, 1979.
56. Sturdee DW, Wilson KA, Pipili E, Crocker AD. Physiological aspects of menopausal hot flush. Br Med J 2:79, 1978.
57. Sturdee DW, Reece BL. Thermography of menopausal hot flushes. Maturitas 1:201, 1979.
58. Tataryn IV, Lomax P, Bajorek JG, et al. Postmenopausal hot flushes: A disorder of thermoregulation. Maturitas 2:101, 1980.
59. Meldrum DR, Tataryn IV, Frumar AM, et al. Gonadotropins, estrogens and adrenal steroids during the menopausal hot flush. J Clin Endocrinol Metab 50:685, 1980.
60. Tataryn IV, Meldrum DR, Lu KH, et al. LH, FSH, and skin temperature during the menopausal hot flash. J Clin Endocrinol Metab 49:152, 1979.
61. Casper RF, Yen SSC, Wilkes MM. Menopausal flushes: A neuroendocrine link with pulsatile luteinizing hormone secretion. Science 205:823, 1979.
62. Genazzani AR, Petraglia F, Fucchinetti F, et al. Increase of proopiomelanocortin-related peptides during subjective menopausal flushes. Am J Obstet Gynecol 149:775, 1984.
63. Nordin BEC. Clinical significance and pathogenesis of osteoporosis. Br Med J 1:571, 1971.
64. Rogers J. Estrogens in the menopause and postmenopause. N Engl J Med 280:364, 1969.
65. Eriksen EF, Colvard DS, Berg NJ, et al. Evidence of estrogen receptors in normal human osteoblast-like cells. Science 241:84, 1988.
66. Komm BS, Terpening CM, Benz DJ, et al. Estrogen binding receptor on RNA, and biologic response in osteoblast-like osteosarcoma cells. Science 241:81, 1988.
67. Globus R, Plovet J, Gospodarowicz D. Cultured bovine bone cells synthesize basic fibroblast growth factor and store it in their extracellular matrix. Endocrinology 124:1539, 1989.
68. Meema S, Meema HE. Menopausal bone loss and estrogen replacement. Isr J Med Sci 12:601, 1976.
69. Aitken JM, Hart DM, Lindsay R, et al. Prevention of bone loss following oophorectomy in premenopausal women. A retrospective assessment of the effects of oophorectomy and a prospective controlled trial of the effects of mestranol therapy. Isr J Med Sci 12:607, 1976.
70. Riggs BJ, Jowsey J, Kelley PJ, Arnaud CD. Role of hormonal factors in the pathogenesis of postmenopausal osteoporosis. Isr J Med Sci 12:615, 1976.
71. Chesnut CH III, Baylin OJ, Sison K, et al. Basal plasma immunoreactive calcitonin in postmenopausal osteoporosis. Metabolism 29:559, 1980.
72. Taggart HM, Chesnut CH III, Ivey JL, et al. Deficient calcitonin response to calcium stimulation in postmenopausal osteoporosis? Lancet 1:473, 1982.
73. Tiegs RD, Body JJ, Wahner HW, et al. Calcitonin secretion in postmenopausal osteoporosis. N Engl J Med 312:1097, 1985.
74. Laitinen O. Relation to osteoporosis of age- and hormone-induced changes in the metabolism of collagen and bone. Isr J Med Sci 12:620, 1976.
75. Daniell HW. Osteoporosis of the slender smoker. Arch Intern Med 136:298, 1976.
76. Knowelden J, Buhr J, Dunbar O. Incidence of fractures in persons over 35 years of age. Br J Prev Soc Med 18:130, 1964.
77. Lindsay R, Hart DM, MacLean A, et al. Bone response to termination of oestrogen treatment. Lancet 1:1325, 1978.
78. Lindsay R, Coutts JR, Hart DM. The effect of endogenous oestrogen on plasma and urinary calcium and phosphate in oophorectomized women. Clin Endocrinol (Oxf) 6:87, 1977.
79. Pullan BR, Roberts TE. Bone mineral measurements using an EMI scanner and standard methods: A comparative study. Br J Radiol 51:24, 1978.
80. Madsen M, Peppler W, Mazess RB. Vertebral and total body mineral content by dual photon absorptiometry. *In* Pors-Nielsen S, Hjorting-Hansen E (eds). Calcified Tissues 1975. Copenhagen, FADL Publishing, 1976, p 361.
81. Cann CE, Genant HK, Ettinger B, Gordon GS. Spinal mineral loss in oophorectomized women: Determination by quantitative computed tomography. JAMA 244:2056, 1980.
82. Stampfer MJ, Colditz GA, Willett WC, et al. Postmenopausal estrogen therapy and cardiovascular disease: Ten-year follow-up from the Nurses' Health Study. N Engl J Med 325:756, 1991.
82a. Hulley S, Grady D, Bush T, et al. Randomized trial of estrogen

plus progestin for secondary prevention of coronary heart disease in postmenopausal women. JAMA 280:605, 1998.
83. Lieberman E, Gerhard M, Uehata A, et al. Estrogen improves endothelium-dependent, flow-mediated vasodilation in postmenopausal women. Ann Intern Med 121:936, 1994.
84. Ylikorkala O, Orpana A, Puolakka J, et al. Postmenopausal hormonal replacement decreases plasma levels of endothelin-1. J Clin Endocrinol Metab 80:3384, 1995.
85. Henden S. Ischaemic heart disease in women. *In* Schettler FG, Boyd GS (eds). Atherosclerosis. New York, American Elsevier, 1971, p 289.
86. Armstrong A, Duncan B, Oliver MF, et al. Natural history of acute coronary heart attacks. A community study. Br Heart J 34:67, 1972.
87. Oliver MF, Boyd GS. Effect of bilateral ovariectomy on coronary artery disease and serum lipid levels. Lancet 2:690, 1959.
88. Snajderman M, Oliver MF. Spontaneous premature menopause, ischaemic heart disease and serum lipids. Lancet 1:962, 1963.
89. Tang M-X, Jacobs D, Stern Y, et al. Effects of oestrogen during menopause on risk and age of onset of Alzheimer's disease. Lancet 348:429, 1996.
90. Sohrabji F, Miranda RC, Toran-Allerand CD. Estrogen differentially regulates estrogen and nerve growth factor receptor mRNAs in adult sensory neurons. J Neurosci 14:459, 1994.
91. Jaffe AB, Toran-Allerand CD, Greengard P, Gandy SE. Estrogen regulates metabolism of Alzheimer amyloid beta precursor protein. J Biol Chem 269:13065, 1994.
92. Newcomb PA, Storer BE. Postmenopausal hormone use and risk of large bowel cancer. J Natl Cancer Inst 87:1067, 1995.
93. Calle EE, Miracle-McMahill HL, Thunb MJ, Heath CW Jr. Estrogen replacement therapy and risk of fatal cancer in a prospective cohort of postmenopausal women. J Natl Cancer Inst 87:517, 1995.
94. Paganini-Hill A. The benefits of estrogen replacement therapy on oral health: The Leisure World cohort. Arch Intern Med 155:2325, 1995.
95. Nevitt MC, Cummings SR, Lane NE, et al. Association of estrogen replacement therapy with the risk of osteoarthritis in elderly women. Arch Intern Med 156:2073, 1996.
96. Smith DC, Prentice R, Thompson DJ, Herrmann WL. Association of exogenous estrogen and endometrial carcinoma. N Engl J Med 293:1164, 1975.
97. Weiss N. Risk and benefits of estrogen use. N Engl J Med 293:1200, 1975.
98. Ziel HK, Finkle WD. Increased risk of endometrial carcinoma among users of conjugated estrogens. N Engl J Med 293:1167, 1975.
99. Hoover RL, Gray A, Cole P, MacMahon B. Menopausal estrogens and breast cancer. N Engl J Med 293:1167, 1976.
100. Bergkvist L, Adami H-O, Persson I, et al. The risk of breast cancer after estrogen and estrogen-progestin replacement. N Engl J Med 321:393, 1989.
101. Grodstein F, Stampfer MJ, Manson JE, et al. Postmenopausal estrogen and progestin use and the risk of cardiovascular disease. N Engl J Med 335:453, 1996.
102. Newcomb PA, Storer BE. Postmenopausal hormone use and risk of large bowel cancer. J Natl Cancer Inst 87:1067, 1995.
103. Genant HK, Cann CE, Ettinger B, Gordon GS. Quantitative computed tomography of vertebral spongiosa: A sensitive method for detecting early bone loss after oophorectomy. Ann Intern Med 97:699, 1982.
104. Ettinger B, Genant HK, Cann CE. Postmenopausal bone loss is prevented by treatment with low-dosage estrogen with calcium. Ann Intern Med 106:40, 1987.
105. The Writing Group for the PEPI (Postmenopausal Estrogen/Progestin Interventions) Trial. Effects of hormone therapy on bone mineral density: Results from the postmenopausal estrogen/progestin interventions (PEPI) trial. JAMA 276:1389, 1996.
106. Felson DT, Zhang Y, Hannan MT, et al. The effect of postmenopausal estrogen therapy on bone density in older women. N Engl J Med 329:1141, 1993.
107. Campbell S, Whitehead M. Oestrogen therapy and the menopausal syndrome. Clin Obstet Gynecol 4:31, 1977.
108. Whitehead MI, McQueen J, Minardi J, Campbell S. Clinical considerations in the management of the menopause: The endometrium. Postgrad Med J (suppl) 54:69, 1978.
109. Whitehead MI, King RJB, McQueen J, Campbell S. Endometrial histology and biochemistry in climacteric women during oestrogen and oestrogen/progestogen therapy. J R Soc Med 72:322, 1979.
110. Paterson MEL, Wade-Evans T, Sturdee DW, et al. Endometrial disease after treatment with estrogens and progestogens in the climacteric. Br Med J 1:822, 1980.
111. Gambrell RD Jr, Massey FM, Castaneda TA, et al. Use of progestogen challenge test to reduce risk of endometrial cancer. Obstet Gynecol 55:732, 1980.
112. Weinstein MC, Schiff I. Cost-effectiveness of hormone replacement therapy in the menopause. Obstet Gynecol Surv 38:445, 1983.
113. Yen SSC, Martin PL, Burnier AM, et al. Circulating estradiol, estrone and gonadotropin levels following the administration of orally active 17-β estradiol in postmenopausal women. J Clin Endocrinol Metab 40:518, 1975.
114. Rigg LA, Millanes B, Villanueva B, Yen SSC. Efficacy of intravaginal and intranasal administration of micronized estradiol-17β. J Clin Endocrinol Metab 95:1261, 1977.
115. Sitruk-Ware R, deLignieres B, Basdevat A, Mauvais-Jarvis P. Absorption of percutaneous oestradiol in postmenopausal women. Maturitas 2:207, 1980.
116. Hsueh AJW, Peck EJ, Clark JH. Progesterone antagonism of estrogen receptor and estrogen induced uterine growth. Nature 254:337, 1975.
117. Reginster JY, Deroisy R, Denis D, et al. Prevention of postmenopausal bone loss by tiludronate. Lancet 2:1469, 1989.
118. Storm T, Thamsborg G, Steiniche T, et al. Effect of intermittent cyclical etidronate therapy on bone mass and fracture rate in women with postmenopausal osteoporosis. N Engl J Med 322:1265, 1990.
119. Watts NB, Harris ST, Genant HK, et al. Intermittent cyclical etidronate treatment of postmenopausal osteoporosis. N Engl J Med 323:73, 1990.
120. Wimalawanse C. Combined therapy with estrogen and etidronate has an additive effect on bone mineral density in the hip and vertebrae: four-year randomized study. Am J Med 99:36, 1995.
121. Liberman UA, Weiss SR, Broll J, et al, for the Alendronate Phase III Osteoporosis Treatment Study Group. Effect of oral alendronate on bone mineral density and the incidence of fractures in postmenopausal osteoporosis. N Engl J Med 333:1437, 1995.
122. Katzenellenbogen BS, Kendra KL, Norman MJ, Berthois Y. Proliferation, hormonal responsiveness, and estrogen receptor content of MCF-7 human breast cancer cells grown in the short-term and long-term absence of estrogens. Cancer Res 47:4355, 1987.
123. Trichopoulos D, MacMahon B, Cole P. Menopause and breast cancer risk. J Natl Cancer Inst 48:605, 1972.
124. Spicer DV, Pike MC. Epidemiology of breast cancer. *In* Lobo RA (ed). Treatment of the Postmenopausal Woman: Basic and Clinical Aspects. New York, Raven Press, 1994, pp 315–324.
125. Henderson BE, Pike MC, Casagrande JT. Breast cancer and the oestrogen window hypothesis. Lancet 2:363, 1981.
126. Henderson BE, Ross RK, Judd HL, et al. Do regular ovulatory cycles increase breast cancer risk? Cancer 56:1206, 1985.
127. Colditz GA, Harkinson SE, Hunter DJ, et al. The use of estrogens and progestins and the risk of breast cancer in postmenopausal women. N Engl J Med 332:1589, 1995.
128. Stanford JL, Weiss NS, Voight LF, et al. Combined estrogen and progestin hormone replacement therapy in relation to risk of breast cancer in middle-aged women. JAMA 274:137, 1995.
129. Col NF, Eckman MH, Karas RH, et al. Patient-specific decisions about hormone replacement therapy in postmenopausal women. JAMA 277:1140, 1997.
130. Grodstein F, Stempfer MJ, Colditz GA, et al. Postmenopausal hormone therapy and mortality. N Engl J Med 336:1769, 1997.
131. Jick H, Derby L, Myers M, et al. Risk of hospital admission for idiopathic venous thromboembolism among users of postmenopausal oestrogens. Lancet 348:983, 1996.
132. Grodstein F, Stampfer M, Goldhaber S, et al. Prospective study of exogenous hormones and risk of pulmonary embolism in women. Lancet 348:983, 1996.
133. Daly E, Vessey M, Hawkins M, et al. Risk of venous thromboembolism in users of hormone replacement therapy. Lancet 348:977, 1996.

134. Conway GS. Clinical manifestations of genetic defects affecting gonadotropins and their receptors. Clin Endocrinol (Oxf) 45:657, 1996.
135. Richardson SJ, Senikas V, Nelson JF. Follicular depletion during the menopausal transition: Evidence for accelerated loss and ultimate exhaustion. J Clin Endocrinol Metab 65:1231, 1987.
136. Luborsky JL, Visintin S, Boyers T, et al. Ovarian antibodies detected by immobilized antigen immunoassay in patients with premature ovarian failure. J Clin Endocrinol Metab 70:69, 1990.
137. Moncayo J, Moncayo R, Benz R, et al. Ovarian failure and autoimmunity. J Clin Invest 84:1857, 1990.
138. Rebar RW, Erickson GF, Yen SSC. Idiopathic premature ovarian failure: Clinical and endocrine characteristics. Fertil Steril 37:35, 1982.
139. Golonka JE, Goodman AD. Coexistence of primary ovarian insufficiency, primary adrenocortical insufficiency, and idiopathic hypoparathyroidism. J Clin Endocrinol Metab 28:79, 1968.
140. Irvine WJ, Chan MMW, Scarth L, et al. Immunological aspects of premature ovarian failure associated with idiopathic Addison's disease. Lancet 2:883, 1968.
141. Rebar RW, Connolly HV. Clinical features of young women with hypergonadotropic amenorrhea. Fertil Steril 53:804, 1990.
142. Hartman ML, Veldhuis JD, Thorner MO. Normal control of growth hormone secretion. Horm Res 40:37, 1993.
143. Daughday WH, Rotwein P. Insulin-like growth factors I and II: Peptide, messenger ribonucleic acid and gene structures, serum, and tissue concentrations. Endocr Rev 10:68, 1989.
144. Hartman ML, Clayton PE, Johnson ML, et al. A low-dose euglycemic infusion of recombinant human insulin-like growth factor-I rapidly suppresses fasting-enhanced pulsatile growth hormone secretion in humans. J Clin Invest 91:2453, 1993.
145. Zadik Z, Chaleu SA, McCarter RJ, et al. The influence of age on 24-hour integrated concentration of growth hormone in normal individuals. J Clin Endocrinol Metab 60:513, 1985.
146. Iranmanesh A, Lizzaralde G, Veldhuis JD. Age and relative adiposity are specific negative determinants of the frequency and amplitude of growth hormone (GH) secretory bursts and the half-life of endogenous GH in healthy men. J Clin Endocrinol Metab 73:1081, 1991.
147. Corpas E, Harman SM, Pineyro MA, et al. Growth hormone (GH)–releasing hormone (1-29) twice daily reverses the decreased GH and insulin-like growth factor-I levels in old men. J Clin Endocrinol Metab 75:530, 1992.
148. Khorram O, Laughlin GA, Yen SSC. Endocrine and metabolic effects of long term administration of [Nle 27] growth-hormone releasing hormone–(1-29)-NH_2 in age-advanced men and women. J Clin Endocrinol Metab 82:1472, 1997.
149. Ho KY, Evans WS, Blizzard RM, et al. Effects of sex and age on the 24-hour profile of growth hormone in man: Importance of endogenous estradiol concentrations. J Clin Endocrinol Metab 64:51, 1987.
150. Dawson-Hughes B, Stern D, Goldman J, Reichlin S. Regulation of growth hormone and somatomedin-C secretion in postmenopausal women: Effect of physiologic estrogen replacement. J Clin Endocrinol Metab 63:424, 1986.
151. Weissberger AJ, Ho KKY, Lazarus L. Contrasting effects of oral and transdermal routes of estrogen replacement therapy on 24-hour growth hormone (GH) secretion, insulin-like growth factor I, and GH-binding protein. J Clin Endocrinol Metab 72:374, 1991.
152. Bowers CY, Sartor AO, Reynolds GA, Badger TM. On the actions of the growth hormone–releasing hexapeptide, GHRP. Endocrinology 128:2027, 1991.
153. Huhn WC, Harman ML, Pezzoli SS, Thorner MO. 24-Hour growth hormone (GH)–releasing peptide (GHRP) infusion enhances pulsatile GH secretion and specifically attenuates the response to a subsequent GHRP bolus. J Clin Endocrinol Metab 76:1202, 1993.
154. Ghigo E, Arvat E, Giamotti L, et al. Growth hormone–releasing activity of hexarelin, a new synthetic hexapeptide, after intravenous, subcutaneous, intranasal, and oral administration in man. J Clin Endocrinol Metab 78:693, 1994.
155. Pong SS, Chaung LYP, Dean DC, et al. Identification of a new G-protein–linked receptor for growth hormone secretagogues. Mol Endocrinol 10:57, 1996.
156. de Boer H, Blok G-J, Van der Veen EA. Clinical aspects of growth hormone deficiency in adults. Endocr Rev 16:63, 1995.
157. Chapman IM, Bach MA, Van Cauter E, et al. Stimulation of the growth hormone (GH)/insulin-like growth factor-I axis by daily oral administration of a GH secretagogue (MK-677) in healthy elderly subjects. J Clin Endocrinol Metab 81:4249, 1996.
158. Holloway L, Butterfield G, Hintz RL, et al. Effects of recombinant human growth hormone on metabolic indices, body composition, and bone turnover in healthy elderly women. J Clin Endocrinol Metab 79:470, 1994.
159. Morales AJ, Nolan JJ, Nelson JC, Yen SSC. Effects of replacement doses of dehydroepiandrosterone in men and women of advancing age. J Clin Endocrinol Metab 78:1360, 1994.
160. Berr C, Lafont S, Debaire B, et al. Relationships of dehydroepiandrosterone sulfate in the elderly with functional, psychological, and mental status, and short-term mortality: A French community-based study. Proc Natl Acad Sci USA 93:13410, 1996.
161. Wolkowitz O, Reus VI, Roberts E, et al. Dehydroepiandrosterone (DHEA) treatment of depression. Biol Psychiatry 41:311, 1997.
162. Mellon SH, Deschepper SF. Neurosteroid biosynthesis: Genes for adrenal steroidogenic enzymes are expressed in the brain. Brain Res 629:283, 1993.
163. Mellon SH. Neurosteroids: Biochemistry, modes of action, and clinical relevance. J Clin Endocrinol Metab 78:1003, 1994.
164. Compagne NA, Bulfone A, Rubenstein JLR, Mellon SH. Steroidogenic enzyme p450c17 is expressed in the embryonic central nervous system. Endocrinology 136:5212, 1995.
165. Corpechot C, Robel P, Axelson M, et al. Characterization and measurement of dehydroepiandrosterone sulfate in rat brain. Proc Natl Acad Sci USA 78:4704, 1981.
166. Baulieu E-E. Neurosteroids: A new function in the brain. Biol Cell 71:3, 1991.
167. Flood JF, Smith GE, Roberts E. Dehydroepiandrosterone and its sulfate enhance memory retention in mice. Brain Res 447:269, 1988.
168. Mortola J, Yen SSC. The effects of oral dehydroepiandrosterone on endocrine-metabolic parameters in postmenopausal women. J Clin Endocrinol Metab 71:696, 1990.
169. Robel P, Baulieu E-E. Dehydroepiandrosterone (DHEA) is a neuroactive neurosteroid. Ann N Y Acad Sci 774:82, 1995.
170. Robel P, Baulieu E-E. Neurosteroids: Biosynthesis and function. Trends Endocrinol Metab 5:1, 1994.
171. Reus VI, Wolkowitz OW, Roberts E, et al. Dehydroepiandrosterone (DHEA) and memory in depressed patients. Neuropsychopharmacology 9:665, 1993.
172. Wolkowitz OM, Reus VI, Roberts E, et al. Antidepressant and cognition-enhancing effects of DHEA in major depression. Ann NY Acad Sci 774:337, 1995.
173. Van Cauter E, Leproult R, Kupfer DJ. Effects of gender and age on the levels and circadian rhythmicity of plasma cortisol. J Clin Endocrinol Metab 81:2468, 1996.

Part II

Pathophysiology

Chapter 12

CYTOGENETICS IN REPRODUCTION

Cynthia C. Morton • Patricia Miron

■ CHAPTER OUTLINE

KEY POINTS

- Chromosome abnormalities are a common cause of infertility, pregnancy loss, and birth defects.
- Classical cytogenetics has been successful in identifying many chromosome abnormalities, particularly abnormalities involving chromosome number and gross chromosome rearrangements.
- The advent of molecular cytogenetics has further increased the number of diagnosable abnormalities because it allows detection of smaller deletions and lower levels of mosaicism.
- Unlike a general karyotype, which provides information about all the chromosomes, molecular diagnostic tests are specific and are generally recommended only after clinical suspicion of a specific abnormality.
- Chromosome analysis is indicated in both the prenatal and postnatal settings.
- In the prenatal setting, classical chromosome analysis is generally performed for pregnancies at risk for a chromosomal abnormality because of advanced maternal age, abnormal triple panel, or a familial chromosomal abnormality.
- Postnatally, chromosome analysis is performed for individuals with a clinical phenotype indicative of a chromosome abnormality and for phenotypically normal individuals with reproductive problems including infertility, multiple spontaneous abortions, or a chromosomally abnormal child.
- Table 12–1 lists the major indications for chromosome analysis in reproductive endocrinology.

Cytogenetics is the area of biology that deals with the study of chromosomes. Classical cytogenetics provides an overview of the genome and allows the identification of chromosome rearrangements and numerical abnormalities. Molecular cytogenetics permits a finer examination of specific areas of the genome and has been a powerful tool in gene mapping. Application of molecular cytogenetic techniques, particularly fluorescence in situ hybridization (FISH), in the clinical laboratory now makes possible routine diagnosis of microdeletion syndromes and cryptic chromosome rearrangements. Further, FISH provides a means to assess ploidy of any chromosome both in uncultured cells largely for rapid diagnosis of trisomy and in archival materials, which previously were not easily evaluated.

Cytogenetics is a critical component of reproductive endocrinology. Chromosome abnormalities are a common cause of infertility and pregnancy loss as well as of sexual dysmorphology. Most chromosomally abnormal conceptions arise de novo after a meiotic nondisjunction event, but chromosomal anomalies in some conceptuses are inherited from a chromosomally abnormal parent. The chromosome abnormality in these conceptuses may or may not be identical to that of the parent, depending on recombination and segregation of chromosomes during gametogenesis. Although some chromosome aberrations cause clear phenotypic abnormalities, other aberrations have no apparent phenotypic effect. Carriers of these apparently phenotypically neutral chromosome aberrations may still produce chromosomally unbalanced gametes and, as such, may be identified after multiple pregnancy losses or the birth of an abnormal child.

ORGANIZATION OF HUMAN CHROMOSOMES AND METHODS OF STUDY

The human chromosome is a complex structure that consists of deoxyribonucleic acid (DNA), ribonucleic acid

■ TABLE 12–1
Reasons to Request a Patient's Karyotype or Fluorescence In Situ Hybridization

CLINICAL INDICATION	TEST*	POSSIBLE CHROMOSOME ABNORMALITY
Couple with 3 or more spontaneous abortions	K	Balanced structural rearrangement
Parent of child with structural chromosome abnormality	K	Balanced structural rearrangement
First-degree relative with structural chromosome abnormality	K	Balanced structural rearrangement
Female expressing X-linked disorder	K	X;autosome translocation or 45,X
Female below 10th percentile in height	K	45,X—possibly mosaic
Female with elevated gonadotropins	K	45,X—possibly mosaic
Female with infertility/ ?ovarian dysgenesis	K	Structural rearrangement of X
Male with elevated gonadotropins, whether		
Tall	K	47,XXY
Short	K	45,X/46,XY
Normal height	K	46,XX (follow up with PCR for Y material)
Gynecomastia	K	47,XXY
Azoospermia or oligospermia	K	Balanced structural rearrangements, particularly involving sex chromosomes; deletions in Yq
Sexual ambiguity	K	
Associated with Wilms' tumor, aniridia	F	11p13 deletion
Hypogonadism and other features of Prader-Willi syndrome	F	15q11q13 deletion

*K, karyotype; F, fluorescence in situ hybridization; PCR, polymerase chain reaction.

(RNA), and protein. A single helix of DNA is bounded on each end by a structure known as a telomere. Each normal human chromosome has one centromere. The centromere is the site at which the kinetochore forms for attachment of the mitotic spindle, which is required for proper segregation of the chromosome during cell division. The centromere divides the chromosome into two arms that are identified as p (petit) for the short arm and q for the long arm. In human chromosomes, the position of the centromere is central (metacentric), distal (acrocentric), or somewhere in between (submetacentric), providing a useful landmark in the identification of a particular chromosome. At the tip of the short arms of the acrocentric chromosomes (13, 14, 15, 21, and 22) are satellites, variably sized structures composed of heterochromatin. Satellites are attached to the chromosome through a secondary constriction known as a satellite stalk. These satellite stalks contain the genes for 18S, 5.8S, and 28S ribosomal RNA. At the end of every chromosome arm is a telomere, a structure composed of tandemly repeated short nucleotide sequences (Fig. 12–1).

Human chromosomes vary in size, with the largest chromosome designated number 1. In 1956, Tjio and Levan[1] determined the total number of human chromosomes to be 46 with 22 pairs of autosomes and 1 pair of sex chromosomes. With the exception of pairs 21 and 22, the numerical designation reflects the size of the chromosome (e.g., chromosome 4 is the fourth largest chromosome in the human complement). Although chromosome 21 is smaller than chromosome 22, this inconsistency in nomenclature has been perpetuated to avoid confusion due to historical references to Down syndrome as trisomy 21.

A karyotype is a display of chromosomes from largest to smallest (except for pairs 21 and 22) with the chromosomes oriented so that the p arm is on top (Fig. 12–2). In humans, the female is the homogametic sex, and a normal female karyotype is designated 46,XX. The male is the heterogametic sex, and a normal male karyotype is described as 46,XY. Excluding chromosome abnormalities and variants, karyotypes of two unrelated males or females may appear virtually identical; furthermore, excluding sex chromosomes, karyotypes of males and females are indistinguishable.

Methods in Classical Cytogenetics

Metaphase Preparations of Cultured Cells

Most cytogenetic analyses are performed on chromosomes that are in metaphase of mitosis. The metaphase cell can reveal both numerical and structural abnormalities. At this stage of the cell cycle, condensation of chromosomal DNA results in distinguishable entities that are characteristic for each species. Special studies to investigate a particular region of a chromosome may require less condensed chromosomes such as those found in prometaphase.

The most frequently used tissues for cytogenetic evaluation, primarily because of their accessibility, are peripheral

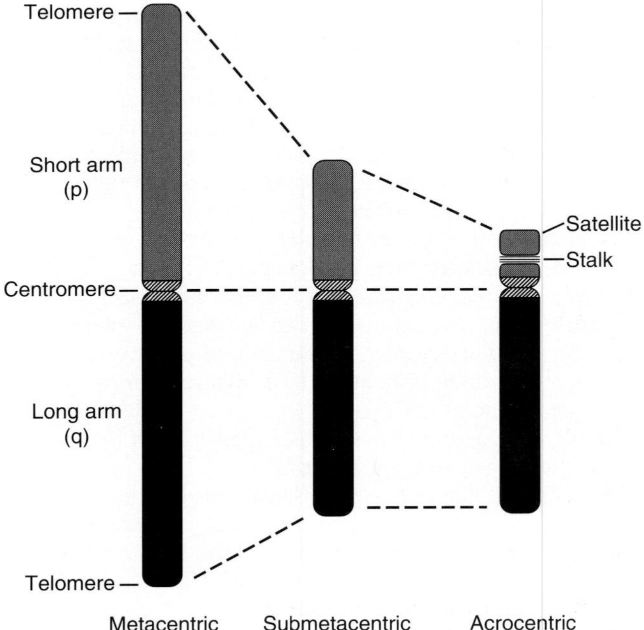

Figure 12–1 ■ Schematic diagram of prototypic human chromosomes demonstrating metacentric, submetacentric, and acrocentric chromosomes. The locations of the telomere, centromere, short arm (p), and long arm (q) are indicated. The locations of the satellite and stalk, characteristic of a human acrocentric chromosome, are indicated on the acrocentric chromosome.

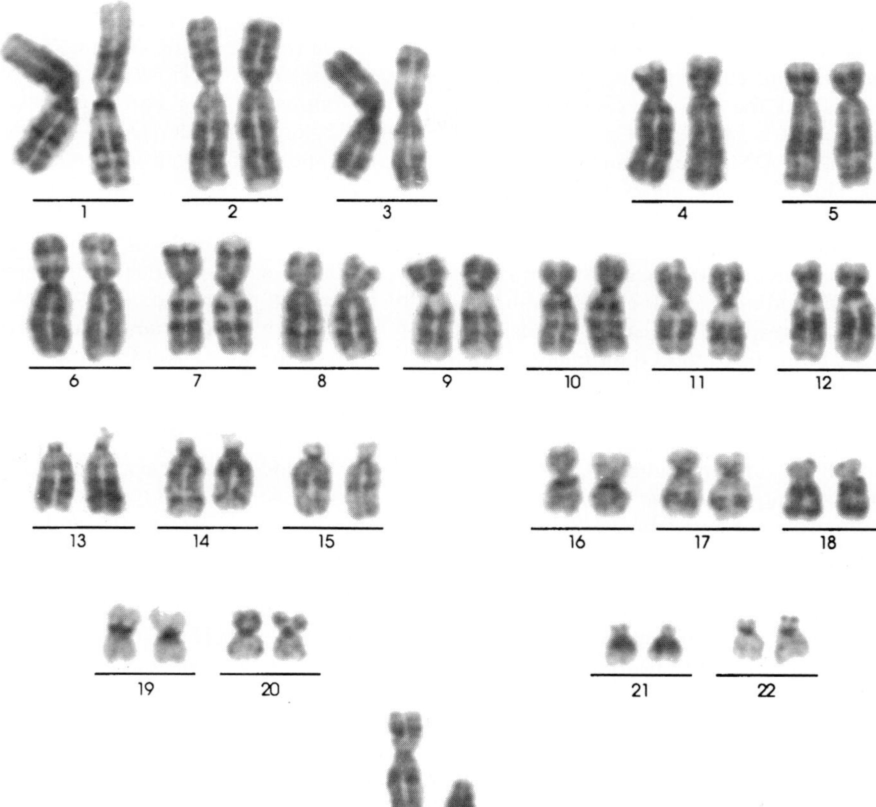

Figure 12–2 ■ A representative normal human male GTG-banded karyotype (46,XY).

blood lymphocytes, amniotic fluid cells, chorionic villi, skin fibroblasts, bone marrow, and solid tumors. The process of preparing chromosomes for analysis is known as a harvest. Chromosomes are harvested either after culture of the tissue or, in the case of bone marrow, some solid tumors, cytotrophoblast and cord blood, after direct harvest of mitotic cells. The harvest itself may be performed in solution, as is commonly done for lymphocyte cultures and for other cultures in which attached cells have been released from the tissue culture vessel, or it may be performed in situ, that is, attached to the tissue culture surface. The in situ procedure is frequently used for amniotic fluid cultures when it is desirable to evaluate colonies of cells to ascertain possible chromosomal mosaicism.

In all cases, dividing cells must be arrested during mitosis. This is accomplished by addition of colchicine to the culture. Colchicine destroys the mitotic spindle and thus arrests cells in metaphase. After incubation in colchicine, the harvest proceeds with a hypotonic treatment, which swells the cells. Several rounds of fixation complete the harvest. Depending on the type of harvest that has been performed, metaphases will now be either dropped onto slides if they have been harvested in solution or spread on a coverslip or slide if they have been harvested in situ. Preparation of slides or coverslips after the harvest is one of the most crucial steps in obtaining quality material for analysis. Factors that influence surface tension such as temperature and humidity are doubtless critical variables in slide making.

Banding Techniques

Before the development of banding techniques, not all chromosomes could be distinguished, and they were grouped according to their size and centromere position. Today, several different banding techniques are used routinely in cytogenetics and allow the unequivocal identification of each (normal) chromosome. The most popular banding techniques are GTG-banding, QFQ-banding, and RHG-banding (Fig. 12–3).

In the United States, GTG-banding, also known as G-banding, is the most commonly used method. This method of banding produces a pattern of alternating light and dark bands that allows identification of each chromosome pair by bright field microscopy. Investigations of chromosome banding patterns with antinucleotide antibodies indicate

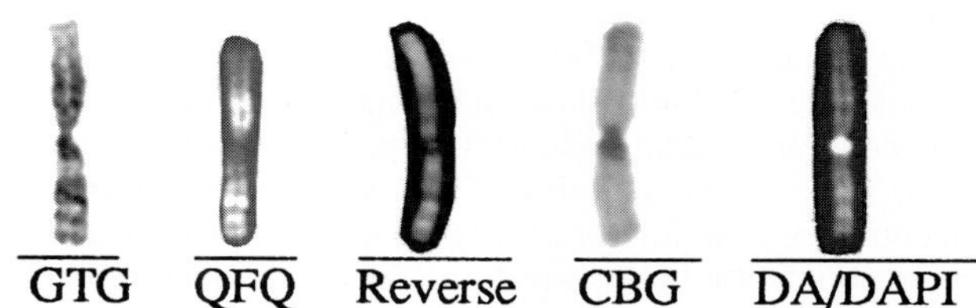

Figure 12–3 ■ Chromosome 1 shown after various banding techniques—GTG, QFQ, reverse, CBG, and DA/DAPI. The three letter code banding designations refer to the type of banding, the method used, and the stain employed (e.g., GTG = G-banding by trypsin with Giemsa).[25]

that light G bands are predominantly GC rich and that dark G bands are AT rich.[2] Light G bands are believed to contain more euchromatin, DNA that is replicated early in S phase of the cell cycle and is transcribed. In contrast, dark G bands are thought to be composed largely of heterochromatin, DNA that is more condensed and late replicating. Housekeeping genes reside in the light G bands and most tissue-specific genes appear to be situated in the dark G bands.[3–5]

Q-banding, a fluorescent staining procedure, produces a pattern similar to that of G-banding; brightly fluorescent bands correspond to G dark bands, and dully fluorescent bands correspond to G light bands. Q-banding is one of the most commonly used techniques for studying chromosomal heteromorphisms associated with the centromeres of chromosomes 3, 4, 13, and 22, the short arms and satellites of acrocentric chromosomes (13, 14, 15, 21, and 22), and the distal region of the Y chromosome. In general, these polymorphisms are stable heritable markers without clinical significance.[6–8] In the past, they were valuable tools in the determination of both paternity[9] and the parental origin of the extra chromosome in a trisomy,[10, 11] but much more informative molecular markers are now used to make these determinations. Chromosome polymorphisms are still useful today, particularly because they may indicate maternal cell admixture in a culture of amniotic fluid cells or a tissue sample from an abortus.[12]

Reverse banding or R-banding produces a banding pattern that is essentially the opposite of that seen with G-banding or Q-banding. In other words, a light G band will be a dark R band and vice versa. Terminal regions of many chromosomes tend to be pale by G-banding or Q-banding, and small deletions or rearrangements in these regions may be difficult to detect. In such cases, an R-banded preparation may make such an aberration visible. Protocols exist for both bright field and fluorescent R-banding.

Special Stains

Special staining techniques have been developed to assist in analysis of particular chromosomes or regions of particular chromosomes. For example, C-banding or centric banding is particularly useful in analysis of centromeres.[13] This technique involves acid treatment of metaphase chromosomes followed by incubation in alkali (e.g., barium hydroxide), then staining in Giemsa. The basis of the banding is that a different type of chromatin, known as constitutive heterochromatin, is present in the centromeric regions of all normal chromosomes and the distal portion of the Y chromosome. Constitutive heterochromatin consists of DNA that remains condensed and genetically inactive. A second, special type of heterochromatin present in the X chromosome, facultative heterochromatin, may decondense and become genetically active. Chromosomes 1, 9, and 16 tend to have larger amounts of C-banded material in the pericentromeric region; considerable variation exists in the human population.[14] An inversion in the pericentromeric region of chromosome 9 is another common polymorphism, and C-banding may be used to show that such an inversion is limited to heterochromatin.[15] C-banding is also commonly used to elucidate the structure of unidentified marker chromosomes or derivative chromosomes.

Other special stains are silver staining, also known as NOR staining,[16] which identifies active nucleolar organizer regions (i.e., sites of the ribosomal RNA genes) on acrocentric chromosomes; and distamycin A/diamidinophenylindole (DA/DAPI) staining,[17] which reacts with centromeres of chromosomes 1, 9, and 16, the short arm of chromosome 15, and the distal end of the Y chromosome. More recently, banding patterns have been produced with a combination of molecular genetic and cytogenetic techniques. For example, enzymatic digestion of chromosomes with restriction endonucleases[18] and hybridization with repetitive DNA sequences[19] have produced banding patterns reminiscent of G and C bands and of R bands, respectively.

High-Resolution Banding

In general, clinical laboratories perform banding techniques on chromosomes in mid-metaphase, at which time 350 to 400 bands can be resolved. Other techniques that enrich for chromosomes in earlier stages of metaphase or in prophase provide higher resolution banding methods and are used when a particular region of a chromosome is being studied. High-resolution methods in practice include amethopterin synchronization of cell cultures with thymidine release[20] and addition of actinomycin D (dactinomycin)[21, 22] or ethidium bromide[23] to the final hours of culture before harvest.

Idiograms and Chromosome Nomenclature

An idiogram is a schematic standardized karyotype that is derived from measured band sizes (Fig. 12–4). The idiogram and chromosome nomenclature have been designed by an international committee that has met periodically since 1960 to establish uniform language for describing chromosome bands and chromosome aberrations.[24] Chromosome regions are subdivided into bands and, at higher resolution, into subbands. For example, the designation 14q24 indicates chromosome 14, the long arm, region 2, band 4. On the idiogram, chromosome bands are numbered in an ascending manner from centromere to telomere on each arm of the chromosome.

A fairly sophisticated set of rules governs the description of chromosome abnormalities; these rules are set out in the 1995 International System for Human Cytogenetic Nomenclature.[25] Basically, the total number of chromosomes is specified first, followed by the sex chromosomes (e.g., the normal male karyotype is given as 46,XY). Chromosome aberrations are listed with sex chromosome aberrations first, in the position of the normal sex chromosome, followed by abnormalities of the autosomes in numerical order irrespective of aberration type. For each chromosome, numerical abnormalities are listed before structural changes. Multiple structural changes of homologous chromosomes are presented in alphabetical order according to the abbreviated term of the abnormality.

Fluorescence In Situ Hybridization (FISH)

In situ hybridization was first used to determine the chromosomal location of particular DNA sequences.[26–30] Still a powerful tool for gene mapping, FISH is employed routinely in the clinical cytogenetics laboratory as well. It is

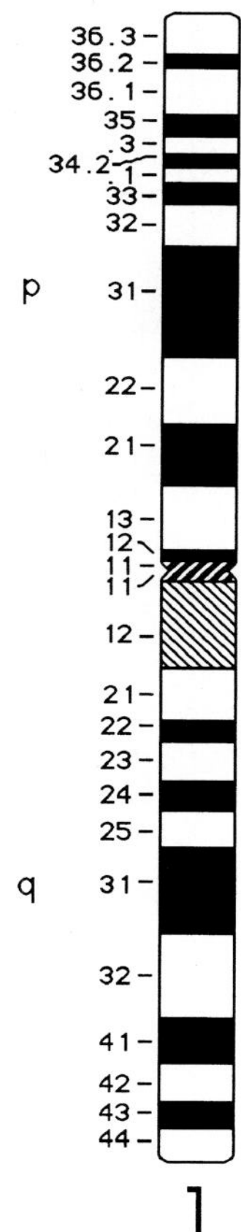

Figure 12–4 ■ Standardized idiogram of human chromosome 1 at the 400-band stage.

used on uncultured, interphase cells as a quick screen for detection of aneuploidy and on metaphase cells to detect a growing number of microdeletion syndromes. This methodology is also applied on metaphase chromosomes to characterize subtle chromosome rearrangements and to identify marker chromosomes, by definition unidentifiable by classical cytogenetics (Fig. 12–5).

Although in situ hybridization was first developed with isotopic probes, clinical laboratories now frequently use commercially available nonisotopic fluorescent probes. Probes are typically labeled with biotin or digoxigenin, which can be detected by highly specific fluorochrome-conjugated antibodies. Probes in which fluorochromes are directly conjugated to DNA are also currently available. Single-copy sequence probes, repetitive-element probes, and whole-chromosome paints can be visualized successfully with FISH. In general, repetitive-element probes hybridizing to particular centromere sequences are used in the detection of aneuploidy, single-sequence probes are used to detect microdeletions, and whole-chromosome paints are used to detect cryptic rearrangements and to identify marker chromosomes. Chromosome-specific centromeric probes are available for most chromosomes. However, the centromeric sequences of chromosome pairs 13 and 21 and pairs 14 and 22 are similar, and a commercially available probe has not yet been developed that selectively hybridizes to only one of the two chromosomes. Thus, to detect aneuploidy of these chromosomes, cosmid (unique sequences) probes are used. The disadvantage of cosmid probes relative to repetitive-element probes is that the intensity of the signal is generally weaker.

CHROMOSOME ABERRATIONS AND REPRODUCTION

Chromosome aberrations are common in humans and account for a large proportion of pregnancy loss and congenital malformations. Chromosome aberrations, especially aberrations of the X and Y chromosomes, can also be a cause of infertility. Common clinical practice for couples who have experienced two, three, or more spontaneous abortions includes full cytogenetic analysis. For the reproductive specialist, chromosome abnormalities can be divided into the following two clinically distinct groups: (1) chromosomally normal patients in whom a reproductive error results in a chromosomally abnormal conceptus, and (2) patients who have either a de novo or inherited constitutional chromosome anomaly with reproductive implications and perhaps other phenotypic effects.

Chromosome abnormalities arising during reproduction are fairly common; an estimated 8 percent of conceptuses possess a chromosome abnormality.[31–33] Most of these chromosomally abnormal products of conception are not viable, but an estimated 0.7 percent of livebirths are chromosomally abnormal.[34] Errors in gametogenesis are the most common cause of chromosomally abnormal conceptuses, but fertilization and post-fertilization errors also occur.

Gametogenesis Errors

Review of Oogenesis and Spermatogenesis

Meiosis, the cell division process producing haploid germ cells from diploid germ cell precursors, is the fundamental event in both oogenesis and spermatogenesis. The overall sequence of meiotic events is the same in oogenesis and spermatogenesis, but several key differences exist between these two processes.

In both female and male gametogenesis, the chromosome number is reduced by half, producing haploid gametes with 23 chromosomes. To produce haploid gametes, diploid germ cell precursor cells replicate their DNA and then undergo two successive cell divisions. The first cell division, meiosis I, is termed the reduction division, because it is here that the number of chromosomes is halved. Homologous chromosomes pair or synapse and then exchange material by recombination or crossing over. Recombination greatly increases the genetic diversity in gametes by reassorting paternally and maternally inherited genetic information. After recombination, homologous chromosomes, whose chromatids now contain segments of both paternally and maternally derived DNA, segregate to opposite poles and form two cells with 23 chromosomes. At this point, each chromosome is composed of two sister chromatids. Sister chromatids remain together until meiosis II, during which time they separate in a manner analogous to mitosis. The end result of meiosis in both spermatogenesis and oogenesis is the production of haploid germ cells carrying 23 chromosomes composed of one chromatid each.

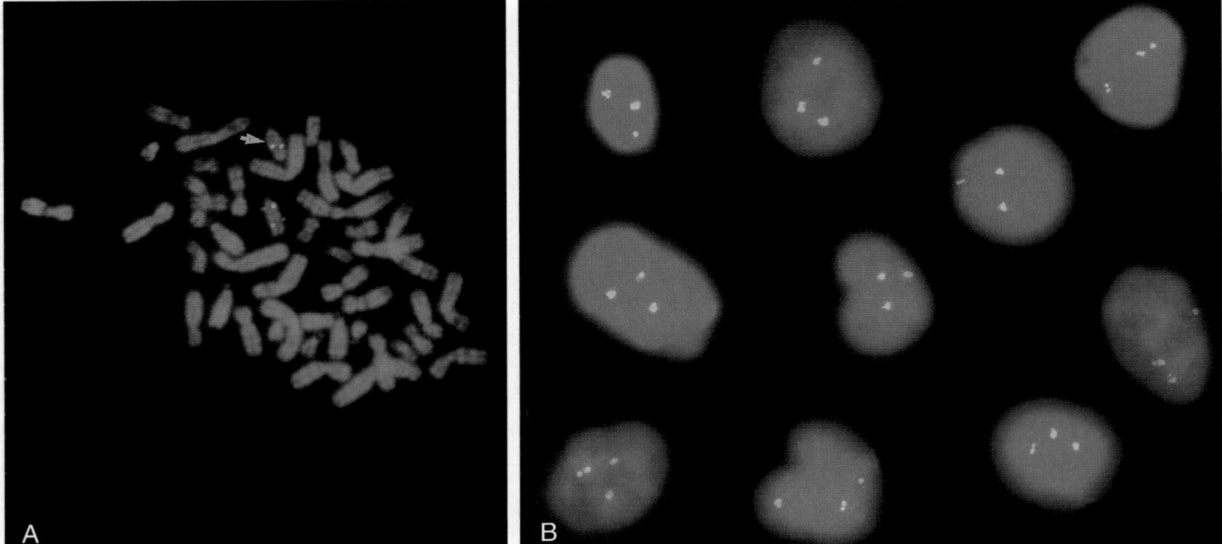

Figure 12–5 ■ *A,* Metaphase chromosome spread showing a microdeletion in one chromosome 15 in the Prader-Willi/Angelman syndrome region. Metaphase chromosomes were hybridized with a fluorescently labeled GABRB3 probe and, as a control for chromosome 15, a fluorescently labeled PML probe. After hybridization, chromosomes were counterstained with DAPI. The chromosome 15 showing hybridization with only the PML probe has a deletion of the GABRB3 probe, which maps to the Prader-Willi/Angelman syndrome region *(arrow). B,* Interphase amniotic fluid cells with trisomy 21. Cells were hybridized with a fluorescently labeled probe to chromosome 21 and counterstained with DAPI.

Although meiosis produces haploid germ cells in both female and male gametogenesis, these two processes differ in several critical ways. One crucial difference is in the timing of events in gametogenesis. In spermatogenesis, the production of mature haploid sperm from diploid spermatogonia does not begin until puberty but then continues throughout life. Production of haploid sperm from diploid spermatogonia requires approximately 64 days and involves a continuing series of both mitotic and meiotic divisions. In oogenesis, the mitotic divisions that precede meiosis are completed during fetal development and do not continue throughout life as in spermatogenesis. The onset of meiosis in females occurs during fetal development but is not completed at this time and arrests, before birth, at the end of prophase I. Meiosis does not proceed again until ovulation. At ovulation, one oocyte completes meiosis I and proceeds to meiosis II. Meiosis II is completed only if fertilization occurs.

The difference in timing of both mitotic and meiotic divisions is thought to play a significant role in the susceptibility of oocytes and spermatocytes to mutation and reproductive errors. Spermatogenesis, which involves continual cell division and hence replication of DNA, is more vulnerable to DNA damage and replication errors. Thus, de novo point mutations are more commonly of paternal than of maternal origin. Conversely, the protracted meiotic arrest in oogenesis is thought to contribute to nondisjunction errors, and the extra chromosome in trisomies is usually of maternal origin.

Female and male gametogenesis also differ in the manner in which cytoplasm is divided during meiosis. In spermatogenesis, a primary spermatocyte divides its cytoplasm equally to produce four functionally equivalent sperm. By contrast, a primary oocyte divides its cytoplasm unequally, with one product in each meiotic division containing most of the cytoplasm. In the first meiotic division, a primary oocyte divides to produce one secondary oocyte that retains most of the cytoplasm and one polar body. If the secondary oocyte is fertilized, it will complete meiosis II, producing a fertilized ovum that again retains most of the cytoplasm and a second polar body. This unequal division of cytoplasmic contents is important because the ovum contributes most of the non-nuclear cytoplasmic contents to the fertilized product. Thus, mitochondria and other cytoplasmic components are essentially exclusively of maternal origin.

A third important difference between oogenesis and spermatogenesis is the synapsis configuration of sex chromosomes during meiosis. In female meiosis, the two X chromosomes pair and recombine over the entire length of the chromosomes,[35, 36] whereas in male meiosis, the morphologically dissimilar X and Y chromosomes pair and recombine in only two regions.[37–41] The first of these regions identified is located on the distal short arms of the X and Y and is now known as pseudoautosomal region 1 (PAR1). Markers in this region can be transferred from one sex chromosome to the other[38, 39, 42, 43] and presumably do not contain genes required for specific male or female sexual differentiation. This region is probably important for initiating chromosome pairing and forming a synaptonemal complex in male meiosis, and it appears that one recombination event is required in this region for proper disjunction of the XY bivalent.[44, 45] More recently, it has been shown that the X and Y can occasionally pair and recombine at a second region on the long arm of each chromosome, at a region termed pseudoautosomal region 2 (PAR2).[40, 41]

Meiotic Nondisjunction

Meiotic nondisjunction errors are common in humans. Aneuploidy, the result of a meiotic nondisjunction event involving usually a single but rarely more than one chromosome, is seen in approximately 0.3 percent of newborns and 35 percent of spontaneous abortions.[46] Trisomy for all chromosomes has been observed in spontaneous abortions, indicating that nondisjunction for each of these chromosomes does occur.[46–48]

Meiotic nondisjunction can involve only one chromosome or the whole chromosome set. In either event, nondisjunction leads to a germ cell product whose chromosome number deviates from the normal haploid number of 23. Nondisjunction of a single chromosome will produce germ cells that carry either two or zero copies of the specific chromosome. If a germ cell carrying an extra chromosome is fertilized with a chromosomally normal germ cell, the product will be trisomic with 47 chromosomes. If a germ cell missing a chromosome is fertilized with a chromosomally normal germ cell, the product will be monosomic with 45 chromosomes. Nondisjunction of the entire chromosome set will lead to germ cells with two copies of every chromosome and to empty germ cells with no chromosomes. The clinical phenotype and histopathology of products that can result from diploid or nullisomic gametes depend both on the total number of chromosomes and on the relative number of paternal versus maternal chromosomes.

Nondisjunction can take place in either meiosis I or meiosis II. If nondisjunction occurs in meiosis I, all four products of meiosis will be chromosomally abnormal. Two of the four products of meiosis will carry two copies of the chromosome involved in the nondisjunction event, and two of the four products of meiosis will carry no copies of that particular chromosome. Of further note, in germ cells carrying two copies of the chromosome, the copies, although homologous, will not be identical. Homologous chromosomes fail to separate in nondisjunction errors in meiosis I, but sister chromatids separate properly in meiosis II. Thus, each of the germ cells with an extra chromosome will have a maternally derived chromosome and a paternally derived chromosome. In the absence of recombination, one chromosome would be entirely of maternal origin and the other entirely paternal. If nondisjunction occurs in meiosis II, two of the four products will be unaffected by the event and two of the products will be abnormal. One abnormal product will carry an extra chromosome, and the other abnormal product will be missing that chromosome. With nondisjunction errors in meiosis II, homologous chromosomes separate properly in meiosis I, but sister chromatids fail to separate in meiosis II. Thus, in contrast to meiotic I nondisjunction errors, the two nondisjoined chromosomes will be genetically identical (Fig. 12–6). This perhaps seemingly trivial difference between meiotic I and meiotic II errors can have important clinical consequences that are discussed later in the section on uniparental disomy. Furthermore, study of the parental origin of chromosomes involved in aneuploidies has led to important observations about the origin and meiotic stage of nondisjunction.

It is difficult to study meiotic nondisjunction for all chromosomes directly in gametes and even indirectly in products of conception, because many aneuploid products of conception are lost early in pregnancy and are never brought to clinical attention. However, conceptuses with trisomies for some chromosomes survive long enough to be clinically recognized, and several studies have used DNA polymorphisms to analyze the source of the extra chromosome in these cases of trisomy. These studies have shown that maternal nondisjunction accounts for signifi-

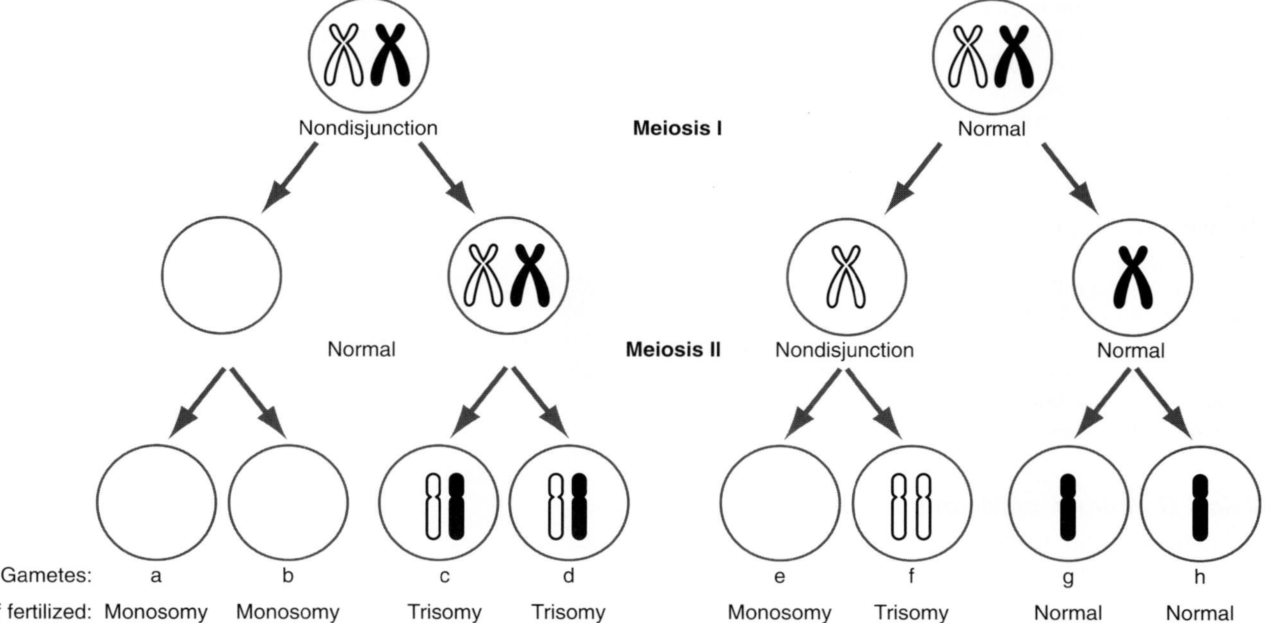

Figure 12–6 ■ Comparison of nondisjunction in meiosis I and meiosis II. With an error in meiosis I, all four gametes (a, b, c, d) are aneuploid. Two gametes (a, b) are nullisomic, potententially resulting in a monosomic conceptus. Two gametes (c, d) are disomic, potentially resulting in a trisomic conceptus. The two homologous chromosomes in the nonreduced, disomic gametes (c, d) are of biparental inheritance. With an error in meiosis II, only two gametes (e, f) are aneuploid. One gamete (e) is nullisomic, and the other aneuploid gamete (f) is disomic. The two homologous chromosomes in the nonreduced gamete (e) are of uniparental inheritance.

cantly more cases of autosomal trisomy than does paternal nondisjunction. For trisomies 13, 14, 15, 16, 18, 21, and 22, maternal nondisjunction accounted for 88, 83, 88, 100, 93, 91, and 89 percent, respectively.[49–54] More difficult and smaller scale direct studies of aneuploidy in gametes gave conservative estimates of 1.4 percent meiotic nondisjunction in sperm[46] and 13 percent meiotic I nondisjunction in oocytes,[55] indicating that the excess of maternal nondisjunction relative to paternal nondisjunction seen in trisomic conceptuses does indeed reflect differences in the rate of nondisjunction in oocytes and spermatocytes. It is still possible, however, that selection against aneuploid sperm occurs after spermatogenesis as well.

Not only is the rate of aneuploidy higher in oocytes than in spermatocytes, but the rate of aneuploidy increases significantly with maternal, but not paternal, age.[56, 57] Although the relationship between increased maternal age and Down syndrome was first described in 1933,[58] the mechanism for this aging effect is still unclear. Most nondisjunction errors in oocytes occur in meiosis I, and it has been hypothesized that the prolonged arrest in meiosis I contributes to these errors.[59]

Paternal nondisjunction is more common in cases of aneuploidy involving sex chromosomes than in cases involving autosomes, and it has been hypothesized that the XY bivalent is more susceptible to nondisjunction than are the homologous bivalents. Eighty percent of 45,X karyotypes can be attributed to paternal nondisjunction, although some of these cases may be caused by early loss of the Y chromosome through mitotic nondisjunction in the zygote.[60, 61] Cases of 47,XXY are divided approximately equally between maternal and paternal nondisjunction.[62, 63] However, like the autosomal trisomies, the extra X chromosome is of maternal origin in 90 percent of cases of 47,XXX.[63]

Studies have demonstrated that recombination is crucial for proper separation of homologous chromosomes. Studies in yeast have shown that recombination is required for formation of the synaptonemal complex and for complete pairing of homologous chromosomes; from this, it has been suggested that in the absence of recombination and hence pairing, nondisjunction would be increased.[64] In humans, studies of trisomies 15, 16, 18, and 21 as well as of XXY and XXX trisomies have shown that, on average, the particular chromosomes involved in a specific nondisjunction event participated in fewer recombinations than usual.[44, 65–69] Interestingly, the overall rate of recombination is higher in female gametogenesis than in male gametogenesis, although some specific chromosomal regions including the telomeric regions of many chromosomes have higher recombination rates in males.[70, 71]

Clinical Outcomes of Meiotic Nondisjunction

Most numerical chromosome abnormalities caused by meiotic nondisjunction errors result in spontaneous abortion. As a group, chromosome abnormalities are the most common cause of pregnancy loss, accounting for 50 percent of spontaneous losses. Triploidy, tetraploidy, trisomy, and monosomy have been reported in spontaneous abortions. The most common chromosome abnormalities in chromosomally abnormal spontaneous abortions are 45,X (20 percent), trisomy 16 (16 percent), and triploidy (16 percent). Trisomy 21 accounts for about 5 percent of chromosomally abnormal spontaneous abortions.[33]

The overall incidence and distribution of numerical chromosome abnormalities differ in newborns and spontaneous abortions, reflecting the differential viabilities of the abnormalities. Trisomies 13, 18, and 21 are compatible with life, although most of these conceptuses result in spontaneous abortion (Table 12–2). No other nonmosaic autosomal trisomy and, with the exception of monosomy 21,[72] no autosomal monosomy has ever been reported in a liveborn. In newborn surveys, trisomy 21 is the most common autosomal aneuploidy, with an overall incidence of 1 in 800. Estimates of trisomy 18 range from 1 in 3500 to 1 in 7000 newborns, and estimates of trisomy 13 range from 1 in 7000 to 1 in 21,000.[73–75]

Trisomy 21, the least severe of the autosomal trisomies, results in Down syndrome, a well-defined and familiar syndrome. This syndrome was first described by Langdon Down in 1866 and is the single most common cause of moderate mental retardation. In addition to mental impairment, patients frequently have other serious clinical phenotypes including cardiac defects and increased risk for both childhood leukemia and early-onset Alzheimer's disease. Approximately 95 percent of Down syndrome cases result from free trisomy or a chromosome constitution of 47,+21, reflecting parental nondisjunction. Approximately 3 percent result from a translocation in which one of the three copies of chromosome 21 is joined in a head-to-head manner to another acrocentric chromosome, usually through repetitive sequences in the p arms; such rearrangements are known as Robertsonian translocations. The remaining 2 percent result from a mosaic chromosome constitution in which one normal cell line has 46 chromosomes and a second abnormal line carries an additional copy of chromosome 21. In these cases, the original conceptus may have been trisomic for chromosome 21 with a postzygotic mitotic nondisjunction event resulting in an additional cell line disomic for chromosome 21, or the original conceptus may have been disomic for chromosome 21 with a postzygotic mitotic nondisjunction event resulting in an additional cell line trisomic for chromosome 21.

■ TABLE 12–2

Probability of Survival to Birth for Viable Aneusomic Conceptuses

KARYOTYPE	PROBABILITY OF SURVIVAL TO BIRTH (%)*
47,+13	2.8
47,+18	5.4
47,+21	22.1
45,X	0.3
47,XXX	70.0
47,XXY	55.3
47,XYY	100.0

*Based on incidence of chromosome abnormalities in spontaneous abortions, stillbirths, and livebirths, assuming an overall 15 percent rate of spontaneous abortion and 1 percent rate of stillbirth in the population.

Adapted from Jacobs PA, Hassold TJ. The origin of numerical chromosome abnormalities. Adv Genet 33:101–133, 1995.

Trisomy 13, first described by Patau in 1960, is much less common than trisomy 21 and clinically much more severe. Approximately 45 percent of liveborns are deceased within the first month after birth and 90 percent by the age of 6 months. The phenotype of trisomy 13 involves severe central nervous system malformations, including severe mental retardation, holoprosencephaly, and arrhinencephaly. Cleft lip and cleft palate are frequently seen in these individuals. Eye anomalies ranging from microphthalmia to anophthalmia are also common. Postaxial polydactyly, clenched fists, and rocker-bottom feet are further features of this syndrome. Like trisomy 21, trisomy 13 occurs both as a free trisomy and in conjunction with a Robertsonian translocation.

The clinical phenotype of trisomy 18 is also severe. Only 10 percent of these individuals survive beyond the first year of life.[76] Failure to thrive and mental retardation are seen in all individuals trisomic for chromosome 18. Prominent occiput, recessed jaw, short sternum, low-set and malformed ears, clenched fists with a characteristic overlapping of the fingers, and rocker-bottom feet are features of this syndrome. Approximately 80 percent of trisomy 18 cases result from free trisomy, approximately 10 percent are mosaic, and the remainder involve a translocation or other rare karyotype.[77]

Recurrence risks for free (nontranslocation) trisomy are based on empirical data that are abundant for trisomy 21 but scanty for trisomies 13 and 18 because of the rarity of these conditions. For trisomy 21, the recurrence risk is increased above the normal age-related risk for mothers who are younger than 35 years but not for mothers who are age 35 years or older. For mothers younger than 35 years, the recurrence risk is approximately 0.5 percent for a subsequent trisomy 21 and 1 percent for any chromosome abnormality. For mothers older than 35 years, in whom the age-related risk of trisomy 21 is equal to or greater than 0.5 percent, the recurrence risks are equivalent to the general population age-related risks.[78] The reasons for the additional risk to young mothers are not entirely clear and may be due to individual differences in rates of nondisjunction or to cases of parental gonadal mosaicism (discussed in further detail later) for trisomy 21; in such instances, a phenotypically normal individual carries a cell line trisomic for chromosome 21 in gonadal but not somatic tissue.

Recurrence for trisomies 13 and 18 is rare, but the risk for trisomy 21 may be increased after the occurrence of one of these other trisomies. All of these recurrence risks are based on a liveborn index case. As already mentioned, nonviable autosomal trisomies are common in spontaneous abortions, and it is unclear whether such an event increases the risk of trisomy in subsequent pregnancies. If a trisomy is detected in a late abortion or in a stillbirth, it is probably prudent to use the same risk figures as for a livebirth.[78] Finally, recurrence risks after a translocation trisomy (not a result of meiotic nondisjunction) depend on the particular translocation (discussed later in the section on translocations; see also Table 12–4).

Trisomies of the sex chromosomes XXX, XXY, and XYY are viable and have a much lower rate of spontaneous abortion than do the autosomal trisomies (see Table 12–2). In newborn surveys, 47,XXX, 47,XXY, and 47,XYY are all found at an approximate incidence of 1 per 1000.[34] Monosomy for the X chromosome, unlike autosomal monosomy, can be viable. However, approximately 99 percent of monosomic X conceptuses result in spontaneous abortion, and its frequency in newborns, approximately 1 per 10,000, is much lower than that of the other numerical sex chromosome abnormalities.[34] In general, phenotypes of sex chromosome aneuploidies are more subtle than those of the autosomal aneuploidies (discussed further in the section on sex chromosome abnormalities). Recurrence for any of the sex chromosome abnormalities is exceedingly rare.[78]

Infrequently, meiotic nondisjunction for the complete chromosome set can occur. One outcome of such an event is a benign cystic teratoma. In the absence of fertilization, an unreduced egg with 46 chromosomes can develop into a benign cystic teratoma. Benign cystic teratomas represent a duplication of the maternal genome with no contribution from a paternal genome. These teratomas can also arise after endoreduplication of a haploid egg.

Like benign cystic teratomas, complete hydatidiform moles are also diploid but, with rare exceptions, are composed of chromosomal DNA solely of paternal origin.[79, 80] (Mitochondrial DNA in complete moles is of maternal origin.) Studies of molecular polymorphisms have shown that 75 to 85 percent of complete moles are homozygous at every locus and thus developed from duplication of the haploid paternal genome in an egg containing no maternal chromosomes.[80–82] Duplication of the haploid paternal genome must be caused either by nondisjunction in meiosis II or by endoreduplication of a haploid sperm after fertilization. The mechanism by which an egg becomes devoid of maternal chromosomes is unclear; possibilities include meiotic nondisjunction, enucleation of the oocyte, or exclusion of the maternal chromosomes in cell divisions after fertilization.[83] An estimated 4 to 15 percent of complete moles are 46,XY and are thought to arise from fertilization of a chromosomally empty egg with two sperm.[81, 84] This same mechanism is believed to account for the 5 percent of complete moles that are 46,XX but not genetically identical at every locus.[81] Note that 46,YY moles are not seen, presumably because this chromosomal constitution is not compatible with development.

Comparing the pathophysiology of benign cystic teratomas and complete hydatidiform moles provided some of the first evidence for imprinting, the differential effect of genetic material depending on whether the inheritance is of maternal or paternal origin. Although both benign cystic teratomas and complete hydatidiform moles are diploid entities with genetic contribution from only one parent, their development is dissimilar. Benign cystic teratomas have little trophoblast development but do have some embryonic development. Complete moles, on the other hand, have no embryonic development but do have placental trophoblast development, albeit abnormal.

Another outcome involving unreduced gametes is triploidy. Although dispermy is thought to be the most common cause of triploidy, fertilization with either an unreduced (diploid) egg or sperm also leads to triploidy. Triploidy almost always results in spontaneous abortion, although it is seen in approximately 1 in 57,000 births. Most of these newborns die within the first day; some isolated cases reportedly have survived for several months.[85, 86]

The phenotype of triploidy differs, depending on whether the origin of the extra chromosome set is paternal (diandric) or maternal (digynic). Although both diandric and digynic triploid products can be associated with a fetus, the diandric triploid is associated with a less developed fetus, and no diandric triploid surviving to term has ever been reported. Diandric triploids are associated with excessive placental growth and partial hydatidiform moles; digynic triploids are associated with smaller, nonmolar placentas. Thus, diandric triploids have increased placental growth but decreased fetal development in comparison to digynic triploids.[87] These placental and fetal developmental differences between diandric triploids and digynic triploids are similar to the developmental differences between complete moles and benign cystic teratomas, in which paternal chromosomes are associated with placental but no embryonic development whereas maternal chromosomes are associated with embryonic but little placental development.

Errors of Recombination

As already mentioned, not only is meiotic recombination crucial for genetic diversity, but its frequency also appears to influence rates of meiotic nondisjunction. Accuracy of recombination is no less important and is critical in maintaining the fidelity of genetic information. Recombination between mispaired chromosomes or misaligned chromatids, known as unequal crossing over, can lead to duplication or deletion of genetic material. On occasion, the resulting rearrangements are large enough to be detectable through classical cytogenetics, but more commonly they can be detected only through high-resolution cytogenetics, FISH, or other molecular methods. The number of genetic diseases known to be caused by microdeletions or microduplications is growing, as is the number of commercially available probes used for their detection. Included among currently commercially available FISH probes are those for detection of Prader-Willi syndrome, Angelman's syndrome, DiGeorge/velocardiofacial syndrome, and Williams syndrome (Table 12–3).

Fertilization and Post-fertilization Errors

In addition to meiotic errors of gametogenesis, a variety of errors can occur at the time of fertilization. Normally, penetration of the zona pellucida by one sperm triggers a series of events leading to prevention of penetration by another sperm, resumption of meiosis II in the egg, and extrusion of the second polar body. Failure of any of these processes can lead to numerical chromosome aberrations, most notably triploidy. As previously mentioned, fertilization of one egg by two sperm is the most common cause of triploidy and results in a partial hydatidiform mole. Fertilization of the first polar body or retention of the second polar body may also result in triploidy.

Post-fertilization errors occur as well. Cleavage errors, resulting in chromosome duplication without subsequent cell division, produce tetraploidy. If a cleavage error occurs during the first division, nonmosaic tetraploidy, which is incompatible with life, results. A cleavage error at a later, multicellular stage produces mosaicism for tetraploid and diploid cell lines.

Mosaicism

Just as cleavage errors at a multicellular stage produce mosaicism for tetraploidy and diploidy, mitotic nondisjunction errors at a multicellular stage produce mosaicism for individual chromosomes. Technically, a mitotic nondisjunction error should create two new cell lines, one monosomic for the nondisjoined chromosome and one trisomic for the nondisjoined chromosome. However, not all cell lines are capable of development; the monosomic cell line usually does not survive.

The three autosomal trisomies, trisomies 13, 18, and 21, which can result in liveborns, can also occur as mosaics in conjunction with a diploid cell line. Two additional autosomal trisomies, trisomy 8 and trisomy 9, are viable as mosaics. Although the presence of a normal cell line can allow the otherwise lethal trisomies 8 and 9 to be viable, the presence of a normal cell line does not appear to improve the phenotype for trisomy 21. The prognosis for trisomies 13 and 18 may be slightly improved when they are present in conjunction with a normal cell line. These are, however, sufficiently severe phenotypes that even the mosaic form does not have a favorable prognosis. Thus, in the setting of prenatal diagnosis, a mosaic result for these trisomies is usually given a prognosis equivalent to that for a complete trisomy. Mosaic trisomy for the other autosomes, like the respective complete trisomy, almost always results in spontaneous abortion, although rare cases of trisomy mosaicism have been diagnosed postnatally for chromosomes 3, 7, 10, 12, 14, 15, 17, 19, and 22.[75] Prognosis for mosaicism involving sex chromosomes, particularly 45,X/46,XY, is more variable (discussed in the section on sex chromosome abnormalities).

Tissue-Limited Mosaicism and Uniparental Disomy

Tissue-limited mosaicism is a specialized form of mosaicism in which some but not all tissues in an individual have two or more cell lines. This type of mosaicism arises when mitotic nondisjunction occurs in a cell type that is a precursor for a subset of tissues. Gonadal mosaicism occurs when the abnormal cell line is confined to the gonadal tissue. This type of mosaicism becomes apparent only when an individual has multiple offspring carrying the same chromosome abnormality and is one reason that recurrence risks are increased after diagnosis of an abnormality. Confined placental mosaicism (CPM) occurs when the abnormal cell line is confined to the placenta with the fetus being karyotypically normal. CPM is suspected most often after cytogenetic studies of tissue obtained from chorionic villus sampling; results of this procedure may indicate a mosaic karyotype reflecting an abnormal placenta and normal fetus. Subsequent chromosome studies of amniotic fluid cells may be performed to confirm that the abnormal cell line is confined most likely to the placenta.

Theoretically, CPM could arise through at least two possible mechanisms. Because the embryo derives from a relatively small number of progenitor cells,[88, 89] one possibility is that CPM could occur after a postzygotic nondisjunction event in a cell lineage that contributes only to extraembryonic tissues. Alternatively, CPM may arise through a mechanism in which the original conceptus is

■ TABLE 12–3

Microdeletions and Microduplications: Chromosomal Location and Availability of Commercial Fluorescence In Situ Hybridization Probes

SYNDROME	LOCATION	DELETION OR DUPLICATION	COMMERCIALLY AVAILABLE FISH PROBE
Williams	7q11.23	Deletion	Yes
Langer-Giedeon/trichorhinophalangeal 2	8q24.1	Deletion	No
WAGR*	11p13	Deletion	No
Retinoblastoma	13q14	Deletion	Yes
Angelman	15q11q13	Deletion	Yes
Prader-Willi	15q11q13	Deletion	Yes
α-Thalassemia/mental retardation	16p13.3	Deletion	No
Rubinstein-Taybi	16p13.3	Deletion	No
Smith-Magenis	17p11.2	Deletion	Yes
Miller-Dieker	17p13.3	Deletion	Yes
Neurofibromatosis type 1	17q11.2	Deletion	No
Alagille	20p11.23p12.2	Deletion	No
DiGeorge/velocardiofacial	22q11.2	Deletion	Yes
Beckwith-Wiedemann	11p15	Duplication	No
Charcot-Marie-Tooth 1A	17p11.2p12	Duplication	No
Cat-eye	22q11	Duplication	No

*Wilms' tumor, aniridia, genital abnormalities, and mental retardation.
Also available are FISH probes for the usually classically detectable deletions associated with cri du chat (5p15) and Wolf-Hirschhorn (4p16) syndromes.

trisomic but then undergoes a nondisjunction event leading to loss of the aneuploid chromosome in some but not all daughter cells. Those pregnancies with a resulting diploid fetal karyotype may be more likely to progress.

To complicate matters further, this second mechanism leading to CPM places the fetus at risk for uniparental disomy (UPD), a condition in which both homologues of a given chromosome are inherited from one parent. This risk for UPD arises because the three chromosomes involved in the original trisomy are not equivalent. Two of the three chromosomes are inherited from one parent, and one of the three chromosomes is inherited from the other parent. Thus, if one of the three chromosomes is randomly lost in the mitotic nondisjunction event, the remaining chromosomes will be of biparental inheritance two thirds of the time but of uniparental inheritance one third of the time.

UPD occurs in two types: heterodisomy, in which the two chromosomes, although homologous, are not genetically identical; and isodisomy, in which the two chromosomes are identical. Heterodisomy results when the nondisjunction error occurs in meiosis I, and isodisomy results when the error occurs in meiosis II.

Clinical Outcomes of Confined Placental Mosaicism and Uniparental Disomy

CPM has a wide range of clinical phenotypes depending on the extent of aneuploidy in the placenta, the particular chromosome involved in the aneuploidy, the presence or absence of UPD, and the type of UPD. UPD always carries the risk of "unmasking" a recessive gene and in fact was first identified in an individual with cystic fibrosis and short stature who had inherited two identical copies of chromosome 7.[90] Both heterodisomic UPD and isodisomic UPD are problems for chromosomes with imprinted regions, regions in which gene expression is not equivalent for maternally and paternally inherited genes. UPD for chromosome 15 has been studied extensively; maternal disomy results in Angelman's syndrome, and paternal disomy results in Prader-Willi syndrome. Imprinted genes also exist on chromosome 11, and paternal disomy for a specific region on this chromosome results in Beckwith-Wiedemann syndrome.[91, 92] Rare cases of UPD for other chromosomes and associated phenotypes are beginning to be reported.[93] Paternal UPD for chromosome 21 and maternal UPD for chromosome 22 do not appear to have any phenotypic effect. Maternal UPD for chromosome 14 probably does have a phenotypic effect; however, this effect is not clinically well defined as yet.[94]

CONSTITUTIONAL CHROMOSOME ANOMALIES AFFECTING REPRODUCTION

Constitutional chromosome anomalies affecting reproduction can be divided into two classes: abnormalities involving autosomes and abnormalities involving one or more of the sex chromosomes. Within each of these groups, chromosome abnormalities can be numerical or structural.

In practice, numerical abnormalities affecting reproduction are limited to sex chromosome abnormalities, although issues of reproduction do affect individuals with trisomy 21. Males with trisomy 21 are usually subfertile or sterile and rarely reproduce, although cases of affected males fathering a pregnancy have been reported.[95, 96] Although females with trisomy 21 are fertile, they also rarely reproduce, so data for the risk of trisomy 21 in offspring are limited. According to Harper,[78] a risk of one in three is most likely.

A variety of structural chromosome rearrangements can affect reproductive outcome. Structural chromosome rearrangements can be considered either balanced or unbalanced. For balanced rearrangements, chromosomes contain the normal complement of genetic information; for unbalanced rearrangements, genetic information is either duplicated or missing. Like the numerical abnormalities, unbalanced rearrangements with significant reproductive concerns are basically limited to the sex chromosome rearrangements because unbalanced autosomal rearrangements produce fairly severe and frequently inviable phenotypes. Balanced chromosome rearrangements usually do not have a phenotypic effect because essentially all the genetic information is present, although the rearrangement may occasionally disrupt a gene or result in a cryptic duplication or deletion. However, even in the absence of any associated phenotype, carriers of presumably balanced structural rearrangements can produce unbalanced gametes, that is, gametes in which genetic information is duplicated or deleted. Because of this, carriers of balanced rearrangements are at increased risk of having abnormal offspring with unbalanced karyotypes. Balanced rearrangements also increase the risk for both spontaneous abortions, which are presumably chromosomally unbalanced, and male infertility.[97–99]

Structural Chromosome Rearrangements

Translocations

Translocations, which involve transfer of one piece of a chromosome to another chromosome, are divided into two classes, reciprocal and Robertsonian. Reciprocal translocations, as the name implies, involve presumably reciprocal exchange of a piece of one chromosome with a piece of another chromosome. Robertsonian translocations, the most common chromosome rearrangements in humans, involve whole-arm exchange of the acrocentric chromosomes. Most Robertsonian translocations involve two nonhomologous chromosomes and appear to result from recombination between homologous DNA sequences present in the proximal short arms of the acrocentric chromosomes.[100–102] The resulting rearrangement is a bicentric chromosome composed of the two long arms of the acrocentric chromosomes with loss of most of the short arm material. One of the two centromeres is inactivated, and the Robertsonian fusion is stable throughout the cell cycle. Homologous Robertsonian translocations are much less common than nonhomologous Robertsonian translocations and, in fact, are usually isochromosomes, cytogenetically indistinguishable from homologous translocations.[94, 103–105] Carriers of either homologous or nonhomologous Robertsonian translocations have a balanced karyotype containing 45 chromosomes.

Carriers of reciprocal translocations can produce both balanced and unbalanced gametes. Because homologous chromosome segments pair in meiosis, the two translocation chromosomes and the two normal chromosomes form a quadriradial figure (Fig. 12–7). If the chromosomes segregate in such a way as to keep the two normal chromosomes together and the two translocation chromosomes together, the resulting gametes will be either karyotypically normal or balanced. Of normal offspring, 50 percent will be translocation carriers and 50 percent will be karyotypically normal. On the other hand, if a normal chromosome segregates with a translocation chromosome, the resulting gametes will be unbalanced. Chromosomes from these quadriradial figures can also undergo abnormal 3:1 segregation, which always produces unbalanced gametes.

The risk to reciprocal translocation carriers of having an unbalanced liveborn offspring depends on several factors. Clearly, some unbalanced products are viable whereas others are not. As a result, the risk of having a chromosomally abnormal offspring is different for carriers ascertained by chance and for those ascertained through a previous unbalanced liveborn offspring. In general, viability is more likely if the chromosome duplication or deletion is small. Duplicated material is usually more easily tolerated than deleted material. If the imbalance is a subset of a known viable imbalance, for example, duplication of a chromosome 21 segment, viability is a possibility and the phenotype is likely to include some if not all of the features of the complete trisomy. Some translocations undergo 3:1 segregation more often than others do; one common translocation t(11;22)(q23;q22) almost always segregates in a 3:1 manner. Finally, for reasons that remain to be elucidated, female carriers of chromosome rearrangements are more likely than male carriers to have unbalanced offspring.

The risk to carriers of Robertsonian translocations for having unbalanced offspring depends both on the specific translocation and on the sex of the carrier. Presumably, unbalanced gametes produced by carriers of Robertsonian translocations lead to conceptuses that are either monosomic or trisomic for one of the acrocentric chromosomes involved in the translocation. However, in assessing the risk of unbalanced offspring, only viable outcomes need be considered. Among Robertsonian translocations involving chromosome 21, rob(14;21) is the most common. Theoretically, carriers of this translocation would produce, in equal proportion, six types of gametes, two of which would be balanced. Of the other four gametes, two would be nullisomic for either 14 or 21, and two would be disomic for one of these chromosomes. The two nullisomic gametes would lead to inviable monosomy, whereas the two disomic gametes would lead to trisomy for either 14 or 21. Because trisomy 14 is inviable, only three of the gametes could lead to viable offspring, and the risk of Down syndrome might be assumed to be approximately one in three (Fig. 12–8). In actuality, empirical risks to rob(14;21) carriers and other carriers of nonhomologous Robertsonian translocation are much lower (Table 12–4). As for reciprocal translocation carriers, the risks of unbalanced offspring are greater for female carriers of Robertsonian translocations than for male carriers.

When a rearrangement involves whole-arm exchanges between two homologous acrocentric chromosomes, the risk of an abnormal trisomic conceptus is virtually 100 percent. Most of these conceptuses will end in spontaneous abortion, but because trisomies 13 and 21 are viable, carriers of rob(13;13) and rob(21;21) can have liveborn offspring with trisomy. Thus, for genetic counseling purposes, a carrier of a homologous Robertsonian translocation will have only spontaneous abortions or abnormal offspring.

However, rare exceptions of offspring carrying the same homologous Robertsonian translocation without an additional copy of the chromosome inherited from the second parent have been reported. These exceptions arise either from fertilization with a monosomic gamete or from a postzygotic loss of the normal, nontranslocated chromosome. These rare individuals, although karyotypically identical to the phenotypically normal carrier parent, have UPD because both copies of the chromosome have been inher-

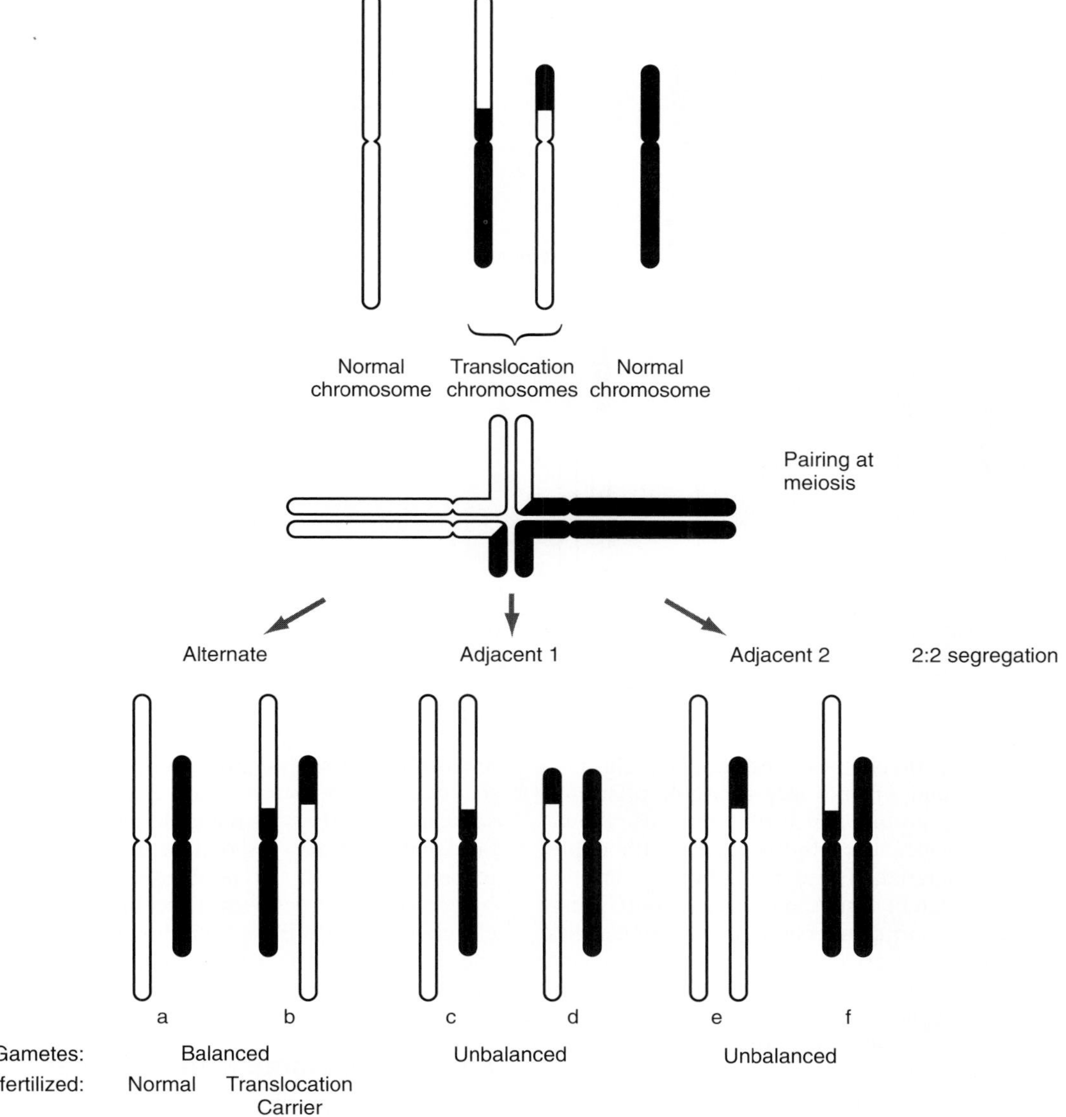

Figure 12–7 ■ Meiotic segregation with a reciprocal translocation. Of six possible gametes after 2:2 segregation, two will be balanced (a, b) and four will be unbalanced (c, d, e, f). After fertilization with a normal haploid gamete, gamete a will produce a chromosomally normal conceptus and gamete b will produce a balanced carrier of the translocation.

ited from the parent with the Robertsonian translocation. Some of these individuals are phenotypically normal; maternal UPD for chromosome 22 and paternal UPD for chromosome 21 appear to have no unusual phenotype.[94] However, UPD for chromosome 15, whether maternally or paternally inherited, has severe phenotypic consequences resulting in either Prader-Willi syndrome or Angelman's syndrome.

In addition to the risk of producing unbalanced gametes, male carriers of balanced translocations are at increased risk of infertility. The incidence of balanced autosomal translocations is approximately sixfold higher in infertile men than in the general population,[98] and translocations involving the X or Y chromosome almost always cause sterility.[106–108]

Inversions

Apparently balanced inversions, like balanced translocations, most often have no phenotypic effect; but also like translocations, they are associated with an increased risk for the production of abnormal gametes in the carrier. Two types of inversions exist: paracentric inversions, in which the inverted segment does not include the centromere; and pericentric inversions, in which the inverted segment includes the centromere. These two types of inversions carry different risks for chromosomally unbalanced offspring. For both types of inversions, the risk for chromosome imbalance is due to meiotic recombination within the inverted segment. For a paracentric inversion, structural rearrangement resulting from recombination will lead to a dicentric chromosome and an acentric chromosome frag-

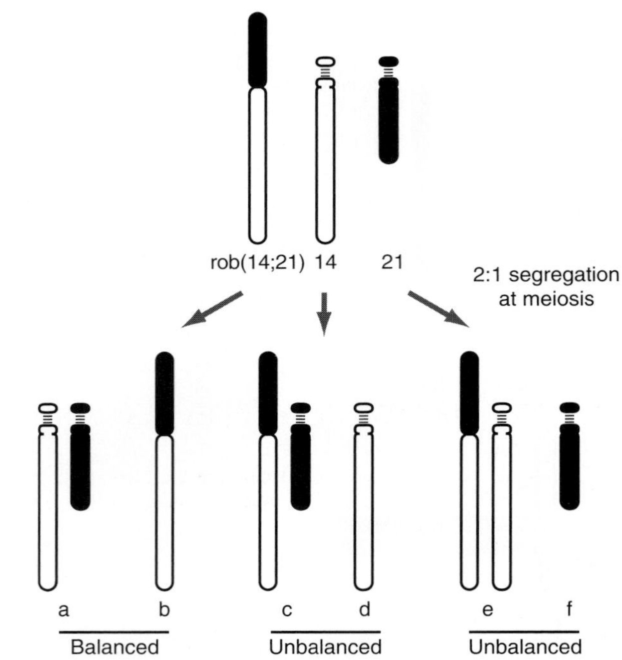

Figure 12–8 ■ Meiotic segregation in a Robertsonian t(14;21) carrier. Of six possible gametes after 2:1 segregation, two (a, b) will be balanced and four (c, d, e, f) will be unbalanced. Of the unbalanced gametes, only one (c) has the potential to result in a liveborn offspring.

ment. With rare exceptions, these recombinant chromosomes are not stable and will not lead to viable offspring. Pericentric inversions are more of a problem; recombination can produce monocentric chromosomes with duplicated and deleted material. These recombinant chromosomes are stable and can be found in unbalanced offspring. Carriers of large pericentric inversions are at higher risk than are carriers of small pericentric inversions for having unbalanced offspring for two reasons. First, a larger inverted chromosome segment is more likely than a small inverted segment to be involved in a recombination event. Second, the resulting duplication and deletion will be smaller if the inverted segment is bigger, and thus it is more likely to be viable.

Insertions

Balanced insertions are another type of rearrangement that rarely have a phenotypic effect on the carrier but portend an increased risk for production of abnormal gametes. If the two chromosomes involved in the insertion do not segregate together in meiosis, gametes with duplication or deletion of the inserted segment will result. Meiotic recombination can also produce recombinant chromosomes by crossing over between a specific region of a rearranged chromosome with the normal homologue. Risks for unbalanced liveborn offspring depend on the viability of the duplication or deletion.

Sex Chromosome Abnormalities

In humans, as in all mammals, the Y chromosome is the key determinant of sex. In the embryo, the human gonad is undifferentiated until approximately 6 to 7 weeks of development. The presence of a normal Y chromosome causes the indifferent gonad to develop into a testis. Testes produce two effectors responsible for subsequent male sex-

■ TABLE 12–4
Probabilities of Unbalanced and Balanced Carrier Offspring for Robertsonian Carriers

TRANSLOCATION	SEX OF CARRIER	PROBABILITY (RISK) OF UNBALANCED OFFSPRING (%)	PROBABILITY OF BALANCED CARRIER OFFSPRING (%)
rob(13;14)*	Female	<1	50
	Male	Very low	50
rob(13;13)	Either sex	100	0
rob(14;21)*	Female	10	50
	Male	2.5	50
rob(21;22)	Female	6.8	50
	Male	<2.9	50
rob(21;21)	Either sex	100	0

*The risks for rob(13;15) are probably similar to those for rob(13;14); rob(13;21) and rob(15;21) risks are probably similar to those for rob(14;21). These translocations are much less common, so risk data are less extensive.

Adapted from Therman E, Susman M. Human Chromosomes: Structure, Behavior, and Effects, 3rd ed. New York, Springer-Verlag, 1993, p 295.

ual differentiation, testosterone and antimüllerian hormone. In the absence of a Y chromosome, the male differentiation pathway is not initiated, the indifferent gonad develops into an ovary, and female differentiation ensues. The Y-encoded gene critical for testes development, the *SRY* gene, has been cloned and characterized,[109–112] but the complete story of sexual differentiation still remains to be elucidated. Clearly, additional gene products are required for normal sexual differentiation in both males and females. This observation has been evident for a long time on the basis of phenotypes of individuals with sex reversal and individuals whose chromosomes differ from the normal 46,XX or 46,XY.

The Y Chromosome

The structure of the Y chromosome has been studied extensively at the cytogenetic and molecular levels (Fig. 12–9). The Y chromosome is easy to distinguish cytogenetically on the basis of its small size and its extraordinarily bright fluorescence with quinacrine staining. This brightly staining region of the Y chromosome, found on the distal segment of the long arm, is composed of heterochromatin, and its size varies greatly in the human population without any apparent phenotypic effect. An essentially complete physical map of the Y chromosome has been constructed; it is estimated to contain 60 million base pairs of DNA.[113]

Two regions on the Y chromosome can pair and recombine with the X chromosome during male meiosis. These two homologous regions are known as the pseudoautosomal regions because DNA sequences in these regions undergo homologous recombination and hence do not show strictly sex-linked inheritance. These two regions, PAR1 and PAR2, are found respectively at the tips of the short and long arms. PAR1 is the major pseudoautosomal region and the site of an obligate crossing over between the X

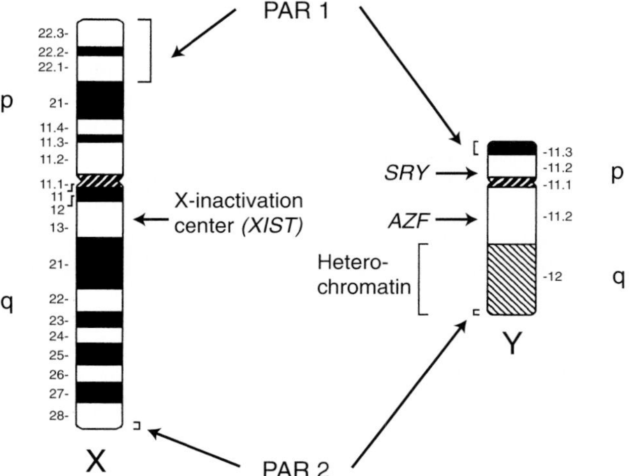

Figure 12–9 ■ Idiograms of G-banded human X and Y chromosomes at the 400-band stage. Approximate locations of the two pseudoautosomal regions (PAR1 and PAR2) are indicated on the X and Y chromosomes. On the X chromosome, the location of the X-inactivation center that contains the *XIST* gene is indicated. On the Y chromosome, the locations of the heterochromatic region, the putative azoospermic factor *AZF*, and the testis-determining gene *SRY* are indicated.

and Y chromosomes during male meiosis. PAR2 is the minor pseudoautosomal region; crossing over in this region is neither necessary nor sufficient for successful male meiosis. On the short arm, just proximal to PAR1, is the *SRY* gene. In rare cases, recombination outside of PAR1 occurs and can produce XX males and XY females. XX males carry the *SRY* gene on one of their X chromosomes, whereas XY females have a Y chromosome deleted for the *SRY* gene. DNA analysis of these sex-reversed individuals was instrumental in mapping the *SRY* gene to an approximately 140-kilobase segment of the Y chromosome.[114] The *SRY* gene was cloned several years later[109]; its identity was verified by female 46,XY individuals with point mutations at this locus.[115, 116]

A unique feature of the Y chromosome is its apparent paucity of genes, even considering that it is a small chromosome with a significant proportion of heterochromatin. The few functional genes mapped to the Y chromosome include genes with homologous copies on the X chromosome and genes unique to the Y chromosome. Genes within PAR1, with homologous copies on the X chromosome, include *MIC2*, encoding a cell surface antigen; *ANT3*, encoding an adenosine diphosphate/adenosine triphosphate translocase; and *CSF2RA*, encoding a receptor involved in regulation of hematopoiesis.[117–119] Genes outside PAR1, some of which are unique to the Y chromosome and some of which have homologous copies on the X chromosome, include the *SRY* gene and two other genes once thought to be sex determining, the *ZFY* gene[114] and a gene involved in regulation of H-Y antigen.[120] The Y chromosome also encodes pseudocopies of several genes, including *STS* (steroid sulfatase), which have functional copies on the X chromosome.[121]

Deletions of the euchromatic portion of the long arm of the Y chromosome have been associated with azoospermia and short stature, and a putative gene or gene complex required for the production of sperm (termed *AZF* for azoospermic factor) and a putative growth control gene have been mapped to the long arm of the Y chromosome.[122–125] Studies of azoospermia have localized the region containing *AZF* to Yq11.23 within a region known as Yq deletion interval 6.[126–128] Approximately 13 percent of men with nonobstructive azoospermia have deletions of this region, and new data have shown that some patients with severe oligospermia are also deleted for this region.[129, 130] Several candidate genes for *AZF* have been proposed, but the identity of the critical gene has not been established firmly.[129, 131, 132] Furthermore, the *AZF* factor, although perhaps necessary for successful spermatogenesis, is not likely to be sufficient; studies of men with translocations involving the Y and an autosome or with large deletions of the long arm of the Y chromosome suggest that most of the euchromatic portion of the Y chromosome must be present for normal germ cell development.[108, 132]

In addition to sterility, structural aberrations of the Y chromosome can have other phenotypic effects including intersex and Turner-like females. Correlations between specific structural aberrations and phenotypes have been difficult to make because the abnormal Y chromosome is frequently present in one of multiple cell lines within an individual. The second cell line may be normal male, normal female, or 45,X or even have an additional abnormal sex chromosome. Whenever the possibility of Y chromosome material in a phenotypic female exists, molecular testing to determine the presence of Y material is important because these females are at increased risk for gonadoblastoma.

Y chromosome structural aberrations with no phenotypic effect exist as well. Large portions of the heterochromatic region can be deleted without any phenotypic effect, and large variations in the size of this region are common polymorphisms. Also fairly prevalent is a pericentric inversion present in approximately 1 in 200 males that moves the centromere to the border of the heterochromatic region. More rare, but still considered a normal variant, is the presence of satellites on the long arm of the Y chromosome, resulting from a translocation between the Y chromosome and an acrocentric chromosome (usually chromosome 15).

The X Chromosome

The structure of the X chromosome has also been studied extensively at the cytogenetic and molecular levels (see Fig. 12–9). The X chromosome is estimated to be 185 cM[133] and to contain 160 million base pairs of DNA. Dosage compensation of X-linked genes in mammals is accomplished through inactivation of essentially one X chromosome in females. The theory of X inactivation[134] developed from studies in cats in which condensed chromatin was detected in females but not in males. Subsequently, it was shown that humans with numerical sex chromosome abnormalities always had one fewer Barr body than the number of X chromosomes.

Inactivation of the X chromosome requires, in *cis*, a region termed the X-inactivation center, which maps to band Xq13.[135, 136] Only one gene, the *XIST* gene, has been mapped within this region. This gene is transcriptionally active only on the inactive X chromosome and, as such, is considered to play a key role in the initiation of X chromosome inactivation.[137, 138] The product of the *XIST* gene, although important in initiation of X inactivation, does not appear to be required for maintenance of inactivation.[139] Interestingly, *XIST* does not encode a protein product; it is thought that its RNA product regulates gene expression by binding DNA.

X inactivation occurs early in development and is considered to be random for maternal and paternal X chromosomes. However, nonrandom X inactivation is seen in females with structural abnormalities and with single-gene disorders (e.g., Duchenne muscular dystrophy) of the X chromosome. In such females, cells with the normal active X may survive preferentially. Conversely, in females with balanced translocations between an X chromosome and an autosome, the normal X may appear to be inactivated preferentially. Presumably, this reflects survival of cells with active autosomal material; inactivation can spread into autosomal material in X;autosome rearrangements. Once X inactivation occurs, it appears to be irreversible, except in oogenesis, during which time reactivation of the inactive X occurs at some point before meiosis.

Inactivation does not abrogate transcription of all genes on the X chromosome. The first genes discovered to escape X inactivation were located within PAR1, and it was once thought that all genes escaping inactivation would be located in this region, thus maintaining equal dosage between males and females for genes with functional copies on the Y chromosome. Now genes escaping inactivation have been identified throughout the X chromosome. Some of these genes have functional copies on the Y chromosome outside the pseudoautosomal regions (e.g., *ZFX* and *RPS4X*), and thus, like genes in the pseudoautosomal region, equal dosage between males and females is maintained by absence of X inactivation in females. However, some of the genes escaping X inactivation do not have homologues on the Y chromosome (e.g., *UBE1* and *SB1.8*); these genes may have higher expression in females than in males. Most likely, it is the activity of genes escaping X inactivation that leads to some of the abnormalities seen in individuals with an abnormal number of X chromosomes (reviewed in reference 140). The mechanism whereby specific genes escape X inactivation remains enigmatic and is an area of intense study.

Numerous aberrations of the X chromosome have been identified and used to define regions of the chromosome. Just distal to the inactivation center is the "critical region" that appears to be required on both X chromosomes for normal ovarian function.[141] Although many balanced rearrangements of the X chromosome have no phenotype, this critical region must remain intact for normal female sexual development. In addition to this critical region, specific ovarian maintenance determinants may exist on both arms of the X chromosome because a variety of deletions in either the short or long arm are associated with ovarian dysgenesis in Turner syndrome. However, it is also possible that the ovarian dysgenesis seen with deletions of the X chromosome is caused not by specific deletions but by the inability of the X chromosomes to pair completely during meiosis.[142]

X;autosome translocations have a variety of phenotypes. They may occasionally disrupt an X-linked gene, resulting in X-linked recessive diseases both in males and in females. Males manifest the recessive disease because they are hemizygous for the X chromosome; females may be affected because of preferential inactivation of their normal X chromosome. X;autosome translocations may also impair fertility in both sexes and, like any translocation, may segregate improperly and result in unbalanced offspring. Individuals with translocations between an X and a Y chromosome may be either phenotypically female or male, depending on the breakpoints of the translocation, the pattern of X inactivation, and the remaining chromosome constitution.

Numerical Abnormalities of Sex Chromosomes

Numerical abnormalities of sex chromosomes are much more prevalent than numerical abnormalities of autosomes, with an overall frequency of 1 per 500 births. Individuals with as many as five sex chromosomes (penta-X syndrome) have been identified, but the most common abnormalities are the trisomies XXX, XXY, and XYY. The viability of these abnormalities is good, as evidenced not only by the fairly high frequency among liveborns but also by the low frequency among spontaneous abortions. Conversely, monosomy for the X chromosome is much less common among liveborns, but it is the most frequent chromosome abnormality in spontaneous abortions.[33, 60] For all sex chromosome abnormalities, mosaicism with normal and abnormal cell lines is often observed.

TURNER SYNDROME/45,X AND VARIANTS

Turner syndrome is widely known as 45,X, although approximately 50 percent of individuals with Turner syndrome have a variation of this karyotype. About 15 percent of patients carry one normal X chromosome and one structurally aberrant X chromosome. These structural abnormalities of the X chromosome include deletions of portions of the short and long arm as well as isochromosomes. Approximately 25 to 30 percent of patients are mosaic with one 45,X cell line and a second cell line that might contain, among others, either two normal X chromosomes (i.e., 45,X/46,XX), one normal and one abnormal X chromosome (i.e., 45,X/46,X, i(Xq)), or one X and one Y chromosome (i.e., 45,X/46,XY).

In apparent nonmosaic 45,X individuals, the single X is maternal in origin 80 percent of the time; in other words, the meiotic error is usually paternal.[143] The basis for the unusually high frequency of X or Y chromosome nondisjunction in paternal meiosis is unknown but may relate to limited meiotic recombination between the X and Y chromosomes. Whether paternal age is a risk factor for Turner syndrome is unclear; advanced maternal age, however, is not correlated with this disorder.

A number of phenotypic abnormalities are pathognomonic for Turner syndrome. The most characteristic findings are short stature (under 5 feet or 150 cm) and gonadal dysgenesis (usually streak gonads). Fetal cystic hygroma, resulting from lymphedema and leading to postnatal neck webbing, is common. Other associated anomalies include low posterior hairline, shield chest with widely spaced nipples, cubitus valgus, cardiac anomalies (frequently coarctation of the aorta), and renal anomalies. Although mental retardation is not any more common in patients with Turner syndrome than in females with two X chromosomes, deficiency in spatial perception, perceptual motor organization, and fine motor skills is frequent. Turner syndrome is fully compatible with life, and it is puzzling why the 45,X karyotype is usually lethal in utero. 45,X is the most common chromosome abnormality in spontaneous abortions; more than 99 percent of 45,X conceptuses are spontaneously aborted.[60]

Obtaining the karyotype of patients with Turner syndrome is clinically important. Although many of the individual symptoms of Turner syndrome seem to be randomly distributed with respect to different deletions throughout the X chromosome, some correlations with phenotype can be made.[142] Most individuals with breakpoints distal to Xq25 have few abnormalities except occasional secondary amenorrhea or premature menopause. Short stature is almost always associated with deletions of the distal portion of the short arm; it is seen less often with long arm deletions. Determination of the presence of Y chromosomal material is of critical medical importance because its presence leads to an increased risk for gonadoblastoma in sex-reversed individuals. Routine cytogenetic testing for individuals with a suspected sex chromosome disorder includes a count of 30 metaphase preparations, which rules out greater than 10 percent mosaicism at a 95 percent confidence level.[144] Even with this level of classical cytogenetic work-up, some individuals with a nonmosaic 45,X karyotype may have an undetected cell line with Y chromosomal material. As such, molecular studies for detection of Y chromosomal DNA should be performed. In addition, rare patients with features of Turner syndrome are determined to have a 46,XY karyotype missing a portion of the Y chromosome.[145] These individuals also have an increased risk for gonadoblastoma.

Infertility in Turner syndrome results from increased germ cell attrition. In the absence of a Y chromosome, the gonad develops into an ovary in which germ cells are initially present. However, germ cells rapidly degenerate during the fetal period, and the resulting lack of oocytes leads to streak gonads and amenorrhea. Most patients carrying deletions of either the short or long arm of the X chromosome suffer from ovarian dysgenesis[141]; thus, two complete X chromosomes are necessary for normal ovarian development and function.

Mosaicism for 45,X and a second cell line is not uncommon. 45,X/46,XX mosaicism is the most common sex chromosome mosaicism diagnosed from genetic amniocentesis. Of 114 cases reviewed,[75] approximately 10 percent had some features of Turner syndrome and approximately 4 percent had other anomalies. Although the majority of these cases were phenotypically normal at either birth or termination, many of the features of Turner syndrome might not be recognized until puberty, and prenatal counseling remains difficult. For 45,X/46,XY individuals, the phenotype ranges from normal, fertile males to individuals with ambiguous genitalia to females with Turner syndrome. Presumably different phenotypes reflect different tissue distributions of the various cell lines. In a compilation of prenatally diagnosed cases,[75] 90 to 95 percent of 45,X/46,XY cases resulted in a normal male phenotype. When a karyotype of 45,X/46,XY is detected at prenatal diagnosis, detailed ultrasonography of the genitalia is recommended. If genitalia appear to be normal male, prognosis is fairly good for a phenotypically normal male. If genitalia appear to be female, Turner syndrome or ambiguous genitalia are more likely to be present at birth.

In both normal females and males, loss of a sex chromosome in peripheral blood cells can occur, leading to apparent mosaicism for 45,X. Although it was once suggested that this type of X chromosome aneuploidy was more frequent in women with multiple pregnancy losses, it is now recognized that 45,X aneuploidy in peripheral blood increases with age and is not associated with reproductive loss.[146, 147]

47,XXX

Individuals with three X chromosomes, or triple-X syndrome, appear physically normal, although by adolescence many are taller than average. Sexual development and fertility are usually normal. Although it might be expected that 50 percent of offspring would carry an extra X chromosome, the actual empirical risk to offspring is low. Prospective studies with long-term follow-up of 47,XXX individuals indicate that although mental retardation is not present, the IQ of many of these patients is 10 to 15 points below that of their siblings. Language delay, learning disabilities, and impaired gross motor skills are common. Also common are psychosocial disorders, particularly depression.[148–151]

In patients with three X chromosomes, 90 percent have two maternal X chromosomes and 10 percent have two paternal X chromosomes. In cases with two maternal X chromosomes, 66 percent are due to meiosis I errors, 18 percent to meiosis II errors, and 16 percent to postzygotic errors. In two reported informative cases in which two paternally derived X chromosomes were found, both were due to postzygotic errors.[143] Increased maternal age is a risk factor for 47,XXX.

KLINEFELTER SYNDROME/47,XXY

Males with the 47,XXY karyotype have a fairly well defined phenotype known as Klinefelter syndrome; they are tall and thin with long legs. Physical appearance is fairly normal until puberty, during which a characteristic eunuchoid habitus develops. Secondary sexual characteristics are underdeveloped and testes remain small, with azoospermia and subsequent infertility. Gynecomastia can be a feature of this syndrome. IQ is reduced in this population of patients, and two thirds of patients have educational problems, particularly dyslexia.

Approximately 50 percent of 47,XXY individuals have two paternally derived sex chromosomes, and approximately 50 percent have two maternally inherited X chromosomes.[63, 143] In all cases with two paternally derived sex chromosomes (one X and one Y chromosome), the error must have occurred in meiosis I. In cases with two maternal sex chromosomes (two X chromosomes), approximately 70 percent are due to a meiosis I error, 25 percent to a meiosis II error, and 5 percent to postzygotic nondisjunction.[143] Increased maternal age is associated only with the maternal meiosis I errors.

47,XYY

The most consistent phenotype in individuals with a 47,XYY chromosome constitution is increased height. Increased risk of behavioral problems and perhaps some decrease in intelligence may be associated with this karyotype. Fertility is normal, and these individuals are not found to be at increased risk of having a chromosomally abnormal child. All 47,XYY cases result from either a paternal meiosis II error or a postzygotic error.

SEX CHROMOSOME TETRASOMY AND PENTASOMY

Although studies of the phenotype of sex chromosome tetrasomy and pentasomy do not exist from unbiased ascertainment (i.e., all information is based on case reports of postnatally identified individuals), it is generally assumed that with an increasing number of supernumerary sex chromosomes comes an increasingly severe phenotype. Supernumerary X chromosomes are clinically more severe than supernumerary Y chromosomes, presumably because the Y chromosome encodes so few genes. Even though supernumerary X chromosomes are inactivated essentially, some genes escape X inactivation, and increased dosage of these gene products presumably leads to the clinical phenotype. Mental capacity is increasingly diminished with each supernumerary X chromosome, with an estimated drop of 15 IQ points for each additional X chromosome. In males, supernumerary X chromosomes lead not only to infertility but also to malformed genitalia. The effect on fertility in females with supernumerary X chromosomes is unclear at present. Fewer cases of supernumerary Y chromosomes have been reported, but additional Y chromosomes also appear to lead to decreased mental capacity, although the effect is less pronounced than with supernumerary X chromosomes (reviewed in reference 150).

Chromosome Abnormalities and Sex Reversal

Although the testis-determining factor on the Y chromosome is now identified, elucidation of the human sex determination pathway is far from complete. *SRY* itself is expressed in both a temporal and tissue-specific manner, indicating interaction of upstream regulatory genes.[109, 152] The presence of downstream genes is also strongly implicated because the *SRY* gene product binds DNA sequences in vitro and presumably exerts its effect by regulating transcription of other genes.[109] Furthermore, not all individuals with XY gonadal dysgenesis have mutations in the *SRY* gene, indicating the presence of additional genes involved in testis formation. The existence of several chromosome abnormalities associated with sex reversal provides further evidence of additional genes involved in sex determination as well as information about their physical map location.

Both deletions of 9p and 10q and duplications of Xp21 have been associated with XY sex reversal.[153–155] The crucial genes missing in the 9p and 10q deletions have not been identified, but the sex reversal seen with these deletions must be caused by haploinsufficiency of one or more genes in these regions. Conversely, the sex reversal seen in patients with duplications of Xp21 must be caused by overexpression of a crucial gene or genes known as *DSS* (dosage-sensitive sex reversal). Improper dosage of this gene product prevents normal testis development despite the presence of an intact *SRY* gene. Because duplications of the *DSS* critical region lead to XY sex reversal, whereas supernumerary X chromosomes do not, it is presumed that *DSS* is subject to X inactivation. Of further interest, the presence on the X chromosome of a dosage-sensitive gene involved in sex determination may provide a link between sex determination and X inactivation.

DSS has been mapped to a 160-kilobase region within Xp21. Also mapping within this region is a gene in which point mutations cause adrenal hypoplasia congenita (AHC). This gene, *DAX1* (DSS-AHC critical region on the X), encodes a member of the nuclear hormone receptor family.[155, 156] Because of its map location and presumed function, *DAX1* is a candidate gene for *DSS*, although no *DAX1* mutations have been associated with sex reversal. However, because overexpression, not inactivity, of *DSS* leads to sex reversal, mutations for adrenal hypoplasia congenita and dosage-sensitive sex reversal would not be overlapping. Whereas inactivating mutations cause adrenal hypoplasia congenita, regulatory mutations leading to increased expression would be predicted to cause dosage-sensitive sex reversal.

Haploinsufficiency of another gene identified in sex determination, *SOX9*, also prevents male development despite the presence of an intact *SRY* gene. This gene was first mapped to 17q24–q25 in patients with apparently balanced translocations and campomelic dysplasia. Approximately two thirds to three quarters of XY individuals with campomelic dysplasia are sex reversed, and some of these cases involve gonadal dysgenesis, indicating that the gene must play a role in testis formation.[157] Although the translocation breaks could have disrupted two separate genes, one involved in campomelic dysplasia and one involved in sex reversal, mutations in *SOX9* have now been shown to cause both campomelic dysplasia and sex reversal.[158] A portion of the *SOX9* gene has significant homology to the DNA binding domain of *SRY* (high-mobility group box) and has been shown to bind to the same DNA sequences in vitro.[159]

Any phenotypic female with the *SRY* gene is susceptible to gonadoblastoma. At risk are not only Turner syndrome patients but also XY individuals with gonadal dysgenesis or an androgen insensitivity syndrome. As more of the genes involved in sex determination are identified, it will remain important to identify all phenotypic females carrying the *SRY* gene.

CYTOGENETICS AND INFERTILITY TREATMENTS

Preimplantation genetic diagnosis for determination of chromosomal sex and detection of chromosomal disorders is ongoing in several clinical centers. Risk for X-linked disease is one of the main indications for diagnosis. In early trials, determination of chromosomal sex was performed by use of the polymerase chain reaction (PCR) to amplify both X- and Y-specific sequences from biopsied blastomeres. Subsequent trials have used FISH with X and Y chromosome–specific probes to analyze blastomeres and have found that FISH may be more accurate than PCR for determination of sex chromosome constitution because both 45,X and 47,XXY embryos misdiagnosed as normal female and normal male, respectively, by PCR have been detected through the use of FISH.[160]

FISH analysis has also been employed to detect specific chromosome aneuploidies. This single-cell analysis has been used successfully to enumerate chromosomes both in blastomeres and in polar bodies. Because of the significant risk of chromosome aneuploidy associated with advanced maternal age, FISH analysis for the viable chromosome aneuploidies may become used more routinely in assisted reproduction procedures. However, initial data from preimplantation diagnoses suggest a high rate of chromosomal mosaicism at the cleavage stage; thus, FISH (or any other) analysis of a single blastomere may not be representative of the whole embryo.[161, 162] Similarly, FISH analysis of the polar bodies may be useful in ensuring that the prefertilized egg does not carry one of the common aneuploidies, but it does not test the conceptus directly. As such, prenatal chromosome analysis may still be recommended at a later stage in a successful pregnancy.

References

1. Tjio JH, Levan A. The chromosome number of man. Hereditas 42:1–6, 1956.
2. Schreck RR, Warburton D, Miller OJ, et al. Chromosome structure as revealed by a combined chemical and immunochemical procedure. Proc Natl Acad Sci USA 70:804–807, 1973.
3. Goldman MA, Holmquist GP, Gray MC. Replication timing of genes and middle repetitive sequences. Science 224:686–692, 1984.
4. Holmquist GP. Evolution of chromosome bands: Molecular ecology of noncoding DNA. J Mol Evol 28:469–496, 1989.
5. Bickmore WA, Sumner AT. Mammalian chromosome banding—an expression of genome organization. Trends Genet 5:144–148, 1989.
6. Robinson JA, Buckton KE, Spowart G. The segregation of human chromosome polymorphisms. Ann Hum Genet 40:113–121, 1976.
7. Phillips RB. Inheritance of Q and C band polymorphisms. Can J Genet Cytol 19:405–413, 1977.
8. Morton CC, Corey LA, Nance WE, et al. Quinacrine mustard and nucleolar organizer region heteromorphisms in twins. Acta Genet Med Gemellol (Roma) 30:39–49, 1981.
9. de la Chapelle A, Fellman J, Unnerus V. Determination of human paternity from the length of the Y chromosome. Ann Hum Genet 10:60–64, 1967.
10. Robinson JA. Origin of extra chromosome in trisomy 21. Lancet 1:131–133, 1973.
11. Mikkelsen M, Hallberg A, Pulsen H. Maternal and paternal origin of extra chromosome in trisomy 21. Hum Genet 32:17–21, 1976.
12. Hauge M, Poulsen H, Halberg A, et al. The value of fluorescence markers in the distribution between maternal and fetal chromosomes. Humangenetik 26:187–191, 1975.
13. Arrighi F, Hsu TC. Localization of heterochromatin in human chromosomes. Cytogenetics 10:81–86, 1971.
14. Brown T, Robertson FW, Dawson BM, et al. Individual variation of centric heterochromatin in man. Hum Genet 55:367–373, 1980.
15. de la Chapelle A, Schroder J, Stenstrand K, et al. Pericentric inversions of human chromosomes 9 and 10. Am J Hum Genet 26:746–766, 1974.
16. Bloom SE, Goodpasture C. An improved technique for selective silver staining of nucleolar organizer regions in human chromosomes. Hum Genet 34:199–206, 1976.
17. Schweizer D. Simultaneous fluorescent staining of R bands and specific heterochromatic regions (DA-DAPI bands) in human chromosomes. Cytogenet Cell Genet 27:190–193, 1980.
18. Miller DA, Choi Y-C, Miller OJ. Chromosome localization of highly repetitive human DNA's and amplified ribosomal DNA with restriction enzymes. Science 219:395–397, 1983.
19. Korenberg JR, Rykowski MC. Human genome organization: Alu, lines and the molecular structure of metaphase chromosome bands. Cell 53:391–400, 1988.
20. Yunis JJ. High resolution of human chromosomes. Science 191:1268–1270, 1976.
21. Yu RL, Aronson MM, Nichols WW. High resolution bands in human fibroblast chromosomes induced by actinomycin D. Cytogenet Cell Genet 31:111–114, 1981.
22. Rybak J. A simple reproducible method for prometaphase chromosome analysis. Hum Genet 60:328–333, 1982.
23. Ikeuchi T. Inhibitory effect of ethidium bromide on mitotic chromosome condensation and its application to high-resolution chromosome banding. Cytogenet Cell Genet 38:56–61, 1984.
24. Denver Conference. A proposed standard system of nomenclature of human mitotic chromosomes. Lancet 1:1063–1065, 1960.
25. Mitelman F (ed). ISCN 1995: An International System for Human Cytogenetic Nomenclature. Basel, S Karger, 1995.
26. Pardue ML, Gall JG. Nucleic acid hybridization to the DNA of cytological preparations. *In* Prescott DM (ed). Methods in Cell Biology, Vol 10. New York, Academic Press, 1975, pp 1–16.
27. Gerhard DS, Kawasaki ES, Bancroft FC, et al. Localization of a unique gene by direct hybridization in situ. Proc Natl Acad Sci USA 78:3755–3759, 1981.
28. Malcolm S, Barton P, Murphy C, et al. Chromosomal localization of a single copy gene by in situ hybridization—human beta globin genes on the short arm of chromosome 11. Ann Hum Genet 45:135–141, 1981.
29. Harper ME, Saunders GF. Localization of single copy DNA sequences on G-banded human chromosomes by in situ hybridization. Chromosoma 83:431–439, 1981.
30. Morton CC, Kirsch IR, Taub RA, et al. Localization of the beta-

globin gene by chromosomal in situ hybridization. Am J Hum Genet 36:576–585, 1984.
31. Jacobs PA, Hassold TJ. Chromosome abnormalities: origin and etiology in abortions and livebirths. *In* Vogel F, Sperling K (eds). Human Genetics: Proceedings of the 7th International Congress, Berlin 1986. Berlin, Springer-Verlag, 1987, pp 233–244.
32. Hassold T. Chromosome abnormalities in human reproductive wastage. Trends Genet 2:105–110, 1986.
33. Boue A, Boue J, Gropp A. Cytogenetics of pregnancy wastage. *In* Harris H, Hirschhorn K (eds). Advances in Human Genetics, Vol 14. New York, Plenum Publishing, 1985, pp 1–57.
34. Hook EB, Hamerton JL. Population cytogenetics: studies in humans. *In* Hook EB, Porter IH (eds). Population Cytogenetics: Studies in Humans. New York, Academic Press, 1977, pp 63–79.
35. Renwick JH. Progress in mapping human autosomes. Br Med Bull 25:65–73, 1969.
36. Weissenbach J, Levilliers J, Petit C, et al. Normal and abnormal interchanges between the human X and Y chromosomes. Development 101:67–74, 1987.
37. Chandley AC, Goetz P, Hargreave TB, et al. On the nature and extent of XY pairing at meiotic prophase in man. Cytogenet Cell Genet 38:241–247, 1984.
38. Cooke HJ, Brown WRA, Rappold GA. Hypervariable telomeric sequences from the human sex chromosomes are pseudoautosomal. Nature 317:687–697, 1985.
39. Simmler MC, Rouyer F, Vergnaud G, et al. Pseudoautosomal DNA sequences in the pairing region of the human sex chromosomes. Nature 317:692–697, 1985.
40. Speed RM, Chandley AC. Prophase of meiosis in human spermatocytes analyzed by EM microspreading in infertile men and their controls and comparisons with human oocytes. Hum Genet 84:547–554, 1990.
41. Freije D, Helms C, Watson MS, et al. Identification of a second pseudoautosomal region near the Xq and Yq telomeres. Science 258:1784–1787, 1992.
42. Rouyer F, Simmler MC, Johnsson C, et al. A gradient of sex linkage in the pseudoautosomal region of the human sex chromosomes. Nature 319:291–295, 1986.
43. Page DC, Bieker K, Brown LG, et al. Linkage, physical mapping, and DNA sequence analysis of pseudoautosomal loci on the human X and Y chromosomes. Genomics 1:243–256, 1987.
44. Hassold TJ, Sherman SL, Pettay D, et al. XY chromosome nondisjunction in man is associated with diminished recombination in the pseudoautosomal region. Am J Hum Genet 49:253–260, 1991.
45. Mohandas TK, Speed RM, Passage MB, et al. Role of the pseudoautosomal region in sex-chromosome pairing during male meiosis: Meiotic studies in a man with a deletion of distal Xp. Am J Hum Genet 51:526–533, 1992.
46. Jacobs PA. The chromosome complement of human gametes. *In* Milligan SR (ed). Oxford Review of Reproductive Biology, Vol 14. New York, Oxford University Press, 1992, pp 47–72.
47. Watt JL, Templeton AA, Messinis I, et al. Trisomy 1 in an eight cell human pre-embryo. J Med Genet 24:60–64, 1987.
48. Hanna JS, Shires P, Matile G. Trisomy 1 in a clinically recognized pregnancy. Am J Med Genet 68:98, 1997.
49. Antonarakis SE. The Down Syndrome Collaborative Group. Parental origin of the extra chromosome in trisomy 21 as indicated by analysis of DNA polymorphisms. N Engl J Med 324:872–876, 1991.
50. Sherman SL, Takaesu N, Freeman SB, et al. Trisomy 21: Association between reduced recombination and nondisjunction [see comments]. Am J Hum Genet 49:608–620, 1991.
51. Fisher JM, Harvey JF, Lindenbaum RH, et al. Molecular studies of trisomy 18. Am J Hum Genet 52:1139–1144, 1993.
52. Hassold T, Sherman S. The origin of non-disjunction in humans. *In* Sumner AT, Chandley AC (eds). Chromosomes Today, Vol 11. London, Chapman & Hall, 1993, pp 313–322.
53. Nothen MM, Eggermann T, Erdmann J, et al. Retrospective study of the parental origin of the extra chromosome in trisomy 18 (Edwards syndrome). Hum Genet 92:347–349, 1993.
54. Zaragoza MV, Jacobs PA, James RS, et al. Nondisjunction of human acrocentric chromosomes: Studies of 432 trisomic fetuses and liveborns. Hum Genet 94:411–417, 1994.
55. Pellester F. Frequency and distribution of aneuploidy in human female gametes. Hum Genet 86:283–288, 1991.
56. Hassold T, Jacobs PA. Trisomy in man. Annu Rev Genet 18:69–97, 1994.
57. Angell RR. Aneuploidy in older women: Higher rates of aneuploidy in oocytes from older women. Hum Reprod 9:199–200, 1994.
58. Penrose LS. The relative effects of paternal and maternal age in mongolism. J Genet 27:219–224, 1933.
59. Hawley RS, Frazier J, Rasooly R. Separation anxiety: The biology of nondisjunction in flies and people. Hum Mol Genet 3:1521–1528, 1994.
60. Jacobs PA, Betts PR, Cockwell AE, et al. A cytogenetic and molecular reappraisal of a series of patients with Turner syndrome. Ann Hum Genet 54:209–223, 1990.
61. Hassold T, Pettay D, Robinson A, et al. Molecular studies of parental origin and mosaicism in 45,X conceptuses. Hum Genet 89:647–652, 1992.
62. Lorda-Sanchez I, Binkert F, Maechler M, et al. Reduced recombination and paternal age effect in Klinefelter syndrome. Hum Genet 89:524–530, 1992.
63. MacDonald M, Hassold T, Harvey J, et al. The origin of 47,XXY and 47,XXX aneuploidy: Heterogeneous mechanisms and role of aberrant recombination. Hum Mol Genet 3:1365–1371, 1994.
64. Roeder GS. Chromosome synapsis and genetic recombination. Trends Genet 6:385–389, 1990.
65. Morton NE, Wu D, Jacobs PA. Origin of sex chromosome aneuploidy. Ann Hum Genet 52:85–92, 1988.
66. Robinson WP, Bernasconi F, Mutirangura A, et al. Nondisjunction of chromosome 15: Origin and recombination. Am J Hum Genet 53:740–751, 1993.
67. Sherman SL, Petersen MB, Freeman SB, et al. Non-disjunction of chromosome 21 in maternal meiosis I: Evidence for a maternal age-dependent mechanism involving reduced recombination. Hum Mol Genet 3:1529–1535, 1994.
68. Hassold T, Merrill M, Adkins K, et al. Recombination and maternal age-dependent nondisjunction: Molecular studies of trisomy 16. Am J Hum Genet 57:867–874, 1995.
69. Fisher JM, Harvey JF, Morton NE, et al. Trisomy 18: Studies of the parent and cell division of origin and the effect of aberrant recombination on nondisjunction. Am J Hum Genet 56:669–675, 1995.
70. Blouin JL, Christie DH, Gos A, et al. A new dinucleotide repeat polymorphism at the telomere of chromosome 21q reveals a significant difference between male and female rates of recombination. Am J Hum Genet 57:388–394, 1995.
71. Rouyer F, de la Chapelle A, Anderson M, et al. An interspersed repeated sequence specific for human subtelomeric regions. EMBO J 9:505–514, 1990.
72. Pellissier MC, Philip N, Voelckel-Baeteman MA, et al. Monosomy 21: A new case confirmed by in situ hybridization. Hum Genet 75:95–96, 1987.
73. Jacobs PA, Melville M, Ratcliffe S, et al. A cytogenetic survey of 11,680 newborn infants. Ann Hum Genet 37:359–376, 1974.
74. Hook EB. Rates of 47, + 13 and 46 translocation D/13 Patau syndrome in live births and comparison with rates in fetal deaths and at amniocentesis. Am J Hum Genet 32:849–858, 1980.
75. Hsu LYF. Prenatal diagnosis of chromosomal abnormalities through amniocentesis. *In* Milunsky A (ed). Genetic Disorders and the Fetus. Baltimore, Johns Hopkins University Press, 1992, pp 155–210.
76. Gorlin RJ. Classical chromosome disorders. *In* Yunis JJ (ed). New Chromosomal Syndromes. New York, Academic Press, 1977, pp 59–117.
77. de Grouchy J. Clinical cytogenetics: autosomal disorders. *In* Busch H (ed). The Cell Nucleus. New York, Academic Press, 1974, pp 371–414.
78. Harper PS. Chromosomal abnormalities. *In* Practical Genetic Counselling. Oxford, UK, Butterworth-Heinemann, 1993, pp 60–62.
79. Kajii T, Ohama K. Androgenetic origin of hydatidiform mole. Nature 268:633–634, 1977.
80. Lawler S, Fisher R, Dent J. A prospective genetic study of complete and partial hydatidiform moles. Am J Obstet Gynecol 164:1270–1277, 1991.
81. Fisher RA, Povey S, Jeffreys AJ, et al. Frequency of heterozygous complete hydatidiform moles, estimated by locus-specific

minisatellite and Y chromosome–specific probes. Hum Genet 82:259–263, 1989.
82. Wake N, Fujino T, Hoshi S, et al. The propensity to malignancy of dispermic heterozygous moles. Placenta 8:319–326, 1987.
83. Roberts DJ, Mutter GL. Advances in the molecular biology of gestational trophoblastic disease. J Reprod Med 39:201–207, 1994.
84. Ohama K, Kajii T, Okamoto E, et al. Dispermic origin of XY hydatidiform moles. Nature 292:551–552, 1981.
85. Fryns JP, van de Kerckhove A, Goddeeris P, et al. Unusually long survival in a case of full triploidy of maternal origin. Hum Genet 38:147–155, 1977.
86. Schröcksnadel H, Guggenbichler P, Rhomberg K, et al. Complete triploidy (69,XXX) surviving until the age of 7 months [in German]. Wien Klin Wochenschr 94:309–315, 1982.
87. Lindor NM, Ney JA, Gaffey TA, et al. A genetic review of complete and partial hydatidiform moles and nonmolar triploidy. Mayo Clin Proc 67:791–799, 1992.
88. Crane JP, Cheung SW. An embryogenic model to explain cytogenetic inconsistencies observed in chorionic villus versus fetal tissue. Prenat Diagn 8:119–129, 1988.
89. Markert CI, Peters RM. Manufactured hexaparental mice show that adults are derived from three embryonic cells. Science 202:56–58, 1978.
90. Spence JE, Perciaccante RG, Greig GM, et al. Uniparental disomy as a mechanism for human genetic disease. Am J Hum Genet 42:217–226, 1988.
91. Henry I, Bonaiti-Pellie C, Chehensse V, et al. Uniparental paternal disomy in a genetic cancer-predisposing syndrome [see comments]. Nature 351:665–667, 1991.
92. Grundy P, Telzerow P, Paterson MC, et al. Chromosome 11 uniparental isodisomy predisposing to embryonal neoplasms (Letter). Lancet 338:1079–1080, 1991.
93. Ledbetter DH, Engel E. Uniparental disomy in humans: Development of an imprinting map and its implications for prenatal diagnosis. Hum Mol Genet 4:1757–1764, 1995.
94. Robinson WP, Bernasconi F, Basaran S, et al. A somatic origin of homologous Robertsonian translocations and isochromosomes. Am J Hum Genet 54:290–302, 1994.
95. Sheridan R, Llerena J Jr, Matkins S, et al. Fertility in a male with trisomy 21 [see comments]. J Med Genet 26:294–298, 1989.
96. Zuhlke C, Thies U, Braulke I, et al. Down syndrome and male fertility: PCR-derived fingerprinting, serological and andrological investigations. Clin Genet 46:324–326, 1994.
97. Davis JR, Weinstein L, Veomett IC, et al. Balanced translocation karyotypes in patients with repetitive abortion. Case study and literature review. Am J Obstet Gynecol 144:229–233, 1982.
98. Zuffardi O, Tiepolo L. Frequencies and types of chromosome abnormalities associated with human male infertility. *In* Crosignani PG, Rubin BL (eds). Genetic Control of Gamete Production and Function. London, Academic Press, 1982, pp 261–273.
99. Fryns JP, Kleczkowska A, Kubien E, et al. Cytogenetic survey in couples with recurrent fetal wastage. Hum Genet 65:336–354, 1984.
100. Cheung SW, Sun L, Featherstone T. Molecular cytogenetic evidence to characterize breakpoint regions in Robertsonian translocations. Cytogenet Cell Genet 54:97–102, 1990.
101. Gravolt CH, Friedrich U, Caprani M, et al. Breakpoints in Robertsonian translocations are localized to satellite III DNA by fluorescence in situ hybridization. Genomics 14:924–930, 1992.
102. Han J-Y, Choo KHA, Shaffer LG. Molecular cytogenetic characterization of 17 rob(13q14q) Robertsonian translocations by FISH, narrowing the region containing the breakpoints. Am J Hum Genet 55:960–967, 1994.
103. Grasso M, Giovannucci Uzielli ML, Pierluigi M, et al. Isochromosome not translocation in trisomy 21q21q. Hum Genet 84:63–65, 1989.
104. Antonarakis SE, Adelsberger PA, Petersen MB, et al. Analysis of DNA polymorphisms suggests that most de novo dup(21q) chromosomes in patients with Down syndrome are isochromosomes and not translocations. Am J Hum Genet 47:968–972, 1990.
105. Shaffer LG, Jackson-Cook CK, Meyer JM, et al. A molecular genetic approach to the identification of isochromosomes of chromosome 21. Hum Genet 86:375–382, 1991.
106. Bernstein R. X;Y chromosome translocations and their manifestations. *In* Sandberg AA (ed). The Y Chromosome, Part B: Clinical Aspects of Y Chromosome Abnormalities. New York, Alan R Liss, 1985, pp 171–206.
107. Chandley AC. Normal and abnormal meiosis in man and other mammals. *In* Crosignani PG, Rubin BL (eds). Genetic Control of Gamete Production and Function. London, Academic Press, 1982, pp 229–237.
108. Maraschio P, Tupler R, Dainotti E, et al. Molecular analysis of a human Y;1 translocation in an azoospermic male. Cytogenet Cell Genet 65:256–260, 1994.
109. Sinclair AH, Berta P, Palmer MS, et al. A gene from the human sex-determining region encodes a protein with homology to a conserved DNA-binding motif [see comments]. Nature 346:240–244, 1990.
110. Su H, Lau Y-F. Identification of the transcriptional unit, structural organization, and promoter sequence of the human sex-determining region Y *(SRY)* gene, using a reverse genetic approach. Am J Hum Genet 52:24–38, 1993.
111. Harley VR, Lovell-Badge R, Goodfellow PN. Definition of a consensus DNA binding site for *SRY.* Nucleic Acids Res 22:1500–1501, 1994.
112. Harley VR, Goodfellow PN. The biochemical role of *SRY* in sex determination. Mol Reprod Dev 39:184–193, 1994.
113. Foote S, Vollrath D, Hilton A, et al. The human Y chromosome: Overlapping DNA clones spanning the euchromatic region. Science 258:60–66, 1992.
114. Page DC, Mosher R, Simpson EM, et al. The sex-determining region of the human Y chromosome encodes a finger protein. Cell 51:1091–1104, 1987.
115. Berta P, Hawkins JR, Sinclair AH, et al. Genetic evidence equating *SRY* and the testis-determining factor. Nature 348:448–450, 1990.
116. Jager RJ, Anvert M, Hall K, et al. A human XY female with a frameshift mutation in the candidate testis-determining gene *SRY.* Nature 348:452–454, 1990.
117. Goodfellow PJ, Darling SM, Thomas NS, et al. A pseudoautosomal gene in man. Science 234:740–743, 1986.
118. Gough NM, Gearing DP, Nicola NA. Localization of the human GM-CSF receptor gene to the X-Y pseudoautosomal region. Nature 345:734–736, 1990.
119. Slim R, Levilliers J, Ludecke HJ, et al. A human pseudoautosomal gene encodes the ANT3 ADP/ATP translocase and escapes X-inactivation. Genomics 16:26–33, 1993.
120. Wolf U. Genetic aspects of H-Y antigen. Hum Genet 58:25–28, 1981.
121. Yen PH, Marsh B, Allen E, et al. The human X-linked steroid sulfatase gene and a Y-encoded pseudogene: Evidence for an inversion of the Y chromosome during primate evolution. Cell 55:1123–1135, 1988.
122. Tiepolo L, Zuffardi O. Localization of factors controlling spermatogenesis in the nonfluorescent portion of the human Y chromosome long arm. Hum Genet 34:119–124, 1976.
123. Alvesalo L, de la Chapelle A. Tooth size in two males with deletions of the long arm of the Y chromosome. Ann Hum Genet 45:49–54, 1981.
124. Chandley AC, Gosden JR, Hargreave TB, et al. Deleted Yq in the sterile son of a man with a satellited Y chromosome (Yqs). J Med Genet 26:145–153, 1989.
125. Salo P, Kääriäinen H, Page DC, et al. Deletion mapping of stature determinants on the long arm of the Y chromosome. Hum Genet 95:283–286, 1995.
126. Andersson M, Page DC, Pettay D, et al. Y;autosome translocations and mosaicism in the aetiology of 45,X maleness: Assignment of fertility factor to distal Yq11. Hum Genet 79:2–7, 1988.
127. Ma K, Sharkey A, Kirsch S. Towards the molecular localization of the *AZF* locus: Mapping of microdeletions in azoospermic men within 14 subintervals of interval 6 of the human Y chromosome. Hum Mol Genet 1:29–33, 1992.
128. Vogt P, Chandley AC, Hargreave TB, et al. Microdeletions in interval 6 of the Y chromosome of males with idiopathic sterility point to disruption of *AZF,* a human spermatogenesis gene. Hum Genet 89:491–496, 1992.
129. Reijo R, Lee TY, Salo P, et al. Diverse spermatogenic defects in humans caused by Y chromosome deletions encompassing a novel RNA-binding protein gene. Nat Genet 10:383–393, 1995.
130. Reijo R, Alagappan RK, Patrizio P, et al. Severe oligozoospermia

resulting from deletions of azoospermia factor gene on Y chromosome. Lancet 347:1290–1293, 1996.
131. Ma K, Inglis JD, Sharkey A, et al. A Y chromosome gene family with RNA-binding protein homology: Candidates for the azoospermia factor AZF controlling human spermatogenesis. Cell 75:1287–1295, 1993.
132. Najmabadi H, Huang V, Yen P, et al. Substantial prevalence of microdeletions of the Y-chromosome in infertile men with idiopathic azoospermia and oligozoospermia detected using a sequence-tagged site-based mapping strategy. J Clin Endocrinol Metab 81:1347–1352, 1996.
133. Drayna D, White R. The genetic linkage map of the human X chromosome. Science 230:753–758, 1985.
134. Lyon MF. Mechanisms and evolutionary origins of variable X-chromosome activity in mammals. Proc R Soc Lond B 187:243–268, 1961.
135. Therman E, Sarto GE, Palmer CG, et al. Position of the human X inactivation center on Xq. Hum Genet 50:59–64, 1979.
136. Brown CJ, Ballabio A, Rupert JL, et al. A gene from the region of the human X inactivation centre is expressed exclusively from the inactive X chromosome. Nature 349:38–44, 1991.
137. Brown CJ, Lafreniere RG, Powers VE, et al. Localization of the X inactivation centre on the human X chromosome in Xq13. Nature 349:82–84, 1991.
138. Brown CJ, Hendrich BD, Rupert JL, et al. The human *XIST* gene: Analysis of a 17 kb inactive X-specific RNA that contains conserved repeats and is highly localized within the nucleus. Cell 71:527–542, 1992.
139. Brown CJ, Willard HF. The human X-inactivation centre is not required for maintenance of X-chromosome inactivation. Nature 368:154–156, 1994.
140. Disteche CM. Escape from X inactivation in human and mouse. Trends Genet 11:17–22, 1995.
141. Therman E, Laxova B, Susman B. The critical region on the human Xq. Hum Genet 85:455–461, 1990.
142. Therman E, Susman B. The similarity of phenotypic effects caused by Xp and Xq deletions in the human female: A hypothesis. Hum Genet 85:175–183, 1990.
143. Jacobs PA, Hassold TJ. The origin of numerical chromosome abnormalities. Adv Genet 33:101–133, 1995.
144. Hook EB. Exclusion of chromosomal mosaicism: Tables of 90 percent, 95 percent, and 99 percent confidence limits and comments on use. Am J Hum Genet 29:94–97, 1977.
145. Levilliers J, Quack B, Weissenbach J, et al. Exchange of terminal portions of X− and Y− short arms in human XY females. Proc Natl Acad Sci USA 86:2296–3000, 1989.
146. Nowinski GP, Van Dyke DL, Tilley BC, et al. The frequency of aneuploidy in cultured lymphocytes is correlated with age and gender but not with reproductive history. Am J Hum Genet 46:1101–1111, 1990.
147. Stone JF, Sandberg AA. Sex chromosome aneuploidy and aging. Mutat Res 338:107–113, 1995.
148. Linden MG, Bender BG, Harmon RJ, et al. 47,XXX: What is the prognosis? [published erratum appears in Pediatrics 83:239, 1989]. Pediatrics 82:619–630, 1988.
149. Bender BG, Harmon RJ, Linden MG, et al. Psychosocial adaptation of 39 adolescents with sex chromosome abnormalities. Pediatrics 96:302–308, 1995.
150. Linden MG, Bender BG, Robinson A. Sex chromosome tetrasomy and pentasomy. Pediatrics 96:672–682, 1995.
151. Linden MG, Bender BG, Robinson A. Intrauterine diagnosis of sex chromosome aneuploidy. Obstet Gynecol 87:468–475, 1996.
152. Koopman P, Munsterberg A, Capel B, et al. Expression of a candidate sex-determining gene during mouse testis differentiation. Nature 348:450–452, 1990.
153. Bennett CP, Docherty Z, Robb S. Deletion of 9p and sex reversal. J Med Genet 30:518–520, 1993.
154. Wilkie AO, Campbell FM, Daubeney P, et al. Complete and partial XY sex reversal associated with terminal deletion of 10q: Report of 2 cases and literature review. Am J Med Genet 46:597–600, 1993.
155. Bardoni B, Zanaria E, Guioli S, et al. A dosage sensitive locus at chromosome Xp21 is involved in male to female sex reversal. Nature Genet 7:497–501, 1994.
156. Zanaria E, Muscatelli F, Bardoni B. An unusual member of the nuclear hormone receptor superfamily responsible for X-linked adrenal hypoplasia congenita. Nature 372:635–641, 1994.
157. Houston CS, Opitz JM, Spranger JW, et al. The campomelic syndrome: Review, report of 17 cases, and follow-up on the currently 17-year-old boy first reported by Maroteaux et al. in 1971. Am J Med Genet 15:3–28, 1983.
158. Foster JW, Dominguez-Steglich MA, Guioli S, et al. Campomelic dysplasia and autosomal sex reversal caused by mutations in an *SRY*-related gene. Nature 372:525–530, 1994.
159. Sudbeck P, Schmitz ML, Baeuerle PA, et al. Sex reversal by loss of the C-terminal transactivation domain of human *SOX9*. Nat Genet 13:230–232, 1996.
160. Verlinsky Y, Handyside A, Grifo J, et al. Preimplantation diagnosis of genetic and chromosomal disorders. J Assist Reprod Genet 11:236–243, 1994.
161. Munné S, Grifo J, Cohen J, et al. Chromosome abnormalities in human arrested preimplantation embryos: A multiple-probe FISH study. Am J Hum Genet 55:150–159, 1994.
162. Munné S, Weier HUG, Grifo J, et al. Chromosome mosaicism in human embryos. Biol Reprod 51:373–379, 1994.

Chapter 13

REPRODUCTIVE IMMUNOLOGY AND ITS DISORDERS

Aydin Arici • Harvey J. Kliman • David L. Olive

CHAPTER OUTLINE

KEY POINTS

- The immune system is a complex entity designed to eliminate foreign intruding antigens and consists of both cellular and humoral components.
- The immune system is influenced by and in turn influences the function of the reproductive system.
- The immune system has known effects on ovulatory function and implantation physiology.
- Disorders of immune function have been linked to such diverse gynecologic abnormalities as endometriosis, antisperm antibody–induced infertility, recurrent pregnancy loss, and premature ovarian failure.

It has long been suggested that for every unexplained aspect of medicine there exists an immunologic theory. Indeed, the mysteries of reproduction have made this field ripe for speculation regarding possible immune-reproductive interactions. Poorly substantiated theories and incorrect or illogical extrapolations have led to many disastrous attempts to provide an intimate link between these two critical systems, frequently leading to overt skepticism regarding any immunologic role in reproductive success.

Despite such an inauspicious beginning, numerous reputable scientists began the painstaking process of piecing together the building blocks of the immunologic-reproductive foundation. Today, it is clear that the two are intimately interrelated, with immunologic cells, molecules, and processes playing crucial roles in many reproductive functions.

This chapter reviews the basics of modern immunology, including immunologic aspects unique to the reproductive organs. The role of the immune system in normal reproduction is also explored, with particular emphasis on separating facts from hypotheses. Finally, we review what is known about immunogenesis of reproductive disorders.

BASIC IMMUNOLOGY REVIEW

General Review

The aim of the immune system is the elimination of foreign intruding antigens. In general, two systems can be discerned: the innate immune system and the adaptive immune system, each with specific cellular and humoral factors. The cells involved are B lymphocytes, T lymphocytes, granulocytes, monocytes, macrophages, and natural killer (NK) cells (Table 13–1). The soluble factors include cytokines, lysozyme, acute-phase proteins, complement, and the immunoglobulins. The intruding antigen is presented by antigen-presenting cells (macrophages and monocytes) to T-helper lymphocytes, which are central to the development of immune responses. The processing of the antigen gives rise to the production of cytokines such as interleukins. These help B cells to produce antibodies and modulate the actions of other effector cells. One of the first lines of defense against aberrant cells is mediated by NK cells.

The specific immunologic response has two components and three essential characteristics. The two components are

1. Primary immune response. Initial exposure to a particular infectious agent, or immunogen, is followed by an induction phase, during which precommitted lymphocytes proliferate and mature into antibody-secreting plasma cells (humoral immune responses) or specifically reactive T cells that secrete various mediators (cytokines) on subsequent contact with that agent (cell-mediated immune responses).
2. Secondary (anamnestic) immune response. On further contact with that same immunogen, increased

■ TABLE 13–1
Cells of the Immune System

SPECIFIC	
B lymphocytes	Precursors of antibody-producing cells
T lymphocytes	Recognize and act on antigens originating from within cells of the host; different populations exist
Helper T cells ($CD4^+$)	Help B cells to divide, differentiate, and produce antibody
Cytotoxic T cells ($CD8^+$)	Capable of destroying target cells
Suppressor T cells	Down-regulate the actions of other T cells and B cells
NONSPECIFIC	
Monocytes	Circulating, nonspecific phagocytotic, antigen-presenting cells
Macrophages	Monocytes that migrated into tissues
Granulocytes	Phagocytic cells with short life span (2–3 days), migrating into the tissues under the influence of chemotactic stimuli
Natural killer cells	Nonspecific, cytotoxic cells able to lyse various tumor or virus-infected cells without prior sensitization

resistance develops through the abundant production of specific antibodies or sensitized lymphocytes.

Three essential characteristics of the specific immunologic response are (1) the ability to distinguish self from non-self; (2) specificity, which is the selectivity shown by antibodies and lymphocytes of the specific immune system reacting only with matching (homologous) immunogens; and (3) immunologic memory, which allows antibodies and sensitized lymphocytes to remember their homologous immunogen (sometimes referred to as an antigen) and react with it later.

Specific immunity may be acquired by natural or artificial processes. Examples of naturally acquired immunity include the immunity that develops during convalescence from an infection and the placental passage of antibody from mother to fetus. Examples of artificially acquired immunity include vaccination and the injection of gamma globulin for the induction of an immune state.

Specific immune responses are mediated by two interrelated and interdependent mechanisms. *Humoral immunity* primarily involves bursa- or bone marrow–derived B lymphocytes, or B cells. Immunoglobulins, as proteins in the plasma fraction of the blood, constitute the humoral (i.e., soluble) component of the specific immune system. The B cell expresses specific immunoglobulin on its surface. When this surface immunoglobulin (sIgM) interacts with its homologous antigen, the B cell is triggered to proliferate and differentiate into plasma cells. The plasma cells excrete vast quantities of immunoglobulin that is specific for the same antigen that originally triggered the B cell.

Cellular immunity primarily involves thymus-derived T lymphocytes, or T cells. The T cell expresses on its surface a receptor molecule that is structurally similar to an immunoglobulin and is similarly specific for its particular homologous immunogen but is not secreted from the cell. When the T-cell receptor contacts its homologous immunogen, proliferation and differentiation of the T cell and its progeny are stimulated. The end product of this developmental process is a variety of T-cell subsets with different functions. Molecules on the T-cell membrane that function chiefly as receptors have been identified by monoclonal antibody techniques and include class I and class II major histocompatibility complex (MHC) molecules and CD

■ TABLE 13–2
Characteristics of T Cells

T-CELL SUBTYPE	SYMBOL	IDENTIFYING SURFACE ANTIGEN	MHC RESTRICTION	TARGET CELL	FUNCTION
Cytotoxic	Tc	CD8	Class I	Tumors Virally infected cells Allografts	Kills foreign cells or cells with new surface antigens
Helper	Th	CD4	Class II	B cells Tc cells	Interleukin secretion
Inducer	Th	CD4	Class II	B cells Tc-cell precursors Macrophages	Interleukin secretion
Suppressor	Ts	CD8	Class II	B cells Th cells Tc cells	Down-regulates cell growth
Delayed-type hypersensitivity	Tdth	CD4	Class II	Langerhans cells Macrophages Tc cells	Releases MAF, MIF, and other cytokines
Memory	Tm	CD8 CD4	Both	B cells T cells	Anamnesis

MAF, macrophage-activating factor; MHC, major histocompatibility complex; MIF, migration-inhibiting factor.

(cluster of differentiation) antigens (e.g., CD4, CD8). These cell surface molecules are used to differentiate T-cell subsets (Table 13–2). These T cells, which reside in the peripheral blood and lymphoid tissues, constitute the cellular (i.e., T-cell–mediated) component of the specific immune system. Interaction of these specifically sensitized lymphocytes with their homologous ligand (antigen) triggers the release of a variety of cytokines. After activation by antigen, $CD4^+$ T-helper (Th) cells produce one of two distinctive cytokine profiles, leading to their classification as Th1 and Th2 cells.[1] The Th1 cells primarily secrete interferon-γ (IFN-γ), interleukin (IL)–2, and tumor necrosis factor (TNF) and induce cellular immunity. The Th2 cells primarily secrete IL-4, IL-5, and IL-10 and down-regulate cellular immunity while inducing heightened antibody production.[2–4]

Cells that contribute to nonspecific immunity include granulocytes, monocytes, macrophages, and NK cells. These cells are phagocytic or cytotoxic against a variety of targets in the absence of any previous exposure to the targets. *Neutrophils* are granulocytes that circulate in the blood and migrate quickly in response to local invasion by microorganisms. *Monocytes* also circulate in the blood, but in much lower number than neutrophils. They migrate to the tissues, where they differentiate into macrophages, which reside in all body tissues. *Macrophages*, the major antigen-presenting cells of the body, interact with antigen as a primary step in the induction of an immune response. In addition to presenting antigen to T and B cells, macrophages release soluble mediators such as cytokines, hydrolytic enzymes, oxygen radicals, and prostaglandins[5] (Table 13–3).

NK cells are granular lymphocytes that appear to function in immune surveillance. These cells are naturally occurring cytotoxic lymphocytes that exist in the body at birth. They are not induced by immunologic insult, although their numbers and activity can be increased by various cytokines (e.g., IL-2). NK cells arise from bone marrow precursors but are of a lineage distinct from that of either T or B cells; they represent 10 to 15 percent of the lymphocytes in peripheral blood, but they are absent from lymph nodes. Endometrial large granulated lymphocytes are believed to be specialized NK cells, and they are present in large numbers in the late secretory phase of the cycle and in early pregnancy decidua. NK cells are cytotoxic for tumor cells and virally infected autologous cells. Recent evidence suggests that NK cells, as well as some T cells, may be responsible for antibody-dependent cell-mediated cytotoxicity. These cells have membrane receptors for the Fc portion of immunoglobulin G and therefore can interact effectively with antibody-coated targets. NK cells have a broad target range, and they are not subject to MHC restriction. That is, cytotoxicity by NK cells does not require that it recognize MHC molecules on the target cells. NK cells do not possess antigenic specificity and do not acquire immunologic memory after exposure to virus-infected cells or tumor cells. Lymphokine-activated killer (LAK) cells are other naturally occurring cytotoxic cells. LAK cells are quiescent lymphocytes that are induced into an active cytotoxic state by IL-2. The LAK cell is similar in many ways to the NK cell but has an even broader target cell range.

■ TABLE 13–3
Secreted Products of Macrophages

PRODUCTS	EXAMPLES
Enzymes	Plasminogen activator Collagenase Lysozyme Lipase Phosphatase Glycosidase
Plasma proteins	α_2-Macroglobulin α_1-Antitrypsin Fibronectin
Coagulation factors	Tissue thromboplastin Factors V, VII, IX, X
Complement components	C1, C2, C3, C4, C5 Properdin Factors B, D, I, H
Oxygen metabolites	Superoxide anion Hydrogen peroxide Hydroxyl radical Singlet oxygen
Arachidonic acid metabolites	Prostaglandin E_2 Thromboxane B_2 Leukotriene C_4 (i.e., slow-reacting substance of anaphylaxis)
Nucleotide metabolites	Cyclic adenosine monophosphate Thymidine
Cell growth and function regulators	Growth factors Interleukins Interferons Erythropoietin

The MHC became relevant when its association with the susceptibility to many diseases was recognized. The MHC molecule on the antigen-presenting cell must be recognized by the appropriate CD membrane component on the T cell, either CD4 of the helper T cell or CD8 of the cytotoxic T cell. This phenomenon is referred to as MHC restriction and is required for T-cell activation. The MHC comprises tightly linked genes for three major classes of human leukocyte antigen (HLA) molecules and is located on the short arm of chromosome 6 in the human[6, 7] (Fig. 13–1).

The HLA class I region may contain as many as 17 gene loci, but only three, HLA-A, HLA-B, and HLA-C, have been well characterized. These molecules have a polymorphic, transmembrane heavy chain noncovalently linked to nonpolymorphic, nontransmembrane β_2-microglobulin (encoded on chromosome 15) whose sequence is homologous with one of the constant region domains of the immunoglobulin molecule[8] (Fig. 13–2). Classic HLA class I molecules are expressed on the surface of virtually all nucleated cells as well as platelets. These antigens act primarily as vehicles for presenting foreign peptides to cytotoxic $CD8^+$ T cells. In contrast, the nonclassic HLA class I molecules are monomorphic, or at most oligomorphic, and do not encode tissue allogeneity but are linked to β_2-microglobulin. These nonpolymorphic class I molecules, also known

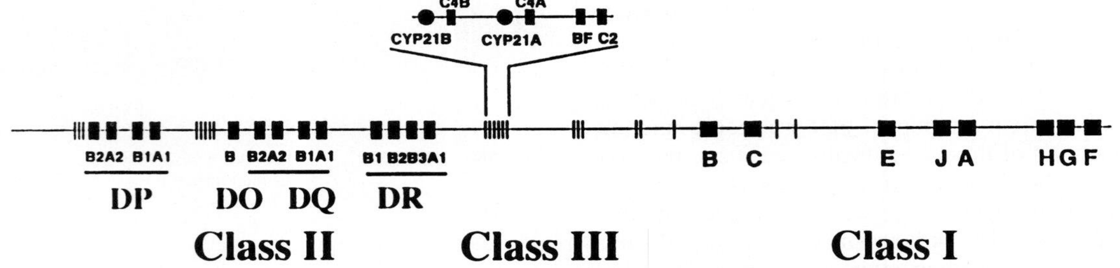

Figure 13–1 ■ Organization of the HLA system on the short arm of chromosome 6.

as class Ib antigens, are HLA-E, HLA-F, and HLA-G. Invasive human cytotrophoblasts express HLA-G, which is trophoblast cell specific.[9, 10] Expression of HLA-G has been suggested as a mechanism that may protect trophoblasts against killing by NK cells.[11, 12]

HLA class II antigens (DP, DQ, and DR) are also heterodimers consisting of noncovalently associated transmembrane heavy α and β chains. The external domains of these chains are the main sites for polymorphic determinants. Class II antigens are expressed on B lymphocytes, macrophages, and activated T lymphocytes.[13] The expression of class II molecules can be up-regulated by certain cytokines such as interferon and TNF. These cell surface molecules present foreign peptides to receptors on T cells capable of undergoing clonal expansion and of producing cytokines. HLA-DR antigens contain epitopes that can stimulate T cells from other individuals in mixed lymphocyte culture (alloreactive response). T cells can recognize even subtle differences within molecules.

Class III antigens are not cell surface molecules but represent complement components (C2, Bf [properdin factor B], C4A, and C4B). TNF and two 21-hydroxylase genes are also encoded in this region.

Soluble products of the immune response include immunoglobulins, the complement system, and cytokines. *Immunoglobulins* are produced by B cells or plasma cells in response to exposure to an immunogen. They react specifically with that antigen in vivo or in vitro; thus, they are a part of the adaptive immune response. The basic structural unit of an immunoglobulin molecule consists of four polypeptide chains linked covalently by disulfide bonds (Fig. 13–3). The four-chain, monomeric immunoglobulin structure is composed of two identical heavy (H) polypeptide chains and two identical light (L) polypeptide chains. The carboxyl end of L chains and the carboxyl end of H chains are extremely homologous (Fc [fragment crystallizable] fragment), a feature that is common to other mammalian immunoglobulins. The amino end of L and H chains has greater heterogeneity within certain areas, resulting in hypervariable regions (Fab [fragment antigen-binding] fragments).

The *complement system* plays a major role in host defense and in the inflammatory process. Complement consists of a complex series of at least 15 proteins that normally are functionally inactive in plasma. Complement is activated sequentially in a cascading manner after antibody-antigen binding. Activation of the complement cascade causes sensitization for phagocytosis (opsonization), lysis of target cells, and release of inflammatory substances (chemotaxis for granulocytes, i.e., C5a, and release of histamine).

Cytokine is a generic term that can be applied to the soluble product of any cell type, as long as its release affects the behavior of other cells. Many cytokines and

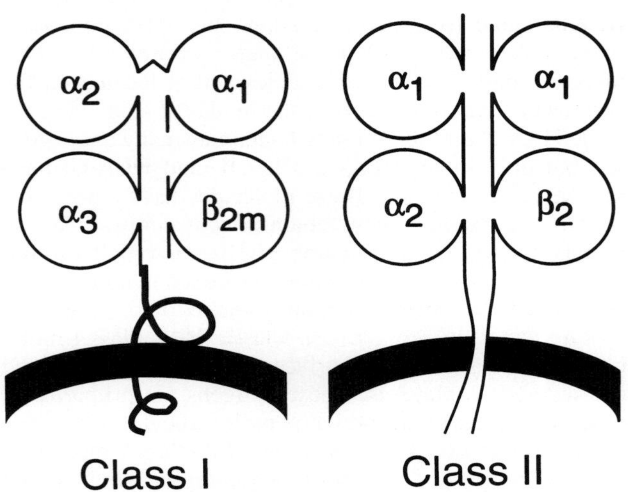

Figure 13–2 ■ Molecular structure of class I and class II molecules of the HLA system.

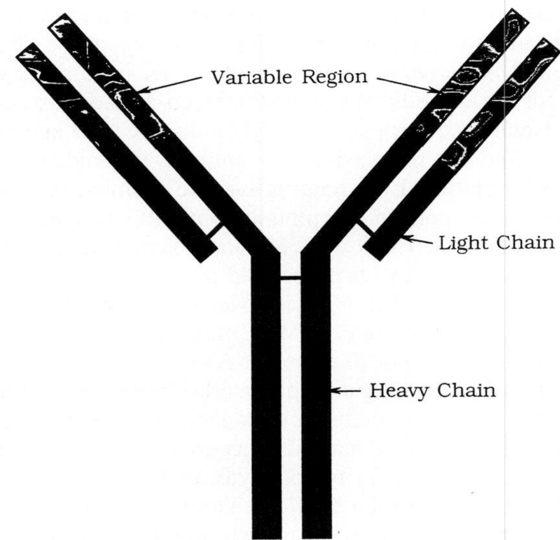

Figure 13–3 ■ Basic immunoglobulin structure.

growth factors are proteins found in a wide variety of tissues where they are produced locally and work by paracrine or autocrine mechanisms. Although these peptides are named after their originally observed biologic action, they are generally involved in a wide range of other actions including stimulation of cell growth, inhibition of cellular proliferation, and alteration of cell functions. Cytokines exert their effects at concentrations between 10^{-9} and 10^{-12} M by binding to cell surface receptors on target cells (Table 13–4).

Effects of Reproductive Hormones on the Immune System

A significant body of data establishes that many aspects of immune response differ between males and females. Women have higher plasma immunoglobulin M levels than men do, a difference that becomes more significant at the time of puberty.[14, 15] Cell-mediated immune responses are also sexually dimorphic, and there are quantitative differences in relative numbers of functional T cells.[16, 17] Higher CD4:CD8 ratios are generally seen in women and hypogonadal men because of relatively lower numbers of circulating $CD8^+$ T cells.[18, 19] A variety of autoimmune diseases are much more likely to occur in women than in men, and sex hormones have been proposed as a reason for this preponderance[20, 21] (Table 13–5). Systemic lupus erythematosus (SLE) exacerbation in women taking estrogens, decreased testosterone levels in men with SLE, and occurrence of SLE in men with Klinefelter's syndrome all implicate estrogen to testosterone ratios as a risk factor.[18, 22] A single estrogen injection induces profound thymic atrophy 10 days later in mice and stimulates extrathymic T-cell maturation, a characteristic finding of autoimmunity.[23] Expression of both estrogen[24] and progesterone[25] receptors has been demonstrated in the human thymus.

Gonadal steroid hormones also affect the cytokines, soluble mediators of the immune system. This influence on cytokines may occur at three levels: (1) alteration of expression of a given cytokine at the transcriptional or post-transcriptional level, (2) modulation of the expression of the cytokine receptor, or (3) modification of the effect of the cytokine in the target cells.[26] Estradiol and progesterone down-regulate the expression of IL-1 in human peripheral monocytes.[27] After oophorectomy, an increased production of IL-1 by peripheral monocytes is observed in women, and estrogen treatment blocks this increase.[28] Consistent with these findings, it was reported that monocyte expression of secretory IL-1 receptor antagonist messenger ribonucleic acid (mRNA) was significantly elevated in the presence of physiologic levels of estradiol and progesterone.[29] Gonadal steroids also modulate TNF-α,[30] IFN-γ,[31] colony-stimulating factor 1 (CSF-1),[32] transforming growth factor-β (TGF-β),[33] and IL-8[34] in responsive cells.

Besides gonadal steroids, a direct role for the gonadotropins and other reproductive peptide hormones in alteration of immune function has been shown. Human lymphocytes express luteinizing hormone (LH) receptor on their surface[35] and also produce both LH[36] and gonadotropin-releasing hormone (GnRH) on activation.[37, 38] GnRH agonist was found to diminish NK cell activity, stimulate T-cell proliferation, and increase T-cell IL-2 receptor expression independent of gonadal steroid production.[39–41] Another reproductive hormone that may affect the immune system is prolactin; hyperprolactinemia is associated with some autoimmune diseases,[42] and the GnRH gene in rat T cells is regulated by prolactin.[43]

THE ROLE OF THE IMMUNE SYSTEM IN REPRODUCTION

Fertility

In many animals, an intact functioning immune system is necessary for normal reproductive function. Thymectomy in mice is accompanied by gonadal degeneration, which can be prevented by thymocyte or spleen cell transplantation.[44] The effects of immune cells and cytokines are observed at all levels of the reproductive system including the hypothalamus, pituitary, gonads, and uterus. At the level of the hypothalamus, IL-1 inhibits the release of GnRH in rats.[45] IL-1 binding, action, and receptor mRNA have been shown in a variety of pituitary cell preparations.[46] In rats, IL-1 inhibits the ovarian steroid-induced LH surge.[45] In dispersed rat pituitary cells, IL-1 and IL-6 induce significant release of follicle-stimulating hormone (FSH), LH, and prolactin comparable to that induced by GnRH and thyrotropin-releasing hormone.[47] In these same cells, TNF-α causes a rapid increase in the release of LH, prolactin, and adrenocorticotropic hormone.[48]

Immune cells and molecules may well serve to modulate ovulation.[49] The number and the type of leukocytes in the ovary vary throughout the phase of the ovulatory cycle.[50] Macrophages are present in both the stroma[51] and the follicle itself.[52] Finally, just before ovulation, there is an infiltration of additional leukocytes into the area surrounding the dominant follicle.[53]

Experimental evidence supports a role for immune components in the ovulatory process. Peripheral blood leukocytes added to the in vitro perfused rat ovary increase the number of LH-induced ovulations.[54] IL-1 stimulates prostaglandin biosynthesis in rat ovary incubations[55] and induces oocyte maturation and ovulation in the in vitro perfused rabbit ovary.[56]

Luteal function, too, may be affected by the immune system. There is an orderly immigration of leukocytes in the early corpus luteum. In addition, substances secreted by macrophages may stimulate the angiogenic process prominent with luteinization.

Cytokines have been shown by a number of investigators to have significant effects on granulosa and luteal cell steroidogenesis,[57–59] but the actions depend on the species studied, the endocrine background, and the degree of differentiation of the steroidogenic cell. In the human, IL-1 stimulates production of progesterone synthesis in granulosa cells[60] and maintains the progesterone synthesis in granulosa-lutein cells.[61] In contrast, IL-1 inhibits FSH-stimulated estradiol synthesis in luteinized granulosa cells.[61] An intraovarian IL-1 system complete with ligands, receptors, and a receptor antagonist in humans is well established.[62] Somewhat similar results have been observed with TNF-α. Progesterone synthesis is enhanced by TNF-α in granulosa cells;[63] however, there is a lack of effect on gonadotropin-stimulated granulosa-lutein cells.[61, 64] TNF-α inhibits estra-

■ TABLE 13–4
Cytokines of Importance in Immune Response

CYTOKINE	SOURCES	TARGETS	EFFECTS
IL-1	Macrophages B cells NK cells	T cells B cells Macrophages	Lymphocyte activation Macrophage stimulation Pyrexia Acute-phase reaction
IL-2	T cells NK cells	B cells T cells NK cells Macrophages	Lymphocyte activation Macrophage activation Stimulation of lymphokine secretion
IL-3	T cells	Stem cells	Proliferation
IL-4	T cells	B cells Macrophages	Lymphocyte proliferation Macrophage activation Influence on immunoglobulin class switching
IL-5	T cells	B cells Stem cells Eosinophils	Proliferation Differentiation Promotion to switch to IgA Eosinophilia
IL-6	Numerous	B cells Macrophages	Proliferation Stimulation of immunoglobulin secretion Acute-phase reaction
IL-7	Stromal cells	Pre-B cells T cells	Proliferation
IL-8	Numerous	Neutrophils T cells	Chemotaxis of leukocytes
IL-9	T cells	Th cells Mast cells	Proliferation
IL-10	T cells	T cells	Inhibition of lymphokine synthesis
IL-11	Stromal cells	Progenitor cells	Hematopoiesis
IL-12	Macrophages	NK cells	Stimulation
IL-13	Activated T cells	Monocytes B cells	B-cell proliferation
IL-14	T cells	B cells	Inhibition of immunoglobulin synthesis
IL-15	Numerous	T cells	Proliferation
GM-CSF	T cells Monocytes	Stem cells Monocytes Granulocytes	Proliferation Differentiation
MCP-1	Numerous	Monocytes	Chemotaxis Activation
TNF-α	Macrophages T cells NK cells	B cells	Growth and differentiation
LIF	Numerous	Progenitor cells Embryonic cells Trophoblasts	Proliferation Differentiation
IFN-γ	T cells NK cells	Macrophages B cells	Differentiation

IL, interleukin; NK, natural killer; GM-CSF, granulocyte-macrophage colony-stimulating factor; MCP, monocyte chemotactic protein; TNF, tumor necrosis factor; LIF, leukemia inhibitory factor; IFN, interferon.

■ TABLE 13–5
Prevalence of Autoimmune Diseases in Women and Men

DISEASE	WOMEN : MEN
Hashimoto's thyroiditis	40 : 1
Systemic lupus erythematosus	9 : 1
Primary biliary cirrhosis	9 : 1
Graves' disease	6 : 1
Rheumatoid arthritis	3 : 1

diol synthesis in luteinized granulosa cells.[65] IFN-γ, on the other hand, inhibits both progesterone and estrogen synthesis in luteinized granulosa cells.[66]

In nonpregnancy cycles, involution of the corpus luteum is characterized by extensive leukocyte infiltration.[67] In fact, macrophages[68] and neutrophils[69] have been proposed as major players in luteolysis; studies show that immunosuppression by dexamethasone blocks functional luteolysis in the rat.[70] The expression of monocyte chemotactic protein 1 (MCP-1) in rat corpus luteum was recently shown to precede the luteal regression and may be one of the signals for timely chemoattraction for monocytes.[71]

Implantation and Early Pregnancy

Cytokines and Growth Factors Relevant to Implantation

Growth factors and cytokines may serve three roles in the implantation process: first, in an autocrine manner, they may mediate the proliferative and secretory actions of steroids in preparing the endometrial receptivity; second, by acting on the embryo, they may mediate implantation and trophoblast invasion; and third, by recruiting selected lymphocytes and macrophages into the endometrium/decidua, they may mediate immunologic acceptance of the pregnancy. Although the maternal immune system has been viewed as antagonistic to placental function, there is evidence that cytokines produced by the uterus may promote trophoblast development.[72] The numbers of cytokines and growth factors expressed in the endometrium are remarkable, and most likely they are integrated into a vast and intricate network (Table 13–6). We review here only those that are believed to play an important role in implantation.

Leukemia inhibitory factor (LIF), a cytokine that regulates the proliferation and differentiation of cells from hematopoietic, embryonal, neural, and other cell lineages, is expressed in mouse uterine endometrial glands, most prominently on the fourth day of pregnancy when implantation occurs. Stewart and coworkers[72a] have shown that well-timed expression of LIF in the endometrium of mice is crucial for successful implantation of the embryo. LIF is expressed in the human endometrium in a menstrual cycle–dependent manner; maximal expression is observed between days 19 and 25 of the menstrual cycle, coinciding with the time of human implantation.[73] A possible mechanism by which LIF could promote implantation was demonstrated by Nachtigall and colleagues,[74] who showed that LIF acts on human trophoblasts to shift their differentiation toward anchoring phenotype by increasing the synthesis of fibronectin and decreasing the production of human chorionic gonadotropin (Fig. 13–4).

Colony-stimulating factor (CSF-1) is also expressed in the uterus, and its synthesis during the early part of pregnancy is regulated in part by estrogen and progesterone.[75] This cytokine enhances the rate of blastocyst development in culture. CSF-1–deficient mice are known to have reduced fertility.[76]

Interleukin-1 is produced by the endometrial cells. Several studies suggest that the expression of IL-1 in the uterus and other tissues may be affected by estrogen and progesterone.[77, 78] Simon and colleagues[79] have shown in mice that the blockade of the type I IL-1 receptor prevented implantation without interfering with embryonic attachment and without any adverse effect on blastocyst formation, hatching, fibronectin attachment, outgrowth, and migration. Immunohistochemical findings also suggest a role for IL-1 in human implantation.[80]

TGF-β is expressed by human endometrium/decidua and promotes the deposition of extracellular matrix by inhibiting the production of matrix metalloproteinases. This suggests that this cytokine may play a role in trophoblast invasion.[81]

Epidermal growth factor (EGF) is a potential mediator of the proliferative action of estradiol in the uterus.[82, 83] EGF is also produced in the uterus during the peri-implantation period, and EGF promotes mouse trophoblast outgrowth. Despite these findings, however, in mice lacking EGF receptors, implantation of blastocyst is not blocked.

A number of proteins have been isolated from the human endometrium and decidua. Some of these proteins are relevant to the implantation period. *Pregnancy-associated endometrial protein*, also known as placental protein 14 (PP14), is the major secretory product of the endometrium and is measurable in the serum. This protein appears in the endometrium 5 days after ovulation and reaches peak levels in the serum during the last 2 or 3 days of the cycle; in conception cycles, the rise continues. The regulation of synthesis and function of PP14 are not known in detail, but PP14 has been suggested to have a local immunoregulatory role at the site of implantation.[84] The endometrium synthesizes both *insulin-like growth factors* (IGF-I and IGF-II). There is a preferential expression of IGF-I during the proliferative phase and of IGF-II in the secretory phase.[85] IGFBP-1, a binding protein for the IGFs, is pro-

■ TABLE 13–6
Endometrial Growth Factors and Cytokines That May Regulate Implantation

Leukemia inhibitory factor
Colony-stimulating factor 1
Granulocyte-macrophage colony-stimulating factor
Interleukin-1 and interleukin-6
Interferon-α and interferon-γ
Tumor necrosis factor-α
Transforming growth factor-β
Transforming growth factor-α
Epidermal growth factor
Fibroblast growth factor
Insulin-like growth factor types I and II
Insulin-like growth factor–binding proteins
Platelet-derived growth factor

Data from Tabibzadeh,[218] Haimovici and Anderson,[219] Giudice,[86] and Arici et al.[73a]

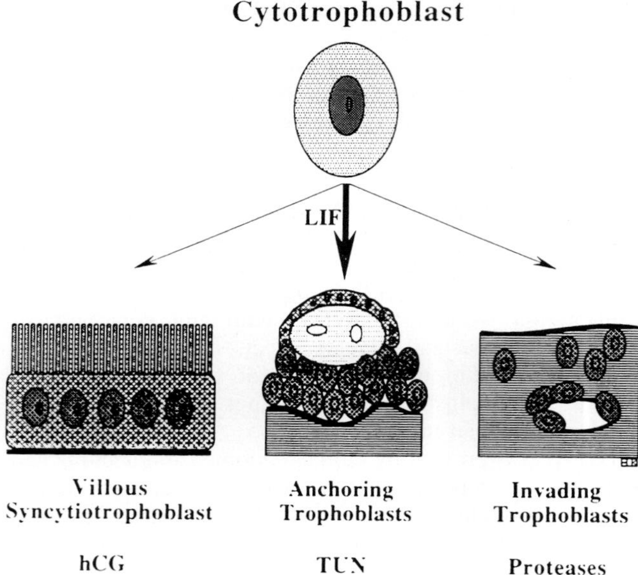

Figure 13–4 ■ Pathways of trophoblast differentiation. Just as the undifferentiated basal layer of the skin gives rise to differentiated keratinocytes, the cytotrophoblast (the stem cell of the placenta) gives rise to the differentiated forms of trophoblasts.

Left, Within the chorionic villi, cytotrophoblasts fuse to form the overlying syncytiotrophoblast. The villous syncytiotrophoblast makes the majority of the placental hormones, the most studied being human chorionic gonadotropin (hCG). Cyclic adenosine monophosphate and its analogues, and more recently hCG itself,[220] have been shown to direct cytotrophoblast differentiation toward a hormonally active syncytiotrophoblast phenotype.

Center, At the point where chorionic villi make contact with external extracellular matrix (decidual stromal extracellular matrix in the case of intrauterine pregnancies), a population of trophoblasts proliferates from the cytotrophoblast layer to form the second type of trophoblast—the junctional trophoblast. These cells form the anchoring cell columns that can be seen at the junction of the placenta and endometrium throughout gestation. Similar trophoblasts can be seen at the junction of the chorion layer of the external membranes and the decidua. The junctional trophoblasts make a unique fibronectin, trophouteronectin (TUN), that appears to mediate the attachment of the placenta to the uterus. TGF-β and now, from our current work, leukemia inhibitory factor (LIF) have been shown to down-regulate hCG synthesis and up-regulate TUN secretion.

Right, Finally, a third type of trophoblast differentiates toward an invasive phenotype and leaves the placenta entirely—the invasive intermediate trophoblast. In addition to making human placental lactogen, these cells also make gelatinases, urokinase-type plasminogen activator, and type 1 plasminogen activator inhibitor. LIF, in addition to up-regulating TUN production and down-regulating hCG secretion, has recently been shown to also down-regulate trophoblast gelatinolytic activity.[221] (From Nachtigall MJ, Kliman HJ, Feinberg RF, et al. The effect of leukemia inhibitory factor on trophoblast differentiation: A potential role in human implantation. J Clin Endocrinol Metab 81:801–806, 1996. © The Endocrine Society.)

duced by decidualized stromal cells. It has been hypothesized that decidual IGFBP-1 competes for the binding of IGFs and thus provides a physiologic mechanism to limit IGF-II–induced mitogenesis. It is believed that this is one of the factors controlling trophoblastic invasion.[86]

Endometrial Leukocytes Relevant to Implantation

Leukocytes form a substantial proportion of the constituent cells of human endometrium, accounting for around 7 percent of stromal cells in proliferative endometrium and increasing to more than 30 percent in early pregnancy, characteristic of an immunologically active tissue. However, organization of the endometrial lymphoid system is atypical in several aspects: there are no intraepithelial B cells, only a few B cells can be identified in the stroma, and no plasma cells are found in normal endometrium. The endometrial leukocyte population primarily consists of macrophages, T cells, and granulated lymphocytes.[87]

Macrophages are present in nonpregnant endometrium, increasing in number premenstrually and in both decidua basalis and decidua parietalis throughout gestation. Macrophages produce cytokines such as CSF-1 or granulocyte-macrophage colony-stimulating factor and regulate the synthesis of growth factors that may have a role in placental growth.[88]

T lymphocytes show little variation in number and distribution during the menstrual cycle and early pregnancy. In contrast with peripheral blood T cells, most endometrial T cells express the CD8 suppressor/cytotoxic subset marker.[89] The function of T cells in human endometrium is not known.

Large granular lymphocytes, a form of NK cell, represent the most abundant lymphoid cell population in human endometrium in the late luteal phase and early pregnancy. The in vivo role of large granular lymphocytes is unknown. They increase around the time of expected implantation, and they persist during the first trimester of pregnancy, after which there is a rapid decline. This pattern suggests that these cells may play a role in implantation and placental development. Clark and associates[90] have shown that human large granular lymphocytes are responsible for the release of the immunosuppressive TGF-β in vitro.

THE ROLE OF THE IMMUNE SYSTEM IN REPRODUCTIVE DISORDERS

Infertility

Endometriosis

Endometriosis is a common condition among women of reproductive age. During the last 70 years, at least a dozen theories have been proposed to explain the histogenesis and etiology of endometriosis. None of the theories alone can explain the entire spectrum and anatomic distribution of the lesions. It appears that the etiology is multifactorial, and a composite theory of retrograde menstruation with implantation of endometrial fragments in conjunction with peritoneal factors to stimulate cell growth is most widely accepted today for peritoneal endometriosis.[91] Retrograde menstruation is a well-established phenomenon, present in 76 to 90 percent of women.[92–94] It may be that the inability to remove retrograde menstrual debris is the mechanism by which endometrial tissue is allowed to implant and grow ectopically. Thus, an altered immune response to shed endometrium would be a primary target for investigation into the pathogenesis of this disease.

In recent years, various data have suggested alterations in both cell-mediated and hormonal immunity in women with endometriosis. In two unrelated studies in which the immune system was suppressed in rhesus monkeys, by proton radiation[95] and by polychlorinated biphenyls,[96] endometriosis developed more frequently than in control subjects. In baboons, immunosuppression with methylprednisolone and azathioprine increased the progression of endometriosis.[97] In humans, most of the research on the immunology of endometriosis is observational and involves studies on the various aspects of immune function in infertile women who have been diagnosed with this disease. A significant trend toward a certain pattern of immune dysfunction can be identified from these studies. Women with endometriosis appear to exhibit increased humoral immune responsiveness and macrophage activation as well as diminished cell-mediated immunity with decreased T-cell and NK cell responsiveness.

CELLULAR IMMUNITY IN ENDOMETRIOSIS

Cellular immunity to autologous endometrium has been shown to be suppressed, secondary to diminished T-cell reactivity, in rhesus monkeys with spontaneous endometriosis.[98] Similarly, T-cell–mediated cytotoxicity to autologous endometrial cells was reported to be significantly reduced in infertile women with endometriosis compared with infertile women without the disease.[98] Peripheral blood leukocyte profiles in women with endometriosis have been investigated with conflicting results. More important, however, may be immune status within the peritoneal cavity, the site of ectopic implantation. T-helper lymphocyte concentrations have been observed to be elevated in women with endometriosis.[99] An increased concentration of both helper and suppressor T lymphocytes has also been demonstrated in ectopic endometrium compared with eutopic endometrium.[100] However, at present, these findings merely represent phenomenology; no cause-effect relationship has been demonstrated.

Another alteration in cellular immunity suggested in endometriosis patients is that of NK cells. Several investigators have observed decreased cytotoxicity of peripheral and peritoneal fluid NK cells from patients with endometriosis to K562 cells (a target cell lysed by NK cells in vitro) and to autologous and heterologous endometrium.[101, 102] In addition, the treatment of normal peripheral blood lymphocytes with sera or peritoneal fluids from endometriosis patients decreased natural killing activity.[103] These data suggest that women with endometriosis have decreased cytotoxicity to endometrial cells attributable to a defect in NK cells, and as a result, endometrial cells implant and grow more easily in ectopic sites. Actual experimentation is needed to confirm this theory.

HUMORAL IMMUNITY IN ENDOMETRIOSIS

Investigators have described increased levels of a variety of autoantibodies in the sera of patients with endometriosis. However, not all investigators have been able to duplicate these findings. In addition, the specificity of these antibodies is questionable, because they are found in women with diverse gynecologic disorders. Moreover, when found, autoantibodies in endometriosis decrease with the severity of the disease. Finally, even if such antibodies do exist, it is unclear whether they precede the disease or follow as a consequence.

PERITONEAL FLUID INFLAMMATION IN ENDOMETRIOSIS

Macrophages are known to be the cell type found in greatest quantity in the peritoneal fluid.[104] The number of these cells and other leukocytes varies throughout the menstrual cycle, being greater in the follicular phase, immediately after menses. Infertile women with endometriosis appear to possess a greater number of peritoneal macrophages than do normal fertile women.[105, 106] There is evidence to suggest that peritoneal macrophages from women with endometriosis possess activation characteristics resulting in enhanced phagocytic activity and secretion of several soluble substances (e.g., proteolytic enzymes, cytokines, prostaglandins, and growth factors).[107–109] Complement components C3 and C4, mediators of host responses to inflammation, have also been reported to be increased in the peritoneal fluids of patients with endometriosis. In addition to complement components, an increase in prostaglandin levels has been reported by some but not by all investigators.[110–112] What role these secretory products may play in the pathogenesis of endometriosis is not yet known.

The findings summarized here are compelling evidence that the peritoneal fluid in women with endometriosis is proinflammatory. Whereas this fact is now widely accepted, investigators have remained divided on whether these changes precede the disease or follow endometriosis as a consequence, because both macrophages and granulocytes may be chemotactically attracted to the peritoneal cavity in response to the disease. Two proinflammatory chemoattractant cytokines for monocyte-macrophages (MCP-1) and for granulocytes (IL-8) have recently been identified in the peritoneal fluid.[113–116] Not only are concentrations of both IL-8 and MCP-1 elevated in peritoneal fluids of women with endometriosis compared with those without endometriosis, but the levels correlate with the severity of the disease. In the peritoneal cavity, several tissues can account for the increased levels of IL-8 and MCP-1. Besides mesothelial cells that form the majority of the cells, peritoneal macrophages and endometrial cells themselves are potential sources of these chemoattractant cytokines.[117, 118] One theory for the pathogenesis of endometriosis uses these findings, placing them into a complex scheme.

THE ROLE OF GROWTH FACTORS AND CYTOKINES

Several studies have documented that the increased macrophage activation in endometriosis is accompanied by their production of growth factors that includes but is not limited to fibroblast growth factor, platelet-derived growth factor, EGF, and TGF-β.[109] These growth factors have been shown to stimulate the proliferation of endometrial stromal cells in vitro, and it has been speculated that they may enhance the ectopic implantation of endometrial cells.[119] Many investigators have shown that viable endometrial cells can be cultured from the peritoneal fluid of virtually all normally ovulating women with patent fallopian tubes.[93, 94] More specifically, macrophage-derived growth factor (MDGF) enhances endometrial stromal cell proliferation, with maximal stimulation of growth when MDGF and estrogen are both present in the culture medium.[120] These data suggest that a combination of factors, including the hormonal milieu and the number and secretory capacity of cells residing in the peritoneal cavity, might be required to sustain the growth of ectopic endometrium and thus induce clinical endometriosis.

The number of cytokines such as IL-1, TNF-α, IL-2, IL-8, MCP-1, and IFN-γ is also elevated in the peritoneal fluid of women with endometriosis.[121] Peritoneal fluid has been shown to have a toxic effect on sperm mobility and survival,[122] sperm-oocyte interaction,[123] and embryonic development.[124] Among the cytokines tested, TNF-α and IFN-γ[125] and prostaglandins adversely affect in vitro reproductive events. Cytokine levels in peritoneal fluid from women with endometriosis have also been reported to be reduced after medical treatment.[126] A reduction in embryotoxicity was associated with this drop in cytokine concentration as determined by use of mouse two-cell embryos. In summary, there is convincing evidence that increased concentrations of growth factors/cytokines found in the peritoneal fluid of patients with endometriosis display a dual effect: while inducing proliferation of the endometrial implants, they may be inhibiting early reproductive events.

Antisperm Antibodies

Antisperm antibodies have been detected in the serum of both men and women, in cervical mucus of women, in seminal plasma of men, and attached to sperm. Numerous investigations have demonstrated that antisperm antibodies are capable of inhibiting the fertility process at various steps. These steps include a decrease in sperm mobility through cervical mucus and the upper reproductive tract and impairment of oocyte fertilization. The incidence of antisperm antibodies in fertile men and women is estimated to be less than 2 percent. Among infertile couples, it is estimated to be in the range of 5 to 25 percent.[127–129] In the seminal plasma, the immobilizing antibodies to sperm are usually of the immunoglobulin G class, and the agglutinating antibodies are immunoglobulin A. Although antisperm antibodies of the immunoglobulin M class have been found in the circulation of men, they are not found in genital tract secretions.

Because spermatozoa are not produced in women and are not present in men until puberty, spermatozoal antigens are foreign to the immune systems of both adult men and women. In adult men, tight inter–Sertoli cell junctions form a blood-testis barrier that blocks autoimmunization to sperm antigens. T-suppressor cells may also play a role in the defense against autoimmunization.[130] There are four possible mechanisms whereby antisperm antibodies may be formed in men as summarized by Witkin:[131] (1) decrease in number or activity of T-suppressor cells; (2) decrease in seminal fluid factors that recruit T-suppressor cells; (3) altered sperm antigenicity that results in an inadequate suppression of immune responses; or (4) breakdown of the blood-testis barrier, resulting in inoculation with spermatozoal antigens. Antibodies against sperm appear in the serum of at least 50 percent of vasectomized men. Studies indicate that the higher the antibody titer before vasectomy reversal, the poorer the subsequent fertility outcome.[132, 133]

Despite exposure to millions of spermatozoa with every episode of intercourse, most women do not develop immune reaction to sperm. Immunosuppressive factors in the seminal plasma, such as TGF-β or prostaglandins, have been claimed to protect against such an immune reaction.[134–136] Why some women do develop such antibodies is obscure. Sperm cells injected directly into the peritoneum for artificial insemination appear to induce an immune response in some women.[137] Women with genital tract infections such as sexually transmitted diseases are more likely to develop circulating antisperm antibodies than are women in a control group.[138, 139] Finally, oral sex or deposition of sperm within the rectum during intercourse has been hypothesized to increase the risk of immunization to sperm antigens.

Proposed treatments for subfertility secondary to antisperm antibodies have included short-term condom use, immunosuppressive therapy with corticosteroids for both men and women, intrauterine insemination of washed sperm, in vitro fertilization–embryo transfer (IVF-ET), and intracytoplasmic sperm injection (ICSI). Short-term condom use has not improved rates of conception. The role of corticosteroid immunosuppression is controversial because some studies have indicated success with this therapy,[140] whereas other studies have failed to validate that the use of corticosteroids in antisperm antibody–positive men improves fertility.[141] Intrauterine insemination of washed sperm may help up to 15 percent of couples with antisperm antibodies to achieve pregnancy.[142]

Several studies have examined the effect of antisperm antibodies on conception by IVF-ET. One large retrospective study found that abnormal semen quality was responsible for a much lower fertilization rate than the presence of antibodies and concluded that IVF provides an equal chance of conception in couples with antisperm antibodies compared with couples with no antibodies if the other semen parameters are normal.[143] Other smaller retrospective studies have concluded that IVF-ET is a viable treatment for infertile couples with antisperm antibodies.[144–146] The role of ICSI in the treatment of such patients is currently unknown.

Implantation and Early Pregnancy Failure

Antiplacental Immune Reaction and Abnormal Trophoblast-Maternal Interaction

In spite of the fact that the placenta and fetus are "foreign" to the mother,[147] most pregnancies show no evidence of "immunologic rejection."[148] When immunologic reactions do occur, they can be against any of the components of the gestation (placenta and fetus).[149–152] These reactions can occur at all stages of pregnancy and can occur repeatedly, pregnancy after pregnancy.

A gestation consists of a fetus and its attached placenta. The placenta consists of the cotyledons, attached membranes, umbilical cord, junctional trophoblasts, and invasive intermediate trophoblasts.[153, 154] Immunologic reactions against all of these components have been described or are at least theoretically possible. The clinical manifestations of these immunologic reactions depend on the severity and which component is under attack.

REACTIONS AGAINST THE VILLOUS CORE: CHRONIC VILLITIS

In approximately 1 to 2 percent of all gestations, mononuclear cells can be seen infiltrating the chorionic villi of the placenta. In situ hybridization for Y and X markers in male gestations has demonstrated that the lymphocytes present in cases of chronic villitis are maternally derived. Immunohistochemistry of such cases has shown that the cells within the villous core are T cells and macrophages.[155] Chronic villitis has been linked to poor fetal growth.

REACTIONS AGAINST VILLOUS SYNCYTIOTROPHOBLASTS: INTERVILLOSITIS

Placentas occasionally manifest an intervillous space that is filled with mononuclear cells.[156–158] When immunohistochemically stained, these cells are revealed to be monocytic-macrophage in origin. This monocytic intervillositis has been associated with intrauterine growth retardation, preeclampsia, recurrent pregnancy loss, and intrauterine fetal demise.

REACTIONS AGAINST THE ANCHORING TROPHOBLASTS

Although no clinical cases of immune reactions against the anchoring trophoblasts have been described, it is theoretically possible. These specialized trophoblasts make a unique fibronectin, trophouteronectin,[159] that may be capable of eliciting an immune response. Such an immune reaction might lead to placental–uterine separation and subsequent abruption.[160, 161] If this occurs early in pregnancy, it is unlikely that histologic evidence for this reaction would be available, possibly explaining why it has not yet been clinically documented.

IMMUNE REACTION AGAINST INVASIVE TROPHOBLASTS

Soon after implantation, invasive populations of extravillous trophoblasts attach to and interdigitate through the extracellular spaces of the endometrium and myometrium.[154] The endpoint for this invasive behavior is penetration of maternal spiral arteries within the uterus.[162] Histologically, trophoblast invasion of maternal blood vessels results in disruption of extracellular matrix components and development of dilated capacitance vessels within the uteroplacental vasculature. Biologically, trophoblast-mediated vascular remodeling within the placental bed allows marked distensibility of the uteroplacental vessels, thus accommodating the increased blood flow needed during gestation. In addition to the presence of markers of extracellular matrix interactions and proteases needed for cell movement and invasion, these trophoblasts also appear to express a unique monomorphic histocompatibility antigen: HLA-G.[163] Abnormalities in this invasive process have been correlated with early and midtrimester pregnancy loss, preeclampsia and eclampsia, and intrauterine growth retardation.[164]

One of the most frequent findings in preeclampsia is decreased or absent trophoblast invasion of the maternal spiral arteries.[165, 166] Decreased or absent trophoblast invasion may be a consequence of primary defects in the invasive trophoblasts or in the environment that the trophoblasts are attempting to invade. Many cases of preeclampsia appear to be related to maternal immunologic reaction against the invading trophoblasts.[149] A common clinical finding in these cases is that the spiral arteries are not converted and instead are surrounded by lymphocytes, presumably attacking the foreign-appearing invasive trophoblasts.[154]

Recurrent Pregnancy Loss

Recurrent pregnancy loss is defined as three or more spontaneous consecutive pregnancy losses. Compared with sporadic abortion, it is relatively uncommon, affecting 1 to 3 percent of couples during pregnancy.[167] The same term is occasionally used to include those with two consecutive spontaneous abortions. Indeed, observations have shown that the greatest change in risk of losing a subsequent pregnancy occurs after two consecutive abortions, and there is no difference in the prevalence of etiologic factors between couples with three or more abortions.[168, 169]

Conventionally identifiable etiologic factors can be shown in about 60 percent of the couples who suffer from recurrent spontaneous abortion.[170] Because the developing embryo and trophoblasts are immunologic targets owing to their paternally inherited genetic products, numerous immunologic theories have been suggested for the unexplained recurrent pregnancy losses. Proposed mechanisms include both alloimmune rejection and autoimmune disruption of the pregnancy.

ALLOIMMUNITY

HLA class I molecules are present on almost every cell in the body and are crucial for defining the self. They are recognized by $CD8^+$ T cells. Exogenous antigens such as proteins and bacteria are exhibited by antigen-presenting cells to the immune system by class II molecules that are recognized by $CD4^+$ T cells.[171] There are no HLA molecules on the spermatozoa,[172] oocyte, and embryo at early cleavage and blastocyst stages.[173, 174]

Trophoblasts are the only fetal cells exposed directly to the maternal blood. Although they do not carry classic HLA molecules, it has been shown that villous and nonvillous cytotrophoblasts of the placenta and cytotrophoblasts of the amniochorion express HLA-G, which is a type of class I antigen.[9] The lack of expression of HLA and presence of nonclassic HLA-G on the trophoblasts were thought to prevent the occurrence of immune attack by hindering the corecognition of any other form of surface antigen that the trophoblasts express.

Trophoblasts also carry so-called trophoblast-lymphocyte cross-reactive antigens, which are presumably near HLA molecules.[175] They were proposed to be important in some kind of maternal recognition and protection of blastocyst by production of blocking factors. According to one hypothesis, their lack of recognition through antigen sharing leads to absence of blocking antibodies, resulting in abortion. It was noted that a recurrent abortion problem resolved in some women after they had changed sexual partners.[176] However, in a series of patients who had been pregnant with two different partners, it was concluded that recurrent abortion is not partner specific, although there may be a strong familial disposition in families in which recurrent miscarriage has occurred.[177] Another study in an ethnically homogeneous Chinese population showed that there was an excess of HLA sharing between husband

and wife in couples experiencing primary and secondary recurrent spontaneous abortions.[178] Recurrent aborters were reported to develop less antipaternal lymphocytotoxic antibody than the control subjects did.[179] This knowledge has been used to identify patients for whom immunotherapy might be beneficial. However, in a prospective study, the development of this antibody was found to be dependent on gestational age of pregnancy.[180] Because antipaternal lymphocytotoxic antibodies were rare before 28 weeks of gestation, it could not be used as a diagnostic test for recurrent aborters. Antibody levels were also shown to diminish between pregnancies. Prospective population-based control studies in Hutterites, a religious isolate that lives communally and proscribes contraception, have demonstrated that sharing HLA does not preclude normal pregnancy.[181] On the other hand, more recent data from the same population suggest that HLA-DR–linked genes may affect fertilization or implantation and HLA-B–linked genes may contribute toward recognized fetal loss.[182]

The blocking factor deficiency as a cause of recurrent abortion is based on pathophysiologic assumptions. According to those assumptions, there is an antifetal cell–mediated immune response that must be blocked during the pregnancy. The blocking antibodies that develop in successful pregnancies are thought to prevent immune attack by blocking antigenic sites.

Immunotherapeutic procedures were invented to induce the production of blocking factors, complement-dependent antipaternal lymphocytotoxic antibodies, or suppressor cells to prevent maternal rejection of the fetus. Types of antigens used for this purpose were paternal or third-party leukocytes, placental syncytiotrophoblast plasma membrane, and immunoglobulin. Numerous prospective, randomized trials have been carried out in an attempt to determine the efficacies of these interventions in couples with recurrent pregnancy loss. Scott[183] has published a meta-analysis reviewing the results of these trials. Criteria for inclusion were randomized controlled trials involving women with three or more prior miscarriages, no more than one prior livebirth, all nonimmunologic causes ruled out, and no simultaneous treatment cointerventions. The analysis included both published and unpublished studies. Results indicated that donor white cell immunization (three trials), trophoblast membrane immunization (one study), and intravenous immune globulin (three trials) do not significantly improve the chance of a livebirth in women with recurrent miscarriages.

Paternal white cell immunization is more controversial. Scott's analysis indicated a small but nonstatistically significant increase in the livebirth rate after treatment; these results are similar to those seen with earlier meta-analyses,[184–187] which all showed a small effect, some achieving statistical significance and some not. These data must be balanced against the risks of such transfusions, including transmission of hepatitis B virus or human immunodeficiency virus, pain and fever, maternal platelet alloimmunization, blood group sensitization, and graft-versus-host–like reaction.[185, 188] In addition, the small improvement in livebirth rate (6.6 percent) suggests that 15 women would require leukocyte immunization to achieve one additional livebirth; thus, the cost of one additional pregnancy is approximately $30,000. Whether this marginally (at best) effective treatment is of value given the risks and expense is highly doubtful.

AUTOIMMUNITY

Autoimmune diseases occur in an overwhelming preponderance in women.[189] In studies of pregnancy among women with SLE, the pregnancy loss rates were higher.[190] Lubbe and colleagues[191] were the first to suggest that abnormal autoimmunity in clinically asymptomatic women may be associated with reproductive failure.

Antiphospholipid antibodies are directed to the negatively charged phospholipids that are constituents of all cell membranes. Their presence has been linked to adverse maternal and fetal outcome including spontaneous abortion, stillbirth, intrauterine growth retardation, preeclampsia, thromboembolism, and thrombocytopenia.

Lupus anticoagulant (LA) was first described in patients with SLE who displayed false-positive serologic test results for syphilis and a plasma inhibitor of in vitro clotting assays.[192] The term is a misnomer because many patients with these antibodies do not have lupus, and it is mostly associated with thrombotic events.[193] It interferes with the binding between the platelet wall phospholipid and activated factors V and X to form prothrombin activator complex.[194] The definitive diagnosis of LA activity requires three criteria: (1) prolongation of a phospholipid-dependent clotting assay, (2) documentation that prolongation is not due to a clotting factor deficiency, and (3) confirmation that the prolongation is phospholipid specific.[195] The initial test should contain a low phospholipid concentration; an activated partial thromboplastin time (aPTT) with platelet-poor plasma is the most sensitive such test.[196] To rule out a factor deficiency in the presence of a prolonged aPTT, test material is mixed with plasma, observing the normalization of the test. If there is no correction with plasma, the test is repeated with an excessive amount of platelet phospholipid for final confirmation. In strongly suspected cases with normal aPTT, a second screening test should be employed.[197] These include dilute Russell viper venom test, kaolin clotting time, and plasma clot time.[198]

Other antiphospholipid antibodies of clinical interest are the anticardiolipin antibodies (ACA). They are quantified by either radioimmunonoassay or enzyme-linked immunosorbent assay. The results of LA tests are more reproducible than those for ACA.[199] Investigators in some laboratories have separated LA and ACA activities, suggesting that these two antiphospholipid antibodies are different immunoglobulins.[200, 201] Therefore, both tests should be obtained when the diagnosis of antiphospholipid syndrome is considered.

Previous pregnancy history is important in determining the significance of a positive laboratory test result for antiphospholipid antibody. The reported incidence of antiphospholipid antibodies among recurrent aborters varies from 5 to 50 percent.[202] A significantly higher rate of positive test results are noted in women with recurrent losses and a history of thrombosis or in women who have documented SLE. The precise pathophysiologic mechanisms of these antibodies are not so clear. Inhibition of prostacyclin generation,[203] diminished protein C activity,[204] inhibition of antithrombin III,[205] alteration of platelet-endothelium interactions,[206] and interference with postreceptor signal transduction processes[207] have been suggested by in vitro experiments.

The availability of treatment for patients with recurrent pregnancy loss and antiphospholipid antibodies necessitated the screening and identification of at-risk patients early in pregnancy. Treatment is clearly indicated for pregnant patients with a history of previous thrombosis, recurrent fetal loss, or thrombocytopenia if they have correctly diagnosed LA activity or medium to high concentrations of ACA confirmed on two occasions more than 6 weeks apart.[195, 208] The need for treatment of patients without previous pregnancy losses or thrombosis but incidentally found LA activity or ACA is controversial.

Treatment options for antiphospholipid syndrome are based on two approaches. The first is to reduce the antibody burden. This includes treatment with prednisone or, in refractory cases, azathioprine or plasmapheresis with or without immunoglobulin therapy. A second approach is to counteract the procoagulant effects of antiphospholipid antibodies. For this, low-dose aspirin (50 to 81 mg/day) and heparin (10,000 to 20,000 U/day subcutaneously) are used. In a comparative trial of prednisone (10 to 40 mg/day) plus low-dose aspirin (81 mg/day) versus low-dose aspirin alone in the treatment of ACA-positive patients, the coadministration of prednisone with low-dose aspirin failed to improve the outcome.[209] A similar study compared aspirin (80 mg/day) plus prednisone (40 mg/day) with aspirin plus heparin (10,000 U twice a day) and revealed similar livebirth rates (around 75 percent). In both studies, however, preterm deliveries were more common in the prednisone-treated groups.[210]

Other treatments have recently been suggested. Intravenous immunoglobulins have been administered in women in whom other therapies have failed.[211, 212] It has been documented in experimental antiphospholipid syndrome in mice that in vivo administration of recombinant IL-3 was beneficial.[213] The pregnancy loss rates dropped from 32 to 4 percent after administration of IL-3, which also corrected the antiphospholipid syndrome–associated thrombocytopenia.

Premature Ovarian Failure

Premature ovarian failure is usually defined by amenorrhea, estrogen deficiency, and elevated plasma concentrations of FSH (>40 mIU/ml) in women younger than 40 years. It has been estimated that 5 to 10 percent of women with secondary amenorrhea have premature ovarian failure and that the risk of experiencing menopause before age 40 years is less than 1 percent.[214] In some women with premature ovarian failure, there is evidence that autoimmune mechanisms may be the cause: (1) circulating antibodies against ovarian tissue are seen in the sera of some women with premature ovarian failure; (2) lymphocyte infiltration is seen histologically in selected cases; (3) premature ovarian failure is seen more frequently in conjunction with other autoimmune diseases.[215]

As much as 15 to 20 percent of premature ovarian failure may be associated with autoimmune disease; higher percentages have been reported in studies in which patients with abnormal karyotypes were excluded.[214, 216] Although various conclusions can be drawn from different studies, a familial tendency has generally been observed among patients with premature ovarian failure. There is evidence that the HLA-DR antigens, especially HLA-DR3, can be associated with this disorder, implying a genetically associated aspect of the disease.[217]

Several investigators have reported circulating immunoglobulins that bind to various ovarian proteins in the sera of patients with premature ovarian failure. Reported ovarian antibodies include those to developing follicles, oocytes, corpus luteum, theca, and granulosa. In some cases, antibodies to multiple endocrine tissues are detected. It is not clear whether these multiple reactions indicate multiple antibody populations or the presence of a particular antigen that is shared by multiple endocrine sites.

There are several reports of women with multiple autoimmune endocrine syndromes, including premature ovarian failure, who had resumption of menses after treatment with corticosteroids.[215] In addition, resumption of ovarian function may occur in women with systemic lupus and premature ovarian failure during quiescent periods of the disease.

Conclusions

The immune system is a complex entity designed to eliminate foreign intruding antigens and consists of both cellular and humoral components. This system is influenced by and in turn influences the function of the reproductive system. The immune system has known effects on ovulatory function and implantation physiology. Disorders of immune function have been linked to such diverse gynecologic abnormalities as endometriosis, antisperm antibody–induced infertility, recurrent pregnancy loss, and premature ovarian failure.

Despite the widespread associations between immunology and reproductive medicine, the study of system interactions remains in its infancy. Although many facts are accumulating, sufficient pieces of the puzzle are rarely available to provide a complete and unambiguous picture. Our limited understanding of these disorders has for the most part failed to translate into effective immune-targeted therapy. Thus our mission is clear: we must strive to better understand reproductive physiologic and pathophysiologic processes, including the contributions made by components of the immune system. If this can be accomplished, more scientific, effective diagnostic and therapeutic schemes can be anticipated.

References

1. Mosmann TR, Coffman RL. TH1 and TH2 cells: Different patterns of lymphokine secretion lead to different functional properties. Annu Rev Immunol 7:145–173, 1989.
2. Kurt-Jones EA, Hamberg S, Ohara J, et al. Heterogeneity of helper/inducer T lymphocytes, I: Lymphokine production and lymphokine responsiveness. J Exp Med 166:1774–1787, 1987.
3. Abbas AK, Urioste S, Collins TL, et al. Heterogeneity of helper/inducer T lymphocytes, IV: Stimulation of resting and activated B cells by TH1 and TH2 clones. J Immunol 144:2031–2037, 1990.
4. Powrie F, Coffman RL. Cytokine regulation of T cell function: Potential for therapeutic intervention. Immunol Today 14:270–274, 1993.
5. Nathan CF. Secretory products of macrophages. J Clin Invest 79:319–326, 1987.

6. Bodmer WF, Albert ED. Nomenclature for factors of the HLA system. Tissue Antigens 24:73, 1984.
7. Trowsdale J, Ragoussis J, Campbell RD. Map of the human MHC. Immunol Today 12:443–446, 1991.
8. Farid NR, Bear JC. Autoimmune endocrine disorders and the major histocompatibility complex. *In* Davies TF (ed). Autoimmune Endocrine Disease. New York, John Wiley & Sons, 1983, p 59.
9. Kovats S, Main EK, Librach C, et al. A class I antigen, HLA-G, expressed in human trophoblast. Science 248:220–223, 1990.
10. Ellis SA, Palmer MS, McMichael AJ. Human trophoblast and the choriocarcinoma cell line BeWo express a truncated HLA class I molecule. J Immunol 144:731–735, 1990.
11. Burt D, Johnston D, RinkedeWit T, et al. Cellular immune recognition of HLA-G–expressing choriocarcinoma cell line Jeg-3. Int J Cancer 6:117–122, 1991.
12. Deniz G, Christmas SE, Brew R, et al. Phenotypic and functional cellular differences between human $CD3^-$ decidual and peripheral blood leukocytes. J Immunol 152:4255–4261, 1994.
13. Kaufman JF, Auffray C, Korman FJ, et al. The class II molecules of the human and murine major histocompatibility complex. Cell 36:1–13, 1984.
14. Butterworth M, McClellan B, Allansmith M. Influence of sex in immunoglobulin levels. Nature 214:1224–1225, 1967.
15. Grundbacher FJ. Human X chromosome carries quantitative genes for immunoglobulin. Science 176:311–312, 1972.
16. Nagel JE, Chrest FJ, Adler WH. Enumeration of T lymphocyte subsets by monoclonal antibodies in young and aged humans. J Immunol 127:2086–2088, 1981.
17. Mylvaganam R, Ahn YS, Harrington WJ, et al. Differences in T cell subsets between men and women with idiopathic thrombocytopenic purpura. Blood 66:967–972, 1985.
18. Bizzarro A, Valentini G, DiMartino G, et al. Influence of testosterone therapy on clinical and immunological features of autoimmune diseases associated with Klinefelter's syndrome. J Clin Endocrinol Metab 64:32–36, 1987.
19. Amadori A, Zamarchi R, DeSilvestro G, et al. Genetic control of the CD4/CD8 T-cell ratio in humans. Nat Med 1:1279–1283, 1995.
20. Talal N, Ahmed SA. Sex hormones, $CD5^+$ (Lyl^+) B cells, and autoimmune diseases. Isr J Med Sci 24:725–728, 1988.
21. Lahita RG. Sex steroids and the rheumatic diseases. Arthritis Rheum 28:121–126, 1985.
22. Lahita RG, Bradlow HL, Fishman J, et al. Abnormal estrogen and androgen metabolism in the human with systemic lupus erythematosus. Am J Kidney Dis 2:206–211, 1982.
23. Okuyama R, Abo T, Seki S, et al. Estrogen administration activates extrathymic T cell differentiation in the liver. J Exp Med 175:661–669, 1992.
24. Nilsson B, Bergqvist A, Lindblom D, et al. Characterization and localization of specific oestrogen binding in the human thymus. Gynecol Obstet Invest 21:150–157, 1986.
25. Nilsson B, Ferno M, von Schoultz B. Estrogen and progesterone receptors in the human thymus. Gynecol Obstet Invest 29:289–291, 1990.
26. Tabibzadeh S. Cytokines and the hypothalamic-pituitary-ovarian-endometrial axis. Hum Reprod 9:947–967, 1994.
27. Polan ML, Loukides J, Nelson P, et al. Progesterone and estradiol modulate interleukin-1 beta messenger ribonucleic acid levels in cultured human peripheral monocytes. J Clin Endocrinol Metab 69:1200–1206, 1989.
28. Pacifici R, Rifas L, McCracken R, et al. Ovarian steroid treatment blocks a postmenopausal increase in blood monocyte interleukin-1 release. Proc Natl Acad Sci USA 86:2398–2402, 1989.
29. Lee BY, Huynh T, Pritchard LE, et al. Gonadal steroids modulate interleukin-1 receptor antagonist mRNA expression in cultured human monocytes. Biochem Biophys Res Commun 209:279–285, 1995.
30. Loy RA, Loukides JA, Polan ML. Ovarian steroids modulate human monocyte tumor necrosis factor alpha messenger ribonucleic acid levels in cultured human peripheral monocytes. Fertil Steril 58:733–739, 1992.
31. Fox HS, Bond BL, Parslow TG. Estrogen regulates the IFN-gamma promoter. J Immunol 146:4362–4367, 1991.
32. Azuma C, Saji F, Kimura T, et al. Steroid hormones induce macrophage colony-stimulating factor (MCSF) and MCSF receptor messenger RNAs in the human endometrium. J Mol Endocrinol 5:103–108, 1990.
33. Arici A, MacDonald PC, Casey ML. Modulation of the levels of transforming growth factor-β mRNA in human endometrial stromal cells. Biol Reprod 54:463–469, 1996.
34. Arici A, Oral E, Bukulmez O, et al. Interleukin-8 expression and modulation in human preovulatory follicles and ovarian cells. Endocrinology 137:3762–3769, 1996.
35. Lin J, Lojun S, Lei ZM, et al. Lymphocytes from pregnant women express human chorionic gonadotropin/luteinizing hormone receptor gene. Mol Cell Endocrinol 111:R13–R17, 1995.
36. Smith EM, Ebaugh MJ. Luteogenic activity from human lymphocytes. Ann N Y Acad Sci 594:492–593, 1990.
37. Mohagheghpour N, Abel K, LaPaglia N, et al. Signal requirements for production of luteinizing hormone releasing-hormone by human T cells. Cell Immunol 163:280–288, 1995.
38. Azad N, LaPaglia N, Jurgens KA, et al. Immunoactivation enhances the concentration of luteinizing hormone–releasing hormone peptide and its gene expression in human peripheral T-lymphocytes. Endocrinology 133:215–223, 1993.
39. Blalock JE, Harbour-McMenamin A, Smith EM. Peptide hormones shared by the neuroendocrine and immunologic systems. J Immunol 135:858–861, 1985.
40. Marchetti B, Guarcello V, Morale MC, et al. Luteinizing hormone–releasing hormone binding sites in the rat thymus: Characteristics and biological function. Endocrinology 125:1025–1036, 1989.
41. Batticane N, Morale MC, Gallo F, et al. Luteinizing hormone–releasing hormone signalling at the lymphocyte involves stimulation of interleukin-2 receptor expression. Endocrinology 129:277–286, 1991.
42. Walker SE, Allen SH, McMurray RW. Prolactin and autoimmune disease. Trends Endocrinol Metab 4:147–150, 1993.
43. Wilson TM, Yu-Lee LY, Kelley MR. Coordinate gene expression of luteinizing hormone–releasing hormone (LHRH) and the LHRH-receptor after prolactin stimulation in the rat Nb2 T-cell line: Implications for a role in immunomodulation and cell cycle gene expression. Mol Endocrinol 9:44–53, 1995.
44. Sakakuva T, Nishizuela Y. Thymic control mechanisms in ovarian development: Reconstitution of ovarian dysgenesis in thymectomized mice by replacement with thymic or other lymphoid tissues. Endocrinology 90:431–437, 1972.
45. Kalra PS, Sahu A, Kalra SP. Interleukin-1 inhibits the ovarian steroid induced luteinizing hormone surge and release of hypothalamic luteinizing hormone–releasing hormone in rats. Endocrinology 126:2145–2152, 1990.
46. Ban E, Haour F, Lenstra R. Brain interleukin-1 gene expression induced by peripheral lipopolysaccharide administration. Cytokine 4:48–54, 1992.
47. Yamaguchi M, Matsuzaki N, Hirota K, et al. Interleukin 6 possibly induced by interleukin 1β in the pituitary gland stimulates the release of gonadotropins and prolactin. Acta Endocrinol 122:201–205, 1990.
48. Yamaguchi M, Sakata M, Matsuzaki N, et al. Induction by tumor necrosis factor-alpha of rapid release of immunoreactive and bioactive luteinizing hormone from rat pituitary cells in vitro. Neuroendocrinology 52:468–472, 1990.
49. Adashi EY. The potential relevance of cytokines to ovarian physiology: The emerging role of resident ovarian cells of the white blood series. Endocr Rev 11:454–464, 1990.
50. Brannstrom M, Pascoe V, Norman RJ, et al. Localization of leukocyte subsets in the follicle wall and in the corpus luteum throughout the human menstrual cycle. Fertil Steril 61:488–495, 1994.
51. Katabuchi H, Fukumatsu Y, Okamura H. Immunohistochemical and morphological observations of macrophages in the human ovary. *In* Growth Factors and the Ovary. Proceedings of the Seventh Ovarian Workshop on Paracrine Communication in the Ovary, Ontogenesis and Growth Factors. New York, Plenum Press, 1989, pp 409–413.
52. Polan ML, Loukides JA, Nelson P. The role of IL-1 in the ovary. *In* Signaling Mechanisms and Gene Expression in the Ovary. Proceedings of the Eighth Ovarian Workshop on Regulatory Processes and Gene Expression in the Ovary. New York, Springer-Verlag, 1991, pp 163–169.
53. Parr EL. Histological examination of the rat ovarian follicle wall prior to ovulation. Biol Reprod 11:483–503, 1974.

54. Hellberg P, Thomson P, Janson PO, et al. Leukocyte supplementation increases the luteinizing hormone–induced ovulation rate in the in vitro–perfused rat ovary. Biol Reprod 44:791–797, 1991.
55. Kokia E, Hurwitz A, Ricciarelli E, et al. Interleukin-1 stimulates ovarian prostaglandin biosynthesis: Evidence for heterologous contact-independent cell-cell interaction. Endocrinology 130:3095–3097, 1992.
56. Takehara Y, Dharmarajan AM, Kaufman G, et al. Effect of interleukin-1β on ovulation in the in vitro perfused rabbit ovary. Endocrinology 134:1788–1793, 1994.
57. Roby KF, Terranova PF. Tumor necrosis factor alpha alters follicular steroidogenesis in vitro. Endocrinology 123:2952–2954, 1988.
58. Adashi EY, Resnick CE, Packman JN, et al. Cytokine-mediated regulation of ovarian function: Tumor necrosis factor-α inhibits gonadotropin-supported progesterone accumulation by differentiating and luteinized murine granulosa cells. Am J Obstet Gynecol 162:889–899, 1990.
59. Benyo DF, Pate JL. Tumor necrosis factor-α alters bovine luteal cell synthetic capacity and viability. Endocrinology 130:845–860, 1992.
60. Sjogren A, Holmes PV, Hillensjo T. Interleukin-1α modulates luteinizing hormone stimulated cyclic AMP and progesterone release from human granulosa cells in vitro. Hum Reprod 6:910–913, 1991.
61. Fukuoka M, Yasuda K, Emi N, et al. Cytokine modulation of progesterone and estradiol secretion in cultures of luteinized human granulosa cells. J Clin Endocrinol Metab 75:254–258, 1992.
62. Hurwitz A, Loukides J, Ricciarelli E, et al. The human intraovarian interleukin-1 (IL-1) system: Highly-compartmentalized and hormonally-dependent regulation of the genes encoding IL-1, its receptor, and its receptor antagonist. J Clin Invest 89:1746–1754, 1992.
63. Yan Z, Hunter VJ, Weed J, et al. Tumor necrosis-α alters steroidogenesis and stimulates proliferation of human ovarian granulosa cells in vitro. Fertil Steril 59:332–338, 1993.
64. Wang LJ, Brannstrom M, Robertson SA, et al. Tumor necrosis factor-α in the human ovary: Presence in follicular fluid and effects on cell proliferation and prostaglandin production. Fertil Steril 58:934–940, 1992.
65. Best CL, Pudney J, Anderson DJ, et al. Modulation of human granulosa cell steroid production in vitro by tumor necrosis factor alpha: Implications of white blood cells in culture. Obstet Gynecol 84:121–127, 1994.
66. Best CL, Griffin PM, Hill JA. Interferon gamma inhibits luteinized human granulosa cell steroid production in vitro. Am J Obstet Gynecol 172:1505–1510, 1995.
67. Lei ZM, Chegini N, Rao CV. Quantitative cell composition of human and bovine corpora lutea from various reproductive states. Biol Reprod 44:1148–1156, 1991.
68. Bagavandoss P, Wiggins RC, Kunkel SL, et al. Tumor necrosis factor production and accumulation of inflammatory cells in the corpus luteum of pseudopregnancy and pregnancy in rabbits. Biol Reprod 42:367–376, 1990.
69. Pepperell JR, Wolcott K, Behrman HR. Effects of neutrophils in rat luteal cells. Endocrinology 130:1001–1008, 1992.
70. Wang F, Riley JCM, Behrman HR. Immunosuppressive levels of glucocorticoid block extrauterine luteolysins in the rat. Biol Reprod 49:66–73, 1993.
71. Townson DH, Warren JS, Flory CM, et al. Expression of monocyte chemoattractant protein-1 in the corpus luteum of the rat. Biol Reprod 54:513–520, 1996.
72. Lea RG, Clark DA. Macrophages and migratory cells in endometrium relevant to implantation. Baillieres Clin Obstet Gynaecol 5:25–29, 1991.
72a. Stewart CL, Kaspar P, Brunet LJ, et al. Blastocyst implantation depends on maternal expression of leukemia inhibitory factor. Nature 359:76–79, 1992.
73. Arici A, Engin O, Attar E, et al. Modulation of leukemia inhibitory factor gene expression and protein biosynthesis in human endometrium. J Clin Endocrinol Metab 80:1908–1915, 1995.
74. Nachtigall MJ, Kliman HJ, Feinberg RF, et al. The effect of leukemia inhibitory factor on trophoblast differentiation: A potential role in human implantation. J Clin Endocrinol Metab 81:801–806, 1996.
75. Arceci RC, Shanahan F, Stanley ER, et al. The temporal expression and location of colony stimulating factor-1 (CSF-1) and its receptor in the female reproductive tract are consistent with CSF-1 regulated placental development. Proc Natl Acad Sci USA 86:8818–8822, 1989.
76. Pollard JW, Hunt JS, Wiktor-Jedrzejczak W, et al. A pregnancy defect in the osteopetrotic (op/op) mouse demonstrates the requirement for CSF-1 in female fertility. Dev Biol 148:273–283, 1991.
77. Flynn A. Expression of Ia and the production of the interleukin 1 by peritoneal exudate macrophages activated in vivo by steroids. Life Sci 38:2455–2460, 1986.
78. Polan ML, Daniele A, Kuo A. Gonadal steroids modulate human monocyte interleukin-1 (IL-1) activity. Fertil Steril 49:964–968, 1988.
79. Simon C, Frances A, Piquette GN, et al. Embryonic implantation in mice is blocked by interleukin-1 receptor antagonist. Endocrinology 134:521–528, 1994.
80. Simon C, Frances A, Piquette G, et al. Interleukin-1 system in the materno-trophoblast unit in human implantation: Immunohistochemical evidence for autocrine/paracrine function. J Clin Endocrinol Metab 78:847–854, 1994.
81. Selick CE, Horowitz GM, Gratch M, et al. Immunohistochemical localization of transforming growth factor-β in human implantation sites. J Clin Endocrinol Metab 78:592–596, 1994.
82. Nelson KG, Takahashi T, Bossert NL, et al. Epidermal growth factor replaces estrogen in the stimulation of female genital tract growth and differentiation. Proc Natl Acad Sci USA 88:1–5, 1991.
83. Mukku VR, Stancel GM. Regulation of epidermal growth factor by estrogen. J Biol Chem 260:9820–9824, 1985.
84. Bell SC. Decidualization and insulin-like growth factor (IGF) binding protein: Implications for its role in stromal cell differentiation and the decidual cell–haemochorial placentation. Hum Reprod 4:125–130, 1989.
85. Giudice LC, Dsupin BA, Jin IH, et al. Differential expression of mRNAs encoding insulin-like growth factors and their receptors in human uterine endometrium and decidua. J Clin Endocrinol Metab 76:1115–1122, 1993.
86. Giudice LC. Growth factors and growth modulators in human uterine endometrium: Their potential relevance to reproductive medicine. Fertil Steril 61:1–17, 1994.
87. Bulmer JN, Sunderland CA. Immunohistological characterization of lymphoid cell populations in the early human placental bed. Immunology 52:349–357, 1984.
88. Tsoukatos D, Skarpelis G, Athanassakis I. Placenta-specific growth factor production by splenic cells during pregnancy. Placenta 15:467–476, 1994.
89. Tabibzadeh S, Sun XZ, Kong QF, et al. Induction of a polarized microenvironment by human T cells and interferon-gamma in three-dimensional spheroid cultures of human endometrial epithelial cells. Hum Reprod 8:182–192, 1993.
90. Clark DA, Vince G, Flanders KC, et al. $CD56^+$ lymphoid cells in human first trimester pregnancy decidua as a source of novel transforming growth factor-β2–related immunosuppressive factors. Hum Reprod 9:2270–2277, 1994.
91. Olive DL, Schwartz LB. Endometriosis. N Engl J Med 328:1759–1769, 1993.
92. Blumenkrantz JM, Gallagher N, Bashore RA, et al. Retrograde menstruation in women undergoing chronic peritoneal dialysis. Obstet Gynecol 57:667–670, 1981.
93. Halme J, Hammond MG, Hulka JF, et al. Retrograde menstruation in healthy women and in patients with endometriosis. Obstet Gynecol 64:151–154, 1984.
94. Kruitwagen RFPM, Poels LG, Willemsen WNP, et al. Endometrial epithelial cells in peritoneal fluid during early follicular phase. Fertil Steril 55:297–303, 1991.
95. Wood DH, Yochmowitz MG, Salmon YL, et al. Proton irradiation and endometriosis. Aviat Space Environ Med 54:718–724, 1983.
96. Rier SE, Martin DC, Bowman RE, et al. Endometriosis in rhesus monkeys *(Macaca mulatta)* following chronic exposure to 2,3,7,8-tetrachlorodibenzo-*p*-dioxin. Fundam Appl Toxicol 21:433–441, 1993.

97. D'Hooghe TM, Bambra CS, Raeymaekers BM, et al. The effects of immunosuppression on development and progression of endometriosis in baboons *(Papio anubis)*. Fertil Steril 64:172–178, 1995.
98. Dmowski WP, Steele RW, Baker GF. Deficient cellular immunity in endometriosis. Am J Obstet Gynecol 141:377–383, 1981.
99. Hill JA, Faris HMP, Schiff I, et al. Characterization of leukocyte subpopulations in the peritoneal fluid of women with endometriosis. Fertil Steril 50:216–222, 1988.
100. Witz CA, Montoya IA, Dey TD, et al. Characterization of lymphocyte subpopulations and T cell activation in endometriosis. Am J Reprod Immunol 32:173–179, 1994.
101. Oosterlynck DJ, Cornillie FJ, Waer M, et al. Women with endometriosis show a defect in natural killer cell activity resulting in a decreased cytotoxicity to autologous endometrium. Fertil Steril 56:45–51, 1991.
102. Wilson TJ, Hertzog PJ, Angus D, et al. Decreased natural killer cell activity in endometriosis patients: Relationship to disease pathogenesis. Fertil Steril 62:1086–1088, 1994.
103. Kanzaki H, Wang H-S, Kariya M, et al. Suppression of natural killer cell activity by sera from patients with endometriosis. Am J Obstet Gynecol 167:257–261, 1992.
104. Haney AF, Muscato JJ, Weinberg JB. Peritoneal fluid cell populations in infertility patients. Fertil Steril 35:696–698, 1981.
105. Halme J, Becker S, Hammond MG, et al. Pelvic macrophages in normal and infertile women: The role of patent tubes. Am J Obstet Gynecol 142:890–895, 1982.
106. Dunselman GA, Hendrix MG, Bouckaert PX, et al. Functional aspects of peritoneal macrophages in endometriosis of women. J Reprod Fertil 82:707–710, 1988.
107. Halme J, Becker S, Hammond MG, et al. Increased activation of pelvic macrophages in infertile women with mild endometriosis. Am J Obstet Gynecol 145:333–337, 1983.
108. Halme J, Becker S, Haskill S. Altered maturation and function of peritoneal macrophages: Possible role in pathogenesis of endometriosis. Am J Obstet Gynecol 156:783–789, 1987.
109. Halme J, White C, Kauma S, et al. Peritoneal macrophages from patients with endometriosis release growth factor activity in vitro. J Clin Endocrinol Metab 66:1044–1049, 1988.
110. Drake TS, O'Brien WF, Ramwell PW, et al. Peritoneal fluid thromboxane B_2 and 6-keto-prostaglandin F1 in endometriosis. Am J Obstet Gynecol 140:401–404, 1981.
111. Badawy SZA, Marshall L, Cuenca V. Peritoneal fluid prostaglandins in various stages of the menstrual cycle: Role in infertile patients with endometriosis. Int J Fertil 30:48–53, 1985.
112. Chacho KJ, Chacho MS, Andresen PJ, et al. Peritoneal fluid in patients with and without endometriosis: Prostanoids and macrophages and their effect on the spermatozoa penetration assay. Am J Obstet Gynecol 154:1290–1296, 1986.
113. Ryan IP, Tseng JF, Schriock ED, et al. Interleukin-8 concentrations are elevated in peritoneal fluid of women with endometriosis. Fertil Steril 63:929–932, 1995.
114. Arici A, Tazuke SI, Attar E, et al. Interleukin-8 concentration in peritoneal fluid of patients with endometriosis and modulation of interleukin-8 expression in human mesothelial cells. Mol Hum Reprod 2:40–45, 1996.
115. Akoum A, Lemay A, McColl S, et al. Elevated concentration and biologic activity of monocyte chemotactic protein-1 in the peritoneal fluid of patients with endometriosis. Fertil Steril 66:17–23, 1996.
116. Arici A, Oral E, Attar E, et al. Monocyte chemotactic protein-1 concentration in peritoneal fluid in patients with endometriosis and its modulation in human mesothelial cells. Fertil Steril 67:1065–1072, 1997.
117. Arici A, Head JR, MacDonald PC, et al. Regulation of interleukin-8 gene expression in human endometrial cells in culture. Mol Cell Endocrinol 94:195–204, 1993.
118. Arici A, MacDonald PC, Casey ML. Regulation of monocyte chemotactic protein-1 gene expression in human endometrial cells in culture. Mol Cell Endocrinol 107:189–197, 1995.
119. Hammond MG, Oh ST, Anners J, et al. The effect of growth factors on the proliferation of human endometrial stromal cells in culture. Am J Obstet Gynecol 168:1131–1136, 1993.
120. Olive DL, Montoya I, Riehl RM, et al. Macrophage-conditioned media enhance endometrial stromal cell proliferation in vitro. Am J Obstet Gynecol 164:953–958, 1991.
121. Oral E, Olive DL, Arici A. The peritoneal environment in endometriosis. Hum Reprod Update 2:385–396, 1996.
122. Curtis P, Jackson AE. Adverse effects on sperm movement characteristics in women with minimal and mild endometriosis. Br J Obstet Gynaecol 100:165–169, 1993.
123. Sueldo CE, Lambert H, Steinleitner A, et al. The effect of peritoneal fluid from patients with endometriosis on murine sperm-oocyte interaction. Fertil Steril 48:697–699, 1987.
124. Marcos RN, Gibbons WE, Findley WE. Effect of peritoneal fluid on in vitro cleavage of 2-cell mouse embryos: Possible role in infertility associated with endometriosis. Fertil Steril 44:678–683, 1985.
125. Hill JA, Haimovici F, Anderson DJ. Products of activated lymphocytes and macrophages inhibit mouse embryo development in vitro. J Immunol 139:2250–2254, 1987.
126. Taketani Y, Kuo TM, Mizuno M. Comparison of cytokine levels and embryo toxicity in peritoneal fluid in infertile women with untreated or treated endometriosis. Am J Obstet Gynecol 167:265–270, 1992.
127. Clarke GN, Elliott PJ, Smaila C. Detection of sperm antibodies in semen using the immunobead test: A survey of 813 consecutive patients. Am J Reprod Immunol Microbiol 7:118–123, 1985.
128. Witkin SS, David SS. Effect of sperm antibodies on pregnancy outcome in a subfertile population. Am J Obstet Gynecol 158:59–62, 1988.
129. Kutteh WH, McAllister D, Byrd W, et al. Antisperm antibodies: Current knowledge and new horizons. Mol Androl 4:183–193, 1992.
130. El-Demiry MIM, Hargreave TB, Busuttil A, et al. Lymphocyte subpopulations in the male genital tract. Br J Urol 57:769–774, 1985.
131. Witkin SS. Mechanisms of active suppression of the immune response to spermatozoa. Am J Reprod Immunol Microbiol 17:61–64, 1988.
132. Sullivan MJ, Howe GE. Correlation of circulating antisperm antibodies to functional success in vasovasostomy. J Urol 117:189–191, 1977.
133. Royle MG, Parslow JM, Kingscott MMB, et al. Reversal of vasectomy: The effects of sperm antibodies on subsequent fertility. Br J Urol 53:654–659, 1981.
134. Tarter T, Cunningham-Rundles S, Koide S. Suppression on natural killer cell activity by human seminal plasma in vitro: Identification of 19-OH-PGE as the suppressor factor. J Immunol 136:2862–2867, 1986.
135. Thaler C. Immunologic role for seminal plasma in insemination and pregnancy. Am J Reprod Immunol 21:147–150, 1989.
136. Nocera M, Chu T. Transforming growth factor-beta as an immunosuppressive protein in human seminal plasma. Am J Reprod Immunol 30:1–8, 1993.
137. Livi C, Coccia E, Versari L, et al. Does intraperitoneal insemination in the absence of prior sensitization carry with it a risk of subsequent immunity to sperm? Fertil Steril 53:137–142, 1990.
138. Cunningham DS, Fulgham DL, Rayl DL, et al. Antisperm antibodies to sperm surface antigens in women with genital tract infection. Am J Obstet Gynecol 164:791–796, 1991.
139. Bahraminejad R, Kadanali S. Reproductive failure and anti-sperm antibody production among prostitutes. Acta Obstet Gynecol Scand 70:483–485, 1991.
140. Hendry WF, Hughes L, Scammell G, et al. Comparison of prednisolone and placebo in subfertile men with antibodies to spermatozoa. Lancet 1:85–88, 1990.
141. Haas GG Jr, Manganiello P. A double-blind, placebo-controlled study of the use of methylprednisolone in infertile men with sperm-associated immunoglobulins. Fertil Steril 47:295–301, 1987.
142. Margalloth EJ, Sauter E, Bronson RA, et al. Intrauterine insemination as treatment for antisperm antibodies in the female. Fertil Steril 50:441–446, 1988.
143. Janssen HJG, Bastiaans BA, Goverde HJM, et al. Antisperm antibodies and in vitro fertilization. J Assist Reprod Genet 9:345–349, 1992.
144. Mandelbaum SL, Diamond MP, DeCherney AH. Relationship of antisperm antibodies to oocyte fertilization in in vitro fertilization–embryo transfer. Fertil Steril 47:644–651, 1987.
145. Daitoh T, Kamada M, Yamano S, et al. High implantation rate and

consequently high pregnancy rate by in-vitro fertilization–embryo transfer treatment in infertile women with antisperm antibody. Fertil Steril 63:87–91, 1995.
146. Vazquez-Levin M, Kaplan P, Guzman I, et al. The effect of female antisperm antibodies on in vitro fertilization, early embryonic development, and pregnancy outcome. Fertil Steril 56:84–88, 1991.
147. Tangri S, Wegmann TG, Lin H, et al. Maternal anti-placental reactivity in natural, immunologically-mediated fetal resorptions. J Immunol 152:4903–4911, 1994.
148. Toder V, Carp H, Strassburger D. Maternal immune recognition of pregnancy. Isr J Med Sci 30:922–927, 1994.
149. Vinatier D, Monnier JC. Pre-eclampsia: Physiology and immunological aspects. Eur J Obstet Gynecol Reprod Biol 61:85–97, 1995.
150. Gersell DJ. Chronic villitis, chronic chorioamnionitis, and maternal floor infarction. Semin Diagn Pathol 10:251–266, 1993.
151. Redline RW, Patterson P. Patterns of placental injury. Correlations with gestational age, placental weight, and clinical diagnoses. Arch Pathol Lab Med 118:698–701, 1994.
152. Redline RW, Patterson P. Villitis of unknown etiology is associated with major infiltration of fetal tissue by maternal inflammatory cells [see comments]. Am J Pathol 143:473–479, 1993.
153. Kliman HJ, Feinberg RF. Trophoblast differentiation. *In* Barnea ER, Hustin J, Jauniaux E (eds). The First Twelve Weeks of Gestation. New York, Springer-Verlag, 1992, pp 3–25.
154. Kliman HJ. Trophoblast infiltration. Reprod Med Rev 3:137–157, 1994.
155. Altemani AM. Immunohistochemical study of the inflammatory infiltrate in villitis of unknown etiology. A qualitative and quantitative analysis. Pathol Res Pract 188:303–309, 1992.
156. Jacques SM, Qureshi F. Chronic intervillositis of the placenta. Arch Pathol Lab Med 117:1032–1035, 1993.
157. Labarrere C, Mullen E. Fibrinoid and trophoblastic necrosis with massive chronic intervillositis: An extreme variant of villitis of unknown etiology. Am J Reprod Immunol Microbiol 15:85–91, 1987.
158. Doss BJ, Greene MF, Hill J, et al. Massive chronic intervillositis associated with recurrent abortions. Hum Pathol 26:1245–1251, 1995.
159. Feinberg RF, Kliman HJ, Lockwood CJ. Is oncofetal fibronectin a trophoblast glue for human implantation? Am J Pathol 138:537–543, 1991.
160. Guller S, Wozniak R, Kong L, et al. Opposing actions of transforming growth factor-beta and glucocorticoids in the regulation of fibronectin expression in the human placenta. J Clin Endocrinol Metab 80:3273–3278, 1995.
161. Guller S, Wozniak R, Krikun G, et al. Glucocorticoid suppression of human placental fibronectin expression: Implications in uterine-placental adherence. Endocrinology 133:1139–1146, 1993.
162. Pijnenborg R. Establishment of uteroplacental circulation. Reprod Nutr Dev 28:1581–1586, 1988.
163. Kovats S, Main EK, Librach C, et al. A class I antigen, HLA-G, expressed in human trophoblasts. Science 248:220–223, 1990.
164. Pijnenborg R, Anthony J, Davey DA, et al. Placental bed spiral arteries in the hypertensive disorders of pregnancy. Br J Obstet Gynaecol 98:648–655, 1991.
165. Pijnenborg R, Robertson WB, Brosens I, et al. Review article: Trophoblast invasion and the establishment of haemochorial placentation in man and laboratory animals. Placenta 2:71–91, 1981.
166. Robertson WB, Brosens I, Pijnenborg R, et al. The making of the placental bed. Eur J Obstet Gynecol Reprod Biol 18:255–266, 1984.
167. Hill JA. Immunological contributions to recurrent pregnancy loss. Baillieres Clin Obstet Gynaecol 6:489–505, 1992.
168. Roman E. Fetal loss rates and their relation to pregnancy order. J Epidemiol Commun Health 38:29–35, 1984.
169. Coulam CB. Epidemiology of recurrent spontaneous abortion. Am J Reprod Immunol 26:23–27, 1991.
170. Stray-Pedersen B, Stray-Pedersen S. Etiological factors and subsequent reproductive performance in 195 couples with a prior history of habitual abortion. Am J Obstet Gynecol 148:140–146, 1984.
171. Lanzavecchia A. Receptor mediated antigen uptake and its effect on antigen presentation to class II–restricted T lymphocytes. Annu Rev Immunol 8:773–793, 1990.
172. Billington WD. The normal fetomaternal immune relationship. Baillieres Clin Obstet Gynaecol 6:417–438, 1992.
173. Desoye G, Dohr GA, Motter W, et al. Lack of HLA class I and class II antigens on the human preimplantation embryos. J Immunol 140:4157–4159, 1988.
174. Roberts JM, Taylor CT, Melling GC, et al. Expression of the CD46 antigen and the absence of class I MHC antigen on the human oocyte and preimplantation blastocyst. Immunology 75:202–205, 1992.
175. McIntyre JA, Faulk WP, Verhulst SJ, Colliver JA. Human trophoblast-lymphocyte cross-reactive (TLX) antigens define a new alloantigen system. Science 222:1135–1137, 1983.
176. Beer AE. New horizons in the diagnosis, evaluation and therapy of recurrent spontaneous abortion. Clin Obstet Gynecol 13:115–124, 1986.
177. Christiansen OB, Mathieson O, Lauritsen JG, et al. Idiopathic recurrent spontaneous abortion. Acta Obstet Gynecol Scand 69:597–601, 1990.
178. Ho HN, Gill TJI, Hsieh RP, et al. Sharing of human leukocyte antigens in primary and secondary recurrent spontaneous abortions. Am J Obstet Gynecol 163:178–188, 1990.
179. Carp HJA, Toder V, Mashiach S, et al. Recurrent miscarriage: A review of current concepts, immune mechanisms, and results of treatment. Obstet Gynecol Surv 45:657–669, 1990.
180. Regan L, Braude PR, Hill DP. A prospective study of the incidence, time of appearance and significance of anti-paternal lymphocytotoxic antibodies in human pregnancy. Hum Reprod 6:294–298, 1991.
181. Ober CL, Martin AO, Simpson JL, et al. Shared HLA antigens and reproductive performance among Hutterites. Am J Hum Genet 35:994–1004, 1983.
182. Ober C. Current topic: HLA and reproduction: Lessons from studies in the Hutterites. Placenta 16:569–577, 1995.
183. Scott JR. Recurrent miscarriage: Immunotherapy. The Cochrane Database of Systematic Reviews. Pregnancy and Childbirth Module. London, BMJ Publishing Group, 1996.
184. Fraser EJ, Grimes DA, Schulz KF. Immunization as therapy for recurrent spontaneous abortion: A review and meta-analysis. Obstet Gynecol 82:854–859, 1993.
185. Coulam CB, Clark DA, Collins J, et al. Worldwide collaborative observational study and meta-analysis on allogenic leukocyte immunotherapy for recurrent spontaneous abortion. Am J Reprod Immunol 32:55–72, 1994.
186. Jeng GT, Scott JR, Burmeister LF. A comparison of meta-analytic results using literature vs. individual patient data: Paternal cell immunization for recurrent miscarriage. JAMA 274:830–836, 1995.
187. Collins J, Roberts R. Immunotherapy for recurrent spontaneous abortion: Analysis 1. Am J Reprod Immunol 32:275–280, 1994.
188. Clark DA, Daya S. Trials and tribulations in the treatment of recurrent spontaneous abortion. Am J Reprod Immunol 25:18–24, 1991.
189. Talal N. Sex factors, steroid hormones and the host response. Proceedings of the Kroc Foundation Conference. Arthritis Rheum 22:1153, 1979.
190. Dudley DJ, Branch DW. Antiphospholipid syndrome. A model for autoimmune pregnancy loss. Infertil Reprod Med Clin North Am 2:149–164, 1991.
191. Lubbe WF, Butler WS, Palmer SJ, et al. Lupus anticoagulant in pregnancy. Br J Obstet Gynaecol 91:357–363, 1984.
192. Conley CL, Hartman RC. Hemorrhagic disorder caused by circulating anticoagulant in patients with disseminated lupus erythematosus. J Clin Invest 31:621–622, 1952.
193. Lubbe WF, Liggins GC. Lupus anticoagulant and pregnancy. Am J Obstet Gynecol 153:322–327, 1985.
194. Thiagarajan P, Shapiro S, Marco LD. Monoclonal immunoglobulin M coagulation inhibitor with phospholipid specificity. J Clin Invest 66:397–405, 1980.
195. Lockwood CJ, Rand JH. The immunobiology and obstetrical consequences of antiphospholipid antibodies. Obstet Gynecol Surv 49:432–441, 1994.
196. Triplett DA. Screening for the lupus anticoagulant. Res Clin Lab 19:379–389, 1989.
197. Triplett DA. Obstetrical implications of antiphospholipid antibodies. Baillieres Clin Obstet Gynaecol 6:507–518, 1992.

198. Kutteh WH, Carr BR. Recurrent pregnancy loss. *In* Carr BR, Blackwell RE (eds). Textbook of Reproductive Medicine. Norwalk, CT, Appleton & Lange, 1993, pp 559–570.
199. Peaceman A, Silver RK, MacGregor SN, et al. Interlaboratory variation in antiphospholipid antibody testing. Am J Obstet Gynecol 166:1780–1787, 1992.
200. Exner T, Sahan N, Trudinger B. Separation of anticardiolipin antibodies from lupus anticoagulant on a phospholipid-coated polystyrene column. Biochem Biophys Res Commun 155:1001–1007, 1988.
201. Chamley LW, Pattison NS, McKay EJ. Separation of lupus anticoagulant from anticardiolipin antibodies by ion-exchange and gel filtration chromatography. Haemostasis 21:25–29, 1991.
202. Regan L. Recurrent early pregnancy failure. Curr Opin Obstet Gynecol 4:220–228, 1992.
203. Wolf FD, Carreras LO, Moerman P, et al. Decidual vasculopathy and extensive placental infarction in a patient with repeated thromboembolic accidents, recurrent fetal loss, and a lupus anticoagulant. Am J Obstet Gynecol 142:829–834, 1982.
204. Cariou R, Tobelem G, Bellucci S, et al. Effect of lupus anticoagulant of antithrombogenic properties of endothelial cells—Inhibition of thrombomodulin-dependent protein C activation. Thromb Haemost 60:54–58, 1988.
205. Cosgriff TM, Martin BA. Low functional and high antigenic antithrombin III level in a patient with the lupus anticoagulant and recurrent thrombosis. Arthritis Rheum 24:94–96, 1981.
206. Harris EN, Ghavari AE, Hedge U, et al. Anticardiolipin antibodies in autoimmune thrombocytopenic purpura. Br J Haematol 59:231–234, 1985.
207. Gleicher N, Harlow L, Zilberstein M. Regulatory effect of antiphospholipid antibodies on signal transduction: A possible model for autoantibody-induced reproductive failure. Am J Obstet Gynecol 167:637–642, 1992.
208. Harris EN. Syndrome of the black swan. Br J Rheumatol 26:324–326, 1987.
209. Silver RK, MacGregor SN, Sholl JS, et al. Comparative trial of prednisone plus aspirin versus aspirin alone in the treatment of anticardiolipin antibody–positive obstetric patients. Am J Obstet Gynecol 169:1411–1417, 1993.
210. Cowchock FS, Reece A, Balaban D, et al. Repeated fetal losses associated with antiphospholipid antibodies: A collaborative randomized trial comparing prednisone with low-dose heparin treatment. Am J Obstet Gynecol 166:1318–1323, 1992.
211. Wapner RJ, Cowchock FS, Shaprio SS. Successful treatment in two women with antiphospholipid antibodies and refractory pregnancy losses with intravenous immunoglobulin infusions. Am J Obstet Gynecol 161:1271–1272, 1989.
212. Spinnato JA, Clark AL, Pierangeli SS, Harris EN. Intravenous immunoglobulin therapy for the antiphospholipid syndrome in pregnancy. Am J Obstet Gynecol 172:690–694, 1995.
213. Fishman P, Falach-Vaknine E, Zigelman R, et al. Prevention of fetal loss in experimental antiphospholipid syndrome by in vivo administration of recombinant interleukin-3. J Clin Invest 91:1834–1837, 1993.
214. Rebar RW, Cedars MI. Hypergonadotropic forms of amenorrhea in young women. Endocrinol Metab Clin North Am 21:173–191, 1992.
215. LaBarbera AR, Miller MM, Ober C, et al. Autoimmune etiology in premature ovarian failure. Am J Reprod Immunol Microbiol 16:115–122, 1988.
216. Coulam C. Immunology of ovarian failure. Am J Reprod Immunol 25:169–174, 1991.
217. Walfish PG, Gottesman IS, Shewchuk AB, et al. Association of premature ovarian failure with HLA antigens. Tissue Antigens 21:168–169, 1983.
218. Tabibzadeh S. Human endometrium: An active site of cytokine production and action. Endocr Rev 12:272–290, 1991.
219. Haimovici F, Anderson DJ. Cytokines and growth factors in implantation. Microsc Res Tech 25:201–207, 1993.
220. Shi Q, Lei Z, Rao C, et al. Novel role of human chorionic gonadotropin in differentiation of human cytotrophoblasts. Endocrinology 132:1387–1395, 1993.
221. Bischof P, Halnggeli L, Campana A. Effects of leukemia inhibitory factor on human cytotrophoblast differentiation along the invasive pathway. Am J Reprod Immunol 34:225–230, 1995.

Chapter 14

DISORDERS OF SEXUAL DEVELOPMENT

Robert B. Jaffe

CHAPTER OUTLINE

KEY POINTS

- The sex-determining region on the Y chromosome (SRY) contains the genetic determinants for testicular development.
- Mutational analysis, other genetic approaches, and information about SRY have furnished new insights into various forms of gonadal dysgenesis, male pseudohermaphroditism, and true hermaphroditism.
- The phenotype of gonadal dysgenesis is consonant with Jost's studies demonstrating that intrauterine fetal castration of both sexes leads to phenotypic female development; i.e., in the absence of male gonadal secretions (testosterone and müllerian-inhibiting substance [MIS]), a female phenotype results.
- Male pseudohermaphroditism results from (1) a disorder of androgen formation, (2) a disorder of androgen action, or (3) a disorder of the formation or action of MIS.
- Increased information concerning the genes encoding the steroid-metabolizing enzymes and their regulation, and detailed genetic analysis of abnormalities of these genes, has shed light on the various forms of congenital adrenal hyperplasia.

Molecular genetic studies are providing new insights into the biology of sex determination as well as mutational and other genetic alterations leading to various forms of gonadal dysgenesis, pseudohermaphroditism, and true hermaphroditism. In addition, further elucidation of the genes involved in adrenal steroid hormone biosynthesis and their regulation, and unraveling of mutational aberrations in these genes and their regulatory elements, are enhancing our understanding of the various forms of congenital adrenal hyperplasia. Some of these advances are discussed in this chapter and others are described in Chapters 1 and 15.

Advances in the disciplines of genetics, experimental endocrinology, molecular biology, and biochemistry have provided a matrix for understanding normal sexual development. In the interstices of this matrix can be found a rational explanation for the aberrations in genetic and hormonal function that are encountered clinically.

This chapter presents the embryonic and biochemical aspects of sexual differentiation. With this substratum of understanding of the physiologic aspects of sexual development, the pathologic alterations in the developmental pattern with which the clinician must deal are discussed.

EMBRYOLOGIC AND BIOCHEMICAL ASPECTS OF SEXUAL DEVELOPMENT

Embryology

The primordial germ cells originate in the endoderm of the yolk sac; migrate, during the fourth and fifth weeks of gestation, through the dorsal mesentery; and finally reach the primordial gonad in the urogenital ridge. The primitive undifferentiated gonad arises from coelomic epithelium on the border of the urogenital ridge, adjacent to the kidney and the adrenal gland. The primary sex cords grow down from the coelomic epithelium into the primitive gonad. With the arrival into the gonad of the germ cells, now approximately 300 to 1300 in number, further development and differentiation of the gonad into the testis or the ovary can occur. Without these germ cells, differentiation and development of the gonad cannot take place, resulting in gonadal agenesis. It is not until after the first 6 weeks of gestation that the male testis and the female ovary are distinguishable. Embryologic studies show that recognizable testicular development antecedes that of the ovary by approximately 5 to 6 weeks.

In the male, the first sign of primary sexual differentiation is the appearance of Sertoli cells that aggregate to form testicular cords, which later enclose the germ cells. In the testis, the epithelial cords and the germ cells, forerunners of the seminiferous tubules, can be discerned in the 43- to 50-day-old embryo. Subsequently, the Leydig cells form in the interstices between the seminiferous tubules and can first be distinguished at approximately 60 days. There is rapid proliferation of the Leydig cells during the 12th through 18th weeks,[1, 2] so that they become a prominent feature of the developing testis at this time. This correlates well with the progressively increasing production of testosterone by the Leydig (interstitial) cells of the fetal testis,[3] which plays a key role in male sexual development (see later).

In the seminiferous tubules, the Sertoli cells can be found lying on the basement membrane of the tubules. These cells appear to be the site of production of an androgen-binding protein[4] as well as müllerian-inhibiting substance (MIS), which inhibits müllerian ductal development in the normal male fetus.[5, 6] The mature Sertoli cells are also the site of production of inhibin, which preferentially inhibits follicle-stimulating hormone (FSH) secretion. Earlier in gestation, inhibin subunits are also found in the interstitial cells.[7]

The development of the ovary occurs later than does that of the testis. Although the gonad destined to be an ovary enlarges, not until the 11th or 12th week are there discernible oocytes derived from the primitive oogonia. The envelopment of the oocyte by a single layer of flattened granulosa cells to form the primordial follicles occurs at about the 14th week and is maximal by the 20th to 25th week, by which time some of the primordial follicles have developed into primary follicles. (For details of this process, see Chapter 6.) At this time, the morphologic features of the ovary can be recognized clearly.

The differentiation of the duct system into the internal genitalia begins before the establishment of definitive gonadal identity. However, development of functional activity of the fetal testis is essential for normal male ductal development (see later). The wolffian ducts give rise to the vasa deferentia, the seminal vesicles, and the epididymis; whereas in the female, the müllerian ducts grow caudal and fuse in the midline to form the fallopian tubes, the uterus, and the upper portion of the vagina (Fig. 14–1). The wolffian ducts regress in the female, apparently without gonadal influence; in the male, müllerian duct regression is the result of the action of MIS originating in the testis.[5, 6, 8]

Although anatomically separate precursor structures give rise to the internal genitalia, the external genitalia are derived from common anlagen (Fig. 14–2). Understanding of the common origins of the external genitalia during normal development facilitates understanding of the ambiguities of abnormal sexual development with which the clinician must deal. The genital tubercle of the primitive

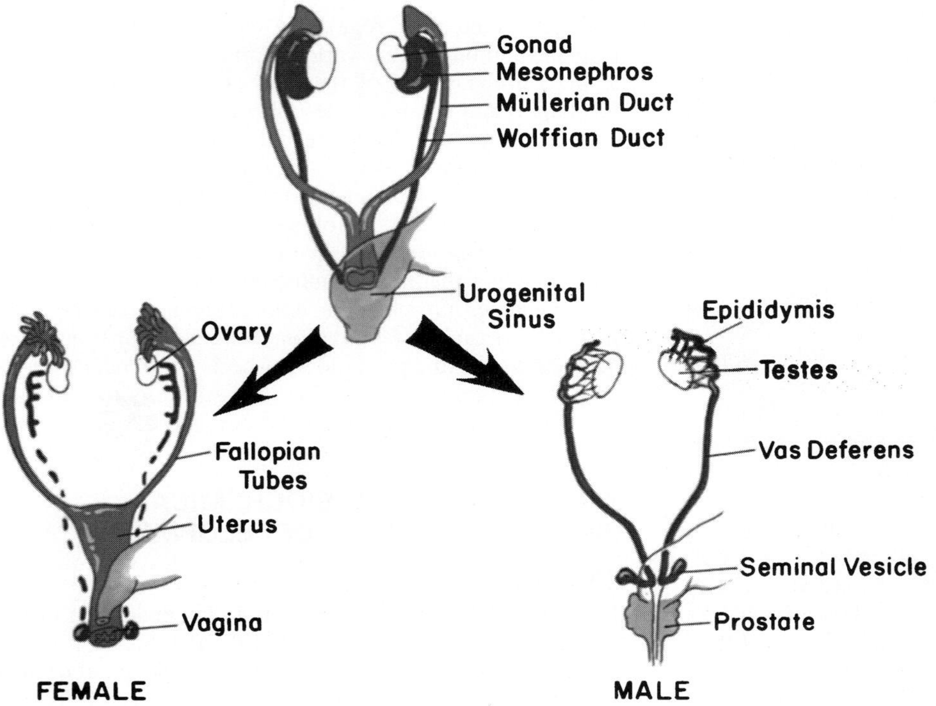

Figure 14–1 ■ Internal genital development in the male and female. (Courtesy of Dr. J. Wilson, University of Texas, Southwestern Medical School, Dallas, TX.)

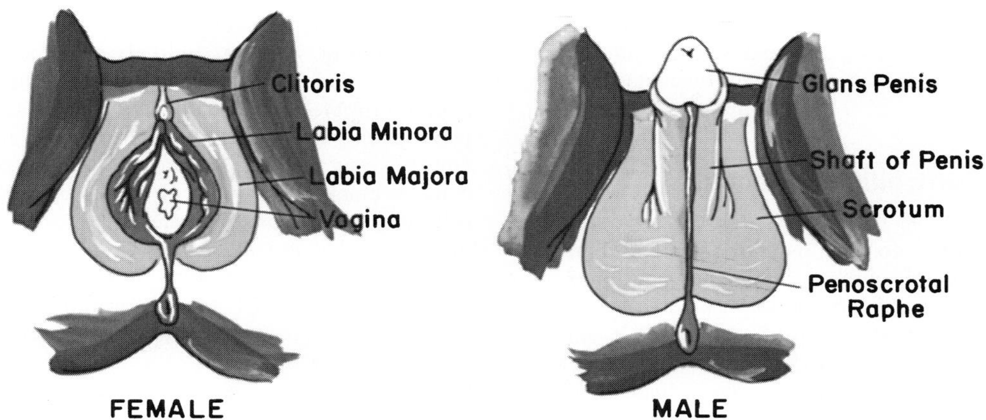

Figure 14–2 ■ External genital development, demonstrating homologies and common anlagen in the male and female. (Courtesy of Dr. J. Wilson, University of Texas, Southwestern Medical School, Dallas, TX.)

embryo gives rise to the glans penis in the male and the clitoris in the female. The paired genital, or urethral, folds give rise to the labia minora in the female (in whom they remain separated) and to the shaft of the penis in the male (in whom they fuse to form a corpus spongiosum and displace the urethral orifice to the tip of the penis). The genital swellings remain separated in the female to form the labia majora, whereas they fuse in the male to form the scrotum and the ventral covering of the penis.

The upper portion of the vagina is formed from the müllerian ducts; the lower portion is derived from the urogenital sinus. In the male, the prostate gland and the bulbourethral (Cowper's) gland are outgrowths of the urogenital sinus. The homologues in the female are Bartholin's and Skene's glands.

The classic work of Jost and associates,[9, 10] the subsequent work of Wilson and colleagues,[11–13] the work of Ohno and Wachtel and others concerning the H-Y antigen,[14–17] subsequent studies concerning the testis-determining factor[18] and the cloning of a putative testis-determining factor gene named *ZFY*[19] that encodes a zinc finger protein, and most importantly the identification of the sex-determining region on the Y chromosome *(SRY)*[20, 21] contributed to the understanding of the principal humoral factors influencing genital differentiation.

In an elegant series of experiments using the rabbit fetus as a model, Jost demonstrated that the fetal testis was necessary for masculine genital development (Fig. 14–3). Jost[9, 10] castrated fetuses at different stages of development, then allowed the pregnancies to continue. If he castrated a male fetus before wolffian duct maturation could occur, the fetus developed female internal and external genitalia, and the müllerian ducts did not regress. Castration of the female fetus, on the other hand, had no appreciable effect, and müllerian development proceeded along normal female lines. Thus, the presence of the ovary is not essential for the development of the fallopian tubes and the uterus.

Unilateral removal of the testis resulted in female duct development on that side, but external virilization proceeded. Bilateral castration and testosterone administration resulted in essentially normal development of the wolffian ducts but failed to cause müllerian regression. Thus, although testosterone could restore wolffian development and was particularly effective when it was implanted as a crystal locally, it was unable to cause müllerian regression. A testicular product other than testosterone was postulated to be responsible for regression of the müllerian ducts. This was a prescient observation, but the characterization of MIS did not occur for many years.

The studies of Josso and colleagues[5, 6, 22] and of Donahoe and associates[8, 23] indicated that MIS is not a steroid but a macromolecular substance originating in the Sertoli cell. MIS has now been characterized and cloned.[22, 23] It is a member of the transforming growth factor-β superfamily, the members of which are involved in various aspects of development. As noted before, the Sertoli cell is also the site of production of androgen-binding protein, and it is possible that this substance maintains the presence of high concentrations of testosterone locally, so that adequate androgen effect can be exerted on the developing wolffian ducts as well as perhaps on the seminiferous tubules.

Wilson[11–13, 24] and others[25] showed that part of the action

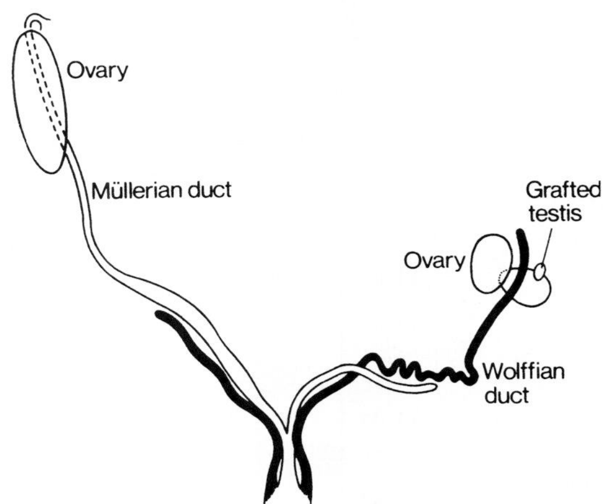

Figure 14–3 ■ The classic experiment of Alfred Jost, in which he grafted a piece of testis against the right ovary of a rabbit fetus. The testis produced local stimulation of the wolffian duct and inhibition of the müllerian duct, but the effect did not extend to the other side of the body. (From Austin C, Short RV [eds]. Embryonic and Fetal Development [Reproduction in Mammals, Book 2]. New York, Cambridge University Press, 1972, p 58.)

of testosterone in certain target tissues, particularly the external genitalia and prostate, is exerted by intracellular conversion to a reduced metabolite of testosterone, 5α-dihydrotestosterone.

The Factors Controlling Testicular Development

In each preceding iteration of this textbook, the identification of putative products of the genes on the Y chromosome responsible for male sex determination has undergone modifications. Initially, it was proposed that the H-Y antigen directed testicular development. Subsequently, it was suggested that a gene for a zinc finger protein located on the Y chromosome *(ZFY)* subsumed this role. It is unlikely that either of these gene products plays a role in sex determination for reasons extensively discussed by Conte and Grumbach.[26]

In 1987, Page and colleagues[19] reported the cloning of a putative testis-determining factor gene named *ZFY* that encoded a zinc finger protein of unknown function. Although *ZFY* was initially regarded as a candidate for testis-determining factor because of its location on the Y chromosome, subsequent findings indicated that this may not be the case. These findings include the observations that (1) a homologue of *ZFY* called *ZFX* is located on the X chromosome[18, 19]; (2) *ZFY* sequences are not found in marsupials that have Y-dependent sex-determining mechanisms[27]; (3) XX male patients possess Y-linked sequences but not *ZFY*[28]; and (4) the sites of expression of *ZFY* during mouse embryogenesis are in germ cells and are not, as expected, in Sertoli cells.[29] Thus, on the basis of current understanding, it seems unlikely that the development of the gonad is dependent on the presence or genetic expression of primordial germ cells in the gonadal ridge. Selective pharmacologic destruction of primordial germ cells in rat embryos[30] as well as surgical excision of primordial germ cells in chick embryos[31] before they reached the gonadal ridge did not inhibit adequate chromosomal differentiation of germ cell–deficient gonads.

Most recently, a region on the Y chromosome (Fig. 14–4) known as *SRY* (sex-determining region on the Y chromosome) has emerged as the most likely candidate for the sex-determining locus.

The studies leading to the conclusion that *SRY* is the sex-determining locus are intriguing and were based on molecular genetic analyses of translocation and deletion sequences in 46,XX and 46,XY sex-reversed patients. The sex-determining region was initially narrowed down to a 35-kilobase segment close to the pseudoautosomal boundary[32] (see Fig. 14–4). Only one of about 50 probes generated from this segment was both Y specific and male specific. It was this unique sequence on the Y chromosome that led to the characterization of *SRY*. Data supporting the thesis that *SRY* is the testis-determining factor were obtained from genetic analyses of 46,XY and 46,XX sex-reversed patients, including 46,XY gonadal dysgenesis (Swyer's syndrome), 46,XY true hermaphroditism, 46,XX males, and 46,XX true hermaphrodites, all of whom are discussed subsequently. In each of these types of sex reversal, at least some of the patients demonstrated mutations in *SRY*.[33–41] In the aggregate, analyses of the gain of function

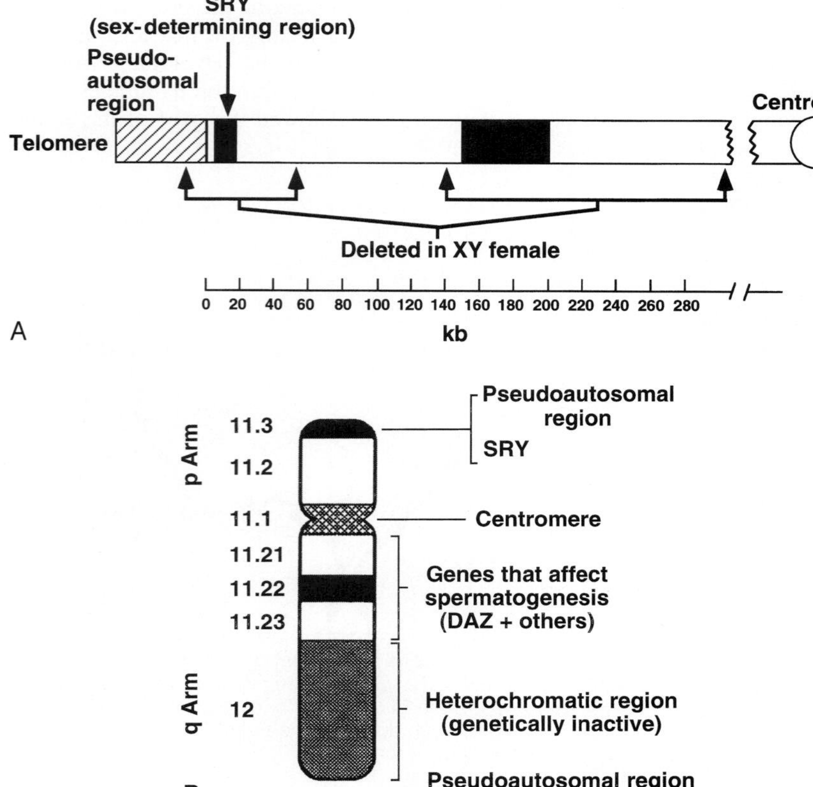

Figure 14–4 ■ *A* and *B*, Approximate location of the *SRY* (sex-determining region of the Y chromosome) gene and the *DAZ* (deleted in azoospermia) gene on the Y chromosome. (Adapted from Grumbach MM, Conte FA. Disorders of sexual differentiation. *In* Wilson JW, Foster DW [eds]. Textbook of Endocrinology, 9th ed. Philadelphia, WB Saunders, 1997.)

(46,XX males and hermaphrodites) and loss of function (46,XY gonadal dysgenesis and true hermaphroditism) patients point to the critical role played by *SRY* in sex determination.

A direct line of evidence linking the mouse homologue of *SRY (Sry)* to sex determination was provided in a transgenic mouse experiment in which testis determination and male development occurred in XX mice made transgenic for *Sry*. These XX, *Sry* transgenic mice were phenotypically male with a normal male reproductive tract and mating behavior.[42]

Müllerian-Inhibiting Substance

MIS mediates müllerian duct regression in males during the course of embryogenesis. It is secreted by the Sertoli cells. Female embryos do not produce MIS during intrauterine life (although they do after birth); therefore, müllerian ducts persist in females and develop into the fallopian tubes, uterus, and upper portion of the vagina. Secretion of MIS by Sertoli cells occurs shortly after testis differentiation, making MIS one of the earliest markers of Sertoli cell differentiation and male development.[43] In 1916, Lillie[44] proposed the existence of a müllerian-inhibiting–like substance to explain the development of freemartins. In freemartins, the female with a male co-twin in a monozygotic twin gestation is masculinized, with regression of müllerian ducts. Therefore, Lillie proposed that an MIS from the male twin inhibited müllerian ductal development in the female twin. Subsequently, as noted previously, Jost proposed that a hormonal substance from the testis, other than testosterone, inhibited müllerian ductal development. Thus, he postulated dual hormonal regulation of male sexual development: testosterone, which masculinizes many male reproductive tract structures, and a müllerian inhibitor, which leads to müllerian duct regression.[10]

Using a bioassay, Josso, a pupil of Jost, and colleagues localized MIS production to Sertoli cells.[6, 45] Biologic purification of MIS[46] led to the cloning of the MIS genes and complementary deoxyribonucleic acid (cDNA).[22, 23, 47] MIS is a 140-kDa homodimeric glycoprotein that is a member of the transforming growth factor-β family.[48] More recently, receptors for MIS were identified.[49] However, the precise mechanism of action of MIS awaits complete elucidation. The orphan receptor, steroidogenic factor 1, appears to play a role in the transcriptional regulation of MIS.[50]

With this substratum of understanding of normal genital development, attention turns to the various pathophysiologic abnormalities encountered clinically. For purposes of description, these abnormalities are discussed under the following topics: gonadal dysgenesis, Klinefelter's syndrome, male pseudohermaphroditism, female pseudohermaphroditism, and true hermaphroditism. A more detailed classification, in which etiologic and clinical mechanisms have been integrated, is contained in an excellent, extensive review by Grumbach and Conte.[51]

GONADAL DYSGENESIS (TURNER SYNDROME)

A group of phenotypic females with short stature, primary amenorrhea, and sexual infantilism was described by the late Henry Turner in 1938,[52] and the classic form of the disorder still bears his name. Other somatic abnormalities were also described. Since then, extensive study as well as progress in the fields of genetics and developmental embryology has led to enhanced understanding of this disorder. Conversely, the thorough evaluation of patients with this interesting syndrome and its variants has greatly enhanced the understanding of sexual differentiation.

In the typical form of the syndrome (Fig. 14–5), the most frequently encountered feature is shortness of stature, present in virtually all patients. The patients are usually less than 58 inches tall. They have a variety of other physical abnormalities: webbed neck (pterygium colli), high-arched palate, low-set prominent ears and low posterior hairline, epicanthal folds, and a tendency to micrognathia. In addition, they may have an increased carrying angle of the arms (cubitus valgus); a shield-like chest with wide-set nipples; a tendency to cardiovascular anomalies, particularly coarctation of the aorta; and frequent hearing loss. They may have shortening of the fourth or fifth digits and hypoplastic nail beds. Increased pigmented nevi, beginning in childhood, are common. So, too, are a variety of renal anomalies; therefore, intravenous pyelograms should be included in the patient's work-up. Lymphedema of the upper and lower extremities (Fig. 14–6) is present

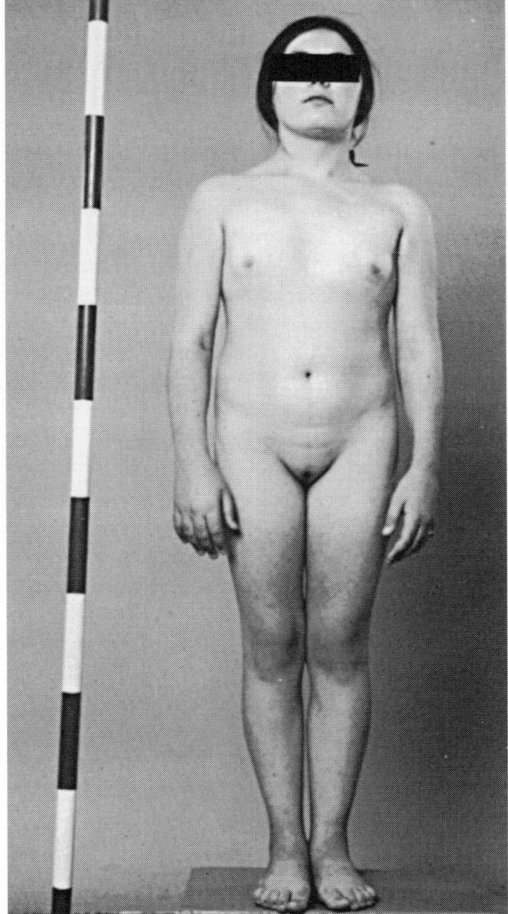

Figure 14–5 ■ Patient with Turner syndrome. Note the shortness of stature, sexual infantilism, and slight webbing of neck.

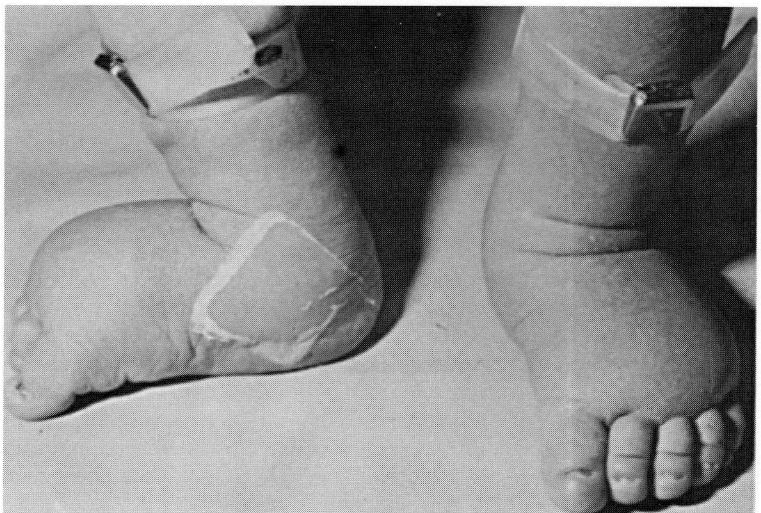

Figure 14–6 ■ Lymphedema of feet in an infant with Turner syndrome.

at birth in approximately 30 percent of cases and alerts the astute clinician to the possibility of genetic abnormality in the newborn nursery when puffiness of the hands or feet is seen in a phenotypic female.

As a group, individuals with gonadal dysgenesis have mean birth weights that are less than the mean for normal newborns at comparable gestational ages; intrauterine growth retardation is not infrequent. The majority of fetuses with gonadal dysgenesis do not reach viability. This is the most common chromosome abnormality found in spontaneous abortions.[53] Many of these abortuses have been found to have lymphedematous collars,[54] and it was postulated that these are the forerunners of the webbed necks in those who survive. It has been estimated that the XO karyotype typical of gonadal dysgenesis occurs in 0.8 percent of zygotes, making this probably the most common human chromosome abnormality. However, less than 3 percent of these fetuses survive to term. Of those that do, there is a higher than normal mortality rate in infancy. The incidence of the XO karyotype is approximately 1 in 2700 live newborn phenotypic females.

Because gonads of these individuals do not develop, either because the primordial germ cells do not reach the gonad or because they are lost after the gonad has been seeded with germ cells initially, gonadal sex hormone production at puberty fails to occur, resulting in sexual infantilism and primary amenorrhea. The gonads appear as streaks or nubbins of white tissue lying subjacent or adjacent to the fallopian tubes—the "streak gonads" characteristic of this syndrome. On histologic section, they appear to contain whorls of primitive connective tissue stroma, lacking primary follicles.

Of interest is the high incidence of diabetes mellitus in these patients; the frequency of diabetes in the families of patients with gonadal dysgenesis equals that of diabetes in the families of known diabetics.[55] There is also an increased incidence of antithyroid antibodies and of Hashimoto's thyroiditis.[55, 56] Red–green color blindness, a trait that is carried on the X chromosome, occurs with increased frequency in patients with Turner syndrome.

Genetic and Developmental Aspects

With the knowledge of the increased incidence of red–green color blindness and coarctation of the aorta, both of which are more commonly found in males, reports accumulated that patients with this disease were sex chromatin–negative.[57] Subsequent studies showed that slightly more than half of the patients with gonadal dysgenesis are sex chromatin–negative. Those who are not have an interesting array of variations in their nuclear chromatin composition. Many of these patients have quantitative and qualitative differences from normal; some have a low percentage of sex chromatin–positive cells, others have a relatively higher percentage. Few affected individuals have normal counts and normal-appearing chromatin (Barr) bodies. There may be two chromatin bodies in the nuclei of some individuals and chromatin bodies that are smaller or larger than normal in those of others. As noted by Federman[58] in his classic monograph, the unifying factor is that there is something wrong with the second sex chromosome in at least some of the person's cells. Twenty-two pairs of autosomes and one normal X chromosome seem necessary for survival. When the second sex chromosome is defective or absent, gonadal dysgenesis or one of its variants may result.

The largest group of patients with gonadal dysgenesis is sex chromatin–negative. They have a total of 45 rather than 46 chromosomes, and there is no Y chromosome present. Because they are sex chromatin–negative, they are also lacking a second X chromosome. Therefore, they are referred to as 45,XO; the O designates the lack of a second sex chromosome.

There are several chromosomal errors that can give rise to an XO karyotype. It may arise from nondisjunction or chromosome loss during spermatogenesis or oogenesis, resulting in a sperm or an egg that lacks any sex chromosome. It may arise at the first cleavage division from anaphase lag during meiosis with loss of a sex chromosome, although errors in mitosis often lead to mosaicism.

Several factors suggest that in many of these patients the second chromosome is lost after fertilization has established an XX or an XY zygote as a result of the abnormality of the missing chromosome and its loss during cell division: (1) mosaicism, a postzygotic event, is frequent in patients with gonadal dysgenesis; (2) the mothers of children with gonadal dysgenesis are not older than the norm, as they are in many cases of chromosome abnormalities in which there is a definite error of meiosis; (3) there is an excess of monozygotic twinning; and (4) the occurrence of an XY monozygotic twin of a patient with XO gonadal dysgenesis has been reported.

As can be seen, the pattern of genital development in patients with typical gonadal dysgenesis is consonant with the experimental data of Jost. Thus, in the absence of a Y chromosome and a functional gonad, as is the case in gonadal dysgenesis, phenotypic development proceeds along female lines, and an immature uterus, fallopian tubes, and vagina are observed. Because there is no functional gonad at puberty and ovarian steroids are not produced, secondary sexual development and menstruation do not occur. As might be expected, levels of gonadotropins are elevated in patients with this disorder as a result of lack of steroid feedback. In fact, FSH levels were found to be increased beginning in infancy in some patients with gonadal dysgenesis,[59] and a diphasic pattern has been reported, with high values during the first 3 years of life, low values until the age of puberty, and high values thereafter.

Treatment

The two facets of gonadal dysgenesis with which the patient is most frequently concerned are shortness of stature and lack of secondary sexual development. In one sense, the clinician must "titrate" these two conditions in deciding on appropriate treatment, because the use of sex steroids to effect secondary sexual development can cause fusion of the epiphyses of the long bones, thus terminating growth. Because these patients frequently have a bone age that lags behind their chronologic age by several years, the decision about when to initiate therapy has been a difficult one.

Alexander and colleagues[60] described a regimen of low-dose estrogen administration that does not appear to hasten epiphyseal fusion. They initiate therapy with 0.3 mg of conjugated estrogen when the patient is 12 to 13 years of age. This is given orally during the first 3 weeks of each month. On the 12th through the 21st day of the month, 5 mg of oral medroxyprogesterone acetate, a progestin, is given with the estrogen. This dosage of estrogen is associated with an initial growth spurt without accelerating skeletal maturation or causing a reduction in final height. Starting therapy at this age allows the patient to have secondary sexual development at approximately the normal age. The superimposition of progestin has two beneficial effects: it effects regular withdrawal bleeding that more closely simulates a normal cycle, and it can potentially reduce the risk of endometrial carcinoma as the result of long-term exposure to unopposed estrogen. Because endometrial carcinoma occurs more frequently in patients with gonadal dysgenesis receiving estrogen therapy than in the general population, the latter effect would be salutary. Subsequently, the estrogen dose can be increased to 0.6 or 1.25 mg if this is necessary to maintain secondary sexual development and to effect regular withdrawal bleeding.

Gonadal Dysgenesis Variants

In addition to the typical form of this disorder, a number of variants of the syndrome occur as a result of chromosome abnormalities, including mosaicism, structural abnormalities of the second sex chromosome, and so-called pure gonadal dysgenesis.

Genetic mosaicism is responsible for the majority of cases of gonadal dysgenesis variants. In fact, some investigators have suggested that some degree of mosaicism may occur in many patients with Turner syndrome. Mosaicism results in the development of two or more cell lines in one individual (see Chapter 12). It is a result of mitotic error. Most likely, it is caused by anaphase lag of an X chromosome or the early mitosis of an XX zygote. The most common form of mosaicism in this syndrome, usually presenting as sex chromatin–positive gonadal dysgenesis, is XO/XX mosaic.

It should be apparent that using only chromatin smears for diagnosis will result in misdiagnosis of a number of patients with mosaicism. Karyotypic analysis is the method of choice in the evaluation of patients with suspected gonadal dysgenesis. It is my opinion that karyotype analysis should always be employed in patients with primary amenorrhea without readily apparent cause, because the incidence of genetic anomalies in patients with primary amenorrhea exceeds 40 percent.[61] Although the chromatin count may be in the normal female range (greater than 25 percent) in XO/XX mosaicism, it is often between the normal female and male ranges, suggesting the admixture of XO and XX cell lines. On occasion, if there are no 46,XX cells sampled, the patient may be found to be sex chromatin–negative. Mosaicism usually "dilutes" the frequency of abnormalities associated with this syndrome. Thus, as indicated in Table 14–1, when the frequency of disorders in a group of patients with XO gonadal dysgenesis is compared with that in a group with XO/XX mosaicism, there is a higher frequency of almost every abnormality in the XO group compared with patients with XO/

■ TABLE 14–1

Incidence of Physical Stigmata Associated with Gonadal Dysgenesis in Patients with XO Karyotype and with XO/XX Mosaicism

XO (%)		XO/XX (%)
100	Short stature	80
80	Shield chest	75
54	Webbed neck	16
39	Lymphedema	12
58	Short IV metacarpal	44
77	Hypoplastic nails	55
52	Multiple nevi	37
21	Congenital heart disease	7
8	Menstruation	21
92	Streak gonads	90
0	Testicular differentiation	0
3	Phallic hypertrophy	5
0	Other masculinization	0

From Ferguson-Smith MA. J Med Gen 2:142, 1965.

XX mosaicism. Patients with this form of mosaicism are not always short, may menstruate, and may even become pregnant. Other variants of this type of mosaicism are individuals with XO/XXX and XO/XX/XXX karyotypes. In the chromatin smears of those groups in which there is an XXX cell line, nuclei with duplicate chromatin bodies may be seen.

Although the sex chromatin–positive group of mosaic variants is more frequent, sex chromatin–negative variants of gonadal dysgenesis are also encountered. This group includes those patients with mosaicism with a normal Y chromosome as well as those with a structurally abnormal Y chromosome in their genetic make-up. Because of its effect on gonadal development, the Y-bearing cell line usually alters the female phenotype of the syndrome, with the result that varying degrees of male differentiation of the genital tract may be encountered. In this group of patients, mosaicism may be seen as an XO/XY, an XO/XYY, or an XO/XY/XYY karyotype; the XO/XY karyotype is most frequently reported. Patients with these forms of mosaicism represent a phenotypic spectrum ranging from those with findings of typical gonadal dysgenesis, those with "diluted" forms of the syndrome, and those with marked ambiguity of the external genitalia (Fig. 14–7) to those presenting as phenotypic males. Most patients have at least one fallopian tube and a uterus. Many have ambiguous genitalia. The development of the duct system and the external genitalia usually correlates well with the extent of testicular differentiation and its location. As might be expected when there is a "dysgenic" Y chromosome, the frequency of gonadal malignant neoplasms is increased, with an incidence of approximately 20 percent in this group of patients.[62]

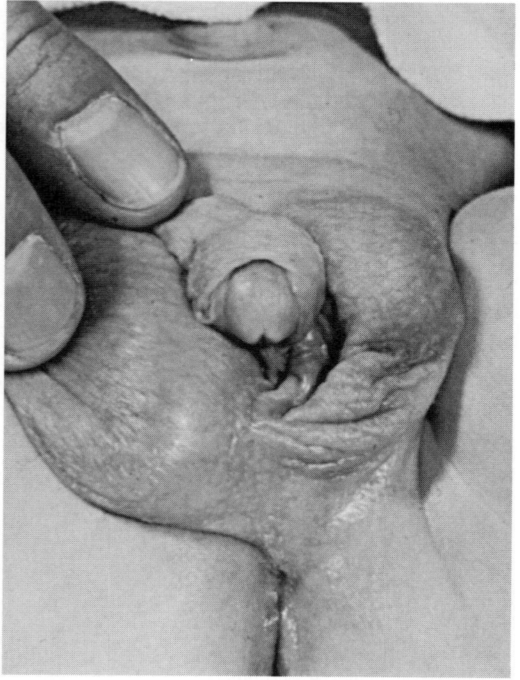

Figure 14–7 ■ External genitalia of infant with XO/XY mosaicism. Note enlarged phallus, labioscrotal fusion, and gonadal bulges (histologically, testes) in labioscrotum.

Some of these patients have asymmetric gonadal development, with a testis on one side and a streak gonad on the other. This subgroup of disorders has been referred to as mixed gonadal dysgenesis. The profound local action of the testis on ductal development is well exemplified in these patients. The development of the wolffian ducts, when it occurs in these individuals, usually takes place on the side on which the testis is located. However, because male external genital development is mediated through circulating androgens, a fetal testis on either side could secrete testosterone into the circulation in amounts capable of masculinizing the external genitalia. Although müllerian duct regression, brought about by the nonsteroidal MIS from the testis, is also purported to occur on the side on which the testis is present, fallopian tubes have been found on the same side as the testis in some of these patients.

Structural Abnormalities Involving the Second Sex Chromosome

Almost half of the patients with some stigmata of gonadal dysgenesis are sex chromatin–positive. Most of these have some form of mosaicism. In addition, structural abnormalities of the X chromosome are found in some of these sex chromatin–positive patients, either with or without associated mosaicism. The study of patients who have a structurally abnormal X chromosome without associated mosaicism can shed light on the specific locus of certain genes on the X chromosome. The two most frequently encountered structural abnormalities of the X chromosome are deletion of a portion of the X and an isochromosome for the long arm of the X.

Deletion of a portion of the X is said to occur when some of the DNA of the chromosome is missing. There may be deletion of a short arm (XXp−) or of a long arm (XXq−). Both of these unusual abnormalities are often associated with mosaicism (XO/XXp− and XO/XXq−, respectively).

In patients with deletion of the short arm, the abnormal X is acrocentric and similar in size to an O group chromosome. The clinical findings in this group of patients, regardless of whether there is or is not an XO cell line, are similar to those in patients with an XO karyotype: shortness of stature, webbed neck, and other somatic abnormalities. The abnormal X chromosome in this group of patients is the late DNA-replicating X chromosome, which is the source of the small chromatin body seen in the karyotype.

The few patients described with deletion of the long arm without mosaicism have normal stature and relatively few of the stigmata of Turner syndrome. They do have streak gonads, primary amenorrhea, and sexual infantilism.

Taken together, the findings in these groups of patients suggest that the shortness of stature and congenital anomalies in Turner syndrome are caused by monosomy of loci on the short arm of the X chromosome and that genes on both the short and long arms of the X are involved in ovarian development.

With the advent of the techniques of Q-banding and G-banding and autoradiography,[63, 64] a small group of patients with X;autosome translocations and X/giant X chromosome karyotypes were identified and studied. Primary amenorrhea was found in some of those with X;autosome translocations, and the patients with X/giant X karyotype have many clinical stigmata of gonadal dysgenesis. The studies of the formation of the giant X support the concept that this is a result of fusion of two X chromosomes.[65]

Another abnormality of the second sex chromosome, usually found in association with mosaicism, is the ring chromosome.[66] This is a round or oval chromosome with no terminal segments. It varies in size from cell to cell. The ring is formed when a chromosome that has had a deletion curves into a shape and a position that allow its free ends to join each other.

Structural abnormalities of the Y chromosome that reach the clinical horizon are much less common than those of the X. Several patients with isochromosome of the long arm of the Y (XYqi) have been described.[67] They are phenotypic females with primary amenorrhea, sexual infantilism, and bilateral streak gonads. They have normal stature and few of the somatic abnormalities associated with the syndrome of gonadal dysgenesis but varying degrees of lymphedema. Studies using quinacrine fluorescence suggested that the testicular determinants are located on the short arm of the Y and that genetic loci on the long arm prevent development of shortness of stature and many of the somatic abnormalities found in Turner syndrome.

Several patients have been described with a dicentric chromosome for the long arm of the Y (XYdic).[68] This is usually associated with mosaicism and an XO cell line. In this group of disorders, varying phenotypes can be seen, including normal males, individuals with ambiguous genitalia and male pseudohermaphroditism, and patients with many of the stigmata of gonadal dysgenesis.

Pure Gonadal Dysgenesis

There are patients who have streak gonads and persistent sexual infantilism but who are of normal stature and lack the other physical stigmata of Turner syndrome. This disorder has been referred to as pure gonadal dysgenesis.[69] A eunuchoid habitus is common, and primary amenorrhea is a frequent presenting complaint. At puberty, gonadotropin concentrations rise, as in individuals with prepubertal castration. The patients may be sex chromatin–negative or sex chromatin–positive, and the karyotype may be XY, XX, or that of mosaicism. Patients in this group tend to develop gonadal malignant neoplasms, either dysgerminomas or gonadoblastomas. This must be kept in mind in their management as well as in treatment of all patients with stigmata of gonadal dysgenesis and the presence of a Y chromosome.

Some authors restrict the term pure gonadal dysgenesis to the disorder of individuals with an XX or an XY karyotype, excluding partial sex chromosome monosomy.

46,XY gonadal dysgenesis is characterized by a 46,XY karyotype without detectable mosaicism, bilateral streak gonads, female internal and external genitalia, and elevated gonadotropins. In essence, 46,XY gonadal dysgenesis represents a developmental abnormality in which the presence of a Y chromosome does not lead to normal testis differentiation. To date, 176 46,XY gonadal dysgenesis patients have been described. Of these, 24 (13.6 percent) showed *SRY* mutations.[70–77]

Like 46,XY gonadal dysgenesis, patients with the 46,XX form of pure gonadal dysgenesis have primitive streak gonads and sexual infantilism but lack other stigmata of classic Turner syndrome.

KLINEFELTER SYNDROME

A disorder of gonadal development that occurs with surprising frequency is Klinefelter syndrome.[78] By screening for sex chromatin–positive, phenotypic males, it has been found in 1 in 400 to 500 newborns. A classic form of the disorder characterizes the majority of the patients, but variant forms have been recognized. The dominant chromosomal feature in almost all patients is at least an XXY chromosomal pattern in at least some of their cells.[58]

The classic form of Klinefelter syndrome is characterized by small, firm testes with hyalinization of seminiferous tubules, azoospermia, gynecomastia, and elevated serum and urinary gonadotropin levels. Mental retardation and other evidence of impairment of social and mental function are frequent concomitants.

It is usually difficult to make the diagnosis of Klinefelter syndrome on clinical grounds before puberty. However, the disorder is sometimes suspected in prepubertal boys with abnormally small testes and in boys with relatively long legs and small external genitalia who have behavioral disorders.

In the postpubertal individual, one finds small, firm testes, usually less than 1.5 cm in largest dimension, that on biopsy reveal extensive hyalinization of the seminiferous tubules, lacking in appreciable spermatogenesis, between which frequently are clumps of adenomatous-appearing interstitial cells. Testosterone concentrations are usually below normal or in the lower part of the normal range, with reported plasma concentrations between 5 and 8 ng/dl in one series.[79] It is possible that a discrepancy exists between circulating levels of total testosterone and those of free, or unbound, testosterone. Levels of gonadotropin, both luteinizing hormone (LH) and FSH, are usually elevated. Reflecting the decreased levels of circulating androgens, there may be a decrease in the size of the penis and sparse pubic hair, although these are often fairly normal.

In many patients, there is characteristically excessive growth of the long bones, to a greater extent in the lower extremities than in the upper (Fig. 14–8). This is in contrast with the usual form of eunuchoidism caused by failure of closure of the epiphyses as a result of deficiency of sex steroids. Further, the bone age in patients with Klinefelter syndrome is usually commensurate with the chronologic age. The span:height ratio in these patients is usually less than 1; in other forms of eunuchoidism, the span is usually more than 2 inches greater than the height, and the long bones of the upper and lower extremities grow in a comparable manner.

Bilateral gynecomastia is a usual feature, the cause of which remains to be elucidated. On histologic examination, it is characterized by hyperplasia of the interductal tissue, whereas in gynecomastia secondary to estrogen excess, the ducts themselves are usually hyperplastic.

Not only is decreased intellectual function frequently encountered in patients with Klinefelter syndrome, but also aberrant social behavior and personality disorders often are

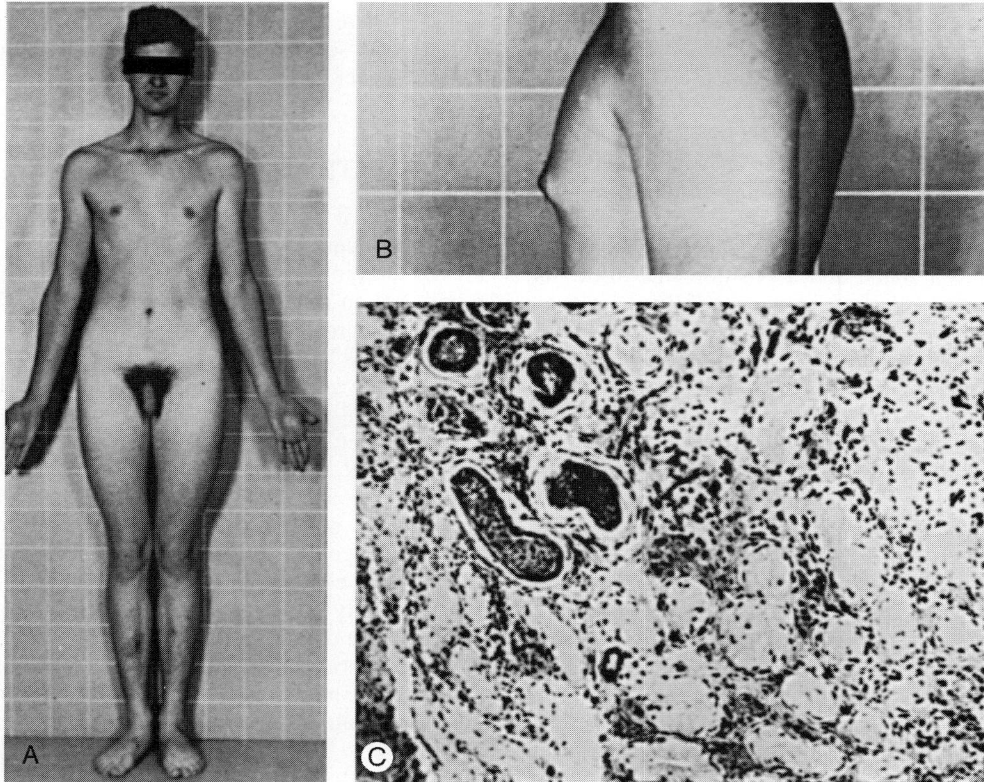

Figure 14–8 ■ Klinefelter syndrome.
A, Phenotypic male with seminiferous tubule dysgenesis.
B, Well-virilized patient with long extremities with eunuchoidal proportions and gynecomastia.
C, Testicular biopsy of patient in *B*. Note marked hyalinization of seminiferous tubules and Leydig cell hyperplasia. (From Grumbach MM, Conte FA. Disorders of sex differentiation. *In* Wilson JD, Foster DW [eds]. Williams Textbook of Endocrinology. Philadelphia, WB Saunders, 1992, p 881).

seen. There is also delayed emotional development and defective gross motor control.[80]

There is an increased incidence of major and minor congenital anomalies and lower birth weight in patients with this syndrome compared with control individuals.[80] For reasons that are not clear, decreased thyroid function assays were reported in many of these patients, with decreased radioactive iodine uptake and a poor response to thyroid-stimulating hormone. Also found in some of these patients with a greater prevalence than expected were chronic pulmonary disease, venous varicosities, abnormal glucose tolerance test results, and an increased risk of breast cancer.

The chromosomal hallmark of Klinefelter syndrome is the presence of an extra sex chromosome, with a 47-chromosome XXY karyotype. Both meiotic and mitotic errors can give rise to the XXY male. The fertilization of an XX ovum by a Y-containing sperm or of an X ovum by an XY-containing sperm could result in an XXY zygote. Mitotic nondisjunction of the sex chromosomes in an XY zygote could result in XXY and YO daughter cells; the latter are nonviable, and only the XXY survive. By use of X-linked markers, such as color vision, pedigree studies revealed both X chromosomes to be of maternal origin in approximately three of four cases, with one X of paternal origin in the remainder.[81]

Several geneticists found an association with advanced maternal gestational age,[82] although not as frequently as is encountered with Down syndrome. This suggests that a high percentage of the cases may result from nondisjunction during oogenesis rather than from mitotic nondisjunction in the first cell division of an XY zygote.

Variant forms of Klinefelter syndrome also occur, as noted earlier. However, it should also be borne in mind when this group is considered that there is at least an XXY cell line in at least some tissues. There may be superimposition of additional X chromosomes, resulting in 48,XXXY and 49,XXXXY karyotypes. In the latter, there is often severe mental retardation, prepubertal testicular damage, small phallic size, and cryptorchidism. These patients often have abnormalities of the elbow joint, with proximal radioulnar synostosis or overgrowth of the radial or ulnar heads. The disorder in patients with 48,XXXY karyotypes is usually somewhere in severity between that in patients with the classic form of Klinefelter syndrome and that in 49,XXXXY individuals. Although they frequently have severe mental retardation, cryptorchidism, and radioulnar synostosis, their testes resemble those seen in patients with the classic form of Klinefelter syndrome. Mosaicism has also been reported as a variant, and here the clinical picture is highly variable, although the majority of patients have less severe changes than do those with the classic form, particularly if a normal XY stem cell line is present. In fact, fertility has been demonstrated in individuals in this group.

An uncommon variant of this syndrome is the 48,XXYY karyotype. These individuals resemble those with the classic form of the disorder in most respects, but they tend to be taller, probably a reflection of the double Y chromosome. There has also been a suggestion of mental instability associated with delinquent and aggressive behavior.

In both the classic and variant forms of Klinefelter syndrome, early detection is important to provide early help for both the androgen deficiency and the social and emotional maladjustments.

MALE PSEUDOHERMAPHRODITISM

In pseudohermaphroditism, the gonadal sex is at variance with the genital sex. The use of the term male or female denotes the corresponding gonadal sex, which is also the genetic sex. Thus, the male pseudohermaphrodite is an individual whose gonads are exclusively testes, whose karyotype is XY, and whose phenotypic characteristics are to varying degrees female. Stated another way, the male pseudohermaphrodite has male gonads and a male karyotype but varying degrees of failure of virilization. One can understand many forms of male pseudohermaphroditism by understanding the biosynthetic pathways and enzymes involved in testosterone formation and the mechanism and sites of androgen action.

The biosynthesis of androgens is detailed in Chapter 4 and illustrated in Figure 14–9. The description of defects in androgen formation (see later) relies on Figure 14–9. As described in detail in Chapter 4 and illustrated in Figure 14–10, the classic concept of steroid hormone action is that steroid hormones, including testosterone, exert their action in target tissues by first becoming attached to an intracellular receptor. The steroid may exert its action as is, or it may be further transformed (in the case of testosterone, to dihydrotestosterone by the 5α-reductase enzyme) before exerting its action. In addition to the enzyme deficiencies in the formation of testosterone, deficiencies in the mechanism of testosterone action may also lead to male pseudohermaphroditism. The mechanism involves (1) formation of the steroid-receptor complex, (2) translocation of the complex into the nucleus, and (3) 5α-reduction of testosterone and its subsequent effect in protein synthesis. There may be abnormalities of each of these components. (Whether there are steroid receptors in the cytoplasm in vivo has been a subject of controversy.)

Knowledge of the biosynthesis of steroids and this brief overview of the mechanisms of testosterone action aid in understanding the majority of the alterations encountered in the various forms of male pseudohermaphroditism. There can be (1) deficient androgen formation, (2) deficient responses to androgen (i.e., deficiencies in androgen action), and (3) defects in formation or action of MIS.

Deficient Androgen Formation

Deficiencies of the enzymes involved in testosterone formation may be manifested in the adrenal gland as well as in the testis (refer to Fig. 14–9).

Cholesterol P450 Side Chain–Cleaving Enzyme (P450scc) Deficiency

The P450scc is the single mitochondrial enzyme, formerly called 20,22-desmolase, that catalyzes the 20- and 22-hydroxylation of cholesterol and cleavage of the C20–22 bond that results in the formation of pregnenolone. This is the principal step in steroidogenesis regulated by adrenocorticotropic hormone (ACTH) and angiotensin II in the adrenal gland and by gonadotropins in the testis and ovary. When there is a deficiency in this enzyme, probably a result of one or more point mutations in the gene encoding the StAR protein (see below), rather than for P450scc as formerly believed, there may be a deficiency of all classes of adrenal steroids (mineralocorticoids, glucocorticoids, and sex steroids).

The rate-limiting step in steroidogenesis in the adrenal gland (and the gonads) is the transport of cholesterol, which is hydrophobic, from the outer to the inner mitochondrial membrane so that it can be acted upon by the P450scc enzyme. This enzyme is located on the inner mitochondrial membrane, where it converts cholesterol to pregnenolone. The movement of cholesterol is mediated by the steroidogenic acute regulatory protein (StAR), which can be stimulated by trophic hormones such as ACTH, acting via cAMP. Trophic hormones trigger StAR expression rapidly. In humans, StAR is a 285 amino acid-containing protein about 30 kDa in size. In patients with lipoidal adrenal hyperplasia (see below), the deficiency is not of P450scc but rather there is a mutation in the gene encoding StAR.[82a]

A group of infants has been described with severe adrenal insufficiency, marked lipid accumulation in both the adrenal gland and the testis, and, in males, female external genitalia and a male duct system. Because of lack of adequate testosterone formation, there is impaired masculinization of the external genitalia and the urogenital sinus. There is little circulating androgen, and there are no 17-ketosteroids in the urine. (Females with this disorder have no abnormality of their genitalia.) This disorder is usually not compatible with life. It is often referred to as congenital lipoid adrenal hyperplasia.

In those few patients who do survive infancy, there is severe adrenal insufficiency with addisonian-like electrolyte imbalance. Because of the early block in steroid biosynthesis, cortisol is not found in the circulation, nor would aldosterone or testosterone be present in appreciable amounts. The conversion of cholesterol to pregnenolone necessitates hydroxylation of cholesterol at the 20 and 22 positions and requires the enzyme cytochrome P450scc. Decreased content of this enzyme in the adrenal mitochondria from a patient with this syndrome has been reported.[83] The cDNA of the gene for human P450scc has been cloned.[84] It is a single gene located on chromosome 15. Urinary steroid analysis has shown the absence of 17-ketosteroids, 17-hydroxycorticosteroids, pregnanediol, and pregnanetriol or the 3β-hydroxysteroid analogues of these compounds in one patient studied with this disorder.[85] Incubations of adrenal tissue obtained at autopsy from these patients indicated deficient 20α-hydroxylation of cholesterol, a key step in the conversion of cholesterol to pregnenolone. The disorder is transmitted in an autosomal recessive manner, as is the case with other forms of

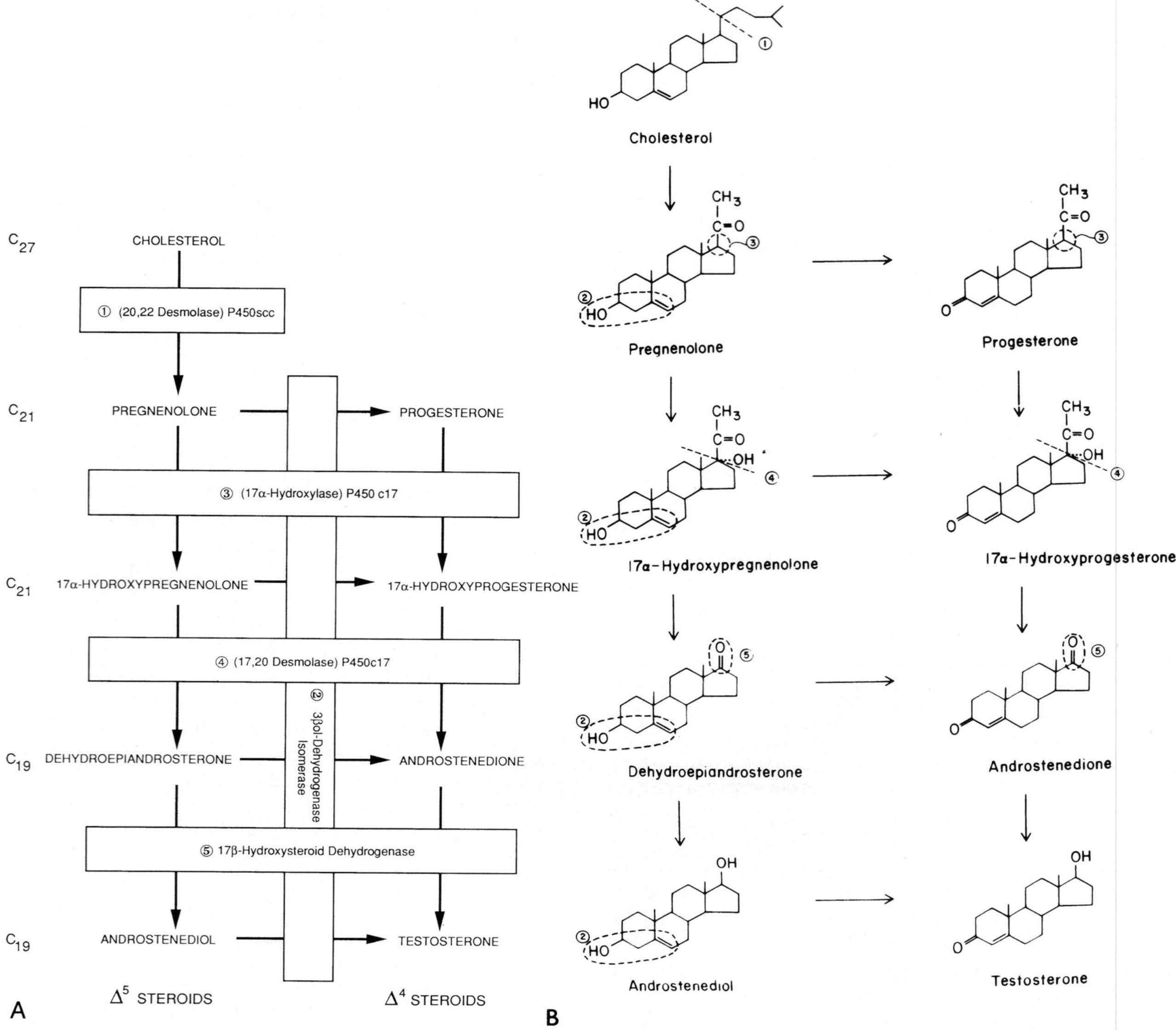

Figure 14–9 ■ Biosynthetic pathways in testosterone formation.

A, The steroids and enzymes involved at each step. Enzymes are named and numbered in boxes. The classic names of the enzymes are given in parentheses, and the newer nomenclatures are presented adjacent to these. There may be an enzyme deficiency at each step, although in the case of P450scc, the defect is in the StAR protein, which transports cholesterol from the outside of the mitochondrial membrane to the inside, where the enzyme is located, rather than in P450scc itself (see text for details).

B, The structural formulas of the steroids involved. The sites of action of the numbered enzymes are shown by dashed lines. Those steroids on the left (with HO— configuration) are shown as Δ^5-steroids because there is a double bond originating in the 5 position. Those steroids on the right (with O= configuration) are known as Δ^4-steroids because there is a double bond originating in the 4 position. These enzymes are present in both the adrenal gland and the testis. Enzymatic defects can affect both glands.

congenital adrenal hyperplasia. Treatment of surviving patients includes administration of mineralocorticoids, glucocorticoids, and, at puberty, androgens.

3β-Hydroxysteroid Dehydrogenase/Isomerase Deficiency

This is a rare disorder that also affects both adrenal and gonadal function. There is often a severe block in the conversion of the Δ^5 steroids to the Δ^4 steroids (Δ^5-3β-hydroxysteroids to Δ^4-3-ketosteroids; see Fig. 14–9) because of the deficiency of the enzyme complex necessary for this conversion. Deficient activity of 3β-hydroxysteroid dehydrogenase causes decreased synthesis of cortisol, aldosterone, and the adrenal sex steroids synthesized beyond dehydroepiandrosterone in the biosynthetic pathway. Male pseudohermaphroditism, with incomplete masculinization of the external genitalia in the face of normal internal male genital ducts and the absence of müllerian ducts, is common in males with this syndrome. It lends further support to the concept of the nonsteroidal nature of MIS in the fetal testis. Most patients with this disorder have died in infancy. However, a few have survived through puberty and have demonstrated excessive amounts of Δ^5-3β-hy-

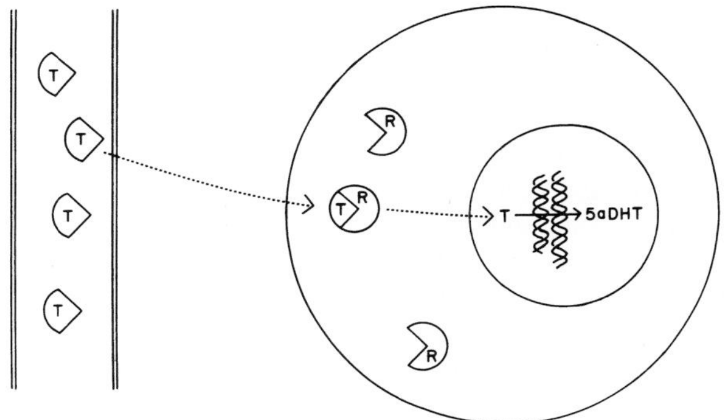

Figure 14–10 ■ Mechanism of testosterone action. Testosterone (T) from the circulation gains entrance to the cell of a target tissue, where it combines with a specific receptor (R). This steroid-receptor complex is translocated into the nucleus, where it may act directly to cause new protein synthesis, or it may be further transformed by a 5α-reductase enzyme associated with the chromatin to form dihydrotestosterone (5α-DHT) and then exert its action on protein synthesis. Data suggest that steroid-receptor interactions may be entirely intranuclear and that cytoplasmic receptors may be an artifact of experimental preparation.

droxysteroid precursors of testosterone but decreased amounts of testosterone itself. Adrenal insufficiency also persists. In the surviving patients, gynecomastia is common at puberty.[86–88]

Heterogeneity of the clinical and biochemical features of 3β-hydroxysteroid dehydrogenase deficiency has been described.[89–94] In addition to the severe, congenital form, a less severe form with onset of hirsutism in pubertal or postpubertal females and without clinical stigmata of adrenal hormone deficiency has been noted.[90, 95–97]

17α-Hydroxylase (P450c17) Deficiency

When there is a deficiency in the 17α-hydroxylase enzyme, there is a deficiency of both the C_{21} steroids derived from pregnenolone and progesterone and the C_{19} steroids from the 17-hydroxylated derivatives 17α-hydroxypregnenolone and 17α-hydroxyprogesterone. Males with this disorder would have pseudohermaphroditism with deficiency in development of secondary sexual characteristics. A spectrum of disorders ranging from normal-appearing female external genitalia and a blind vaginal pouch to hypospadias and a small phallus has been described. The degree of abnormality reflects the severity of the enzymatic block.[98–100] In the case of the female with this disorder described by Biglieri and associates,[101] secretory rates of steroids not dependent on 17-hydroxylated precursors were elevated. These included progesterone, 11-deoxycorticosterone, and corticosterone. Although the presence of these steroids permitted the patient's survival, hypertension and hypokalemic alkalosis were sequelae. As would be expected in the female, there was negligible estrogen production with ensuing sexual infantilism. The cDNA of the gene encoding the 17-hydroxylase enzyme has been characterized,[102–104] cloned, and localized to human chromosome 10.[103] The same enzyme is responsible for both 17-hydroxylation and 17,20-desmolase activity (see following). For excellent reviews of the molecular biology of steroid hormone synthesis, see references 105, 106, and 107.

17,20-Desmolase or Lyase (P450c17) Deficiency

Because both 17α-hydroxylase and 17,20-lyase activity are encoded by the same gene, deficiencies of these enzymes are probably different manifestations of defects affecting the same gene.

Unlike the three enzyme deficiencies described earlier, which affect the synthesis of adrenal corticosteroids as well as androgens, deficiency of the 17,20-desmolase component of the P450c17 enzyme affects only androgen (and subsequent estrogen) formation. The family member with this disorder, described by Zachman and colleagues,[108] had ambiguous external genitalia, inguinal or intra-abdominal testes, and severe hypospadias with a male-type urethra and male duct development. Two cousins with the disorder were studied at approximately 2 years of age. Although the excretion of 17-ketosteroids and 17-hydroxycorticosteroids was normal, excretion of pregnanetriol and 11-ketopregnanetriol was increased. After ACTH administration, excretion increased in a normal manner. Administration of human chorionic gonadotropin (hCG) did not result in an increase in testosterone glucuronide excretion, although 11-ketopregnanetriol excretion increased markedly. Incubation of testicular tissue with C_{21} precursors demonstrated deficient conversion to testosterone. The pattern of inheritance in this family suggested that genetic transmission was as an autosomal dominant or X-linked recessive trait. Goebelsmann and colleagues[109] described another patient suspected of having this disorder. There were normal female external genitalia, a blind-ending vagina, no müllerian derivatives, atrophic wolffian derivatives, and bilateral abdominal testes. Levels of circulating gonadotropins were increased, and testosterone and estradiol concentrations were low.

An additional 46,XY child with ambiguous genitalia most likely due to incomplete 17,20-desmolase activity has been described.[110] The child had a microphallus, perineal hypospadias, chordee, and cryptorchidism. Serum C_{19} steroid levels were abnormally low in the basal state and after adrenal and testicular stimulation. Levels of C_{21} steroids were elevated in the basal state and increased further after adrenal but not after gonadal stimulation. Urinary excretion of pregnanetriolone, a metabolite of 17-hydroxypregnenolone and 17-hydroxyprogesterone, normally present in the urine, was increased in the basal and stimulated states. Cortisol production was normal, and all steroid hormone levels were suppressed by dexamethasone. A significant increase in phallic length occurred after treatment with exogenous androgen.

If the diagnosis can be made in infancy, treatment with testosterone should result in adequate growth of the penis and development of male secondary sex characteristics. As noted before, the same enzyme (P450c17) catalyzes 17-hydroxylation and 17,20-lyase activity.

17β-Hydroxysteroid Dehydrogenase Deficiency

As can be seen in Figure 14–9, a 17β-hydroxysteroid dehydrogenase enzyme is required for the conversion of androstenedione to testosterone and for the conversion of estrone to estradiol. Thus, males who have a deficiency of this enzyme are expected to have a deficiency in the biosynthesis of testosterone and, therefore, abnormalities of those structures that depend on androgens for their development. Indeed, Saez and coworkers[111, 112] and Goebelsmann and associates[113] described such patients.

The well-studied patient of Goebelsmann and colleagues was a married phenotypic female with hirsutism. The patient appeared to be a normal girl until puberty. At that time, however, breast development, clitoral enlargement, and male-type growth of body hair began; menstruation failed to occur. Physical examination at the time revealed a blind-ending vagina and an absent uterus. A clitoridectomy was performed. Subsequent examination of the patient as an adult revealed a typical male body habitus with well-developed musculature of the trunk and extremities, some recession of the hairline, and moderate facial hair. There was a male escutcheon, prominent thyroid cartilage, and a low-pitched voice. In addition, there was normal female breast development and areolar pigmentation.

Gonads were present in the upper lateral parts of both labia majora, which, at histologic examination, were found to be testes with uniformly small seminiferous tubules having markedly thickened, hyalinized lamina propria and an abundance of mature Leydig cells. Mature Sertoli cells predominated within the tubules, which contained only a few spermatogonia and spermatocytes but neither spermatids nor spermatozoa. There was a normal 46,XY karyotype. The serum LH concentration was elevated, and the serum testosterone level was well below that of normal men but considerably above that of normal women. Urinary 17-ketosteroid concentrations were significantly elevated. The androstenedione concentration was 10 times normal. Although androstenedione and estrone concentrations doubled after hCG stimulation, little change in serum testosterone levels was noted. Studies of blood production, metabolic clearance, and androstenedione-to-testosterone conversion rates indicated that 91 percent of circulating testosterone was derived from androstenedione. Studies of testicular arteriovenous differences demonstrated testicular secretion of both androstenedione and estrone but minimal secretion of testosterone and estradiol.

A sibship with 17β-hydroxysteroid dehydrogenase (17-ketosteroid reductase) deficiency, which was associated with hypothyroidism, has been described.[114] No linkage between human leukocyte antigen (HLA) and 17β-hydroxysteroid dehydrogenase loci was found.

Thus, the 17β-hydroxysteroid dehydrogenase deficiency syndrome is a form of male pseudohermaphroditism associated with pubertal gynecomastia and virilism. It is entirely possible that many patients previously classified as exhibiting the "incomplete" form of testicular feminization may, in reality, have this deficiency. (Testicular feminization is described later.) In contrast with individuals with classic testicular feminization, these patients have a defect in testicular testosterone formation, but the sensitivity of target tissues to androgens is normal. Because of the block in the formation of testosterone and estradiol, the testes secrete androstenedione and estrone at increased rates. The conversion of androstenedione to testosterone at extratesticular sites occurs less efficiently than within the testis, but such increased amounts of androstenedione are produced that the resulting amounts of testosterone are sufficient to cause virilization. The arrest in spermatogenesis and the small tubules may be the result of deficient intratesticular androgen. The lack of fetal virilization in utero may be a result of placental aromatization of androstenedione, obviating its extratesticular conversion to testosterone. The LH levels that are increased after puberty would stimulate increased androstenedione and estrone, which, by peripheral conversion to testosterone and estradiol, could cause simultaneous virilization and gynecomastia.

As Goebelsmann[113] pointed out, because feminization in this syndrome is the result of increased amounts of estrogen directly or indirectly originating in the testis, perhaps the name testicular feminization syndrome would be a more appropriate term for the 17β-hydroxysteroid dehydrogenase deficiency than for the entity it was initially used to describe.

Defects in Androgen Action

At least four inherited syndromes that result from androgen resistance, owing to some defect in the mechanism of androgen action, have been described. As noted by Wilson and Goldstein[115] in an excellent classification of hereditary disorders of sexual development, these disorders embrace a spectrum of deficiencies of masculinization, presumably reflecting either discrete biochemical errors in androgen action during sexual differentiation or a smaller number of mutations, some of which may be variably expressed.

Testicular Feminization: Complete Form

This is the most common form of male pseudohermaphroditism. In the spectrum of deficiencies of virilization, it is the most severe. Its mode of inheritance is either X-linked recessive or X-linked dominant. The disorder is often found in several members of the same family, who have almost invariably been reared as females, even though they have male gonads (testes) and genetic constitution (XY). These individuals have a female habitus and, at puberty, develop abundant breast tissue (Fig. 14–11). However, they have scant or absent pubic and axillary hair, and the vagina ends as a blind pouch, although they have unambiguous female external genitalia. There is an absence of internal female genital structures (i.e., uterus, fallopian tubes, and ovaries). This would be expected, because the testes produce MIS. Although the breasts of these individuals are often large, the nipples and areolae frequently are pale and immature in appearance. The enlarged breasts are presumably the result of the action of estrogen uninhibited by active androgen. The testes may be either in the pelvis or in an inguinal hernia. Before puberty, they appear similar to normal prepubertal testes. After puberty, the seminiferous tubules are decreased in size and spermatogonia are scant. Because of an increased risk of malignant change in these gonads, they should be removed. I favor delaying removal until after secondary sexual development has occurred, even though there have been occasional reports of malignant neoplasms developing in the gonads before puberty. After postpubertal gonadectomy, exogenous estrogen therapy should be instituted.

A key to the understanding of this disorder was the observation that patients with testicular feminization syn-

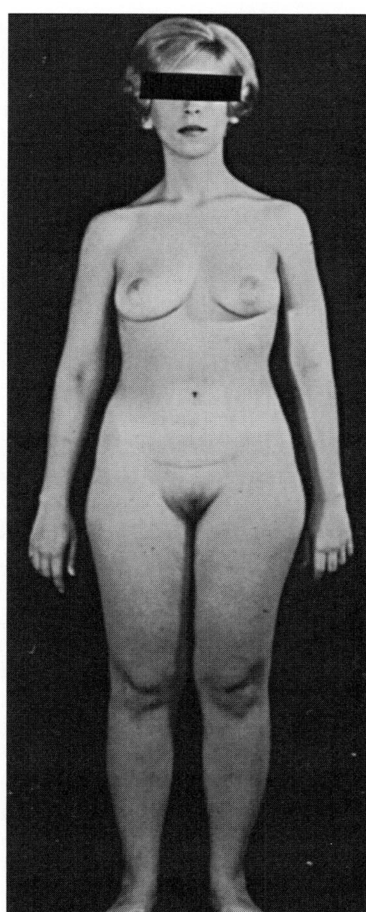

Figure 14–11 ■ Patient with testicular feminization syndrome. Note paucity of pubic hair and abundant breast development.

drome did not have growth of sexual hair after administration of methyltestosterone. This led Wilkins[116] to speculate that the failure of sexual differentiation was the result of target organ insensitivity to androgen. This hypothesis is supported by the observation that the circulating level and the production rate of testosterone by the testes of these individuals are the same as or higher than those of normal men.[117, 118] The circulating estradiol concentration and the estradiol production rate are also higher than in normal men. The concentrations of circulating LH are increased, presumably as a result of the resistance of the hypothalamic-pituitary system to androgen inhibition. This increased LH, then, can stimulate the testis to increase production of testosterone. The increased androgen, both within and outside the testis, can serve as a substrate for increased estrogen formation. In addition, in mice with testicular feminization trait, there is evidence that the failure of male sexual differentiation is the result of primary androgen insensitivity during embryogenesis.[119] As Wilson and Goldstein[115] pointed out, many of the studies that have been performed in patients with this disorder are difficult to interpret, because they have used mature target tissues rather than embryonic cell lines. However, the preponderance of evidence places the site of the disorder in the cellular androgen receptor (see Fig. 14–10). The best-characterized defect is the absence of the binding protein that is required for the initial step in dihydrotestosterone interaction with the cell.[120]

There is another group of individuals in whom binding of dihydrotestosterone is normal and who are indistinguishable phenotypically from the group with absent or low amounts of binding protein.[121, 122] This may represent a postreceptor abnormality (i.e., a defect in the mechanism of androgen action after steroid-receptor binding has occurred) or an as yet undetectable abnormality in the receptor itself. A thermolabile androgen receptor, suggesting an aberrant, unstable form, has been described in patients with the testicular feminization syndrome.[123]

Testicular Feminization: Incomplete or Partial Form

There remains some difference in opinion as to whether this entity constitutes a defect in androgen action, as classified here, or is more appropriately a 17β-hydroxysteroid dehydrogenase defect in androgen formation (described before).

Clinically, these patients resemble individuals with the complete form of testicular feminization in having a male genotype, bilateral intra-abdominal or inguinal testes, and breast development at puberty. However, in contrast with the complete form, there may be phallic enlargement at birth, and some degree of virilization occurs at puberty. The extent of masculinization is variable, and the mode of inheritance remains to be elucidated. Because the circulating androgens are those of normal males, some investigators believed that this entity also results from androgen resistance.[124]

A number of other forms of hereditary male pseudohermaphroditism have been described in which the failure of virilization is incomplete and understanding of the pathogenesis is lacking. On a genetic basis, these disorders of incomplete male pseudohermaphroditism have been divided into two groups: (1) those inherited as an apparent X-linked recessive trait, and (2) those inherited as an autosomal recessive trait.

Incomplete Male Pseudohermaphroditism: X-Linked Recessive Type

This group encompasses a spectrum of disorders from almost complete lack of virilization to almost complete masculinization. The common thread in this group is that all affected males are sterile. The syndrome described by Lubs and colleagues[125] is at the more extreme "lack of virilization" end of the spectrum. Although the majority of family members with this syndrome were reared as females (as in testicular feminization), these individuals had partial wolffian duct development, pubic and axillary hair, partial labioscrotal fusion, and masculine skeletal development (unlike patients with testicular feminization).

One step further toward the masculinized end of the spectrum is the family described by Gilbert-Dreyfus and colleagues.[126] In this family, a masculine habitus with a small phallus, hypospadias, gynecomastia, and incompletely developed wolffian duct derivatives were present.

Still further toward the masculinized end of the spectrum

is Reifenstein syndrome.[127] The dominant feature of this entity is perineoscrotal hypospadias, often associated with a bifid scrotum or incomplete fusion of the scrotal folds. At puberty, gynecomastia often develops. This is the most common and probably the best studied of the incomplete forms of familial male pseudohermaphroditism. The affected individuals often have sufficient virilization to be reared as males.

In the cases studied by Wilson and associates,[128] the phenotype ranged from a minimal defect of virilization with microphallus and bifid scrotum to a more severe abnormality with perineoscrotal hypospadias to almost complete male pseudohermaphroditism with absent vasa deferentia, perineoscrotal hypospadias, and a vaginal orifice. Wilson suggested that this abnormality, as well as the syndromes of defective virilization described by Reifenstein, Lubs, Gilbert-Dreyfus, and Rosewater (noted later) and their associates, represents variable degrees of expression of a single genetic defect. In addition, evidence that this form of incomplete male pseudohermaphroditism, like testicular feminization, derives from an inherited resistance to androgen action was provided by studies of androgen and estrogen dynamics in several members of the pedigree studied by Wilson and colleagues.[128, 129] They found that some patients manifest reduced binding of dihydrotestosterone to the androgen receptor. (There were other individuals and families in whom no qualitative or quantitative alterations in androgen receptor could be demonstrated.) Similar findings were reported by Migeon's group.[130] Further supporting this relationship is the finding that circulating testosterone concentrations are higher, on the average, in affected than in unaffected men. This suggests that the capacity to form testosterone is adequate and that there is impaired feedback regulation of LH. These findings, as well as elevated estrogen secretion, resemble those in the testicular feminization syndrome. The feminization of the breasts at puberty probably represents a combination of increased estrogen secretion and impaired androgen action.

At the most fully masculinized end of the spectrum (or the mildest expression of male pseudohermaphroditism) is the family reported by Rosewater and associates.[131] The affected males exhibited gynecomastia and sterility but did not have defective development of the internal or external genitalia.

Incomplete Male Pseudohermaphroditism: Autosomal Recessive Type (5α-Reductase-2 Deficiency)

This entity, also referred to as pseudovaginal perineoscrotal hypospadias, is characterized by severe hypospadias and variable development of the vagina, usually so marked that affected individuals are called females at birth.[132, 133] This disorder bears a resemblance to the most extensive form of the X-linked recessive type described before, except that gynecomastia does not develop at puberty and inheritance is autosomal recessive. At puberty, these individuals undergo marked although not complete masculinization.

The studies of Peterson and associates[134] and of Walsh and colleagues[135] demonstrated that structures derived from the wolffian ducts (seminal vesicles, ejaculatory ducts, epididymides, and vasa deferentia) are male in character, whereas those structures that develop from the urogenital sinus and the anlagen of the external genitalia are female in nature. Thus, the failure of male differentiation is limited to the urogenital sinus and the urogenital fold, tubercle, and swelling, because these structures are under the influence of dihydrotestosterone, which cannot be formed adequately in patients with the 5α-reductase-2 deficiency (there are two isoenzymes of the 5α-reductase enzyme). There is evidence that dihydrotestosterone formation is deficient in the tissues of the urogenital tract in these patients. Several abnormalities of the 5α-reductase-2 enzyme have been identified biochemically. In one of these, the enzyme is deficient in its ability to bind the testosterone substrate.[136] This was the first abnormality described. Subsequently, instability of the enzyme with low affinity for the cofactor reduced nicotinamide adenine dinucleotide phosphate (NADPH) was found.[137] A third type has been described in which both of these abnormalities are present. Normal male circulating testosterone and estrogen levels, production rates, and interconversions are present. The normal estrogen production rate may explain the lack of development of gynecomastia. After puberty, the testosterone:dihydrotestosterone ratio in peripheral blood is markedly increased in these individuals compared with that in normal men.[136] Although this ratio may be normal in affected children before puberty in the basal state, the increased ratio can be demonstrated readily after hCG stimulation.[138]

In the 17 families from Santo Domingo initially studied by Peterson and colleagues,[134] the affected patients were 46,XY males who had bilateral inguinal or labioscrotal testes. A single perineal opening was present in 29 of the 30 patients in the 17 families studied. Although a vaginal pouch was present, there were no müllerian derivatives. The wolffian duct derivatives were well differentiated. At puberty, a striking degree of virilization occurred in the affected males owing to the increased concentration of testosterone. The voice deepened, the muscle mass increased, the phallus enlarged to functional size, the testes descended, and the scrotum became hyperpigmented and rugose. In contrast, prostatic enlargement, acne, facial hair growth, temporal recession, and gynecomastia did not occur. Of great interest was that the psychosexual orientation was male postpubertally, although all of these patients in this isolated community had been raised as females before puberty.

Imperato-McGinley and associates[139] demonstrated decreased urinary C_{19} and C_{21} steroid 5α metabolites in parents of male pseudohermaphrodites with 5α-reductase-2 deficiency. These studies demonstrated a generalized defect in 5α-reductase-2 activity involving C_{19} and C_{21} steroid metabolism in obligate carrier parents and provided confirmation of an autosomal recessive mode of inheritance in this condition.

In addition to the pseudovaginal perineoscrotal hypospadias in males who are homozygous for the disorder, these patients usually have separate urethral and vaginal openings within a urogenital sinus and a clitoris-appearing phallus. The deficiency in dihydrotestosterone production impairs development and secretory function of the prostate gland and seminal vesicles.[140, 141] As a consequence, adults have a rudimentary prostate and underdeveloped seminal vesicles. This results in viscous semen and volume of ejaculate, although they may have normal sperm counts. Recently, Imperato-McGinley and associates[142] described the use of intrauterine insemination with sperm from a man with this disorder to achieve fertilization. Among other considerations, this lends support to the concept of raising these individuals as males.

Lack of Müllerian Duct Regression

In addition to the syndromes arising from defects in androgen action as detailed, the failure of müllerian duct regression in otherwise normal males has also been described.[143] Patients are usually seen with bilateral cryptorchidism and inguinal hernias but otherwise normal external genitalia. When herniorrhaphy is performed, a uterus and fallopian tubes are found in the inguinal canals. No ovaries are present, because the gonads are testes and the wolffian ductal derivatives are those of the normal male. Thus, this disorder is the result of abnormal synthesis or secretion of MIS by the fetal Sertoli cells or of some defect in its mechanism of action. The cases that have been described suggest a recessive mode of inheritance that is either autosomal or X-linked.[144, 145]

Leydig Cell Hypoplasia

The intersitial, or Leydig, cells are the site of testicular testosterone production. The de novo synthesis of testosterone by the human fetal testis has been demonstrated[3] and is necessary for development of the internal and external male genitalia. Hypoplasia of testicular Leydig cells resulting in male pseudohermaphroditism has been described.[146, 147] As might be predicted, these patients have sexual infantilism, immature testes containing few spermatogonia in infantile seminiferous tubules (in either an inguinal or an abdominal location), and a female phenotype. Gonadotropin concentrations are increased. No müllerian duct derivatives are present, and there are discrete vaginal and urethral orifices. Plasma testosterone concentrations are low and unstimulable by hCG. Although this disorder may be the result of hypoplasia or agenesis of the Leydig cells, as originally suggested, it may also represent a Leydig cell receptor defect for hCG and LH, as suggested by Grumbach[148] and a preliminary report by Perez-Palacios and associates.[149]

The phenotype of inherited Leydig cell hypoplasia ranges from severe forms presenting as 46,XY females to milder forms in which males have hypergonadotropic hypogonadism and a very small penis.[150, 151] Binding of LH in the testes of these individuals can be decreased or absent, which may be the cause or result of Leydig cell hypoplasia.[152] A family with a missense mutation of the LH receptor gene resulting in Leydig cell hypoplasia in two siblings has been described.[153]

Androgen Insensitivity as a Cause of Male Infertility

Although perhaps it cannot strictly be classified as a form of male pseudohermaphroditism, an entity described by Aiman and colleagues[154] warrants comment. This is a form of androgen insensitivity responsible for male infertility. It is a result of a partial deficiency of the androgen receptor. One of the three patients described initially had mild gynecomastia, some reduction in testicular size, and decreased body hair. The other two each had a normal male habitus. They had marked oligospermia or azoospermia. Circulating testosterone concentrations were elevated, and LH levels were normal or increased. Biochemical studies demonstrated a decrease in high-affinity cytosol binding of dihydrotestosterone, a reflection of androgen resistance. Presumably, because high concentrations of testosterone are necessary for normal spermatogenesis, this deficient androgen action resulted in oligospermia or azoospermia and resultant infertility.

(Note: A gene [*DAZ*, *d*eleted in *az*oospermia] has been described on the Y chromosome [see Fig. 14–4], the absence of which is associated with some cases of azoospermia and oligospermia.[155])

FEMALE PSEUDOHERMAPHRODITISM

Patients with female pseudohermaphroditism have a female gonad (ovary) and karyotype (XX) and varying degrees of external genital virilization. There is no karyotypic abnormality in this disorder, no major abnormality of the ovary or its functional capacity, and no abnormality of internal genital development. Thus, the uterus, the tubes, and the ovaries are normal, and in contrast with the case in most of the other abnormalities of sexual development discussed in this chapter, reproductive function is often possible after appropriate treatment has been instituted. However, because adequate control of these patients and infertility can be a problem, bilateral adrenalectomy with adrenal corticosteroid therapy was recently suggested.[156] Female pseudohermaphroditism is usually due to enzyme abnormalities involved in adrenal steroid biosynthesis resulting in congenital adrenal hyperplasia. Less frequently, it may result from maternal ingestion of steroid-containing preparations with androgenic properties.

Congenital Adrenal Hyperplasia

Cortisol and aldosterone are key hormonal products secreted by the adrenal cortex. Clinical manifestations of abnormalities in steroid production result both from the degree of deficiency of cortisol and aldosterone formation and from the biologic activity of steroid precursors produced in excess as a result of the enzymatic block involved.

An understanding of the various forms of congenital adrenal hyperplasia and their manifestations depends on an understanding of the pathways of adrenal steroid biosynthesis and the enzymes involved. These are presented in Figure 14–12. As indicated earlier, the genes encoding most of the steroid-metabolizing enzymes have been identified. An overview of the molecular aspects is presented in references 105 to 107.

ACTH acts principally at the step between cholesterol and pregnenolone to stimulate adrenal steroidogenesis, although it also acts at additional steps in the pathway. The production of ACTH is regulated by the amount of cortisol in the circulation through a negative feedback mechanism. The action of cortisol may be directly on the pituitary or

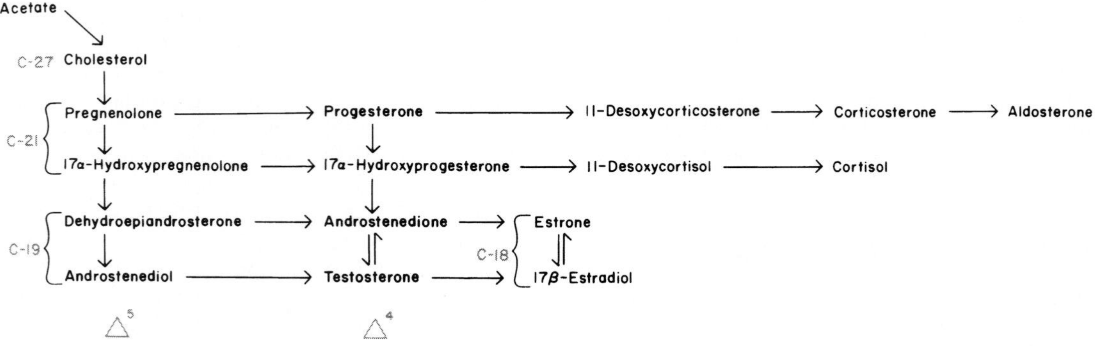

Figure 14–12 ■ Pathways of adrenal steroid hormone biosynthesis. The formation of the C-18 estrogens does not occur to an appreciable extent in the adrenals.

indirectly by way of corticotropin-releasing hormone from the hypothalamus. Thus, when the amount of cortisol is decreased, ACTH production increases. In all of the forms of congenital adrenal hyperplasia in which genital tract abnormalities occur, there is a decreased capacity to produce cortisol, with compensatory ACTH overproduction. With excessive ACTH secretion, there is increased production of steroids in the steps in the biosynthetic pathway up to the enzymatic block. There is a "damming up" of those steroids immediately preceding the block, and these are present in the circulation in increased concentrations.

Decreased cortisol levels stimulate the production of ACTH, and impaired mineralocorticoid formation increases renin-angiotensin production.

Enzyme deficiencies at each step of the biosynthetic pathway have been described. They may occur in males or in females. All are transmitted as autosomal recessive characteristics. When the male is involved and there is abnormal genital tract development, male pseudohermaphroditism results, as described earlier. When the female is involved and masculinization of the external genitalia occurs to varying degrees, female pseudohermaphroditism is a consequence. Five forms of congenital adrenal hyperplasia that may affect genital tract development have been identified, three of which have been discussed in the section on male pseudohermaphroditism (P450scc, 3β-hydroxysteroid dehydrogenase-isomerase, and P450c17 deficiencies). There may be a rare sixth form, P450 aldosterone synthase deficiency, which leads to deficient aldosterone production but does not affect genital tract development. The other two enzyme defects are 21-hydroxylase and 11-hydroxylase deficiencies.

Factors that may be involved in fetal adrenal growth, and hence adrenal hyperplasia, have recently been suggested. Two growth factors, insulin-like growth factor type II (IGF-II) and basic fibroblast growth factor (bFGF), have been demonstrated in the human fetal adrenal gland, and the expression of IGF-II and bFGF is enhanced by ACTH.[157, 158] The increased ACTH levels in congenital adrenal hyperplasia cause an increase in IGF-II and bFGF, which may be responsible for the hyperplasia of the gland. However, markedly increased mitogenesis in the human fetal adrenal gland has not been demonstrated when the glandular tissue is exposed to IGF-II in vitro. In contrast, bFGF is a potent mitogen for the human fetal adrenal gland,[159] and its expression is also increased by ACTH.[158] Basic FGF has been characterized as a "competence" factor, which brings the resting cell into the cell cycle, whereas the IGFs are considered "progression" factors, which drive the cell to mitosis. Therefore, it has been postulated that ACTH stimulates both the competence factor bFGF and the progression factor IGF-II to function in a coordinate manner to increase adrenal growth.[158] Because ACTH levels are increased in congenital adrenal hyperplasia as a result of decreased amounts of cortisol, the resultant increase in bFGF and IGF-II, and perhaps other locally produced growth factors or their receptors, acting in an autocrine or a paracrine manner, could bring about the hyperplasia and hypertrophy seen in this disorder.

21-Hydroxylase (P450c21) Deficiency

The most common form of congenital adrenal hyperplasia is the 21-hydroxylase deficiency.[106] This may be of varying severity, from partial to almost complete absence of the 21-hydroxylating enzyme system. Hydroxylation at C-21 is a key step in the formation of glucocorticoids and mineralocorticoids. Because patients with this disorder cannot form cortisol in normal amounts, there is a compensatory increase in ACTH, leading to hyperplasia of the adrenal gland. The excessive ACTH drives steroid production to the point of the enzymatic block, with a resultant increase in the amount of 17-hydroxyprogesterone produced. An increase in circulating levels of 17-hydroxyprogesterone with increased excretion of its urinary metabolite, pregnanetriol, is a pathognomonic finding. Further, the increased ACTH stimulates increased production of the adrenal androgen dehydroepiandrosterone, and perhaps androstenedione and testosterone, because the enzyme deficiency does not affect this portion of the biosynthetic pathway. It has been shown that increased concentrations of 17-hydroxyprogesterone and androstenedione can be found in the saliva of these patients as well as in the plasma.[160] If the enzymatic defect is severe and present in the zona glomerulosa, the site of aldosterone production, as well as in the zona fasciculata, in which cortisol is synthesized, there will be markedly decreased production of aldosterone also.

As is true with the other forms of adrenal hyperplasia, the disorder is inherited as an autosomal recessive trait. It has been shown that the gene coding for the P450c21 enzyme is on the short arm of chromosome 6, which is close to the HLA-B histocompatibility gene locus.[161] New and colleagues[162] studied this area extensively. HLA typing of cells has been used for amniotic fluid of mothers who previously had children with the adrenogenital syndrome to identify fetuses with heterozygous or homozygous forms of 21-hydroxylase deficiency.[163] Concentrations of 17α-hydroxyprogesterone can also be quantified in amniotic fluid.

New and associates[164] proposed prenatal treatment of congenital adrenal hyperplasia by administration of synthetic glucocorticoids to mothers at risk for having an affected fetus in utero because of previous delivery of an affected infant. If the diagnosis is confirmed after chorionic villus sampling or amniocentesis, treatment is continued. Whether treatment can be initiated early enough in pregnancy to be effective in the majority of cases remains to be ascertained.

In the milder forms of the disorder, the primary manifestations are those of excessive androgen production. The androgen excess is first expressed in utero, resulting in masculinization of the external genitalia to varying degrees (Fig. 14–13). The extent of the masculinization is probably dependent on the stage of intrauterine development of the external genitalia at which the effect of androgen excess is first manifested. It is also probably commensurate with the severity of the enzymatic defect. Most commonly, at birth, there is enlargement of the phallus, which is larger than that of the normal female but smaller than that of the normal male. Instead of a separate external orifice for the urethra and the vagina, there is a common urogenital sinus into which both the bladder and the uterus empty. The vaginal orifice is frequently covered by tissue resulting from posterior fusion of the labioscrotal folds. Any degree of external genital anomaly, from an almost normal-appearing perineum to a phallic urethra, may be encountered.

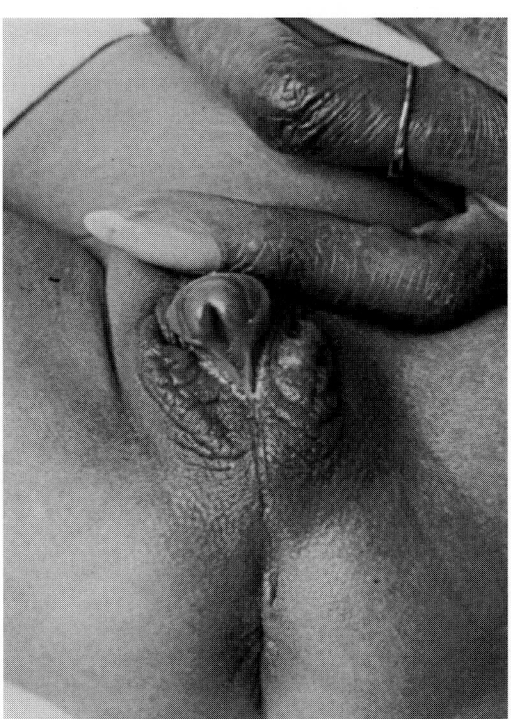

Figure 14–13 ■ Genitalia of female infant with adrenogenital syndrome. Note enlarged phallus (common urogenital sinus below) and wrinkled fused labioscrotal folds.

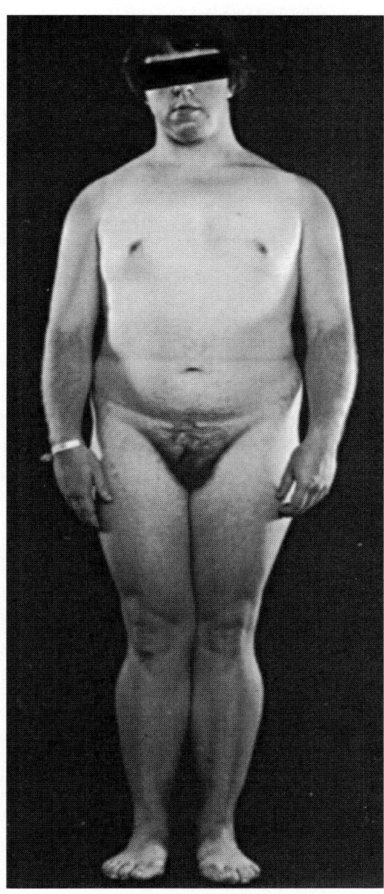

Figure 14–14 ■ Adult female with untreated adrenogenital syndrome due to 21-hydroxylase deficiency. Note masculinized habitus, short stature, and lack of female secondary sexual development.

If the disorder is unrecognized or not treated appropriately, the increased androgen concentration will cause excessive long bone growth and heterosexual precocity. Thus, in childhood, the patient will be taller than her peers, with pubic and axillary hair development and phallic hypertrophy. In the presence of continuing androgen excess, the epiphyses will fuse prematurely, so that the patient will be shorter than her peers in adulthood. In addition, she will have a masculinized body habitus (Fig. 14–14). Because of the excessive androgen, pituitary gonadotropins will be suppressed; as a result, ovarian function will not be stimulated, and the patient will have neither female secondary sexual development nor menstrual periods.

A form of congenital adrenal hyperplasia that first becomes manifest in the peripubertal period, often associated with hirsutism and sometimes mistaken for polycystic ovary syndrome, has been recognized and characterized.[95, 165, 166] This may be a result of 21-hydroxylase,[165, 166] 11β-hydroxylase,[167, 168] or 3β-hydroxysteroid dehydrogenase deficiency.[95]

In the most severe forms of the enzymatic defect, there is

a frank deficiency of deoxycorticosterone and aldosterone because of deficient 21-hydroxylation of progesterone, in addition to the androgen excess. The lack of mineralocorticoid leads to the "salt-losing" form of the disorder with severe hyponatremia, hyperkalemia, and marked dehydration. If not recognized and treated appropriately, this can be fatal.

Close linkage has been demonstrated between the HLA complex and the 21-hydroxylase gene in both its classic and nonclassic forms.[165, 166, 168–170]

11β-Hydroxylase (P450c11) Deficiency

11-Hydroxylation represents the final step in the biosynthesis of cortisol and corticosterone. Two forms of the enzyme have been described. Type 1 catalyzes the interconversion of cortisol and cortisone, while Type 2 catalyzes the conversion of cortisol to cortisone, but not the reverse. The 11β-hydroxylase enzyme has been purified,[171] and the cDNA from the gene encoding it has been cloned.[172] Because a deficiency of 11β-hydroxylase activity leads to decreased secretion of cortisol, there is a compensatory increase in ACTH secretion. As a result of the increased ACTH secretion, there is an increase in the biosynthesis and secretion of 11-deoxysteroids. This is a relatively uncommon form of congenital adrenal hyperplasia, accounting for less than 5 percent of reported cases. It is more common in Jews of North African origin.

The following chemical aberrations can result: (1) decreased plasma cortisol, urinary tetrahydrocortisol, and urinary tetrahydrocortisone levels; (2) increased plasma 11-deoxycortisol and 11-deoxycorticosterone levels and increased urinary excretion of the tetrahydro- derivatives of these steroids; (3) increased excretion of 11-deoxy-17-ketosteroids (these are derived primarily from dehydroepiandrosterone and are excreted in the urine as androsterone and etiocholanolone; total urinary 17-ketosteroid levels are increased even though the concentrations of 11-oxygenated 17-ketosteroids are diminished); and (4) increased plasma ACTH and melanocyte-stimulating hormone-β levels and decreased plasma renin activity and aldosterone secretion rates.

As a result of the 11β-hydroxylase deficiency, virilization and hypertension are encountered clinically. The virilization is the result of adrenal androgen overproduction and may be manifested as rapid somatic growth initially but early closure of the epiphyses, phallic enlargement, premature appearance of pubic and axillary hair, breast hypoplasia, and amenorrhea. The hypertension results from overproduction of deoxycorticosterone. Unlike the gene for 21-hydroxylase, the gene for 11β-hydroxylase is not associated with the HLA loci.[173, 174] Familial combined 21- and 11β-hydroxylase deficiencies have been described.[175] Zachmann[176] and others called attention to the clinical and biochemical variability of congenital adrenal hyperplasia due to 11β-hydroxylase deficiency.

Treatment of the 11β-hydroxylase deficiency consists of the administration of exogenous glucocorticoids in sufficient amounts to inhibit the secretion of ACTH, thereby suppressing the secretion of adrenal androgens and deoxycorticosterone. As with other forms of congenital adrenal hyperplasia, excessive glucocorticoid administration may inhibit linear growth. In addition, although aldosterone production is decreased, deoxycorticosterone production compensates for this. Therefore, mineralocorticoid substitution is not necessary in this form of congenital adrenal hyperplasia.

Maternal Ingestion of Steroids with Androgenic Potential

In 1959 and 1960, several reports suggested that maternal ingestion of synthetic progestins and testosterone during the first trimester of pregnancy was associated with masculinization of the external genitalia of newborn girls.[177–180] This is usually manifested by fusion of the labioscrotal folds and, less commonly, by clitoromegaly. These progestins were usually administered in an attempt to prevent abortion. Because many of these compounds have at least some androgenic activity and are not completely aromatized on passage across the placenta, masculinization of the female fetus can occur. Since knowledge of this condition became widespread, its occurrence has correspondingly diminished. The use of progestins during pregnancy is currently proscribed in the United States. Simple surgical correction of this disorder is usually accomplished easily.

TRUE HERMAPHRODITISM

The diagnosis of true hermaphroditism should be made only if the coexistence of ovarian and testicular tissue can be demonstrated definitively. There may be ovarian and testicular tissue either within the same gonad or in opposite gonads. Germ cells of both sexes as well as evidence of other gonadal elements should be demonstrated. Thus, the presence of gonadal stroma or streak gonads without an appreciable number of oocytes is not adequate to classify gonadal tissue as ovarian. Further, the nature of the internal or external genitalia, regardless of their ambisexual appearance, should not form the basis of classification as a true hermaphrodite.

True hermaphroditism may be further classified according to the location of the gonadal tissue as unilateral, lateral, or bilateral. The unilateral form is the most common, occurring in almost half of the cases, and refers to patients who have testicular and ovarian tissue on one side and either an ovary or a testis on the other. The lateral form refers to an ovary on one side and a testis on the other and occurs in approximately one third of the cases. The bilateral form, which occurs in approximately one fifth of the cases, refers to the presence of both ovarian and testicular tissue on both sides.

A wide spectrum of disorders of genital tract differentiation and secondary sexual development is seen clinically in true hermaphroditism (Fig. 14–15). Although the external genitalia are often ambiguous, the majority of the patients are reared as males because of the size of the phallus. Most have hypospadias, which may vary from perineal to penile, accompanied by incomplete fusion of the labioscrotal folds. A penile urethra may occasionally be present. Cryptorchidism is encountered commonly. Many patients have inguinal hernias, which may contain a gonad or a uterus. There is almost always a uterus, and ductal development is usually correlated with the nature of the gonads. In the lateral

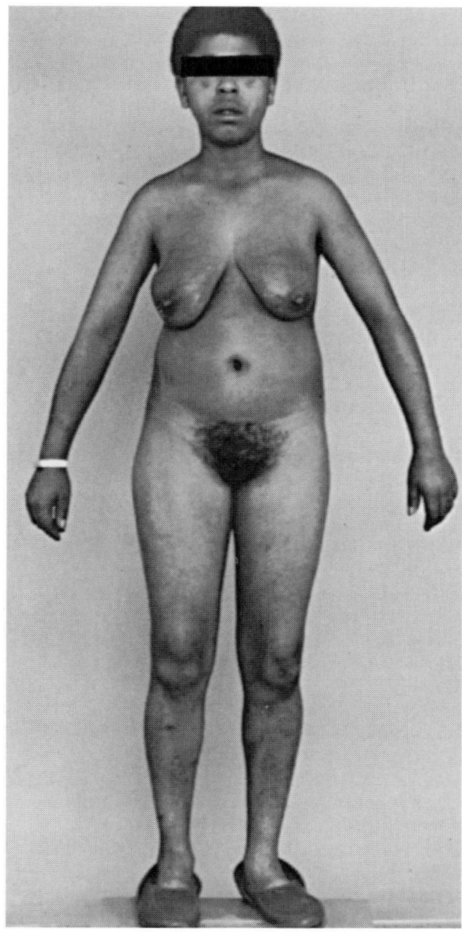

Figure 14–15 ■ True hermaphrodite, XX karyotype.

form, the duct on each side usually develops according to the nature of the gonad on that side.

Approximately 70 percent of patients with true hermaphroditism are sex chromatin–positive, the majority having an XX karyotype.[181] About two thirds of patients menstruate, and the majority have significant breast development. Menstruation has not been reported in sex chromatin–negative cases. Cyclic hematuria may occur. Ovulation occurs frequently, but spermatogenesis is rare.

In XX true hermaphrodites, an ovary is more likely to be found on the left side and the inappropriate gonad (either ovotestis or testis) on the right. The puzzle is why patients who do not have a Y chromosome have testicular tissue and elements of masculinization. The answer may lie in the observation, to which reference was made earlier, of the presence of the H-Y antigen in XX true hermaphrodites[25] or, perhaps more likely, of the sex-determining gene portion of the Y chromosome. In an analysis of 119 patients with true hermaphroditism, Benirschke and colleagues[181] found that 61 were 46,XX, 23 were 46,XY, and 35 were mosaics or chimeras, including 10 XX/XY chimeras and 6 XY/XYY mosaics.

The true hermaphrodite with a 46,XY karyotype, like 46,XY gonadal dysgenesis discussed previously, represents a developmental abnormality in which the presence of a Y chromosome fails to lead to normal testicular development. Postzygotic point mutations in the *SRY* gene were identified in a 46,XY true hermaphrodite with ambiguous genitalia and ovotestes.[182]

In 46,XX true hermaphrodites, *SRY* sequences have been found in 17 of 40 cases reported to date.[39, 183, 184] These studies suggest that the translocation of *SRY* onto either the X chromosome or autosomes is the basis for at least some cases of 46,XX true hermaphroditism.

GENERAL CLINICAL CONSIDERATIONS

It is crucial that the clinician who deals with patients with genital ambiguities be sensitive to the emotional as well as the physical needs of the patient. The patients frequently have a great deal of confusion and anxiety about their sexual roles. Whereas genetic, gonadal, hormonal, and genital sex may be of prime importance to the physician, the gender identity (that is, how the patient views himself or herself) and the sex of rearing are paramount in determining the patient's sexual identity. The correct diagnosis should optimally be made at birth, and appropriate sex assignation and therapy should be instituted at that time. Often, however, the correct diagnosis is not made at birth, and the clinician is faced with a teenage patient with sexual infantilism, precocious pubertal development, primary amenorrhea, or ambiguous genitalia.

At birth, definite sex assignment should be made as rapidly as possible. All hormonal, surgical, and psychologic steps should be taken to reinforce that assignment. After the first 1 to 2 years of life, attempts at reversing the gender identity and the sex of rearing can be catastrophic, other than for some patients with 5α-reductase-2 deficiency, and the clinician should do everything feasible to make the genital structures conform to the patient's perception of his or her sexual identity. Although there are instances in which an accurate pathophysiologic explanation is appropriate for a given patient, it is seldom necessary to give detailed anatomic and genetic explanations to the patient. Rather, discussion should be tailored to the perceived needs, age, and psychologic makeup of the patient. Thus, for example, if the patient has been reared as a female and views herself as a female, there is frequently little to be gained by telling the patient that there is some aspect of "maleness" about her chromosomes or gonads, even though the clinician knows that the individual is a male pseudohermaphrodite.

From a practical point of view, the only disorders of sexual development in which fertility is possible are the XX female pseudohermaphrodites with 21- and 11-hydroxylase deficiencies and an occasional patient with XO/XX mosaicism or 5α-reductase-2 deficiency. In XX female pseudohermaphrodites, it is important that the correct diagnosis be made and appropriate corticosteroid and surgical management be instituted, so that minimal deviations from normal occur and maximal potential for later fertility is ensured.

References

1. Jirasek JE. Development of the Genital System and Male Pseudohermaphroditism. Baltimore, Johns Hopkins University Press, 1971.

2. Van Wagenen G, Simpson ME. Embryology of the Ovary and Testis, *Homo sapiens* and *Macaca mulatta*. New Haven, Yale University Press, 1965.
3. Serra GB, Perez-Palacios G, Jaffe RB. De novo testosterone biosynthesis in the human fetal testis. J Clin Endocrinol Metab 30:128, 1970.
4. Ritzen EMS, Neyfeh SN, French FS, Dobbins MV. Demonstration of androgen-binding components in rat epididymis cytosol and comparison with binding components in prostate and other tissues. Endocrinology 89:143, 1971.
5. Josso N. Permeability of membranes to the müllerian-inhibiting substance synthesized by the human fetal testis in vitro: A clue to its biochemical nature. J Clin Endocrinol Metab 34:265, 1972.
6. Blanchard M, Josso N. Source of the anti-müllerian hormone synthesized by the fetal testis: Müllerian-inhibiting activity of fetal bovine Sertoli cells in tissue culture. Pediatr Res 8:968, 1974.
7. Rabinovici J, Goldsmith P, Roberts V, et al. Localization and secretion of inhibin/activin subunits in the human and subhuman primate fetal gonads. J Clin Endocrinol Metab 73:1141, 1991.
8. Donahoe PK, Budzik GP, Trelstad R, et al. Müllerian-inhibiting substance: An update. Recent Prog Horm Res 38:279, 1982.
9. Jost A. Problems of fetal endocrinology: The gonadal and hypophyseal hormones. Recent Prog Horm Res 8:379, 1953.
10. Jost A, Vigier B, Prepin J, Perchellet JP. Studies on sex differentiation in mammals. Recent Prog Horm Res 29:1, 1973.
11. Wilson JD. Recent studies on the mechanisms of action of testosterone. N Engl J Med 287:1284, 1972.
12. Wilson JD. Testosterone uptake by the urogenital tract of the rabbit embryo. Endocrinology 92:1192, 1973.
13. Wilson JD, Gloyna RE. The intranuclear metabolism of testosterone in the accessory organs of reproduction. Recent Prog Horm Res 26:309, 1970.
14. Wachtel SS, Ohno S. The immunogenetics of sexual development. *In* Steinberg AG (ed). Progress in Medical Genetics, Vol III. Philadelphia, WB Saunders, 1979, pp 109–142.
15. Wachtel SS, Koo GC, Boyse EA. Evolutionary conservation of H-Y ("male") antigen. Nature 254:272, 1975.
16. Ohno S, Nagai Y, Ciccares S, Iwata H. Testis-organization, H-Y antigen and the primary sex-determining mechanism of mammals. Recent Prog Horm Res 35:449, 1979.
17. Ohno S, Nagai Y, Ciccares S. Testicular cells lysostripped of H-Y antigen organize ovarian follicle-like aggregates. Cytogenet Cell Genet 20:351, 1978.
18. McClaren A. Sex determination in mammals. Trends Genet 4:153, 1988.
19. Page DC, Mosher R, Simpson EM, et al. The sex determining region of the human Y chromosome encodes a finger protein. Cell 51:1091, 1987.
20. Sinclair AH, Berta P, Palmer MS, et al. A gene from the human sex-determining region encodes a protein with homology to a conserved DNA-binding motif. Nature 346:240, 1990.
21. Gubbay J, Collignon J, Koopman P, et al. A gene mapping to the sex-determining region of the mouse Y-chromosome is a member of a novel family of embryonically expressed genes. Nature 346:245, 1990.
22. Ricard JY, Benarous R, Guerrier D, et al. Cloning and expression of cDNA for anti-müllerian hormone. Proc Natl Acad Sci USA 83:5464, 1986.
23. Cate RL, Mattalians PJ, Hession C, et al. Isolation of the bovine and human genes for müllerian inhibiting substance and expression of the human gene in animal cells. Cell 45:685, 1986.
24. Siiteri PK, Wilson JD. Testosterone formation and metabolism during male sexual differentiation in the human embryo. J Clin Endocrinol Metab 38:113, 1974.
25. Anderson KM, Liao S. Selective retention of dihydrotestosterone by prostatic nuclei. Nature 219:277, 1968.
26. Conte FA, Grumbach MM. Recent insights into sex determination. *In* Sizonenko PC, Aubert ML (eds). Developmental Endocrinology, Serono Symposium, Vol 67. New York, Raven Press, 1990, pp 49–55.
27. Sinclair AH, Foster JW, Spencer JA, et al. Sequences homologous to *ZFY*, a candidate human sex-determining gene, are autosomal in marsupials. Nature 33:780, 1988.
28. Palmer MS, Sinclair AH, Berta P, et al. Genetic evidence that *ZFY* is not the testis-determining factor. Nature 342:937, 1989.
29. Koopman P, Gubbay J, Collignon J, Lovell-Badge R. *ZFY* gene expression patterns are not compatible with a primary role in mouse sex determination. Nature 342:940, 1989.
30. Merchant H. Rat gonadal and ovarian organogenesis with and without germ cells. An ultrastructural study. Dev Biol 44:1, 1975.
31. McCarrey JR, Abbott UK. Chick gonadal differentiation following excision of primordial germ cells. Dev Biol 66:256, 1978.
32. Sinclair AH, Berta P, Palmer MS, et al. A gene from the human sex-determining region encodes a protein with homology to a conserved DNA-binding motif. Nature 346:240, 1990.
33. Berta P, Hawkins JR, Sinclair AH, et al. Genetic evidence equating *SRY* and the testis-determining factor. Nature 348:448, 1990.
34. Vilain E, McElreavey K, Jaubert F, et al. Familial case with sequence variant in the testis-determining region associated with two sex phenotypes. Am J Hum Genet 50:1008, 1992.
35. Affara NA, Chalmers IJ, Ferguson SM. Analysis of the *SRY* gene in 22 sex-reversed XY females identifies four new point mutations in the conserved DNA binding domain. Hum Mol Genet 2:785, 1993.
36. Braun A, Kammerer S, Cleve H, et al. True hermaphroditism in a 46,XY individual caused by a postzygotic somatic point mutation in the male gonadal sex-determining locus (*SRY*): Molecular genetics and histological findings in a sporadic case. Am J Hum Genet 52:578, 1993.
37. Hawkins JR, Taylor A, Berta P, et al. Mutational analysis of *SRY*: Nonsense and missense mutations in XY sex reversal. Hum Genet 88:471, 1992.
38. Harley VR, Jackson DI, Hextall PJ, et al. DNA binding activity of recombinant *SRY* from normal males and XY females. Science 255:453, 1992.
39. McElreavey KD, Vilain E, Boucekkine C, et al. XY sex reversal associated with a nonsense mutation in *SRY*. Genomics 13:838, 1992.
40. Jager RJ, Anvret M, Hall K, Scherer G. A human XY female with a frame shift mutation in the candidate testis-determining gene *SRY*. Nature 348:452, 1990.
41. Schmitt NM, Thiele H, Kaltwasser P, et al. Two novel *SRY* missense mutations reducing DNA binding identified in XY females and their mosaic fathers. Am J Hum Genet 56:862, 1995.
42. Koopman P, Munsterberg A, Capel B, et al. Expression of a candidate sex-determining gene during mouse testis differentiation. Nature 348:450, 1990.
43. Munsterberg A, Lovell-Badge R. Expression of the mouse anti-müllerian hormone gene suggests a role in both male and female sexual differentiation. Development 113:613, 1991.
44. Lillie F. Theory of freemartin. Science 43:611, 1916.
45. Picon R. Action au testicule foetal sur le development in vitro des canaux de Müller chez le rat. Anat Micro Morph Exp 58:1, 1969.
46. Swann D, Donahoe P, Ito Y, et al. Extraction of müllerian inhibiting substance from newborn calf testes. Dev Biol 69:73, 1979.
47. Hagg C, Lee MM, Tizard R, et al. Isolation of the rat gene for müllerian inhibiting substance. Genomics 12:665, 1992.
48. Lee MM, Donahoe PK. Müllerian inhibiting substance: A gonadal hormone with multiple functions. Endocr Rev 14:152, 1993.
49. di Clemente C, Wilson C, Faure E, et al. Cloning, expression, and alternative splicing of the receptor for anti-müllerian hormone. Mol Endocrinol 8:1006, 1994.
50. Shen W-H, Moore CC, Ikeda Y, et al. Nuclear receptor steroidogenic factor 2 regulates the müllerian inhibiting substance gene: A link to the sex determination cascade. Cell 77:651, 1994.
51. Grumbach MM, Conte FA. Disorders of sexual differentiation. *In* Wilson JW, Foster DW (eds). Textbook of Endocrinology, 8th ed. Philadelphia, WB Saunders, 1992, pp 853–952.
52. Turner HH. A syndrome of infantilism, congenital webbed neck, and cubitus valgus. Endocrinology 23:566, 1938.
53. Carr DH. Chromosome studies in selected spontaneous abortions and early pregnancy loss. Obstet Gynecol 37:570, 1971.
54. Singh RF, Carr DH. The anatomy and histology of XO human embryos and fetuses. Anat Rec 155:369, 1966.
55. Van Campenhout J, Antaki A, Rasio E. Diabetes mellitus and thyroid autoimmunity in gonadal dysgenesis. Fertil Steril 24:1, 1973.
56. Fialkow PJ, Uchida IA. Antibodies in Down's syndrome and gonadal dysgenesis. Ann N Y Acad Sci 155:759, 1968.

57. Wilkins L, Grumbach MM, van Wyk JJ. Chromosomal sex in "ovarian agenesis." J Clin Endocrinol Metab 14:270, 1954.
58. Federman DD. Abnormal Sexual Development. Philadelphia, WB Saunders, 1967.
59. Conte FA, Grumbach MM, Kaplan SL. A diphasic pattern of gonadotropin secretion in patients with syndrome of gonadal dysgenesis. J Clin Endocrinol Metab 40:670, 1975.
60. Alexander RL, Conte FA, Kaplan SL, Grumbach MM. The effect of estrogen treatment on height in patients with gonadal dysgenesis (Abstract). Clin Res 26:174a, 1978.
61. Ross GT, Vande Wiele RL. The ovaries. *In* Williams RH (ed). Textbook of Endocrinology, 5th ed. Philadelphia, WB Saunders, 1974, p 401.
62. Simpson JL. Male pseudohermaphroditism: Genetics and clinical delineation. Hum Genet 44:1, 1978.
63. Dutrillaux B, Lejeune J. New techniques in the study of human chromosomes. Adv Hum Genet 5:119, 1975.
64. Schwarzacher HG, Wolf V, Passarge E (eds). Methods in Human Cytogenetics. New York, Springer-Verlag, 1974, chapters VI and VII.
65. Disteche C, Hagemeijer A, Frederic J, Prognaux J. An abnormal large human chromosome identified as an end-to-end fusion of two X's by combined results of the new banding techniques and microdensitometry. Clin Genet 3:338, 1972.
66. Hagemeijer A, Hoovers J, Harper-Voogt L, et al. Late replicating ring X-chromosomes identified by R-banding after BrdU pulse: Three new examples of mosaicism 45,XO/46Xr(X). Hum Genet 34:35, 1976.
67. Jacobs PA, Ross A. Structural abnormalities of the Y chromosome in man. Nature 210:352, 1966.
68. Robinson JA, Buckton RE. Quinacrine fluorescence of variant and abnormal human Y chromosomes. Chromosoma 35:342, 1971.
69. Sohval AR. The syndrome of pure gonadal dysgenesis. Am J Med 38:615, 1965.
70. Jager RJ, Anvret M, Hall K, Scherer G. A human XY female with a frame shift mutation in the candidate testis-determining gene *SRY.* Nature 348:452, 1990.
71. Muller J, Schwartz M, Skakkebaek NE. Analysis of the sex-determining region of the Y chromosome (SRY) in sex reversed patients: Point-mutation in *SRY* causing sex-reversion in a 46,XY female. J Clin Endocrinol Metab 750:331, 1992.
72. Hawkins JR, Taylor A, Berta P, et al. Mutational analysis of *SRY*: Nonsense and missense mutations in XY sex reversal. Hum Genet 88:471, 1992.
73. Harley VR, Jackson DI, Hextall PJ, et al. DNA binding activity of recombinant *SRY* from normal males and XY females. Science 255:453, 1993.
74. Zeng YT, Ren ZR, Zhang ML, et al. A new de novo mutation (A113T) in HMG box of the *SRY* gene leads to XY gonadal dysgenesis. J Med Genet 30, 655, 1993.
75. Affara NA, Chalmers IJ, Ferguson SM. Analysis of the *SRY* gene in 22 sex-reversed XY females identifies four new point mutations in the conserved DNA binding domain. Hum Mol Genet 2:785, 1993.
76. Schmitt NM, Thiele H, Kaltwasser P, et al. Two novel *SRY* missense mutations reducing DNA binding identified in XY females and their mosaic fathers. Am J Hum Genet 56:862, 1995.
77. Iida T, Nakahori Y, Komaki R, et al. A novel nonsense mutation in the HMG box of the *SRY* gene in a patient with XY sex reversal. Hum Mol Genet 3:1437, 1994.
78. Klinefelter HF Jr, Reifenstein EC Jr, Albright F. Syndrome characterized by gynecomastia, aspermatogenesis without a-leydigism and increased excretion of follicle-stimulating hormone. J Clin Endocrinol Metab 2:615, 1942.
79. Bardin CW, Paulsen CA. The testes. *In* Williams RH (ed). Textbook of Endocrinology, 6th ed. Philadelphia, WB Saunders, 1981, pp 293–351.
80. Robinson A, Lubs HA, Nielson J, Sorensen K. Summary of clinical findings: Profiles of children with 47,XXY, 47,XXX, and 47,XYY karyotypes. Birth Defects 15:1, 261, 1979.
81. De la Chapelle A. Analytic review: Nature and origin of males with XX sex chromosomes. Am J Hum Genet 24:71, 1972.
82. Ferguson-Smith MA, Mack WS, Ellis PM, et al. Parental age and the source of the X chromosomes in XXY Klinefelter's syndrome. Lancet 1:46, 1964.
82a. Bose HS, Sugawara T, Strauss JF III, Miller WL. The pathophysiology and genetics of congenital lipid adrenal hyperplasia. N Engl J Med 335:1870, 1996.
83. Koizumi S, Kyoya S, Miyananki T, et al. Cholesterol side-chain cleavage enzyme activity and cytochrome P450 content in adrenal mitochondria of a patient with congenital lipoid adrenal hyperplasia (Prader disease). Clin Chim Acta 77:301, 1977.
84. Chung B, Matteson KJ, Voutilainen R, et al. Human cholesterol side-chain cleavage enzyme, P450scc: cDNA cloning assignment of the gene to chromosome 15, and expression in the placenta. Proc Natl Acad Sci USA 83:8962, 1986.
85. Prader A, Anders GJPA. Zur Genetik der Kongenitalen Lipoidhyperplasie der Nebennieren. Helvet Paediatr Acta 17:285, 1962.
86. Janne O, Perheentupa J, Vikho R. Plasma and urinary steroids in an eight-year-old boy with 3β-hydroxysteroid dehydrogenase deficiency. J Clin Endocrinol Metab 31:162, 1970.
87. Parks GA, Bermudez JA, Anast CS, et al. Pubertal boy with 3β-hydroxysteroid dehydrogenase defect. J Clin Endocrinol Metab 33:269, 1971.
88. Janne O, Perheentupa J, Viinkka L, Vikho R. Testicular endocrine function in a pubertal boy with 3β-hydroxysteroid dehydrogenase deficiency. J Clin Endocrinol Metab 39:206, 1974.
89. New MI, White PC, Pang S, et al. The adrenal hyperplasias. *In* Scrivner R, Beaudet AL, Sly WS, Valle D (eds). The Metabolic Basis of Inherited Disease, 6th ed. New York, McGraw-Hill, 1989, pp 1881–1917.
90. Bongiovanni AM. Acquired adrenal hyperplasia: With special reference to 3β-hydroxysteroid dehydrogenase. Fertil Steril 35:599, 1981.
91. Rosenfeld RL, Rich BH, Wolfsdorf JI, et al. Pubertal presentation of congenital Δ^5-3β-hydroxysteroid dehydrogenase deficiency. J Clin Endocrinol Metab 51:345, 1980.
92. Lobo RA, Goebelsmann U. Evidence for reduced 3β-ol-hydroxysteroid dehydrogenase activity in some hirsute women thought to have polycystic ovary syndrome. J Clin Endocrinol Metab 53:394, 1981.
93. Forest MG. Inborn errors of testosterone biosynthesis. Pediatr Adolesc Endocrinol 8:133, 1981.
94. Pang S, Levine LS, Stoner E, et al. Nonsalt-losing congenital adrenal hyperplasia due to 3β-hydroxysteroid dehydrogenase deficiency with normal glomerulosa function. J Clin Endocrinol Metab 56:808, 1983.
95. Pang S, Lerner AJ, Stoner E, et al. Late-onset adrenal steroid 3β-hydroxysteroid dehydrogenase deficiency. I. A cause of hirsutism in pubertal and postpubertal women. J Clin Endocrinol Metab 60:428, 1985.
96. Eldar-Geva T, Hurwitz A, Vecsei P, et al. Secondary biosynthetic defects in women with late-onset congenital adrenal hyperplasia. N Engl J Med 323:855, 1990.
97. Siegel SF, Finegold DN, Lanes R, Lee PA. ACTH stimulation tests and plasma dehydroepiandrosterone sulfate levels in women with hirsutism. N Engl J Med 323:849, 1990.
98. Bricaire H, Luton JP, Laudat P, et al. A new male pseudohermaphroditism associated with hypertension due to a block of 17α-hydroxylation. J Clin Endocrinol Metab 35:67, 1972.
99. Tournaire J, Audi-Parera L, Laras B, et al. Male pseudohermaphroditism with hypertension due to a 17α-hydroxylation deficiency. Clin Endocrinol (Oxf) 5:53, 1976.
100. Kershnar AK, Borut D, Kogut MD, et al. Studies in phenotypic female with 17α-hydroxylase deficiency. J Pediatr 89:395, 1976.
101. Biglieri EG, Herron MA, Brust N. 17-Hydroxylation deficiency in man. J Clin Invest 45:1946, 1966.
102. Nakajin S, Shinoda M, Haniu M, et al. C_{21} steroid side chain cleavage enzyme from porcine adrenal microsomes: Purification and characterization of the 17α-hydroxylase/$C_{17,20}$ lyase cytochrome P450. J Biol Chem 259:3971, 1984.
103. Chung B, Picado-Leonard J, Chung B, et al. Cytochrome P450c17 (steroid 17α-hydroxylase/17,20 lyase): Cloning of human adrenal and testis cDNAs indicate the same gene is expressed in both tissues. Proc Natl Acad Sci USA 84:407, 1987.
104. Matteson KJ, Picado-Leonard J, Chung B, et al. Assignment of the gene for adrenal P450c17 (17α-hydroxylase/17,20 lyase) to human chromosome 10. J Clin Endocrinol Metab 63:789, 1986.
105. Miller WL. Molecular biology of steroid hormone synthesis. Endocr Rev 9:195, 1988.

106. Morel Y, Miller WL. Clinical and molecular genetics of congenital adrenal hyperplasia due to 21-hydroxylase deficiency. Adv Hum Genet 20:1, 1991.
107. Miller WL, Levine LS. Molecular and clinical advances in congenital adrenal hyperplasia. J Pediatr 11:1, 1987.
108. Zachmann M, Vollmin JA, Hamilton W, Prader A. Steroid 17,20-desmolase deficiency: A new cause of male pseudohermaphroditism. Clin Endocrinol 1:369, 1972.
109. Goebelsmann U, Zachmann M, Davajan V, et al. Male pseudohermaphroditism due to 17,20-desmolase deficiency. Gynecol Invest 7:138, 1976.
110. Kaufman FR, Costin G, Goebelsmann U, et al. Male pseudohermaphroditism due to 17,20-desmolase deficiency. J Clin Endocrinol Metab 57:32, 1983.
111. Saez JM, de Peretti E, Morera AM, et al. Familial male pseudohermaphroditism with gynecomastia due to a testicular 17-ketosteroid reductase defect. I. Studies in vivo. J Clin Endocrinol Metab 32:604, 1971.
112. Saez JM, Morera AM, de Peretti E, Bertrand J. Further in vivo studies in male pseudohermaphroditism with gynecomastia due to a testicular 17-ketosteroid reductase defect (compared to a case of testicular feminization). J Clin Endocrinol Metab 34:598, 1972.
113. Goebelsmann U, Horton R, Mestmant JM, et al. Male pseudohermaphroditism due to testicular 17β-hydroxysteroid dehydrogenase deficiency. J Clin Endocrinol Metab 36:867, 1973.
114. Lanes R, Brown TR, de Bustos EG, et al. Sibship with 17-ketosteroid reductase (17-KSR) deficiency and hypothyroidism: Lack of linkage of histocompatibility leucocyte antigen and 17-KSR loci. J Clin Endocrinol Metab 57:190, 1983.
115. Wilson JD, Goldstein JL. Classification of hereditary disorders of sexual development. Birth Defects 11:1, 1975.
116. Wilkins LM. The Diagnosis and Treatment of Endocrine Disorders in Childhood and Adolescence, 2nd ed. Springfield, IL, Charles C Thomas, 1957, p 278.
117. Southern AT, Ross H, Sharma DC, et al. Plasma concentration and biosynthesis of testosterone in the syndrome of feminizing testes. J Clin Endocrinol Metab 25:518, 1965.
118. Judd HL, Hamilton CR, Barlow JJ, et al. Androgen and gonadotropin dynamics in testicular feminization syndrome. J Clin Endocrinol Metab 34:229, 1972.
119. Goldstein JT, Wilson JD. Studies on the pathogenesis of the pseudohermaphroditism in the mouse with testicular feminization syndrome. J Clin Endocrinol Metab 34:229, 1972.
120. Keenan BS, Meyer WJ III, Hadjian AJ, et al. Syndrome of androgen insensitivity in man: Absence of 5α-dihydrotestosterone binding protein in skin fibroblasts. J Clin Endocrinol Metab 38:1143, 1974.
121. Amrhein JA, Meyer WJ III, Jones HW Jr, Migeon CJ. Androgen insensitivity in man: Evidence for genetic heterogeneity. Proc Natl Acad Sci USA 73:891, 1976.
122. Kaufman M, Pinsky L, Baird PA, McGillivray BC. Complete androgen insensitivity with a normal amount of 5α-dihydrotestosterone–binding activity in labium majus skin fibroblasts. Am J Med Genet 4:401, 1979.
123. Griffin JE. Testicular feminization associated with a thermolabile androgen receptor in cultured fibroblasts. J Clin Invest 64:1624, 1979.
124. Rosenfield RL, Lawrence AM, Liao S, Landau RL. Androgens and androgen responsiveness in the feminizing testes syndrome; comparison of complete and "incomplete" forms. J Clin Endocrinol Metab 36:625, 1971.
125. Lubs HA Jr, Vilar O, Bergenstal DM. Familial male pseudohermaphroditism with labial testes and partial feminization: Endocrine studies and genetic aspects. J Clin Endocrinol Metab 19:1110, 1959.
126. Gilbert-Dreyfus S, Sebaoun CA, Belaish J. Etude d'un cas familial d'androgynoidisme avec hypospadias grave, gynecomastie et hyperoestrogenie. Ann Endocrinol 18:93, 1957.
127. Reifenstein EC Jr. Hereditary familial hypogonadism. Clin Res 3:86, 1947.
128. Wilson JD, Harrod MJ, Goldstein JL, et al. Familial incomplete male pseudohermaphroditism, type I. Evidence for androgen resistance and variable clinical manifestations in a family with the Reifenstein syndrome. N Engl J Med 290:1097, 1974.
129. Griffin JE, Punyashthiti K, Wilson JD. Dihydrotestosterone binding by cultured human fibroblasts: Comparison of cells from control subjects and from patients with hereditary male pseudohermaphroditism due to androgen resistance. J Clin Invest 57:1342, 1976.
130. Amrhein JA, Klingensmith GJ, Walsh PC, et al. Partial androgen insensitivity: The Reifenstein syndrome revisited. N Engl J Med 297:350, 1977.
131. Rosewater S, Gwinup G, Hamwi GJ. Familial gynecomastia. Ann Intern Med 63:377, 1965.
132. Simpson JL, New M, Peterson RE, German J. Pseudovaginal perineoscrotal hypospadias in sibs. Birth Defects 7:140, 1971.
133. Apitz JM, Simpson JL, Sarto GE, et al. Pseudovaginal perineoscrotal hypospadias. Clin Genet 3:1, 1972.
134. Peterson RE, Imperato-McGinley J, Gautier T, Sturla E. Male pseudohermaphroditism due to steroid 5α-reductase deficiency. Am J Med 62:170, 1977.
135. Walsh PC, Madden JD, Harrod MJ, et al. Familial incomplete male pseudohermaphroditism, type 2. Decreased dihydrotestosterone formation in pseudovaginal perineoscrotal hypospadias. N Engl J Med 291:944, 1974.
136. Peterson RE, Imperato-McGinley J, Gautier T, Sturla E. Hereditary steroid 5α-reductase deficiency: A newly recognized cause of male pseudohermaphroditism. *In* Vallet HL, Porter IH (eds). Genetic Mechanisms of Sexual Development. New York, Academic Press, 1979, pp 149–167.
137. Griffin JE, Wilson JD. The syndrome of androgen resistance. N Engl J Med 302:198, 1980.
138. Pang S, Levine LS, Chou D, et al. Dihydrotestosterone and its relationship to testosterone in infancy and childhood. J Clin Endocrinol Metab 48:821, 1979.
139. Imperato-McGinley J, Petersen RE, Gautier T, et al. Decreased urinary C_{19} and C_{21} steroid 5α-metabolites in parents of male pseudohermaphrodites with 5α-reductase deficiency: Detection of carriers. J Clin Endocrinol Metab 60:533, 1985.
140. Cai L-Q, Fratianni CM, Gautier T, Imperato-McGinley J. Dihydrotestosterone regulation of semen in male pseudohermaphrodites with 5α-reductase-2 deficiency. J Clin Endocrinol Metab 79:409, 1994.
141. Imperato-McGinley J, Gautier T, Zirinsky K, et al. Prostate visualization studies in males homozygous and heterozygous for 5α-reductase deficiency. J Clin Endocrinol Metab 75:1022, 1992.
142. Katz MD, Kligman I, Cai L-Q, et al. Paternity by intrauterine insemination with sperm from a man with 5α-reductase-2 deficiency. N Engl J Med 336:994, 1997.
143. Nilson O. Hernia uteri inguinalis. Acta Chir Scand 83:231, 1939.
144. Morillo-Cucci G, German J. Males with a uterus and fallopian tubes, a rare disorder of sexual development. Birth Defects 7:229, 1971.
145. Brook CGD, Wagner H, Zachmann M, et al. Familial occurrence of persistent müllerian structures in otherwise normal males. Br Med J 1:771, 1973.
146. Berthezene F, Forest MG, Grimaud JA, et al. Leydig cell agenesis: A cause of male pseudohermaphroditism. N Engl J Med 295:969, 1976.
147. Brown DM, Markland C, Dehner LP. Leydig cell hypoplasia: A cause of male pseudohermaphroditism. J Clin Endocrinol Metab 46:1, 1978.
148. Grumbach MM. Genetic mechanisms of sex differentiation. *In* Vallet HL, Porter IH (eds). Genetic Mechanisms of Sexual Development. New York, Academic Press, 1979, 33–74.
149. Perez-Palacios G, Scaglia H, Kofman AS, et al. Inherited deficiency of gonadotropin receptor in Leydig cells: A new form of male pseudohermaphroditism (Abstract). Am J Hum Genet 27:71a, 1975.
150. Toledo SPA, Arnhold IJ, Luthold W, et al. Leydig cell hypoplasia determining familial hypergonadotropic hypogonadism. Prog Clin Biol Res 200:311, 1985.
151. Toledo SPA. Leydig cell hypoplasia leading to two different phenotpyes: Male pseudohermaphroditism and primary hypogonadism not associated with this. Clin Endocrinol (Oxf) 36:521, 1992.
152. Martinez-Mora J, Saez JM, Toran N, et al. Male pseudohermaphroditism due to Leydig cell agenesia and absence of testicular LH receptors. Clin Endocrinol (Oxf) 34:485, 1991.
153. Kremer H, Kraaij R, Toledo SPA, et al. Male

pseudohermaphroditism due to a homozygous missense mutation of the luteinizing hormone gene. Nat Genet 9:160, 1995.
154. Aiman J, Griffin JE, Gazak JM, et al. Androgen insensitivity as a cause of infertility in otherwise normal men. N Engl J Med 300:223, 1979.
155. Reijo R, Alagappan R, Patrizio P, Page DC. Severe oligospermia resulting from deletions of the azoospermia factor gene on the Y chromosome. Lancet 347:1290, 1996.
156. Van Wyk JJ, Gunther DF, Ritzen EM, et al. The use of adrenalectomy as a treatment for congenital adrenal hyperplasia. J Clin Endocrinol Metab 81:3180, 1996.
157. Mesiano S, Mellon SH, Jaffe RB. Mitogenic action, regulation and localization of insulin-like growth factors in the human fetal adrenal gland. J Clin Endocrinol Metab 76:968, 1993.
158. Mesiano S, Mellon SH, Gospodarowicz D, et al. Basic fibroblast growth factor is regulated by corticotropin in the human fetal adrenal: A model for adrenal growth regulation. Proc Natl Acad Sci USA 88:5428, 1991.
159. Crickard K, Ill CR, Jaffe RB. Control of proliferation of human fetal adrenal cells in vitro. J Clin Endocrinol Metab 53:790, 1981.
160. Otten BJ, Wellen JJ, Rijken CW, et al. Salivary and plasma androstenedione and 17-hydroxyprogesterone levels in congenital adrenal hyperplasia. J Clin Endocrinol Metab 57:1150, 1983.
161. Levine L, Zachmann SM, New MI, et al. Genetic mapping of the 21-hydroxylase deficiency gene within the HLA linkage group. N Engl J Med 299:911, 1978.
162. New MI, Dupont B, Pang S, et al. An update of congenital adrenal hyperplasia. Recent Prog Horm Res 37:105, 1981.
163. Pollack MS, Levine LS, Duchon M, et al. Prenatal diagnosis of CAH due to 21-hydroxylase deficiency by HLA typing of cultured amniotic cells (Abstract). Pediatr Res 13:384, 1979.
164. Spieser PW, Laforgia N, Kato K, et al. First trimester prenatal treatment and molecular genetic diagnosis of congenital adrenal hyperplasia (21-hydroxylase deficiency). J Clin Endocrinol Metab 70:838, 1990.
165. Kohn B, Levine LS, Pollack MS, et al. Late-onset steroid 21-hydroxylase deficiency: A variant of classical congenital hyperplasia. J Clin Endocrinol Metab 55:817, 1982.
166. Levine LS, Dupont B, Lorenzen F, et al. Cryptic 21-hydroxylase deficiency in families of patients with classical congenital adrenal hyperplasia. J Clin Endocrinol Metab 51:1316, 1980.
167. Newmark S, Dluhy RG, Williams GF, et al. Partial 11- and 21-hydroxylase deficiencies in hirsute women. Am J Obstet Gynecol 127:594, 1977.
168. New MI, Dupont B, Grumbach MM, Levine LS. Congenital adrenal hyperplasia and related conditions. *In* Stanbury JB, Wyngaarden JB, Frederickson DS, et al (eds). The Metabolic Basis of Inherited Disease, 5th ed. New York, McGraw-Hill, 1982, p 273.
169. Dupont B, Oberfield SE, Smithwick EM, et al. Close genetic linkage between HLA and congenital adrenal hyperplasia (21-hydroxylase deficiency). Lancet 2:1309, 1977.
170. Libber SM, Migeon CJ, Bias WB. Ascertainment of 21-hydroxylase deficiency in individuals with HLA-B14 haplotype. J Clin Endocrinol Metab 60:727, 1985.
171. Lakshmi V, Monder C. Purification and characterization of the corticosteroid 11β-dehydrogenase component of the rat liver 11β-hydroxysteroid-dehydrogenase complex. Endocrinology 123:2390, 1988.
172. Chua SC, Szabo P, Vitek A, et al. Cloning of cDNA encoding steroid 11 beta-hydroxylase (P450c11). Proc Natl Acad Sci USA 84:7193, 1987.
173. Brautbar C, Rosler A, Landau H, et al. No linkage between HLA and congenital adrenal hyperplasia due to 11β-hydroxylase deficiency. N Engl J Med 300:205, 1979.
174. Glenthoj A, Nielsen MD, Starup J, Svejgaard A. HLA and congenital hyperplasia due to 11-hydroxylase deficiency. Tissue Antigens 14:181, 1979.
175. Hurwitz A, Brautbar C, Milwidsky A, et al. Combined 21- and 11β-hydroxylase deficiency in familial congenital adrenal hyperplasia. J Clin Endocrinol Metab 60:631, 1985.
176. Zachmann M, Tassinari D, Prader A. Clinical and biochemical variability of congenital adrenal hyperplasia due to 11β-hydroxylase deficiency: A study of 25 patients. J Clin Endocrinol Metab 56:222, 1983.
177. Jones HW Jr, Wilkins L. The genital anomaly associated with prenatal exposure to progestogens. Fertil Steril 11:148, 1960.
178. Grumbach MM, Ducharme JR, Moloshak RE. On the fetal masculinizing action of certain oral progestins. J Clin Endocrinol Metab 19:1369, 1959.
179. Grumbach MM, Ducharme JR. The effects of androgens on fetal sexual development: Androgen-induced female pseudohermaphroditism. Fertil Steril 11:157, 1960.
180. Wilkens L. Masculinization of the female fetus due to the use of orally given progestins. JAMA 172:1028, 1960.
181. Benirschke K, Naftolin F, Gittes R, et al. True hermaphroditism and chimerism. Am J Obstet Gynecol 113:449, 1972.
182. Braun A, Kammeres S, Cleve H, et al. True hermaphroditism in a 46,XY individual caused by a postzygotic somatic point mutation in the male gonadal sex-determining locus *(SRY)*: Molecular genetics and histological findings in a sporadic case. Am J Hum Genet 52:578, 1993.
183. Berkovitz GD, Fechner PY, Marcantonio SM, et al. The role of the sex determining region of the Y chromosome *(SRY)* in the etiology of 46,XX true hermaphroditism. Hum Genet 88:411, 1992.
184. Boucekkine C, Toublanc JE, Abbas N, et al. Clinical and anatomical spectrum in XX sex reversed patients. Relationship to the presence of Y specific DNA-sequences. Clin Endocrinol (Oxf) 40:733, 1994.

Chapter 15

FEMALE PUBERTY AND ITS DISORDERS

Walter L. Miller • Dennis M. Styne

■ CHAPTER OUTLINE

KEY POINTS

- Puberty is the activation of the hypothalamic-pituitary-gonadal axis, generally beginning at age 8 to 10 years and culminating in menarche at 12 to 13 years.
- Puberty may be early (precocious) or delayed.
- Although disorders of the onset of puberty by definition refer to hypothalamic disorders, diseases of gonadal development (e.g., Turner syndrome) or of gonadal and adrenal steroid hormone biosynthesis (e.g., the congenital adrenal hyperplasias) often come to attention as disorders of "puberty."
- True precocious puberty may be caused by central nervous system tumors but is most commonly idiopathic or caused by hamartomas of the tuber cinereum, which are readily treated with superactive gonadotropin-releasing hormone (GnRH) agonists.
- Isosexual GnRH-independent sexual precocity (feminization) is generally due to primary ovarian disease; contrasexual precocity (virilization) is usually due to adrenal hyperplasia.
- Delayed puberty with low serum gonadotropins is most commonly due to idiopathic constitutional delay, which is a benign condition. Hypogonadotropic hypogonadism may be due to tumors or malformations of the central nervous system or be secondary to other diseases, malnutrition, or emotional disorders.
- Delayed development of the signs of puberty associated with hypergonadotropic hypogonadism is most commonly due to Turner syndrome and other variants of the syndrome of gonadal dysgenesis, but it may also be due to primary ovarian failure or to rare disorders of steroid hormone biosynthesis that do not cause virilization.
- The evaluation, diagnosis, and treatment of disorders presenting as early or late puberty are the particular expertise of the pediatric or reproductive endocrinologist.

ENDOCRINOLOGY OF PUBERTY

Physiology of Puberty

Puberty reiterates endocrine activity seen in the fetus.[1–3] Gonadotropins released in response to gonadotropin-releasing hormone (GnRH) are high in the fetus at midgestation but decrease toward term, partly owing to the maturation of hypothalamic inhibition and partly due to negative feedback from high concentrations of circulating estrogens. At birth, with the elimination of placental estrogens, serum gonadotropins rise in an episodic pattern to higher than pubertal values. These pulses of gonadotropin and estrogen secretion persist in a diminishing pattern until about the age of 4 years, when the central nervous system (CNS) inhibits hypothalamic GnRH release. During this "juvenile pause," pulsatile gonadotropin secretion and ovarian estradiol production remain at low but detectable levels. Puberty is initiated by the release of this CNS inhibition, allowing increasing gonadotropin secretion and the induction of ovarian estrogen synthesis. At the onset of puberty, the amplitude of serum luteinizing hormone (LH) and follicle-stimulating hormone (FSH) pulses first increases at night and later establishes a consistent pattern without diurnal variation. The diurnal rhythm of gonadotropin secretion can be detected by 6 years in males; puberty simply increases the amplitude of these pulses rather than creating them de novo.[4] As puberty progresses, urinary gonadotropin excretion increases in parallel with the rise in serum gonadotropins.[5] Ovarian estrogen secretion follows gonadotropin pulses by a few hours, resulting in estrogen levels in early puberty that may vary from the high midpubertal range to nondetectable within a few hours. The first hormonal evidence of the onset of puberty is a rise in LH of greater than 7.6 IU/L after intravenous administration of 100 μg of GnRH, which may precede the first physical signs of puberty by up to a year. New, extremely sensitive assays for LH, FSH, and estradiol may allow prediction of the onset of secondary sexual development with a single blood sample.[6] Estrogen can stimulate gonadotropin secretion by a positive feedback mechanism as well as suppress gonadotropins by negative feedback. The onset of this positive feedback is a late pubertal event in which the LH to FSH ratio rises, stimulating the monthly increase in estrogen secretion that triggers the midcycle LH surge that induces ovulation and menstruation.

The sex steroids of puberty also increase the secretion of growth hormone (GH), augmenting the production of insulin-like growth factor type I (IGF-I).[7] The estrogen and GH-induced bone growth raise serum alkaline phosphatase and galanin. Insulin resistance increases during puberty, making the management of insulin-dependent diabetes mellitus more difficult.[8]

Genetics of Steroidogenesis

Ovarian Steroidogenesis

Ovarian, placental, and adrenal steroidogenesis employ subsets of a common group of biosynthesis pathways (Fig. 15–1). The steroidogenic enzymes fall into two classes: cytochrome P450 oxidases and hydroxysteroid dehydrogenases. Cytochrome P450 designates a large number of oxidative enzymes, most of which are found in the liver, where they metabolize drugs and xenobiotics. Three P450 enzymes are involved in ovarian steroidogenesis; additional P450 enzymes participate in adrenal steroidogenesis (for review, see reference 9). P450scc, found in the mitochondria of both granulosa and theca cells, is the cholesterol side-chain cleavage enzyme that converts cholesterol to pregnenolone. P450c17, found in the endoplasmic reticulum of theca but not granulosa cells, mediates both 17α-hydroxylase and 17,20-lyase activities. P450arom, found in the endoplasmic reticulum of granulosa but not theca cells, catalyzes the conversion of androgens to estrogens.

Hydroxysteroid dehydrogenases fall into two groups of 35- to 45-kDa nonheme enzymes, the short-chain dehydrogenases and the aldo-keto reductases (for review, see refer-

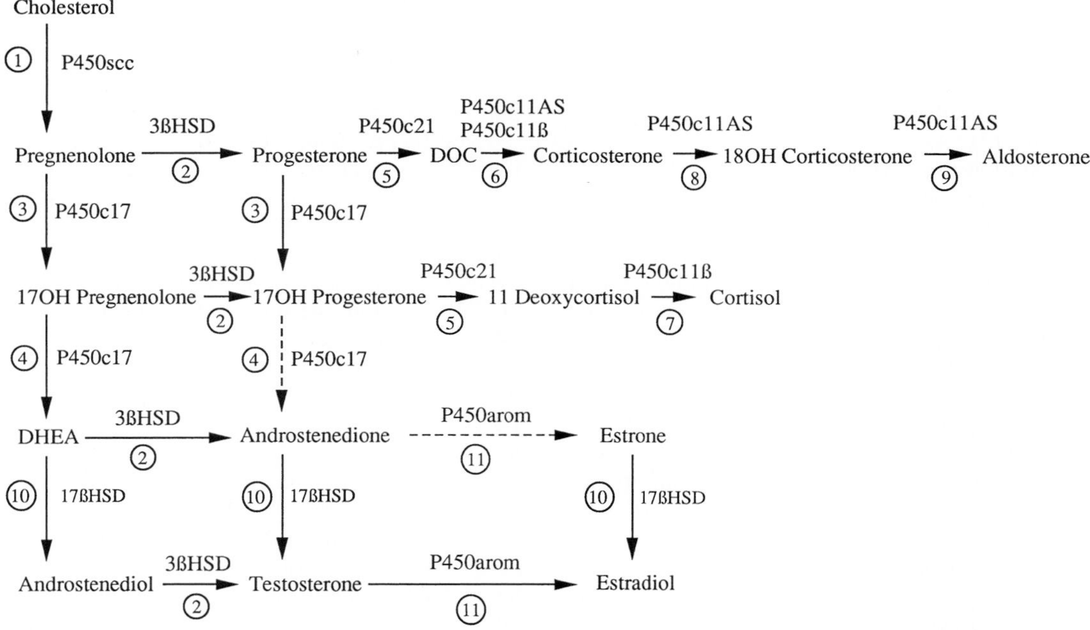

Figure 15–1 ■ Principal pathways of steroid hormone synthesis. Reaction 1: Mitochondrial cytochrome P450scc catalyzes 20α-hydroxylation, 22-hydroxylation, and scission of the C20–22 bond, thus converting cholesterol to pregnenolone. Reaction 2: 3βHSD type II catalyzes 3β-hydroxysteroid dehydrogenase and isomerase activities. Reaction 3: P450c17 catalyzes the 17α-hydroxylation of pregnenolone to 17-hydroxypregnenolone and of progesterone to 17-hydroxyprogesterone. Reaction 4: The 17,20-lyase activity of P450c17 converts 17-hydroxypregnenolone to dehydroepiandrosterone (DHEA), but little 17-hydroxyprogesterone is converted to Δ^4-androstenedione. Reactions 5 to 9 are found only in the adrenal, but disorders of these enzymes can affect sex steroid synthesis. Reaction 5: P450c21 catalyzes the 21-hydroxylation of progesterone to deoxycorticosterone (DOC) and of 17-hydroxyprogesterone to 11-deoxycortisol. Reaction 6: DOC is converted to corticosterone, by both P450c11β and P450c11AS. Reaction 7: P450c11β converts 11-deoxycortisol to cortisol. Reactions 8 and 9: Corticosterone is converted to 18-hydroxycorticosterone and aldosterone by a single enzyme, P450c11AS. Reaction 10: Several forms of 17βHSD mediate 17β-hydroxysteroid dehydrogenase activities, converting DHEA to androstenediol (type III), androstenedione to testosterone (type III), and estrone to estradiol (type I). The reverse 17-ketosteroid reductase activities are catalyzed by the type II and IV enzymes. Reaction 11: Testosterone is converted to estradiol and androstenedione is converted to estrone by P450arom (aromatase).

ence 10). The short-chain dehydrogenase family includes ovarian and placental 3β-hydroxysteroid dehydrogenase/isomerase (3βHSD) and ovarian 17β-hydroxysteroid dehydrogenase/17-ketosteroid dehydrogenase (17βHSD). Aldo-keto reductase enzymes include ovarian 20α-hydroxysteroid dehydrogenase and the hepatic and testicular forms of 17βHSD, which, even though they have activities similar to ovarian 17βHSD, belong to a different family of genes and proteins. Whereas each ovarian P450 is a single enzyme encoded by a single gene that is similar in all mammals, the hydroxysteroid dehydrogenases are characterized by having multiple isozymes encoded by different genes, whose numbers and activities vary substantially among different mammals.

Sources, Storage, and Delivery of Cholesterol. Ovarian granulosa cells can synthesize cholesterol de novo from acetate, but most ovarian steroidogenesis derives from cholesterol taken up from circulating high- and low-density lipoproteins by receptor-mediated endocytosis (for review, see references 9 and 11). Gonadotropins will stimulate, and cholesterol metabolites and precursors will inhibit, the transcription of the genes for the low-density lipoprotein receptor and for hydroxymethylglutaryl–coenzyme A reductase, the rate-limiting step in cholesterol synthesis. Low-density lipoprotein cholesterol is the single most important source of substrate for ovarian steroidogenesis. Cellular cholesterol is esterified by acyl coenzyme A:cholesterol acyltransferase (ACAT) and stored in lipid droplets; free cholesterol for steroidogenesis is liberated from cholesterol esters by one or more cholesterol ester hydrolases. Gonadotropins stimulate hydrolase activity and inhibit ACAT. The movement of cholesterol from lipid droplets to the outer membrane appears to require vimentin intermediate filaments of the cytoskeleton (for review, see references 12 and 13).

The first steroidogenic enzyme, P450scc, lies on the inner mitochondrial membrane. The movement of free cholesterol from the outer to the inner mitochondrial membrane is the rate-limiting step in steroid hormone synthesis. In the ovaries, testes, and adrenals, this intramitochondrial cholesterol flux is stimulated by the 30-kDa steroidogenic acute regulatory (StAR) protein. This protein is synthesized rapidly in response to cyclic adenosine monophosphate and has a short half-life, permitting rapid, finely tuned control of steroidogenesis. StAR protein is not found in the placenta or brain, where the regulation of steroidogenesis is more chronic.[13a] The gonads and adrenals exhibit basal, StAR protein–independent steroidogenesis and StAR protein–dependent, acutely regulated steroidogenesis.[14, 15]

P450scc. Conversion of cholesterol to pregnenolone in mitochondria is the first, rate-limiting and hormonally regulated step in the synthesis of all steroid hormones. The sequential 20α-hydroxylation, 22-hydroxylation, and scission of the cholesterol side chain to yield pregnenolone are catalyzed by the single active site of a single protein, termed P450scc (scc refers to the side-chain cleavage of cholesterol), encoded by a single gene on chromosome 15. P450scc functions as the terminal oxidase in a mitochondrial electron transport system. Electrons from reduced nicotinamide adenine dinucleotide phosphate (NADPH) are accepted by a flavoprotein, termed adrenodoxin reductase, which transfers the electrons to an iron-sulfur protein termed adrenodoxin, which then transfers the electrons to P450scc.

3β-Hydroxysteroid Dehydrogenase/$\Delta^5 \rightarrow \Delta^4$ Isomerase. Once pregnenolone is produced from cholesterol, it may undergo 17α-hydroxylation by P450c17 to yield 17-hydroxypregnenolone, or it may be converted to progesterone by 3β-hydroxysteroid dehydrogenase/$\Delta^5 \rightarrow \Delta^4$ isomerase (3βHSD). This single 42-kDa enzyme can convert pregnenolone to progesterone, 17α-hydroxypregnenolone to 17α-hydroxyprogesterone; dehydroepiandrosterone (DHEA) to androstenedione; and androstenediol to testosterone. As is typical of hydroxysteroid dehydrogenases, there are at least two human isozymes of 3βHSD, encoded by separate genes. The enzyme catalyzing 3βHSD activity in the ovaries, testes, and adrenals is the type II enzyme; the type I enzyme, encoded by a closely linked gene with identical intron/exon organization, catalyzes 3βHSD activity in placenta, breast, and "extraglandular" tissue.

17α-Hydroxylase/17,20-Lyase (P450c17). Both pregnenolone and progesterone may undergo 17α-hydroxylation to 17α-hydroxypregnenolone and 17α-hydroxyprogesterone. These 17-hydroxylated steroids may then undergo scission of the C17–20 bond to yield DHEA and androstenedione, respectively. All four of these reactions are mediated by a single enzyme, P450c17. This P450 is bound to smooth endoplasmic reticulum, where it accepts electrons from P450 oxidoreductase, a flavoprotein structurally distinct from the adrenodoxin reductase employed in mitochondria, and without benefit of an iron-sulfur protein. P450c17 is expressed in ovarian theca cells, where it is needed to produce the androgens that serve as substrate for aromatization to estrogens in human granulosa cells, but P450c17 is not expressed in human granulosa cells, consistent with the two-cell model of ovarian steroidogenesis.[16]

Even though both 17α-hydroxylase and 17,20-lyase activities are catalyzed by a single enzyme, encoded by a single gene on chromosome 10q24.3, these activities are regulated independently (for review, see reference 17). This appears to occur by regulating the availability of electrons (reducing equivalents). P450c17 receives electrons from NADPH through the intermediacy of a flavoprotein termed P450 oxidoreductase; cytochrome b_5 may augment 17,20 lyase activity but does not serve as an alternative electron donor.[17a] Increasing the molar ratio of electron donor to P450c17 increases the ratio of lyase to hydroxylase activity, and serine phosphorylation of P450c17, which is required for lyase activity,[18] may also increase the enzyme's affinity for electron donors.

17β-Hydroxysteroid Dehydrogenase. The conversion of estrone to estradiol, Δ^4-androstenedione to testosterone, and DHEA to androstenediol is catalyzed by a group of enzymes termed 17β-hydroxysteroid dehydrogenase (17βHSD), also sometimes termed 17-ketosteroid reductase because they can also catalyze the reverse reaction (for review, see reference 10). There are at least four human forms of 17βHSD. Type I, encoded by a gene on 17q21, is found in placenta, ovary, endometrium, liver, prostate, testis, and adipose tissue, where it favors conversion of estrone and estradiol. Type II, encoded by a gene on 16q24, is found primarily in liver, placenta, small intestine, and endometrium, where it inactivates circulating estradiol to estrone and testosterone to Δ^4-androstenedione. Type III, encoded by a gene on 9q22, is expressed only in the testis, where it converts Δ^4-androstenedione to testosterone. Type IV, which is a large 80-kDa protein containing domains not found in other 17βHSDs, appears to inactivate estradiol and testosterone, similar to type II.

Aromatase (P450arom). The aromatization of the steroid A ring is catalyzed by microsomal P450arom, which converts Δ^4-androstenedione to estrone, testosterone to estradiol, and, in the placenta, 16α-hydroxy-DHEA to estriol. P450arom is encoded by a single, large gene on chromosome 15q21.1. This gene uses several different promoter sequences, transcriptional start sites, and alternatively chosen first exons to encode aromatase messenger ribonucleic acid in different tissue under different hormonal regulation.

Steroidogenic Enzymes Not Found in the Ovary

The adrenal cortex contains additional steroidogenic enzymes involved in mineralocorticoid and glucocorticoid synthesis.[9, 19] These are not expressed in the ovary but are germane because disorders in these enzymes can result in excessive production of adrenal androgens, which can cause virilizing syndromes.

21-Hydroxylase (P450c21). After the synthesis of progesterone and 17α-hydroxyprogesterone, P450c21 in the adrenal cortex can hydroxylate these steroids at the 21 position to yield deoxycorticosterone and 11-deoxycortisol, respectively. Adrenal 21-hydroxylation is catalyzed by microsomal P450c21, which is encoded in a complex gene locus on chromosome 6p21.3. P450c21 employs the same P450 oxidoreductase used by P450c17 to receive electrons from NADPH. 21-Hydroxylase activity has also been described in a broad range of fetal and adult extra-adrenal tissues. However, extra-adrenal 21-hydroxylation is not mediated by the P450c21 enzyme found in the adrenal, but the nature of the enzyme responsible for extra-adrenal 21-hydroxylation is unknown.[20] As a result, patients having absent adrenal 21-hydroxylase activity may still have appreciable concentrations of 21-hydroxylated steroids in their plasma. P450c21 is of major importance because it is responsible for more than 90 percent of all cases of congenital adrenal hyperplasia (CAH; see later).

11β-Hydroxylase (P450c11β) and Aldosterone Synthase (P450c11AS). Two closely related enzymes, P450c11β and P450c11AS, catalyze the final steps in the synthesis of glucocorticoids and mineralocorticoids, respectively. These two isozymes are 93 percent identical and are encoded by tandemly duplicated genes on 8q22 (for review, see reference 19). Like P450scc, these mitochondrial enzymes use adrenodoxin and adrenodoxin reductase to receive electrons from NADPH. P450c11β is the classic 11β-hydroxylase that converts 11-deoxycortisol to cortisol and 11-deoxycorticosterone to corticosterone. P450c11AS is found in small amounts only in the zona glomerulosa, where it has 11β-hydroxylase, 18-hydroxylase, and 18-methyl oxidase (aldosterone synthase) activities; thus, P450c11AS is able to catalyze all the reactions needed to convert deoxycorticosterone to aldosterone.

Adrenarche

Normal Adrenarche

Adrenarche is a developmentally programmed increase in the secretion of adrenal androgens, principally DHEA and dehydroepiandrosterone sulfate (DHEA-S), that begins in girls at about age 6 to 8 years, preceding the onset of puberty by about 2 years (Fig. 15–2). Adrenarche is independent of GnRH and pituitary gonadotropins or ovarian function[21]; the secretion of adrenal androgens continues to increase after puberty, peaks at 20 to 30 years, then slowly falls, returning to preadrenarchal levels in the elderly.[22]

The physiologic trigger to adrenarche is unknown; some have suggested that an adrenal androgen–stimulatory hormone specifically stimulates DHEA production in the adrenal zona reticularis, but no such factor has been found. Current attention focuses on intra-adrenal events. Measurements of the serum ratios of 17-hydroxypregnenolone to pregnenolone and of DHEA to 17-hydroxypregnenolone indicate that the adrenal 17α-hydroxylase activities of normal cycling women and postmenopausal women are equivalent but that 17,20-lyase activity is reduced in postmenopausal women, suggesting that the diminution in serum DHEA with advancing age is due to an intra-adrenal event.[23] The report that phosphorylation of P450c17 selectively increases 17,20-lyase activity without altering 17α-hydroxylase activity suggests a mechanism for adrenarche[18] that may assist in identifying the physiologic trigger.

Premature Adrenarche and the Polycystic Ovary Syndrome

Polycystic ovary syndrome (PCOS), which is discussed in detail in Chapter 17, may include hirsutism, virilism, hyperandrogenism, menstrual irregularities, chronic anovulation, hyperinsulinism, insulin resistance, obesity, acanthosis nigricans, high serum concentrations of LH, high ratios of LH to FSH, and ultrasonographically detectable ovarian cysts, although it is unusual to find all of these features in a single patient. The 1990 National Institute of Child

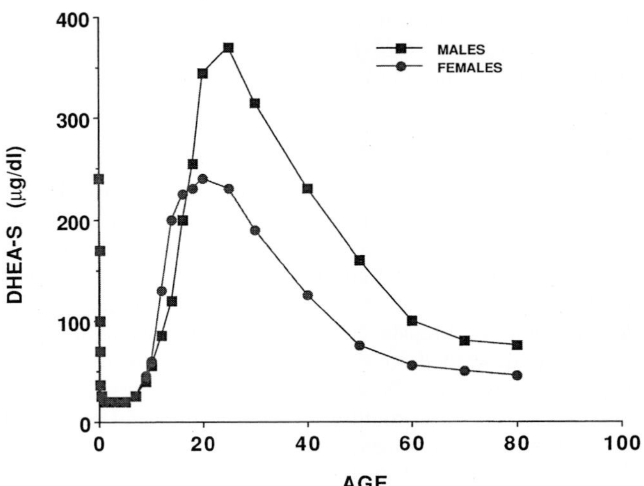

Figure 15–2 ■ Concentrations of serum dehydroepiandrosterone sulfate (DHEA-S) as a function of age in females and males. Values are high in cord blood and immediately after birth, falling rapidly in the first month of life and remaining low until the onset of adrenarche. In girls, adrenarche begins at about age 8 years (generally a bit earlier in girls of African ancestry than in those of European ancestry), and values rise earlier than in males but do not reach values as high as in males. In both sexes, the values decline slowly during adult years. Redrawn from the data of Orentreich et al.[22]

Health and Human Development conference on PCOS emphasized hyperandrogenism, chronic anovulation, and hyperinsulinism in the diagnosis.[24] The hyperandrogenism of PCOS is not due to mild forms of CAH. Although polycystic ovaries are found in many women with the mild, nonclassic form of 21-hydroxylase deficiency, these patients lack insulin resistance; conversely, the majority of patients with the PCOS phenotype do not have molecular lesions in their genes for 21-hydroxylase or 3βHSD.[25–27] The hyperandrogenism of PCOS is of both ovarian and adrenal origin, suggesting that the adrenal component is an exaggerated form of adrenarche.[28, 29] Although prospective data are lacking, cross-sectional data indicate that girls with premature adrenarche already have insulin resistance[30] and are at a substantially higher risk for developing PCOS[31] (see also Chapter 17: Exaggerated Adrenarche in PCOS, p. 456).

The physiologic connection between the hyperandrogenism and insulin resistance of PCOS has never been explained adequately. The insulin resistance in PCOS appears to be clinically distinct from that in typical non–insulin-dependent diabetes mellitus. Insulin binding to the insulin receptor is not changed, suggesting a postreceptor defect in signal transduction.[24, 32] Insulin action is initiated by tyrosine autophosphorylation of the β chain of the insulin receptor in response to the binding of insulin by the α chain. Serine phosphorylation of the β chain can diminish or block the insulin-induced tyrosine autophosphorylation needed for insulin signal transduction.[33] Such a receptor-based mechanism would be consistent with the suggestion that PCOS may be an autosomal dominant disorder.[34] About half of PCOS women have insulin receptors with 3.7-fold higher levels of β chain serine phosphorylation, which strongly suggests that this mechanism accounts for the insulin resistance of a substantial portion of the PCOS population.[35] Zhang and colleagues hypothesized that an activating (and hence dominant) mutation in a single serine kinase can cause hyperphosphorylation of both the insulin receptor (causing insulin resistance) and P450c17 (causing hyperandrogenism), thus accounting for the two principal clinical features and the observed genetics of PCOS.[18]

Physical Changes of Female Puberty

Ovarian estrogens are principally responsible for breast development and female body habitus (feminization); ovarian and adrenal androgens are responsible for development of pubic and axillary hair and axillary sebaceous gland development (virilization). The physical changes in the development of breasts (Fig. 15–3) and pubic hair (Fig. 15–4) are described in five stages.[36] Whereas most girls undergo coordinated breast and pubic hair development, these can occur discordantly in both normal and abnormal development; thus, breast and pubic hair development should be documented separately. Although increased growth rate is the first measurable sign of female puberty, breast development is usually noted first. The onset of breast development generally precedes the onset of menses by about 2½ years. The age of menarche in the United States is 12.8 ± 1.2 (SD) years for white girls and 0.3 months earlier for African-American girls.[37a] The age of menarche in the United States has been stable for the last five decades, in contrast to a decrease of 2 to 3 months per decade during the 150 years before World War II. This stabilization in the age of menarche suggests an optimal state of health and nutrition in the Western world allowing expression of the genetically determined optimal age of menarche. Genetic influences are seen within individual families and ethnic groups. Completion of secondary sexual development (from onset of breast development to cessation of growth) takes 1.5 to 6 years in girls (mean, 4.2 years)[38] (Fig. 15–5). Irregular, anovulatory cycles are typical in the first years after menarche,[39] but by 5 years after menarche, 90 percent of girls have regular, ovulatory periods.

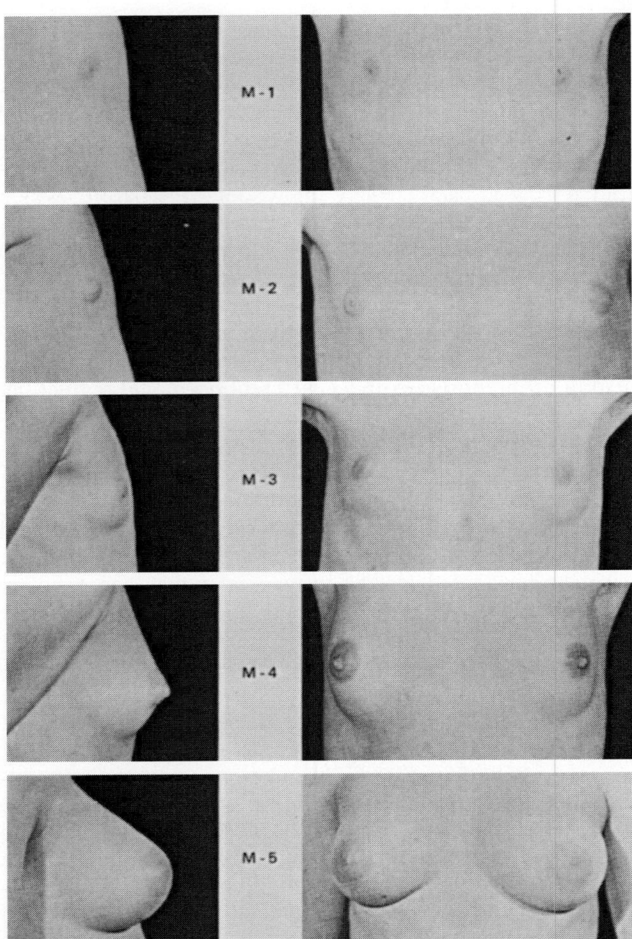

Figure 15–3 ■ Stages of breast development. Stage 1, preadolescent; elevation of papilla only. Stage 2, breast bud stage; elevation of breast and papilla as a small mound, enlargement of areolar diameter. Stage 3, further enlargement of breast and areola with no separation of their contours. Stage 4, projection of areola and papilla to form a secondary mound above the level of the breast. Stage 5, mature stage; projection of papilla only, resulting from recession of the areola to the general contour of the breast. (From Van Wieringen JD, Wafelbakker F, Verbrugge HP, et al. Growth Diagrams 1965 Netherlands: Second National Survey on 0–24 Year Olds. Netherlands Institute for Preventative Medicine TNO. Groningen, Wolters-Noordhoff, 1971. © Wolters-Noordhoff, Groningen.)

Other effects of estrogen include increased production of extracellular matrix ("cornification") of the vaginal mucosa, leading to the pink color typical of adult females in

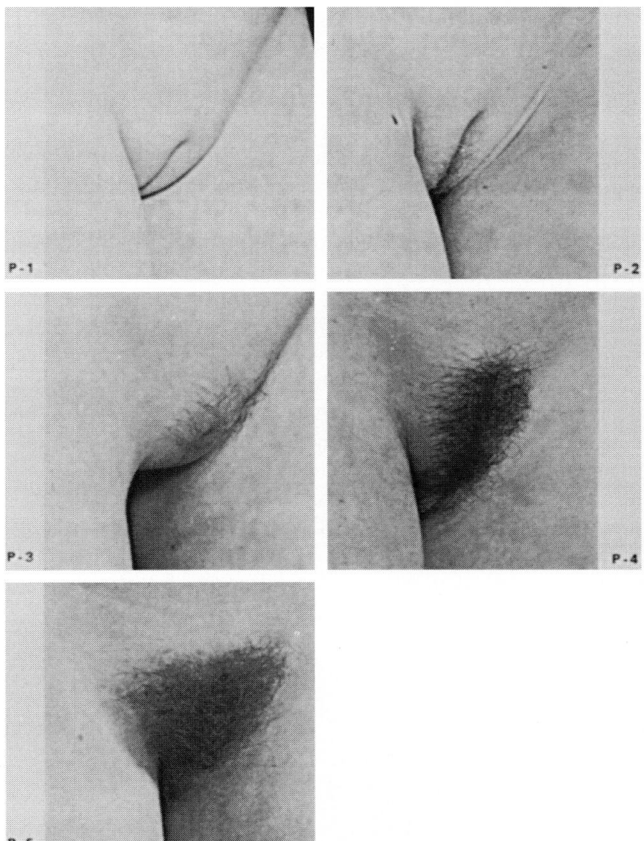

Figure 15–4 ■ Stages of female pubic hair development. Stage 1, preadolescent; the vellus over the superior junction of the labia is not further developed than that over the anterior abdominal wall; that is, there is no pubic hair. Stage 2, sparse growth of long, slightly pigmented, downy hair, straight or only slightly curled, appearing chiefly along the labia. This stage is difficult to see on photographs. Stage 3, hair is considerably darker, coarser, and curlier. The hair spreads sparsely over the junction of the labia. Stage 4, hair is now adult in type, but the area covered by it is still considerably smaller than in most adults. There is no spread to the medial surface of the thighs. Stage 5, hair is adult in quantity and type, distributed as an inverse triangle of the classic feminine pattern. The spread is to the medial surface of the thighs but not up the linea alba or elsewhere above the base of the inverse triangle. (From Van Wieringen JD, Wafelbakker F, Verbrugge HP, et al. Growth Diagrams 1965 Netherlands: Second National Survey on 0–24 Year Olds. Netherlands Institute for Preventative Medicine TNO. Groningen, Wolters-Noordhoff, 1971. © Wolters-Noordhoff, Groningen.)

contrast to the bright reddish prepubertal color. Estrogen also induces enlargement of the labia majora and minora, enlargement of the uterus, and an increase in the sonographically measured fundal to cervical ratio. Increased fat distribution in parts of the body having high aromatase activity (e.g., hips) leads to an adult female body habitus.

The pubertal growth spurt in girls generally begins 2 years before that in boys. This difference accounts for about 50 percent of the 12-cm difference in average adult height between men and women; the other 50 percent is due to the smaller amount of growth that occurs in the female growth spurt compared with the male growth spurt.[40] Only about 1 to 2 inches of growth remains after menarche in most (but not all) girls. Progress toward the cessation of growth that marks the end of puberty can be monitored by "bone age." Radiographs of the left hand and wrist are compared with standard radiographs[41] at various ages to determine bone age. Assessment of bone age cannot make a diagnosis but indicates the state of physiologic development and how much time is left for the child to grow. Furthermore, menarche is more closely associated with a bone age of 13 years than it is with a chronologic age. Thus, bone age is an important adjunct in the assessment of disorders of growth and adolescence.

Although prepubertal boys and girls have equal lean body mass, skeletal mass, and body fat, adult men have 1.5 times the lean body mass, skeletal mass, and muscle mass of women, but women have twice the body fat of men.[42] Bone density increases during puberty, and delayed pubertal development will decrease bone density. Osteopenia from pubertal delay may have serious consequences in later life. Calcium intake during puberty is important in determining adult bone mass; while calcium supplementation may increase bone accretion, the effect may be reversed by discontinuing the supplement.[43, 44]

SEXUAL PRECOCITY

True Precocious Puberty

Definitions

Sexual precocity is the appearance of the secondary sexual characteristics before age 8 years and can be isosexual feminization (including true precocious puberty) or contrasexual virilization (Table 15–1). Sexual precocity will arise from any source of sex steroids, but the term *true precocious puberty* properly applies only to sexual precocity mediated by premature activation of the hypothalamic-pituitary-ovarian axis usually before the age of 8 years.

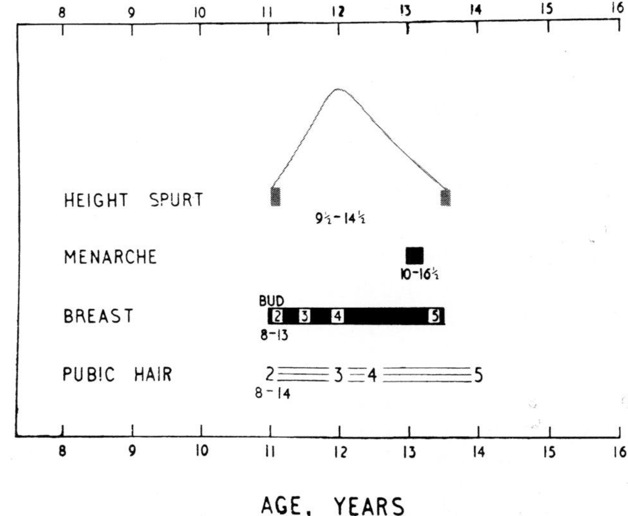

Figure 15–5 ■ The sequence of events at puberty in females. An average age is represented in relation to the scale of age in years; the age range within which the changes occur is indicated by the figures below each bar. (From Marshall WA, Tanner JM. Variations in pattern of pubertal changes in girls. Arch Dis Child 44:291–303, 1969.)

■ TABLE 15–1
Classification of Sexual Precocity

True Precocious Puberty or Complete Isosexual Precocity

Idiopathic true precocious puberty
Central nervous system
  Hamartomas
  Other tumors
True precocious puberty after late treatment of congenital virilizing adrenal hyperplasia

Incomplete Isosexual Precocity (GnRH-Independent Sexual Precocity)

Estrogen-secreting ovarian or adrenal neoplasms
Ovarian cysts
McCune-Albright syndrome
Primary hypothyroidism
Peutz-Jeghers syndrome

Iatrogenic Sexual Precocity

Variations of Pubertal Development

Premature thelarche
Premature menarche
Premature adrenarche

Contrasexual Precocity

Virilization in females
  Congenital adrenal hyperplasia
    21-hydroxylase deficiency
    11β-hydroxylase deficiency
    3β-hydroxysteroid dehydrogenase deficiency
  Virilizing adrenal neoplasms
  Virilizing ovarian neoplasms (e.g., arrhenoblastomas)

The sine qua non of true precocious puberty has been a rise in serum LH to greater than 7.6 IU/L 1 hour after 100 μg of GnRH is given intravenously. However, one study showed that the same results are obtained 40 minutes after the GnRH is given subcutaneously, facilitating the testing procedure.[45] Estrogen accelerates both the linear growth rate and the rate of epiphyseal fusion. Thus, girls with sexual precocity may be tall for their age as children but become short adults. Untreated girls with true precocious puberty reach final heights of 151 to 155 cm, well below the U.S. mean of 163 cm.[46, 47]

Idiopathic True Precocious Puberty

Many girls aged 6 to 8 years with precocious puberty simply represent the early end of the normal spectrum for the age at onset of puberty.[37a] Some will have a family history of early puberty, but most have no familial tendency and no organic disease. The age at onset is 6 to 7 years in about 50 percent of cases, 2 to 6 years in about 25 percent, and in infancy in 18 percent.[48]

Idiopathic true precocious puberty usually presents with breast development, enlargement of the labia minora, and maturational changes in the vaginal mucosa (Fig. 15–6). In true precocious puberty, ultrasound examination shows that both the uterus and ovaries are enlarged for age.[49] Pubic hair may or may not be present initially. Progression of secondary sexual maturation is usually rapid but may wax and wane. GH secretion is increased because of stimulation by gonadal steroids, and serum IGF-I rises during the rapid growth.[50] More mildly affected children have lower IGF-I and estradiol levels, have less advanced bone age, progress less rapidly, and tend to reach their target height; these children usually do not require therapy. Normal pregnancies have occurred in women who previously had precocious puberty.[47] Ovulation and fertility are possible; patients with true or central precocious puberty have become pregnant as early as 5 years or age, an unfortunate combination of premature sexual development and childhood sexual abuse. Girls with precocious puberty appear to be at a significantly higher risk of such abuse. True precocious puberty does not lead to premature menopause, but there is increased risk for the development of carcinoma of the breast in adulthood. Psychosexual development is not advanced by precocious puberty per se but depends on the child's surrounding environment. Serum gonadotropin and estrogen concentrations, the LH response to GnRH, and the amplitude and frequency of LH pulses are in the normal pubertal range.[51] Adrenarche usually does not accompany puberty in girls younger than 6 years, but it may be early when the onset of puberty occurs after age 6 years.[21]

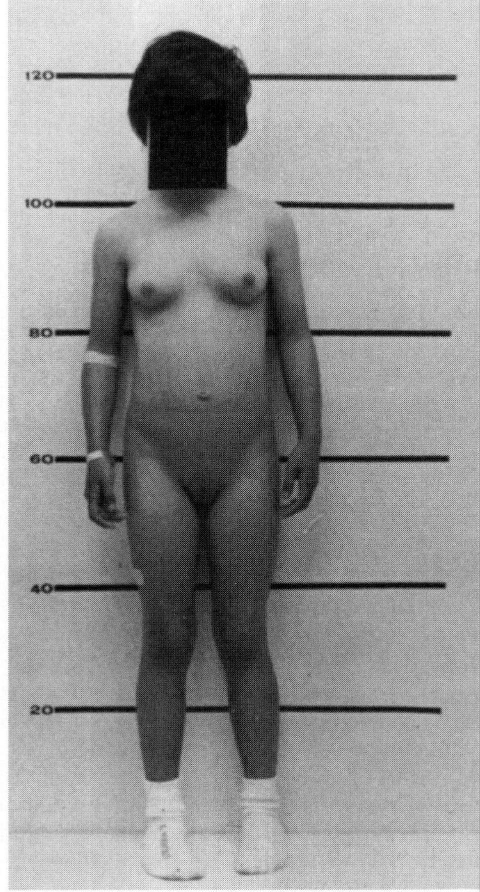

Figure 15–6 ■ A 5-year-old girl with idiopathic precocious puberty. Enlargement of breasts and vaginal discharge were noted at 10 months, with the appearance of pubic hair soon after. At 1 year 9 months, her bone age was 3½ years and treatment was begun. (From Styne DM, Kaplan SL. Normal and abnormal puberty in the female. Pediatr Clin North Am 26:123–148, 1979.)

Central Nervous System Tumors Causing True Precocious Puberty

CNS tumors must be considered in any patients with true precocious puberty, because this can be a manifestation of any neoplasm in or near the posterior hypothalamus. A magnetic resonance imaging (MRI) evaluation is usually indicated.[52] Astrocytomas, ependymomas, and, rarely, craniopharyngiomas may cause true precocious puberty. True precocious puberty may occur after cranial irradiation for local tumors or leukemia.[53] Optic and hypothalamic gliomas associated with neurofibromatosis type 1 (von Recklinghausen's disease) may cause precocious puberty,[54] especially if they involve the optic tracts.[55] This dominant disorder caused by a gene on 17q11.2 has a prevalence of 1 in 3000 to 4000. Patients with neurofibromatosis have multiple café au lait spots that have smoother borders than those of the McCune-Albright syndrome. Most affected children have some manifestations of the disease by 1 year of age.

GH deficiency may accompany central precocious puberty in some children receiving radiation therapy to a CNS neoplasm or trauma. The increased growth resulting from elevated gonadal steroid levels may hide GH deficiency; GH-deficient children with precocious puberty grow more slowly than GH-sufficient children with central precocious puberty but faster than GH-deficient children without sexual precocity.[56] Treatment of CNS tumors causing true precocious puberty is usually conservative, consisting of biopsy of the neoplasm followed by radiation, chemotherapy, or both, depending on the cell type.

Hamartoma of the tuber cinereum is a congenital malformation consisting of fiber bundles, glial cells, and ectopic GnRH neurosecretory cells similar to the GnRH-containing neurons in the medial basal hypothalamus that cause normal puberty. These hamartomas, which are not neoplasms, are usually connected to the posterior portion of the tuber cinereum or mamillary body or the floor of the third ventricle by a distinct stalk. They appear on a computed tomographic (CT) or MRI scan as an isodense, abnormal fullness of the interpeduncular, prepontine, and posterior suprasellar cisterns, occasionally with distortion of the anterior third ventricle[57–59] (Fig. 15–7). MRI provides the best imaging, but these lesions do not enhance with contrast material. Hamartomas of the tuber cinereum are often detected on MRI in children previously thought to have idiopathic central precocious puberty.[59] In a series of 87 girls with true precocious puberty, 16 percent had a hypothalamic hamartoma, 40 percent had other CNS abnormalities, and 60 percent had idiopathic true precocious puberty.[48]

However, hypothalamic hamartomas do not grow with time and require no surgery or radiation because the precocious sexual development can be controlled by treatment with GnRH agonists.[58, 59] Although some favor neurosurgical removal of these hamartomas, the sensitive location of the hamartomas militates against extirpation, unless tumor growth is seen on MRI or there is an associated complication such as intractable seizures or hydrocephalus.

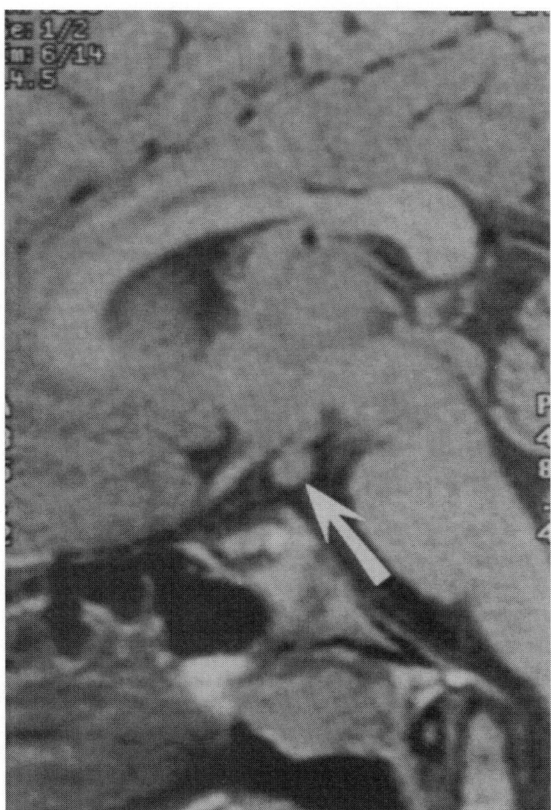

Figure 15–7 ■ Sagittal magnetic resonance scan showing a large, 8-mm isodense hypothalamic hamartoma *(arrow)* attached to the tuber cinereum. (From Mahachoklertwattana P, Kaplan SL, Grumbach MM. The luteinizing hormone–releasing hormone–secreting hypothalamic hamartoma is a congenital malformation: Natural history. J Clin Endocrinol Metab 77:118–124, 1993. © The Endocrine Society.)

Other Central Nervous System Conditions

True precocious puberty may be secondary to hydrocephalus, encephalitis, static cerebral encephalopathy, brain abscess, head trauma, or hypothalamic granulomas (sarcoid or tuberculous).[60] Arachnoid cysts can cause sexual precocity that can be reversed by decompression and extirpation of the cyst.[1] Other neurologic disorders including epilepsy and mental retardation may be associated with true precocious puberty, but the basis of this is unknown.

Correction of a long-standing virilizing condition may be followed by development of true precocious puberty.[61] The withdrawal of the virilizing androgens removes their inhibition of the hypothalamus, allowing increased secretion of GnRH and gonadotropins, stimulating the ovary. This is most commonly seen in children with CAH who are begun on glucocorticoid replacement therapy after age 4 to 8 years.[61] Girls with severe primary hypothyroidism may develop true precocious puberty with hyperprolactinemia and galactorrhea (but without a pubertal growth spurt) apparently because of the cross-reaction of high concentrations of thyroid-stimulating hormone with the FSH receptor.[62]

Management of True Precocious Puberty

For GnRH to stimulate gonadotropin synthesis and release, the pituitary must be exposed to GnRH in a pulsatile manner; continuous infusion of GnRH into the blood or cerebral ventricles will stimulate the pituitary only transiently, followed by profound inhibition.[63] Potent GnRH agonists that have long biologic half-lives and extended receptor occupancy times will mimic the effect of continuous GnRH infusion, shutting down pituitary gonadotropin synthesis and release; this essentially produces a reversible medical gonadectomy.[64] GnRH agonists are the treatment of choice for true precocious puberty. Changes in the amino acid sequence of GnRH can make it resistant to enzymatic degradation and increase the receptor binding affinity. These agonists have about 15 to 200 times the potency of natural GnRH, prolonged action, and low toxicity. Depot formulations of GnRH agonists can provide continuous treatment with a single monthly intramuscular injection.

GnRH agonist therapy initially increases circulating LH, FSH, and estradiol concentrations for a few days to weeks; chronic therapy suppresses the pulsatile gonadotropin secretion and blocks the LH response to administration of native GnRH.[65] Suppression must be monitored by serum gonadotropin measurements, because urinary determinations are insufficiently sensitive.[66] Estradiol concentrations are reduced to prepubertal levels within 2 to 4 weeks and remain low for the duration of treatment. Plasma estradiol concentrations below 36 pmol/L (10 pg/ml) indicate adequate gonadal suppression. GnRH therapy reduces the size of the enlarged ovaries of girls with true precocious puberty, although they do not return to prepubertal size. After treatment, some girls develop the sonographic characteristics of polycystic ovaries.[67] GnRH agonist therapy does not affect the secretion of adrenal androgens and hence does not affect adrenarche. Reduction in breast size and pubic hair, cessation of menses, and decreased size of the uterus and ovaries occur within the first 6 months of therapy. Some girls have hot flashes and moodiness because of estrogen withdrawal. Height velocity decreases about 60 percent during the first year of therapy and skeletal maturation slows dramatically during the first 3 years, often to a rate less than the progression in chronologic age, so that ultimate adult height is improved.[65] GH secretion increases in true precocious puberty to levels comparable to those in normal puberty, and GnRH agonists usually decrease GH secretion. GnRH agonist therapy permits girls with precocious puberty to reach a greater adult height, especially if therapy is begun at an early age. Girls treated before age 5 years reached an average final height of 164 cm, whereas girls who began treatment after age 5 years reached an average adult height of 158 cm, which was still considerably taller than untreated girls.[68] Plasma IGF-I is high for chronologic age in girls with true precocious puberty, consistent with increased estrogen secretion and comparable to the typically elevated IGF-I levels of normal puberty. GnRH agonists reduce IGF-I to the normal range for bone age but not for chronologic age.[50]

Irregular treatment and poor compliance increase estrogen concentrations and may facilitate the worst outcome: suppression of growth with continued advancement of the bone age. Regular assessment, initially at 1-month intervals and eventually extending to 3 months, should include measurement of serum estradiol, the LH response to GnRH, height, and bone age; assessment of secondary sexual characteristics; and occasional evaluation of ovarian morphology and uterine size by pelvic sonography. GnRH agonist therapy slows the pubertal accretion of bone density, apparently by the suppression of estrogen secretion.[69] Untoward reactions to GnRH agonists include local and systemic allergic reactions in a few patients, including rare asthmatic episodes. When therapy is discontinued in 11-year-old girls, menarche occurs, on average, 1.2 years later. After menarche, 50 percent of treated girls ovulated within 1 year, and 90 percent had ovulated after 2 years.[70] This pattern is similar to that of normal pubertal maturation.

Treatment with GnRH agonists is effective in all patients with true precocious puberty who have a pubertal pattern of pulsatile LH secretion and a pubertal response of LH to GnRH, including those with hamartomas of the tuber cinereum. GnRH agonists may be used in conjunction with GH in patients having both GH deficiency and true precocious puberty, usually as a result of radiation of the brain.[56] This regimen may allow a longer period of GH treatment before epiphyseal fusion. Before treatment is begun, it is essential to establish the progressive nature of the sexual precocity. In some girls, the tempo of puberty is relatively slow, so that sexual precocity may not be sustained.[71] Many such girls have clinical and hormonal features intermediate between those of premature thelarche and true precocious puberty that are typical of neither condition. Thus, girls who progress through puberty slowly and who do not have elevated estradiol and IGF-I concentrations may not require GnRH treatment to achieve normal height.[72]

GnRH-Independent Sexual Precocity

Iso-Sexual Precocity

Sexual precocity may be independent of GnRH when estrogen is secreted independently (e.g., from an ovarian cyst or tumor), causing hypogonadotropic hypergonadism (Table 15–2). Although these girls present with premature feminization and may be referred for precocious puberty, these GnRH-independent syndromes are not forms of puberty and usually produce incomplete isosexual precocity.

Autonomous Ovarian Follicular Cysts. Autonomous ovarian follicular cysts are the most common childhood estrogen-secreting ovarian mass. Ovarian follicles up to 8 mm in diameter are common in normal prepubertal girls and may appear and regress spontaneously.[73, 74] Enlarged follicles or cysts are also found in true precocious puberty. Large follicular cysts may be discovered in patients with an abdominal mass or abdominal pain (especially after torsion) or as an unexpected finding on pelvic sonography performed for other reasons. These follicles may secrete estrogen and may resolve and recur, causing reappearing signs of sexual precocity and vaginal bleeding with anovulatory cycles. Plasma estradiol concentrations in girls with recurrent cysts may range from high levels, indistinguishable from those in granulosa cell tumors, down to the early pubertal range, usually correlating with changes in the size of the cyst. Gonadotropin concentrations are suppressed, a pubertal pattern of pulsatile LH secretion is absent, and the LH response to GnRH is prepubertal.[75]

GnRH agonists are not effective in autonomous cysts, although they are effective in treating cysts associated with true precocious puberty. Medroxyprogesterone acetate may be used for therapy to prevent recurrence and accelerate

■ TABLE 15–2
Differential Diagnosis of Isosexual Precocity

	SERUM GONADOTROPIN CONCENTRATION	LH RESPONSE TO GnRH	SERUM SEX STEROID CONCENTRATIONS	GONADAL SIZE	MISCELLANEOUS
True Precocious Puberty (premature reactivation of hypothalamic GnRH pulse generator)	Prominent LH pulses, initially during sleep	Pubertal LH response	Pubertal values of estradiol	Normal pubertal ovarian and uterine enlargement by sonography	MRI scan of brain to rule out CNS tumor or other abnormality; skeletal survey for McCune-Albright syndrome
Incomplete Sexual Precocity (GnRH-Independent Sexual Precocity)					
Granulosa cell tumor (follicular cysts may present similarly)	Low	Suppressed LH response	Very high estradiol	Ovarian enlargement on physical examination, MRI, CT, or sonography	Tumor often palpable on abdominal examination
Follicular cyst	Low	Suppressed LH response	Prepubertal to very high estradiol values	Ovarian enlargement on physical examination, MRI, CT, or sonography	Single or repetitive episodes; exclude McCune-Albright syndrome
Feminizing adrenal tumor	Low	Suppressed LH response	High estradiol and DHEA-S values	Ovaries prepubertal	Unilateral adrenal mass
Premature thelarche	Prepubertal	Prepubertal LH response	Prepubertal or early pubertal estradiol	Ovaries prepubertal	Onset usually before age 3 yr
Premature adrenarche	Prepubertal	Prepubertal LH response	Prepubertal estradiol; DHEA-S or urinary 17-ketosteroid values appropriate for pubic hair stage 2	Ovaries prepubertal	More frequent in African-American children

LH, luteinizing hormone; GnRH, gonadotropin-releasing hormone; MRI, magnetic resonance imaging; CT, computed tomography; CNS, central nervous system; hCG, human chorionic gonadotropin; DHEA-S, dehydroepiandrosterone sulfate.

involution of the follicular cysts. The size of the cyst can be monitored by pelvic sonography. Surgical intervention is rarely indicated; a large or persistent cyst can be reduced by puncture at laparoscopy.

Juvenile Granulosa Cell Tumors of the Ovary. Juvenile granulosa cell tumors of the ovary are rare in childhood, and theca cell tumors are even less common.[76] Their size can vary from 2.5 to 25 cm with a mean diameter of 12 cm. Approximately 80 percent of granulosa cell tumors can be palpated on bimanual examination. Sonograms of the ovary facilitate diagnosis. The concentration of plasma estradiol may increase to high levels, suppressing gonadotropin concentrations. About 3 percent of patients die of the disease; less than 5 percent are bilateral or clinically malignant. After surgical removal of the tumor, measurement of plasma estradiol levels is a useful screen for metastases; if the patient is younger than 8 to 9 years, elevated estradiol concentrations suggest recurrence or metastasis.

On occasion, gonadoblastomas in streak gonads, rare lipoid tumors, cystadenomas, and ovarian carcinomas may secrete estrogens, androgens, or both.[77] Some of these neoplasms secrete α-fetoprotein and other tumor markers.

Peutz-Jeghers syndrome is mucocutaneous pigmentation and gastrointestinal polyposis associated with rare sex cord tumors having annular tubules.[78] Epithelial tumors of the ovary are occasionally found in Peutz-Jeghers syndrome.

McCune-Albright Syndrome. McCune-Albright syndrome consists of irregularly edged and hyperpigmented café au lait spots, slowly progressive polyostotic fibrous dysplasia of the bones, and GnRH-independent sexual precocity.[79] At least two of these features should be present to consider the diagnosis. McCune-Albright syndrome is caused by activating mutations in the guanosine triphosphate–activated $G_s\alpha$ signal transduction protein that is linked to many peptide hormone receptors.[80] The mutations are postzygotic somatic cell mutations that occur at various times in fetal development, accounting for the patchy tissue distribution of affected cells. Such somatic cell mutations are not heritable. The café au lait macules may not be conspicuous in infancy, usually do not cross the midline, and are often located on the same side as the main bone lesions. Other endocrinopathies include nodular thyroid hyperplasia with thyrotoxicosis, multiple hyperplastic adrenal nodules with Cushing's syndrome, pituitary adenomas or mammosomatotroph hyperplasia with gigantism and acromegaly or hyperprolactinemia, and parathyroid adenoma or hyperplasia with hyperparathyroidism. Hypophosphatemic vitamin D–resistant rickets and osteomalacia can also occur in this syndrome. The cystic skeletal lesions, which often result in pathologic fractures and deformities, may be detected by a bone scan before they are visible radiographically. Skull involvement may include compression of optic or auditory nerve foramina, which can lead to blindness, deafness, facial asymmetry, and ptosis.

The sexual precocity is due to autonomously functioning luteinized follicular cysts, often causing asymmetric enlargement. However, when the bone age approaches 12 years, there is pulsatile GnRH secretion and ovulatory cycles ensue. Thus, an affected girl may progress from GnRH-independent puberty to GnRH-dependent puberty. GnRH agonists are not effective, but testolactone, an aromatase inhibitor, and medroxyprogesterone acetate may be useful.[81]

Iatrogenic Sexual Precocity. Prepubertal girls may show signs of sexual maturation including breast development, pigmentation of the areolae and the linea alba, and appearance of pubic hair from exposure to tonics, lotions, or creams that contain or are contaminated with an estrogen.[82] Epidemics of gynecomastia in boys and thelarche in girls have occurred in children in Italy and Puerto Rico apparently as a result of estrogen contamination of meat.

Variations of Normal Pubertal Development

Premature Thelarche. Unilateral or bilateral breast enlargement without other signs of sexual maturation is fairly common; this premature thelarche usually occurs by age 2 years, rarely after age 4 years, and usually regresses by 6 months to 6 years after diagnosis.[83] No negative effects on later health, growth, or fertility occur. Other signs of estrogen action, such as significant nipple development, estrogen-induced thickening and dulling of the vaginal mucosa, enlargement of the uterus, and increased growth rate, are rare. Plasma estrogen levels may be undetectable to slightly elevated for age. Increased nocturnal FSH pulsatility and an elevated FSH response to GnRH for chronologic age may be seen.[84] The LH response remains prepubertal, with higher FSH to LH ratios than in normal individuals or girls with central precocious puberty.[85] Sonograms of the ovary may show cysts larger than 0.5 cm that disappear and reappear, usually correlating with changes in the size of the breasts. The uterus remains prepubertal in size.[86] Thus, this is usually a benign self-limited disorder compatible with normal pubertal development at an appropriate age, and hence reassurance and follow-up are usually all that is necessary. However, in one study, 14 percent of girls with typical premature thelarche progressed to true precocious puberty[87]; thus, continued surveillance is necessary. Because the development may be unilateral, it is important to ensure that unnecessary surgical procedures are not performed in a futile search for a pathologic process. Breast sonography may be useful in distinguishing unilateral premature thelarche from cysts or tumors.

Premature Isolated Menarche. Girls may rarely begin periodic vaginal bleeding at age 1 to 9 years without any other signs of secondary sexual development.[88] The bleeding can recur for 1 to 6 years and then cease. At the normal age of puberty, secondary sexual development and menses ensue and follow a normal pattern. Normal puberty and fertility have been described in this pubertal variant of uncertain etiology. Isolated menarche may appear before other manifestations of sexual precocity in the McCune-Albright syndrome and in the precocious sexual maturation that can occur in juvenile hypothyroidism. All other causes of vaginal bleeding and precocious estrogen secretion and of exposure to exogenous estrogens should be excluded, including neoplasms, granulomas, infection of the vagina or cervix, or a foreign body, before one considers the diagnosis of premature menarche. Vaginal bleeding from tumors or trauma should not be cyclic. Among 50 girls who had vaginal bleeding before age 10 years, about 50 percent had a local lesion, of which half had a malignant neoplasm (usually a rhabdomyosarcoma).[89] A foreign body may be found in 25 percent of prepubertal girls with vaginal bleeding. A careful examination for trauma, such as that caused by sexual abuse, is indicated.

Virilizing Disorders

P450c21 (21-Hydroxylase) Deficiency

Physiology. 21-Hydroxylase deficiency accounts for 90 to 95 percent of the genetic disorders of steroidogenesis. The severe forms occur in about 1 in 12,000 persons, but the mild, nonclassic form probably affects more than 1 in 1000 persons (for review, see references 90 and 91). In severe P450c21 deficiency, inability to convert progesterone to deoxycorticosterone causes aldosterone deficiency, and inability to convert 17-hydroxyprogesterone to 11-deoxycortisol causes cortisol deficiency. In the absence of aldosterone, the kidney cannot retain sodium normally and instead retains K^+ and H^+, resulting in hyponatremia, hyperkalemia, acidosis, hypertension, shock, cardiovascular collapse, and death. Because the control of fluids and electrolytes in the fetus can be maintained by the placenta and the mother's kidneys, this "salt-losing crisis" develops only after birth, usually during the second week of life. However, the cortisol deficiency is manifested in fetal life. Fetal hypocortisolism stimulates fetal adrenocorticotropic hormone (ACTH) production, causing adrenal growth and increased steroidogenic enzyme synthesis and activity. This results in accumulation of 17-hydroxyprogesterone and other adrenal steroids, which in the absence of 21-hydroxylase are metabolized to androstenedione and testosterone. This fetal adrenal testosterone can have profound effects in the female fetus, ranging from mild clitorimegaly, with or without posterior fusion of the labioscrotal folds, to complete labioscrotal fusion including a urethra traversing the enlarged clitoris. At birth, these female infants, who retain normal ovaries, fallopian tubes, and a uterus, may have "ambiguous" genitalia or may be sufficiently virilized to appear to be male, resulting in errors of sex assignment at birth (Fig. 15–8).

The diagnosis of 21-hydroxylase deficiency is easily suspected in newborns with ambiguous genitalia, but it must be suspected in any phenotypic male (which includes males and profoundly virilized females) with a salt-losing crisis in the first month of life. Plasma 17-hydroxyprogesterone is markedly elevated (>2000 ng/dl after 24 hours of age) and hyperresponsive to stimulation with ACTH. Measurement of other steroids, such as 11-deoxycortisol, 17-hydroxypregnenolone, DHEA, and androstenedione, is important, because adrenal or testicular tumors can also produce abundant 17-hydroxyprogesterone, and high 17-hydroxyprogesterone values that rise further after ACTH can also be seen in 3βHSD and P450c11 deficiencies. 17-Hydroxyprogesterone is normally high in cord blood but falls to "normal" levels in the normal newborn after 12 to 24 hours; endocrinologically normal premature infants and stressed term infants (e.g., cardiac and pulmonary disease) may have persistently elevated concentrations of 17-hydroxyprogesterone with normal 21-hydroxylase.

Clinical Forms of 21-Hydroxylase Deficiency. There is a wide range of clinical variants of CAH. These are often described as different diseases but should be considered part of a continuous spectrum of manifestations of this

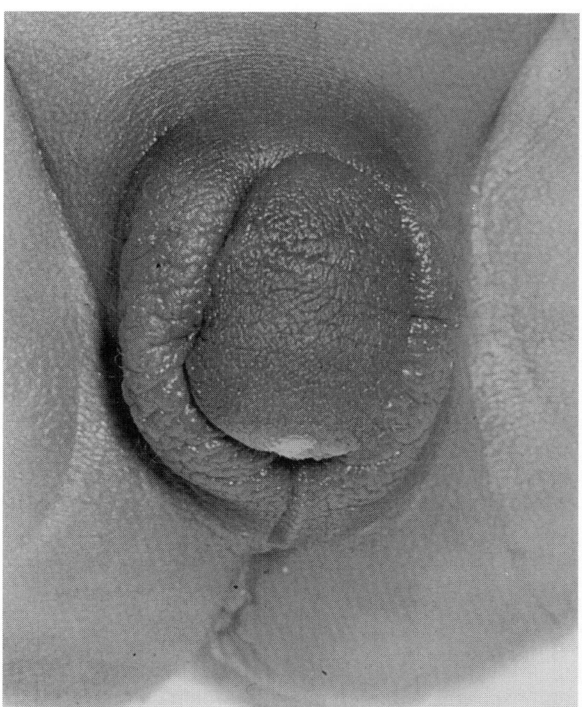

Figure 15–8 ■ Genitalia of a severely virilized 2-week-old 46,XX female with severe salt-losing 21-hydroxylase deficiency. At birth, this infant was incorrectly thought to be a male with undescended testes and mild hypospadias. Presenting symptoms included vomiting, dehydration, Na^+ = 107 mEq/L, K^+ = 10.1 mEq/L, pH 7.4. (From Miller WL, Tyrrell JB. The adrenal cortex. *In* Felig P, Baxter JD, Frohman L [eds]. Endocrinology and Metabolism, 3rd ed. New York, McGraw-Hill, 1995, pp 555–717. Reproduced with permission of The McGraw-Hill Companies.)

disease, ranging from the severe "salt-losing form" to clinically inapparent forms that may be normal variants.

Salt-Losing CAH. The clinical picture described before is that of a patient with salt-losing 21-hydroxylase deficiency. Girls with this disorder are frequently diagnosed at birth because of virilized "ambiguous" genitalia, although some are incorrectly assigned a male gender and are discharged from the newborn nursery only to develop salt loss and life-threatening shock within 2 weeks. In such cases, the mineralocorticoid and glucocorticoid deficiencies can be replaced orally, and the virilized genitalia can be corrected by a series of plastic surgical procedures. Untreated or poorly treated children with CAH may fail to undergo normal puberty, as the high androgen concentrations will suppress gonadotropins and consequently ovarian estrogen production and feminization. The replacement steroid management is difficult, especially in the rapidly growing child, and these patients frequently have decreased fertility, short stature, and psychosexual adjustment problems as adolescents and adults. Females with CAH marry with a lower frequency, have fewer children when they do marry, and have a higher incidence of lesbian behavior[92]; they also tend to have a more negative body image, less sexual activity, and less interest in sexual activity.[93] The potential contributions of androgenization of the fetal brain as opposed to the contributions of parental uncertainty about the sex assignment and of the possible psychologic trauma of genital surgery have not been distinguished. The diagnosis and management of severe forms of CAH in the newborn are difficult and complex and should be undertaken only by experienced pediatric endocrinologists.

Simple Virilizing CAH. Girls with virilized, ambiguous genitalia and increased concentrations of 17-hydroxyprogesterone who do not experience a salt-losing crisis have the simple virilizing form of CAH. Because the adrenal normally produces 100 to 200 times as much cortisol as aldosterone, mild defects (point mutations) in P450c21 are much less likely to affect mineralocorticoid secretion than cortisol secretion. Thus, patients with simple virilizing CAH simply have a less severe disorder of P450c21. This is reflected physiologically by increased plasma renin activity, after moderate salt restriction, which reflects hyperstimulation of the mineralocorticoid pathway.

Nonclassic CAH. Mild forms of 21-hydroxylase deficiency are extremely common, occurring in 1 in 100 to 1 in 1000 persons, depending on the population. Nonclassic CAH, also mistermed late-onset, cryptic, or acquired CAH, may present in the same manner as premature adrenarche, polycystic ovary disease, hirsutism, virilism, or menstrual irregularities. These patients are distinguished from those with premature adrenarche or PCOS by mild basal elevations in 17-hydroxyprogesterone (≥200 ng/dl) and a characteristically elevated response of 17-hydroxyprogesterone to greater than 1000 ng/dl (and usually greater than 1500 ng/dl) after ACTH (for review, see reference 94). Although about one third of these patients will have sonographically detectable polycystic ovaries, they lack the insulin resistance characteristic of PCOS.

Genetics of CAH. The genetics of the 21-hydroxylase locus are complex and atypical (for review, see references 90 and 91). Adrenal 21-hydroxylase activity is catalyzed by cytochrome P450c21, encoded by a gene termed *CYP21B* or P450c21B. This gene, the gene for the fourth component of serum complement *(C4)*, and a gene for the extracellular matrix protein tenascin-X are duplicated in tandem in an array *(C4A, 21A, XA, C4B, 21B, XB)* lying in the midst of the HLA locus on chromosome 6. Both *C4* genes encode active complement protein, but only the *21B* and *XB* genes encode 21-hydroxylase and tenascin-X, respectively.[95]

Random gene deletions, insertions, and point mutations, which cause virtually all other genetic disorders, are extremely rare in CAH. About 15 percent of severely affected *21B* genes have unusual gene deletions that extend from various locations between exons 3 and 8 of the *21A* gene to the precisely corresponding base in the *21B* gene, resulting in a perfectly spliced but nonfunctional *21A/B* hybrid gene. The remaining 85 percent of severely affected alleles and all alleles causing nonclassic CAH are due to gene conversions. About 10 percent of alleles causing severe disease have large macroconversions that change all of the *21B* gene sequence into a *21A* sequence. The remaining 75 percent of severely affected alleles have microconversions. These look like ordinary point mutations, but the point mutations identified to date change a small region of the *21B* gene to the sequence of the corresponding defected *21A* gene. This is unique in human genetics but simplifies the study and understanding of defective genes causing CAH, because there is only a small array of likely defects in the *21B* gene, defined by those preexisting in the *21A* gene. Because individuals normally carry two *21B* alleles (one from each parent), the severity of the disease in a compound heterozygote is determined by the activity of the less severely affected of the two alleles.

11β-Hydroxylase (P450c11β) Deficiency: The Hypertensive Form of CAH

Disorders of P450c11β cause a virilizing and often hypertensive form of CAH, whereas disorders of the similar P450c11AS gene cause the corticosterone methyl oxidase deficiencies, which do not affect sex steroid synthesis (for review, see reference 19). Disorders of P450c11β account for about 15 percent of CAH in both Arab and Jewish Middle Eastern populations but are rare elsewhere. P450c11β deficiency reduces cortisol production, causing CAH and virilization of affected females as described for P450c21 deficiency. The diagnosis is usually made by high basal concentrations of 11-deoxycortisol and its hyperresponsiveness to ACTH. Unlike the typical salt-losing syndrome seen in 21-hydroxylase deficiency, patients with 11-hydroxylase deficiency are able to retain sodium normally because the substrate for 11-hydroxylation in the mineralocorticoid pathway, deoxycorticosterone, is a mineralocorticoid, and older children often produce enough deoxycorticosterone to become hypertensive.

Other rare virilizing disorders include Cushing's syndrome due to adrenal carcinoma or to multinodular adrenal hyperplasia. Arrhenoblastoma, the most common virilizing ovarian tumor in adults, is rare in children; gonadoblastoma and lipoid cell tumors are even rarer.

Diagnosis

Many diagnoses can be made from the patient's history and physical examination (see Table 15–2). One should search for a history of perinatal abnormalities or injuries, CNS infections, exposure to gonadal steroids, and a family history of sexual precocity. A growth chart should determine when the growth rate began to increase. The physical examination should note the Tanner stages of secondary sexual development; the presence of acne and oily skin; facial, body, pubic, and axillary hair development; apocrine gland odor; muscle development; and galactorrhea. Examination of the external genitalia should be done with a nonrelated chaperone present, because the performance of such an examination has occasionally been interpreted as sexual abuse by some patients. The visual fields and optic discs should be assessed and signs of increased intracranial pressure sought. Skin is examined for lesions of the McCune-Albright syndrome or neurofibromatosis. Abdominal, gonadal, or adnexal masses and coexisting endocrine disease are noted. Bone age is determined, and brain MRI is performed if central precocious puberty is suspected. Ultrasonography will determine the shape and volume of the uterus and the ovaries and the presence and size of ovarian cysts; the upper limit of uterine length in the prepubertal state is 3.5 cm. Measurements of plasma gonadotropin concentrations (by a highly sensitive assay), estradiol levels, and the LH response to administration of GnRH are important in diagnosis of central precocious puberty. Only laboratories able to measure the low hormone values of early puberty should be used. Determination of thyroxine concentration is indicated when hypothyroidism is suspected.

Pubertal serum gonadotropin concentrations, pubertal pulsatile LH secretion (initially during sleep), or pubertal LH response to GnRH confirms the diagnosis of central precocious puberty. A CNS tumor must be considered a potential cause of this premature activation of the hypothalamic GnRH pulse generator. MRI is more sensitive than CT scanning for the detection of small tumors in the hypothalamus, such as a hamartoma of the tuber cinereum.

Virilized girls having pubic hair, clitoral enlargement, acne, deepening voice, muscle development, or a growth spurt might have CAH or a virilizing adrenal or ovarian tumor. Cushing's syndrome can cause virilization but is associated with growth failure, weight gain, and other signs rather than a growth spurt. Virilizing ovarian tumors may be palpated by bimanual examination or detected by pelvic ultrasound examination. Pubic hair without other signs of puberty is usually a result of premature adrenarche but may be the first sign of either isosexual or contrasexual precocity.

Breast development, dulling and thickening of the vaginal mucosa, and enlargement of the labia minora indicate significant estrogen exposure. If the plasma gonadotropin concentrations are pubertal, if pubertal LH pulses are detected, or if there is a pubertal LH response to GnRH, true precocious puberty is present. Estrogen concentrations in girls with normal or true precocious puberty vary considerably, so a single determination may not be adequate. Elevated plasma estradiol with low gonadotropins indicates an estrogen-secreting cyst or neoplasm. Ovarian tumors of moderate size can be palpated by bimanual examination, but an ultrasound evaluation is warranted if a tumor is suspected. High estradiol values usually accompany estrogen-secreting ovarian neoplasms, but some ovarian cysts produce estradiol concentrations as high as those in granulosa cell tumors; the differential diagnosis can usually be resolved by ultrasonography. Breast development in the absence of other estrogen effects is almost always a result of premature thelarche.

DELAYED PUBERTY

At 13 years of age, only 0.4 percent of white American girls and no African-American girls lack all secondary sexual development.[38] Thus, 13 years is a convenient cutoff for identifying patients who need evaluation for delayed puberty (Table 15–3). Delayed puberty may be due to (1) constitutional (idiopathic) delay in puberty, a variation of normal that usually includes delay in growth in stature; (2) disorders of the hypothalamus or pituitary causing hypogonadotropic hypogonadism; and (3) disorders of the gonad causing hypergonadotropic hypogonadism.

Constitutional Delay

Healthy girls who eventually enter puberty spontaneously after the age of 13 years have idiopathic or constitutional delay in puberty. They are physically and hormonally prepubertal; the absence of pathologic history, signs, and

■ TABLE 15–3
Classification of Delayed Puberty and Sexual Infantilism

Constitutional Delay in Growth and Puberty

Hypogonadotropic Hypogonadism

Central nervous system disorders
- Tumors
- Congenital malformations
- Radiation therapy
- Other causes

Isolated gonadotropin deficiency
- Kallmann syndrome
- Other disorders

Idiopathic and genetic forms of multiple pituitary hormone deficiencies

Miscellaneous disorders
- Prader-Willi syndrome
- Laurence-Moon and Bardet-Biedl syndromes
- Functional gonadotropin deficiency
  - Chronic systemic disease and malnutrition
  - Hypothyroidism
  - Cushing's disease
  - Diabetes mellitus
  - Hyperprolactinemia
  - Anorexia nervosa
  - Psychogenic amenorrhea
  - Exercise-induced amenorrhea

Hypergonadotropic Hypogonadism

Syndrome of gonadal dysgenesis and its variants (Turner syndrome)

Other forms of primary ovarian failure

XX and XY gonadal dysgenesis
- Familial and sporadic XX gonadal dysgenesis and its variants
- Familial and sporadic XY gonadal dysgenesis and its variants

Pseudo-Turner syndrome

Galactosemia

symptoms can suggest a diagnosis of constitutional delay, but this is a diagnosis of exclusion (Fig. 15–9). Significant pathologic conditions (e.g., CNS tumors) must be ruled out before the diagnosis is made and the patient is observed without intervention.

These girls typically have a long-standing history of being shorter than their classmates, although their growth velocity and height are appropriate for their bone age. The mother often had delayed menarche or the father entered puberty late. These girls have a slow tempo of maturation in all stages of endocrine and physical development; GnRH secretion is deficient for chronologic age but appropriate for bone age. Adrenarche may also occur later in subjects with constitutional delay in puberty, in contrast to the normal age of adrenarche in patients with isolated gonadotropin deficiency.[21] Bone age is usually retarded at presentation, but these girls will usually begin to enter puberty on achieving a bone age of about 12 years and will usually have menarche at a bone age of 13 years. Estradiol concentrations will be low at presentation but rise as bone age advances, concordant with maturation of the hypothalamic-pituitary axis. Thus, all stages of pubertal development occur at a later than usual age.

Girls with constitutional delay in growth and puberty usually do not reach their predicted adult height.[96–98] Because the growth rate before puberty is appropriate for bone age but not chronologic age, it may be suboptimal, and GH secretion after provocative stimuli may be decreased for chronologic age, suggesting GH deficiency. However, growth velocity and GH secretion in girls with constitutional delay return to normal after the onset of puberty. As GH secretion and GH responses to GH secretagogues increase with the administration of estrogens, girls with constitutional delay in puberty may have a state of functional, temporary GH insufficiency for chronologic age but not for bone age.[99] However, treatment with GH does not increase final height, even if growth velocity temporarily increases in some girls.

Hypogonadotropic Hypogonadism

Deficient pulsatile GnRH, LH, and FSH secretion leads to delayed puberty and sexual infantilism. GnRH deficiency may be due to genetic or developmental defects of the hypothalamus or to destructive lesions such as tumors, inflammatory processes, vascular lesions, or trauma. Gonadotropin deficiency may also be due to lesions in the pituitary itself. Patients with isolated gonadotropin deficiency are usually of normal height for age in early adoles-

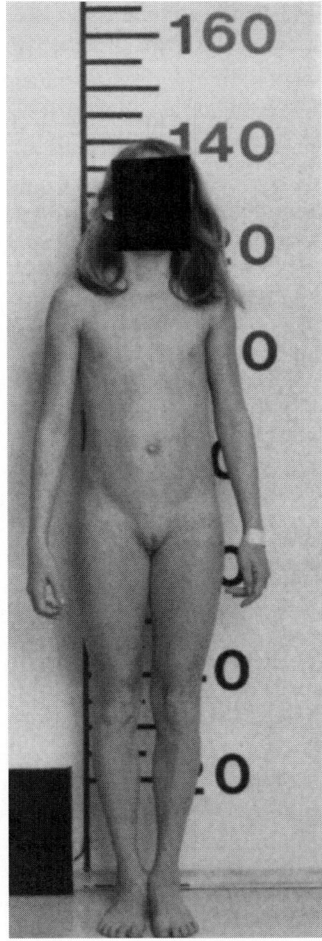

Figure 15–9 ■ Constitutional delay of growth and puberty in a girl who had a normal growth rate but short stature throughout her childhood. In this photograph at 13 years 4 months, her height was 138 cm (−4.5 SD), and weight was 28.6 kg (−3 SD); she had 1 to 2 cm of palpable breast tissue (stage 2), and her bone age was 10 years. She subsequently progressed through puberty normally. (From Styne DM, Kaplan SL. Normal and abnormal puberty in the female. Pediatr Clin North Am 26:123–148, 1979.)

cent years, whereas patients with constitutional delay are usually short for chronologic age. In contrast to girls with constitutional delay, gonadotropin-deficient girls usually have subnormal LH responses to GnRH stimulation, commensurate with bone age, and the serum concentrations of LH, FSH, and estradiol are low.[2] However, the differential diagnosis between hypogonadotropic hypogonadism and constitutional delay of puberty remains difficult in many patients, and watchful waiting is often required.

Central Nervous System Tumors

CNS tumors may delay or eliminate pubertal development; more rarely, they may cause precocious puberty. The tumors causing delayed puberty are usually extrasellar, interfering with GnRH synthesis or secretion. Almost all patients with hypothalamic-pituitary tumors and gonadotropin deficiency are also deficient for additional pituitary hormones. Tumors causing gonadotropin and GH deficiency cause a later onset of growth failure than is seen in congenital hypopituitarism. Associated posterior pituitary disease manifested by diabetes insipidus suggests an expanding lesion in childhood or a developmental defect in infancy. Thus, the late onset of anterior pituitary deficiencies, especially in conjunction with diabetes insipidus, is an ominous sign suggesting a CNS tumor.

Craniopharyngioma. Craniopharyngioma, a congenital tumor of Rathke's pouch, is the most common neoplasm causing hypothalamic-pituitary dysfunction and hypogonadotropic hypogonadism. Craniopharyngiomas usually become symptomatic before age 20 years, with a peak incidence between 6 and 14 years.[100] The presentation may include headache, visual disturbances, short stature, delayed puberty, polyuria and polydipsia, and weakness of one or more limbs. Visual defects (bilateral temporal field deficits, optic atrophy, papilledema), GH deficiency, delayed puberty, and hypothyroidism are common. Most patients have short stature, delayed bone age, and hormonal deficiencies. Skull radiographs detect suprasellar or intrasellar calcification or an abnormal sella turcica in about 70 percent of patients with craniopharyngioma but in less than 1 percent of normal subjects. These radiographic findings may be detected in asymptomatic patients being evaluated for other reasons. CT scans may reveal fine calcifications that are not apparent on routine skull radiographs. CT or MRI scans can determine whether the tumor is solid or cystic and indicate the presence of hydrocephalus. Treatment consists of surgery and radiotherapy. Small intrasellar craniopharyngiomas can be resected or decompressed by transsphenoidal microsurgery, but larger or suprasellar masses may require craniotomy.[101, 102] The recurrence rate is high when complete surgical removal is attempted, and further damage to the optic nerves may occur. The combination of limited tumor removal and radiation therapy leads to as satisfactory a neurologic outcome as attempts at complete removal, and the endocrine outcome is often better.

Other Pituitary Tumors. Other pituitary tumors, such as chromophobe adenomas and prolactin-secreting adenomas, are rare in childhood but may occur in the later teenage years, leading to delayed puberty or secondary amenorrhea.[103] Hyperprolactinemia is associated with delayed puberty and galactorrhea without gynecomastia; bromocriptine suppresses the elevated prolactin secretion and the galactorrhea and allows progression of puberty.

Germinomas. Germinomas are the extrasellar tumors that most commonly cause sexual infantilism, even though these tumors are a minority of all primary CNS tumors. Polydipsia and polyuria are the most common symptoms, followed by visual difficulties and abnormalities of growth and puberty.[104] Vasopressin and GH deficiencies are common, but gonadotropin deficiency and hyperprolactinemia are also frequent. Germinomas may be located in the suprasellar hypothalamus, the pineal, or other areas of the CNS. Subependymal spread along the lining of the third ventricle is common, and seeding of the cerebrospinal fluid may lead to involvement of the lower spinal cord and cauda equina. CT and MRI scans are useful in the diagnosis of tumors greater than 0.5 cm in diameter.[105] Radiation is the preferred treatment; the clinical features and excellent response to radiation therapy are so characteristic that surgery is rarely indicated except for biopsy to establish a tissue diagnosis. Hypothalamic and optic gliomas or astrocytomas in the hypothalamic area, occurring independently or as part of neurofibromatosis (von Recklinghausen's disease), can also cause sexual infantilism.[54]

Langerhans Cell Histiocytosis. Langerhans cell histiocytosis, also called Hand-Schüller-Christian disease or histiocytosis X, is characterized by the infiltration of lipid-laden histiocytic cells or foam cells in the skin, viscera, and bone.[106] Whereas histiocytosis is not a tumor, its capacity to invade adjacent tissues and response to chemotherapeutic agents, especially vinblastine, are behaviors reminiscent of tumors. Diabetes insipidus is the most common endocrine manifestation, but GH deficiency and delayed puberty occur; the lungs, liver, and spleen may also be involved. Characteristic radiographic findings include cyst-like areas in flat bones of the skull, ribs, pelvis, scapula, long bones of the arms and legs, and dorsolumbar spine. Such lesions of the mandible lead to the radiographic impression of "floating teeth" within rarefied bone and the clinical finding of absent or loose teeth. Infiltration of the orbit may lead to exophthalmos, and mastoid or temporal bone involvement may lead to chronic otitis media. The natural waxing and waning course of this disease makes evaluation of therapy difficult.

Congenital Central Nervous System Disorders

Developmental Defects. Midline malformations of the CNS and optic dysplasia are caused by abnormal development of the prosencephalon. Small, dysplastic, pale optic discs, often with a partial ring of pigmentation around the border and associated pendular nystagmus, are characteristic of optic dysplasia. Visual defects may extend to blindness. The hypothalamic defect may cause deficiency of any or all pituitary hormones; hence, short stature and delayed puberty frequently result, although precocious puberty may occur. An absent septum pellucidum is often demonstrable by imaging techniques (septo-optic dysplasia).[107] Other congenital midline defects ranging from complete dysraphism and holoprosencephaly to cleft lip and palate can also be associated with hypothalamic-pituitary dysfunction.

Isolated Gonadotropin Deficiency. Isolated gonadotropin deficiency may occur sporadically or in familial clusters.[108] In contrast to patients with CNS tumors, who usually have associated GH deficiency and growth failure, and to patients with constitutional delay in growth and adolescence, who are short for chronologic age, patients with isolated gonadotropin deficiency are usually of appropriate height for their chronologic age (Fig. 15–10). Deficient gonadal steroids prevent normal epiphyseal closure, so these patients develop eunuchoid proportions, with increased arm span for height and decreased upper to lower ratios. If untreated, these patients become tall adults.

Kallmann Syndrome. Kallmann syndrome, the most common form of isolated hypogonadotropic hypogonadism, consists of GnRH deficiency associated with hyposmia and hypoplasia of the olfactory lobes. Kallmann syndrome appears to be due to failure of fetal GnRH neurosecretory neurons to migrate from the olfactory placode, where they arise, to the medial basal hypothalamus. About half of Kallmann syndrome patients have mutations in the *KAL* gene on chromosome Xp22.3. This gene encodes an extracellular matrix protein that appears to regulate cellular adhesion and axonal pathfinding.[109, 110] Because half the patients have an X-linked disorder, Kallmann syndrome is more common in boys than in girls. The impaired olfaction may go unnoticed and requires careful evaluation.

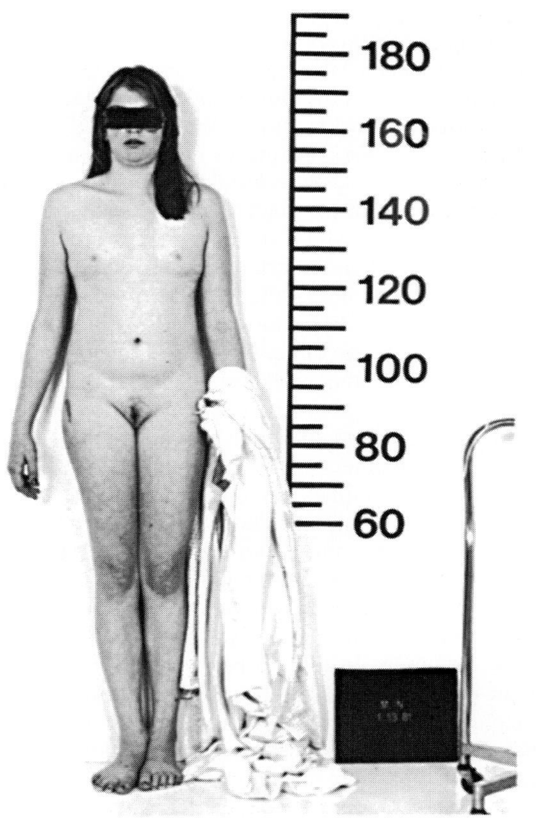

Figure 15–10 ■ Isolated gonadotropin deficiency in a patient 18 years 8 months with a height of 173 cm (+1 SD), weight of 66.5 kg (+1 SD), and bone age of 13 years. Adrenarche and pubic hair developed at age 13½ years, showing the dissociation between adrenarche and puberty. Her slight breast development is from a previous short course of estrogen therapy. Estradiol was undetectable, and there was only an early pubertal response of LH to GnRH.

Associated defects include cleft lip, cleft palate, imperfect facial fusion, unilateral renal agenesis, epilepsy, bimanual synkinesis, short metacarpals, developmental delay, and neurosensory hearing loss. As-yet uncharacterized autosomal disorders can also cause Kallmann syndrome. MRI imaging of the brain may show hypoplasia of the olfactory sulci.[110a]

Idiopathic Hypopituitarism. Idiopathic hypopituitarism is caused by a deficiency of hypothalamic releasing factors. Patients with isolated GH deficiency often undergo spontaneous but delayed puberty when the bone age reaches 11 to 13 years, but those who have associated gonadotropin deficiency do not undergo spontaneous puberty. Breech delivery and perinatal trauma are associated with idiopathic hypopituitarism and pituitary stalk malformations. Familial forms of multiple pituitary hormone deficiencies are rare. Early growth failure is common in patients with idiopathic hypopituitary dwarfism; by contrast, late growth failure suggests a CNS tumor.

Other Central Nervous System Disorders

Cranial radiation for treatment of CNS tumors, leukemia, or neoplasms may result in the gradual onset of hypothalamic-pituitary failure, usually more than 18 months after therapy.[111] Radiation therapy may reduce gonadotropin secretion and delay puberty, or it may advance the age at onset of puberty.[112] GH deficiency is the most common hormone disorder resulting from radiation, but gonadotropin deficiency also occurs when radiation doses are high.

Postinfectious inflammatory lesions of the CNS, vascular abnormalities, and head trauma are unusual causes of hypogonadotropic hypogonadism. Hydrocephalus may cause delayed puberty that can be reversed with decompression.

Functional Gonadotropin Deficiencies

Chronic Disease and Malnutrition. Chronic disease and malnutrition to less than 80 percent of ideal weight can lead to delayed or arrested puberty[113]; weight regain usually restores hypothalamic-pituitary-gonadal function during a variable period. If adequate nutrition and body weight are maintained in patients with regional enteritis or chronic pulmonary disease, gonadotropin secretion is usually adequate, whereas impaired nutrition inhibits pubertal development. Chronic renal disease delays pubertal development, but successful renal transplantation usually restores gonadotropin secretion.[114] Children with early-onset leukemia in long-term remission experience puberty at an appropriate age or with only slight delay, but onset of leukemia in late childhood may delay puberty considerably.[115] CNS irradiation may cause hypogonadotropic hypogonadism; radiation to the gonads and certain types of chemotherapy, especially during puberty, may cause primary hypergonadotropic hypogonadism.

Other Endocrine Disorders. Other endocrine disorders, especially poorly controlled diabetes mellitus, can lead to poor growth, fatty infiltration of the liver, and sexual infantilism (Mauriac's syndrome) probably related to poor nutrition. Adolescents with even moderately poor diabetic control usually have some degree of growth impairment and delayed puberty or irregular menses. Young patients with Cushing's disease[115a] and with hypothyroidism may have delayed or arrested puberty, which is usually corrected after appropriate treatment.

Anorexia Nervosa. Anorexia nervosa, characterized by a distorted body image, obsessive fear of obesity, and food avoidance, can cause severe, even fatal weight loss.[116, 117] Primary or secondary amenorrhea is found in virtually all patients. Anatomic disease, such as a macroprolactinoma, may present as anorexia nervosa. Anorexia nervosa is more common in girls with gonadal dysgenesis. Hypogonadotropic hypogonadism is found in most patients with anorexia nervosa and, at least in part, is related to weight loss, but the onset of amenorrhea can precede the onset of severe weight loss. Functional amenorrhea can also occur in women of normal weight, leading to effects ranging in severity from severe estrogen deficiency to anovulation to a short luteal phase.

Affected women may revert to the circadian rhythm of LH secretion characteristic of early puberty and have blunted or absent LH responses to GnRH, but GnRH administration at 90- to 120-minute intervals can restore a pubertal pattern of LH secretion, demonstrating the role of GnRH deficiency in the amenorrhea of anorexia nervosa.[118] Other hormonal changes include increased GH and decreased IGF-I (as found in malnutrition); low cortisol, DHEA-S, and triiodothyronine levels; and normal thyroxine and thyroid-stimulating hormone levels. The response of prolactin to thyrotropin-releasing hormone or insulin-induced hypoglycemia is blunted, and urine concentrating capacity is diminished. Recovery of normal weight will normalize most endocrine and metabolic functions, but amenorrhea may persist for months. Bulimia nervosa, a variant of anorexia nervosa, is common among high-school and college students and is associated with food gorging, induced vomiting, and laxative and diuretic abuse leading to amenorrhea but not weight loss.[119]

Intensive Exercise and Athletic Training. Intensive exercise and athletic training may delay or arrest puberty and cause amenorrhea due to inhibition of GnRH secretion, especially among long-distance runners, gymnasts, and ballerinas.[120] Interruption of intensive training (e.g., by injury) advances puberty and menarche before body composition or weight change significantly, suggesting a direct effect of physical activity on GnRH secretion. Female athletes with normal weight but less fat and more muscle than nonathletic girls (e.g., ice skaters or swimmers) are also at risk for delayed puberty and for primary and secondary amenorrhea, but adrenarche is not delayed.[121]

Although it has been suggested that female gymnasts are small because small girls seek careers in gymnastics, a prospective Swiss study demonstrated decreased growth velocity, stunting of leg growth, and decreased height in 22 gymnasts compared with 21 swimmers.[122] The conclusion that heavy training in gymnastics during childhood leads to a decrease in ultimate height is supported by a Swedish study showing decreased growth spurts and final adult heights of female gymnasts compared with nonathletic control subjects.[123] Some have even suggested that the intensive training of competitive female gymnasts should be considered a ritualized form of child abuse.[124]

Hyperprolactinemia. Hyperprolactinemia is a rare cause of delayed puberty.[125] Galactorrhea may not be apparent, but manipulation of the nipples may cause the release of fluid. Hyperprolactinemia may be due to a tumor or to a functional defect; tumors usually develop after the onset of puberty.[103] Bromocriptine may decrease serum prolactin concentrations and the size of the tumors and allow pubertal progression and the resumption of menses, but transsphenoidal excision of the larger tumors is necessary. Prolactin levels may be elevated in women athletes and may contribute to their delayed menarche.[126]

Hypergonadotropic Hypogonadism

The Syndrome of Gonadal Dysgenesis

Primary gonadal failure and decreased or absent gonadal steroid secretion eliminate negative feedback, causing elevated serum LH and FSH. The syndrome of gonadal dysgenesis (Turner syndrome) and its variants, characterized by short stature and ovarian failure, is the most common form of hypergonadotropic hypogonadism, occurring in 1 in 2500 to 10,000 liveborn girls (for review, see reference 127). About 50 percent of cases of Turner syndrome have the 45,X karyotype. However, up to 99 percent of 45,X conceptuses abort spontaneously, and 1 in 15 spontaneous abortions has the 45,X karyotype. Mosaicism or structural abnormalities of sex chromosomes may modify the clinical features. Turner syndrome may be viewed on a continuum ranging from the typical 45,X phenotype to a normal male or female phenotype. Typical features include lymphedema of the extremities and loose posterior cervical skinfolds in the newborn (which later develop into the webbed neck), micrognathia, fishmouth, high-arched palate, dental abnormalities, epicanthal folds, ptosis, low-set or deformed ears, broad shield-like chest leading to the appearance of wide-spaced nipples, hypoplastic areolae, short neck with low hairline, recurrent otitis media, short fourth metacarpals and cubitus valgus (which develop after birth), extensive nevi, tendency to keloid formation, and hypoplastic nails (Fig. 15–11). Anomalies of the left side of the heart include coarctation of the aorta, aortic stenosis, bicuspid aortic valves, and a risk for dissecting aortic aneurysms. Renal anomalies include abnormal pelvicaliceal collecting systems, abnormal renal position or alignment (including horseshoe kidney), and abnormal vascular supply. Gastrointestinal defects include intestinal telangiectasias and hemangiomatoses (sometimes causing massive gastrointestinal bleeding) and a higher incidence of inflammatory bowel disease. The uterus and fallopian tubes are present but remain infantile in the absence of estrogen, because the ovaries are streaks of connective tissue. Autoimmune disease, including Hashimoto's thyroiditis and Graves' disease, are common. Insulin resistance and glucose intolerance are common after the age of puberty, and serum cholesterol values are higher than normal.[128] Intelligence is normal, but spatiotemporal processing, visuomotor coordination, and mathematical ability (particularly in geometry) may be impaired. Gender identity and sexual orientation are female.

Patients are usually small for gestational age, grow slowly after the age of 3 years, fail to have a pubertal growth spurt, and have adult heights of about 143 cm, depending on parental height. Specific growth curves are available for plotting the growth of affected children.[129]

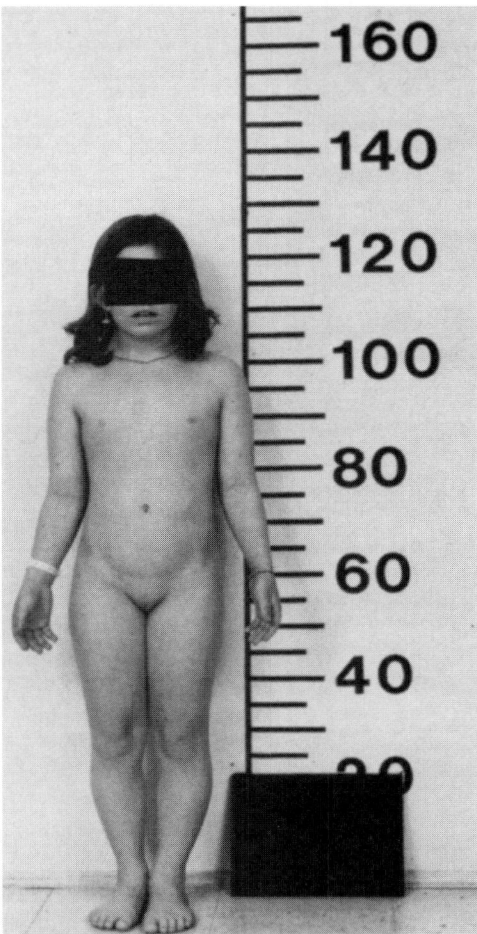

Figure 15–11 ■ Turner syndrome in a girl 12 years 5 months with a 45,X karyotype. Height was 126.7 cm (−4.6 SD), weight was 31.2 kg (−1.9 SD), and bone age was 11 years. Note the down-turned mouth, cubitus valgus, and widely spaced nipples; she also had a low posterior hairline, edema of the dorsum of the hands, and dystrophic nails. She had stage 2 pubic hair from adrenal androgens, but estradiol was undetectable, and both LH and FSH were high. (From Styne DM, Kaplan SL. Normal and abnormal puberty in the female. Pediatr Clin North Am 26:123–148, 1979.)

Bone density is decreased, partly owing to hypogonadism at puberty. Patients who discontinue or do not receive estrogen replacement may have severe osteopenia. The defect in growth appears to be related to haploinsufficiency of the gene termed PHOG or SHOX, which appears to encode a transcription factor expressed in osteoblasts.[129a,b]

The biphasic pattern of gonadotropin secretion in normal infancy and childhood is exaggerated in Turner syndrome, although the basic pattern is the same. Basal and GnRH-induced LH and FSH values are above normal between birth and 4 years of age and again after age 10 years. Baseline FSH values are 3 to 10 times higher than LH values. Between 4 and 10 years, gonadotropin concentrations are similar to those in normal girls and are lower than those before age 4 years, but the amount of pubic hair is sparse.

Patients with mosaicism (45,X/46,XX, 45,X/47,XXX, or 45,X/46,XX/47,XXX karyotypes) or with structural abnormalities usually have fewer phenotypic manifestations. Mosaicism with the Y chromosome (45,X/46,XY) may result in phenotypes ranging from classic gonadal dysgenesis to ambiguous genitalia even to normal males. Gonadal structure ranges from a streak gonad to functional testes. Patients with a Y cell line or abnormalities of the Y chromosome are at risk for neoplastic transformation of the dysgenetic testes. Benign nonmetastasizing gonadoblastomas may arise within the gonad and produce either testosterone or estrogens; these tumors can become sufficiently calcified to be detected on an abdominal radiograph.[130] Malignant germ cell tumors may arise within dysgenetic gonads or gonadoblastomas, especially after puberty. As in all patients with an abnormal Y cell line, the dysgenetic gonads should be removed.

The term pure gonadal dysgenesis refers to phenotypic females with sexual infantilism and a 46,XX or 46,XY karyotype without detectable chromosomal abnormalities. Autosomal recessive sporadic 46,XX gonadal dysgenesis and its variants will present with normal stature, sexual infantilism, bilateral streak gonads, normal female internal and external genitalia, and primary amenorrhea, sometimes associated with sensorineural deafness.[127] Malignant transformation of the streak gonads is rare. Familial and sporadic 46,XY gonadal dysgenesis and its variants may present with female genitalia with or without clitoral enlargement, normal or tall stature, bilateral streak gonads, normal müllerian structures, sexual infantilism, and a eunuchoid body habitus. If the dysgenetic testes produce some testosterone, there may be slight clitoral enlargement at birth and virilization at puberty. Incomplete 46,XY gonadal dysgenesis may involve any degree of genital ambiguity. The dysgenetic testes may undergo neoplastic transformation, so gonadectomy is indicated. Transmission is usually X-linked or sex-limited autosomal dominant and less commonly autosomal recessive.

Noonan syndrome (pseudo-Turner syndrome, Ullrich syndrome) is characterized by webbed neck, ptosis, short stature, cubitus valgus, and lymphedema and hence resembles the phenotype of Turner syndrome.[131] Noonan syndrome also includes triangular facies, pectus excavatum, right-sided heart disease (e.g., pulmonic stenosis or atrial septal defect), and an increased incidence of mental retardation. Females with Noonan syndrome have normal ovarian function.

Genetic Disorders of Ovarian Steroidogenesis

Autosomal recessive disorders have been described in each step of the steroidogenic pathway. The disorders of ovarian steroidogenesis are also manifested as disorders of adrenal steroidogenesis. Because disruption of adrenal mineralocorticoid and glucocorticoid synthesis can be life threatening in the newborn, the adrenal, rather than the gonad, is the usual center of attention; hence, these disorders are generally termed the congenital adrenal hyperplasias. From the perspective of disorders of puberty, we classify the disorders of steroidogenesis as those that result in sexual infantilism and those that cause virilization; there are no disorders of steroidogenesis that cause premature feminization.

Congenital Lipoid Adrenal Hyperplasia (Lipoid CAH). Lipoid CAH is the most severe form of CAH. Affected newborns have a severe defect in the conversion of cholesterol to pregnenolone in both the adrenal and gonad; hence, they have little or no circulating adrenal or gonadal steroids. Lipoid CAH is most common among the Japanese and Palestinians.[15] Absent adrenal steroidogenesis leads to profound glucocorticoid and mineralocorticoid deficiency, causing salt loss, hyponatremia, hyperkalemia, acidosis, hypotension, and death within the first few weeks or months of life. Adequate glucocorticoid and mineralocorticoid replacement is compatible with normal life to adulthood.[132] In genetic XX female fetuses, the ovaries normally do not produce steroidogenic enzymes or steroids[133]; hence, the disrupted gonadal steroidogenesis in lipoid CAH has no effect on the external genitalia. In genetic XY male fetuses, absent testicular steroidogenesis results in a failure to develop male external genitalia; hence, XY males with lipoid CAH are born with wholly normal female genitalia.[15] The diagnosis can be made only by suspecting it in a normal-looking female infant with a salt-losing syndrome.

Lipoid CAH was formerly thought to be due to a mutation in P450scc and was mistermed 20,22-desmolase deficiency. However, the P450scc genes in these patients are normal[134]; the disorder is due to mutations in the StAR protein.[15, 135, 136] A disruption of human P450scc is probably incompatible with life, because the placenta uses P450scc to synthesize the progesterone needed to maintain pregnancy after the 8th to 10th week. Thus, a deletion in the rabbit P450scc gene is compatible with term delivery,[137] because the corpus luteum of pregnancy suffices for progesterone synthesis in the rabbit (and maternal ovariectomy causes abortion), whereas the human corpus luteum does not suffice for progesterone production (and ovariectomy after the 12th week is compatible with normal pregnancy). Not surprisingly, cord blood progesterone is normal in lipoid CAH fetuses, but the affected fetal adrenal cannot produce DHEA, and maternal estriol is nil.[138]

Although newborns with lipoid CAH have wholly normal-appearing female external genitalia, they can show substantial variation in the age at onset of salt loss (from newborn to 6 months),[15] and affected 46,XX females may feminize and experience vaginal bleeding at the time of puberty.[139] This reflects the biology of the StAR protein, which facilitates acute ACTH-induced and gonadotropin-induced steroidogenesis but is not required for basal steroidogenesis. Thus, the lipoid CAH phenotype is due to two cellular events. First, StAR protein mutations ablate the acute steroidogenic response but permit StAR protein–independent steroidogenesis to persist. Second, with continued trophic stimulation of the StAR protein–depleted cell, cholesterol esters and cholesterol auto-oxidation products accumulate, eventually killing the cell and thus eliminating StAR protein–independent steroidogenesis. Hence, in the fetus, Leydig cells and fetal zone adrenal cells, which normally make huge quantities of steroids, are destroyed before birth. However, cells of the definitive zone of the fetal adrenal are relatively unstimulated and undamaged at birth, leading to a variable capacity to produce aldosterone and thus preventing a salt-losing crisis for days to months, depending on the severity of the StAR protein mutation.[15] Similarly, because even the StAR protein–deficient ovary has experienced no trophic stimulation until puberty, it can still make the small amounts of estradiol needed to induce breast development. With each cycle, a new cohort of previously unstimulated follicles is recruited; hence, these StAR protein–deficient follicular cells, which have not been damaged by accumulated cholesterol auto-oxidation products, can still produce basal StAR protein–independent levels of estradiol. These anovulatory cycles can persist for years, leading to fairly normal feminization (but without much pubic hair from adrenal androgens), including monthly cycles. However, because these patients are profoundly hypergonadotropic, they also develop cystic ovaries.

3β-Hydroxysteroid Dehydrogenase Deficiency. Severe 3βHSD deficiency is a rare disorder presenting with signs and symptoms of glucocorticoid and mineralocorticoid deficiency; it is usually fatal if it is not diagnosed in infancy. 3βHSD deficiency is due to mutations in the type II gene that is expressed in the adrenals and gonads; mutations in the type I gene have not been described.[140] Type I but not type II is expressed in the placenta; hence, type I mutations would interfere with placental production of progesterone and would presumably be incompatible with term pregnancy. Disruption of 3βHSD activity interferes with adrenal production of 17-hydroxyprogesterone; however, the high concentrations of adrenal-produced 17-hydroxypregnenolone may be converted to 17-hydroxyprogesterone by hepatic 3βHSD type I, so that circulating concentrations of 17-hydroxyprogesterone may be paradoxically elevated in 3βHSD deficiency, approaching the levels seen in 21-hydroxylase deficiency. This 17-hydroxyprogesterone may be peripherally converted to low levels of androgens, causing partial virilization.[141] Thus, the persistence of extraglandular 3βHSD type I activity when gonadal-adrenal 3βHSD type II is mutated may complicate and obscure the diagnosis of 3βHSD deficiency.

Hormone values suggesting a mild or partial defect in 3βHSD have been described in large numbers of young women with premature adrenarche, hirsutism, and virilism. However, the overwhelming majority of these patients with elevated ACTH-stimulated ratios of Δ^5 to Δ^4 steroids have no 3βHSD mutations, and it is now clear that this ratio must exceed 850 above the mean before it is suggestive of true 3βHSD deficiency.[26, 27, 140] The basis for these mild changes in steroid hormone profiles is not yet known.

17α-Hydroxylase/17,20-Lyase (P450c17) Deficiency. P450c17 deficiency has been reported in more than 120 patients.[142] Deficient 17α-hydroxylase activity results in decreased cortisol synthesis, with consequent overproduction of ACTH and stimulation of the steps proximal to P450c17. These patients may have mild symptoms of glucocorticoid deficiency, but this is not life threatening because the lack of P450c17 results in the overproduction of corticosterone, a weak glucocorticoid. These patients typically overproduce deoxycorticosterone in the zona fasciculata, which results in sodium retention and hypertension but also suppresses aldosterone secretion from the zona glomerulosa. Absence of 17α-hydroxylase and 17,20-lyase activities means that adrenal and gonadal sex steroids are not produced. As a result, genetic males may have completely female external genitalia or may have incomplete development (male pseudohermaphroditism). Affected females are phenotypically normal but fail to undergo adrenarche and puberty. The classic presentation is that of a teenage phenotypic female (who may be XX or XY) with sexual infantilism and hypertension. The diagnosis is readily made by finding low or absent 17-hydroxylated C_{21} and C_{19} plasma steroids and low urinary 17-hydroxycorticosteroids and 17-ketosteroids, which respond poorly to stimulation with ACTH. Serum levels of deoxycorticosterone, corticosterone, and 18-hydroxycorticosterone will be elevated and show hyperresponsiveness to ACTH and suppression after treatment with glucocorticoids. Many different P450c17 mutations can cause severe 17α-hydroxylase/17,20-lyase deficiency.[143]

Isolated 17,20-lyase deficiency, in which 17α-hydroxylase activity is retained, is very rare. It can present in infancy or adolescence with female or ambiguous genitalia, low plasma sex steroids, low urinary 17-ketosteroids, and normal plasma cortisol and urinary 17-hydroxycorticosteroids. The disease is due to amino acid replacements in P450c17 that impair electron transfer but not substrate binding.[143a]

Other Causes of Primary Ovarian Failure

Radiation to the Ovaries. Radiation to the ovaries can cause primary ovarian failure[144]; thus, before radiation therapy, the ovaries should be moved out of the radiation field surgically. Some chemotherapeutic regimens, especially with nitroso compounds or procarbazine, are associated with primary gonadal failure.[145] Suppressing the pituitary-gonadal axis with gonadal steroids or GnRH agonists does not protect the gonads from radiotherapy or chemotherapy.

Autoimmune Oophoritis. Autoimmune oophoritis, often associated with other autoimmune endocrinopathies, can cause premature ovarian failure, primary or secondary amenorrhea, oligomenorrhea, arrested puberty, and occasionally ovarian cysts. Ovarian failure occurred before age 20 years in 36 percent of women with type I autoimmune polyglandular insufficiency (hypoparathyroidism, adrenal insufficiency, gonadal failure, diabetes mellitus, pernicious anemia, hypothyroidism, chronic hepatitis, mucocutaneous candidiasis, dystrophic nail hypoplasia, vitiligo, alopecia, keratinopathy, and intestinal malabsorption).[146] Autoimmune oophoritis is found in more than 20 percent of patients with autoimmune Addison's disease. Glucocorticoid therapy may temporarily improve ovarian function.

Resistant Ovary. Resistant ovary syndrome is a heterogeneous disorder. Most cases appear to be autosomal recessive, caused by mutations of the FSH receptor in its extracellular ligand-binding domain. Such mutations can result in either delayed or temporally normal onset of puberty, but with primary amenorrhea, elevated gonadotropins and hypergonadotropic ovarian dysgenesis with arrest of ovarian follicular development at the primary follicle stage, and continued atresia.[146a] Estrogen therapy can suppress the elevated gonadotropin levels and restore spontaneous ovarian cycles. Resistance to LH/hCG may similarly be due to mutations in the gene for the LH/hCG receptor, which, like the FSH receptor, is a G-protein–linked, seven-transmembrane receptor. In affected females, LH/hCG resistance does not influence pubertal maturation but leads to amenorrhea with high serum LH levels but normal FSH and estradiol levels.[146b]

Diagnosis

Girls who lack secondary sexual development at age 13 years, who fail to progress through puberty, or who do not menstruate within 5 years after the onset of puberty should be evaluated. A thorough history should especially note the details of growth and development and any history of chronic illness or disorders of olfaction (Table 15–4). Disorders of pregnancy and delivery may suggest a congenital or neonatal event. Poor growth and poor nutrition reflect long-standing abnormalities of development. Family history may reveal delayed or disordered puberty, infertility, anosmia, or hyposmia in parents or siblings.

The physical examination should include measurements of height, weight, the upper to lower body segment ratio, and arm span as qualitative and quantitative indices of growth. A growth chart including prior measurements should be plotted to assess growth velocity from birth. The signs of puberty should be noted carefully, and the Tanner stages of breast and pubic hair development are recorded, including the diameter of glandular breast tissue, areolar size, and possible presence of galactorrhea. The neurologic examination should include particular attention to the optic discs, the visual fields, and the olfaction, abnormalities of which may suggest the presence of a CNS neoplasm or a developmental defect (e.g., Kallmann syndrome). The stigmata of gonadal dysgenesis should be sought.

Laboratory determinations should include basal and GnRH-induced plasma LH and FSH concentrations, estradiol (not total estrogen), thyroxine, and prolactin. A lateral skull radiograph, bone age determination, and, depending on the clinical findings, MRI and CT scan of the brain should be done. Ultrasonography of the uterus and ovaries can be useful but is not routinely included in an initial evaluation. A karyotype should be done in all short girls, even in the absence of signs of Turner syndrome.

Many tests have been proposed for differentiating hypogonadotropic hypogonadism from constitutional delay in puberty, but the results are far too variable to allow a specific diagnosis. A presumptive diagnosis of constitutional delay in growth and adolescence may be made if the history and growth chart reveal short stature but consistent growth rate for skeletal age, if the family history includes parents or siblings with delayed puberty, if the findings on physical examination (including assessment of the olfactory threshold) are normal, if optic discs and visual fields are normal, if the bone age is delayed, and if a lateral skull film is normal. A decrease in growth velocity occurs in some normal children just before the appearance of secondary sexual characteristics. The onset at puberty correlates better with bone age than with chronologic age. Increased plasma gonadotropins and estradiol precede pubertal development by several months; thus, these measurements may help to predict future developments. A GnRH-induced increase in LH of more than 7.6 IU/L usually precedes the first sign of sexual maturation by about 1 year.

Patients with isolated gonadotropin deficiency usually have normal height but eunuchoid body proportions. Plasma estradiol, LH, and FSH are low and exhibit little or no response to GnRH. The sense of smell is absent or impaired in Kallmann syndrome, but in the absence of hyposmia, differentiation of Kallmann syndrome from iso-

■ TABLE 15–4
Diagnostic Features of Delayed Puberty and Sexual Infantilism

	STATURE	PLASMA GONADOTROPINS	GnRH TEST: LH RESPONSE	PLASMA GONADAL STEROIDS	PLASMA DHEA-S	KARYOTYPE	OLFACTION
Constitutional delay in growth and adolescence	Short for chronologic age, usually appropriate for bone age	Prepubertal, later pubertal	Prepubertal, later pubertal	Low, later normal	Low for chronologic age, appropriate for bone age	Normal	Normal
Hypogonadotropic Hypogonadism							
Isolated gonadotropin deficiency	Normal, absent pubertal growth spurt	Low	Prepubertal or no response	Low	Appropriate for chronologic age	Normal	Normal
Kallmann syndrome	Normal, absent pubertal growth spurt	Low	Prepubertal or no response	Low	Appropriate for chronologic age	Normal	Anosmia or hyposmia
Idiopathic multiple pituitary hormone deficiencies	Short stature and poor growth since early childhood	Low	Prepubertal or no response	Low	Usually low	Normal	Normal
Hypothalamic pituitary tumors	Decrease in growth velocity of late onset	Low	Prepubertal or no response	Low	Normal or low for chronologic age	Normal	Normal
Primary Gonadal Failure							
Turner syndrome and its variants	Short stature since early childhood	High	Hyperresponse for age	Low	Normal for chronologic age	XO or variant	Normal
Familial XX or XY gonadal dysgenesis	Normal	High	Hyperresponse for age	Low	Normal for chronologic age	XX or XY	Normal

GnRH, gonadotropin-releasing hormone; LH, luteinizing hormone; DHEA-S, dehydroepiandrosterone sulfate.

lated gonadotropin deficiency or constitutional delay is difficult. Gonadotropin-deficient patients may be as short as those with constitutional delay, and concentrations of LH and FSH in hypogonadotropic hypogonadism may be indistinguishable from those of normal prepubertal children or children with constitutional delay. Sometimes, years of observation are necessary to detect the signs of secondary sexual development or to document rising concentrations of gonadotropins or gonadal steroids before the diagnosis is clear.

Patients with combined deficiency of gonadotropins and other pituitary hormones require careful evaluation for a CNS neoplasm. Even if the visual fields and optic discs appear normal, radiographic examination of the skull should be done to evaluate the sella turcica and the suprasellar region for calcification or erosion; MRI may reveal a mass lesion or developmental abnormalities of the hypothalamic-pituitary region.

Treatment

Patients with constitutional delay in growth and adolescence ultimately have spontaneous onset of and progression through puberty. Reassurance and continued observation to ensure that the expected sexual maturation occurs may be sufficient, but the stigma of appearing less mature than one's peers can cause psychologic stress. Some children feel such intense peer pressure and low self-esteem that only the appearance of signs of puberty will reassure them and enable them to participate in sports and social activities with their peers. For girls age 13 years or older, a 3-month course of ethinyl estradiol (5 to 10 μg/day orally) or conjugated estrogens (0.3 mg/day orally) may be used to initiate breast development without unduly advancing bone age or limiting final height.[147] If spontaneous puberty does not ensue or the concentrations of plasma gonadotropins and plasma estradiol do not increase during the 3 to 6 months after gonadal steroid therapy is discontinued, the treatment may be repeated. Only one or two courses of therapy are usually necessary. When treatment is discontinued after bone age has advanced to the pubertal range, patients with constitutional delay continue pubertal development on their own, whereas those with gonadotropin deficiency do not progress and may, in fact, regress.

Gonadotropin deficiency requires gonadal steroid replacement therapy at the normal age of puberty. An exception may occur when GH and gonadotropin deficiencies coexist; adult height will be compromised if estradiol-induced bone age advancement and epiphyseal fusion occur before GH therapy causes adequate linear growth. To achieve adequate growth without the psychologic stress of severely delayed puberty, treatment with low-dose estrogen should begin by age 13 years regardless of the definitive diagnosis of gonadotropin deficiency. Thus, these children with GH deficiency would be treated in a manner similar to those with isolated delayed puberty. By contrast, artificially delaying puberty with GnRH agonists for 2 years in 31 patients with constitutional short stature resulted in only a minimal effect that did not justify their use to increase final height in this condition.[148] Similarly, estrogen replacement therapy should be initiated in Turner syndrome at age 12 to 13 years to allow secondary sexual development at an appropriate chronologic age; delaying treatment has little effect on final adult height. Clinical trials of hGH therapy in gonadal dysgenesis suggest an increased growth rate and final height when therapy is initiated in early childhood[149];

GH therapy may also ameliorate the loss in bone density characteristic of Turner syndrome.[150]

Episodic administration of GnRH by portable pumps can elicit pulsatile LH and FSH release and gonadal stimulation in prepubertal children or hypogonadotropic patients.[108] Pulsatile GnRH therapy can induce puberty and promote the progression of secondary sexual characteristics and ovulation, and pregnancy has been achieved with this regimen in women with hypogonadotropic hypogonadism. However, this approach is not practical for the routine induction of pubertal maturation in adolescent girls with gonadotropin deficiency. Human chorionic gonadotropin and human menopausal gonadotropin can be used as substitutes for LH and FSH, respectively, to produce full gonadal maturation, but these preparations are expensive and frequent injections are required. Thus, long-term estrogen replacement therapy is the treatment of choice for hypothalamic or pituitary gonadotropin deficiency until fertility is desired.

The estrogen replacement regimen is the same in both hypogonadotropic and hypergonadotropic hypogonadism. Girls age 12 to 13 years are given ethinyl estradiol, 5 to 10 μg/day orally, or conjugated estrogens, 0.3 mg/day by mouth, initially administered daily and after 6 months changed to only the first 21 days of the month. The dose is gradually increased during 2 to 3 years to 10 to 20 μg of ethinyl estradiol or 0.6 to 1.25 mg of conjugated estrogen for the first 21 days of the month. The maintenance dose should be the minimal amount needed to maintain secondary sexual characteristics, sustain withdrawal bleeding, and prevent osteoporosis. After breakthrough bleeding occurs, or no later than 6 months after the start of cyclic therapy, a progestogen (e.g., medroxyprogesterone acetate, 5 to 10 mg/day) is added on days 12 through 21 of the month to guard against the neoplastic effects of unopposed estrogens on the breast and uterus. Undesirable effects are uncommon but may include weight gain, headache, nausea, peripheral edema, and mild hypertension.

References

1. Kaplan SL, Grumbach MM. The neuroendocrinology of human puberty: An ontogenic perspective. *In* Grumbach MM, Sizonenko PC, Aubert ML (eds). Control of the Onset of Puberty. Baltimore, Williams & Wilkins, 1990, pp 1–62.
2. Grumbach MM, Styne DM. Puberty: Ontogeny, neuroendocrinology, physiology, and disorders. *In* Wilson JD, Foster DW (eds). Williams Textbook of Endocrinology. Philadelphia, WB Saunders, 1992, pp 1139–1221.
3. Grumbach MM, Gluckman PD. The human fetal hypothalamus and pituitary gland: The maturation of neuroendocrine mechanisms controlling the secretion of fetal pituitary growth hormone, prolactin, gonadotropin, adrenocorticotropin-related peptides, and thyrotropin. *In* Tulchinsky D, Little AB (eds). Maternal-Fetal Endocrinology. Philadelphia, WB Saunders, 1994, pp 193–261.
4. Wu FC, Butler GE, Kelnar CJ, et al. Ontogeny of pulsatile gonadotropin releasing hormone secretion from midchildhood, through puberty, to adulthood in the human male: A study using deconvolution analysis and an ultrasensitive immunofluorometric assay. J Clin Endocrinol Metab 81:1798–1805, 1996.
5. Demir A, Dunkel L, Stenman UH, Voutilainen R. Age-related course of urinary gonadotropins in children. J Clin Endocrinol Metab 80:1457–1460, 1995.
6. Neely EK, Hintz RL, Wilson DM, et al. Normal ranges for immunochemiluminometric gonadotropin assays. J Pediatr 127:40–46, 1995.
7. Attie KM, Ramirez NR, Conte FA, et al. The pubertal growth spurt in eight patients with true precocious puberty and growth hormone deficiency: Evidence for a direct role of sex steroids. J Clin Endocrinol Metab 71:975–983, 1990.
8. Amiel SA, Caprio S, Sherwin RS, et al. Insulin resistance of puberty: A defect restricted to peripheral glucose metabolism. J Clin Endocrinol Metab 72:277–282, 1991.
9. Miller WL, Tyrrell JB. The adrenal cortex. *In* Felig P, Baxter J, Frohman L (eds). Endocrinology and Metabolism. New York, McGraw-Hill, 1995, pp 555–717.
10. Penning TM. Molecular endocrinology of hydroxysteroid dehydrogenases. Endocr Rev 18:281–305, 1997.
11. Strauss JF III, Miller WL. Molecular basis of ovarian steroid synthesis. *In* Hillier S (ed). Ovarian Endocrinology. Oxford, UK, Blackwell Scientific Publications, 1991, pp 25–72.
12. Hall PF. The roles of microfilaments and intermediate filaments in the regulation of steroid synthesis. J Steroid Biochem Mol Biol 55:601–605, 1995.
13. Hall PF. The roles of calmodulin, actin and vimentin in steroid synthesis by adrenal cells. Steroids 62:187–191, 1997.

13a. Pollack SE, Furth EE, Kallen CB, et al. Localization of the steroidogenic acute regulatory protein in human tissues. J Clin Endocrinol Metab 82:4243–4251, 1997.

14. Arakane F, Sugawara T, Nishino H, et al. Steroidogenic acute regulatory protein (StAR) retains activity in the absence of its mitochondrial import sequence: Implications for the mechanism of StAR action. Proc Natl Acad Sci USA 93:13731–13736, 1996.
15. Bose HS, Sugawara T, Strauss JF III, Miller WL. The pathophysiology and genetics of congenital lipoid adrenal hyperplasia. N Engl J Med 335:1870–1878, 1996.
16. Voutilainen R, Tapanainen J, Chung B, et al. Hormonal regulation of P450scc (20,22-desmolase) and P450c17 (17α-hydroxylase/17,20-lyase) in cultured human granulosa cells. J Clin Endocrinol Metab 63:202–207, 1986.
17. Miller WL, Auchus RJ, Geller DH. The regulation of 17,20 lyase activity. Steroids 62:135–144, 1997.

17a. Auchus RJ, Lee TC, Miller WL. Cytochrome b_5 augments the 17,20 lyase activity of human P450c17 without direct electron transfer. J Biol Chem 273:3158–3165, 1998.

18. Zhang L, Rodriguez H, Ohno S, Miller WL. Serine phosphorylation of human P450c17 increases 17,20-lyase activity: Implications for adrenarche and for the polycystic ovary syndrome. Proc Natl Acad Sci USA 92:10619–10623, 1995.
19. Fardella CE, Miller WL. Molecular biology of mineralocorticoid metabolism. Annu Rev Nutr 16:443–470, 1996.
20. Mellon SH, Miller WL. Extra-adrenal steroid 21-hydroxylation is not mediated by P450c21. J Clin Invest 84:1497–1502, 1989.
21. Sklar CA, Kaplan SL, Grumbach MM. Evidence for dissociation between adrenarche and gonadarche: Studies in patients with idiopathic precocious puberty, gonadal dysgenesis, isolated gonadotropin deficiency, and constitutionally delayed growth and adolescence. J Clin Endocrinol Metab 51:548–556, 1980.
22. Orentreich N, Brind JL, Rizer RL, Vogelman JH. Age changes and sex differences in serum dehydroepiandrosterone sulfate concentrations throughout adulthood. J Clin Endocrinol Metab 59:551–555, 1984.
23. Liu CH, Laughlin GA, Fischer VG, Yen SSC. Marked attenuation of ultradian and circadian rhythms of dehydroepiandrosterone in postmenopausal women: Evidence for a reduced 17,20-desmolase enzymatic activity. J Clin Endocrinol Metab 71:900–906, 1990.
24. Dunaif A, Segal DR, Shelley DR, et al. Evidence for distinctive and intrinsic defects in insulin action in polycystic ovary syndrome. Diabetes 41:1257–1266, 1992.
25. Azziz R, Wells G, Zacur HA, Acton RT. Abnormalities of 21-hydroxylase gene ratio and adrenal steroidogenesis in hyperandrogenic women with an exaggerated 17-hydroxyprogesterone response to acute adrenal stimulation. J Clin Endocrinol Metab 73:1327–1331, 1991.
26. Chang YT, Zhang L, Alkaddour HS, et al. Absence of molecular defect in the type II 3β-hydroxysteroid dehydrogenase (3β-HSD) gene in premature pubarche children and hirsute female patients with moderately decreased adrenal 3β-HSD activity. Pediatr Res 37:820–824, 1995.
27. Sakkal-Alkaddour H, Zhang L, Yang X, et al. Studies of 3β-hydroxysteroid dehydrogenase genes in infants and children

manifesting premature pubarche and increased adrenocorticotropin-stimulated Δ^5-steroid values. J Clin Endocrinol Metab 81:3961–3965, 1996.

28. Lachelin GCL, Barnett M, Hopper BR, et al. Adrenal function in normal women and women with the polycystic ovary syndrome. J Clin Endocrinol Metab 62:840–848, 1979.
29. Lucky AW, Rosenfield RL, McGuire J, et al. Adrenal androgen hyperresponsiveness to ACTH in women with acne and/or hirsutism: Adrenal enzyme defects and exaggerated adrenarche. J Clin Endocrinol Metab 62:840–848, 1986.
30. Oppenheimer E, Linder B, DiMartino-Nardi J. Decreased insulin sensitivity in prepubertal girls with premature adrenarche and acanthosis nigricans. J Clin Endocrinol Metab 80:614–618, 1995.
31. Ibãnez L, Potau N, Virdis R, et al. Postpubertal outcome in girls diagnosed of premature pubarche during childhood: Increased frequency of functional ovarian hyperandrogenism. J Clin Endocrinol Metab 76:1599–1603, 1993.
32. Ciaraldi TP, El-Roeiy A, Madar Z, et al. Cellular mechanisms of insulin resistance in polycystic ovarian syndrome. J Clin Endocrinol Metab 75:577–583, 1992.
33. Takayama S, White MF, Kahn CR. Phorbol ester–induced serine phosphorylation of the insulin receptor decreases its tyrosine kinase activity. J Biol Chem 263:3440–3447, 1988.
34. Carey AH, Chan KL, Short F, et al. Evidence for a single gene effect in polycystic ovaries and male pattern baldness. Clin Endocrinol (Oxf) 38:653–658, 1992.
35. Dunaif A, Xia J, Book C-B, et al. Excessive insulin receptor serine phosphorylation in cultured fibroblasts and in skeletal muscle. J Clin Invest 96:801–810, 1995.
36. Marshall WA, Tanner JM. Variations in the pattern of pubertal changes in girls. Arch Dis Child 44:291–303, 1969.
37. MacMahon B. Age at menarche. *In* National Health Survey. Washington, DC, US Government Printing Office, 1973, p 1. US Department of Health, Education, and Welfare publication (HRA) 74–1615.
37a. Herman-Giddens ME, Slora EJ, Wasserman RC et al. Secondary sexual characteristics and menses in young girls seen in office practice: A study from the Pediatric Research in Office Settings Network. Pediatrics 99:505–512, 1997.
38. Harlan WR, Harlan EA, Grillo GP. Secondary sex characteristics of girls 12 to 17 years of age: The US Health Examination Survey. J Pediatr 96:1074–1078, 1980.
39. Apter D, Vihko R. Serum pregnenolone, progesterone, 17-hydroxyprogesterone, testosterone and 5α-dihydrotestosterone during female puberty. J Clin Endocrinol Metab 45:1039–1048, 1977.
40. Largo RH, Gasser T, Prader A, et al. Analysis of the adolescent growth spurt using smoothing spline functions. Ann Hum Biol 5:421–434, 1978.
41. Greulich WS, Pyle SI. Radiographic Atlas of Skeletal Development of the Hand and Wrist. Stanford, CA, Stanford University Press, 1959.
42. Forbes GB. Body composition in adolescence. *In* Falkner F, Tanner JM (eds). Human Growth. New York, Plenum Publishing, 1986, pp 119–145.
43. Chan GM, Hoffman K, McMurry M. Effects of dairy products on bone and body composition in pubertal girls. J Pediatr 126:551–556, 1995.
44. Lee WT, Leung SS, Leung DM, Cheng JC. A follow-up study on the effects of calcium-supplement withdrawal and puberty on bone acquisition of children. Am J Clin Nutr 64:71–77, 1996.
45. Eckert KL, Wilson DM, Bachrach LK, et al. A single-sample, subcutaneous gonadotropin-releasing hormone test for central precocious puberty. Pediatrics 97:517–519, 1996.
46. Thamdrup E. Precocious Sexual Development: A Clinical Study of 100 Children. Springfield, IL, Charles C Thomas, 1961, p 50.
47. Murram D, Dewhurst J, Grant DB. Precocious puberty: A follow-up study. Arch Dis Child 59:77–78, 1984.
48. Kaplan SL, Grumbach MM. Clinical review 14: Pathophysiology and treatment of sexual precocity. J Clin Endocrinol Metab 71:785–789, 1990.
49. Haber HP, Wollmann HA, Ranke MB. Pelvic ultrasonography: Early differentiation between isolated premature thelarche and central precocious puberty. Eur J Pediatr 154:182–186, 1995.
50. Harris DA, Van Vliet G, Egli CA, et al. Somatomedin-C in normal puberty and in true precocious puberty before and after treatment with a potent LRF agonist: Evidence for an effect of estrogen and testosterone on somatomedin-C concentrations. J Clin Endocrinol Metab 61:152–159, 1985.
51. Jenner MR, Kelch RP, Kaplan SL, Grumbach MM. Hormonal changes in puberty. IV. Plasma estradiol, LH, and FSH in prepubertal children, pubertal females, and in precocious puberty, premature thelarche, hypogonadism, and in a child with a feminizing ovarian tumor. J Clin Endocrinol Metab 34:521–530, 1972.
52. Robben SG, Oostdijk W, Drop SL, et al. Idiopathic isosexual central precocious puberty: Magnetic resonance findings in 30 patients. Br J Radiol 68:34–38, 1995.
53. Rappaport R, Brauner R. Growth and endocrine disorders secondary to cranial irradiation. Pediatr Res 25:561–567, 1989.
54. Laue L, Comite F, Hench K, et al. Precocious puberty associated with neurofibromatosis and optic gliomas. Treatment with luteinizing hormone releasing hormone analogue. Am J Dis Child 139:1097–1100, 1985.
55. Habiby R, Silverman B, Listernick R, Charrow J. Precocious puberty in children with neurofibromatosis type 1. J Pediatr 126:364–367, 1995.
56. Cara JF, Kreiter ML, Rosenfield RL. Height prognosis of children with true precocious puberty and growth hormone deficiency: Effect of combination therapy with gonadotropin releasing hormone agonist and growth hormone. J Pediatr 120:709–715, 1992.
57. Hahn FJ, Leibrock LG, Huseman CA, Makos MM. The MR appearance of hypothalamic hamartoma. Neuroradiology 30:65–68, 1988.
58. Turjman F, Xavier JL, Froment JC, et al. Late MR follow-up of hypothalamic hamartomas. Childs Nerv Syst 12:63–68, 1996.
59. Mahachoklertwattana P, Kaplan SL, Grumbach MM. The luteinizing hormone–releasing hormone–secreting hypothalamic hamartoma is a congenital malformation: Natural history. J Clin Endocrinol Metab 77:118–124, 1993.
60. Lopponen T, Saukkonen AL, Serlo W, et al. Accelerated pubertal development in patients with shunted hydrocephalus. Arch Dis Child 74:490–496, 1996.
61. Pescovitz OH, Comite F, Cassorla F, et al. True precocious puberty complicating congenital adrenal hyperplasia: Treatment with a luteinizing hormone–releasing hormone analog. J Clin Endocrinol Metab 58:857–861, 1984.
62. Anasti JN, Flack MR, Froehlich J, et al. A potential novel mechanism for precocious puberty in juvenile hypothyroidism. J Clin Endocrinol Metab 80:276–279, 1995.
63. Knobil E. The neuroendocrine control of the menstrual cycle. Recent Prog Horm Res 36:53–88, 1980.
64. Boepple PA, Mansfield MJ, Wierman ME, et al. Use of a potent, long acting agonist of gonadotropin-releasing hormone in the treatment of precocious puberty. Endocr Rev 7:24–33, 1986.
65. Styne DM, Harris DA, Egli CA, et al. Treatment of true precocious puberty with a potent luteinizing hormone–releasing factor agonist: Effect on growth, sexual maturation, pelvic sonography, and the hypothalamic-pituitary-gonadal axis. J Clin Endocrinol Metab 61:142–151, 1985.
66. Witchel SF, Baens-Bailon RG, Lee PA. Treatment of central precocious puberty: Comparison of urinary gonadotropin excretion and gonadotropin-releasing hormone (GnRH) stimulation tests in monitoring GnRH analog therapy. J Clin Endocrinol Metab 81:1353–1356, 1996.
67. Bridges NA, Cooke A, Healy MJ, et al. Ovaries in sexual precocity. Clin Endocrinol (Oxf) 42:135–140, 1995.
68. Paul D, Conte FA, Grumbach MM, Kaplan SL. Long-term effect of gonadotropin-releasing hormone agonist therapy on final and near-final height in 26 children with true precocious puberty treated at a median age of less than 5 years. J Clin Endocrinol Metab 80:546–551, 1995.
69. Verrotti A, Chiarelli F, Montanaro AF, Morgese G. Bone mineral content of girls with precocious puberty treated with gonadotropin-releasing hormone analog. Gynecol Endocrinol 9:277–281, 1995.
70. Manasco PK, Pescovitz OH, Feuillan PP, et al. Resumption of puberty after long term luteinizing hormone–releasing hormone agonist treatment of central precocious puberty. J Clin Endocrinol Metab 67:368–372, 1988.

71. Fontoura M, Brauner R, Prevot C, Rappaport R. Precocious puberty in girls: Early diagnosis of a slowly progressing variant. Arch Dis Child 64:1170–1176, 1989.
72. Bar A, Linder B, Sobel EH, et al. Bayley-Pinneau method of height prediction in girls with central precocious puberty: Correlation with adult height. J Pediatr 126:955–958, 1995.
73. Peters H, Byskov AG, Grinsted J. Follicular growth in fetal and prepubertal ovaries of humans and other primates. Clin Endocrinol Metab 7:469–485, 1978.
74. Millar DM, Blake JM, Stringer DA, et al. Prepubertal ovarian cysts formation: 5 years' experience. Obstet Gynecol 81:434–438, 1993.
75. Lyon AJ, De Bruyn R, Grant DB. Transient sexual precocity and ovarian cysts. Arch Dis Child 60:819–822, 1985.
76. Biscotti CV, Hart WR. Juvenile granulosa cell tumors of the ovary. Arch Pathol Lab Med 113:40–46, 1989.
77. Gribbon M, Ein SH, Mancer K. Pediatric malignant ovarian tumors: A 43-year review. J Pediatr Surg 27:480–484, 1992.
78. Young RH, Dickersin GR, Scully RE. A distinctive ovarian sex cord–stromal tumor causing sexual precocity in the Peutz-Jeghers syndrome. Am J Surg Pathol 7:233–243, 1983.
79. Lee PA, Van Dop C, Migeon CJ. McCune-Albright syndrome. Long-term follow-up. JAMA 256:2980–2984, 1986.
80. Schwindinger WF, Francomano CA, Levine MA. Identification of a mutation in the gene encoding the alpha subunit of the stimulatory G protein of adenylyl cyclase in McCune-Albright syndrome. Proc Natl Acad Sci USA 89:5152–5156, 1992.
81. Feuillan PP, Jones J, Cutler GB. Long-term testolactone therapy for precocious puberty in girls with the McCune-Albright syndrome. J Clin Endocrinol Metab 77:647–651, 1993.
82. Cook CD, McArthur JW, Berenberg W. Pseudoprecocious puberty in girls as a result of estrogen ingestion. N Engl J Med 248:671–674, 1953.
83. Mills JL, Stolley PD, Davies J, Moshang TJ. Premature thelarche. Natural history and etiologic investigation. Am J Dis Child 135:743–745, 1981.
84. Pescovitz OH, Hench KD, Barnes KM, et al. Premature thelarche and central precocious puberty: The relationship between clinical presentation and the gonadotropin response to luteinizing hormone–releasing hormone. J Clin Endocrinol Metab 67:474–479, 1988.
85. Garibaldi LR, Aceto TJ, Weber C. The pattern of gonadotropin and estradiol secretion in exaggerated thelarche. Acta Endocrinol 128:345–350, 1993.
86. Stanhope R, Abdulwahid NA, Adams J, Brook CG. Studies of gonadotrophin pulsatility and pelvic ultrasound examinations distinguish between isolated premature thelarche and central precocious puberty. Eur J Pediatr 145:190–194, 1986.
87. Pasquino AM, Pucarelli I, Passeri F, et al. Progression of premature thelarche to central precocious puberty. J Pediatr 126:11–14, 1996.
88. Murram D, Dewhurst J, Grant DB. Premature menarche: A follow-up study. Arch Dis Child 58:142–143, 1983.
89. Hill NC, Oppenheimer LW, Morton KE. The aetiology of vaginal bleeding in children. A 20-year review. Br J Obstet Gynaecol 96:467–470, 1989.
90. Morel Y, Miller WL. Clinical and molecular genetics of congenital adrenal hyperplasia due to 21-hydroxylase deficiency. Adv Hum Genet 20:1–68, 1991.
91. Miller WL. Genetics, diagnosis, and management of 21-hydroxylase deficiency. J Clin Endocrinol Metab 78:241–246, 1994.
92. Mulaikal RM, Migeon CJ, Rock JA. Fertility rates in female patients with congenital adrenal hyperplasia due to 21-hydroxylase deficiency. N Engl J Med 316:178–182, 1987.
93. Kuhnle U, Bollinger M, Schwarz HP, Knorr D. Partnership and sexuality in adult female patients with congenital adrenal hyperplasia. First results of a cross-sectional quality-of-life evaluation. J Steroid Biochem Mol Biol 45:123–126, 1993.
94. Azziz R, Dewailly D, Owerbach D. Nonclassic adrenal hyperplasia: Current concepts. J Clin Endocrinol Metab 78:810–815, 1994.
95. Bristow J, Tee MK, Gitelman SE, et al. Tenascin-X. A novel extracellular matrix protein encoded by the human XB gene overlapping P450c21B. J Cell Biol 122:265–278, 1993.
96. Crowne EC, Shalet SM, Wallace WH, et al. Final height in girls with untreated constitutional delay in growth and puberty. Eur J Pediatr 150:708–712, 1991.
97. LaFranchi S, Hanna CE, Mandel SH. Constitutional delay of growth: Expected versus final adult height. Pediatrics 87:82–87, 1991.
98. Bramswig JH, Fasse M, Holthoff ML, et al. Adult height in boys and girls with untreated short stature and constitutional delay of growth and puberty: Accuracy of five different methods of height prediction. J Pediatr 117:886–891, 1990.
99. Marin G, Domene HM, Barnes KM, et al. The effects of estrogen priming and puberty on the growth hormone response to standardized treadmill exercise and arginine-insulin in normal girls and boys. J Clin Endocrinol Metab 79:537–541, 1994.
100. Thomsett MJ, Conte FA, Kaplan SL, Grumbach MM. Endocrine and neurologic outcome in childhood craniopharyngioma: Review of effect of treatment in 42 patients. J Pediatr 97:728–735, 1980.
101. Baskin DS, Wilson CB. Surgical management of craniopharyngiomas. A review of 74 cases. J Neurosurg 65:22–27, 1986.
102. Fischer EG, Welch K, Shillito JJ, et al. Craniopharyngiomas in children. Long-term effects of conservative surgical procedures combined with radiation therapy. J Neurosurg 73:534–540, 1990.
103. Mindermann T, Wilson CB. Pediatric pituitary adenomas. Neurosurgery 36:259–268, 1995.
104. Sklar CA, Grumbach MM, Kaplan SL, Conte FA. Hormonal and metabolic abnormalities associated with central nervous system germinoma in children and adolescents and the effect of therapy: Report of 10 patients. J Clin Endocrinol Metab 52:9–16, 1981.
105. Wara WM, Fellows FC, Sheline GE. Radiation therapy for pineal tumors and suprasellar germinomas. Radiology 124:221–223, 1977.
106. Sims DG. Histiocytosis X; follow-up of 43 cases. Arch Dis Child 52:433–440, 1977.
107. Hanna CE, Mandel SH, LaFranchi SH. Puberty in the syndrome of septo-optic dysplasia. Am J Dis Child 143:186–189, 1989.
108. Santoro N, Filicori M, Crowley WF. Hypogonadotropic disorders in men and women: Diagnosis and therapy with pulsatile gonadotropin releasing hormone. Endocr Rev 7:11–23, 1986.
109. Franco B, Guioli S, Pragliola A, et al. A gene deleted in Kallmann's syndrome shares homology with neural cell adhesion and axonal path-finding molecules. Nature 353:529–536, 1991.
110. Legouis R, Hardelin J-P, Levilliers J, et al. The candidate gene for the X-linked Kallmann syndrome encodes a protein related to adhesion molecules. Cell 67:423–435, 1991.
110a. Quinton R, Duke VM, deZoysa PA, et al. The neuroradiology of Kallmann's syndrome: A genotypic and phenotypic analysis. J Clin Endocrinol Metab 81:3010–3017, 1996.
111. Richards GE, Wara WM, Grumbach MM, et al. Delayed onset of hypopituitarism: Sequelae of therapeutic irradiation of central nervous system, eye, and middle ear tumors. J Pediatr 89:553–559, 1976.
112. Sklar CA, Constine LS. Chronic neuroendocrinological sequelae of radiation therapy. Int J Radiat Oncol Biol Phys 31:1113–1121, 1995.
113. Kulin HE, Bwibo N, Mutie D, Santner SJ. Gonadotropin excretion during puberty in malnourished children. J Pediatr 105:325–328, 1984.
114. Van Diemen-Steenvoorde R, Donckerwolcke RA. Growth and sexual maturation in paediatric patients treated by dialysis and following kidney transplantation. Acta Paediatr Scand Suppl 343:109–117, 1988.
115. Siris ES, Leventhal BG, Vaitukaitis JL. Effects of childhood leukemia and chemotherapy on puberty and reproductive function in girls. N Engl J Med 294:1143–1146, 1976.
115a. Devoe DJ, Miller WL, Conte FA, et al. Long-term outcome in children and adolescents after transsphenoidal surgery for Cushing disease. J Clin Endocrinol Metab 82:3196–3202, 1997.
116. Crisp AH. The dyslipophobias: A view of the psychopathologies involved and the hazards of construing anorexia nervosa and bulimia nervosa as "eating disorders." Proc Nutr Soc 54:701–709, 1996.
117. Schwabe AD, Lippe BM, Chang RJ, et al. Anorexia nervosa. Ann Intern Med 94:371–381, 1981.
118. Marshall JC, Kelch RP. Low dose pulsatile gonadotropin-releasing hormone in anorexia nervosa: A model of human pubertal development. J Clin Endocrinol Metab 49:712–718, 1979.

119. Russell GFM. Bulimia nervosa: An ominous variant of anorexia nervosa. Psychol Med 9:429–448, 1979.
120. Warren MP. Metabolic factors and the onset of puberty. *In* Grumbach MM, Sizonenko PC, Aubert ML (eds). Control of the Onset of Puberty. Baltimore, Williams & Wilkins, 1990, pp 553–573.
121. Laughlin GA, Yen SSC. Nutritional and endocrine-metabolic aberrations in amenorrheic athletes. J Clin Endocrinol Metab 81:4301–4309, 1996.
122. Theintz GE, Howald H, Weiss U, Sizonenko PC. Evidence for a reduction of growth potential in adolescent female gymnasts. J Pediatr 122:306–313, 1993.
123. Lindholm C, Hagenfeldt K, Ringertz BM. Pubertal development in elite juvenile gymnasts. Effects of physical training. Acta Obstet Gynecol Scand 73:269–273, 1994.
124. Tofler IR, Stryer BK, Micheli LJ, Herman LR. Physical and emotional problems of elite female gymnasts. N Engl J Med 335:281–283, 1996.
125. Patton ML, Woolf PD. Hyperprolactinemia and delayed puberty: A report of three cases and their response to therapy. Pediatrics 71:572–575, 1983.
126. Brisson GR, Volle MA, Desharnais M, et al. Exercise induced dissociation of the blood prolactin response in young women according to their sports habits. Horm Metab 21:201–205, 1980.
127. Grumbach MM, Conte FA. Disorders of sexual differentiation. *In* Wilson JD, Foster DW (eds). Williams Textbook of Endocrinology. Philadelphia, WB Saunders, 1992, pp 853–952.
128. Ross JL, Feuillan P, Long LM, et al. Lipid abnormalities in Turner syndrome. J Pediatr 126:242–245, 1995.
129. Lyon AJ, Preece MA, Grant DB. Growth curve for girls with Turner syndrome. Arch Dis Child 60:932–935, 1985.
129a. Ellison JW, Wardak Z, Young MF, et al. PHOG, a candidate gene for involvement in the short stature of Turner syndrome. Hum Mol Genet 6:1341–1347, 1997.
129b. Rao E, Weiss B, Fukami M, et al. Pseudoautosomal deletions encompassing a novel homeobox gene cause growth failure in idiopathic short stature and Turner syndrome. Nature Genet 16:54–63, 1997.
130. Scully RE. Gonadoblastoma: A review of 74 cases. Cancer 25:1340–1356, 1970.
131. Ranke MB, Heidemann P, Knupfer C, et al. Noonan's syndrome: Growth and clinical manifestations in 144 cases. Eur J Pediatr 148:220–227, 1988.
132. Hauffa BP, Miller WL, Grumbach MM, et al. Congenital adrenal hyperplasia due to deficient cholesterol side-chain cleavage activity (20,22-desmolase) in a patient treated for 18 years. Clin Endocrinol (Oxf) 23:481–493, 1985.
133. Voutilainen R, Miller WL. Developmental expression of genes for the steroidogenic enzymes P450scc (20,22-desmolase), P450c17 (17α-hydroxylase/17,20-lyase) and P450c21 (21-hydroxylase) in the human fetus. J Clin Endocrinol Metab 63:1145–1150, 1986.
134. Lin D, Gitelman SE, Saenger P, Miller WL. Normal genes for the cholesterol side chain cleavage enzyme, P450scc, in congenital lipoid adrenal hyperplasia. J Clin Invest 88:1955–1962, 1991.
135. Lin D, Sugawara T, Strauss JF III, et al. Role of steroidogenic acute regulatory protein in adrenal and gonadal steroidogenesis. Science 267:1828–1831, 1995.
136. Tee MK, Lin D, Sugawara T, et al. T → A transversion 11 bp from a splice acceptor site in the gene for steroidogenic acute regulatory protein causes congenital lipoid adrenal hyperplasia. Hum Mol Genet 4:2299–2305, 1995.
137. Yang X, Iwamoto K, Wang M, et al. Inherited congenital adrenal hyperplasia in the rabbit is caused by a deletion in the gene encoding cytochrome P450 cholesterol side-chain cleavage enzyme. Endocrinology 132:1977–1982, 1993.
138. Saenger P, Klonari Z, Black SM, et al. Prenatal diagnosis of congenital lipoid adrenal hyperplasia. J Clin Endocrinol Metab 80:200–205, 1995.
139. Bose HS, Pescovitz OH, Miller WL. Spontaneous feminization in a 46,XX female patient with congenital lipoid adrenal hyperplasia due to a homozygous frameshift mutation in the steroidogenic acute regulatory protein. J Clin Endocrinol Metab 82:1511-1515, 1997.
140. Morel Y, Mebarki F, Rhéaume E, et al. Structure-function relationships of 3β-hydroxysteroid dehydrogenase: Contributions made by the molecular genetics of 3β-HSD deficiency. Steroids 62:178–186, 1997.
141. Cara JF, Moshang T Jr, Bongiovanni AM, Marx BS. Elevated 17-hydroxy-progesterone and testosterone in a newborn with 3β-hydroxysteroid dehydrogenase deficiency. N Engl J Med 313:618–621, 1985.
142. Yanase T, Simpson ER, Waterman MR. 17α-Hydroxylase/17,20-lyase deficiency: From clinical investigation to molecular definition. Endocr Rev 12:91–108, 1991.
143. Fardella CE, Hum DW, Homoki J, Miller WL. Point mutation Arg440 to His in cytochrome P450c17 causes severe 17α-hydroxylase deficiency. J Clin Endocrinol Metab 79:160–164, 1994.
143a. Geller DH, Auchus RJ, Mendonca BB, Miller WL. The genetic and functional basis of isolated 17,20-lyase deficiency. Nature Genet 17:201–205, 1997.
144. Barrett A, Nicholls J, Gibson B. Late effects of total body irradiation. Radiother Oncol 9:131–135, 1987.
145. Mackie EJ, Radford M, Shalet SM. Gonadal function following chemotherapy for childhood Hodgkin's disease. Med Pediatr Oncol 27:74–78, 1996.
146. Ahonen P, Myllarniemi S, Sipila I, et al. Clinical variation of autoimmune polyendocrinopathy–candidiasis–ectodermal dystrophy (APECED) in a series of 68 patients. N Engl J Med 322:1829–1836, 1990.
146a. Aittomäki K, Herva R, Stenman U-H, et al. Clinical features of primary ovarian failure caused by a point mutation in the follicle-stimulating hormone receptor gene. J Clin Endocrinol Metab 81:3722–3726, 1996.
146b. Latronico AC, Anasti J, Arnold IP. Testicular and ovarian resistance to luteinizing hormone caused by inactivating mutations of the luteinizing hormone receptor gene. N Engl J Med 344:507–512, 1996.
147. Rosenfield RL. Clinical review 6: Diagnosis and management of delayed puberty. J Clin Endocrinol Metab 70:559–562, 1990.
148. Carel JC, Hay F, Coutant R, et al. Gonadotropin-releasing hormone agonist treatment of girls with constitutional short stature and normal pubertal development. J Clin Endocrinol Metab 132:699–704, 1996.
149. Rosenfeld RG, Frane J, Attie KM, et al. Six-year results of a randomized, prospective trial of human growth hormone and oxandrolone in Turner syndrome. J Pediatr 121:49–55, 1992.
150. Neely EK, Marcus R, Rosenfeld FG, Bachrach LK. Turner syndrome adolescents receiving growth hormone are not osteopenic. J Clin Endocrinol Metab 76:861–866, 1993.

Chapter 16

THE THYROID GLAND AND REPRODUCTION

Silvio E. Inzucchi • Gerard N. Burrow

■ CHAPTER OUTLINE

KEY POINTS

- The essentials of thyroid anatomy and physiology are briefly summarized.
- The most common functional and anatomic thyroid diseases are discussed.
- With this background, the notable changes in maternal and fetal thyroid function during gestation are presented.
- The effects of hypothyroidism on both fertility and pregnancy are reviewed, with particular attention to iodine deficiency and thyroid autoimmunity.
- The corresponding effects of hyperthyroidism are delineated, with a discussion of the various causes of thyrotoxicosis during pregnancy, their diagnosis, therapy, and possible complications.
- Thyroid dysfunction in the postpartum setting is reviewed.
- Brief mention is made of the effects of radioiodine on reproductive health and the relationship of thyroid dysfunction and osteoporosis.

For reasons that are not fully understood, both functional and anatomic diseases of the thyroid are 5 to 10 times more common in females than in males at all ages. Many of these conditions are autoimmune in nature and, as such, peak in incidence during childbearing years. Thus, thyroid disease is frequently encountered in the practice of reproductive medicine. Hypothyroidism, in particular, is common in adult women. During reproductive years, substantial effects on menstrual function, fertility, and gestational outcome are observed. In later years, treatment of hypothyroidism carries with it certain precautions during the menopause. Hyperthyroidism also has profound effects on reproductive physiology. Although fertility is not affected as in hypothyroidism, abnormalities of the menstrual cycle are encountered. In the pregnant woman, the diagnosis and management of hyperthyroidism may be particularly complex, because gestation affects the clinical manifestations of thyrotoxicosis as well as the approaches available to diagnosis and therapy. In addition, during pregnancy, thyrotoxicosis may itself have significant effects on both the mother and the fetus. Finally, the approach to other thyroid conditions such as nodular disease must also be modified during pregnancy. For these reasons, among others, familiarity with the thyroid gland and its functions, diseases, and relationships with other hormonal axes is necessary for an optimal understanding of reproduction.

THE THYROID: BASIC CONCEPTS

Anatomy

The thyroid gland is a bilobed structure with an interconnecting isthmus, whose center lies directly anterior to the second or third tracheal ring, just below the cricoid cartilage. The normal adult thyroid weighs 15 to 20 gm; each lobe measures 4 to 5 cm in length, 2 to 3 cm in width, and 1 to 2 cm in thickness. A vestigial pyramidal lobe is often present, emanating from the isthmus, adjacent to the left lobe.

Essentials of Iodine Metabolism

Thyroid hormone production is, in part, dependent on the supply of iodine, which is solely derived from dietary sources. The recommended intake of iodine is 100 to 150 μg/day for adults and 200 μg/day in pregnant women. Iodine-deficient areas, predominantly in Africa and Asia, have average intakes of less than 50 μg/day. Areas with borderline iodine supply, including regions of central Europe, have average intakes of 60 to 90 μg/day. When the physiologic requirements for iodine are met only marginally by a population's dietary habits, increased frequency of hypothyroidism and euthyroid goiter (both diffuse and nodular) occurs.[1] When dietary iodine supply is severely deficient, especially if other intrinsic diseases of the thyroid are present or if the diet contains other goitrogens, functional and anatomic abnormalities of the thyroid become more manifest. Endemic goiter and cretinism, endemic mental retardation, decreased fertility rates, and increased perinatal death rates and infant mortality are seen. At least 1 billion people may be at risk for iodine deficiency, by far the most common preventable cause of cognitive impairment in the world.[1]

The thyroid's responses to alterations in iodine supply have been well studied. When iodine intake is low, the gland's 24-hour radioiodine uptake increases above the usual 15 to 30 percent. Similarly, when the supply is abundant, as may be seen in patients taking iodine-containing medications, uptake is usually low. Indeed, a decrease in thyroid hormone production, known as the Wolff-Chaikoff effect, occurs acutely.[2] Such a homeostatic mechanism ensures a steady supply of thyroid hormones in the face of significant alterations in substrate availability. In certain thyroid disease states, however, the gland's response to a change in iodine supply may have a negative impact on thyroid hormone metabolism. For instance, the normal thyroid, after 2 to 3 weeks, "escapes" from the Wolff-Chaikoff effect, and thyroid hormone production is eventually normalized. Failure to escape, with prolonged hypothyroidism, however, may be seen in autoimmune thyroid disease. When iodine supply is abruptly increased to an autonomous thyroid that is rendered independent of hypothalamic-pituitary control, as in multinodular goiter, unrestrained overproduction of thyroid hormone may occur.[3] This phenomenon is known as jodbasedow, after the German physician von Basedow, who first made this observation in the 19th century (*jod* is the German word for iodine).

Normal Thyroid Physiology

The chief, perhaps sole function of the thyroid is to produce thyroid hormones. It is responsible for the production of all circulating thyroxine (T_4) and 20 percent of triiodothyronine (T_3). Most of the body's supply of T_3 results from the peripheral conversion of T_4 through a variety of deiodinases, which demonstrate interesting tissue specificity.

The functional unit of the thyroid gland is the thyroid follicle, composed of a spherical alignment of cuboid epithelial cells surrounding a core of colloid. Colloid consists primarily of thyroglobulin, which provides tyrosine residues for serial iodination that results, through a complex series of biochemical and biophysical alterations, in the production of the terminal hormones T_4 and T_3.[4] The follicular cell is responsible for the production of thyroglobulin, the uptake of inorganic iodide from the circulation and its organification into iodinated thyronine compounds, the reuptake of formed thyroid hormone at its juxtacolloidal apical membrane, the transcellular diffusion of this hormone, and its ultimate release into the systemic circulation at its basolateral surface. Follicular cell activity is under the direct control of the pituitary gland, by the secretion of thyrotropin or thyroid-stimulating hormone (TSH), whose production is modulated by the hypothalamic secretion of thyrotropin-releasing hormone (TRH).

Thyroid hormones circulate in a mostly bound form, distributed among thyroid-binding globulin (TBG) and, to a lesser extent, albumin and prealbumin. T_4 and T_3, whose total serum concentrations are approximately 5 to 12 μg/dl and 80 to 200 ng/dl, respectively, circulate greater than 99 percent bound to plasma proteins.[5] As in most endocrine systems, the free fractions of these hormones, *not* the total concentrations, are physiologically important.

The Control of Thyroid Hormone Secretion

The control of the secretion of thyroid hormones is diagrammed in Figure 16–1. In normal circumstances, the circulating concentration of T_4, the most abundant and commonly measured thyroid hormone, is maintained within a narrow range varying little from day to day.

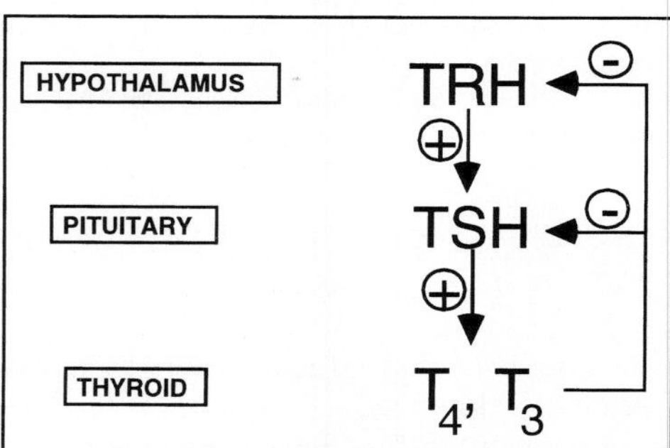

Figure 16–1 ■ Diagrammatic relationship of the hypothalamic-pituitary-thyroid axis.

Iodine uptake, thyroid hormone production, and thyroid follicle growth are under the control of the hypothalamic-pituitary axis. The hypothalamus elaborates TRH, a tripeptide. TRH enters the portal circulation of the infundibular stalk and travels to the anterior lobe of the pituitary, where it stimulates specific cells (thyrotrophs) to produce TSH. TSH, a glycoprotein, is a more complex structure than TRH. It is composed of two chains, α and β, similar in structure to the glycoproteins luteinizing hormone, follicle-stimulating hormone, and human chorionic gonadotropin (hCG). Indeed, all these share a common α-subunit, with the β chain lending specificity. (The importance of the similarity in structure between hCG and TSH becomes obvious when pregnancy-related thyrotoxicosis is discussed later.) As with other glycoprotein hormones, the activity and metabolic clearance of TSH is altered by post-translational glycosylation. TSH secretion varies diurnally, with peak secretion occurring between 11 PM and 4 AM.[6] It interacts with a specific receptor at the basolateral surface of thyroid follicular cells, a member of the superfamily of G protein–linked transmembrane receptors.[7] Interaction with TSH results in a complex series of second messenger steps and, ultimately, the production and release of thyroid hormones.

Through a classical endocrine negative feedback loop, decreased circulating concentrations of thyroid hormones (probably T_4, which is converted to T_3 within pituitary cells) lead to an increase in TRH and TSH secretion, which in turn stimulate increased thyroid growth and activity. Thus, in primary hypothyroid states, TRH and TSH secretion is augmented, and measured TSH concentrations are elevated. In situations of thyroid hormone excess, such as Graves' hyperthyroidism, TRH and TSH secretion is suppressed; TSH serum levels are almost invariably undetectable in reliable assays.

The Physiologic Role of Thyroid Hormone

The exact role of thyroid hormone remains incompletely understood, although it clearly interacts with numerous biologic systems. This importance is demonstrated by the myriad signs and symptoms involving multiple organs in patients with altered thyroid hormone metabolism. T_3, which is the "active" hormone, is transported into cells and interacts with a specific nuclear receptor. The T_3-receptor complex functions as a transcription factor, working with other nuclear proteins to regulate gene expression.[8] Thyroid hormone response elements are located adjacent to many genes. T_3 interaction with thyroid hormone response elements serves to enhance or diminish protein transcription. In addition, thyroid hormone appears to have important extranuclear actions, such as regulation of deiodinase activity and, perhaps, mitochondrial function.

The reproductive system requires normal amounts of thyroid hormone for adequate functioning. Disturbances in menstrual function are commonly seen in women with either hypothyroidism or hyperthyroidism, with menometrorrhagia occurring in the former and oligomenorrhea reported in the latter. The association between hyperthyroidism and menstrual disturbance may be overstated, however, on the basis of one study.[9] Infertility is also commonly reported in women with severe hypothyroidism, whereas fertility is usually maintained in most hyperthyroid women. Once conception has occurred, thyroid hormone remains important not only for the development of the fetus but for the viability of the pregnancy itself; increased incidence of fetal loss is observed in both hypothyroid and hyperthyroid pregnancies.[10] It has been shown, in an organ culture system of early-term human placentas, that both T_3 and T_4 stimulate steroid hormone production, with no such effect observed in term placentas. These effects were diminished with both increasing and decreasing concentrations of thyroid hormones. Therefore, the increased incidence of spontaneous abortion in dysthyroid states might result from inadequate trophoblast endocrine function secondary to thyroid hormone imbalance.[11]

Diagnosis of Abnormal Thyroid Function

The diagnosis of functional abnormalities of the thyroid has been simplified by the availability of excellent immunoassays in the modern laboratory. In hypothyroidism, as thyroid hormone levels begin to fall, a compensatory increase in the pituitary secretion of TSH occurs, which in turn maintains T_4 and T_3 within normal range, often for a period of years. As progressive thyroid failure ensues, despite increasing concentrations of TSH, further decreases in thyroid hormone levels occur, with an accompanying clinical syndrome. Thus, an elevated TSH with normal free T_4 (fT_4) or free thyroxine index (FTI) is termed subclinical hypothyroidism (although certain subtle symptoms may indeed be present). When TSH is elevated and fT_4 or FTI is low, frank hypothyroidism is said to be present. Total and free T_3 (fT_3) fall to subnormal levels only in the very late stages of the disease and are not useful for making the diagnosis of hypothyroidism. The measurement of TSH alone, when elevated, is sufficient to secure the diagnosis of primary hypothyroidism. Secondary or tertiary hypothyroidism (i.e., due to pituitary or hypothalamic disease) is a more difficult diagnosis, because thyroid hormone levels are not as dramatically low as they may become in primary thyroid failure, and TSH is usually low (although it may be "inappropriately normal" or even minimally elevated in certain situations).[12]

Similarly, thyrotoxicosis is easily diagnosed after clinical evaluation of the patient, with a few concise biochemical tests. The response of pituitary TSH secretion to elevated concentrations of thyroid hormones is the reciprocal of that which occurs in primary hypothyroidism. That is, TSH secretion falls in this setting, almost always to undetectable levels, depending on the sensitivity of the assay used. In modern third-generation assays using chemoluminescence, sensitivity approaches 0.01 mU/L, a marked improvement from earlier assays that had difficulty distinguishing the truly thyrotoxic from those with low TSH levels yet normal thyroid function or those patients with the "euthyroid sick syndrome." Today, when fT_4 or FTI is elevated and TSH is below the detection limits of the assay, the patient can be considered at least biochemically thyrotoxic.

THYROID DISEASE STATES

Functional Disorders of the Thyroid

Hypothyroidism

The differential diagnosis of hypothyroidism is listed in Table 16–1. Common signs and symptoms are noted in

■ TABLE 16–1
Differential Diagnosis of Hypothyroidism

Primary Hypothyroidism

Iodine deficiency
Chronic autoimmune thyroiditis (Hashimoto's)
Silent/postpartum thyroiditis (hypothyroid phase)
Subacute thyroiditis (hypothyroid phase)
Thyroid dysgenesis/agenesis
Organification enzyme defects
Drugs (thioamides, lithium)
Dietary goitrogens
Radioiodine ablation
External-beam neck irradiation (high-dose)
Thyroidectomy

Secondary/Tertiary Hypothyroidism

Pituitary adenoma
Pituitary necrosis/hemorrhage
Lymphocytic hypophysitis
Central nervous system sarcoidosis
Histiocytosis
Hypophysectomy
Cranial irradiation
Suprasellar/parasellar neoplasms
Traumatic injury to pituitary/hypothalamus

Table 16–2. The majority of cases in the United States result from chronic autoimmune thyroiditis (Hashimoto's disease).[13] The majority of patients affected have elevated circulating titers of thyroid autoantibodies, such as those directed against microsomal thyroid peroxidase or to thyroglobulin itself. This disorder consists of two forms, one goitrous and one atrophic, based on the clinical appearance of the gland. Patients experience a variable but typically lengthy period of subclinical hypothyroidism, with absent or minimal symptoms. Free thyroid hormone levels remain within normal range, yet at the expense of increased TSH secretion. The majority of these patients eventually develop progressive thyroid failure, with fT_4 becoming frankly low, and symptoms eventually become more manifest. Biochemical and symptomatic improvement occurs with thyroid hormone replacement therapy, usually in the form of levothyroxine, in doses typically between 75 and 200 μg/day, as titrated to a normal TSH.

Thyrotoxicosis

Causes of thyrotoxicosis are listed in Table 16–3. Signs and symptoms of this common disorder are included in

■ TABLE 16–2
Common Clinical Features of Hypothyroidism

Weight gain	Bradycardia
Fatigue	Congestive heart failure
Cold intolerance	Pleural effusions
Constipation	Hoarseness
Cool, dry skin	Cognitive deficits
Coarsened hair	Anemia
Periorbital edema	Macroglossia
Generalized edema	Menorrhagia
Muscle weakness	Infertility

■ TABLE 16–3
Differential Diagnosis of Thyrotoxicosis

Graves' disease
Thyroiditis
  Silent/postpartum (lymphocytic)
  Subacute (granulomatous)
  Suppurative (bacterial)
Toxic multinodular goiter
Solitary toxic nodule
Exogenous thyroid hormone ingestion
Iodine-induced thyrotoxicosis
Thyroid-stimulating hormone–secreting pituitary adenoma
Pituitary resistance to thyroid hormone
Struma ovarii
Gestational trophoblastic disease
(?Hyperemesis gravidarum)

Table 16–4. The term thyrotoxicosis refers to a clinical syndrome marked by excess circulating levels of both fT_4 and fT_3 and encompasses a broad range of disorders. Hyperthyroidism, on the other hand, should be used to define those causes of thyrotoxicosis that are attributable to an overactive thyroid gland, as occurs in Graves' disease or nodular goiter. Acute thyroiditis, for example, may lead to thyrotoxicosis but is not truly a "hyperthyroid" state, because hormone production by the thyroid is actually decreased secondary to active glandular inflammation.

The most common cause of thyrotoxicosis in the United States is Graves' disease, an autoimmune multisystem disorder that may involve abnormalities of the thyroid, the orbits, and the skin.[14] In this condition, hyperthyroidism results from the unregulated stimulation of an intrinsically normal thyroid by thyroid-stimulating immunoglobulin (TSI), which activates the TSH receptor.[15] Extrathyroidal manifestations often clearly set Graves' disease apart from other forms of hyperthyroidism. It may also be seen in conjunction with a personal or family history of other autoimmune conditions, such as myasthenia gravis or collagen-vascular disease. Graves' disease is usually associated with a small or moderate-sized goiter. Thyroid function test results are elevated to a variable degree, and TSH is suppressed. When a patient is truly thyrotoxic with an elevated fT_4 yet the TSH concentration is either normal or elevated, the possibility of much rarer diagnoses, such as a TSH-secreting pituitary adenoma or pituitary resistance to thyroid hormone, is raised.[16] The diagnosis of Graves' disease is supported by a 24-hour radioiodine uptake and a nuclear thyroid scan showing increased and diffusely homogeneous uptake. Various treatment options are avail-

■ TABLE 16–4
Common Clinical Features of Thyrotoxicosis

Weight loss	Hyperdefecation
Fatigue	Diaphoresis
Increased appetite	Heat intolerance
Palpitations	Lid lag, "stare"
Supraventricular arrhythmias	Dyspnea on exertion
Anxiety	Congestive heart failure
Tremor	Proximal myopathy
Hyperreflexia	Oligomenorrhea

able, including subtotal thyroidectomy, antithyroid drug therapy with agents of the thioamide class (propylthiouracil [PTU], methimazole [MMI]), or radioablation with ^{131}I; each has its advantages and disadvantages. Antithyroid drug therapy is typically chosen initially in most patients, because this results in a rapid normalization of thyroid hormone levels. Once a euthyroid state is achieved, radioiodine may then be administered. Thioamide therapy may be continued for longer periods, with radioiodine reserved for those cases in which remission does not occur after 1 to 2 years. The natural history of Graves' disease is for hypothyroidism to eventually develop, as progressive inflammatory changes lead to fibrosis and gland dysfunction. However, this may take decades to occur and does not obviate the need to treat the thyrotoxicosis when it is present.

Anatomic Disorders of the Thyroid

Anatomic disorders of the thyroid include nodular disease and goiter. The term goiter refers to enlargement of the entire thyroid, with either a diffuse or nodular character; it is often misused, however, to describe any enlargement, even of portions of the thyroid, such as occurs in solitary nodules.

Thyroid Nodules

Nodules of the thyroid are common; they are palpable in 5 percent of the general population,[17] depending on the population, sex, and geographic region examined, being more common in areas of relative iodine deficiency. Attention must be paid to the careful evaluation of thyroid nodules because of the small but real potential of malignant transformation. Although this occurs in only 5 percent of clinically detectable lesions, greater risk occurs at the extremes of the life cycle, in the largest nodules, in those nodules whose growth is progressive, and in patients with other risks for thyroid malignant neoplasia such as a prior history of neck irradiation. The actual incidence of thyroid cancer is not appreciably different between the sexes. However, because benign nodules are much more common in women, an individual nodule discovered in a man carries with it an apparently greater risk of malignancy.

The majority of nodules are found, by pathologic examination, to be either hyperplastic or adenomatous in origin. Benign and malignant neoplasms of the thyroid are listed in Table 16–5; papillary and follicular carcinomas represent the majority of the cancers. Diagnosis of the thyroid nodule is most rapidly performed with the fine-needle aspiration technique.[17] Specimens are interpreted by the cytologist as benign, suspicious for malignancy (usually papillary carcinoma), or indeterminate. This last category includes follicular neoplasms, with the distinction between follicular adenoma and carcinoma by definition requiring examination of the surgical specimen in toto. Ultrasound examination may be helpful in distinguishing simple cysts from solid nodules and in determining if other nonpalpable lesions exist, as in multinodular goiter. In addition, serial ultrasound examinations may be useful in the follow-up of lesions, although the cost-effectiveness of this approach is questionable. Because it is a purely anatomic study and does not yield any functional or histologic information, ultrasonography is not routinely helpful in the initial evaluation of thyroid nodules. Scintigraphy, with either technetium or radioiodine, will provide functional information that may be important because, with few exceptions, functional ("hot") nodules are rarely malignant, and virtually all carcinomas are nonfunctional ("cold"). With the advent of the fine-needle aspiration technique, however, nuclear medicine studies are becoming less relevant during the initial evaluation of thyroid nodules. In the United States, most (>90 percent) nodules are nonfunctional (i.e., cold by scintigraphy), but only a small minority of these are actually malignant. Thus, the cost-effectiveness of a diagnostic procedure that only confirms an a priori clinical impression has been called into question.[17] In iodine-deficient regions of the world, such as in parts of Europe, the percentage of hot nodules is increased. Here, scintigraphy may be of greater usefulness, because a greater percentage of patients may be safely excluded from further evaluation. Most experts agree that in the United States, nuclear studies are most useful for those nodules with indeterminate cytology by fine-needle aspiration, because hot or warm nodules reside overwhelmingly in this category. Figure 16–2 outlines a rational diagnostic approach for the evaluation of the thyroid nodule. The treatment and follow-up of thyroid malignant neoplasms and a detailed discussion of the utility of thyroid hormone suppression therapy for nodules are outside the scope of this text.

■ TABLE 16–5
Most Common Causes of Thyroid Nodules

Benign
Follicular adenoma
Colloid nodule
Hürthle cell adenoma
Multinodular goiter
Simple cyst
Nodular autoimmune thyroiditis
Marine-Lenhart nodule (in Graves' disease)
Malignant
Papillary carcinoma
Follicular carcinoma
Hürthle cell carcinoma
Medullary carcinoma
Anaplastic carcinoma
Lymphoma
Metastases to the thyroid

Goiter

Goiter may be distinguished into several categories on the basis of the functional status of the gland (hypothyroid, hyperthyroid, or euthyroid) or on the basis of its clinical or scintigraphic appearance (diffuse or multinodular). A classification schema is listed in Table 16–6.

Euthyroid goiter may be either diffuse or nodular, the latter of which may indeed represent an evolution of the former.[18] In diffuse goiter, a trial of thyroid hormone suppression may be warranted if there are cosmetic concerns, although conservative follow-up suffices in most cases. In multinodular goiter, progressive autonomous function of

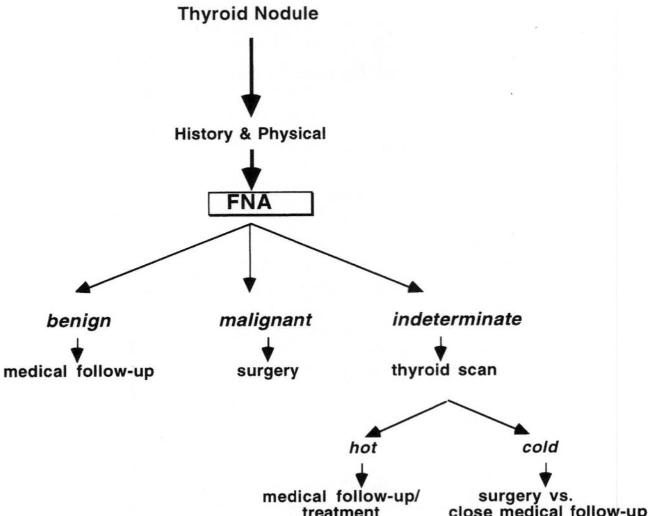

Figure 16–2 ■ Diagnostic algorithm for the evaluation of thyroid nodules. FNA, fine-needle aspiration.

groups of follicles develops over a period of years; hot nodules develop in a sizable subset of patients, sometimes progressing to thyrotoxicosis. This is typically seen in the largest goiters, with nodules greater than 2.5 cm in size, and in older patients, particularly after a cold iodine load, such as occurs with radiocontrast studies.[18] The approach to the multinodular goiter is similar to that of the solitary thyroid nodule, although the risk of malignancy in any one nodule may be comparatively less. Large, dominant nodules should undergo fine-needle aspiration, however, because malignant neoplasms may coexist with this typically benign condition. A trial of thyroid hormone suppression is reasonable in most patients, although less than 50 percent of nodules respond by decreasing in size.[19] It should be avoided in the older patient and in those with clinical or biochemical evidence of hyperthyroidism. The approach to therapy in the patient with a toxic multinodular goiter includes radioiodine ablation, thioamides, and thyroidectomy.

■ TABLE 16–6
Most Common Causes of Goiter

- Endemic goiter (iodine deficiency)
- Sporadic goiter
  - Diffuse nontoxic goiter
  - Multinodular goiter
- Diffuse toxic goiter (Graves' disease)
- Thyroiditis
  - Chronic autoimmune (Hashimoto's disease)
  - Subacute
  - Silent/postpartum
  - Suppurative
- Drugs
  - Thioamides
  - Iodides
  - Lithium
- Dietary/environmental goitrogens
- Organification enzyme defects
- Diffuse malignant disease
  - Lymphoma
  - Anaplastic carcinoma
- Infiltrative diseases
  - Riedel's thyroiditis
  - Sarcoidosis
  - Amyloidosis

MATERNAL AND FETAL THYROID FUNCTION DURING PREGNANCY

Pregnancy induces substantial alterations in maternal thyroid function. Simultaneously, the fetal hypothalamic-pituitary-thyroid axis is maturing in utero. Investigation into the physiology of the maternal and fetal thyroid units during gestation has shown their interrelationship to be highly complex. To rapidly and accurately assess aberrations of thyroid function during pregnancy, the physician must have sufficient familiarity with the changes in thyroid function that occur as part of normal pregnancy.

Maternal Changes

An elevated circulating amount of thyroid hormone was first appreciated in 1948, when researchers precipitated iodine in increased concentrations from the sera of pregnant women.[20] The explanation for this was elucidated in 1956, when the increased T_4 binding of such sera was disclosed.[21] With modern radioimmunoassay techniques, elevated total serum concentrations of both T_4 and T_3 are the rule in pregnancy; mean concentrations increase by 10 to 30 percent in most longitudinal studies,[22–24] usually into a range considered elevated for the general population (Fig. 16–3). Most of these changes occur in the first and second trimesters. The cause is an even more impressive rise in thyroid hormone–binding capacity, as assessed by the direct measurement of TBG, which increases by 75 to 100 percent (the T_3 resin uptake decreases proportionately). These changes are related to the effects of the hyperestrogenemic state on hepatocytes, with stimulation of TBG synthesis and alteration of TBG glycosylation, resulting in prolongation of its metabolic half-life.[25] With an increased number of total serum binding sites for both T_4 and T_3, total concentrations of both these hormones rise. The *free* fractions, however, are within the normal range and do not progressively increase.

Longitudinal studies[22–24] have actually shown *decreases* in maternal fT_4, fT_3, and FTI during pregnancy, most of the decline occurring in the first two trimesters (see Fig. 16–3). Short-lived and minor increases in free thyroid hormone levels have been observed early in the first trimester, correlating temporally with a rise in hCG concentration,[26] which has direct thyrotropic activity.[27] The thyroid-stimulating activity of maternal sera has been documented in normal pregnancy, hyperemesis gravidarum, and gestational trophoblastic disease.[28] Sera from women in early pregnancy have been shown to stimulate cyclic adenosine monophosphate production[29] and iodide uptake[30] in fetal rat thyroid cell culture, with a potency that correlates with hCG concentration in most[29, 30] but not all[31] studies. In addition, anti-hCG antibodies block this effect.[29] After termination of pregnancy, thyroid-stimulating activity of serum declines rapidly in conjunction with the fall in serum hCG,[30] although residual thyrotropic effect has been dem-

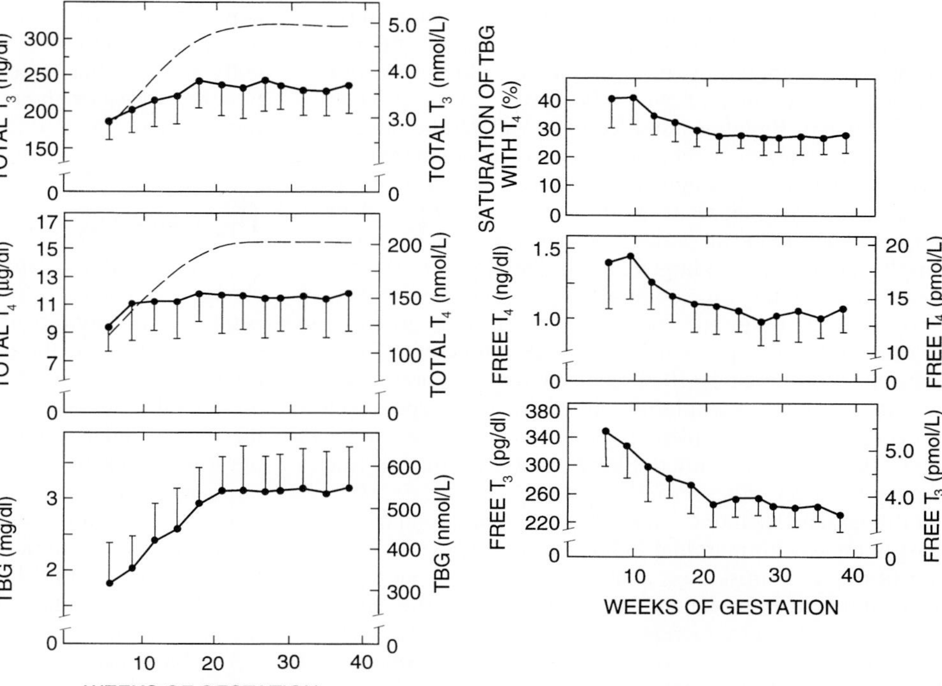

Figure 16–3 ■ Serum T_4, T_3, fT_4, fT_3, TBG, and TBG saturation as a function of gestational age in 606 healthy pregnant women. (Adapted from Glinoer D, de Nayer P, Bourdoux P, et al. Regulation of maternal thyroid during pregnancy. J Clin Endocrinol Metab 71:276–287, 1990. © The Endocrine Society.)

onstrated, despite the disappearance of hCG immunoactivity.[32] Thus, hCG itself may not be solely responsible for the thyrotropic activity of pregnant serum. Taken together, these data do suggest, however, that the physiologic stimulation of the thyroid seen in early pregnancy is at least partially attributable to rises in hCG concentration. In the sera of women in their first trimester, 25,000 U/L of hCG has been shown to have the stimulatory power roughly equivalent to 1 mU/L of TSH.[30] Under normal circumstances, this effect is of a trivial degree, especially in light of the homeostatic mechanisms that control TSH secretion. However, when hCG concentrations rise to greater than 1 million U/L, as they may in molar pregnancy, uncontrolled thyroid stimulation may occur, resulting in thyrotoxicosis. As stated, hCG from such pathologic pregnancies may have enhanced potency, probably owing to altered glycosylation.[33]

Pituitary secretion of TSH remains normal during gestation; the slight suppression noted in the first trimester is presumably due to the same mechanism that stimulates thyroid hormone production (Fig. 16–4). In the second and third trimesters, TSH tends to increase marginally, always staying well within normal range for the nonpregnant population,[22–24] unless another stress such as iodine deficiency or autoimmune thyroiditis supervenes.[34, 35]

Because of the increased glomerular filtration rate that accompanies normal pregnancy, iodine clearance is increased, leading to a reduction in circulating plasma inorganic iodide levels.[36] As a consequence, radioiodine uptake increases.

In addition to the changes in laboratory testing of maternal thyroid function during pregnancy, the clinical diagnosis of thyroid disease, particularly hyperthyroidism, is rendered more difficult by certain physiologic changes that occur at this time. These include an increased metabolic rate of 20 percent[37] attributed to the fetus itself as well as to the circulatory and metabolic changes that enable the mother to support its demands. Certain symptoms of thyrotoxicosis, such as tachycardia, widened pulse pressure, nausea, fatigue, heat intolerance, hyperphagia, and emotional changes, are also frequently encountered during the course of a normal pregnancy. Similarly, symptoms commonly associated with hypothyroidism, such as fatigue, weight gain, and edema, may also represent nothing more than the expected sequelae of a normal gestation. Therefore, the diagnosis of thyroid disease must be, in substantial part, based on biochemical testing, which, as previously stated, requires cautious interpretation at this time.

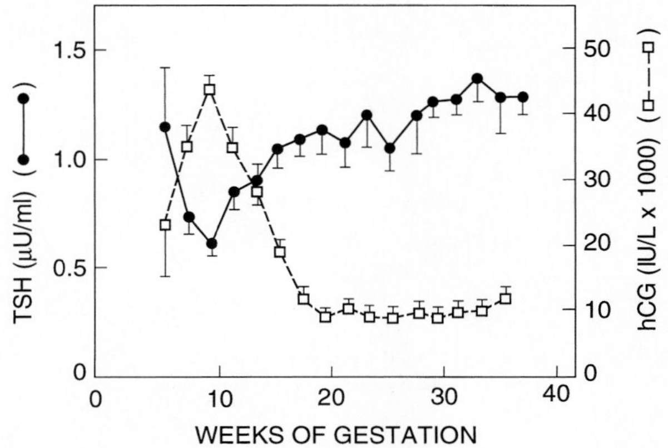

Figure 16–4 ■ Serum TSH and hCG as a function of gestational age from a cohort of 606 healthy pregnant women. (Adapted from Glinoer D, de Nayer P, Bourdoux P, et al. Regulation of maternal thyroid during pregnancy. J Clin Endocrinol Metab 71:276–287, 1990. © The Endocrine Society.)

Anatomic changes in the thyroid may also occur during pregnancy. Such changes may be a reflection more of dietary iodine intake or the predisposition to autoimmune thyroid disease than of any inherent effect of gestation itself. Ancient Egyptians and Romans viewed the development of a goiter as a reliable indicator of pregnancy.[38] In medieval paintings, pregnant women are sometimes portrayed with thyromegaly (Fig. 16–5). The actual prevalence of pregnancy-induced goiter correlates with local iodine supply. Gestational enlargement of the thyroid has been noted in the relatively iodine-deficient countries of Scotland, Ireland, Belgium, and Denmark, with a growth in volume of 20 to 30 percent[22, 39–41] and development of frank goiter in approximately 10 percent.[42] Growth is presumably due to increased vascularity and follicular hypertrophy. However, in iodine-replete regions, such as the Netherlands, Iceland, the United States, and Canada, no such change has been noted.[39, 43, 44]

Glinoer and Lemone[42] have argued that pregnancy, at least in areas with marginal iodine supply such as Belgium, constitutes a "stress" on maternal thyroid economy. In their study cohorts, functional stimulation of the thyroid was demonstrated by increases in thyroglobulin, the preferential secretion of T_3 over T_4, rises in basal overnight TSH secretion, and volumetric increases in thyroid size by ultrasound examination. Such alterations were attenuated when dietary iodine was increased.[42] Changes appeared to be even more acute in Belgian women with underlying autoimmune or nodular thyroid disease; a significant proportion of these experienced goiter growth, an increased number and size of nodules, or both.[45] The suggestion has been made that fetal changes in thyroid function, such as the slight decrease in fT_4 and a rise in reverse T_3, resemble changes seen in the euthyroid sick syndrome, possibly representing a physiologic adaptation enabling energy conservation in the face of the high metabolic demands of pregnancy.[43]

Where iodine supply is sufficient, changes in maternal thyroid function are mild and presumably serve to saturate new serum binding sites. Overall, T_4 turnover during pregnancy is essentially unchanged when it is corrected for body surface area.[46] However, the thyroid with underlying functional abnormalities, such as iodine deficiency or thyroiditis, may find it difficult to adapt to the stress imposed by gestation.

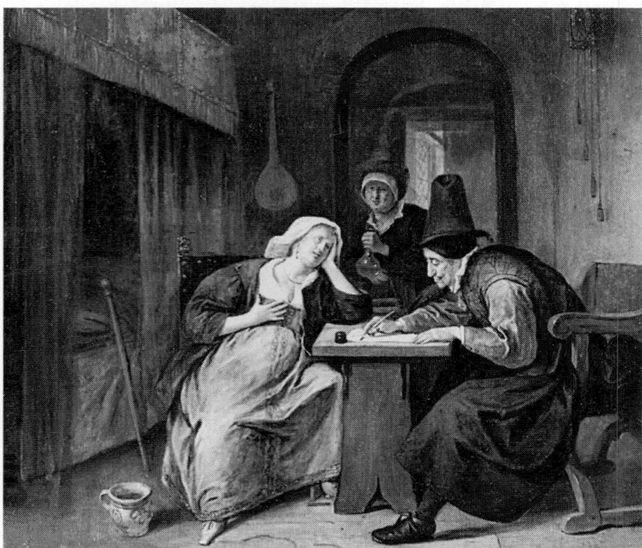

Figure 16–5 ■ *A Pregnant Woman in a Medical Consultation,* by Jan Steen (mid-17th century). (National Gallery, Prague.)

The Fetal Thyroid

Superimposed on and often working in concert with changes in maternal thyroid function is a developing independent fetal thyroid unit. During the fifth or sixth week of embryogenesis, the ultimobranchial bodies arising from diverticuli of the fourth or fifth pharyngeal pouches form the lateral lobes of the thyroid. These ultimately fuse with the medial anlage and migrate caudally, finally resting in the lower neck by the eighth week.[47] This development is intimately linked to the adjacent formation of the parathyroid glands, thymus, and thyroglossal ducts, accounting for frequent rests of these tissues within normal thyroid. By week 12, the thyroid begins to organify iodine; the entire hypothalamic-pituitary-thyroid axis, however, is not fully mature until week 20 to 22.

Cordocentesis has been developed in the past decade as a tool for the diagnosis of a variety of fetal diseases. It has also allowed extensive investigation into fetal thyroid physiology. In the second and third trimesters, fetal T_4, fT_4, T_3, fT_3, TSH, and TBG concentrations increase progressively, with little correlation with the corresponding maternal concentrations, suggesting independent control of the fetal thyroid.[48, 49] Fetal TSH is usually higher than the adult range after the second trimester. T_3 and fT_3 are always lower, whereas T_4 and fT_4 approach the level of an adult by late gestation. Thus, as in the adult, T_4 production in the fetus appears to be driven by TSH, although the sensitivity of the fetal pituitary gland to negative feedback is limited or is offset by other, possibly hypothalamic, stimuli.[49] The fetal TSH:T_4 ratio decreases during gestation, suggesting a fluctuating pituitary set-point or changing thyroid responsiveness.[50] Thus, the fetal thyroid shares both similarities and differences with the adult thyroid.

On the basis of investigations involving newborns with congenital hypothyroidism, maternal-fetal transfer of thyroid hormone clearly occurs during gestation. In one study, thyroid hormone kinetics were analyzed in the first few days of life in neonates with congenital hypothyroidism, half of whom suffered from a complete enzymatic block of thyroid hormone organification and half of whom had thyroid agenesis. T_4 disappeared from the sera of both these groups of children, suggesting that transfer from mother to fetus had occurred ante partum.[51] In a related study of athyreotic neonates, the T_4 at birth was low but decreased further to an undetectable concentration when it was sampled again before treatment was initiated. TSH was elevated, and bone maturation was significantly delayed. The authors concluded that some maternal-fetal thyroid hormone transfer occurs in late gestation, although not to a degree sufficient to prevent the effects of hypothyroidism.[52] Although it is of potential importance in fetuses without other endogenous sources of T_4, late-gestation transfer of thyroid hormones from the mother is probably of little significance in the euthyroid setting.

For obvious reasons, less is known about the early stages of fetal thyroid metabolism. The question of whether maternal thyroid hormone is available to the fetus during early gestation has been addressed by several investigators. Thyroid hormone receptors have been isolated from the brains of 9- to 10-week-old fetuses, before the development of a functioning fetal thyroid apparatus, suggesting the existence of some degree of early maternal-fetal transfer.[53, 54] In embryonic cavity sampling studies during the first trimester, T_4 was detected in coelomic fluid as early as the sixth week of gestation, with concentrations increasing with gestational age and with rising maternal thyroid hormone levels. Amniotic fluid T_4 was markedly lower than that in coelomic fluid.[55] These data would suggest that maternal T_4 traverses the placenta at least as early as the second month of pregnancy. This raises the possibility that the observed rise in maternal thyroid hormone levels during the first trimester may have functional importance for the developing embryo, at a time when the fetal thyroid is not yet mature.[55] In the long-term follow-up of congenitally hypothyroid infants, no consistent deficits in physical development or cognitive function are reported, as long as thyroid hormone is adequately replaced soon after birth.[56] Thus, early in gestation, the fetal concentrations of thyroid hormone may be more dependent on maternal supply than previously suspected. The true significance of this supply and its adequacy is difficult to assess.

The fetal thyroid is also capable of adaptive responses. In two settings marked by fetal hypoxia, intrauterine growth retardation, and red cell isoimmunization, fetal hypoxia, acidemia, and indices of the adequacy of fetal circulation correlated with fetal thyroid function in that fT_4 and fT_3 were lowest in those fetuses in the most severe distress.[57, 58] Because these fetuses were born to euthyroid mothers and, when born, were themselves found to have no abnormality of thyroid function, this was considered an adaptive response of fetal thyroid function to a hostile uterine environment and not a primary abnormality of their thyroid function. Such a response may be similar in part to that observed in adults with nonthyroidal illness. Conversely, when faced with mild or moderate maternal iodine deficiency, compensatory and seemingly protective increases in fetal T_3 have been observed, despite a decrease in maternal T_3.[59]

In sum, the fetal thyroid unit appears to have the capacity to be autonomous and even sophisticated by the middle of the second trimester. Earlier, a complex relationship with the maternal thyroid exists but is not fully elucidated.

Interactions of the Maternal and Fetal Thyroid Units

The changes in fetal and maternal thyroid function during gestation are obviously complex, especially when transplacental communication between the mother and the fetus is additionally considered. This relationship is summarized in Figure 16–6.

The placenta allows the free passage of inorganic iodide, which is necessary for the fetal thyroid to produce thyroid hormones. Whether TRH passes the placenta is still unsettled. TRH administered pharmacologically to women in the third trimester of pregnancy results in increases in

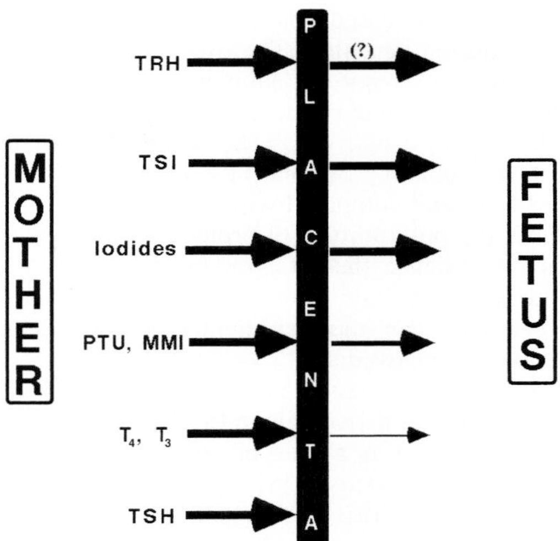

Figure 16–6 ■ Schematic of the placental transfer of maternal factors to the fetus.

TSH and prolactin in the fetus, as measured by cordocentesis,[60, 61] with the TSH response actually more exuberant than that which occurs simultaneously in the mother.[61] Because maternal TSH is known not to cross the placenta, it had been presumed that maternal TRH, a small peptide, had easy access to the fetal circulation. However, a study that used ex vivo perfused human term placentas showed that the placenta may act as an enzymatic barrier to the free passage of TRH to the fetus.[62] The placenta allows the passage of maternal antibodies, including TSI and thyrotropin-binding inhibitory immunoglobulin, which may lead to thyroid stimulation or inhibition, respectively, in the fetus. Both PTU and MMI cross the placenta with relative ease, MMI less so than PTU, as reported in a study[63] that measured fetal concentrations after a single injection of radiolabeled drug to women undergoing therapeutic abortion in early pregnancy. More recently, however, significant concentrations of PTU were measured in the blood of fetuses of mothers receiving PTU chronically for documented thyrotoxicosis in the second half of pregnancy.[64] β-Adrenergic receptor blocking drugs also easily pass the placental circulation, with the degree correlating with a specific agent's lipophilic characteristics.[65] T_4 and T_3 traverse the placental circulation with difficulty, although apparently in a physiologically important amount, on the basis of the aforementioned studies of fetal brain thyroid hormone receptors[53, 54] and of congenitally hypothyroid neonates[52] previously discussed. Five tissue-specific deiodinases have been described, each responsible for the conversion of T_4 to T_3 and the inactive reverse T_3 in equimolar amounts. The type 3 deiodinase is highly expressed in the placenta and appears to be responsible for the deactivation of both T_4 and T_3 and may regulate fetal circulating free thyroid hormone levels in early pregnancy.[66] Access of maternal TSH to the fetal circulation is completely blocked by the placenta.

The presence of T_4 and T_3 sulfates adds another layer of complexity to our understanding of gestational thyroid physiology. These compounds, which circulate in small quantities in the nonpregnant, euthyroid woman, are found in dramatically increased concentrations in both mother[67] and fetus[68] during gestation. The exact function of thyroid hormone sulfates is not yet known. Fetal T_3 sulfate has been shown to correlate positively with gestational age but not with fetal fT_4, fT_3, or TSH. In hypothyroid fetuses, despite low circulating fT_4 and fT_3, the T_3 sulfate concentrations are normal compared with those in control fetuses. This raises the possibility of a protective function for this substance.[69] Because the fetal rat brain can desulfate T_3 sulfate to T_3, T_3 sulfate may serve as a reservoir of T_3, which can attenuate the detrimental cerebral effects of intrauterine hypothyroidism.[69]

In summary, pregnancy is characterized by marked changes in maternal thyroid gland function, which has been interpreted by some as a state of controlled hyperthyroidism, without thyrotoxicosis. When additional stress supervenes, because of either iodine deficiency or underlying thyroid autoimmunity, normal augmentation may not proceed as planned, with potential detrimental effects. Simultaneously, a second, distinct, and autonomous hypothalamic-pituitary-thyroid axis develops in the fetus. These combined systems interrelate throughout gestation. Various placental and fetal mechanisms appear to be in place that safeguard the fetus from unexpected alterations in maternal thyroid function. Much of the remainder of this chapter serves to discuss those situations in which such protection is lacking or insufficient.

REPRODUCTIVE AND GESTATIONAL CONSIDERATIONS IN HYPOTHYROIDISM

Effects of Hypothyroidism on Fertility

Hypothyroidism is associated with menstrual abnormalities, anovulation, and infertility. Hypothyroidism may interfere with normal gonadotropin secretion, but direct effects of thyroid hormone on ovarian steroidogenesis are also apparent. Experimental studies have shown that T_4 increases the secretion of both estradiol and progesterone from granulosa cells maintained in vitro.[70] In hypothyroid men, alterations in sperm count and motility and mild abnormalities of gonadotropic axis (mild hypergonadotropism, low concentrations of serum sex hormone–binding globulin, and subnormal testosterone response to hCG injections) have been described, with amelioration after hormone replacement.[71] In one study, a large cohort of women without known thyroid disease, being evaluated in an infertility clinic, were screened for subclinical abnormalities of thyroid function. TRH testing conducted during the early follicular phase distinguished the subjects into three groups: euthyroid (normal response to TRH), those with latent hyperthyroidism (inadequate response), and those with latent hypothyroidism (supranormal response). Subsequent pregnancy rates were highest in women with normal TSH responses to TRH.[72] Rates were diminished in both those with latent hyperthyroidism and those with latent hypothyroidism.

In a population of women with decreased fertility, antithyroid antibodies (antithyroglobulin or antimicrosomal) are found with increased frequency and may be a marker for women at greater risk for miscarriage. In one study of 487 patients at a university-based reproductive health clinic, 106 women were positive for either or both antibodies, with an overall rate of 22 percent, higher than that seen in age- and sex-matched control subjects.[73] The antibody-positive group suffered from a miscarriage rate twice that of the antibody-negative group, despite not being biochemically or clinically hypothyroid. Therefore, antithyroid antibodies may be a marker of reproductive failure, although a cause and effect relationship is not apparent. Because the most common cause of hypothyroidism is autoimmune thyroid disease, the decreased fertility rates in women with hypothyroidism may have less to do with the thyroid functional status than a generalized autoimmune state.

Primary hypothyroidism has also been associated with elevated prolactin levels, resulting from increased infundibular concentrations of TRH, a prolactin-releasing factor. Hyperprolactinemia interferes with normal hypothalamic pulsatile secretion of gonadotropin-releasing hormone and its ability to stimulate pituitary gonadotropin secretion. Galactorrhea and amenorrhea may follow, with a diagnosis of prolactinoma sometimes made in error. In addition, severe hypothyroidism has been associated with pituitary enlargement, resulting from thyrotroph hyperplasia.[74] Such a finding may also mislead the clinician into considering a primary pituitary disease. Whether such changes within the pituitary gland lead secondarily to failure of gonadotropin secretion has not been thoroughly investigated. Careful assessment of thyroid function is therefore imperative in any patient with hyperprolactinemia or pituitary mass.

Hypothyroidism During Pregnancy

Whereas hypothyroidism is usually easily treated in the nonpregnant woman, the management may not be as straightforward during gestation. Hypothyroidism during pregnancy, particularly when it is profound, may be associated with serious effects on both the mother and fetus, as listed in Table 16–7.

Because severe hypothyroidism is associated with infertility, it is rarely seen in pregnancy. Hypothyroid women who become pregnant are at increased risk for low-birth-weight or stillborn infants.[75] The effects of subclinical maternal hypothyroidism on the fetus are not well defined, although it would seem logical to achieve euthyroidism as quickly as possible in all individuals.

In a study of 43 pregnancies in which the mother was either biochemically hypothyroid or receiving replacement therapy for previously diagnosed hypothyroidism, the incidence of fetal distress during labor correlated with the severity of the maternal hypothyroidism in early pregnancy. More than half of the infants born to mothers with severe hypothyroidism during the first trimester experienced fetal distress at delivery, requiring cesarean section. Thus, mater-

■ TABLE 16–7
Obstetric Complications of Hypothyroidism

Maternal Complications	Fetal Complications
Miscarriage	Low birth weight
Preterm delivery	Stillbirth
Hypertensive disorders	Prematurity
Postpartum hemorrhage	Mental retardation

nal thyroid status in the first trimester may exert prolonged effects on the fetoplacental unit and the maternal adaptation to pregnancy.[76]

In another study of 68 pregnant women with either overt or subclinical hypothyroidism during pregnancy, gestational hypertensive disorders (eclampsia, preeclampsia, and pregnancy-induced hypertension) were twofold to threefold more common than in a control pregnant population. Rates were even higher for a subgroup of women who remained hypothyroid at delivery date. Lower birth weights were also observed, but these appeared to correlate with the degree of prematurity, resulting directly from the effects of the hypertension. There was, however, no statistical association with other adverse fetal or neonatal outcomes. Normalization of thyroid function during pregnancy in hypothyroid women could decrease the risks associated with hypertensive disorders and, perhaps, improve fetal outcomes.[77]

After birth, it has been difficult to demonstrate any significant long-term detrimental effects on the physical or intellectual development of children of hypothyroid mothers, even if the maternal thyroid dysfunction was known to be present during early pregnancy, before the initiation of fetal thyroid function. In one study, children of such pregnancies were compared with their siblings who enjoyed a normal in utero environment, and no adverse effect on cognitive function was apparent.[78] Most but not all[79] studies have reported similar findings. Abnormalities in later intellectual development have been more consistently observed in children with congenital hypothyroidism in whom thyroid hormone replacement does not occur soon after birth.[56] Such a distinction suggests a greater importance to the fetus/neonate of its own thyroid status, as opposed to that of its mother during gestation. In the situation of iodine deficiency when the inability of the fetal thyroid to produce adequate amounts of thyroid hormone is combined with mild to severe maternal hypothyroidism, the more obvious and graver consequences of cretinism and mental retardation may occur. It is therefore important to optimize maternal and fetal thyroid function throughout gestation.

Requirements for exogenous thyroid hormone increase in most hypothyroid women receiving thyroxine replacement therapy during pregnancy. Mandel and colleagues[80] reported that 75 percent of previously hypothyroid women required an average levothyroxine dosage increase of greater than 50 percent during gestation. Most of the subjects who did not require an increase had pre-pregnancy TSH levels in a low range, suggesting overreplacement at that time. Post partum, a decrease toward the pre-pregnancy requirements was observed.[80] In another study, levothyroxine dosage increase was required in five of eight pregnant women who had previously undergone thyroidectomy. Interestingly, both women who were taking desiccated thyroid, which contains both T_4 and T_3, along with other substances, required no change.[81] In the largest study of this type, thyroid function was analyzed serially in 77 pregnancies of women with primary hypothyroidism resulting from Hashimoto's thyroiditis or from thyroid ablation. Less than half of the women in the first group required levothyroxine dosage increase, whereas more than three quarters of those in the second group required upward titration.[82] Most of the increase occurs during the first half of gestation.

Causes of fetal goitrous hypothyroidism include iodine deficiency; iodine excess; thioamide therapy provided to the mother[83]; the antiarrhythmic amiodarone, which has large amounts of iodine[84, 85]; or, rarely, the passage of thyrotropin-binding inhibitory immunoglobulin from mother to fetus in Graves' disease.[86] In such cases, unless a sizable goiter is seen by ultrasonography, it may be difficult to make a diagnosis. Other clinical features may include intrauterine growth retardation, fetal bradycardia, and polyhydramnios. In certain situations, a precise diagnosis may be required, particularly in pregnancies complicated by Graves' disease. Amniotic thyroid hormone or TSH levels appear not to correlate well with the actual thyroid status of the fetus.[83] Cordocentesis (funipuncture), an invasive technique that carries with it a considerable risk of miscarriage, has been used to measure the actual circulating fetal concentrations of T_4, T_3, and TSH.[87] Because of the inability to provide thyroid hormones reliably to the fetus by maternal administration (without inducing maternal thyrotoxicosis), weekly intra-amniotic injections of thyroxine have been successful in isolated cases of fetal hypothyroidism.[83, 86] Follow-up cordocentesis has demonstrated adequate delivery of thyroid hormone with this technique, which may theoretically result in overtreatment of the fetus.

Iodine Deficiency and Pregnancy

Severe iodine deficiency is a monumental public health problem in many underdeveloped regions of the world. This condition is associated with a variety of fetal and neonatal effects, including congenital hypothyroidism, cretinism, and mental deficiency. As previously mentioned, there is relative sparing of permanent cognitive effects in newborns with congenital hypothyroidism born to euthyroid mothers or in euthyroid newborns born to hypothyroid mothers. However, the combination of insufficient thyroid hormone supply from both maternal and fetal sources, as seen in severe endemic iodine deficiency, has disastrous consequences.

The exact clinical expression of endemic cretinism results from the variable admixture of two distinct pathophysiologic events, both sharing a common etiology—iodine deficiency. Deficiency in the mother, and secondarily in the fetus, results in inadequate thyroid hormone supply to the developing fetal nervous system, with profound impact on neurologic outcome.[88] A superimposed syndrome of myxedema, accompanied by abnormal somatic development in the form of dwarfism and sexual immaturity, results if iodine deficiency persists postnatally and for which inadequate thyroid compensation occurs.[88] Thus, the purely neurologic form, as opposed to the myxedematous form of cretinism, occurs when the mother is iodine deficient but the fetus' hypothyroidism is corrected postnatally by either an improvement in iodine supply or other compensatory factors.

More moderate iodine deficiency during pregnancy has been associated with other difficulties, including the development of maternal hypothyroidism. Up to 50 percent of euthyroid pregnant women from an iodine-deficient area of

Sicily have been shown to develop either overt or borderline hypothyroidism during gestation, manifested by a fall in both T_4 and fT_4, an increase in the T_3:T_4 molar ratio representing preferential T_3 secretion, and an increase in TSH.[89] In the face of this stress, the fetus may develop protective mechanisms, as demonstrated by studies in Nigeria that have compared pregnancy outcomes in two regions, one with moderate iodine deficiency and one that is iodine sufficient. Maternal T_4, FTI, and T_3 were significantly lower in the iodine-deficient group, with TSH being higher. Corresponding fetal cord blood samples showed a similar decrement in T_4 and FTI but not in T_3, which was actually higher in this group, as was TSH, compared with the iodine-sufficient fetuses. Maternal and fetal blood levels were significantly correlated, except for T_3. These data provide support to the previously discussed notion that fetal T_3 serves as a main form of defense for the fetus to safeguard itself against maternal hypothyroidism or iodine deficiency.[59]

Marginal iodine supply during pregnancy leads to evidence of a similar stimulation of the maternal thyroid. Thyroglobulin, the T_3:T_4 ratio, and TSH all increase, although the last remains within the normal range. In addition, goiter develops in 10 percent of mothers.[34] In the offspring of these pregnancies, although there is no evidence of hypothyroxinemia at term, TSH and thyroglobulin are elevated, significantly higher than maternal values, and appear to increase in parallel with corresponding maternal levels. It therefore appears that the changes in maternal thyroid function induced by marginal iodine supply are, in part, amplified in the fetus,[34] although circulating fetal thyroid hormone levels, in contrast to the maternal levels, appear to be safeguarded.

Prophylactic maternal iodine repletion blunts many of these changes. In one study of iodine supplementation to pregnant women from a moderately iodine deficient area, thyroid size was stabilized, whereas thyroid volume increased by one sixth in untreated patients.[90] In a randomized trial of placebo, iodine alone, or iodine plus levothyroxine in 180 euthyroid women from an area of Belgium with marginal iodine supply, improved thyroid function and economy were observed in both treatment groups. Those patients in the combination therapy group enjoyed the greatest improvement. The placebo group experienced a significant incidence of deteriorating thyroid function, as manifested by decreases in fT_4; increases in TSH (above normal range in 20 percent of this group), thyroglobulin, and the T_3:T_4 ratio; and the development of goiter in almost 1 in 5 patients.[91]

Thyroid Autoimmunity and Reproduction

An interesting relationship between thyroid autoimmunity and pregnancy has developed in the past decade. Thyroid autoantibodies include antimicrosomal (or antithyroid peroxidase [anti-TPO]) and antithyroglobulin antibodies. These antibodies are commonly present in low titer in many thyroid conditions, particularly if cellular injury has occurred. When they circulate in high titer, however, they almost invariably represent autoimmune thyroid disease (i.e., Hashimoto's thyroiditis).

Pregnancy in women with autoimmune thyroid disease in the relatively iodine deficient area of Denmark has been associated with a 20 to 30 percent increase in thyroid volume but no change in thyroid hormone levels.[92] In a larger study, in an area of marginal iodine supply, the risk of the future development of clinical or subclinical hypothyroidism was assessed prospectively in 87 women with autoimmune thyroid disease but normal thyroid function.[35] At baseline, mean TSH was significantly higher than in control subjects although still within normal range. During subsequent gestations, antibody titers fell approximately 60 percent, yet TSH remained significantly higher than in control subjects. An exaggerated response to TRH was seen in 50 percent of cases, with free thyroid hormone levels within a hypothyroid range in a surprising 42 percent of women. The authors theorized that this hypothyroidism resulted from the reduced ability of these subjects' thyroids to adjust appropriately to the increased demands of pregnancy. Obstetric sequelae were also observed in this cohort, with increased rates of miscarriage and premature labor.[35]

As previously mentioned, autoimmune thyroid disease, even when it is not accompanied by any alteration in thyroid hormone levels, has also been associated with recurrent early pregnancy loss.[93] In a group of 42 women with a history of three or more miscarriages, the disease was present in almost one third. In addition, two thirds of patients who experienced first-trimester abortions were antibody-positive.[94] A control group of 30 nonaborting women had an antibody prevalence of only 17 percent. Thus, the presence of autoimmune thyroid disease identifies a subgroup of women at significantly increased risk for fetal loss. Most authorities suspect that the antibodies are not directly causative of the miscarriages. Instead, they may be a marker for generalized autoimmunity, perhaps an underlying T-lymphocyte defect, that essentially results in intolerance of foreign fetal antigens.

The possibility of long-term effects on offspring associated with maternal thyroid autoimmunity has also been raised. Offspring of women with thyroid antibodies, although having no difference in birth weight, gestational age at birth, and Apgar scores, have been shown to have decreased neonatal growth rates compared with control subjects.[95] In a larger study involving nearly 300 pregnancies, children of women with positive titers of anti-TPO antibodies during late gestation had significantly lower scores on cognitive function testing than did those children of anti-TPO–negative women.[96]

In sum, thyroid autoimmunity is associated with (1) mildly decompensated maternal thyroid function during pregnancy, in the setting of simultaneous marginal iodine intake; (2) increased risk of fetal loss, especially during early gestation; and (3) developmental abnormalities in offspring. (The association with postpartum thyroiditis is discussed later.) Explanations for most of these observations remain unclear. However, systematic screening for thyroid autoantibodies during pregnancy has been recommended by some.[35]

REPRODUCTIVE AND GESTATIONAL CONSIDERATIONS IN HYPERTHYROIDISM

Effects of Hyperthyroidism on Fertility

The frequency of menstrual disturbance in thyrotoxicosis has been overstated. In a study of 214 premenopausal women with hyperthyroidism, more than 75 percent reported normal menstrual function. The less than 25 percent with irregular menses had a significantly higher T_4 level. Amenorrhea was not reported.[9] In contradistinction to the notable effects of hypothyroidism on reproductive capacity, mild to moderate thyrotoxicosis does not have a substantial impact on fertility. Indeed, pregnancy commonly occurs in even severely hyperthyroid women. The lack of reproductive failure in thyrotoxicosis and the frequency of hyperthyroid disorders in women of childbearing age make a thorough understanding of the diagnosis and treatment of gestational hyperthyroidism important for anyone who cares for women during pregnancy.

Hyperthyroidism During Pregnancy

Both diagnosis and management of hyperthyroidism during pregnancy are notoriously difficult.[97] First, many women develop signs or symptoms during pregnancy that are suggestive of a thyrotoxic state, such as fatigue, nausea, heat intolerance, palpitations, widened pulse pressure, and dyspnea on exertion. Second, as previously described, various changes in the laboratory evaluation of thyroid function during normal gestation suggest, at first glance, hyperthyroidism. Because a thyrotoxic pregnancy is associated with significant maternal and fetal morbidities, the distinction between true thyrotoxicosis and the hyperdynamic changes of normal pregnancy must be made expeditiously so that treatment in the case of the former may be initiated. Fortunately, in most situations, thyrotoxicosis during pregnancy can usually be distinguished with the aid of the modern laboratory.

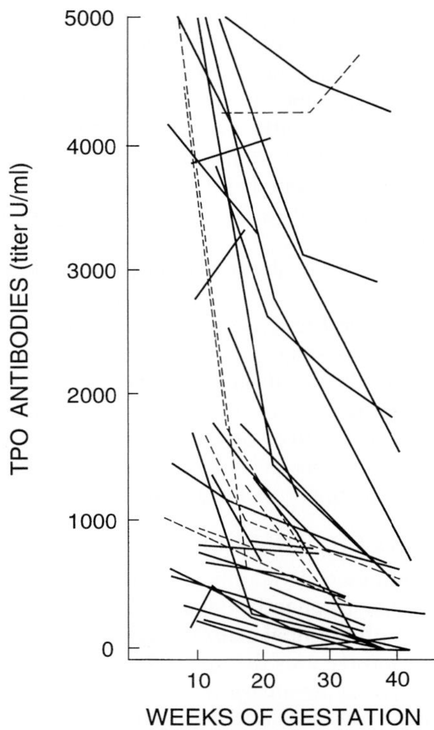

Figure 16–7 ■ Individual changes in anti-TPO antibody titers in 87 pregnant women with asymptomatic autoimmune thyroid disease. (Adapted from Glinoer D, Riahi M, Grun JP, Kinthaert J. Risk of subclinical hypothyroidism in pregnant women with asymptomatic autoimmune thyroid disorders. J Clin Endocrinol Metab 79:197–204, 1994. © The Endocrine Society.)

Etiology

Whereas pregnant women may experience any of the causes of thyrotoxicosis listed in Table 16–3, Graves' disease is responsible for more than 95 percent of cases.

GRAVES' DISEASE

The incidence of Graves' thyrotoxicosis during pregnancy is approximately 2 per 1000.[98] The disorder carries with it several special considerations at this time. An exacerbation of thyrotoxicosis during the early first trimester is sometimes observed, corresponding to the thyrotropic effects of increased circulating concentrations of hCG.[99] During the second and particularly the third trimesters, however, hyperthyroidism frequently abates,[100] associated with a decline in TSH receptor antibody titers. A similar decline in antimicrosomal antibodies occurs in pregnant women with autoimmune thyroid disease, although without an apparent resulting clinical significance (Fig. 16–7).

Progressive immune tolerance is a manifestation of normal pregnancy, presumably allowing the mother to accept the new antigen load provided by the fetus.[101] Similarly, improvement in various autoimmune diseases, such as lupus and multiple sclerosis, is known to occur during pregnancy. In Graves' disease, the dosage of antithyroid medication is often able to be substantially decreased or even discontinued altogether during the last few months of gestation. In individual patients, however, the course of Graves' disease during pregnancy may be variable. In a study of 32 pregnancies complicated by maternal hyperthyroidism, half of patients required no change in antithyroid drug dosage during pregnancy; one quarter required a decrease, and one quarter required an increase.[102] The diagnosis and treatment of Graves' disease during pregnancy, as well as special considerations that involve the fetus, are described later.

GESTATIONAL TROPHOBLASTIC DISEASE

Gestational trophoblastic disease spans the spectrum from molar pregnancy to metastatic choriocarcinoma.[103] These neoplastic tissues of placental derivation elaborate large quantities of hCG, which may have enhanced thyrotropic activity compared with hCG from normal placentas because of alteration in oligosaccharide side-chain composition.[28, 33] Purified hCG from the urine of women with gestational trophoblastic disease has a much greater TSH-like activity in human thyroid follicular cell culture, with an equivalency of 37 to 84 μU hTSH per milligram protein, compared with 468 μU in a patient with choriocarcinoma, compared with the usually trivial TSH activity of hCG from normal pregnancy (19.7 μU hTSH per milligram hCG).[104] Glycosylation of glycoprotein hormones is known to substantially affect their metabolic clearance and bioactivity[26]; those isoforms with decreased sialic acid content demonstrate the highest bioactivity to immunoactivity ratio.[28]

Whereas thyroid hormone levels may be significantly elevated in these patients, often greater than twice normal and accompanied by the expected suppression of TSH, those affected are typically not severely thyrotoxic clinically and there is usually no goiter. This observation is perhaps a manifestation of the relatively brief duration of the hyperthyroidism or due to other circulating factors associated with general medical illness that impair T_4 to T_3 conversion.

In such cases, surgical extirpation of the abnormal uterine tissue will result in the eventual normalization of thyroid function. Persistent elevation may indicate residual neoplasm, and this may be corroborated by a remeasurement of serum hCG. If general anesthesia is required, hemodynamic stabilization is necessary preoperatively, with β-blockers effective in the treatment of tachycardia. Thioamide therapy, because of its delayed action, has little role in the management of most cases.

HYPEREMESIS GRAVIDARUM

The exact etiology of hyperemesis gravidarum is unknown. Women affected frequently develop evidence of dehydration and electrolyte imbalance, sometimes requiring hospitalization for intravenous therapy.[105] Concentrations of hCG are statistically higher in women with hyperemesis gravidarum relative for the stage of gestation in some but not all studies.[106]

Abnormally elevated levels of free thyroid hormones are seen in up to 67 percent of women with hyperemesis gravidarum,[107–109] with concurrent TSH suppression. In one large series of 67 patients, two thirds had biochemical evidence of hyperthyroidism. All were self-limited, abating by the 18th week. Those with biochemical hyperthyroidism tend to be more seriously ill, with increased severity of hyperemesis and a greater frequency of having abnormal electrolytes.[107]

In an interesting study of 51 pregnancies, women were divided into three categories on the basis of the degree of emesis they experienced during gestation (no emesis, some emesis, and hyperemesis). Serum fT_4 and fT_3 were higher and TSH was lower in both emetic groups, but hCG was not different. However, the thyroid-stimulating activity of the serum, measured by use of fetal rat thyroid cell culture, was much higher in the hyperemetic women; this activity was abolished by anti-hCG antibodies, raising the possibility of enhanced bioactivity of hCG in this group.[106] However, the enhanced bioactivity of hCG in this condition, unlike the situation with trophoblastic disease, has not yet been demonstrated in human thyroid cell culture.[110]

Whether these patients are hyperemetic because of their hyperthyroxinemia or whether both the hyperemesis and the thyrotoxicosis originate from a single physiologic process (i.e., excess hCG, increased estrogen levels) remains controversial. Most women with hyperemesis gravidarum and biochemical hyperthyroxinemia have no other signs or symptoms of thyrotoxicosis. Thus, it would appear that they are not truly thyrotoxic. Indeed, most studies have not been able to document a beneficial effect from treatment of the hyperthyroidism. However, in one small study, the majority of patients with hyperemesis gravidarum had low red blood cell zinc levels, a measure of thyroid hormone action on carbonic anhydrase, which has been reported in Graves' hyperthyroidism.[108] If hyperemesis continues in the face of climbing thyroid hormone levels, consideration should be given to a brief therapeutic trial of antithyroid drugs.

TOXIC NODULES

There is a paucity of published experience with this phenomenon. In women with toxic multinodular goiter or toxic adenoma, treatment should be based on clinical symptoms and biochemical indices. If thyroid hormone elevation is mild and the woman is asymptomatic or minimally symptomatic, because no antibody-mediated process places the fetus at risk for thyrotoxicosis, conservative follow-up may be indicated. However, if thyroid hormone levels continue to rise, especially if clinical symptoms of maternal thyrotoxicosis supervene, treatment with antithyroid drugs should be initiated.

Diagnosis

The diagnosis of hyperthyroidism must first depend on a careful clinical evaluation of the patient, with appropriate laboratory confirmation. As mentioned, many of the features of normal pregnancy may also be signs of thyrotoxicosis. However, a goiter (in iodine-replete regions) and a pulse persistently above 100 beats per minute should be considered strong supporting evidence of true thyroid dysfunction. Biochemical assessment indicates thyrotoxicosis when the TSH, in a reliable assay, is fully suppressed, with the T_4, fT_4, free throxine index, T_3, or fT_3 near or above the upper limit of normal range. Because of the slight drop in TSH and rise in thyroid hormone levels early in the first trimester, such a biochemical diagnosis may be difficult to make at this time. On occasion, when the clinical diagnosis is not secured, nothing can substitute for careful clinical and laboratory follow-up assessments. Because of the high predictive value of currently available third-generation TSH assays, a detectable level, even if it is below the statistical mean for the nonpregnant population, indicates euthyroidism. To our knowledge, a case of a TSH-secreting pituitary adenoma has not yet been reported during pregnancy. In particularly vexing cases, the measurement of TSI titers may be helpful. In addition, erythrocyte zinc levels may rarely be useful.[111]

Once biochemical confirmation is secured, unless a dominant nodule is palpated on examination of the thyroid or other features of an abnormal pregnancy are manifested, such as hyperemesis gravidarum or trophoblastic disease, the diagnosis is almost always Graves' disease. An elevated TSI titer is helpful in confirming the diagnosis but usually not necessary when the entire clinical context is considered. Although most TSI bioassays are extremely specific, they lack the sensitivity to rule out the diagnosis in a significant proportion of cases.[15] TSI may be used as a predictor for the development of fetal or neonatal complications (see later). Whereas radionuclide uptakes and scans are often helpful in nonpregnant individuals, they are absolutely contraindicated during pregnancy.

Therapy

Therapeutic options for Graves' hyperthyroidism during pregnancy are similarly limited. The treatment of choice continues to be drugs of the thioamide class, either PTU or MMI in the United States or carbimazole, which is converted to MMI by the liver, in other parts of the world.

THIOAMIDES

Depending on the degree of hyperthyroidism, PTU is begun with doses of 100 to 200 mg orally every 8 hours until biochemical control is achieved, with subsequent gradual dosage reduction to 100 to 300 mg/day, considered an extremely safe range during pregnancy. Although it was once believed that PTU passed the placenta with difficulty,[63] more recent data show that oral administration to the mother results in therapeutic blood levels in the fetus.[64] The risk of inducing hypothyroidism in the fetus is low, especially if the PTU dose is maintained at the lowest possible effective dose without causing maternal hypothyroidism. Once the mother is receiving PTU, clinical and biochemical monitoring should be performed at least monthly during gestation, more frequently if warranted by the clinical situation. An open dialogue between the obstetrician, endocrinologist, and fetal specialist is necessary to ensure a good outcome. Fetal heart rate and parameters of fetal growth and development should additionally be monitored closely. The main adverse reactions to PTU include rashes, hepatitis, and agranulocytosis; the last is of particular concern but is rare.

Because MMI has been thought to traverse the placenta more easily than PTU, it has been used less often in the treatment of Graves' disease during pregnancy. Few data support this distinction, however. Perhaps more important, there have been several reports of an unusual skin defect, aplasia cutis congenita, in neonates exposed to MMI in early gestation (before 12 weeks)[112] (Fig. 16–8). There is insufficient evidence to either establish or eliminate a direct causal relationship between aplasia cutis and gestational use of MMI.[113] However, because PTU has not been associated with such a complication, it would appear to be the safer drug, at least as first-line therapy. In certain circumstances, such as with fetal thyrotoxicosis, the use of MMI may be advantageous, because its presumed enhanced availability to the fetal circulation may be exploited. Because fetal thyrotoxicosis always occurs well into the second trimester, the risk of aplasia cutis from MMI is minimized. MMI is administered in doses of 2.5 to 40 mg/day. Its longer metabolic half-life makes daily or twice-daily dosing possible, whereas PTU should be given every 6 to 8 hours, with more frequent intervals used for the most severely thyrotoxic patients. MMI, however, does lack PTU's additional benefit of blocking T_4 to T_3 conversion.

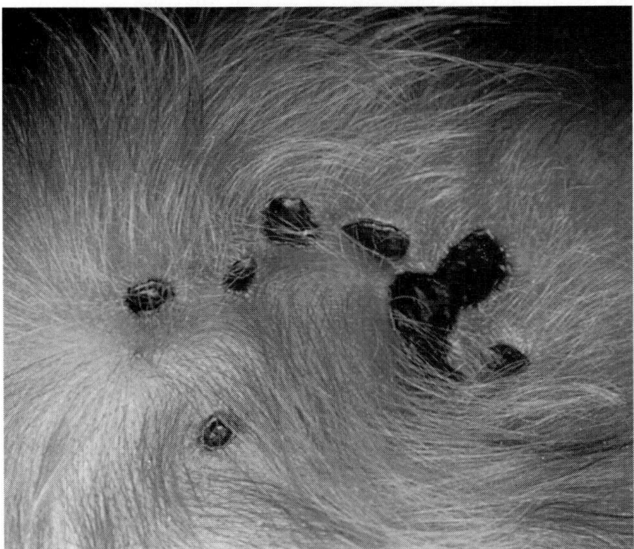

Figure 16–8 ■ Aplasia cutis in a child whose mother had received methimazole during early pregnancy. (From Burrow GN, Klatskin EH, Genel M. Intellectual development in children whose mothers received propylthiouracil during pregnancy. Yale J Biol Med 51:151–156, 1978.)

Despite the historical tendency to favor PTU over MMI during pregnancy, both appear to be equally safe and efficacious. In a retrospective analysis of 185 pregnancies complicated by Graves' disease, the average time to normalization of thyroid indices was equivalent in those treated with PTU or MMI (7 to 8 weeks). In addition, there was no difference in the frequency of congenital malformations in either group compared with the frequency in the general population.[114]

There appear to be no particular long-term effects on the offspring of mothers treated with thioamides during pregnancy for Graves' disease.[115]

OTHER TREATMENTS

β-Adrenergic receptor blocking agents are useful in the nonpregnant patient with thyrotoxicosis, particularly in the control of hyperadrenergic symptoms and for the control of cardiac rate. They easily pass the placenta, however, and their long-term use during pregnancy has been associated with intrauterine growth retardation. Thus, β-blockers should be used when their potential benefits outweigh their risks, and only for brief periods during gestation.

Iodine, which is occasionally useful in rapidly decreasing thyroid hormone production in Graves' disease, is considered relatively contraindicated during pregnancy. In cases involving indiscriminate use of iodine during pregnancy, profound fetal hypothyroidism and goiter have been described.[116] Such reports raise the possibility that the fetal thyroid may be unable to escape from the Wolff-Chaikoff effect. However, Momotani and colleagues[117] have demonstrated both efficacy and safety when iodine is used in modest doses during hyperthyroid pregnancies. In their cohort of mildly to moderately thyrotoxic patients, 6 to 40 mg/day of iodine administered between weeks 11 and 37 resulted in biochemical improvement of maternal thyroid hormone levels in all patients, with normalization in more than one third. Fetal cord thyroid hormone levels measured during week 35 were also either normal or slightly elevated and correlated with maternal values. No fetus was biochemically hypothyroid.[117]

Surgery, for obvious reasons, is restricted to those women who are noncompliant or in whom drug therapy is contraindicated or ineffective. Although preferably performed during the second trimester, at which time some have suggested lower rates of spontaneous abortions, surgery may be performed at any time during gestation when it is warranted by the clinical condition. Reports of satisfactory surgical outcomes exist for all trimesters.

The clinical experience with inadvertent radioiodine

treatment during an unrecognized pregnancy is limited. Depending on the stage of gestation, the fetal thyroid may receive an ablative dose.[118] In this light, and because of the potential for other adverse fetal consequences, radioiodine is *absolutely* contraindicated during gestation.

Complications

Potential maternal and fetal complications related to uncontrolled thyrotoxicosis during pregnancy are listed in Table 16–8. In a landmark study[119] from 1984 of more than 600 pregnancies in women with Graves' disease, a 14-fold increase in the incidence of congenital malformations was reported in those with uncontrolled hyperthyroidism during gestation. Use of antithyroid drugs, if anything, appeared to decrease this risk. The incidence of other complications is also substantial on the basis of some more recent studies. In an analysis of 230 pregnancies in women with active Graves' disease, 6.5 percent of newborns were small for gestational age.[120] This risk was positively correlated with the presence of clinical thyrotoxicosis for 30 or more weeks of gestation, elevated TSH receptor antibody titers at delivery, a history of Graves' disease for more than 10 years before pregnancy, and onset of disease before the age of 20 years. Somewhat surprisingly, no significant correlation could be found with the degree of hyperthyroxinemia. Neonatal thyroid dysfunction was found in 38 infants (16.5 percent), with the risk positively correlating with the mother's total antithyroid drug dose, the duration of thyrotoxicosis during the pregnancy, and the TSH receptor antibody titers at delivery.[120]

In a retrospective review of 181 pregnancies complicated by active maternal Graves' disease, 20 percent of patients were controlled at the onset of pregnancy, 50 percent became controlled during pregnancy, and 30 percent remained uncontrolled during pregnancy. The relative risk of low birth weight was 9.2 and 2.4 in the third and second groups, respectively. In addition, preeclampsia was significantly more common in the uncontrolled group, with a relative risk of 4.7. Maternal thioamide therapy did not have any adverse impact on neonatal outcomes.[121]

In another study of 32 gestations complicated by maternal hyperthyroidism (with 6 cases newly diagnosed during the pregnancy), an increased frequency of both maternal and fetal complications including preterm labor, pregnancy-induced hypertension, thyroid crisis, and intrauterine growth retardation and an almost 10 percent incidence of neonatal thyroid abnormalities were observed.[102]

■ TABLE 16–8
Obstetric Complications of Thyrotoxicosis

Maternal Complications	Fetal/Neonatal Complications
Miscarriage	Congenital malformations
Preterm delivery	Intrauterine growth retardation
Abruptio placentae	Stillbirth
Hypertensive disorders	Prematurity
Congestive heart failure	Fetal/neonatal thyrotoxicosis
Thyroid storm	

THYROID STORM

Thyroid storm is a rare and life-threatening complication of hyperthyroidism, almost invariably associated with Graves' disease. In this syndrome, moderately to severely increased thyroid hormone levels are associated with significant tachycardia and hypertension in addition to fever and mental status changes.

Immediate treatment is important in these patients, being particularly crucial if thyroid storm develops in the pregnant woman. This typically occurs at the time of delivery, when it is associated with significant obstetric morbidity.[122] In such cases, the rapid administration of drugs that will result in a prompt fall in thyroid hormone levels is mandatory. PTU should be started as soon as possible. Whereas it primarily works on blocking organification of new thyroid hormone, which may take several weeks to become apparent, it has a more rapid effect on peripheral T_4 to T_3 conversion. β-Blockers quickly ameliorate many of the hyperadrenergic signs and circulatory abnormalities. In high doses, they, too, block peripheral conversion, as do corticosteroids. Both of these drugs are reasonably safe if they are used for short periods during pregnancy. Iodine is also effective in rapidly decreasing thyroid hormone levels in thyroid storm. Although generally not advisable during pregnancy, it has a role in the treatment of thyroid storm, particularly if it occurs at delivery. In addition, by decreasing thyroid gland vascularity, iodine is particularly useful in the preoperative setting. In addition to these therapies, standard supportive care with intravenous hydration, antipyretics, and the treatment of any precipitating events, such as infection, are mandatory. In a woman who develops thyroid storm or severe hyperthyroidism in late pregnancy, attempts at natural labor or induction should best be avoided and the child should be delivered by cesarean section. In early pregnancy, thyroid storm poses a significant management problem. In individual severe cases, particularly if the thyroid storm has resulted from the patient's noncompliance, proceeding to urgent thyroidectomy after medical stabilization may be the most prudent approach.[122]

FETAL AND NEONATAL THYROTOXICOSIS

The diagnosis and treatment of Graves' disease during pregnancy are made particularly challenging by the possible simultaneous occurrence of fetal or neonatal thyrotoxicosis.[123] By week 22 to 24 of gestation, the fetal thyroid is of sufficient size and maturity to be stimulated by maternally derived TSI, resulting in fetal goiter and excess concentrations of thyroid hormones in the fetal circulation. Signs of fetal thyrotoxicosis include tachycardia, thyroid enlargement (Fig. 16–9), oligohydramnios, and craniosynostosis.[124] Many cases of fetal Graves' disease presumably go undiagnosed, because the mother is often already receiving thioamides, with the fetus inadvertently treated. Therefore, it is typically diagnosed during a pregnancy involving a euthyroid woman with a past history of Graves' disease previously treated with radioiodine or surgery. Because maternal TSI still circulates and no antithyroid drugs are being administered to the mother, the fetal thyroid remains susceptible to thyroid stimulation in such situations. In these cases, thioamides may be given to the mother, who acts as a conduit for ultimate fetal administration.[86, 125–127]

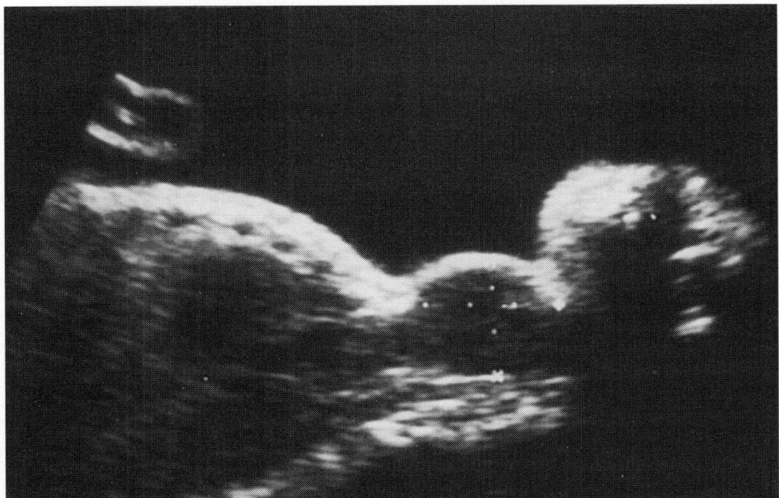

Figure 16–9 ■ Ultrasound examination demonstrating fetal goiter. (From Nelson M, Wickus G, Caplan R, Beguin E. Thyroid gland size in pregnancy. J Reprod Med 32:888–890, 1987.)

If not already receiving levothyroxine replacement, the mother may require it to avoid the development of drug-induced hypothyroidism. In difficult cases, when the actual thyroid status of the fetus is in question, cordocentesis will provide direct measurement of fetal thyroid hormone levels, and TSH and may be helpful in delineating the appropriate treatment. In the neonatal setting, because Graves' disease antibodies are still present in the newborn's blood stream for up to 2 months, thyrotoxicosis may also present at this time. Neonatal signs may include low birth weight associated with advanced bone age, failure to gain weight, hyperactivity, and "thyroid stare."[124] Such infants can and should be treated with small doses of antithyroid drugs and observed closely for the gradual disappearance of TSI and the normalization of thyroid function.

Maternal TSI titers measured during the 26th week of gestation have been shown to correlate with the risk for development of either fetal or neonatal thyrotoxicosis.[128] Little is known about the passage of maternal TSH receptor antibodies from mother to fetus. Because of the frequent presence of thyrotropin-binding inhibitory immunoglobulin, which blocks thyroid activity, in women with Graves' disease, the net result on the fetal thyroid, when it is considered in combination with maternal TSI, may vary from patient to patient. Cases of fetal and neonatal hypothyroidism due to thyrotropin-binding inhibitory immunoglobulin have also been reported.[124] Nothing substitutes, therefore, for a careful clinical assessment of both mother and fetus in these particularly challenging cases.

OTHER THYROID DISORDERS DURING PREGNANCY

Thyroid diseases other than hypothyroidism and hyperthyroidism are rarely encountered during pregnancy. When they are, however, as in the case of Graves' disease, the diagnostic and therapeutic approach must weigh the risks and benefits to both mother and fetus.

Thyroid Nodules

Because fine-needle aspiration biopsy has taken the place of radionuclide scanning as the initial work-up step for thyroid nodules, the evaluation of such in the pregnant woman should not be appreciably different from that in the nonpregnant woman.[17] Certainly, however, if a malignant neoplasm is discovered, further staging and treatment necessarily need to be altered.

If a nodule is discovered during late pregnancy, depending on its size, character, and growth rate, it may be reasonable to defer any evaluation until after delivery.[129] If, however, one is discovered during early pregnancy or midpregnancy, the diagnostic approach should approximate that in the nonpregnant state, save for the absolute contraindication for nuclear thyroid studies.[130] Cases of rapid growth of papillary carcinoma of the thyroid have been described during pregnancy.[131] These data are consistent with evidence of a thyroid-stimulatory milieu of early pregnancy, although a true association at this point remains speculative. A reasonable approach would be to proceed with biopsy of any solitary thyroid nodule greater than 2 cm in size before 30 weeks of gestation or in any patient with a nodule that is increasing in size rapidly or has other clinical findings suggestive of a malignant process.

Thyroid Cancer

If a thyroid malignant process (i.e., papillary carcinoma) is discovered by fine-needle aspiration during pregnancy, depending on the tumor type and stage of the pregnancy, the surgical and anesthetic risks to both mother and fetus must be weighed against the risks of an untreated malignant neoplasm. Most cases of well-differentiated thyroid cancer are slow-growing tumors, and a delay of several weeks should not prejudice the ultimate outcome. If it is discovered in early pregnancy or midpregnancy, surgical intervention is the most reasonable option. If it is discovered in late gestation, delaying therapy until after delivery is justified, depending on the tumor type and clinical stage. In such cases, supplemental levothyroxine to lower any possible TSH stimulation should be considered. If the cytologic interpretation is that of a "follicular neoplasm" (i.e., indeterminate), there is an approximately 20 percent chance of malignancy, that is, follicular carcinoma, which tends to behave a bit more aggressively than follicular adenoma.

However, because the great majority of such diagnoses are only follicular adenomas, particularly late in pregnancy, it would appear prudent to wait until after delivery to surgically resect any such tumor. If this occurs early in pregnancy, especially if the lesion has any other sign that would place it at higher risk for malignancy (such as recent growth, associated cervical lymphadenopathy, hoarseness, or firm mass) or if the patient received any form of radiation exposure to the neck, a more aggressive approach will be necessary, including surgical resection during pregnancy. A similar approach has proved safe and effective.[132] Other authors have suggested a more conservative approach, that is, to delay any surgical intervention until after delivery in most cases.[133]

In the case of actual thyroid cancer discovered and resected during pregnancy, postoperative radioablation is absolutely contraindicated. In particularly aggressive tumors with significant metastatic disease, the therapeutic options must obviously be carefully considered in light of the stage of pregnancy and viability of the fetus.

POSTPARTUM THYROID DYSFUNCTION

Thyroid dysfunction during the puerperium is common; approximately 5 to 10 percent of women are affected in the 12 months post partum,[134] an incidence that has been observed in studies in which thyroid function was determined at fixed intervals post partum.[134] Actual clinical thyroid dysfunction occurs less frequently.

Graves' Disease Post Partum

Up to 30 percent of patients with Graves' disease will experience a clinical flare of their hyperthyroidism within 1 to 2 months after delivery,[135] consistent with an increase in immune surveillance at this time. This is in sharp contrast to the immune tolerance that develops during pregnancy and that has been thought to be responsible for the usual attenuation of Graves' disease activity during the second and third trimesters. In some cases, the postpartum flare of Graves' disease may be its first manifestation. In up to half of such cases, the thyrotoxicosis may be transient.[136] Elevated TSI titers during early pregnancy may be able to predict the postpartum onset of Graves' disease.[136] In patients with gestational hyperthyroidism, combination treatment with antithyroid drugs and levothyroxine may decrease the incidence of postpartum recurrence. Hashizume and colleagues[135] have reported that this treatment results in a reduction in the postpartum rise of anti-TSH receptor antibodies, accompanied by an ultimate decrease in the postpartum recurrence rate of hyperthyroidism from 31 percent to 5 percent within the first year after delivery. This group has also reported similar beneficial effects of combined therapy on the future recurrence rate of Graves' disease in nonpregnant individuals.[137] However, this effect has not been confirmed by other investigators.[138]

Diagnosis and Treatment of Hyperthyroidism in the Nursing Woman

In the postpartum setting, issues surrounding diagnosis and treatment of hyperthyroidism must be considered in light of the patient's desire to breast feed. Both PTU and MMI are excreted in breast milk, PTU somewhat less than MMI.[139] Therefore, PTU is considered the drug of choice for the nursing woman who requires treatment of her thyrotoxicosis in the puerperium. Breast milk concentrations of PTU are low, and exposure of the neonate is small, although periodic monitoring of the child is indicated, particularly if high doses are used. In one study, infants with fetal hypothyroidism born to mothers with Graves' disease experienced no delay in the recovery of their thyroid function despite exposure to PTU postnatally during breast feeding.[140]

More serious effects to the neonate may occur when nursing mothers receive radioiodine compounds, because these isotopes are readily excreted in breast milk. Scintigraphic evidence of radioiodine breast uptake has been seen in up to 6 percent of non–breast feeding women receiving radioiodine.[141] Certainly, even diagnostic doses of ^{131}I with its long half-life should lead to an immediate cessation of nursing. Neonatal exposure to this isotope may lead to ablation of its thyroid gland, although there are few experiential data on this matter. Whether nursing can be safely resumed is not at all clear. An analysis of breast milk after diagnostic doses of ^{131}I has indicated a longer duration of radioactivity than previously suspected.[142] Thus, ^{131}I may not be suitable if nursing is to be resumed. ^{123}I with its shorter half-life is safer; an interruption of nursing for 7 days may be sufficient. Technetium pertechnetate has an even shorter half-life than either radioiodine, and an interlude in breast feeding of 24 hours would suffice after a diagnostic dose.[97]

Postpartum Thyroiditis

Analogous to silent thyroiditis, which by definition occurs outside of the puerperium, postpartum thyroiditis (PPT) classically involves an initial hyperthyroid stage beginning 1 to 2 months after delivery and lasting 2 to 3 months. Immune-mediated lymphocytic infiltration of the thyroid leads to parenchymal inflammation and follicular destruction, with uncontrolled release of preformed hormone stores. During this time, radioiodine uptake is expectedly low, and thyroid indices are mild to moderately elevated. In PPT, the gland is mildly enlarged and painless. There is a strong association with thyroid autoantibodies, which are present in more than 75 percent of cases.[134] TSH receptor antibodies are usually absent, however.

After the initial hyperthyroid phase, affected patients may pass through a hypothyroid phase, because the healing thyroid is not yet able to produce sufficient quantities of hormone. Affected patients may clinically experience only the hyperthyroid or hypothyroid phase. Almost half of affected women will require some treatment of their thyroid dysfunction during this time.[143] At the end of 6 to 12 months, 95 percent of patients are fully recovered, with a small percentage proceeding to permanent hypothyroidism. Up to one quarter of women with PPT, however, may become hypothyroid after 3 to 4 years; predictive factors include the severity of the initial hypothyroidism, the degree of elevation of antimicrosomal antibodies at the 16th week of gestation, and multiparity.[144] PPT recurs with future pregnancies in approximately 50 percent of patients.[145]

It would seem reasonable to screen high-risk individuals for dysfunction periodically during the first postpartum year or at least be particularly cognizant of associated symptoms, such as unusual changes in weight, lability of mood, palpitations, and depression.

The incidence of PPT appears to be approximately 5 to 10 percent in the general population. However, in selected groups of patients, it may be higher. Women with elevated antimicrosomal antibodies measured at 32 weeks of gestation have a 20-fold greater risk of developing PPT.[146] In women with insulin-dependent diabetes mellitus, the incidence may approach 25 percent.[143] Prophylactic therapy during the puerperium with either levothyroxine or iodide in high-risk patients with presence of anti-TPO antibodies has no effect on the incidence of PPT in high-risk women.[147]

A possible association between PPT and postpartum depression has been suggested in the past.[148] Recent studies, however, have raised doubts concerning any true relationship.[146, 149]

Distinguishing PPT from the postpartum "onset" of (or flare of previously unrecognized) Graves' disease may be difficult. The serial measurement of thyroid hormone levels will eventually show normalization or progression to hypothyroidism within several months in PPT. In contradistinction, in Graves' disease, hyperthyroidism usually persists, but not always. Scintigraphic studies are helpful, with the demonstration of absent or markedly reduced isotope uptake in thyroiditis and increased uptake in Graves' disease. However, these studies may pose some problems for the nursing mother (see earlier). A progressive increase in serum thyroglobulin level may also distinguish postpartum thyroiditis from a flare of Graves' disease.[150]

Postpartum Hypothyroidism

Hypothyroidism may also occur in the postpartum setting. In most situations, a prior subclinical thyrotoxic phase of PPT was missed. Alternatively, the etiology may be the onset of chronic lymphocytic thyroiditis (Hashimoto's disease). One should additionally be wary of the unlikely possibility of two forms of central (or secondary) hypothyroidism that may occur in the postpartum setting.

Sheehan's Syndrome

Sheehan's syndrome, or postpartum pituitary necrosis, usually occurs in the setting of obstetric hemorrhage.[151] Pituitary size increases appreciably during normal gestation, predominantly owing to lactotroph hyperplasia. Its blood supply, however, remains somewhat tenuous, and the gland is prone to infarction if hypotension occurs.

Lymphocytic Hypophysitis

Autoimmune inflammation of the pituitary, known as lymphocytic hypophysitis, may also occur in the peripartum setting.[152] Infiltration of lymphocytes in the pituitary and its stalk may cause substantial pituitary enlargement, which may be mistaken for an adenoma, with a diagnosis being made by the neuropathologist after transsphenoidal exploration. In the majority of cases, associated pituitary dysfunction is transient, with partial or full recovery in most cases. Patients with lymphocytic hypophysitis are at risk for the development of other autoimmune conditions, such as primary hypothyroidism and premature ovarian failure. It is rarely reported in males.

The first manifestation in either lymphocytic hypophysitis or Sheehan's syndrome may be the failure to lactate post partum because of insufficient prolactin secretion. Hypothyroxinemia may be demonstrated on laboratory testing. In marked contrast to primary hypothyroidism, however, TSH concentrations are low or inappropriately normal. In addition, other anterior pituitary hormones may be deficient, including growth hormone, cortisol, and gonadotropins. Posterior pituitary dysfunction occurs uncommonly.

SPECIAL TOPICS

Reproductive Factors and the Epidemiology of Thyroid Cancer

Epidemiologic surveys have revealed modest effects of reproductive history on the incidence of thyroid cancer. In Norway, a slight increased risk of well-differentiated thyroid cancer was seen in multiparous women, with a greater influence on the incidence of follicular carcinoma than papillary carcinoma.[153] In another study, a long reproductive history as well as late last birth was mildly associated with an increased risk of papillary carcinoma; a decreased risk of follicular carcinoma was seen in women with early menarche and late menopause.[154] It is obviously difficult to make any firm conclusions from these data.

Effects of Radioiodine on Reproductive Health

Radioiodine is frequently used for the treatment of hyperthyroidism, usually administered as ^{131}I. It is considered the treatment of choice in older individuals and is becoming increasingly popular for those of reproductive age.[155] Small doses of 5 to 15 mCi used for Graves' disease have not been associated with any definable long-term effect on secondary tumor formation, subsequent fertility, or congenital anomalies in offspring.[156] With higher doses used for radioablation of thyroid remnants after thyroidectomy for well-differentiated carcinomas, most studies have also not been able to demonstrate any significant impact on ultimate fertility in women.[157, 158] Subtle and reversible effects have been observed in spermatogenesis in males, however.[159] Slight increases in the incidence of certain secondary neoplasms have been detected, however, most commonly for salivary gland tumors and melanoma.[158] Hematologic malignant neoplasms have been reported after very high doses.[159]

The Effect of Estrogenic Drugs on the Laboratory Assessment of Thyroid Function

Similar to that which occurs during pregnancy, the use of oral contraceptives or other estrogenic drugs is associated with an increase in thyroid hormone–binding capacity and decrease in T_3 resin uptake. Total T_4 and T_3 are therefore increased, because thyroid hormone production is transiently augmented to saturate newly available binding sites. Free thyroid hormone levels remain normal, however.

Thyroid Disease, Thyroid Hormone Replacement Therapy, and Osteoporosis

Bone mineral density is diminished in hyperthyroid patients.[160] Thyroid hormone is known to stimulate bone turnover.[161] Because thyroid hormone is a frequently used medication in older women, questions regarding the possible exacerbation of an underlying predisposition toward osteopenia have been raised. Initial studies pointed toward a potential deleterious effect.[162] More recent data, however, suggest that when thyroid hormone is given in replacement doses, no significant effect on bone density occurs.[163] In a carefully designed study of thyroxine therapy in 87 premenopausal and postmenopausal women, levothyroxine therapy alone did not appear to represent a significant risk factor for bone loss.[163] In those postmenopausal women with a prior history of thyrotoxicosis treated with radioiodine, however, substantial decreases in bone mineral density were observed. Importantly, the bone density did not correlate with the duration or dosage of levothyroxine therapy or with the degree of suppression of TSH. Thus, it must be concluded that thyroxine therapy by itself is not a risk factor for osteoporosis, although women who take L-thyroxine may have an underlying predisposition toward osteopenia, such as previous hyperthyroidism, from which full skeletal recovery has not occurred.

References

1. Delange F. The disorders induced by iodine deficiency. Thyroid 4:107, 1994.
2. Hershman J. Inhibition of organic binding of iodide with graded doses of iodide in euthyroid men. J Clin Endocrinol Metab 27:1607, 1967.
3. Fradkin J, Wolf J. Iodide-induced thyrotoxicosis. Medicine (Baltimore) 62:1, 1983.
4. Ekholm R. Biosynthesis of thyroid hormone. Int Rev Cytol 120:243, 1990.
5. Bartalena L, Robbins J. Thyroid hormone transport proteins. Clin Lab Med 13:583, 1993.
6. Caron P, Nieman L, Rose S, Nisula B. Deficient nocturnal surge of thyrotropin in central hypothyroidism. J Clin Endocrinol Metab 62:960, 1983.
7. Parmentier M, Libert F, Maenhunt C, et al. Molecular cloning of the thyrotropin receptor. Science 284:1620, 1989.
8. Samuels H, Forman B, Horowitz Z, Ye Z. Regulation of gene expression by thyroid hormone. J Clin Invest 81:957, 1988.
9. Krassas GE, Pontikides N, Kaltsas T, et al. Menstrual disturbances in thyrotoxicosis. Clin Endocrinol (Oxf) 40:641, 1994.
10. Burrow G. Thyroid function and hyperfunction during gestation. Endocr Rev 14:194, 1993.
11. Maruo T, Matsuo H, Mochizuki M. Thyroid hormone as a biological amplifier of differentiated trophoblast function in early pregnancy. Acta Endocrinol (Copenh) 125:58, 1991.
12. Beck-Peccoz P. Decreased receptor binding of biologically inactive thyrotropin in central hypothyroidism: Effect of treatment with thyrotropin releasing hormone. N Engl J Med 312:1085, 1985.
13. Dayan C, Daniels G. Chronic autoimmune thyroiditis. N Engl J Med 335:99, 1996.
14. Hurley D, Gharib H. Detection and treatment of hypothyroidism and Graves' disease. Geriatrics 60:41, 1995.
15. McKenzie J, Zakarija M. The clinical use of thyrotropin receptor antibody measurements. J Clin Endocrinol Metab 69:1093, 1989.
16. Magner J. TSH-mediated hyperthyroidism. Endocrinologist 3:289, 1993.
17. Inzucchi S, Burrow G. Thyroid nodules and goiter. *In* Conn RB, Borer WZ, Snyder JW (eds). Current Diagnosis 9. Philadelphia, WB Saunders, 1997, pp 761–767.
18. Thomas C, Croon R. Current management of the patient with autonomously functioning nodular goiter. Surg Clin North Am 67:315, 1987.
19. Mandel S, Brent G, Larsen P. Levothyroxine therapy in patients with thyroid disease. Ann Intern Med 119:492, 1993.
20. Heinman M, Johnson C, Man E. Serum precipitable iodine correlations during pregnancy. J Clin Invest 27:91, 1948.
21. Dowling J, Freinkle N, Ingbar S. Thyroxin-binding by sera of pregnant women, newborn infants and women with spontaneous abortion. J Clin Invest 35:1263, 1956.
22. Glinoer D, de Nayer P, Bourdoux P, et al. Regulation of maternal thyroid during pregnancy. J Clin Endocrinol Metab 71:276, 1990.
23. Nissim M, Giorda G, Ballabio M, et al. Maternal thyroid function in early and late pregnancy. Horm Res 36:196, 1991.
24. O'Leary PC, Boyne P, Atkinson G, et al. Longitudinal study of serum thyroid hormone levels during normal pregnancy. Int J Gynaecol Obstet 38:171, 1992.
25. Kaplan M. Assessment of thyroid function during pregnacy. Thyroid 2:57, 1992.
26. Thotakura NR, Blithe DL. Glycoprotein hormones: Glycobiology of gonadotrophins, thyrotrophin and free alpha subunit. Glycobiology 5:3, 1995.
27. Kennedy RL, Darne J. The role of hCG in regulation of the thyroid gland in normal and abnormal pregnancy. Obstet Gynecol 78:298, 1991.
28. Yoshimura M, Hershman JM. Thyrotropic action of human chorionic gonadotropin. Thyroid 5:425, 1995.
29. Kimura M, Amino N, Tamaki H, et al. Physiologic thyroid activation in normal early pregnancy is induced by circulating hCG. Obstet Gynecol 75:775, 1990.
30. Kennedy RL, Darne J, Griffiths H, et al. Thyroid-stimulatory effects of human chorionic gonadotrophin in early pregnancy. In vivo and in vitro studies. Horm Res 33:177, 1990.
31. Ballabio M, Poshychinda M, Ekins RP. Pregnancy-induced changes in thyroid function: Role of human chorionic gonadotropin as putative regulator of maternal thyroid. J Clin Endocrinol Metab 73:824, 1991.
32. Kennedy RL, Darne J, Cohn M, et al. Human chorionic gonadotropin may not be responsible for thyroid-stimulating activity in normal pregnancy serum. J Clin Endocrinol Metab 74:260, 1992.
33. Pekary AE, Jackson IM, Goodwin TM, et al. Increased in vitro thyrotropic activity of partially sialated human chorionic gonadotropin extracted from hydatidiform moles of patients with hyperthyroidism. J Clin Endocrinol Metab 76:70, 1993.
34. Glinoer D, Delange F, Laboureur I, et al. Maternal and neonatal thyroid function at birth in an area of marginally low iodine intake. J Clin Endocrinol Metab 75:800, 1992.
35. Glinoer D, Riahi M, Grun JP, Kinthaert J. Risk of subclinical hypothyroidism in pregnant women with asymptomatic autoimmune thyroid disorders. J Clin Endocrinol Metab 79:197, 1994.
36. Abdoul-Khair S, Crooks J, Turnbull A. The physiologic changes in thyroid function during pregnancy. Clin Sci 27:195, 1964.
37. Mussey R. The thyroid gland in pregnancy. Am J Obstet Gynecol 36:529, 1938.
38. Medvei V. A History of Endocrinology. Lancaster, UK, MTP Press, 1982, p 58.
39. Crooks J, Tulloch M, Turnbull AC, et al. Comparative incidence of goitre in pregnancy in Iceland and Scotland. Lancet 2:635, 1967.
40. Drury M. Hyperthyroidism in pregnancy. J R Soc Med 79:317, 1986.
41. Rasmussen NG, Hornnes PJ, Hegedus L. Ultrasonographically determined thyroid size in pregnancy and post partum: The goitrogenic effect of pregnancy. Am J Obstet Gynecol 160:1216, 1989.
42. Glinoer D, Lemone M. Goiter and pregnancy: A new insight into an old problem [see comments]. Thyroid 2:65, 1992.
43. Berghout A, Endert E, Ross A, et al. Thyroid function and thyroid size in normal pregnant women living in an iodine replete area. Clin Endocrinol (Oxf) 41:375, 1994.

44. Murray T. Goiter in Canada. Can J Public Health 68:431, 1977.
45. Glinoer D, Soto MF, Bourdoux P, et al. Pregnancy in patients with mild thyroid abnormalities: Maternal and neonatal repercussions. J Clin Endocrinol Metab 73:421, 1991.
46. Dowling J, Appleton W, Nicoloff J, et al. Thyroxine turnover during human pregnancy. J Clin Endocrinol Metab 27:1749, 1967.
47. Pintar JE, Toran-Allerand CD. Normal development of the hypothalamic-pituitary-thyroid axis. *In* Braverman LE, Utiger R (eds). Werner and Ingbar's The Thyroid, 6th ed. Philadelphia, JB Lippincott, 1991.
48. Radunovic N, Dumez Y, Nastic D, et al. Thyroid function in fetus and mother during the second half of normal pregnancy. Biol Neonate 59:139, 1991.
49. Thorpe-Beeston JG, Nicolaides KH, Felton CV, et al. Maturation of the secretion of thyroid hormone and thyroid-stimulating hormone in the fetus [see comments]. N Engl J Med 324:532, 1991.
50. Ballabio M, Nicolini U, Jowett T, et al. Maturation of thyroid function in normal human foetuses. Clin Endocrinol (Oxf) 31:565, 1989.
51. Vulsma T, Gons MH, de Vijlder JJ. Maternal-fetal transfer of thyroxine in congenital hypothyroidism due to a total organification defect or thyroid agenesis [see comments]. N Engl J Med 321:13, 1989.
52. Sack J, Kaiserman I, Siebner R. Maternal-fetal T_4 transfer does not suffice to prevent the effects of in utero hypothyroidism. Horm Res 39:1, 1993.
53. Ferreiro B, Bernal J, Goodyer G, Branchard C. Estimation of nuclear thyroid hormone receptor saturation in human fetal brain and lung during gestation. J Clin Endocrinol Metab 67:853, 1988.
54. Bernal J, Pekonen F. Ontogenesis of the nuclear 3,5,3′-triiodothyronine receptor in the human fetal brain. Endocrinology 114:677, 1984.
55. Contempre B, Jauniaux E, Calvo R, et al. Detection of thyroid hormones in human embryonic cavities during the first trimester of pregnancy. J Clin Endocrinol Metab 77:1719, 1993.
56. LaFranchi S. Congenital hypothyroidism: A newborn screening success story? Endocrinologist 4:477, 1994.
57. Thorpe-Beeston JG, Nicolaides KH, Snijders RJ, et al. Relations between the fetal circulation and pituitary-thyroid function. Br J Obstet Gynaecol 98:1163, 1991.
58. Thorpe-Beeston JG, Nicolaides KH, Snijders RJ, et al. Thyroid function in small for gestational age fetuses. Obstet Gynecol 77:701, 1991.
59. Das SC, Isichei UP. The "feto-maternal" thyroid function interrelationships in an iodine-deficient region in Africa—the role of T_3 in possible fetal defence. Acta Endocrinol (Copenh) 128:116, 1993.
60. Moya F, Mena P, Foradori A, et al. Effect of maternal administration of thyrotropin releasing hormone on the preterm fetal pituitary-thyroid axis. J Pediatr 119:966, 1991.
61. Thorpe-Beeston JG, Nicolaides KH, Snijders RJ, et al. Fetal thyroid-stimulating hormone response to maternal administration of thyrotropin-releasing hormone. Am J Obstet Gynecol 164:1244, 1991.
62. Bajoria R, Oteng-Ntim E, Fisk N. Transfer and metabolism of thyrotropin releasing hormone across the perfused human term placenta. J Clin Endocrinol Metab 81:3476, 1996.
63. Marchant B, Brownlie B, Hart D, et al. The placental transfer of propylthiouracil, methimazole and carbimazole. J Clin Endocrinol Metab 45:1187, 1977.
64. Gardner D, Cruikshank D, Hays P, Cooper D. Pharmacology of maternal propylthiouracil (PTU) in pregnant hyperthyroid women: Correlation of maternal PTU concentration with cord serum thyroid function tests. J Clin Endocrinol Metab 62:217, 1986.
65. Schneider H, Proegler M. Placental transfer of beta-adrenergic antagonists studied in an in vitro perfusion system of human placental tissue. Am J Obstet Gynecol 159:42, 1988.
66. Salvatore D, Low SC, Berry M, et al. Type 3 iodothyronine deiodinase: Cloning, in vitro expression, and functional analysis of the placental selenoenzyme. J Clin Invest 96:2421, 1995.
67. Wu SY, Polk DH, Chen WL, et al. A 3,3′-diiodothyronine sulfate cross-reactive compound in serum from pregnant women. J Clin Endocrinol Metab 78:1505, 1994.
68. Chopra IJ, Wu SY, Teco GN, Santini F. A radioimmunoassay for measurement of 3,5,3′-triiodothyronine sulfate: Studies in thyroidal and nonthyroidal diseases, pregnancy, and neonatal life. J Clin Endocrinol Metab 75:189, 1992.
69. Santini F, Cortelazzi D, Baggiani AM, et al. A study of the serum 3,5,3′-triiodothyronine sulfate concentration in normal and hypothyroid fetuses at various gestational stages. J Clin Endocrinol Metab 76:1583, 1993.
70. Wakim AN, Polizotto SL, Burholt DR. Influence of thyroxine on human granulosa cell steroidogenesis in vitro. J Assist Reprod Genet 12:274, 1995.
71. Jaya Kumar B, Khurana ML, Ammini AC, et al. Reproductive endocrine functions in men with primary hypothyroidism: Effect of thyroxine replacement. Horm Res 34:215, 1990.
72. Gerhard I, Becker T, Eggert-Kruse W, et al. Thyroid and ovarian function in infertile women. Hum Reprod 6:338, 1991.
73. Singh A, Dantas ZN, Stone SC, Asch RH. Presence of thyroid antibodies in early reproductive failure: Biochemical versus clinical pregnancies. Fertil Steril 63:277, 1995.
74. Ahmed M, Banna M, Sakati N, Woodhouse N. Pituitary gland enlargement in primary hypothyroidism: A report of 5 cases with follow-up data. Horm Res 32:188, 1989.
75. American College of Obstetricians and Gynecologists. Thyroid disease in pregnancy. ACOG Technical Bulletin Number 181—June 1993. Int J Gynaecol Obstet 43:82, 1993.
76. Wasserstrum N, Anania CA. Perinatal consequences of maternal hypothyroidism in early pregnancy and inadequate replacement. Clin Endocrinol (Oxf) 42:353, 1995.
77. Leung AS, Millar LK, Koonings PP, et al. Perinatal outcome in hypothyroid pregnancies. Obstet Gynecol 81:349, 1993.
78. Liu H, Momotani N, Noh JY, et al. Maternal hypothyroidism during early pregnancy and intellectual development of the progeny. Arch Intern Med 154:785, 1994.
79. Man EB, Brown JF, Serunian SA. Maternal hypothyroxinemia: Psychoneurological deficits of progeny. Ann Clin Lab Sci 21:227, 1991.
80. Mandel SJ, Larsen PR, Seely EW, Brent GA. Increased need for thyroxine during pregnancy in women with primary hypothyroidism [see comments]. N Engl J Med 323:91, 1990.
81. Tamaki H, Amino N, Takeoka K, et al. Thyroxine requirement during pregnancy for replacement therapy of hypothyroidism. Obstet Gynecol 76:230, 1990.
82. Kaplan MM. Monitoring thyroxine treatment during pregnancy [see comments]. Thyroid 2:147, 1992.
83. Van Loon AJ, Derksen JT, Bos AF, Rouwe CW. In utero diagnosis and treatment of fetal goitrous hypothyroidism, caused by maternal use of propylthiouracil. Prenat Diagn 15:599, 1995.
84. Magee LA, Downar E, Sermer M, et al. Pregnancy outcome after gestational exposure to amiodarone in Canada. Am J Obstet Gynecol 172:1307, 1995.
85. De Catte L, De Wolf D, Smitz J, et al. Fetal hypothyroidism as a complication of amiodarone treatment for persistent fetal supraventricular tachycardia. Prenat Diagn 14:762, 1994.
86. Hadi HA, Strickland D. Prenatal diagnosis and management of fetal goiter caused by maternal Graves' disease. Am J Perinatol 12:240, 1995.
87. Abuhamad AZ, Fisher DA, Warsof SL, et al. Antenatal diagnosis and treatment of fetal goitrous hypothyroidism: Case report and review of the literature. Ultrasound Obstet Gynecol 6:368, 1995.
88. Boyages SC, Halpern JP. Endemic cretinism: Toward a unifying hypothesis. Thyroid 3:59, 1993.
89. Vermiglio F, Lo Presti VP, Scaffidi Argentina G, et al. Maternal hypothyroxinaemia during the first half of gestation in an iodine deficient area with endemic cretinism and related disorders. Clin Endocrinol (Oxf) 42:409, 1995.
90. Romano R, Jannini EA, Pepe M, et al. The effects of iodoprophylaxis on thyroid size during pregnancy. Am J Obstet Gynecol 164:482, 1991.
91. Glinoer D, de Nayer P, Delange F, et al. A randomized trial for the treatment of mild iodine deficiency during pregnancy: Maternal and neonatal effects. J Clin Endocrinol Metab 80:258, 1995.
92. Rasmussen NG, Hornnes PJ, Hoier-Madsen M, et al. Thyroid size and function in healthy pregnant women with thyroid autoantibodies. Relation to development of postpartum thyroiditis. Acta Endocrinol (Copenh) 123:395, 1990.
93. Lejeune B, Grun JP, de Nayer P, et al. Antithyroid antibodies

underlying thyroid abnormalities and miscarriage or pregnancy induced hypertension [see comments]. Br J Obstet Gynaecol 100:669, 1993.

94. Pratt D, Novotny M, Kaberlein G, et al. Antithyroid antibodies and the association with non–organ-specific antibodies in recurrent pregnancy loss [see comments]. Am J Obstet Gynecol 168:837, 1993.
95. Bech K, Hoier-Madsen M, Feldt-Rasmussen U, et al. Thyroid function and autoimmune manifestations in insulin-dependent diabetes mellitus during and after pregnancy. Acta Endocrinol (Copenh) 124:534, 1991.
96. Pop VJ, de Vries E, van Baar AL, et al. Maternal thyroid peroxidase antibodies during pregnancy: A marker of impaired child development? J Clin Endocrinol Metab 80:3561, 1995.
97. Inzucchi S, Comite F, Burrow G. Graves' disease and pregnancy. Endocr Pract 1:186, 1995.
98. Niswander K, Gordon M. The Collaborative Perinatal Study: The Women and Their Pregnancies. Philadelphia, WB Saunders, 1972.
99. Tamaki H, Itoh E, Kaneda T, et al. Crucial role of serum human chorionic gonadotropin for the aggravation of thyrotoxicosis in early pregnancy in Graves' disease. Thyroid 3:189, 1993.
100. Abs R, Martin M, Blockx P. Changes in serum thyroid hormone autoantibody concentrations during pregnancy: A case report. Horm Res 35:205, 1991.
101. Froelich C, Goodwin J, Bankhurst A, et al. Pregnancy, a temporary fetal graft of suppressor cells in autoimmune disease? Am J Med 69:329, 1980.
102. Kriplani A, Buckshee K, Bhargava VL, et al. Maternal and perinatal outcome in thyrotoxicosis complicating pregnancy. Eur J Obstet Gynecol Reprod Biol 54:159, 1994.
103. Desai R, Norman R, Jialal I, et al. Spectrum of thyroid function abnormalities in gestational trophoblastic neoplasia. Clin Endocrinol 298:583, 1988.
104. Yamazaki K, Sato K, Shizume K, et al. Potent thyrotropic activity of human chorionic gonadotropin variants in terms of ^{125}I incorporation and de novo synthesized thyroid hormone release in human thyroid follicles. J Clin Endocrinol Metab 80:473, 1995.
105. Bouillon R, Naesens M, Assch FV, et al. Thyroid function in patients with hyperemesis gravidarum. Am J Obstet Gynecol 143:992, 1982.
106. Kimura M, Amino N, Tamaki H, et al. Gestational thyrotoxicosis and hyperemesis gravidarum: Possible role of hCG with higher stimulating activity [see comments]. Clin Endocrinol (Oxf) 38:345, 1993.
107. Goodwin TM, Montoro M, Mestman JH. Transient hyperthyroidism and hyperemesis gravidarum: Clinical aspects. Am J Obstet Gynecol 167:648, 1992.
108. Chin RK, Lao TT, Swaminathan R, Mak YT. A longitudinal study of changes in erythrocyte zinc concentration in hyperemesis gravidarum. Gynecol Obstet Invest 29:22, 1990.
109. Wilson R, McKillop JH, MacLean M, et al. Thyroid function tests are rarely abnormal in patients with severe hyperemesis gravidarum [see comments]. Clin Endocrinol (Oxf) 37:331, 1992.
110. Kennedy RL, Darne J, Davies R, Price A. Thyrotoxicosis and hyperemesis gravidarum associated with a serum activity which stimulates human thyroid cells in vitro. Clin Endocrinol (Oxf) 36:83, 1992.
111. Lao TT, Chin RK, Mak YT, Swaminathan R. Second-trimester thyroid function and pregnancy outcome in mothers with hyperthyroidism. Birth weight related to mid-trimester triiodothyronine and RBC zinc. Gynecol Obstet Invest 32:78, 1991.
112. Mujtaba Q, Burrow G. Treatment of hyperthyroidism in pregnancy with propylthiouracil and methimazole. Obstet Gynecol 46:282, 1975.
113. Mandel SJ, Brent GA, Larsen PR. Review of antithyroid drug use during pregnancy and report of a case of aplasia cutis. Thyroid 4:129, 1994.
114. Wing DA, Millar LK, Koonings PP, et al. A comparison of propylthiouracil versus methimazole in the treatment of hyperthyroidism in pregnancy. Am J Obstet Gynecol 170:90, 1994.
115. Messer PM, Hauffa BP, Olbricht T, et al. Antithyroid drug treatment of Graves' disease in pregnancy: Long-term effects on somatic growth, intellectual development and thyroid function of the offspring. Acta Endocrinol (Copenh) 123:311, 1990.
116. Crepin G, Delahousse G, Decocq J, et al. Dangers of iodine drugs in the pregnant woman. Phlebologie 31:279, 1978.
117. Momotani N, Hisaoka T, Noh J, et al. Effects of iodine on thyroid status of fetus versus mother in treatment of Graves' disease complicated by pregnancy. J Clin Endocrinol Metab 75:738, 1992.
118. Arndt D, Mehnert WH, Franke WG, et al. Radioiodine therapy during an unknown remained pregnancy and radiation exposure of the fetus. A case report. Strahlenther Onkol 170:408, 1994.
119. Momotani N, Ito K, Hamada N, et al. Maternal hyperthyroidism and congenital malformations in the offspring. Clin Endocrinol (Oxf) 20:695, 1984.
120. Mitsuda N, Tamaki H, Amino N, et al. Risk factors for developmental disorders in infants born to women with Graves disease. Obstet Gynecol 80:359, 1992.
121. Millar LK, Wing DA, Leung AS, et al. Low birth weight and preeclampsia in pregnancies complicated by hyperthyroidism. Obstet Gynecol 84:946, 1994.
122. Prihoda JS, Davis LE. Metabolic emergencies in obstetrics. Obstet Gynecol Clin North Am 18:301, 1991.
123. Perelman AH, Clemons RD. The fetus in maternal hyperthyroidism. Thyroid 2:225, 1992.
124. McKenzie JM, Zakarija M. Fetal and neonatal hyperthyroidism and hypothyroidism due to maternal TSH receptor antibodies [see comments]. Thyroid 2:155, 1992.
125. Wallace C, Couch R, Ginsberg J. Fetal thyrotoxicosis: A case report and recommendations for prediction, diagnosis, and treatment. Thyroid 5:125, 1995.
126. Wenstrom KD, Weiner CP, Williamson RA, Grant SS. Prenatal diagnosis of fetal hyperthyroidism using funipuncture. Obstet Gynecol 76:513, 1990.
127. Porreco RP, Bloch CA. Fetal blood sampling in the management of intrauterine thyrotoxicosis. Obstet Gynecol 76:509, 1990.
128. Mortimer RH, Tyack SA, Galligan JP, et al. Graves' disease in pregnancy: TSH receptor binding inhibiting immunoglobulins and maternal and neonatal thyroid function. Clin Endocrinol (Oxf) 32:141, 1990.
129. Choe W, McDougall IR. Thyroid cancer in pregnant women: Diagnostic and therapeutic management. Thyroid 4:433, 1994.
130. Walker RP, Lawrence AM, Paloyan E. Nodular disease during pregnancy. Surg Clin North Am 75:53, 1995.
131. Kobayashi K, Tanaka Y, Ishiguro S, Mori T. Rapidly growing thyroid carcinoma during pregnancy. J Surg Oncol 55:61, 1994.
132. Doherty C, Shindo M, Rice D, et al. Management of thyroid nodules during pregnancy. Laryngoscope 105:251, 1995.
133. Herzon FS, Morris DM, Segal MN, et al. Coexistent thyroid cancer and pregnancy. Arch Otolaryngol Head Neck Surg 120:1191, 1994.
134. Learoyd DL, Fung HY, McGregor AM. Postpartum thyroid dysfunction. Thyroid 2:73, 1992.
135. Hashizume K, Ichikawa K, Nishii Y, et al. Effect of administration of thyroxine on the risk of postpartum recurrence of hyperthyroid Graves' disease. J Clin Endocrinol Metab 75:6, 1992.
136. Hidaka Y, Tamaki H, Iwatani Y, et al. Prediction of post-partum Graves' thyrotoxicosis by measurement of thyroid stimulating antibody in early pregnancy [see comments]. Clin Endocrinol (Oxf) 41:15, 1994.
137. Hashizume K, Ichikawa K, Sakurai A, et al. Administration of thyroxine in treated Graves' disease. Effects on the level of antibodies to thyroid-stimulating hormone receptors and on the risk of recurrence of hyperthyroidism. N Engl J Med 324:947, 1991.
138. McIver B, Rae P, Beckett G, et al. Lack of effect of thyroxine in patients with Graves' hyperthyroidism who are treated with an antithyroid drug. N Engl J Med 334:220, 1996.
139. Cooper D. Antithyroid drugs: To breast-feed or not to breast-feed. Am J Obstet Gynecol 157:234, 1987.
140. Momotani N, Yamashita R, Yoshimoto M, et al. Recovery from foetal hypothyroidism: Evidence for the safety of breast-feeding while taking propylthiouracil. Clin Endocrinol (Oxf) 31:591, 1989.
141. Hammami MM, Bakheet S. Radioiodine breast uptake in nonbreastfeeding women: Clinical and scintigraphic characteristics. J Nucl Med 37:26, 1996.
142. Dydek G, Blue P. Human breast milk excretion of iodine-131 following diagnostic and therapeutic administration to a lactating mother with Graves' disease. J Nucl Med 29:407, 1988.
143. Alvarez-Marfany M, Roman SH, Drexler AJ, et al. Long-term

prospective study of postpartum thyroid dysfunction in women with insulin dependent diabetes mellitus [see comments]. J Clin Endocrinol Metab 79:10, 1994.
144. Othman S, Phillips DI, Parkes AB, et al. A long-term follow-up of postpartum thyroiditis. Clin Endocrinol (Oxf) 32:559, 1990.
145. Jansson R, Dahlberg P, Karlsson F. Postpartum thyroiditis. Baillieres Clin Endocrinol Metab 2:619, 1988.
146. Pop VJ, de Rooy HA, Vader HL, et al. Microsomal antibodies during gestation in relation to postpartum thyroid dysfunction and depression. Acta Endocrinol (Copenh) 129:26, 1993.
147. Kampe O, Jansson R, Karlsson FA. Effects of L-thyroxine and iodide on the development of autoimmune postpartum thyroiditis. J Clin Endocrinol Metab 70:1014, 1990.
148. Kaplinsky N, Pines A, Olchovsky D, Frankl O. Transient post-partum hypothyroidism. Acta Obstet Gynecol Scand 62:91, 1983.
149. Harris B, Fung H, Johns S, et al. Transient post-partum thyroid dysfunction and postnatal depression. J Affect Disord 17:243, 1989.
150. Hidaka Y, Nishi I, Tamaki H, et al. Differentiation of postpartum thyrotoxicosis by serum thyroglobulin: Usefulness of a new multisite immunoradiometric assay. Thyroid 4:275, 1994.
151. Sheehan H, Stanfield J. The pathogenesis of postpartum necrosis of the anterior lobe of the pituitary gland. Acta Endocrinol (Copenh) 37:479, 1961.
152. Patel M, Guneratne N, Haq N, et al. Peripartum hypopituitarism and lymphocytic hypophysitis. Q J Med 88:571, 1995.
153. Kravdal O, Glattre E, Haldorsen T. Positive correlation between parity and incidence of thyroid cancer: New evidence based on complete Norwegian birth cohorts. Int J Cancer 49:831, 1991.
154. Akslen LA, Nilssen S, Kvale G. Reproductive factors and risk of thyroid cancer. A prospective study of 63,090 women from Norway. Br J Cancer 65:772, 1992.
155. Farrar J, Toft A. Iodine-131 treatment of hyperthyroidism: Current issues. Clin Endocrinol (Oxf) 35:207, 1991.
156. Safa A, Schumacher O, Rodriguez-Antunez A. Long-term followup results in children and adolescents treated with radioactive iodine for hyperthyroidism. N Engl J Med 292:167, 1975.
157. Sarkar S, Beierwaltes W, Gill S, Cowley B. Subsequent fertility and birth histories of children and adolescents treated with ^{131}I for thyroid cancer. J Nucl Med 17:460, 1976.
158. Dottorini ME, Lomuscio G, Mazzucchelli L, et al. Assessment of female fertility and carcinogenesis after iodine-131 therapy for differentiated thyroid carcinoma. J Nucl Med 36:21, 1995.
159. Freitas J, Gross M, Ripley S, Shapiro B. Radionuclide diagnosis and therapy of thyroid cancer: Current status report. Semin Nucl Med 15:106, 1985.
160. Ross D, Neer R, Ridgeway E, Daniels G. Subclinical hyperthyroidism and reduced bone density as a possible result of prolonged suppression of the pituitary-thyroid axis with L-thyroxine. Am J Med 82:1167, 1987.
161. Melsen F, Mosekilde L. Morphometric and dynamic studies of bone changes in hyperthyroidism. Acta Pathol Microbiol Scand 85A:141, 1977.
162. Paul T, Kerrigan J, Kelly A, et al. Long-term L-thyroxine therapy is associated with decreased hip bone density in premenopausal women. JAMA 259:3137, 1988.
163. Franklyn J, Betteridge J, Holder R, et al. Bone mineral density in thyroxine treated females with or without a previous history of thyrotoxicosis. Clin Endocrinol (Oxf) 41:425, 1994.

Chapter 17

POLYCYSTIC OVARY SYNDROME (Hyperandrogenic Chronic Anovulation)

S. S. C. Yen

CHAPTER OUTLINE

KEY POINTS

- Polycystic ovary syndrome (PCOS), the most common cause of hyperandrogenic chronic anovulation and infertility, involves accelerated GnRH pulsatile activity, insulin resistance, hyperinsulinemia, and downstream metabolic dysregulation and is discernible peripubertally.
- Abnormalities of the reproductive axis are manifested as hypersecretion of LH, theca-stromal cell hyperactivity, and hypofunction of the FSH–granulosa cell axis resulting in hyperandrogenism, hirsutism, follicular arrest, and ovarian acyclicity.
- Obesity is a common feature of PCOS but not a prerequisite for its development. The degree of insulin resistance is amplified in obese women with PCOS, resulting in overt hyperinsulinemia, dyslipidemia, and fibrinolytic defects. Neuroendocrine-metabolic disturbances are distinct between obese and nonobese women with PCOS.
- GH–IGF-I and insulin are pro-gonadotropins; in synergy with LH, they act on the ovarian theca-stromal cells to stimulate the expression of cytochrome P450c17 and excessive androgen production. The relative input of each is modified by the presence of obesity.
- The functional integrity of granulosa cells of polycystic ovaries is fully intact when it is assessed in vitro. The arrested follicles are probably due to inadequate FSH input and to the effects of intrafollicular IGFBPs as inhibitors of IGF and FSH actions.
- The propensity for the development of insulin resistance and obesity in PCOS may reside in the marked impairment of catecholamine-induced lipolysis due to a reduced β_2-adrenoceptor density on adipocytes from nonobese women with PCOS.
- The long-term sequelae of PCOS include the development of endometrial cancer, type II diabetes, and cardiovascular abnormalities.
- Chronic anovulation can be rectified by several modes of treatment. Improvement of insulin sensitivity and hyperinsulinemia can be achieved by using insulin-sensitizing agents with subsequent amelioration of metabolic and hormonal derangements of the syndrome.

AN EVOLUTIONARY PERSPECTIVE

The polycystic ovary syndrome (PCOS) is by far the most common cause of hyperandrogenic anovulatory infertility. Although this syndrome was described more than half a century ago, the underlying cause of this disorder remains uncertain. However, cumulative information, coupled with important recent advances addressing neuroendocrine-metabolic derangements and the intraovarian autocrine/paracrine regulators in this syndrome, has afforded a better understanding of its pathophysiology and long-term consequences and provided approaches for effective management.

Between the years of 1925 and 1935, Stein and Leventhal recognized an association between the presence of bilateral polycystic ovaries and signs of amenorrhea, oligomenorrhea, hirsutism, and obesity. These manifestations represented the criteria rigidly applied to the diagnosis of what was then known as the *Stein-Leventhal syndrome*. Later, in 1964, Stein reported the reversal to normal menstrual cycles and conceptions after bilateral ovarian wedge resection in a significant number of patients diagnosed by the foregoing criteria.[1] On the basis of this result, a primary ovarian defect was inferred and the disorder was commonly referred to as the *polycystic ovarian disease*. Subsequent clinical, morphologic, biochemical, and endocrinologic studies have recognized an array of underlying abnormalities. The term *polycystic ovary syndrome* was then introduced to reflect the heterogeneity of this disorder.

During the ensuing two decades, interconnected functional abnormalities at all levels of the hypothalamic-pituitary-ovarian axis in patients with PCOS were described; hyperfunction of the luteinizing hormone (LH)–theca cell axis with excessive production of androgens and hypofunction of the follicle-stimulating hormone (FSH)–granulosa cell axis resulting in acyclic estrogen production and chronic anovulation were characterized.[2–5] Together with the extraglandular formation of estrogen and its impact on the functionality of the hypothalamic-pituitary-ovarian axis, the existence of a vicious circle in the pathophysiology of PCOS was recognized.[6, 7]

Perhaps most important was the disclosure of a unique form of insulin resistance and associated hyperinsulinemia in women with PCOS,[8–10] which may serve to link the abnormalities within and outside the hypothalamic-pituitary-ovarian axis. This coupling includes the ability of insulin to synergize the trophic effect of LH on theca cell androgen production and to inhibit hepatic production of insulin-like growth factor (IGF)–binding protein 1 (IGFBP-1) and sex hormone–binding globulin (SHBG), high-affinity binding proteins that, respectively, modulate the bioavailability of IGFs and sex steroids to target cells.[11, 12] The demonstration of lipolysis defects due to a reduced β_2-adrenoceptor density in abdominal adipocytes of nonobese women with PCOS, an event favoring the development of obesity, constitutes a major lead to the pathogenesis of insulin resistance in this syndrome.[13] Expanding knowledge now includes insulin and growth hormone (GH) as putative co-gonadotropins that act synergistically with LH to stimulate excessive ovarian androgen production, and the relative input of each is adiposity dependent.[14–16] Parallel advances in understanding neuroendocrine-metabolic signals that govern the maturational events of adrenarche and puberty, including physiologic insulin resistance, and the identification of endocrine-metabolic similarities between adolescent hyperandrogenism and adult women with PCOS have affirmed the peripubertal onset of this syndrome.[17–22] Moreover, accumulated evidence supports the proposal that an exaggerated adrenarche contributes to adrenal hyperandrogenism, hypersecretion of LH, and ovarian hyperandrogenism at puberty.[23–25]

In recent years, the putative role of intraovarian growth factors, neuropeptides, and cytokines as autocrine and paracrine regulators of the coordinated and gonadotropin-dependent functions of theca and granulosa cells in the development or maintenance of polycystic ovary phenotype has been widely considered.[26–28] The identification of increased expression of cytochrome P450c17, an androgen-synthesizing enzyme, in both the ovary and adrenal of women with PCOS accounts for the genesis of hyperandrogenism by both glands in this syndrome.[29] Evidence has also emerged that nearly half of follicular testosterone can be derived from circulating dehydroepiandrosterone sulfate (DHEA-S), establishing the prehormone-hormone relationship and the link between adrenal and ovarian androgenesis.[30, 31] However, it has been recognized that the array of abnormalities ascribed to PCOS are mimicked by several endocrine dysfunctions of diverse etiology, particularly late-onset congenital adrenal hyperplasia. Peripubertal onset of menstrual irregularities, increased hair growth, excess body weight, and androgen excess as well as insulin resistance are common to both PCOS and congenital adrenal hyperplasia.[32, 33] Further, the high incidence (25 percent) of ultrasound-detected "polycystic ovaries" reported in the adult female population[34, 35] complicates the diagnosis of the "classical form" of PCOS. It is clear that several new pathways in the understanding of PCOS have emerged during the last decade. At the moment of this writing, we are at the crossroads of producing a cohesive picture of this complex syndrome, the elucidation of which is reminiscent of the torturous course during a period of 50 years leading to the characterization of Cushing's syndrome.

PATHOPHYSIOLOGY AND CLINICAL FEATURES

PCOS is manifested clinically by a combination of hyperandrogenism with chronic anovulation and an elevated LH:FSH ratio. Hyperandrogenism is manifested by hirsutism and acne and, rarely, androgen-dependent alopecia and by elevated serum concentrations of testosterone and androstenedione. Chronic anovulation is associated with oligomenorrhea or amenorrhea and the presence of bilateral polycystic ovaries on ultrasound examination. Obesity is common but is not a prerequisite for the development of PCOS because 50 percent of PCOS women are not obese. Obesity per se is a disease entity, and its association with insulin resistance/hyperinsulinemia and impaired GH secretion is well established. Thus, neuroendocrine-metabolic dysfunction in PCOS in the absence of the confounding influence of obesity may be viewed as the pathophysiologic process underlying the *authentic syndrome,* and obesity constitutes a *modifier of the syndrome*. This basic tenet should facilitate assessments and interpretation of clinical manifestations, laboratory results, and long-term sequelae in women with PCOS.

Inappropriate Gonadotropin Secretion

In 1970, it was reported that inappropriate gonadotropin secretion is associated with the classic form of PCOS. Compared with the follicular phase of the normal menstrual cycle, women with PCOS exhibit a disproportionately high LH secretion with relatively constant low FSH secretion.[2]

Accelerated GnRH/LH Pulsatile Activity

An increased LH pulse frequency in PCOS women, independent of body mass index (BMI) or adiposity, is now well established.[36, 37] Whereas hypersecretion of LH, an elevated LH:FSH ratio, and heightened LH responses to gonadotropin-releasing hormone (GnRH) are evident in nonobese PCOS, the presence of obesity attenuates these neuroendocrine abnormalities.[37–39] In a study of PCOS subjects with widely separated adiposity, normal weight PCOS displayed increased LH pulse amplitude together with accelerated LH pulse frequency, resulting in a threefold increase in 24-hour mean LH levels.[37] In contrast, in obese PCOS, LH pulse amplitude and the LH response to GnRH were attenuated in parallel with the degree of adiposity, and increased pulse frequency alone accounted for a twofold increase in 24-hour mean LH levels[37] (Fig. 17–1). These differences between nonobese and obese PCOS *do not* represent subsets of PCOS. Rather, they constitute two ends of a *continuous spectrum* of adiposity-related attenuation.[38, 39] Thus, increased LH pulse frequency is a feature specific for PCOS, independent of obesity. The presence of obesity in PCOS serves as a modifier with a negative influence on LH pulse amplitude but not pulse frequency. That increased LH pulse frequency and amplitude are already evident in peripubertal girls with ovarian hyperandrogenism[21, 22] supports the proposition that acceleration of the GnRH pulse generator is an intrinsic defect of PCOS and reinforces the peripubertal onset of PCOS.[5]

The mechanism to account for the accelerated GnRH/LH pulse frequency in PCOS is unclear. It does not appear to be related to α_1-adrenergic mechanisms.[40] Chronic inappropriate (nonlinear) feedback action of estrogen, particularly in the face of prolonged deprivation of progesterone, may play a role. Indeed, in PCOS patients, LH pulse frequency can be reduced by the administration of progestin,[41] and the LH response to GnRH, LH levels, and the LH:FSH ratio are nearly normalized by the administration of estradiol and progesterone in doses that produce midluteal-phase levels.[42, 43] These findings are consistent with the concept that chronic progesterone deficiency plays a *facilitory role* in the development of accelerated GnRH/LH pulsatile activity, but it is unlikely that progesterone deprivation is the cause of this dysfunction (see Pathogenesis).

Disparity of LH and FSH Secretion

The disproportionately low and constant FSH levels in PCOS women may be the critical abnormality leading to

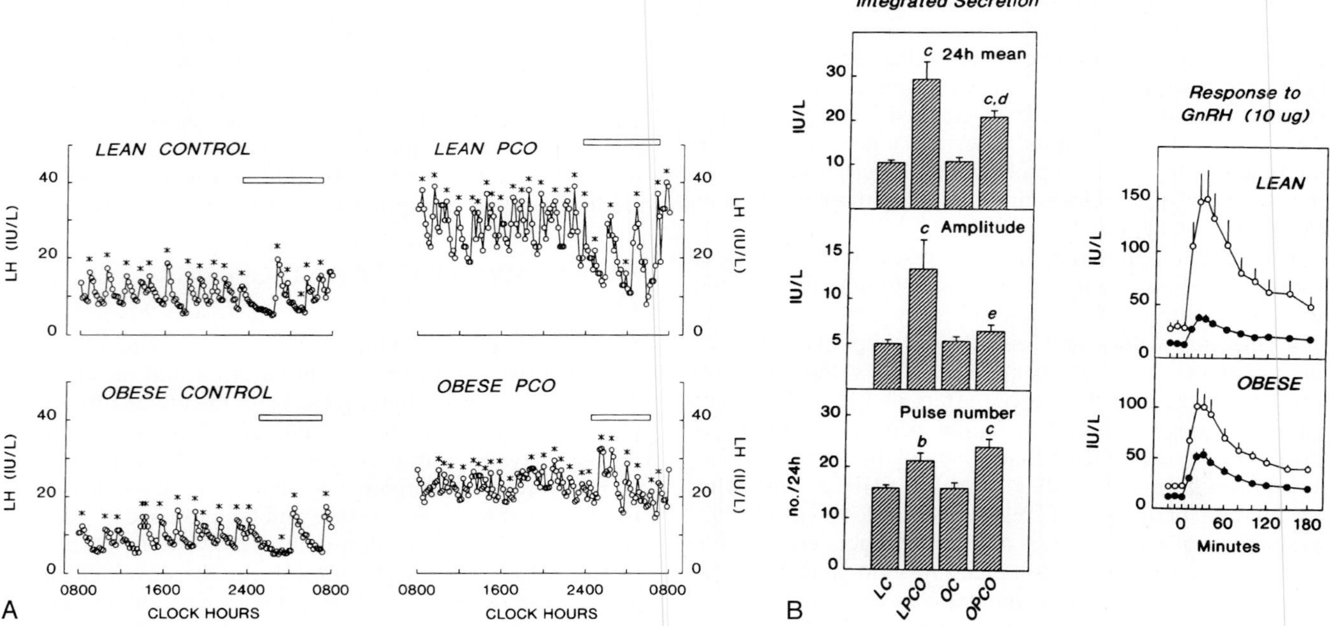

Figure 17–1 ■ *A*, Representative 24-hour LH pulsatile patterns in lean and obese control women during the follicular phase of the menstrual cycle and in lean and obese women with PCOS. Asterisks indicate LH pulses. Open bars signify sleep times. (From Morales AJ, Laughlin GA, Bützow T, et al. Insulin, somatotropic, and LH axes in lean and obese women with polycystic ovary syndrome: Common and distinct features. J Clin Endocrinol Metab 81:2854–2864, 1996. © The Endocrine Society.)

B, Twenty-four hour mean (±SE) LH levels, pulse amplitude, pulse frequency, and LH responses to GnRH in lean and obese women with PCOS (LPCO, OPCO) and their respective controls (LC, OC; n = 8 for each group). *a*, $P < .001$ versus corresponding control group; *b*, $P < .01$; *c*, $P < .001$ versus corresponding lean group. ○, PCOS; ●, normal control subjects. (From Morales AJ, Laughlin GA, Bützow T, et al. Insulin, somatotropic, and LH axes in lean and obese women with polycystic ovary syndrome: Common and distinct features. J Clin Endocrinol Metab 81:2854–2864, 1996. © The Endocrine Society.)

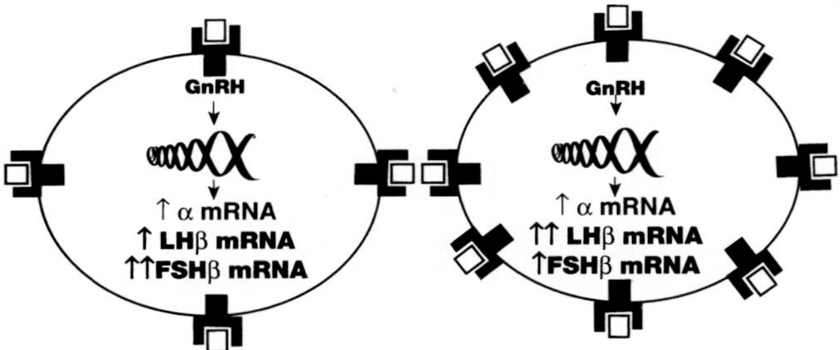

Figure 17–2 ■ Diagrammatic depiction of mechanisms of differential regulation of gonadotropin subunit genes by GnRH. When GnRH binds to its receptor on gonadotrophs, a signal transduction pathway is activated that results in the stimulation of the expression of all three subunit genes, α, LH-β, and FSH-β. Low GnRH pulse frequency increases FSH-β expression preferentially *(left)*, and high GnRH pulse frequency up-regulates the GnRH receptor and selectively increases LH-β expression without affecting α and FSH-β subunits *(right)*. (Modified from Kaiser UB, Conn M, Chin WW. Studies of gonadotropin-releasing hormone [GnRH] action using GnRH receptor–expressing pituitary cell lines. Endocr Rev 18:46–70, 1997.)

follicular arrest in this syndrome. Compared with the early follicular phase, FSH levels in PCOS women are reduced about 30 percent.[2] Because an increment of FSH levels of 30 percent above luteal-phase levels is necessary to initiate folliculogenesis,[44] the unvarying FSH levels in PCOS may be instrumental for the development of the follicular arrest, which can be easily rescued by the administration of small doses of exogenous FSH.[45, 46] Evidence suggests that the relatively fixed FSH levels are also linked to the *high frequency of GnRH pulses.* In this context, gonadotropin subunit genes are differentially regulated by GnRH. GnRH up-regulates the GnRH receptor, thereby increasing the GnRH signal. High-frequency GnRH pulses induce a preferential increase in LH-β messenger ribonucleic acid (mRNA) without influencing FSH-β mRNA, resulting in a higher secretory rate for LH than for FSH. By contrast, a slower GnRH frequency selectively enhances FSH-β mRNA, resulting in a higher rate of secretion of FSH than of LH (Fig. 17–2). In addition, a high frequency of GnRH pulses induces an increase in the intrapituitary high-affinity activin-binding protein *follistatin*, thereby reducing the FSH-releasing activity of activin[47–49] (Fig. 17–3). Thus, the disparity of LH and FSH secretion in PCOS is a consequence of the accelerated GnRH pulse frequency.

LH Levels as Diagnostic Marker (Influence of Adiposity)

When basal LH measurements are used as clinical markers of PCOS, a significant number of patients fail to exhibit an elevated LH level and hence LH:FSH ratio. This issue prompted a National Institute of Child Health and Human Development–sponsored consensus conference on diagnostic criteria for PCOS in 1990 and the recommendation that LH and the LH:FSH ratio are not required for the diagnosis of PCOS.[50] Several studies have observed that in women with PCOS, there is a negative influence of obesity on basal LH values.[51–53] This issue was recently evaluated across a wide range of BMI by more intensive studies, which demonstrated that obesity exerts a negative impact on LH pulse amplitude at the pituitary level without affecting LH pulse frequency. Accordingly, the LH:FSH ratio also decreased.[38, 39] When the degree of adiposity is taken into consideration, PCOS women with BMI of 30 kg/m^2 or less had significantly higher 24-hour mean LH levels than did matched normal women, whereas LH levels failed to discriminate PCOS from normal women in about 50 percent of obese subjects with BMI greater than 30 kg/m^2 (Fig. 17–4). Of clinical significance is the finding that the *mean of two LH values* in samples collected at a 30-minute interval, but not a single determination, had a discriminatory power equal to that of the 24-hour mean LH value.[38] The negative influence of adiposity on LH pulse amplitude, but not pulse frequency, may account for the heterogeneity of LH values observed in PCOS women across a wide range of BMI or adiposity. It is therefore suggested that assessments of LH levels and LH:FSH ratios determined in two samples at 30-minute intervals are of diagnostic value when BMI and adiposity are taken into consideration.[38]

Gonadotropin-Ovarian Axis

Polycystic Ovary Phenotype

In morphologic appearance, polycystic ovaries are enlarged bilaterally, and each has a smooth but thickened avascular capsule (Fig. 17–5). On cut section, the ovary exhibits 8 to 10 discrete subcapsular follicles, varying from 4 to 8 mm in diameter and peripherally arrayed with a necklace appearance. On occasion, a corpus luteum or corpus albicans may be found. The cysts are usually lined with a few layers of granulosa cells and are not atretic.[54] The most striking

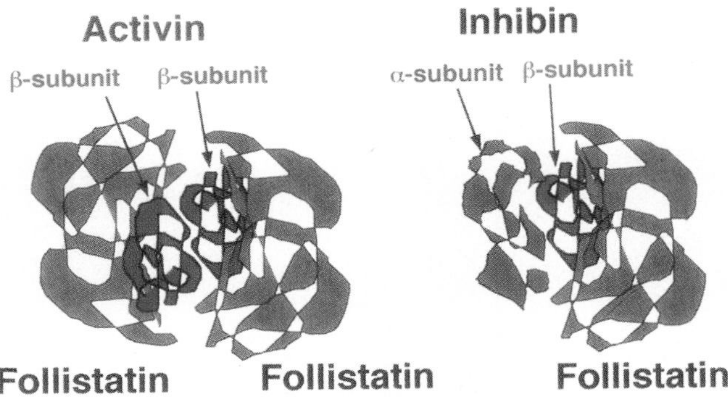

Figure 17–3 ■ Computer-generated structures of follistatin, the high-affinity binding protein for ββ activin with low-affinity binding for the single β-subunit of inhibin. (Courtesy of Dr. Nicholas Ling.)

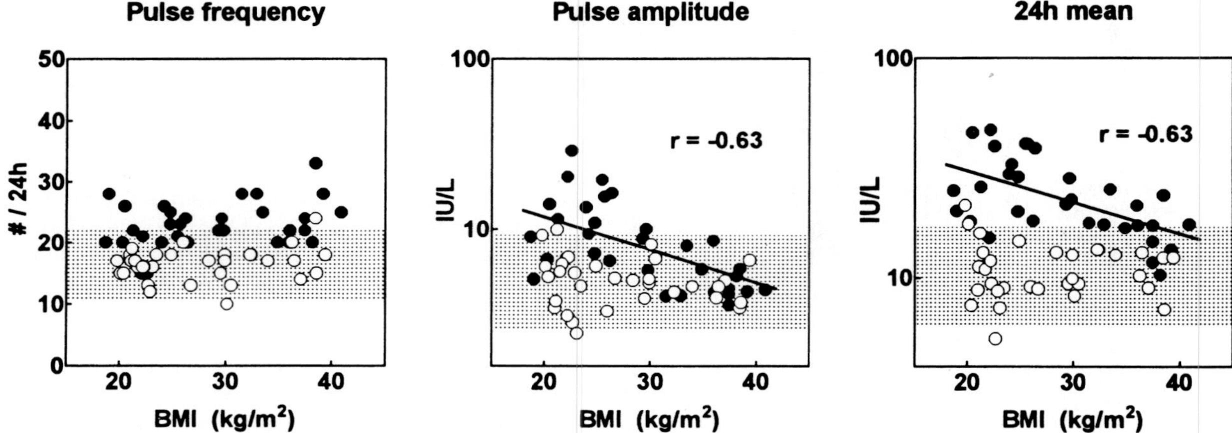

Figure 17–4 ■ Regression of BMI for PCOS (●) and normal control (NC) (○) women against LH pulse frequency (PCOS and NC, P = ns), LH pulse amplitude (PCOS: r = −0.63, $P < .001$; NC: P = ns), and 24-hour mean LH levels (PCOS: r = −0.63, $P < .001$; NC: P = ns). Values for LH pulse amplitude and 24-hour mean are $\log_{10}$ transformed. Shaded area represents 95 percent confidence interval for NC (frequency, 11–22 pulses/24-hours; amplitude, 2.6–9.2 IU/L; 24-hour mean, 6.1–18.2 IU/L). (From Arroyo A, Laughlin GA, Morales AJ, Yen SSC. Inappropriate gonadotropin secretion in polycystic ovary syndrome: Influence of adiposity. J Clin Endocrinol Metab 82:3728–3733, 1997. © The Endocrine Society.)

feature of the PCOS ovary is the hyperplasia of the theca-stromal cells surrounding arrested follicles and an increased stromal area. Microscopic examination reveals islands of luteinized theca cells indicative of hyperstimulation by LH and other trophic factors such as insulin and IGF-I (see co-gonadotropins). In addition to an increased number of small antral follicles, there is also an increased number of primary and secondary follicles in polycystic ovaries. These features suggest that there is an underlying disorder of folliculogenesis in PCOS with increased follicular recruitment but an arrest of follicular development at the small antral stage, a phenomenon related to the presence of inhibitors of FSH action on granulosa cells (see FSH–Granulosa Cell Axis).

The polycystic morphology is not unique to PCOS. It has been observed in a variety of anovulatory states including women receiving exogenous androgen and reproductively normal women.[34, 55, 56] However, the functional behavior of these ovaries with polycystic morphology has not been fully evaluated,[34, 56] whereas polycystic ovaries in PCOS function abnormally; steroidogenic hyperactivity of the theca cells and hypofunction of the granulosa cells are salient features of the syndrome.[4, 29, 56] Spontaneous ovulation and associated hormonal changes resembling those of

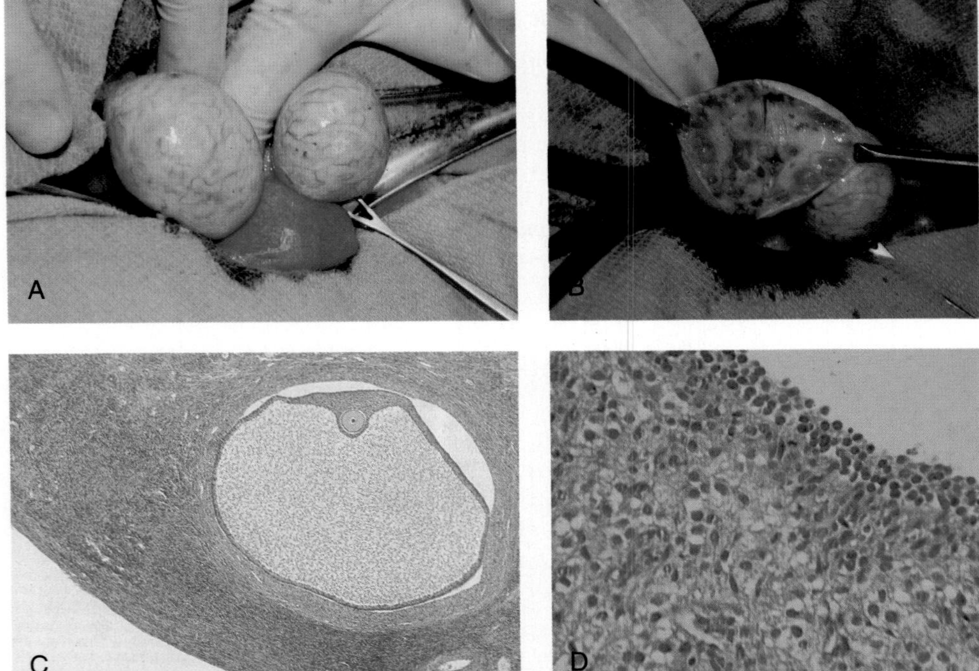

Figure 17–5 ■ The gross and microscopic characteristics of the polycystic ovaries. *A,* Bilateral enlarged ovaries with a smooth and thickened capsule. *B,* On cut section, multiple follicular cysts surrounded by abundant ovarian stroma are found throughout the cortex of the ovary. *C,* The subcapsular cysts are lined with granulosa cells, with early stages of antrum formation. *D,* Hyperplasia of theca interna with luteinization.

the normal menstrual cycle do occur occasionally (Fig. 17–6). Given these attributes, the author maintains that the presence of bilateral polycystic ovaries represents a component of the syndrome, and therefore its inclusion for the diagnosis of PCOS is required.

LH–Theca Cell Axis

Chronic LH stimulation in PCOS induces sustained hypersecretion of androgens by the theca compartment. The hyperactivity of theca cells is manifested in vivo by hyperresponsiveness of 17-hydroxyprogesterone to GnRH agonist challenge[29] and to human chorionic gonadotropin (hCG) stimulation.[57] When the *steroidogenic capacity* of theca cells from PCOS women was examined, 17-hydroxyprogesterone and androstenedione responses to a physiologic dose of LH on a per cell basis were respectively 8-fold and 20-fold greater in theca cells from PCOS compared with normal ovaries.[58] Further, the 17-hydroxyprogesterone response to hCG stimulation after suppression of endogenous LH by GnRH agonist for 4 weeks is also significantly greater in PCOS than in normal women.[57] Thus, the in vitro data are consistent with the in vivo results supporting the proposed primary "dysregulation of ovarian P450c17" in theca cell steroidogenesis in PCOS.[29] This issue is by no means settled. However, a persistent effect of an antecedent LH excess cannot be ruled out. Moreover, the experiments cited have two important limitations in the implication of primary ovarian P450c17 dysfunction; first, the LH suppression by GnRH agonist is incomplete, and second, they do not exclude the synergistic effect of insulin excess and increased IGFs[29, 59] on preexisting LH-mediated theca cell hyperfunction. As such, the multiple trophic inputs may be instrumental for the maintenance of the increased expression of P450c17 activities in theca cells of PCOS (Fig. 17–7).

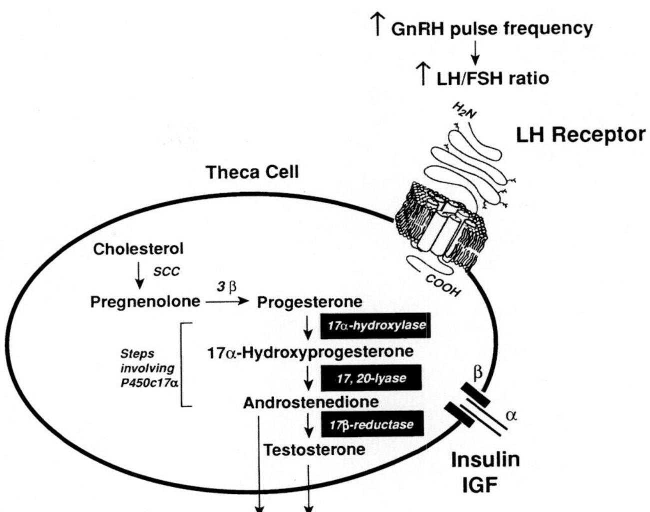

Figure 17–7 ■ Augmentation of LH–theca cell androgen biosynthesis by insulin/IGF-I. Diagrammatic depiction linking the accelerated GnRH/LH pulsatile activities and extraovarian factors (insulin/IGF-I) in the development of hyperandrogenism by ovarian theca cells. The trophic effect of LH, the indispensable regulator of theca cell steroidogenesis through the LH receptor, is augmented by insulin and IGF-I (as co-gonadotropins), inducing overexpression of P450c17, the rate-limiting enzyme for androgen biosynthesis. This bifunctional enzyme catalyzes progesterone to 17α-hydroxyprogesterone by 17α-hydroxylase activity and downstream to androstenedione by 17,20-lyase activity. Androstenedione serves as substrate for formation of testosterone by 17β-reductase and estrogen biosynthesis by granulosa cells, as well as being secreted into the circulation for biotransformation to estrone by peripheral target tissues. scc, side-chain cleavage enzyme; 3β, 3β-hydroxysteroid dehydrogenase, which converts Δ^5 to Δ^4 steroids. The α- and β-subunits of insulin and IGF-I receptors and the LH receptors are endowed on the cell surface of theca cells as shown.

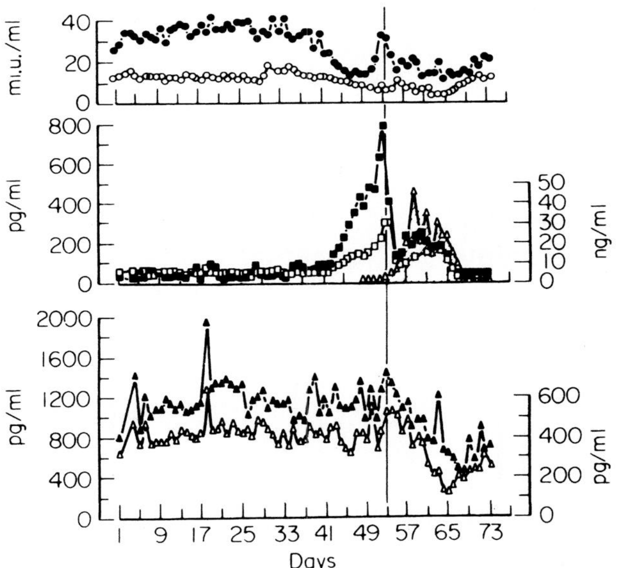

Figure 17–6 ■ Daily fluctuations of circulating gonadotropin (*top;* ●, LH; ○, FSH), estrogens and progesterone (*middle;* ■, estradiol; □, estrone; △, progesterone) and androgens (*bottom;* ▲, androstenedione; △, testosterone) monitored during a period of 74 days in a patient with PCOS. Within the period of study, spontaneous ovulation occurred with concomitant reduction of LH and androgen levels during the luteal phase.

FSH–Granulosa Cell Axis

The follicular cysts in the ovaries of PCOS patients do not mature fully, and the absence of mature follicles results in low estradiol production. Granulosa cells in these arrested follicles are few in number and are virtually devoid of P450arom (aromatase) activity. However, when granulosa cells are examined in vitro, these cells are not apoptotic, expressing high levels of FSH receptors, and they are highly responsive to FSH in vitro[54] as well as in vivo.[46] As such, the functional integrity of granulosa cells from PCOS ovaries is fully maintained complete with the FSH signaling mechanism to stimulate the aromatization of androstenedione to estradiol. Thus, the low aromatase activity in PCOS implicates inadequate FSH or a blockade of FSH action in vivo. Because follicular fluids from PCOS patients contain saturating concentrations of IGF-I and FSH, the hypothesis of the presence of FSH and IGF-I inhibitors has been proposed.[60] Although this issue is under intense investigation, available evidence suggests a reduced bioavailability of IGFs due to the quenching effects of increased follicular IGFBPs resulting in follicular arrest in PCOS (see later).[61]

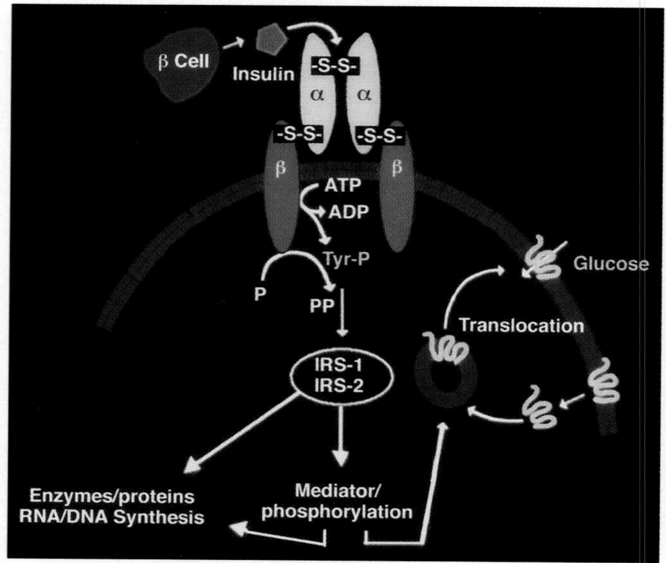

Figure 17–8 ■ The pathways of insulin action. The extramembrane domain of the α-subunit of the insulin receptor is the binding site for insulin. The transmembrane and intracellular domains of the β-subunits express tyrosine kinase (Tyr) activity and undergo autophosphorylation when activated by signals from α-subunits. Subsequent intracellular action involves IRS-1, initiating signal cascades that lead to stimulation of enzymatic systems, protein synthesis, and gene expression. In the fat and muscle, insulin induces recruitment of specific glucose transporters (the yellow loops depicted on the right) from the intracellular vesicle pool to the cell membrane, thereby mediating glucose transport. IRS-1 and IRS-2, insulin receptor substrates; ADP, adenosine diphosphate; ATP, adenosine triphosphate.

Metabolic Aberrations

Insulin

INSULIN ACTION

Insulin, a polypeptide hormone secreted by the β cells of the pancreas, plays a dominant role in maintaining glucose homeostasis. Its classic target tissues include the liver, muscle, and fat. Insulin suppresses hepatic glucose output, inhibits glycogenolysis and gluconeogenesis, and promotes glycogen synthesis. Insulin stimulates peripheral glucose uptake in muscle and fat and induces protein synthesis, cell growth, and differentiation. It also inhibits lipolysis.[62]

Figure 17–8 shows insulin binding to its cell surface receptor and its downstream signaling pathways. The insulin receptor is a transmembrane glycoprotein containing two αβ dimers connected by disulfide bonds. The extracellular α-subunits contain the insulin binding sites, whereas the intracellular components of the membrane-spanning β-subunits contain intrinsic protein tyrosine kinase activity. After insulin binds to and activates its receptor, the ligand-receptor complex is internalized through endocytosis. Insulin is then degraded, and most of the receptors are returned to the cell surface. This action, which results in insulin clearance, may be responsible for the insulin receptor down-regulation seen in chronic hyperinsulinemia.[62] Insulin binding results in phosphorylation of the β-subunit on specific tyrosine residues. This autophosphorylation increases the intrinsic tyrosine kinase activity of the β-subunit and results in activation of endogenous substrates that mediate insulin action.[63] Although not all mediators responsible for downstream signaling have been clearly defined, the apparent *proximate mediator, insulin receptor substrate-1 (IRS-1),* and IRS-2 have been cloned, sequenced, and characterized.[64, 65] IRS-1 is required for insulin-mediated translocation of the intracellular pool of glucose transporters (GLUT-4) to the cell surface and thereby increases glucose uptake in response to insulin.[66] The insulin and IGF-I receptors are remarkably similar, whereas the IGF-II receptor consists of an unusually long sequence of extracellular domain and short cytoplasmic domain (Fig. 17–9). The IGF-I receptor binds insulin with low affinity and can be activated by insulin, and *IRS-1 is a substrate* of both the insulin and IGF-I receptors.[67] Hybrid insulin/IGF-I receptors have been reported, but their biologic function is unknown.

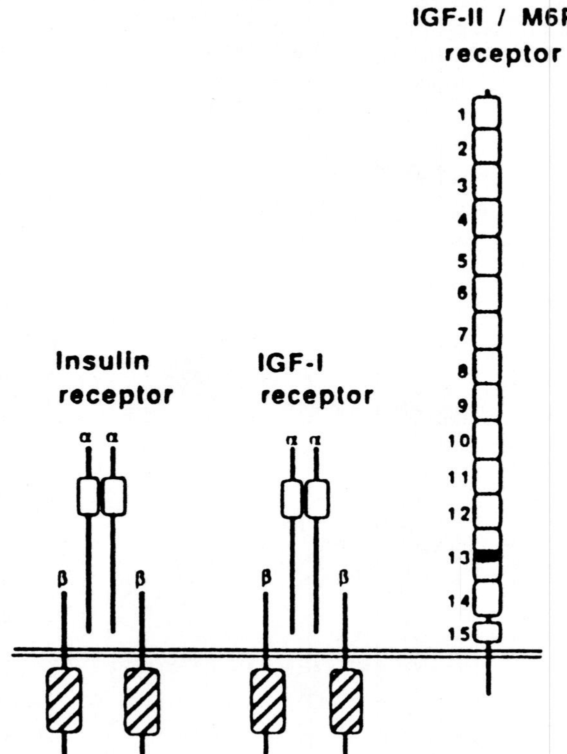

Figure 17–9 ■ There is a striking resemblance between receptors for insulin and IGF-I; both possess dimers of α- and β-subunits. The IGF-II receptor (same as the mannose-6-phosphate [M6P] receptor) structure is in marked contrast to both the insulin and IGF-I receptors.

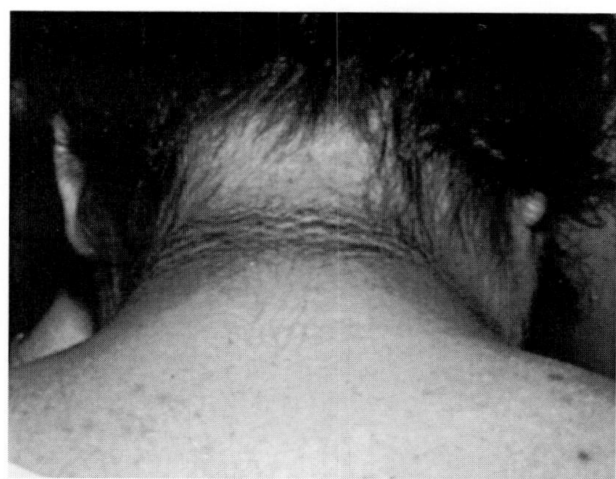

Figure 17–10 ■ Acanthosis nigricans—hyperpigmentation in the neck region in a patient with severe insulin resistance, hirsutism, and polycystic ovaries.

INSULIN RESISTANCE

Long before the identification of the association of insulin resistance with PCOS, several clinical models of rare syndromes of extreme insulin resistance had been described. In these syndromes, manifestations of androgen excess, amenorrhea, bilateral polycystic ovaries, and acanthosis nigricans were observed. The underlying defects reside in the insulin receptor. *Type A syndrome* of insulin resistance is due to a point mutation in the DNA sequence coding for the α-subunit and β-subunit of the insulin receptor.[68, 69] *Leprechaunism* is a rare genetic syndrome with a point mutation of the α-subunit.[70] *Type B syndrome* is due to the presence of autoantibodies against the insulin receptor associated with autoimmune diseases.

These diverse syndromes share a remarkable commonality of insulin resistance, hyperinsulinemia, and hyperandrogenism and a resemblance to PCOS.[71] In these syndromes, hirsutism is a marker for increased androgen production and acanthosis nigricans is a cutaneous marker of insulin resistance (Fig. 17–10). In PCOS, however, insulin resistance is not due to defects in insulin binding to the insulin receptor; rather, it involves post-binding signaling pathways.

INSULIN RESISTANCE IN PCOS

PCOS is associated with peripheral insulin resistance and hyperinsulinemia, and the degree of both abnormalities is amplified by the presence of obesity[37] (Fig. 17–11). Studies of insulin-mediated glucose disposal have shown that women with PCOS have peripheral insulin resistance similar in magnitude to that seen in patients with non–insulin-dependent diabetes mellitus (NIDDM).[10] Hyperinsulinemia consequent to peripheral insulin resistance represents a mechanism to overcome the impaired insulin-mediated glucose use in women with PCOS. Obesity, commonly associated with PCOS (50 percent of cases), has an additive negative effect on insulin resistance as indicated by the reduced hepatic insulin sensitivity in obese PCOS women beyond that associated with obesity alone.[37, 72] A positive correlation between the degree of hyperinsulinemia and hyperandrogenism has been observed. Reduction of ovarian androgen secretion does not alter insulin resistance, but reduction of hyperinsulinemia results in a substantial decrease in serum testosterone concentrations.[73] Impaired glucose tolerance is seen in obese but rarely in lean women with PCOS.[74] The presence of β-cell dysfunction as evidenced by the decreased first-phase insulin release in response to glucose stimulation occurs more commonly in PCOS women.[37, 74, 75] Thus, PCOS women are *insulin resistant* and have *β-cell dysfunction.*

The cellular mechanism of insulin resistance in PCOS was investigated in adipocytes, a classic insulin target tissue. It was found that the insulin receptor number and affinity are normal. In contrast, the dose-response curve for insulin-mediated glucose use is markedly shifted to the right in PCOS adipocytes independent of obesity[72, 76] (Fig. 17–12). This impaired glucose use is accompanied by a reduced abundance of GLUT-4 glucose transporter in adipocytes.[77] Autophosphorylation of insulin receptors in adipocytes is also decreased. Further, PCOS adipocytes are threefold (EC_{50}) less sensitive to the antilipolytic effect of insulin similar to the defect seen in glucose transport, and both events can be normalized by treatment with adenosine analogue in vitro.[78] Collectively, these findings suggest that insulin resistance in PCOS is associated with defects of both glucose transport and antilipolysis and that these events occur at an early step in insulin signaling common for glucose transport stimulation and the antilipolysis pathway.

Excessive *insulin receptor serine phosphorylation* in fibroblast and skeletal muscle has been found in a subset of PCOS.[79] Because serine phosphorylation has been shown

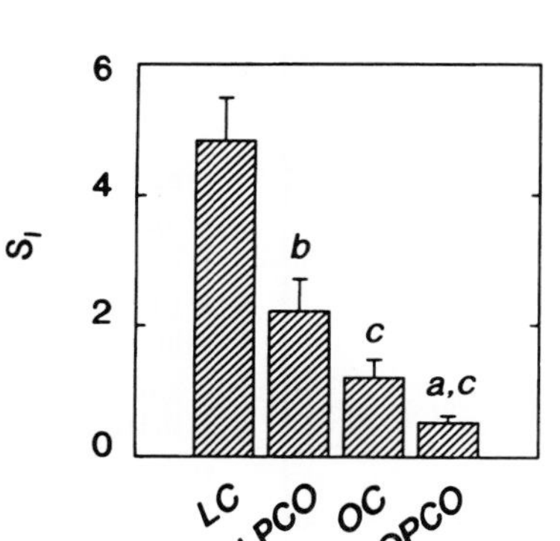

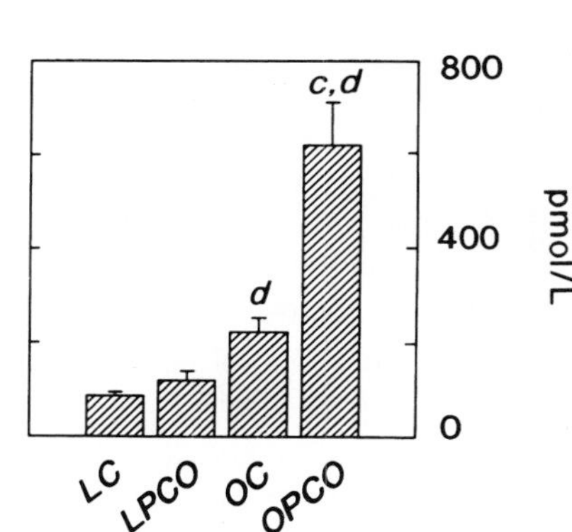

Figure 17–11 ■ Mean (±SE) insulin sensitivity (S_I) as determined by the modified rapid intravenous glucose tolerance test and 24-hour mean insulin levels in lean and obese women with PCOS (LPCO, OPCO) and their respective controls (LC, OC; n = 8 for each group). *a*, $P < .05$; *b*, $P < .01$; *c*, $P < .001$ versus corresponding control group; *d*, $P < .001$ versus corresponding lean group. S_I and 24-hour insulin levels (both log transformed) were inversely correlated for the groups considered together ($r = -0.75$; $P = .00001$). (From Morales AJ, Laughlin GA, Bützow T, et al. Insulin, somatotropic, and LH axes in lean and obese women with polycystic ovary syndrome: Common and distinct features. J Clin Endocrinol Metab 81:2854–2864, 1996. © The Endocrine Society.)

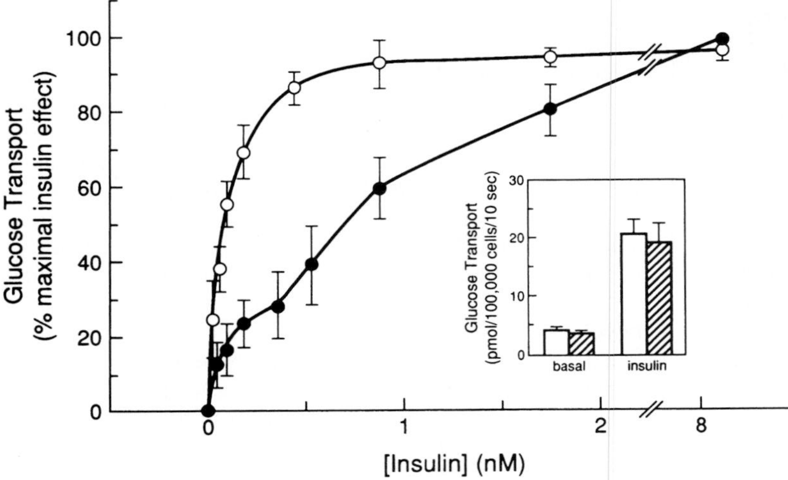

Figure 17–12 ■ Dose-response curves for insulin stimulation of glucose transport in isolated adipocytes from control (○) and PCOS (●) subjects. Cells were incubated with insulin for 60 minutes before measurements of initial rates of 3-*O*-methylglucose transport. Results are normalized against maximal activity for each subject, average ± SEM. *Inset,* Absolute rates of glucose transport in normal control *(open bars)* and PCOS *(hatched bars)* subjects, average ± SEM. (From Ciaraldi TP, el-Roeiy A, Madar Z, et al. Cellular mechanisms of insulin resistance in polycystic ovary syndrome. J Clin Endocrinol Metab 75:577–583, 1992. © The Endocrine Society.)

experimentally to inhibit insulin receptor signaling and is activated by factors extrinsic to the insulin receptor, a serine-threonine kinase may be implicated. These preliminary findings suggest that the presence of insulin resistance may reflect a genetic defect in a subset of PCOS women.[79]

GH–IGF-I System

The somatotropic axis is critical in the regulation of mitogenic and metabolic homeostasis. This axis is primarily driven by pituitary GH and nutritional status.[80] As depicted in Figure 17–13, the GH-IGF system has multiple levels of control including GH-binding protein (GHBP), IGFBPs, and IGFBP proteases and has widespread functions. GH is secreted in discrete pulses throughout the day. The hypothalamic regulation of the episodic secretion of GH is detailed in Chapter 2. Circulating GH is delivered to the liver as well as to numerous target tissues where GH receptors are abundant. In the liver, GH stimulates the gene expression and synthesis of the metabolic and mitogenic mediator IGF-I and to a lesser extent IGF-II.[80]

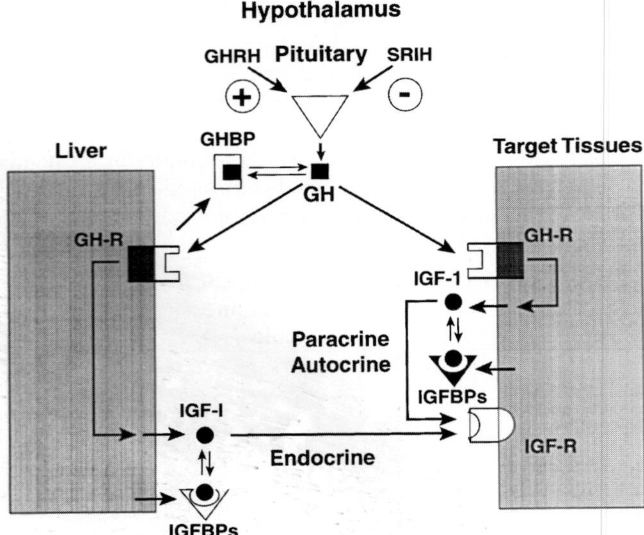

Figure 17–13 ■ Schematic depiction of the GH–IGF-I axis and its downstream modes of action and modulation by GHBP for GH and by IGFBPs for IGF-I both at the hepatic level (endocrine) and in peripheral tissues (paracrine/autocrine). (Modified from Thissen J-P, Ketelslegers J-M, Underwood LE. Nutritional regulation of the insulin-like growth factors. Endocr Rev 15:80–101, 1994.)

The relative biologic action of GH is modulated by a high-affinity GHBP in circulation that is derived from the extracellular domain of the GH receptor by proteolytic cleavage. Approximately 40 to 50 percent of circulating GH is bound to GHBP, and the complex serves to prolong the half-life of GH and hence modulate its bioactivity.[81] Regulation of GHBP production is not entirely clear. Both GH and adiposity appear to play a role.[82]

IGF-I and IGF-II are multifunctional polypeptides with mitogenic and insulin-like activities. The biologic and structural characteristics of IGFs compared with insulin are shown in Table 17–1. IGFs possess both endocrine (circulating compartment) and tissue-specific paracrine/autocrine (locally produced) modes of action (see Fig. 17–13). Circulating concentrations for IGF-II are two to three times higher than for IGF-I (Fig. 17–14). IGFs are also synthesized in multiple extrahepatic tissues, including granulosa cells of the ovary where they are under the control of FSH and play a role in folliculogenesis.[83] Unlike insulin, circulating and tissue IGFs are associated with high-affinity IGFBPs that serve to modulate the bioavailability of IGFs at receptor sites (see Fig. 17–13).

Six IGFBPs that differ in molecular size, hormonal control, and functional significance have been characterized.[84] Circulating concentrations of IGFBPs are highest for IGFBP-3 and lower for IGFBP-1 (see Fig. 17–14). Among them, IGFBP-1 and IGFBP-3 are the best studied. IGFBP-3, a major binding moiety in serum, possesses the highest binding affinity for IGFs and is in a *saturated state*. Circulating concentrations of IGFBP-3 are regulated by GH and IGF-I levels.[85] IGFBP-1 is a relatively low affinity binding protein and is *unsaturated*. Increments of circulating IGFs that occur are bound by IGFBP-1. Thus, IGFBP-1 serves as an *acute modulator* of the bioactivity of IGFs, whereas IGFBP-3 functions as a *reservoir* for long-term monitoring of IGF levels.[85–87] Proteolysis of IGFBPs increases free IGF levels, and the presence of proteases in target tissues represents the final step in control of IGF bioavailability.

■ TABLE 17–1
Comparison of Characteristics Between IGF-I, IGF-II, and Insulin in Humans

	IGF-I	IGF-II	INSULIN
Molecular mass	7649 daltons	7471 daltons	5734 daltons
Structure	1 chain; E-peptide is cleaved off	1 chain; E-peptide is cleaved off	2 chains; C-peptide is cleaved off
Origin	Mainly liver, widespread	Liver; widespread	β cells of pancreatic islets
Secretion	Constant slow release	Constant slow release	Pulsatile release
Production rate	10 mg/day	13 mg/day	2 mg/day
Circulating forms	Mostly bound	Mostly bound	Free
Binding proteins	6 distinct forms	6 distinct forms	None
Concentrations in adults	200 ng/ml (30 nmol/L) (1 U/ml)	700 ng/ml (85 nmol/L)	0.5–5 ng/ml (35–170 pmol/L)
Daily variations	Little or none	Little or none	Yes
Half-life	12–15 hr	15 hr	10 min
Affinity for receptors*	Type 1 > 2 > Ins.	Type 2 > 1 > Ins.	Ins. > type 1
Action	Endocrine Paracrine/autocrine	Endocrine Paracrine/autocrine	Endocrine
Growth hormone dependence†	+ + + +	+	0

*Receptors: type 1, IGF type 1 receptor; type 2, IGF type 2 receptor; Ins., insulin receptor.
†Growth hormone dependence: + + + +, strong; +, weak; 0, nul.
From Thissen J-P, Ketelslegers J-M, Underwood LE. Nutritional regulation of the insulin-like growth factors. Endocr Rev 16:80–101, 1994.

Insulin is a major regulator of hepatic IGFBP-1 production, and it enhances IGFBP-1 translocation to the extravascular space.[85–87] In humans, rapidly fluctuating serum insulin concentrations in response to meals result in inverse changes in serum IGFBP-1 levels but not in serum IGFBP-2 or IGFBP-3 levels.[80] These dynamics of serum IGFBP-1 and its *relatively unsaturated state* account for most of the binding activity of newly delivered free IGF in the circulation. IGFBP-1 sequesters free IGF-I and inhibits its metabolic (insulin-like) activity (Fig. 17–15*A*). IGF-I is also a potent anabolic growth factor; reduced circulating IGF-I levels during fasting are accompanied by pronounced catabolic events as indicated by the negative nitrogen balance (Fig. 17–15*B*). Thus, insulin regulation of hepatic IGFBP-1 production may coordinate insulin and IGF action with nutritional signals[80] and provide a link to reproductive function.

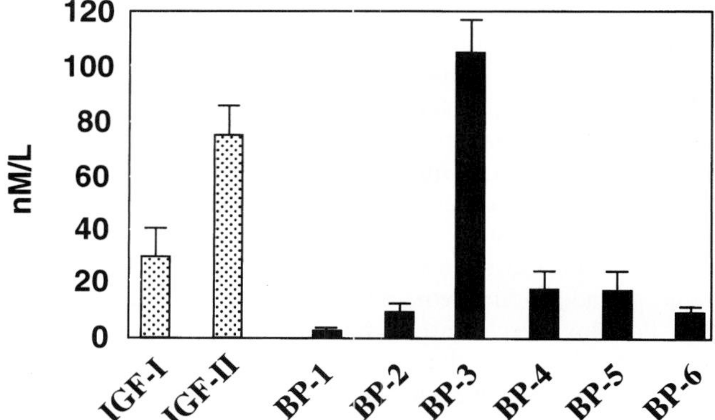

Figure 17–14 ■ Concentrations of IGFs and IGFBPs in adult human serum. Values are the mean ± SD. (From Mohan S, Baylink DJ, Pettis JL. Insulin-like growth factor (IGF)–binding proteins in serum—do they have additional roles besides modulating the endocrine IGF actions? [Editorial] J Clin Endocrinol Metab 81:3817–3820, 1996. © The Endocrine Society.)

GH AND THE OVARY

Increasing evidence suggests that GH augments gonadotropin action on ovarian function.[14] The localization and gene expression of the hGH receptor gene in human granulosa cells of antral and dominant follicles and corpus lutea[88] afforded the critical link supporting an endocrine role for circulating GH in the augmentation of FSH-mediated cytodifferentiation and steroidogenesis of ovarian granulosa cells.[89, 90] Cotreatment with rhGH and gonadotropin for induction of ovulation in women with anovulatory infertility induced a rise in serum IGF-I levels and a significant reduction in the effective dose and duration of gonadotropin treatment, indicating an augmented ovarian response to the combined regimen.[91] Thus, both in vivo and in vitro data support a corporate, but not indispensable, function of GH with FSH in the regulation of follicular development and steroidogenesis.

GH action in the ovary probably occurs in a cascading manner. GH through GH receptor enhances FSH-mediated cytodifferentiation and induces IGF-II expression in the granulosa cells. IGFs in turn promote granulosa cell steroidogenesis. Ultimately, IGFs and estrogen from granulosa cells may extend to the theca cell and synergize with LH to promote P450c17 activity, a paracrine action for androgen biosynthesis with downstream estrogen formation in the granulosa cells.[60, 92] Thus, an interacting loop of endocrine (GH/FSH), autocrine (IGF–granulosa cell), and paracrine (IGF–theca cell) actions appears to be operative in the control of follicular growth and steroidogenesis. *GH plays a permissive role* rather than serving an indispensable function.

GH AND PCOS

From the foregoing, it is apparent that characterization of the endocrine impact of GH on ovarian function in PCOS requires simultaneous assessment of the *entire somatotropic axis*. A study using 24-hour frequent sampling (10-minute) revealed remarkable differences in the somatotropic axis between lean and obese women with PCOS and

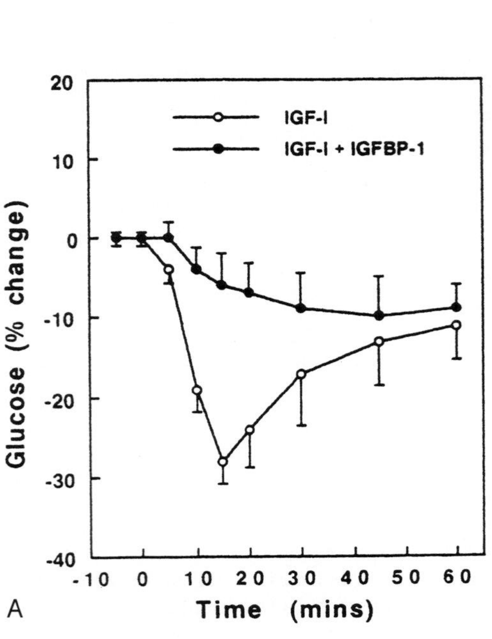

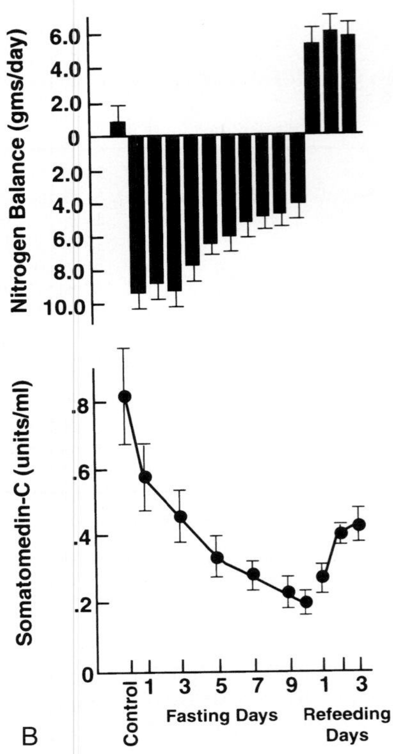

Figure 17–15 ■ *A,* Effect of IGFBP-1 to attenuate the hypoglycemic action of IGF-I, illustrating the inhibitory effect of IGFBP-1 on the metabolic action of free IGF-I. (From Lewitt MS, Denyer GS, Cooney GJ, Baxter RC. Insulin-like growth factor–binding protein-1 modulates blood glucose levels. Endocrinology 129:2254–2256, 1991.)

B, Nitrogen balance and plasma somatomedin-C/IGF-I levels in seven fasted and refed subjects. Nitrogen balance *(top)* was determined as the nitrogen intake minus daily urinary urea nitrogen plus 2 gm nitrogen (2 gm nitrogen was estimated to be the loss in stool, in skin, and as urinary non-urea nitrogen). Plasma somatomedin-C/IGF-I values are depicted in the lower panel. Values are expressed as mean ± SEM. The control day sample represents the mean values for all subjects on three consecutive control days. (From Thissen J-P, Ketelslegers J-M, Underwood LE. Nutritional regulation of the insulin-like growth factors. Endocr Rev 15:80–101, 1994.)

their respective controls. In lean PCOS, 24-hour mean GH pulse amplitude was *selectively increased by 30 percent*[37] (Fig. 17–16), as are GH responses to hypoglycemia,[93] without changes in 24-hour mean GH pulse frequency. Serum modulators for GH (GHBP), IGF-I (IGFBP-1 and IGFBP-3), and the feedback regulator of GH release (IGF-I) were unaltered from those of control subjects.[37] The selective increase in GH pulse amplitude in nonobese PCOS may be an expression of altered hypothalamic inputs in favor of release versus inhibition, because the pituitary response to exogenous growth hormone–releasing hormone (GHRH) remained unchanged.[37] This increased episodic exposure of granulosa cells to GH should in theory enhance FSH action and stimulate production of IGFs, which in turn would induce proliferation and aromatase activity.[94] These events do not occur because of the presence of FSH inhibitors (see FSH–Granulosa Cell Axis). However, GH-induced IGFs in granulosa cells may target to theca cells by a paracrine mode to promote androgenesis.[95]

By marked contrast, *obese PCOS* exhibited *a state of hyposomatotropinism*, with a *50 percent reduction* of GH pulse amplitude, 24-hour mean GH levels, and GH responses to GHRH without altering GH pulse frequency (see Fig. 17–16). The development of hyposomatotropinism in obese women with PCOS is obesity dependent because identical events occur in obese control subjects.[37, 96, 97] Serum levels of high-affinity GHBP were elevated twofold in both obese control subjects and obese women with PCOS, which may reduce free GH availability to target tissue[81] and thereby amplify the state of hyposomatotropinism. Obese subjects are more hyperinsulinemic, and insulin excess may up-regulate hepatic production of GHBP[81] and inhibit hepatic production of IGFBP-1,[98] resulting in reduced GH availability and a *10-fold elevation in the IGF-I:IGFBP-1 ratio.* As a consequence, there occurs an increased bioavailability of IGF-I[99] to theca tissue. In contrast to a *paracrine action* of IGFs from granulosa cells to theca cells in lean PCOS, an increased *endocrine input* of *IGF-I* in concert with insulin excess and elevation of *24-hour mean LH levels* in obese PCOS may jointly through their respective receptors[100, 101] enhance androgen production by the theca cell. Finally, the antilipolytic effect of hyposomatotropinism in concert with hyperinsulinemia affords a metabolic setting favoring increased adiposity in this syndrome.

THE LINK OF SOMATOTROPH AND GONADOTROPH

There exists in nonobese PCOS a strong positive association between the augmented pulse amplitude for LH and GH ($r = 0.95$; $P < .001$),[37] an observation suggesting that a common neuroendocrine mechanism may be involved. It has been shown that mRNAs for GH and for LH-β and FSH-β subunits are colocalized in a subset of GH-producing cells,[102] suggesting that coproduction and release of GH and gonadotropin by a common cell might serve to augment gonadotropin-mediated regulation of ovarian function. Perhaps more informative is the finding that intrapituitary GH stimulates the expression of follistatin, thereby reducing the FSH-releasing property of activin in the same cells that contain LH-β or FSH-β and follistatin mRNA.[103] Together with the evidence that accelerated GnRH pulse frequency enhances follistatin gene expression (see earlier), these observations serve as a basis for future elucidation of the overlapping neuroendocrine mechanisms accountable for the exaggerated LH and GH pulsatile secretion and

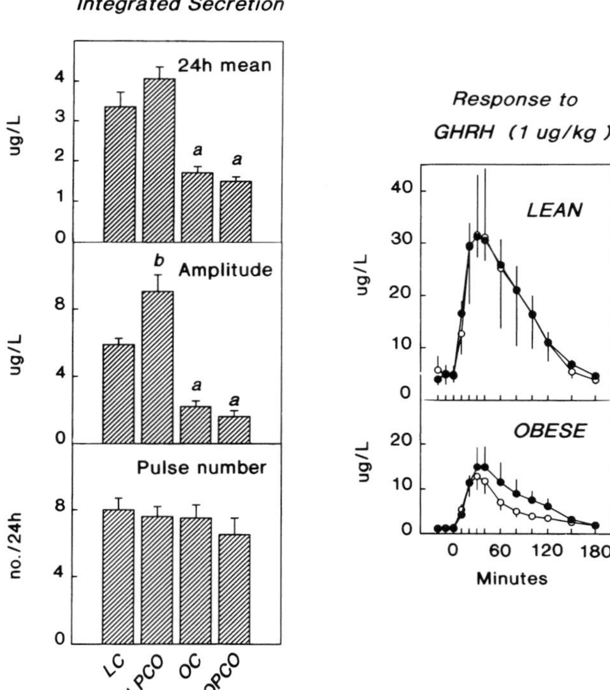

Figure 17–16 ■ Twenty-four-hour mean (±SE) GH levels, pulse amplitude, pulse frequency, and GH responses to GHRH for lean and obese women with PCOS (LPCO, OPCO) and their respective controls (LC, OC; n = 8 for each group). *a*, *P* < .001 versus corresponding lean group; *b*, *P* < .01 versus corresponding control group. ○, PCOS; ●, normal control subjects. (From Morales AJ, Laughlin GA, Bützow T, et al. Insulin, somatotropic, and LH axes in lean and obese women with polycystic ovary syndrome: Common and distinct features. J Clin Endocrinol Metab 81:2854–2864, 1996. © The Endocrine Society.)

disproportionately low FSH release in PCOS. These events are specific to PCOS in the absence of the confounding influence of obesity. Attenuation of both LH and GH pulse amplitude occurs in obese PCOS, suggesting that adiposity and associated factors are modifiers of the neuroendocrine-metabolic systems involved.

Obesity

Approximately 50 percent of women with PCOS are obese, which is significantly greater than the 30 percent incidence of obesity in the general population. When intake of energy chronically exceeds energy expenditure, most of excess energy is stored in the form of triglycerides in adipose tissue. Insulin and glucocorticoids promote lipogenesis, whereas lipolysis is regulated by β-adrenergic stimulation as well as by reductions in the lipogenic properties of insulin and glucocorticoid. Advances have been made in defining the molecular mechanisms that regulate preadipocyte growth, adipocyte differentiation, and lipogenesis.

LIPOGENESIS: PPARγ NUCLEAR HORMONE RECEPTOR

Central to the progress in the understanding of the biology of fat cells is the discovery of PPARγ, a member of the peroxisome proliferator-activated receptor (PPAR) subfamily of nuclear hormone receptors. PPARγ is found predominantly in the adipose tissue and appears to function as a transcription factor and *a key regulator of adipogenesis*. The adipogenic activity of PPARγ is markedly enhanced by the presence of insulin.[104] Insulin also stimulates PPARγ phosphorylation and enhances the transcriptional activity of PPAR. As such, insulin-mediated phosphorylation of this nuclear hormone receptor may function in the coordinated regulation of adipocyte differentiation and metabolism (lipid metabolism, glucose transport).[105] A new class of insulin-sensitizing compounds, thiazolidinediones, has been found to be a specific ligand for PPARγ and enhance insulin action. In recent clinical trials, troglitazone, a member of the thiazolidinedione family, has been shown to be successful in improving insulin resistance states in patients with NIDDM and PCOS[106–108] (see Management).

LIPOLYSIS: ADRENERGIC DYSREGULATION

An imbalance between the uptake and breakdown of triglycerides in abdominal adipocytes leads to the accumulation of fat and the development of upper body obesity. In human adipose tissue, catecholamines stimulate lipolysis through β_1- and β_2-adrenoceptors and inhibit lipolysis through α_2-adrenoceptors. A third β-adrenoceptor (namely, β_3-adrenoceptors) has recently been found to be specific for adipocytes in humans, especially in the omental fat depot.[109] The possibility of altered omental fat cell–specific β_3-adrenoceptor sensitivity in women with PCOS has not been determined. However, nonobese women with PCOS display marked impairment of cathecholamine-induced lipolysis due to a *reduced β_2-adrenoceptor density* and decreased activity of the protein kinase, hormone-sensitive lipase complex.[13] These lipolytic defects are similar to those found in women with upper body obesity and features of insulin resistance syndrome[110] and could be a primary mechanism for the development of this syndrome. As a consequence of catecholamine resistance, a compensatory increase in sympathetic activity may induce insulin resistance and hyperinsulinemia with resulting secondary hyperandrogenemia. Further, the primary lipolytic defect favors the development of obesity. The adrenergic dysfunction in adipocytes may antedate to early ages because adolescent girls with PCOS display endocrine-metabolic defects similar to those of adult PCOS.[21, 111] Experimental data showing that activation of sympathetic nerves innervating the ovary precedes the development of the polycystic ovary phenotype in rats[112] support the proposition that adrenergic dysfunction plays a role in the development of PCOS.

LEPTIN: ADIPOCYTES AS ENDOCRINE CELLS

Leptin is derived from the Greek word *leptos*, meaning thin. It is a 167–amino acid peptide product of the *ob* gene identified in *ob/ob* mice by Zhang and colleagues in 1994.[113] Leptin is produced exclusively in the fat cells across a wide range of animal species including the human, and in humans there is a close association among serum leptin levels, body fat, and leptin mRNA[114, 115] (Fig. 17–17). The discovery of leptin as a hormone secreted by fat cells has provided a new feedback loop between peripheral signals and hypothalamic sites in the regulation of feeding behavior, energy expenditure, and reproductive function.

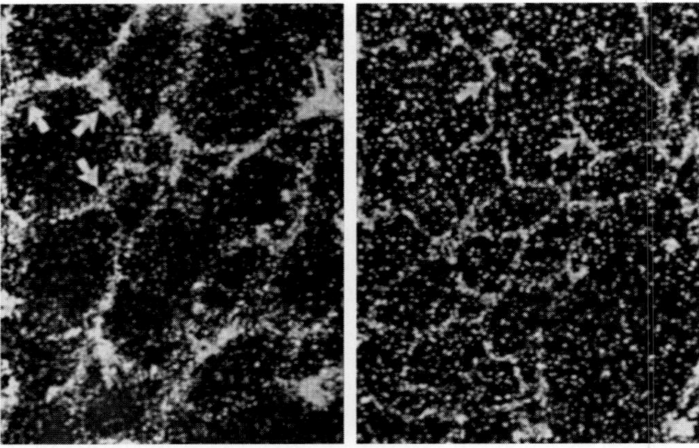

Figure 17–17 ■ In situ hybridization labeling *ob* mRNA *(arrows)* in adipose tissue taken from an obese person *(left)* and from a person of normal weight *(right)*; *ob* is overexpressed in the fat cells of the obese person, which are also enlarged. (From Lonnqvist F, Arner P, Nordfors L, Schalling M. Overexpression of the obese *[ob]* gene in adipose tissue of human obese subjects. Nat Med 1:950–953, 1995.)

Circulating leptin from the fat cell appears to bind to one or more binding proteins in the circulation including a splice variant of the leptin receptor (Rc) that has a short cytoplasmic domain (34 amino residues) and is soluble.[116] The percentage of free leptin in circulation is higher in obese than in lean individuals[116] (Fig. 17–18). Plasma leptin levels are higher in women than in men, and this sex difference in leptin levels appears to be a reflection of the suppressive influence of testosterone, not genetic sex.[117–119] The correlation between circulating leptin levels and adiposity or BMI is maintained during pubertal development in girls and in aging women. Leptin secretion is composed of a series of high-frequency pulses with greater amplitude in obese than in lean individuals[120, 121] (Fig. 17–19). A diurnal rhythm with nighttime elevation of leptin levels is evident in both sexes and appears to be entrained to meal timing rather than to the light-dark cycle or sleep.[122]

Glucocorticoids have been shown, both in vivo and in

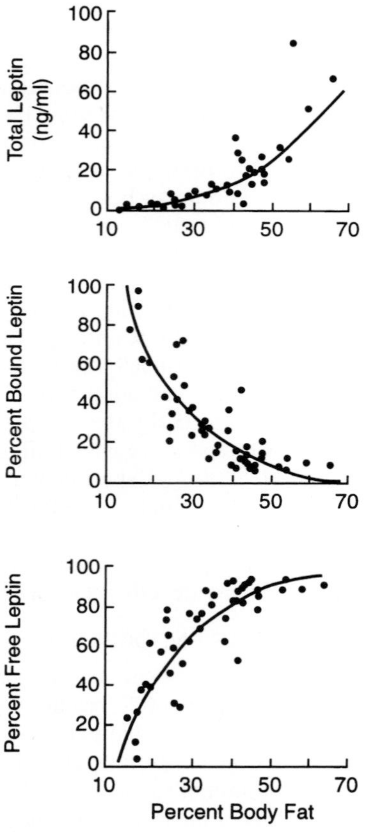

Figure 17–18 ■ Circulating leptin and the relative percentage in free form in 16 lean and 30 obese subjects. Total *(top)*, percentage bound *(middle)*, and percentage free *(bottom)* leptin levels are plotted against percentage of body fat. (From Sinha MK, Opentanova I, Ohannesian JP, et al. Evidence of free and bound leptin in human circulation. J Clin Invest 98:1277–1282, 1996.)

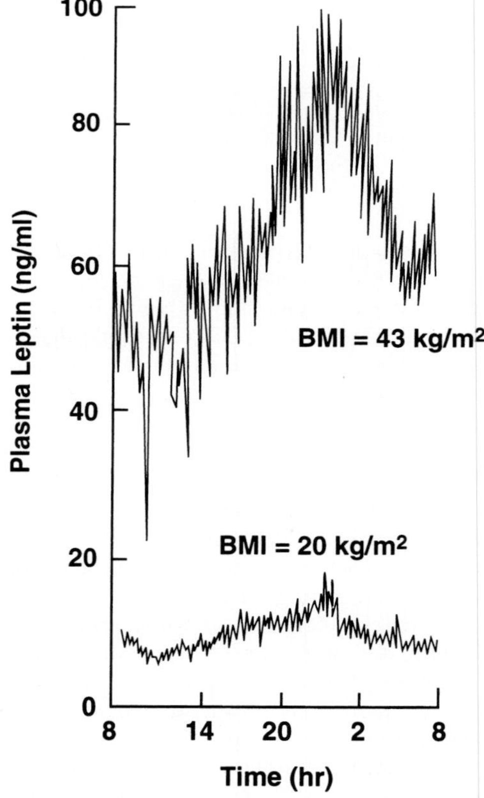

Figure 17–19 ■ Leptin levels and pulse amplitude are higher in an obese than in a nonobese woman. High-frequency pulsatile secretory activity occurs throughout the day with increased amplitude at night and peaks around 1 to 2 AM; thus, leptin levels exhibit a diurnal pattern. (From Licinio J, Mantzoros C, Negrao AB, et al. Human leptin levels are pulsatile and inversely related to pituitary-adrenal function. Nat Med 3:575–579, 1997.)

vitro, to enhance leptin gene transcription and leptin levels in human adipocytes.[123, 124] *Insulin* also stimulates leptin production, but its effect has a lag time of at least 24 hours.[125] Leptin secretion is regulated by changes in *energy balance*, falling during long-term fasting and increasing during overfeeding.[126] It is well known that counterregulatory responses to deficits in energy availability involve catecholaminergic activation. *Catecholamines inhibit leptin* secretion. In white adipose tissue, adrenergic activation through β_2-adrenoceptor induces lipolysis and decreases leptin expression. In brown adipose tissue (omental fat), adrenergic activation through β_3-adrenoceptor triggers thermogenesis as well as inhibiting leptin expression[127] (Fig. 17–20). The resulting low leptin levels will signal hypothalamic sites regulating feeding behavior.[109] Chronic negative energy balance is associated with a reduction in leptin secretion as seen in women athletes, with a selective absence of the diurnal rhythm in hypoinsulinemic amenorrheic athletes.[128] Thus, leptin secretion is regulated by nutritional status and associated changes in insulin, glucocorticoids, and catecholaminergic activities.

Leptin Receptors and Targets in Hypothalamus. Leptin receptors have been cloned and found to be members of the cytokine receptor family. Several forms of leptin receptors have been identified; *a short form (Ra)* lacks the intracellular signal domain, and *a long form (Rb)* represents the functional leptin receptor with transmembrane and cytoplasmic domains of 302 amino residues.[129] A mutation of the intracellular signal domain of the receptor was identified in *db/db* mice and provided a molecular basis for the failure of these mice to respond to either endogenous or exogenous leptin. This is in distinct contrast to *ob/ob* mice with leptin deficiency due to mutation of the *ob* gene itself.[126] In this case, exogenous leptin administration reduces food intake, increases metabolic rate, and restores fertility.[130–132] In humans, a decreased cerebrospinal fluid to serum leptin ratio was found in obesity, a finding that suggests leptin resistance as the mechanism in the genesis of obesity.[126]

Twins, adoption, and population-based segregation analysis indicate that up to 80 percent of the risk for human obesity is conferred by genes. Until most recently, no instance of human obesity had been proved to result from a mutation in any gene. Now two studies have found a genetic basis for human obesity. (1) A *homozygous frameshift mutation* involving the deletion of a single guanine nucleotide in codon 133 of the gene for leptin was found. These individuals have congenital leptin deficiency, severe obesity, and presumed infertility.[133] (2) *Mutations in the human prohormone convertase 1 (PC1) gene* were found to cause failure of post-translational processing of prohormones and preproneuropeptides. This defect led to the secretion of proinsulin instead of insulin, accounting for glucose intolerance; impaired processing of pro-opiomelanocortin (POMC), which may underlie the abnormal adrenal function; and impaired processing of neuropeptide GnRH, resulting in hypothalamic hypogonadism. In the *PC1* gene mutation, serum leptin levels are appropriate for obesity.[134] Undoubtedly, more genetic defects of human obesity will be uncovered. The proposal of leptin resistance as a cause of human obesity[126] may not be applicable to all obesity syndromes.

The long form of the leptin receptor (Rb) has been identified in several brain regions including human hypothalamus and may also be present in peripheral tissues including liver, pancreas,[135] and possibly ovaries. However, the predominant form in peripheral tissue is the short variant (Ra). The high level of expression of Ra in the choroid plexus in humans led to the proposition that Ra functions to transport leptin into the brain.[129] Within the hypothalamus, Rb receptors are found in the regions that have been associated with the regulation of feeding behavior, energy balance, and reproduction including the arcuate nucleus and the ventromedial and paraventricular nuclei of the hypothalamus.[136–139]

Targets for leptin in the hypothalamus are neurons expressing *neuropeptide Y (NPY)* and *POMC*. Leptin receptors have been identified and are expressed in both neuronal systems in the arcuate nucleus, and exogenous leptin increases arcuate nucleus mRNA levels for POMC and

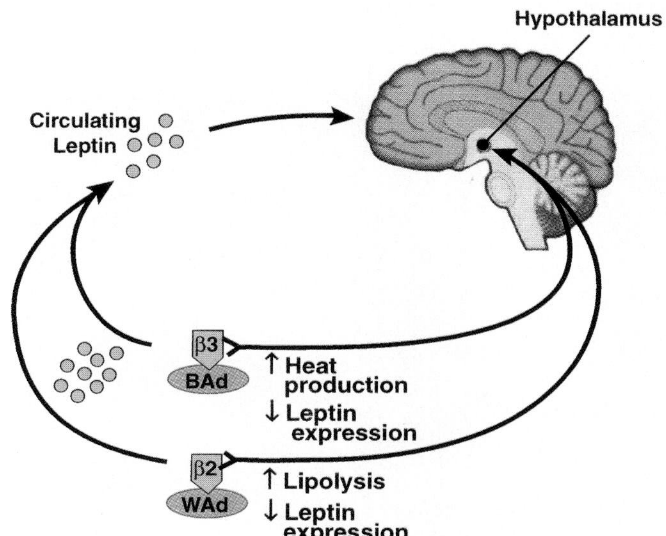

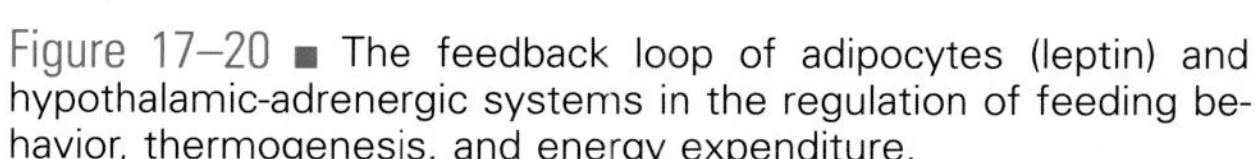
Figure 17–20 ■ The feedback loop of adipocytes (leptin) and hypothalamic-adrenergic systems in the regulation of feeding behavior, thermogenesis, and energy expenditure.

NPY.[137–140] Moreover, NPY and POMC gene products are involved in the regulation of body weight and reproduction.[136] NPY gene expression is increased by insulin and glucocorticoid and decreased by leptin. Central administration of NPY or β-endorphin increases food intake and inhibits GnRH release.[136, 141, 142] Leptin feedback on the paraventricular nucleus can inhibit corticotropin-releasing factor (CRF) release.[143] As such, resistance to leptin, as suggested in human obesity, or inadequate production of leptin, as in the case of hypoleptinemic women with nutritional amenorrhea, could result in hypercortisolemia by a compensatory increase in CRF secretion and adrenergic activation.[143] Thus, communication exists between adipocytes (leptin), hypothalamic neuronal systems (NPY, POMC, and CRF), and central adrenergic pathways in the regulation of adiposity, food intake, and reproduction (Fig. 17–21). This feedback loop would be disrupted if obese individuals are leptin resistant.[115, 143]

Leptin in PCOS. An earlier report suggested that a substantial proportion of women with PCOS have leptin levels that are higher than expected for their BMI.[144] However, subsequent studies have provided evidence that circulating leptin levels are fully accounted for by the degree of adiposity and BMI in PCOS patients compared with matched control subjects[145–148] (Fig. 17–22*A*), and a parallel reduction of percentage of body fat and leptin levels occurred in response to programmed weight loss in obese PCOS patients and control subjects (Fig. 17–22*B*). Serum leptin levels in PCOS patients are unaffected by improvement of insulin resistance and hyperinsulinemia by troglitazone administration.[148] At the ovarian level, leptin appears to inhibit the synergistic action of IGF-I on FSH-dependent estradiol-17β production by rat ovarian granulosa cells in vitro.[149] There are confounding issues regarding these preliminary results, and a clearer picture of leptin dynamics in PCOS must await further studies. For example, leptin circulates in bound and free form[116]; therefore, the relative proportion of these forms needs to be defined. Further, functional leptin receptors in the ovary have yet to be characterized. Analyses of the circadian rhythm and pulsatile pattern of leptin levels must also be conducted.[120] Finally, characterization of the sensitivity to exogenous leptin of the metabolic-reproductive axes in PCOS versus controls must be investigated before any conclusion can be made.

ADIPOSE TISSUE AS AN ENDOCRINE COMPARTMENT

Several studies have extended understanding of the role of adipose tissue in the storage and metabolism of sex steroid hormones. Active uptake of circulating androgens for *in situ estrogen biosynthesis* occurs in fat cells.[150, 151] Aromatase and 17β-hydroxysteroid dehydrogenase (17βHSD)—two enzymes that, to a large extent, determine extragonadal estrogen formation—are highly active in fat cells from both sexes.[150, 151] The intracellular biosynthesis of estrogens from androgens with local action through estrogen receptors constitutes a highly economic means of hormone action—*intracrinology.*[152] Aromatase activity is stimulated by glucocorticoids.[153] Further, obesity is associated with a decrease in 2-hydroxylation and 17β-oxidation of C_{18} estrogen, altered *metabolic pathways* favoring a relative hyperestrogenic state.[154] The relationship between sex steroids and lipid metabolism is supported by the presence of estrogen receptors in adipocytes[155] and the fact that the triglyceride storage process is under the influence of estrogen.[156] *Testosterone* also plays a role in the control of lipolysis in fat cells by *promoting α_2-adrenergic (antilipolytic) activity*, an effect mediated through androgen receptors that can be reversed by the administration of antiandrogens in vivo.[157, 158] Androgens also exert an inhibitory action on leptin secretion by adipocytes,[119] an effect that may account for the sex difference in leptin concentrations with lower leptin levels in men than in women.[118]

That *differing phenotypes of obesity* are associated with opposite hormonal environments is well established. In women with upper body obesity, such as in PCOS, there are higher androgen production rates and elevated free testosterone levels; whereas in women with lower body obesity, there are increased amounts of estrone from aromatization of androstenedione.[151] Adipocyte P450arom transcript levels increase in direct proportion to advancing age; they are highest in buttocks, followed by thigh, and are lowest in the abdomen. Aromatase expression in adipocytes is mainly under local control by a number of cytokines

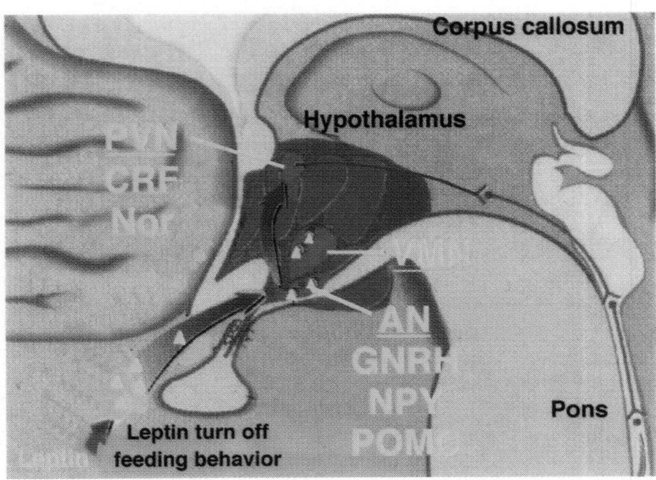

Figure 17–21 ■ Diagrammatic illustration of communications between leptin, hypothalamic neuronal systems (POMC, NPY, and CRF), and central adrenergic pathways in the regulation of feeding behavior, adipose tissue, and reproduction. PVN, paraventricular nucleus; AN, arcuate nucleus; VMN, ventromedial nucleus.

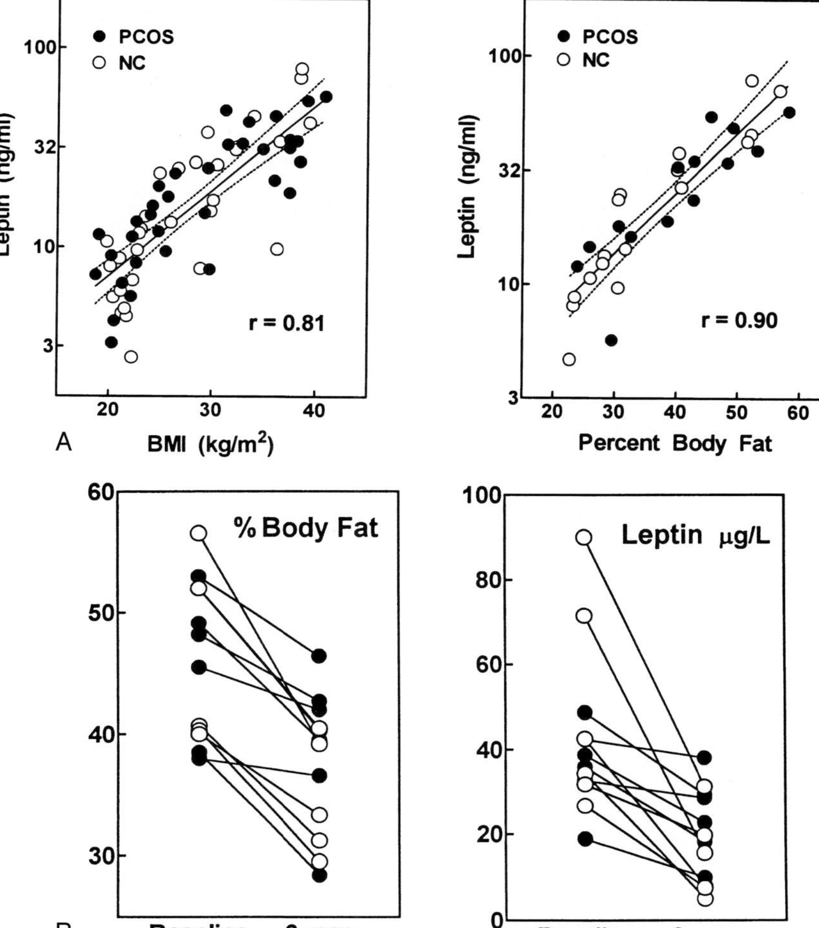

Figure 17–22 ■ *A*, Regression of serum leptin levels (log transformed) versus BMI *(left)* and percentage body fat *(right)* for PCOS (●) and normal control (NC) (○) women (both $P < .0001$). Values on the y-axis are antilogs. Dashed lines indicate 95 percent confidence intervals. (From Laughlin GA, Morales AJ, Yen SSC. Serum leptin levels in women with polycystic ovary syndrome: The role of insulin resistance/hyperinsulinemia. J Clin Endocrinol Metab 82:1692–1696, 1997. © The Endocrine Society.)

B, Effects of weight reduction on leptin concentrations in obese PCOS (●) and normal control (○) women (unpublished data).

through paracrine/autocrine mechanisms in the presence of systemic glucocorticoids.[159]

The *GH–IGF-I system* also plays a role in the regulation of adipocytes. GH treatment leads to an increase in IGF-I production and stimulates adipocyte proliferation and differentiation. Importantly, GH *inhibits glucose uptake and lipogenesis* and *stimulates lipolysis*. Thus, GH has a *direct antiadipogenic activity* and acting indirectly through IGF-I *enlarges the human adipocyte precursor pool*.[160, 161] Fat cells are devoid of receptors for IGFs, and IGF actions are mediated through insulin receptors.[161]

In sum, adipose tissue constitutes a dynamic endocrine-metabolic compartment and is influenced by and contributes to the biologic expression of estrogens, androgens, dehydroepiandrosterone (DHEA), glucocorticoids, insulin, and GH-IGFs as well as to the production of the hormone leptin. Although not all PCOS patients are obese, these characteristics of adipocyte physiology may be causally related to the propensity for the development of obesity in this syndrome.

ABERRATIONS OF LIPOPROTEIN LIPID PROFILE

Impaired insulin action due to peripheral insulin resistance results in aberrations of glucose metabolism and defects in activation of antilipolytic activities in women with PCOS. Several studies with relatively large samples have shown an abnormal lipoprotein lipid profile in PCOS women with insulin resistance.[162–164] Lipid profiles in PCOS were found, to a large extent, to be related to the degree of *insulin resistance/hyperinsulinemia*, independent of androgen levels and BMI.[164] However, free fatty acid levels are elevated only in obese PCOS and are correlated with adiposity and androgen levels.[165] Compared with a BMI-matched control population, the aberrations of lipoprotein lipid profiles are

↑ triglycerides
↑ low-density lipoprotein (LDL) cholesterol
↓ high-density lipoprotein (HDL) cholesterol
↑ very low density lipoprotein (VLDL) cholesterol
↑ apolipoprotein A1, B
↑ free fatty acids

These findings are similar to those for individuals with insulin resistance syndrome and increased cardiovascular disease risk. Further, plasminogen activator inhibitor (PAI) levels are elevated[108, 166, 167] and together with the alterations of lipids are responsible for the increased incidence of hypertension, coronary heart disease, and thrombosis in PCOS women.[162–164] The major underlying cause appears to be insulin resistance, hyperinsulinemia, and altered lipoprotein lipase activity. The degree of alterations of lipids in PCOS can be influenced by *lifestyle*, *diet*, and *exercise* regimens.

Ovarian Modulators

Extraovarian Modulators (Co-gonadotropins)

Co-gonadotropin or pro-gonadotropin is the term applied to extraovarian hormonal molecules that exhibit a potentiating or synergistic effect through their specific receptors on gonadotropin-mediated follicular growth and steroidogenesis. Substantial evidence suggests that *GH* and *insulin* can play an augmenting role in ovarian function, and thus they are referred to as co-gonadotropins.[14, 59, 168] As alluded to earlier, the relative inputs of GH and insulin to the ovary and their downstream effect on IGFs are remarkably different among PCOS women with varying adiposity. It is emphasized that in nonobese PCOS, the 30 percent increase in GH pulse amplitude represents an important co-gonadotropin input in synergy with markedly elevated LH in the augmentation of theca cell androgenesis through enhanced expression of P450c17, a setting that is viewed as *the authentic syndrome*. In obese women with PCOS, *a shift of co-gonadotropin from GH to insulin occurs*. Insulin, through its potent inhibitory influence on hepatic production of IGFBP-1 and SHBG, may increase respectively free IGF-I and unbound sex steroid levels. In this setting, insulin and IGF-I may act in synergy with LH to stimulate P450c17 activity and androgenesis, as depicted in Figure 17–23. Thus, *GH and IGF-I* in nonobese PCOS and *insulin and IGF-I* in obese PCOS are extraovarian factors in concert with the common regulator of LH to produce hyperandrogenism by the theca cells. The relative input of LH is greater in nonobese than in obese PCOS.

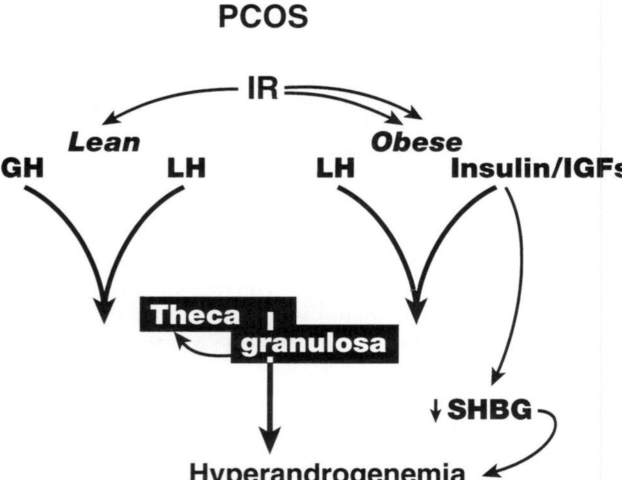

Figure 17–23 ■ Schematic depiction of distinct and common neuroendocrine-metabolic variables between lean PCOS and obese PCOS. (Note the two arrows between insulin resistance [IR] and obese representing the two components of insulin resistance in obese PCOS.) Although insulin resistance and LH hyperpulsatility are common features of PCOS, the coupling of enhanced GH pulsatility in lean PCOS and of insulin and the insulin-mediated increase in bioavailability of IGFs as co-gonadotropins in obese PCOS may contribute to the genesis and maintenance of hyperandrogenic chronic anovulation and polycystic ovary morphology. (From Morales AJ, Laughlin GA, Bützow T, et al. Insulin, somatotropic, and LH axes in lean and obese women with polycystic ovary syndrome: Common and distinct features. J Clin Endocrinol Metab 81:2854–2864, 1996. © The Endocrine Society.)

Intraovarian Modulators

During the transition from the luteal to the follicular phase, a cohort of follicles is recruited that grow to the 4- to 6-mm stage in the early follicular phase under the control of FSH. As FSH levels decline in the midfollicular phase, selection of the dominant follicle takes place and the remainder of the cohort begins to undergo atresia.[169, 170] It is the growth of dominant follicles in the presence of declining FSH levels that has generated the hypothesis of intraovarian modulators as enhancers of FSH action.[171]

The concept has been advanced that locally produced substances may serve as signals to enhance or to inhibit extraovarian sources of gonadotropic hormonal actions. Several classes of intraovarian modulators have been identified. For authenticity as an intraovarian regulator to be established, evidence of local production, reception, and action is required. Moreover, a functional role should be established. Few putative intraovarian regulators appear to have fulfilled these requirements, and others remain tentative. Among them, the IGF system as an amplifier of gonadotropin action is best characterized.

INTRAOVARIAN IGF SYSTEM

The presence of an intrinsic IGF system in the human ovarian follicle is established. Physiologic levels of IGF-I and IGF-II are found in the follicular fluid, and IGF-II is synthesized by follicular cells. Receptors for IGF-I and IGF-II are expressed in the follicle cells,[100, 169, 172] and IGFs are highly active in enhancing LH and FSH actions on theca and granulosa cells, respectively.[173–176] Thus, human ovarian follicles contain an intrinsic IGF system replete with ligands, receptors, and biologic responses. In addition, regulators of the IGF system, IGFBP and IGFBP proteases, are also expressed.[177] Human granulosa cells have been shown to express GH receptors,[88] and GH acts together with FSH to enhance estradiol production in vitro[89] (see preceding section on co-gonadotropins). IGF-I levels in follicular fluid from estrogen-dominant follicles are similar to those from androgen-dominant follicles, whereas follicular fluid IGF-II levels are significantly higher in estrogen- than in androgen-dominant follicles and correlate with follicular size[178] (Table 17–2). This is consonant with the parallel increase in IGF-II gene expression with follicular maturation and suggests that follicular fluid IGF-II levels are derived primarily from granulosa cells with possible contributions from theca cells and the general circulation.[179] IGF-II is the major intraovarian IGF; it enhances LH-mediated P450scc mRNA and activity levels, up-regulates P450c17 production and androgenesis by the theca cell, increases aromatase activity and estrogen production by the granulosa cell, and enhances oocyte maturation (Table 17–3). Altogether, the evidence supports the proposition that the mechanism by which FSH evokes dominant follicle development involves interactions with an intrinsic IGF system.

IGFBPs. Of the six IGFBPs, five (IGFBPs 1, 2, 3, 4,

■ TABLE 17–2
IGF-I and IGF-II Concentrations in Androgenic Versus Estrogenic Follicular Fluid

	IGF-I	IGF-II
Androgenic follicular fluid	149 ng/ml (22–232)	474 ng/ml (272–603)
Estrogenic follicular fluid	192 ng/ml (20–265)	630 ng/ml (212–1000)*

*P = .002 versus androgenic follicular fluid.
From Thierry van Dessel HJ, Chandrasekher YA, Yap OW, et al. Serum and follicular fluid levels of insulin-like growth factor I (IGF-I), IGF-II, and IGF-binding protein-1 and -3 during the normal menstrual cycle. J Clin Endocrinol Metab 81:1224–1231, 1996.

and 5) have been identified in human ovaries.[100, 172] IGFBPs 1, 2, 3, and 4 have been found in the follicular fluid[180, 181] and are likely to be derived from a combination of local production and the circulation. The IGFBP profile in follicular fluid is dependent on the functional status of the follicle. Androgen-dominant follicles are found to have high levels of IGFBP-2 and IGFBP-4 and low levels of IGFBP proteases compared with growing estrogen-dominant follicles[181, 182] (Table 17–4). It would appear that intrafollicular levels of bioavailable IGF peptides are reduced in androgen-dominant follicles owing to sequestration by high levels of IGFBPs, thereby leading to arrested follicular development. Withdrawal of intrafollicular IGFs (i.e., quenching by IGFBPs) may be implicated in follicular atresia through apoptotic processes.[183] In vitro apoptosis can be prevented by exposure to IGF-I or gonadotropin and is enhanced by the presence of IGFBPs.[184] The production of IGFBP by the ovary is inhibited by gonadotropin and IGF peptides.[185, 186] The final step in the control of bioavailability of IGFs is *IGFBP proteases,* which lower the affinity of IGFBPs for IGFs, thereby increasing free IGFs (see Table 17–4).

IGF System in PCOS Follicles. In the PCOS follicle, FSH and IGF-I are in the physiologic range.[176, 187] In the presence of abundant androstenedione substrate, aromatase activity and estradiol production by granulosa cells are very low, resulting in a higher androgen to estrogen ratio and follicular arrest. However, when PCOS granulosa cells are removed from their ovarian environment, these cells respond normally or hyperrespond to IGF-I and FSH in the stimulation of aromatase activity and estradiol production.[4, 60, 94] These findings indicate that the functional integrity of granulosa cells in PCOS is fully retained and lead to the proposal of the presence of inhibitors of FSH or IGF actions in the in vivo environment of PCOS follicles.

■ TABLE 17–3
Effects of IGF-I and IGF-II in Human Ovary

Theca	↑ DNA synthesis ↑ Androgenesis (synergy with LH)
Granulosa	↑ DNA synthesis ↑ E_2 and P_4 production (synergy with FSH) ↑ P450 aromatase activity and mRNA
Oocytes	↑ Maturation

From Giudice LC, van Dessel HJ, Cataldo NA, et al. Circulating and ovarian IGF binding proteins: Potential roles in normo-ovulatory cycles and in polycystic ovarian syndrome. Prog Growth Factor Res 6:397–408, 1995.

■ TABLE 17–4
Follicular Fluid Concentrations of IGFBPs in Androgen- and Estrogen-Dominant Follicles

ESTROGEN-DOMINANT	ANDROGEN-DOMINANT
↓ IGFBPs ↑ IGFBP proteases	↑ IGFBPs ↓ IGFBP proteases

A direct inhibitory effect of IGFBPs on FSH-induced estradiol secretion has been demonstrated in human granulosa cells in vitro.[175] As such, the IGFBPs may act as FSH antagonists in arrested follicles of PCOS. Indeed, it has been demonstrated that PCOS follicular fluid contains high levels of IGFBP-2 through IGFBP-4, similar to those found in androgen-dominated follicles from normally cycling women.[176] This is in marked contrast to the near absence of these IGFBPs in estrogen-dominated follicles. The arrested follicles in PCOS, like the androgenic follicles, have low levels of IGF-II expression, a finding consonant with abundant expression of IGF-II occurring mainly in matured follicles.[100] Further, IGFBP-4 protease is present in estrogenic follicles, thereby enhancing the synergistic action of IGF-II and FSH on granulosa cells by reducing IGFBP activities. This is not the case in the androgenic follicles of PCOS.[176] Thus, high levels of IGFBPs and the absence of IGFBP protease in PCOS follicles would sequester the IGF-I and thereby reduce its synergistic action with FSH. Accordingly, follicle development would be arrested (Fig. 17–24).

TGF-β FAMILY (INHIBIN/ACTIVIN/FOLLISTATIN)

Ovarian inhibin, a granulosa cell–derived glycoprotein, is a heterodimer composed of covalently linked α- and β-subunits. There are two distinct β-subunits, β_A and β_B,

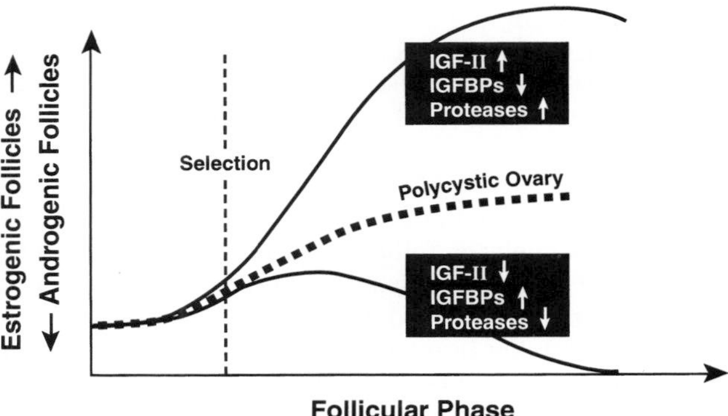

Figure 17–24 ■ Diagrammatic depiction of the role of the intraovarian IGF system in gonadotropin-dependent follicular maturation and atresia *(solid lines).* Follicular arrest in PCOS *(dotted line)* appears to be an intermediate event. (Modified from Giudice LC, van Dessel HJ, Cataldo NA, et al. Circulating and ovarian IGF binding proteins: Potential roles in normo-ovulatory cycles and in polycystic ovarian syndrome. Prog Growth Factor Res 6:397–408, 1995.)

which show 85 percent identity. Combination of an α-subunit with either of the β-subunits (i.e. $\alpha\beta_A$ or $\alpha\beta_B$) forms inhibin A and inhibin B. Activin, a homodimer of the β-subunits (i.e., $\beta_A\beta_A$, $\beta_A\beta_B$, or $\beta_B\beta_B$) has bioactivity opposite that of inhibin.[188] Follistatin, a glycoprotein, is also produced by human granulosa cells. It binds activin with high affinity comparable to that of the activin receptor and binds inhibin with lower affinity.[189, 190] In situ hybridization/immunohistochemistry studies revealed that both theca and granulosa cells in human ovarian follicles are endowed with the ability to synthesize inhibin, activin, and follistatin.[191]

Human theca cells pretreated with LH/IGF-I display *augmentation* of androgen synthesis in response to inhibin A, whereas activin inhibits androgen production.[192, 193] The stimulatory action of inhibin was achieved at lower concentrations than the inhibitory effects of activin were. The relative preponderance of C_{19} steroids compared with progesterone in the inhibin-treated cell culture was considered to indicate stimulation of 17α-hydroxylase activity.[194] Furthermore, androgens and inhibin seem to have a reciprocal interaction with a significant enhancement of FSH-stimulated inhibin production in human granulosa cells in vitro by testosterone and dihydrotestosterone (DHT), but not estrogen.[194] The mechanisms of inhibin and activin action have yet to be defined because receptors for these peptides in the human ovary are unknown at this time.

To date, most of the data obtained in clinical studies investigating the role of inhibin are based on the use of the first-generation inhibin immunoassays. These assays are unable to distinguish between inhibin A and inhibin B and may also detect unprocessed precursor forms and free α-subunits.[195] Two-site enzyme-linked immunosorbent assays using specific antibodies directed against the β_A and β_B inhibin subunits have been developed that can measure serum levels of dimeric inhibin A or B.[196, 197] Initial results obtained with these assays indicate that inhibin A and inhibin B display different secretory patterns during the menstrual cycle; inhibin A is mainly secreted in the preovulatory phase and peaks during the luteal phase, whereas inhibin B rises in the early follicular phase and increases in parallel with estradiol. After a short midcycle peak, inhibin B declines to low levels in the luteal phase.[196, 198]

Inhibin System in PCOS. The underlying cause of the relative deficiency of FSH in women with PCOS is not entirely clear. Both estradiol and inhibin are capable of negatively regulating FSH secretion. In PCOS women, estradiol levels are comparable to those of the midfollicular phase and are derived mainly from peripheral conversion of androgen. Because the administration of the antiestrogen clomiphene stimulates follicular development in women with PCOS,[199] an extraglandular source of estrogen may play an important role in suppressing FSH.

A role for inhibin in the negative feedback regulation of FSH secretion in PCOS has been postulated for a long time, but solid evidence supporting this notion is lacking.[200, 201] Jaatinen[202] and Roberts[191] and their colleagues, using in situ hybridization, have demonstrated that both granulosa cells and theca cells of normal and polycystic ovaries express inhibin subunits mRNA. Moreover, α-subunit mRNA levels were higher in theca cells than in granulosa cells of polycystic ovaries, a finding opposite from that of the normal ovary.[191] Using two-site enzyme-linked assay measurements of dimeric serum inhibin A and inhibin B in PCOS women, Anderson and coworkers[203] have shown that concentrations of inhibin B and to a lesser extent inhibin A are consistently higher in PCOS than in normal follicular-phase women. Treatment of PCOS women with low-dose FSH stimulated the development of a single dominant follicle, which had a rate of growth and secretion of estradiol and inhibin A identical to that observed in spontaneous cycles in normal women. In contrast to the normal cycle, the concentration of inhibin B rose sevenfold after FSH treatment, indicating that inhibin B production is FSH dependent.[203, 204] These preliminary findings are of interest, but the functionality of the intraovarian inhibins and their feedback regulation of FSH remain to be clarified, particularly regarding the role of activin and its binding protein follistatin in the regulation of folliculogenesis and FSH secretion in PCOS as well as in normal cycling women.

Transforming Growth Factor-β. TGF-β1 and TGF-β2 are homodimer polypeptides with structural homology to inhibin/activin and müllerian-inhibiting substance. Members of the TGF-β superfamily of peptide growth factors have profound inhibitory or stimulatory effects on the growth and differentiation of many cell types. Two types of TGF-β receptors were recently cloned, providing a basis for defining the sites and mechanisms of action. Type II receptor has been shown to be a member of the serine-threonine kinase receptor family, which also includes two homologous activin receptors.[205] TGF-β has an extremely short biologic half-life in vivo and is cleared from plasma with a half-life of less than 3 minutes. This indicates that the actions of TGFs-β are mainly local, occurring at their site of production through autocrine or paracrine regulating mechanisms.

TGF-β–like activity is present in human ovarian follicular fluid. Immunocytochemistry confirms the presence of both TGF-β1 and TGF-β2 in theca, granulosa, and luteal cells. TGF-β1 is more predominant in theca cells,[206, 207] whereas TGF-β2 is more abundant in granulosa cells. In the oocytes, TGF-β1 but not TGF-β2 is detected. The mRNA is more abundant for TGF-β2 than for TGF-β1 in the theca cells, whereas only TGF-β2 mRNA was detected in granulosa cells.[208] Although TGF-β1 appears to exert an inhibitory action on androgen biosynthesis, probably through suppression of P450c17 activity, its precise function in theca cells as well as in granulosa cells is unclear.[209] However, the changes in human TGF-β1 immunostaining in follicles of different sizes during the menstrual cycle suggest a physiologic role for TGF-β1 in human ovarian function.[206] The role, if any, of TGF-β in the follicular arrest of PCOS is unknown.

TGF-α

TGF-α and epidermal growth factor (EGF) share 20 percent structural homology and a common receptor. TGF-α and EGF are produced in the ovary and are present in follicular fluid in sufficient quantities to exert an effect. Both TGF-α and EGF concentrations are inversely correlated with follicular size and have inhibitory effects on estrogen production by granulosa cells in vitro.[210, 211] TGF-α also inhibits LH-stimulated androgen production by blocking 17α-hydroxylase/17,20-lyase activity in ovarian theca-interstitial cells. Similar findings were obtained in normal and PCOS granulosa and theca cells,[211] suggesting that TGF-α and EGF do not play a role in follicular arrest in PCOS.

CYTOKINES

Cytokines, immunoregulatory molecules derived from resident macrophage or ovarian cells, may have a role as paracrine regulators. *Tumor necrosis factor-α (TNF-α)* is a cytokine mediator of the inflammatory reaction induced by macrophages. The human ovary contains immunocytochemically detectable TNF-α in follicular fluid, granulosa cells, and the luteal compartment.[212] This cytokine has been shown to *inhibit* hCG-stimulated androsterone production by rat ovaries,[213] and theca-interstitial cells appear to be the target.[214, 215] On the other hand, TNF-α has been shown to exert a *stimulatory* effect on theca cells in culture from preovulatory follicles with production of 17α-hydroxyprogesterone and androstenedione.[214] The precise functional role of TNF-α is unknown. Another aspect of TNF-α that may be of interest is that *TNF-α is overexpressed in adipose tissue,* and its levels are highly correlated with adiposity and insulin resistance. The possibility exists that TNF-α may serve as a link between hyperandrogenism and insulin resistance in PCOS. *Interleukin-1 (IL-1)* in the human ovary is derived from resident macrophages as well as granulosa cells.[216] Human ovarian IL-1 and its receptors are highly compartmentalized in the granulosa cells. The genes encoding IL-1 and IL-1 receptor are regulated by gonadotropin, and transcription of IL-1 can be induced by gonadotropin in human ovary at midcycle.[216] IL-1 inhibits androgen production in vitro, but the relevance of these findings in ovarian physiology and in PCOS remains unknown.

IMPLICATIONS IN PCOS

Most of the putative intraovarian factors appear to exert an inhibitory effect on androgen production with the notable exception of the IGFs. Given the stimulatory effect of IGFs (and insulin) on ovarian androgen synthesis by theca cells and enhancement of FSH action on granulosa cells, alterations of these growth factors and their binding proteins represent the most promising intraovarian regulators leading to follicular arrest in PCOS.

Adrenal Hyperandrogenism in PCOS

P450c17 Hyperfunction

The pathways of adrenal steroidogenesis are shown in Figure 17–25. Functional adrenal hyperandrogenism occurs in approximately 50 percent of women with PCOS. Serum levels of the adrenal sex steroid precursors DHEA-S and 11β-hydroxyandrostenedione are elevated, reflecting enhanced steroidogenesis by the zona reticularis.[217–219] For the most part, the nature of the adrenal hyperandrogenism in PCOS is unclear, but evidence supports an increase of P450c17 activities in the zona reticularis of the adrenal cortex. Studies conducted under basal conditions and in response to a sustained adrenocorticotropic hormone (ACTH) stimulation revealed significantly higher increments of 17-hydroxyprogesterone in PCOS women compared with normal control subjects.[220] In a prospective study of 40 consecutive hyperandrogenic anovulatory women undergoing both an ACTH-stimulated and a GnRH agonist challenge, 55 percent had functional adrenal hyperandrogenism–ACTH-dependent 17-ketosteroid excess, that is, hyperresponsiveness of DHEA and androstenedione from dexamethasone-suppressed basal states.[221] Adrenal androgen abnormalities occur *concurrently* in more than 50 percent of women with ovarian hyperandrogenism. Several studies showed a lack of evidence for increased adrenal P450c17 activity in PCOS,[222–224] but these experiments were conducted without dexamethasone suppression and therefore lack baseline uniformity.

Increased IGFs, insulin, or both may amplify ACTH-mediated P450c17 expression and adrenal androgen synthesis,[225, 226] resembling closely the synergistic effect of LH, IGFs, and insulin on ovarian P450c17 expression in theca cells of PCOS[29, 168] (see co-gonadotropins). The salient feature of hypersecretion of androgen involves primarily the Δ^5 pathway in the case of the adrenal, whereas Δ^4 pathways predominate in the ovary (Fig. 17–26). This functional dichotomy occurs only in human and higher primate adrenals wherein the C_{19} steroids DHEA and DHEA-S are the major sex steroids synthesized in the

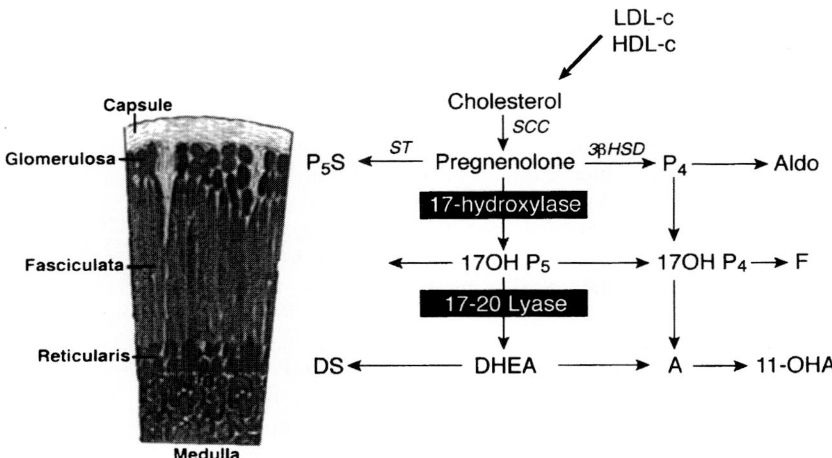

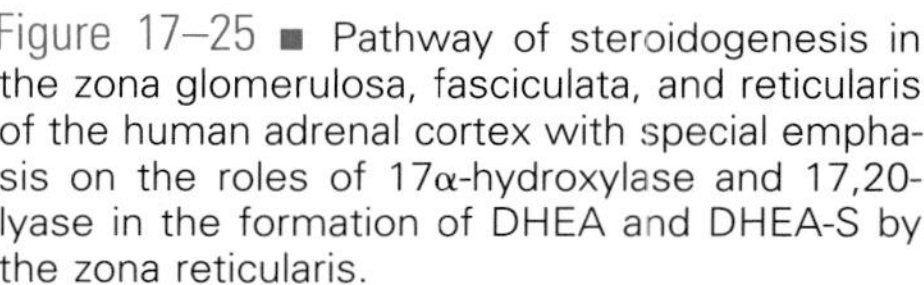
Figure 17–25 ■ Pathway of steroidogenesis in the zona glomerulosa, fasciculata, and reticularis of the human adrenal cortex with special emphasis on the roles of 17α-hydroxylase and 17,20-lyase in the formation of DHEA and DHEA-S by the zona reticularis.

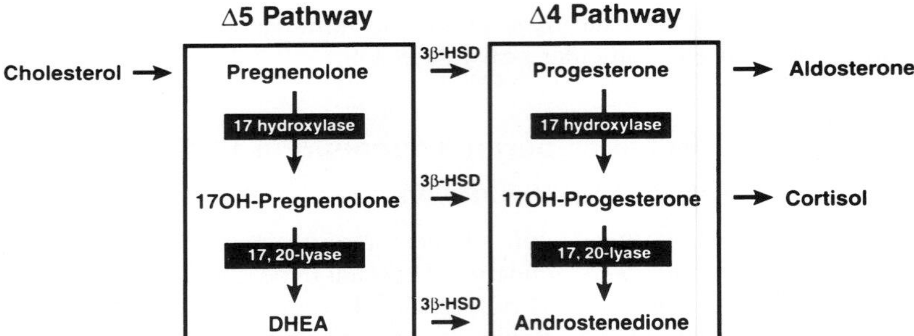

Figure 17–26 ■ Biosynthesis of adrenal DHEA by the Δ^5 pathway and ovarian androgen production by the Δ^4 pathway. 3β-HSD, 3β-hydroxysteroid dehydrogenase.

reticularis and testosterone synthesis cannot be accomplished because of the relative deficiency of 17βHSD. In contrast, the ovary is endowed with abundant 3βHSD, 17βHSD, and aromatase and thereby produces mainly testosterone and estrogen. This critical enzymatic difference is designed to maintain the functional distinction between adrenal and gonads in humans and higher primates.[227] In lower species, adrenal C_{19} steroid biosynthesis is not possible because P450c17 expression is restricted to the gonads.[227]

Exaggerated Adrenarche Hypothesis

Lucky and colleagues[25] have demonstrated that in women with PCOS, there is a prompt and excessive responsiveness of DHEA and androstenedione to ACTH stimulation. These responses resemble *an exaggerated adrenarche* confirming our original proposal[6] (Fig. 17–27). In this scheme, exaggerated adrenarche, before the activation of ovarian function, triggers the onset of PCOS by providing a substrate, androstenedione, from which extraglandular conversion to estrone occurs (estrone hypothesis). The subsequent conversion of estrone to estradiol at the target cells may exert a trophic effect prematurely on the reproductive axis. Several reports have shown that children with premature or exaggerated adrenarche are at high risk of developing PCOS-like functional ovarian hyperandrogenism at puberty.[20, 228, 229] These findings, together with the observation that hyperandrogenemia in adolescent girls is accompanied by neuroendocrine-metabolic features closely akin to those found in adult PCOS,[21, 22] support the exaggerated adrenarche hypothesis.

Because relative hyperestrogenemia exists in PCOS, the impact of estrogen on adrenal androgen sensitivity to ACTH has been evaluated in PCOS women with elevated basal DHEA-S levels; suppression of estrogen levels by GnRH agonist treatment normalized the adrenal hyperandrogenism, but androgens returned to pretreatment levels after estrogen was added back.[223] Whereas these findings support the notion that estrogen may influence adrenal androgen production, the major confounding issue is why only 50 percent of PCOS women display adrenal hyperandrogenism. Clearly, additional critical evaluations are required.

Hirsutism and Acne

Hirsutism in women, with or without acne, is a common clinical condition manifested by excessive hair growth toward a male pattern (Fig. 17–28). It is frequently associated with chronic anovulation and reflects increased androgenic stimulation (through excessive glandular secretion, extraglandular production, or local biotransformation).

Hirsutism can be a distressing symptom for most patients

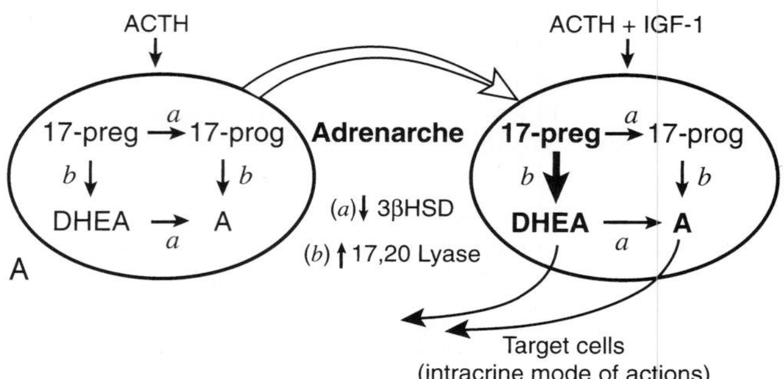

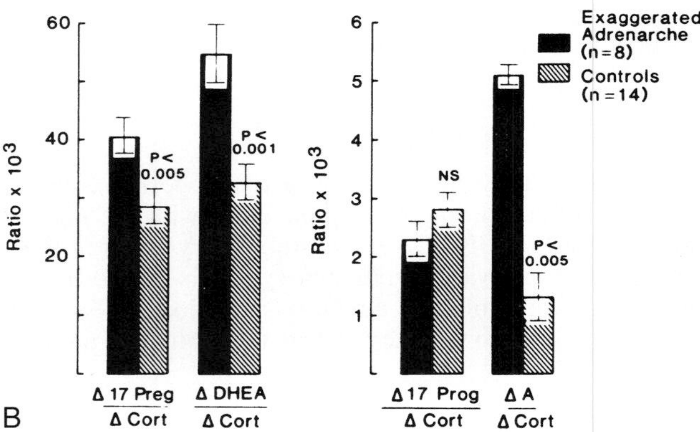

Figure 17–27 ■ *A,* Diagrammatic depiction of changes in enzymatic efficiency during adrenarche. There is a relative decrease in 3β-HSD and a relative increase in 17,20-lyase efficiency resulting in increased synthesis of 17-hydroxypregnenolone (17-preg), DHEA, and androstenedione. (Modified from Lucky AW, Rosenfield RL, McGuire J, et al. Adrenal androgen hyperresponsiveness to ACTH in women with acne and/or hirsutism: Adrenal enzyme defects and exaggerated adrenarche. J Clin Endocrinol Metab 62:840–848, 1986. © The Endocrine Society.)

B, Mean (±SE) ratios of incremental responses to ACTH at 60 minutes of the androgen precursors 17-preg, DHEA, 17-prog, and androstenedione to that of the cortisol response. There are significantly greater increments in 17-prog/cortisol, DHEA/cortisol, and androstenedione/cortisol ratios, resembling an exaggerated pattern during normal adrenarche. (From Lucky AW, Rosenfield RL, McGuire J, et al. Adrenal androgen hyperresponsiveness to ACTH in women with acne and/or hirsutism: Adrenal enzyme defects and exaggerated adrenarche. J Clin Endocrinol Metab 62:840–848, 1986. © The Endocrine Society.)

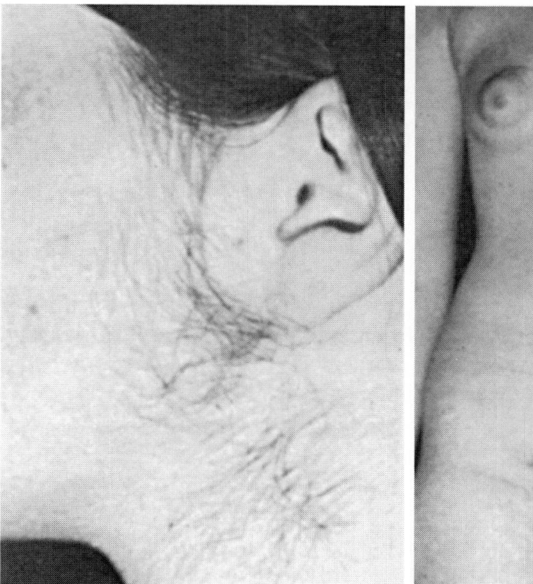

Figure 17–28 ■ Moderately severe hirsutism in a young woman. Note the male pattern of hair distribution.

seeking medical advice. In addition to worrying about cosmetic problems, the patient is also concerned with more serious endocrine disorders. The most common (95 percent) underlying causes are PCOS and idiopathic hirsutism.[230] When *virilization* is evident, the attending physician must consider hyperplasia or tumors of the adrenal or ovary as the underlying cause, and prompt diagnostic work-up should be initiated. To provide a rational approach for the evaluation and management of both hirsutism and less frequent virilizing syndromes, an understanding of the biology of hair growth and its endocrine regulation is imperative.

Biology of the Hair Follicle

Types of Hair Follicles. Human hair follicles are distinguishable into three main types according to the size and depth of the follicle and the characteristics of the hair.

- *Vellus hair follicles* are small in structure and shallow in depth and produce fine and poorly pigmented hairs. Vellus follicles are found in most body regions except the scalp, eyebrow, and eyelashes.
- *Medium follicles* are larger in caliber and extend deeper into the dermis than vellus follicles do. These follicles produce pigmented hair and are present in the upper arms, the lower legs, and the transitional zone between thick-hair and fine-hair regions such as the scalp hairline.
- *Terminal follicles* are large hair follicles and produce thick and pigmented hairs. During the growing phase, they are rooted in the entire skin layer with bulbs extended to the cutaneous adipose layer. Terminal follicles are found in the scalp, in the axillary and pubic regions of adult men and women, and on the face and chest of men.

Cyclic Activity of Hair Follicles. All hair follicles undergo a cyclic pattern of growth and regression. There are three distinct phases of hair follicle activity: (1) *anagen* (growth phase), (2) *catagen* (involution phase), and (3) *telogen* (resting phase). Each follicle has an intrinsic cycle characteristic of its region and its sensitivity to hormonal influences[231–233] (Fig. 17–29).

During the resting (telogen) phase, the initiation of anagen can be profoundly influenced by hormonal factors and can be advanced or retarded by several weeks. There are marked variations in the duration of anagen and telogen phases with the cyclic activity of the hair follicles being a mosaic in a given anatomic region.[232] For example, the duration of anagen and telogen phases averages, respectively, 3 years and 3 months in the scalp and 4 months and 2 months for the face. It is therefore important that such cycle variations be taken into account when one attempts to interpret hair changes, or the lack thereof, that result from hormonal or other manipulative treatments. Androgen sensitivity varies with region and age among normal individuals. Hair follicles are richly vascularized and innervated. The sensory nerve endings remain intact during remodeling.[232]

Endocrinology of the Pilosebaceous Unit

The sebaceous glands and sexual hair follicles together form a functional unit, the pilosebaceous unit, the activity of which is governed by the inherent cyclicity of the hair follicle in a given region. The dermal papilla is central to hair growth. Damage or degeneration of the dermal papilla is the crucial factor in permanent hair loss. After any injury, including skin graft, the hair follicle will regenerate and hair growth will initiate if the dermal papilla survives. Human skin and hair follicles are endowed with specific androgen and estrogen receptors.[234, 235] The pilosebaceous unit possesses the enzymatic capability of converting the inactive prehormones DHEA and androstenedione to the potent androgens testosterone and DHT and estrogens.[235, 236] The activity of the pilosebaceous apparatus is reflective of the balance of androgenic, estrogenic, and enzymatic activities (Fig. 17–30*A*). Sexual hair growth on

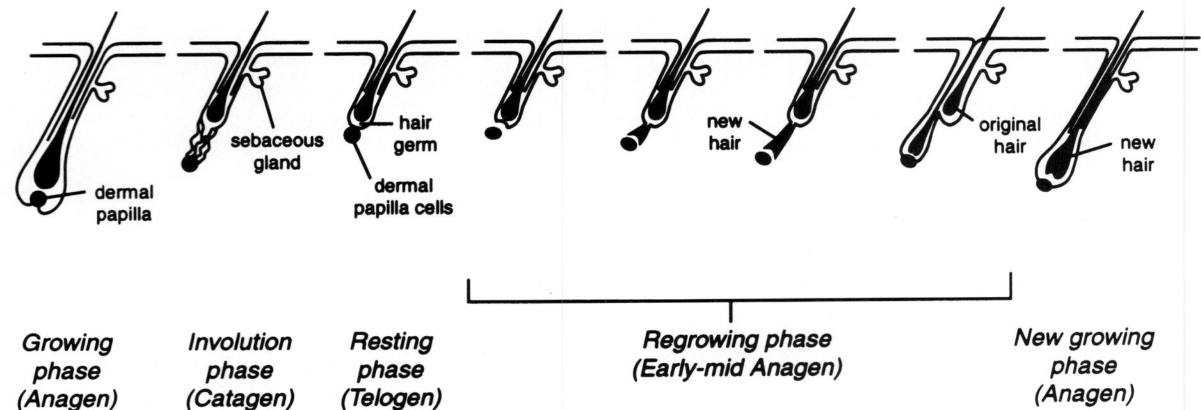

Figure 17–29 ■ Cyclic activity of human hair follicles. (Modified from Randall VA. Androgens and human hair growth. Clin Endocrinol 40:439–457, 1997.)

the face, lower abdomen, anterior thighs, chest, breasts, and pubic area and in the axilla is determined by sex steroids, the intrinsic rhythms of activity and inactivity, and genetic factors.[232] In addition, human hair follicles are influenced by seasonal variation probably related to circannual changes in androgen levels. The color of the hair is determined by the pigment produced by the melanocytes and their ability to transfer it to cortical cells of the hair. Loss of hair and reduced diameter is encountered in hypothyroidism and hypopituitarism.[237]

In hirsute women, the metabolic conversion of DHEA, testosterone, and Δ^4-androstenedione to DHT appears to be accelerated.[238] As a consequence, the vellus follicles develop into terminal hair follicles in large numbers in areas of androgen-sensitive skin, thereby increasing the diameter and density of hairs. Local estrogen formation in the hair follicle may play a modulating role in determining the degree of hirsutism. Thus, the hair follicle is a sex steroid target with its own microenvironment, capable of local transformation and actions (Fig. 17–30*A*). After exposure to androgen dominance beyond the individual and genetic threshold for a sufficient time, the manifestation of hirsutism will become apparent. However, high androgen levels are neither essential nor sufficient for the development of hirsutism or acne. A prerequisite for the cellular action of androgens on the pilosebaceous unit is the in situ conversion of testosterone to DHT through the enzymatic action of *5α-reductase*.[231, 239, 240] It has been shown that androgen induction of 5α-reductase activity is mediated by *IGF-I*.[241] Increased bioavailable IGF-I in hyperinsulinemic/hyperandrogenic women with PCOS may amplify the manifestation of hirsutism.

After nuclear receptor binding of DHT, androgenic expression takes place within the pilosebaceous unit. Local formation of testosterone from other C_{19} steroid precursors occurs; 3βHSD converts Δ^5-DHEA to Δ^4-androstenedione; and 17βHSD transforms Δ^4-androstenedione to testosterone. Δ^4-Androstenedione also metabolizes to form andros-

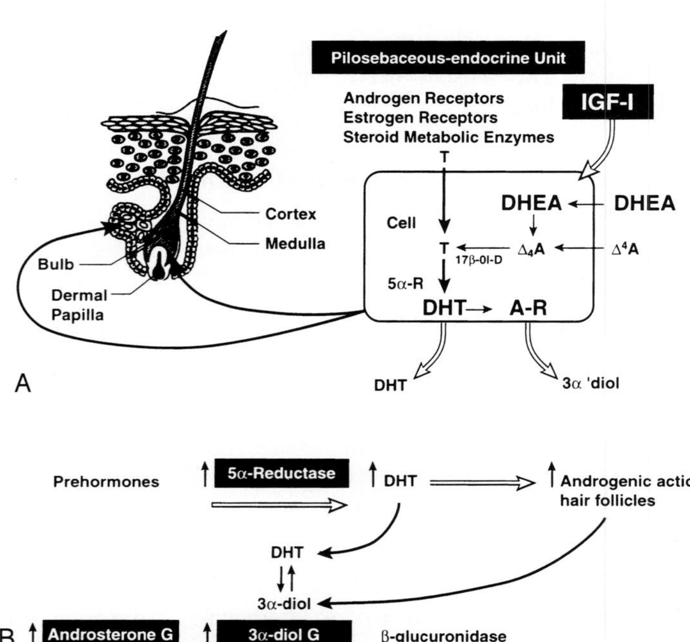

Figure 17–30 ■ *A*, Diagram of the pilosebaceous unit as an endocrine target as well as local modulation of endocrine microenvironments by enzymatic conversion of androgens to more potent androgen and to estrogens. Both DHEA and Δ^4-androstenedione (Δ^4-A) can be converted to testosterone (T) within the hair follicle. 3β-ol-D, 3β-hydroxysteroid dehydrogenase; 5α-R, 5α-reductase. *B*, The sensitivity of androgenic action in the skin is dependent on the activity of 5α-reductase and the quantitative formation of DHT. Thus, hirsutism can develop when 5α-reductase is increased in the absence of an elevated androgen level. The metabolic production of 3α-androstenediol (3α-diol) and androsterone, with their final conjugation products 3α-androstenediol glucuronide (3α-diol G) and androsterone glucuronide, represent sensitive markers of peripheral androgen action.

terone (Fig. 17–30*B*). The necessary metabolizing enzymes 3α- and 3β-ketoreductase are also present, resulting in the formation of 3α- and 3β-androstenediol, the ultimate end product of DHT metabolism in the skin.[240] These metabolites then enter the plasma pool, and levels of 3α-androstenediol may reflect androgenic events in the peripheral target tissue.[231, 239, 240] Elevated levels of 3α-androstenediol glucuronide in blood have been reported in hirsute women; consequently, 3α-androstenediol glucuronide levels reflect 5α-reductase activity and may be informative in delineating the underlying mechanism for the development of hirsutism.[242] Serum androsterone glucuronide and sulfate determinations may also be markers of 5α-reductase activity in women with PCOS.[243]

Acne

The activity of the sebaceous gland appears to be stimulated by DHEA and DHEA-S.[244] In patients with cystic acne, serum levels of DHEA-S are consistently elevated, and remission can be achieved by lowering DHEA-S levels by means of a low-dose (0.25 mg) nighttime dexamethasone suppression.[245]

Acne occurs frequently in hyperprolactinemic patients with elevated DHEA and DHEA-S levels, and remission can be achieved by lowering prolactin (PRL) levels with bromocriptine treatment. The demonstration that PRL acts directly to stimulate adrenal androgen secretion in the presence of ACTH explains this association.[246, 247] The role of adrenal androgen precursors DHEA and DHEA-S and their impact on the sebaceous gland are illustrated by the appearance of acne during adrenarche. The elevation of serum IGF-I levels and increased 5α-reductase activity at puberty in combination with adrenal androgen precursors serve as a physiologic model to account for the activation of sebaceous gland activity during sexual maturation.[244]

Idiopathic Hirsutism (End-Organ Hypersensitivity)

Hirsutism in women with relatively normal testosterone levels and regular menstrual cycles is a common clinical entity. Until recently, its cause was unclear and the disorder was called idiopathic hirsutism. It is not due to increased androgen receptors, and androgen receptors are not regulated by androgens in the skin.[248] It has now been clarified that 5α-reductase activity in the skin—the major determinant of androgenic (DHT) action on the hair follicle—is increased in these patients.[248, 249] Enhanced DHT formation in the hair follicle in the face of normal androgen levels accounts for the development of hirsutism. Suppression of normal ovarian production of androgen by contraceptive pills frequently results in improvement of hirsutism. Because increased 5α-reductase activity is determined by *genetic and ethnic* background, some patients may elect *not* to be treated.

Evaluation

The initial evaluation of hirsutism should include the following:

1. Quantitation of the degree of hirsutism by the method of Ferriman and Gallwey[250] in which the regions of androgen-sensitive pilosebaceous unit are graded and added; a score of 8 or more is considered beyond normal hair growth in adult women. An analysis by Barth[251] revealed that there are many pitfalls in all methods of scoring hair growth in women and concluded that it is unlikely that there will ever be a consensus about its definition. A classification of mild, moderate, or severe, based on distribution and textures of hair, would be practical clinically.
2. Chronology of the appearance of increased hair growth is of critical importance in dictating the direction of evaluation; implications of peripubertal versus recent onset and rapid versus slow progression are obvious.
3. Exclusion of drugs as a cause. Many drugs have a direct effect on SHBG production, and other drugs may possess androgenic properties.
4. Initial hormonal screening by measuring serum levels of testosterone, DHEA-S, and PRL is of value. Determination of 17α-hydroxyprogesterone levels may be informative, depending on the chronology of hirsutism (especially pubertal onset), to exclude the late onset of congenital adrenal hyperplasia (see Disorder of Puberty, Chapter 15). When chronic anovulation is present, determination of serum LH, FSH, and androgen levels may be helpful.

Repeated hormonal measurements are both costly and impractical. The properly developed rationale for each hormonal index would limit the number of determinations and would afford maximal information.

The chronology in women with hirsutism is commonly peripubertal or adolescent onset, with or without progression, with the majority having chronic anovulation. The results of initial hormonal screening frequently provide an answer. Measurements of prostate-specific antigen and 3α-androstenediol glucuronide or androsterone glucuronide may jointly provide diagnostic value in assessing 5α-reductase activity because they are highly correlated.[252, 253] However, the ultimate treatment is *independent* of these results, and these measurements are unnecessary for clinical management. When laboratory values and clinical manifestations dictate further evaluations as to the underlying cause of hirsutism, such as *adrenal* versus *ovarian* sources of hyperandrogenism and *functional* versus *neoplastic*, the procedures to be performed are detailed in the appropriate section in Chapter 26.

Management

The goal of treatment is to interrupt the steps leading to the increased androgen expression of the pilosebaceous unit. Several strategies are available. Mechanical hair removal (shaving, tweezing, waxing, and depilatory creams) can improve hirsutism, but it is a temporary measure. However, medical treatments in combination with a mechanical method such as electrolysis offer a better prospect for improvement.

OVARIAN SUPPRESSION

Oral Contraceptives. Low-dose oral contraceptive pills have been shown to be modestly effective in reducing circulating androgen levels and in alleviating hirsutism.[254] Oral contraceptive treatment is most effective in women with ovarian hyperandrogenism, especially those with PCOS. The benefits of oral contraceptive treatment have been attributed to the following effects[230]:

- suppression of gonadotropin secretion[254]
- reduction of ovarian androgen secretion[215]
- increased SHBG synthesis, thus decreased androgen action
- inhibition of DHT binding to androgen receptors[255]
- enhancement of antiandrogen effectiveness

The attempt to alleviate hirsutism caused by androgen excess with oral contraceptives represents a temporary measure. The preferred treatment is to target the pathogenic sites of hyperandrogenism or the site of action, thereby providing a long-term therapeutic measure.

GnRH Agonists. Suppression of ovarian function by the use of GnRH agonists has also been successful in the improvement of hirsutism, particularly in women with ovarian hyperandrogenism, including ovarian hyperthecosis. The availability of the long-acting GnRH agonist leuprolide (Lupron) has afforded an alternative in the management of hirsutism. The associated hypoestrogenism and its sequelae can be effectively prevented by concurrently adding back estrogen and progestin.[256, 257] The cost-effectiveness in the use of long-term GnRH agonist treatment should be discussed with the patient.

ANTIANDROGENS

Cyproterone Acetate. Originally known as a progestin, cyproterone acetate (CPA) has been found to possess antiandrogen and antigonadotropin properties. It acts as a competitive inhibitor of DHT binding to its specific receptors, reduces 5α-reductase in the skin, and lowers ovarian androgen secretion by inhibiting gonadotropin release.[258] Thus, CPA is effective in the treatment of hirsutism that is due to both androgen excess and hypersensitivity to androgen.[259]

Administered orally at a daily dose of 50 mg from days 5 to 25 of the cycle, CPA has induced a remarkable improvement in hirsutism after 3 to 6 months of treatment. Further reduction of hirsutism has been noted after up to 12 months of treatment. The undesirably low estradiol levels induced by CPA treatment can be corrected by topical daily application of 17β-estradiol.[259] This combined treatment is widely used in Europe, but CPA is not available in the United States.

Spironolactone. An aldosterone antagonist traditionally used as a diuretic in treatment of mild hypertension, spironolactone has been found to possess antiandrogenic properties. The steroid molecule of spironolactone is remarkably similar to that of testosterone (Fig. 17–31). It has the ability to inhibit the cytochrome P450c17 enzyme, which is required for biosynthesis of androgens in gonadal and adrenal steroid-producing cells.[260] It also inhibits the androgenic action of DHT by occupying the androgen receptors in target tissues including hair follicles.[261] Several clinical studies have shown remarkable improvements of hirsutism that was due to both androgen excess and hypersensitivity to androgen after 6 months of spironolactone treatment.[262–264] The maximal effectiveness of this inhibitory action of spironolactone on androgen secretion occurs at 3 to 6 months (Fig. 17–32). Regression of hirsutism, in terms of decreased hair diameter and density plus a reduced rate of facial hair growth, can be achieved and maintained for the duration of treatment (Fig. 17–33).

Spironolactone Testosterone

Figure 17–31 ■ Similarities in steroid molecules between spironolactone and testosterone.

A daily dose of 100 mg of spironolactone is recommended. The lack of adrenal suppression is a distinct advantage for long-term use of the agent. Spironolactone appears to induce cyclic menses in most amenorrheic patients with PCOS and in anovulatory hyperandrogenic women.[263, 264]

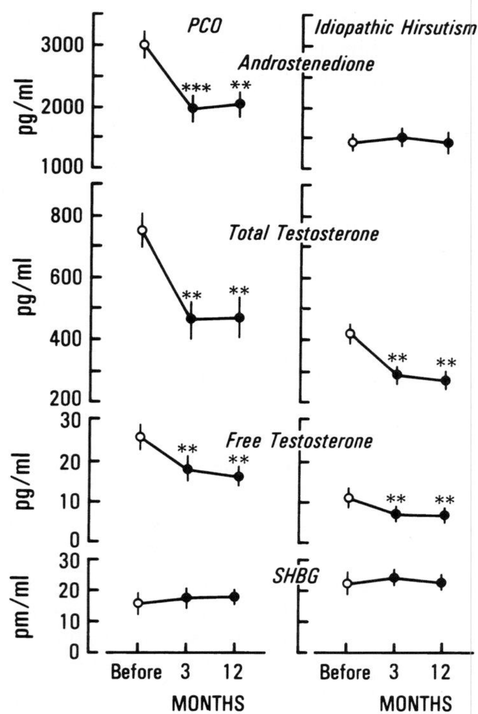

Figure 17–32 ■ Serum concentrations (mean ± SE) of androstenedione, total testosterone, free testosterone, and sex hormone–binding globulin (SHBG) before and after 3 and 12 months of therapy with spironolactone in polycystic ovarian (PCO) syndrome and idiopathic hirsutism. Double asterisk, $P < .01$; triple asterisk, $P < .001$. (From Cumming DC, Yang JC, Rebar RW, Yen SSC. Treatment of hirsutism with spironolactone. JAMA 247:1295–1298, 1982. © 1982, American Medical Association.)

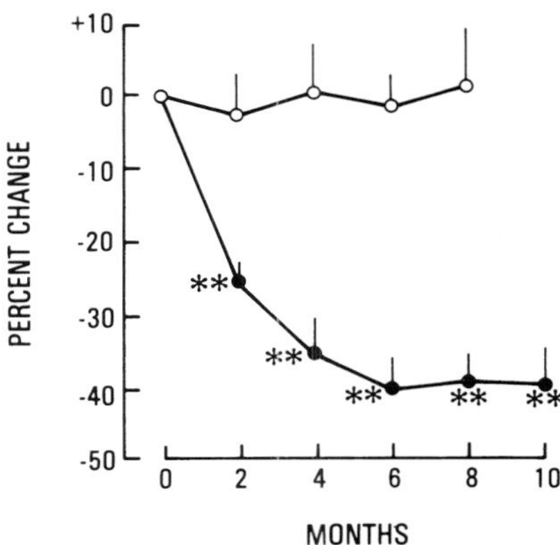

Figure 17–33 ■ Percentage (mean ± SE) change in hair shaft diameter in 11 patients receiving spironolactone compared with 7 untreated hirsute control subjects. Double asterisk, $P < .01$. (From Cumming DC, Yang JC, Rebar RW, Yen SSC. Treatment of hirsutism with spironolactone. JAMA 247:1295–1298, 1982. © 1982, American Medical Association.)

Flutamide. Flutamide is a potent, nonsteroidal, selective antiandrogen that acts by blockade of the androgen receptor, without progestational, estrogenic, glucocorticoid, or antigonadotropic activities. In doses of 250 mg twice daily, flutamide has been shown to be beneficial in the improvement of hirsutism.[265] Prospective studies comparing the efficacy of flutamide and spironolactone have shown that flutamide is superior to spironolactone in the improvement of hirsutism and endocrine parameters.[266] A long-term clinical trial (12 months) confirmed its efficacy, but careful monitoring of liver function is required.[230, 266]

Finasteride. Finasteride is a specific competitive inhibitor of 5α-reductase, targeted to type 2 isoenzyme. Several studies have shown that the administration of a 5-mg daily dose of finasteride is safe and effective in the improvement of both idiopathic hirsutism and hirsutism in association with PCOS.[267–269] The relative effectiveness in reducing hirsutism is similar to that of spironolactone[270] and flutamide[271] in comparison studies. Finasteride administration (5-mg dose) did not alter LH pulsatility and serum levels of testosterone, androstenedione, estradiol, or SHBG, but serum concentration of DHT and 3α-androstenediol glucuronide decreased significantly, indicating an inhibition of 5α-reductase activity.[272] Thus, finasteride appears to be a relatively specific therapeutic agent to reduce DHT formation and thereby improve hirsutism independent of underlying causes.

Glucocorticoids. In patients with functional adrenal hyperandrogenism (e.g., partial enzymatic defects), the use of dexamethasone in small doses (e.g., 0.25 mg at bedtime) is both effective and specific. At this dose, dexamethasone selectively suppresses adrenal androgen without interfering with cortisol secretion.[273]

ADJUNCT THERAPY

The improvement of hirsutism in response to antiandrogen administration is facilitated by electrolysis to remove old hair because antiandrogens inhibit only the growth of new hair.

WEIGHT REDUCTION

Weight reduction is an effective means of reducing androgen and increasing SHBG levels in obese women with hirsutism. This effect is probably due to improvement of hyperinsulinemia, which has a direct stimulatory action on ovarian androgen production. Failure to respond to appropriate management is commonly a result of noncompliance.

PATHOGENESIS

The cause of PCOS is unknown. The intense interest in this multifunctional disorder is evident from the overwhelming amount of literature on this topic. The emphasis is variously focused on

- insulin resistance/hyperinsulinemia, obesity
- hypothalamic GnRH pulse generator dysregulation
- functional derangements of the GH–IGF-I axis
- P450c17 dysregulation
- adrenergic dysfunction
- hereditary and genetic factors

Although all elements may be involved in the pathogenesis of this syndrome, the precise link that entails the array of abnormalities cannot be made. There are, however, several interrelated events that have pathogenic significance, which are highlighted.

Extraovarian Factors (Co-gonadotropins)

PCOS, in its classic form, may not be evolved solely from inherent defects of the hypothalamic-pituitary-ovarian system, including intraovarian autocrine/paracrine regulators.[26, 175] Rather, regulators outside the reproductive axis may be involved in the genesis and maintenance of hypersecretion of LH, theca-stromal cell hyperactivity, and hypofunction of the FSH–granulosa cell axis, resulting in hyperandrogenism and ovarian acyclicity.[168] In recent years, substantial evidence has accumulated suggesting that insulin[16] and GH[14, 90, 274] may have gonadotropin-augmenting effects on ovarian function. The localization of receptors and their gene expression for GH,[88] insulin, and IGFs[100, 172, 179] in ovarian compartments have afforded critical links supporting an endocrine role for these extraovarian factors as co-gonadotropins. Thus, they may play a corporate function with gonadotropins in the regulation of cyclic ovarian follicle development and steroidogenesis. Alterations of these putative co-gonadotropins may, therefore, contribute to hypothalamic-pituitary-ovarian dysfunction.

Given these considerations, the author has postulated that aberrations of gonadotropic and putative co-gonadotropic inputs to ovarian androgenesis and follicular arrest together with a marked impairment of catecholamine-induced lipolysis[13] in PCOS in the absence of obesity may represent *the authentic syndrome*. It follows that PCOS in combination with obesity may constitute a *modified version of the syndrome*.[37]

Insulin resistance is a common defect in PCOS independent of obesity, and obesity contributes an additive effect to insulin resistance in obese women with PCOS[37, 73] with a parallel increase in the degree of compensatory hyperinsulinemia. Insulin resistance in obese PCOS is, therefore, composed of dual contributions, one unique to PCOS and the other obesity specific. As a co-gonadotropin, insulin is capable of stimulating androgen secretion directly and enhances LH-mediated responses in isolated theca tissue to a greater degree in PCOS than in normal ovaries.[16, 58, 59, 275–277]

GH pulse amplitude is selectively increased by 30 percent in lean PCOS and thus GH input to the ovary is enhanced and the intraovarian production of IGFs may be increased, and thereby augmented LH-mediated theca cell androgenesis may ensue. By contrast, obese PCOS exhibited a state of *hyposomatotropinism* with a 50 percent reduction of GH pulse amplitude, 24-hour mean GH levels, and GH responses to GHRH and an unaltered GH pulse frequency. These events are entirely obesity dependent,[94–97, 275] resulting in a substantial decrease in GH input to the ovary. The link between insulin and functional activity of the somatotropic axis is evident by the ability of insulin excess to inhibit hepatic production of IGFBP-1,[98] with a marked suppression of IGFBP-1 levels in obese PCOS resulting in a more than 10-fold increase in the IGF-I:IGFBP-1 ratio and elevated free IGF-I levels.[275] As a consequence, increased bioavailability of IGF-I[99] to theca tissue through the IGF-I receptor[100] may serve a pro-gonadotropin role inducing hyperandrogenism in obese PCOS.[175, 276–278] Thus, there is a *shift of co-gonadotropin from GH to insulin/IGF-I with increasing adiposity.* These co-gonadotropins may provide *unremitting inputs* in concert with the *common influence of LH* in the genesis of ovarian hyperandrogenism and chronic anovulation. Further, the combined antilipolytic effects of hyperinsulinemia and hyposomatotropinism together with reduced β_2-adrenergic–stimulated lipolysis afford a *metabolic setting favoring increased adiposity in this syndrome.*

Dysregulation of P450c17

Exaggerated Adrenarche Hypothesis

The origin of this syndrome as an adrenal disorder manifested during the early phase of sexual maturation in the form of an *exaggerated adrenarche* was proposed some time ago.[6] A host of reports have shown that children with premature or exaggerated adrenarche are at high risk of developing PCOS-like functional ovarian hyperandrogenism at puberty.[20, 23, 24, 228, 229, 279–282] These findings, together with the observation that hyperandrogenemia in adolescent girls is accompanied by neuroendocrine-metabolic features closely akin to those found in adult PCOS,[21, 22] strongly support the exaggerated adrenarche hypothesis. The key event of adrenarche is the initiation of adrenal androgen secretion of DHEA, DHEA-S, and androstenedione through the activation of 17,20-lyase activity of the P450c17.[283, 284] Premature hypersecretion of adrenal androgen precursors provides substrate for transformation to potent androgens and estrogens in the target cells of the reproductive axis where they act locally through androgen and estrogen receptors.[285] Free IGF-I levels have recently been shown to increase during childhood and peak at puberty in girls[286] (Fig. 17–34). This event occurs during the transition from adrenarche to early puberty and together with concurrent elevations of GH, insulin, and gonadotropin secretion and

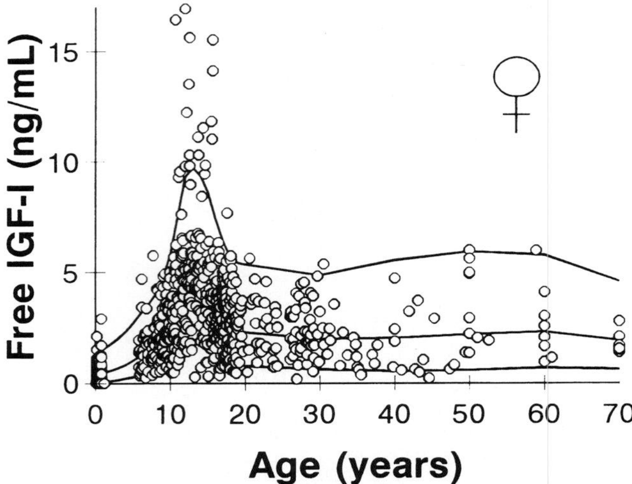

Figure 17–34 ■ Serum levels of free IGF-I in 1430 healthy children and adults in relationship to age. The lines represent the mean (±SE) value and upper and lower limits. (From Juul A, Holm K, Kastrup KW, et al. Free insulin-like growth factor I serum levels in 1430 healthy children and adults, and its diagnostic value in patients suspected of growth hormone deficiency. J Clin Endocrinol Metab 82:2497–2502, 1997. © The Endocrine Society.)

the development of insulin resistance[287] may augment androgen biosynthesis by the adrenal as well as by the ovary. It is speculated that such events may be responsible for the development of hyperandrogenism of both adrenal and ovarian origin. Whether this enzymatic hyperfunction is inherent to both adrenal and ovary or whether DHEA/DHEA-S from the adrenal acts as a prehormone to initiate premature ovarian androgenesis is unclear. Although both mechanisms are compatible with the exaggerated adrenarche hypothesis, other factors may be involved, such as *insulin excess.*

Insulin Resistance at Puberty

Insulin resistance normally develops during the process of puberty in association with the rise in the secretion of insulin, IGF-I, GH, and gonadotropin[17–19, 286–288] (Fig. 17–35). These changes may synergistically enhance gonadotropic action on the ovary (see Fig. 17–23). Thus, physiologic pubertal insulin resistance, among other biologic roles, may contribute to the transition of hyperandrogenism from the adrenal to the ovary. Insulin resistance and hyperinsulinemia appear to extend beyond puberty in women who have inherent cellular defects of insulin resistance and are thus destined to develop PCOS. The demonstration of increased insulin resistance and hyperinsulinemia in hyperandrogenic girls with an endocrine-metabolic profile akin to adult women with PCOS supports this hypothesis[21, 22] (Fig. 17–36).

Dysregulation of GnRH Pulse Generator

The inappropriate gonadotropin secretion with disproportionately high LH and relatively low FSH is a unique feature in PCOS. As discussed earlier, the underlying cause of this pattern of gonadotropin secretion is linked to an

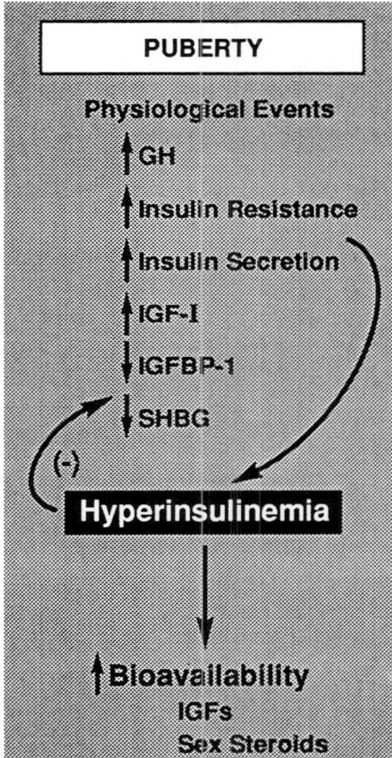

Figure 17–35 ■ Activation of GH–IGF-I axis and the development of physiologic insulin resistance during puberty. The resulting relative hyperinsulinemia is accompanied by a host of changes in growth-promoting hormones and their binding proteins and the bioavailability of IGF-I and sex steroids. This transient dynamic change in normal girls may persist in individuals with inherent insulin resistance who are destined to develop PCOS.

accelerated GnRH pulse generator activity and heightened pituitary responses to GnRH. High-frequency GnRH pulsatile input to the gonadotroph induces up-regulation of LH β-subunit and down-regulation of FSH β-subunit expressions, resulting in relatively greater synthesis and secretion of LH than of FSH. Regulation of the intrapituitary activin/follistatin system is also linked to GnRH pulse frequency. Fast-frequency GnRH pulses are associated with an increase in follistatin mRNA, thereby reducing the FSH-releasing property of activin and decreasing FSH secretion. Thus, GnRH pulse frequency may differentially regulate LH and FSH secretion both directly and through follistatin, and heightened pituitary sensitivity to GnRH may reflect increased GnRH receptor on the gonadotroph.[47–49] In addition, chronically elevated levels of unbound estrogen can augment pituitary sensitivity to GnRH both by a direct action on gonadotropin synthesis and by enhancing GnRH-induced GnRH receptors.[289, 290]

Chronic inappropriate (nonlinear) feedback action of estrogen, particularly in the face of prolonged deprivation of progesterone, may play a role in the altered GnRH neuronal activity in PCOS. Indeed, in PCOS patients, LH pulse frequency can be reduced by the administration of progestin,[41] and the LH response to GnRH, LH levels, and the LH:FSH ratio are nearly normalized by the administration of estradiol and progesterone in doses that produce midluteal-phase levels.[42, 43] This progesterone deprivation hypothesis may also be related to a reduction of dopaminergic and opioidergic inhibitory actions[291–294] on GnRH pulse frequency because administration of progesterone restores the opioidergic activity in PCOS.[41] However, it is unlikely that chronic progesterone deficiency is the cause of accelerated GnRH/LH pulsatile activity in PCOS; rather, it plays a *facilitory role* in the maintenance of this dysfunction.

Thus, the precise mechanism to account for the GnRH pulse generator dysregulation in PCOS is not entirely clear. However, strong evidence supports a role for insulin, IGFs, and estrogen in the modulation of GnRH neuronal activities.[295–298] Receptors for insulin, IGF-I, IGF-II,[299, 300] and the α and β estrogen receptor (unpublished observation) are expressed in GnRH neuronal cell lines. Activation of the IGF-I receptor induces cell proliferation and growth-independent GnRH gene expression[295] and secretion.[296] IGF-I immunoreactivity has been found in the astrocytes of the arcuate nucleus and at a higher density in androgenized than in normal female rats. Further, IGF-I immunoreactivity in arcuate nucleus glial cells showed a dose-dependent increase in ovariectomized rats treated with 17β-estradiol.[298] Thus, the GnRH neuron appears to be a target for insulin, IGFs, and sex steroids in the regulation of its functional activities. These findings are complemented by the demonstration that IGF-I of peripheral origin acts centrally to accelerate the initiation of female puberty in rats[297] and rhesus monkeys.[301]

Given these experimental data, it was postulated that altered inputs to the GnRH neuronal system by one or all of these factors during the critical development phase of adrenarche/puberty may induce dysregulation of GnRH

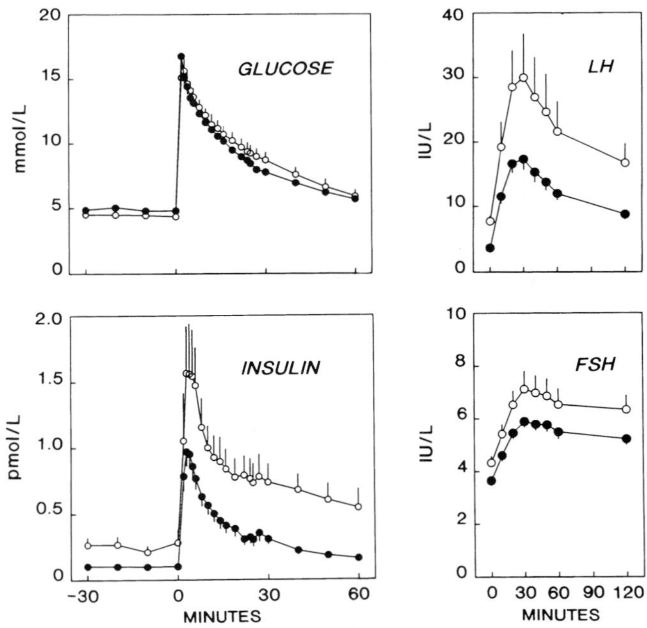

Figure 17–36 ■ Mean ± SE plasma glucose and serum insulin concentrations after intravenous administration of 0.3 gm/kg glucose *(left)* and serum LH and FSH responses to 10 μg GnRH for 13 hyperandrogenic (○) and 23 normal (●) girls. (From Apter D, Bützow T, Laughlin GA, et al. Metabolic features of polycystic ovary syndrome are found in adolescent girls with hyperandrogenism. J Clin Endocrinol Metab 80:2966–2973, 1995; and Apter D, Bützow T, Laughlin GA, et al. Accelerated 24-hour luteinizing hormone pulsatile activity in adolescent girls with ovarian hyperandrogenism: Relevance to the developmental phase of polycystic ovarian syndrome. J Clin Endocrinol Metab 79:119–125, 1994. © The Endocrine Society.)

pulse generator activities, a proposition consonant with observations in peripubertal girls with PCOS.[21, 22] In these girls, GnRH/LH pulsatility is accelerated, and the shift from the pubertal pattern of LH pulsatility (sleep-related augmentation) to the adult pattern (augmentation during waking hours) occurs 2 years earlier than in normal girls, suggesting an untimely activation of the GnRH-gonadotropin axis resulting in ovarian hyperandrogenism.[21, 22] That hypersecretion of LH is of paramount importance in the development of PCOS is complemented by the recently developed transgenic mouse model with hypersecretion of LH secondary to targeted expression of a transgene encoding a chimeric LH β-subunit. These mice exhibit elevated androgens, anovulation, and the polycystic ovary phenotype with hypertrophy of theca-stromal cells.[302] Collectively, peripubertal hyperactivity of the GnRH/LH axis may be a major component in the pathogenesis of PCOS, a view compatible with the exaggerated adrenarche hypothesis in which adrenal androgens provide substrates for peripheral conversion to estrogens resulting in untimely feedback impacts on the hypothalamic-pituitary unit.

Hereditary and Genetic Factors

Familial clustering of PCOS has been reported. Both autosomal and X-linked patterns have been invoked to explain the familial nature of this disorder, but the available pedigree data do not distinguish between these modes of inheritance.[303–305] The major problems of previous studies were the lack of specificity of phenotype and the use of ultrasonography for the detection of polycystic ovaries, which can be misleading.[306] Thus, the issues of the familial nature of PCOS and potential genetic abnormalities in patients with PCOS are yet to be defined.[72, 73, 307]

LONG-TERM SEQUELAE AND RISKS

Abnormalities associated with PCOS suggest that women with PCOS are at risk for the development of NIDDM, hypertension, coronary artery disease, intravascular thrombosis, and endometrial cancer. Some of these risks are established and others are less substantiated.

Endometrial Cancer

Much evidence has accumulated to suggest that chronic exposure to unopposed estrogen, as in the case of PCOS patients, may lead to the development of endometrial hyperplasia and carcinoma. Epidemiologic studies have shown an increased risk for endometrial cancer in women with chronic anovulation.[308] Because fat depots represent a large compartment for peripheral conversion of androgen to estrogen, the high incidence of obesity in PCOS patients may represent the key factor in the genesis of endometrial neoplasia.[308] The increased incidence of endometrial carcinoma in these patients is usually classified as type 1, and the prognosis is highly favorable.[309]

The choice of surgery or a treatment with a progestational agent for stage I endometrial cancer in PCOS patients depends on age. In young women, the use of a potent progestational agent, such as medroxyprogesterone acetate, as an initial therapeutic approach is both logical and effective. If no improvement is observed in 4 to 6 months, hysterectomy should be considered.

Diabetes Mellitus (NIDDM)

Substantial evidence indicates that 20 to 40 percent of obese PCOS women have impaired glucose tolerance or NIDDM by the end of their fourth decade of life. However, although it is uncommon, abnormal glucose tolerance can occur as early as adolescence.[74] Fasting glucose levels are typically within the normal range, and impairments are detected only during glucose tolerance testing. Thus, NIDDM in women with PCOS is usually not diagnosed until later in life. A study of postmenopausal women with a history of PCOS revealed a 13 percent prevalence of NIDDM compared with 2 percent in the control population.[310] Legro and colleagues[311] reported that insulin resistance persists in older PCOS women, whereas hyperandrogenemia tends to be resolved. Thus, one would anticipate an increased prevalence of NIDDM in PCOS women with advancing age. Because pregnancy is associated with insulin resistance, it is reasonable to anticipate an increase in the incidence of gestational diabetes in PCOS women during pregnancy.[312] Studies involving larger populations are required to establish this proposition.

Cardiovascular Disease

The presence of obesity in PCOS women has a synergistic impact on the metabolic consequences of the syndrome.[313] BMI (weight in kilograms divided by the square of the height in meters) is easy to calculate and is sufficiently correlated with direct measures of body fatness to be useful in defining obesity clinically. A BMI greater than 28 kg/m^2 is defined as obese and is associated with a significant increase in morbidity. Dyslipidemia in PCOS women has been reported by several studies; elevated free fatty acid, triglyceride, and LDL levels and reduced HDL or HDL_2 levels relative to age-, sex-, and weight-matched control subjects were found.[163, 314–316] Insulin rather than androgen levels are correlated with lipid abnormalities, and suppressing androgen levels does not alter lipid profiles in PCOS women.[317] Thus, insulin resistance and hyperlipidemia constitute the basis for an increase in cardiovascular risks.[318] In addition, impaired fibrinolytic activity with increased circulating levels of plasminogen activator inhibitor (PAI-1) is found in PCOS women.[167, 319] Elevated PAI-1 levels are related to insulin resistance and are considered to be an added independent cardiovascular risk factor by increasing the incidence of intravascular thrombosis. Improved insulin resistance is accompanied by a decrease in PAI-1 levels.[108] Thus, women with PCOS have an increased risk of cardiovascular disease including myocardial infarction and atherosclerosis.[320–323]

DIAGNOSIS

The diagnosis of PCOS requires a *combination* of clinical, ultrasonographic, and biochemical features that include

- oligomenorrhea and amenorrhea
- polycystic ovaries by ultrasonography

- hyperandrogenemia or hirsutism, or both
- increased LH:FSH ratio >2.0 (for BMI <30 kg/m^2)
- peripubertal onset of symptoms

Clinical Presentation

A detailed history concerning the chronologic development of symptoms and signs is crucial in establishing the direction of evaluations for the diagnosis. Reliable assessment of hormonal disturbances can be made by careful and systematic physical examination, with the patient in a sense acting as her own bioassay system.

Hirsutism and Acne

Patients with PCOS usually give a history of peripubertal onset of increased hair growth, irregularity of menses, and overweight. Hirsutism and acne are common symptoms, reflecting hyperandrogenism that may or may not be progressive. However, overt signs of *virilization* usually reflect the presence of an androgen-producing tumor or ovarian hyperthecosis. The time course of development of the androgenic signs is of great importance; a recent, rapid onset of androgenization requires urgent and special diagnostic testing for distinguishing PCOS from other more serious underlying causes of androgen excess.

Menstrual Disorder and Infertility

In most cases, a history of menstrual disturbance dates back to menarche.[5] Oligomenorrhea, amenorrhea, or dysfunctional uterine bleeding and infertility are common presenting symptoms. Primary amenorrhea can occur but is uncommon.

Metabolic Disorders

Rarely, patients present themselves as having problems of obesity and related disorders. The association of obesity with PCOS in 50 percent of patients constitutes an *important modifier* of the biochemical changes seen in lean/normal weight PCOS. This must be taken into account in the interpretation of laboratory results. The relative degree of obesity can be assessed semiquantitatively by calculating BMI (see Fig. 17–37 for determining the BMI). The presence of *acanthosis nigricans* is a cutaneous marker of insulin resistance and hyperinsulinemia (see later).

Body fat distribution has significant impacts on the long-term consequences of PCOS. A central distribution of body fat estimated by a ratio of waist circumference to hip circumference greater than 0.90 in women and greater than 1.0 in men is associated with a higher risk of morbidity and mortality than a more peripheral distribution of body fat (waist to hip ratio less than 0.75 in women and less than 0.85 in men). Pasquali and colleagues[324] have shown that central as opposed to peripheral fat distribution in women with PCOS is associated with

- a progressive increase of LH, androstenedione, and estrone concentrations
- higher fasting and glucose-stimulated insulin levels
- higher levels of triglycerides, VLDL, and apolipoprotein B and lower values of HDL cholesterol (without differences in total cholesterol and apolipoprotein A1)
- higher diastolic blood pressure, a greater degree of obesity, and a lower prevalence of acne

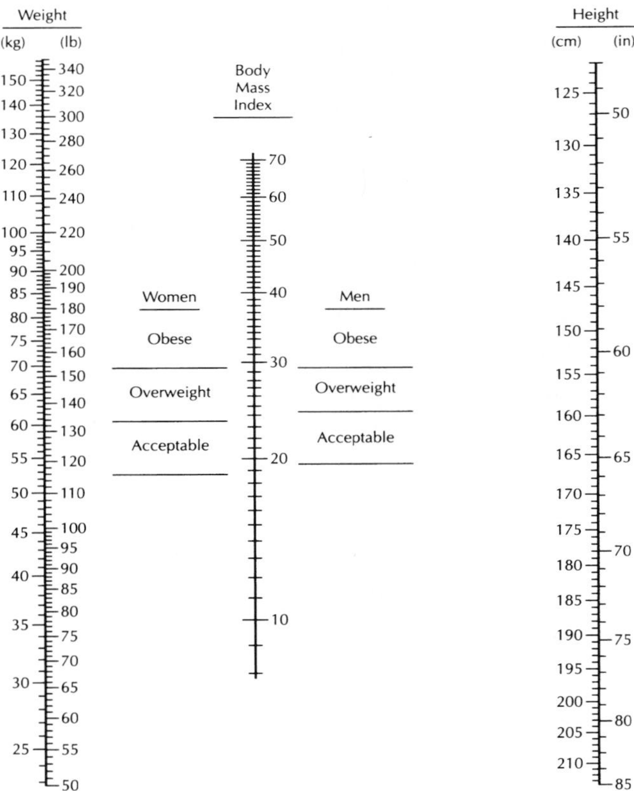

Figure 17–37 ■ The chart for clinical assessments of relative adiposity by calculating body mass index (BMI).

Laboratory Diagnosis

There is no clear consensus on hormonal tests that can be expected to fully discriminate women with PCOS from normal cycling women. This is in part due to the heterogeneity of the syndrome, and in large measure the influence of obesity or BMI has not been included as a factor in the assessment of the relative diagnostic usefulness of a given set of hormonal parameters.

It is recommended that the diagnosis of PCOS be made on the basis of a *combination of clinical, ultrasonographic,* and *biochemical criteria.* For a woman presenting with oligomenorrhea or amenorrhea and polycystic ovary on ultrasound examination (Fig. 17–38), an optimal and cost-effective hormonal discrimination between PCOS and non-PCOS may be achieved by measuring serum levels of LH, FSH, and androstenedione. Interpretation of these values must take into account the presence of obesity or BMI greater than 28 kg/m^2, because it negatively influences LH levels. Because of the pulsatility of LH levels, the author recommends averaging the values of two samples drawn 30 minutes apart, which provides a diagnostic accuracy of 95 percent of cases in nonobese PCOS.[38] Consistent with

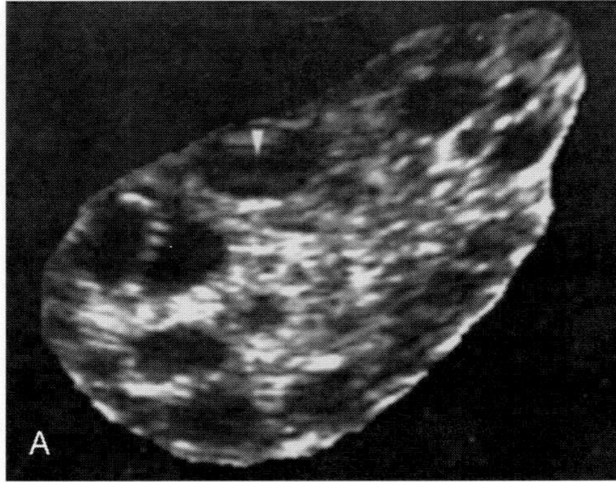

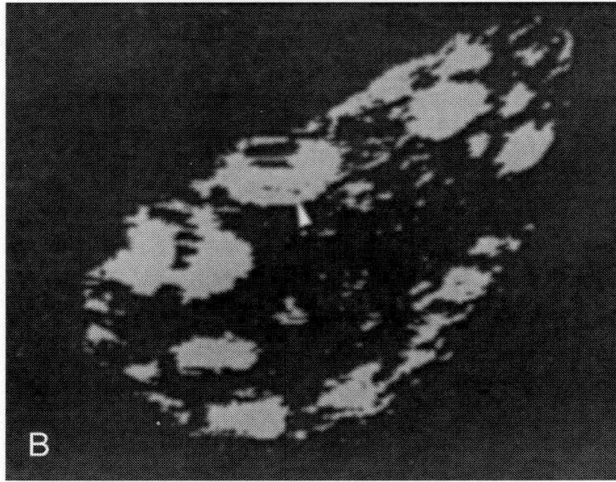

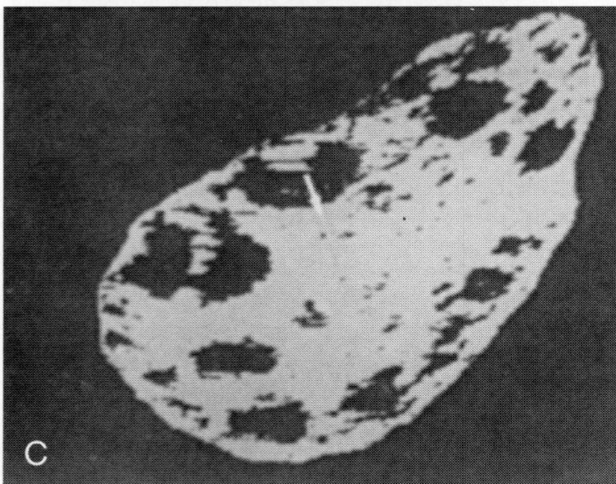

Figure 17–38 ■ Computerized analysis of a typical polycystic ovary. Longitudinal cut at the middle part of the ovary was selected from the videotape record and acquired on a microcomputer. *A,* After shaping of the outline, the ovary was pasted on a calibrated image. *B,* Selection of the range values on a gray-level scale and automatic calculation of the microcyst *(arrowhead)* area. *C,* Selection of the stroma *(arrow)* by setting the range values, just up to the maximal threshold obtained for the microcysts, and automatic calculation of the stroma area. (From Robert Y, Dubrulle F, Gaillandre L, et al. Ultrasound assessment of ovarian stroma hypertrophy in hyperandrogenism and ovulation disorders: Visual analysis versus computerized quantification. Fertil Steril 64:307–312, 1995. Reproduced with permission of the American Society for Reproductive Medicine.)

this approach, Koskinen and colleagues,[325] using logistic regression analysis in a large population of women with PCOS and matched normal cycling control subjects (without polycystic ovaries), showed LH, FSH, and androstenedione levels, when used in combination, attained a diagnostic sensitivity, specificity, and overall concordance of 98, 93, and 96 percent, respectively.

Clinical Diagnosis of Insulin Resistance

There are major constraints to determining insulin resistance in a clinical setting. First, there is a wide range of insulin sensitivity in normal individuals, and approximately 25 percent overlap with those of insulin resistance individuals. Second, fasting or glucose-stimulated insulin values do not correlate well with results of more frequent and well-timed measurements of insulin responses during, for example, a rapid intravenous glucose tolerance test used in research settings.[326] However, extensive data support the association of PCOS and insulin resistance with additive effects of obesity; thus, early detection of metabolic abnormalities is imperative. The combination of hyperinsulinemia and hyperandrogenism is the basis for development of cardiovascular disease, dyslipidemia, fibrinolytic abnormalities, and NIDDM. It is recommended that lipid and lipoprotein profiles be obtained in all patients with PCOS; and in obese women with PCOS, plasma glucose levels should be measured at fasting and 2 hours after a 75-gm glucose load as a screen for glucose intolerance according to the World Health Organization criteria[327]:

- Fasting glucose levels: ≥126 mg/dl
- 2-hour glucose value: <140 mg/day, *normal*
140–199 mg/dl, *impaired*
≥200 mg/dl, *NIDDM*

It is of paramount importance that the clinician acquire a full understanding of several polycystic ovary–like syndromes, some of which are serious illnesses, in order not to delay the diagnosis and institution of prompt treatment.

MANAGEMENT

Aside from establishing fertility, inducing ovulatory cycles, and improving hirsutism, the aim in the treatment of patients with PCOS is to reduce the long-term consequences of metabolic sequelae. Establishing cyclic ovulation can be accomplished in most cases and hirsutism and metabolic abnormalities can be attenuated effectively by medical treatments.

Anovulation

Ovulation Induction

CLOMIPHENE CITRATE

In women with infertility, the effectiveness of clomiphene, an antiestrogen, in inducing ovulation is well established. The success rate, especially in patients with substantial endogenous estrogen, as in PCOS, is high (75 to 80 percent) with a cumulative conception rate that approaches normal.[328, 329] Previous failure to induce ovulation by dexamethasone suppression, ovarian wedge resection, or both is not a contraindication to clomiphene treatment. The majority of PCOS patients respond to a 5-day course of 50- to 100-mg daily doses of clomiphene. If an ovulatory cycle does not ensue within 3 months of the last clomiphene treatment, the same course of treatment can be repeated.

Clomiphene induces an increase in FSH secretion that is crucial to the initiation of cyclic ovarian function. Although there is a concomitant and unwanted increase in LH levels, follicular maturation occurs, resulting in an increase in circulating estradiol levels. By a positive feedback effect on the hypothalamic-pituitary unit, the increased estradiol levels result in an ovulatory surge of LH and FSH (Fig. 17–39). This event usually occurs, on an average, 7 days after the completion of treatment. Twins, but not multiple ovulation, can occur, and ultrasonographic monitoring of the ovarian response is informative. The use of commercially available urinary LH measurement kits offers a practical and reliable means for the detection of an LH surge as an indicator of ovulation. The mechanisms and sites of clomiphene action in the reversal of anovulatory states remain to be fully clarified. Available evidence suggests that the clomiphene citrate–initiated ovulatory events may represent the sum of direct effects at all levels of the hypothalamic-pituitary-ovarian axis.[330, 331]

COMBINED CLOMIPHENE AND DEXAMETHASONE

Patients taking clomiphene combined with 0.5 mg of dexamethasone nightly have achieved a significantly higher rate of ovulation and conception than with clomiphene alone.[332, 333] This combined therapeutic approach may prove to be more effective in patients with both adrenal and ovarian sources of androgen excess. However, it has been demonstrated that a 0.5-mg dose may be excessive. Because adrenal androgen secretion is more sensitive than cortisol to small doses of dexamethasone, a 0.25-mg dose may be effectively employed to suppress adrenal androgen to normal levels without attendant changes in cortisol secretion.[273]

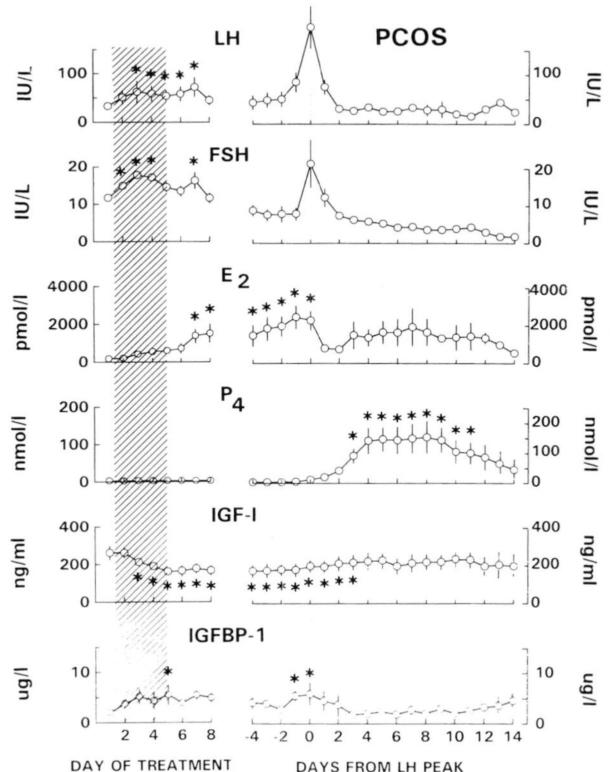

Figure 17–39 ■ Ovulation induction with clomiphene citrate in patients with PCOS. Mean (±SE) serum gonadotropin, steroid, IGF-I, and IGFBP-1 levels before, during *(shaded area)*, and after 5 days of clomiphene citrate treatment (150 mg/day) in seven women with PCOS. The data during treatment are plotted with treatment day 1 as the reference point, and the subsequent hormonal data are plotted with the LH surge as the reference point. Note that the key event may reside in the ~35 percent increment of FSH levels on days 3 and 4 of treatment (unpublished data).

EXOGENOUS GONADOTROPIN

For PCOS patients who do not conceive after clomiphene citrate, induction of ovulation with the administration of human menopausal gonadotropin or pure FSH has been used for a long time and is highly successful with an overall pregnancy rate on the order of 50 percent.[334, 335] Because of the side effects attending overstimulation, the cost, and the demand on patients, this mode of treatment should be reserved for cases that failed clomiphene treatment.

On the premise that the chronically low levels of FSH may be an important underlying factor in the arrested follicular maturation, judicious use of small doses (52.5 to 75 IU) of a urinary "pure" FSH or recombinant FSH preparations has achieved highly favorable results.[45] In a large series of patients (225 women) during a 10-year period, pregnancies occurred in 109 patients with an overall conception rate of 45 percent and miscarriage rate of 20 percent, approaching that observed in the general population. Most remarkable was the occurrence of single ovulatory cycles in the majority of cases, thus limiting multiple pregnancies and hyperstimulation syndrome. High LH levels did not have a significant impact on the outcome of treatment. Excess body weight and age had a negative impact, probably related to the presence of hyperinsulinemia.[336]

GnRH AND GnRH AGONIST

The notion that the high frequency and amplitude of LH pulses in PCOS patients may be overridden by programmed pulsatile GnRH administration at a lower frequency has not proved to be the case. Several trials using a variety of doses and frequencies of GnRH pulses (by automatic pump) have yielded a relatively low rate of ovulation and even lower pregnancy rate compared with other medical regimens.[337] The hypersensitivity of the pituitary to GnRH in PCOS patients is likely to be the reason for poor responses to pulsatile GnRH administration.

However, when endogenous gonadotropin secretion is *down-regulated by a GnRH agonist*, thus rendering a hypogonadotropic state in PCOS patients, a remarkable improvement of the ovulation rate with normal corpus luteum function can be achieved by pulsatile GnRH administration.[338] When exogenous gonadotropin administration with low-dose step-up or step-down protocols[46] is used instead of GnRH pulsatile regimens, the conception rate is increased and the risk of multiple pregnancies and ovarian hyperstimulation is reduced.[339]

Surgical Induction of Ovulation

WEDGE RESECTION OF THE OVARIES

It has been known since 1906 that wedge resection of the ovaries in PCOS patients is usually followed by the initiation of ovulatory cycles. The results of this treatment, as reported in the literature, are highly variable. For restoration of regular menses, the average success rate is about 80 percent, and only 63 percent of patients subsequently become pregnant.[340] In a retrospective cohort study of 96 consecutive cases of PCOS from Johns Hopkins Hospital, bilateral ovarian wedge resection resulted in the resumption of menstrual cyclicity in 91 percent (82 of 90) of the cases observed for up to 10 years.[341] As expected, the conception rate was higher in patients who had regular cycles (60.3 percent) than in those who had irregular ovulatory cycles (29.2 percent).

The mechanism by which wedge resection induces or initiates ovulation and regular cycles is not clear. Our studies have demonstrated a marked but transient reduction of ovarian androstenedione production and a persistent decrease in testosterone secretion after this treatment[342] (Fig. 17–40). An accompanying transient decline of estrone and estradiol levels is also observed. It is possible that changes in the acute local production of androgen result in a decrease of its inhibitory effect on follicular maturation or that autocrine and paracrine effects of intraovarian growth factors are altered, thereby permitting a more favorable follicular microenvironment for the initiation of folliculogenesis.

Ovarian wedge resection is now performed only rarely because of the ease and success of clomiphene and low-dose FSH treatments and more importantly because of the frequent occurrence of postoperative adhesions that result in infertility.

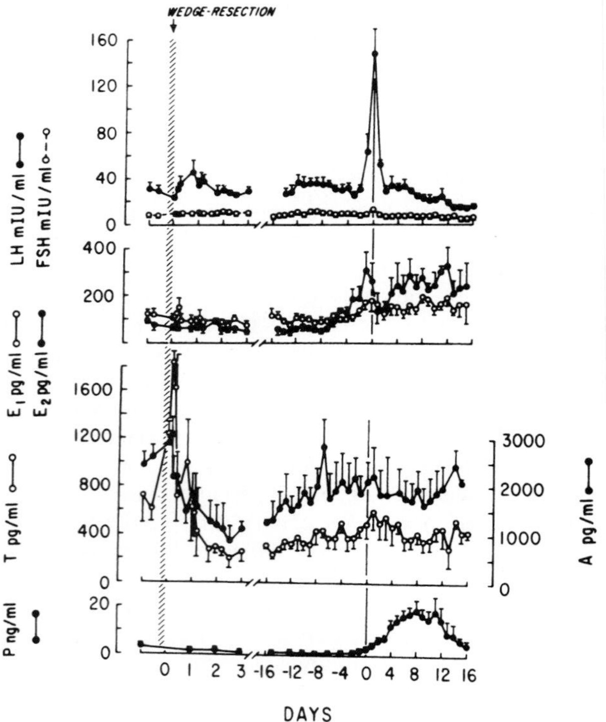

Figure 17–40 ■ The changes in hormonal levels before and after bilateral wedge resection of the ovary in five polycystic ovarian disease patients who ovulated. The data during the first three operative days are plotted with surgery as the reference point, and the subsequent hormonal data are plotted with the LH surge as the reference point. (From Judd HL, Rigg LA, Anderson DC, Yen SSC. The effects of ovarian wedge resection on circulating gonadotropin and ovarian steroid levels in patients with polycystic ovary syndrome. J Clin Endocrinol Metab 43:347–355, 1976. © The Endocrine Society.)

OVARIAN ELECTROCAUTERY

One approach to surgical induction of ovulation in women with PCOS who failed medical means of treatment has been reported by Gjonnaess.[343] The cystic follicles were electrocauterized with subsequent ovulation occurring in significant numbers of patients. Further studies have confirmed the efficacy of this procedure and demonstrate hormonal changes closely resembling those observed after wedge resection.[344–346] In a critical review of surgically induced ovulation in PCOS patients, Donesky and Adashi[347] provided pros and cons of this mode of management and recommended that controlled trials be conducted before the procedure can be viewed as efficacious and safe.

Dysfunctional Uterine Bleeding

Dysfunctional uterine bleeding is the term applied to out-of-phase uterine bleeding that is not caused by evident organic disease. It is manifested by episodic, excessive bleeding or varying frequency and its diagnosis requires exclusion of local and systemic diseases.

To counteract effects of unopposed estrogen, treatment with a synthetic progestin is required, and medroxyprogesterone acetate (Provera) appears to be the drug of choice. A daily dose of 5 to 10 mg for 10 days in a cyclic manner is recommended. If progestin alone fails to control the bleeding, a combination estrogen-progestin preparation may be used in a cyclic schedule for 2 to 3 months and treatment may be continued, if desired, particularly in PCOS women not desiring fertility. However, progestins with androgenic effects, such as norgestrel or norethindrone, should be avoided.

Metabolic Abnormalities

Diet and Exercise

The association of obesity with PCOS (50 percent) constitutes a negative impact in all medical and surgical treatment modalities. Weight reduction by dietary restriction in obese PCOS reduces insulin resistance and hyperinsulinemia. Improvement of endocrine-metabolic parameters occurs after 4 to 12 weeks of dietary restriction; a twofold increase in SHBG is accompanied by a fall in free testosterone levels with parallel changes in serum insulin and IGF-I concentrations. In addition, serum concentrations of IGFBP-1 rise significantly with a negative correlation with serum insulin and a positive correlation with serum SHBG levels. In accord with these findings, weight loss in obese PCOS patients is attended by a substantial reduction of hyperandrogenism and a return of the ovulatory cycle in 30 percent of patients.[348–352]

Moderate exercise, a process of increased fuel expenditure, has also been shown to induce a rise in serum IGFBP-1 concomitant with a decrease (20 percent) in serum IGF-I concentrations.[353] Thus, when combined with dietary restriction, exercise serves as an important adjunct to therapeutic success in PCOS patients (see later).

Improvement of Endocrine-Metabolic Derangements

It is evident that insulin resistance and concomitant hyperinsulinemia impart hyperandrogenemia and chronic anovulation as well as a high risk for the development of metabolic abnormalities in women with PCOS. Therefore, the attenuation of hyperinsulinemia may have a salutary effect on the metabolic and hormonal sequelae of PCOS.[29] The recent availability of two insulin-sensitizing agents, metformin and troglitazone, has afforded a new option with specific therapeutic goals to improve insulin resistance and hyperinsulinemia and its associated sequelae of *dyslipidemia, glucose intolerance,* and *hyperandrogenemia.*

Metformin. Metformin (dimethylbiguanide) is an orally active drug used to lower blood glucose in NIDDM. It improves insulin sensitivity and thus reduces insulin resistance and hyperinsulinemia. Its major action on glucose homeostasis is suppression of hepatic glucose output.[354] This drug is approved for the treatment of type II diabetes and is being used worldwide.[355]

Results of studies using metformin for the treatment of the insulin resistance state of PCOS have not been consistent. Some report improvement of insulin resistance, decreased serum insulin levels, improved dyslipidemia and hyperandrogenemia,[356, 357] and reversal of irregular menstrual cycles with improved fertility.[357] Other studies have found no specific improvement of the aforementioned clinical features.[358, 359]

Troglitazone. Troglitazone is a novel insulin-sensitizing agent that improves oral glucose tolerance, insulin resistance, and defects in β-cell function in obese patients with impaired glucose tolerance.[106] In assessing the beneficial effect of troglitazone in the insulin resistance state of PCOS, Dunaif and colleagues[107] have shown an improvement of total body insulin action resulting in lower circulating insulin and androgen levels. In addition, a decline in DHEA-S and estrogen levels was observed. These beneficial effects were evident at a *daily dose of 400 mg* troglitazone for 12 weeks of treatment.

In obese PCOS women with impaired glucose tolerance, Ehrmann and colleagues[108] have shown that troglitazone treatment (400 mg × 12 weeks) resulted in remarkable improvements in all endocrine-metabolic parameters:

- Both fasting and 2-hour plasma glucose concentrations during the oral glucose tolerance test declined significantly with a concordant reduction of glycosylated hemoglobin.
- Insulin sensitivity increased, as did the insulin secretion rate and disposition index.
- Total and free testosterone declined significantly, and GnRH agonist–stimulated 17-hydroxyprogesterone, androstenedione, and total testosterone levels were lowered. The reduction of androgen levels occurred independently of any change in gonadotropin levels.
- Functional activity of PAI-1 in blood was markedly reduced, which could be expected to improve the fibrinolytic response to thrombosis.

Thus, administration of troglitazone to women with PCOS with impaired glucose tolerance ameliorates the metabolic and hormonal derangements characteristic of the syndrome. It is proposed that troglitazone may prove to be a primary or adjunctive treatment for women with PCOS.[108] This drug is in phase III clinical trial at this time.

Mechanism of Action. Troglitazone is a member of the thiazolidinedione family of compounds. Although the mechanism of action of troglitazone remains incompletely defined, it has a unique mode of action that is dependent on the presence of insulin for activity. Troglitazone decreases hepatic glucose output and enhances insulin-dependent glucose disposal in skeletal muscle. It acts as a selective ligand for PPARγ, a nuclear receptor that regulates the transcription of a number of insulin-responsive genes crucial to the control of glucose and lipid metabolism and plays a central role in the regulation of adipocyte gene expression and differentiation.[360–363]

OVARIAN HYPERTHECOSIS

In 1943, Fraenkel described a non-neoplastic pathologic lesion of the human ovary characterized by the presence of islands of luteinized theca cells in the ovarian stroma at a distance from follicles; he coined the term hyperthecosis. Clinical, hormonal, and histologic studies of the ovarian hyperthecosis syndrome have revealed features in common with and distinct from those seen in PCOS.[364–370]

1. The degree of androgen excess of ovarian origin, including testosterone, androstenedione, and DHT, is greater in hyperthecosis; consequently, androgenization is more severe and virilization may occur.
2. The rate of estrone formation is greater, as might be expected, because of the higher rate of androgen production.
3. Levels of LH and FSH are either normal or (frequently) lower than in normal women, but postmenopausal women with hyperthecosis have high FSH levels.[251]
4. Islets of luteinized theca cells in the ovarian stroma are not present in the ovaries of PCOS patients. The hyperthecosis patient fails to respond to usual treatments, such as clomiphene citrate, but the reversal of chronic anovulation occurs after wedge resection.
5. Most striking is the presence of insulin resistance and hyperinsulinism. There are positive correlations between insulin levels and ovarian vein testosterone, androstenedione, and DHEA levels, suggesting that hyperinsulinism is causally related to the hyperandrogenism produced by the large nests of luteinized cells in the ovarian stroma.[371]
6. As for PCOS, a familial occurrence has been documented for ovarian hyperthecosis.[365]
7. Ovarian hyperthecosis *in postmenopausal women* frequently manifests more severe hirsutism or virilism, hypergonadotropism, and ovarian hyperandrogenism, which frequently responds to GnRH agonist treatment with normalization of serum androgen levels. Most remarkable is the frequent association of NIDDM, hyperlipidemia, and cardiovascular diseases. Insulin resistance and hyperinsulinemia are common underlying abnormalities. Whereas GnRH agonist treatment can effectively reduce androgen levels, it does not improve metabolic abnormalities.[251, 371, 372]

These findings are highly consistent with the retrospective analyses of premenopausal women with PCOS 20 to 30 years previously. They showed a higher incidence of hyperinsulinemia, diabetes, and cardiovascular disease,[320] and Birdsall and Farquhar[373] reported a 37 percent prevalence of polycystic ovaries diagnosed by ultrasound examination in postmenopausal women with ischemic heart disease. It is highly probable that ovarian hyperthecosis represents a variant of PCOS. The diagnosis of ovarian hyperthecosis cannot be made by ultrasonography or responses to GnRH agonist because hilar cell tumor, granulosa cell tumor, and Sertoli-Leydig cell tumor are also responsive to GnRH treatment.[370, 374, 375] The definitive diagnosis as well as treatment is bilateral ovariectomy, which does not improve hyperinsulinemia. The use of troglitazone as adjunct therapy should be considered.

References

1. Stein IF. Duration of infertility following ovarian wedge resection. West J Surg 72:237, 1964.
2. Yen SSC, Vela P, Rankin J. Inappropriate secretion of follicle-stimulating hormone and luteinizing hormone in polycystic ovarian disease. J Clin Endocrinol Metab 30:435, 1970.
3. Rebar R, Judd HL, Yen SSC, et al. Characterization of the inappropriate gonadotropin secretion in polycystic ovary syndrome. J Clin Invest 57:1320, 1976.
4. Erickson GF, Hsueh AJW, Quigley ME, et al. Functional studies of aromatase activity in human granulosa cells from normal and polycystic ovaries. J Clin Endocrinol Metab 49:514, 1979.
5. Yen SSC. The polycystic ovary syndrome. Clin Endocrinol 12:177, 1980.
6. Yen SSC, Chaney C, Judd HL. Functional aberrations of the hypothalamic-pituitary system in polycystic ovary syndrome: A consideration of the pathogenesis. *In* Serio M. The Endocrine Function of the Human Ovary. New York, Academic Press, 1976, pp 373–383.
7. McKenna TJ. Pathogenesis and treatment of polycystic ovary syndrome. N Engl J Med 318:558, 1988.
8. Burghen GA, Givens JR, Kitabchi AE. Correlation of hyperandrogenism with hyperinsulinism in polycystic ovarian disease. J Clin Endocrinol Metab 50:113, 1980.
9. Chang RJ, Nakamura RM, Judd HL, et al. Insulin resistance in nonobese patients with polycystic ovarian disease. J Clin Endocrinol Metab 57:356, 1983.
10. Dunaif A, Segal KR, Futterweit W, et al. Profound peripheral insulin resistance, independent of obesity, in polycystic ovary syndrome. Diabetes 38:1165, 1989.
11. Nestler JE, Powers LP, Matt DW, et al. A direct effect of hyperinsulinemia on serum sex hormone–binding globulin in obese women with the polycystic ovary syndrome. J Clin Endocrinol Metab 72:83, 1991.
12. Conover CA, Lee PDK, Kanaley JA, et al. Insulin regulation of insulin-like growth factor binding protein-1 in obese and nonobese humans. J Clin Endocrinol Metab 74:1355, 1992.
13. Ek I, Arner P, Bergqvist A, et al. Impaired adipocyte lipolysis in nonobese women with the polycystic ovary syndrome: A possible link to insulin resistance? J Clin Endocrinol Metab 82:1147, 1997.
14. Katz E, Ricciarelli E, Adashi EY. The potential relevance of growth hormone to female reproductive physiology and pathophysiology. Fertil Steril 59:8, 1993.
15. Pasquali R, Casimirri F. The impact of obesity on hyperandrogenism and polycystic ovary syndrome in premenopausal women. Clin Endocrinol (Oxf) 39:1, 1993.
16. Nestler JE, Clore JN, Blackard WG. The central role of obesity (hyperinsulinemia) in the pathogenesis of the polycystic ovary syndrome. Am J Obstet Gynecol 161:1095, 1989.
17. Holly JMP, Smith CP, Dunger DB, et al. Relationship between the pubertal fall in sex hormone binding globulin and insulin-like growth factor binding protein-1. A synchronized approach to pubertal development? Clin Endocrinol (Oxf) 31:277, 1989.
18. Smith CP, Dunger DB, Williams AJK, et al. Relationship between insulin, insulin-like growth factor-I and dehydroepiandrosterone sulfate concentrations during childhood, puberty, and adult life. J Clin Endocrinol Metab 68:932, 1989.
19. Bloch CA, Clemons P, Sperling MA. Puberty decreases insulin sensitivity. J Pediatr 110:481, 1987.
20. Ibãnez L, Potau N, Virdis R, et al. Postpubertal outcome in girls diagnosed with premature pubarche during childhood: Increased frequency of functional ovarian hyperandrogenism. J Clin Endocrinol Metab 76:1599, 1993.
21. Apter D, Bützow T, Laughlin GA, et al. Metabolic features of polycystic ovary syndrome are found in adolescent girls with hyperandrogenism. J Clin Endocrinol Metab 80:2966, 1995.
22. Apter D, Bützow T, Laughlin GA, et al. Accelerated 24-hour luteinizing hormone pulsatile activity in adolescent girls with ovarian hyperandrogenism: Relevance to the developmental phase of polycystic ovarian syndrome. J Clin Endocrinol Metab 79:119, 1994.
23. Ibañez L, Potau N, Zampolli M, et al. Hyperinsulinemia in postpubertal girls with a history of premature pubarche and functional ovarian hyperandrogenism. J Clin Endocrinol Metab 81:1237, 1996.
24. Ibañez L, Potau N, Zampolli M, et al. Hyperinsulinemia and decreased insulin-like growth factor–binding protein-1 are common features in prepubertal and pubertal girls with a history of premature pubarche. J Clin Endocrinol Metab 82:2283, 1997.
25. Lucky AW, Rosenfield RL, McGuire J, et al. Adrenal androgen hyperresponsiveness to ACTH in women with acne and/or hirsutism: Adrenal enzyme defects and exaggerated adrenarche. J Clin Endocrinol Metab 62:840, 1986.
26. Adashi EY, Rohan M. Intraovarian regulation: Peptidergic signaling systems. Trends Endocrinol Metab 3:243, 1992.
27. Franks S, Hamilton-Fairley D, Kiddy D, et al. Growth factors and the polycystic ovary. *In* Sjöberg N-O. Local Regulation of Ovarian Function. Park Ridge, NJ, The Parthenon Publishing Group, 1992, pp 97–106.
28. Hillier SG, Miró F. Inhibin, activin, and follistatin. *In* Tolis G. Intraovarian Regulators and Polycystic Ovary Syndrome. New York, New York Academy of Science, 1993, pp 29–38.
29. Ehrmann DA, Barnes RB, Rosenfield RL. Polycystic ovary syndrome as a form of functional ovarian hyperandrogenism due to dysregulation of androgen secretion. Endocr Rev 16:322, 1995.
30. Haning RV Jr, Hackett RJ, Flood CA, et al. Testosterone, a follicular regulator: Key to anovulation. J Clin Endocrinol Metab 77:710, 1993.
31. Haning RV Jr, Hua JJ, Hackett RJ, et al. Dehydroepiandrosterone sulfate and anovulation increase serum inhibin and affect follicular function during administration of gonadotropins. J Clin Endocrinol Metab 78:145, 1994.
32. Azziz R, Zacur HA. 21-Hydroxylase deficiency in female hyperandrogenism: Screening and diagnosis. J Clin Endocrinol Metab 69:577, 1989.
33. Speiser PW, Serrat J, New MI, et al. Insulin insensitivity in adrenal hyperplasia due to nonclassical steroid 21-hydroxylase deficiency. J Clin Endocrinol Metab 75:1421, 1992.
34. Polson DW, Wadsworth J, Adams J, et al. Polycystic ovaries—a common finding in normal women. Lancet 16:870, 1988.
35. Conway GS, Honour JW, Jacobs HS. Heterogeneity of the polycystic ovary syndrome: Clinical, endocrine and ultrasound features in 556 patients. Clin Endocrinol (Oxf) 30:459, 1989.
36. Waldstreicher J, Santoro NF, Hall JE, et al. Hyperfunction of the hypothalamic-pituitary axis in women with polycystic ovarian disease: Indirect evidence for partial gonadotroph desensitization. J Clin Endocrinol Metab 66:165, 1988.
37. Morales AJ, Laughlin GA, Bützow T, et al. Insulin, somatotropic, and LH axes in lean and obese women with polycystic ovary syndrome: Common and distinct features. J Clin Endocrinol Metab 81:2854, 1996.
38. Arroyo A, Laughlin GA, Morales AJ, Yen SCC. Inappropriate gonadotropin secretion in polycystic ovary syndrome: Influence of adiposity. J Clin Endocrinol Metab 82:3728, 1997.
39. Taylor AE, McCourt B, Martin KA, et al. Determinants of abnormal gonadotropin secretion in clinically defined women with polycystic ovary syndrome. J Clin Endocrinol Metab 82:2248, 1997.

40. Paradisi R, Venturoli S, Capelli M, et al. Effects of α_1-adrenergic blockade on pulsatile luteinizing hormone, follicle-stimulating hormone, and prolactin secretion in polycystic ovary syndrome. J Clin Endocrinol Metab 65:841, 1987.
41. Berga SL, Yen SSC. Opioidergic regulation of LH pulsatility in women with polycystic ovary syndrome. Clin Endocrinol (Oxf) 30:177, 1989.
42. Fiad TM, Cunningham SK, McKenna TJ. Role of progesterone deficiency in the development of luteinizing hormone and androgen abnormalities in polycystic ovary syndrome. Eur J Endocrinol 135:335, 1996.
43. Christman GM, Randolph JF, Kelch RP, et al. Reduction of gonadotropin-releasing hormone pulse frequency is associated with subsequent selective follicle-stimulating hormone secretion in women with polycystic ovarian disease. J Clin Endocrinol Metab 72:1278, 1991.
44. Brown JB. Pituitary control of ovarian function–concepts derived from gonadotrophin therapy. Aust N Z J Obstet Gynaecol 18:46, 1978.
45. White DM, Polson DW, Kiddy D, et al. Induction of ovulation with low-dose gonadotropins in polycystic ovary syndrome: An analysis of 109 pregnancies in 225 women. J Clin Endocrinol Metab 81:3821, 1996.
46. Fauser BCJM, Van Heusden AM. Manipulation of human ovarian function: Physiological concepts and clinical consequences. Endocr Rev 18:71, 1997.
47. Weiss J, Crowley WF Jr, Halvorson LM, et al. Perfusion of rat pituitary cells with gonadotropin-releasing hormone, activin, and inhibin reveals distinct effects on gonadotropin gene expression and secretion. Endocrinology 132:2307, 1993.
48. Kirk SE, Dalkin AC, Yasin M, et al. Gonadotropin-releasing hormone pulse frequency regulates expression of pituitary follistatin messenger ribonucleic acid: A mechanism for differential gonadotrope function. Endocrinology 135:876, 1994.
49. Kaiser UB, Sabbagh E, Katzenellenbogen RA, et al. A mechanism for the differential regulation of gonadotropin subunit gene expression by gonadotropin-releasing hormone. Proc Natl Acad Sci USA 116:2113, 1995.
50. Zawadzki JK, Dunaif A. Diagnostic criteria: Towards a rational approach. *In* Hershmann JM. Current Issues in Endocrinology and Metabolism. Boston, Blackwell Scientific Publications, 1992, pp 377–384.
51. Dale PO, Tanbo T, Vaaler S, et al. Body weight, hyperinsulinemia, and gonadotropin levels in the polycystic ovarian syndrome: Evidence of two distinct populations. Fertil Steril 58:487, 1992.
52. Grulet H, Hecart AC, Delemer B, et al. Roles of LH and insulin resistance in lean and obese polycystic ovary syndrome. Clin Endocrinol (Oxf) 38:621, 1993.
53. Holte J, Bergh T, Gennarelli G, et al. The independent effects of polycystic ovary syndrome and obesity on serum concentrations of gonadotrophins and sex steroids in premenopausal women. Clin Endocrinol (Oxf) 41:473, 1994.
54. Almahbobi G, Anderiesz C, Hutchinson P, et al. Functional integrity of granulosa cells from polycystic ovaries. Clin Endocrinol (Oxf) 44:571, 1996.
55. Futterweit W, Deligdisch L. Effects of androgens on the ovary. Fertil Steril 46:343, 1986.
56. Franks S. Polycystic ovary syndrome. N Engl J Med 333:1435, 1995.
57. Gilling-Smith C, Story H, Rogers V, et al. Evidence for a primary abnormality of thecal cell steroidogenesis in the polycystic ovary syndrome. Clin Endocrinol (Oxf) 47:93, 1997.
58. Gilling-Smith C, Willis DS, Beard RW, et al. Hypersecretion of androstenedione by isolated thecal cells from polycystic ovaries. J Clin Endocrinol Metab 79:1158, 1994.
59. Barbieri RL, Makris A, Randall RW, et al. Insulin stimulates androgen accumulation in incubations of ovarian stroma obtained from women with hyperandrogenism. J Clin Endocrinol Metab 62:904, 1986.
60. Erickson GF, Magoffin DA, Cragun JF, et al. The effects of insulin and insulin-like growth factors-I and II on estradiol production by granulosa cells of polycystic ovaries. J Clin Endocrinol Metab 70:894, 1990.
61. Giudice LC, Morales AJ, Yen SSC. Growth factors and polycystic ovarian syndrome. Semin Reprod Endocrinol 14:203, 1996.
62. Cheatham B, Kahn CR. Insulin action and the insulin signaling network. Endocr Rev 16:117, 1995.
63. Kahn CR, White MF, Shoelson SE, et al. The insulin receptor and its substrate: Molecular determinants of early events of insulin action. Recent Prog Horm Res 48:291, 1993.
64. Sun XJ, Rothenberg P, Kahn CR, et al. Structure of the insulin receptor substrate IRS-1 defines a unique signal transduction protein. Nature 352:73, 1991.
65. Sun XJ, Wang LM, Zhang Y, et al. Role of IRS-2 in insulin and cytokine signalling. Nature 377:173, 1995.
66. Rose DW, Saltiel AR, Majumdar M, et al. Insulin receptor substrate 1 is required for insulin-mediated mitogenic signal transduction. Proc Natl Acad Sci USA 91:797, 1994.
67. Myers MG Jr, Sun XJ, Cheatham B, et al. IRS-1 is a common element in insulin and insulin-like growth factor-I signaling to the phosphatidylinositol 3′-kinase. Endocrinology 132:1421, 1993.
68. Kahn CR, Goldstein BJ. Molecular defects in insulin action. Science 245:13, 1989.
69. Kadawaki T, Bevins C, Cama A, et al. Two mutant alleles of the insulin receptor gene in a patient with extreme insulin resistance. Science 240:787, 1988.
70. D'Ercole AJ, Underwood LE, Grokle J. Leprechaunism: Studies on the relationship among hyperinsulinemia, insulin resistance and growth retardation. J Clin Endocrinol Metab 48:495, 1979.
71. Barbieri RL, Ryan KJ. Hyperandrogenism, insulin resistance, and acanthosis nigricans syndrome. A common endocrinopathy with distinct pathophysiologic features. Am J Obstet Gynecol 147:90, 1983.
72. Dunaif A, Segal KR, Shelley DR, et al. Evidence for distinctive and intrinsic defects in insulin action in polycystic ovary syndrome. Diabetes 41:1257, 1992.
73. Dunaif A. Insulin resistance and the polycystic ovary syndrome: Mechanism and implications for pathogenesis. Endocr Rev 18:774, 1997.
74. Dunaif A, Finegood DT. Beta-cell dysfunction independent of obesity and glucose intolerance in the polycystic ovary syndrome. J Clin Endocrinol Metab 81:942, 1996.
75. Ehrmann DA, Sturis J, Byrne MM, et al. Insulin secretory defects in polycystic ovary syndrome. Relationship to insulin sensitivity and family history of non–insulin-dependent diabetes mellitus. J Clin Invest 96:520, 1995.
76. Ciaraldi TP, el-Roeiy A, Madar Z, et al. Cellular mechanisms of insulin resistance in polycystic ovarian syndrome. J Clin Endocrinol Metab 75:577, 1992.
77. Rosenbaum D, Haber RS, Dunaif A. Insulin resistance in polycystic ovary syndrome: Decreased expression of GLUT-4 glucose transporters in adipocytes. Am J Physiol 264:E197, 1993.
78. Ciaraldi TP, Morales AJ, Hickman MG, et al. Cellular insulin resistance in adipocytes from obese polycystic ovary syndrome subjects involves adenosine modulation of insulin sensitivity. J Clin Endocrinol Metab 82:1421, 1997.
79. Dunaif A, Xia J, Book CB, et al. Excessive insulin receptor serine phosphorylation in cultured fibroblasts and in skeletal muscle. A potential mechanism for insulin resistance in the polycystic ovary syndrome. J Clin Invest 96:801, 1995.
80. Thissen JP, Ketelslegers JM, Underwood LE. Nutritional regulation of the insulin-like growth factors. Endocr Rev 15:80, 1994.
81. Baumann G. Growth hormone–binding proteins: State of the art. J Endocrinol 141:1, 1994.
82. Fisker S, Vahl N, Jorgensen JOL, et al. Abdominal fat determines growth hormone–binding protein levels in healthy non-obese adults. J Clin Endocrinol Metab 81:123, 1997.
83. Giudice LC. Insulin-like growth factors and ovarian follicular development. Endocr Rev 13:641, 1992.
84. Shimasaki S, Ling N. Identification and molecular characterization of insulin-like growth factor binding proteins (IGFBP-1, -2, -3, -4, 5, -6). Prog Growth Factor Res 3:243, 1991.
85. Jones JI, Clemmons DR. Insulin-like growth factors and their binding proteins: Biological action. Endocr Rev 16:1, 1995.
86. Holly JMP. The physiological role of IGFBP-1. Acta Endocrinol (Copenh) 124:55, 1991.
87. Lee PDK, Conover CA, Powell DR. Regulation and function of insulin-like growth factor–binding protein-1. Proc Soc Exp Biol Med 204:4, 1993.
88. Sharara FI, Nieman LK. Identification and cellular localization of

growth hormone receptor gene expression in the human ovary. J Clin Endocrinol Metab 79:670, 1994.
89. Jia X-C, Kalmijn J, Hsueh AJW. Growth hormone enhances follicle-stimulating hormone–induced differentiation of cultured rat granulosa cells. Endocrinology 118:1041, 1986.
90. Mason HD, Martikainen H, Beard RW, et al. Direct gonadotrophic effect of growth hormone on oestradiol production by human granulosa cells in vitro. J Endocrinol 126:R1, 1990.
91. Homburg R, West C, Torresani T, et al. Cotreatment with human growth hormone and gonadotropins for induction of ovulation: A controlled clinical trial. Fertil Steril 53:254, 1990.
92. Gilling-Smith C, Willis DS, Franks S. Oestradiol feedback stimulation of androgen biosynthesis by human theca cells. Hum Reprod 12:1621, 1997.
93. Gennarelli G, Holte J, Stridsberg M, et al. The counterregulatory response to hypoglycaemia in women with the polycystic ovary syndrome. Clin Endocrinol (Oxf) 46:167, 1997.
94. Erickson GF, Garzo G, Magoffin DA. Insulin-like growth factor-I regulates aromatase activity in human granulosa and granulosa luteal cells. J Clin Endocrinol Metab 69:716, 1989.
95. Cara JF. Insulin-like growth factors, insulin-like growth factor binding proteins and ovarian androgen production. Horm Res 42:49, 1994.
96. Kopelman PG. Hormones and obesity. Baillieres Clin Endocrinol Metab 8:549, 1994.
97. Slowinska-Srzednicka J, Zgliczynski W, Makowska A, et al. An abnormality of the growth hormone/insulin-like growth factor-1 axis in women with polycystic ovary syndrome due to coexistent obesity. J Clin Endocrinol Metab 74:1432, 1992.
98. Suikkari A-M, Koivisto VA, Koistinen R, et al. Dose-response characteristics for suppression of low molecular weight plasma insulin-like growth factor–binding protein by insulin. J Clin Endocrinol Metab 68:135, 1989.
99. Cohen P, Fielder PJ, Hasegawa Y, et al. Clinical aspects of insulin-like growth factor binding proteins. Acta Endocrinol (Copenh) 124:74, 1991.
100. el-Roeiy A, Chen X, Roberts VJ, et al. Expression of the genes encoding the insulin-like growth factors (IGF-I and II), the IGF and insulin receptors, and IGF-binding proteins-1–6 and the localization of their gene products in normal and polycystic ovary syndrome ovaries. J Clin Endocrinol Metab 78:1488, 1994.
101. el-Roeiy A, Chen X, Roberts VJ, et al. Expression of insulin-like growth factor-I (IGF-I) and IGF-II and the IGF-I, IGF-II, and insulin receptor genes and localization of the gene products in the human ovary. J Clin Endocrinol Metab 77:1411, 1993.
102. Childs GV, Unabia G, Rougeau D. Cells that express luteinizing hormone (LH) and follicle-stimulating hormone (FSH) β-subunit messenger ribonucleic acids during the estrous cycle: The major contributors contain LHβ, FSHβ, and/or growth hormone. Endocrinology 134:990, 1994.
103. Kaiser UB, Lee BL, Carroll RS, et al. Follistatin gene expression in the pituitary: Localization in gonadotropes and folliculostellate cells in diestrous rats. Endocrinology 130:3048, 1992.
104. Hu E, Tontonoz P, Spiegelman BM. Transdifferentiation of myoblasts by the adipogenic transcription factors PPARγ and C/EBPα. Proc Natl Acad Sci USA 92:9856, 1995.
105. Shalev A, Siegrist-Kaiser CA, Yen PM, et al. The peroxisome proliferator-activated receptor is a phosphoprotein: Regulation by insulin. Endocrinology 137:4499, 1996.
106. Nolan J, Ludvik B, Beerdsen P, et al. Improvement in glucose tolerance and insulin resistance in obese subjects treated with troglitazone. N Engl J Med 331:1188, 1994.
107. Dunaif A, Scott D, Finegood D, et al. The insulin-sensitizing agent troglitazone improves metabolic and reproductive abnormalities in the polycystic ovary syndrome. J Clin Endocrinol Metab 81:3299, 1996.
108. Ehrmann DA, Schneider DJ, Sobel BE, et al. Troglitazone improves defects in insulin action, insulin secretion, ovarian steroidogenesis, and fibrinolysis in women with polycystic ovary syndrome. J Clin Endocrinol Metab 82:2108, 1997.
109. Lönnqvist F, Thörne A, Nilsell K, et al. A pathogenic role of visceral fat beta$_3$-adrenoceptor in obesity. J Clin Invest 95:1109, 1995.
110. Reynisdottir S, Ellerfeldt K, Wahrenberg H, et al. Multiple lipolysis defects in insulin resistance (metabolic) syndrome. J Clin Invest 93:2590, 1994.
111. Apter D, Bützow T, Laughlin GA, et al. Hyperandrogenism During Puberty and Adolescence, and Its Relationship to Reproductive Function in the Adult Female. Serono Symposium, Vol 93. New York, Raven Press, 1993, pp 265–275.
112. Barria A, Leyton V, Ojeda SR, et al. Ovarian steroidal response to gonadotropins and beta-adrenergic stimulation is enhanced in polycystic ovary syndrome: Role of sympathetic innervation. Endocrinology 133:2696, 1993.
113. Zhang Y, Proenca R, Maffei M, et al. Positional cloning of the mouse obese gene and its human homologue. Nature 372:425, 1994.
114. Lönnqvist F, Arner P, Nordfors L, et al. Overexpression of the obese (*ob*) gene in adipose tissue of human obese subjects. Nat Med 1:950, 1995.
115. Considine RV, Sinha MK, Heiman ML, et al. Serum immunoreactive-leptin concentrations in normal-weight and obese humans. N Engl J Med 334:292, 1996.
116. Sinha MK, Opentanova I, Ohannesian JP, et al. Evidence of free and bound leptin in human circulation: Studies in lean and obese subjects and during short-term fasting. J Clin Invest 98:1277, 1996.
117. Rosenbaum M, Nicolson M, Hirsch J, et al. Effects of gender, body composition, and menopause on plasma concentrations of leptin. J Clin Endocrinol Metab 81:3424, 1996.
118. Saad MF, Damani S, Gingerich RL, et al. Sexual dimorphism in plasma leptin concentrations. J Clin Endocrinol Metab 82:579, 1997.
119. Wabitsch M, Blum WF, Muche R, et al. Contribution of androgens to the gender difference in leptin production in obese children and adolescents. J Clin Invest 100:808, 1997.
120. Licinio J, Mantzoros C, Negrao AB, et al. Human leptin levels are pulsatile and inversely related to pituitary-adrenal function. Nat Med 3:575, 1997.
121. Sinha MK, Sturis J, Ohannesian J, et al. Ultradian oscillations of leptin secretion in humans. Biochem Biophys Res Commun 228:733, 1996.
122. Schoeller DA, Cella LK, Sinha MK, et al. Entrainment of the diurnal rhythm of plasma leptin to meal timing. J Clin Invest 100:1882, 1997.
123. DeVos P, Saladin R, Auwerx J, et al. Induction of *ob* gene expression by corticosteroids is accompanied by body weight loss and reduced food intake. J Biol Chem 270:15958, 1995.
124. Papaspyrou-Rao S, Schneider SH, Petersen RN, et al. Dexamethasone increases leptin expression in humans in vivo. J Clin Endocrinol Metab 82:1635, 1997.
125. Boden G, Chen X, Kolaczynski JW, et al. Effects of prolonged hyperinsulinemia on serum leptin in normal human subjects. J Clin Invest 100:1107, 1997.
126. Caro JF, Sinha MK, Kolaczynski JW, et al. Leptin: The tale of an obesity gene. Diabetes 45:1455, 1996.
127. Giacobino J-P. Role of the β$_3$-adrenoceptor in the control of leptin expression. Horm Metab Res 28:633, 1996.
128. Laughlin GA, Yen SSC. Hypoleptinemia in women athletes: Absence of a diurnal rhythm with amenorrhea. J Clin Endocrinol Metab 82:318, 1997.
129. Tartaglia LA, Dembrski M, Weng X, et al. Identification and expression cloning of a leptin receptor, OB-R. Cell 83:1263, 1995.
130. Chelab FF, Lim ME, Lu R. Correction of the sterility defect in homozygous obese female mice by treatment with the human recombinant leptin. Nat Genet 12:318, 1996.
131. Barash IA, Cheung CC, Weigle DS, et al. Leptin is a metabolic signal to the reproductive system. Endocrinology 137:3144, 1996.
132. Phillips MS, Liu QY, Hammond HA, et al. Leptin receptor missense mutation in the fatty Zucker rat. Nat Genet 13:18, 1996.
133. Montague CT, Farooqi IS, Whitehead JP, et al. Congenital leptin deficiency is associated with severe early-onset obesity in humans. Nature 387:903, 1997.
134. Jackson RS, Creemers JW, Ohagi S, et al. Obesity and impaired prohormone processing associated with mutations in the human prohormone convertase 1 gene. Nat Genet 16:303, 1997.
135. Emilsson V, Liu Y-L, Cawthorne MA, et al. Expression of the functional leptin receptor mRNA in pancreatic islets and direct inhibitory action of leptin on insulin secretion. Diabetes 46:313, 1997.
136. Kalra SP, Kalra PS. Nutritional infertility: The role of the

interconnected hypothalamic neuropeptide Y–galanin–opioid network. Front Neuroendocrinol 17:371, 1996.
137. Mercer JG, Hoggard N, Williams LM, et al. Coexpression of leptin receptor and preproneuropeptide Y mRNA in arcuate nucleus of mouse hypothalamus. J Neuroendocrinol 8:733, 1997.
138. Cheung CC, Clifton DK, Steiner RA. Proopiomelanocortin neurons are direct targets for leptin in the hypothalamus. Endocrinology 138:4489, 1997.
139. Hakansson M, Hulting A, Meister B. Expression of leptin receptor mRNA in the hypothalamic arcuate nucleus—relationship with NPY neurons. Neuroreport 7:3087, 1996.
140. Thornton JE, Cheung CC, Clifton DK, et al. Regulation of hypothalamic proopiomelanocortin mRNA by leptin in *ob/ob* mice. Endocrinology 138:5063, 1997.
141. Rosenbaum M, Leibel RL, Hirsch J. Obesity. N Engl J Med 337:396, 1997.
142. Kalra SP, Sahu A, Kalra PS, et al. Hypothalamic neuropeptide Y: A circuit in the regulation of gonadotropin secretion and feeding behavior. Ann N Y Acad Sci 611:273, 1990.
143. Heiman ML, Ahima RS, Craft LS, et al. Leptin inhibition of the hypothalamic-pituitary-adrenal axis in response to stress. Endocrinology 138:3859, 1997.
144. Brzechffa PR, Jakimiuk AJ, Agarwal SK, et al. Serum immunoreactive leptin concentrations in women with polycystic ovary syndrome. J Clin Endocrinol Metab 81:4166, 1996.
145. Chapman IM, Wittert GA, Norman RJ. Circulating leptin concentrations in polycystic ovary syndrome: Relation to anthropometric and metabolic parameters. Clin Endocrinol (Oxf) 46:175, 1997.
146. Rouru J, Anttila L, Koskinen P, et al. Serum leptin concentrations in women with polycystic ovary syndrome. J Clin Endocrinol Metab 82:1697, 1997.
147. Laughlin GA, Morales AJ, Yen SS. Serum leptin levels in women with polycystic ovary syndrome: The role of insulin resistance/hyperinsulinemia. J Clin Endocrinol Metab 82:1692, 1997.
148. Mantzoros CS, Dunaif A, Flier JS. Leptin concentrations in the polycystic ovary syndrome. J Clin Endocrinol Metab 82:1687, 1997.
149. Zachow RJ, Magoffin DA. Direct intraovarian effects of leptin: Impairment of the synergistic action of insulin-like growth factor-I on follicle-stimulating hormone–dependent estradiol-17β production by rat ovarian granulosa cells. Endocrinology 138:847, 1997.
150. Deslypere JP, Verdonck L, Vermeulen A. Fat tissue: A steroid reservoir and site of steroid metabolism. J Clin Endocrinol Metab 61:564, 1985.
151. Kirschner MA, Samojlik E, Drejka M, et al. Androgen-estrogen metabolism in women with upper body versus lower body obesity. J Clin Endocrinol Metab 70:473, 1990.
152. Labrie F. Intracrinology. Mol Cell Endocrinol 78:C113, 1991.
153. Simpson ER, Merrill JC, Hollub AJ, et al. Regulation of estrogen biosynthesis by human adipose cells. Endocr Rev 10:136, 1989.
154. Schneider J, Bradlow HL, Strain G, et al. Effects of obesity on estradiol metabolism: Decreased formation of nonuterotropic metabolites. J Clin Endocrinol Metab 56:973, 1983.
155. Gray JM, Dudley SD, Wade GN. In vivo cell nuclear binding of 17β-[^{3}H]-estradiol in rat adipose tissues. Am J Physiol 240:E43, 1981.
156. Rebuffe-Scrive M, Enk L, Crona N, et al. Fat cell metabolism in different regions in women: Effect of menstrual cycle, pregnancy and lactation. J Clin Invest 75:1973, 1985.
157. Pecquery R, Leneveu M-C, Giudicelli Y. Influence of androgenic status on the α_2/β-adrenergic control of lipolysis in white fat cells: Predominant α_2-antilipolytic response in testosterone-treated castrated hamsters. Endocrinology 122:2590, 1988.
158. Pecquery R, Dieudonne M-N, Leneveu M-C, et al. Evidence that testosterone modulates in vivo the adenylate cyclase activity in fat cells. Endocrinology 126:241, 1990.
159. Agarwal VR, Ashanullah CI, Simpson ER, et al. Alternatively spliced transcripts of the aromatase cytochrome P450 (CYP19) gene in adipose tissue of women. J Clin Endocrinol Metab 82:70, 1997.
160. Wabitsch M, Hauner H, Heinze E, et al. The role of growth hormone/insulin-like growth factors in adipocyte differentiation. Metabolism 44:45, 1995.
161. Bolinder J, Lindblad A, Engfeldt P, et al. Studies of acute effects of insulin-like growth factors I and II in human fat cells. J Clin Endocrinol Metab 65:732, 1987.
162. Wild RA, Painter PC, Coulson PB, et al. Lipoprotein lipid concentrations and cardiovascular risk in women with polycystic ovary syndrome. J Clin Endocrinol Metab 61:946, 1985.
163. Talbott E, Guzick D, Clerici A, et al. Coronary heart disease risk factors in women with polycystic ovary syndrome. Arterioscler Thromb Vasc Biol 15:821, 1995.
164. Norman RJ, Hague WM, Masters SC, et al. Subjects with polycystic ovaries without hyperandrogenaemia exhibit similar disturbances in insulin and lipid profiles as those with polycystic ovary syndrome. Hum Reprod 10:2258, 1995.
165. Holte J, Bergh T, Berne C, et al. Serum lipoprotein lipid profile in women with the polycystic ovary syndrome: Relation to anthropometric, endocrine and metabolic variables. Clin Endocrinol (Oxf) 41:463, 1994.
166. Dahlgren E, Janson PO, Johansson S, et al. Hemostatic and metabolic variables in women with polycystic ovary syndrome. Fertil Steril 61:455, 1994.
167. Sampson M, Kong C, Patel A, et al. Ambulatory blood pressure profiles and plasminogen activator inhibitor (PAI-1) activity in lean women with and without the polycystic ovary syndrome. Clin Endocrinol (Oxf) 45:623, 1996.
168. Yen SSC, Laughlin GA, Morales AJ. Interface between extra- and intraovarian factors in polycystic ovarian syndrome. Ann N Y Acad Sci 687:98, 1993.
169. Adashi EY, Resnick CE, Hurwitz A, et al. Insulin-like growth factors: The ovarian connection. Hum Reprod 6:1213, 1991.
170. Hsueh AJ, Billig H, Tsafriri A. Ovarian follicle atresia: A hormonally controlled apoptotic process. Endocr Rev 15:707, 1994.
171. Davoren JB, Hsueh AJW. Growth hormone increases ovarian levels of immunoreactive somatomedin/insulin-like growth factor-1 in vivo. Endocrinology 118:888, 1986.
172. Zhou J, Bondy C. Anatomy of the human ovarian insulin-like growth factor system. Biol Reprod 43:467, 1993.
173. Rosenfeld R, Barnes RB, Cara JF, et al. Dysregulation of cytochrome P450c17a as the cause of polycystic ovarian syndrome. Fertil Steril 53:785, 1990.
174. Mason HD, Margara R, Winston RM, et al. Insulin-like growth factor-I (IGF-I) inhibits production of IGF-binding protein-1 while stimulating estradiol secretion in granulosa cells from normal and polycystic human ovaries. J Clin Endocrinol Metab 76:1275, 1993.
175. Giudice LC. The insulin-like growth factor system in normal and abnormal human ovarian follicle development. Am J Med 98:48S, 1995.
176. Giudice LC, van Dessel HJ, Cataldo NA, et al. Circulating and ovarian IGF binding proteins: Potential roles in normo-ovulatory cycles and in polycystic ovarian syndrome. Prog Growth Factor Res 6:397, 1995.
177. Mason HD, Cwyfan-Hughes SC, Heinrich G, et al. Insulin-like growth factor (IGF) I and II, IGF-binding proteins, and IGF-binding protein proteases are produced by theca and stroma of normal and polycystic human ovaries. J Clin Endocrinol Metab 81:276, 1996.
178. Thierry van Dessel HJ, Chandrasekher YA, Yap OW, et al. Serum and follicular fluid levels of insulin-like growth factor I (IGF-I), IGF-II, and IGF-binding protein-1 and -3 during the normal menstrual cycle. J Clin Endocrinol Metab 81:1224, 1996.
179. el-Roeiy A, Chen X, Roberts VJ, et al. Expression of insulin-like growth factor-I (IGF-I) and IGF-II and the IGF-I, IGF-II, and insulin receptor genes and localization of the gene products in the human ovary. J Clin Endocrinol Metab 77:1411, 1993.
180. Holly JMP, Eden JA, Alaghband-Zadeh J, et al. Insulin-like growth factor binding proteins in follicular fluid from normal dominant and cohort follicles, polycystic and multicystic ovaries. Clin Endocrinol (Oxf) 33:53, 1990.
181. Cataldo NA, Giudice LC. Insulin-like growth factor binding protein profiles in human ovarian follicular fluid correlate with follicular functional status. J Clin Endocrinol Metab 74:821, 1992.
182. San Roman GA, Magoffin DA. Insulin-like growth factor–binding proteins in healthy and atretic follicles during natural menstrual cycles. J Clin Endocrinol Metab 76:625, 1993.
183. Parrizas M, LeRoith D. Insulin-like growth factor-1 inhibition of

apoptosis is associated with increased expression of the bcl-xL gene product. Endocrinology 138:1355, 1997.
184. Chun SY, Billig H, Tilly JL, et al. Gonadotropin suppression of apoptosis in cultured preovulatory follicles: Mediatory role of endogenous insulin-like growth factor I. Endocrinology 135:1845, 1994.
185. Suikkari A-M, Ruutiainen K, Erkkola R, et al. Low levels of low molecular weight insulin-like growth factor–binding protein in patients with polycystic ovarian disease. Hum Reprod 4:136, 1989.
186. Poretsky L, Chun B, Liu HC, et al. Insulin-like growth factor II (IGF-II) inhibits insulin-like growth factor binding protein I (IGFBP-1) production in luteinized human granulosa cells with a potency similar to insulin-like growth factor I (IGF-I) and higher than insulin. J Clin Endocrinol Metab 81:3412, 1996.
187. Eden JA, Jones J, Carter GD, et al. Follicular fluid concentrations of insulin-like growth factor 1, epidermal growth factor, transforming growth factor-alpha and sex-steroids in volume matched normal and polycystic human follicles. Clin Endocrinol (Oxf) 32:395, 1990.
188. Vale W, Rivier C, Hsueh AJ, et al. Chemical and biological characterization of the inhibin family of protein hormones. Recent Prog Horm Res 44:1, 1988.
189. Nakamura T, Takio K, Eto Y, et al. Activin-binding protein from rat ovary is follistatin. Science 247:836, 1990.
190. Shimonaka M, Inouye S, Shimasaki S, et al. Follistatin binds to both activin and inhibin through the common subunit. Endocrinology 128:3313, 1991.
191. Roberts VJ, Barth S, el-Roeiy A, et al. Expression of inhibin/activin system messenger ribonucleic acids and proteins in ovarian follicles from women with polycystic ovarian syndrome. J Clin Endocrinol Metab 79:1434, 1994.
192. Hillier SG, Yong EL, Illingworth PJ, et al. Effect of recombinant activin on androgen synthesis in cultured human thecal cells. J Clin Endocrinol Metab 72:1206, 1991.
193. Hillier SG, Yong EL, Illingworth PJ, et al. Effect of recombinant inhibin on androgen synthesis in cultured human thecal cells. Mol Cell Endocrinol 75:R1, 1991.
194. Hillier SG. Regulatory functions for inhibin and activin in human ovaries. J Endocrinol 131:171, 1991.
195. Woodruff TK, Mather JP. Inhibin, activin and the female reproductive axis. Annu Rev Physiol 57:219, 1995.
196. Groome NP, Illingworth PJ, O'Brien M, et al. Detection of dimeric inhibin throughout the human menstrual cycle by two-site enzyme immunoassay. Clin Endocrinol (Oxf) 40:717, 1994.
197. Groome NP, Illingworth PJ, O'Brien M, et al. Measurement of dimeric inhibin B throughout the human menstrual cycle. J Clin Endocrinol Metab 81:1401, 1996.
198. Illingworth PJ, Groome NP, Duncan WC, et al. Measurement of circulating inhibin forms during the establishment of pregnancy. J Clin Endocrinol Metab 81:1471, 1996.
199. Yen SSC, Vela CP, Ryan KJ. Effect of clomiphene citrate in polycystic ovary syndrome: Relationship between serum gonadotropin and corpus luteum function. J Clin Endocrinol Metab 31:7, 1970.
200. Buckler HM, McLachlan RI, MacLachlan VB, et al. Serum inhibin levels in polycystic ovary syndrome: Basal levels and responses to luteinizing hormone–releasing hormone agonist and exogenous gonadotropin administration. J Clin Endocrinol Metab 66:798, 1988.
201. Reddi K, Wickings EJ, McNeilly AS, et al. Circulating bioactive follicle stimulating hormone and immunoreactive inhibin levels during the normal human menstrual cycle. Clin Endocrinol (Oxf) 33:547, 1990.
202. Jaatinen TA, Penttila TL, Kaipia A, et al. Expression of inhibin alpha, beta A and beta B messenger ribonucleic acids in the normal human ovary and in polycystic ovarian syndrome. J Endocrinol 143:127, 1994.
203. Anderson RA, Groome NP, Baird DT. Inhibin A and inhibin B in women with polycystic ovarian syndrome during treatment with FSH to induce mono-ovulation. Clin Endocrinol (in press).
204. Welt CK, Martin KA, Taylor AE, et al. Frequency modulation of follicle-stimulating hormone (FSH) during the luteal-follicular transition: Evidence for FSH control of inhibin B in normal women. J Clin Endocrinol Metab 82:2645, 1997.
205. Lin HY, Lodish HF. Receptors for TGF-β superfamily: Multiple polypeptides and serine threonine kinases. Trends Cell Biol 3:14, 1992.
206. Chegini N, Flanders KC. Presence of transforming growth factor β and their selective cellular localization in human ovarian tissue of various reproductive stages. Endocrinology 130:1707, 1992.
207. Hernandez ER, Hurwitz A, Payne DW, et al. Transforming growth factor-β1 inhibits ovarian androgen production: Gene expression, cellular localization, mechanism(s), and site(s) of action. Endocrinology 127:2804, 1990.
208. Mulheron GW, Bossert NL, Lapp JA, et al. Human granulosa-luteal and cumulus cells express transforming growth-factors-beta type 1 and type 2 mRNA. J Clin Endocrinol Metab 74:458, 1992.
209. Fournet N, Weitsman SR, Zachow RJ, et al. Transforming growth factor-β inhibits ovarian 17α-hydroxylase activity by a direct noncompetitive mechanism. Endocrinology 137:166, 1996.
210. Mason HD, Margara R, Winston RML, et al. Inhibition of oestradiol production by epidermal growth factor in human granulosa cells of normal and polycystic ovaries. Clin Endocrinol (Oxf) 33:511, 1990.
211. Mason HD, Carr L, Leake R, et al. Production of transforming growth factor-alpha by normal and polycystic ovaries. J Clin Endocrinol Metab 80:2053, 1995.
212. Roby KF, Terranova PF. Immunological evidence for a human ovarian tumor necrosis factor-α. J Clin Endocrinol Metab 71:1096, 1990.
213. Andreani CL, Payne DW, Packman JN, et al. Cytokine-mediated regulation of ovarian function. Tumor necrosis factor-α inhibits gonadotropin-supported ovarian androgen biosynthesis. J Biol Chem 266:6761, 1991.
214. Roby KE, Terranova PF. Effects of tumor necrosis factor-α in vitro on steroidogenesis of healthy and atretic follicles of the rat: Theca as a target. Endocrinology 126:2711, 1990.
215. Wild RA, Umstot ES, Andersen RN, et al. Adrenal function in hirsutism: II. Effect of an oral contraceptive. J Clin Endocrinol Metab 54:676, 1982.
216. Hurwitz A, Loukides J, Ricciarelli E, et al. Human intraovarian interleukin-1 (IL-1) system: Highly compartmentalized and hormonally dependent regulation of the genes encoding IL-1, its receptor, and its receptor antagonist. J Clin Invest 89:1746, 1992.
217. Hoffman DI, Klive K, Lobo RA. The prevalence and significance of elevated dehydroepiandrosterone sulfate levels in anovulatory women. Fertil Steril 42:76, 1984.
218. Lobo RA, Paul WL, Goebelsmann U. Dehydroepiandrosterone sulfate as an indicator of adrenal androgen function. Obstet Gynecol 51:69, 1981.
219. Hudson RW, Lochnan HA, Danby FW, et al. 11β-Hydroxyandrostenedione: A marker of adrenal function in hirsutism. Fertil Steril 54:1065, 1990.
220. Lachelin GCL, Barnett M, Hopper BR, et al. Adrenal function in normal women and women with the polycystic ovary syndrome. J Clin Endocrinol Metab 49:892, 1979.
221. Ehrmann DA, Rosenfield RL, Barnes RB, et al. Detection of functional ovarian hyperandrogenism in women with androgen excess. N Engl J Med 327:157, 1992.
222. Azziz R, Bradley EJ, Potter H, et al. Adrenal androgen excess in women: Lack of a role for 17-hydroxylase and 17,20-lyase dysregulation. J Clin Endocrinol Metab 80:400, 1995.
223. Ditkoff EC, Fruzzetti F, Chang L, et al. The impact of estrogen on adrenal androgen sensitivity and secretion in polycystic ovary syndrome. J Clin Endocrinol Metab 80:603, 1995.
224. Sahin Y, Ayata D, Kelestimur F. Lack of relationship between 17-hydroxyprogesterone response to buserelin testing and hyperinsulinemia in polycystic ovary syndrome. Eur J Endocrinol 136:410, 1997.
225. Mesiano S, Katz SL, Lee JY, et al. Insulin-like growth factors augment steroid production and expression of steroidogenic enzymes in human fetal adrenal cortical cells: Implications for adrenal androgen regulation. J Clin Endocrinol Metab 82:1390, 1997.
226. L'Allemand D, Penhoat A, Lebrethon MC, et al. Insulin-like growth factors enhance steroidogenic enzyme and corticotropin receptor messenger ribonucleic acid levels and corticotropin steroidogenic responsiveness in cultured human adrenocortical cells. J Clin Endocrinol Metab 81:3892, 1996.
227. Conley AJ, Bird IM. The role of cytochrome P450 17 alpha-

hydroxylase and 3 beta-hydroxysteroid dehydrogenase in the integration of gonadal and adrenal steroidogenesis via the delta 5 and delta 4 pathways of steroidogenesis in mammals. Biol Reprod 56:789, 1997.
228. Lazar L, Kauli R, Bruchis C, et al. Early polycystic ovary–like syndrome in girls with central precocious puberty and exaggerated adrenal response [see comments]. Eur J Endocrinol 133:403, 1995.
229. Oppenheimer E, Linder B, DiMartino-Nardi J. Decreased insulin sensitivity in prepubertal girls with premature adrenarche and acanthosis nigricans. J Clin Endocrinol Metab 80:614, 1995.
230. Rittmaster RS. Hirsutism. Clin Endocrinol 47:29, 1997.
231. Wilson JD, Walker J. The conversion of testosterone to 5α-androstan-17β-ol-3-one (dihydrotestosterone) by skin slices of man. J Clin Invest 48:371, 1969.
232. Randall VA. Androgen and human hair growth. Clin Endocrinol 40:439, 1997.
233. Ebling FJ. Hair. J Invest Dermatol 67:98, 1976.
234. Hasselquist MB, Goldberg N, Schroeter A, et al. Isolation and characterization of the estrogen receptor in human skin. J Clin Endocrinol Metab 50:76, 1980.
235. Schweikert HU, Wilson JD. Regulation of human hair growth by steroid hormones: I. Testosterone metabolism in isolated hairs. J Clin Endocrinol Metab 38:811, 1974.
236. Schweikert HU, Milewich L, Wilson JD. Aromatization of androstenedione by isolated human hairs. J Clin Endocrinol Metab 40:413, 1975.
237. Freinkel RK, Freinkel N. Hair growth and alopecia in hypothyroidism. Arch Dermatol 106:349, 1972.
238. Horton R, Hawks D, Lobo R. 3α,17β-Androstanediol glucuronide in plasma: A marker of androgen action in idiopathic hirsutism. J Clin Invest 69:1203, 1982.
239. Kaufman FR, Gentzschein E, Stancyzk FZ, et al. Dehydroepiandrosterone and dehydroepiandrosterone sulfate metabolism in human genital skin. Fertil Steril 54:251, 1990.
240. Kuttenn F, Mowszowicz G, Schaison G, et al. Androgen production and skin metabolism in hirsutism. J Clin Endocrinol Metab 75:83, 1977.
241. Horton R, Pasupuletti V, Antonipillai I. Androgen induction of steroid 5α-reductase may be mediated via insulin-like growth factor-I. Endocrinology 133:447, 1993.
242. Lobo RA, Paul WL, Gentzchein E, et al. Production of 3α-androstanediol glucuronide in human genital skin. J Clin Endocrinol Metab 65:711, 1987.
243. Matteri RK, Stancyzk FZ, Gentzchein E, et al. Androgen sulfate and glucuronide conjugates in nonhirsute and hirsute women with polycystic ovarian syndrome. Am J Obstet Gynecol 161:1704, 1989.
244. Stewart ME, Downing DT, Cook JS, et al. Sebaceous gland activity and serum dehydroepiandrosterone sulfate levels in boys and girls. Arch Dermatol 128:1345, 1992.
245. Marynick SP, Chakmakjian ZH, McCaffree DL, et al. Androgen excess in cystic acne. N Engl J Med 308:981, 1983.
246. Higuchi K, Nawata H, Maki T, et al. Prolactin has a direct effect on adrenal androgen secretion. J Clin Endocrinol Metab 59:714, 1984.
247. Serafini P, Lobo RA. Prolactin modulates peripheral androgen metabolism. Fertil Steril 45:41, 1986.
248. Mowszowicz I, Melanitou E, Doukani A, et al. Androgen binding capacity and 5α-reductase activity in pubic skin fibroblasts from hirsute patients. J Clin Endocrinol Metab 56:1209, 1983.
249. Serafini P, Lobo RA. Increased 5α-reductase activity in idiopathic hirsutism. Fertil Steril 43:74, 1985.
250. Ferriman D, Gallwey JD. Clinical assessment of body hair in women. J Clin Endocrinol Metab 24:1440, 1961.
251. Barth JH. How hairy are hirsute women? Clin Endocrinol 47:255, 1997.
252. Melegos DN, Mala HY, Wang AC, et al. Prostate-specific antigen in female serum, a potential new marker of androgen excess. J Clin Endocrinol Metab 82:777, 1997.
253. Carmina E, Gonzalez F, Chang L, et al. Reassessment of adrenal androgen secretion in women with polycystic ovary syndrome. Obstet Gynecol 85:971, 1995.
254. Givens JR, Andersen RN, Wiser WL, et al. Dynamics of suppression and recovery of plasma FSH, LH, androstenedione and testosterone in polycystic ovarian disease using an oral contraceptive. J Clin Endocrinol Metab 38:727, 1974.
255. Eil C, Edelson SK. The use of human skin fibroblasts to obtain potency estimates of drug binding to androgen receptors. J Clin Endocrinol Metab 59:51, 1984.
256. Rittmaster RS, Thompson DL. Effect of leuprolide and dexamethasone on hair growth and hormone levels in hirsute women: The relative importance of the ovary and the adrenal in the pathogenesis of hirsutism. J Clin Endocrinol Metab 70:1096, 1990.
257. Adashi EY. Potential utility of gonadotropin-releasing hormone agonists in the management of ovarian hyperandrogenism. Fertil Steril 53:765, 1990.
258. Neumann F, Von Berswordt-Wallrabe R, Eiger W, et al. Aspects of androgen-dependent events as studied by antiandrogens. Recent Prog Horm Res 26:337, 1970.
259. Kuttenn F, Rigaud C, Wright F, et al. Treatment of hirsutism by oral cyproterone acetate and percutaneous estradiol. J Clin Endocrinol Metab 51:1107, 1980.
260. Menard RH, Guenther TM, Kon H, et al. Studies on the destruction of adrenal and testicular cytochrome P450 by spironolactone. J Biol Chem 254:1726, 1979.
261. Corvol P, Michaud A, Menard J. Antiandrogenic effect of spironolactones: Mechanism of action. Endocrinology 97:52, 1975.
262. Shapiro G, Evron S. A novel use of spironolactone: Treatment of hirsutism. J Clin Endocrinol Metab 51:429, 1980.
263. Cumming DC, Yang JC, Rebar RW, Yen SCC. Treatment of hirsutism with spironolactone. JAMA 247:1295, 1982.
264. Evron S, Shapiro G, Diamant YZ. Induction of ovulation with spironolactone (aldactone) in anovulatory oligomenorrheic and hyperandrogenic women. Fertil Steril 36:468, 1981.
265. Cusan L, Dupont A, Gomez J-L, et al. Comparison of flutamide and spironolactone in the treatment of hirsutism: A randomized controlled trial. Fertil Steril 61:281, 1994.
266. Moghetti P, Castello R, Negri C, et al. Flutamide in the treatment of hirsutism: Long-term clinical effects, endocrine changes, and androgen receptor behavior. Fertil Steril 64:511, 1995.
267. Tolino A, Petrone A, Sarnacchiaro F, et al. Finasteride in the treatment of hirsutism: New therapeutic perspectives. Fertil Steril 66:61, 1996.
268. Castello R, Tosi F, Perrone F, et al. Outcome of long-term treatment with the 5α-reductase inhibitor finasteride in idiopathic hirsutism: Clinical and hormonal effects during a 1-year course of therapy and 1 year follow-up. Fertil Steril 66:734, 1996.
269. Moghetti P, Castello R, Magnani CM, et al. Clinical and hormonal effects of the 5α-reductase inhibitor finasteride in idiopathic hirsutism. J Clin Endocrinol Metab 79:1115, 1994.
270. Wong IL, Morris RS, Chang L, et al. A prospective randomized trial comparing finasteride to spironolactone in the treatment of hirsute women. J Clin Endocrinol Metab 80:233, 1995.
271. Falsetti L, DeFusco D, Eleftheriou G, et al. Treatment of hirsutism by finasteride and flutamide in women with polycystic ovary syndrome. Gynecol Endocrinol 11:251, 1997.
272. Fruzzetti F, DeLorenzo D, Parrini D, et al. Effects of finasteride, a 5α-reductase inhibitor, on circulating androgens and gonadotropin secretion in hirsute women. J Clin Endocrinol Metab 79:831, 1994.
273. Rittmaster RS, Loriaux DL, Cutler GB Jr. Sensitivity of cortisol and adrenal androgens to dexamethasone suppression in hirsute women. J Clin Endocrinol Metab 61:462, 1985.
274. Barreca A, Artini PG, DelMonte P, et al. In vivo and in vitro effects of growth hormone on estradiol secretion by human granulosa cells. J Clin Endocrinol Metab 77:61, 1993.
275. Nam SY, Lee EJ, Kim KR, et al. Effect of obesity on total and free insulin-like growth factor (IGF)-1, and their relationship to IGF-binding protein (BP)–1, IGFBP-2, IGFBP-3, insulin, and growth hormone. Int J Obes 21:355, 1997.
276. Barbieri RL, Smith S, Ryan KJ. The role of hyperinsulinemia in the pathogenesis of ovarian hyperandrogenism. Fertil Steril 50:197, 1988.
277. Bergh C, Carlsson B, Olsson J-H, et al. Regulation of androgen production in cultured human thecal cells by insulin-like growth factor I and insulin. Fertil Steril 59:323, 1993.
278. Nahum R, Thong KJ, Hillier SG. Metabolic regulation of androgen production by human thecal cells in vitro. Hum Reprod 10:75, 1995.
279. Likitmaskul S, Cowell CT, Donaghue K, et al. "Exaggerated adrenarche" in children presenting with premature adrenarche. Clin Endocrinol 42:265, 1995.

280. Barnes RB, Rosenfield RL, Ehrmann DA, et al. Ovarian hyperandrogenism as a result of congenital adrenal virilizing disorders: Evidence for perinatal masculinization of neuroendocrine function in women. J Clin Endocrinol Metab 79:1328, 1994.
281. Nobels F, Dewailly D. Puberty and polycystic ovarian syndrome: The insulin/insulin-like growth factor I hypothesis. Fertil Steril 58:655, 1992.
282. Ibãnez L, Potau N, Georgopoulos N, et al. Growth hormone, insulin-like growth factor-I axis, and insulin secretion in hyperandrogenic adolescents. Fertil Steril 64:1113, 1995.
283. Schiebinger RJ, Albertson BD, Cassorla FG, et al. The developmental changes in plasma adrenal androgens during infancy and adrenarche are associated with changing activities of adrenal microsomal 17-hydroxylase and 17,20-desmolase. J Clin Invest 67:1177, 1981.
284. Dickerman Z, Grant D, Faiman C, et al. Intraadrenal steroid concentrations in man: Zonal differences and developmental changes. J Clin Endocrinol Metab 59:1031, 1984.
285. Labrie F, Luu-The V, Lin S-X, et al. The key role of 17β-hydroxysteroid dehydrogenases in sex steroid biology. Steroids 62:148, 1997.
286. Juul A, Holm K, Kastrup KW, et al. Free insulin-like growth factor I serum levels in 1430 healthy children and adults, and its diagnostic value in patients suspected of growth hormone deficiency. J Clin Endocrinol Metab 82:2497, 1997.
287. Amiel SA, Sherwin RS, Simonson DC, et al. Impaired insulin action in puberty: A contributing factor to poor glycemic control in adolescents with diabetes. N Engl J Med 315:215, 1986.
288. Luna AM, Wilson DM, Wibbelsman CJ, et al. Somatomedins in adolescence: A cross-sectional study of the effect of puberty on plasma insulin-like growth factor I and II levels. J Clin Endocrinol Metab 57:268, 1983.
289. Lobo RA, Granger L, Goebelsmann U, et al. Elevations in unbound serum estradiol as a possible mechanism for inappropriate gonadotropin secretion in women with PCO. J Clin Endocrinol Metab 52:156, 1981.
290. Frager MS, Pieper DR, Tonetta SA, et al. Effects of castration, steroid replacement, and the role of gonadotropin-releasing hormone in modulating receptors in the rat. J Clin Invest 67:615, 1981.
291. Reid RL, Quigley ME, Yen SSC. The disappearance of opioidergic mechanism in the control of gonadotropin secretion in postmenopausal women. J Clin Endocrinol Metab 52:1179, 1981.
292. Quigley ME, Rakoff JS, Yen SSC. Increased luteinizing hormone sensitivity to dopamine inhibition in polycystic ovary syndrome. J Clin Endocrinol Metab 52:231, 1981.
293. Cumming DC, Reid RL, Quigley ME, et al. Evidence for decreased endogenous dopamine and opioid inhibitory influences on LH secretion in polycystic ovary syndrome. Clin Endocrinol 20:643, 1984.
294. Reid RL, Hoff JD, Yen SSC, et al. Effects of exogenous β_h-endorphin on pituitary hormone secretion and its disappearance rate in normal human subjects. J Clin Endocrinol Metab 52:1179, 1981.
295. Zhen S, Zakaria M, Wolfe A, et al. Regulation of gonadotropin-releasing hormone (GnRH) gene expression by insulin-like growth factor I in a cultured GnRH-expressing neuronal cell line. Mol Endocrinol 11:1145, 1997.
296. Olson BR, Scott DC, Wetsel WC, et al. Effects of insulin-like growth factors I and II and insulin on the immortalized hypothalamic GT1-7 cell line. Neuroendocrinology 62:155, 1995.
297. Hiney JK, Srivastava V, Nyberg CL, et al. Insulin-like growth factor 1 of peripheral origin acts centrally to accelerate the initiation of female puberty. Endocrinology 137:3717, 1996.
298. Duenas M, Luquin S, Chowen JA, et al. Gonadal hormone regulation of insulin-like growth factor-I–like immunoreactivity in hypothalamic astroglia of developing and adult rats. Neuroendocrinology 59:528, 1994.
299. Zhen S, Zakaria M, Wolfe A, et al. Regulation of gonadotropin-releasing hormone (GnRH) gene expression by insulin-like growth factor I in a cultured GnRH-expressing neuronal cell line. Mol Endocrinol 11:1145, 1997.
300. Olson BR, Scott DC, Wetsel WC, et al. Effects of insulin-like growth factors I and II and insulin on the immortalized hypothalamic GT1-7 cell line. Neuroendocrinology 62:155, 1995.
301. Wilson ME. IGF-I administration advances the decrease in hypersensitivity to oestradiol negative feedback inhibition of serum LH in adolescent female rhesus monkeys. J Endocrinol 145:121, 1995.
302. Risma KA, Hirshfield AN, Nilson JH. Elevated luteinizing hormone in prepubertal transgenic mice causes hyperandrogenemia, precocious puberty, and substantial ovarian pathology. Endocrinology 138:3540, 1997.
303. Cooper HE, Spellacy WN, Prem KA, et al. Hereditary factors in the Stein-Leventhal syndrome. Am J Obstet Gynecol 100:371, 1968.
304. Ferriman D, Purdie AW. The inheritance of polycystic ovarian disease and a possible relationship to premature balding. Clin Endocrinol 11:291, 1979.
305. Wilroy RS, Givens JR, Wiser WL, et al. Hyperthecosis: An inheritable form of polycystic ovarian disease. Birth Defects 11:81, 1975.
306. Hague WM, Adams J, Reeders ST, et al. Familial polycystic ovaries: A genetic disease? Clin Endocrinol 29:593, 1988.
307. Legro RS. The genetics of polycystic ovary syndrome. Am J Med 98:9S, 1995.
308. Coulam CB, Anegers JF, Kranz JS. Chronic anovulation syndrome and associated neoplasia. Obstet Gynecol 61:403, 1983.
309. Rose PG. Endometrial carcinoma. N Engl J Med 335:640, 1996.
310. Dahlgren E, Johansson S, Lindstedt G. Women with polycystic ovary syndrome wedge resected in 1956 to 1965: A long-term follow-up focusing on natural history and circulating hormones. Fertil Steril 57:505, 1992.
311. Legro RS, Coleman KH, Irwin L, et al. Polycystic ovary syndrome over age 40: Age related differences in phenotype. Proceedings of the 42nd Annual Meeting of the Society for Gynecologic Investigation; March 15–18, 1995; Chicago, IL.
312. Lanzone A, Caruso A, DiSimone N, et al. Polycystic ovary disease. A risk factor for gestational diabetes? J Reprod Med 40:312, 1995.
313. DeFronzo RA, Ferrannini E. Insulin resistance. A mulifaceted syndrome responsible for NIDDM, obesity, hypertension, dyslipidemia, and atherosclerotic cardiovascular disease. Diabetes Care 14:173, 1991.
314. Wild RA. Obesity, lipids, cardiovascular risk, and androgen excess. Am J Med 98:27S, 1995.
315. Wild RA, Bartholomew MJ. The influence of body weight on lipoprotein lipids in patients with polycystic ovary syndrome. Am J Obstet Gynecol 159:423, 1988.
316. Conway GS, Agrawal R, Betteridge DJ, et al. Risk factors for coronary artery disease in lean and obese women with the polycystic ovary syndrome. Clin Endocrinol (Oxf) 37:119, 1992.
317. Wild RA, Alaupovic P, Parker IJ. Lipid and apolipoprotein abnormalities in hirsute women. Am J Obstet Gynecol 166:1191, 1992.
318. Goode GK, Miller JP, Haegerty AM. Hyperlipidaemia, hypertension, and coronary heart disease. Lancet 345:362, 1995.
319. Andersen P, Ingebjørg S, Abdelnoor M, et al. Increased insulin sensitivity and fibrinolytic capacity after dietary intervention in obese women with polycystic ovary syndrome. Metabolism 44:611, 1995.
320. Dahlgren E, Janson PO, Johansson S, et al. Polycystic ovary syndrome and risk for myocardial infarction. Evaluated from a risk factor model based on a prospective population study of women. Acta Obstet Gynecol Scand 71:599, 1992.
321. Birdsall MA, Farquhar CM, White HD. Association between polycystic ovaries and extent of coronary artery disease in women having cardiac catheterization. Ann Intern Med 126:32, 1997.
322. Guzick DS, Talbott EO, Sutton-Tyrrell K, et al. Carotid atherosclerosis in women with polycystic ovary syndrome: Initial results from a case-control study. Am J Obstet Gynecol 174:1224, 1996.
323. Graf M, Brown V, Richards C, et al. The independent effects of hyperandrogenemia, hyperinsulinemia, and obesity on lipid and lipoprotein profiles in women. Clin Endocrinol (Oxf) 33:119, 1990.
324. Pasquali R, Casimirri F, Venturoli S, et al. Body fat distribution has weight-independent effects on clinical, hormonal, and metabolic features of women with polycystic ovary syndrome. Metabolism 43:706, 1994.

325. Koskinen P, Penttila TA, Anttila L, et al. Optimal use of hormone determinations in the biochemical diagnosis of the polycystic ovary syndrome. Fertil Steril 65:517, 1996.
326. Bergman RN, Hope ID, Yang YJ, et al. Assessment of insulin sensitivity in vivo: A critical review. Diabetes Metab Rev 5:411, 1989.
327. Modan M, Harris MI, Halkin H. Evaluation of WHO and NDDG criteria for impaired glucose tolerance. Diabetes 38:1603, 1989.
328. Hull MGR. The causes of infertility and relative effectiveness of treatment. *In* Templeton AA, Drife JO. Infertility. London, Springer-Verlag, 1992, pp 33–62.
329. Franks S, Adams J, Mason H, et al. Ovulatory disorders in women with polycystic ovary syndrome. Clin Obstet Gynecol 12:605, 1985.
330. Adashi EY. Clomiphene citrate: Mechanism(s) and site(s) of action—a hypothesis revisited. Fertil Steril 42:331, 1984.
331. Kerin JF, Liu JH. Evidence for a hypothalamic site of action of clomiphene citrate in women. J Clin Endocrinol Metab 61:265, 1985.
332. Lobo RA, Paul W, March CM, et al. Clomiphene and dexamethasone in women unresponsive to clomiphene alone. Obstet Gynecol 60:497, 1982.
333. Daly DC, Walters CA, Soto-Albors CE, et al. A randomized study of dexamethasone in ovulation induction with clomiphene citrate. Fertil Steril 41:844, 1984.
334. Lunenfeld B, Insler V. Diagnosis and Treatment of Functional Infertility. Berlin, Grosse Verlag, 1978.
335. Wang CF, Gemzell C. The use of human gonadotropins for induction of ovulation in women with polycystic ovarian disease. Fertil Steril 33:479, 1980.
336. Fulghesu AM, Villa P, Pavone V, et al. The impact of insulin secretion on the ovarian response to exogenous gonadotropins in polycystic ovary syndrome. J Clin Endocrinol Metab 82:644, 1997.
337. Kelly AC, Jewelewicz R. Alternate regimens for ovulation induction in polycystic ovarian disease. Fertil Steril 54:195, 1990.
338. Filicori M, Flamigni C, Campaniello E, et al. The abnormal response of polycystic ovarian disease patients to exogenous pulsatile gonadotropin-releasing hormone: Characterization and management. J Clin Endocrinol Metab 69:825, 1989.
339. Filicori M. Gonadotropin-releasing hormone analogs in ovulation induction: Current status and perspectives. J Clin Endocrinol Metab 81:2413, 1996.
340. Goldzieher JW, Green JA. The polycystic ovary: I. Clinical and histologic features. J Clin Endocrinol Metab 22:325, 1962.
341. Adashi EY, Rock JA, Guzick D, et al. Fertility following bilateral ovarian wedge resection: A critical analysis of 90 consecutive cases of the polycystic ovary syndrome. Fertil Steril 36:320, 1981.
342. Judd HL, Rigg LA, Anderson DC, Yen SCC. The effects of ovarian wedge resection on circulating gonadotropin and ovarian steroid levels in patients with polycystic ovary syndrome. J Clin Endocrinol Metab 43:347, 1976.
343. Gjonnaess H. Polycystic ovary syndrome treated by ovarian electrocautery through the laparoscope. Fertil Steril 41:20, 1984.
344. Greenblatt E, Casper RF. Endocrine changes after laparoscopic ovarian cautery in polycystic ovarian syndrome. Am J Obstet Gynecol 156:279, 1987.
345. Sakata M, Terakawa N, Tasaka K, et al. Changes of bioactive luteinizing hormone after laparoscopic ovarian cautery in patients with polycystic ovarian syndrome. Fertil Steril 53:610, 1990.
346. Gadir AA, Khatim MS, Mowafi RS, et al. Hormonal changes in patients with polycystic ovarian disease after ovarian electrocautery or pituitary desensitization. Clin Endocrinol 32:749, 1990.
347. Donesky BW, Adashi EY. Surgically induced ovulation in the polycystic ovary syndrome: Wedge resection revisited in the age of laparoscopy [see comments]. Fertil Steril 63:439, 1995.
348. Jakubowicz DJ, Nestler JE. 17α-Hydroxyprogesterone responses to leuprolide and serum androgens in obese women with and without polycystic ovary syndrome offer dietary weight loss. J Clin Endocrinol Metab 82:556, 1997.
349. Holte J, Bergh T, Berne C, et al. Restored insulin sensitivity but persistently increased early insulin secretion after weight loss in obese women with polycystic ovary syndrome. J Clin Endocrinol Metab 80:2586, 1995.
350. Guzick DS, Wing R, Smith D, et al. Endocrine consequences of weight loss in obese, hyperandrogenic, anovulatory women. Fertil Steril 61:598, 1994.
351. Hamilton-Fairley D, Kiddy D, Anyaoku V, et al. Response of sex hormone binding globulin and insulin-like growth factor binding protein-1 to an oral glucose tolerance test in obese women with polycystic ovary syndrome before and after calorie restriction. Clin Endocrinol (Oxf) 39:363, 1993.
352. Kiddy DS, Hamilton-Fairley D, Bush A, et al. Improvement in endocrine and ovarian function during dietary treatment of obese women with polycystic ovary syndrome. Clin Endocrinol (Oxf) 36:105, 1992.
353. Suikkari A-M, Sane T, Seppala M, et al. Prolonged exercise increases serum insulin-like growth factor–binding protein concentrations. J Clin Endocrinol Metab 68:141, 1989.
354. Stumvoll M, Nurjhan N, Perriello G, et al. Metabolic effects of metformin in non–insulin-dependent diabetes mellitus. N Engl J Med 333:550, 1995.
355. Bailey CJ, Turner RC. Metformin. N Engl J Med 334:574, 1996.
356. Nestler JE, Jakubowicz DJ. Decreases in ovarian cytochrome P450c17 alpha activity and serum free testosterone after reduction of insulin secretion in polycystic ovary syndrome [see comments]. N Engl J Med 335:617, 1996.
357. Velazquez EM, Mendoza S, Hamer T, et al. Metformin therapy in polycystic ovary syndrome reduces hyperinsulinemia, insulin resistance, hyperandrogenemia, and systolic blood pressure, while facilitating normal menses and pregnancy. Metabolism 43:647, 1994.
358. Crave J-C, Fimbel S, Lejeune H, et al. Effects of diet and metformin administration on sex hormone–binding globulin, androgens, and insulin in hirsute and obese women. J Clin Endocrinol Metab 80:2057, 1995.
359. Ehrmann DA, Cavaghan MK, Imperial J, et al. Effects of metformin on insulin secretion, insulin action, and ovarian steroidogenesis in women with polycystic ovary syndrome. J Clin Endocrinol Metab 82:524, 1997.
360. Keller H, Wahli W. Peroxisome proliferator-activated receptors: A link between endocrinology and nutrition? J Clin Endocrinol Metab 80:2586, 1993.
361. Ibrahimi A, Teboul L, Gaillaird D, et al. Evidence for a common mechanism of action for free fatty acids and thiazolidinedione antidiabetic agents on gene expression in preadipose cells. Mol Pharmacol 46:1070, 1994.
362. Brandes R, Arad R, Bar-Tana J. Inducers of adipose conversion activate transcription promoted by a peroxisome proliferators response element in 3T3-L1 cells. Biochem Pharmacol 50:1949, 1995.
363. Kliewer S, Lenhard J, Willson T, et al. A prostaglandin J2 metabolite binds peroxisome proliferator-activated receptor gamma and promotes adipocyte differentiation. Cell 83:813, 1995.
364. Bardin CW, Lipsett MB, Edgcomb JH, et al. Studies of testosterone metabolism in a patient with masculinization due to stromal hyperthecosis. N Engl J Med 277:399, 1967.
365. Judd HL, Scully RE, Herbst AL, et al. Familial hyperthecosis: Comparison of endocrinologic and histologic findings with polycystic ovarian disease. Am J Obstet Gynecol 117:976, 1973.
366. Braithwaite SS, Erkmann-Balis B, Avila TD. Postmenopausal virilization due to ovarian stromal hyperthecosis. J Clin Endocrinol Metab 46:295, 1978.
367. Dunaif A, Hoffman AR, Scully RE, et al. The clinical, biochemical and ovarian morphologic features in women with acanthosis nigricans and masculinization. Obstet Gynecol 66:545, 1985.
368. Leedman PJ, Bierre AR, Martin FIR. Virilizing nodular ovarian stromal hyperthecosis, diabetes mellitus and insulin resistance in a postmenopausal woman: Case report. Br J Obstet Gynaecol 96:1095, 1989.
369. Nuovo GJ. Virilizing stromal thecosis of the ovary associated with multiple corpora atretica. Am J Clin Pathol 92:505, 1989.
370. Pascale M-M, Pugeat M, Roberts M, et al. Androgen suppressive effect of GnRH agonist in ovarian hyperthecosis and virilizing tumors. Clin Endocrinol (Oxf) 41:571, 1994.
371. Nagamani M, Dinh TV, Kelver ME. Hyperinsulinemia in hyperthecosis of the ovaries. Am J Obstet Gynecol 154:384, 1986.

372. Rittmaster RS. Polycystic ovary syndrome, hyperthecosis and the menopause [comment]. Clin Endocrinol (Oxf) 46:129, 1997.
373. Birdsall MA, Farquhar CM. Polycystic ovaries in pre and post-menopausal women. Clin Endocrinol (Oxf) 44:269, 1996.
374. Kennedy L, Traub AI, Atkinson AB, et al. Short term administration of gonadotropin-releasing hormone analog to a patient with a testosterone-secreting ovarian tumor. J Clin Endocrinol Metab 64:1320, 1987.
375. Steingold KA, Judd HL, Nieberg RK, et al. Treatment of severe androgen excess due to ovarian hyperthecosis with a long-acting gonadotropin-releasing hormone agonist. Am J Obstet Gynecol 154:1241, 1986.

Chapter 18

CHRONIC ANOVULATION CAUSED BY PERIPHERAL ENDOCRINE DISORDERS

S. S. C. Yen

■ CHAPTER OUTLINE

KEY POINTS

- Disruptions of the integrated hypothalamic-pituitary-ovarian (HPO) axis secondary to peripheral endocrine disorders represent an important cause of menstrual disorders and infertility.
- An inappropriate extraglandular contribution of estrogen derived through the peripheral conversion of androgens by P450arom occurs with increased substrate, enzymatic activity, or conversion sites and represents a common basis in the development of chronic anovulation.
- Syndromes of aromatase excess and deficiency due to mutations of the P450arom gene (*CYP19*) as underlying causes of dysfunction of the HPO axis have characteristic clinical manifestations.
- Cushing's syndrome includes adrenal adenomas and ectopic ACTH or CRF secretion by a variety of tumors that are important causes of menstrual disorders.
- Gonadal tumors producing excessive amounts of androgens or estrogens interfere with the feedback signal of the neuroendocrine axis regulating menstrual cyclicity. Inhibin and müllerian-inhibiting substance are markers for these tumors.
- Hypoadrenalism and hypothyroidism due to a variety of causes including autoimmune bases, thyroid hormone resistance syndrome (mutation of the β-subunit of TSH receptor), and congenital lipoid adrenal hyperplasia are frequently associated with reproductive disorders.
- Ectopic production of prolactin and glycoprotein hormones by tumors disrupts the HPO axis, leading to menstrual disorders; hCG-β is a unique marker for these tumors.
- Gene mutations of FSH, LH, and estrogen receptors are novel causes of ovarian failure and estrogen deficiency.

The most notable feature of the female reproductive system is the total absence of a steady state. By virtue of its ever-changing morphologic, biochemical, and functional states, the female reproductive cycle must be viewed as a dynamic system with a long-term (monthly) rhythm and short-term (minute to minute) fluctuations. Thus, from the operational viewpoint, when the system attains a steady-state condition, chronic anovulation occurs. This principle may be the most important one in the clinical assessment of pathophysiologic changes in patients with menstrual disorders.

THE CONCEPT OF CHRONIC ANOVULATION

Chronic anovulation refers to conditions with repeated ovulation failure and is manifested clinically as amenorrhea or menstrual acyclicity. In principle, these menstrual disorders can be traced physiopathologically to the disruption of the integrated function of the hypothalamic-pituitary-ovarian (HPO) axis, either within or secondary to the perturbation of the system by peripheral endocrine dysfunction.

As is the case for all self-regulated systems, feedback control is a critical element in the regulation of female reproductive cyclicity. Such control is entrained in the "ovarian clock," whereby a nonlinear feedback signal (i.e., incremental estradiol) is generated during a well-defined time course. This timekeeping signal is expressed as sequential but interdependent negative and positive feedback actions and is functionally coupled with the ever-changing secretory capacity of cellular components of the neuroendocrine axis. When the normal pattern of the feedback signal is blurred, disrupted, or modified, either quantitatively or qualitatively, the dynamic state of the cyclic reproductive function ceases.

Abnormalities of reproductive function, including precocious and delayed puberty, amenorrhea, and irregular menstrual bleeding, can result from an inappropriate extraglandular contribution of estrogen derived through the peripheral conversion of androgen.[1] This mode of estrogen production, which is not under direct control of pituitary gonadotropin, is apulsatile in nature. As a consequence, the cyclic feedback signal is masked and chronic anovulation ensues, despite the absence of abnormalities within the HPO system. In fact, it is the understanding of this precept that led Dr. Gregory Pincus and associates to develop the "contraceptive pill."

This chapter covers a variety of causes of chronic anovulation, including hyperfunction and hypofunction of the *adrenal glands* and *thyroid glands.*

Chronic Anovulation and Amenorrhea

Primary Versus Secondary Amenorrhea

In the past, great significance was assigned to the difference between primary and secondary amenorrhea; the former has been considered more serious than the latter. Although the incidence of genetic and anatomic abnormalities is higher in patients with primary amenorrhea, this distinction between primary and secondary forms is less informative and, indeed, can be misleading. For example, patients with gonadal dysgenesis who have had prior cyclic menses are classified as having *secondary amenorrhea;* on the other hand, women with chronic functional anovulation of pubertal onset are regarded as having *primary amenorrhea.* For these reasons, we emphasize the assessment of degrees of secondary sex characteristics to denote the presence or absence of ovarian steroid influence on target tissues in the past. This basic premise—that the patient's body functions as *a bioassay system*—provides an axiomatic reference for subsequent investigation.

Secondary Sex Characteristics

It is essential to determine whether normal secondary sex characteristics are present or absent in postpubertal patients with amenorrhea. Inappropriate development of these characteristics should direct the clinician to carefully assess possible failure within the HPO system. Gonadal dysgenesis can be identified or ruled out promptly by measuring serum concentrations of follicle-stimulating hormone (FSH) and luteinizing hormone (LH). Elevated levels are a most reliable index of gonadal failure. On occasion, even patients with XO gonadal dysgenesis have fully developed secondary sex characteristics owing to a limited but functional gonadal remnant. When normal or low gonadotropin levels are found, systemic evaluation of hypothalamic-pituitary function is the next step.

Definition of Amenorrhea

There is no uniform agreement on the length of menstruation absence required to define amenorrhea. My definition is the absence of menstruation for 3 months or more in individuals who previously had experienced periodic menstruation, whatever the frequency or regularity. In addition, the term amenorrheic may be applied to individuals in whom menarche does not become established by the age of 16 years, regardless of the presence or absence of secondary sex characteristics. Independent of its pathophysiologic basis, amenorrhea, then, is the failure of HPO interaction to produce cyclic expression of the appropriate hormones at the chronologic age at which sexual maturation should normally occur.

Classification of Amenorrhea

To gain an overview of the causes of amenorrhea and to acquire proper perspectives of the menstrual disorders resulting from inappropriate feedback systems, a classification of causes of amenorrhea is necessary. A simple and unified classification is impossible. Although some overlap is evident, the following is based on pathophysiologic considerations, distinguishing between dysfunctions caused by defects within and without the central nervous system–hypothalamic-pituitary-uterine axis (Table 18–1).

Anatomic Causes. This group includes a variety of anatomic defects that prevent menstrual bleeding; examples include abnormal differentiation of the genital tract and endometrial adhesions.

Primary Ovarian Failure. In this category, patients commonly, but not exclusively, have *hypergonadotropism,* in which the FSH:LH ratio exceeds unity. The presence of secondary sex characteristics indicates that there has been some ovarian activity in the past. The most common type of this disorder is gonadal dysgenesis. Premature ovarian failure due to autoimmune disorders and gonadotropin receptor abnormalities are included in this category.

Chronic Anovulation Syndrome. This is by far the most common type of amenorrhea and involves an acyclic HPO system associated with three patterns of pituitary gonadotropin secretion: (1) *hypogonadotropic,* (2) *normo-*

■ TABLE 18–1
Causes of the Chronic Anovulation Syndrome

Hypothalamic Chronic Anovulation*

Dysfunction of pulsatile GnRH secretion
Aberration of the integrated function of the integrated function of the central nervous system–hypothalamic element of the hypothalamic-pituitary-ovarian system

Pituitary Chronic Anovulation*

Defects or dysfunction of the gonadotroph*

Chronic Anovulation Due to Inappropriate Feedback

Use of contraceptive steroids or exposure to constant doses of estrogen
Excessive extraglandular estrogen production
Abnormal buffering system
Functional androgen excess (adrenal or ovarian)
Androgen- or estrogen-producing tumor
Aromatase excess and deficiency syndromes
Gene mutations of FSH, LH, and estrogen receptors
Autoimmune disorders

Chronic Anovulation Due to Inappropriate Feedback Secondary to Combined Central-Peripheral Dysfunctions

Polycystic ovary syndrome†
Excessive cortisol and androgen production (ectopic/eutopic) in Cushing's syndrome
Deficiency or excess of thyroid hormone and thyroid hormone resistance syndrome
Excess of prolactin or growth hormone (ectopic and eutopic)
Malnutrition

*See Chapter 19.
†See Chapter 17.

gonadotropic, and (3) *hypergonadotropic.* Chronic anovulation syndrome includes the ovary as an etiologic factor in the development of amenorrhea and effects in the hypothalamic-pituitary system or disturbance in the secretion and metabolism of steroid and protein hormones. Under these circumstances, a variety of clinical manifestations occur, including androgen and estrogen imbalance, that are reflections of functional changes of the ovaries or are extraovarian in origin.

PHYSIOLOGY OF ANDROGENS IN WOMEN

Secretion and Action

The normal ovary, in addition to the adrenal gland, produces and secretes three major C_{19} steroid androgens: (1) androstenedione, (2) testosterone, and (3) dehydroepiandrosterone (DHEA). The ovarian androgens are primarily androstenedione and testosterone, secreted by the stroma (interstitial tissue) and by the theca interna cells. DHEA and its sulfate (DHEA-S) are the principal androgens secreted by the zona reticularis of the adrenal cortex. The relative androgenic potencies of these steroids are given in Table 18–2. The relative contributions of the adrenal and ovary may vary during the course of the menstrual cycle.

Intracrine Action

A significant extraglandular contribution to the total androgen pool in the body results from the conversion of biologically inactive "prehormone" steroids to potent androgens in tissues such as fat, muscle, skin, and brain. The formation of potent androgens within the cells may be a mechanism by which high concentrations of hormones can be achieved locally and their action mediated by binding to nuclear receptors in target tissues without the attendant need of high concentrations in the systemic circulation: the so-called *intracrinology.* By this means, a specific hormone action may be enhanced manyfold over amounts delivered by circulation. Another aspect of the intracrine concept is the conversion of androgen to estrogen, especially androstenedione to estrone. This conversion provides a significant source of estrogen and functions as a sink for the androgen pool.[1] The pathways for biosynthesis of androgens and the necessary enzymatic systems required are detailed in Chapter 4.

Δ^4-Androstenedione

As an androgen, Δ^4-androstenedione has several distinctive features in women:

- It is the only circulating androgen that is higher in premenopausal women than in men.
- Only 4 percent or less of circulating Δ^4-androstenedione is bound to sex steroid–binding globulin (SHBG).
- Its androgenic potency is only 10 percent of that of testosterone.
- Serving as a prohormone, Δ^4-androstenedione is readily converted to testosterone and estrone, and both products are convertible to estradiol.

The contribution of Δ^4-androstenedione production between the ovary and adrenal appears to vary with time of day and phase of the ovarian cycle.[2, 3] The adrenal output of Δ^4-androstenedione is responsive to adrenocorticotropic hormone (ACTH) stimulation and exhibits a circadian rhythm with peaks in the morning and nadir in the evening coincident with that of cortisol.[4] Thus, in the morning hours, the adrenal contribution to the circulating pool may account for more than 80 percent of the total Δ^4-androstenedione production, with a substantial reduction in the evenings (Fig. 18–1). When measurements are made for assessment of abnormalities, the time of sampling would obviously become important. In the early follicular phase, the daily secretion of the adrenals (1.2 mg) exceeds that of both ovaries (0.8 mg). The mature graafian follicle secretes increasing amounts of Δ^4-androstenedione, which is reflected by an elevation of the circulating concentrations and a twofold increase in the daily production near the midcycle.[3, 5] This increase is maintained during the luteal

■ TABLE 18–2
Relative Androgenic Activity of Androgens

STEROID	ACTIVITY*
Dihydrotestosterone	300
Testosterone	100
Androstenedione	10
DHEA, DHEA-S	5

DHEA, dehydroepiandrosterone; DHEA-S, DHEA sulfate.
*Testosterone serves as a reference = 100.
Adapted from Nelson DH. The Adrenal Cortex: Physiological Function and Disease. Philadelphia, WB Saunders, 1980, p 1122.

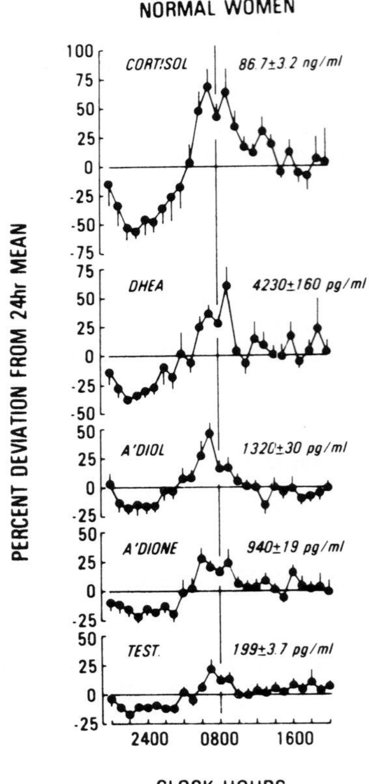

Figure 18–1 ■ The circadian rhythm of circulating androgens coincident with that of cortisol in women during the early follicular phase of the cycle (N = 9). Hormone concentrations are determined in hourly samples obtained around-the-clock for 24 hours. The data (mean ± SE) are expressed as percent deviation from the 24-hour mean concentrations; 0800 hours is used as the reference point. The excursion between morning peaks and evening nadir for all androgens measured are synchronized with the cortisol rhythm and represent adrenal contributions. (Data from Lachelin GCL, Barnett M, Hopper G, et al. Adrenal function in normal women and women with the polycystic ovary syndrome. J Clin Endocrinol Metab 49:892–898, 1979. © The Endocrine Society.)

phase by secretion from the corpus luteum. The average blood production rate of Δ^4-androstenedione in men is 1.4 mg/day; in cycling women, it is 3.4 mg/day; and in postmenopausal women, it is 1.6 mg/day.

The cyclic fluctuation in ovarian secretion of androstenedione becomes more apparent when the adrenal source is absent, as in adrenalectomized subjects,[6] during suppression with dexamethasone,[2] or in Addison's disease.[3] Under these circumstances, a normal cyclic pattern of LH, FSH, estradiol, and progesterone secretion may be maintained, implying that the adrenal source of androgen does not contribute significantly to the integrity of ovarian function.

Testosterone and 5α-Dihydrotestosterone

Testosterone is considered the most potent androgen. Its hormonal action can be exerted either directly or indirectly, depending on the target tissues. In the muscle, it acts directly on the androgen receptors to produce growth-promoting and anabolic effects. However, the expression of androgenicity in sexual target cells requires the formation of dihydrotestosterone (DHT) by the reduction of testosterone at position 5 (through 5α-reductase); this reduction takes place in tissues such as hair follicle, prostate, and external genitalia.[7] In the process of sex differentiation of the genital tract in the male fetus, but not in the female fetus, testosterone is responsible for stimulation of the development of internal genitalia, whereas the differentiation of external genitalia is dependent exclusively on DHT.

The relative contributions of testosterone from ovarian and adrenal sources and peripheral conversion of prehormone are presented schematically in Figure 18–2. On the basis of testosterone concentrations in the ovarian and adrenal venous blood from normal women, it is estimated that approximately 25 percent of total testosterone production is of adrenal origin and another 25 percent is contributed by the ovaries.[8, 9] The remaining 50 to 60 percent arises from peripheral metabolism of prehormones, principally Δ^4-androstenedione, which is transformed at several sites (including the liver, fat, and skin) and re-enters the circulation as testosterone.[9, 10] The adrenal component of circulating testosterone exhibits a discernible circadian rhythm suppressible by the administration of dexamethasone[2] and increased by ACTH (see Fig. 18–1).

The average daily metabolic clearance rate for testosterone in women is 370 L/24 hr, which is about one third that for Δ^4-androstenedione (about 1100 L/24 hr) (Table 18–3). A daily production rate of 250 μg for testosterone is found in normal women, which is many orders of magnitude lower than that in a man (7 mg/day).[10]

Testosterone and Δ^4-androstenedione are precursors (prehormones) for plasma DHT. Testosterone conversion accounts for at least 70 percent of plasma DHT in the male but for less than 20 percent in the normal female. Δ^4-Androstenedione appears to be the major prehormone for plasma DHT in adult women, accounting for at least two thirds of plasma DHT formed by peripheral conversion.[11] Thus, in women there is little direct ovarian secretion of DHT; instead, DHT is derived from the peripheral conversion of both testosterone and Δ^4-androstenedione. It is suggested, therefore, that the plasma DHT concentration

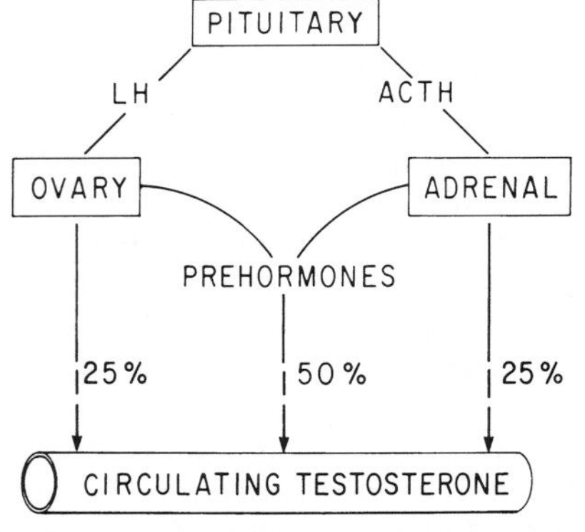

Figure 18–2 ■ The multiple sources of circulating testosterone, showing the relative contribution of ovarian and adrenal secretion and the peripheral conversion of prehormone (principally androstenedione) to the circulating pool of testosterone in normal women. (Modified from Kirschner MA, Zucker IR, Jesperson DL. Ovarian and adrenal vein catheterization studies in women with idiopathic hirsutism. In James VHT, Serio M, Giusti G (eds). The Endocrine Function of the Ovary. New York, Academic Press, 1976, pp 443–456.)

■ TABLE 18–3

Relationship Between Metabolic Clearance Rates of Steroid Hormones and Their Binding Affinity to Sex Hormone–Binding Globulin

STEROID	MCR ($L/m^2/24$ hr) Male	Female	RELATIVE SHBG BINDING*
5α-DHT	340	150	290
Testosterone	635	370	100
Estradiol	1000	800	30
Androstenedione	1300	1100	4

DHT, dihydrotestosterone; SHBG, sex hormone–binding globulin; MCR, metabolic clearance rate.

*Testosterone serves as a reference = 100.

in normal women may reflect activity in peripheral target tissues for androgen.

The metabolic clearance rate for DHT is relatively low, with a mean of 150 L/day. This slow clearance is related, at least in part, to the high binding affinity to SHBG (see Table 18–3). The mean daily production rate is 56 μg in normal women, which is about one sixth that in adult men (300 μg/day).

Δ^5-Androstenediol

Androstenediol is a moderately androgenic steroid that is an intermediate metabolite in the formation of testosterone from DHEA in humans.[12] The Δ^5-androstenediol concentration in men averages 20 percent of the testosterone level, but in women it is nearly twice the testosterone value.[13] Like other C_{19} steroids, Δ^5-androstenediol exhibits a diurnal rhythm (see Fig. 18–1). It has a strong affinity for albumin but binds much less strongly to SHBG.[14] The mean metabolic clearance rate for men and women is 1300 and 850 L/day, respectively. The calculated blood production rates are 1300 μg/day for men and 1000 μg/day for women.[14] Estrogen treatment in men has been shown to decrease the metabolic clearance rate toward the value found in women.[14] In hirsute women, the production of Δ^5-androstenediol is twofold higher than normal, and this is associated with an increased metabolic clearance rate of Δ^5-androstenediol.[14] In normal women, peripheral metabolism of DHEA contributes one third of Δ^5-androstenediol production; in hirsute women, it accounts for half of the total production. The remainder of the circulating Δ^5-androstenediol appears to be secreted by the ovary and adrenal.[15] Thus, the circulating concentrations of Δ^5-androstenediol reflect DHEA and DHEA-S metabolism.

DHEA and DHEA-S

DHEA and DHEA-S represent the major androgen precursors secreted by the adrenal, with small amounts of DHEA derived from the ovary. It has been estimated that in young adult women, 16 mg of DHEA is produced daily, of which less than 10 percent can be accounted for by ovarian secretion.[16] DHEA-S is exclusively adrenal in origin with a production rate of 19 mg/day. The circulating half-life for DHEA is approximately 25 minutes. This relatively short half-life is due, in large measure, to its extensive transformation to DHEA-S through sulfotransferase in the liver and peripheral tissues. The plasma half-life for DHEA-S, in contrast, is about 10 hours.[12] The metabolic clearance rate for DHEA is 1600 L/day, whereas the metabolic clearance rate for DHEA-S is only 15 L/day. DHEA-S appears to be hydrolyzed continuously, thus contributing about 28 percent to the pool of free DHEA. This may explain why circulating DHEA levels are maintained at relatively high basal levels despite a short half-life. Likewise, free DHEA is constantly sulfated to DHEA-S (~ 31 percent).[17, 18] Circulating concentrations for normal adult women range from 1.5 to 6 ng/ml for DHEA and 0.75 to 2.5 μg/ml for DHEA-S.

The metabolic pathways and interconversions of DHEA and DHEA-S are shown in Figure 18–3. Many of these conversions take place in peripheral tissues, such as the formation of androstenediol, testosterone, DHT, and estrogens. The relative degree of conversions and interconversions is substrate dependent; when circulating levels of DHEA are increased, the precursor-product transformations increase manyfold, indicating that the enzymatic systems are present in abundance in peripheral tissues.[19] Thus, as relatively impotent androgens, DHEA and DHEA-S may serve as a reserved pool of precursors for peripheral conversion to potent androgens and estrogens when concentrations exceed physiologic ranges.

Circulating levels of DHEA and DHEA-S at birth are higher than those in the upper limits of adult range and fall rapidly until adrenarche, when a marked increase occurs for both sexes.[20, 21] Concentrations of DHEA and DHEA-S peak during the third decade, reaching levels at least 15-fold that of the prepubertal nadir, and thereafter progressively decline to low levels in senescence.[22, 23] The marked decrease in adrenal secretion of androgen during aging, with small but significant increase in cortisol secretion, is reflected by a marked attenuation of pulsatile secretion (Fig. 18–4). An increase followed by a decrease of 17,20-lyase activity of the 17α-hydroxylase enzyme in the reticularis zone of the adrenal cortex during the periods of "switch on" and "switch off" of DHEA and DHEA-S production from adrenarche to aging,[24–26] together with a 30 percent reduction of the adrenal zona reticularis with aging,[27] may account for the age-related decline.

The importance of the age-related decline in DHEA and DHEA-S is unclear but underscored by observations of

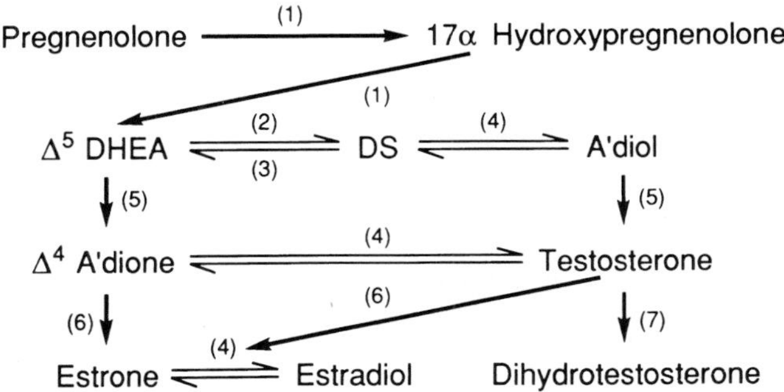

Figure 18–3 ■ Synthesis and biotransformation of DHEA and DHEA-S. Enzymes: (1) bifunctional P450c17 (17-hydroxylase and 17,20-lyase); (2) steroid sulfotransferase; (3) steroid sulfatase; (4) 17-ketosteroid reductase; (5) 3β-hydroxysteroid dehydrogenase/ Δ^5,Δ^4 -isomerase; (6) aromatase; (7) 5α-reductase.

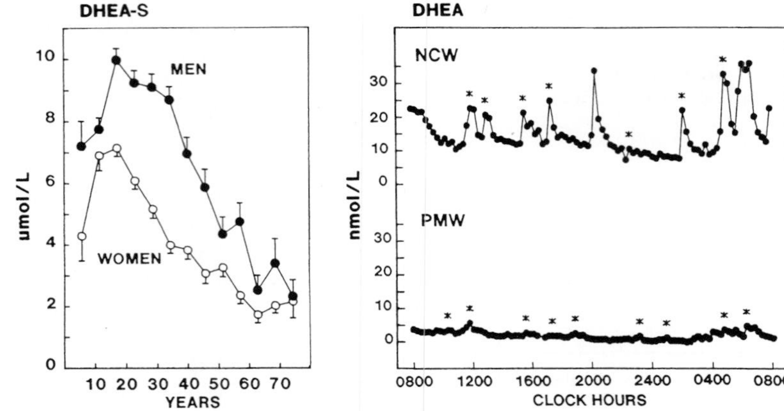

Figure 18–4 ■ Circulating levels of DHEA and DHEA-S according to aging and to the 24-hour day.

Left, Mean serum DHEA-S concentrations decline with chronologic age in men and women. (Modified from Orentreich N, Brind JL, Rizer RL, Vogelman JH. Age changes and sex differences in serum dehydroepiandrosterone sulfate concentration throughout adulthood. J Clin Endocrinol Metab 59:551–555, 1984.)

Right, Representative 24-hour pulsatile secretion of adrenal DHEA in cycling women during the early follicular phase (NCW) and in aged postmenopausal women (PMW). (From Liu CH, Laughlin GA, Fischer UG, Yen SSC. Marked attenuation of circadian pulsatile secretion of dehydroepiandrosterone in postmenopausal women: Evidence for a reduced 17,20-desmolase enzymatic activity. J Clin Endocrinol Metab 71:900–906, 1990. © The Endocrine Society.)

protective effects of DHEA on diabetes, cancer, aging, and autoimmune diseases in experimental animals. These multifunctional properties of DHEA have led to recent clinical trials. Replacement of DHEA in aging populations using different doses, duration, route of administration, experimental designs, and endpoints have generated favorable results in the context of restoration of serum DHEA and DHEA-S to youthful levels and improvement of cognitive and well-being effects.[28–32] Serum DHEA and DHEA-S are negatively correlated with IL-6, a cytokine that is one of the pathogenetic factors in age-related diseases. In vitro, DHEA and androstenedione inhibited IL-6 production from peripheral blood mononuclear cells of both men and women.[33] These findings are highly suggestive that DHEA provides immunomodulatory properties with potentials to improve immunosenescence.[33] A multicenter trial is required to define the role of DHEA in aging and age-related diseases.

Androstanediol (3α-diol)

Of particular relevance to androgen action in the target cells is the formation of DHT and 3α-diol from testosterone and other prehormones (Δ^4-androstenedione, Δ^5-androstenediol, and DHEA). This process requires the enzyme 5α-reductase, the activity of which is increased by the presence of testosterone and DHT.[34] The subsequent conjugation of 3α-diol to glucuronide with the formation of 3α-diol glucuronide occurs not in the usual sites (liver and gut) but in the sexual target tissue, such as skin and sebaceous glands, where β-glucuronidase enzyme has been identified.[35, 36] The circulating levels of this conjugated metabolite reflect closely the utilization of androgens by the target tissues.

Specific Hormone-Binding Globulins

The bulk of steroid and thyroid hormones that circulate in the plasma are bound by albumin and globulins. Albumin is present in abundance, and it is the principal steroid binder in circulation. It is of low affinity and readily dissociable, and therefore the albumin-bound fraction is bioavailable for target cells.[37] Specific binding globulins exist for all biologically potent hormones (Table 18–4): (1) corticoid-binding globulin, or transcortin, has high-affinity binding for cortisol and progesterone; (2) thyroid-binding globulin, for thyroid hormones; and (3) SHBG, or testosterone-estradiol–binding globulin, for androgens and estrogens. In the globulin-bound form, these steroids are not readily available for target tissue action. The transport and bioavailability of steroid hormone action on target cells depend on the following dynamics[37–39]:

- The free (non–SHBG-bound) and the albumin-bound fractions are available for target cells.
- The balance between capillary transit time (blood flow) and the rate of dissociation from binding proteins determines the delivery of free hormones to receptors of the target cells.
- The relative binding of SHBG and corticoid-binding globulin to their specific membrane receptors determines the degree of steroid hormone action without interaction with the intracellular nuclear steroid receptor (see later).

Quantitative changes in these parameters as well as circulating levels of the binding proteins occur in certain disease states and provide valuable information for endocrine manifestations of the several types of apparent hormone excess or deficiency.

Properties of Sex Hormone–Binding Globulin

Synthesized in the liver, SHBG exists as a homodimeric glycoprotein with a 20 to 30 percent carbohydrate moiety and a molecular weight of approximately 90 kDa. The homodimer is formed by the association of two identical subunits that are differentially glycosylated.[40, 41] The bind-

■ TABLE 18–4

Relative Distribution of Steroid and Thyroid Hormones to Plasma Binding Proteins and Their Half-Time Dissociation in Seconds ($d^{t1/2}$) at 37°C

HORMONE	PERCENT GLOBULIN-BOUND	$d^{t1/2}$	PERCENT ALBUMIN-BOUND	$d^{t1/2}$	PERCENTAGE FREE
Sex Hormone–Binding Globulin					
DHT	78	100	21	4	1
T	66	20	33	4	2
E_2	37	7	61	4	2
Thyroid-Binding Globulin					
T_4	70	40	20	4	0.03
T_3	40	4	35	4	0.4
Corticoid-Binding Globulin					
Cortisol	90	1	7		4
P_4	17	<1	80		2

DHT, dihydrotestosterone; T, testosterone; E_2, estradiol; T_4, thyroxine; T_3, triiodothyronine; P_4, progesterone.
Data from Pardridge WM. Transport of protein-bound hormones into tissues in vivo. Endocr Rev 2:103–123, 1981; and Anderson DC. Sex-steroid-binding globulin. Clin Endocrinol (Oxf) 3:69–96, 1974.

ing affinity of SHBG for testosterone at 37°C (10^9 $mole^{-1}$) is one or two orders of magnitude less than that of the intracellular receptor protein and 30,000 times greater than that of serum albumin.[40]

SHBG has one binding site per mole. Synthetic steroids may compete with endogenous steroid for the SHBG steroid-binding site.[42] The percentages of SHBG and of albumin-bound and free testosterone in plasma and the rates of dissociation relative to other hormones are presented in Table 18–4. SHBG has a rapid rate of dissociation, with a half-time of about 20 seconds for testosterone and 7 seconds for estradiol. In comparison to the binding affinity for testosterone, SHBG has three times the affinity for DHT but about one third that for estradiol. Δ^5-Androstenediol binds less strongly than does testosterone, and there is virtually no SHBG binding of Δ^4-androstenedione or DHEA. The metabolic clearance rate of sex steroids is inversely related to their relative binding affinity to SHBG (see Table 18–3), and therefore alterations of SHBG concentrations influence sex steroid metabolism and action.[37–41, 43]

Although the non–SHBG-bound (free) testosterone in blood correlates with the manifestation of androgenicity,[44] the functionality of SHBG may be more complex than previously appreciated. SHBG is an allosteric protein with both steroid and membrane binding sites. When free SHBG is bound to its membrane receptor, it activates the intracellular second messenger but retains the ability to bind sex steroids.[38, 45] Moreover, SHBG itself can enter the cell, and the steroid-SHBG–membrane receptor complex can be internalized.[38] Although the physiologic significance is under study, these new insights have already provided a broader view of SHBG function.

Hormonal Influence of SHBG Concentrations: Estrogens and Androgens

The plasma concentration of SHBG is twice as high in adult women as in adult men. This sex difference is due to the fact that SHBG production is promoted by estrogen and inhibited by androgen. Thus, hirsute women with elevated androgen levels have lower SHBG concentrations than do normal women (Fig. 18–5). Conversely, estrogen administration to normal adult men within 2 weeks induces an elevation of SHBG, with a resulting increase in the percentage of SHBG-bound plasma testosterone to levels comparable with those found in normal women.

Because of this high sensitivity of SHBG synthesis to *estrogen augmentation* and *androgen inhibition*, the level of circulating SHBG is viewed as a major controlling factor in the balance between biologically active androgens and estrogens.[43] This relationship is an important factor in the interpretation of circulating hormone levels and biologic action at target tissues.

Other Hormonal Influences

Low SHBG concentrations may also result from administration of progestogens with the exception of medroxy-

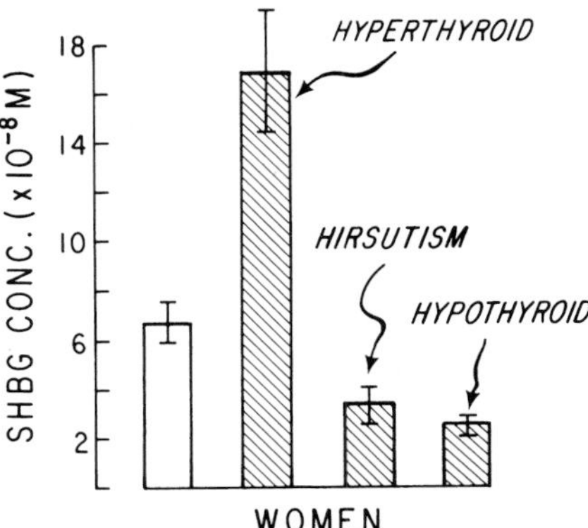

Figure 18–5 ■ Effects of thyroid hormone excess (hyperthyroid) and deficiency (hypothyroid) and hirsutism (androgen excess) on sex hormone–binding globulin (SHBG) concentrations. The open bar represents SHBG concentrations in normal women. Not shown here is the inhibitory effect of hyperinsulinemia on hepatic SHBG production. (Modified from Anderson DC. Sex-hormone-binding globulin. Clin Endocrinol [Oxf] 3:69–96, 1974.)

progesterone; from glucocorticoid excess, as in Cushing's syndrome; from growth hormone excess, as in acromegaly; and from thyroid hormone deficiency.[43, 46, 47] Thyroid hormone excess from either exogenous or endogenous sources is associated with a marked elevation of SHBG levels (see Fig. 18–5). Men of advancing age[48] show a modest increase in SHBG levels, and both men and women with obesity[46] show a modest decrease. *Hyperinsulinemia* has a direct *inhibitory* effect on hepatic SHBG production.[49] Prepubertal girls show high levels of SHBG, with a 30 percent decrease at the time of puberty.[50] Conditions and drugs that influence SHBG concentrations are listed in Table 18–5.

EXTRAGLANDULAR FORMATION OF ESTROGEN

Physiology

In cycling women, most of the estrogen in the body is derived from ovarian secretion of estradiol; however, a significant portion comes also from the extraglandular conversion of androstenedione to estrone and, to a lesser extent, testosterone and estrone conversions to estradiol. It is estimated that 1.3 percent of androstenedione is converted to estrone and only 0.15 percent of testosterone is converted to estradiol.[51]

Although the percentage of conversion is small, the relatively high daily production rate of androstenedione (3 mg) by the adrenal and the ovary results in a significant amount of estrone formation by this route. It is estimated that up to *40 μg of estrone* comes from androstenedione precursor in adult women each day (Fig. 18–6). The contribution of estrone derived from conversion of androstenedione is substantially increased in anovulatory states owing to increased substrate availability (Fig. 18–7).

The aromatization of androgens to estrogens has been demonstrated in several tissue sites where P450 aromatase enzyme (P450arom) is found. The human P450arom gene *(CYP19)* contains 10 exons and is located on chromosome 15q21. It is expressed in the placenta, ovary, testis, brain, muscle, skin, adipocytes, and epithelial and stromal cells of the breast.[52]

■ TABLE 18–5

Factors Having an Impact on the Concentration of Sex Hormone–Binding Globulin (SHBG) in Plasma

INCREASED SHBG	DECREASED SHBG
Increased thyroid hormone	Obesity/hyperinsulinemia
Increased estrogens	Syndrome of androgenization in women (polycystic ovary syndrome, hirsutism, hyperinsulinemia, acne)
Pregnancy	Testosterone administration
Luteal phase of menstrual cycle	Hyperprolactinemia
Exogenous estrogens	Increased growth hormone
Cirrhosis of the liver	Puberty/menopause
Phenytoin (Dilantin)	Progestational agents
Tamoxifen	Danazol
Prolonged stress	Glucocorticoids
Carcinoma of the prostate	
Anorexia nervosa	
Aging in men	
High-carbohydrate diet	

From Rosner W. The functions of corticosteroid-binding globulin and sex hormone–binding globulin: Recent advances. Endocr Rev 11:80–91, 1990.

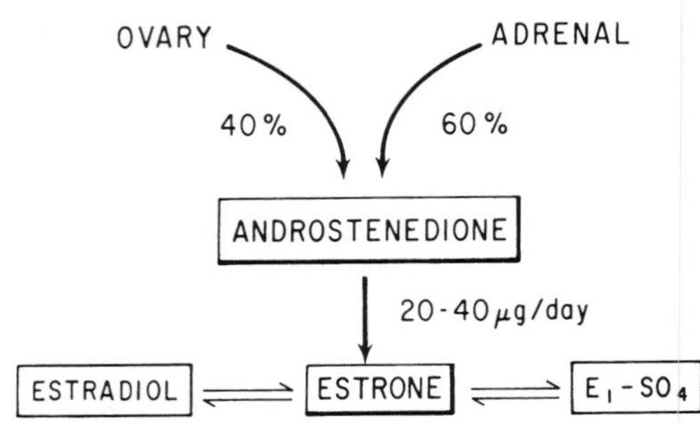

Figure 18–6 ■ Circulating estrone is derived from multiple sources. In addition to ovarian and adrenal contribution of androstenedione, peripheral conversion of androstenedione to estrone represents a major contribution to the circulating pool of estrone. The metabolism of estradiol to estrone and the continuously hydrolyzed estrone sulfate (E_1SO_4) results in additional sources of circulating estrone.

- Muscle and adipose tissue are the major sites of aromatization; muscle tissue accounts for 25 to 30 percent and adipose tissue for 10 to 15 percent of the total extraglandular aromatization of androgens to estrogens.[53, 54] The greater capacity of muscle for this process may explain the higher rate of aromatization observed in men than in women.[51] On the other hand, when there is an increase in the fat compartment, as in obese individuals, adipose tissue constitutes a greater rate of aromatization than does muscle. The fractional conversion of androstenedione is greater than the fractional conversion of testosterone, suggesting that the binding affinity of aromatase is higher for the former than for the latter.
- Although the liver is well known as the major site of metabolism of steroids, the aromatizing process in this organ is limited. In adults, it is responsible for less than 4 percent of overall peripheral aromatization of androgens to estrogens.[55]
- The skin fibroblasts and hair follicles are capable of aro-

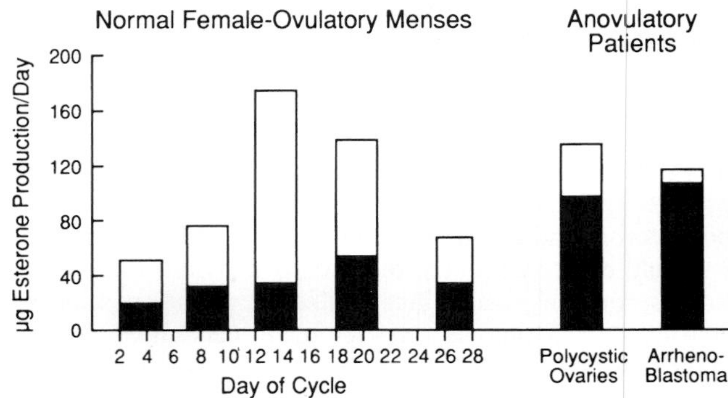

Figure 18–7 ■ The extent of circulating androstenedione conversion to estrone in normal ovulating women is 1.3 percent. The variation of estrone production (μg/day) derived from this route depends on the availability of precursor androstenedione during the menstrual cycle, and it is markedly increased in anovulatory patients with polycystic ovary syndrome and arrhenoblastoma *(right)*. The open portion of each bar represents ovarian secretion, and the black portion represents estrone production derived from utilization of plasma Δ^4-androstenedione. (From MacDonald PC, et al. Progress in Endocrinology. International Congress Series 184. Amsterdam, Excerpta Medica, 1968.)

matizing androgens to estrogens[56, 57] and exert a paracrine action on these target sites rather than contribute to the circulating pool of estrogen.

- The brain, especially the hypothalamus, contains aromatase enzyme, which is responsible for the in situ formation of estrogens from androgen.[58]
- Bone marrow also exhibits aromatizing activity,[59] but the biologic significance is unclear.

Pathophysiology

Under several pathophysiologic conditions, the extraglandular production of estrogen may be excessive, resulting in a relatively constant and elevated level of circulating estrogen. Such acyclic extraglandular estrogen production may occur under circumstances of increased precursors (androgens), enhanced P450arom activity, and enlarged tissue sites for conversion (Fig. 18–8):

- Increased precursor availability, as in congenital adrenal hyperplasia, polycystic ovary syndrome, androgen-producing tumors, and some cases of Cushing's syndrome.[1]
- Aging in men and women, which is associated with a twofold to fourfold increase in extraglandular formation of estrone. This is due, in large measure, to the increase in aromatase enzyme activity in the adipose tissue.[60]
- Increased extraglandular tissue for conversion, as in simple obesity. In the case of obesity associated with Cushing's syndrome, both the increased numbers of adipose cells and the elevated cortisol level may be involved, because the latter has been shown in vitro to induce aromatase activity in human adipose stromal cells.[61]
- Increased conversion of androgens to estrogens, which also occurs in hypothyroidism and hyperthyroidism as a result of alterations of sex steroid metabolism and the enzymatic systems involved in interconversions (see later).
- Estrogen formation in the ovarian follicle (Fig. 18–9). The interaction between the granulosa and theca compartments, which results in accelerated estrogen formation, does not appear to be fully functional until the late stage of antral development. The granulosa cells

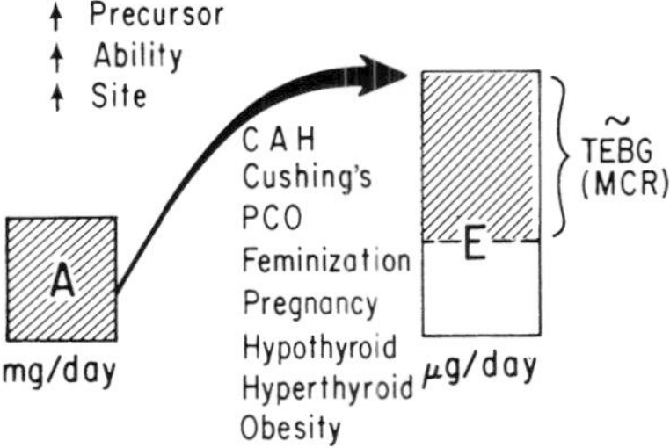

Figure 18–8 ■ Conditions associated with increased extraglandular estrogen production (μg/day). The rate of conversion depends on the size of the androgen (A) pool (mg/day), increased amounts of aromatase (ability), and the mass of conversion site. The shaded are represents the contribution of estrogen pool (E) from androgen pool (A), and it is influenced by the level of testosterone-estradiol–binding globulin (TEBG) and metabolic clearance rate (MCR). CAH, congenital adrenal hyperplasia: PCO, polycystic ovary.

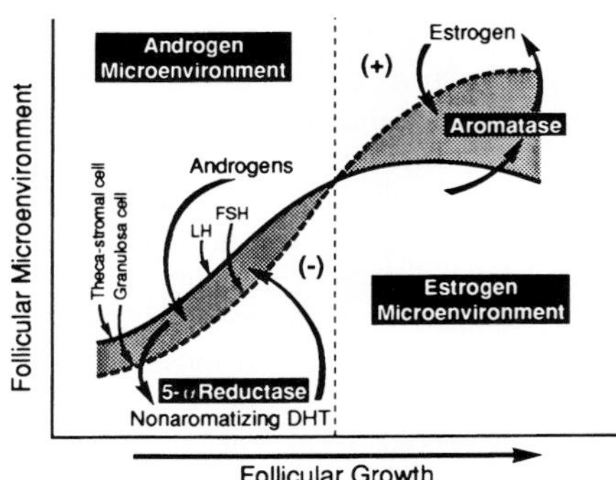

Figure 18–9 ■ Diagrammatic illustration of a shift of microenvironment from androgenic dominance (through 5α-reductase activity) to estrogenic dominance (through aromatase) during the course of follicular maturation.

from human preantral follicles possess the ability to convert Δ^4-androstenedione to more potent androgens rather than estrogens.[62] This process is mediated by the presence of 5α-reductase, which catalyzes the formation of the nonaromatized androgen DHT from testosterone. In contrast, granulosa cells isolated from large antral follicles exhibit marked aromatase activity, which converts androgens to estrogens. Thus, a shift from the androgenic microenvironment to an estrogenic microenvironment may be the major determinant for the autoregulation in the gonadotropin-dependent selection and maintenance of the dominant follicle[62, 63] (see Fig. 18–9).

In chronic anovulation states, follicle maturation does not occur, and consequently the microenvironment of the ovarian apparatus is shifted from the cyclic estrogen dominance to a relatively linear process of expression with androgen dominance. Under this hyperandrogenic microenvironment, multiple small follicles may be present as a result of a normal rate of recruitment coupled with follicular arrest.

Because estrone is the principal estrogen formed in extraglandular production, an increase in the estrone to estradiol ratio (E_1:E_2) would be anticipated in patients with an increased peripheral conversion of androstenedione. In addition, the decreased ovarian secretion of E_2, occasioned by the follicular arrest in anovulatory states, can likewise contribute to increased E_1:E_2 ratio in these patients. Thus, analysis of the E_1:E_2 ratio provides clues to the relative contribution of acyclic peripheral versus ovarian sources of estrogens and may reflect the state of chronic anovulation or out-of-phase (functional) uterine bleeding.

Aromatase Excess Syndrome

Increased extraglandular aromatization was first reported in a boy with prepubertal gynecomastia in 1977[64] and subsequently in five members of an African-American kindred in 1985.[65] Pubertal gynecomastia has been associated with an elevated ratio of serum estrogen to androgen[66] and excessive aromatase activity in cultured pubic skin fibroblast from these patients with gynecomastia.[67]

AROMATASE GENE *(CYP19)*

Aromatase, also known as estrogen synthetase, is the key enzyme in estrogen biosynthesis. It is an enzymatic complex composed of the aromatase cytochrome P450 (P450arom) and the flavoprotein NADPH–P450 reductase, which catalyzes the conversion of androgens to estrogens[52] (Fig. 18–10). The human P450arom gene *(CYP19)* contains 10 exons and is located on chromosome 15q21.[68] Tissue-specific regulation of the P450arom messenger ribonucleic acid (mRNA) is ensured by alternative splicing of exon 1 and part of exon 2, driven by at least five major promoter regions located in the 5′ untranslated end of the gene. A number of additional minor complementary deoxyribonucleic acid (cDNA) species have been identified in various tissues, although their functional significance remains uncertain. Both sequences with enhancing and silencing function as well as known responsive elements to a variety of transcription factors have been identified in the regulatory region upstream of the P450arom gene. Because of its complex regulation of function, the 5′ end of the P450arom gene has long been considered a candidate for disorders in which inappropriate aromatase activity is encountered.[68]

AROMATASE EXCESS SYNDROME IS ASSOCIATED WITH FEMINIZATION OF BOTH SEXES

A family with the aromatase excess syndrome has recently been described in which the condition was inherited in an autosomal dominant manner and led to feminization in both sexes. This was associated with the aberrant utilization of a novel transcript of the P450arom gene.[69] In this family, there are a boy with pubertal gynecomastia and a girl with isosexual precocious puberty with elevated estrogen levels. The source of estrogen appeared to be extragonadal with increased conversion of adrenal androgen (androstenedione and testosterone) to estrogen (estrone and estradiol, respectively). Indeed, symptoms were manifested shortly after *adrenarche*. Although aromatase excess syndrome has been described in prepubertal boys (see earlier), this is the first report of aromatase excess syndrome in girls. In this kindred, the aromatase excess syndrome was transmitted to the two children from their father, who had peripubertal gynecomastia, elevated serum estrogen levels as an adult, and evidence of increased aromatase activity in vitro. The male to male transmission and expression of the syndrome in a female are compatible with autosomal dominant inheritance in this family.

- Despite increased estrogen levels, males with aromatase excess syndrome appear to be fertile with normal libido despite a small testicular volume (15 ml bilaterally) and low testosterone levels. In general, the inhibitory effects of estrogen on reproductive function appear to be milder in males with this syndrome than in patients receiving exogenous estrogen or with estrogen-producing tumors. This difference may be related to the relatively lower elevation of estrogen levels in aromatase excess syndrome.
- Increased aromatase activity in females appears to be associated with *isosexual precocity* at a young age and a variable degree of *macromastia* in adulthood. These findings are consistent with the major functions of estrogens, that is, the growth and maturation of female secondary sex characteristics, including the breast. Sexual function, fertility, and menstrual periods were normal in the paternal grandmother of these two children, who had increased aromatase activity in vitro. These findings should be contrasted with the dramatic effects of aromatase deficiency in female patients, which include virilization at birth, followed by hypergonadotropic hypogonadism, and sexual infantilism at puberty (see later).
- Both the boy and the girl with the aromatase excess syndrome had greatly advanced bone age; their degree of skeletal maturity was disproportionate to their height (chronologic age $<$ height for age $<$ skeletal age) despite accelerated growth. This situation is seen frequently in untreated precocious puberty, when the rate of skeletal maturation overcomes linear growth. The short stature of their father was also indicative of the potent effect of estrogens on accelerating premature epiphyseal closure. These findings are in sharp contrast with the tall stature and delayed epiphyseal closure of patients with aromatase deficiency (see later). Because of their predicted final height, these patients were treated with an aromatase inhibitor and a gonadotropin-releasing hormone (GnRH) analogue; although the 3-year evaluation indicated an improvement in their final height prediction, the final outcome of this therapy remains to be seen.

In sum, aromatase excess syndrome is a genetically heterogeneous disorder that can be inherited in an autosomal dominant mode and leads not only to heterosexual precocity and gynecomastia in males but also to isosexual precocity and macromastia in females. Increased aromatase

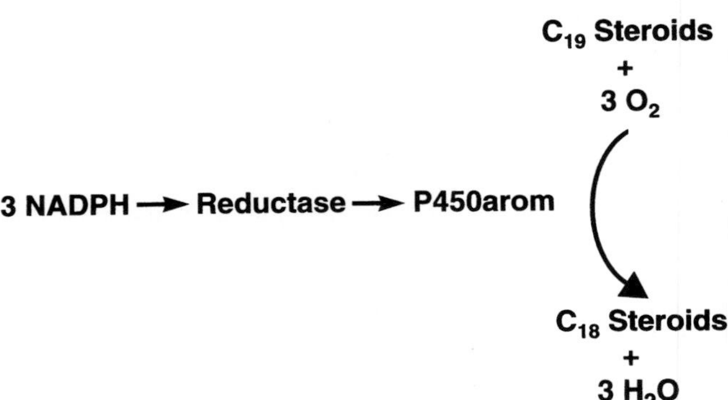

Figure 18–10 ■ Pathways for the conversion of C_{19} steroids to C_{18} steroids by P450arom enzyme.

expression can be shown in skin fibroblast in vitro and appears to be associated with the utilization of a normal exon 1 of the P450arom cDNA. The genetic defect is likely to be located in the 5′ end of the P450arom gene.

Aromatase Deficiency Syndrome

There have been several recent reports in the world literature describing aromatase deficiency, following the first description in 1991 of a Japanese newborn girl with an aromatase P450 (P450arom) gene defect.[70, 71] Until then, aromatase deficiency had been considered incompatible with life, and this dogma may have undermined the efforts of investigators to entertain this diagnosis in suspected cases. To date, one female infant,[70] one adolescent girl,[72] and two adult siblings, a woman and a man,[73] have been found to have P450arom gene defects. Convincingly, *estrogen biosynthesis in all of these patients was virtually absent,* giving rise to a number of anticipated as well as unexpected symptoms. As a result, it is known now that aromatase deficiency is an autosomal recessive condition manifested in 46,XX fetuses by *female pseudohermaphroditism* and, in the case of *adult men, extreme tallness due to unfused epiphyses.* In two of three cases, transient maternal virilization during pregnancy was noted.

GENOTYPE VERSUS PHENOTYPE

Estrogen biosynthesis is catalyzed by an enzyme located in the endoplasmic reticulum of estrogen-producing cells. This enzyme is a member of the cytochrome P450 superfamily, namely, aromatase P450 (P450arom), the product of the *CYP19* gene.[52] P450arom has the capacity to metabolize the three precursors androstenedione, testosterone, and 16α-hydroxydehydroepiandrosterone sulfate (after conversion to 16α-hydroxyandrostenedione) into estrone, estradiol, and estriol, respectively.[74] In humans, the *CYP19* gene and its product P450arom are expressed in ovary, testis, placenta, adipose tissue, and brain. Estrogen levels in the circulation are primarily maintained by aromatase activity in the ovarian granulosa cells of ovulatory women and adipose tissue of men[75] and postmenopausal women.[76] Examination of genomic DNA from the Japanese patient[70, 71] revealed that a consensus splice acceptor site between the coding exon 6 and intron 6 was mutated, resulting in the use of a cryptic acceptor site further downstream in intron 6. This homozygous mutation added an insert of 87 base pairs to P450arom mRNA, resulting in translation of an *abnormal protein with 29 extra amino acids.*[71] The Japanese infant was born with severely virilized external genitalia. At this time, it is not known whether she will have pubertal failure at the expected age. It is possible that in tissues other than the placenta (e.g., the ovary), the original splice site would be recognized despite the point mutation in intron 6.[71] This might lead to normal estrogen production in the ovary.

The second case was an 18-year-old girl with primary amenorrhea and female pseudohermaphroditism.[72] She was found to be a compound heterozygote for two different missense mutations in the heme-binding region of the P450arom gene,[52] one of which comprises the fifth coordinating ligand of the heme iron and is conserved in all P450 family members. Finally, studies of a 27-year-old woman and her 24-year-old brother, both affected by aromatase deficiency, have been reported.[73] Both were found to have the same homozygous missense mutation in a highly conserved region of the P450arom gene believed to guard the substrate access channel. In all of these cases, in vitro transient expression of the mutant cDNAs gave rise to only trace amounts of aromatase activity. Various point mutations in the *CYP19* (P450arom) gene have given rise to certain common phenotypic features (Table 18–6). In the female, clinical findings include congenital genital ambiguity, pubertal failure, *hypergonadotropic hypogonadism*, and *multicystic ovaries*. The male phenotype for aromatase deficiency is similar in many respects to the previously described case of estrogen receptor deficiency,[77] namely, *extremely tall stature* due to incomplete epiphyseal closure, continued growth into adulthood, and osteoporosis (see later). Laboratory findings in aromatase deficiency are listed in Table 18–7.

■ TABLE 18–6
Clinical Findings in Aromatase Deficiency

	FEMALE	MALE
Fetal life	Virilization of the mother during second half of pregnancy	Virilization of the mother during second half of pregnancy
Genitalia at birth	Clitorimegaly and posterior labioscrotal fusion	Normal male
Childhood	Unremarkable	Unremarkable
Puberty	Absent growth spurt, absent breast development, primary amenorrhea, further enlargement of clitoris, normal development of pubic and axillary hair	Normal pubertal development
Adult	Severe estrogen deficiency, virilization, multicystic ovaries, tallness	Extremely tall (>3 SD) with continued linear growth into adulthood, osteoporosis, macro-orchidism, infertility?

LESSONS FROM AROMATASE DEFICIENCY SYNDROMES

First, aromatase deficiency is not a universally lethal defect as once believed. This pertains, because two homozygous

■ TABLE 18–7
Laboratory Findings in Aromatase Deficiency

Mother (pregnant woman)	Extremely low maternal serum estradiol or estriol, markedly elevated maternal serum testosterone
Infancy (girls)	Elevated FSH and undetectable serum estradiol
Puberty (girls)	Sonographic examination: multicystic ovaries, retarded bone age, markedly elevated FSH and LH, mildly elevated levels of testosterone and androstenedione
Adult (man)	Undetectable estrone or estradiol in serum despite markedly elevated FSH and LH, severely retarded bone age with unfused epiphyses, densitometric and biochemical evidence of osteoporosis, elevated basal insulin level, decreased HDL to LDL cholesterol ratio, abnormal semen analysis?

siblings were conceived. Estrogens may not be necessary for successful implantation or embryonic or fetal development. On the other hand, aromatase expression in human placenta appears to be necessary for the clearance of DHEA-S from fetal and maternal adrenals by conversion into estrogens. Otherwise, placental sulfatase, 3β-hydroxysteroid dehydrogenase/Δ^{4-5}-isomerase, and 17β-hydroxysteroid dehydrogenase have the capacity to convert this precursor into testosterone. This results in enough testosterone production to create severe virilization of female genitalia in early embryonic life. The same level of androgen exposure of the aromatase-deficient male fetus does not cause any genital abnormalities at birth, which is consistent with the findings in male fetuses affected by congenital adrenal hyperplasia.

Aromatase-deficient girls at puberty[72, 73] revealed the presence of multiple large ovarian cysts. This is probably due to high levels of gonadotropins in the absence of estrogen and possibly inhibin feedback. The ovarian biopsy from one of the aromatase-deficient girls at puberty was reported to have findings similar to the polycystic ovary syndrome.[73] Comparable histologic features were found in the ovaries of estrogen receptor–disrupted transgenic mice.[78]

ADRENAL DYSFUNCTION

Hyperfunction and hypofunction of the adrenal gland are frequently associated with chronic anovulation and amenorrhea. Hormones produced by the adrenal gland—both androgens and cortisol—have potent biologic effects on virtually all tissues in the body, including the brain. The development of abnormal HPO interaction secondary to dysfunction of adrenal hormones, therefore, may be multifactorial. The site of disturbance may be central or peripheral, but it is usually a combination of both. A discussion of normal and abnormal adrenal functions as well as the mechanisms of associated chronic anovulation follows.

Regulation of Adrenal Cortical Function

The adrenal cortex in an adult makes up about 90 percent of the gland and surrounds the centrally located medulla. It is composed of three zones:

1. The zona glomerulosa, the outer layer, produces aldosterone (mineralocorticoids) and constitutes about 15 percent of the cortex.
2. The zona fasciculata, the middle layer, produces cortisol and constitutes about 75 percent of the cortex.
3. The zona reticularis, the inner layer, produces mainly androgens but also produces small amounts of cortisol and constitutes about 10 percent of the cortex.

Actions of ACTH on the Adrenal Cortex

Steroidogenesis. The primary action of ACTH on the adrenal cortex is to increase cortisol secretion by increasing its synthesis: intra-adrenal cortisol storage is minimal.[79, 80] ACTH depletes adrenal cholesterol content,[81] which correlates with enhanced steroid synthesis.[82]

- ACTH acts by binding to specific cell surface receptors.[83, 84] There is a single class of high-affinity receptors with an apparent dissociation constant (K_a) of 1.6 nmol/L. About 9600 sites are present on each adrenocortical cell. Extracellular calcium is required for optimal ACTH binding[83] but not ACTH-induced steroidogenesis. Release of intracellular calcium may play a role in steps subsequent to ACTH binding.[80, 84] ACTH binding promotes adenylate cyclase activation, which increases cyclic adenosine monophosphate (cAMP) concentration, which in turn activates cAMP-dependent protein kinase (protein kinase A) and phosphorylation of a number of proteins.[85] Most if not all of the actions of ACTH appear to be mediated through cAMP.[86–88]
- The effects of ACTH on steroidogenesis can be divided into acute effects, which occur within minutes, and chronic effects, which require hours or days.[89, 90] The acute effect of ACTH is to increase conversion of cholesterol to Δ^5-pregnenolone, the initial and rate-limiting step in cortisol biosynthesis.[80, 89, 90] As discussed later, this effect is mediated by activation of existing side-chain cleavage enzyme P450scc. In contrast, the chronic effects of ACTH involve increased synthesis of most of the enzymes of the steroidogenic pathway and more general actions of adrenocortical cell protein RNA and DNA synthesis and cell growth.[80, 89, 90] When ACTH levels are low such as after hypophysectomy or during glucocorticoid administration, steroid biosynthesis declines and there is a dramatic decrease in the levels of all steroidogenic P450 enzymes[89] and in protein and RNA synthesis.[85, 90] With prolonged ACTH deficiency or suppression, the adrenal glands become small and atrophic. These changes are reversed by ACTH administration, although steroidogenesis may take several days to return to normal and return of adrenal size to normal takes even longer. ACTH is essential for normal steroidogenesis, and it is required but is not sufficient, by itself, to maintain normal adrenal size.[91, 92]
- ACTH also increases the synthesis of other proteins required for steroidogenesis, such as the low-density lipoprotein (LDL) receptor, which is required for uptake of circulating cholesterol; adrenodoxin,[93] which is needed for transfer of reducing equivalents; sterol carrier protein 2,[94, 95] which is required for transport of cholesterol from intracellular lipid stores to mitochondria; and in fetal but not adult adrenals, hydroxymethylglutaryl–coenzyme A (HMG-CoA) reductase,[96] which catalyzes the rate-limiting step in *de novo* cholesterol biosynthesis. The increase in HMG-CoA reductase synthesis and part of the increase in LDL receptor synthesis are thought to be secondary to cholesterol depletion rather than to a direct action of ACTH or cAMP.[94, 96] HDL can also provide cholesterol for steroidogenesis in the adrenal cortex (see Chapter 7 for details).

Extra-adrenal Actions of ACTH

Large doses of ACTH increase glucose and amino acid transport into muscle cells,[97] increase hepatic protein synthesis,[98] and increase cAMP concentration and stimulate lipolysis in adipocytes.[99] Physiologic levels of ACTH do not cause these effects, but markedly elevated plasma ACTH concentrations, such as those observed in some patients with *Nelson's syndrome* or untreated *Addison's disease*, may do so. ACTH has weak melanotropic activity and, alone or together with β-lipotropin, may be the major cause of *hyperpigmentation* when plasma pro-opiomelanocortin (POMC) peptide levels are elevated as in Nelson's syndrome or Addison's disease.

Normal Patterns of ACTH and Cortisol Secretion

Pulsatile Secretion. ACTH is secreted in brief episodic bursts, which cause rises in plasma cortisol concentrations, followed by slower declines because of cortisol's prolonged clearance from plasma. The normal diurnal rhythm results from changes in ACTH secretory episodes in amplitude but not in frequency. ACTH pulse amplitudes reach a maximum during the last few hours before and the hour after awakening and then decline throughout the morning and are minimal in the evening.[100] Consequently, plasma ACTH and cortisol levels are highest at about the time of waking in the morning, are low in the late afternoon and evening, and reach a nadir an hour or two after sleep begins. Additional secretory episodes frequently coincide with lunch and sometimes with dinner and are dependent on the protein content of the meal.[101, 102]

Regulation of Glucocorticoid Secretion

THE HYPOTHALAMIC-PITUITARY-ADRENAL AXIS

Glucocorticoid secretion is regulated by hormonal interactions among the hypothalamus, the pituitary, and the adrenal glands and by neural and other stimuli.[103–105] Neural stimuli from the brain, as in the response to stress, cause the release into the hypothalamic-hypophysial portal blood of corticotropin-releasing factor (CRF), arginine vasopressin (AVP), and other agents from hypothalamic neurons. They are carried to the pituitary where they stimulate ACTH secretion into the systemic blood. ACTH acts on the adrenal cortex to cause secretion of cortisol and other steroids. The negative feedback loop is completed by the inhibitory effect of glucocorticoids on CRF, AVP, and ACTH synthesis and secretion (see Chapter 2 for details).

PRO-OPIOMELANOCORTIN

Structure, Synthesis, and Processing. ACTH is synthesized as part of a large precursor (241 amino acids in humans), POMC, which also contains the sequences for other peptides, including the lipotropins, melanocyte-stimulating hormones, and β-endorphin[106–108] (Fig. 18–11). The human POMC gene is located on chromosome 2[109] and consists of three exons separated by two large introns.[106–108] The gene structure is the same in different species, and there is considerable sequence homology. Exon 3 codes for most of the translated sequence, and exon 2 codes for the signal peptide and the 18 NH_2-terminal amino acids of POMC. Multiple peptides are produced from the POMC precursor by enzymatic cleavage (see Fig. 18–11).

ACTH is processed from POMC within the corticotroph of the anterior pituitary gland. The topograph of corticotrophs in the human adult pituitary, as determined by immunoreactive POMC fragments, reveals that cells staining with β-endorphin, β-lipotropin, and ACTH are confined mainly around the junction of pars intermedia–like cells and the posterior lobe. Only a paucity of cells stain with a specific melanocyte-stimulating hormone antiserum. It therefore appears that the human pituitary contains subtypes of corticotrophs.[110] The synthesis and secretion of ACTH are under control of hypothalamic CRF. Administration of hCRF at a dose of 1 μg/kg causes a prompt release of ACTH and cortisol resembling those physiologic secretory episodes (see Chapter 2 for details).[111]

Glucocorticoid exerts a negative feedback action at both the hypothalamic CRF neurons and the pituitary corticotrophs; it inhibits synthesis and release of POMC-related peptides of the corticotroph mediated through glucocorticoid receptors, and it also inhibits CRF release by acting at the specific receptors in the paraventricular nuclei as demonstrated both in vivo and in vitro (see Chapter 2).

Regulation of Mineralocorticoid Secretion

The major circulating mineralocorticoid is aldosterone, which is synthesized exclusively in the zona glomerulosa.

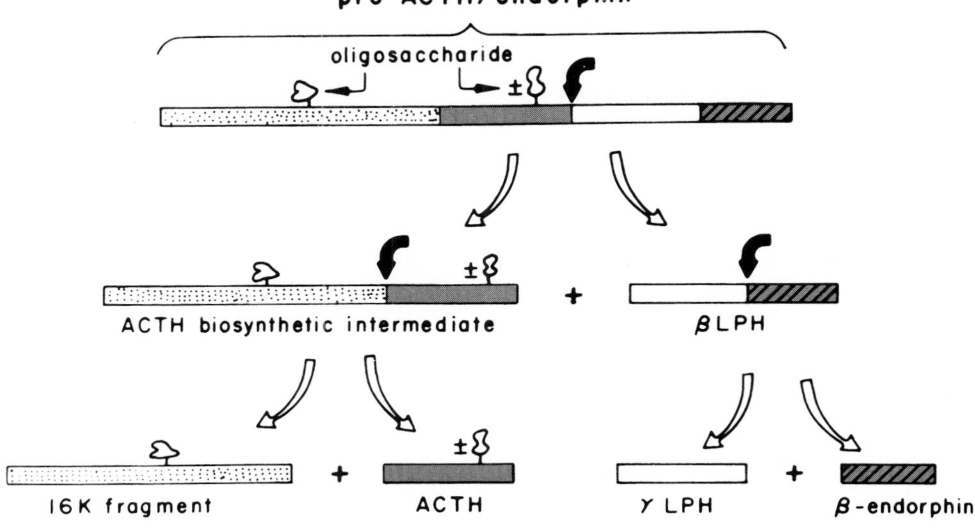

Figure 18–11 ■ Schematic drawing of the 31-kDa precursor for both ACTH and β-lipotropin (BLPH) and for other polypeptides thought to be derived from β-lipotropin. (From Mains RE, Eipper BA. Synthesis and secretion of corticotropins, melanotropins, and endorphins by rat intermediate pituitary cells. J Biol Chem 254:7885–7894, 1979. Used by permission.)

Its precursors, 18-hydroxycorticosterone, corticosterone, and deoxycorticosterone, also have weak mineralocorticoid activity. The three precursors are synthesized in all three zones of the adrenal cortex, but 18-hydroxycorticosterone is produced predominantly in the zona glomerulosa, so its secretion correlates with that of aldosterone. Much more corticosterone and deoxycorticosterone are produced in the zona fasciculata than in the zona glomerulosa. Their secretion correlates with that of cortisol and is ACTH dependent.[112, 113] Cortisol also has modest mineralocorticoid activity, which becomes significant during the hypercortisolemia of Cushing's syndrome. Secretion of 18-oxygenated cortisol derivatives, which have weak mineralocorticoid activity and are implicated in the hypertension of glucocorticoid-suppressible aldosteronism, is also ACTH dependent.[114] 19-Nordeoxycorticosterone is a potent mineralocorticoid that is produced by extraglandular conversion of 19-oxygenated deoxycorticosterone precursors and may be involved in the pathogenesis of some forms of hypertension.[115]

Although acute ACTH administration increases the plasma concentration,[115] aldosterone secretion, unlike that of cortisol, is governed by multiple factors that have complex regulatory interactions.[116, 117] The renin-angiotensin system and potassium ion are the major regulators; ACTH and other POMC-derived peptides, sodium ion, and other agents such as AVP, dopamine, atrial natriuretic factor, β-adrenergic agents, serotonin, and somatostatin are minor modulators. These factors regulate aldosterone secretion by modulating one or more biosynthetic steps. The early step is the conversion of corticosterone to aldosterone,[116] catalyzed by a single mitochondrial enzyme, cytochrome P450c11AS.[118]

Regulation of Adrenal Androgen and Estrogen Secretion

ADRENAL ANDROGENS

The major androgens secreted by the adrenal cortex are DHEA, DHEA-S, and androstenedione.[119, 120] They are not effective androgens (see Table 18–2), but they can be converted to the potent androgens testosterone and 5α-dihydrotestosterone in peripheral tissues. Peripheral conversion contributes significantly to circulating testosterone levels in women but not in men, in whom testosterone is produced predominantly by the testis. Peripheral tissues also interconvert DHEA and DHEA-S through sulfotransferase and sulfatase, respectively. During the follicular phase of the menstrual cycle, the adrenal glands of women secrete 3 to 4 mg of DHEA, 7 to 14 mg of DHEA-S, 1 to 1.5 mg of androstenedione, and 50 μg of testosterone per day.[119] This accounts for about 50 percent, more than 90 percent, and about 50 percent of circulating DHEA, DHEA-S, and androstenedione, respectively. An additional 30 percent of circulating DHEA arises from peripheral conversion of DHEA-S. In women, about 67 percent and 50 percent of the plasma testosterone and 5α-dihydrotestosterone, respectively, come from androstenedione.[2, 119] The ovaries produce the remainder. Androstenedione and testosterone levels rise at midcycle because of increased ovarian secretion. Adrenal secretion of androgens in men is similar to that in women during the follicular phase.

Possible Stimulators of Adrenal Androgen Secretion

ACTH. Control of adrenal androgen secretion is less well understood than that of glucocorticoids and mineralocorticoids. ACTH clearly plays a role. Plasma DHEA, androstenedione, and testosterone concentrations closely parallel the circadian rhythm in plasma cortisol levels[4, 121] (see Fig. 18–1). Plasma DHEA-S does not exhibit a circadian rhythm because of its longer half-life in the circulation.[120] Similarly, ACTH acutely increases circulating DHEA and androstenedione levels, but 1 or 2 days of treatment is needed before an increase in DHEA-S level can be detected.[22, 119] Dexamethasone administration lowers plasma adrenal androgen levels.[22, 119]

Other Possible Factors. *Prolactin* has been suggested as an androgen-stimulating hormone because of the increase in circulating adrenal androgen levels in some patients with hyperprolactinemia[22, 119] and subsequent fall during bromocriptine treatment.[122, 123] Synergism between prolactin and ACTH stimulation of DHEA and DHEA-S, but not cortisol or androstenedione, secretion of human adrenal cells in vitro was reported by one group[123] but not by others.[22, 124] It seems unlikely that prolactin has a physiologically important effect on adrenal androgen secretion, but an extra-adrenal effect on androgen metabolism has not been excluded.

Insulin-like growth factor type I (IGF-I) has been demonstrated in vitro as an adrenal androgen stimulator. In addition, an increase in IGF-I levels precedes that of androgens during weight gain in patients with anorexia nervosa.[125] Growth hormone and gonadotropins appear to have no direct effect on adrenal androgen secretion.[22]

ADRENAL ESTROGENS

The adrenal cortex secretes estrone and estradiol, but the amounts are minimal compared with those secreted by the ovary. Most adrenal estrogens are derived indirectly from peripheral conversion of androstenedione, mainly in adipose tissue and muscle.[126]

Adrenal Cortical Steroidogenesis. Accumulating evidence indicates that HDL cholesterol may also serve as substrate for human adrenal steroidogenesis. First, in clinical conditions in which delivery of LDL cholesterol to the adrenal is impaired as in the case of abetalipoproteinemia, a hereditary deficiency of apolipoprotein B production associated with absence of LDL from plasma, basal adrenal steroid production is unimpaired.[127, 128] Patients with familial hypercholesterolemia caused by defects in the LDL receptor system also have normal basal steroidogenesis, although the increased rate of steroidogenesis caused by prolonged ACTH administration cannot be sustained by de novo synthesis of cholesterol alone.[127, 129] Second, a receptor for HDL[130] is expressed in steroidogenic tissues, including the adrenal.[131, 132] This receptor, called SR-BI (scavenger receptor, class B, type I), is capable of binding modified lipoproteins of several kinds[130] and mediates the transfer of cholesterol into cells from HDL without the endocytosis of the entire lipoprotein particle, as occurs with LDL (see Chapter 7 for details).[130] The role of the SR-BI in steroidogenesis and its importance in relation to the LDL pathway remain to be elucidated. The adrenal cortex can also synthesize cholesterol de novo from cholesterol formed locally.[133–135]

Steroidogenic Enzymes. Four CYP enzymes (Table 18–8) are involved in adrenal steroid biosynthesis. The CYPs are a large family of oxidative enzymes with a characteristic 450-nm absorbance maximum when reduced with carbon monoxide that serve a variety of biologic functions.[136] These enzymes transfer electrons from NADPH, provided by an electron transport protein intermediary, to molecular oxygen with concomitant oxygenation of a variety of substrates. The steroidogenic CYPs act on various ring carbons of cholesterol. For example, CYP11A1 (side-chain cleavage enzyme) cleaves the side chain from C-21 of cholesterol in adrenal mitochondria. A second mitochondrial enzyme, CYP11B1 (11β-hydroxylase), catalyzes the β-hydroxylation at C-11. Two enzymes of the smooth endoplasmic reticulum, CYP17 (17α-hydroxylase) and CYP21A2 (21-hydroxylase), catalyze hydroxylations at C-17 and C-21, respectively.[136] A fifth enzyme required for adrenal steroidogenesis, 3β-hydroxysteroid dehydrogenase, is also associated with the smooth endoplasmic reticulum and catalyzes the conversion of Δ^5-pregnenolone to Δ^4-progesterone. The biosynthetic pathways for adrenal steroidogenesis are detailed in Chapter 4. SF-1 (steroidogenic factor 1), acting through conserved elements in the proximal promoter regions of all *CYP* genes, is a major but not exclusive regulator of their expression.[137]

Effects of Glucocorticoids. As the first step of action in target cells, glucocorticoids enter the cells through a passive process. They bind to a cytoplasmic glucocorticoid receptor to form a complex that is capable of activating transcription of target genes. The mRNA is translated into new proteins that initiate the biologic action (Fig. 18–12). The cysteine-rich region of the central DNA binding domain forms a finger-like loop structure of 12 amino acids at the base by a zinc ion chelated between two cysteine and histidine residues (see Fig. 18–12).

Effects on Metabolism

Glycogen Metabolism. It was known by the mid-19th century that the adrenal glands are essential for life, but their role in intermediary metabolism was not established

■ TABLE 18–8
Nomenclature for Steroidogenic Enzymes and Their Genes

TRIVIAL NAME	PAST	CURRENT	GENE
Cholesterol side-chain cleavage enzyme; desmolase	P450scc	CYP11A1	*CYP11A1*
3β-Hydroxysteroid dehydrogenase	3βHSD	3βHSD II	*HSD3B2*
17α-Hydroxylase/17,20-lyase	P450c17	CYP17	*CYP17*
21-Hydroxylase	P450c21	CYP21A2	*CYP21A2*
11β-Hydroxylase	P450c11	CYP11B1	*CYP11B1*
Aromatase	P450arom	CYParom	*CYP19*
Aldosterone synthase; corticosterone 18-methylcorticosterone oxidase/lyase	P450c11AS	CYP11B2	*CYP11B2*

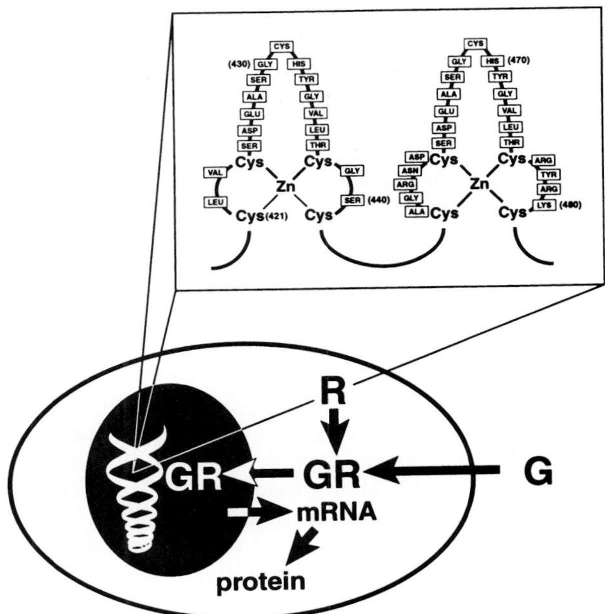

Figure 18–12 ■ Diagrammatic depiction of glucocorticoid (G) action in target cells. After entering the cell by a passive process, G binds to cytoplasmic G receptor (GR) to form a complex. GR enters the nucleus and is capable of activating transcription of target genes. The mRNA is then translated into new proteins that express biologic activity. The putative zinc finger structure in the DNA binding domain functions as a transcriptional regulatory factor.

until 1927 when it was noted that adrenalectomized animals cannot maintain hepatic glycogen stores.[138] Replacement of adrenocortical steroids reversed both glycogen depletion and hypoglycemia in fasting adrenalectomized animals.[139] Glucocorticoids both activate glycogen synthase[140, 141] and inactivate the glycogen-mobilizing enzyme glycogen phosphorylase.[141] The total amount of glycogen synthase remains unchanged, but the enzyme is activated by dephosphorylation. It is unknown whether glucocorticoids achieve this effect directly by activating a hepatic phosphatase or indirectly by inactivating glycogen phosphorylase, a phosphatase inhibitor.

Gluconeogenesis. Glucocorticoids increase hepatic glucose production in part by increasing substrate availability and stimulating release of glucogenic amino acids from peripheral tissues, such as skeletal muscle.[142] The effect is most apparent when a physiologic replacement dose is administered to adrenalectomized animals.[139] Glucocorticoids also directly activate key hepatic gluconeogenic enzymes, such as glucose-6-phosphatase and phosphoenolpyruvate carboxykinase (PEPCK).[142] The increased PEPCK activity results from glucocorticoid-induced activation of PEPCK gene transcription[143, 144] mediated by interaction of the glucocorticoid type II receptor complex with a specific glucocorticoid response element located in the 5′ flanking region of the PEPCK gene.[144, 145]

Other gluconeogenic hormones such as glucagon and epinephrine are effective without the permissive effect of glucocorticoids.[142, 146] Glucocorticoids enhance the sensitivity of lipolysis to catecholamines in target tissues.[142] The glycerol released during lipolysis provides a substrate for glucose production, and released fatty acids provide an energy source for the process. Glucocorticoids also enhance the sensitivity of lactate production to catecholamine stimulation in muscle. Increased sensitivity also underlies the permissive effect of glucocorticoids on glucagon action, but the mechanism is unknown.[142]

Peripheral Glucose Utilization. In addition to mobilizing substrate for hepatic gluconeogenesis, glucocorticoids inhibit glucose uptake and utilization by peripheral tissues,[147–150] in part by direct inhibition of glucose transport into the cells.[151, 152] The number of glucose transporters and mRNA levels in adipocytes are decreased by glucocorticoids.[153]

Lipid Metabolism. Glucocorticoids acutely activate lipolysis in adipose tissue.[150] Lipolytic activity and, consequently, plasma free fatty acid levels are reduced in adrenalectomized animals and return to normal within 2 hours after glucocorticoid administration.[154, 155] This permissive effect may be mediated by altered sensitivity to other lipolytic hormones, such as catecholamines and growth hormone,[154–156] but the molecular mechanisms are not known.

Glucocorticoids also exert chronic effects on lipid metabolism. One of the most striking in humans is the redistribution of body fat after chronic glucocorticoid excess. There is relative sparing of the extremities, whereas the dorsocervical and supracervical regions, the trunk, and the anterior mediastinum and mesentery are sites of marked fat deposition. Animals exposed to excess glucocorticoids generally do not exhibit similar fat distribution and may lose weight, although protein loss exceeds that of fat.[157] Hyperinsulinemia resulting from glucocorticoid effects on glucose metabolism may underlie the lipogenic effect,[158] but the reason for the central predisposition for fat deposition is unknown.

Effects on Immunologic Function and Inflammatory Processes

Endogenous glucocorticoid excess suppresses immunologic responses,[159] and reactivation of latent infections, such as tuberculosis, may result from administration of pharmacologic doses of glucocorticoids. Various effects on components of the immunologic and inflammatory responses have been described in vitro, but their relevance to a physiologic role for glucocorticoids in normal immunomodulation is not clear. Immune cells have high-affinity glucocorticoid receptors, but in vitro results have usually been characterized as supraphysiologic hormone concentrations. Moreover, the clinical immunosuppressive and anti-inflammatory properties of glucocorticoids are, in general, observed only when pharmacologic amounts of the hormones are administered.

Hyperadrenalism

Cushing's syndrome is a generic term applied to the manifestation of chronic glucocorticoid excess regardless of the underlying causes (Table 18–9). *Cushing's disease,* originally described in 1912 by Harvey Cushing,[160] refers to the disorder of hypercortisolism resulting from pituitary ACTH hypersecretion (details are presented in Chapter 19). It is imperative that reproductive endocrinologists be familiar with the pathophysiology, clinical manifestations, and laboratory findings of Cushing's syndrome to provide an appropriate diagnosis. Although Cushing's syndrome is a relatively uncommon disorder, it must be considered in the differential diagnosis of polycystic ovary syndrome and other conditions that have common manifestations such as obesity, diabetes, weakness, hirsutism, and menstrual disorders. Among adult patients with Cushing's syndrome, approximately 70 percent have Cushing's disease due to ACTH-secreting microadenoma.[161] There is a female to male ratio of 10 to 1, and the disease is most frequently encountered during the reproductive years (ages 20 to 40 years).[162]

■ TABLE 18–9
Endocrine Laboratory Abnormalities in Cushing's Syndrome of Any Cause

Increased cortisol secretory rate
Increased 24-hr urinary excretion of free cortisol and its metabolites (17-hydroxycorticosteroid or 17-ketogenic steroids)
Loss of normal diurnal rhythm in plasma cortisol concentration with increased late evening and mean daily plasma cortisol concentrations
Relative or absolute resistance to glucocorticoid negative feedback suppression of cortisol secretion

Cushing's disease is covered in Chapter 19. In this chapter, the causes and clinical manifestations of Cushing's syndrome other than pituitary ACTH-secreting adenoma are discussed. During the past decade, it became apparent that nonendocrine tumors secrete hormones and prehormone molecules with clinical manifestations resembling Cushing's disease (Table 18–10). The effects of these hormone-producing tumors are referred to as *ectopic hormone syndromes.*

Ectopic Hormone Syndromes

ECTOPIC ACTH SYNDROME

In the ectopic ACTH syndrome,[163] the nonpituitary tumor secretes ACTH, which stimulates bilateral adrenal hyperplasia and hyperfunction (Fig. 18–13*A*). Increased plasma cortisol concentration suppresses hypothalamic CRF syn-

■ TABLE 18–10
Classification of Cushing's Syndrome

ACTH Dependent
Pituitary ACTH excess
  Nontumor
  Tumor
Ectopic ACTH-secreting tumors
Ectopic CRF-producing tumors

ACTH Independent
Adrenal adenoma
Adrenal carcinoma
Adrenal nodular hyperplasia
Adrenal rest tumor of the ovary
Exogenous corticoid administration

ACTH, adrenocorticotropic hormone (adrenocorticotropin); CRF, corticotropin-releasing factor.

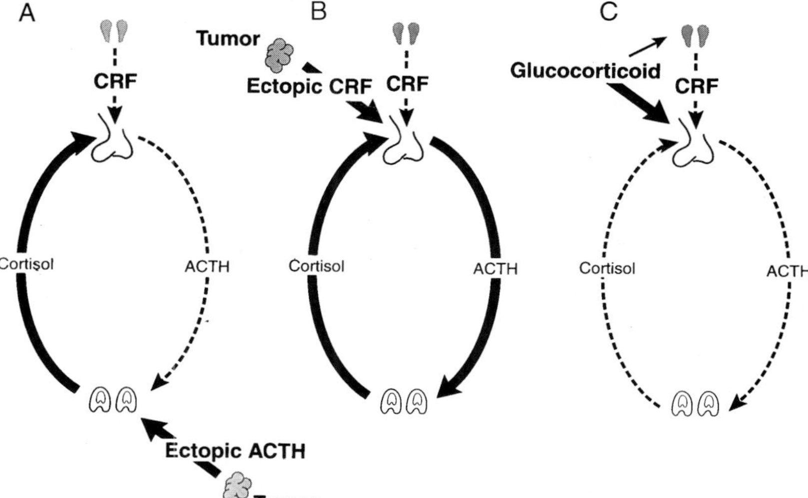

Figure 18–13 ■ Cushing's syndrome caused by hormones outside the CRF-ACTH-adrenal axis: ectopic ACTH-producing tumors *(A)*, ectopic CRF-producing tumors *(B)*, and iatrogenic by pharmacologic doses of glucocorticoids *(C)*. The paraventricular nuclei are shown on top of each panel; solid thick lines depict excessive production; the dotted lines depict inhibitions.

thesis and secretion and blocks CRF action on the normal pituitary corticotrophs, suppressing pituitary ACTH secretion. Except in some bronchial carcinoid tumors,[164–166] tumor secreting ACTH is not regulated by plasma glucocorticoid concentrations. As in Cushing's disease, urinary excretion of cortisol and its precursors is increased proportionately.

ECTOPIC CRF SYNDROME

The ectopic CRF syndrome[167] is similar to the ectopic ACTH syndrome, except that secretion of CRF by the nonhypothalamic tumor stimulates hyperplasia of anterior pituitary corticotrophs[167] and hypersecretion of ACTH (Fig. 18–13*B*). The ACTH stimulates bilateral adrenocortical hyperplasia and hypersecretion of cortisol,[167] which presumably suppresses hypothalamic CRF secretion. Somewhat surprisingly, ACTH secretion is often not suppressed by high glucocorticoid concentrations.[167, 168] This may be related to the fact that the majority of these tumors also produce ACTH,[169–174] and hypercortisolism is actually induced by ectopic ACTH, not CRF. When CRF alone is produced, dosages of dexamethasone higher than 8 mg/day may be required to suppress ACTH secretion.[175]

An interesting variant of this syndrome was produced by a CRF-secreting gangliocytoma composed of hypothalamic-like neurons within the sella turcica and adjacent to the pituitary gland.[176] There was partial (i.e., 40 percent) suppression with low-dose dexamethasone; the high-dose test was not performed. There was also a fourfold increase in urinary 17-hydroxycorticosteroid excretion in response to metyrapone, further indicating that ACTH secretion was responsive to glucocorticoid negative feedback. The corticotrophs were hyperplastic, and the patient recovered normal hypothalamic-pituitary-adrenal function after the tumor was removed.[176] One CRF-producing prostatic carcinoma metastasized to the median eminence and pituitary stalk.[167] ACTH was not suppressed by high-dose dexamethasone, presumably because of high local concentrations of CRF.

ACTH-Independent Cushing's Syndrome

PRIMARY ADRENOCORTICAL HYPERFUNCTION

In Cushing's syndrome caused by primary adrenocortical disease (i.e., adrenocortical tumor, micronodular dysplasia, or ACTH-independent macronodular hyperplasia), increased cortisol secretion suppresses CRF synthesis, release, and action, thereby suppressing POMC synthesis and ACTH secretion (Fig. 18–14). Pituitary corticotrophs atrophy, as does the normal adrenal cortex.

Adrenal carcinomas produce excessive adrenal steroids only because of their size; they are usually inefficient per unit weight in converting cholesterol to cortisol, and

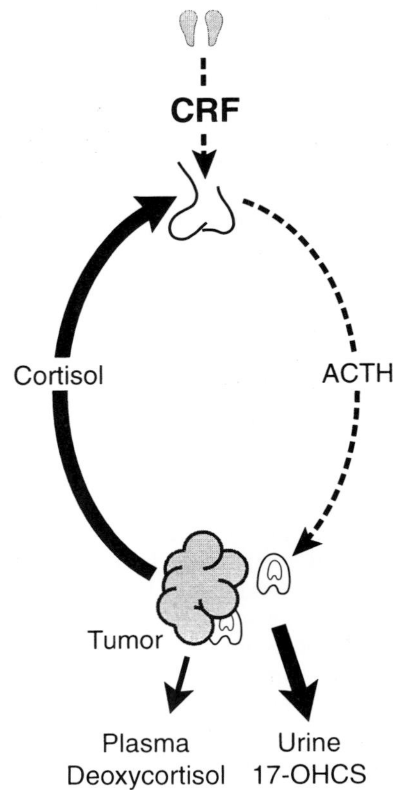

Figure 18–14 ■ Excessive production of cortisol by adrenal adenomas causes inhibition of CRF and ACTH secretion by neurons of the paraventricular nuclei and pituitary corticotrophs, respectively. Plasma and urinary cortisol and its metabolite 17-OHCS are markedly elevated.

production of cortisol precursors is disproportionately high. In contrast, adrenal adenomas can exhibit efficient steroidogenesis, and urinary excretion of DHEA-S and 17-ketosteroids is often low in relation to that of 17-hydroxycorticosteroid or free cortisol and may even be normal. The occasional adenoma may produce relatively large amounts of androgen because of increased expression of cytochrome b_5 with consequent increased 17,20-lyase activity of CYP17.[177] Low aldosterone levels and normal or increased plasma concentrations of aldosterone precursors (i.e., deoxycorticosterone, 18-hydroxydeoxycorticosterone, corticosterone, and 18-hydroxycorticosterone) are found in most adrenal carcinomas but not in adenomas.[178]

On rare occasions, Cushing's syndrome may become evident or more pronounced during pregnancy and may improve or remit spontaneously post partum.[179–181] Most of these patients have adrenal adenomas.[182] The role of placental ACTH and CRF in these cases is unclear. One patient had apparent estrogen-dependent bilateral nodular adrenal hyperplasia.[183]

IATROGENIC CUSHING'S SYNDROME

Iatrogenic Cushing's syndrome is usually caused by administration of excessive amounts of potent synthetic glucocorticoids, rarely by ACTH administration. The exogenous steroid inhibits hypothalamic synthesis and secretion of CRF, suppresses pituitary ACTH synthesis and secretion (Fig. 18–13*C),* and results in bilateral adrenocortical atrophy. Levels of *both* plasma ACTH and cortisol are suppressed.

Endocrine Laboratory Findings

The laboratory findings in endogenous Cushing's syndrome of all causes (see Table 18–9) reflect increased synthesis and secretion of cortisol. The early morning plasma cortisol level may be normal, but the normal circadian rhythm is lost and the late evening plasma cortisol concentration is increased. This leads to increased excretion of free cortisol in saliva[184] and of free cortisol and 17-hydroxycorticosteroid in urine. Urinary and salivary free cortisol reflect plasma free cortisol concentration and are more sensitive indicators of increased cortisol secretion than is urinary 17-hydroxycorticosteroid excretion because they increase more rapidly after plasma cortisol exceeds the binding capacity of corticoid-binding globulin at about 690 nmol/L (25 μg/dl). Similarly, the normal hepatic metabolic pathway becomes saturated at high plasma cortisol concentrations, shunting metabolism toward 6β-hydroxycortisol, which is disproportionately increased in the urine.[185]

Because almost all POMC peptides have been measured in blood and a perfect correlation between lipotropin and ACTH has been found, assessments of lipotropin values in the differential diagnosis for Cushing's syndrome can be made with an equal degree of diagnostic accuracy as with ACTH (Fig. 18–15). The advantages are that no extraction of serum or plasma is needed, serum is stable at room temperature, and only 50-μl samples are required.

Incidentalomas

The incidentally discovered adrenal mass (incidentaloma) is a newly recognized clinical entity disclosed with the advent of high-resolution imaging techniques such as computed tomography (CT) and magnetic resonance imaging (MRI). Most such tumors are benign, and most do not secrete hormones in sufficient amounts to be of clinical importance. However, incidentally discovered adrenal masses may require therapeutic intervention if they are caused by infectious agents; if they secrete excess glucocorticoids, androgens, mineralocorticoids, estrogens, or catecholamines; or if they represent primary or metastatic tumors that can be treated.[186–188]

Studies of the function of adrenal "incidentalomas" have revealed that a proportion of those tumors secrete cortisol insufficiently to produce overt clinical Cushing's syndrome but that their autonomous cortisol production can suppress the hypothalamic-pituitary-adrenal axis to various degrees; this needs to be recognized to avoid acute adrenal insufficiency after adrenalectomy. Several diagnostic approaches have been used to identify the partially autonomous cortisol-secreting adenomas. It has been suggested that a lack of normal suppression of cortisol (>140 nmol/L) on the morning after 1 mg oral dexamethasone at bedtime would identify most functional autonomous cortisol-secreting tumors. On the basis of this criterion, approximately 18 percent of published cases of incidentalomas would secrete cortisol autonomously. However, other test results indicating alterations of the hypothalamic-pituitary-adrenal axis, such as abnormal adrenal iodocholesterol uptake or decreased plasma levels of DHEA-S, were found to be present in up to 79 to 86 percent of incidentalomas. After laparoscopic adrenalectomy, the response of plasma cortisol to 250 μg intravenous $ACTH_{1-24}$ was frequently subnormal and was restored to normal within 2 months. The reader is referred to two excellent reviews in which recommendations for evaluation and treatment are presented.[186, 187]

Prevalence. Adrenal nodules are found at autopsy in about 1 to 10 percent of cases in most series; the prevalence increases with age.[186] CT reveals adrenal masses in 0.35 to 4.36 percent of all such examinations.[188, 189] Approximately 50 percent of incidentally discovered adrenal masses occur in the setting of a known or prior malignant neoplasm or are obviously metastatic lesions.[189] With the further exclusion of cases in which a clinical or biochemical endocrinopathy has already been documented, approximately 0.4 percent of CT scans reveal an unanticipated adrenal nodule.[189]

Pathophysiology. Incidentally discovered adrenal masses may be pheochromocytomas, or adrenocortical adenomas secreting excess glucocorticoids, mineralocorticoids, or androgens. In accumulated series, each of these hypersecreting states has been reported to occur in no more than 10 percent of incidentally discovered nodules.[188] Estrogen secretion in such a setting is extremely rare.

Autonomous cortisol biosynthesis occurs in about 18 percent of incidentally discovered adrenal adenomas.[187] These patients have no overt clinical evidence of glucocorticoid excess and have normal urinary cortisol excretion; however, they demonstrate incomplete suppression of cortisol in the overnight low-dose (3-mg) dexamethasone suppression test, blunted ACTH and cortisol responses to CRF, and loss of circadian rhythm of cortisol secretion.[190] Further evidence of the functional significance of this autonomy is

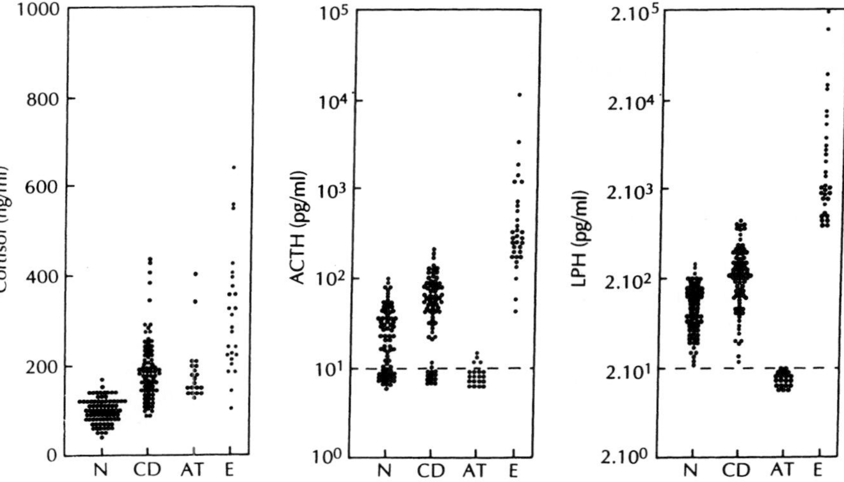

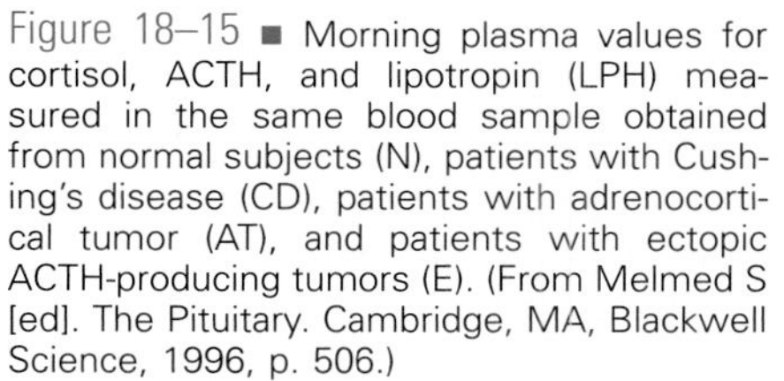

Figure 18–15 ■ Morning plasma values for cortisol, ACTH, and lipotropin (LPH) measured in the same blood sample obtained from normal subjects (N), patients with Cushing's disease (CD), patients with adrenocortical tumor (AT), and patients with ectopic ACTH-producing tumors (E). (From Melmed S [ed]. The Pituitary. Cambridge, MA, Blackwell Science, 1996, p. 506.)

the fact that adrenal insufficiency occurs in some of these patients after removal of the adenoma.[187]

Biochemical evidence of mild CYP21A2 deficiency is seen in patients with incidentally discovered adrenal nodules.[190, 191] The abnormality is defined by an exaggerated 17α-hydroxyprogesterone response to stimulation with cosyntropin and is not accompanied by evidence of diminished cortisol response[191]; it can occur independent of the secretory autonomy described earlier[190] and reverts to normal after removal of the adrenal nodule.

Plasma DHEA-S levels are reduced in as many as 87 percent of patients with incidentally discovered adrenal nodules.[192] This finding can occur in the absence of any evidence of autonomous adrenal function and is sometimes observed in association with the mild CYP21A2 deficiency.

Management. Two central issues guide the management of an incidentally discovered adrenal nodule: whether it secretes excess hormones and whether the mass is malignant. The biochemical evaluation should include measurement of plasma renin activity and aldosterone in patients with hypertension and hyperkalemia and measurements of urinary metanephrine or catecholamine excretion in all patients. An overnight low-dose (1-mg) dexamethasone suppression test is the most sensitive screen for autonomous cortisol production of these nodules. DHEA-S measurements may show evidence of androgen overproduction, although the levels are frequently low (see previous discussion). Larger adrenal masses are usually considered more likely to be adrenocortical carcinomas,[193] and the conventional approach has been adrenalectomy for masses larger than 4 to 6 cm.[189, 193] However, this reliance on size has been questioned,[188] and the use of adrenal scintigraphy with NP-59 has been advocated for identification of benign nodules by virtue of their avid iodocholesterol uptake.[188] Surgical removal is indicated for adrenals with aldosterone-producing adenomas, pheochromocytomas, adenomas causing Cushing's syndrome, and lesions suspected of being malignant. Patients with autonomous cortisol secretion but not hypersecretion may be observed for development of more overt evidence of cortisol excess.[194]

Hypoadrenalism

Although hypofunction of the adrenal cortex may be associated with various causes, the common clinical feature is *failure of adequate cortisol secretion* and extremely low DHEA and DHEA-S levels. Because cortisol is needed to sustain life, an early diagnosis is imperative. All physicians, particularly endocrinologists, should be able to identify such cases, and dramatically successful therapy is available.

Hypofunction of the adrenal cortex resulting from destruction of cortical tissue constitutes *primary adrenal insufficiency.* Deficiency of pituitary ACTH secretion or hypothalamic CRF secretion is referred to as *secondary* or *tertiary* adrenal insufficiency, respectively.

Primary Adrenal Insufficiency (Addison's Disease)

In this condition, all three layers of the adrenal cortex are usually involved by a destructive process, the most common of which is autoimmune disease (75 percent). It occurs either as an isolated deficiency or, more commonly, as a component of the polyglandular autoimmune syndrome. The onset of manifestations is usually gradual with progressive impairment of glucocorticoid, mineralocorticoid, and androgen secretion. Full expression of these deficiencies does not occur until 90 percent of the adrenal cortical tissue is destroyed. Clinical and laboratory features are presented in Table 18–11.

The lack of cortisol negative feedback increases hypothalamic CRF synthesis and secretion, which in turn stimulates the synthesis and secretion of pituitary ACTH and other POMC-related peptides (Fig. 18–16). These other peptides are responsible for the hyperpigmentation of the skin and mucous membranes; decrease or absence of aldosterone causes hypotension, hyponatremia, and hyperkalemia. Excessive CRF stimulation results in corticotroph hyperplasia, which in the absence of glucocorticoid replacement may be evident on CT scan and rarely can lead to the development of adenoma. Whereas ACTH secretion is increased, the circadian rhythm is usually maintained, but it is suppressed by glucocorticoid administration.

Secondary and Tertiary Adrenal Insufficiency

The underlying causes of adrenal hypofunction are either defects in pituitary ACTH (secondary) or impairment of

■ TABLE 18–11
Major Manifestations in Patients with Primary Adrenal Insufficiency

SYMPTOM, SIGN, OR LABORATORY FINDING	FREQUENCY (%)
Symptom	
Weakness, tiredness, fatigue	100
Anorexia	100
Gastrointestinal symptoms	92
Nausea	86
Vomiting	75
Constipation	33
Abdominal pain	31
Diarrhea	16
Salt craving	16
Postural dizziness	12
Muscle or joint pains	6–13
Sign	
Weight loss	100
Hyperpigmentation	94
Hypotension (<110 mm Hg systolic)	88–94
Vitiligo	10–20
Auricular calcification	5
Laboratory Finding	
Electrolyte disturbances	92
Hyponatremia	88
Hyperkalemia	64
Hypercalcemia	6
Azotemia	55
Anemia	40
Eosinophilia	17

hypothalamic CRF release resulting in a reduced synthesis and secretion of ACTH and other POMC-related peptides. Thus, the basic cause of adrenal hypofunction is ACTH deficiency, but *hyperpigmentation is absent.* Glucocorticoid and androgen deficiencies are clinically evident. Mineralocorticoid secretion usually remains normal because it is regulated by the renin-angiotensin system. Hence, hypotension, dehydration, and shock are not present. With prolonged and more profound ACTH deficiency, the adrenal fasciculata and reticularis zones atrophy and lose their ability to respond acutely to ACTH. However, with continuous stimulation by ACTH for a few days or a week, recovery does occur.

CLINICAL PRESENTATIONS

Adrenal Crisis. Acute adrenal insufficiency or *adrenal crisis* usually presents as shock in a previously undiagnosed patient with Addison's disease who has been subjected to major stresses or infection and in patients with an established diagnosis who do not increase glucocorticoid replacement during episodes of infection or major illness. Adrenal cortical hypofunction may also occur secondary to the reduction of ACTH secretion that results from a destructive lesion of the pituitary or hypothalamus, such as *Sheehan's syndrome* and *pituitary apoplexy* (see Chapter 19). More frequently, it occurs in conditions in which ACTH secretion is chronically suppressed and the recovery is slow, such as after removal of a corticosteroid-producing tumor of the adrenal cortex or an ACTH-producing pituitary adenoma. In addition, it can be induced iatrogenically as a consequence of corticoid withdrawal after long-term treatment. In secondary adrenal insufficiency, the function of the zona glomerulosa is preserved.

The clinical picture of acute adrenal cortical insufficiency is dominated by nausea, vomiting, hypotension, and shock; symptoms and signs are presented in Table 18–12. Although hyperthermia is a usual finding, hypothermia may be present. Hypoglycemia, hyponatremia, and hyperkalemia are commonly associated with this condition.

The possibility of acute adrenal cortical insufficiency must be considered when any patient is in shock if an obvious cause is not immediately discernible. In this situation, the intravenous administration of hydrocortisone, 100 to 300 mg, may produce a dramatic response.

Chronic Adrenal Insufficiency. The clinical manifesta-

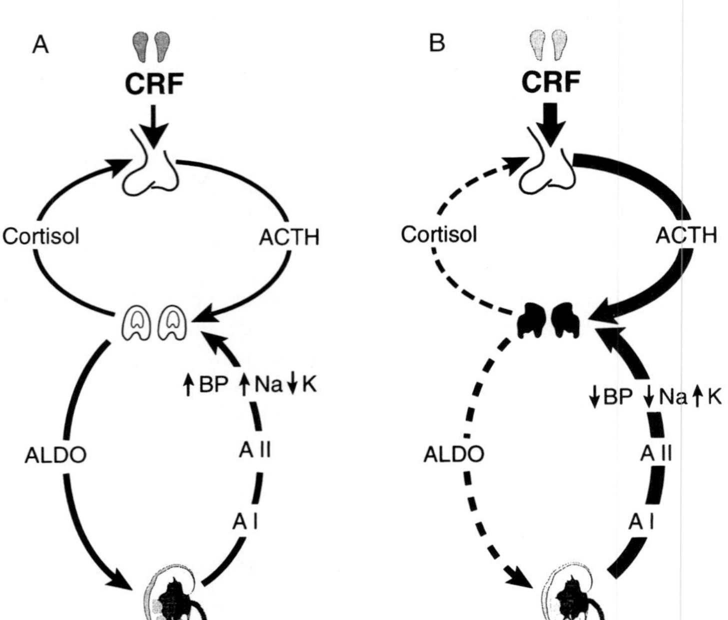

Figure 18–16 ■ Diagrammatic depiction of hypothalamic CRF–pituitary ACTH–adrenal axis in normal subjects *(A)* and in patients with primary adrenal insufficiency *(B)* in which inadequate secretion of glucocorticoids, mineralocorticoids (i.e., aldosterone) (ALDO), and androgens results in the disruption of negative feedback regulation with marked increase in CRF/AVP and ACTH (thick lines). The loss of aldosterone activates the renin-angiotensin system resulting in hypotension, hyponatremia, and hyperkalemia (see text).

■ TABLE 18–12

Clinical and Laboratory Features Suggesting Adrenal Crisis in a Patient with Chronic Primary Adrenal Insufficiency

Dehydration, hypotension, or shock out of proportion to severity of current illness
Nausea and vomiting with a history of weight loss and anorexia
Abdominal pain, so-called acute abdomen
Unexplained hypoglycemia
Unexplained fever
Hyponatremia, hyperkalemia, azotemia, hypercalcemia, or eosinophilia
Hyperpigmentation or vitiligo
Other autoimmune endocrine deficiencies, such as hypothyroidism or gonadal failure

Adapted from Burke CW. Adrenocortical insufficiency. Clin Endocrinol Metab 14:947–976, 1985. © The Endocrine Society.

tion of chronic adrenal insufficiency varies from complete adrenal cortical failure to modest impairment. The principal symptoms and signs are weakness, weight loss, hyperpigmentation, hypotension, and gastrointestinal symptoms (see Table 18–11). Hyperpigmentation is often the first clinical sign that raises the suspicion of primary hypoadrenalism. The most common sites of pigmentation are areas exposed to light and to pressure. The gums and oral mucosa, the conjunctiva, and the vagina may also become pigmented. Vitiligo (patches of depigmentation) occurs in 10 to 20 percent of patients with Addison's disease.

Hypotension is almost always present. The homeostatic mechanism for maintaining blood pressure is impaired, and normal peripheral vasoconstriction as a compensatory response to hypotension fails to occur. Dizziness and syncopal attacks are frequent consequences of postural hypotension.

Hypoglycemia, usually after a carbohydrate meal, is another frequent finding and is due to the absence of the antagonistic effect of cortisol on insulin action. Hypoglycemia is frequently responsible for fatigue and lethargy, commonly manifested as difficulty in getting up in the morning.

Loss of hair, especially in the female, is occasionally found. It is generally less marked than in hypopituitarism. The loss of androgen secretion by the adrenal and ovary would account for this clinical event.

Menstrual disorders are found in more than 25 percent of women with idiopathic forms of Addison's disease. Primary or secondary amenorrhea, menorrhagia, and anovulatory cycles may occur. Some patients have apparently normal cycles. It is of interest that the development of amenorrhea is frequently associated with evidence of premature ovarian failure involving low estrogen and elevated gonadotropin levels. The cause of premature ovarian failure in this condition appears to be related to the presence of circulating antibodies against steroidogenic enzymes (see later).

PATHOGENESIS

It is now apparent that the enzymes involved in steroidogenesis are the primary autoantigens in idiopathic Addison's disease. Immunoassays demonstrate autoantibodies to 17α-hydroxylase,[195] 21α-hydroxylase, and the side-chain cleavage enzymes,[196] which are highly specific for this disease and correlate well with the presence of antibodies to adrenal cortical cells detected by immunofluorescence.[196, 197] There is also evidence of cellular sensitization to adrenal antigens as demonstrated by lymphocyte proliferation in response to homogenates of adrenal tissue.[198] This disorder has been associated with HLA class II antigens DR3 and DR4, but the significance of this association is not clear. The association of Addison's disease and premature ovarian failure has also been clarified, at least in part.[199]

It now seems clear that two P450 cytochrome enzymes, 17α-hydroxylase (P450c17) and side-chain cleavage enzyme (P450scc), are the major targets of steroid cell antibodies. Both are present in adrenal, ovary, testis, and placental trophoblast. The enzyme distribution within these organs corresponds to the immunofluorescence patterns found in earlier studies, and the presence of antibodies to P450c17 or P450scc is *strongly associated with premature ovarian failure*[196, 197, 200] (Table 18–13). In contrast, isolated Addison's disease is associated with autoantibodies against P450c21.

DIAGNOSIS AND TREATMENT

Idiopathic Addison's disease is diagnosed by symptoms of hypoadrenalism in the presence of inappropriately low serum cortisol levels and elevated ACTH concentrations. Tumor, tuberculosis, or other granulomatous disorders of the adrenal glands must be eliminated from the differential. The presence of autoantibodies may assist in making this diagnosis; however, this test should not be performed without also doing imaging studies to rule out an adrenal tumor or infection, because positive test results have also been reported in patients with these disorders.

Congenital Lipoid Adrenal Hyperplasia (Combined Adrenal and Gonadal Failure)

Patients with congenital lipoid adrenal hyperplasia, the most severe genetic disorder of steroid hormone biosynthesis, have a severe defect in the conversion of cholesterol to pregnenolone, the first step in adrenal and gonadal steroidogenesis. Deficient fetal testicular steroidogenesis in patients with a 46,XY karyotype results in phenotypically normal genitalia. The adrenal cortex becomes engorged

■ TABLE 18–13

Incidence of Other Endocrine and Autoimmune Diseases in Patients with Autoimmune Adrenal Insufficiency (N = 448)

DISEASE	INCIDENCE (%)
Thyroid disease	
Hypothyroidism	8
Nontoxic goiter	7
Thyrotoxicosis	7
Gonadal failure	
Ovarian	20
Testicular	2
Insulin-dependent diabetes mellitus	11
Hypoparathyroidism	10
Pernicious anemia	5
None	53

with cholesterol and cholesterol esters; deficient adrenal steroidogenesis leads to salt wasting, hyponatremia, hypovolemia, hyperkalemia, acidosis, and death in infancy,[201] although patients can survive to adulthood with appropriate mineralocorticoid and glucocorticoid replacement therapy.[202] Some affected infants have intermediate signs of mineralocorticoid deficiency, but others remain asymptomatic for months; furthermore, affected 46,XX females may undergo feminization and have vaginal bleeding at puberty.[203] Thus, initially it was not known whether the congenital lipoid adrenal hyperplasia syndrome was a single disease or how a single genetic defect could account for these clinical variations.

Affected adrenal or testicular tissues cannot convert cholesterol to pregnenolone in vitro, suggesting a defect in the cholesterol side-chain cleavage system, which consists of cytochrome P450scc and its electron transfer proteins adrenodoxin reductase and adrenodoxin.[136] Adrenodoxin reductase, adrenodoxin, and several factors thought to participate in the transport of cholesterol to mitochondria are normal in patients with congenital lipoid adrenal hyperplasia.[204, 205] A 30-kDa mitochondrial protein that appears to be a rapidly inducible, cycloheximide-sensitive mediator of the acute steroidogenic response has been cloned in the human and named the steroidogenic acute regulatory protein (StAR).[206] Messenger RNA for this protein was expressed in the adrenal glands and gonads but not in the placenta or brain, as expected for a factor that might cause congenital lipoid adrenal hyperplasia but spare placental steroidogenesis. StAR protein was found in 14 patients with 15 different mutations.[207] This study explains the different phenotype, such as the secretion of some steroid hormones by the ovaries after puberty before the affected cells accumulate large amounts of cholesterol esters. Thus, the congenital lipoid adrenal hyperplasia phenotype is the result of two separate events, an initial genetic loss of steroidogenesis that is dependent on StAR protein and a subsequent loss of steroidogenesis that is independent of the protein but due to cellular damage from accumulated cholesterol esters.[207]

THYROID DYSFUNCTION

Substantial evidence indicates that both deficiency and excess of thyroid hormone induce significant changes in the metabolism and interconversion of androgens and estrogens. Thus, chronic anovulation with or without dysfunctional uterine bleeding may result from inappropriate feedback in patients with thyroid abnormalities.

Regulation of Hypothalamic-Pituitary-Thyroid Axis

The physiologic control of the hypothalamic-pituitary-thyroid axis is fully covered in Chapter 16. It is important for the reader to be familiarized with the hypothalamic-pituitary control of thyroid function and its feedback regulation as depicted in Figure 18–17. Thyrotropin-releasing hormone (TRH) and somatostatin (SS) are regulators located in the paraventricular nuclei. The pathways descend to the median eminence and portal circulation where they exert positive (TRH) and negative (SS) influences on thyroid-stimulating hormone (TSH) synthesis and secretion (Fig. 18–18). A brief account of the metabolism of thyroid hormones and their impact on reproductive function is provided.

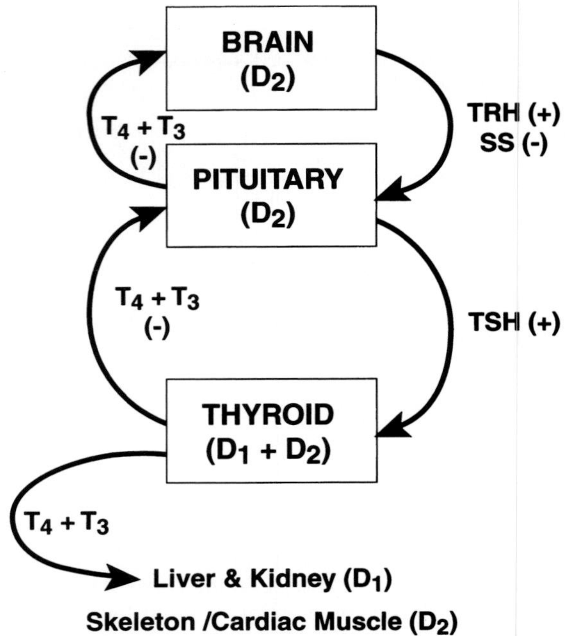

Figure 18–17 ■ Diagrammatic illustration of the hypothalamic-pituitary-thyroid axis and its feedback loops; thyroid hormones, T_4 and T_3, exert negative feedback regulation of TRH and TSH, and their action requires conversion of T_4 to T_3 through tissue-specific deiodinases (D_1, D_2, and D_3) (see text).

Thyroid Hormone Activation and Inactivation by the Selenodeiodinases

The metabolic transformation of thyroid hormones in peripheral tissues determines their biologic potency and regulates their biologic effects. Consequently, an understanding of thyroid physiopathology requires a knowledge of the pathways of thyroid hormone metabolism. The production rate, relative potency, and half-life of triiodothyronine (T_3) and thyroxine (T_4) are given in Table 18–14.

A wide variety of iodothyronines and their metabolic derivatives exist in plasma. Of these, T_4 is highest in concentration and the only one that arises solely from direct secretion by the thyroid gland. In normal humans, T_3 is also released from the thyroid, but most T_3 is derived from the peripheral tissues by the enzymatic removal of a single iodine atom (monodeiodination) from T_4 (Fig. 18–19). Further deiodination reaction deactivates the hormones, and their derivatives are almost entirely generated in the peripheral tissues from T_4 and T_3. Principal among them are 3,3′,5′-triiodothyronine (rT_3) and 3,3′-diiodo-L-thyronine (3,3′-T_2).

The deiodination processes are regulated by three deiodinase enzymes that are relatively tissue specific:

- Type 1 deiodinase (D_1) appears to provide T_3 in the circulation and to deiodinate 3,3′,5′-triiodothyronine (rT_3) to produce 3,3′-diiodothyronine (3,3′-T_2). Because rT_3 and T_2 are biologically inactive, these processes of deio-

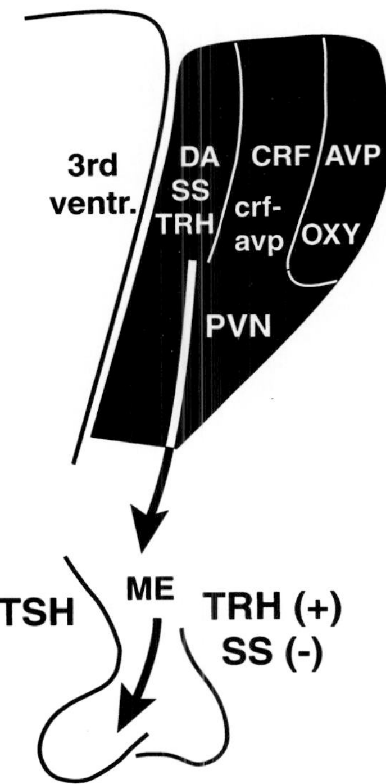

Figure 18–18 ■ Neural pathways regulating pituitary TSH secretion emanating from the paraventricular nucleus (PVN) with stimulatory function of TRH and inhibitory action of somatostatin (ss). ME, median eminence.

dination appear to be responsible for the inactivation of T_3 in the circulation.

- Type 2 deiodinase (D_2) is present in the brain, pituitary gland, brown fat, and placenta. The affinity is lower than for the type 1 enzyme, and the type 2 enzyme can deiodinate only the outer ring of iodothyronine. This enzyme acts to maintain intracellular T_3 concentrations at constant levels. Thus, a reduction of T_4 concentration leads to an increase in the activity of this enzyme and vice versa. The type 2 enzyme may thus provide the mechanism whereby the thyrotroph of the pituitary monitors the concentration of T_4 and T_4 inhibition of TSH secretion[208]—low T_4 concentrations signal an increase in TSH release serving to maintain stable levels of serum T_3 concentrations.
- Type 3 deiodinase (D_3) provides inactivation of T_3 and T_4. It increases in response to T_3, suggesting that it is part of the homeostatic mechanism for maintaining appropriate T_3 concentrations in the brain and skin.[209] A decrease in D_3 activity in hypothyroid states blocks T_3 and T_4 inactivation and facilitates the adaptation by the conservation of biologically active thyroid hormones.

■ TABLE 18–14
Comparison of T_3 and T_4 in Humans

	T_3	T_4
Production rate (nmol/d)	50	100
Fraction from thyroid	0.2	1.0
Relative metabolic potency	1.0	0.3
Serum concentration		
Total (nmol/L)	1.8	100
Free (pmol/L)	5	20
Fraction of total hormone in free form ($\times 10^{-2}$)	0.3	0.02
Distribution volume (L)	40	10
Fraction intracellular	0.64	0.15
Half-life (d)	0.75	7.0

To convert T_4 from nmol/L to μg/dl (total) or pmol/L to ng/dl (free), divide by 12.87. To convert T_3 from nmol/L to ng/dl (total) or pmol/L to pg/dl (free), multiply by 65.1.

Hyperthyroidism

Thyroid hormones amplify the actions of catecholamines in numerous target tissues.[210] In thyrotoxicosis, several

3,5,3',5'-tetraiodol-thyronine (thyroxine, T_4)

D_2, D_1 / - I (5') → 3,5,3',5'-triiodol-thyronine (T_3)

D_3, D_1 \ - I (5') → 3,5,3',5'-triiodol-thyronine (reverse T_3)

D_3, (D_1) \ - I (5') ; - I (5') / D_1, D_2 → 3,3'-diiodothyronine

Figure 18–19 ■ Pathways of thyroid hormone activation and inactivation catalyzed by human iodothyronine deiodinases. Numbers refer to the iodine positions in the iodothyronine nucleus. The iodothyronine deiodinases are abbreviated D_1, D_2, and D_3 for type 1, 2, and 3 deiodinases, respectively. Arrows refer to nondeiodination of the outer or inner ring of the iodothyronine nucleus, which is termed 5′ or 5 by convention. Parentheses reflect the fact that D_3 is very likely the major enzyme catalyzing inner ring deiodination of T_4 and T_3.

signs and symptoms suggest increased adrenergic activity, which can be efficiently inhibited by β-adrenoceptor blocking drugs. Moreover, in hypothyroidism, a large number of changes are opposite those in hyperthyroidism,[210] mimicking a low adrenergic activity state.

In hyperthyroidism, excess thyroid hormones have marked metabolic effects, such as enhancement of oxygen consumption and thermogenesis as well as increased lipid mobilization, all factors that promote weight loss. The enhanced lipolytic response to catecholamines found in fat cells of hyperthyroid subjects has been attributed to an increase in the expression of β_2-adrenergic receptors and enhanced cAMP-activated hormone-sensitive lipase activity without changes in enzyme capacity.[211] This thyroid hormone and catecholamine interaction represents an important mechanism of clinical manifestations of hyperthyroidism and hypothyroidism.

Thyrotoxicosis, whether spontaneous or induced by T_3, is accompanied by an increase in the concentration of SHBG in plasma. Thyroid hormones represent one of the most potent stimulators of hepatic production of SHBG (see Fig. 18–5). As a result, the plasma concentrations of total testosterone, DHT, and estradiol are increased, but their unbound fractions are normal or transiently decreased. The increased binding in plasma is responsible for the decreased metabolic clearance rate of testosterone and DHT. In the case of estradiol, however, the metabolic clearance rate is normal, suggesting that tissue metabolism of the hormone is increased. Conversion rates of androstenedione to testosterone, estrone, and estradiol and of testosterone to DHT are increased (Fig. 18–20). The increased rate of conversion of androgens to estrogens may be the mechanism for gynecomastia in some 10 percent of thyrotoxic men and one mechanism for menstrual irregularities in women.

In some patients, menstrual cycles are predominantly *anovulatory with oligomenorrhea,* but in most, ovulation occurs, as indicated by a secretory endometrium. In the former, a subnormal midcycle surge of LH may be responsible. In premenopausal women with thyrotoxicosis, basal plasma concentrations of LH and FSH are reportedly normal but may display enhanced responsiveness to GnRH stimulation.

Thyrotoxicosis in early life may cause delayed sexual maturation, although physical development is normal and skeletal growth may be accelerated. Thyrotoxicosis after puberty influences reproductive function, especially in women. An increase in libido sometimes occurs in both sexes. The intermenstrual interval may be prolonged or shortened, and menstrual flow is initially diminished and ultimately ceases. Fertility may be reduced, and if conception takes place, there is an increased risk of miscarriage. The association of thyroid autoantibodies and increased pregnancy loss is not related to changes in thyroid function[212]; the thyroid autoantibodies are thought to represent a marker of immune instability predisposing to pregnancy interruption (see Chapter 13 for details).

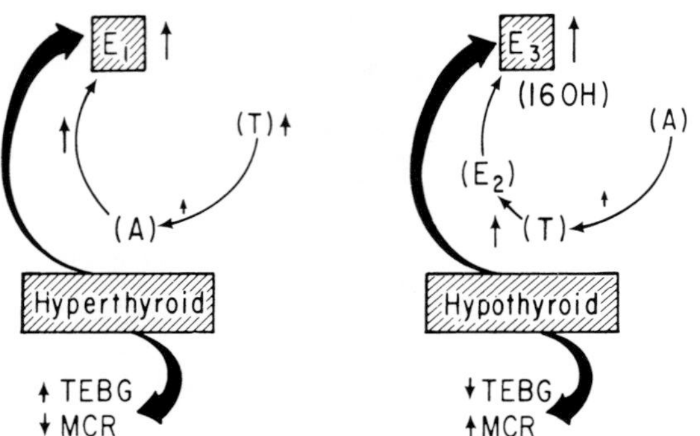

Figure 18–20 ■ Alterations in interconversion and metabolism of androgens and estrogen in hyperthyroidism and hypothyroidism. TEBG, testosterone-estradiol–binding globulin; MCR, metabolic clearance rate; A, androstenedione; T, testosterone; 16-OH, 16-hydroxylation. Arrows indicate increase or decrease.

■ TABLE 18–15
Symptoms of Hypothyroidism

SYMPTOM	PERCENT OF CASES
Weakness	99
Dry skin	97
Coarse skin	97
Lethargy	91
Slow speech	91
Edema of eyelids	90
Sensation of cold	89
Decreased sweating	89
Cold skin	83
Thick tongue	82
Edema of face	79
Coarseness of hair	76
Pallor of skin	67
Memory impairment	66
Constipation	61
Gain in weight	59
Loss of hair	57
Pallor of lips	57
Dyspnea	55
Peripheral edema	55
Hoarseness or aphonia	52
Anorexia	45
Nervousness	35
Menorrhagia	32
Palpitation	31
Deafness	30
Precordial pain	25

Data from Means JH. The Thyroid and Its Diseases, 2nd ed. Philadelphia, JB Lippincott, 1948, p 233.

Hypothyroidism

In adult women, severe hypothyroidism represents a hypometabolic state (Table 18–15) and is commonly associated with reproductive dysfunction such as diminished libido and failure of ovulation. Secretion of progesterone is inadequate, and endometrial proliferation persists, resulting in excessive and irregular breakthrough menstrual bleeding (menorrhagia). These changes may be due to deficient secretion of LH. Rarely, in primary hypothyroidism, secondary depression of pituitary function may lead to ovarian functional arrest and amenorrhea. Fertility is reduced, and spontaneous abortion may result, although many pregnancies are successful.[213, 214] Hypothyroidism in men may cause diminished libido, impotence, and oligospermia.

The metabolism of both androgens and estrogens is altered in hypothyroidism. Secretion of androgens is decreased, and the metabolism of testosterone is shifted toward etiocholanolone rather than androsterone. With respect to estradiol and estrone, hypothyroidism favors metabolism of these steroids through 16α-hydroxylation over that through 2-oxygenation, with the result that formation of estriol is increased and that of 2-hydroxyestrone and its derivative, 2-methoxyestrone, is decreased. The hepatic production of SHBG is decreased with the result that the plasma concentrations of both testosterone and estradiol are decreased, but the unbound fractions are increased (see Fig. 18–20). The alterations in steroid metabolism are corrected by restoration of the euthyroid state.[215]

In both sexes, thyroid hormones influence sexual development and reproductive function. Infantile hypothyroidism, if untreated, leads to sexual immaturity, and juvenile hypothyroidism causes a delay in the onset of puberty followed by anovulatory cycles. As indicated before, hypothyroidism is associated with a decreased adrenergic activity, a reduced basal metabolic rate, and a hypometabolic state.

Syndrome of Thyroid Hormone Resistance

Clinical Features. The syndromes of resistance to thyroid hormone (RTH) are characterized by reduced clinical and biochemical manifestations of thyroid hormone action relative to the circulating hormone levels. In practice, most patients are identified by the persistent elevation of serum levels of T_4 and T_3 with "inappropriately" nonsuppressed TSH, in the absence of intercurrent acute illness, drugs, or alterations of thyroid hormone binding to serum proteins. More important, administration of supraphysiologic doses of thyroid hormone fails to produce the expected suppressive effect on the secretion of pituitary TSH or to induce the expected metabolic responses in the peripheral tissues. Since the publication of the index cases in 1967,[216] 347 subjects have been reported who exhibit the characteristics of the syndrome.

Pathophysiology. This syndrome is recognized by mild to marked elevations in T_3 levels and inappropriately normal or elevated TSH levels resulting from pituitary resistance to T_3. The molecular cause of RTH was first linked to the thyroid hormone receptor (TR)–β gene in 1988[217]; subsequently, point mutations in the hinge region and ligand binding domains of the TR-β gene have been found in more than 100 families with RTH.[218] In contrast, no patients with RTH have been found with mutations in the TR-α gene. Recent data from the TR-β "knockout" mouse provide an explanation for this curious finding in patients with RTH.[219] Mice lacking the TR-β gene on both alleles had evidence of significant pituitary resistance to thyroid hormone, indicating that the TR-α gene could not substitute for the function-specific regulation of the anterior pituitary. Thus, given the TR isoform-specific regulation of the anterior pituitary, it is not surprising that TR mutations in patients with RTH are found only in the TR-β gene.

RTH mutations in the TR-β gene usually reduce or eliminate T_3 binding. RTH mutations causing the most severe clinical phenotype (generalized resistance, GRTH) are usually those with the most dramatic reductions in T_3 binding. By repressing transcription on genes containing positive thyroid hormone response elements, regardless of the T_3 level, the mutant TR interferes with normal gene activation by the wild-type TR.[220] Conversely, by activating gene transcription on genes containing negative thyroid hormone response elements, regardless of the T_3 level, the mutant TR interferes with normal gene repression by the wild-type TR. But RTH mutations that do not affect or minimally affect T_3 binding have also been reported.[221, 222] Such mutations tend to cause a milder form of RTH that is *limited to the pituitary (PRTH).* Mutations in the latter category have challenged somewhat the simple view that RTH phenotype can be directly correlated with the impairment in T_3 binding exhibited by the TR. Alternatively, these RTH mutations suggest that certain RTH mutations interfere with the ability of TR-β to transmit its signal through cofactors to the transcriptional machinery.

Weiss and colleagues[223] have demonstrated that fibroblasts in affected patients exhibit significant tissue resistance to T_3 action. They further showed that in addition to TR-β mutation, a postreceptor defect in T_3 action is also present to account for the underlying molecular mechanism of the GRTH syndrome.

Diagnosis. The diagnosis of thyroid hormone resistance is still based on clinical findings and standard laboratory tests. The current classification of the various forms of thyroid hormone resistance reflects the paucity of available methods to determine the degree of hormone responsiveness at the level of each target tissue. With the exception of the pituitary gland, measurements of thyroid hormone responses in other tissues are insensitive and relatively nonspecific. For this reason, all tissues exclusive of the pituitary are only roughly assessed by a combination of tests providing a poorly defined index of thyroid hormone action on peripheral tissues. It is therefore important to keep in mind that the currently used classification of syndromes of resistance to thyroid hormone is biased by practical constraints. Because the mode of action of thyroid hormone on the pituitary may not be different from that on other target tissues, the only possible justification of singling out the pituitary gland is its role in regulating the level of thyroid gland activity. In fact, through secretion of TSH, the pituitary thyrotrophs determine the level of thyroid hormone in blood. All other tissues have to comply with the amount of hormone provided at the discretion of the thyrotrophs, which is that required to down-regulate TSH secretion.[208] Autoregulation of active thyroid hormone supply in tissues other than the pituitary is limited to hormone entry and the effectiveness of generating T_3 from T_4 by 5′-monodeiodination.[224, 225]

Generalized Resistance to Thyroid Hormone

The majority of reported cases with thyroid hormone resistance belong to this category. The participation of the pituitary thyrotrophs in the global tissue hyposensitivity to thyroid hormone provides a mechanism for the partial compensation of the defect. Untreated subjects usually achieve a normal metabolic state at the expense of high levels of circulating thyroid hormone maintained by the secretion of TSH in response to hypothalamic TRH. This compensation appears, however, to be variable among individuals and in different tissues so that clinical and laboratory evidence of thyroid hormone excess and deficiency can often coexist. Supraphysiologic doses of exogenous hormone are required to suppress the basal TSH secretion and its response to TRH and can do so without inducing the combined biochemical and clinical changes of thyrotoxicosis. Consistent with the global hyposensitivity to thyroid hormone, reduction of its level through ablative thyroid therapy or by antithyroid drugs results in an increase in serum TSH concentration and the appearance of clinical and laboratory changes suggestive of hypothyroidism while thyroid hormone levels remain elevated or well within the normal range.

SEX HORMONE–PRODUCING TUMORS

Androgen-Producing Tumors

Several types of ovarian and adrenal tumors produce androgen autonomously and cause chronic anovulation and virilization. These tumors—which include hilus cell tumors, arrhenoblastomas (Sertoli-Leydig cell tumors), benign cystic teratomas, luteinized thecoma, gynandroblastoma in which both granulosa and Leydig cell elements coexist, adrenal rest tumors of the ovary, ovarian sex cord tumor in which both granulosa and Sertoli cells coexist, and adrenal adenoma and carcinoma—may simulate the polycystic ovary syndrome. Normal ovulatory cycles can be restored after removal of these tumors. Although the degree of androgenization and elevated levels of serum testosterone frequently are more pronounced in patients with tumors, differentiation among the tumors may be difficult. For example, arrhenoblastoma and lipid cell tumor of the ovary have been shown to produce both Δ^5-androgens (DHEA and DHEA-S) and Δ^4-androgens.[226, 227] Virilization, with clinical manifestations of clitorimegaly, temporal balding, excessive muscle mass, and a deepening of the voice, occurs only when the plasma concentration of testosterone approaches male levels (Fig. 18–21).

Adrenal adenomas and *carcinomas* are rare and usually produce large amounts of 17-ketosteroids: DHEA and Δ^4-androstenedione as well as cortisol. Although these tumors usually are not responsive to dexamethasone suppression, in isolated cases some tumors are. Circulating ACTH levels are persistently low in these patients, in contradistinction to patients with an ectopic ACTH-producing tumor, in whom the level is markedly elevated.

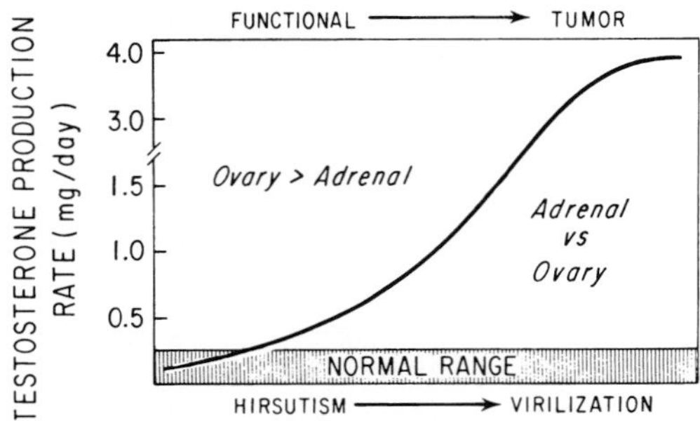

Figure 18–21 ■ The clinical and pathophysiologic relationship between the degree of testosterone overproduction and the progression from hirsutism to virilization. Small to modest increases usually reflect ovarian sources of overproduction of a functional nature. Large elevations are frequently an indication of the presence of androgen-producing tumors in either adrenal or ovarian sites.

In suspected cases, immediate work-up and treatment are mandatory. MRI, CT, and ultrasonography may be helpful in localizing the tumor. Retrograde venous catheterization to determine the site (adrenal versus ovary) and the side (left or right) of hormonal excess has been used extensively before surgical removal. Scan with ^{131}I-6β-iodomethylnorcholesterol (NP-59) has been successful in establishing the precise location of the tumor preoperatively. Stimulation and suppression tests in different combinations may be misleading because a wide range of responses for both ovarian and adrenal tumors has been observed.[228, 229]

Tumor Markers. Inhibin and müllerian-inhibiting substances are markers for sex cord tumors, germ cell tumors in XY individuals, and possibly granulosa and Leydig cell tumor.[230, 231]

Estrogen-Producing Tumors

Granulosa-theca cell tumors are the most common hormone-producing neoplasms of the ovary and account for 15 to 20 percent of all solid ovarian tumors. They commonly produce estrogen, but these tumors also frequently produce androgens, which is not surprising, considering the theca cell component of the tumor. In either case, autonomous production of estrogen and androgen, together with peripheral conversion of androgen to estrogen, accounts for the chronic anovulation that is due to acyclic ovarian steroid feedback. When these tumors develop before sexual maturation, they cause precocious puberty; when they occur after menopause, they cause postmenopausal bleeding. Cyclic menses are restored after surgical removal of the tumor. Germinomas of the hypothalamus secrete human chorionic gonadotropin (hCG) and express aromatase enzyme in the germ cell component of this type tumor, and the development of precocious puberty in this condition may be related to estrogen production in the hypothalamus[232] in addition to ovarian activation by hCG. Müllerian-inhibiting substance is a reliable tumor marker.[233]

ECTOPIC PROLACTIN- AND GLYCOPROTEIN HORMONE–SECRETING TUMORS

Ectopic Prolactin

Relatively few patients with tumors ectopically secreting TSH, FSH, LH, and prolactin have been described. Galactorrhea, menstrual dysfunction, impotence, altered libido, and gynecomastia have been described among patients with markedly elevated prolactin levels.[167] Those tumors that are most likely to secrete prolactin ectopically are bronchogenic carcinomas and hypernephromas. Prolactin secretion may increase in response to stress as well as in response to a wide variety of drugs, including phenothiazines, methyldopa, and haloperidol. Prolactin concentrations do not exceed 30 ng/ml under basal conditions. If a tumor secreted low concentrations of prolactin ectopically, circulating prolactin levels could still remain within normal limits. Moreover, even if tumor secretion resulted in low-grade, increased circulating prolactin levels, more than likely no signs or symptoms of that relative hormone excess would be apparent.

Ectopic Pituitary Glycoprotein Hormone

Ectopic TSH secretion has been associated with tumors of the lung and breast with clinically apparent symptoms of excess thyroid stimulation.[234] Relatively few cases of ectopic TSH have been documented. Menstrual aberrations may be expected to be present among women with significant hyperthyroidism secondary to excessive thyroid stimulation with TSH. Moreover, men with clinically significant hyperthyroidism may present with gynecomastia because of altered peripheral sex steroid metabolism in that state. Consequently, one may observe gynecomastia among men with tumors secreting significant quantities of biologically active TSH ectopically. Fortunately, clinically significant ectopic TSH secretion is extremely rare. No well-documented cases of ectopic LH or FSH secretion exist. In those cases in which ectopic LH or FSH secretion has been described, the experimental data do not support the investigators' conclusions.

Ectopic Human Chorionic Gonadotropin

Human chorionic gonadotropin (hCG) and human luteinizing hormone (hLH) share extensive structural homologies, accounting for their similar biologic and immunologic activities.[235] The placenta normally secretes hCG, whereas hLH is physiologically secreted by the pituitary gland; hCG circulates physiologically at readily detectable levels only during pregnancy. Most clinical assays cannot discern immunologically between hLH and hCG. With use of an antiserum directed to hCG-β, a specific hCG assay was developed to measure hCG selectively in plasma or serum samples containing LH, hCG, or both hormones. Since the initial description, a host of other "β-subunit" assays have been developed. Extracts of several normal tissues, including the pituitary, testis, and upper gastrointestinal tract, contain an hCG-like substance.[235] Low concentrations of an hCG-like substance have been reported in extracts of almost all tumors described.[236] However, other investigators have not confirmed those observations. This disparity may be the result of proteases in tissue extracts. Proteases may induce artifacts in bioassays and immunoassays for hCG, resulting in spuriously high hCG concentrations in those assays.[237] Patients with tumors secreting gonadotropins ectopically were initially recognized by clinical syndromes attributed to excessive gonadotropin secretion.[238, 239] Before specific immunologic and physical techniques, it was impossible to discern whether LH or hCG was secreted by those tumors.

The syndrome of precocious puberty was initially described in boys with hepatoblastomas and teratomas secreting gonadotropin.[238] Precocious puberty resulted from hCG stimulation of Leydig cells and secretion of testosterone, which in turn induced development of secondary sex characteristics. Some boys may have midline intracranial teratomas or pinealomas that secrete hCG. Low levels of hCG secretion are sufficient to induce the signs of sexual precocity in boys.[240, 241] In men, ectopic gonadotropin secretion has been associated with gynecomastia. Tumors secreting hCG may secrete sex steroids as well.[242] Estrogen secretion by those tumors may be responsible for the gynecomastia observed in men and dysfunctional uterine bleeding in women.[243] Levels of hCG in excess of concentrations found in the first trimester of pregnancy have been observed in patients without any clinical manifestations of excess circulating hCG.[243] Adenocarcinomas of the stomach are most likely to secrete high levels of hCG.

Table 18–16 summarizes the distribution of tumors secreting hCG ectopically. Tumors of the stomach, pancreas, liver, and gonads are among those most commonly associated with ectopic hCG secretion. The incidence of ectopic hCG secretion ranges between 17 and 40 percent among patients with that subset of tumors. Most tumors secrete levels of hCG too low to be detected by conventional pregnancy tests. Sensitivity of the specific hCG assay is usually of the order of 5 mIU/ml (Second International Standard for hCG) for a 200-μl sample. The sensitivity of conventional urinary pregnancy tests is of the order of 300 to 500 mIU/ml.

Several tumors may secrete hCG eutopically. Choriocarcinomas of the testis and the ovary, as well as teratomas, secrete hCG.[235, 244, 245] In contrast to the prognosis of patients with gestational trophoblastic disease, the prognosis of patients with nongestational choriocarcinomas or teratomas of midline structures is relatively poor in spite of aggressive chemotherapy. On the other hand, women with gestational trophoblastic disease show a greater than 90 percent cure rate with conventional chemotherapy, even in the presence of lung metastases at the onset of therapy.[246] The cure rate approaches only 50 percent in women with gestational trophoblastic disease who have liver or brain metastases, or both, in spite of aggressive chemotherapy. Unfortunately, if therapy of women with gestational trophoblastic disease is delayed for several months, the survival rate declines precipitously and approaches that of patients

■ TABLE 18–16

Incidence of Immunoreactive Human Chorionic Gonadotropin in Sera of Patients with Malignant Tumors

TISSUE	NUMBER EXAMINED		PERCENTAGE	
Breast	163		21	
Gastrointestinal system	363		18	
Esophagus		12		0
Stomach		73		22
Small intestine		23		13
Pancreas		42		33
Biliary tract		9		11
Liver		92		21
Large bowel/rectum		112		12
Lung	158		10	
Pigment cells (melanoma)	99		9	
Ovary (adenocarcinoma)	45		40	
Testis	102		62	
Embryonal cell carcinoma		55		58
Seminoma		16		38
Choriocarcinoma		9		100
Unspecified or mixed		22		73
Miscellaneous	573		3	
Total	1503		15	

with nongestational trophoblastic disease as well as that of patients with tumors secreting hCG ectopically. Germinal cell tumors of the testes are the most common neoplasia among 20- to 34-year-old men and account for 11.4 percent of all cancer deaths in that age group.[247] In approximately 10 to 30 percent of men with seminomas, circulating hCG levels are abnormally high; in approximately two thirds of men with embryonal cell carcinomas, serum hCG concentrations are abnormally high.[235] All choriocarcinomas secrete hCG, and a variable percentage of men with teratomas demonstrate abnormal circulating hCG levels. Persistently high tumor marker levels in the absence of any other evidence of tumor usually herald occult neoplastic disease.

Ectopic Human Placental Lactogen

Human placental lactogen (hPL), also known as human chorionic somatomammotropin (hCS), like hCG is a trophoblastic hormone that is not present normally in peripheral blood at readily detectable levels except during pregnancy. Ectopic hPL secretion was initially documented in a man with gynecomastia and an anaplastic large cell carcinoma of the lung.[248] In addition to hPL, the patient's tumor produced gonadotropin ectopically (probably hCG). In a study of 128 patients with nontrophoblastic tumors, 10 of the patients' serum samples contained immunoreactive hPL.[248] Half of the patients in that study had lung tumors, and of those individuals, seven showed immunoreactive hCS in the sera. Five of the seven had gynecomastia as well as increased estradiol secretory rates. Four of the five individuals with gynecomastia also had presumptive evidence of hCG secretion by the tumors. Whether the gynecomastia was attributable solely to increased estradiol secretory rates, to hCS, to hCG, or to combinations thereof could not be ascertained.

Clinical Usefulness of Tumor Markers

Tumor markers may be useful in monitoring selected patients during chemotherapy, after surgery, or during remission after medical or surgical therapy has been completed. Monitoring hCG levels of women with gestational trophoblastic disease is imperative, because persistent hCG secretion heralds occult tumor. Men with hCG-secreting germinal cell tumors of the testis should be monitored with serial hCG levels during and after therapy. Monitoring of hCG and α-fetoprotein levels among men with nonseminomatous germinal cell testicular tumors has been an invaluable adjunct to staging of the tumor. Discordance of tumor markers has been demonstrated in a variety of situations. When possible, it is best to monitor several tumor markers, both hormonal and nonhormonal. With tumor therapy, two of three markers may disappear and only one (for example, α-fetoprotein) may be secreted in excess, reflecting persistent tumor activity or tumor growth.

In summary, monitoring of serial hCG levels among women with gestational trophoblastic disease and men with hCG-secreting germinal cell tumors of the testis is an invaluable adjunct to conventional diagnostic techniques for ascertaining the response to therapy or the recurrence of a tumor. However, a high incidence of discordance between the response of the tumor to chemotherapy and circulating levels of hormone or nonhormonal tumor markers is commonly observed among other hCG-secreting tumors.

GENE MUTATIONS OF GONADOTROPIN AND ESTROGEN RECEPTORS

Mutations of LH Receptor Gene

Missense and Nonsense Mutations

Several novel homozygous (inactivating) nonsense and missense mutations of the LH-receptor (LHR) gene have been reported.[249–253] All mutations causing inactivation (loss of function) of human LHR are located at highly conserved amino acids of the G protein–coupled receptors with seven transmembrane domains.[254] The sites of mutation are varied, with one located in the extracellular domain of the receptor directly adjacent to the first transmembrane domain[253] and others located in transmembrane domains 5 and 6[249, 251, 255] and in the intracellular domain.[252]

In males, defects in LHR result in abnormal Leydig cell differentiation and function at a crucial period of sexual differentiation in affected 46XY individuals. Inadequate testosterone (T) and dihydrotestosterone (DHT) production results in the development of abnormal male external genitalia. The phenotype of 46XY subjects with LHR defects is variable. At one end of the spectrum are phenotypic males with micropenis and primary hypogonadism and at the other end are males with female external genitalia or severe ambiguity of the genitalia. The phenotypic variations can be explained, at least in part, by varying defects of LHR gene with mutations that can cause either complete[251, 253] or partial[252, 256] loss of LH receptor function.

Hormonal evaluation in 46XY persons with LHR defects revealed low levels of T and DHT, which failed to respond to hCG stimulation. LH levels were markedly elevated with a normal or borderline rise of FSH.

Females with LHR defects present with primary amenorrhea and normal pubertal breast development. This finding indicates LH is not required for pubertal development in genetic females. However, LH action is necessary for follicular development and ovulation. Normal primordial, preantral, and antral follicles are present in these ovaries; findings are consistent with the initial follicular growth that is independent of LH stimulation.[257]

Laboratory findings revealed an elevated LH and high normal FSH levels in association with low estradiol and pregnenolone levels. As expected, androgens, testosterone, and androstenedione levels were very low.

The disclosure of LHR gene mutation as a cause of primary amenorrhea added a new dimension in the differential diagnosis of ovarian failure.

Activating Mutation of LH Receptor Gene

Familial male precocious puberty (FMPP) is a gonadotropin-independent disorder that is inherited in an autosomal dominant, male-limited pattern.[258, 259] Affected males generally exhibit signs of puberty by age 4 years. Testosterone production and Leydig cell hyperplasia occur in the context of prepubertal levels of LH.[259, 260] FMPP provides the first example of an inherited human disease that is due to a constitutively activating mutation in a G-protein-coupled hormone receptor.[261] A single A → G base change that results in substitution of glycine for aspartate at position 578 in the sixth transmembrane helix of the LH receptor was found in affected individuals from eight different families. Linkage of the mutation to FMPP was supported by restriction-digest analysis. COS-7 cells expressing the mutant LH receptor exhibited markedly increased cAMP production in the absence of ligand, suggesting that autonomous Leydig cell activity in FMPP is caused by a constitutively activated LH receptor.[261] Point mutations with changes of Ala to Val in codon 373 in the first transmembrane domain[262] and Leu to Arg in codon 457 in the third transmembrane domain[255] have also been demonstrated to be constitutively activating LHR causing FMPP.

Constitutively activating point mutations have been described in other classes of transmembrane receptors.[263, 264] Inactivating mutations of G protein–coupled receptors can serve as a mechanism of human disease,[265, 266] and the identification of amino acid substitutions that cause constitutive activation of adrenergic receptors in vitro led to the prediction that such mutations might also be pathogenic.[267, 268] Activating mutations of the melanocyte-stimulating hormone receptor have been found in mice with dominantly inherited hyperpigmentation[269] and activating mutations of rhodopsin described in severe retinitis pigmentosa[270] and in congenital stationary night blindness.

Mutations of FSH Receptor Gene

Given the crucial role of FSH in reproduction, mutations in the FSH receptor (FSHR) could severely affect gametogenesis and result in infertility. Based on this premise, screening programs have been initiated. The FSHR gene can be mapped to chromosome 2 p21, a position identical to that of the human LHR.[271, 272] The similarity of exon sizes between the LHR, TSHR, and FSHR and adjacent chromosomal localization of the FSHR and LHR support the hypothesis that the three receptors may have evolved by gene duplication from a common ancestral gene. The human FSHR gene, which spans a region of 54 kb, consists of 10 exons and 9 introns. The extracellular domain is encoded by 9 exons ranging in length between 69 bp to 251 bp, while the C-terminal parts of the extracellular domain, the transmembrane, and the intracellular domain are encoded by exons with 1251 bp. Overall the gene encodes 695 amino acids including a signal peptide of 18 amino acids. The mature FSHR consists of 678 amino acids with a molecular weight of 75 kDa, the extracellular domain alone containing 349 amino acids.[273]

Inactivating Mutation of FSH Receptor. Aittomäki and colleagues[274] identified 75 patients with hypergonadotropic ovarian failure characterized by primary or secondary amenorrhea before the age of 20 years and XX gonadal dysgenesis in Finland and showed that segregation ratios were compatible with recessive inheritance.[275] The locus of ovarian dysgenesis was mapped to chromosome 2p in six multiplex families of the patient series, and a C → T point mutation was detected in nucleotide 566 of exon 7 of the FSHR gene, predicting an alanine to valine substitution at residue 189 of FSHR protein.[274] The mutation segregated perfectly with the disease, and by functional assays, the mutated FSHR protein expressed in transfected cells was shown to be defective. This mutation was thus thought to cause this ovarian failure.

The same group of investigators subsequently characterized the phenotypic features of patients with this mutation (designated FSH-resistant ovary or FSHRO). A major phenotypic feature that evokes FSHRO is the presence of ovarian follicles. Because some pubertal development was observed in all FSHRO cases, the authors suggested that low-level residual FSHR function is present in the ovaries with mutated receptor.[276] In addition, normal adrenarche with appropriate DHEA-S values occurred, explaining in part the pubertal development in these patients. These observations may be important in managing infertility—instead of ovum donation, large doses of FSH stimulation may benefit those with residual FSHR function.

Inactivating FSHR gene mutations described above resemble phenotypically those caused by inactivating FSHβ subunit mutations (see Review[277]). The females have hypergonadotropic amenorrhea with complete arrest of follicular maturation. Males homozygous for mutations display normal virilization with variable reduction of testicular size and suppression of spermatogenesis. As with isolated FSH deficiency, some of the men may have normal phenotype and fertility. Consequently, men who are homozygous for inactivating FSHR show no clinical manifestations and could be traced only through siblingship with receptor defects and phenotype. Thus, both FSH ligand and receptor defects indicate that FSH is more crucial for female than male fertility, suggesting male contraceptive methods of suppression of FSH secretion are not likely to be successful.

Activating Mutation of FSH Receptor. In the male, FSH is needed for pubertal proliferation of Sertoli cells, but the distinct effects of FSH on initiation and maintenance of spermatogenesis are still a matter of discussion. Whereas production of mature, fertile sperm can be induced in gonadotropin-deficient rats with testosterone alone and in hamsters with FSH alone, it seems that primate spermatogenesis requires both hormones. In hypogonadotropic patients, fertility cannot be achieved by testosterone treatment only, and both LH and FSH are necessary to restore normal spermatogenesis.

A patient who underwent hypophysectomy because of a pituitary tumor was prescribed substitution with glucocorticoids and thyroxine as well as with testosterone to maintain normal androgenization. This treatment normally results in a drop of spermatogenesis, and if the patient wants to regain fertility, treatment has to include LH and FSH. Surprisingly, the patient had ongoing normal spermatogenesis and, despite gonadotropin deficiency, fathered three children. The recent description of activating mutations in G protein–coupled receptors prompted investigation of whether *constitutive activation of the FSHR* could be the cause of his unexplained fertility. Screening of the FSHR gene led to the identification of a heterozygous mutation changing Ala to Gly at position 567, located in the third intracellular loop. Functional studies showed a similar marked increase in cAMP production in both receptors. Transfection of different concentrations of FSHR cDNA in the absence of FSH resulted in no increase in basal cAMP production in the wild-type receptor, whereas a 1.5-fold increase was observed for the mutated receptor. The amino acid substitution Ala to Gly therefore leads to a *ligand-independent constitutive activation of FSHR.*[278] The mutation is localized in a crucial region of the transmembrane domain, highly conserved in all glycoprotein hormone receptors and within the FSHR of different species.

This patient provides an exceptional model of nature defining the role of FSH in human spermatogenesis. Mutations of the FSHR might have differential effects in each gender. Activating mutations have not been described in women at the time of this writing; therefore, it is not clear whether the constitutive activity of the receptor could disturb normal follicular development, resulting in infertility.

Mutations in the Estrogen Receptor Gene

The actions of adrenal and gonadal steroids, thyroid hormone, and vitamin D are mediated by receptors encoded by a family of related genes. Mutations of glucocorticoid, androgen, thyroid hormone, and vitamin D receptors leading to syndromes of hormone resistance have been reported.[279–281] Mutations in the estrogen receptor gene have been thought to be lethal. A 28-year-old man whose estrogen resistance was caused by a disruptive mutation in the estrogen receptor gene underwent studies of pituitary-gonadal function and bone density and received transdermal estrogen for 6 months. Estrogen receptor DNA, extracted from lymphocytes, was evaluated by analysis of single-stranded conformation polymorphisms and by direct sequencing.[282]

The patient was tall (204 cm [80.3 in]) and had incomplete epiphyseal closure, with a history of continued linear growth into adulthood despite otherwise normal pubertal development. He was normally masculinized and had bilateral axillary acanthosis nigricans. Serum estradiol and estrone concentrations were elevated, and serum testosterone concentrations were normal. Serum FSH and LH concentrations were increased. Glucose tolerance was impaired, and hyperinsulinemia was present. The bone mineral density of the lumbar spine was 0.745 g/cm^2, 3.1 SD below the mean for age-matched normal women; there was biochemical evidence of increased bone turnover.

The patient had *no detectable response to estrogen administration,* despite a 10-fold increase in the serum free estradiol concentration. Conformation analysis of his estrogen receptor gene revealed a variant banding pattern in exon 2. Direct sequencing of exon 2 revealed a cytosine to thymine transition at codon 157 of both alleles, resulting in a premature stop codon. The patient's parents were heterozygous carriers of this mutation, and pedigree analysis revealed consanguinity.[282]

The case illustrates that disruption of the estrogen receptor in humans need not be lethal. Estrogen is important for bone maturation and mineralization in men as well as in women.[77]

DYSFUNCTIONAL UTERINE BLEEDING

Dysfunctional uterine bleeding is a term loosely applied to out-of-phase uterine bleeding that is not caused by evident organic disease. It is manifested as episodic, excessive bleeding of varying frequency, and its diagnosis requires the exclusion of local and systemic disease.

Pathophysiology

Investigations designed to define the pathophysiology of dysfunctional uterine bleeding have been disappointingly limited. Thus, the underlying mechanism for the seemingly out-of-phase bleeding is obscure. The association of dysfunctional uterine bleeding with anovulation has been recognized for a long time through analysis of endometrial biopsy specimens and the study of urinary excretion of estrogens and pregnanediol.

Investigations of circulating gonadotropins and of ovarian steroid patterns have confirmed the anovulatory nature of this condition. Studying adolescent girls with dysfunctional uterine bleeding, Fraser and colleagues[283] found that the blood concentrations of circulating estrone and estradiol are in the normal range for mature cycling women but that normal positive feedback effect on the induction of the LH surge is absent, and consequently ovulation fails to occur. Clomiphene treatment is effective in these adolescent patients. Furthermore, in a study of perimenopausal dysfunctional bleeding, Sherman and associates[284] indicated that both the variability of cycle length and the bleeding are due to a diminished ovarian responsiveness to gonadotropin stimulation, resulting in irregular maturation of ovarian follicles.

These two studies indicate that the primary defect in anovulatory bleeding of adolescents is a failure of the hypothalamic-pituitary system to respond to the positive feedback effect of estrogen. In contrast, the anovulatory bleeding in the menopausal transition is due primarily to the declining functional capacity of the ovary.

When dysfunctional bleeding occurs during the reproductive phase, the hormonal patterns exhibit marked random episodic fluctuations in levels of LH, estrogens, and androgens. The mean levels of both LH and estrone are inappropriately elevated. Testosterone and androstenedione levels are within the normal range for women, and adrenal androgens do not appear to play a role in the pathophysiologic process of this syndrome. The aberrant gonadotropin and ovarian steroid patterns do not provide a clue to the site of the primary defect. A hypothalamic-pituitary dysfunction resulting in the failure of a positive feedback effect of estrogen seems likely as the initiating cause, but an equally attractive hypothesis includes abnormal peripheral conversion of androgen to estrogen or a defect in endometrial prostaglandin release. Obviously, more work is needed to define this common disorder.

The mechanism by which the out-of-phase bleeding from the endometrium occurs is not entirely clear. In most instances, inappropriate estrogen levels or estrogen to progesterone ratios are accountable for endometrial regression and bleeding. Acute fluctuations of estrogen levels in the endometrium exposed to constant levels of estrogen stimulation result in an *estrogen withdrawal* type of bleeding. Alternatively, the increased cellularity and thickness of endometrium under chronic estrogen stimulation demand additional estrogen to maintain growth. Consequently, *breakthrough bleeding* would occur in the absence of estrogen decline. In the ovulatory type of dysfunctional bleeding, the ratio of progesterone to estrogen required to maintain the secretory endometrium may be inappropriate. Under these circumstances, alteration of estrogen or progesterone receptor populations, or of both, would occur in the endometrium; as a consequence, local prostaglandin release would be induced, which may be mechanistically responsible for the vasospasm, ischemia, and bleeding. (See Chapters 5 and 8.)

Organic disease must be ruled out before treatment of dysfunctional bleeding. Uterine curettage is required for the diagnosis and frequently results in a therapeutic success. The relatively high incidence of submucous myoma, endometrial polyps, endometrial hyperplasia, and, possibly, endometrial carcinoma in association with this condition renders endometrial biopsy or hysteroscopic examination imperative.

Management

Treatment with synthetic progestin is both rational and successful. Medroxyprogesterone acetate (MPA) appears to be the drug of choice because it has a much greater progestational effect than does progesterone and dissociates more slowly than does progesterone from the receptors.[285] Moreover, progestin induces, within the endometrial cells, 17-hydroxysteroid dehydrogenase enzyme, which converts estradiol to less active estrone in situ (see Chapter 8). Thus, administration of MPA, at a daily dose of 5 to 10 mg for 10 days in a cyclic manner to patients with dysfunctional uterine bleeding, is recommended. If progestin treatment alone fails to control the bleeding, a combined estrogen-progestin preparation may be used in a cyclic schedule for 2 to 3 months and repeated, if necessary.

If menstrual bleeding persists in spite of medical treatment, the presence of submucous myoma should be suspected. After confirmation by hysteroscopic examination, the patient may be managed by the suppression of the gonadotropin-ovarian axis through the administration of long-acting progestin—depot medroxyprogesterone (Provera), 150 mg intramuscularly given every 3 to 4 weeks. Induction of reversible "medical ovariectomy" by a GnRH agonist constitutes another approach in the management of these patients.

References

1. Siiteri PK, MacDonald PC. Role of extraglandular estrogen in human endocrinology. *In* Greep RO, Astwood E (eds). Handbook of Physiology: Endocrinology. Washington, DC, American Physiological Society, 1973, p 615.
2. Abraham GE. Ovarian and adrenal contribution to peripheral androgens during the menstrual cycle. J Clin Endocrinol Metab 39:340, 1974.
3. Baird DT. Ovarian steroid secretion and metabolism in women. *In* James VHT, Serio M, Giusti G (eds). The Endocrine Function of the Human Ovary. New York, Academic Press, 1976, pp 125–133.
4. Lachelin GC, Barnett M, Hopper BR, et al. Adrenal function in normal women and women with the polycystic ovary syndrome. J Clin Endocrinol Metab 49:892, 1979.
5. Judd HL, Yen SS. Serum androstenedione and testosterone levels during the menstrual cycle. J Clin Endocrinol Metab 36:475, 1973.
6. Abraham GE, Chakmakjian ZH. Serum steroid levels during the menstrual cycle in a bilaterally adrenalectomized woman. J Clin Endocrinol Metab 37:581, 1973.
7. Wilson JD, Gloyna RE. The intranuclear metabolism of testosterone in the accessory organs of reproduction. Recent Prog Horm Res 26:309, 1970.
8. Kirschner MA, Zucker IR, Jesperson DL. Ovarian and adrenal vein catheterization studies in women with idiopathic hirsutism. *In* James VHT, Serio M, Giusti G (eds). The Endocrine Function of the Ovary. New York, Academic Press, 1976, pp 443–456.
9. Horton R, Tait JF. Androstenedione production and interconversion rates measured in peripheral blood and studies on the possible site of its conversion to testosterone. J Clin Invest 45:301, 1966.
10. Bardin CW, Lipsett MB. Testosterone and androstenedione blood production rates in normal women and women with idiopathic hirsutism or polycystic ovaries. J Clin Invest 46:891, 1967.
11. Ito T, Horton R. The source of plasma dihydrotestosterone in man. J Clin Invest 50:1621, 1971.
12. Baulieu EE, Corpechot C, Dray F, et al. An adrenal-secreted "androgen": Dehydroisoandrosterone sulfate—its metabolism and tentative generalization on the metabolism of other steroid conjugates in man. Recent Prog Horm Res 21:411, 1965.
13. Rosenfield RL, Otto P. Androstenediol levels in human peripheral plasma. J Clin Endocrinol Metab 35:818, 1972.
14. Bird CE, Morrow L, Fukumoto Y, et al. Δ^5-Androstenediol: Kinetics of metabolism and binding to plasma proteins in normal men and women. J Clin Endocrinol Metab 43:1317, 1976.
15. Kirschner MA, Sinhamahapatra S, Zucker IR, et al. The production, origin and role of dehydroepiandrosterone and Δ^5-androstenediol as androgen prehormones in hirsute women. J Clin Endocrinol Metab 37:183, 1973.
16. Lipsett MB, Migeon CJ, Kirschner MA, et al. Physiologic basis of disorders of androgen metabolism. Ann Intern Med 68:1327, 1968.
17. Bird CE, Murphy J, Boroomand K, et al. Dehydroepiandrosterone: Kinetics of metabolism in normal men and women. J Clin Endocrinol Metab 47:818, 1978.
18. Haning RJ, Chabot M, Flood CA, et al. Metabolic clearance rate of dehydroepiandrosterone sulfate (DS), its metabolism to dehydroepiandrosterone, androstenedione, testosterone, and dihydrotestosterone, and the effect of increased plasma DS concentration on DS metabolic clearance rate in normal women. J Clin Endocrinol Metab 69:1047, 1989.
19. Mortola JF, Yen SS. The effects of oral dehydroepiandrosterone on endocrine-metabolic parameters in postmenopausal women. J Clin Endocrinol Metab 71:696, 1990.
20. Hopper BR, Yen SS. Circulating concentrations of dehydroepiandrosterone and dehydroepiandrosterone sulfate during puberty. J Clin Endocrinol Metab 40:458, 1975.
21. de Peretti E, Forest MG. Unconjugated dehydroepiandrosterone plasma levels in normal subjects from birth to adolescence in human: The use of a sensitive radioimmunoassay. J Clin Endocrinol Metab 43:982, 1976.
22. Parker LN, Odell WD. Control of adrenal androgen secretion. Endocr Rev 1:392, 1980.
23. Orentreich N, Brind JL, Rizer RL, et al. Age changes and sex differences in serum dehydroepiandrosterone sulfate concentrations throughout adulthood. J Clin Endocrinol Metab 59:551, 1984.
24. Schiebinger RJ, Albertson BD, Cassorla FG, et al. The developmental changes in plasma adrenal androgens during infancy and adrenarche are associated with changing activities of adrenal microsomal 17-hydroxylase and 17,20-desmolase. J Clin Invest 67:1177, 1981.
25. Couch RM, Muller J, Winter JS. Regulation of the activities of 17-hydroxylase and 17,20-desmolase in the human adrenal cortex: Kinetic analysis and inhibition by endogenous steroids. J Clin Endocrinol Metab 63:613, 1986.
26. Liu CH, Laughlin GA, Fischer UG, et al. Marked attenuation of ultradian and circadian rhythms of dehydroepiandrosterone in postmenopausal women: Evidence for a reduced 17,20-desmolase enzymatic activity. J Clin Endocrinol Metab 71:900, 1990.
27. Parker CR Jr, Mixon RL, Brissie RM, et al. Aging alters zonation in the adrenal cortex of men. J Clin Endocrinol Metab 82:3898, 1997.
28. Morales AJ, Nolan JJ, Nelson JC, et al. Effects of replacement dose of dehydroepiandrosterone in men and women of advancing age. J Clin Endocrinol Metab 78:1360, 1994.
29. Friess E, Trachsel L, Guldner J, et al. DHEA administration increases rapid eye movement sleep and EEG power in the sigma frequency range. Am J Physiol 268:E107, 1995.
30. Diamond P, Cusan L, Gomez JL, et al. Metabolic effects of 12-month percutaneous dehydroepiandrosterone replacement therapy in postmenopausal women. J Endocrinol 150:S43, 1996.
31. Labrie F, Diamond P, Cusan L, et al. Effect of 12-month

dehydroepiandrosterone replacement therapy on bone, vagina, and endometrium in postmenopausal women. J Clin Endocrinol Metab 82:3498, 1997.
32. Morales AJ, and Yen, SSC. The effect of 6 months' treatment with a 100 mg daily dose of dehydroepiandrosterone on circulating sex steroids, body composition and muscle strength in age-advanced men and women. Clin Endocrinol. In press.
33. Straub, RH, Konecna L, Hrach S, et al. Serum dehydroepiandrosterone (DHEA) and DHEA sulfate are negatively correlated with serum interleukin-6 (IL-6), and DHEA inhibits IL-6 secretion from mononuclear cells in man in vitro: Possible link between endocrinosenescence and immunosenescence. J Clin Endocrinol Metab 83:2012, 1998.
34. Mowszowicz I, Melanitou E, Kirchhoffer MO, et al. Dihydrotestosterone stimulates 5α-reductase activity in pubic skin fibroblasts. J Clin Endocrinol Metab 56:320, 1983.
35. Moghissi E, Ablan F, Horton R. Origin of plasma androstanediol glucuronide in men. J Clin Endocrinol Metab 59:417, 1984.
36. Gibbs GE, Friffin GD. Quantitative determination of beta-glucuronidase in sweat gland and other skin components in cystic fibrosis. J Invest Dermatol 51:200, 1968.
37. Pardridge WM. Transport of protein-bound hormones into tissues in vivo. Endocr Rev 2:103, 1981.
38. Rosner W. The functions of corticosteroid-binding globulin and sex hormone–binding globulin: Recent advances. Endocr Rev 11:80, 1990.
39. Siiteri PK, Murai JT, Hammond GL, et al. The serum transport of steroid hormones. Recent Prog Horm Res 38:457, 1982.
40. Hammond GL. Molecular properties of corticosteroid binding globulin and the sex-steroid binding proteins. Endocr Rev 11:65, 1990.
41. Danzo BJ, Bell BW, Black JH. Human testosterone-binding globulin is a dimer composed of two identical protomers that are differentially glycosylated. Endocrinology 124:2809, 1989.
42. Pugeat MM, Dunn JF, Nisula BC. Transport of steroid hormones: Interaction of 70 drugs with testosterone-binding globulin and corticosteroid-binding globulin in human plasma. J Clin Endocrinol Metab 53:69, 1981.
43. Anderson DC. Sex-hormone-binding globulin. Clin Endocrinol (Oxf) 3:69, 1974.
44. Vermeulen A, Stoica T, Verdonck L. The apparent free testosterone concentration, an index of androgenicity. J Clin Endocrinol Metab 33:759, 1971.
45. Hryb DJ, Khan MS, Romas NA, et al. The control of the interaction of sex hormone–binding globulin with its receptor by steroid hormones. J Biol Chem 265:6048, 1990.
46. Vermeulen A, Verdonch M, VanderStraeten M, et al. Capacity of the testosterone-binding globulin in human plasma and influence of specific binding of testosterone on its metabolic clearance rate. J Clin Endocrinol Metab 29:1470, 1969.
47. DeMoor P, Heyns W, Bouillon R. Growth hormone and the steroid binding β-globulin of human plasma. J Steroid Biochem 3:593, 1972.
48. Vermeulen A, Rubens R, Verdonck L. Testosterone secretion and metabolism in male senescence. J Clin Endocrinol Metab 34:730, 1972.
49. Nestler JE, Powers LP, Matt DW, et al. A direct effect of hyperinsulinemia on serum sex hormone–binding globulin levels in obese women with the polycystic ovary syndrome. J Clin Endocrinol Metab 72:83, 1991.
50. Apter D, Vihko R. Serum sex hormone–binding globulin and sex steroids in relation to pubertal and postpubertal development of the menstrual cycle. Prog Reprod Biol Med 14:58, 1990.
51. Longcope C, Kato T, Horton R. Conversion of blood androgens to estrogens in normal adult men and women. J Clin Invest 48:2191, 1969.
52. Simpson ER, Mahendroo MS, Means GD, et al. Aromatase cytochrome P450, the enzyme responsible for estrogen biosynthesis. Endocr Rev 15:342, 1994.
53. Longcope C, Pratt JH, Schneider SH, et al. Aromatization of androgens by muscle and adipose tissue in vivo. J Clin Endocrinol Metab 46:146, 1978.
54. Matsumine H, Hirato K, Yanaihara T, et al. Aromatization by skeletal muscle. J Clin Endocrinol Metab 63:717, 1986.
55. Longcope C, Sato K, McKay C, et al. Aromatization by splanchnic tissue in men. J Clin Endocrinol Metab 58:1089, 1984.
56. Schweikert HU, Milewich L, Wilson JD. Aromatization of androstenedione by cultured human fibroblasts. J Clin Endocrinol Metab 43:785, 1976.
57. Schweikert HU, Milewich L, Wilson JD. Aromatization of androstenedione by isolated human hairs. J Clin Endocrinol Metab 40:413, 1974.
58. Naftolin F, Ryan KJ, Petro Z. Aromatization of androstenedione by the diencephalon. J Clin Endocrinol Metab 33:368, 1971.
59. Frisch RE, Canick JA, Tulchinsky D. Human fatty marrow aromatizes androgen to estrogen. J Clin Endocrinol Metab 51:394, 1980.
60. Cleland WH, Mendelson CR, Simpson ER. Effects of aging and obesity on aromatase activity of human adipose cells. J Clin Endocrinol Metab 60:174, 1985.
61. Simpson ER, Merrill JC, Hollub AJ, et al. Regulation of estrogen biosynthesis by human adipose cells. Endocr Rev 10:136, 1989.
62. McNatty KP, Makris A, Reinhold VN, et al. Metabolism of androstenedione by human ovarian tissues in vitro with particular reference to reductase and aromatase activity. Steroids 34:429, 1979.
63. Hillier SG, van den Boogaard AM, Reichert LJ, et al. Intraovarian sex steroid hormone interactions and the regulation of follicular maturation: Aromatization of androgens by human granulosa cells in vitro. J Clin Endocrinol Metab 50:640, 1980.
64. Hemsell DL, Edman CD, Marks JF, et al. Massive extraglandular aromatization of plasma androstenedione resulting in feminization of a prepubertal boy. J Clin Invest 60:455, 1977.
65. Berkovitz GD, Guerami A, Brown TR, et al. Familial gynecomastia with increased extraglandular aromatization of plasma carbon 19–steroids. J Clin Invest 75:1763, 1985.
66. Moore DC, Schlaepfer LV, Paunier L, et al. Hormonal changes during puberty: V. Transient pubertal gynecomastia: Abnormal androgen-estrogen ratios. J Clin Endocrinol Metab 58:492, 1984.
67. Bulard J, Mowszowicz I, Schalson G. Increased aromatase activity in pubic skin fibroblasts from patients with isolated gynecomastia. J Clin Endocrinol Metab 64:618, 1987.
68. Simpson ER, Zhao Y, Agarwal VR, et al. Aromatase expression in health and disease. Recent Prog Horm Res 52:185, 1997.
69. Stratakis CA, Vottero A, Brodie A, et al. The aromatase excess syndrome is associated with feminization of both sexes and autosomal dominant transmission of aberrant P450 aromatase gene transcription. J Clin Endocrinol Metab 83:1348, 1998.
70. Shozu M, Akasofu K, Harada T, et al. A new cause of female pseudohermaphroditism: Placental aromatase deficiency. J Clin Endocrinol Metab 72:560, 1991.
71. Harada N, Ogawa H, Shozu M, et al. Biochemical and molecular genetic analyses on placental aromatase (P-450AROM) deficiency. J Biol Chem 267:4781, 1992.
72. Conte FA, Grumbach MM, Ito Y, et al. A syndrome of female pseudohermaphrodism, hypergonadotropic hypogonadism, and multicystic ovaries associated with missense mutations in the gene encoding aromatase P450arom. J Clin Endocrinol Metab 78:1287, 1994.
73. Morishima A, Grumbach MM, Simpson ER, et al. Aromatase deficiency in male and female siblings caused by a novel mutation and the physiological role of estrogens. J Clin Endocrinol Metab 80:3689, 1995.
74. Corbin CJ, Graham-Lorence S, McPhaul M, et al. Isolation of a full-length cDNA insert encoding human aromatase system cytochrome P-450 and its expression in nonsteroidogenic cells. Proc Natl Acad Sci USA 85:8948, 1988.
75. MacDonald PC, Madden JD, Brenner PF, et al. Origin of estrogen in normal men and in women with testicular feminization. J Clin Endocrinol Metab 49:905, 1979.
76. Grodin JM, Siiteri PK, MacDonald PC. Source of estrogen production in postmenopausal women. J Clin Endocrinol Metab 36:207, 1973.
77. Smith EP, Boyd J, Frank GR, et al. Estrogen resistance caused by a mutation in the estrogen-receptor gene in a man [see comments] (published erratum appears in N Engl J Med 332:131, 1995). N Engl J Med 331:1056, 1994.
78. Lubahn DB, Moyer JS, Golding TS, et al. Alteration of reproductive function but not prenatal sexual development after insertional disruption of the mouse estrogen receptor gene. Proc Natl Acad Sci USA 90:11162, 1993.

79. Yamaguchi H, Liotta AS, Krieger DT. Simultaneous determination of human plasma immunoreactive β-lipotropin, γ-lipoprotein, and β-endorphin using immune-affinity chromatography. J Clin Endocrinol Metab 51:1002, 1980.
80. Bertagna XY, Stone WJ, Nicholson WE, et al. Simultaneous assay of immunoreactive β-lipoprotein, γ-lipotropin, and β-endorphin in plasma of normal human subjects, patients with ACTH/lipotropin hypersecretory syndromes, and patients undergoing chronic hemodialysis. J Clin Invest 67:124, 1981.
81. Richter WO, Schwandt P. Physiologic concentrations of β-lipotropin stimulate lipolysis in rabbit adipocytes. Metabolism 34:539, 1985.
82. O'Connell Y, McKenna TJ, Cunningham SK. Effects of pro-opiomelanocortin–derived peptides on adrenal steroidogenesis in guinea-pig adrenal cells in vitro. J Steroid Biochem 44:77, 1993.
83. Carter RJ, Shuster S, Morley JS. Melanotropin potentiating factor is the C-terminal tetrapeptide of human β-lipotropin. Nature 279:74, 1979.
84. Schioth HB, Muceniece R, Wikberg JE, et al. Characterisation of melanocortin receptor subtypes by radioligand binding analysis. Eur J Pharmacol 288:317, 1995.
85. Lowry PJ, Silas L, McLean C, et al. Pro-γ-melanocyte–stimulating hormone cleavage in adrenal gland undergoing compensatory growth. Nature 306:70, 1983.
86. Mountjoy KG. The human melanocyte stimulating hormone receptor has evolved to become "super-sensitive" to melanocortin peptides. Mol Cell Endocrinol 102:R7, 1994.
87. Suzuki I, Cone RD, Im S, et al. Binding of melanotropic hormones to the melanocortin receptor MC1R on human melanocytes stimulates proliferation and melanogenesis. Endocrinology 137:1627, 1996.
88. Shenker Y, Villareal JZ, Sider RS, et al. α-Melanocyte–stimulating hormone stimulation of aldosterone secretion in hypophysectomized rats. Endocrinology 116:138, 1985.
89. Robba C, Rebuffat P, Mazzocchi G, et al. Long-term trophic action of α-melanocyte–stimulating hormone on the zona glomerulosa of the rat adrenal cortex. Acta Endocrinol (Copenh) 112:404, 1986.
90. Reid RL, Ling N, Yen SSC. Gonadotropin-releasing activity of α-melanocyte–stimulating hormone in normal subjects and in subjects with hypothalamic-pituitary dysfunction. J Clin Endocrinol Metab 58:773, 1984.
91. Monkhouse WS, Khalique A. The adrenal and renal veins of man and their connections with azygos and lumbar veins. J Anat 146:105, 1986.
92. Catania A, Lipton JM. α-Melanocyte stimulating hormone in the modulation of host reactions. Endocr Rev 14:564, 1993.
93. Saito E, Iwasa S, Odell W. Widespread presence of large molecular weight adrenocorticotropin-like substances in normal rat extrapituitary tissues. Endocrinology 113:1010, 1983.
94. Yanigabashi K, Hall PF. Role of electron transport in the regulation of lyase activity of C_{21} side-chain cleavage P450 from porcine adrenal and testicular microsome. J Biol Chem 261:8429, 1986.
95. DeBold CR, Menefee JK, Nicholson WE, et al. Proopiomelanocortin gene is expressed in many normal human tissues and in tumors not associated with ectopic adrenocorticotropin syndrome. Mol Endocrinol 2:862, 1988.
96. Lacaze-Masmonteil T, de Keyzer Y, Luton J-P, et al. Characterization of proopiomelanocortin transcripts in human nonpituitary tissues. Proc Natl Acad Sci USA 84:7261, 1987.
97. Peron FG, Koritz SB. On the location of the stimulation in vitro by Ca^{++} and freezing of corticoid production by rat adrenal homogenates. J Biol Chem 235:1625, 1960.
98. Mountjoy KG, Robbins LS, Mortrud MT, et al. The cloning of a family of genes that encode the melanocortin receptors. Science 257:1248, 1992.
99. Cone RD, Mountjoy KG. Molecular genetics of the ACTH and melanocyte-stimulating hormone receptors. Trends Endocrinol Metab 4:242, 1993.
100. Veldhuis JD, Iranmanesh A, Johnson ML, et al. Amplitude, but not frequency, modulation of adrenocorticotropin secretory bursts gives rise to the nyctohemeral rhythm of the corticotropic axis in man. J Clin Endocrinol Metab 71:452, 1990.
101. Quigley ME, Yen SS. A mid-day surge in cortisol levels. J Clin Endocrinol Metab 49:945, 1979.
102. Slag MF, Ahmed M, Gannon MC, et al. Meal stimulation of cortisol secretion: A protein induced effect. Metabolism 30:1104, 1981.
103. Taylor AL, Fishman LM. Corticotropin-releasing hormone. N Engl J Med 319:213, 1988.
104. Jones MT, Gillham B. Factors involved in the regulation of adrenocorticotropic hormone/beta-lipotropic hormone. Physiol Rev 68:743, 1988.
105. Antoni FA. Hypothalamic control of adrenocorticotropin secretion: Advances since the discovery of 41-residue corticotropin-releasing factor. Endocr Rev 7:351, 1986.
106. Takahasi I, Teranishi Y, Nakanishi S, et al. Isolation and structural organization of the human corticotropin–β-lipotropin precursor gene. FEBS Lett 135:97, 1981.
107. Whitfeld PL, Seeburg PH, Shine J. The human pro-opiomelanocortin gene: Organization, sequence, and interspersion with repetitive DNA. DNA 1:133, 1982.
108. Lundblad JR, Roberts JL. Regulation of proopiomelanocortin gene expression in pituitary. Endocr Rev 9:135, 1988.
109. Owerbach D, Rutter WJ, Roberts JL, et al. The proopiocortin adrenocorticotropin/beta-lipoprotein gene is located on chromosome 2 in humans. Somat Cell Genet 7:359, 1981.
110. Krieger DT. Physiopathology of Cushing's disease. Endocr Rev 4:22, 1983.
111. Scheurmeyer TH, Avgerinos PC, Gold PW, et al. Human corticotropin-releasing factor in man: Pharmacokinetic properties and dose-response of plasma adrenocorticotropin and cortisol secretion. J Clin Endocrinol Metab 59:1103, 1984.
112. Tan SY, Mulrow PJ. The contribution of the zona fasciculata and glomerulosa to plasma 11-deoxycorticosterone levels in man. J Clin Endocrinol Metab 41:126, 1975.
113. Kater CE, Biglieri EG, Brust N, et al. Stimulation and suppression of the mineralocorticoid hormones in normal subjects and adrenocortical disorders. Endocr Rev 10:149, 1989.
114. Gomez-Sanchez CE, Montgomery M, Ganguly A, et al. Elevated urinary excretion of 18-oxocortisol in glucocorticoid-suppressible aldosteronism. J Clin Endocrinol Metab 59:1022, 1984.
115. Griffing GT, Dale SL, Holbrook MM, et al. The regulation of urinary free 19-nor-deoxycorticosterone and its relation to systemic arterial pressure in normotensive and hypertensive subjects. J Clin Endocrinol Metab 56:99, 1983.
116. Quinn SJ, Williams GH. Regulation of aldosterone secretion. Annu Rev Physiol 50:409, 1988.
117. Williams GH, Dluhy RG. Control of aldosterone secretion. *In* Genest J, Kuchel O, Hamet P, Doe J (eds). Hypertension: Physiopathology and Treatment. New York, McGraw-Hill, 1983, pp 320–337.
118. Yanagibashi K, Haniu M, Shively JE, et al. The synthesis of aldosterone by the adrenal cortex. Two zones (fasciculata and glomerulosa) possess one enzyme for 11β-, 18-hydroxylation, and aldehyde synthesis. J Biol Chem 261:3556, 1986.
119. Longcope C. Adrenal and gonadal androgen secretion in normal females. Clin Endocrinol Metab 15:213, 1986.
120. Nelson DH. The Adrenal Cortex: Physiological Function and Disease. Philadelphia, WB Saunders, 1980.
121. Rosenfeld RS, Rosenberg BJ, Fukushima D, et al. 24-Hour secretory pattern of dehydroisoandrosterone and dehydroisoandrosterone sulfate. J Clin Endocrinol Metab 40:850, 1975.
122. Lobo RA, Kletzky OA, Kaptein EM, et al. Prolactin modulation of dehydroepiandrosterone sulfate secretion. Am J Obstet Gynecol 138:632, 1980.
123. Higuchi K, Nawata H, Maki T, et al. Prolactin has a direct effect on adrenal androgen secretion. J Clin Endocrinol Metab 59:714, 1984.
124. Feher T, Szalay KS, Szilagyi G. Effect of ACTH and prolactin on dehydroepiandrosterone, its sulfate ester and cortisol production by normal and tumorous human adrenocortical cells. J Steroid Biochem 23:153, 1985.
125. Winterer J, Gwirtsman HE, George DT, et al. Adrenocorticotropin-stimulated adrenal androgen secretion in anorexia nervosa: Impaired secretion at low weight with normalization after long-term weight recovery. J Clin Endocrinol Metab 61:693, 1985.
126. James VHT, Few JD. Adrenocorticosteroids: Chemistry, synthesis and disturbances in diseases. Clin Endocrinol Metab 14:867, 1985.

127. Illingworth DR, Kenny TA, Orwoll ES. Adrenal function in heterozygous and homozygous hypobetalipoproteinemia. J Clin Endocrinol Metab 54:27, 1982.
128. Illingworth DR, Orwoll ES, Connor WE. Impaired cortisol secretion in abetalipoproteinemia. J Clin Endocrinol Metab 50:977, 1980.
129. Illingworth DR, Lees AM, Lees RS. Adrenal cortical function in homozygous familial hypercholesterolemia. Metabolism 32:1045, 1983.
130. Acton S, Rigotti A, Landschulz KT, et al. Identification of a scavenger receptor SR-BI as a high density lipoprotein receptor. Science 271:518, 1996.
131. Plump AS, Erickson SK, Weng W, et al. Apolipoprotein A-1 is required for cholesteryl ester accumulation in steroidogenic cells and for normal adrenal steroid production. J Clin Invest 97:2660, 1996.
132. Landschulz KT, Pathak RK, Rigotti A, et al. Regulation of scavenger receptor, class B, type I, a high density lipoprotein receptor, in liver and steroidogenic tissues of the rat. J Clin Invest 98:984, 1996.
133. Borkowski AJ, Levin S, Delcroix C, et al. Blood cholesterol and hydrocortisone production in man: Quantitative aspects of the utilization of circulating cholesterol by the adrenals at rest and under adrenocorticotropin stimulation. J Clin Invest 46:797, 1967.
134. Bolte E, Coudert S, Lefebvre Y. Steroid production from plasma cholesterol. II. In vivo conversion of plasma cholesterol to ovarian progesterone and adrenal C^{19} and C^{21} steroids in humans. J Clin Endocrinol Metab 38:394, 1967.
135. Gwynne JT, Strauss JF III. The role of lipoprotein in steroidogenesis and cholesterol metabolism in steroidogenic glands. Endocr Rev 3:299, 1982.
136. Miller WL. Molecular biology of steroid hormone synthesis. Endocr Rev 9:295, 1988.
137. Parker KL, Chimmer BP. Transcriptional regulation of the genes encoding the cytochrome P450 steroid hydroxylases. Vitam Horm 51:339, 1995.
138. Cori CF, Cori GT. Fate of sugar and animal body: Carbohydrate metabolism of adrenalectomized rats and mice. J Biol Chem 74:473, 1927.
139. Long CNH, Katzin B, Fry EG. The adrenal cortex and carbohydrate metabolism. Endocrinology 26:309, 1940.
140. Hornbrook KR, Burch HB, Lowry OH. The effects of adrenalectomy and hydrocortisone on rat liver metabolites and glycogen synthetase activity. Mol Pharmacol 2:106, 1966.
141. Stalmans W, Laloux M. Glucocorticoids and hepatic glycogen metabolism. *In* Baxter JD, Rousseau GG (eds). Glucocorticoid Hormone Action. New York, Springer-Verlag, 1979, pp 518–533.
142. Exton JH. Regulation of gluconeogenesis by glucocorticoids. *In* Baxter JD, Rousseau GG (eds). Glucocorticoid Hormone Action. New York, Springer-Verlag, 1979, pp 535–546.
143. Yoo-Warren H, Cimbala MA, Felz K, et al. Identification of a DNA clone to phosphoenolpyruvate carboxykinase (GTP) from rat cytosol. Alterations in phosphoenolpyruvate carboxykinase RNA levels detectable by hybridization. J Biol Chem 256:10224, 1981.
144. Magnuson MA, Quinn PG, Granner DK. Multihormonal regulation of phosphoenolpyruvate carboxykinase–chloramphenicol acetyltransferase fusion genes. J Biol Chem 262:14917, 1987.
145. Petersen DD, Magnuson MA, Granner DK. Location and characterization of two widely separated glucocorticoid response elements in the phosphoenolpyruvate carboxykinase gene. Mol Cell Biol 8:96, 1988.
146. Friedmann N, Exton JH, Parker CR Jr. Interaction of adrenal steroids and glucagon on gluconeogenesis in perfused rat liver. Biochem Biophys Res Commun 29:113, 1967.
147. Munck A. Studies on the mode of action of glucocorticoids in rats. II. The effects in vivo and in vitro on net glucose uptake by isolated adipose tissue. Biochim Biophys Acta 57:318, 1962.
148. LeBoeuf B, Renold AE, Cahill GF. Studies on rat adipose tissue in vitro. IX. Further effects of cortisol on glucose metabolism. J Biol Chem 237:988, 1962.
149. Fain JN, Scow RO, Chernick SS. Effects of glucocorticoids on metabolism of adipose tissue in vitro. J Biol Chem 238:54, 1963.
150. Fain JH. Inhibition of glucose transport in fat cells and activation of lipolysis by glucocorticoids. *In* Baxter JD, Rousseau GG (eds). Glucocorticoid Hormone Action. New York, Springer-Verlag, 1979, pp 547–560.
151. Olefsky JM. Effect of dexamethasone on insulin binding, glucose transport, and glucose oxidation of isolated rat adipocytes. J Clin Invest 56:1499, 1975.
152. Livingston JN, Lockwood DH. Effect of glucocorticoids on the glucose transport system of isolated fat cells. J Biol Chem 250:8353, 1975.
153. Garvey WT, Huecksteadt TP, Lima FB, et al. Expression of a glucose transporter gene cloned from brain in cellular models of insulin resistance: Dexamethasone decreases transporter mRNA in primary cultured adipocytes. Mol Endocrinol 3:1132, 1989.
154. Goodman HM, Knobil E. Some endocrine factors in regulation of fatty acid mobilization during fasting. Am J Physiol 201:1, 1961.
155. Fain JH. Effects of dexamethasone and growth hormone on fatty acid mobilization and glucose utilization in adrenalectomized rats. Endocrinology 71:633, 1962.
156. Havel R. Transport and metabolism of chylomicrons. Am J Clin Nutr 6:662, 1958.
157. Rudman D, DiGirolamo M. Effects of adrenal cortical steroids on lipid metabolism. *In* Christy NP (ed). The Human Adrenal Cortex. New York, Harper & Row, 1971, pp 241–255.
158. Hausberger FX. Influence of insulin and cortisone on hepatic and adipose tissue metabolism of rats. Endocrinology 63:14, 1958.
159. Graham BS, Tucker WS Jr. Opportunistic infection in endogenous Cushing's syndrome. Ann Intern Med 101:334, 1984.
160. Cushing H. The Pituitary Body and Its Disorders. Philadelphia, JB Lippincott, 1912.
161. Huff TA. Clinical syndromes related to disorders of adrenocorticotrophic hormone. *In* Allen BM, Makesh VB. The Pituitary: A Current Review. New York, Academic Press, 1977, pp 153–168.
162. Plotz CM, Knowlton AL, Ragan C. The natural history of Cushing's syndrome. Am J Med 13:597, 1952.
163. Orth DN. Ectopic hormone production. *In* Felig P, Baxter JD, Broadus AE, Doe J (eds). Endocrinology and Metabolism. New York, McGraw-Hill, 1987, pp 1692–1735.
164. Strott CA, Nugent CA, Tyler FH. Cushing's syndrome caused by bronchial adenomas. Am J Med 44:97, 1968.
165. Mason AMS, Ratcliff JG, Buckle RM, et al. ACTH secretion by bronchial carcinoid tumours. Clin Endocrinol (Oxf) 1:3, 1972.
166. Flack MR, Oldfield EH, Cutler GJ, et al. Urine free cortisol in the high-dose dexamethasone suppression test for the differential diagnosis of the Cushing syndrome. Ann Intern Med 116:211, 1992.
167. Carey RM, Varma SK, Drake CR Jr, et al. Ectopic secretion of corticotropin-releasing factor as a cause of Cushing's syndrome. A clinical, morphologic, and biochemical study. N Engl J Med 311:13, 1984.
168. Belsky JL, Cuello B, Swanson LW, et al. Cushing's syndrome due to ectopic production of corticotropin-releasing factor. J Clin Endocrinol Metab 60:496, 1985.
169. Orth DN. Corticotropin-releasing hormone in humans. Endocr Rev 13:164, 1992.
170. Schteingart DE, Lloyd RV, Akil H, et al. Cushing's syndrome secondary to ectopic corticotropin-releasing hormone–adrenocorticotropin secretion. J Clin Endocrinol Metab 63:770, 1986.
171. Zarate A, Kovacs K, Flores M, et al. ACTH and CRF-producing bronchial carcinoid associated with Cushing's syndrome. Clin Endocrinol 24:523, 1986.
172. Jessop DS, Cunnah D, Miller JG, et al. A phaeochromocytoma presenting with Cushing's syndrome associated with increased concentrations of circulating corticotrophin-releasing factor. J Endocrinol 113:133, 1987.
173. Gerl H, Knappe G, Rohde W, et al. Cushing-Syndrom bei CRF-produzierendem mediastinalem Karzinoid. Dtsch Med Wochenschr 115:332, 1990.
174. O'Brien T, Yoiung WF Jr, Davila DG, et al. Cushing's syndrome associated with ectopic production of corticotrophin-releasing hormone, corticotrophin and vasopressin by a phaeochromocytoma. Clin Endocrinol (Oxf) 37:460, 1992.
175. Kruimel JW, Smals AGH, Beex LV, et al. Favourable response of a virilizing adrenocortical carcinoma to preoperative treatment with ketoconazole and postoperative chemotherapy. Acta Endocrinol (Copenh) 124:492, 1991.
176. Asa SL, Kovacs K, Tindall GT, et al. Cushing's disease associated

with an intrasellar gangliocytoma producing corticotrophin-releasing factor. Ann Intern Med 101:789, 1984.
177. Sakai Y, Yanase T, Takayanagi R, et al. High expression of cytochrome b_5 in adrenocortical adenomas from patients with Cushing's syndrome associated with high secretion of adrenal androgens. J Clin Endocrinol Metab 76:1286, 1993.
178. Aupetit-Faisant B, Battaglia C, Zenatti M, et al. Hypoaldosteronism accompanied by normal or elevated mineralocorticosteroid pathway steroid: A marker of adrenal carcinoma. J Clin Endocrinol Metab 76:38, 1993.
179. Buescher MA. Cushing's syndrome in pregnancy. Endocrinology 6:357, 1996.
180. DaMotta LA, Motta LD, Barbosa AM, et al. Two pregnancies in a Cushing's syndrome: Case report. Panminerva Med 33:44, 1991.
181. Close CF, Mann MC, Watts JF, et al. ACTH-independent Cushing's syndrome in pregnancy with spontaneous resolution after delivery: Control of the hypercortisolism with metyrapone. Clin Endocrinol 39:375, 1993.
182. Buescher MA, McClamrock HD, Adashi EY. Cushing syndrome in pregnancy. Obstet Gynecol 79:130, 1992.
183. Caticha O, Odell W, Wilson DE, et al. Estradiol stimulates cortisol production by adrenal cells in estrogen-dependent primary adrenocortical nodular dysplasia. J Clin Endocrinol Metab 77:494, 1993.
184. Evans PJ, Peters JR, Dyas J, et al. Salivary cortisol levels in true and apparent hypercortisolism. Clin Endocrinol 20:709, 1984.
185. Voccia E, Saenger P, Peterson RE, et al. 6β-Hydroxycortisol excretion in hypercortisolemic states. J Clin Endocrinol Metab 48:467, 1979.
186. Latronico AC, Chrousos GP. Extensive personal experience: Adrenocortical tumors. J Clin Endocrinol Metab 82:1317, 1997.
187. Lavoie H, Lacroix A. Partially autonomous cortisol secretion by incidentally discovered adrenal adenomas. TEM 6:191, 1995.
188. Kloos RT, Gross MD, Francis IR, et al. Incidentally discovered adrenal masses. Endocr Rev 16:460, 1995.
189. Herrera MF, Grant CS, vanHeerden JA, et al. Incidentally discovered adrenal tumors: An institutional perspective. Surgery 110:1014, 1991.
190. Terzolo M, Osella G, Ali A, et al. Different patterns of steroid secretion in patients with adrenal incidentaloma. J Clin Endocrinol Metab 81:740, 1996.
191. Seppel T, Schlaghecke R. Augmented 17α-hydroxyprogesterone response to ACTH stimulation as evidence of decreased 21-hydroxylase activity in patients with incidentally discovered adrenal tumours ('incidentalomas'). Clin Endocrinol 41:445, 1994.
192. Flecchia D, Mazza E, Carlini M, et al. Reduced serum levels of dehydroepiandrosterone sulphate in adrenal incidentalomas: A marker of adrenocortical tumour. Clin Endocrinol (Oxf) 42:129, 1995.
193. Copeland PM. The incidentally discovered adrenal mass. Ann Intern Med 98:940, 1983.
194. Rosen HN, Swartz SL. Subtle glucocorticoid excess in patients with adrenal incidentaloma. Am J Med 92:213, 1992.
195. Krohn K, Uibo R, Aavik E, et al. Identification by molecular cloning of an autoantigen associated with Addison's disease as steroid 17α-hydroxylase [see comments]. Lancet 339:770, 1992.
196. Chen S, Sawicka J, Betterle C, et al. Autoantibodies to steroidogenic enzymes in autoimmune polyglandular syndrome, Addison's disease, and premature ovarian failure. J Clin Endocrinol Metab 81:1871, 1996.
197. Uibo R, Aavik E, Peterson P, et al. Autoantibodies to cytochrome P450 enzymes P450scc, P450c17, and P450c21 in autoimmune polyglandular disease types I and II and in isolated Addison's disease. J Clin Endocrinol Metab 78:323, 1994.
198. Winqvist O, Seoderbergh A, Keampe O. The autoimmune basis of adrenocortical destruction in Addison's disease. Mol Med Today 2:282, 1996.
199. Wheatcroft N, Weetman AP. Is premature ovarian failure an autoimmune disease? Autoimmunity 25:157, 1997.
200. Winqvist O, Gustafsson J, Rorsman F, et al. Two different cytochrome P450 enzymes are the adrenal antigens in autoimmune polyendocrine syndrome type I and Addison's disease. J Clin Invest 92:2377, 1993.
201. Sandison AT. A form of lipoidosis of the adrenal cortex in an infant. Arch Dis Child 30:538, 1955.
202. Kirkland RT, Kirkland JL, Johnson CM, et al. Congenital lipoid adrenal hyperplasia in an eight-year-old phenotypic female. J Clin Endocrinol Metab 36:488, 1973.
203. Matsuo N, Tsuzaki S, Anzo M, et al. The phenotypic definition of congenital lipoid adrenal hyperplasia: Analysis of the 67 Japanese patients (Abstract). Horm Res 41:(suppl 106), 1994.
204. Lin D, Chang YJ, Strauss JF, et al. The human peripheral benzodiazepine receptor gene: Cloning and characterization of alternative splicing in normal tissues and in a patient with congenital lipoid adrenal hyperplasia. Genomics 18:643, 1993.
205. Lin D, Gitelman SE, Saenger P, et al. Normal genes for the cholesterol side chain cleavage enzyme, P450scc, in congenital lipoid adrenal hyperplasia. J Clin Invest 88:1955, 1991.
206. Sugawara T, Lin D, Holt JA, et al. Structure of the human steroidogenic acute regulatory protein StAR gene: StAR stimulates mitochondrial cholesterol 27-hydroxylase activity. Biochemistry 34:12506, 1995.
207. Bose HS, Sugawara T, Strauss JF, et al. The pathophysiology and genetics of congenital lipoid adrenal hyperplasia. International Congenital Lipoid Adrenal Hyperplasia Consortium. N Engl J Med 335:1870, 1996.
208. Larsen PR, Dick TE, Markowitz MM, et al. Inhibition of intrapituitary thyroxine to 3,5,3′-triiodothyronine conversion prevents the acute suppression of thyrotropin release by thyroxine in hypothyroid rats. J Clin Invest 64:117, 1979.
209. Campos-Barros A, Hoell T, Musa A, et al. Phenolic and tyrosyl ring iodothyronine deiodination and thyroid hormone concentrations in the human central nevous system. J Clin Endocrinol Metab 81:2179, 1996.
210. Bilezikian JP, Loeb JN. The influence of hyperthyroidism and hypothyroidism on α- and β-adrenergic receptor systems and adrenergic responsiveness. Endocr Rev 4:378, 1983.
211. Hellström L, Wahrenberg H, Reynisdottir S, et al. Catecholamine-induced adipocyte lipolysis in human hyperthyroidism. J Clin Endocrinol Metab 82:159, 1997.
212. Stagnaro-Green A, Roman SH, Cobin RH, et al. Detection of at-risk pregnancy by means of highly sensitive assays for thyroid autoantibodies. JAMA 264:1422, 1990.
213. Montoro M, Collea JV, Frasier SD, et al. Successful outcome of pregnancy in women with hypothyroidism. Ann Intern Med 94:31, 1981.
214. Davis LE, Leveno KJ, Cunningham FG. Hypothyroidism and thyrotoxicosis. Obstet Gynecol 72:108, 1988.
215. Gordon GG, Southren AL. Thyroid-hormone effects on steroid-hormone metabolism. Bull N Y Acad Med 53:241, 1977.
216. Refetoff S, DeWint LT, DeGroot LJ. Familial syndrome combining deaf-mutism, stippled epiphyses, goiter, and abnormally high PBI: Possible target organ refractoriness to thyroid hormone. J Clin Endocrinol Metab 27:279, 1967.
217. Usala SJ, Bale AE, Gesundheit N, et al. Tight linkage between the syndrome of generalized thyroid hormone resistance and the human c-erbA-β gene. Mol Endocrinol 2:1217, 1988.
218. Refetoff S, Weiss RE, Usala SJ. The syndromes of resistance to thyroid hormone. Endocr Rev 14:348, 1993.
219. Forrest D, Hanebuth E, Smeyne RJ, et al. Recessive resistance to thyroid hormone in mice lacking thyroid hormone receptor β: Evidence for tissue-specific modulation of receptor function. EMBO J 15:3006, 1996.
220. Baniahmad A, Tsai SY, O'Malley BW, et al. Kindred S thyroid hormone receptor is an active and constitutive silencer and a repressor for thyroid hormone and retinoic acid responses. Proc Natl Acad Sci USA 89:10633, 1992.
221. Flynn TR, Hollenberg AN, Cohen O, et al. A novel C-terminal domain in the thyroid hormone receptor selectively mediates thyroid hormone inhibition. J Biol Chem 269:32713, 1994.
222. Adams M, Matthews C, Collingwood TN, et al. Genetic analysis of 29 kindreds with generalized and pituitary resistance to thyroid hormone. J Clin Invest 94:506, 1994.
223. Weiss RE, Hayashi Y, Nagaya T, et al. Dominant inheritance of resistance to thyroid hormone not linked to defects in the thyroid hormone receptor alpha or beta genes may be due to a defective co-factor. J Clin Endocrinol Metab 81:4196, 1996.
224. Larsen PR, Silva JE, Kaplan MM. Relationships between circulating and intracellular thyroid hormones: Physiological and clinical implications. Endocr Rev 2:87, 1981.

225. Kohrle J, Hesch RD, Leonard JL. Intracellular pathways of iodothyronine metabolism. *In* Braverman LE, Utiger RD (eds). Werner's and Ingbar's The Thyroid. Philadelphia, JB Lippincott, 1991, pp 144–186.
226. Nagamani M, Stuart CA, VanDinth T. Steroid biosynthesis in the Sertoli-Leydig cell tumor: Effects of insulin and luteinizing hormone. Am J Obstet Gynecol 161:1738, 1989.
227. Shenker Y, Malozowski SN, Ayers J, et al. Steroid secretion by a virilizing lipoid cell ovarian tumor: Origins of dehydroepiandrosterone sulfate. Obstet Gynecol 74:502, 1989.
228. Adashi EY, Rosenwaks Z, Lee PA, et al. Endocrine features of an adrenal-like tumor of the ovary. J Clin Endocrinol Metab 48:241, 1979.
229. Werk EJ, Sholiton LE, Kalejs L. Testosterone-secreting adrenal adenoma under gonadotropin control. N Engl J Med 289:767, 1973.
230. Gustafson ML, Lee MM, Scully RE, et al. Müllerian inhibiting substance as a marker for ovarian sex-cord tumor. N Engl J Med 326:466, 1992.
231. Matzuk MM, Finegold MJ, Mishina Y, et al. Synergistic effects of inhibins and müllerian-inhibiting substance on testicular tumorigenesis. Mol Endocrinol 9:1337, 1995.
232. O'Marcaigh AS, Ledger GA, Roche PC, et al. Aromatase expression in human germinomas with possible biological effects. J Clin Endocrinol Metab 80:3763, 1995.
233. Rey RA, Lhommae C, Marcillac I, et al. Antimüllerian hormone as a serum marker of granulosa cell tumors of the ovary: Comparative study with serum alpha-inhibin and estradiol. Am J Obstet Gynecol 174:958, 1996.
234. Anderson G. Paramalignant syndrome. *In* Baron DN, Compston NH, Dawson AM (eds). Recent Advances in Medicine. Edinburgh, Churchill Livingstone, 1973, pp 1–23.
235. Vaitukaitis JL, Ross GT, Braunstein GD, et al. Gonadotropins and their subunits: Basic and clinical studies. Recent Prog Horm Res 32:289, 1976.
236. Odell W, Wolfsen A, Yoshimoto Y, et al. Ectopic peptide synthesis: A universal concomitant of neoplasia. Trans Assoc Am Physicians 90:204, 1977.
237. Maruo T, Segal SJ, Koide SS. Studies on the apparent human chorionic gonadotropin-like factor in the crab *Ovalipes ocellatus.* Endocrinology 104:932, 1979.
238. Hung W, Blizzard RM, Migeon CJ, et al. Precocious puberty in a boy with hepatoma and circulating gonadotropin. J Pediatr 63:895, 1963.
239. Fusco FD, Rosen SW. Gonadotropin-producing anaplastic large-cell carcinomas of the lung. N Engl J Med 275:507, 1966.
240. Sklar CA, Conte FA, Kaplan SL, et al. Human chorionic gonadotropin-secreting pineal tumor: Relation to pathogenesis and sex limitation of sexual precocity. J Clin Endocrinol Metab 53:656, 1981.
241. Ahmed SR, Shalet SM, Price DA, et al. Human chorionic gonadotrophin secreting pineal germinoma and precocious puberty. Arch Dis Child 58:743, 1983.
242. Kirschner MA, Cohen FB, Jespersen D. Estrogen production and its origin in men with gonadotropin-producing neoplasms. J Clin Endocrinol Metab 39:112, 1974.
243. Vaitukaitis JL. Immunologic and physical characterization of human chorionic gonadotropin hCG secreted by tumors. J Clin Endocrinol Metab 37:505, 1973.
244. Lange PH, McIntire KR, Waldmann TA, et al. Serum alpha fetoprotein and human chorionic gonadotropin in the diagnosis and management of nonseminomatous germ-cell testicular cancer. N Engl J Med 295:1237, 1976.
245. Braunstein GD, Vaitukaitis JL, Carbone PP, et al. Ectopic production of human chorionic gonadotrophin by neoplasms. Ann Intern Med 78:39, 1973.
246. Hammond CB, Parker RT. Diagnosis and treatment of trophoblastic disease. A report from the Southeastern Regional Center. Obstet Gynecol 35:132, 1970.
247. MacKay EN, Sellers AH. A statistical review of malignant testicular tumours based on the experience of the Ontario Cancer Foundation Clinics, 1938–1961. Can Med Assoc J 94:889, 1966.
248. Weintraub BD, Rosen SW. Ectopic production of human chorionic somatomammotropin by nontrophoblastic cancers. J Clin Endocrinol Metab 32:94, 1971.
249. Kremer H, Kraaij R, Toledo SP, et al. Male pseudohermaphroditism due for homozygous missense mutation of the luteinizing hormone receptor gene. Nat Genet 9:160, 1995.
250. Latronico AC, Anasti J, Arnhold IJ, et al. Brief report: Testicular and ovarian resistance to luteinizing hormone caused by inactivating mutations of the luteinizing hormone–receptor gene. N Engl J Med 334:507, 1996.
251. Toledo SP, Brunner HG, Kraaij R, et al. An inactivating mutation of the LH receptor causes amenorrhea in a 46XX female. J Clin Endocrinol Metab 81:3850, 1996.
252. Misrahi M, Meduri G, Piccard S, et al. Comparison of immunocytochemical and molecular features with the phenotype in a case of incomplete male pseudohermaphroditism associated with a mutation of the luteinizing hormone receptor. J Clin Endocrinol Metab 82:2159, 1997.
253. Stavrou SS, Zhu Y-S, Cai L-Q, et al. A novel mutation of the human luteinizing hormone receptor in 46XY and 46XX sisters. J Clin Endocrinol Metab 83:2091, 1998.
254. Minegish T, Nakamura K, Takakura Y, et al. Cloning and sequencing of the human LH/hCG receptor cDNA. Biochem Biophys Res Commun 172:1049, 1990.
255. Latronico AC, Abell AN, Arnhold IJP, et al. A unique constitutively activating mutation in third transmembrane helix of luteinizing hormone receptor causes sporadic male gonadotropin-independent precocious puberty. J Clin Endocrinol Metab 83:2435, 1998.
256. Laue L, Wu SM, Kudo M, et al. Compound heterozygous mutations of the LHR gene in Leydig cell hypoplasia. Mol Endocrinol 10:987, 1996.
257. Meduri G, Mai TVL, Jovlet A, et al. New functional zonation in the ovary as shown by immunobiochemistry of the luteinizing hormone receptor. Endocrinology 131:366, 1992.
258. Stone RK. Am J Med Sci. 24:561, 1852.
259. Holland FJ. Gonadotropin-independent precocious puberty. Endocrinol Metab Clin North Am 20:191, 1991.
260. Schedewie HK, Reiter EO, Beitins IZ, et al. Testicular Leydig cell hyperplasia as a cause of familial sexual precocity. J Clin Endocrinol Metab 52:271, 1981.
261. Shenker A, Laue L, Kosugi S, et al. A constitutively activating mutation of the luteinizing hormone receptor in familial male precocious puberty (see comments). Nature 365:652, 1993.
262. Gromoll J, Partsch CJ, Simoni M, et al. A mutation in the first transmembrane domain of the lutropin receptor causes male precocious puberty. J Clin Endocrinol Metab 83:476, 1998.
263. Bargmann CI, Hung MC, Weinberg RA. Multiple independent activations of the *neu* oncogene by a point mutation altering the transmembrane domain of p185. Cell 45:649, 1986.
264. Yaghmai R, Hazelbauer GL. Ligand occupancy mimicked by single residue substitutions in a receptor: Transmembrane signaling induced by mutation. Proc Natl Acad Sci USA 89:7890, 1992.
265. Dryja TP, McGee TL, Hahn LB, et al. Mutations within the rhodopsin gene in patients with autosomal dominant retinitis pigmentosa. N Engl J Med 323:1302, 1990.
266. Rosenthal W, Seibold A, Antaramian A, et al. Molecular identification of the gene responsible for congenital nephrogenic diabetes insipidus. Nature 359:233, 1992.
267. Allen LF, Lefkowitz RJ, Caron MG, et al. G-protein–coupled receptor genes as protooncogenes: constitutively activating mutation of the alpha 1β-adrenergic receptor enhances mitogenesis and tumorigenicity. Proc Natl Acad Sci USA 88:11354, 1991.
268. Kjelsberg MA, Cotecchia S, Ostrowski J, et al. Constitutive activation of the alpha 1β-adrenergic receptor by all amino acid substitutions at a single site. Evidence for a region which constrains receptor activation. J Biol Chem 267:1430, 1992.
269. Robbins LS, Nadeau JH, Johnson KR, et al. Pigmentation phenotypes of variant extension locus alleles result from point mutations that alter MSH receptor function. Cell 72:827, 1993.
270. Robinson PR, Cohen GB, Zhukovsky EA, et al. Constitutively active mutants of rhodopsin. Neuron 9:719, 1992.
271. Rousseau-Merck MF, Misrahi M, Atger M, et al. Localization of the human luteinizing hormone/choriogonadotropin receptor gene LHCGR to chromosome 2p21. Cytogenet Cell Genet 54:77, 1990.
272. Gromoll J, Ried T, Holtgreve-Grez H, et al. Localization of the human FSH receptor to chromosome 2 p21 using a genomic probe comprising exon 10. J Mol Endocrinol 12:265, 1994.

273. Gromoll J, Pekel E, Nieschlag E. The structure and organization of the human follicle-stimulating hormone receptor FSHR gene. Genomics 35:308, 1996.
274. Aittomeaki K, Lucena JL, Pakarinen P, et al. Mutation in the follicle-stimulating hormone receptor gene causes hereditary hypergonadotropic ovarian failure. Cell 82:959, 1995.
275. Aittomeaki K. The genetics of XX gonadal dysgenesis. Am J Hum Genet 54:844, 1994.
276. Aittomeaki K, Herva R, Stenman UH, et al. Clinical features of primary ovarian failure caused by a point mutation in the follicle-stimulating hormone receptor gene. J Clin Endocrinol Metab 81:3722, 1996.
277. Huhtaniemi I, Pettersson K. Mutations and polymorphisms in the gonadotrophin genes; clinical relevance. Clin Endocrinol 48:675, 1998.
278. Gromoll J, Simoni M, Nieschlag E. An activating mutation of the follicle-stimulating hormone receptor autonomously sustains spermatogenesis in a hypophysectomized man. J Clin Endocrinol Metab 81:1367, 1996.
279. Chrousos GP, Detera-Wadleigh SD, Karl M. Syndromes of glucocorticoid resistance (see comments). Ann Intern Med 119:1113, 1993.
280. McDermott MT, Ridgway EC. Thyroid hormone resistance syndromes (see comments). Am J Med 94:424, 1993.
281. Brown TR, Lubahn DB, Wilson EM, et al. Functional characterization of naturally occurring mutant androgen receptors from subjects with complete androgen insensitivity. Mol Endocrinol 4:1759, 1990.
282. Smith EP, Boyd J, Graeme RF, et al. Estrogen resistance caused by mutation in the estrogen receptor gene in a man. N Engl J Med 331:1056, 1994.
283. Fraser IS, Michie EA, Wide L, et al. Pituitary gonadotropins and ovarian function in adolescent dysfunctional uterine bleeding. J Clin Endocrinol Metab 37:407, 1973.
284. Sherman BM, West JH, Korenman SG. The menopausal transition: analysis of LH, FSH, estradiol, and progesterone concentrations during menstrual cycles of older women. J Clin Endocrinol Metab 42:629, 1976.
285. Mann WJ, Feil PD, Demers L, et al. Factors affecting biologic action of progestins in human endometrium. Gynecol Invest 8:49, 1977.

Chapter 19

CHRONIC ANOVULATION DUE TO CNS-HYPOTHALAMIC-PITUITARY DYSFUNCTION

S. S. C. Yen • with the assistance of Gail Laughlin

CHAPTER OUTLINE

KEY POINTS

- GnRH neurons are unique because they are seeded outside the brain—in the nasal placode. Migration from the nose to the hypothalamus occurs during fetal development. When migration fails, hypogonadotropic hypogonadism ensues.
- All cell types of the anterior pituitary gland are capable of developing adenomatous lesions due to monoclonal proliferations. Hormonal hypersecretions and suprasellar extensions cause disruption of reproductive integrity.
- The biologic essentials are *feeding, mating,* and *sleeping.* These innate behaviors are dictated by neural and metabolic networks to sustain life and perpetuate the species. Derangement of neural communications and metabolic fuel deficit, when sustained, disrupt the reproductive axis.
- The reproductive axis involves ultradian and circadian rhythmicity and the sleep-wake cycle, dynamic processes that are properties of the hypothalamic pulse generator, circadian pacemaker, and environmental cues.
- Neuronal networks governing mood and behavior (cognitive being) are the foundation of psychoneuroendocrinology. Negative impacts of life events and environmental factors cause reproductive disorder.
- Functional hypothalamic amenorrhea syndromes are the most common form of clinical disorders. Both psychogenic and exercise-related types are associated with nutritional deficits with a remarkable commonality of multiple neuroendocrine-metabolic adaptations.
- Anorexia nervosa, an extraordinary psychoneuroendocrinologic disorder, is associated with dysfunctions involving virtually all the neuroendocrine-metabolic systems and profound psychologic aberrations—management of these patients is highly complex.
- Premenstrual dysphoria is associated with affective disorders, and mounting evidence supports the impact of cyclic ovarian steroids on the alterations of serotoninergic neurotransmission in the manifestation of symptoms. During the late luteal phase, selective serotonin reuptake inhibitors offer symptomatic improvements.

To be fully versed in centrally initiated reproductive disorders in women, an understanding of hypothalamic control of reproductive (follicle-stimulating hormone [FSH], luteinizing hormone [LH], and prolactin) and metabolic (thyroid-stimulating hormone [TSH], corticotropin [ACTH], and the growth hormone–insulin-like growth factor I [GH–IGF-I] system) hormones as well as of neurohypophysial hormones is required. For example, reproductive dysfunction may be associated with GH excess (acromegaly), ACTH excess (Cushing's syndrome), and thyroid hormone deficiency and excess. In fact, patients with amenorrhea due to hypothalamic lesions may have abnormal hormone secretion by both adenohypophysial and neurohypophysial systems. Further, neuroendocrine regulation of reproductive homeostasis has been recognized to involve circadian rhythmicity and sleep-wake cycles within the 24-hour biologic clock. These dynamic processes are properties of a hypothalamic pacemaker (the suprachiasmatic nucleus), and they invoke cyclic changes of almost all clinically discernible physiologic variables such as body temperature, blood pressure, and pituitary hormone release. Frequent sequential measurement of plasma hormone concentrations has led to the recognition that most hormones are secreted episodically (ultradian rhythm); several have prominent circadian rhythmicity; some are linked to the sleep-wake cycle; and others are synchronized with food ingestion and the dark-light cycle. These entrained neuroendocrine rhythms have emerged as critical indices of "glandular" function of the brain. There is growing appreciation that desynchronization of these rhythms may underlie a number of important reproductive disorders. On the basis of these premises, chronic anovulation resulting from dysfunction of the CNS-hypothalamic-pituitary system can be divided pathophysiologically into two broad categories, as presented in Table 19–1.

■ TABLE 19–1

Pathophysiologic Bases of Chronic Anovulation Secondary to Dysfunction of the CNS-Hypothalamic-Pituitary System

Defects Within Hypothalamic-Pituitary Unit

- Hypothalamic lesions—primary and secondary
- Isolated hypothalamic GnRH deficiency
- Inappropriate prolactin secretion
- Interruption of vascular link of the unit (Sheehan's syndrome and pituitary apoplexy)
- Cellular and anatomic defects of the pituitary gland
  - Pituitary adenoma
  - Pituitary tumors
  - Empty sella syndrome
  - Lymphocytic hypophysitis (autoimmune diseases)

Aberrations of CNS-Hypothalamic Interaction

- Physiologic models
  - Initiation of puberty
  - Amenorrhea
  - Postpartum lactational amenorrhea
- Psychoneuroendocrinologic disorders
  - Pseudocyesis ("phantom pregnancy")
  - Functional hypothalamic amenorrhea syndrome (psychogenic, nutritional, exercise-related)
  - Anorexia nervosa
  - Premenstrual dysphoria

HYPOTHALAMIC-PITUITARY DYSREGULATION

Isolated GnRH Deficiency

Kallmann's Syndrome

Isolated gonadotropin-releasing hormone (GnRH) deficiency is a genetic defect characterized by a functional deficit in hypothalamic GnRH production and secretion. A syndrome involving hypogonadotropic hypogonadism associated with anosmia or hyposmia was described by Kallmann and associates[1] in 1944. Included in the original observations were families in which members were afflicted with additional disorders such as color blindness, synkinesis, mental retardation, and a series of congenital midline defects.[2] Subsequent studies in familial cases of Kallmann's syndrome demonstrated several modes of inheritance—autosomal dominant, autosomal recessive, and X-linked.

In the search for the genetic basis of this syndrome, the crucial lead to the understanding of GnRH deficiency came from observations that patients with ichthyosis, known to be caused by a steroid sulfatase gene deletion on the distal portion of the Xp region, also had Kallmann's syndrome. This association prompted investigators to identify the locus of steroid sulfatase and Kallmann's gene defects to adjacent regions of the X chromosome, near the tip of the short arm (Xp22.3); this was named the *KAL* gene.[3–5]

This finding, together with earlier studies of the developmental biology of GnRH-secreting neurons,[6] showed that the hypothalamic GnRH neurons are not of CNS origin embryonically. Rather, they migrate into the hypothalamus from an epithelial cluster of cells derived from the olfactory placode outside the developing brain. GnRH neuronal migration appears to follow the pathway of the olfactory bulb and olfactory tract before entering the brain, where a sharp turn is required to localize in the arcuate nucleus of the mediobasal hypothalamus[7, 8] (Fig. 19–1). Identification of the *KAL* gene as a *neural adhesion molecule* involved in the migration of GnRH neurons provided a potential basis for explaining the migration process of GnRH neurons.[4, 5]

Whereas the X-linked *KAL* gene is clearly established in the pathogenesis of Kallmann's syndrome, subsequent studies have demonstrated that this mode of inheritance is relatively uncommon (18 to 36 percent). The syndrome is sporadic in most cases, and autosomal modes of inheritance are far more common than the X-lineage in familial cases of Kallmann's syndrome.[9]

Idiopathic Hypogonadotropic Hypogonadism

Patients without anosmia and other associated abnormalities are described as having idiopathic hypogonadotropic hypogonadism (IHH).[10, 11] Whether IHH and Kallmann's syndrome represent a spectrum of manifestations of GnRH deficiency rather than two distinct syndromes remains unsettled.

In a murine model of hypogonadotropic hypogonadism (the hpg mouse), GnRH deficiency was found to be caused by a deletion of the GnRH gene.[12] Transgenic insertion of a normal GnRH gene or hypothalamic implants of GT-1 GnRH neural cells[13] restore reproductive function in the hpg mouse, confirming that GnRH gene deletion is the

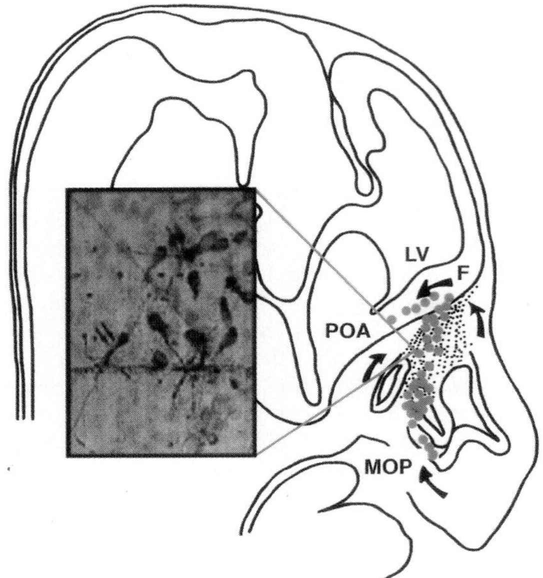

Figure 19–1 ■ Microprojection drawing of an 8-μm sagittal section of a 14-day-old embryonic mouse head, showing diagrammatically the migration route of immunoreactive GnRH neurons from the nose into the forebrain. Immunoreactive GnRH neurons are indicated by brown dots; the dashed lines represent central processes of the olfactory, vomeronasal, and terminalis nerves. MOP, medial olfactory pit; POA, preoptic area; F, forebrain; LV, lateral ventricle. GnRH neurons originate in the epithelium of the medial olfactory pit, the same part of the pit that gives origin to the vomeronasal and terminalis nerves. The GnRH neurons migrate across the developing nasal septum and into the brain along the central processes of these nerves. Arrows indicate the direction of GnRH cell migration.

Inset: Immunoreactive GnRH neurons from a 12-day-old embryo. The proliferation of non-neuronal cells is evident by the sheet of violet stain cells that cover the field. Note the direction of upward migration of GnRH neurons. (Modified from Schwanzel-Fukuda M, Jorgenson KL, Bergen HT, et al. Biology of normal luteinizing hormone–releasing hormone neurons during and after their migration from olfactory placode. Endocr Rev 13:623–634, 1992. © The Endocrine Society.)

cause of hypogonadism and providing a dramatic example of gene replacement therapy. In contrast, humans with the GnRH deficiency and IHH do not have an analogous deletion of the GnRH gene.[14, 15] Moreover, point mutations or frameshifts in the coding sequence have been eliminated as a genetic cause of IHH in humans.[15, 16]

On the basis of the GnRH neuronal migration arrest found in patients with Kallmann's syndrome, it was hypothesized that residual GnRH neurons would be found in the upper nasal epithelium of patients with Kallmann's syndrome but not in patients with IHH with normal olfaction or in eugonadal subjects. Biopsies of nasal mucosa in these subjects revealed the *presence of immunoreactive GnRH neurons in all groups of individuals*. Thus, GnRH-synthesizing cells persist in the upper nasal epithelium into adult life in normal human subjects and in both anosmic Kallmann's syndrome and normosmic IHH patients. Consequently, IHH cannot be distinguished from Kallmann's syndrome by the presence of vestigial GnRH neurons in the nasal mucosa.[17] In any case, the management of IHH patients is the same as that of Kallmann's patients, that is, hormone replacement or pulsatile GnRH stimulation in selective cases of infertility.

Hypogonadotropic Hypogonadism Due to GnRH Receptor Gene Mutations

On the basis of the foregoing, it is clear that the underlying cause of IHH has not been characterized. One possible candidate is the gene for GnRH, especially because hypogonadal mice with the deletion of this gene have been identified. However, no such abnormality has been found in patients with IHH. The gene for the *GnRH receptor* is another candidate in this disease. This gene has been cloned, and it is a G protein–coupled receptor with seven transmembrane segments and an extracellular amino terminus but no intracellular carboxy terminus. Activation of this receptor results in increased activity of phospholipase C and mobilization of calcium by means of the Gq/G_{11} group of G proteins. The gene comprises three exons and maps to the long arm of chromosome 4. A family with IHH with compound heterozygous *mutations of the GnRH receptor gene* has recently been described. One mutation, in the first extracellular loop of the receptor, dramatically decreased the binding of GnRH to its receptor. The other mutation, in the third intracellular loop, did not modify the binding of the hormone but decreased the activation of phospholipase C.[18] These loss-of-function mutations of the GnRH receptor in a man and his sister are associated with partial hypogonadotropic hypogonadism. Both patients are compound heterozygotes, and their parents and one sister have normal phenotype. The disorder was thus transmitted as an autosomal recessive trait. It is likely that additional genetic loci will be found in patients with IHH.

CLINICAL FEATURES

The salient feature of Kallmann's syndrome and IHH is gonadotropin deficiency and hypogonadism, which includes failure of both gametogenic function and sex steroid production. Because the appearance of secondary sex characteristics is dependent on sex steroids, *sexual infantilism is the prominent manifestation of this syndrome*. The degree of hypogonadism in male patients varies over a wide range, from complete testicular immaturity and Leydig cell atrophy (aleydigism) to a mild syndrome principally involving hypoleydigism, with testicular size approaching normal and with spermatid formation. In the latter clinical situation, the disparity between the development of gametogenic function and deficient testosterone production was considered to be a consequence of isolated LH deficiency in the face of normal circulating levels of FSH.[19] The term *fertile eunuch syndrome* was introduced for patients with normal spermatogenesis with androgen insufficiency due to isolated LH deficiency.

In women, the clinical features also vary widely, with secondary sex characteristics ranging from classic eunuchoid features to moderate breast development.[20] Primary amenorrhea is common. The ovaries of these patients rarely contain follicles past the primordial stage, suggesting that early stages of follicular maturation require amounts of gonadotropin beyond those secreted in these patients.[21] These immature ovaries respond readily to exogenous gonadotropin or pulsatile GnRH stimulation, and ovulation and pregnancy may result.[22] Thus, in both males and females, this syndrome is characterized by a high degree of clinical, biochemical, developmental, and genetic heterogeneity.

PATHOPHYSIOLOGY

Circulating levels of LH and FSH are usually undetectable, although low-normal values are occasionally found. Most patients exhibit subnormal LH and FSH release in response to GnRH stimulation. Complete unresponsiveness to GnRH is relatively uncommon.[23–25] The varying degrees of gonadotroph responsiveness to GnRH in these patients include failure of both LH and FSH to rise, appropriate rise of both LH and FSH, and an increase in FSH only or in LH only.[22, 26] These findings are consistent with those observed in patients with isolated monohormonal deficiency of LH or FSH.[27]

Crowley and coworkers[28] demonstrated the heterogeneity of LH secretory episodes in these patients; it varied from complete absence of pulsatile LH activity to low-frequency and low-amplitude pulses to nearly normal patterns of pulsatile LH secretory episodes. In the last group, the defect appears to be the secretion of biologically inactive LH molecules, the majority of which are the uncoupled α-subunit. The heterogeneous nature of this syndrome may reflect the degree of migration failure of GnRH neurons from the olfactory placode to the arcuate nucleus in the hypothalamus during development.

MANAGEMENT

The diagnosis of Kallmann's syndrome or IHH can be made *only when a mass lesion* of the hypothalamic-pituitary sites is excluded by either magnetic resonance imaging (MRI) scan or the presence of otherwise normal pituitary function.[25] A careful assessment as to the presence or absence of anosmia and hyposmia, pubertal development, and clinical manifestations of sexual infantilism and eunuchoid features is imperative.

In female patients, induction of ovulation and resulting pregnancy can be accomplished readily by administration of exogenous gonadotropin. In male patients, exogenous gonadotropin induces prompt Leydig cell function, but spermatogenesis is rarely restored to the final stage of maturation. The use of *pulsatile modes of GnRH administration*, with an average dose of 5 μg per pulse, has been remarkably successful in the activation of gonadotropin secretion and ovarian cyclicity.[25, 28] Ovulation resulting in normal pregnancies occurred in a high percentage of patients. Thus, the defective GnRH secretory activity can be effectively replaced by the use of an automatic portable pump GnRH delivery system with a frequency of 60 to 90 minutes for women. Slower or faster frequency tends to induce abnormal follicular development and luteal-phase defects. Higher doses of GnRH (i.e., 10 μg per pulse) can override the negative feedback control system, as evidenced by an increased amplitude of LH pulses, resulting in development of multiple follicles and ovulation.[29] In male patients, *long-term subcutaneous delivery of GnRH* at 2-hour intervals has been successful in inducing puberty and stimulating sustained testosterone secretion and spermatogenesis, with the ability to impregnate in a limited number of cases.[29, 30]

Hypothalamic Hypopituitarism

The introduction of hypothalamic releasing hormones into clinical medicine made it possible to evaluate pituitary secretory reserve in patients with subnormal circulating pituitary hormone levels (hypopituitarism). In this section, the features that distinguish the failure of pituitary cells *(primary hypopituitarism)* from a lack of appropriate hypothalamic releasing factors (secondary or hypothalamic hypopituitarism) in patients with pituitary hypofunction are discussed. Both types of hypopituitarism may involve a single pituitary hormone (monotropic deficiency) or several and even all pituitary hormones *(panhypopituitarism)*[31] (Fig. 19–2).

Tumors of the Hypothalamic Area

CRANIOPHARYNGIOMA

Craniopharyngioma is a tumor of nonpituitary origin and accounts for approximately 3 percent of intracranial neoplasms. This tumor is more commonly suprasellar rather than intrasellar in location. Craniopharyngiomas are composed of an admixture of epithelial cells and are considered to arise from remnants of Rathke's pouch. The pathologic features of craniopharyngioma were described in 1932 by Cushing to include those tumors originating from epithelial nests ascribable to an incomplete closure of the hypophysial or craniopharyngeal duct.[32] These tumors are more often cystic (54 percent) than solid (14 percent), but frequently both components are present (32 percent). Anatomically, they are usually present along the anterior surface of the infundibulum of the pituitary stalk; consequently, the location of these tumors may be above or below the diaphragma sellae.[32]

Clinical Features. Craniopharyngiomas are more common in men than in women. The tumor occurs in all age groups, with prevalence highest in the second decade and decreasing with advancing age. Because craniopharyngiomas are frequently suprasellar in location, a variety of clinical manifestations may be noted, depending on whether the expanding tumor compresses the hypothalamus or the pituitary stalk. Thus, the rate of expansion of the tumor obviously influences the clinical picture.[33]

Visual Impairment. The common presenting feature in both sexes is visual impairment (70 percent). Bitemporal hemianopia is the most common visual field defect, whereas impairment ranging from total blindness to optic atrophy and papilledema occurs only rarely.[33]

Endocrine Dysfunction. Some degree of hypopituitarism is found in most cases of craniopharyngioma.[33, 34] The degree of impairment of pituitary function depends on the extent of hypothalamic or pituitary stalk involvement. Deficiencies of GH (75 percent) and gonadotropin (40 percent) are common, and pituitary-adrenal dysfunction occurs in half of the patients. Depressed thyroid function also occurs (25 percent). Prolactin levels are either normal or moderately elevated. Gonadotropin response to GnRH is usually impaired. Diabetes insipidus occurs in 10 percent

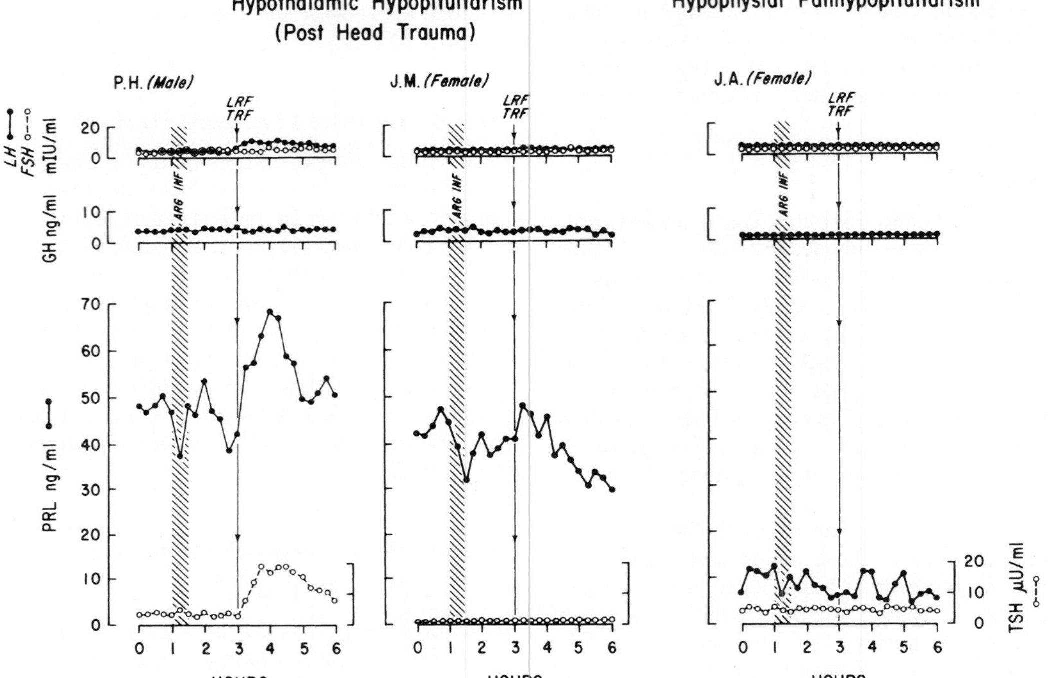

Figure 19–2 ■ Basal and stimulated pituitary hormone release by sequential administration of arginine infusion *(shaded area)* and GnRH (LRF) plus TRF in patients with hypopituitarism. *Left,* Hypopituitarism with relative hyperprolactinemia in two patients with whiplash after automobile collisions (stalk resection). *Right,* In contrast, a patient with pituitary panhypopituitarism.

and somnolence in about 20 percent of patients before treatment.[35]

Radiologic Findings. Enlargement of the pituitary fossa occurs in 70 percent of children and 50 percent of adults with craniopharyngioma.[36] Suprasellar extension and calcification are common, especially in children.

Management. Suprasellar extension of the tumor should be assessed by computed tomography (CT) or MRI in determining the anatomic extent of the tumor. Surgical relief of local compression, particularly of the optic chiasm, is frequently necessary. Total excision of the tumor is technically difficult, and surgery often results in damage to the hypothalamus. The degree of hypothalamic damage can be determined by MRI.[37] Conservative surgical excision followed by intensive radiotherapy has yielded good results, with a 70 to 80 percent 10-year survival rate. Severe pituitary deficiency and hyperphagia are common sequelae of surgical treatment.[37] Appropriate endocrine replacement therapy, including the use of synthetic vasopressin for the management of diabetes insipidus, both before and after tumor treatment, is of obvious importance. *GH replacement* is both sound and important. Guidelines for and complications of GH replacement are well established.[38, 39]

GERMINOMA

Germinoma, previously known as *ectopic pinealoma* or *atypical teratoma* of the pineal gland, is another relatively common lesion. The histologic features of this tumor are the same as in seminoma of the testis and dysgerminoma of the ovary. Thus, the term germinoma has been adopted to emphasize identity with its gonadal counterparts.

ENDODERMAL SINUS TUMOR

Endodermal sinus tumor, a rare but highly malignant tumor of the hypothalamus, requires some emphasis; it is a germ cell tumor and is also found in the testes and ovaries, as well as in the cervix and vagina, of infants and children. To date, a few such tumors have also been identified in the pineal gland region.[40, 41] The endodermal sinus tumor has a typical "honeycomb" pattern and is believed to be derived from antecedents of the yolk sac ("yolk sac carcinoma"). It is a highly vascular tumor capable of producing α-fetoprotein, and it metastasizes early to various regions of the CNS.

HAND-SCHÜLLER-CHRISTIAN DISEASE

Hand-Schüller-Christian disease (histiocytosis X), a condition with multifocal eosinophilic granulomas, is a rare cause of a hypothalamic destructive lesion in children, producing hypopituitarism with delayed puberty, growth retardation, and diabetes insipidus (40 percent).[42, 43] It has been more than 30 years since Lichtenstein's concept linked eosinophilic granuloma of bone, Letterer-Siwe disease, and Hand-Schüller-Christian syndrome under the category histiocytosis X,[44] now more correctly called Langerhans cell histiocytosis. Reassessment of these and other distinctive histiocytosis syndromes in children has revealed mononuclear phagocytes (histiocytes) and their interactions with other cells; the Langerhans cell, a unique histiocyte, has been clearly associated with Lichtenstein's histiocytosis X.[45] Other infiltrating lesions include *sarcoidosis*, *Wegener's granulomatosis,* and *hemochromatosis.*

Clinically, several classic features suggest a hypothalamic basis for hypopituitarism in histiocytosis X: (1) the presence of diabetes insipidus, (2) the modest elevation of prolactin levels along with reduced levels of other pituitary hormones, and (3) visual disturbances.[46] Other symptoms suggesting hypothalamic involvement are obesity, psychiatric disturbances, and hypersomnolence. Growth retardation in children may be the first presenting complaint in those seeking medical evaluation.[46] A definitive diagnosis by biopsy is essential. When the diagnosis is established, radiation therapy has been shown to be effective. GH deficiency in children has serious consequences, and either therapy with recombinant GH or frequent injection of GH-releasing hormone (GHRH) is indicated. Restoration of GH secretion is accompanied by a prompt rise in serum levels of insulin-like growth factor-I (IGF-I).[47]

Head Injury

Head injuries, especially those sustained in head-on automobile collisions, can cause hypothalamic damage resulting in hypopituitarism with elevated prolactin levels that may or may not respond to thyrotropin-releasing hormone (TRH) stimulation (see Fig. 19–2). The presence of hyperprolactinemia provides crucial evidence of the hypothalamic site of damage and serves to discriminate from pituitary panhypopituitarism. It is believed that automobile accidents resulting in whiplash injury may cause *transection of the pituitary stalk* during the acute forward motion of the head. Patients with such injuries may have permanent diabetes insipidus, a feature consistent with stalk transection (see Fig. 19–2). Prolonged hypotension, hypovolemia, and unconsciousness may precipitate either hypothalamic ischemia or portal vein thrombosis, which represents another mechanism for the development of hypopituitarism that sometimes follows head injury.

Irradiation

External irradiation can cause damage to the hypothalamus and impair its function. Pituitary cells are relatively radioresistant, whereas the brain and its nerves are more radiosensitive. Thus, changes in pituitary function after radiation therapy for pituitary tumor may be attributable to an indirect effect of hypothalamic damage. In this circumstance, hypopituitarism develops slowly but progressively and is frequently associated with modest elevation of prolactin levels.[48, 49]

Irradiation of the head and neck for the treatment of cancer of the nasopharynx frequently results in hypopituitarism. In two prospective studies in which the time course and relative deficiency of hypothalamic-pituitary function after cranial irradiation (1200 to 6000 cGy) were evaluated, the progressive impairment of the hypothalamic-pituitary function became evident as early as 1 year after radiotherapy, and further impairments of GH, FSH/LH, TSH, and ACTH occurred with time and dose.[50, 51]

Pituitary Hypopituitarism (Primary Hypopituitarism)

Primary hypopituitarism may result from surgical or radiologic ablation. It also occurs as a result of large pituitary tumors or infarction or from infiltrating and granulomatous lesions. Among these, pituitary infarction represents one of the most important problems in reproductive endocrinology. It can occur spontaneously; idiopathic pituitary infarction usually occurs in late reproductive or menopausal age groups. More commonly, it is associated with postpartum hemorrhage and shock *(Sheehan's syndrome).* Rarely, it can occur in patients with diabetic vasculitis, lymphocytic hypophysitis, or sickle cell anemia. The destruction of the pituitary gland may reach 70 percent before the clinical manifestations of hypopituitarism occur. However, with the use of hypothalamic releasing hormones (TRH, GnRH, corticotropin-releasing factor [CRF], GHRH) as diagnostic tools, lesser degrees of pituitary hypofunction can be detected earlier.

Recent investigations have revealed mutation of the POU-specific domain of Pit-1 resulting in hypopituitarism with deficiencies of GH, prolactin, and TSH. In contrast to individuals with POU-1 mutations, those with PROP-1 mutations cannot produce LH and FSH at a sufficient level and thus do not enter puberty spontaneously. In general, the combined pituitary hormone deficiencies in these individuals with both POU-1 and PROP-1 mutations do not respond to hypothalamic-releasing factor stimulation.[51a, 51b]

Sheehan's Syndrome

In 1939, Sheehan[52] described a syndrome of hypopituitarism resulting from acute necrosis of the anterior pituitary gland secondary to postpartum hemorrhage and shock. The neurohypophysis is usually involved, and the osmoregulation by arginine vasopressin is frequently impaired, although overt symptoms of diabetes insipidus are not common.[53] Clinical manifestations of hypopituitarism in patients surviving the period of postpartum shock are rapid and dramatic. Mammary involution and failure of lactation are the earliest signs; fatigue, loss of vigor, and hypotension are common findings during the puerperium. Loss of pubic and axillary hair and other features common to hypopituitarism follow. Failure to establish the diagnosis and to institute replacement therapy promptly may have lethal consequences.

The *pathophysiologic* basis for pituitary necrosis in patients with postpartum hemorrhage is not entirely clear. The anterior (but not the posterior) pituitary gland nearly doubles in size during the course of pregnancy (from 500 to 1000 mg), owing primarily to the hypertrophy and hyperplasia of the lactotrophs.[54] The enlarged gland with low pressure in the portal vein is vulnerable to ischemia resulting from postpartum hemorrhage with its attendant hypotension and shock. Interruption or rapid reduction of blood flow in the superior hypophysial vessels not only curtails arterial blood supply but also stops portal venous flow. The marked increase in the size of the anterior pituitary gland requires high oxygen consumption and thus demands an increased blood supply, which serves to explain the vulnerability to pituitary infarction during hypotensive-hypovolemic shock in postpartum women. In addition, the frequent coagulation abnormalities encountered during pregnancy may be important predisposing factors.[55]

The degree of hypopituitarism in Sheehan's syndrome is highly variable. Partial or complete spontaneous recovery does take place in some cases, and subsequent pregnancy in these patients has been reported.[56] The pituitary response to GnRH stimulation may be normal, diminished, or absent.[57] This is to be expected, because the extent of the infarction and the rate of regeneration are variable from patient to patient. In 23 patients evaluated by Imura,[58] the frequency of impaired GH secretion was 100 percent; this was followed in frequency by impairments in gonadotropin, ACTH, prolactin, and TSH secretory capacity. The availability of all hypothalamic releasing hormones today is invaluable in ascertaining the extent of pituitary damage and the prognosis for these patients. In addition to usual hormone replacement, rhGH therapy should be instituted.[38]

Empty Sella Syndrome

The term empty sella was first introduced by Busch in 1951 to describe an incomplete or vestigial diaphragma sellae found at autopsy in individuals without known pituitary disease.[59] In such cases, the pituitary gland tends to be flattened, and the pituitary fossa, at first glance, is empty. This finding is now well characterized as a syndrome in which the sella turcica forms an extension of the subarachnoid space and is partially or completely filled with cerebrospinal fluid (CSF) (Fig. 19–3*A* and *B*). These patients are said to have an idiopathic or primary empty sella syndrome, as distinct from those conditions that follow spontaneous infarction of pituitary adenomas, surgery, or radiation therapy. Radiologic examination of the sella turcica reveals it to be enlarged in most but not all cases; it is often symmetrically enlarged and gives a ballooned appearance.

Primary empty sella syndrome is typically found in middle-aged women[59] who have been investigated for presumed pituitary tumor. The presenting symptoms are generally nonspecific, but spontaneous CSF rhinorrhea has been reported. Headache is the most frequent complaint. Conspicuously absent is any defect in visual fields. Intracranial hypertension may be present.

Although most patients with empty sella syndrome have no discernible endocrine abnormalities, deficiency or hypersecretion of a single or of multiple hormones has been reported. Included are isolated ACTH deficiency, amenorrhea-galactorrhea in association with hyperprolactinemia, and hypersecretion of GH with the associated metabolic derangements.[60–62] The hypersecretion of prolactin and GH is probably due to the presence of microadenomas in these patients (Fig. 19–3*C*). The empty sella syndrome can also occur in children; 48 percent of those affected have GH deficiency or a combination of pituitary hormone deficiencies.[31]

The cause of the empty sella syndrome is unknown. An incomplete or defective diaphragma sellae is a prerequisite. The most generally accepted hypothesis is that transmitted CSF pressure results in flattening of the pituitary, followed by bony remodeling of the sella. CT scanning or MRI should be performed in any patient with a symmetrically enlarged sella turcica and clinical characteristics suggestive of an empty sella. However, children and young women with *primary hypothyroidism* may also have generalized enlargement of the sella turcica, and consequently thyroid function studies are of obvious importance.

3rd ventricle
Subarachnoid space
Anterior pituitary
Arachnoid membrane
Dura
Sphenoid sinus
Posterior pituitary
A

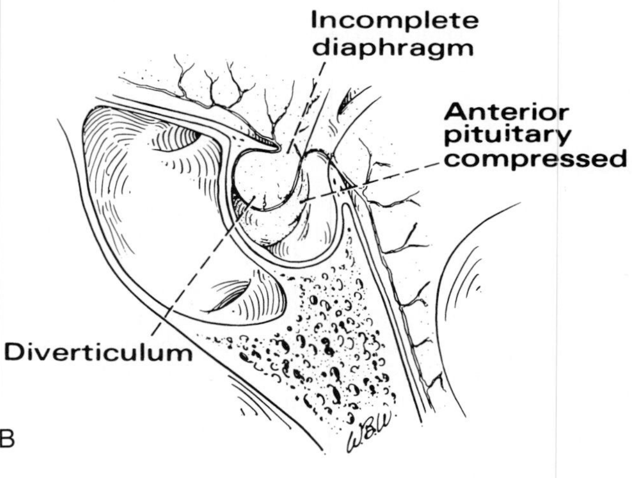

Microadenoma
C

Figure 19–3 ■ *A,* Illustration depicting the normal relationships between the sellar contents and the suprasellar arachnoid space.

B, Illustration of a primary empty sella with herniation of arachnoid space and cerebrospinal fluid and compression of the pituitary gland.

C, Illustration of primary empty sella coexisting with a pituitary microadenoma. (*A* to *C* from Randall RV, Scheithauer BW, Abboud CF. Anterior pituitary in clinical medicine. *In* Spittell JA Jr [ed]. Clinical Medicine, Vol 8. Philadelphia, Harper & Row, 1983, pp 1–97.)

Pituitary Apoplexy

Pituitary apoplexy—acute massive infarction of the pituitary gland—is a rare but life-threatening disorder that requires prompt recognition and timely medical intervention to avoid catastrophe. Reid and associates[63] have reviewed this subject. A variety of pituitary tumors have been associated with pituitary apoplexy. The fact that chromophobe adenomas predominate over eosinophilic adenomas as the tumor cell type most commonly found in cases of pituitary apoplexy merely reflects the relative prevalence of these tumors. Rarely has apoplexy been documented in association with basophilic adenomas, craniopharyngiomas, or primary pituitary carcinomas. Most tumors associated with this condition are endocrinologically "silent," although both acromegaly and Cushing's disease have been recorded. On occasion, the progression of acromegaly and the associated diabetes mellitus have been ameliorated after pituitary apoplexy.[63]

Clinical Manifestations. Dramatic neurologic symptoms and signs may accompany the loss of pituitary function resulting from infarction of a pre-existing pituitary adenoma or tumor. The pattern of tumor growth before the acute episode, combined with the degree of hemorrhage and edema within the pituitary, determines the nature and extent of neurologic findings. Autopsy studies have confirmed that neurologic sequelae are a late phenomenon in individuals with pituitary tumors, for the rate of tumor growth is often so gradual that adjacent nerves are able to accommodate by a process of slow lengthening. In contrast, infarction of such a tumor with secondary hemorrhage and edema causes rapid expansion of the lesion, acute compression of adjacent structures, and compromised neurologic function. In patients who remain conscious, the first symptom is almost always the sudden onset of *excruciating localized retro-orbital headache.* This symptom, thought to result from meningeal irritation or stretching of the dura on the lateral walls of the sella, is frequently accompanied by nausea and vomiting.[63]

Expansion of a tumor that has grown upward may cause visual field defects and impaired visual acuity owing to pressure on the optic chiasm or optic tracts. Expansion within the sella frequently results in compression of the cavernous sinus, which forms the lateral boundary of the pituitary fossa. Occupying vulnerable positions are cranial nerves III, IV, V, and VI; the branches of the sympathetic chain; and the carotid artery, which courses through the cavernous sinus. The oculomotor nerve (cranial nerve III) is most commonly involved, resulting in unilateral (or rarely bilateral) ophthalmoplegia[63] (Fig. 19–4).

Clinical Features. Destruction of adenohypophysial tissue may lead to multiple endocrine deficiencies, as demonstrated by low basal or stimulated levels of GH, ACTH, TSH, and gonadotropins in individual cases. Life-threatening endocrine abnormalities resulting from pituitary apoplexy, however, must involve major destruction of the adenohypophysis, for the functional reserve of this tissue is so great that it has been estimated that survival is possible with as little as 10 percent of the gland remaining intact. Failure to recognize deficiencies of ACTH secretion and to institute prompt cortisol replacement therapy has undoubtedly contributed to the high death rate in previously reported apoplectic episodes. Although pathologic alterations of the pars nervosa are frequently found in cases coming to autopsy, clinically significant neurohypophysial dysfunction in surviving individuals is uncommon.[63]

Management. Limited individual experience and the highly variable clinical course in pituitary apoplexy have led to disagreement on the optimal management of the acute episode. Undoubtedly, the mere suspicion that acute pituitary apoplexy is evolving is reason enough to initiate corticosteroid therapy and other vigorous supportive measures. The fact that some patients deteriorate rapidly and may die within hours to days has led some authors to advocate early transsphenoidal neurosurgical decompression in all cases, with the aim of rapid improvement of pituitary function and reversal of neurologic defects.[64] However, there is considerable evidence to suggest that conservative management is justified when the patient has retained consciousness, despite unilateral ophthalmoplegia and partial visual field defects. There have been numerous reports of complete spontaneous neurologic recovery in these circumstances. Careful evaluation of hormonal status and appropriate replacement therapy are the only interventions necessary. Whether the decompression surgery is more beneficial than conservative management should be evaluated on an individual basis.[63]

Lymphocytic Hypophysitis

Lymphocytic hypophysitis is an uncommon, non-neoplastic cause of hypopituitarism most commonly found in women in relationship to pregnancy (37 of the 39 reported cases). Extensive lymphocytic infiltration confined to the anterior pituitary is the uniform finding. Evidence exists for an autoimmune pathogenesis, including an association with autoimmune thyroiditis, pernicious anemia, and organ-specific antimitochondrial and antinuclear antibodies.[65] Varying degrees of hypopituitarism are present and frequently are associated with modest hyperprolactinemia, which is probably due to compression of the pituitary stalk caused

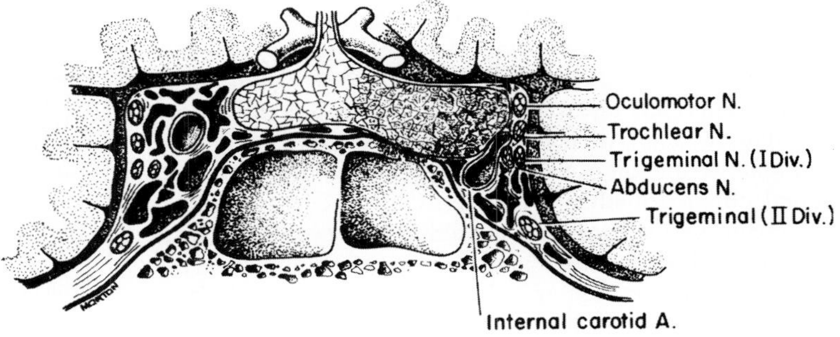

Figure 19–4 ■ Drawing depicts the compression of cranial nerves as a consequence of infarction and expansion of pituitary adenomas or tumors.

by generalized enlargement of the pituitary. The diagnosis remains difficult because CT scanning or MRI shows only generalized enlargement. Definitive diagnosis is based on histologic examination of pituitary tissue at surgical resection or autopsy in most of the cases reported to date.[65, 66]

Pituitary Adenomas

Pituitary tumors in the form of adenomas are frequent. It is estimated that 10 percent of all intracranial tumors are pituitary adenomas, but many are too small or endocrinologically inactive to be discernible clinically. With recent advances in radiographic techniques, especially CT and MRI, early recognition of these adenomas has been achieved.

Hypersecreting pituitary adenomas were thought to involve mainly the simple polypeptide hormone–producing cells and were recognized as three classic endocrinopathies: (1) acromegaly due to GH excess, (2) Cushing's disease due to ACTH excess, and (3) amenorrhea-galactorrhea syndrome due to prolactin hypersecretion. Since 1970, however, clinical and laboratory evidence of hypersecreting adenomas of glycoprotein hormone–producing cells (e.g., TSH, FSH, and LH) has been reported. In addition, a variety of glycoprotein hormone subunit–producing adenomas have recently been described. Thus, it is now established that pituitary cells of all types can form adenomatous lesions.

NONFUNCTIONING PITUITARY ADENOMAS (GONADOTROPH ADENOMA)

More than 25 percent of pituitary adenomas are not associated with overt evidence of hypersecretion of adenohypophysial hormones[67] and are variously called *silent, nonsecreting,* or *nonfunctioning adenomas.* Because these patients are asymptomatic, the majority of detected tumors are macroadenomas. Therefore, patients present with signs of mass effect, such as visual changes, headaches, and symptoms of pituitary insufficiency. Although clinical evidence for hormone hypersecretion is typically absent, hormone synthesis and secretion have been detected in the majority of such tumors with use of histomorphologic and molecular biology techniques. Studies have shown that clinically nonfunctioning tumors reflect a heterogeneous population of anterior pituitary cells, and the majority of such tumors synthesize glycoprotein hormones (FSH, LH) or their free α- and β-subunits. Clonal expansion is the key underlying event in the initiation of tumorigenesis; however, hypothalamic and other hormonal factors are likely to play an important role in promoting tumor growth.[68] For example, expression of receptors for thyroid hormone (TR) and estrogen (ER) in nonfunctioning pituitary adenoma was determined. Expression of all TR variants and ER was reduced from that of normal pituitaries. It was suggested that the reduced expression of TR and ER may account for decreased inhibition of glycoprotein hormone α-subunit gene and may contribute to uncontrolled tumor growth.[69] Moreover, GnRH, GnRH receptor, and receptors for TRH and dopamine are expressed in the cells of nonfunctional adenomas, suggesting autocrine and paracrine roles in tumor growth.[70] Interestingly, inhibin and activin subunits have been localized in all pituitary adenomas, but follistatin was expressed only in gonadotroph adenomas. Thus, *follistatin constitutes a tumor marker for gonadotroph adenoma.*[71]

The heterogeneity of ligands and receptors found in this type of tumor has prompted clinical trials of the dopamine agonist octreotide and of GnRH agonists and antagonists, with tumor shrinkage of up to 10 to 20 percent. In the case of FSH-producing adenoma with elevated FSH levels, the administration of a GnRH antagonist (Nal-Glu) induced a prompt suppression[72] (Fig. 19–5*A*). This observation indicates that hypersecretion of FSH by gonadotroph adenoma, but not its pathogenesis, may be dependent on endogenous GnRH drive. Surgical removal of the adenoma is followed by rapid decline in FSH levels (Fig. 19–5*B*).

Clinical Features and Treatment Options. Gonadotroph adenoma usually comes to clinical attention when the tumor becomes large enough to cause neurologic symptoms, most commonly impaired vision and headache. The large mass lesion may also cause compression resulting in deficient hormone secretion from nonadenomatous pituitary cells. Remarkably, the common pituitary hormone deficiency is of LH. In men, it results in subnormal testosterone levels, which produces symptoms of decreased energy and libido. In premenopausal women, amenorrhea develops. TSH and ACTH deficiencies may also occur. In addition, the use of MRI to determine the extent of the tumor is required. Hormonal and clinical criteria for the diagnosis of gonadotroph adenoma are listed in Table 19–2. Treatment options are limited to observation only or transsphenoidal removal of the tumor followed by radiation therapy. Because of the large size and suprasellar extension, complications such as hypopituitarism, diabetes insipidus, and oculomotor palsy are common.[73] Clinical trials with D_2 receptor dopamine agonists and GnRH antagonists are ongoing.

PROLACTIN-PRODUCING ADENOMAS

Hypersecretion of prolactin by pituitary tumors may occur as an isolated abnormality or in association with overproduction of other pituitary hormones. Hyperprolactinemia occurs in 25 percent of patients with GH-producing adenomas and acromegaly.[74, 75] It has now become clear that this association is expected because the lactotroph is derived from a common progenitor GH-expressing stem cell.[75] The excessive prolactin secretion in the presence of large tumors of any type is thought, in most cases, to be caused

■ TABLE 19–2
Hormonal and Clinical Criteria for the Diagnosis of Gonadotroph Adenoma

	MEN	WOMEN
Supranormal basal concentration	FSH α-subunit LH and testosterone	FSH but not LH α-subunit
Supranormal response to TRH	FSH LH LH-β	FSH LH LH-β
Neurologic and visual defects	Common	Common
Symptoms of gonadotropin excess	None	Menstrual disorders

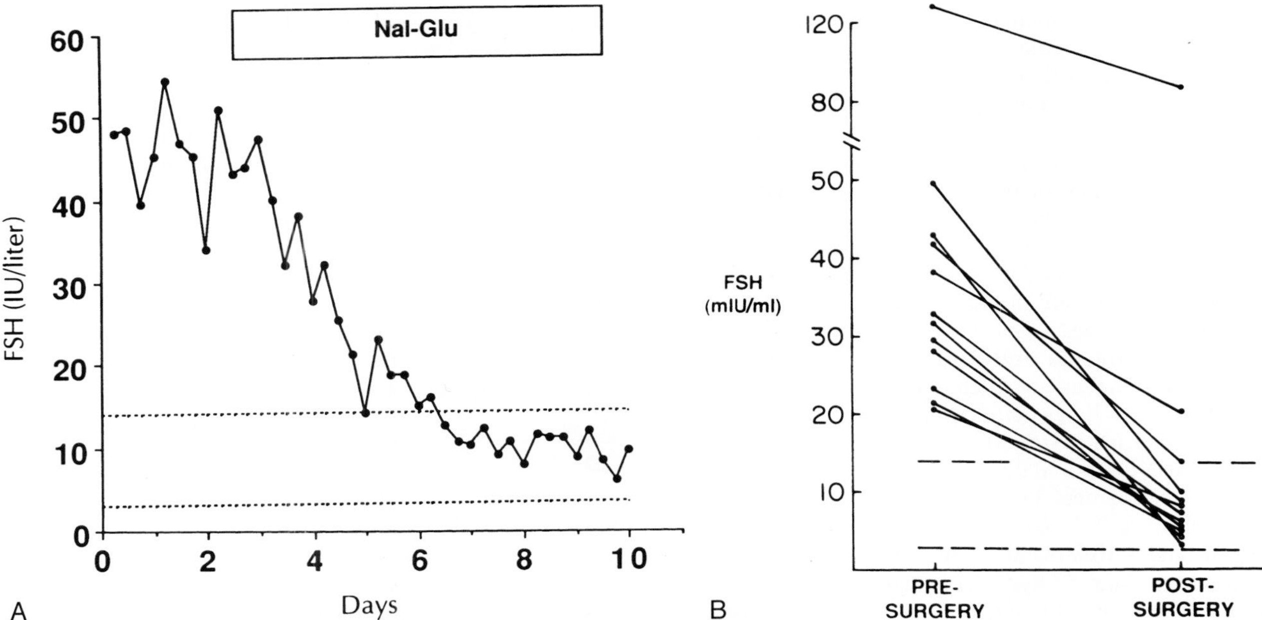

Figure 19–5 ■ *A,* Suppression to normal levels of the initially supranormal serum FSH concentration in a man with a gonadotroph adenoma in response to the administration of the GnRH antagonist Nal-Glu, 5 mg twice a day for 7 days. (From Daneshdoost L, Pavlou S, Molitch ME. Inhibition of follicle-stimulating hormone secretion from gonadotroph adenomas by repetitive administration of a gonadotropin-releasing hormone antagonist. J Clin Endocrinol Metab 71:92–97, 1990. © The Endocrine Society.)
B, Serum FSH concentrations in 12 men with gonadotroph adenomas before and 4 to 6 weeks after transsphenoidal surgery. The decreases in FSH correlated with the decrease in size as determined by imaging. (From Harris RI, Schatz NJ, Gennarelli T, et al. Follicle-stimulating hormone–secreting pituitary adenomas: Correlation of reduction of adenoma size with reduction of hormonal hypersecretion after transsphenoidal surgery. J Clin Endocrinol Metab 56:1288–1293, 1983. © The Endocrine Society.)

by impingement on the pituitary stalk by an upward extension of the adenoma, thereby reducing the delivery of dopamine to the lactotroph.

Pituitary tumors that secrete prolactin only are referred to as prolactin-producing adenomas. This type of adenoma is most common, accounting for at least 70 percent of all pituitary adenomas,[76] and is often associated with galactorrhea and amenorrhea. The prolactin-producing adenomas develop in the lateral wing of the pituitary gland, and they account for the early appearance of the asymmetric distortion of the sella.

Pathophysiology. The prolactin-producing cell (the *lactotroph)* of the adenohypophysis and the hypothalamic mechanism controlling prolactin release are discussed in detail in Chapter 9.

There is evidence that the abnormalities governing the hypersecretion of prolactin in patients with pituitary adenoma are associated with central dysfunction. Pointing to disturbances of hypothalamic regulatory mechanisms shared by prolactin and gonadotropin are the loss of the sleep-entrained prolactin rise[77]; the unresponsiveness of prolactin release after chlorpromazine,[78] metoclopramide (a dopamine receptor antagonist), and arginine infusion[79]; and the attenuation of pulsatile release of gonadotropin.[77, 80]

It has been proposed that a link between pituitary prolactin-secreting adenomas and acyclic gonadotropin secretion involves a dysfunction of hypothalamic dopamine.[81] A specific prolactin-dopamine short-loop feedback system appears to be operative: increased prolactin levels induce a dose-dependent increase in dopamine secretion by the tuberoinfundibular neurons, which in turn inhibits GnRH pulsatile release through the *D_1 receptor on GnRH neurons* and by the activation of the β-endorphin neuronal system that also inhibits GnRH release[81–83] (Fig. 19–6).

The hypersecretion of prolactin by the adenoma appears *not* to be entirely autonomous because dopamine and dopamine agonists induce rapid suppression of prolactin secretion in these patients. Thus, dopamine receptors of D_2

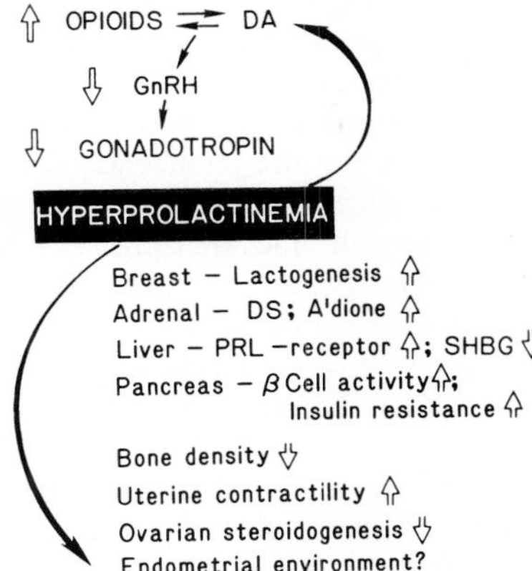

Figure 19–6 ■ Diagrammatic representation of neuroendocrine-metabolic effects of hyperprolactinemia. At the hypothalamic-pituitary level, high prolactin (PRL) levels induce increased dopamine and opioid peptide in the hypothalamus. These inhibitors in turn reduce pulsatile GnRH secretion, resulting in hypogonadotropism. At the peripheral level, prolactin may exert functional changes in many target tissues. (See text.) DA, dopamine; DS, dehydroepiandrosterone sulfate; A'dione, androstenedione; SHBG, sex hormone–binding globulin.

subtype on the adenomatous prolactin-secreting cells are functionally intact. On the other hand, the prompt prolactin release in response to D_2 receptor blockade seen in normal women is markedly attenuated in adenoma patients. It has been suggested that the imbalance between TRH and dopamine content in prolactin-producing adenoma may lead to hypersecretion of prolactin and the growth of adenoma lactotrophs.[84] Although these factors may be responsible for sustaining adenoma growth, *clonal expansion of a genomically altered cell* is found to underlie the initiation of tumorigenesis of pituitary adenomas including the prolactin-producing type.[85]

Hyperprolactinemia and Androgens. Hirsutism in association with the amenorrhea-galactorrhea syndrome is not uncommon. Whereas circulating levels of testosterone, dihydrotestosterone, estradiol, and sex hormone–binding globulin (SHBG) are reduced, the adrenal androgens—dehydroepiandrosterone (DHEA) and its sulfate (DHEAS)—may be elevated.[86, 87] Normalization of elevated adrenal androgens and SHBG occurs in response to dexamethasone or after suppression of hyperprolactinemia by a dopamine agonist.[88] The recent finding of the presence of prolactin receptor in all layers of the human adrenal cortex suggests that prolactin has a direct action on adrenal androgen biosynthesis.[89]

Hyperprolactinemia and Bone Density. Hyperprolactinemic women with amenorrhea have decreased bone density.[90–92] However, decreased bone density in women with hyperprolactinemia is not correlated with estradiol levels, and the spine mineral density remains low 3 to 9 years after restoration of physiologic levels of estrogen,[93] suggesting that prolactin may have a direct bone resorptive action. This association represents the rationale for prolactin suppression without undue delay.

Management. Three major advances have influenced the approach to the management of prolactin-secreting adenoma:

1. Both prospective and retrospective studies have indicated that the natural history of the disorder usually follows a benign clinical course in most women, which serves to advocate a conservative approach to management.[94, 95]
2. Transsphenoidal microsurgical removal of adenomas has been successful, but the recurrence is frequent, particularly of the macroadenomas (80 percent in 3 years).[96] In addition, the fact that prolactin responses to TRH and dopamine agonists are impaired in patients after successful removal of adenomas suggests a defective dopaminergic regulation of prolactin secretion, which may account for the high recurrence rate.[97, 98]
3. A new generation of dopamine agonists has been developed with a high degree of potency, longer duration of action, and lesser incidence of side effects (e.g., *cabergoline* and CV205-502). The efficacy of these new compounds in the treatment of prolactin-secreting adenomas of all sizes has been demonstrated.[99]

It is apparent that medical management with the use of D_2 receptor dopamine agonists for both microadenoma and macroadenoma should be the first choice and constitutes the primary therapeutic modality. In occasional cases that do not respond to oral administration of these agents or when side effects persist, the vaginal route of application should be attempted. Suppression of prolactin levels with dopamine agonists results in the initiation of ovulatory cycles in most patients and a high pregnancy rate. It has been recommended that the drug be withdrawn as soon as pregnancy is diagnosed, although evidence of adverse effects of dopamine agonists on the fetus has not been observed. Primary therapy with dopamine agonists is also recommended in women in whom conception is not an issue. These patients are treated to reverse either the galactorrhea or the distressing symptoms of estrogen deficiency and other sequelae of hyperprolactinemia.

GROWTH HORMONE–HYPERSECRETING ADENOMA (ACROMEGALY)

Chronic GH excess causes reproductive dysfunctions in both men and women. Reproductive endocrinologists should be familiar with this classic syndrome, acromegaly, with its extensive endocrine-metabolic aberrations.

Hypersecretion of pituitary growth hormone (hGH) produces gigantism (proportionate growth) in children and acromegaly (disproportionate growth) in adults and is usually associated with a GH-secreting adenoma. In adults, there is enlargement of the skeleton, especially of the skull, hands, and feet. Thus, an increase in size for hats, gloves, or shoes provides an early diagnostic clue. The progressive facial and acral changes are often gradual and not recognized by the patient, family, or friends until they are well advanced.

When the disease is fully developed, the face appears massive and coarse and the lips and nose are large and thick. The supraorbital ridges bulge, the lower jaw protrudes, the teeth may become separated, and malclosure of the jaw frequently occurs. The skin and subcutaneous tissue become thick and spongy. The larynx and sinuses enlarge, and the voice develops a peculiar resonance and cavernous quality. The tongue is enlarged, and the speech may be thickened. The hair tends to be coarse. *Impotence in men and amenorrhea and hirsutism in women are frequent manifestations.* These clinical symptoms and signs are due to excessive stimulation directly by GH itself and are mediated through the hepatic production of IGF-I. The negative feedback axis of IGF-I and GH is disrupted in patients with acromegaly.[100] This important disease has been the subject of several reviews.[101–103]

Excessive GH secretion causing acromegaly due to autonomous extrahypothalamic (ectopic) GHRH secretion from pancreatic tumors also occurs.[104] Although this is rare, it is important to exclude this possibility by measuring plasma GHRH levels so that unnecessary surgical exploration or irradiation of the pituitary gland may be avoided and specific treatment can be targeted to the tumor site.

Manifestations. The magnitude of hGH excess varies markedly from patient to patient, and the circulating levels range from 5 to 20 ng/ml to more than 1000 ng/ml. The 24-hour secretory patterns are also highly variable; they range from virtually no fluctuation to frequent episodic pulses.[105] The clinical manifestations of acromegaly are given in Table 19–3. In almost all cases, the normal sleep-related peaks of hGH secretion are absent. The normal

■ TABLE 19–3
Clinical Presentation of Acromegaly

PRESENTING CHIEF COMPLAINT	FREQUENCY (%)
Menstrual disorder	13
Change in appearance/acral growth	11
Headache	8
Carpal tunnel syndrome	6
Diabetes mellitus	5
Heart disease	3
Visual impairment	3
Decreased libido/impotence	3
Arthropathy	3
Thyroid disorder	2
Hypertension	1
Chance (e.g., dental x-ray)	40

Based on analyses of 310 patients.
From Molitch ME. Clinical manifestations of acromegaly. Endocrinol Metab Clin North Am 21:597–614, 1992.

episodic secretion of hGH may be altered; the usual fall in hGH in the face of hyperglycemia (after meals) and the rise in response to hypoglycemia may be absent. A paradoxical elevation of hGH in response to glucose is another feature in some patients with acromegaly.[106] Moreover, inappropriate hGH release occurs in response to GnRH and TRH in most patients. These findings suggest that two basic abnormalities exist in these patients: (1) dysfunction of hypothalamic control mechanisms and (2) alteration of the specific membrane receptors on the GH-producing adenoma cells.

Other endocrine disturbances may occur in conjunction with acromegaly: markedly elevated serum IGF-I levels, which may be responsible for excessive tissue growth, as well as paracrine and autocrine effects of IGF-I produced locally in a variety of target tissues. The *ovary* is endowed with the GH receptor and IGF system, and they play a trophic role in folliculogenesis. When they are excessive, the ovarian function is dysregulated and *anovulation ensues*. The occurrence of *galactorrhea* in some women with acromegaly is associated with modest elevation of prolactin secretion. In other cases, hypersecretion of adrenal androgens, causing hirsutism, has been reported. *Low gonadotropin secretion and amenorrhea*, occasioned by altered GnRH secretion, are also frequent findings in patients with active acromegaly. Glucose intolerance and hyperinsulinemia occur in the majority of patients.[100]

Management. The primary treatment modality is transsphenoidal surgery. From recent reviews, it is inferred that the cure is achieved by surgery in approximately 70 percent of patients with microadenomas, whereas macroadenomas, particularly with extrasellar extension, have poor prognosis.[101, 102] Pretreatment with octreotide for 3 to 6 months before surgery for GH-secreting adenomas improved surgical outcome.[107] If this fails, medical treatment with the somatostatin analogue octreotide followed by irradiation is indicated.[108, 109] However, studies indicate that radiotherapy lowers GH levels, but IGF-I levels remain elevated.[110] Thus, attempts should be made to reserve radiotherapy for use only when both surgical and medical treatments have failed.

ADENOMAS OF THE MULTIPLE ENDOCRINE NEOPLASIA TYPE I

This familial disease is transmitted as an autosomal dominant trait and combines tumoral lesions in the parathyroids, the pancreas, and the pituitary. The multiple endocrine neoplasia type I (MEN I) gene, a *putative tumor suppressor gene*, has been mapped to chromosome 11q13 and recently cloned.[111] Pituitary adenomas have been reported to occur in 15 to 50 percent of the cases, with a high predominance of prolactin and GH hypersecretory syndromes and nonfunctioning tumors.[112] On occasion, well-documented pituitary-dependent Cushing's disease has also been reported.[113] Cushing's disease of MEN I must be distinguished from Cushing's syndrome, which often occurs in the sporadic form of Zollinger-Ellison syndrome in which an ectopic ACTH secretion originates from the pancreatic tumor. The interesting feature of MEN I is the insight gained on multifocal clonal tumor formation in association with a *putative tumor suppressor gene*. Because of a high penetrance, careful follow-up of all members of the family is required.[114]

ACTH-HYPERSECRETING PITUITARY ADENOMA (CUSHING'S DISEASE)

Adenomas developed from ACTH-producing pituitary cells described by Harvey Cushing in 1932 represent one of the most devastating endocrinopathies. The accompanying hypercortisolemia exerts widespread impact on a wide range of organs and tissues. Evidence of suppressed hypothalamic CRF in Cushing's disease includes the following: (1) corticotroph hyperplasia outside the adenoma is absent[115]; (2) relative to the adenoma or normal pituitary corticotrophs, low concentrations of pro-opiomelanocortin (POMC) peptides are found in periadenomatous tissue[116]; (3) there is lack of CRF/ACTH response to insulin-induced hypoglycemic stress[117]; and (4) successful removal of the adenoma results in a state of ACTH deficiency and recovery of its activity during months or years.[118]

Within the adenoma, POMC peptides, including ACTH messenger ribonucleic acid (mRNA) and transcripts, are unaltered. The hallmark of ACTH hypersecretion in Cushing's disease is its partial resistance to the normal suppressive effect of glucocorticoids.[119, 120] Because ACTH secretion by the adenoma is unrestrained, ACTH overproduction occurs with the development of chronic hypercortisolism (Fig. 19–7). Since most peripheral tissues have normal sensitivity to the action of cortisol, features of Cushing's disease develop.

To explain the growth of a pituitary corticotroph adenoma, two necessary conditions are required: (1) that the adenoma be sensitive to CRF and (2) that CRF be present, at least some time, during the development of the adenoma. Invoking CRF in the growth of the corticotroph adenoma is paradoxical when much evidence suggests it is suppressed in Cushing's disease. This contradiction can be logically resolved by considering that CRF contributes to (but is not responsible for) the beginning of the disease. The progression to a tumor status and increase in adipose tissue mass are related to the clonal event and are primarily responsible for a set-point negative feedback effect of cortisol with subsequent tumor growth.

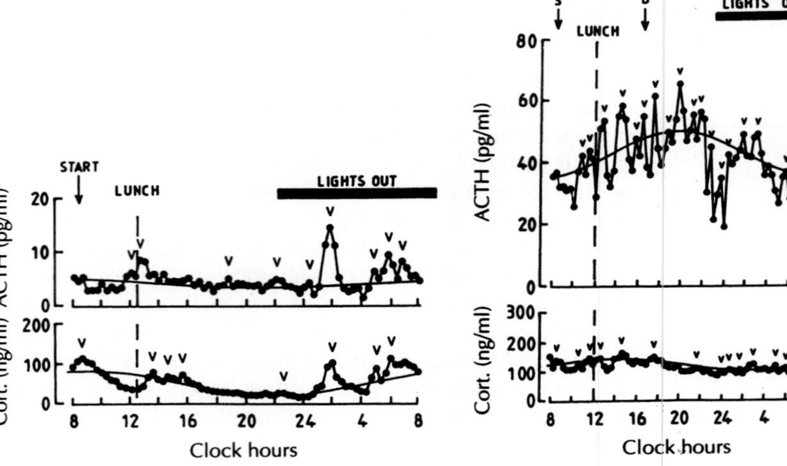

Figure 19–7 ■ The 24-hour profile of cortisol (Cort.) and adrenocorticotropic hormone (ACTH) in a normal woman *(left)* and a woman with Cushing's disease *(right)*. (From Liu JH, Muse K, Contrepas P, et al. Augmentation of ACTH-releasing activity of synthetic corticotropin releasing factor by vasopressin in women. J Clin Endocrinol Metab 57:1087–1089, 1983. © The Endocrine Society.)

Impacts of Hypercortisolemia. Under chronic elevated ACTH, adrenocortical hypersecretion develops with sustained hypercortisolemia and elevated DHEA and DHEA-S levels; 24-hour urinary cortisol levels constitute the best diagnostic marker (Fig. 19–8). In contrast, the action of ACTH on adrenal mineralocorticoids is only transient because the increased intra-adrenal concentration of cortisol inactivates P450 11β-corticosterone methyl oxidase. Thus, aldosterone secretion remains in the normal range.

The typical patient with Cushing's disease is a 30- to 40-year-old woman with obesity, amenorrhea, hypertension, muscle weakness, "moon" facies, and abdominal striae (Fig. 19–9). In addition, a mottled cyanosis of the hands, lower legs, and feet is often seen. These manifestations, plus the results of adrenal function tests, greatly assist in making correct diagnoses. The incidence of the clinical manifestations of Cushing's disease is presented in Table 19–4.

Obesity. The most common manifestation of Cushing's disease, obesity, often antedates the onset of other symptoms by many years. The distribution of fat, which is particularly obvious on the face, trunk (see Fig. 19–9), and cervicodorsal or supraclavicular regions, is a valuable diagnostic sign. Fat on the limbs is less obvious because of simultaneous muscle wasting. *Leptin levels* (*ob* gene product) are increased in both Cushing's disease and Cushing's syndrome,[121, 122] most likely because of the presence of chronic hypercortisolemia and hyperinsulinemia.

Hypertension. In most patients with Cushing's disease (85 percent), both diastolic and systolic blood pressures are elevated. Although the hypertension is rarely severe, congestive heart failure develops in a small percentage of patients. The hypertension appears to be related to altered sodium and potassium distribution.

Decreased Glucose Tolerance. About 70 to 80 percent of patients with Cushing's disease experience decreased glucose tolerance. The presence of hyperinsulinism in these patients represents a compensatory beta cell hyperactivity. Unlike the diabetogenic effect of GH excess (i.e., acromegaly), the hyperinsulinism in Cushing's disease is frequently accompanied by excessive glucagon secretion, which contributes further to the hyperglycemia of Cushing's disease. The mechanism for the hyperglucagonemia is an accelerated mobilization of amino acids (especially alanine) from muscle, which causes a direct stimulation of pancreatic alpha cell secretion of glucagon as well as increased sub-

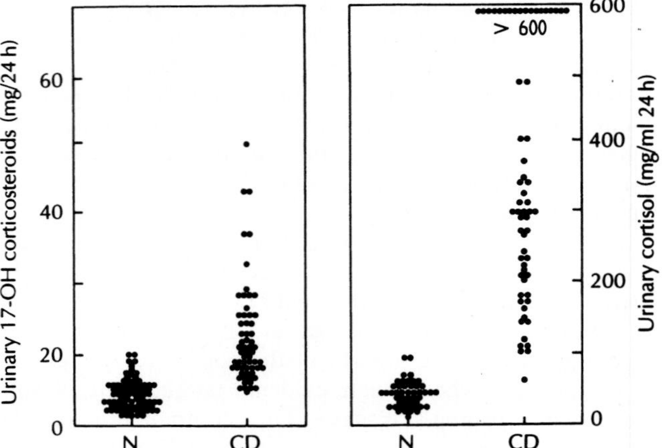

Figure 19–8 ■ Baseline urinary 17-hydroxycorticosteroids and cortisol levels in 61 patients with Cushing's disease (CD) are compared with the values obtained in normal subjects (N). (From Bertagna X, Raux-Demay M-C, Guilhaume B, et al. Cushing's disease. *In* Melmed S [ed]. The Pituitary. Cambridge, MA, Blackwell Scientific Publications, 1995, p 504.)

■ TABLE 19–4
Incidence of Clinical Manifestations in Cushing's Syndrome

SYMPTOM	PERCENT
Obesity	95
Moon face and malar flush	95
Hypertension	85
Glucose intolerance	80
Menstrual and sexual dysfunction	75
Hirsutism and acne	72
Striae	67
Weakness (and muscle wasting)	65
Osteoporosis	55
Easy bruisability	55
Depression	50
Edema of legs	40

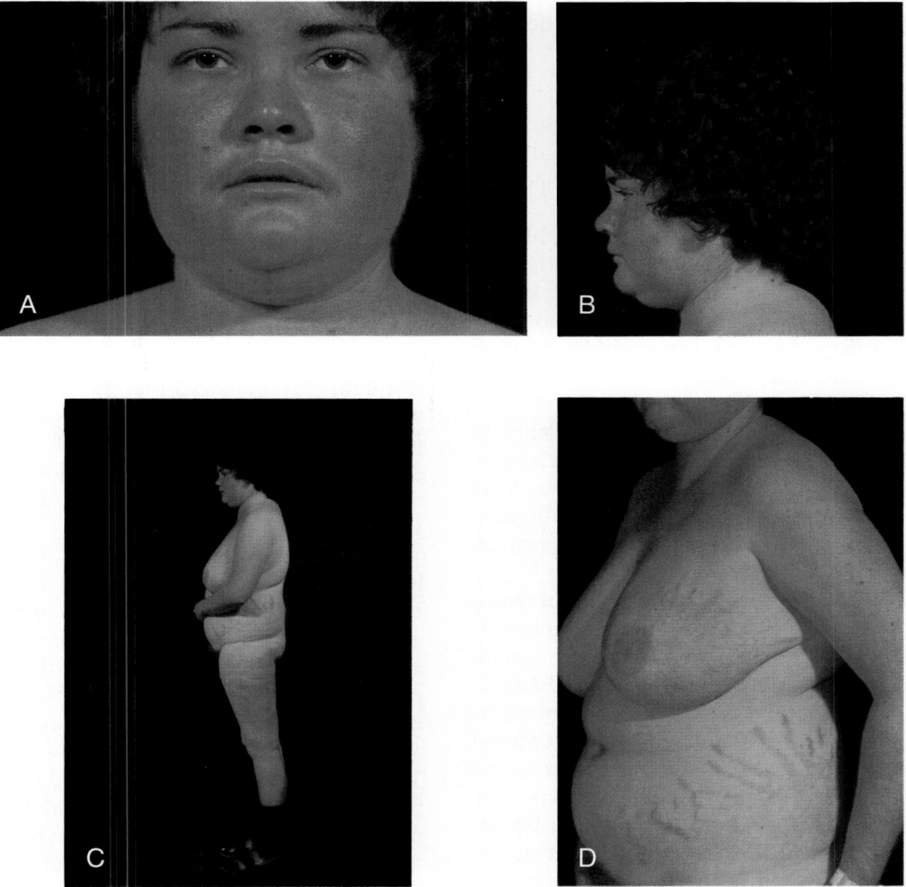

Figure 19–9 ■ Clinical features of a patient with hypothalamic Cushing's disease with pituitary adenoma. *A,* The moon face and malar flush. *B* and *C,* Obesity with the distribution of fat, particularly on the trunk, and the "buffalo hump." *D,* The purple abdominal striae.

strate for gluconeogenesis by the liver. This has been clearly delineated as a catabolic effect of cortisol excess.[123]

Hirsutism. The hirsutism is of two varieties. When the excess adrenal hormone is primarily cortisol, hair growth appears on the sides of the face, the forehead, and the limbs and trunk and has a lanugo-like texture. When there is a coexisting excess of androgen, relatively severe hirsutism can occur with temporal hairline recession and a deepening of the voice.

Striae. Purple striae are noted, especially around the hips and abdomen (see Fig. 19–9), the front of the shoulders, and the upper outer area of the breasts. The development of striae is probably secondary to the catabolic effect of cortisol, resulting in weakness of the subcutaneous tissue and thinning of the skin. The striae are wide and have a purplish hue, reflecting erythrocytosis; this is unlike their appearance in other obesity states, in which striae are either pink or colorless and narrow.

Weakness. Muscle weakness is among the *most frequent signs* in Cushing's disease. It affects the upper legs and arms in particular and occurs secondary to the reduction of *muscle mass* resulting from the cortisol-induced mobilization of amino acid from muscle and the consequent loss of muscle protein. Muscle weakness is greatly aggravated when hypokalemia is also present.

Osteoporosis. From 40 to 80 percent of patients with Cushing's disease are affected by osteoporosis, which is sometimes so serious that spontaneous fractures of the ribs and vertebrae may result. Kyphosis and a loss in truncal height are also common. In children and adolescents, retardation of growth is observed. The osteoporosis caused by glucocorticoid excess differs sharply from most other forms of osteoporosis, in that there is a decrease in bone formation as well as an increase in bone resorption. The impaired bone formation is probably due to the combination of inhibiting effects of cortisol on collagen biosynthesis and bone matrix formation plus interference with calcium absorption. The latter may be related to glucocorticoid antagonism to vitamin D.

Purpura and Easy Bruisability. In Cushing's disease, the capillaries are unduly fragile; purpura and bruises develop spontaneously or after trivial trauma, especially on the dorsal surface of the forearms, thighs, and lower legs. The blood-clotting mechanism is normal.

Psychiatric Disorders. Mental disturbances include euphoria, irritability, insomnia, emotional lability, *and most commonly depression.* This is due to chronic hypercortisolism feedback on the limbic system in the CNS. After satisfactory treatment and despite a return to a normal biochemical and metabolic state, emotional problems may persist. Patients often show marked fluctuations in anxiety and depression for long periods (1 to 3 years).

Management

Transsphenoidal Surgery. The primary treatment modality is surgery. All Cushing's disease patients should have venous sampling from the cavernous sinuses bilaterally with simultaneous peripheral blood sampling. A 2:1 or greater cephalic to peripheral ACTH gradient establishes the diagnosis of Cushing's disease. More importantly, this procedure will frequently enable the location (left versus right lobes) of the tumor to be determined, and removal of the appropriate half of the anterior pituitary will be curative in 80 percent of cases of microadenoma.[124] Macroadenomas, on the other hand, have a lower cure rate.[125]

Radiation and Medical Therapy. In cases of incomplete surgical removal or recurrent tumor, a course of radiotherapy is indicated. Various drugs have been used, such as cyproheptadine, bromocriptine, somatostatin analogues, and RU 486. However, none of these drugs has proven long-term benefits.

Medical and Surgical Adrenalectomy. The observation that dogs treated with the insecticide dichlorodiphenyldichloroethane (DDD) developed adrenal atrophy led to the development of the adrenolytic agent *o,p′*-DDD (mitotane) in the late 1950s. Mitotane causes selective necrosis of the zona fasciculata and reticularis. The most common side effects of mitotane are nausea, anorexia, and dizziness. The effectiveness of this drug in the reduction of hypercortisolemia is established. This mode of therapy can be applied to patients who have failed surgical treatment, for preoperative treatment with the aim of diminishing the cortisol impact on tissue damage, and as an adjunct to radiotherapy.[126]

Surgical Bilateral Adrenalectomy. Surgical bilateral adrenalectomy is reserved for patients with persistent disease despite surgical and medical treatments of the pituitary tumor. This procedure induces rapid reduction of hypercortisolemia and is lifesaving. Careful cortisol replacement may be necessary to deal with the appearance of adrenal crisis.

Nelson's Syndrome. After bilateral adrenalectomy for the management of pituitary-dependent Cushing's disease, an increase in pituitary *tumor size*, *plasma ACTH,* and *hyperpigmentation* develops in 8 to 30 percent of patients. These tumors are highly invasive and difficult to treat and may be the cause of death in some patients despite normal cortisol levels. Hyperpigmentation is due to the stimulation of melanocytes by increased secretion of the POMC product—melanocyte-stimulating hormone.

THYROTROPIN-SECRETING PITUITARY ADENOMA

TSH-secreting pituitary tumors (TSH-omas) are associated with hyperthyroidism. TSH-secreting pituitary adenomas are a rare cause of hyperthyroidism characterized by inappropriate secretion of TSH. Their diagnosis is now facilitated by the recent introduction of ultrasensitive TSH immunoassays as well as free thyroid hormone assays that are not obscured by abnormal serum transport proteins. Increased awareness and early recognition of these tumors will prevent mistreatment, such as thyroid ablation or long-term antithyroid drug administration, which undoubtedly further increases TSH secretion, tumor size, and invasiveness. Although no single diagnostic test is pathognomonic in establishing the diagnosis, the elevation of α-subunit levels and serum SHBG concentrations and the frequently absent or impaired TSH responses to TRH stimulation and triiodothyronine (T_3) suppression are the most useful markers to distinguish patients with TSH-omas from those with thyroid hormone resistance syndrome (Table 19–5). Furthermore, high-resolution CT scanning and MRI may help in detecting tumors as small as 3 mm. Surgery remains the first-line therapeutic approach to the disease, followed by radiotherapy in the case of surgical failure. The finding of measurable TSH levels after a simple T_3 suppression test definitely indicates that the removal of the tumor cells was incomplete, thus requiring a closer follow-up of the patient or additional therapies. If needed, treatment with somatostatin analogues, which allows restoration of euthyroidism and even tumor shrinkage in many cases, is worthwhile.[127]

Hyperplasia of the pituitary as a result of long-standing hypothyroidism is common but is rarely symptomatic. However, when symptoms are present, tumoral signs, amenorrhea-galactorrhea, and even postpartum thyroiditis are frequent presentations in adults, whereas precocious puberty is classic in children. Medical treatment is the rule because of the almost certain regression of pituitary abnormalities with proper thyroid hormone replacement. The evolution should be monitored closely, given the possibility of initial worsening (pseudotumor cerebri) or the possibility of an incidental nonthyrotropic pituitary tumor that will not regress with thyroid hormone replacement. The association of moderate hyperprolactinemia is common; however, if amenorrhea-galactorrhea or hyperprolactinemia does not resolve with thyroid hormone replacement, a prolactinoma should be suspected.

MECHANISM(S) OF TUMORIGENESIS

The current understanding of mechanisms for the pathogenesis and progression of these common pituitary adenomas is incomplete. During recent years, new information on the role of intrinsic pituitary genetic alterations and on disorders of transcription factors, growth factors, and signaling proteins involved in pituitary tumorigenesis of both spo-

■ TABLE 19–5
Laboratory Findings in Patients with TSH-Secreting Tumors

LABORATORY RESULTS	NUMBER OF PATIENTS (%)
Elevated T_4 or T_3	115/121 (95)
Detectable TSH	21/121 (100)
"Normal" TSH	28/121 (23)
Elevated α-subunit	69/72 (96)
Elevated α-subunit/TSH ratio	47/50 (94)
Elevated GH	29
Elevated PRL	37
Elevated FSH	7
Elevated LH	4
TSH response to TRH	24/94 (26)
TSH suppression by T_3	6/32 (19)

Modified from Melmed S (ed). The Pituitary. Cambridge, MA, Blackwell Scientific Publications, 1995, p 550.

radic and hereditary adenomas has been reported. These advances are the subject of a comprehensive review.[85]

Evidence Against Hypothalamic Etiology. Pituitary hormone synthesis and secretion are under tight control by hypothalamic releasing and inhibiting factors. It has been suggested that inappropriate hypothalamic inputs to the pituitary cells may be responsible for tumorigenesis. Evidence against this proposition includes the following:

1. Ectopic GHRH-secreting tumors and hypothalamic GHRH-producing tumors (hamartomas and gangliocytomas) result in *somatotroph hyperplasia* and GH hypersecretion but rarely in the formation of GH-producing adenoma.[128]
2. Patients with Cushing's syndrome caused by ectopic CRF oversecretion from intrasellar gangliocytoma or prostate cancer develop *corticotroph hyperplasia* but not adenoma.[67, 129, 130]
3. Histologic studies of pituitary adenomas clearly reveal distinct tumor borders that are not surrounded by hyperplastic pituitary tissue.[131]
4. Hormonal secretion by adenomatous cells is usually independent of physiologic hypothalamic control, and surgical resection of small, well-defined tumors usually results in functional cure.
5. There is no evidence to suggest that the receptors for hypothalamic hormones are defective to account for adenoma formation.

Oncogenes and Tumor Suppressor Genes. Oncogenes are mutated proteins leading to inappropriate or constitutive signaling of downstream effectors without upstream signals. In recent years, one of the most exciting advances is the discovery that 30 to 40 percent of human pituitary GH-hypersecreting adenomas carry somatic single-base missense mutation of the gene for the α-subunit of the stimulatory guanosine triphosphate–binding protein G_s ($G_s\alpha$). These mutations, termed *gsp* oncogenes,[132] resulting in elevation of intracellular cyclic adenosine monophosphate levels are thought to be responsible for tumor growth and excessive GH secretion. Interestingly, *gsp* oncogenes also occur in nonfunctioning pituitary adenomas and ACTH-producing adenomas.[133, 134] Thus, *gsp* oncogenes appear to play a role in the tumorigenesis of some but not all pituitary hormone–secreting adenomas.

Multiple endocrine neoplasia type I (MEN I) is a hereditary syndrome characterized by the combined occurrence of tumor formation of the parathyroids, anterior pituitary, and pancreatic islets. The *MEN1* gene, a tumor suppressor gene, has been cloned and mapped to chromosome 11q13 (see earlier). Allelic loss of 11q13 was demonstrated in pituitary adenomas obtained from patients with MEN I syndrome[135, 136] and in nonfunctioning pituitary adenomas (20 percent) and other pituitary adenomas. Thus, recessive mutations (11q13) are associated with pituitary tumorigenesis in MEN I and in 10 to 15 percent of all sporadic adenomas.

Monoclonality. Thus, these observations strongly suggest that pituitary tumors are derived from intrinsic pituitary cell defects leading to monoclonal expansion of a single transformed cell, rather than from excessive polyclonal proliferation due to generalized hypothalamic overstimulation. However, the *gsp* oncogene, allelic loss of 11q13 as well as hypothalamic hormones and their receptors, and local growth factors may all have an important role in promoting the *growth* of already transformed cell clones and the expansion of small adenomas into large invasive tumors.[85]

CNS-HYPOTHALAMIC DERANGEMENTS

The biologically essential activities of all species including humans are *feeding, mating,* and *sleeping*. These innate behaviors are dictated by neural and metabolic networks to sustain life and perpetuate the species. Derangement of neural communications and insufficiency of metabolic fuels, when prolonged, may disrupt the functional integrity of the reproductive system.

Complex neural networks governing *mood and behavior (cognitive being)* are the foundation of psychoneuroendocrinology. The negative impact of life events and interpersonal and environmental factors may alter cognitive processes. If this is sustained, *cognitive dysfunction* occurs, resulting in clinical or subclinical manifestations of reproductive dysfunction.

That reproduction is also highly dependent on *metabolic fuel availability* has been recognized since ancient times. Nutritional deficiencies at the cellular level have significant negative impact on the brain-pituitary hormone secretion, with enhanced release of catabolic hormone and reduced output of anabolic factors. These adjustments are innate neuroendocrine mechanisms to conserve metabolic fuel. Reduction of metabolic fuel availability below the crucial level by food restriction, either voluntary or involuntary, or by increased energy expenditure through exercise may result in reproductive dysfunction.

It is likely that these seemingly separate underlying causes of reproductive dysfunction may be mechanistically interdependent and, therefore, inseparable in actuality. The end result of these conditions is expressed centrally by the attenuation of GnRH neuronal activity—the seat of reproduction. This section covers the psychoneuroendocrine-metabolic bases for a variety of hypothalamic amenorrhea syndromes.

Psychoneuroendocrine Concept: Pseudocyesis as a Model

Pseudocyesis has been described as the oldest known psychosomatic condition. Illustrious cases include Mary Tudor, Queen of England (1516–1558), who experienced two episodes. It is a rare condition with a total of 547 cases reported in the English medical literature in women ranging in age from 6 to 79 years.[137] The common theme found in pseudocyesis is the strong belief by the woman that she is pregnant with the full manifestation of the symptoms and signs of pregnancy.

The underlying causes are unresolved grief; the recent loss of a lover or perceived rejection; recent miscarriage, abortion, or infant death; and unrelenting anxiety. Thus, the imagined pregnancy serves to provide a diffuse restitution in response to a real or imagined loss, events suggesting a *reciprocal interplay between mind and body*.[2, 138] The condition of pseudocyesis, therefore, serves as a firm basis for *psychoneuroendocrine aspects of reproduction*.

Evidence of hypersecretion of LH and prolactin with

increased amplitude of pulsatile release has been found.[106, 139, 140] Circulating estradiol and progesterone are elevated to levels comparable with those found during the luteal phase of the normal cycle. Cortisol levels and circadian rhythm are within normal limits, but GH secretion, particularly during sleep, is blunted.[140] The elevated levels of prolactin and LH are high enough to maintain quasi-luteal function and galactorrhea in these patients. Secretion of FSH is reduced in most cases studied. Disparate endocrine findings have been reported.[137, 140, 141] The lack of uniform endocrine profiles is probably due to the timing of investigation during the process of rapid resolution of central mechanisms soon after the patient is told that she is not pregnant.[106]

The psychogenic basis for neuroendocrine abnormalities in pseudocyesis is further suggested by the immediate fall in serum prolactin and LH levels after the diagnosis is revealed to the patient.[106] It has been proposed that depression is critically involved in the genesis of pseudocyesis.[138] The fantasy of pregnancy appears to function as a defense against such depression.[142]

The management of patients with pseudocyesis should be individualized. The psychogenic nature of this disorder should be revealed to the husband or parent. Psychiatric care is frequently necessary in the general management of the patient to prevent the recurrence of the disorder and suicidal tendency.

Physiologic Hypothalamic Hypogonadotropinism

Puberty

Neuroendocrine control of the initiation of human puberty may shed some light on the nature of the defects in hypothalamic chronic anovulation. The limiting factor for increasing amounts of gonadotropin secretion as puberty approaches is hypothalamic GnRH release.[143, 144] The ovary and pituitary of prepubertal girls are not limiting factors because follicular maturation and ovulation can be achieved by the activation of pituitary gonadotropin secretion through the intermittent delivery of exogenous GnRH.[143, 145]

The ontogeny of pulsatile GnRH-mediated gonadotropin secretion appears to conform to a U-shaped curve (Fig. 19–10); the GnRH pulse-generating system is functionally active after 20 weeks of gestation,[146] extends to the first year of life, and then is followed by a progressive decline, reaching a quiescent phase of hypogonadotropic state at ages 6 to 8 years.[147] The fact that this occurs in girls without ovarian function (i.e., XO Turner's syndrome)[148] offers compelling support for the view that prepubertal restraint on gonadotropin secretion is entirely due to a *central mechanism that governs hypothalamic GnRH secretion* (see Chapter 15).

The concept of pubertal activation of the GnRH secretory program (the upswing of the U-shaped curve) implies a decline in hypothalamic inhibitors or an increase in stimulators,[149] which permits a greater increase in GnRH/LH pulse amplitude than frequency.[144] This results in a remarkable 100-fold increase in levels of LH, a 6-fold increase in FSH levels, and a 12-fold rise in estradiol levels.[150] An additional neuroendocrine mechanism results in a switch from sleep-entrained amplification of GnRH/LH pulsatility to a progressive increase in daytime pulsatility[144, 151, 152] (Fig. 19–11); ovarian activation ultimately ensues. Before final synchronization of the hypothalamic-pituitary-ovarian axis, luteal-phase defects and anovulatory cycles are common occurrences in adolescent girls.[153] This simple scheme (see Fig. 19–10) provides an overview of our current knowledge and offers a framework for understanding neuroendocrine mechanisms underlying these transitions. For example, the U-shaped curve may be interrupted by several well-known clinical conditions; premature activation occurs in cases of central precocious puberty with the appearance of amplified GnRH/LH pulses and the sleep-entrained augmentation.[152, 154] Delay of onset of puberty or regression to a prepubertal state can be observed

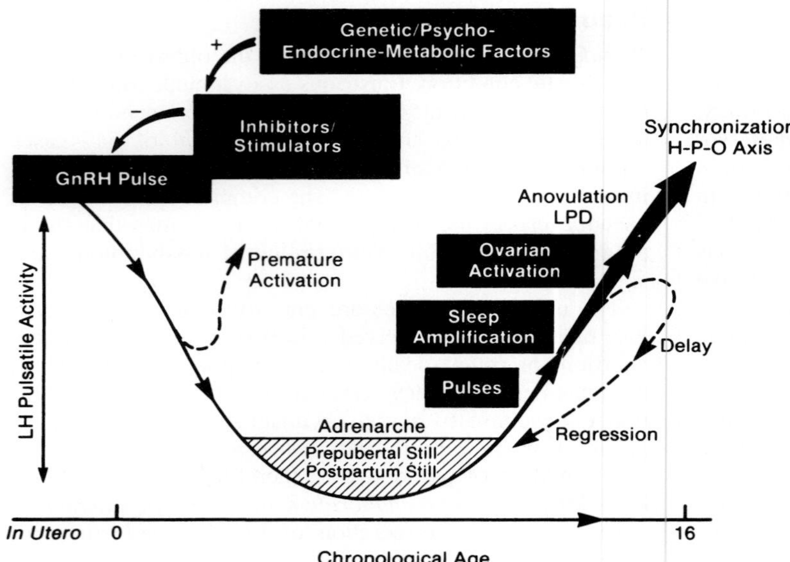

Figure 19–10 ■ Diagrammatic display of the U-shaped curve relating a time-compressed neuroendocrine event of puberty. The prepubertal restraint of GnRH/LH pulses is an expression due either to the increase in hypothalamic inhibitors or to reduced stimulators, resulting in a hypogonadotropic state. The final synchronization of the hypothalamic-pituitary-ovarian (H-P-O) axis in generating ovulatory cycles follows a sequence of decline of inhibitory mechanisms or increase in stimulatory inputs, initiation of GnRH/LH pulsatile activity, and the sleep-entrained amplifications. The time course of these events is determined by nutritional and socioenvironmental factors. The interruption of this sequence of events occurs in several clinical abnormalities, as exemplified by premature activation in central precocious puberty and the delay or regression to prepubertal state in patients with anorexia nervosa. LPD, luteal-phase defect. (From Yen SSC. Reproductive strategy in women: Neuroendocrine basis of endogenous contraception. *In* Rolan R [ed]. Neuroendocrinology of Reproduction. Amsterdam, Excerpta Medica, 1988, pp 231–239.)

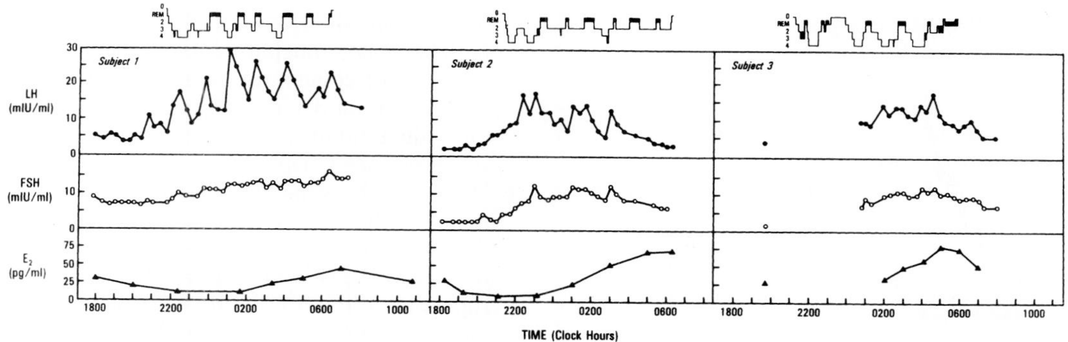

Figure 19–11 ■ Luteinizing hormone (LH), follicle-stimulating hormone (FSH), and 17β-estradiol (E_2) levels are shown with sleep histograms for three subjects with idiopathic precocious puberty who exhibited episodic, nocturnal LH release concomitant with significantly elevated FSH levels. Nocturnal elevation of both gonadotropins was associated with a significant elevation of E_2 levels occurring during the sleep period. Stages of sleep monitored by electroencephalography are displayed at the top of the illustration. (From Matthews MJ, Parker DC, Rebar RW, et al. Sleep associated gonadotropin and oestradiol patterns in girls with precocious sexual development. Clin Endocrinol [Oxf] 17:601–607, 1982.)

with athletic training before menarche and in psychoneuroendocrine disorders such as anorexia nervosa.

Postpartum Amenorrhea (Miniature Puberty)

The *hypogonadotropic state* of the postpartum period provides a unique physiologic model for understanding the neuroendocrine mechanisms responsible for reactivation of the GnRH-gonadotropin-ovarian system. The massive increase in sex steroids during pregnancy may induce hypothalamic GnRH suppression, and the prolonged deprivation of endogenous GnRH may extend into the puerperium to account for the hypogonadotropism and diminished responsiveness to exogenous GnRH resembling that seen in prepubertal quiescence (see Fig. 19–10).

Recovery, either spontaneous[155–157] or prematurely activated by the administration of GnRH,[158, 159] follows a predictable sequence of preferential FSH and then LH secretion, an event closely resembling that of the peripubertal state. Furthermore, the reactivation of cyclic ovarian function during the first 4 weeks post partum appears to involve the appearance of sleep-associated pulsatile release of LH by the pituitary[159] (Fig. 19–12). This compressed event is remarkably reminiscent of the neuroendocrine manifestations that initiate puberty; hence, the concept of *miniature puberty* has been proposed, in which a common neuroendocrine mechanism involves diminished hypothalamic inhibition of GnRH secretory activity to account for the spontaneous recovery from postpartum amenorrhea by the reactivation of gonadotropin-ovarian cyclicity.[160] Both the pubertal model and the postpartum model serve to illustrate the neuroendocrine mechanism that governs activation and suppression of the GnRH pulse generator appropriate to physiologic demands and therefore serve as a basis for the understanding of menstrual disorders under a variety of reduced-GnRH neuronal activities.

Lactational Amenorrhea

Breast feeding results in a variable period of ovarian inactivity that is also related to suppression of the normal pulsatile GnRH release as evidenced by the occurrence of ovulation and corpus luteum formation in response to programmed pulsatile administration of GnRH[161] (Fig. 19–13). The 24-hour pattern of pulsatile LH secretion at 4 weeks post partum revealed occasional LH pulses or the complete absence of LH pulsatile activity. LH pulses were resumed at 8 weeks post partum with a varied pulse frequency of two to eight pulses during 24 hours, and there was no influence of the time of day or sleep on LH pulses (Fig. 19–14). Lactational amenorrhea can be maintained for at least a year or two depending on the duration and intensity of suckling and the nutritional status of the mother. Thus, lactational amenorrhea represents nature's device for spacing the young and represents endogenous hypothalamic contraception. Cessation of lactation is followed by the resumption of LH pulsatility with a *prepubertal pattern of nocturnal amplification*[162] (see Fig. 19–12).

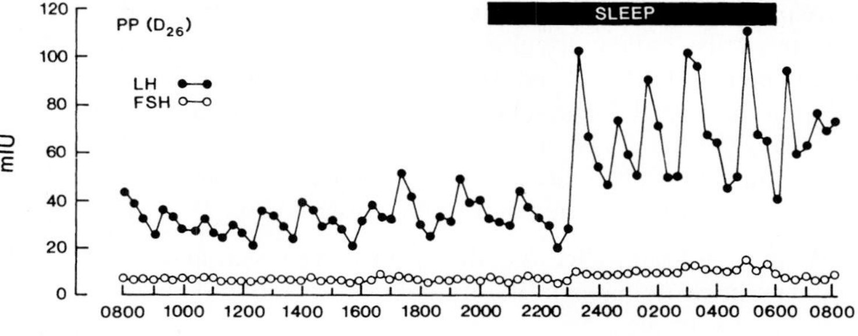

Figure 19–12 ■ Pulsatile activities of LH and FSH secretion in a representative nonlactating woman during wakeful and sleep periods on day 26 post partum (PP). (From Liu JH, Rebar RW, Yen SSC. Neuroendocrine control of the postpartum period. Clin Perinatol 10:723–736, 1983.)

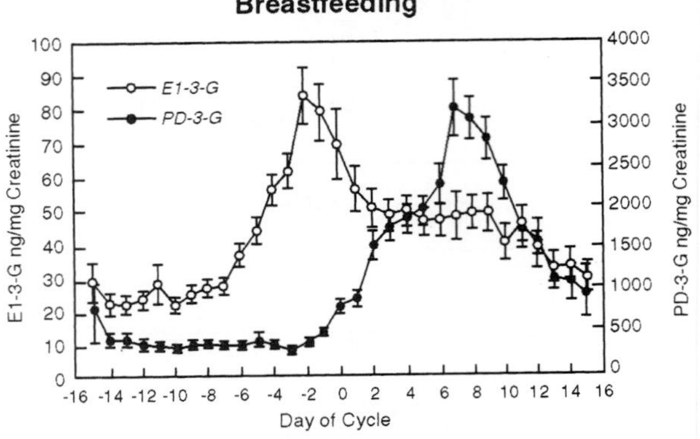

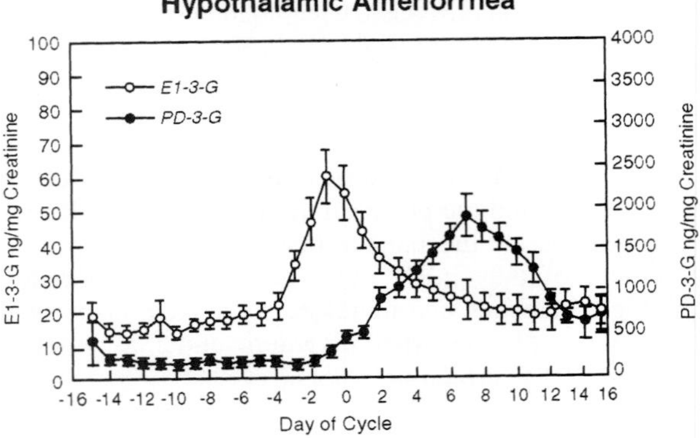

Figure 19–13 ■ Daily urinary estrone and pregnanediol conjugates corrected for creatinine excretion during the first cycle of GnRH administration in eight lactating postpartum women *(upper panel)* and in five women with hypothalamic amenorrhea *(lower panel)*. Individual data sets are aligned so that day 0 represents the peak urinary LH value during that cycle. The values shown are means ± SEM. E1-3-G, estrone-3-glucuronide; PD-3-G, pregnanediol-3-glucuronide. (From Zinaman MJ, Cartledge T, Tomai T, et al. Pulsatile GnRH stimulates normal cyclic ovarian function in amenorrheic lactating postpartum women. J Clin Endocrinol Metab 80:2088–2093, 1995. © The Endocrine Society.)

Psychogenic/Nutritional Hypothalamic Dysfunction

Stress and Reproductive Function

Events evoked by physical (metabolic), psychobiologic (emotional), and psychosocial stresses activate the sympathetic nervous system and the pituitary release of stress hormones—prolactin, GH, and ACTH. The response of the ACTH-adrenal axis with the secretion of glucocorticoids and catecholamines constitutes the most important neuroendocrine-metabolic response to stress.[163, 164] Central to this activational response is the release of CRF by the neuronal system of the paraventricular nucleus (PVN). As detailed in Chapter 2, CRF has multiple sites of action mediated through four pathways: (1) the PVN–median eminence pathway, (2) the PVN–autonomic projections (brain stem and spinal cord), (3) the PVN–arcuate nucleus pathway, and (4) the cerebral cortex and limbic system (Fig. 19–15).

- Within the brain, CRF together with vasopressin and oxytocin participates in the modulation of mood, behavior, and learning.
- CRF stimulates central noradrenergic activity through the PVN–brain stem pathway, which in turn activates peripheral norepinephrine release and adrenomedullary secretion of epinephrine. Catecholamines, a major regulator of the fat depot acting through β_2-adrenergic receptor, induce lipolysis and decrease leptin expression and secretion (see Chapter 17, Fig. 17–20).
- Within the hypothalamus, CRF projects to the arcuate nucleus where it induces the processing of the POMC-derived peptides, such as β-endorphin, ACTH, and α-melanocyte–stimulating hormone. Together with neuropeptide Y (NPY), POMC peptides mediate a direct feedback signal of leptin through leptin receptors on POMC neurons to PVN, thereby regulating eating behavior.
- The PVN–median eminence CRF pathway serves to deliver CRF through the portal circulation to the anterior pituitary where it stimulates ACTH and β-endorphin release. Cortisol secretion in response to ACTH exerts catabolic effects in peripheral tissues, suppresses immune function, and feeds back to the hypothalamus to inhibit CRF gene expression and regulate mood and behavior.

In humans, vasopressin enhances and oxytocin attenuates the CRF-mediated ACTH release.[165, 166] High concentrations of oxytocin and vasopressin are found in the portal blood, and pituitary corticotrophs appear to be the site of these interactions.[167] In addition, both epinephrine and norepinephrine have been shown to potentiate CRF action at the pituitary level.[167] Thus, under stressful conditions, CRF-mediated ACTH release is determined by several modifiers. The relative inputs may vary, depending on the type, intensity, and duration of stressful events.

CRF has been shown to impair the reproductive axis by

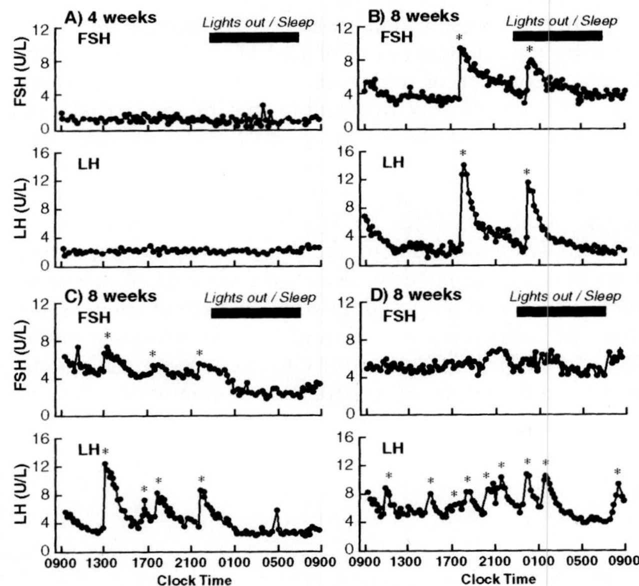

Figure 19–14 ■ Changes in the plasma concentrations of FSH and LH in four fully breastfeeding women, one at 4 weeks *(A)* and three at 8 weeks *(B* to *D)* post partum. The asterisks indicate significant pulses of FSH or LH. (From Tay CCK, Glasier AF, McNeilly AS. The 24-h pattern of pulsatile luteinizing hormone, follicle stimulating hormone and prolactin release during the first 8 weeks of lactational amenorrhoea in breastfeeding women. Hum Reprod 7:951–958, 1992.)

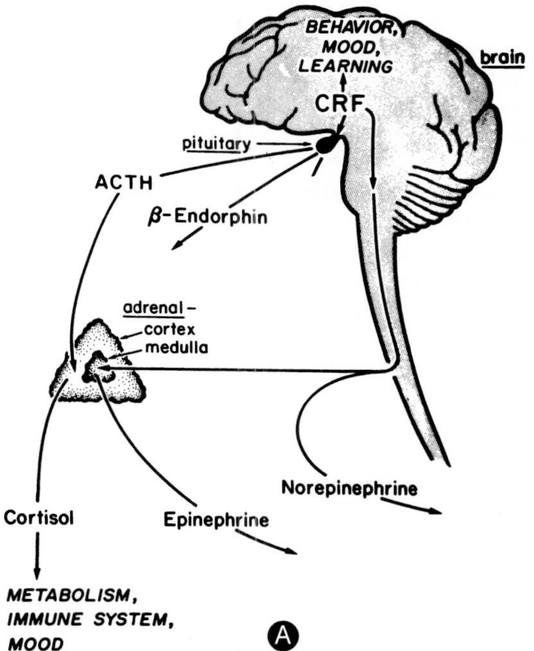

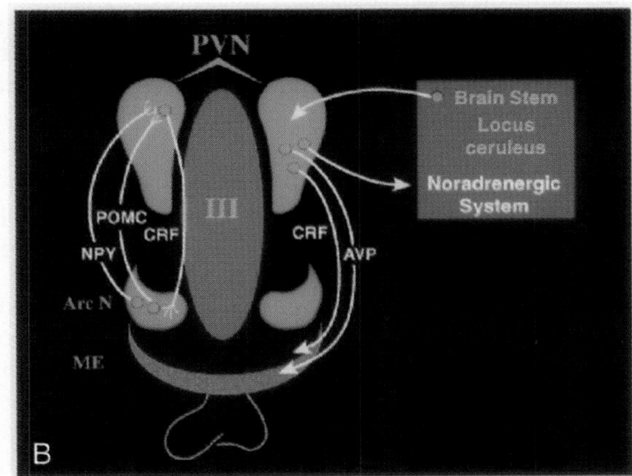

Figure 19–15 ■ *A,* Diagram depicting the multitude of corticotropin-releasing factor (CRF)–mediated peripheral and central neuroendocrine-metabolic responses to stressful stimuli (see text for details). (Courtesy of Dr. Wylie Vale, The Salk Institute, La Jolla, CA.)

B, CRF and arginine vasopressin (AVP) from the paraventricular nucleus (PVN) project to the median eminence (ME) and are secreted into the portal circulation, where they synergistically stimulate pro-opiomelanocortin (POMC)–containing neurons in the arcuate nucleus (Arc N) with the release of ACTH and β-endorphin by the pituitary. The lateral portion of the PVN also contains adrenergic neurons that project to the brain stem. POMC and neuropeptide Y (NPY) in the arcuate nucleus project their fibers to the PVN. When activated, both POMC and NPY inhibit the secretion of CRF and norepinephrine such as occurs with leptin feedback to the arcuate nucleus.

reducing the circulating levels of LH, to attenuate the frequency of pulsatile GnRH secretion, and to bring about a prompt suppression of electrophysiologic activity of the GnRH pulse generator[168–173] (see Chapter 2). The CRF action on GnRH neuronal activities appears to be mediated by the activation of endogenous opioids independent of hypercortisolism, and the effect is reversible by the administration of naloxone.[174–176] Thus, the link of CRF and reproductive dysfunction appears to involve stress-induced elevation of hypothalamic CRF and opioid peptides that inhibit GnRH secretion with curtailment of reproductive function. By inference, the association of hypercortisolism in psychoneuroendocrine-metabolic disorders (see later) may be related to endogenous hypersecretion of CRF.[177]

Nutrition and Reproduction

In affluent sections of Western societies, the availability of food is usually not a factor in determining the nutritional state of an individual. In recent years, however, a number of reproductive disorders have emerged that appear to be related to dieting and a desire for leanness. Weight loss, whether it occurs in the setting of food restriction or exercise, is associated with delayed puberty, delayed menarche, and amenorrhea.

Given the demands of reproduction—to provide nutrients to the fetus and to nurse the newborn infant—female body composition is crucial and reproduction is curtailed when the fat depots and lean body mass are reduced to suboptimal levels. Because of these special needs, women, in contrast to men, are endowed with a significant amount of fat beginning at the time of puberty, an endowment that is maintained throughout adult life[178] (Fig. 19–16). This sex difference in body composition is biologically relevant to ensure sufficient energy storage as a reproductive strategy. However, a growing number of studies have failed to identify a consistent correlation between reproductive function and body status.[179] Rather, reproductive success and failure appear to be responsive to the general availability

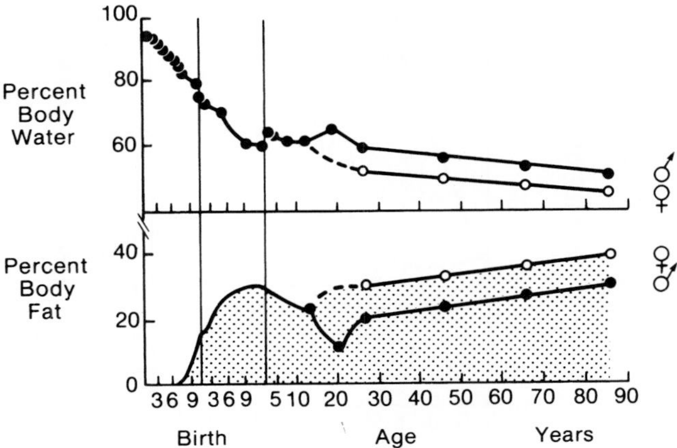

Figure 19–16 ■ Changing body composition from late gestation through adult life. Note the dramatic departure of the amount of body fat in females and males at the time of puberty. (From Friis-Hansen B. Hydrometry of growth and aging. *In* Brozek J [ed]. Human Body Composition: Approaches and Application. Symposia of the Society for the Study of Human Biology, Vol VII. New York, Pergamon Press, 1965, pp 191–209. © 1965, Pergamon Press.)

of metabolic fuels.[180] Thus, reduction of metabolic fuel availability below the crucial level by food restriction, either voluntary or involuntary, is appropriately accompanied by anovulation and amenorrhea, an important device for endogenous contraception in the face of a large calorie demand.

The importance of adequate nutrition for neuroendocrine-metabolic control of ovarian function is seen in primitive desert-dwelling hunter-gatherers of the !Kung San ("Bushman") population of Botswana in the Kalahari Desert, South Africa. In this ecologic environment, seasonal changes of nutrition, body weight, and activity exist and the women have a peak time of giving birth: exactly 9 months after attainment of maximal weight, at which time conception occurs[181] (Fig. 19–17*A*). Thus, seasonal suppression of ovulation and luteal-phase defects, as documented by hormonal studies, occur in these women at a time when they are most active and have the lowest body weight. This corresponds to the winter months, when food availability is most limited and the search for food is most intense, with strenuous physical activity; the Bushwomen often carry children 30 miles or more a day.[182]

The precise causal relationship between food deprivation and cessation of cyclic menstrual function is not entirely clear. Several findings implicate hypothalamic dysfunction as the basis for the onset of amenorrhea: altered temperature regulation and reduced pulsatile LH activity, with a reversion to a peripubertal sleep-entrained episodic LH secretory pattern.[183–186] Moderate dietary restriction and weight loss in normal cycling women are associated with a reduction of estradiol levels and anovulation in the face of normal LH levels,[184] and severe starvation in healthy women for 2½ weeks induces a reversal of LH pulses to prepubertal patterns[185] (Fig. 19–17*B*).

Functional Hypothalamic Amenorrhea Syndrome

Cessation of menstrual cycles in young women without clinically demonstrable abnormalities of the pituitary-ovarian axis or other endocrine functions represents one of the most common types of amenorrhea. The term functional hypothalamic amenorrhea (FHA) indicates a nonorganic origin and a reversible disorder. There are two major types of FHA syndrome; one has a *psychogenic basis,* and the other is *exercise related.* Recent investigations have revealed compelling evidence of nutritional deficits as a common contributing factor to FHA syndrome.[187–189] Equally remarkable is the commonality of neuroendocrine-metabolic aberrations in these patients as revealed by recent investigations. On the basis of this understanding, the pathophysiologic processes of these two types of FHA syndrome are discussed together. Differences, when they exist, are identified.

EXERCISE AND MENSTRUAL CYCLE: CLINICAL ASPECTS

The rapid increase in popularity of physical exercise during the past decade has led to the recognition of deleterious

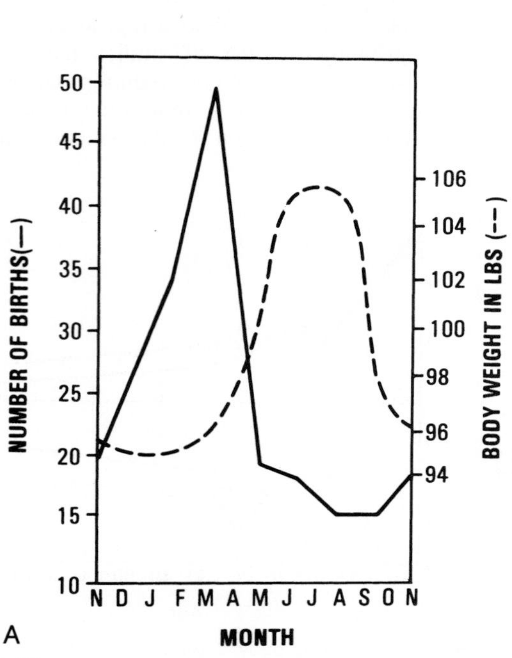

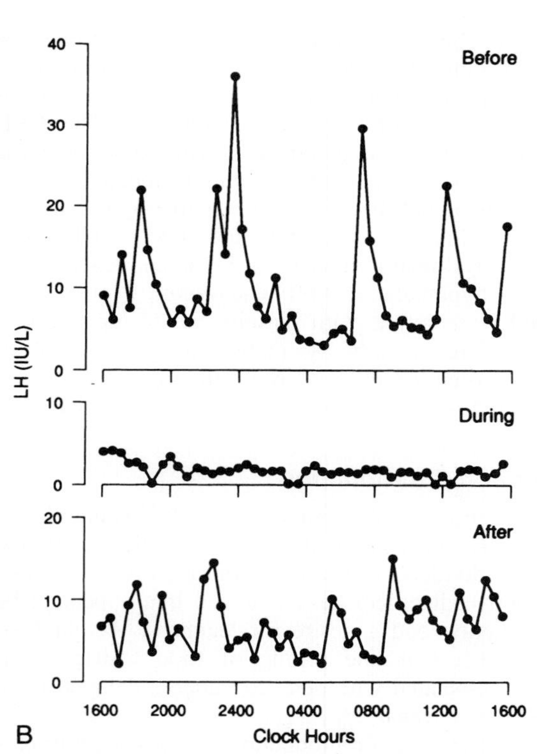

Figure 19–17 ■ *A,* Annual fluctuation of birth and mean body weight of the !Kung San of Botswana. Note that the peak time of birth follows a month after maximal weight gain. (From van der Walt LA, Wilmsen EN, Jenkins T. Unusual sex hormone patterns among desert-dwelling hunter-gatherers. J Clin Endocrinol Metab 46:658–663, 1978. © The Endocrine Society.)

B, Pulsatile LH pattern before (luteal phase), during, and after 2½ weeks of fasting in a healthy cycling woman. (From Fichter MM, Pirke KM. Hypothalamic-pituitary function in starving healthy subjects. *In* Pirke KM, Ploog D [eds]. The Psychobiology of Anorexia Nervosa. Berlin, Springer-Verlag, 1984, pp 124–135.)

effects of strenuous exercise on reproductive function.[190] The cause-effect relationship of this association is difficult to quantify because physiologic responses to various forms of exercise and athleticism have not been fully characterized and because of the presence of individual lifestyle variables, which also influence reproductive function.[191] Thus, confounding factors to be considered in assessing the exercise-related neuroendocrine-metabolic consequences are the type, duration, and intensity of exercise; body composition; psychologic background; and stress factors of individuals participating in exercise programs.[192]

Menstrual abnormalities have been reported in connection with a wide variety of sports, including middle- and long-distance running, swimming, ballet dancing, and field events. Varying degrees of menstrual disorders are related to the length and intensity of the activity.[193] The incidence of such disorders is higher at the end of the athletic season, and there is a positive correlation between weekly training mileage and the incidence of amenorrhea. Even joggers ("slow and easy," 5 to 30 miles/week) have significantly fewer menses per year than their less energetic counterparts.[194]

Of women athletes at the Tokyo Olympics (1964), 90 percent reported normal menstrual function[195]; at Montreal (1976), 59 percent experienced some irregularity.[196] Whether or not this was a real increase, there has certainly been an upsurge in the reporting of menstrual abnormalities associated with physical exercise. It is important to distinguish among the different physical activities and the age at which they are started. When training starts before the menarche, as in gymnastics and ballet dancing, the menarche is delayed by about 3 years and the incidence of secondary amenorrhea or chronic anovulation in later life is also higher.[193] This age-related effect was also found in a group of college swimmers and runners; each year of training before menarche delayed it by an average of 5 months[197] (Fig. 19–18).

Exercise amenorrhea may be sport-specific. The incidence is much higher in high-intensity runners and ballet dancers (40 to 50 percent), whereas it is lower in swimmers independent of training intensity (approximately 12 percent)[198] (Fig. 19–19). This difference may be attributable to the relatively high percentage of body fat among swimmers (approximately 20 percent) compared with runners (15 percent) and ballet dancers (about 15 percent).[199] In addition, runners with amenorrhea have significantly less daily protein intake and greater weight loss compared with runners without amenorrhea.[200] These observations support the hypothesis elaborated by Frisch and McArthur[201] that the integrity of menstrual function depends on crucial levels of body weight, specifically the lean to fat ratio, with a level of at least 22 percent body fat being required for normal menses. This proposed "body composition mechanism" for the development of amenorrhea should be viewed with caution, however, because there are obvious exceptions:

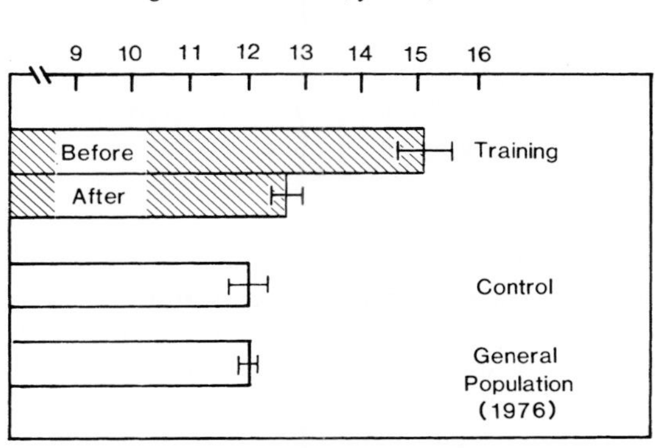

Figure 19–18 ■ Delayed menarche in girls who start exercise training before menarche compared with girls who start after menarche. (From Frisch RE, Gotz-Welbergen AV, McArthur JW, et al. Delayed menarche and amenorrhea of college athletes in relation to age of onset of training. JAMA 246:1559–1563, 1981. © 1981, American Medical Association.)

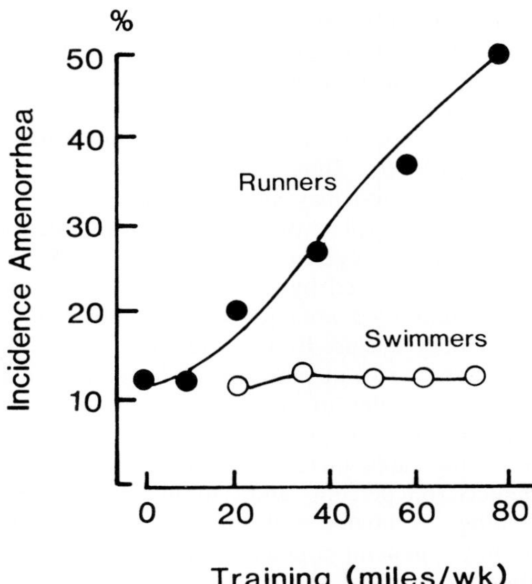

Figure 19–19 ■ Among runners, the frequency of amenorrhea is positively correlated with the number of miles run per week. In contrast, among swimmers in endurance training, the frequency of amenorrhea is about 12 percent and is independent of the intensity of training. (From Sanborn CF, Martin BJ, Wagner WW. Is athletic amenorrhea specific to runners? Am J Obstet Gynecol 143:859–861, 1982.)

1. Athletic amenorrhea can occur with or without weight loss.
2. If training is interrupted in ballet dancers (e.g., through injury), menses return without changes in body weight or in the lean to fat ratio.
3. Although a 10 to 15 percent loss of body weight (reflecting a 30 percent loss of body fat) can produce amenorrhea, the underlying mechanism is likely to be multifactorial rather than reduced extraglandular formation of estrogen from androgen by the fat compartment as proposed.[201] The lean body mass, mainly the muscle, must be taken into account as an important site for aromatization of androgen to estrogen.[202]

Exercise and its associated variables appear to induce a progressive dysfunction of ovarian cyclicity that includes (1) luteal-phase defects, (2) anovulatory cycles and amenorrhea, and (3) a delayed menarche in prepubertal girls.

Defects in pulsatile LH release have also been observed

in "normally menstruating" runners in whom pulsatile LH frequency is reduced and amplitude is increased compared with sedentary control subjects.[203–205] Although these runners have regular menstrual bleeding, the integrity of ovarian function is impaired, as reflected by luteal-phase defects[203] (Fig. 19–20). Thus, altered pulsatile patterns of gonadotropin secretion may lead to impaired folliculogenesis as an initiating cause of a continuum of luteal-phase defects, anovulatory cycles, and amenorrhea.[203, 206] This formulation is supported by a well-controlled prospective study in 28 untrained college women with documented normal ovulatory cycles. Bullen and associates[206] demonstrated that progressive increases in the intensity of exercise (from running 4 miles to 10 miles/day during a 4-week span), particularly if compounded by weight loss, over time induced a remarkable increase in the incidence of luteal-phase defects (63 percent) and anovulation (81 percent). These findings, compared with the incidence of menstrual disorders in the general population (Table 19–6), represent a transition from initial to long-term impacts of vigorous exercise that, with time, can lead to complete functional arrest of the hypothalamic-pituitary-ovarian axis, resulting in hypoestrogenic amenorrhea. Thus, high-intensity endurance exercise is associated with a central inhibition on hypothalamic GnRH secretory function that is discernible even before clinical evidence of altered menstrual cyclicity. Recent evidence, however, indicates that it is the energy cost of exercise and not exercise per se that disrupts menstrual function (see later).

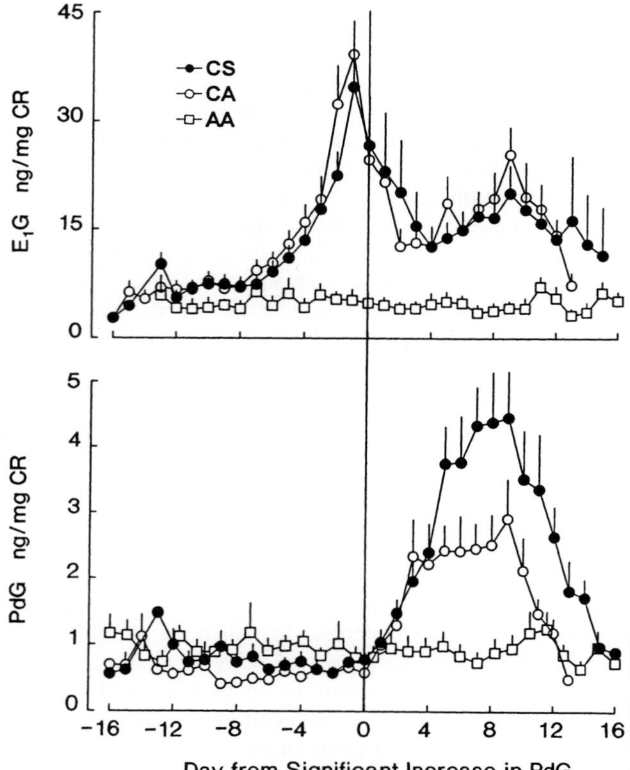

Figure 19–20 ■ Mean (± SE) daily urinary excretion of estrone glucuronide (E_1G, *top)* and pregnanediol glucuronide (PdG, *bottom)* in regularly cycling sedentary women (CS), athletic women with regular menstrual cycles (CA), and athletic women with amenorrhea (AA). Days are oriented from a significant increase in urinary PdG excretion, with day 0 being the day of the first significant increase. (From Loucks AB, Mortola JF, Girton L, Yen SSC. Alterations in the hypothalamic-pituitary-ovarian and the hypothalamic-pituitary-adrenal axes in athletic women. J Clin Endocrinol Metab 68:402–411, 1989. © The Endocrine Society.)

■ TABLE 19–6

Incidence of Luteal-Phase Defects and Anovulation* in the General Population,† and in 28 Young Women Who Participated in a Prospective Study of Progressively Increasing Vigorous Exercise with or without Weight Loss

ABNORMAL CYCLE	GENERAL POPULATION‡	VIGOROUS EXERCISE§ DURING A 4-WEEK SPAN: No Weight Loss	Weight Loss
Luteal-phase defects	15.8%	33%	63%
Anovulation	10.6%	42%	81%

*Loss of luteinizing hormone surge or flat basal body temperature.

†Ages 20 to 30 years, 1004 cycles.

‡Weighted mean from Collet ME, et al: Fertil Steril 5:437, 1954; Doring GK: J Reprod Fertil Suppl 6:77, 1969; and Metcalf MG, et al: J Endocrinol 97:213, 1983.

§Data from Bullen BA, Skrinar GS, Beitins IZ, et al. Induction of menstrual disorders by strenuous exercise in untrained women. N Engl J Med 312:1349–1353, 1985.

PSYCHOGENIC FACTORS AND MENSTRUAL CYCLE: CLINICAL ASPECTS

Over a half-century ago, Reifenstein[207] and others collectively offered indirect evidence for a hypothalamic mechanism by which psychogenic stress impairs ovarian function through reduced pituitary gonadotropin secretion.[23, 28, 189, 208, 209] Since the discovery of GnRH, it became clear that pituitary-ovarian function is intact in such patients[210–212] and that this disorder is a consequence of reduced pulsatile GnRH secretion. Whereas psychogenic dysfunction was assumed to be the underlying cause of hypothalamic amenorrhea, appropriate psychologic assessments were made only in recent years by Berga,[213] Giles,[214] and Laughlin[189] and coworkers. Women with hypothalamic amenorrhea were found to be perfectionistic overachievers with low self-esteem, an overall sense of ineffectiveness or lack of control, and an inability to cope with daily stress. They also score higher than control subjects do on depression and eating disorder inventories, although both conditions are in the subclinical range. These aberrant psychologic traits are not readily apparent clinically but require careful interview to be identified.

PATHOPHYSIOLOGY

Dysfunction of GnRH Pulse Generator. Identification and characterization of pulsatile patterns of LH secretion, which reflect episodic secretory activity of hypothalamic GnRH, have revealed a variety of abnormalities.[28, 208, 213] The degree of impairment of GnRH secretion varies widely, as evidenced by the *diversity of pulsatile LH activity.* In general, the frequency and, in psychogenic amenorrhea, the amplitude of the pulses are diminished; in some cases, a pubertal pattern of amplification of pulsatile LH activity in association with sleep is evident.

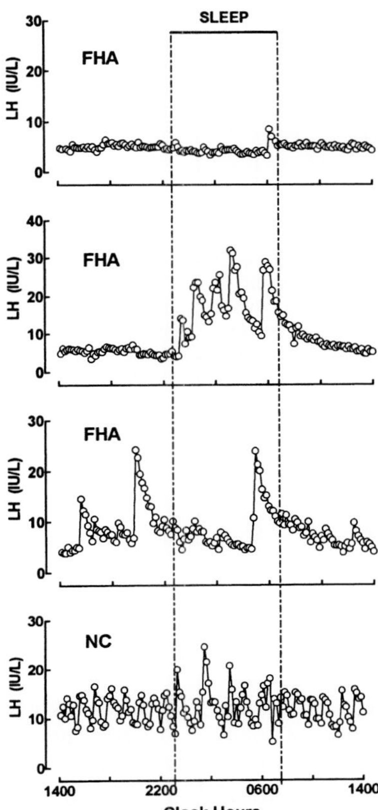

Figure 19–21 ■ Variations of 24-hour LH pulsatility in four women with functional hypothalamic amenorrhea (FHA) syndrome. The salient features are slowing of LH pulses and sleep-entrained amplification of LH pulses. NC, normal cycling women.

The spectrum of abnormalities most likely reflects a *pathophysiologic continuum* and changing hypothalamic GnRH activity with time[215] (Fig. 19–21). In severe cases, when few quasi-pulses of LH are present, ovarian activity virtually ceases, as reflected by markedly reduced levels of estradiol, androstenedione, and testosterone. Thus, the entire reproductive axis—hypothalamic-pituitary-ovarian system—is functionally regressed to the prepubertal state (Fig. 19–22). In contrast, patients with modest LH pulse amplitude but significantly reduced numbers of LH pulses have a substantial degree of ovarian secretion of estradiol and normal levels of androgens (Fig. 19–22). In this setting, spontaneous menses may occur in some cases. The continuum of hypothalamic-pituitary-ovarian dysfunction in psychogenic amenorrhea reflects the deranged GnRH pulse generator activity as well as gonadotropin responses to exogenous GnRH stimulation: low, normal, or exaggerated GnRH responses have been observed.[210] Ovulation and pregnancy can be achieved readily by pulsatile administration of GnRH with appropriate frequency and dose[28, 216–218] (Fig. 19–23*A* and *B*), indicating further that the random or irregular GnRH secretory program is the immediate underlying cause of amenorrhea in this syndrome. FSH levels are unaffected. This is consistent with the evidence that slowing of GnRH pulses preferentially decreases LH-β mRNA and enhances FSH-β mRNA, resulting in a higher FSH to LH ratio (see Chapter 17, Fig. 17–2), and resembles that seen in prepubertal children.

Nutritional Deficit. The psychogenic dysfunctions noted before appear to influence the eating behaviors of women with hypothalamic amenorrhea syndrome, whose dietary intake differed markedly from that of regular cycling women.[189] Although caloric intakes were similar, they consumed 50 percent less fat and more carbohydrates and fiber than did normal cycling women (Fig. 19–24*A*). The same unbalanced dietary intake was found in *exercise-associated amenorrhea*[188] (Fig. 19–24*B*). Thus, unbalanced nutrient intake may contribute to the disruption of menstrual cycle integrity in these patients.[187, 189, 219]

It has been recognized since ancient times that nutrition influences fertility. The energetic investment for reproduction is vastly greater for women than for men to provide an uninterrupted delivery of nutrients to the fetus and to nurse the newborn infant. Given the inordinate demands of reproduction, the development of luteal-phase defects, anovulation, and amenorrhea in the face of limited metabolic fuels is nature's device for *endogenous hypothalamic contraception* by reduced activities of the GnRH-gonadotropin axis.[160] The generally held concept that changes in body weight or composition, particularly body fat, form the basis for the curtailment of reproduction in women has been challenged by a growing number of studies that have failed to identify a clear correlation between reproductive function and body status.[179] Rather, reproductive success and failure appear to be responsive to the general availability of metabolic fuels.[180] Reduction of metabolic fuel availability below the crucial level by food restriction, either voluntary or involuntary, or by increased energy expenditure through exercise without compensating by increased food intake may cause delay of puberty, postponement of menarche, and amenorrhea through reversal of gonadotropin secretion to a prepubertal state—the *miniature puberty concept*.[160] This concept is further supported by the decreased DHEA levels in the face of hypercortisolemia seen in women with FHA syndrome, resulting in an increased cortisol to DHEA ratio (Fig. 19–25) resembling that seen in prepubertal girls.

Low energy availability, not stress of exercise, alters LH pulsatility in exercising women and may contribute to FHA of the psychogenic type as well. Reductions in LH pulse frequency comparable to those seen in women with FHA syndrome have been induced by the imposition of calorie deficits, either by restricting intake[220, 221] or increasing expenditure[222] or a combination of both,[223, 224] and were prevented in exercising women when increased intake compensated for exercise expenditure.[222–224] Thus, the inhibition of LH pulsatility in amenorrheic athletes appears to be related to chronic low energy availability and not to the effects of exercise per se as clearly demonstrated in short-term experiments by Loucks and colleagues.[222] However, the degree of slowing of LH pulse frequency in interventional studies is dependent on the source of the energy restriction: low energy availability caused by dietary restriction reduces LH pulse frequency by 23 percent, whereas an equivalent reduction by increasing exercise energy expenditure slows LH pulse frequency by only 10 percent.[220, 222] The link of nutrition and reproductive function appears to involve hypothalamic NPY.[225] NPY cell

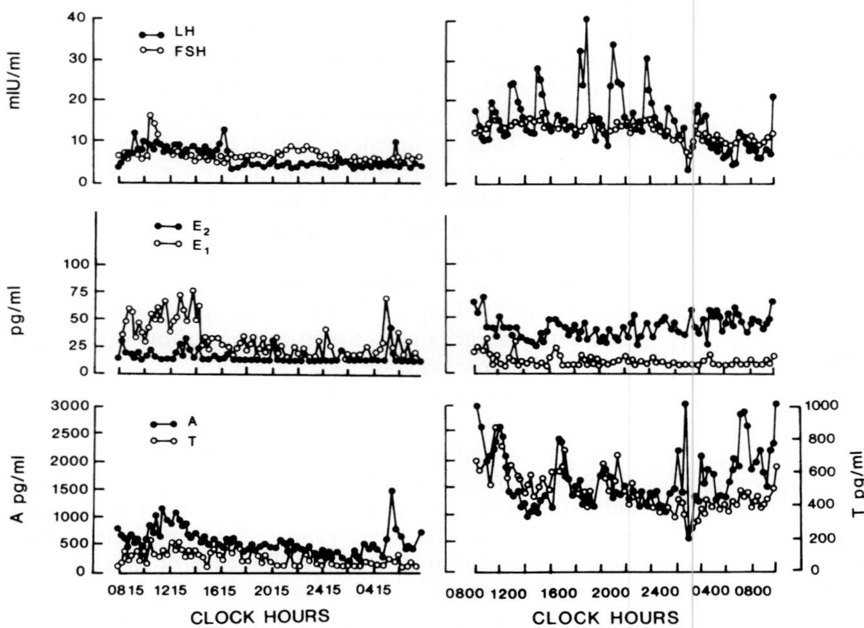

Figure 19–22 ■ Representative patterns of pulsatile LH secretion and corresponding ovarian estrogen and androgen levels determined at 15-minute intervals around the clock in severe *(left)* and mild *(right)* forms of functional hypothalamic amenorrhea.

bodies in the arcuate nucleus are functionally and morphologically linked to hypothalamic galanin and opioid networks, which also play a role in the control of reproduction and eating behavior. Leptin, the hormone of adipocytes, among other nutritional factors, has a direct feedback action on NPY gene expression and thus activates the interconnected NPY-galanin-opioid network. Modification of information flow within this link due to nutritional imbalance may have an adverse impact on reproductive function.[225]

Metabolic Aberrations

Hypoglycemia and Hypoinsulinemia. During the feeding phase of the day, hypothalamic amenorrhea patients exhibit lower glucose and insulin levels than cycling women (see Fig. 19–24). That the severe deficit of fat intake identified in these patients may play a role in determining overall metabolic fuel availability is suggested by the positive relationship between dietary fat intake and circulating insulin levels.[189, 226] Reduced glucose availability, especially to the brain, may represent the metabolic cue transmitting information to the core of the reproductive axis—GnRH neurons. There are, however, several other metabolic alterations (see later) that may act alone or in a synergistic manner to impair the functionality of the reproductive axis.

Hypothyroidemia. Circulating total and free thyronine (T_4) and triiodothyronine (T_3) are significantly reduced without discernible changes in TSH levels[209, 227] (Fig. 19–26). Because thyroid hormones are potent stimulators of peripheral and central cellular metabolism, the reduced thyroid hormone levels together with lower levels of glucose and insulin indicate an overall negative energy balance in patients with hypothalamic amenorrhea syndrome. When the relationship between energy availability (dietary energy intake minus energy expended during exercise) and thyroid hormone metabolism was examined in normal cycling women with controlled exercise and varying amount of energy intake, a *threshold effect* of energy availability was found. Reduction of total T_3 (16 percent) and free T_3 (9 percent) occurred abruptly between 19 and 25 kcal·kg of lean body mass^{-1} · day^{-1}. Thus, energy deficiency suppresses thyroid hormone, resulting in a low T_3 syndrome condition, and may inhibit reproductive function. It was proposed that exercise-associated amenorrhea might be prevented or reversed by increasing energy availability without moderating the exercise regimen.[228] These observations also provided additional evidence that energy deficits, but not high-intensity exercise per se, constitute the underlying disruption of menstrual cyclicity in exercise-associated amenorrhea.

The mechanism to account for reduced thyroid hormones in nutritional deficiency states may be an inhibition of pro-TRH mRNA expression in the hypothalamic paraventricular nucleus where TRH neurons are located. This reduction of pro-TRH gene expression induced by fasting in rats can be prevented by the *administration of leptin*. It was proposed that a fall in circulating leptin levels during fasting or nutritional deficit as in hypothalamic amenorrhea syndrome resets the set-point for feedback inhibition by thyroid hormones on the biosynthesis of hypothalamic pro-TRH, thereby allowing adaptation to starvation or chronic nutritional deficiencies.[229] In patients with hypothyroidism, leptin levels are decreased despite higher body mass index. The low leptin levels in these patients can be normalized by the administration of T_4.[230] Collectively, leptin levels may serve as a marker of nutritional status and thyroid hormone deficiency.

Hypercortisolemia. It is well known that emotional stress and nutritional deficits are associated with activation of the pituitary-adrenal axis and blunting of the circadian rhythm of cortisol secretion.[231, 232] Not unexpectedly, patients with FHA syndrome are found to have hypersecretion of cortisol, with selective increase in the amplitude of secretory episodes during the daytime hours (Fig. 19–27)

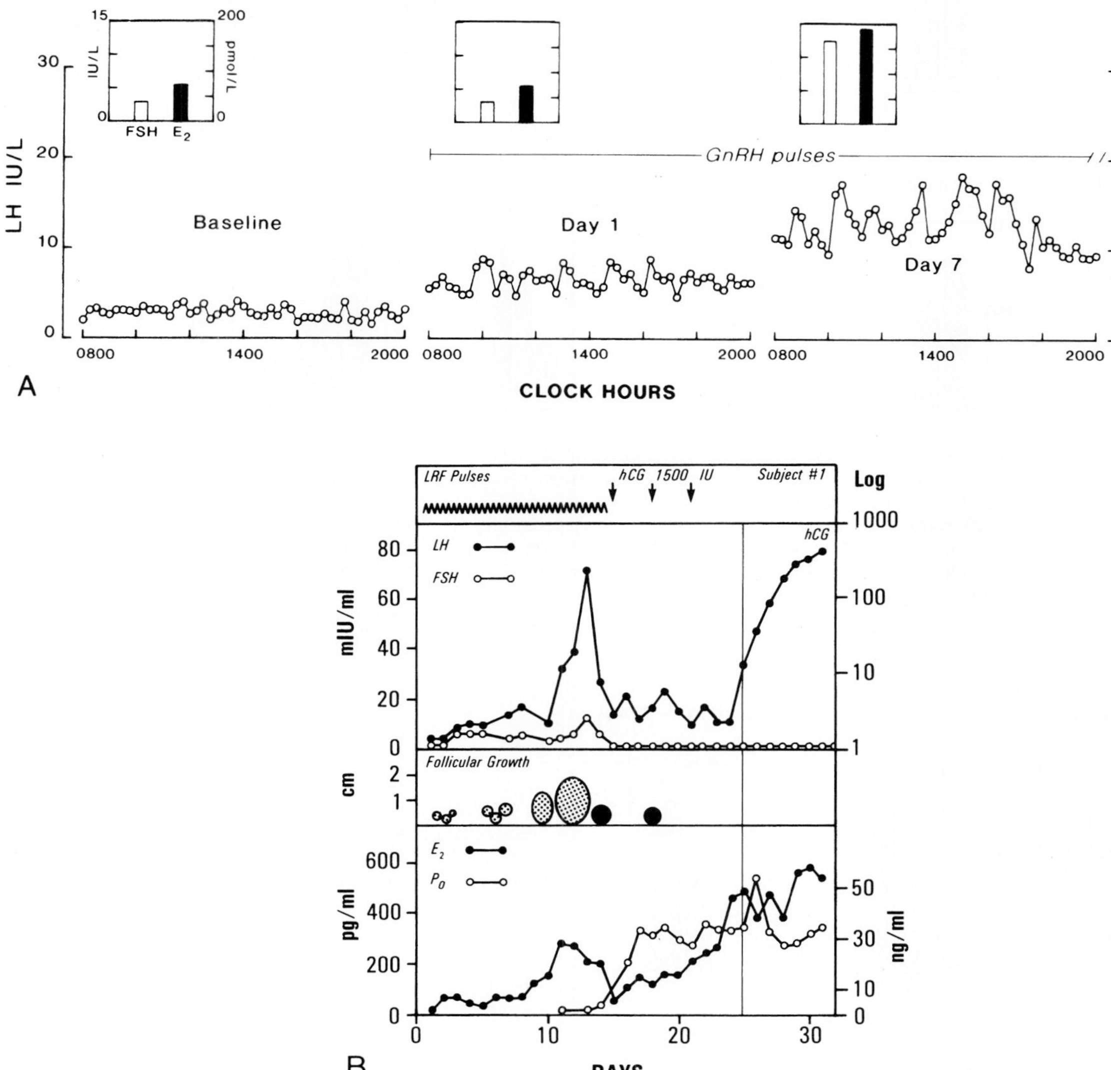

Figure 19–23 ■ *A* and *B*, Activation of cyclic gonadotropin-ovarian function in a patient with apulsatile gonadotropin release by 1-μg-dose pulses of GnRH at 90-minute intervals delivered by an automatic pump. The appearance of progressive increase in LH pulse frequency and amplitude on day 1 and day 7 of treatment is displayed in *A*. FSH and estradiol (E_2) values during the baseline studies and on days 1 and 7 of treatment with GnRH pulses are shown in the insets. The ovulatory events are shown in *B*. After onset of a midcycle surge, the GnRH pump was discontinued and replaced by the administration of human chorionic gonadotropin (hCG) every third day to maintain the corpus luteum function. Ultrasound studies showed follicular development and ovulation, which resulted in pregnancy. Po, progesterone.

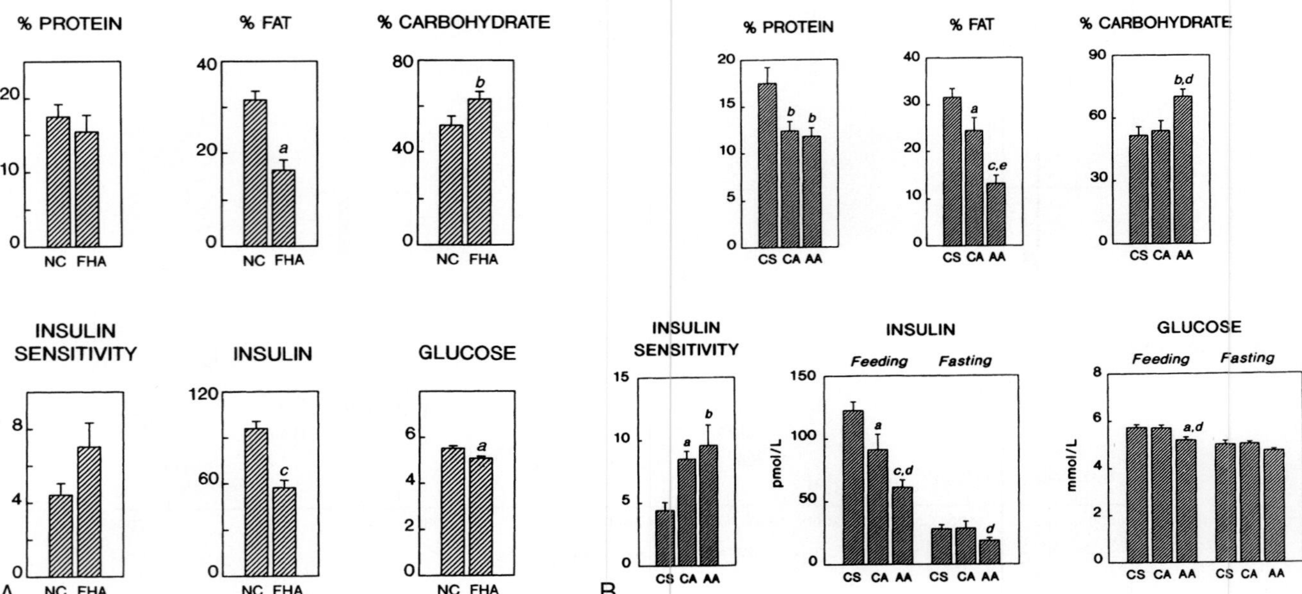

Figure 19–24 ■ *A, Upper panel,* Relative dietary compositions for women with functional hypothalamic amenorrhea (FHA) and normal cycling women (NC). *Lower panel,* Insulin sensitivity and 24-hour mean serum insulin and plasma glucose concentrations for FHA and NC. a, $P < .01$; b, $P < .05$; c, $P < .001$ (versus NC).

B, Upper panel, Relative dietary composition for regularly cycling sedentary women (CS), athletic women with regular menstrual cycles (CA), and athletic women with amenorrhea (AA). *Lower panel,* Insulin sensitivity and mean serum insulin and plasma glucose concentrations during feeding (0800 to 2300 hours) and fasting (2300 to 0800 hours) for CS, CA, and AA. a, $P < .05$; b, $P < .01$; c, $P < .005$ (versus CS) and d, $P < .01$; e, $P < .001$ (versus CA).

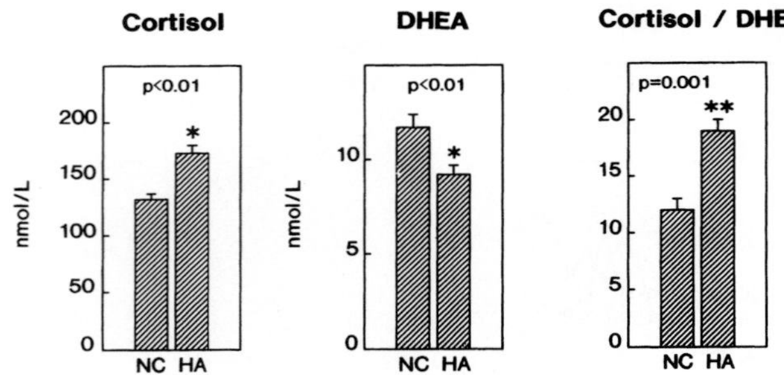

Figure 19–25 ■ The 24-hour mean DHEA and cortisol levels and cortisol to DHEA ratio in women with hypothalamic amenorrhea (HA) syndrome and in normal cycling women (NC).

Figure 19–26 ■ Thyroid hormones are reduced in women with hypothalamic amenorrhea syndrome for both exercise-related and psychogenic types. CS, regularly cycling sedentary women; CA, athletic women with regular menstrual cycles; AA, athletic women with amenorrhea.

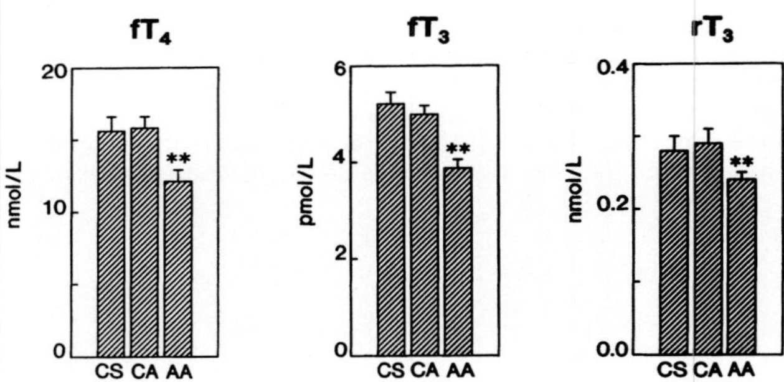

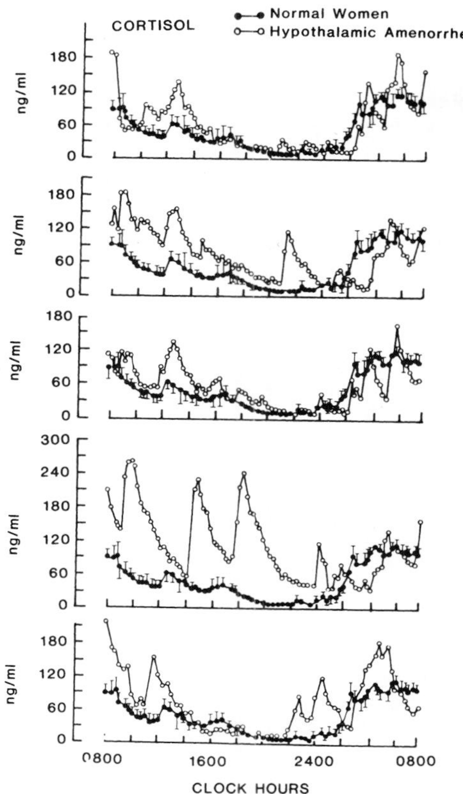

Figure 19–27 ■ Episodic secretory activities of cortisol studied around the clock in five psychogenic amenorrhea patients compared with the mean (± SE) cortisol pattern in eight normal cycling women during early follicular phase. (From Suh BY, Liu JH, Berga SL, et al. Hypercortisolism in patients with functional hypothalamic-amenorrhea. J Clin Endocrinol Metab 66:733–739, 1988. © The Endocrine Society.)

in psychogenic/nutritional amenorrhea and extending to the nighttime in women with exercise-associated amenorrhea.[188, 203, 233] The 24-hour mean cortisol level is increased without alteration of the circadian rhythm of cortisol. The ACTH and cortisol responses to CRF stimulation are blunted, reflecting the appropriate negative feedback effects of hypercortisolism (Fig. 19–28). These findings suggest an increased CRF drive centrally in this syndrome.[203, 230, 231, 233, 234] That CRF can inhibit the GnRH-gonadotropin axis has been demonstrated in a variety of in vivo and in vitro experiments in both rodents and primates. This effect of CRF appears to be mediated by endogenous opioids and can be reversed by naloxone administration[169–174, 235] (Fig. 19–29). This activation of the CRF-adrenal system and its inhibition of the reproductive axis may represent a compensatory mechanism in response to metabolic fuel deficiency.

Hypoprolactinemia. The 24-hour serum prolactin levels in patients with FHA syndrome at all time points are lower than in normally cycling women during the early follicular phase. The 24-hour integrated prolactin value is reduced by 39 percent. However, the sleep-associated increments are greater in patients with the syndrome.[213] The neuroendocrine mechanism accounting for the decreased prolactin secretion is not clear, but the link of a reduced hypothalamic TRH, as described in the hypothyroidemia section, may be considered. The role of a potentially increased dopaminergic activity or of decreased estrogen level has not been established.

GH–IGF-I Axis. Evidence of metabolic adaptation in patients with FHA syndrome extends to the somatotropic axis as well. The reader is referred to Chapters 2 and 17 for detailed orientation to this complex axis. Whereas 24-hour mean GH levels for FHA are in the normal range, the pattern of GH pulsatility is distinctly altered with blunted pulse amplitude, accelerated pulse frequency, and elevated interpulse GH levels throughout the sleep-wake cycle[188, 189] (Fig. 19–30). Increased GH pulse frequency and higher interpulse levels have also been described in states of nutritional deprivation.[236, 237]

Insulin-like growth factor–binding protein 1 (IGFBP-1) levels are elevated, consistent with the well-known negative regulation of hepatic production of IGFBP-1 by insulin[238, 239] and the presence of hypoinsulinemia in FHA. Glucocorticoids have also been shown to increase IGFBP-1 hepatic production and gene expression in conditions with low insulin levels.[239, 240] Regression analysis indicated that the presence of hypercortisolemia in FHA contributed positively to the elevation of IGFBP-1 levels, independent of the negative influence of insulin. Thus, the combined effects of hypoinsulinemia (disinhibition) and hypercortisolemia (stimulation) account for the augmentation of IGFBP-1 in FHA. Although serum levels of IGF-I and IGFBP-3 are not reduced in FHA, as would be expected in an energy-deficient state,[241] the elevation of IGFBP-1 levels resulted in a lower IGF-I to IGFBP-1 ratio for FHA than for cycling control subjects. IGFBP-1 is a potent inhibitor

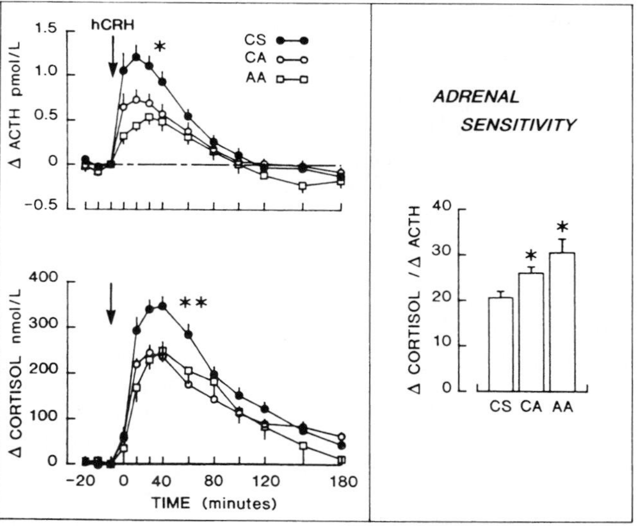

Figure 19–28 ■ ACTH, cortisol, TSH, and thyroid hormones in patients with hypothalamic amenorrhea. *Left,* Mean (± SE) plasma ACTH and serum cortisol responses (Δ, changes from baseline) to administration of 1 μg/kg corticotropin-releasing hormone (hCRH) at time zero in sedentary control subjects (CS), cycling athletes (CA), and amenorrheic athletes (AA). *Right,* Δ Cortisol/Δ ACTH ratios after hCRH administration reflecting adrenal sensitivity. (From Loucks AB, Mortola JF, Girton L, Yen SCC. Alterations in the hypothalamic-pituitary-ovarian and the hypothalamic-pituitary-adrenal axes in athletic women. J Clin Endocrinol Metab 68:402–411, 1989. © The Endocrine Society.)

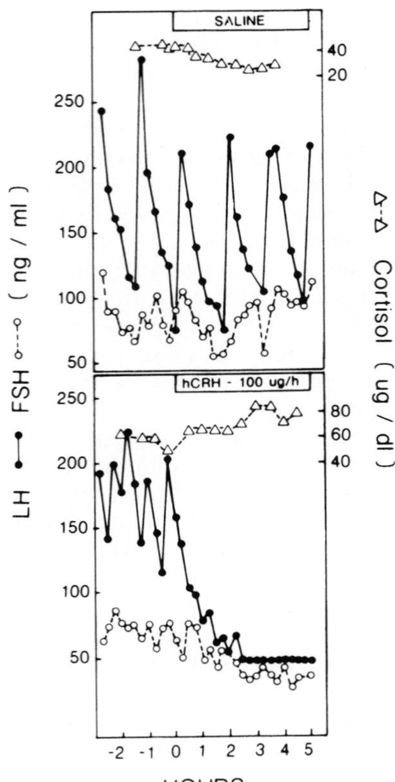

Figure 19–29 ■ Serum LH, FSH, and cortisol concentrations in an ovariectomized monkey for 3 hours before and during a 5-hour infusion of saline *(top)* or corticotropin-releasing factor (hCRF) 100 µg/hr *(bottom)*. (From Olster DH, Ferin M. Corticotropin-releasing hormone inhibits gonadotropin secretion in the ovariectomized rhesus monkey. J Clin Endocrinol Metab 65:262–267, 1987. © The Endocrine Society.)

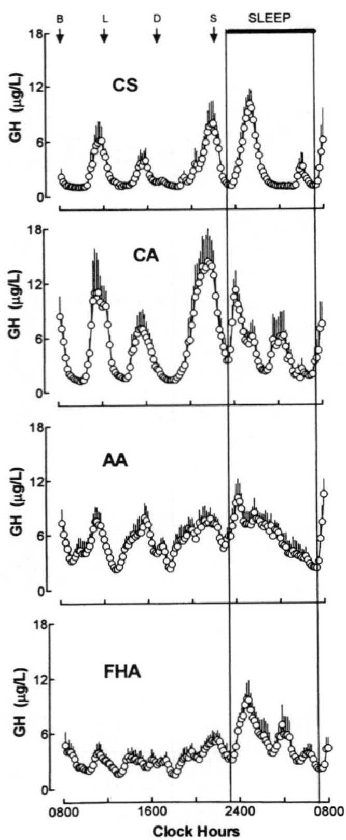

Figure 19–30 ■ Pattern of GH secretory episodes in women with hypothalamic amenorrhea syndrome. CS, sedentary control; CA, cycling athletes; AA, amenorrheic athletes; FHA, psychogenic amenorrhea.

of the insulin-like activity of IGF-I[242]; thus, the reduction in the ratio of IGF-I to IGFBP-1 in FHA may act as an energy-conserving strategy by minimizing the hypoglycemic action of IGF-I. Growth hormone–binding protein (GHBP) concentrations, a reflection of the extracellular domain of hepatic GH receptors,[243] were reduced 40 percent in FHA, consistent with relative resistances of GH action as seen in severe hypometabolic states such as anorexia nervosa[237, 244] and fasting.[243] In sum, the GH–IGF-I axis appears to be altered for both psychogenic and exercise-associated FHA syndrome. The mechanism to account for these alterations is unclear. Alterations of the hypothalamic regulator in response to amplified peripheral nutritional deficiency need to be elucidated.

Amplification of Nocturnal Melatonin Secretion. Nocturnal melatonin secretion in women with FHA syndrome is remarkably amplified.[245, 246] Although daytime melatonin concentrations are similar, the integrated nocturnal melatonin secretion is more than twofold greater in these patients compared with season- and age-matched cycling women. This increase in melatonin is reflected by elevated peak amplitude and extended duration (delayed offset time) and is virtually identical for psychogenic and exercise-associated FHA[246] (Fig. 19–31). The underlying mechanism of the amplified nocturnal melatonin secretion in women with this syndrome is unclear. It is not related to body weight or to seasonal differences, as both patients and control subjects are exposed to the same light-dark environment. Low estrogen levels in these patients have been implicated, because estrogen administration reduced the nocturnal melatonin levels in FHA patients.[247] It remains to be elucidated whether the CRF-mediated activation of catecholaminergic neurons in the brain stem[247] may enhance biosynthesis of melatonin through β-receptors in

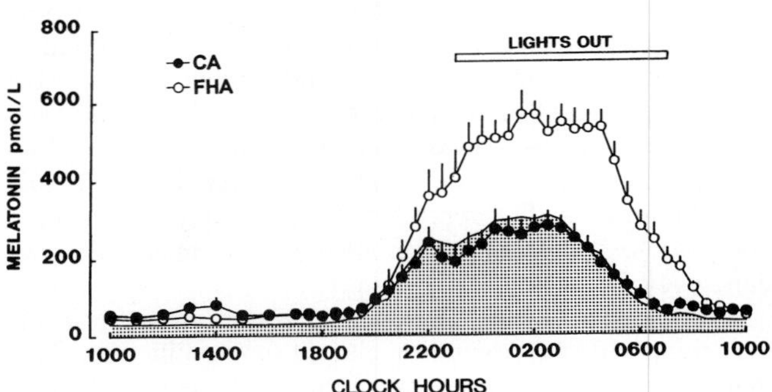

Figure 19–31 ■ Amplification of 24-hour melatonin secretion in women with hypothalamic amenorrhea syndrome (FHA). Cycling athletes (CA) and amenorrheic athletes (AA) with comparable degree of exercise training, psychometric tests, body composition, and dietary consumption. The data (mean ± SE) are plotted against the values of regularly cyclic sedentary women *(shaded area)*.

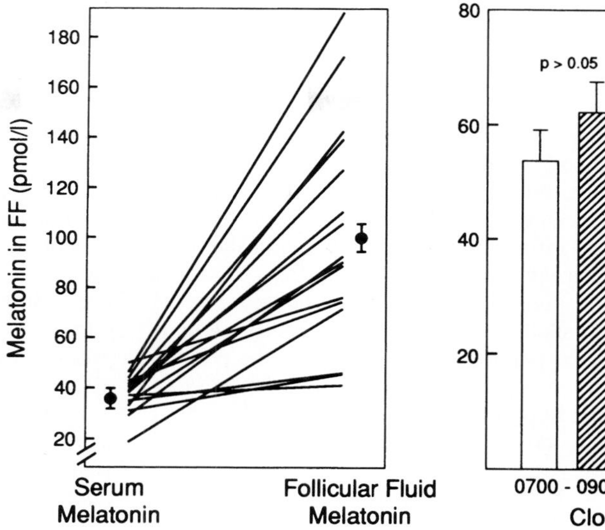

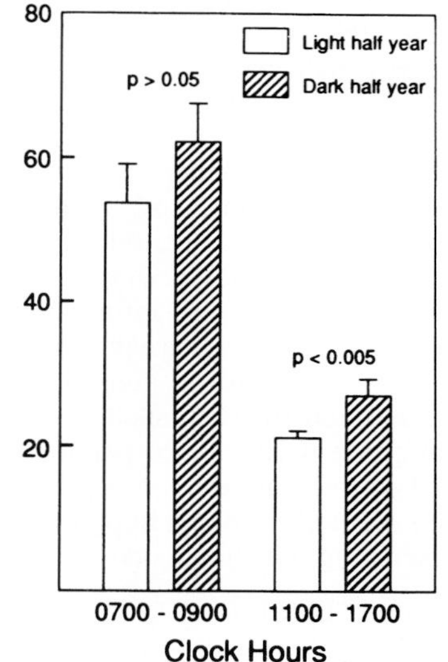

Figure 19–32 ■ Follicular fluid melatonin levels. *Left,* Individual melatonin concentrations in serum and follicular fluid samples taken during laparotomy during a spontaneous cycle in 16 endocrinologically healthy women. The largest (dominant) follicle was chosen for melatonin determination. *Right,* Mean (± SE) follicular fluid melatonin concentrations in the morning (0700 to 0900 hours) and in the daytime (1100 to 1700 hours) during the light and dark seasons of the year. (Redrawn from Rönnberg L, Kauppila A, Leppaluoto J, et al. Circadian and seasonal variation in human preovulatory follicular fluid melatonin concentration. J Clin Endocrinol Metab 71:492–496, 1990. © The Endocrine Society.)

the pineal gland (see Chapter 2 for details). Limited evidence suggests that hypermelatonemia may have a causal role in hypogonadism[248] and may have a direct inhibitory effect on granulosa cell function (Fig. 19–32).

Leptin Levels and Diurnal Rhythm. Leptin levels for FHA of a psychogenic basis and for cycling control subjects exhibit similar diurnal patterns, with lowest levels at 0900 hours after nocturnal fasting, rising gradually to maximal levels at 0100 hours, followed by a rapid fall and return to early morning levels by 0900 hours (Fig. 19–33). The relative excursion of leptin levels from morning nadir to nocturnal peak in FHA (42 ± 19 percent) did not differ from that in cycling control subjects (54 ± 7 percent).[189] The 24-hour mean leptin levels for FHA (7.0 ± 1.5 ng/ml) are lower than those for cycling control subjects (10.1 ± 1.3 ng/ml) and were highly correlated with percentage body fat ($r = .88$; $P < .0001$). The difference in leptin levels can be fully accounted for by the lower percentage body fat in FHA.

In contrast, leptin levels in FHA in association with exercise and low body fat stores are markedly reduced. Moreover, the diurnal rhythm of leptin is no longer discernible in FHA but remains intact in athletes with menstrual cycles.[249] Percentage body fat cannot fully account for the low leptin levels in both groups as well as the absence of diurnal rhythm in the amenorrheic group. Whereas estrogen has been shown to enhance leptin secretion,[250] the reduction of estrogen levels in both groups of FHA were similar and thus unrelated to the absence of a diurnal rhythm in the amenorrheic exercise group. There was a positive association between leptin levels and hypoinsulinemia and hypercortisolemia, a finding consistent with metabolic adaptations to chronic energy deficits and leptin regulation (see Chapter 17 for details). A growing body of evidence sup-

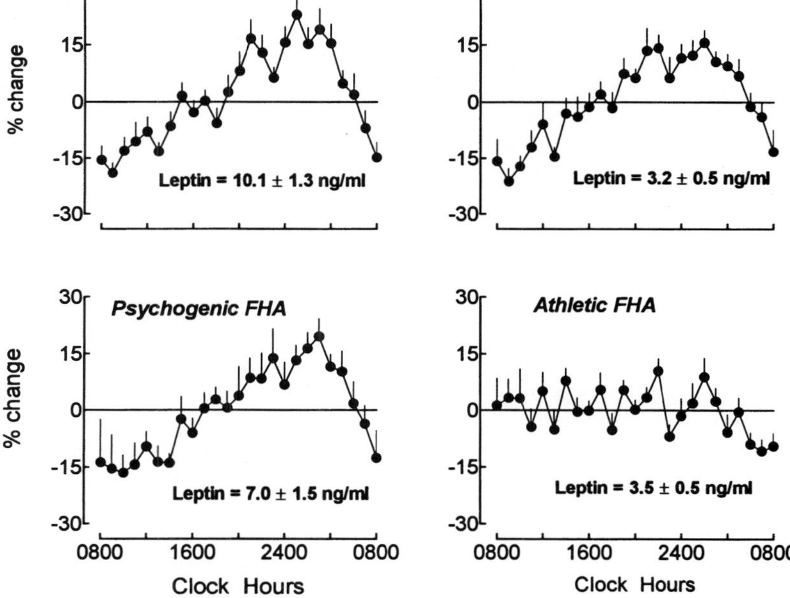

Figure 19–33 ■ Diurnal pattern of leptin levels in normal women and women with functional hypothalamic amenorrhea (FHA). In athletic FHA, diurnal rhythm is uniquely absent (note the 24-hour mean ± SE value in each panel).

ports the contention that leptin is regulated acutely by energy balance independent of body fat stores.[251] Thus, factors other than fat stores influence the interaction of energy status and leptin regulation. Indeed, tumor necrosis factor-α, a cytokine, has been associated with increased energy expenditure and weight loss in humans.[252–254] There may also exist a neural substrate of the interconnected network with NPY pathway as a primary target for receiving and transducing information necessary for sustaining reproductive function and nutritional homeostasis.[225] Consideration should be given to several other *neuropeptides* in addition to NPY, such as CRF and the recently cloned urocortin (CRF-related peptide; see Chapter 2). The potential interaction between peptides, cytokines, and leptin systems could provide important insights into mechanisms regulating nutritional status and reproductive integrity.

MANAGEMENT

The multiple hormonal aberrations and their various forms of expression of nutritional deficiency as a consequence of psychogenic aberration and exercise-associated FHA and occult eating disorders represent a continuum of neuroendocrine adaptations with a time course construct that resembles the U-shaped curve described for the onset of puberty.

Psychogenic FHA Syndrome. Successful management requires establishing rapport between physician and patient. A careful and detailed history concerning parental, sexual,[255] social, environmental, and interpersonal relationships and the availability of support during childhood and adolescence is essential. Dietary evaluation is imperative. When a deficit state is disclosed, guidance by a nutritionist is required. After careful exclusion of organic disease, reassurance and appropriate, timely, and positive reinforcement are effective modes of management. When spontaneous recovery does not ensue within 6 to 8 months after nutritional and psychologic guidance, additional measures may be required, such as estrogen-progestin replacement and clomiphene induction of ovulation if pregnancy is desired. When clomiphene fails, induction of ovulation by pulsatile administration of GnRH is associated with a high degree of success.

Exercise-Associated FHA Syndrome. The rapid increase in popularity of physical exercise during the past decade has led to the recognition of deleterious effects of strenuous exercise on reproductive function.[190] The cause-effect relationship has recently been identified, with nutritional deficit a major factor but not exercise per se.[222]

The approaches to counseling and management of patients with exercise-associated amenorrhea and infertility must take into account the fact that many women include regular exercise as an important part of their lifestyle. Appropriate care in these patients should include providing up-to-date information on the beneficial as well as deleterious effects of strenuous exercise on the reproductive and skeletal systems and on lipoproteins.

Physiologic responses to exercise mainly involve the activation of cellular and compartmental fuel mobilization, redistribution, and utilization. This is accomplished by a multitude of changes in neuroendocrine signals from the brain. Although the mechanisms of these complex activational processes are unclear, the integrity of neuroendocrine-metabolic homeostasis is influenced by the mode, frequency, duration, and intensity of exercise regimens. Perhaps even more important are the quantity and quality of food intake, which determine body composition. Thus, an understanding of *balanced inputs and expenditures is of fundamental importance*.

Guidance and information exchange with the patients may result in moderation of exercise and establishment of optimal nutritional needs. The fact that exercise-associated amenorrhea is reversible adds further incentive for the patient to make rational decisions with respect to major problems of amenorrhea and infertility as well as osteoporosis. Supplementation with estrogen-progestin, multivitamins, and calcium is an important consideration, but the primary aim in management is to provide guidance in terms of exercise moderation and fuel economy.

Bone. Patients with FHA syndrome are at risk for premature bone loss and, if the amenorrhea occurs during the years critical for bone accretion, inadequate bone formation.[256–258] In amenorrheic athletes, bone density is reduced at multiple skeletal sites, including those subjected to impact loading during exercise,[259, 260] and is associated with a higher incidence of fracture.[261, 262] Bone loss in FHA patients is rapid and may not be completely reversible by resumption of menses or estrogen replacement therapy,[263, 264] despite recent reports of improvements of 3 to 8 percent in bone mineral density with hormone replacement therapy.[258, 265] Osteoporosis is most severe in women whose amenorrhea began in adolescence and in those with the longest duration of amenorrhea[257, 266]; thus, early intervention is critical to minimize demineralization.

Anorexia Nervosa

Anorexia nervosa, an extraordinary psychoneuroendocrinologic disorder, was recognized more than two centuries ago. During recent decades, the incidence of eating disorders, particularly anorexia nervosa and bulimia nervosa, has increased at least fivefold in Western society. The prevalence of anorexia nervosa in girls of school age has been estimated in three studies: (1) about 1 in 150 adolescent girls in Sweden,[267] (2) approximately 1 in 200 girls in private schools and 1 in 550 girls in state schools in England,[268] and (3) a similar incidence but an increase in the number of cases to 1 in 90 English schoolgirls aged 16 years or older.[269]

CLINICAL FEATURES

The salient clinical features of anorexia nervosa are

1. a marked predominance in adolescent girls, with only rare cases in prepubertal boys;
2. relentless dieting in an obsessive pursuit of thinness, often leading to marked emaciation (Fig. 19–34), cold intolerance, and occasionally death;
3. a morbid fear of losing control over dietary intake and body weight, marked by episodes of overeating (bulimia) and self-induced vomiting;
4. a desire to maintain or to regress to the prepubertal body habitus in an effort to delay or disguise femininity;
5. amenorrhea, an essential feature, which may occur before, concurrent with, or after significant weight loss;
6. a hyperactive, intense, commonly obsessive-compulsive personality, often leading to overachievement;

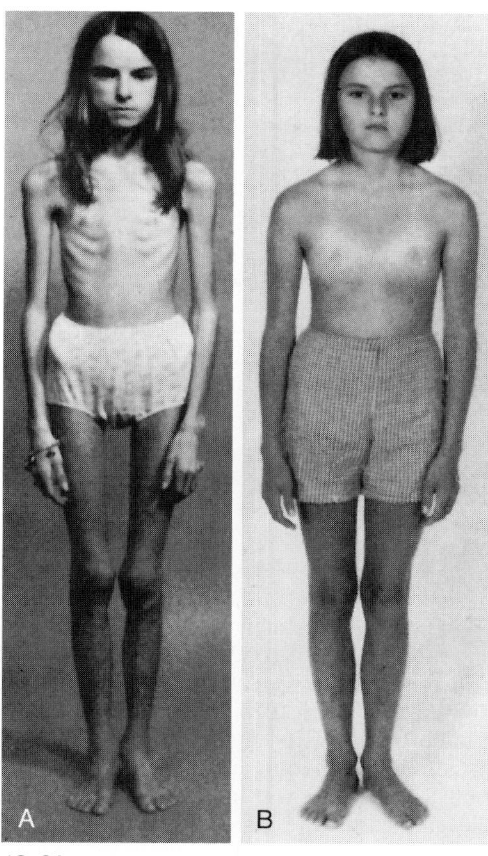

Figure 19–34 ■ A 12-year-old girl with severe anorexia nervosa and marked generalized wasting before *(A)* and after *(B)* recovery following 6 months of psychotherapy. (Courtesy of Dr. Dorothy Hollingsworth, UCSD, La Jolla, CA.)

7. a lack of self-perception and lack of ability to discriminate appropriately between fatness and thinness;
8. a family environment usually characterized as upper middle class, possibly with a domineering or insensitive parent;
9. a history of sexual molestation or incest and physical or emotional abuse.

Physical symptoms include hypothermia, hypotension, lanugo hair, and amenorrhea. These features serve to distinguish anorexia from "simple weight loss" from dieting and weight loss from illness, such as hypopituitarism. Thus, patients with anorexia nervosa are typically compulsive and introverted, with an inner psychosexual conflict and poor adaptation.

PATHOPHYSIOLOGY

To delineate the underlying pathophysiologic mechanism of this syndrome, a separation of the eating behaviors into *restrictor* and *bulimic* subtypes may provide clinically relevant information. "Restrictors" are characterized by their following of a virtually unremitting pattern of dietary deprivation; "bulimics" are characterized by periodic eating binges. It is estimated that 50 percent of patients with primary anorexia nervosa exhibit bulimic behavior, and their disorder tends to have a later onset with more discernible symptoms of anxiety, guilt, and depression.[270, 271] The development of bulimia in anorectic patients may indicate that inheritable and socioenvironmental factors are operating to sustain body weight as a counterregulatory mechanism to combat starvation.

In the assessment of this complex syndrome, three broad interrelated aspects should be considered: (1) malnutrition, (2) neuroendocrine-metabolic aberrations, and (3) psychogenic factors.

Malnutrition. There are no unique features because they occur in other semistarvation conditions. Some of the notable changes are: (1) anemia and occasional pancytopenia appear to be due to hypoplasia of bone marrow; (2) hypokalemia may occur secondary to vomiting and/or laxative use; (3) hypoalbuminemia, hypercholesterolemia (mainly LDL fraction of cholesterol and elevated plasma β-carotene levels; (4) depressed immune cell functions, and (5) interestingly, plasma protein levels are normal.

Neuroendocrine-Metabolic Aberrations. Although the pathogenesis of anorexia nervosa remains unclear, several specific hypothalamic regulatory abnormalities have been described.

Hypothalamic-Pituitary-Ovarian Axis (Central Inhibition of GnRH Secretion). Amenorrhea, a constant feature of anorexia nervosa, is due to marked reduction of gonadotropin secretion to a level comparable with that seen in prepubertal girls. The underlying cause of this hypogonadotropic state is the reduced frequency and amplitude of LH pulsatile release occasioned by the arrest of hypothalamic GnRH pulsatile activity. Pituitary release of LH and FSH in response to exogenous GnRH stimulation varies from complete impairment, to a normal response with delayed peak, to an exaggerated response.[272–275] These discrepant findings may be explained by varying degrees of functional impairment of GnRH secretion, which determines the priming effect and the secretory response to exogenous GnRH.[276] Additional factors, such as the degree of weight loss, the stage of disease, remission, and subtypes of the syndrome, may be important in contributing to the variability of GnRH-mediated gonadotropin secretory states. Melatonin levels and diurnal rhythm are *not* abnormal if patients with depression are excluded. Suppression of gonadotropin secretion is not mediated by melatonin.[277]

Nutritional rehabilitation is accompanied by both increased basal and GnRH-stimulated gonadotropin release,[278] and the resumption of menstrual cyclicity is predicted by the increase in GnRH-induced LH secretion.[279] Restoration of ovulatory cycles is also preceded by the reestablishment of the inhibitory effect of opioids on LH secretion, an effect that is absent in anorexia nervosa patients during the weight loss phase of the disease.[280, 281] The lack of LH response to opioid receptor blockade together with occurrence of sleep-entrained pulsatile LH patterns (Fig. 19–35), the GnRH-gonadotropin axis in patients with anorexia nervosa, represents the *regression* of neuroendocrine control mechanisms to the prepubertal state. The cessation of reproductive function in this syndrome may be viewed as a protective strategy in the face of severe nutritional and psychobiologic deficits.

Altered Sex Steroid Metabolism. In anorexia nervosa, estradiol secretion by the resting ovary is low, but circulating testosterone levels remain in the normal female range. However, the metabolism of both estradiol and testosterone is abnormal. A shift of estradiol metabolism from 16α-hydroxylation to 2-hydroxylation occurs; consequently, the

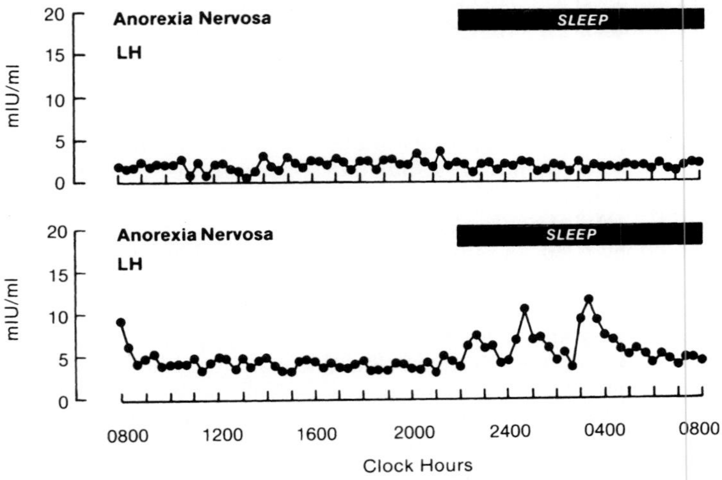

Figure 19–35 ■ Representative pattern of pulsatile LH secretion around the clock in two patients with anorexia nervosa. Complete cessation and the absence of sleep-associated activation of GnRH pulses in one patient *(top)* are contrasted to the presence of the sleep-entrained amplification of LH pulses in another patient *(bottom)*.

formation of estriol is decreased, and catecholestrogen (2-hydroxyestrone) is disproportionately increased.[282] Catecholestrogens are endogenous antiestrogens because they are capable of binding to estrogen receptors without eliciting biologic action. Therefore, this altered metabolic pathway is directed to further estrogen deficiency. These changes in estradiol metabolism are not specific for anorexia nervosa but are related to changes in body weight or composition or nutrition.[283] Nonetheless, the hypoestrogenic state in anorexia nervosa predisposes the patient to osteoporosis. The degree of osteopenia is positively correlated with the duration of amenorrhea and significantly reduced by physical exercise.[284]

In normal women, the metabolism of testosterone is a reductive process, involving 5α-reduction to form androsterone and etiocholanolone. In anorexia nervosa patients, the urinary androsterone to etiocholanolone ratio is decreased, reflecting a *decreased 5α-reductase activity.* The development of lanugo hair may be causally related to the diminished androgenic action on the hair follicle, because the 5α-reductase–dependent formation of dihydrotestosterone from testosterone is essential for androgenic action on the hair follicle. This abnormality is also found in the hypothyroid state. A reversal of the androsterone to etiocholanolone ratio to normal occurs after T_3 treatment in both conditions, and thus the altered testosterone metabolism appears to be secondary to the associated hypothyroid state in this syndrome.[285]

Hypothalamic-Pituitary-Adrenal Axis. In patients with anorexia nervosa, plasma cortisol levels are elevated throughout the 24-hour biologic clock. The circadian pattern, however, is maintained. These findings, first reported by Boyar and colleagues,[286] have been confirmed and expanded. The abnormalities of the ACTH-adrenal axis include the following:

1. The mean 24-hour plasma cortisol levels are significantly elevated during relapse compared with patients in the recovery phase and age-matched control subjects[287] (Fig. 19–36).
2. In the face of a prolonged plasma half-life of cortisol and normal levels of corticosteroid-binding globulin, the daily cortisol production rate is significantly increased in anorexia nervosa patients compared with that of matched control subjects in terms of both body mass and body surface area (24 versus 18 mg/day). Urinary "free" cortisol concentrations are more than three times greater in patients with anorexia nervosa than in normal women (225 versus 65 μg/day).[288] Thus, the elevation of plasma cortisol levels in this syndrome reflects not only a slowing of cortisol metabolism but also a rise in adrenocortical secretion.
3. The elevated cortisol levels exhibit either incomplete suppression or an early escape from suppression by dexamethasone (1.5 mg, single dose), a finding resembling that seen in patients with depression and Cushing's disease.[289]
4. Plasma ACTH levels are within normal range, but ACTH response to CRF is attenuated, the degree of which is negatively correlated with basal cortisol levels.[290, 291] The negative feedback of cortisol at the level of the corticotroph appears to be intact in patients with anorexia nervosa. These findings further implicate a central mechanism in the genesis of hyperactivity of the hypothalamic-pituitary-adrenal axis.[292]

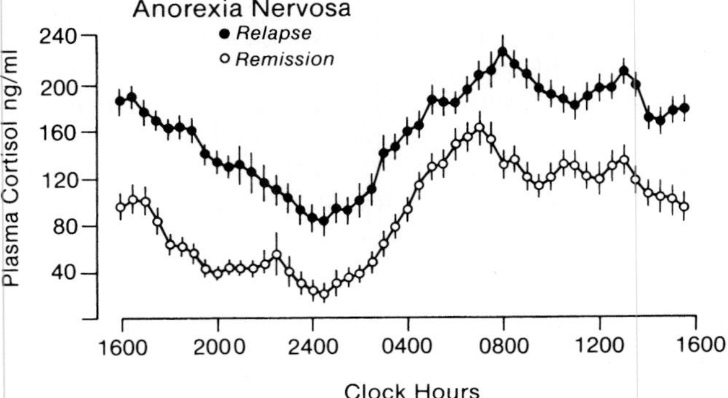

Figure 19–36 ■ The mean (± SE) 24-hour cortisol concentrations during relapse (N = 18) and after recovery (N = 15) in patients with anorexia nervosa. (Redrawn from Doerr P, Fichter M, Pirke KM, Lund R. Relationship between weight gain and hypothalamic pituitary adrenal function in patients with anorexia nervosa. J Steroid Biochem 13:529–537, 1980. Reproduced with permission by Pergamon Press.)

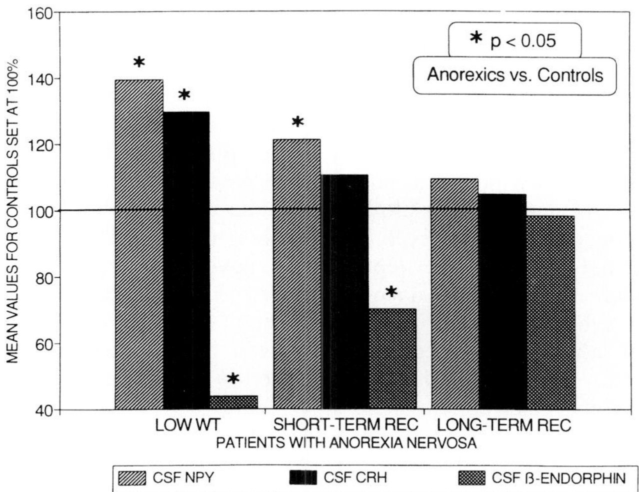

Figure 19–37 ■ CSF concentrations of NPY, CRH, and β-endorphin in patients with anorexia nervosa at 3 stages of treatment. Values of each neuropeptide are expressed as a percent of the values found in matched healthy volunteer women, which are set at 100% for each neuropeptide. *Indicates a significant difference ($p<0.05$) between anorexics and controls. (Reproduced with permission from Kaye WH, Neuropeptide abnormalities in anorexia nervosa. Psychiatry Res 62:65, 1996.)

5. Levels of CRF measured in the CSF are elevated in underweight anorectics but not in weight-restored anorectics independent of depression[291, 293] (Fig. 19–37). Collectively, the appropriate negative feedback effect of hypercortisolemia is consistent with hypersecretion of CRF underlying hypothalamic-pituitary-adrenal activation.
6. The demonstration that cellular glucocorticoid receptors are reduced in many patients with anorexia nervosa[294] may explain the absence of clinical signs of cortisol excess.
7. In contrast to cortisol hypersecretion, levels of adrenal androgens, particularly DHEA, are decreased with a markedly reduced ratio of DHEA to cortisol[295] (Fig. 19–38). Thus, a shift of adrenal steroidogenesis (relative deficiency of 17,20-desmolase) resembling that seen in prepubertal children occurs, representing another hormonal parameter of ontogenic regression in anorexia nervosa patients. The recovery of adrenal androgen secretion during remission is positively correlated with the concomitant rise of IGF-I levels as seen during adrenarche.[296, 297] That IGF-I plays a role in regulating adrenal androgenesis is shown by increases in P450c17 mRNA levels and basal and ACTH-induced steroidogenesis in human adrenocortical cells treated with IGF-I in culture.[298]

In summary, the hypothalamic CRF-ACTH-adrenal axis in anorexia nervosa patients appears to be activated with hypersecretion of cortisol but with a suppression of adrenal androgen secretion. The reduced peripheral metabolism of cortisol is probably due to T_3 deficiency, and a reversal to normal can be observed after T_3 administration. The presence of hypercortisolism is likely to be mediated through an increased hypothalamic CRF drive. All abnormalities are readily reversed after weight gain and remission of symptoms.

Hypothalamic-Pituitary-Thyroid Axis (Low T_3 Syndrome). Serum T_4 and T_3 levels in patients with anorexia nervosa are lower than those in normal women; a proportionately greater decrease in T_3 than in T_4 reflects impaired peripheral deiodination of T_4 to T_3 with increased formation of metabolically inactive rT_3.[299, 300] As indicated earlier, the abnormalities of cortisol and testosterone metabolism are due to the low T_3 and can be reversed to normal by T_3 treatment.

The genesis of low T_3 appears to be primarily a consequence of malnutrition. There is evidence that the peripheral formation of T_3 is related to body weight; it is increased by overeating and reduced after weight loss and starvation.[301, 302] The presence of a clinical and biochemical hypothyroid state (low T_3, decreased body temperature, and slow pulse) without hypersecretion of TSH and with a delayed response to TRH stimulation suggests an altered set-point of endogenous TRH regulation as a component of generalized hypothalamic dysfunction.[272] Reversal of low T_3 occurs after weight gain. Teleologically, the presence of severe malnutrition accompanied by a reduction of thyroid hormone action may subserve a "protective hypometabolic" state for survival in the face of the ongoing catabolic events.

Somatotropic Axis. Patients with anorexia nervosa display abnormalities of the somatotropic axis at the hypothalamic, pituitary, and peripheral levels. GH concentrations are generally elevated in adult patients with anorexia nervosa and are unrelated to either body weight loss or the duration of amenorrhea; adolescent patients with a relatively shorter duration of symptoms may have low, normal, or elevated GH levels.[237, 244, 303, 304] Enhanced GH secretion

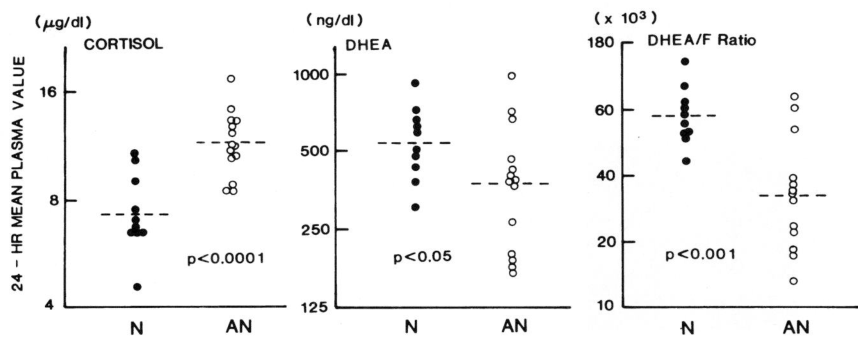

Figure 19–38 ■ The 24-hour mean plasma cortisol and DHEA levels and DHEA to cortisol (F) ratio in young women with anorexia nervosa (AN) and age-matched control subjects (N). (Redrawn from Zumoff B, Walsh BT, Katz JL, et al. Subnormal plasma dehydroisoandrosterone to cortisol ratio in anorexia nervosa: A second hormonal parameter of ontogenic regression. J Clin Endocrinol Metab 56:668–672, 1983. © The Endocrine Society.)

appears to be the result of increased GH pulse frequency superimposed on enhanced tonic secretion.[244, 305] Both high and low GH levels are normalized by weight recuperation.[237, 244] Regardless of age, serum levels of IGF-I, GHBP, and IGFBP-3 are decreased, and IGFBP-1 and IGFBP-2 are increased in anorexia nervosa patients, to a degree relative to the body weight deficit, and return to nearly normal levels after nutritional rehabilitation.[237, 244, 303, 304, 306, 307] Low circulating levels of GHBP reflecting decreased numbers of cellular GH receptors[308, 309] may account for the *GH resistance* of anorexia nervosa. These alterations are similar to those seen with starvation and are consistent with the notion that alteration of the GH–IGF-I axis in anorexia is due to nutritional deprivation, an effect that is reversible with refeeding.

Hypothalamic dysfunction in the control of GH secretion in patients with anorexia nervosa is evident. GH responses to several provocative stimuli are altered, which include defects in response to dexamethasone,[310] insulin-induced hypoglycemia,[311] and α_2-adrenergic stimulation.[312, 313] The blockade of GHRH-stimulated GH secretion by muscarinic cholinergic receptor blockade is also absent,[314, 315] and a paradoxical increase in GH secretion occurs in response to glucose load.[316, 317] GH responses to sequential GHRH stimulations are unaltered,[315] and GH release in response to the synthetic GH secretagogue hexarelin is also maintained. However, desensitization of GHRH stimulation due to prior GH release in response to hexarelin seen in normal subjects is uniquely absent in patients with anorexia nervosa, but not in women with simple weight loss amenorrhea and fasted subjects.[318] Interpretation of this interesting finding requires further understanding of the mechanism of action of the GH secretagogue on GHRH-mediated GH release (see Chapter 2).

Insulin Sensitivity and Insulin/Glucose Dynamics. Consistent with their hypometabolic state, patients with anorexia nervosa have increased insulin sensitivity, reduced glucose effectiveness, and lower fasting plasma glucose and insulin levels.[319, 320] These metabolic alterations as well as impaired glucose tolerance are normalized by weight gain, suggesting that abnormal carbohydrate metabolism is due to underweight and calorie restriction[321] and is not an intrinsic defect of anorexia nervosa. However, higher than normal free fatty acid levels persist in physiologically fully recovered anorexia nervosa patients and may be related to either increased anxiety or enhanced lipolysis.[321]

Leptin. Plasma leptin levels are severely reduced in patients with anorexia nervosa during the active phase of the disease[322–324] to a greater degree than expected on the basis of low body fat alone.[325] The presence of hypercortisolemia and hypoinsulinemia may account for the severe reduction in leptin levels in anorexia nervosa. During nutritional rehabilitation, leptin levels have been reported to increase but remain low,[323] to return to normal before full weight restoration,[252] and to increase to levels beyond those of adiposity-matched control subjects.[325] Only with long-term recovery do leptin levels return to normal.[325] The weight-inappropriate increase in leptin levels in anorexia nervosa patients after treatment may be a response to positive energy balance, an interpretation consistent with experiments showing that leptin secretion is dynamically responsive to changes in energy availability.[251]

Leptin feedback signals through NPY in the arcuate nucleus regulate feeding behavior. CSF levels of NPY are elevated in low-weight anorexia nervosa patients and return to normal only after long-term weight gain[326] (see Fig. 19–37). The lack of increased food intake in the face of low leptin and elevated NPY levels in anorexia nervosa patients is paradoxical according to the current understanding of appetite control by the fat cycle (Fig. 19–39). However, CRF per se has an appetite-inhibitory effect as well as the ability to inhibit NPY-induced feeding[327]; thus, increased CRF drive in anorexia nervosa may antagonize the orexigenic effect of low leptin levels.

Neurotransmitter Abnormalities. Serotonin synthesis, uptake, and turnover as well as postsynaptic receptor sensitivity are reduced in low-weight anorexia nervosa patients, as are CSF serotonin metabolite levels.[328] Postsynaptic adrenergic receptor sensitivity also appears to be reduced as evidenced by reduced responses of GH, β-endorphin, and β-lipoprotein to clonidine, an α_2-adrenergic receptor agonist.[312, 313, 329] Disturbances of serotonin activity seem to persist after long-term weight recovery and may be linked to the pathogenesis of restricted eating and obsessional behaviors in anorexia nervosa patients.[328]

Diabetes Insipidus. Nearly half the patients with an-

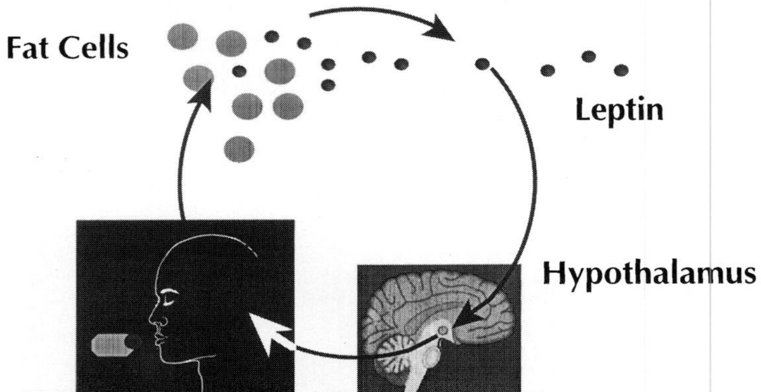

Figure 19–39 ■ The fat cycle: leptin (from the fat cell) feedback to arcuate nucleus of the hypothalamus (where leptin receptor and neuropeptide Y are located) regulates eating behavior appropriate to the leptin signals. In anorexia nervosa, there is an inappropriate feedback relationship between low leptin levels and increased neuropeptide Y levels (see Chapter 17 for details).

orexia nervosa have partial diabetes insipidus. No correlation has been found between the magnitude of response to exogenous vasopressin (ADH) or maximal urinary osmolarities attained after dehydration and the severity of weight loss. These observations suggest primary hypothalamic dysfunction in the regulation of ADH secretion.[330] The demonstration of an erratic or osmotically uncontrolled release of vasopressin or, less commonly, a deficiency of vasopressin secretion adds further support for a central defect.[331]

In addition, the low CSF to plasma vasopressin ratio found in normal subjects is reversed in patients with anorexia nervosa, suggesting an increased central secretion of vasopressin into the CSF compartment.[331] Because vasopressin may influence complex behavior and cognitive function (see Chapter 2), the increased CSF to plasma ratio may be important in the pathophysiology of the syndrome. These abnormalities are not accompanied by electrolyte imbalance, and their reversal is slow after weight gain.

Thermoregulation. Significant abnormalities of thermoregulation in both hot and cold environments have been observed in the majority of patients with anorexia nervosa. Heat intolerance is significantly more severe than cold intolerance, and both are correlated with severity of weight loss.[330] Interestingly, shivering—a hypothalamic function independent of the amount of adipose tissue—typically is absent in these patients.

Psychoneuroendocrine Correlates. Anorexia nervosa is a multidimensional disorder with a wide variety of interacting symptoms and developmental correlates. Although the cause of this eating disorder is unknown, the psychodynamic basis as a major component of this illness is well accepted.[332] The behavioral abnormalities associated with anorexia nervosa include those related to perceptual-cognitive processes and those that involve social standing and position in the family. The role of neuroendocrine aberrations, discussed before, is difficult to assess, because many are integral to anorectic behavior itself and others are secondary to factors such as weight loss and depression. In regard to psychoneuroendocrine correlates of eating disorders, it is both logical and advantageous to view psychogenic obesity and anorexia nervosa as opposing extremes of a single disease with common denominators. The pathogenic processes of eating disorders have been a subject of several critical reviews, and many writers have proposed that both anorexia nervosa and obesity represent *stress syndromes* with failure of psychosocial adaptation to an individual's environment as an important precipitating factor.[333]

MANAGEMENT AND OUTCOME OF ANOREXIA NERVOSA

Although diagnosing anorexia nervosa is relatively easy, managing this often life-threatening illness is difficult, and strikingly diverse approaches have been followed. In severe cases, when 40 percent or more of normal body weight has been lost, immediate force-feeding by parenteral hyperalimentation is required to combat the profound malnutrition and prevent death. The compensatory systemic balance achieved by these severely malnourished patients can be easily upset by too-vigorous refeeding by any route. Complications have resulted from parenteral feeding, including transaminase elevation and electrolyte imbalance, with occasional death. Most patients seek medical attention before the advanced phase of the disease, and such patients frequently respond to treatment. Patients occasionally have spontaneous recovery without medical attention. Therapeutic interventions have included psychoanalysis, psychotherapy, family therapy, force-feeding, behavioral modification, and a combination of these approaches. It is remarkable that regardless of the method of treatment employed, most patients improve, with a weight gain of between 1 and 2 kg/week. Recovery of weight to about 90 percent of standard body weight resulted in a return of menses in 86 percent of 100 adolescent anorexia nervosa patients.[334] However, some patients fare poorly after having received a variety of therapies.

Behavioral modification through positive reinforcement has provided preliminary encouraging results. There is no evidence to suggest that it is superior to other conventional therapies. Furthermore, not all patients with anorexia nervosa require or benefit from behavioral modification.[335]

The use of neuropharmacologic and antidepressant agents with the aim of correcting the assumed involvement of serotoninergic systems in anorexia nervosa has shown little benefit in the acute phase of the disease. However, several open trials of fluoxetine suggest that this drug is effective in preventing relapse in weight-recovered anorexia nervosa patients.[336, 337] Cyproheptadine, a drug with serotoninergic properties, was more efficacious for restrictor anorexics than for bulimics.[328]

The outcome is still controversial. However, one analysis of a consecutive series of 100 female patients with anorexia nervosa observed for at least 4 years has yielded important information.[338] Of the 100 patients, the outcome was good in almost half (48 percent), as judged by nearly normal weight, return of regular menstrual cycles, and satisfactory mental state, including psychosexual and psychosocial adjustments. The outcome was intermediate in 30 percent and poor in 20 percent of patients, with two deaths reported (2 percent). Furthermore, poor outcome is positively associated with factors such as longer duration of illness, the presence of bulimia and vomiting, poor childhood social adjustment, and poor child-parent relationships.

Finally, reductions in bone mineral density, particularly during adolescence when bone accretion should be occurring, represent a critical problem in the management of anorexia nervosa patients. Weight rehabilitation and resumption of menses result in increased bone mineral density[339, 340]; however, osteopenia persists, indicating that the loss of bone mineral during adolescence may not be completely reversible.[340] Hormone replacement therapy is effective for some but not all patients.[258, 339, 341] A report of increases in markers of bone formation in anorexia nervosa patients with osteopenia after short-term treatment with recombinant IGF-I deserves additional study with the hope for an alternative management.[322]

Bulimia Nervosa

Normal-weight bulimia or bulimia nervosa is at least 10 times more prevalent than anorexia nervosa.[328] The eating disorder bulimia nervosa is characterized by binge eating, self-induced vomiting, and intermittent episodes of calorie restriction, but these patients do not lose weight to the point of emaciation. Normal-weight bulimics have multiple neuroendocrine disturbances in a milder form than anorexia nervosa: reduced LH levels[342, 343] due primarily to a slowing of pulse frequency,[343] blunted TSH responses to TRH,[342] low T_3 levels,[344] hypercortisolemia[292, 343] hypoprolactinemia,[342] hypoinsulinemia,[343, 345] and impaired glucose tolerance.[346] Women with bulimia nervosa have disturbances of serotoninergic activity, which may be related to the psychopathology of this disorder.[347] However, the degree of neuroendocrine and, consequently, menstrual dysfunction seems to be related to the intensity of the weight control behavior rather than to depressive symptoms.[342]

Premenstrual Dysphoria

Clinical Features

The premenstrual syndrome (PMS) is a collection of affective, behavioral, and somatic disorders that occurs in a cyclic pattern during the second half of the menstrual cycle. The clinical features are diverse, with prompt resolution at or soon after the onset of menstrual flow. A symptom-free period during the follicular phase of the cycle is a prerequisite for the diagnosis of PMS.[348] In its more severe form, PMS is referred to as premenstrual dysphoric disorder in the *Diagnostic and Statistical Manual of Mental Disorders* (DSM-IV-R) of the American Psychiatric Association.[349]

The symptoms, which usually occur 7 to 10 days before the onset of menses, include breast tenderness, abdominal bloating, edema of the lower extremities, fatigue, mood swings, and depression. Many patients also complain of headache, increased thirst or appetite, and craving for carbohydrates and salty foods. These symptoms increase progressively in some women and suddenly in others. The patient may become increasingly anxious, restless, irritable, and hostile. More severely affected individuals may have impairment of judgment and episodes of violence.[350, 351]

An incidence of up to 5 percent is reported for women of reproductive age who experience PMS.[352, 353] A disruption of the personal and professional lives of PMS victims can result from the predictable premenstrual onset of distressing *physical*, *psychologic*, and *behavioral* changes.[354] There are measurable impacts of this syndrome on social, marital, legal, and political issues. Although marital discord, sexual dysfunction, social isolation, and work inefficiency or absenteeism are common, suicidal and psychotic behavior and criminal acts ranging from child abuse to theft and murder are also possible.[350, 351] PMS is now accepted as a mitigating factor in crimes committed in the United Kingdom. In France, the syndrome is grounds for a plea of temporary insanity.

Physiopathology

Numerous hypotheses have been proposed, but the underlying physiopathologic change of PMS remains to be identified. The limitations and the validity of previous studies have been critically reviewed.[355, 356] The diversity of proposed etiologic factors and the lack of scientific rationale in most instances have been clarified by several controlled clinical studies. Some proposed etiologic factors include

1. progesterone insufficiency or withdrawal
2. vitamin B_6 deficiency
3. hypoglycemia
4. endogenous hormone allergy
5. prolactin excess
6. thyroid dysfunction
7. abnormalities of water- and salt-regulating hormones
8. psychosomatic influences
9. endogenous opioid withdrawal
10. serotonin dysfunction

In a physiologic context, cyclic changes in several target tissues, in synchrony with the ebb and flow of ovarian steroids, occur in the majority of ovulatory women. In women with PMS, these physiologic changes may be exaggerated, either by poorly defined factors or by environmental influences. On the other hand, the behavioral symptoms of this syndrome are likely to be linked to responses of target cells in the brain to ovarian factors. The marked attenuation of both physical and behavioral symptoms after "medical ovariectomy" by the use of a daily injection of a GnRH agonist validates this contention[357] (Fig. 19–40). Just how ovarian steroids induce PMS is far from clear. Proof that steroids, but not other substances secreted by the corpus luteum, are responsible for the manifestation of PMS has recently been demonstrated. In this study, women with a remission during ovarian suppression by GnRH agonist were given replacement with exogenous estrogen and progesterone separately in an attempt to determine the specificity of their effects on symptoms of PMS. It was found that estrogen was as potent as progesterone in reproducing the symptoms after 1 to 2 weeks of treatment. In normal women, similar manipulations have no perturbation.[358] These data suggest that changes in either estradiol or progesterone during the follicular and periovulatory phases may be crucial in the onset of symptoms in the luteal phase.

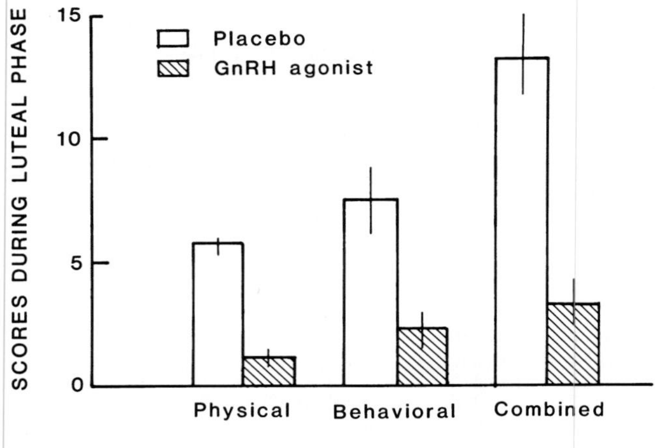

Figure 19–40 ■ A remarkable improvement in both physical and behavioral symptoms in patients with premenstrual syndrome is achieved after "functional ovariectomy" induced by treatment with a GnRH agonist. Experiments were conducted in a double-blind crossover design. (From Muse KN, Celel NS, Futterman LA, Yen SSC. Effects of medical ovariectomy by a GnRH agonist in women with premenstrual syndrome. N Engl J Med 311:1345, 1984. Reproduced by permission of The New England Journal of Medicine. © 1984, Massachusetts Medical Society.)

Research on PMS has been hampered by the difficulty in excluding the effect of psychiatric disorders in the PMS population. Clinically, the majority of patients who present for treatment of PMS can be demonstrated to have other disorders.[359] The incidence of depression in the PMS population has been reported to be more than 50 percent.[359] In these patients, it appears that the mood changes consistent with depression become entrained to the menstrual cycle.[360, 361] However, a subset of patients exists in whom no psychiatric illness can be discerned and whose symptoms are not specifically affected by psychosocial stress.[361] These individuals have a disorder that is distinct from endogenous depression by both psychometric testing and cortisol secretory rhythm.[362] Diagnostic criteria have been established to identify these individuals (Table 9–7). A prospective rating scale, the Calendar of Premenstrual Experiences, has proven utility in differentiating PMS from other disorders.[363]

New Perspectives

CYCLIC OVARIAN STEROIDS ACT AS A TRIGGER

The results of studies in which the preceding factors were critically evaluated either partially or completely have excluded most of them. During the past years, evidence has been mounting in support of serotoninergic and GABAergic dysfunction hypotheses. Because it is impossible to perform some definitive experiments on humans, speculations that ovarian steroids influence neurotransmitter changes in susceptible individuals ultimately are defended by analogies with animal data and by indirect information obtained by clinical investigations.

■ TABLE 19–7

Diagnostic Criteria for Premenstrual Syndrome

The presence by self-report of at least one of the following somatic *and* affective symptoms is noted during the 5 days before menses in each of the three prior menstrual cycles:

Affective	Somatic
Depression	Breast tenderness
Angry outbursts	Abdominal bloating
Irritability	Headache
Anxiety	Swelling of extremities
Confusion	
Social withdrawal	

These symptoms are relieved within 4 days of the onset of menses, without recurrence until at least cycle day 13.

The symptoms are present in the absence of any pharmacologic therapy, hormone ingestion, or drug or alcohol use.

The symptoms occur reproducibly during two cycles of prospective recording.

Identifiable dysfunction in social or economic performance is present by one of the following criteria:

Marital or relationship discord confirmed by partner
Difficulties in parenting
Poor work or school performance, poor attendance, or tardiness
Increased social isolation
Legal difficulties
Suicidal ideation
Seeking medical attention for a somatic symptom

From Mortola JF, Girton L, Beck L, Yen SSC. Depressive episodes in premenstrual syndromes. Am J Obstet Gynecol 161:1682–1687, 1989.

SEROTONIN HYPOTHESIS

The major serotoninergic pathway in humans, as in experimental animals, projects from the median raphe nucleus and terminates in the hypothalamus. Central serotoninergic systems are important in the regulation of several major physiologic functions, such as appetite, locomotor activity, thermoregulation, and mood. Further, dysfunction of serotoninergic neurotransmission may be involved in the pathogenesis of several neuropsychiatric disorders, particularly endogenous depression.[364]

Experimental evidence indicates that ovarian steroids exert influences on the serotoninergic neuronal activity in the hypothalamic nuclei; estrogen induces a diurnal pattern of serotonin rhythm and density of serotonin receptors and serotonin transporter,[365, 366] whereas progesterone increases the turnover rate of serotonin.[367, 368] In monkeys, a transient reduction of serotoninergic function by the administration of fenfluramine induced manifestations of irritability, behavioral alterations, and social withdrawal.[369] Decreased serotoninergic activity in patients with PMS during the week before menstruation is inferred by the observation of a reduced platelet uptake of serotonin and serotonin levels in the peripheral blood.[370, 371] Administration of serotonin agonists such as *m*-chlorophenylpiperazine induces mood elevation.[372, 373] The serotonin hypothesis in the pathophysiology of PMS is further supported by recent controlled clinical trials with the serotonin reuptake inhibitors fluoxetine[374] and sertraline.[375] In both studies, treatments were effective in alleviating tension, irritability, dysphoria, and physical symptoms in PMS. Further, these serotonin reuptake inhibitors do not appear to increase the teratogenic risk when they are used in their recommended doses.[376]

NEUROSTEROIDS AND $GABA_A$ RECEPTOR

In recent years, the biosynthesis of neurosteroids by the brain and their action within the brain have been demonstrated in rodents[377] (see Chapter 2, Neurosteroids). That progesterone metabolites markedly potentiated γ-aminobutyric acid (GABA) transmission through binding to the $GABA_A$ receptor complex at or near the barbiturate-binding site[378] supports the possibility that progesterone metabolites—allopregnanolone and pregnenolone—may have an anxiolytic effect through enhancement of GABAergic transmission. Pertinent to this proposition, Rapkin and colleagues[379] and Freeman and coworkers[380] have tested the potential beneficial effects of alprazolam in the treatment of women with premenstrual dysphoria. In these placebo-controlled studies, comparison of progesterone and alprazolam was made; whereas oral micronized progesterone or placebo was without significant effect, alprazolam (0.25 mg) provided a 50 percent symptom improvement. These observations are welcome in the management of patients with PMS. However, more basic research and adequate testing in controlled clinical trials are needed before these treatment modalities can be promoted for the treatment of PMS. Otherwise, we run the risk of adding more unproven remedies to an already cumbersome therapeutic armamentarium.

References

1. Kallmann FJ, Schoenfeld WA, Barrera SE. The genetic aspects of primary eunuchoidism. Am J Ment Defic 48:203, 1944.

2. White BJ, Rogol AD, Brown KS, et al. The syndrome of anosmia with hypogonadotropic hypogonadism: A genetic study of 18 new families and a review. Am J Med Genet 15:417, 1983.
3. Ballabio A, Bardoni B, Carrozzo R, et al. Contiguous gene syndromes due to deletions in the distal short arm of the human X-chromosome. Proc Natl Acad Sci USA 86:10001, 1989.
4. Franco B, Guioli S, Pragliola A, et al. A gene deleted in Kallmann's syndrome shares homology with neural cell adhesion and axonal pathfinding molecules. Nature 353:529, 1991.
5. Legouis R, Hardelin JP, Levilliers J, et al. The candidate gene for the X-linked Kallmann syndrome encodes a protein related to adhesion molecules. Cell 67:423, 1991.
6. Schwanzel-Fukuda M, Jorgenson KL, Bergen HT, et al. Biology of normal luteinizing hormone–releasing hormone neurons during and after their migration from olfactory placode. Endocr Rev 13:623, 1992.
7. Schwanzel-Fukuda M, Pfaff DW. Origin of luteinizing hormone–releasing hormone neurons. Nature 338:161, 1989.
8. Wray S, Nieburgs A, Elkabes S. Spatiotemporal cell expression of luteinizing hormone–releasing hormone in the prenatal mouse: Evidence for an embryonic origin in the olfactory placode. Dev Brain Res 46:309, 1989.
9. Waldstreicher J, Seminara SB, Jameson JL, et al. The genetic and clinical heterogeneity of gonadotropin-releasing hormone deficiency in the human. J Clin Endocrinol Metab 81:4388, 1996.
10. Spratt DI, Carr DB, Merriam GR, et al. The spectrum of abnormal patterns of gonadotropin-releasing hormone secretion in men with idiopathic hypogonadotropic hypogonadism: Clinical and laboratory correlations. J Clin Endocrinol Metab 64:283, 1987.
11. Santoro N, Filicori M, Crowley WF Jr. Hypogonadotropic disorders in men and women: Diagnosis and therapy with pulsatile gonadotropin-releasing hormone. Endocr Rev 7:11, 1986.
12. Seeburg PH, Mason AJ, Stewart TA, et al. The mammalian GnRH gene and its pivotal role in reproduction. Recent Prog Horm Res 43:69, 1987.
13. Silverman AJ, Roberts JL, Dong KW, et al. Intrahypothalamic injection of a cell line secreting gonadotropin-releasing hormone results in cellular differentiation and reversal of hypogonadism in mutant mice. Proc Natl Acad Sci USA 89:10668, 1992.
14. Weiss J, Crowley WF Jr, Jameson JL. Normal structure of the gonadotropin-releasing hormone (GnRH) gene in patients with GnRH deficiency and idiopathic hypogonadotropic hypogonadism. J Clin Endocrinol Metab 69:299, 1989.
15. Nakayama Y, Wondisford FE, Lash RW, et al. Analysis of gonadotropin-releasing hormone gene structure in families with familial central precocious puberty and idiopathic hypogonadotropic hypogonadism. J Clin Endocrinol Metab 70:1233, 1990.
16. Weiss J, Adams E, Whitcomb RW, et al. Normal sequence of the gonadotropin-releasing hormone gene in patients with idiopathic hypogonadotropic hypogonadism. Biol Reprod 45:743, 1991.
17. Quinton R, Hasan W, Grant W, et al. Gonadotropin-releasing hormone immunoreactivity in the nasal epithelia of adults with Kallmann's syndrome and isolated hypogonadotropic hypogonadism and in the early midtrimester human fetus. J Clin Endocrinol Metab 82:309, 1997.
18. DeRoux N, Young J, Misrahi M, et al. A family with hypogonadotropic hypogonadism and mutations in the gonadotropin-releasing hormone factor. N Engl J Med 22:1597, 1997.
19. Fairman C, Hoffman DL, Ryan RJ, et al. The "fertile eunuch" syndrome: Demonstration of isolated luteinizing hormone deficiency by radioimmunoassay technique. Mayo Clin Proc 43:661, 1968.
20. Spitz IM, Diamant Y, Rosen E, et al. Isolated gonadotropin deficiency: A heterogenous syndrome. N Engl J Med 290:10, 1974.
21. Goldenberg RL, Powell RD, Rosen SW, et al. Ovarian morphology in women with anosmia and hypogonadotropic hypogonadism. Am J Obstet Gynecol 126:91, 1976.
22. Tagatz G, Fialkow PJ, Smith D, et al. Hypogonadotropic hypogonadism associated with anosmia in the female. N Engl J Med 283:1326, 1970.
23. Yen SSC, Rebar R, Vandenberg G, et al. Pituitary gonadotrophin responsiveness to synthetic LRF in subjects with normal and abnormal hypothalamic-pituitary-gonadal axis. J Reprod Fertil 20:137, 1973.
24. Yeh J, Rebar R, Liu JH, et al. Pituitary function in isolated gonadotrophin deficiency. Clin Endocrinol 31:375, 1989.
25. Whitcomb RW, Crowley WF Jr. Clinical review 4: Diagnosis and treatment of isolated gonadotropin-releasing hormone deficiency in men. J Clin Endocrinol Metab 70:3, 1990.
26. Bell J, Spitz IM, Slonim A, et al. Heterogeneity of gonadotropin response to LHRH in hypogonadotropic hypogonadism. J Clin Endocrinol Metab 36:791, 1973.
27. Rabin D, Spitz IM, Bercovici B, et al. Isolated deficiency of follicle-stimulating hormones: Clinical and laboratory features. N Engl J Med 287:1313, 1972.
28. Crowley WF Jr, Filicori M, Spratt D, et al. The physiology of gonadotropin-releasing hormone (GnRH) secretion in men and women. Recent Prog Horm Res 41:473, 1985.
29. Hoffman AR, Crowley WF Jr. Induction of puberty in men by long-term pulsatile administration of low-dose gonadotropin-releasing hormone. N Engl J Med 307:1237, 1982.
30. Finkelstein JS, Spratt D, O'Dea LSL, et al. Pulsatile gonadotropin secretion after discontinuation of long term gonadotropin-releasing hormone (GnRH) administration in a subset of GnRH-deficient men. J Clin Endocrinol Metab 69:377, 1989.
31. Vance ML. Hypopituitarism. N Engl J Med 330:1651, 1994.
32. Banna M. Craniopharyngioma: Based on 160 cases. Br J Radiol 49:206, 1976.
33. Freda PU, Wardlaw SL, Post KD. Unusual causes of sellar/parasellar masses in a large transsphenoidal surgical series. J Clin Endocrinol Metab 81:3455, 1996.
34. Sklar CA. Craniopharyngioma: Endocrine abnormalities at presentation. Pediatr Neurosurg 21:18, 1994.
35. Sklar CA. Craniopharyngioma: Endocrine sequelae of treatment. Pediatr Neurosurg 21:120, 1994.
36. Hoff JT, Patterson RH Jr. Craniopharyngiomas in children and adults. J Neurosurg 36:299, 1972.
37. DeVile CJ, Grant DB, Hayward RD, et al. Growth and endocrine sequelae of craniopharyngioma. Arch Dis Child 75:108, 1996.
38. deBoer H, van der Veen E. Guidelines for optimizing growth hormone replacement therapy in adults. Horm Res 48:21, 1997.
39. Jorgensen JO, Thuesen L, Muller J, et al. Three years of growth hormone treatment in growth hormone–deficient adults: Near normalization of body composition and physical performance. Eur J Endocrinol 130:224, 1994.
40. Bestle J. Extragonadal endodermal sinus tumors originating in the region of the pineal gland. Acta Pathol Microbiol Scand 74:214, 1968.
41. Borit A. Embryonal carcinoma of the pineal region. J Pathol 97:165, 1969.
42. Braunstein GD, Kohler PO. Pituitary function in Hand-Schüller-Christian disease: Evidence for deficient growth hormone release in patients with short stature. N Engl J Med 286:1225, 1972.
43. Dunger DB, Broadbent V, Yeoman E, et al. The frequency and natural history of diabetes insipidus in children with Langerhans-cell histiocytosis. N Engl J Med 321:1157, 1989.
44. Lichtenstein L. Histiocytosis X, integration of eosinophilic granuloma of bone, Letterer-Siwe disease and Schüller-Christian disease as related manifestations of a single nosologic entity. Arch Pathol 56:84, 1953.
45. Nezelof C, Basset F, Rousseau MF. Histiocytosis X: Histogenetic arguments for a Langerhans cell origin. Biomedicine 18:365, 1973.
46. Strauss JH, Yen SSC, Benirschke K, et al. Hypothalamic hypopituitarism in an adolescent girl: Assessment by a direct functional test of the adenohypophysis. J Clin Endocrinol Metab 39:639, 1974.
47. Gelato MC, Loriaux DL, Merriam GR. Growth hormone responses to growth hormone–releasing hormone in Hand-Schüller-Christian disease. Neuroendocrinology 50:259, 1989.
48. Samaan NA, Bakdash MM, Caderao JB, et al. Hypopituitarism after external irradiation: Evidence for both hypothalamic and pituitary origin. Ann Intern Med 83:771, 1975.
49. Larkins RG, Martin FIR. Hypopituitarism after extracranial irradiation: Evidence for hypothalamic origin. Br Med J 1:152, 1973.
50. Lam KSL, Tse VKC, Wang C, et al. Early effects of cranial irradiation on hypothalamic-pituitary function. J Clin Endocrinol Metab 64:418, 1987.

51. Littley MD, Shalet SM, Beardwell CG, et al. Radiation-induced hypopituitarism is dose-dependent. Clin Endocrinol 31:363, 1989.
51a. Pfäffle RW, DiMattia GE, Parks JS, et al. Mutation of the POU-specific domain of Pit-1 and hypopituitarism without pituitary hypoplasia. Science 257:1118, 1992.
51b. Wu W, Cogan JD, Pfäffle RW, et al. Mutations in PROP1 cause familial combined pituitary hormone deficiency. Nature Genet 18:147, 1998.
52. Sheehan HL. Simmond's disease due to postpartum necrosis of the anterior pituitary. Q J Med 8:277, 1939.
53. Iwasaki Y, Oiso Y, Yamauchi K, et al. Neurohypophyseal function in postpartum hypopituitarism: Impaired plasma vasopressin response to osmotic stimuli. J Clin Endocrinol Metab 68:560, 1989.
54. Goluboff LG, Ezrin C. Effect of pregnancy on the somatotroph and the prolactin cell of the human adenohypophysis. J Clin Endocrinol Metab 29:1553, 1969.
55. Kovacs K. Necrosis of anterior pituitary in humans: I. Neuroendocrinology 4:170, 1969.
56. Jackson IMD, Whyte WG, Garrey MM. Pituitary function following uncomplicated pregnancy in Sheehan's syndrome. J Clin Endocrinol Metab 29:315, 1969.
57. Aono T, Mingawa J, Kinugasa T, et al. Response of pituitary LH and FSH to synthetic LH-releasing hormone in normal subjects and patients with Sheehan's syndrome. Am J Obstet Gynecol 117:1046, 1973.
58. Imura H. Hypopituitarism. The Pituitary Gland. New York, Raven Press, 1985, p 501.
59. Kaufman B. The turcica—a manifestation of the intrasellar subarachnoid space. Endocrinology 90:931, 1968.
60. Neelon FA, Goree JA, Lebovitz HE. The primary empty sella: Clinical and radiographic characteristics and endocrine function. Medicine (Baltimore) 52:73, 1973.
61. Nakagawa H, Nagasaka A, Koie K, et al. Isolated adrenocorticotropin deficiency associated with an empty sella. J Clin Endocrinol Metab 55:795, 1982.
62. Bryner JR, Greenblatt RB. Primary empty sella syndrome with elevated serum prolactin. Obstet Gynecol 50:375, 1977.
63. Reid RL, Quigley ME, Yen SSC. Pituitary apoplexy associated with diabetes insipidus: Case report and review of the literature. Arch Neurol 42:712, 1985.
64. Arafah BM, Harrington JF, Madhoun ZT, et al. Improvement of pituitary function after surgical decompression for pituitary tumor apoplexy. J Clin Endocrinol Metab 71:323, 1990.
65. Pestell RG, Best JD, Alford FP. Lymphocytic hypophysitis: The clinical spectrum of the disorder and evidence for an autoimmune pathogenesis. Clin Endocrinol 33:457, 1990.
66. Feigenbaum SL, Martin MC, Wilson CB, et al. Lymphocytic adenohypophysitis: A pituitary mass lesion occurring in association with pregnancy; proposal for medical treatment. Am J Obstet Gynecol 164:1549, 1991.
67. Asa SL, Kovacs K. Histological classification of pituitary disease. Clin Endocrinol Metab 12:567, 1983.
68. Katznelson L, Alexander JM, Klibanski A. Clinically nonfunctioning pituitary adenomas. J Clin Endocrinol Metab 76:1089, 1993.
69. Gittoes NJL, McCabe CJ, Verhaeg J, et al. Thyroid hormone and estrogen receptor expression in normal pituitary and nonfunctioning tumors of the anterior pituitary. J Clin Endocrinol Metab 82:1960, 1997.
70. Sanno N, Jin L, Qian X, et al. Gonadotropin-releasing hormone and gonadotropin-releasing hormone receptor messenger ribonucleic acids: expression in nontumorous and neoplastic pituitaries. J Clin Endocrinol Metab 82:1974, 1997.
71. Alexander JM, Swearingen B, Tindall GT, et al. Human pituitary adenomas express endogenous inhibin subunit and follistatin messenger ribonucleic acids. J Clin Endocrinol Metab 80:147, 1995.
72. Daneshdoost L, Pavlou SN, Molitch ME, et al. Inhibition of follicle-stimulating hormone secretion from gonadotroph adenomas by repetitive administration of a gonadotropin-releasing hormone antagonist. J Clin Endocrinol Metab 71:92, 1990.
73. Liuzzi A, Tassi V, Pirro MT, et al. Nonfunctioning adenomas of the pituitary. Metabolism 45:80, 1996.
74. Franks S, Jacobs HS, Nabarro JDN. Prolactin concentrations in patients with acromegaly: Clinical significance and response to surgery. Clin Endocrinol (Oxf) 5:63, 1976.
75. Zimmerman EA, Defendini R, Frantz AG. Prolactin and growth hormone in patients with pituitary adenomas: A correlative study of hormone in tumor and plasma by immunoperoxidase technique and radioimmunoassay. J Clin Endocrinol Metab 38:577, 1974.
76. Franks S, Jacobs HS, Nabarro JDN. Studies of prolactin in pituitary disease. J Endocrinol 67:55, 1975.
77. Boyar RM, Kapen S, Finkelstein JW, et al. Hypothalamic-pituitary function in diverse hyperprolactinemic states. J Clin Invest 53:1588, 1974.
78. Zarate A, Jacobs LS, Canales ES, et al. Functional evaluation of pituitary reserve in patients with the amenorrhea-galactorrhea syndrome utilizing luteinizing hormone–releasing hormone (LH-RH), L-dopa and chlorpromazine. J Clin Endocrinol Metab 37:855, 1973.
79. Rakoff J, Vandenberg G, Siler T, et al. An integrated direct functional test of the adenohypophysis. Am J Obstet Gynecol 119:358, 1974.
80. Kapen S, Boyer S, Freeman R, et al. Twenty-four-hour secretory patterns of gonadotropins and prolactin in a case of Chiari-Frommel syndrome. J Clin Endocrinol Metab 90:234, 1975.
81. Quigley ME, Judd SJ, Gilland GB, et al. Effects of a dopamine antagonist on the release of gonadotropin and prolactin in normal women and women with hyperprolactinemic anovulation. J Clin Endocrinol Metab 48:718, 1979.
82. Quigley ME, Sheehan KL, Casper RF, et al. Evidence for an increased opioid inhibition of luteinizing hormone secretion in hyperprolactinemic patients with pituitary microadenoma. J Clin Endocrinol Metab 50:427, 1980.
83. Seki K, Kato K, Shima K. Parallelism in the luteinizing hormone responses to opioid and dopamine antagonists in hyperprolactinemic women with pituitary microadenoma. J Clin Endocrinol Metab 63:1225, 1986.
84. LeDafniet M, Blumberg-Tick J, Barret A, et al. Altered balance between thyrotropin-releasing hormone and dopamine in prolactinomas and other pituitary tumors compared to normal pituitaries. J Clin Endocrinol Metab 69:267, 1989.
85. Shimon I, Melmed S. Genetic basis of endocrine disease. Pituitary tumor pathogenesis. J Clin Endocrinol Metab 82:1675, 1997.
86. Vermeulen A, Ando S. Prolactin and adrenal androgen secretion. Clin Endocrinol (Oxf) 8:295, 1978.
87. Glickman SP, Rosenfield RL, Bergenstal RM, et al. Multiple androgenic abnormalities, including elevated free testosterone, in hyperprolactinemic women. J Clin Endocrinol Metab 55:251, 1982.
88. Lobo RA, Kletzky OA. Normalization of androgen and sex hormone–binding globulin levels after treatment of hyperprolactinemia. J Clin Endocrinol Metab 56:562, 1983.
89. Glasow A, Breidert M, Haidan A, et al. Functional aspects of the effect of prolactin (prolactin) on adrenal steroidogenesis and distribution of the prolactin receptor in the human adrenal gland. J Clin Endocrinol Metab 81:3103, 1996.
90. Klibanski A, Neer RM, Beitins IZ, et al. Decreased bone density in hyperprolactinemic women. N Engl J Med 303:1511, 1980.
91. Schlechte JA, Sherman B, Martin R. Bone density in amenorrheic women with and without hyperprolactinemia. J Clin Endocrinol Metab 56:1120, 1983.
92. Koppelman MC, Kurtz DW, Morrish KA, et al. Vertebral body bone mineral content in hyperprolactinemic women. J Clin Endocrinol Metab 59:1050, 1984.
93. Schlechte J, Walkner L, Kathol M. A longitudinal analysis of premenopausal bone loss in healthy women and women with hyperprolactinemia. J Clin Endocrinol Metab 75:698, 1992.
94. Koppelman MC, Jaffe MJ, Rieth KG, et al. Hyperprolactinemia, amenorrhea, and galactorrhea. Ann Intern Med 100:115, 1984.
95. Schlechte J, Dolan K, Sherman B, et al. The natural history of untreated hyperprolactinemia: A prospective analysis. J Clin Endocrinol Metab 68:412, 1989.
96. Serri O, Rasio E, Beauregard H, et al. Recurrence of hyperprolactinemia after selective transsphenoidal adenomectomy in women with prolactinoma. N Engl J Med 309:280, 1983.
97. Camanni F, Ghigo E, Ciccarelli E, et al. Defective regulation of prolactin secretion after successful removal of prolactinomas. J Clin Endocrinol Metab 57:1270, 1983.
98. Tucker HSG, Lankford HV, Gardner DF, et al. Persistent defect in

regulation of prolactin secretion after successful pituitary tumor removal in women with the galactorrhea-amenorrhea syndrome. J Clin Endocrinol Metab 51:968, 1980.
99. Ferrari C, Piscitelli G, Crosignani PG. Cabergoline: A new drug for the treatment of hyperprolactinaemia. Hum Reprod 10:1647, 1995.
100. Melmed S. Acromegaly. N Engl J Med 322:966, 1990.
101. Frohman LA. Acromegaly: What constitutes optimal therapy? J Clin Endocrinol Metab 81:443, 1996.
102. Melmed S, Ho K, Klibanski A, et al. Clinical review 75: Recent advances in pathogenesis, diagnosis, and management of acromegaly. J Clin Endocrinol Metab 80:3395, 1995.
103. Losa M, vonWerder K. Pathophysiology and clinical aspects of the ectopic GH-releasing hormone syndrome. Clin Endocrinol (Oxf) 47:123, 1997.
104. Thorner MO, Frohman LA, Deong dopamine, et al. Extrahypothalamic growth hormone–releasing factor (GRF) secretion is a rare cause of acromegaly: Plasma GRF levels in 177 acromegalic patients. J Clin Endocrinol Metab 59:846, 1984.
105. Lawrence AM, Goldfine ID, Kirstins L. Growth hormone dynamics in acromegaly. J Clin Endocrinol Metab 31:239, 1970.
106. Yen SSC, Rebar RW, Quesenberry W. Pituitary function in pseudocyesis. J Clin Endocrinol Metab 43:132, 1976.
107. Colao A, Ferone D, Cappabianco P, et al. Effect of octreotide pretreatment on surgical outcome in acromegaly. J Clin Endocrinol Metab 82:3308, 1997.
108. Melmed S. Acromegaly. Metabolism 45:51, 1996.
109. Sheppard MC, Stewart PM. Treatment options for acromegaly. Metabolism 45:63, 1996.
110. Barkan AL, Halanz I, Dornfeld KJ, et al. Pituitary irradiation is ineffective in normalizing plasma insulin-like growth factor I in patients with acromegaly. J Clin Endocrinol Metab 82:3187, 1997.
111. Chandrasekharappa SC, Guru SC, Manickam P, et al. Positional cloning of the gene for multiple endocrine neoplasia-type 1. Science 276:404, 1997.
112. Brandi ML, Marx SJ, Aurbach GD, et al. Familial multiple endocrine neoplasia type 1: A new look at pathophysiology. Endocr Rev 8:391, 1987.
113. Maton PN, Gardner JD, Jensen RT. Cushing's syndrome in patients with the Zollinger-Ellison syndrome. N Engl J Med 315:1, 1986.
114. Giraud S, Choplin H, Teh BT, et al. A large multiple endocrine neoplasia type 1 family with clinical expression suggestive of anticipation. J Clin Endocrinol Metab 82:3487, 1997.
115. Martin R, Cetin Y, Fehm GL, et al. Multiple cellular forms of corticotrophs in surgically removed pituitary adenomas and periadenomatous tissue in Cushing's disease. Am J Pathol 106:332, 1982.
116. Suda T, Demura H, Demura R, et al. Anterior pituitary hormones in plasma and pituitaries from patients with Cushing's disease. J Clin Endocrinol Metab 51:1048, 1980.
117. vonWerder K, Smilo RP, Hane S, et al. Pituitary response to stress in Cushing's disease. Acta Endocrinol (Copenh) 67:127, 1971.
118. Guilhaume B, Bertagna X, Thomsen M, et al. Transsphenoidal pituitary surgery for the treatment of Cushing's disease: Results in 64 patients and long term follow-up studies. J Clin Endocrinol Metab 66:1056, 1988.
119. Liddle GW. Tests of pituitary-adrenal suppressibility in the diagnosis of Cushing's syndrome. J Clin Endocrinol Metab 20:1539, 1960.
120. Tyrrell JB, Brooks RM, Fitzgerald PA, et al. Cushing's disease: Selective transsphenoidal resection of pituitary adenomas. N Engl J Med 298:753, 1978.
121. Widjaja A, Schurmeyer TH, Muhlen AV, et al. Determinants of serum leptin levels in Cushing's syndrome. J Clin Endocrinol Metab 83:600, 1998.
122. Masuzaki H, Ogawa Y, Hosoda K, et al. Glucocorticoid regulation of leptin synthesis and secretion in humans: Elevated plasma leptin levels in Cushing's syndrome. J Clin Endocrinol Metab 82:2542, 1997.
123. Wise JK, Hendler R, Felig P. Influence of glucocorticoids on glucagon secretion and plasma amino acid concentrations in man. J Clin Invest 52:2777, 1973.
124. Wilson CB. Surgical management of pituitary tumors. J Clin Endocrinol Metab 82:2381, 1997.
125. Blevins LS Jr, Christy JH, Khajavi M, et al. Outcomes of therapy for Cushing's disease due to adrenocorticotropin-secreting pituitary macroadenomas. J Clin Endocrinol Metab 83:63, 1998.
126. Miller JW, Crapo L. The medical treatment of Cushing's syndrome. Endocr Rev 14:443, 1993.
127. Beck-Peccoz P, Brucker-Davis F, Persani L, et al. Thyrotropin-secreting pituitary tumors. Endocr Rev 17:610, 1996.
128. Sano T, Asa SL, Kovacs K. Growth hormone–releasing hormone–producing tumors: Clinical, biochemical, and morphological manifestations. Endocr Rev 9:357, 1988.
129. Asa SL, Kovacs K, Tindall GT, et al. Cushing's disease associated with an intrasellar gangliocytoma producing corticotropin-releasing factor. Ann Intern Med 101:789, 1984.
130. Carey RM, Varma SK, Drake CR Jr, et al. Ectopic secretion of corticotropin-releasing factor as a cause of Cushing's syndrome. N Engl J Med 311:13, 1984.
131. Molitch ME. Pathogenesis of pituitary tumors. Endocrinol Metab Clin 16:503, 1987.
132. Landis CA, Masters SB, Spada A, et al. GTPase inhibiting mutations activate the α chain of G_s and stimulate adenylyl cyclase in human pituitary tumors. Nature 340:692, 1989.
133. Tordjman K, Stern N, Ouaknine G, et al. Activating mutations of the G_s α-gene in nonfunctioning pituitary tumors. J Clin Endocrinol Metab 77:765, 1993.
134. Williamson EA, Harrison D, Ince PG, et al. Mutations of Gs-alpha in human pituitary adrenocorticotrophin hormone (ACTH)–secreting adenomas. J Clin Invest 16:S14, 1993.
135. Beckers A, Abs R, Reyniers E, et al. Variable regions of chromosome 11 loss in different pathological tissues of a patient with the multiple endocrine neoplasia type 1 syndrome. J Clin Endocrinol Metab 79:1498, 1994.
136. Thakker RV, Pook MA, Wooding C, et al. Association of somatotrophinoma with loss of alleles on chromosome 11 and with *gsp* mutations. J Clin Invest 91:2815, 1993.
137. Whelan CI, Stewart DE. Pseudocyesis—a review and report of six cases. Int J Psychiatry Med 20:97, 1990.
138. Brown E, Barglow P. Pseudocyesis, a paradigm for psychophysiological interaction. Arch Gen Psychiatry 4:221, 1971.
139. Zarate A, Canales ES, Soria J, et al. Gonadotropin and prolactin secretion in human pseudocyesis. Ann Endocrinol (Paris) 35:445, 1974.
140. Starkman MN, Marshall JC, LaFerla J, et al. Pseudocyesis: Psychologic and neuroendocrine interrelationships. Psychosom Med 47:46, 1985.
141. Bray MA, Muneyyirci-Delae O, Kolinas GD, et al. Circadian, ultradian, and episodic gonadotropin and prolactin secretion in human pseudocyesis. Acta Endocrinol (Copenh) 124:501, 1991.
142. Aldrich CK. A case of recurrent pseudocyesis. Perspect Biol Med 16:11, 1972.
143. Wildt L, Marshall G, Knobil E. Experimental induction of puberty in the infantile female rhesus monkey. Science 207:1373, 1980.
144. Apter D, Bhtzow T, Laughlin GA, et al. Gonadotropin-releasing hormone pulse generator during pubertal transition in girls: Pulsatile and diurnal patterns of circulating gonadotropin. J Clin Endocrinol Metab 76:940, 1993.
145. Crowley WF, McArthur JW. Simulation of the normal menstrual cycle in Kallmann's syndrome by pulsatile administration of luteinizing hormone–releasing hormone (LHRH). J Clin Endocrinol Metab 51:173, 1980.
146. Rasmussen DD, Gambacciani M, Swartz W, et al. Pulsatile gonadotropin-releasing hormone release from the human mediobasal hypothalamus in vitro: Opiate receptor–mediated suppression. Neuroendocrinology 49:150, 1989.
147. Conte FA, Grumbach MM, Kaplan SL. A diphasic pattern of gonadotropin secretion in patients with the syndrome of gonadal dysgenesis. J Clin Endocrinol Metab 40:670, 1975.
148. Ross JL, Loriaux DL, Cutler GB Jr. Developmental changes in neuroendocrine regulation of gonadotropin secretion in gonadal dysgenesis. J Clin Endocrinol Metab 57:288, 1983.
149. Plant TM, Gay VL, Marshall G, et al. Puberty in monkeys is triggered by chemical stimulation of the hypothalamus. Proc Natl Acad Sci USA 86:2506, 1989.
150. Apter D, Cacciatore B, Alfthan H, et al. Serum luteinizing hormone concentrations increase 100-fold in females from 7 years of age to adulthood, as measured by time-resolved immunofluorometric assay. J Clin Endocrinol Metab 68:53, 1989.

151. Boyar RM, Finkelstein JS, Roffwarg H, et al. Synchronization of augmented and luteinizing hormone secretion with sleep during puberty. N Engl J Med 287:582, 1972.
152. Matthews MJ, Parker DC, Rebar RW, et al. Sleep-associated gonadotropin and oestradiol patterns in girls with precocious sexual development. Clin Endocrinol 17:601, 1982.
153. Apter D, Viinikka L, Vihko R. Hormonal pattern of adolescent menstrual cycles. J Clin Endocrinol Metab 47:944, 1978.
154. Boyar RM, Finkelstein JW, David R, et al. Twenty-four hour patterns of plasma luteinizing hormone and follicle-stimulating hormone in sexual precocity. N Engl J Med 289:282, 1973.
155. Jeppsson S, Rannevik G, Kullander S. Studies on the decreased gonadotrophin response after administration of LH/FSH-releasing hormone during pregnancy and the puerperium. Am J Obstet Gynecol 120:1029, 1974.
156. Canales ES, Zarate A, Gairido J, et al. Study on recovery of pituitary FSH function during puerperium using synthetic LRH. J Clin Endocrinol Metab 38:1140, 1974.
157. Keye WR Jr, Jaffe RB. Changing patterns of FSH and LH response to gonadotrophin-releasing hormone in the puerperium. J Clin Endocrinol Metab 42:1133, 1976.
158. Sheehan KL, Yen SSC. Activation of pituitary gonadotropic function by an agonist of luteinizing hormone–releasing factor in the puerperium. Am J Obstet Gynecol 135:755, 1979.
159. Liu JH, Rebar RW, Yen SSC. Neuroendocrine control of the postpartum period. Clin Perinatol 10:723, 1983.
160. Yen SSC. Reproductive strategy in women: Neuroendocrine basis of endogenous contraception. *In* Roland R. Neuroendocrinology of Reproduction. Amsterdam, Excerpta Medica, 1988, pp 231–239.
161. Zinaman MJ, Cartledge T, Tomai T, et al. Pulsatile GnRH stimulates normal cyclic ovarian function in amenorrheic lactating postpartum women. J Clin Endocrinol Metab 80:2088, 1995.
162. McNeilly AS, Tay CC, Glasier A. Physiological mechanism underlying lactational amenorrhea. Ann N Y Acad Sci 709:145, 1994.
163. Axelrod J, Reisine TD. Stress hormones: Their interaction and regulation. Science 224:452, 1984.
164. Swanson LW, Mogenson GJ. Neural mechanisms for the functional coupling of autonomic, endocrine and somatomotor responses in adaptive behavior. Brain Res Rev 3:1, 1981.
165. Liu JH, Muse K, Contrepas P, et al. Augmentation of ACTH-releasing activity of synthetic corticotropin releasing factor by vasopressin in women. J Clin Endocrinol Metab 57:1087, 1983.
166. Suh BY, Liu JH, Rasmussen DD, et al. The role of oxytocin in the modulation of ACTH release in women. Neuroendocrinology 44:309, 1986.
167. Vale W, Vaughan J, Smith M, et al. Effects of synthetic ovine corticotropin-releasing factor, glucocorticoids, catecholamines, neurohypophysial peptides, and other substances on cultured corticotropic cells. Endocrinology 113:1121, 1983.
168. Rivier C, Vale W. Influence of corticotropin-releasing factor on reproductive functions in the rat. Endocrinology 114:914, 1984.
169. Petraglia F, Sutton S, Vale W, et al. Corticotropin-releasing factor decreases plasma luteinizing hormone levels in female rats by inhibiting gonadotropin-releasing hormone release into hypophyseal portal circulation. Endocrinology 120:1083, 1987.
170. Gambacciani M, Yen SSC, Rasmussen DD. GnRH release from the medial basal hypothalamus: In vitro inhibition by corticotropin-releasing factor. Neuroendocrinology 43:533, 1986.
171. Olster DH, Ferin M. Corticotropin-releasing hormone inhibits gonadotropin secretion in the ovariectomized rhesus monkey. J Clin Endocrinol Metab 65:262, 1987.
172. Nikolarakis KE, Almeida OFX, Herz A. Corticotropin-releasing factor (CRF) inhibits gonadotropin-releasing hormone (GnRH) release from superfused rat hypothalami in vitro. Brain Res 377:388, 1986.
173. Williams CL, Nishihara M, Thalabard JC, et al. Corticotropin-releasing factor and gonadotropin-releasing hormone pulse generator activity in the rhesus monkey. Electrophysiological studies. Neuroendocrinology 52:133, 1990.
174. Gindoff PR, Ferin M. Endogenous opioid peptides modulate the effect of corticotropin-releasing factor on gonadotropin release in the primate. Endocrinology 121:837, 1987.
175. Petraglia F, Vale W, Rivier C. Opioids act centrally to modulate stress-induced decrease in LH in the rat. Endocrinology 119:2445, 1986.
176. Xiao E, Luckhaus J, Niemann W, et al. Acute inhibition of gonadotropin secretion by corticotropin-releasing hormone in the primate: Are the adrenal glands involved? Endocrinology 124:1632, 1989.
177. Magiakou MA, Mastorakos G, Webster E, et al. The hypothalamic-pituitary-adrenal axis and the female reproductive system. Ann N Y Acad Sci 816:42, 1997.
178. Friis-Hansen B. Hydrometry of growth and aging. *In* Brozek J. Human Body Composition: Approaches and Applications. New York, Pergamon Press, 1965, pp 191–209.
179. l'Anson H, Foster DL, Foxcroft GR, et al. Nutrition and reproduction. Oxford Rev Reprod Biol 13:239, 1991.
180. Wade GN, Schneider JE. Metabolic fuels and reproduction in female mammals. Neurosci Biobehav Rev 16:235, 1991.
181. Van der Walt LA, Wilmsen EN, Jenkins T. Unusual sex hormone patterns among desert-dwelling hunter-gatherers. J Clin Endocrinol Metab 46:658, 1978.
182. Lee RB, San K. Women and Work in a Foraging Society. New York, Cambridge University Press, 1978.
183. Vigersky RA, Andersen AE, Thompson RH, et al. Hypothalamic dysfunction in secondary amenorrhea associated with simple weight loss. N Engl J Med 297:1141, 1977.
184. Pirke K-M, Schweiger U, Lemmel W, et al. The influence of dieting on the menstrual cycle of healthy young women. J Clin Endocrinol Metab 60:1174, 1985.
185. Fichter MM, Pirke K-M. Hypothalamic-pituitary function in starving healthy subjects. *In* Pirke K-M, Ploog D. The Psychobiology of Anorexia Nervosa. Berlin, Springer-Verlag, 1984, pp 124–135.
186. Kapen S, Sternthal E, Braverman L. Case report: A pubertal 24-hour luteinizing hormone (LH) secretory pattern following weight loss in the absence of anorexia nervosa. Psychosom Med 43:177, 1981.
187. Warren MP, Holderness CC, Lesobre V, et al. Hypothalamic amenorrhea and hidden nutritional insults. J Soc Gynecol Invest 1:84, 1994.
188. Laughlin GA, Yen SSC. Nutritional and endocrine-metabolic aberrations in amenorrheic athletes. J Clin Endocrinol Metab 81:4301, 1996.
189. Laughlin GA, Dominguez CE, Yen SSC. Nutritional and endocrine-metabolic aberrations in women with functional hypothalamic amenorrhea. J Clin Endocrinol Metab 83:25, 1998.
190. Cumming DC, Rebar RW. Exercise and reproductive function in women. Am J Ind Med 4:113, 1983.
191. Malina RM, Spirduso WW, Tate C, et al. Age at menarche and selected menstrual characteristics in athletes at different competitive levels and in different sports. Med Sci Sports 10:218, 1978.
192. Loucks AB, Horvath SM. Athletic amenorrhea: A review. Med Sci Sports Exerc 17:56, 1985.
193. Cumming DC, Wheeler GD. Exercise-associated changes in reproduction: A problem common to women and men. *In* Reisch RE. Adipose Tissue and Reproduction. Basel, Karger, 1990, pp 125–135.
194. Dale E, Gerlach DH, Wilhite AL. Menstrual dysfunction in distance runners. Obstet Gynecol 54:47, 1979.
195. Zaharieva E. Survey of sportswomen at the Tokyo Olympics. J Sports Med Phys Fitness 5:215, 1965.
196. Webb JL, Millan DL, Stoltz CJ. Gynecological survey of American female athletes competing at the Montreal Olympic Games. J Sports Med Phys Fitness 19:405, 1979.
197. Frisch RE, Gotz-Welbergen AV, McArthur JW, et al. Delayed menarche and amenorrhea of college athletes in relation to age of onset of training. JAMA 246:1559, 1981.
198. Sanborn CF, Martin BJ, Wagner WW. Is athletic amenorrhea specific to runners? Am J Obstet Gynecol 143:859, 1982.
199. Frisch RE. Body fat, menarche, fitness and fertility. *In* Reisch RE. Adipose Tissue and Reproduction. Basel, Karger, 1990, pp 1–26.
200. Schwartz B, Cumming DC, Riordan E, et al. Exercise-associated amenorrhea: A distinct entity? Am J Obstet Gynecol 141:662, 1981.
201. Frisch RE, McArthur JW. Menstrual cycles: Fatness as a determinant of minimum weight for height necessary for their maintenance or onset. Science 185:949, 1974.
202. Longcope C, Pratt JH, Schneider SH, et al. Aromatization of

androgens by muscle and adipose tissue in vivo. J Clin Endocrinol Metab 46:16, 1978.

203. Loucks AB, Mortola JF, Girton L, et al. Alterations in the hypothalamic-pituitary-ovarian and the hypothalamic-pituitary-adrenal axes in athletic women. J Clin Endocrinol Metab 68:402, 1989.
204. Veldhuis JD, Evans WS, Demers LM, et al. Altered neuroendocrine regulation of gonadotropin secretion in women distance runners. J Clin Endocrinol Metab 61:557, 1985.
205. Cumming DC, Vickovic MM, Wall SR, et al. Defects in pulsatile LH release in normally menstruating runners. J Clin Endocrinol Metab 60:810, 1985.
206. Bullen BA, Skrinar GS, Beitins IZ, et al. Induction of menstrual disorders in untrained women by strenuous exercise. N Engl J Med 312:1349, 1985.
207. Reifenstein EC Jr. Psychogenic or "hypothalamic" amenorrhea. Med Clin North Am 30:1103, 1946.
208. Reame NE, Sauder SE, Case GD, et al. Pulsatile gonadotropin secretion in women with hypothalamic amenorrhea: Evidence that reduced frequency of gonadotropin-releasing hormone secretion is the mechanism of persistent anovulation. J Clin Endocrinol Metab 61:851, 1985.
209. Berga SL, Girton LG. The psychoneuroendocrinology of functional hypothalamic amenorrhea. Psychiatr Clin North Am 12:105–116, 1989.
210. Yen SSC, Rebar R, Vandenberg G, et al. Hypothalamic amenorrhea and hypogonadotropism: Responses to synthetic LRF. J Clin Endocrinol Metab 36:811, 1973.
211. Lachelin GCL, Yen SSC. Hypothalamic chronic anovulation. Am J Obstet Gynecol 130:825, 1978.
212. Rebar RW, Harman SM, Vaitukaitis JL. Differential responsiveness for LRF after estrogen therapy in women with hypothalamic amenorrhea. J Clin Endocrinol Metab 46:48, 1978.
213. Berga SL, Mortola JF, Girton L, et al. Neuroendocrine aberrations in women with functional hypothalamic amenorrhea. J Clin Endocrinol Metab 68:301, 1989.
214. Giles DE, Berga SL. Cognitive and psychiatric correlates of functional hypothalamic amenorrhea: A controlled comparison. Fertil Steril 60:486, 1993.
215. Khoury SA, Reame NE, Kelch RP, et al. Diurnal patterns of pulsatile luteinizing hormone secretion in hypothalamic amenorrhea: Reproducibility and responses to opiate blockade and an $alpha_2$-adrenergic agonist. J Clin Endocrinol Metab 64:755, 1987.
216. Miller DS, Reid R, Cetel N, et al. Pulsatile administration of low dose gonadotropin-releasing hormone (GnRH) for the induction of ovulation and pregnancy in patients with hypothalamic amenorrhea. JAMA 250:2937, 1983.
217. Leyendecker G, Wildt L, Hansmann M. Pregnancies following chronic intermittent (pulsatile) administration of GnRH by means of a portable pump (Zyklomat): A new approach in the treatment of infertility in hypothalamic amenorrhea. J Clin Endocrinol Metab 51:1214, 1980.
218. Reid RL, Leopold GR, Yen SSC. Induction of ovulation and pregnancy with pulsatile luteinizing hormone releasing factor: Dosage and mode of delivery. Fertil Steril 40:18, 1981.
219. Snow RC, Schneider JL, Barbieri RL. High dietary fiber and low saturated fat intake among oligomenorrheic undergraduates. Fertil Steril 54:632, 1990.
220. Loucks AB, Heath EM. Dietary restriction reduces luteinizing hormone (LH) pulse frequency during waking hours and increases LH pulse amplitude during sleep in young menstruating women. J Clin Endocrinol Metab 78:910, 1994.
221. Olson BR, Cartledge T, Sebring N, et al. Short-term fasting affects luteinizing hormone secretory dynamics but not reproductive function in normal-weight sedentary women. J Clin Endocrinol Metab 80:1187, 1995.
222. Loucks AB, Verdun M, Heath EM. Low energy availability, not stress of exercise, alters LH pulsatility in exercising women. J Appl Physiol 84:37, 1998.
223. Williams NI, Young JC, McArthur JW, et al. Strenuous exercise with caloric restriction: Effect on luteinizing hormone secretion. Med Sci Sports Exerc 27:1390, 1995.
224. Loucks AB, Brown R, King K, et al. A combined regimen of moderate dietary restriction and exercise training alters luteinizing hormone pulsatility in regularly menstruating young women (Abstract P3-360). Presented at the 77th Annual Meeting of The Endocrine Society, San Francisco, June 20, 1995.
225. Kalra SP, Kalra PS. Nutritional infertility: The role of the interconnected hypothalamic neuropeptide Y–galanin-opioid network. Front Neuroendocrinol 17:371, 1996.
226. Riccardi G, Parillo M. Comparison of the metabolic effects of fat-modified vs low fat diets. Ann N Y Acad Sci 683:192, 1993.
227. Loucks AB, Laughlin GA, Mortola JF, et al. Hypothalamic-pituitary-thyroidal function in eumenorrheic and amenorrheic athletes. J Clin Endocrinol Metab 75:514, 1992.
228. Loucks AB, Heath EM. Induction of low-T_3 syndrome in exercising women occurs at a threshold of energy availability. Am J Physiol 266:R817, 1994.
229. Legradi G, Emerson CH, Ahima RS, et al. Leptin prevents fasting-induced suppression of prothyrotropin-releasing hormone messenger ribonucleic acid in neurons of the hypothalamic paraventricular nucleus. Endocrinology 138:2569, 1997.
230. Valcavi R, Zini M, Peino R, et al. Influence of thyroid status on serum immunoreactive leptin levels. J Clin Endocrinol Metab 82:1632, 1997.
231. Gold PW, Loriaux DL, Roy A, et al. Responses to corticotropin-releasing hormone in the hypercortisolism of depression and Cushing's disease. N Engl J Med 314:1329, 1986.
232. Rupprecht R, Lesch L-P, Muller U, et al. Blunted adrenocorticotropin but normal β-endorphin release after human corticotropin-releasing hormone administration in depression. J Clin Endocrinol Metab 69:600, 1989.
233. Suh BY, Liu JH, Berga SL, et al. Hypercortisolism in patients with functional hypothalamic amenorrhea. J Clin Endocrinol Metab 66:733, 1988.
234. Biller BMK, Federoff HJ, Koenig JI, et al. Abnormal cortisol secretion and response to corticotropin-releasing hormone in women with hypothalamic amenorrhea. J Clin Endocrinol Metab 70:311, 1990.
235. Rivier C, Rivier J, Vale W. Stress-induced inhibition of reproductive functions: Role of endogenous corticotropin-releasing factor. Science 231:607, 1986.
236. Vance ML, Hartman ML, Thorner MO. Growth hormone and nutrition. Horm Res 38:85, 1992.
237. Counts DR, Gwirtsman H, Carlsson LM, et al. The effect of anorexia nervosa and refeeding on growth hormone–binding protein, the insulin-like growth factors (IGFs), and the IGF-binding proteins. J Clin Endocrinol Metab 75:762, 1992.
238. Suikkari M, Koivisto VA, Koistinen R, et al. Dose-response characteristics for suppression of low molecular weight plasma insulin-like growth factor–binding protein by insulin. J Clin Endocrinol Metab 68:135, 1989.
239. Pao C-J, Farmer PK, Begovic S, et al. Regulation of insulin-like growth factor-I (IGF-I) and IGF-binding protein 1 gene transcription by hormones and provision of amino acids in rat hepatocytes. Mol Endocrinol 7:1561, 1993.
240. Conover CA, Divertie GD, Lee PDK. Cortisol increases plasma insulin-like growth factor binding protein-1 in humans. Acta Endocrinol (Copenh) 128:140, 1993.
241. Thissen J-P, Ketelslegers J-M, Underwood LE. Nutritional regulation of the insulin-like growth factors. Endocr Rev 15:80, 1994.
242. Lewitt MS. Role of the insulin-like growth factors in the endocrine control of glucose homeostasis. Diabetes Res Clin Pract 23:3, 1994.
243. Baumann G. Growth hormone binding proteins: State of the art. J Endocrinol 141:1, 1994.
244. Argente J, Caballo N, Barrios V, et al. Multiple endocrine abnormalities of the growth hormone and insulin-like growth factor axis in patients with anorexia nervosa: Effect of short- and long-term weight recuperation. J Clin Endocrinol Metab 82:2084, 1997.
245. Brzezinski A, Lynch HJ, Seibel MM, et al. The circadian rhythm of plasma melatonin during the normal menstrual cycle and in amenorrheic women. J Clin Endocrinol Metab 66:891, 1988.
246. Berga SL, Mortola JF, Yen SSC. Amplification of nocturnal melatonin secretion in women with functional hypothalamic amenorrhea. J Clin Endocrinol Metab 66:242, 1988.
247. Okatani Y, Sagara Y. Amplification of nocturnal melatonin secretion in women with functional secondary amenorrhoea:

Relation to endogenous oestrogen concentration. Clin Endocrinol (Oxf) 41:763, 1994.
248. Walker AB, English J, Arendt J, et al. Hypogonadotrophic hypogonadism and primary amenorrhoea associated with increased melatonin secretion from a cystic pineal lesion. Clin Endocrinol (Oxf) 45:353, 1996.
249. Laughlin GA, Yen SSC. Hypoleptinemia in women athletes: Absence of a diurnal rhythm with amenorrhea. J Clin Endocrinol Metab 82:318, 1997.
250. Shimizu H, Shimomura Y, Nakanishi Y, et al. Estrogen increases in vivo leptin production in rats and human subjects. J Endocrinol 154:285, 1997.
251. Caro JF, Sinha MK, Kolaczynski JW, et al. Leptin: The tale of an obesity gene. Diabetes 45:2455, 1996.
252. Mantzoros CS, Moschos S, Avramopoulos I, et al. Leptin concentrations in relation to body mass index and the tumor necrosis factor-α system in humans. J Clin Endocrinol Metab 82:3408, 1997.
253. Toomey D, Redmond P, Bouchier-Hayes D. Mechanisms mediating cancer cachexia. Cancer 76:2418, 1995.
254. Staal van den Brekel AJ, Dentener MA, Schols AM, et al. Increased resting energy expenditure and weight loss are related to a systemic inflammatory response in lung cancer patients. J Clin Oncol 13:2600, 1995.
255. DeBellis MD, Chrousos GP, Dorn LD, et al. Hypothalamic-pituitary-adrenal axis dysregulation in sexually abused girls. J Clin Endocrinol Metab 78:249, 1994.
256. Drinkwater BL, Nilson K, Chesnut CH, et al. Bone mineral content of amenorrheic and eumenorrheic athletes. N Engl J Med 311:277, 1984.
257. Biller BMK, Coughlin JF, Saxe V, et al. Osteopenia in women with hypothalamic amenorrhea: A prospective study. Obstet Gynecol 78:996, 1991.
258. Hergenroeder AC, Smith E, Shypailo R, et al. Bone mineral changes in young women with hypothalamic amenorrhea treated with oral contraceptives, medroxyprogesterone, or placebo over 12 months. Am J Obstet Gynecol 176:1017, 1997.
259. Rencken ML, Chesnut CH, Drinkwater BL. Bone density at multiple skeletal sites in amenorrheic athletes. JAMA 276:238, 1996.
260. Myburgh KH, Bachrach LK, Lewis B, et al. Low bone mineral density at axial and appendicular sites in amenorrheic athletes. Med Sci Sports Exerc 25:1197, 1993.
261. Davies MC, Hall ML, Jacobs HS. Bone mineral loss in young women with amenorrhoea. BMJ 301:790, 1990.
262. Myburgh KH, Hutchins J, Fataar AB, et al. Low bone density is an etiologic factor for stress fractures in athletes. Ann Intern Med 113:754, 1990.
263. Gulekli B, Davies MC, Jacobs HS. Effect of treatment on established osteoporosis in young women with amenorrhea. Clin Endocrinol (Oxf) 41:275, 1994.
264. Keen AD, Drinkwater BL. Irreversible bone loss in former amenorrheic athletes. Osteoporos Int 7:311, 1997.
265. Cumming DC. Exercise-associated amenorrhea, low bone density, and estrogen replacement therapy. Arch Intern Med 156:2193, 1996.
266. Drinkwater BL, Bruemner B, Chesnut CH. Menstrual history as a determinant of current bone density in young athletes. JAMA 263:545, 1990.
267. Nylander I. The feeling of being fat and dieting in a schoolgirl population: An epidemiologic interview investigation. Acta Sociomed Scand 3:17, 1971.
268. Crisp AH, Palmer RL, Kalucy RS. How common is anorexia nervosa? A prevalence study. Br J Psychiatry 128:549, 1976.
269. Szmukler GI. Weight and food preoccupation in a population of English schoolgirls. *In* Understanding Anorexia Nervosa and Bulimia: Report of the Fourth Ross Conference on Medical Research. Columbus, OH, Ross Laboratories, 1983, p 21.
270. Casper RC, Eckert ED, Halmi KA. Bulimia: Its incidence and clinical importance in patients with anorexia nervosa. Arch Gen Psychiatry 37:1030, 1980.
271. Gwirtsman HE, Roy-Byrne P, Yager J, et al. Neuroendocrine abnormalities in bulimia. Am J Psychiatry 140:5, 1983.
272. Vigersky RA, Loriaux DL, Andersen AE, et al. Delayed pituitary hormone response to LRF and TRF in patients with anorexia nervosa and with secondary amenorrhea associated with simple weight loss. J Clin Endocrinol Metab 43:893, 1976.
273. Travaglini P, Peccoz P, Ferrari C, et al. Some aspects of hypothalamic-pituitary function in patients with anorexia nervosa. Acta Endocrinol (Copenh) 81:252, 1976.
274. Beumont PJV, George GCW, Pimstone BL, et al. Body weight and the pituitary response to hypothalamic releasing hormones in patients with anorexia nervosa. J Clin Endocrinol Metab 43:487, 1976.
275. Katz JL, Boyar RM, Roffwarg H, et al. LHRH responsiveness in anorexia nervosa: Intactness despite prepubertal circadian LH pattern. Psychosom Med 39:241, 1977.
276. Hoff JD, Lasley BL, Yen SSC. The functional relationship between priming and releasing actions of LRF. J Clin Endocrinol Metab 49:8, 1979.
277. Mortola JF, Laughlin GA, Yen SSC. Melatonin rhythms in women with anorexia nervosa and bulimia nervosa. J Clin Endocrinol Metab 77:1540, 1993.
278. Sherman BM, Halmi KA, Zamuldio R. LH and FSH response to gonadotropin-releasing hormone in anorexia nervosa: Effect of nutritional rehabilitation. J Clin Endocrinol Metab 41:135, 1975.
279. vanBinsbergen CJ, Coelingh Bennink HJ, Odink J, et al. A comparative and longitudinal study on endocrine changes related to ovarian function in patients with anorexia nervosa. J Clin Endocrinol Metab 71:705, 1990.
280. Garcia-Rubi E, Vasquez-Aleman D, Mendez JP, et al. The effects of opioid blockade and GnRH administration upon luteinizing hormone secretion in patients with anorexia nervosa during the stages of weight loss and weight recovery. Clin Endocrinol (Oxf) 37:520, 1992.
281. Baranowska B, Rozbicka G, Jeske W, et al. The role of endogenous opiates in the mechanism of inhibited luteinizing hormone (LH) secretion in women with anorexia nervosa: The effects of naloxone on LH, follicle-stimulating hormone, prolactin and β-endorphin secretion. J Clin Endocrinol Metab 59:412, 1984.
282. Fishman J, Boyar RM, Hellman L. Influence of body weight on estradiol metabolism in young women. J Clin Endocrinol Metab 41:989, 1975.
283. Anderson KE, Keppas A, Conney AH, et al. The influence of dietary protein and carbohydrate on the principal oxidative biotransformations of estradiol in normal subjects. J Clin Endocrinol Metab 59:103, 1984.
284. Rigotti NA, Nussbaum SR, Herzog DB, et al. Osteoporosis in women with anorexia nervosa. N Engl J Med 311:1601, 1984.
285. Bradlow HL, Boyar RM, O'Connor J, et al. Hypothyroid-like alterations in testosterone metabolism in anorexia nervosa. J Clin Endocrinol Metab 43:571, 1976.
286. Boyar RM, Hellmann LD, Roffwarg H, et al. Cortisol secretion and metabolism in anorexia nervosa. N Engl J Med 296:190, 1977.
287. Doerr P, Fichter M, Pirke KM, et al. Relationship between weight gain and hypothalamic pituitary adrenal function in patients with anorexia nervosa. J Steroid Biochem 13:529, 1980.
288. Walsh BT, Katz JL, Levin J, et al. The production rate of cortisol declines during recovery from anorexia nervosa. J Clin Endocrinol Metab 53:203, 1981.
289. Estour B, Pugeat M, Lang F, et al. Rapid escape of cortisol from suppression in response to I.V. dexamethasone in anorexia nervosa. Clin Endocrinol (Oxf) 33:45, 1990.
290. Gold PW, Gwirtsman H, Augerinos PC. Abnormal hypothalamic-pituitary-adrenal function in anorexia nervosa. N Engl J Med 314:1335, 1986.
291. Hotta M, Shibash T, Masurd A, et al. The response of plasma adrenocorticotropin and cortisol to corticotropin-releasing hormone (CRH) and cerebrospinal fluid immunoreactive CRH in anorexia nervosa patients. J Clin Endocrinol Metab 62:319, 1986.
292. Mortola JF, Rasmussen DD, Yen SSC. Alterations of the adrenocorticotropin-cortisol axis in normal weight bulimic women: Evidence for a central mechanism. J Clin Endocrinol Metab 68:517, 1989.
293. Kaye WH, Gwirtsman H, George DT. Elevated cerebrospinal fluid levels of immunoreactive corticotropin-releasing hormone in anorexia nervosa: Relation to state of nutrition, adrenal function, and intensity of depression. J Clin Endocrinol Metab 64:203, 1987.
294. Kontula K, Andersson LC, Huttunen M, et al. Reduced level of cellular glucocorticoid receptors in patients with anorexia nervosa. Horm Metab Res 14:619, 1982.

295. Zumoff B, Walsh BT, Katz JL, et al. Subnormal plasma dehydroisoandrosterone to cortisol ratio in anorexia nervosa: A second hormonal parameter of ontogenic regression. J Clin Endocrinol Metab 56:668, 1983.
296. Devesa J, Perez-Fernandez R, Bokser L, et al. Adrenal androgen secretion and dopaminergic activity in anorexia nervosa. Horm Metab Res 20:57, 1988.
297. Winterer J, Gwirtsman H, George DT, et al. Adrenocorticotropin-stimulated adrenal androgen secretion in anorexia nervosa: Impaired secretion at low weight with normalization after long term weight recovery. J Clin Endocrinol Metab 61:693, 1985.
298. l'Allemand D, Penhoat A, Lebrethon MC, et al. Insulin-like growth factors enhance steroidogenic enzyme and corticotropin receptor messenger ribonucleic acid levels and corticotropin steroidogenic responsiveness in cultured human adrenocortical cells. J Clin Endocrinol Metab 81:3892, 1996.
299. Miyai K, Yamamoto T, Azukizawa M, et al. Serum thyroid hormones and thyrotropin in anorexia nervosa. J Clin Endocrinol Metab 40:334, 1975.
300. Moshang T Jr, Parks JS, Baker L, et al. Low serum triiodothyronine in patients with anorexia nervosa. J Clin Endocrinol Metab 40:470, 1975.
301. Bray GA, Fisher DA, Chopra IJ. Relation of thyroid hormones to body weight. Lancet 1:1206, 1976.
302. Spencer CA, Lum SMC, Wilber JF, et al. Dynamics of serum thyrotropin and thyroid hormone changes in fasting. J Clin Endocrinol Metab 56:883, 1983.
303. Hochberg Z, Hertz P, Colin V, et al. The distal axis of growth hormone (GH) in nutritional disorders: GH-binding protein, insulin-like growth factor-I (IGF-I), and IGF-I receptors in obesity and anorexia nervosa. Metabolism 41:106, 1992.
304. Golden NH, Kreitzer P, Jacobson MS, et al. Disturbances in growth hormone secretion and action in adolescents with anorexia nervosa. J Pediatr 125:655, 1994.
305. Scacchi M, Pincelli AI, Caumo A, et al. Spontaneous nocturnal growth hormone secretion in anorexia nervosa. J Clin Endocrinol Metab 82:3225, 1997.
306. Hall K, Lundin G, Povoa G. Serum levels of the low molecular weight form of insulin-like growth factor binding protein in healthy subjects and patients with growth hormone deficiency, acromegaly and anorexia nervosa. Acta Endocrinol (Copenh) 118:321, 1988.
307. Rappaport R, Prevot C, Czernichow P. Somatomedin activity and growth hormone secretion: Changes related to body weight in anorexia nervosa. Acta Paediatr Scand 69:37, 1980.
308. Daughaday WH, Trivedi B. Absence of serum growth hormone binding protein in patients with growth hormone receptor deficiency (Laron dwarfism). Proc Natl Acad Sci USA 84:4636, 1987.
309. Baumann G, Shaw MA, Winter RJ. Absence of the plasma growth hormone–binding protein in Laron-type dwarfism. J Clin Endocrinol Metab 65:814, 1987.
310. Scacchi M, Invitti C, Pincelli AI, et al. Lack of growth hormone response to acute administration of dexamethasone in anorexia nervosa. Eur J Endocrinol 132:152, 1995.
311. Nakagawa K, Matsubara M, Obara T, et al. Responses of pituitary and adrenal medulla to insulin-induced hypoglycemia in patients with anorexia nervosa. Endocrinol Jpn 32:719, 1985.
312. Brambilla F, Ferrari E, Cavagnini F, et al. Alpha$_2$-adrenoceptor sensitivity in anorexia nervosa: GH response to clonidine or GHRH stimulation. Biol Psychiatry 25:256, 1989.
313. Nussbaum MP, Blethen SL, Chasalow FI, et al. Blunted growth hormone responses to clonidine in adolescent girls with early anorexia nervosa. Evidence for an early hypothalamic defect. J Adolesc Health Care 11:145, 1990.
314. Tamai H, Komaki G, Matsubayashi S, et al. Effect of cholinergic muscarinic receptor blockade on human growth hormone (GH)–releasing hormone-(1–44)–induced GH secretion in anorexia nervosa. J Clin Endocrinol Metab 70:738, 1990.
315. Ghigo E, Arvat E, Gianotti L, et al. Arginine but not pyridostigmine, a cholinesterase inhibitor, enhances the GHRH-induced GH rise in patients with anorexia nervosa. Biol Psychiatry 36:689, 1994.
316. Rolla M, Andreoni A, Belliti D, et al. Failure of glucose infusion to suppress the exaggerated GH response to GHRH in patients with anorexia nervosa. Biol Psychiatry 27:215, 1990.
317. Tamai H, Kiyohara K, Mukuta T, et al. Responses of growth hormone and cortisol to intravenous glucose loading test in patients with anorexia nervosa. Metabolism 40:31, 1991.
318. Popovic V, Micic D, Djurovic M, et al. Absence of desensitization by hexarelin to subsequent GH releasing hormone–mediated GH secretion to patients with anorexia nervosa. Clin Endocrinol (Oxf) 46:539, 1997.
319. Scheen AJ, Castillo M, Lefebvre PJ. Insulin sensitivity in anorexia nervosa: A mirror image of obesity? Diabetes Metab Rev 4:681, 1988.
320. Fukushima M, Nakai Y, Taniguchi A, et al. Insulin sensitivity, insulin secretion, and glucose effectiveness in anorexia nervosa: A minimal model analysis. Metabolism 42:1164, 1993.
321. Casper RC. Carbohydrate metabolism and its regulatory hormones in anorexia nervosa. Psychiatry Res 62:85, 1996.
322. Grinspoon S, Gulick T, Askari H, et al. Serum leptin levels in women with anorexia nervosa. J Clin Endocrinol Metab 81:3861, 1996.
323. Casanueva FF, Dieguez C, Popovic V, et al. Serum immunoreactive leptin concentrations in patients with anorexia nervosa before and after partial weight recovery. Biochem Mol Med 60:116, 1997.
324. Mantzoros C, Flier JS, Lesem MD, et al. Cerebrospinal fluid leptin in anorexia nervosa: Correlation with nutritional status and potential role in resistance to weight gain. J Clin Endocrinol Metab 82:1845, 1997.
325. Hebebrand J, Blum WF, Barth N, et al. Leptin levels in patients with anorexia nervosa are reduced in the acute stage and elevated upon short-term weight restoration. Mol Psychiatry 2:330, 1997.
326. Kaye WH. Neuropeptide abnormalities in anorexia nervosa. Psychiatry Res 62:65, 1996.
327. Heinrichs SC, Menzaghi F, Merlo Pich E, et al. Corticotropin releasing factor in the paraventricular nucleus modulates feeding induced by neuropeptide Y. Brain Res 611:18, 1993.
328. Kaye WH. Persistent alterations in behavior and serotonin activity after recovery from anorexia and bulimia nervosa. Ann N Y Acad Sci 817:162, 1997.
329. Brambilla F, Ferrari E, Petraglia F, et al. Peripheral opioid secretory pattern in anorexia nervosa. Psychiatry Res 39:115, 1991.
330. Vigersky RA, Loriaux DL. Anorexia nervosa as a model of hypothalamic dysfunction. *In* Vigersky RA. Anorexia Nervosa. New York, Raven Press, 1977, p 109.
331. Gold PW, Kaye W, Robertson GL, et al. Abnormalities in plasma and cerebrospinal-fluid arginine vasopressin in patients with anorexia nervosa. N Engl J Med 308:1117, 1983.
332. Tolstrup K. Anorexia nervosa—a typical psychosomatic disease of puberty and adolescence. Triangle 21:85, 1982.
333. Fava M, Copeland PM, Schweiger U, et al. Neurochemical abnormalities of anorexia nervosa and bulimia nervosa. Am J Psychiatry 146:963, 1989.
334. Golden NH, Jacobson MS, Schebendach J, et al. Resumption of menses in anorexia nervosa. Arch Pediatr Adolesc Med 151:16, 1997.
335. Halmi KA, Powers P, Cunningham S. Treatment of anorexia nervosa with behavior modification. Arch Gen Psychiatry 32:93, 1975.
336. Kaye WH. Double-blind fluoxetine study in anorexia nervosa. Presented at the American Psychiatric Association Annual Meeting, Miami, FL, 1995.
337. Kaye WH, Weltzin TE, Hsu LK, et al. An open trial of fluoxetine in patients with anorexia nervosa. J Clin Psychiatry 52:464, 1991.
338. Hsu LKG, Crisp AH, Harding B. Outcome of anorexia nervosa. Lancet 1:61, 1979.
339. Klibanski A, Biller BM, Schoenfeld DA, et al. The effects of estrogen administration on trabecular bone loss in young women with anorexia nervosa. J Clin Endocrinol Metab 80:898, 1995.
340. Bachrach LK, Katzman DK, Litt IF, et al. Recovery from osteopenia in adolescent girls with anorexia nervosa. J Clin Endocrinol Metab 72:602, 1991.
341. Rigotti NA, Neer RM, Skates SJ, et al. The clinical course of osteoporosis in anorexia nervosa. A longitudinal study of cortical bone mass. JAMA 265:1133, 1991.
342. Fichter MM, Pirke K-M, Pollinger J, et al. Disturbances in the hypothalamo-pituitary-adrenal and other neuroendocrine axes in bulimia. Biol Psychiatry 27:1021, 1990.

343. Schweiger U, Pirke K-M, Laessle RG, et al. Gonadotropin secretion in bulimia nervosa. J Clin Endocrinol Metab 74:1122, 1992.
344. Pirke K-M, Pahl J, Schweiger U, et al. Metabolic and endocrine indices of starvation in bulimia: A comparison with anorexia nervosa. Psychiatry Res 15:33, 1985.
345. Schreiber W, Schweiger U, Werner D, et al. Circadian pattern of large neutral amino acids, glucose, insulin and food intake in anorexia nervosa and bulimia nervosa. Metabolism 40:503, 1991.
346. Schweiger U, Pollinger J, Laessle R, et al. Altered insulin response to a balanced test meal in bulimic patients. Int J Eat Disord 6:551, 1987.
347. Weltzin TE, Fernstrom MH, Kaye WH. Serotonin and bulimia nervosa. Nutr Rev 52:399, 1994.
348. Reid RL. Premenstrual syndrome. Am Assoc Clin Chem 5:1, 1987.
349. Gold JH. Historical perspective of premenstrual syndrome. *In* Gold JH, Severino SK. Premenstrual Dysphorias: Myths and Realities. New York, American Psychiatric Association, 1994.
350. Dalton K. Cyclical criminal acts in premenstrual syndrome. Lancet 2:1070, 1980.
351. Reid RL, Yen SSC. Premenstrual syndrome. Am J Obstet Gynecol 139:85, 1981.
352. Woods NF, Most D, Dery GK. Prevalence of perimenstrual symptoms. Am J Public Health 72:1257, 1982.
353. Andersch B, Wendestram C, Huhn L, et al. Premenstrual complaints, I. Prevalence of premenstrual symptoms in a Swedish urban population. J Psychosom Obstet Gynecol 5:39, 1986.
354. Reid RL, Yen SSC. The premenstrual syndrome. Clin Obstet Gynecol 26:710, 1983.
355. Mortola JF. Premenstrual syndrome. Trends Endocrinol Metab 7:184, 1996.
356. Dye L, Blundell JE. Menstrual cycle and appetite control: Implications for weight regulation. Hum Reprod 12:1142, 1997.
357. Muse KN, Cetel N, Futterman LA, et al. The premenstrual syndrome: Effects of "medical ovariectomy." N Engl J Med 311:1345, 1984.
358. Schmidt PJ, Nieman LK, Danaceau MA, et al. Differential behavioral effects of gonadal steroids in women with and in those without premenstrual syndrome. N Engl J Med 338:209, 1998.
359. Diamond SB, Rubenstein AA, Dunner DL, et al. Menstrual problems in women with primary affective illness. Compr Psychiatry 17:541, 1976.
360. Schmidt PJ, Nieman LK, Grover GN, et al. Neurobehavioral effects of late luteal phase endocrine manipulations in women with premenstrual syndrome. Presented at the 72nd Annual Meeting of the Endocrine Society; June 20–23, 1990; Atlanta, GA, p 314.
361. Beck LE, Gervitz R, Mortola JF. Psychosocial stress and symptoms severity in premenstrual syndrome. Psychosom Med 52:536, 1990.
362. Mortola JF, Girton L, Beck L, et al. Depressive episodes in premenstrual syndromes. Am J Obstet Gynecol 161:1682, 1989.
363. Mortola JF, Girton L, Yen SSC. Diagnosis of premenstrual syndrome by a simple, prospective and reliable instrument: The calendar of premenstrual experiences (COPE). Obstet Gynecol 76:302, 1990.
364. Grosser BI. Serotonin: A reappraisal. J Clin Psychiatry 48:3, 1987.
365. Fink G, Sumner BEH. Oestrogen and mental state. Nature 383:306, 1996.
366. McQueen JK, Wilson H, Fink G. Estradiol-17 beta increases serotonin transporter (SERT) mRNA levels and the density of SERT-binding sites in female rat brain. Brain Res Mol Brain Res 45:13, 1997.
367. Cohen IR, Wise PM. Effects of estradiol on the diurnal rhythm of serotonin activity in microdissected brain areas of ovariectomized rats. Endocrinology 122:2619, 1988.
368. Ladisich W. Influence of progesterone on serotonin metabolism: A possible causal factor for mood changes. Psychoneuroendocrinology 2:257, 1977.
369. Raleigh MJ, Brammer GL, McGuire MT. Dominant social status facilitates the behavioral effects of serotonergic agonists. Brain Res 348:274, 1985.
370. Taylor DL, Mathew RJ, Beng TH. Serotonin levels and platelet uptake during premenstrual tension. Neuropsychobiology 12:16, 1984.
371. Rapkin AJ, Edelmuth E, Chang LC, et al. Whole-blood serotonin in premenstrual syndrome. Obstet Gynecol 70:533, 1987.
372. Mueller EA, Murphy DL, Sunderland T. Neuroendocrine effects of *m*-chlorophenylpiperazine, a serotonin agonist, in humans. J Clin Endocrinol Metab 61:1179, 1985.
373. Su T-P, Schmidt PJ, Danaceau M, et al. Effect of menstrual cycle phase on neuroendocrine and behavioral responses to the serotonin agonist *m*-chlorophenylpiperazine in women with premenstrual syndrome and controls. J Clin Endocrinol Metab 82:1220, 1997.
374. Steiner M, Steinberg S, Stewart D, et al. Fluoxetine in the treatment of premenstrual dysphoria. N Engl J Med 332:1529, 1995.
375. Yonkers KA, Halbreich U, Freeman E, et al. Symptomatic improvement of premenstrual dysphoric disorder with sertraline treatment. JAMA 278:983, 1997.
376. Kulin NA, Pastuszak A, Sage SR, et al. Pregnancy outcome following maternal use of the new selective serotonin reuptake inhibitors. A prospective controlled multicenter study. JAMA 279:609, 1998.
377. Baulieu E-E. Neurosteroids: Of the nervous system, by the nervous system, for the nervous system. Recent Prog Horm Res 52:1–32, 1997.
378. Majewska MD, Harrison NJ, Schwartz RD, et al. Steroid hormone metabolites are barbiturate-like modulators of the GABA receptor. Science 232:1004, 1986.
379. Rapkin AJ, Morgan M, Goldman L, et al. Progesterone metabolite allopregnanolone in women with premenstrual syndrome. Obstet Gynecol 90:709, 1997.
380. Freeman E, Rickels K, Sondheimer SJ, et al. A double-blind trial of oral progesterone, alprazolam, and placebo in treatment of severe premenstrual syndrome. JAMA 274:51, 1995.

Chapter 20

INFERTILITY

Robert L. Barbieri

■ CHAPTER OUTLINE

KEY POINTS

- The fertility potential of a couple is best described by an estimate of the chance that the couple will become pregnant in any given menstrual cycle—the fecundability of the couple.
- In infertile couples, the reproductive diseases that are commonly diagnosed include ovulatory disorders (27 percent of couples), abnormal semen parameter (25 percent), tubal defect (22 percent), endometriosis (5 percent), other (4 percent), and unexplained (17 percent).
- A midluteal serum progesterone concentration less than 10 ng/ml is associated with a lower per cycle pregnancy rate than is a midluteal progesterone concentration greater than 10 ng/ml.
- In some women with nonclassic 21-hydroxylase deficiency, treatment with clomiphene will induce ovulation and result in successful pregnancy.
- In women with hypogonadotropic anovulatory infertility, treatment with gonadotropins often results in a monthly fecundability greater than that observed in a normal population.
- The success of both clomiphene and gonadotropin is dependent on the age of the female partner.
- Cycle day 3 serum FSH concentration is an important predictor of fecundability.
- Tubal factor infertility is often treated with either surgical pelvic reconstruction or in vitro fertilization.
- Empirical treatment of infertility involves stimulation of multiple follicles (with clomiphene or gonadotropins) and placement of sperm high in the reproductive tract (intrauterine insemination). Observational studies suggest that empirical treatment of infertility is associated with a higher fecundability than is expectant management.
- Of the fertility treatments available, in vitro fertilization offers the highest fecundability across a wide spectrum of reproductive tract diseases.

Fertility is defined as the capacity to conceive and produce offspring. Infertility is the state of a diminished capacity to conceive and bear offspring. In contrast to sterility, infertility is not an irreversible state. The current *clinical* definition of infertility is the inability to conceive after 12 months of frequent coitus. Among married couples in the United States aged 15 to 44 years, approximately 13 percent reported that they were infertile in surveys conducted in both 1965 and 1985.[1] In the late 1980s, this represented approximately 5 million couples.

A STATISTICAL MODEL OF INFERTILITY

The clinical definition of infertility is relatively crude because it does not reflect the wide range of fertility potential in couples who have not conceived after 12 months. The clinical definition of infertility implies the existence of a dichotomous state: either a pregnancy is achieved in 12 months (infertility is not present) or a pregnancy is not achieved in 12 months and, by definition, infertility is present. The current clinical definition of infertility is similar to analyzing a continuous variable, such as height, by using a dichotomous variable, short and tall. It is clear that height is much better described by a continuous measure, such as centimeters, rather than by a dichotomous variable such as short and tall.

Our clinical approach to fertility and infertility would be best advanced by the use of the concept of fecundability. Fecundability is the probability of achieving a pregnancy in one menstrual cycle (approximately 0.25 in healthy young couples). A related concept, fecundity, is the ability to achieve a pregnancy that results in a livebirth in one menstrual cycle. Fecundability, a population estimate of the probability of achieving pregnancy in one menstrual cycle, is a valuable clinical and scientific concept because it creates a framework for the quantitative analysis of fertility potential. On the basis of the clinical characteristics of an infertile couple, the estimated fecundability may range from 0.00 in the case of a couple with an azoospermic male partner to approximately 0.04 in the case of an infertile couple in which the female partner has early-stage endometriosis. In addition, fecundability provides a convenient quantitative estimate of the efficacy of various fertility treatments. An infertile couple with an estimated fecundability of 0.04 may have the choice of two approaches to the treatment of infertility: a low-cost treatment that will increase fecundability to 0.08, or an expensive treatment that will increase fecundability to 0.25. A clear quantitative presentation of the potential effect of each treatment on fecundability should assist the couple in choosing an optimal treatment plan. Clinical care for the infertile couple would be significantly advanced if all discussions of infertility used the concept of fecundability. In this chapter, the terms fecundability and per cycle pregnancy rate are both used to mean the proportion of couples achieving pregnancy in one cycle. The concept of fecundability can be used to derive a simple statistical description of the fertility process.

Fecundability (f) is defined as the probability of conceiving during any one cycle. The probability of failing to conceive during any one cycle is $1 - f$. During a short period of time, the fecundability of a couple is often stable.[2] For a large group of couples, the probability of conception is f for the first month, $f \times (1 - f)$ for the second month, $f \times (1 - f)^2$ for the third month, and $f \times (1 - f)^{N-1}$ for the nth month. With use of this model, the mean number of months required to achieve conception is 1/f. The cumulative probability of conception, F, through month N is calculated as follows:

$$F = 1 - (1 - f)^N$$

On the basis of this simple statistical model, assuming a normal menstrual cycle fecundability of 0.25 and starting with 100 couples, approximately 98 couples should conceive within 13 cycles. If each cycle is 28 days, then 98 percent of couples should conceive within one calendar year (13 cycles × 28 days/cycle = 364 days).

In a population of infertile couples, the overall population fecundability is a function of the per cycle pregnancy rate of each couple. During short periods of follow-up, the population behaves in a statistically stable manner, with a fixed proportion of the cohort becoming pregnant with each additional cycle of follow-up. However, as the follow-up is extended, the fecundability of most populations appears to decline, and the cumulative pregnancy rate approaches an asymptote that is less than 100 percent. It is likely that this is due to heterogeneity in the fecundability of the initial population. The couples with the highest pregnancy rate are rapidly culled from the population (they became pregnant), leaving the couples with the more severe infertility problem in the residual pool. Conceptually, this issue can be managed by assuming that there is an asymptote to the cumulative pregnancy rate of the population or by using complex mathematical modeling of the population fecundability based on the assumption that couples in the population have a range of per cycle pregnancy rates. This issue is of special importance in the analysis of fertility rates in populations for long periods of time, such as 2 years. This issue is of less practical importance in studies in which the time period for analysis is three cycles or less.

The simple statistical model of fertility presented here assumes that the fecundability of a population is relatively stable during a short time. Many studies suggest that the observed fecundability of a population diminishes with long-term follow-up of the population. For example, Guttmacher[3] assessed the number of months to conception in 5574 women who achieved pregnancy between 1946 and 1956. During the first 3 months of observation, the fecundability was 0.25. During the next 9 months of observation, the fecundability was 0.15. A similar observation has been made by Zinaman and colleagues[4] and Wilcox and associates.[5] Zinaman and colleagues[4] studied 200 healthy couples who desired to conceive. During the first 3 months of observation, the fecundability was 0.25. During the next 9 months of observation, the fecundability was 0.11 (Table 20–1). The drop in fecundability suggests that each large population consists of a heterogeneous mixture of couples.

■ TABLE 20–1

Observational Studies Often Demonstrate That the Fecundability of the Cohort Decreases as Follow-Up Progresses

CYCLE	NUMBER OF WOMEN AVAILABLE FOR STUDY AT START OF CYCLE	NUMBER OF PREGNANCIES IN CYCLE	PER CYCLE PREGNANCY RATE
1	200	59	0.30
2	137	41	0.30
3	95	16	0.17
4	78	12	0.15
5	66	14	0.21
6	52	4	0.08
7	48	5	0.10
8	43	3	0.07
9	40	2	0.05
10	38	1	0.03
11	37	2	0.05
12	35	1	0.03

From Zinaman MJ, Clegg ED, Brown CC, et al. Estimates of human fertility and pregnancy loss. Fertil Steril 65:503–509, 1996. Reprinted with permission of the American Society for Reproductive Medicine.

■ TABLE 20–2

Pregnancy Occurrence and Outcome During 3 Consecutive Menstrual Cycles in 200 Healthy Couples Desiring Pregnancy*

	CYCLE NUMBERS			
CYCLE OUTCOME	1	2	3	TOTAL
Not pregnant at start of cycle	200	137	95	
Pregnant during cycle	59	41	16	116
Chemical pregnancy	7	7	1	15
Spontaneous abortion	12	5	4	21
Livebirths	40	29	10	79
Dropped out, not pregnant	4	1	1	6
Lost to follow-up			1	

* Age of female partner was 30.6 ± 3.3 years (mean ± SD).

From Zinaman MJ, Clegg ED, Brown CC, et al. Estimates of human fertility and pregnancy loss. Fertil Steril 65:503–509, 1996. Reprinted with permission of the American Society for Reproductive Medicine.

Some couples have completely normal fertility and achieve pregnancy at a high rate (0.25 per cycle). The remaining couples have a lower fecundability (ranging from 0.00 to 0.15). Some of the couples in this pool will eventually present to a clinician for the treatment of infertility.

Unfortunately, not all pregnancies produce a livebirth. Many pregnancies are lost soon after implantation. The terms occult pregnancy and chemical pregnancy are often used to describe these early pregnancy losses. Occult pregnancy was defined by Bloch[6] as a pregnancy that terminates so soon after implantation that there was no clinical suspicion of its existence. In one study, approximately 13 percent of pregnancies were occult. A chemical pregnancy typically occurs in the presence of a clinical suspicion that a pregnancy may exist. A blood human chorionic gonadotropin (hCG) assay demonstrates the presence of a pregnancy, but before the loss of the pregnancy, no clinical evidence of the pregnancy is detectable by ultrasound examination. Of all clinical pregnancies, approximately 20 percent result in a spontaneous abortion. Of all pregnancies, approximately 30 percent are lost as occult, chemical, or clinical spontaneous abortions[4] (Table 20–2).

DISEASES THAT CAUSE OR ARE ASSOCIATED WITH INFERTILITY

Pregnancy is the result of the successful completion of a complex series of physiologic events occurring in both the male and female that allows the implantation of an embryo in the endometrium (Fig. 20–1). At a minimum, pregnancy requires ovulation and the production of a competent oocyte, production of a competent sperm, proximity of the sperm and oocyte in the reproductive tract, transport of the embryo into the uterine cavity, and implantation of the embryo into the endometrium. Many disease processes can result in subfertility. Some diseases, such as those that cause azoospermia, clearly have a *cause-effect relationship* with infertility. For other disease processes, such as stage I endometriosis, it is not clear that there is a cause-effect relationship between the disease and the infertile state. In these situations, it is preferable to state that there is an *association* between the disease condition and the infertile state but that causality has not been definitively established. Because of the limits of our current understanding of fertility in humans, it is often difficult to categorize disease conditions as either causal factors (azoospermia) or associated factors (stage I endometriosis) of infertility. Consequently, a discussion of the distribution of reproductive diseases that are diagnosed in infertile couples is not necessarily based on hard scientific data; rather, descriptive observations and assumptions are made about which diseases might *cause* or might be *associated with* infertility.

Most tabulations of the medical conditions that "cause" infertility divide the problem into male factors and female factors. The World Health Organization (WHO) task force on Diagnosis and Treatment of Infertility conducted a study of 8500 infertile couples using a standardized diagnostic protocol.[7] In developed countries, diseases that were identified as contributing to the infertile state were attributed to the female partner in 37 percent of couples, to the male partner in 8 percent of couples, and to both partners in 35 percent of couples. Five percent of the couples had no identifiable cause of infertility (unexplained infertility), and 15 percent of the couples became pregnant during the investigation. The diseases in the female partner most often identified were ovulatory disorders (25 percent), pelvic adhesions (12 percent), tubal occlusion (11 percent), other tubal abnormalities (11 percent), hyperprolactinemia (7 percent), and endometriosis (15 percent); no disease was identifiable in 20 percent. In a review of 21 published reports containing 14,141 infertile couples, Collins[8] reported that the primary diagnoses in the couples were ovulatory disorders (27 percent), abnormal semen parameter (25 percent), tubal defect (22 percent), endometriosis (5 percent), other (4 percent), and unexplained (17 percent) (Fig. 20–2). These observations can be broadly grouped into five major conditions that influence fecundability:

1. abnormalities in the production of a competent oocyte (ovulatory factor or depletion of the oocyte pool);
2. abnormalities in reproductive tract transport of the sperm, oocyte, and embryo (tubal, uterine, cervical, and peritoneal factors);
3. abnormalities in the implantation process including early defects in embryo development and embryo-endometrial interaction (embryo-endometrial factors);
4. abnormalities of sperm production (male factor); and

■ TABLE 20–3

Initial Laboratory Approach to the Infertile Couple

Primary Tests for Infertility

Documentation of competent ovulation
- Midluteal progesterone concentration >10 ng/ml
- Day 3 follicle-stimulating hormone concentration (if female partner >35 yr)

Semen analysis
- Volume 2 to 6 ml
- Concentration >20 million/ml
- Motility >50%
- Morphology >40%

Documentation of tubal patency
- Hysterosalpingogram

Secondary Tests for Infertility

Laparoscopy
Postcoital test
Endometrial biopsy

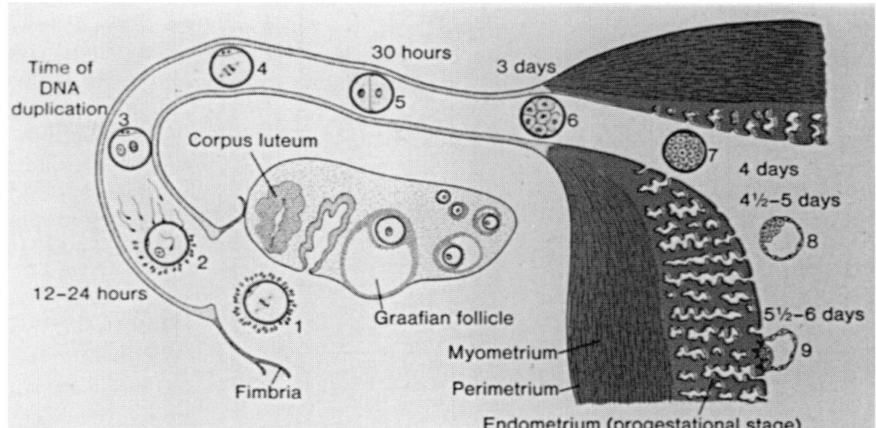

Figure 20–1 ■ Schematic representation of the transport of the oocyte, sperm, and embryo in the female reproductive tract.

5. other conditions including immunologic factors that can affect multiple components of the process.

The initial infertility evaluation focuses on these five major processes (Table 20–3).

ABNORMALITIES IN OOCYTE PRODUCTION

Disorders of oocyte production are the most common cause of female infertility. Anovulation is typically associated with amenorrhea or severe oligomenorrhea. Oligo-ovulation is typically associated with oligomenorrhea (cycle lengths greater than 35 days).

Women who have monthly menses and report moliminal symptoms such as breast tenderness and dysmenorrhea are typically ovulatory. The least expensive "laboratory" method for detecting ovulation is the measurement of the basal body temperature. For most women, the morning basal temperature obtained before rising from bed is below 98°F before ovulation and above 98°F after ovulation. Progesterone production from the ovary appears to raise the hypothalamic set-point for basal temperature by approximately 0.6°F. The normal luteal phase is typically associated with a temperature rise, above 98°F, for at least 10 days in length. On occasion, basal body temperature recordings may appear monophasic even in the presence of ovulation. A biphasic pattern is almost always associated with ovulation. If the pattern is biphasic, coitus can be recommended every other day for a period including the 5 days before and the day of ovulation[9] (Fig. 20–3).

A serum progesterone level greater than 3 ng/ml is diagnostic of ovulation. Luteal-phase progesterone is pulsatile owing to the pulsatile nature of luteinizing hormone (LH) secretion.[10] At a conceptual level, the pulsatile nature of progesterone secretion may make it difficult to reliably use a single progesterone measurement as a marker for the adequacy of ovulation. However, in most clinical situations, a single midluteal progesterone measurement appears to be a useful marker of the adequacy of ovulation. Hull and colleagues[11] have suggested that a midluteal progesterone concentration less than 10 ng/ml is associated with a lower per cycle pregnancy rate than are progesterone levels above 10 ng/ml. Endometrial biopsy that demonstrates secretory changes is another method of definitively diagnosing ovulation and making an estimate of the adequacy of both luteal progesterone secretion and endometrial response to progesterone. Because the endometrial biopsy is invasive, it is typically reserved for the diagnosis of luteal-phase defect or other defects in endometrial receptivity. It is likely that endometrial proteins that can serve as clinically useful markers of endometrial receptivity will be identified in the near future[12] (see Chapter 8).

Some authorities have suggested that a follicle may luteinize and differentiate into a corpus luteum (secreting progesterone and inducing a secretory endometrium) without rupturing and allowing the oocyte to escape the follicle.[13] The "luteinized unruptured follicle syndrome" may occur occasionally, but it is not clear that it is a major cause of infertility.[14, 15]

Sonographic examination of the ovary and measurement of LH can be used as indirect markers of ovulation. During

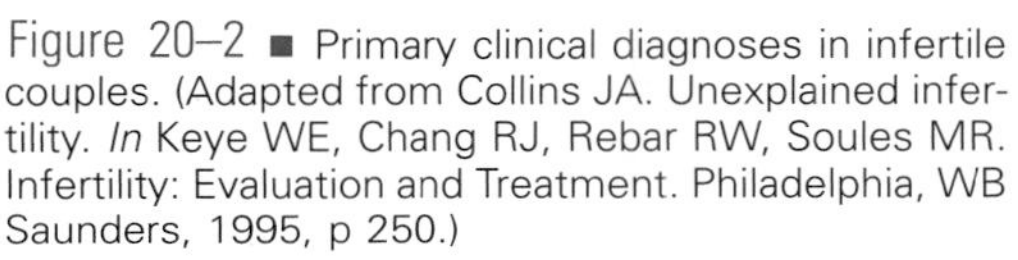

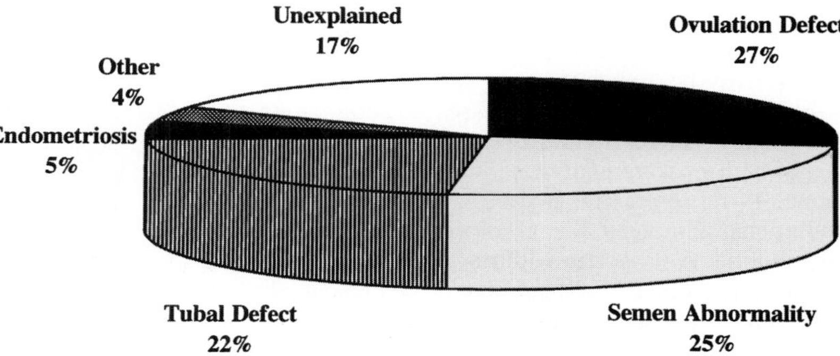

Figure 20–2 ■ Primary clinical diagnoses in infertile couples. (Adapted from Collins JA. Unexplained infertility. *In* Keye WE, Chang RJ, Rebar RW, Soules MR. Infertility: Evaluation and Treatment. Philadelphia, WB Saunders, 1995, p 250.)

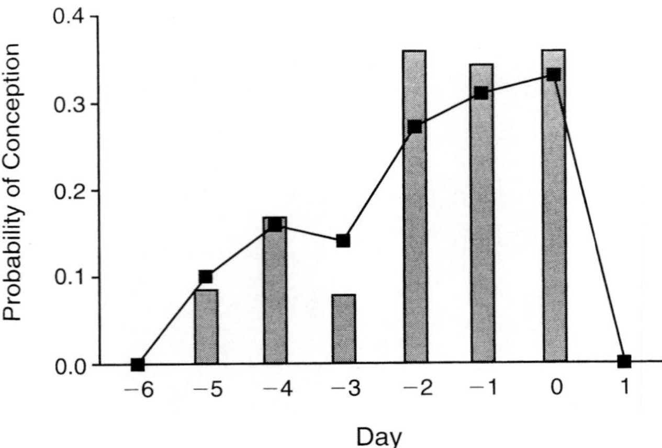

Figure 20–3 ■ Probability of conception on specific days near the day of ovulation. The bars represent data reported by 129 women who had sexual intercourse on only 1 day in the 6-day interval ending on the day of ovulation (day 0). The solid line shows the probability of conception based on a statistical analysis of data from 625 cycles. (From Wilcox AJ, Weinberg CR, Baird DD. Timing of sexual intercourse in relation to ovulation. N Engl J Med 333:1517–1521, 1995. Reproduced by permission of The New England Journal of Medicine. © 1995, Massachusetts Medical Society.)

menses, the follicles in the ovary are approximately 4 mm in diameter. Before ovulation, the dominant follicle reaches a diameter in the range of 20 to 25 mm. Demonstration of follicle growth and rupture of the dominant follicle is presumptive evidence that ovulation has occurred. The demonstration of an LH surge is also presumptive evidence of ovulatory cycles. Ovulation typically occurs 34 to 36 hours after the onset of the LH surge and approximately 10 to 12 hours after the LH peak.

Anovulation

Many diseases can cause anovulation and infertility. The most common causes of adult-onset anovulation are hypothalamic dysfunction (38 percent of cases), pituitary disease (17 percent), and ovarian dysfunction (45 percent).[16, 17] The most common causes of hypothalamic dysfunction are abnormalities in weight and body composition, stress, and strenuous exercise. Less common causes of hypothalamic dysfunction are infiltrating diseases of the hypothalamus such as lymphoma and histiocytosis. The most common pituitary disorder that causes anovulation is prolactinoma, followed by empty sella syndrome, Sheehan's syndrome, and Cushing's disease. The most common ovarian causes of anovulation are ovarian failure (depletion of the oocyte pool) and ovarian hyperandrogenism (polycystic ovary syndrome [PCOS]) (see Chapter 17). Thyroid disease can occasionally be associated with anovulation.

Evaluation of the various causes of anovulation can be complex. Typically, measurement of body weight and height and measurement of serum follicle-stimulating hormone (FSH), prolactin, thyroid-stimulating hormone, and androgens, if indicated, can help identify the cause of the anovulation. A progestin withdrawal test may be helpful to evaluate the degree of hypogonadism present. This may help guide treatment choices.[18]

Patients with anovulation have the greatest success with infertility therapy.[19] Treatment of anovulatory disorders can result in fecundability similar to that observed in normal couples (0.15 to 0.25). The choice of treatment is dependent on the cause of the anovulation. Common treatment choices include (1) dietary interventions to modulate weight, (2) clomiphene citrate, (3) clomiphene plus other hormone adjuvants, (4) gonadotropin treatment, (5) pulsatile gonadotropin-releasing hormone (GnRH), (6) bromocriptine, and (7) glucocorticoids.

Weight Abnormalities Associated with Anovulation

Anovulation, oligo-ovulation, and subfertility are commonly observed in women above or below their ideal body weight.[20] In one study of 597 cases of women with anovulatory infertility and 1695 fertile control subjects, obese women (body mass index greater than 27 kg/m^2) had a relative risk of anovulatory infertility of 3.1 compared with women of body mass index 20 to 25 kg/m^2. Women with a body mass index less than 17 kg/m^2 had a relative risk of anovulatory infertility of 1.6. The investigators concluded that the risk of ovulatory infertility is highest in obese women but is also increased in underweight and moderately obese women.[21]

Anovulatory women far below their ideal body weight often have hypogonadotropic hypogonadism. Anovulatory women far above their ideal body weight often have PCOS. For women who are far below (hypogonadotropic hypogonadism) or far above (PCOS) their ideal body weight, appropriate management of dietary intake may be associated with resumption of ovulation. For example, Pasquali and colleagues[22] demonstrated that anovulation in obese women with PCOS could be successfully treated with weight loss. Obese women with anovulation and PCOS were prescribed a diet of 1000 to 1500 calories for 6 months. The mean weight loss was 10 kg. After weight loss, there was a 45 percent decrease in basal LH concentration and a 35 percent decrease in serum testosterone. Many of the women resumed ovulation and became pregnant. Similar results were reported by Clark and colleagues.[23] Thirteen obese anovulatory infertile women were entered into a program of diet and exercise and lost on average 6.3 kg during 6 months. Fasting insulin and testosterone decreased and sex hormone–binding globulin concentrations increased. Of the 13 subjects, 12 resumed ovulation and 5 became pregnant without any other intervention.

Some women with hypogonadotropic hypogonadism have low body mass index, high-fiber low-fat diets,[24] or intense exercise regimens.[25] When these women present with anovulatory infertility, they are often reluctant to gain weight, alter their diet, or reduce their exercise regimen. It is likely that spontaneous ovulation could be achieved in some of these women by lifestyle changes. Pulsatile GnRH can be used to induce ovulation in these women, and pregnancy rates tend to be high. Abraham and colleagues[26] studied 14 women with hypogonadotropic hypogonadism associated with eating disorders or intensive exercise programs; 12 women became pregnant when they were treated with pulsatile GnRH. One risk of inducing ovulation and pregnancy before correcting body composition is low-birthweight infants. Abraham and colleagues[26] reported that in their study, 20 percent of the newborns had low birth weight (<2500 gm).

CLOMIPHENE

Clomiphene, a nonsteroidal estrogen agonist/antagonist, was synthesized in 1956, reported to be effective in the induction of ovulation by Greenblatt[27] in 1961, and approved by the Food and Drug Administration in 1967. Clomiphene is a triphenylethylene derivative related to tamoxifen and diethylstilbestrol. Clomiphene citrate is marketed as a racemic mixture of *trans* (enclomiphene) and *cis* (zuclomiphene) in a ratio of approximately 3 to 2. The *cis* isomer may have greater ovulation-inducing properties than the *trans* isomer.[28]

Clomiphene has a half-life of approximately 5 days. Clomiphene is metabolized by the liver and excreted in the feces. Fecal clomiphene can be detected up to 6 weeks after discontinuation of the drug. Clomiphene has both estrogen antagonist and agonist effects. In hypoestrogenic women, clomiphene and tamoxifen are associated with an increase in high-density lipoprotein cholesterol concentration, an "estrogen agonist" effect.[29] Clomiphene probably induces ovulation by binding to hypothalamic estrogen receptors, creating a hypoestrogenic state in the hypothalamus that results in an increase in GnRH pulse frequency, in turn increasing FSH and LH secretion. Successful induction of ovulation with clomiphene requires an intact hypothalamic-pituitary-ovarian axis. This contrasts with exogenous gonadotropin treatment, which can be effective in the absence of a functional hypothalamus or pituitary.

Evidence that clomiphene has central nervous system effects includes the observation that clomiphene (1) induces vasomotor symptoms,[30] (2) increases LH pulse frequency,[31] and (3) partially blocks the contraceptive potency of estrogen.[32] Studies in laboratory animals demonstrate that clomiphene can decrease estrogen-stimulated hypothalamic tyrosine hydroxylase[33] and that clomiphene increases GnRH secretion from the rat medial basal hypothalamus.[34]

In addition to a hypothalamic site of action, clomiphene also has biologic effects on the pituitary, ovary, endometrium, and cervix. Adashi and colleagues[35] demonstrated that in incubations of rat pituitary cells, both estradiol and clomiphene augmented GnRH-induced release of FSH and LH. Zhuang and coworkers[36] demonstrated that clomiphene, estradiol, and diethylstilbestrol all augmented gonadotropin induction of aromatase activity in rat granulosa cells. In hypoestrogenic women receiving exogenous estrogen, clomiphene can cause endometrial atrophy.[28] Clomiphene can decrease estrogen-induced cervical mucus quantity and quality, as demonstrated by decreased ferning and spinnbarkeit formation.[37, 38]

For clinical purposes, the WHO classification divides women with anovulation into two major groups. WHO group I consists of those women with anovulation, low levels of endogenous gonadotropins, and little endogenous estrogen production. WHO group II consists of those women with anovulation or oligo-ovulation, a wide variety of menstrual disorders, relatively normal (or elevated) gonadotropin levels, and evidence for significant endogenous estrogen production.[39] Clomiphene is most effective in inducing ovulation in women in WHO group II. In women with severe hypoestrogenism and hypogonadotropic hypogonadism (WHO group I), clomiphene is often ineffective in the induction of ovulation. Failure to have a withdrawal uterine bleed after the administration of progesterone is presumptive evidence of severe hypoestrogenism in women with anovulation and an anatomically normal uterus.[40] In women with no withdrawal uterine bleeding after progesterone administration, clomiphene is unlikely to effectively induce ovulation.[40] Clomiphene citrate induction of ovulation is unlikely to be effective in women with an FSH concentration greater than 20 mIU/ml (depletion of oocyte pool). Clomiphene is relatively contraindicated in women with pituitary tumors. However, clomiphene has been reported to be effective in the induction of ovulation in women with prolactinomas who did not ovulate with bromocriptine treatment.[41] Many physicians prefer to document tubal patency and evaluate semen parameters before initiating ovulation induction.

The Food and Drug Administration–approved dosages for clomiphene are 50 or 100 mg daily for a maximum of 5 days per cycle. After spontaneous menses, or the induction of menses with a progestin withdrawal, clomiphene is started on cycle day 3, 4, or 5 at 50 mg daily for 5 days. Starting clomiphene on cycle day 3 or 5 does not appear to influence the cycle pregnancy rate.[42] In properly chosen women, approximately 50 percent will ovulate at the 50-mg daily dosage. Another 25 percent will ovulate if the dose is increased to 100 mg daily.[43] During each cycle, determination of ovulation should be attempted. In most patients, ovulation occurs approximately 5 to 12 days after the last dose of clomiphene. Measurement of the urinary LH surge is often recommended to assist the couple in prospectively determining the periovulatory interval.

Although the Food and Drug Administration has approved maximal clomiphene doses of 100 mg daily, many clinicians have experience using clomiphene at doses of up to 250 mg daily. Women who fail to ovulate at clomiphene doses of 100 mg daily for 5 days may ovulate if they are treated with clomiphene at doses up to 250 mg daily for up to 14 days. Of the women who fail to ovulate at doses of 100 mg daily, up to 70 percent will ovulate at higher doses, but less that 30 percent become pregnant.[44]

Anovulatory women in WHO group II have a fecundability of 0.00 without treatment. During the first three to six cycles of clomiphene treatment, the fecundability is in the range of 0.08 to 0.25. Infertile couples in which the only infertility factor is anovulation in the female partner have a fecundability with clomiphene treatment in the range of 0.20 to 0.25[45] (Fig. 20–4). A unique advantage of clomiphene is that few fertility treatments are available that increase fecundability from 0.00 to 0.20 at a cost in the range of $100. After 3 to 6 months of clomiphene treatment, fecundability appears to decline.

Preliminary reports suggest that ovulation-inducing medications may be associated with ovarian tumors[46, 47] and that the risk may increase with extended use of ovulation-inducing agents. My current view of these data is that infertility is a more important risk factor for ovarian tumors than is treatment with an ovulation-inducing medication.[48] However, given the reduced fecundability observed in women who fail to achieve pregnancy after six clomiphene cycles and the potential risk of ovarian tumors associated

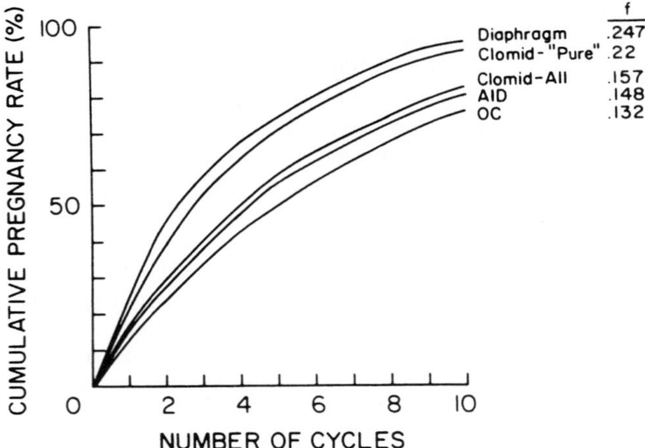

Figure 20–4 ■ Cumulative pregnancy rates in women treated with clomiphene for infertility, women discontinuing contraception with the diaphragm or oral contraceptives (OC), and women treated with donor insemination (AID). f, Fecundability, or pre-cycle pregnancy rate. (From Hammond MG. Monitoring techniques for improved pregnancy rates during clomiphene ovulation induction. Fertil Steril 42:499–509, 1984. Reproduced with permission of the American Society for Reproductive Medicine.)

with prolonged exposure to clomiphene, it is reasonable to limit clomiphene treatment to less than 12 cycles. Failure to achieve pregnancy after six clomiphene treatment cycles should prompt a thorough review of the potential causes of the failure and consideration of a new approach to treatment, such as gonadotropin therapy.

The combination of clomiphene plus a single dose of hCG may increase the efficacy of clomiphene induction of ovulation when women fail to ovulate with standard doses of clomiphene.[49] After administration of the clomiphene, sonography can be used to monitor follicle size. When mean follicle diameter becomes at least 17 mm, hCG can be administered.[50]

Clomiphene treatment can be associated with adverse changes in the reproductive tract including induction of a luteal-phase defect and the creation of a hostile cervical environment due to low quantity and quality of cervical mucus.[51] Some clinicians recommend endometrial biopsy in a test cycle of clomiphene treatment to assess whether clomiphene induces luteal-phase deficiency. Many clinicians recommend that a postcoital test be performed during the first clomiphene cycle.

In one study of 2369 clomiphene-induced pregnancies, 7 percent were twins, 0.5 percent were triplets, 0.3 percent were quadruplets, and 0.13 percent were quintuplets.[52] This demonstrates that the absolute risk of high-order multiple gestation with clomiphene treatment is low. However, because clomiphene is a heavily prescribed medication, the number of triplets resulting from clomiphene treatment is substantial. In one study that reviewed all the high-order multiple gestations at one tertiary care center, more triplets were conceived after clomiphene treatment than after treatment with exogenous gonadotropin therapy.[53] The rate of spontaneous abortion after clomiphene-induced ovulation and pregnancy is approximately 15 percent.[54] The most common symptoms experienced by women taking clomiphene include vasomotor symptoms (20 percent), adnexal tenderness (5 percent), nausea (3 percent), headache (1 percent), and rarely blurring of vision or scotomas. Most clinicians permanently discontinue clomiphene treatment in women with clomiphene-induced visual changes.

CLOMIPHENE PLUS GLUCOCORTICOID INDUCTION OF OVULATION

Anovulatory women in WHO group II with dehydroepiandrosterone sulfate (DHEA-S) levels above the midnormal range (approximately 2 μg/ml) appear to have reduced ovulation and pregnancy rates when they are treated with clomiphene. Some studies suggest that treatment with clomiphene plus glucocorticoid improves pregnancy rates in these women. Daly and colleagues[55] randomized 64 anovulatory infertile women to receive either clomiphene 50 mg daily on cycle days 5 to 9 or clomiphene plus 0.5 mg dexamethasone daily. If ovulation did not occur, clomiphene was increased 50 mg daily per cycle up to 150 mg daily. The investigators observed significantly higher rates of ovulation and conception in the women who received clomiphene plus dexamethasone. The impact of the combined therapy was especially marked in the women with DHEA-S concentrations above 2.0 μg/ml. Of the women with a DHEA-S concentration greater than 2.0 μg/ml, 12 were randomized to receive clomiphene alone, and 13 were randomized to receive clomiphene plus dexamethasone. Among the women receiving clomiphene alone, 6 (50 percent) ovulated and 4 (33 percent) conceived. Among the women receiving clomiphene plus dexamethasone, 13 (100 percent) ovulated and 11 (85 percent) conceived.

INFLUENCE OF THYROID HORMONES ON CLOMIPHENE INDUCTION OF OVULATION

Women with hypogonadotropic hypogonadism and low endogenous production of estrogen are resistant to induction of ovulation with clomiphene. The mechanisms responsible for the low rate of ovulation in response to clomiphene are not fully characterized. Maruo and colleagues[56] have reported that clomiphene induction of ovulation has a low chance of success in women with triiodothyronine levels below 80 ng/ml. In preliminary studies, thyroid hormone supplementation appeared to increase the efficacy of clomiphene induction of ovulation in these women.

CLOMIPHENE AND NONCLASSIC ADRENAL HYPERPLASIA

Many authorities recommend that infertile anovulatory women with nonclassic adrenal hyperplasia receive glucocorticoids for induction of ovulation. However, some women with long-standing nonclassic adrenal hyperplasia also have evidence of ovarian hyperandrogenism and polycystic ovaries by sonographic imaging. Clomiphene alone[57] or clomiphene plus glucocorticoids[58] can be used to induce ovulation and achieve pregnancy in infertile women with nonclassic adrenal hyperplasia.

CLOMIPHENE PLUS GONADOTROPIN INDUCTION OF OVULATION

In women who fail to ovulate with standard doses of clomiphene citrate, gonadotropin injections can be added to clomiphene treatment to induce ovulation.[59] The main benefit of this approach to ovulation induction is that it tends to reduce the quantity of gonadotropins needed to induce ovulation during each cycle. The initial rise in LH and FSH induced by clomiphene increases the sensitivity of the follicles to respond to the gonadotropin injections. Typically, clomiphene at doses of 100 to 200 mg daily is administered for 5 days, followed by the initiation of FSH or LH/FSH injections. Investigators have reported that this regimen is associated with a 50 percent decrease in the dose of gonadotropin required to induce ovulation.[60]

GONADOTROPIN INDUCTION OF OVULATION

In 1958, Gemzell and associates[61] reported the efficacy of pituitary extracts of FSH to induce ovulation. In 1962, Lunenfeld and colleagues[62] described the efficacy of extracts of urinary gonadotropins from menopausal women to induce ovulation. Since these two pioneering reports, the trend in the use of gonadotropin therapy for ovulation induction has been to continually improve the purity of the agents used. Currently, the two agents most commonly used to induce ovulation are highly purified preparations of FSH (Metrodin or Fertinex) and LH plus FSH derived from menopausal urine (Pergonal, Humegon, Repronex). Until recently, these urinary gonadotropin preparations were administered by intramuscular injections. A major advance in gonadotropin therapy has been the development of highly purified preparations of FSH that can be administered by subcutaneous injection. Urofollitropin (Fertinex) is a preparation of FSH purified from the urine of menopausal women by use of immunoaffinity chromatography. Urofollitropin is more than 95 percent pure and has less than 0.1 mIU/ml of LH activity for every 1000 IU of FSH activity. Recently, recombinant FSH (Gonal-F, Follistim) has been released for clinical use. Recombinant FSH is produced using genetically altered Chinese hamster ovary cell lines. The recombinant FSH is purified from the cultures using immunochromatography. The purified recombinant FSH contains a 92 amino acid α subunit and a 111 amino acid β subunit, indistinguishable from the native human FSH amino acid structure. The final purified product has a consistent isoform pattern and contains no LH bioactivity. Advances in DNA pharmacotechnology also make possible the production of novel chimeric gonadotropins with unique properties (e.g., an ultralong-acting FSH).

It is clear that FSH can be used as a single agent to induce ovulation in most women with anovulation. FSH is the primary hormone responsible for follicular recruitment and growth in the human. Experiments in monkeys in which LH is reduced to extremely low levels demonstrate that the administration of FSH stimulates follicular recruitment and growth but that estradiol production is suppressed.[63] It appears that most anovulatory women secrete enough LH so that no exogenous LH is required to achieve successful follicular growth and estradiol production. For most women in WHO group I, administration of exogenous hCG is required to effect final maturation of the follicle and trigger ovulation.

The main indications for gonadotropin induction of ovulation include (1) WHO group I patients with low levels of endogenous gonadotropins and little endogenous estrogen activity, (2) women with PCOS in whom clomiphene induction of ovulation fails, (3) women undergoing empirical ovarian hyperstimulation for treatment of unexplained infertility or early-stage endometriosis, and (4) women in programs of assisted reproduction such as in vitro fertilization (IVF). In anovulatory women treated with FSH, ovulation rates are greater than 80 percent per cycle, and pregnancy rates are in the range of 10 to 40 percent per cycle (Fig. 20–5). In a large group of hypoestrogenic women (WHO group I), Lunenfeld and Eshkol[64] reported a six-cycle cumulative pregnancy rate of 91 percent, which reflects an average fecundability of 0.33 (Fig. 20–6). This fecundability (0.33) is higher than that seen in the normal population in six cycles. The higher cycle fecundability achieved with gonadotropin therapy is probably due, in part, to the multifollicular development and multiple ovulations associated with gonadotropin treatment. The fecundability observed in gonadotropin treatment cycles is dependent on the age of the female partner and the underlying cause of the anovulation (Fig. 20–7; see also Figs. 20–5 and 20–6). Gonadotropin induction of ovulation is not recommended for women with primary ovarian failure and markedly elevated levels of FSH and LH production. In addition, because of the expense of gonadotropin treatment, most clinicians recommend the completion of a thorough infertility evaluation before gonadotropin therapy is initiated.

Ovulation induction with gonadotropin must be individualized to the specific clinical setting. Therapy is usually instituted 2 to 4 days after the completion of a short course of a progestin. In the first treatment cycle, most women in WHO group I are started on FSH or LH/FSH, 75 IU or 150 IU daily. This dosage is administered daily until cycle day 6 or 7, when serum estradiol is measured. If the estradiol level indicates an inadequate follicular response,

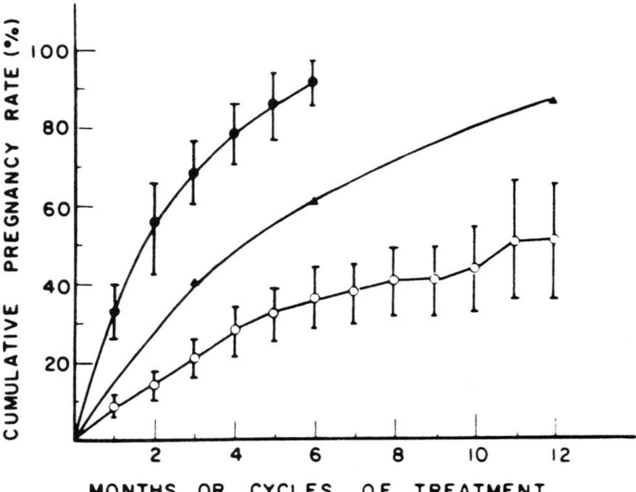

Figure 20–5 ■ Cumulative pregnancy rates for infertile anovulatory women treated with gonadotropins for ovulation induction. Solid circles represent the cumulative pregnancy rate in women in WHO group I. Open circles represent the cumulative pregnancy rate in women in WHO group II who have failed induction of ovulation with clomiphene. For comparison, the triangles represent the cumulative pregnancy rate in normal women. (From Dor J, Itzkowic DJ, Mashiach S. Cumulative pregnancy rates following gonadotropin therapy. Am J Obstet Gynecol 136:102–105, 1980.)

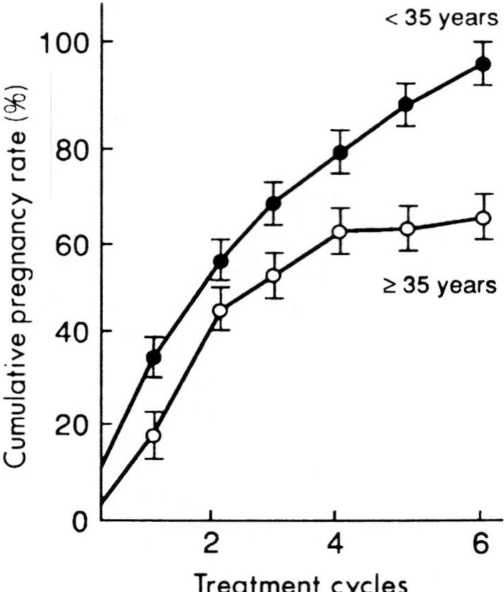

Figure 20–6 ■ Cumulative pregnancy rates for hypogonadotropic anovulatory women (WHO group I) treated with gonadotropins. Solid circles represent the cumulative pregnancy rate in women younger than 35 years. Open circles represent the cumulative pregnancy rate in women older than 35 years. (From Lunenfeld B, Insler V. Human gonadotropins. *In* Wallach EE, Zacur HA [eds]. Reproductive Medicine and Surgery. St. Louis, Mosby–Year Book, 1995, p 617.)

the dose of FSH or LH/FSH can be increased to 150 IU daily. If an adequate follicular response is obtained, no further increase in gonadotropin dose is warranted. Transvaginal ovarian sonography and estradiol measurements are performed sequentially until the mean diameter of the largest follicle is in the range of 16 to 18 mm, with a serum estradiol concentration of 150 to 250 pg/ml per large follicle. The target range for serum estradiol is approximately 500 to 1500 pg/ml[65, 66] (Fig. 20–8). If estradiol levels greater than 1500 pg/ml are achieved, the risk of ovarian hyperstimulation syndrome increases. Many clinicians cancel the cycle and do not administer hCG in this situation. When appropriate follicular size has been achieved, 5000 IU of hCG is administered, and ovulation is expected to occur approximately 36 hours after the injection. Some clinicians administer a second dose of hCG (2500 IU or 5000 IU) in the midluteal phase.[67, 68] Administration of a second dose of hCG in the midluteal phase clearly lengthens the luteal phase compared with a single dose of hCG (11 days versus 16 days), but its impact on fecundability is not clear.[67]

In women with PCOS, induction of ovulation with long-term low-dose FSH treatment appears to result in a high pregnancy rate with a low rate of complications such as high-order multiple gestation or ovarian hyperstimulation.[69] Homburg and coworkers[69] randomized 50 women with PCOS and infertility who failed to conceive with clomiphene to receive either conventional FSH treatment (75 IU daily and increasing by 75 IU every 5 or 6 days until follicle ripening has occurred) or low-dose FSH treatment (75 IU daily for 14 days of treatment and increasing by 37.5 IU every 7 days until follicular ripening was complete). The pregnancy rates were higher in the women who

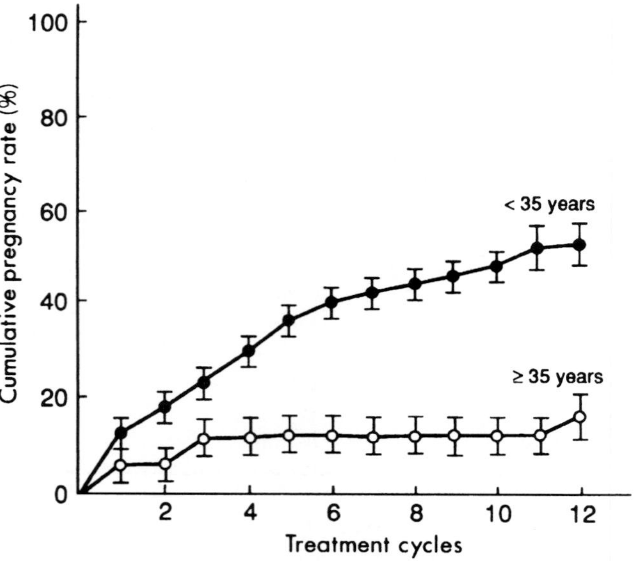

Figure 20–7 ■ Cumulative pregnancy rates after gonadotropin treatment for anovulatory women who did not respond to clomiphene induction of ovulation (WHO group II). Solid circles represent the cumulative pregnancy rate in women younger than 35 years. Open circles represent the cumulative pregnancy rate in women older than 35 years. (From Lunenfeld B, Insler V. Human gonadotropins. *In* Wallach EE, Zacur HA [eds]. Reproductive Medicine and Surgery. St. Louis, Mosby–Year Book, 1995, p 617.)

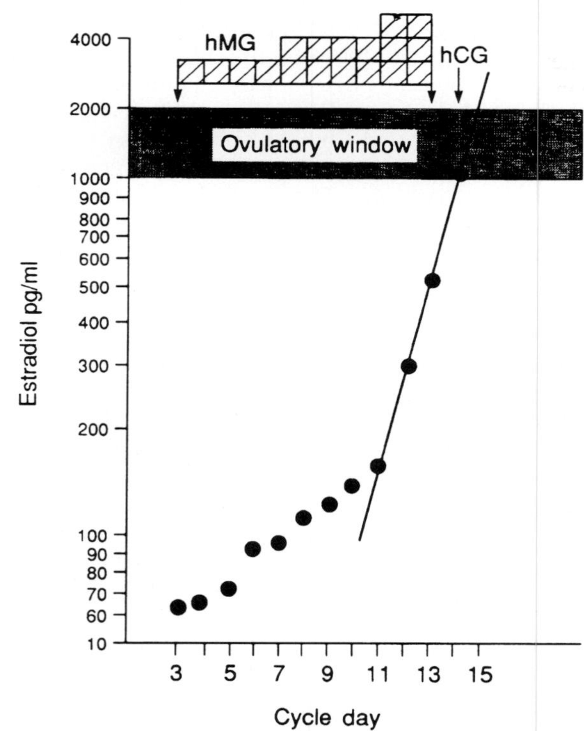

Figure 20–8 ■ Semilog plot of the 8 AM serum estradiol concentration in response to increasing 8 PM doses of gonadotropins. In this example, hCG was administered when the estradiol concentration reached 1000 pg/ml. (From Stillman RJ. Ovulation induction. *In* DeCherney AH [ed]. Reproductive Failure. New York, Churchill Livingstone, 1986.)

received long-term low-dose FSH compared with standard FSH treatment (40 percent versus 24 percent). Monofollicular development was achieved more frequently in the group that received long-term low-dose FSH compared with standard FSH treatment (74 percent vs 27 percent). There were fewer cases of high-order multiple gestation and ovarian stimulation in the group that received low doses of FSH. For women with PCOS who fail to conceive with clomiphene, long-term low-dose FSH treatment is an effective option. Compared with women in WHO group I, infertile anovulatory women with PCOS have lower fecundability with FSH or human menopausal gonadotropin (hMG) treatment. IVF has recently been demonstrated to be effective in treating infertile women with PCOS who fail to become pregnant with FSH or hMG.[70] In preliminary reports, IVF treatment of infertile women with PCOS is associated with a fecundability of 0.24 to 0.27.[71, 72]

During gonadotropin induction of ovulation, mild to moderate enlargement of the ovary occurs in as many as 20 percent of women. Some women treated with gonadotropins develop an increase in vascular permeability, which is associated with the accumulation of fluid in the peritoneal cavity and pleural space, the ovarian hyperstimulation syndrome (OHSS) (Table 20–4). Symptoms of OHSS include abdominal pain, abdominal distention, nausea, vomiting, diarrhea, and dyspnea. Physical and laboratory findings of OHSS include weight gain, ovarian enlargement, ascites, pleural effusion, hemoconcentration, electrolyte imbalances, renal dysfunction, and thrombosis.[73] Treatment includes bed rest, maintenance of intravascular volume, prophylaxis against thrombosis, and surgical correction of ovarian torsion. Before the use of repetitive estradiol measurements and sonographic evaluation of the follicular development, OHSS occurred in as many as 5 percent of women receiving gonadotropin treatment. In recent series, in which intense monitoring with estradiol measurement and sonography have been employed, approximately 0.5 percent of women treated with gonadotropins for ovulation induction have developed OHSS. OHSS may be more severe and have a longer course if a successful pregnancy occurs.

■ TABLE 20–4

A Classification System for Ovarian Hyperstimulation Syndrome

SEVERITY		SYMPTOMS AND SIGNS
Mild form	Stage A	Estradiol >2000 pg/ml
	Stage B	Estradiol >2000 pg/ml; plus enlarged ovaries, up to 6 cm in diameter
Moderate form	Stage A	Estradiol >4000 pg/ml; ovaries 6 to 12 cm
	Stage B	Ascites by ultrasonography; plus findings in stage A
Severe form	Stage A	Estradiol >6000 pg/ml; ovaries >12 cm in diameter; ascites; liver function abnormalities
	Stage B	Tension ascites; adult respiratory distress syndrome; shock; renal failure; thromboembolism

Adapted from Schenker JG. Ovarian hyperstimulation syndrome. *In* Wallach EE, Zacur HA (eds). Reproductive Medicine and Surgery. St. Louis, Mosby–Year Book, 1995, p 650.

Multiple births occur in approximately 15 percent of pregnancies that result after ovulation induction with gonadotropins.

GONADOTROPIN AND GnRH AGONIST ANALOGUE INDUCTION OF OVULATION

In women with PCOS, the elevated circulating concentration of LH may contribute to the growth of an excessive number of follicles and the production of high levels of estradiol during gonadotropin induction of ovulation.[74] The administration of a GnRH agonist analogue can suppress pituitary LH secretion and may be associated with gonadotropin treatment cycles in which the basal levels of androgens are suppressed and there is less premature luteinization of developing follicles.[75] Preliminary studies suggest that the combination of gonadotropin plus GnRH agonist treatment may reduce the spontaneous abortion rate compared with gonadotropin therapy alone.[76] In this study, the spontaneous abortion rate associated with gonadotropin-induced pregnancy was 39 percent. Treatment with gonadotropin plus GnRH agonist analogue was associated with a spontaneous abortion rate of 18 percent. One problem with the studies reported to date is that the doses of GnRH agonist analogue employed do not fully suppress LH secretion.

GONADOTROPIN AND GROWTH HORMONE INDUCTION OF OVULATION

Growth hormone, a major regulator of insulin-like growth factor type I, may be important in sensitizing the ovary to the actions of FSH and LH. Homburg and colleagues[77] reported that the combination of growth hormone (24 IU every other day) plus hMG reduced the number of ampules of hMG needed to induce ovulation compared with a regimen of hMG alone (24 versus 37 ampules). There was no difference in pregnancy rates between the two groups. Because there was no change in fecundability, the high cost of growth hormone does not warrant its widespread use as an adjuvant to gonadotropin treatment.

GnRH INDUCTION OF OVULATION

A key feature of hypothalamic biology is the pulsatile release of the decapeptide GnRH into the pituitary portal circulation. The pulsatile release of GnRH stimulates the pituitary to produce LH and FSH in a pulsatile manner. In turn, pituitary gonadotropin secretion stimulates follicular development, ovulation, and progesterone secretion in the luteal phase. In women with WHO group I anovulation (low levels of endogenous gonadotropins and low levels of endogenous estrogen production), the pulsatile administration of GnRH is effective in inducing ovulation (Fig. 20–9). The advantages of GnRH induction of ovulation include a reduced need for cycle monitoring and a reduced risk of multiple gestation due, in part, to an intact pituitary feedback system.

Santoro and colleagues[78] have proposed eight criteria for identifying women most likely to safely achieve ovulation with pulsatile GnRH: (1) primary or secondary amenorrhea for at least 6 months; (2) absence of hirsutism, galactorrhea, or ovarian enlargement; (3) weight not below 90 percent of ideal body weight; (4) no excessive exercise or

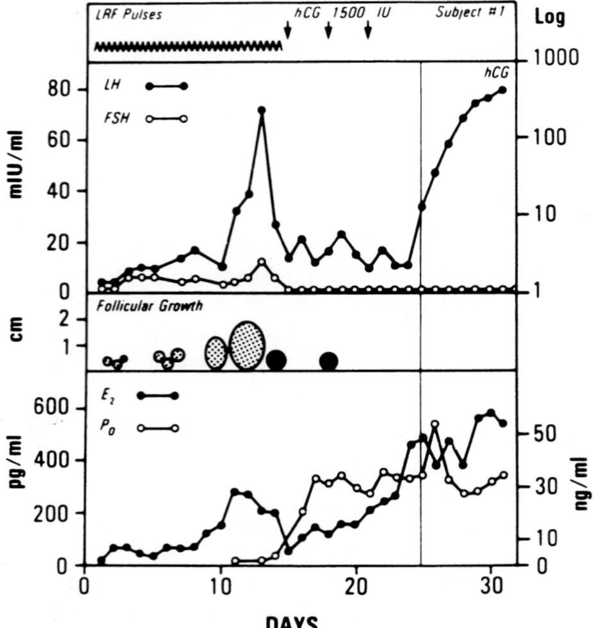

Figure 20–9 ■ Endocrine and ovarian follicular response to induction of ovulation with gonadotropin-releasing hormone, 5 μg intravenous bolus every 2 hours. LRF, gonadotropin-releasing hormone; hCG, human chorionic gonadotropin. (From Reid RL, Leopold GR, Yen SSC. Induction of ovulation and pregnancy with pulsatile luteinizing hormone releasing factor: Dosage and mode of delivery. Fertil Steril 36:553–559, 1981. Reproduced with permission of the American Society for Reproductive Medicine.)

stress; (5) normal serum concentrations of prolactin, thyroid-stimulating hormone, DHEA-S, and testosterone; (6) low gonadotropin concentrations; (7) no evidence for a structural central nervous system lesion; and (8) no recent hormone treatment. The GnRH is administered by use of a computerized pump that delivers one pulse of GnRH every 90 minutes at a dose of 75 to 100 ng/kg per pulse. Interpulse intervals as short as 1 hour[78] or as long as 2 hours[79] have been successfully used. GnRH doses as low as 25 ng/kg per pulse can successfully induce ovulation but are associated with subnormal luteal-phase progesterone secretion.[78] Both intravenous and subcutaneous routes of administration of GnRH have been successfully used to induce ovulation. Intravenous administration probably results in more reliable induction of ovulation but is associated with more technical problems (restarting the intravenous catheter) and a greater risk of infection than is subcutaneous administration.

The intensity of clinical monitoring can range from regular follicle monitoring with sonography plus serum estradiol measurements to basal body temperature measurement with use of an ovulation predictor kit. Low-intensity monitoring is acceptable because the risk of multiple pregnancy or ovarian hyperstimulation is low with pulsatile GnRH therapy. If no response is observed after 2 to 3 weeks of treatment, the GnRH dose per pulse can be increased to the range of 10 to 20 μg per pulse.[80]

Studies that directly compare the efficacy of gonadotropin versus pulsatile GnRH induction of ovulation report equivalent rates of ovulation and pregnancy. However, the risk of multiple gestation is probably higher with gonadotropin treatment (14 percent) than with pulsatile GnRH treatment (8 percent). This is due to a higher rate of multifollicular development with gonadotropin treatment (48 percent of cycles) than with pulsatile GnRH treatment (19 percent of cycles). Pulsatile GnRH may result in a decreased risk of high-order multiple gestation compared with gonadotropin treatment.[81]

Hyperprolactinemia

Infertile women with hyperprolactinemia and anovulation often achieve pregnancy after treatment with bromocriptine. Bromocriptine treatment at doses from 2.5 to 7.5 mg daily is usually sufficient to restore ovulatory cycles in women with anovulation due to hyperprolactinemia. For women with microprolactinomas, there is a low likelihood that a pregnancy will be associated with growth of the prolactinoma. For women with macroprolactinomas, approximately 10 percent will develop clinically significant growth of the tumor during pregnancy, necessitating neurologic or neurosurgical intervention. Before ovulation is induced in women with a macroprolactinoma, consideration should be given to potential approaches to minimize pregnancy-associated complications (surgical treatment, radiotherapy, continuation of bromocriptine during pregnancy).[82]

Luteal-Phase Deficiency

Luteal-phase deficiency is the delayed maturation of the endometrium as determined by histologic dating of tissue obtained by endometrial biopsy that lags appropriate development by at least 2 days. Most commonly, luteal-phase deficiency is caused by abnormal follicular development and ovulation, which results in abnormal estradiol and progesterone production, leading to delayed endometrial maturation.[83] Many authorities believe that the crucial feature of luteal-phase deficiency is a relative deficiency of progesterone production. The effect of progesterone on the endometrium is probably both dose and time dependent. If progesterone concentrations are nearly normal but the length of time of progesterone secretion is subnormal, then luteal-phase deficiency could occur. Alternatively, if progesterone concentrations are subnormal, luteal-phase deficiency could occur, even if the length of the luteal phase is normal. An infrequent cause of luteal-phase deficiency is endometrial resistance to the action of estradiol or progesterone.[84] Theoretically, an endometrium that is repetitively out of phase with the menstrual cycle could result in an embryo arriving in the uterus at a time when the endometrium is not prepared to receive it. This could reduce fecundability. However, up to 40 percent of normal women can have a 2-day lag in endometrial maturation,[85] and sequential endometrial biopsies in normal fertile women demonstrate that approximately 7 percent have delayed endometrial maturation in two consecutive cycles.[86] The rate of out-of-phase endometrial biopsies appears to be dependent on the method used to time the date of ovulation. If the onset of menses is used to "time" ovulation, a large number of endometrial biopsies demonstrate "delayed" maturation. In contrast, if sonography and measurement of the LH surge are used to time ovulation, then few endometrial biopsies demonstrate delayed maturation.[87]

If the definition of luteal-phase deficiency requires an endometrium that demonstrates delayed maturation of 4 days or more, the relationship between the deficiency and reduced fecundability appears to be clinically significant. Treatment of infertile women with luteal-phase endometrial biopsies 4 days or more out of phase appears to significantly increase fecundability.[88]

Two commonly recommended treatments of luteal-phase deficiency are induction of ovulation with clomiphene or gonadotropin injections and supplementation of luteal progesterone production with vaginal progesterone suppositories. Both clomiphene and exogenous gonadotropin stimulation can overcome the abnormal follicular development that is the most likely cause of luteal-phase deficiency. Alternatively, progesterone vaginal suppositories at a dose of 25 to 50 mg twice daily starting 3 days after ovulation can be used to treat the delayed endometrial maturation.[89]

The Aging Ovary: The Aging Follicle

An immutable feature of ovarian physiology is that the number of oocytes, and follicles, is fixed in utero and declines following an exponential curve from the second trimester in utero (Fig. 20–10). At birth, the number of oocytes and follicles in a pair of human ovaries is approximately 2 million. At the completion of puberty, the number of eggs in a pair of human ovaries is in the range of 250,000.[90] During adult reproductive life, it appears that the follicles most sensitive to the growth-promoting effects of FSH are first selected to become the dominant follicle. As the ovary and the follicular apparatus age, it appears that the follicles that are relatively resistant to FSH populate the residual follicular pool. These aging follicles contain oocytes that are less likely to result in a successful pregnancy. It is likely that the decrease in fecundability associated with aging is due to a decline in both the quantity and quality of the oocytes. Data to support the concept that the aging oocyte is less likely to result in a successful pregnancy are based on multiple sources (see Figs. 20–6 and 20–7).

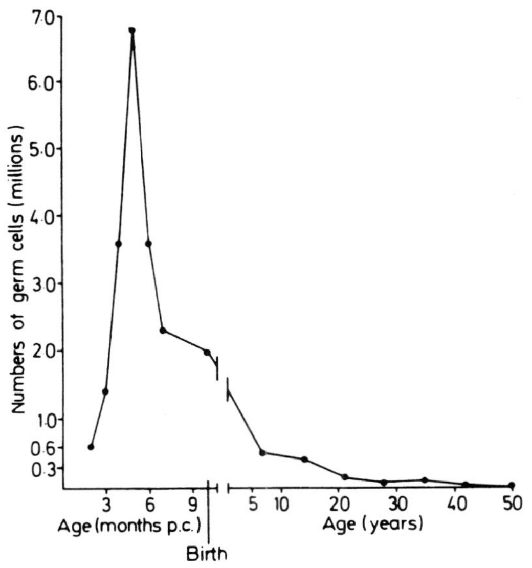

Figure 20–10 ■ Changes in the total number of oocytes (and follicles) in human ovaries before and after birth. The number of germ cells in the ovary peaks in utero during the second trimester. (From Baker TG. Radiosensitivity of mammalian oocytes with particular reference to the human female. Am J Obstet Gynecol 110:746–761, 1971.)

In infertile couples in which the cause of the infertility is azoospermia in the male partner, the success of donor sperm insemination is directly related to the age of the female partner. In women younger than 30 years, the first three cycles of insemination resulted in a per cycle pregnancy rate of 0.10. In women older than 35 years, the first three cycles of insemination were associated with a 0.06 per cycle pregnancy rate.[91] Data from IVF programs also suggest that the age of the female partner is an important determinant of pregnancy rates. In women younger than 30 years, the clinical pregnancy rate per cycle is in the range of 0.25. In women older than 40 years, the pregnancy rate per cycle is in the range of 0.12 with a high rate of spontaneous abortion.[92]

Many factors may account for the relationship between the age of the female partner and fecundability. A major cause of the relationship appears to be the relatively poor quality of the oocytes that compose the terminal follicular pool. A biochemical correlate of the depleted follicular pool is an elevation in the FSH concentration during menses. In the normal menstrual cycle, decreases in estradiol and inhibin during menses are associated with an increase in FSH production during the first 5 days of the menstrual cycle. The increase in FSH stimulates the growth of an ovarian follicle that will be selected to achieve dominance during the cycle. As the selected follicle secretes increasing quantities of estradiol and inhibin, FSH production is suppressed. As the follicular pool ages, ever-increasing quantities of FSH are required to stimulate follicular growth. This results in elevated serum FSH concentrations on cycle days 2, 3, and 4.[93] An elevated serum FSH concentration on cycle day 3 is a good marker of a depleted follicular pool and is associated with decreased fecundability.[94] In one study of the relationship between cycle day 3 FSH concentration and pregnancy rate in an IVF program, Toner and colleagues[92] reported that for women with a day 3 FSH concentration less than 10 mIU/ml, the ongoing pregnancy rate was 18 percent. In contrast, for women with a cycle day 3 FSH concentration greater than 25 mIU/ml, the ongoing pregnancy rate was 0 percent. In addition to predicting the pregnancy rate in IVF cycles, the cycle day 3 FSH concentration also predicts the magnitude of the ovarian response to exogenous gonadotropin stimulation, including the peak estradiol concentration, the number of follicles, and the number of oocytes that are obtained at follicular aspiration.[95] It is clear that the age of the female partner plays a major role in determining fecundability. Unfortunately, many clinical studies of fertility treatment have not explicitly controlled for this important variable.

Cycle day 3 FSH levels are emerging as an important predictor of follicular and oocyte competence and fecundability. In infertile women older than 35 years, cycle day 3 FSH concentration may be helpful in identifying women with a reduced follicular pool. Many genetic and lifestyle factors determine the rate of follicular loss and the age at which the serum FSH level measured during menses begins to rise. For example, cigarette smoking appears to hasten the pace at which the follicular pool is depleted. Menopause occurs significantly earlier in women who smoke.[96] In addition, in women in their mid-30s, cycle day 3 FSH concentration appears to be approximately 25 percent higher in cigarette smokers than in nonsmokers.[97] Chemotherapy with alkylating agents and pelvic radiation are two important exposures that are associated with a diminished follicular pool. Women who are older than 30 years and have completed six courses of chemotherapy for Hodgkin's disease typically lose more than 90 percent of their follicles, and many enter menopause immediately after the chemotherapy.[98] Radiation doses as low as 400 rad to the ovary will induce menopause in women older than 35 years. Girls are much more resistant to the induction of menopause with chemotherapy or pelvic radiation, probably because of their large follicular pool.

As noted before, estradiol and inhibin both exert negative feedback on FSH secretion during the early follicular phase of the cycle. During menses, owing to low levels of both estradiol and inhibin, FSH secretion is elevated in women with a normal follicular pool and is markedly elevated in women with a depleted follicular pool. Investigators have reported that the measurement of FSH after a course of clomiphene citrate is more sensitive for identifying women with diminished ovarian reserve than is the day 3 FSH test.[99, 100] The clomiphene challenge test is performed by administering clomiphene 100 mg daily from cycle day 5 to 9. FSH levels are sampled on cycle days 3 and 10. An elevated FSH level on either cycle day 3 or day 10 is associated with a diminished ovarian follicular pool. In some series, for every 100 women with an elevated day 10 FSH, only 40 have an elevated day 3 FSH. The clomiphene test is probably effective in detecting women with diminished follicular reserve because it blocks the negative feedback of estrogen, leaving only inhibin to suppress FSH production. In women with diminished ovarian reserve, inhibin levels appear to be low and are incapable, on their own, of suppressing FSH production.

Once a diminished ovarian follicular pool has been identified, it is "often too late." Fertility treatments at this point have lower success than do the same treatments in women with a normal follicular pool.[101] Consequently, many authorities are recommending that infertility evaluation and treatment be initiated in women older than 35 years after only 6 months of failure to conceive. Evaluation of day 3 FSH concentration is probably warranted in infertile women older than 30 years. Measurement of a day 3 and a day 10 FSH concentration after a clomiphene challenge is probably warranted in infertile women older than 37 years.

The aging oocyte that is fertilized and implants in the endometrium appears to be associated with a markedly increased rate of spontaneous abortion. The rate of clinically detected spontaneous abortion increases 100 percent between 20 and 40 years of age.[102] In IVF programs, the pregnancy loss rate is approximately 19 percent in women younger than 40 years and greater than 35 percent in women older than 40 years.[103] The increase in spontaneous abortion associated with the aging oocyte also contributes to the decreased fecundity apparent in aging women.

ANATOMIC FACTORS IN THE FEMALE

Tubal Factor Infertility

Tubal disease is identified in approximately 20 percent of the female partners of infertile couples. Pelvic inflammatory disease (PID), appendicitis, septic abortion, previous tubal surgery, and use of an intrauterine device resulting in a pelvic infection are major contributors to tubal disease. The rate of tubal infertility has been reported to be 12 percent, 23 percent, and 54 percent after one, two, or three episodes of PID.[104] Subclinical pelvic infections with *Chlamydia trachomatis* may be another major cause of tubal disease associated with infertility. Patton and colleagues[105] studied tubal biopsy specimens from 25 women with PID and tubal infertility. *C. trachomatis* was detected in 3 of 25 specimens by culture, 12 of 24 specimens by in situ hybridization, 15 of 22 specimens by immunoperoxidase staining, and 2 of 10 specimens by transmission electron microscopy. Serum antibodies against *Chlamydia* were detected in 15 of 21 subjects. In this cohort, *Chlamydia* was identified in 19 of 24 women with PID and infertility.[105] A history of a ruptured appendix appears to increase the risk of developing tubal factor infertility. In one case-control study, a history of ruptured appendix was associated with a 4.8-fold increase in the risk of tubal infertility. Appendicitis without rupture was not associated with an increased risk of tubal infertility.[106]

After pelvic surgery, adhesions develop in approximately 75 percent of women.[107] The mechanism of postoperative adhesion formation is not fully understood but involves invasion of fibroblasts into the postsurgical fibrinous bridges, resulting in the development of adhesive tissue that connects two normally unconnected structures or covers the surface of a structure with de novo adhesions (Fig. 20–11). In the normal peritoneal healing process, a serosanguineous proteinaceous fluid exudes from the site of injury and coagulates into fibrin bands. In the normal healing process, endogenous fibrinolytic activity lyses these fibrin bands within 4 days. If the fibrinous bands are invaded by fibroblasts, angiogenesis occurs and a permanent bridge of tissue (an adhesion) is created. Factors that decrease fibrinolytic activity (ischemia, infection, drying of peritoneal surfaces) or increase fibroblast infiltration of the fibrin clot will increase the chance of adhesions.[108]

Methods reported to minimize postoperative adhesions include the use of dextran, adhesion prevention barriers such as oxidized regenerated cellulose (Interceed) and expanded polytetrafluoroethylene (PTFE, Gore-Tex), heparin, glucocorticoids, fibrinolytic agents, and nonsteroidal anti-inflammatory agents. Most of these agents have been demonstrated to be effective in laboratory models of adhesion formation.[109–111] Interceed, one of the best studied adhesion prevention adjuvant agents, becomes a gel shortly after placement on a surgically traumatized pelvic surface. The gel reduces the chance of formation of fibrin bridges between two opposing structures and thereby reduces the chance of adhesion formation. The material is resorbed within 1 week as it is metabolized into glucose and glucuronic acid. Oxidized regenerated cellulose has been demon-

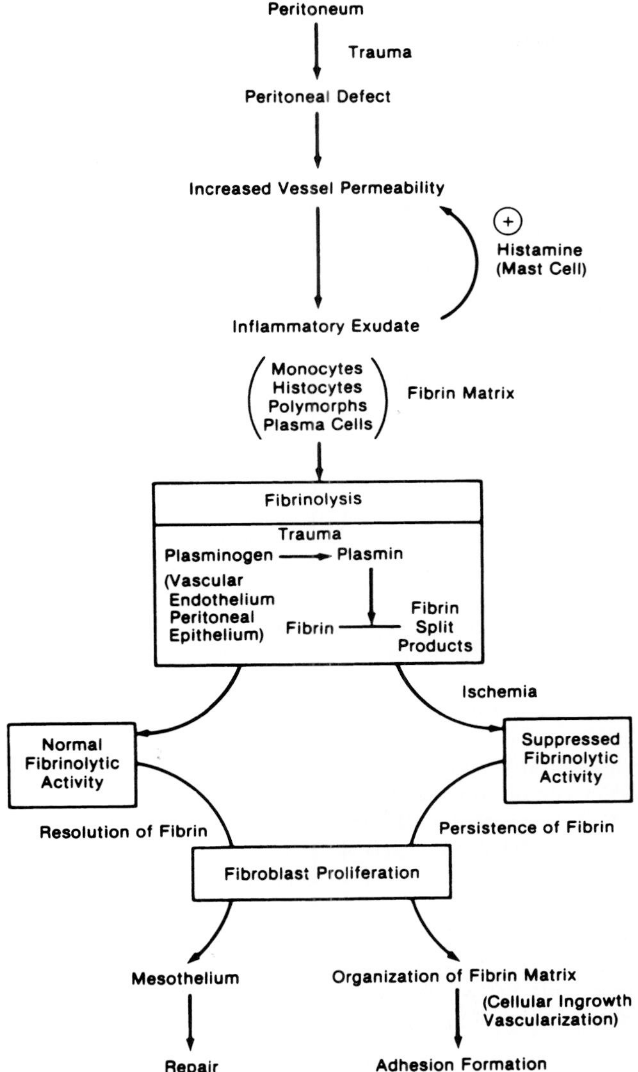

Figure 20–11 ■ Schematic of the normal healing response to a surgical injury in the pelvic peritoneum. (From Montz FJ, Shimanuki T, DiZerega GS. Postsurgical mesothelial re-epithelialization. *In* DeCherney AH, Polan ML [eds]. Reproductive Surgery. St. Louis, Mosby–Year Book, 1987.)

strated to reduce adhesion formation in women in well-controlled randomized prospective studies. In one study of 66 women with bilateral adnexal adhesive disease, the use of Interceed on the adnexa of one side resulted in a 39 percent reduction of postoperative adhesion scores compared with the adnexa that did not receive the Interceed barrier. The use of Interceed resulted in a twofold increase in the number of adnexa without adhesions at the second-look laparoscopy.[112] Similar findings were observed when oxidized regenerated cellulose was used to reduce adhesions after ovarian surgery.[113] However, none of these agents has been demonstrated to be effective in increasing the fecundability of women undergoing infertility surgery.

The two most commonly used tests of tubal patency are hysterosalpingography (HSG) and laparoscopy. The advantages of HSG are that it uses few resources, produces data concerning the shape of the uterine cavity, and may increase fecundability by altering the peritoneal environment. The major disadvantages of HSG are that it causes pain during the performance of the procedure and provides no information concerning the presence of other peritoneal diseases such as endometriosis and ovarian adhesions. HSG is usually performed between cycle days 6 and 12. Many centers prepare women for the procedure with a short course of an antibiotic and an antiprostaglandin agent such as ibuprofen immediately before the procedure. The risk of infection after HSG is in the range of 1 percent.[114] Traditional teaching is that oil-based contrast agents are associated with a higher postprocedure pregnancy rate than that observed with water-based contrast agents.[115] However, some well-designed studies do not support this conclusion.[116, 117] de Boer and colleagues[117] randomized 175 women to undergo HSG with oil-based or water-soluble contrast agents. The oil-based contrast agent gave better resolution of the uterine cavity, the aqueous agent gave better resolution of the tubal mucosa. The postprocedure pregnancy rates were similar in the two groups. The main diagnostic advantage of laparoscopy over HSG is that it has better sensitivity and specificity for diagnosing tubal disease than HSG does. In addition, laparoscopy can diagnose endometriosis and can be used to treat abnormalities observed at the time of the procedure.

Surgery for the treatment of infertility due to tubal disease is most successful if the tubal disease is localized in the distal portion of the tube. Fimbrioplasty is the lysis of fimbrial adhesions or dilatation of fimbrial strictures. Neosalpingostomy is the creation of a new tubal opening in a fallopian tube with a distal occlusion. Dlugi and colleagues[118] evaluated the success of unilateral versus bilateral fimbrioplasty or neosalpingostomy in 113 women with tubal factor infertility. Overall, these procedures were associated with a fecundability of 0.026. Women who had bilateral procedures with major adhesions had the lowest chance of achieving pregnancy. Overall, approximately 20 percent of the patients became pregnant, and approximately 20 percent of the pregnancies achieved were ectopic pregnancies. Similar monthly pregnancy rates after fimbrioplasty or neosalpingostomy have been reported by Canis and colleagues.[119]

Poor prognostic factors for successful pregnancy after surgical treatment of tubal disease include tubal diameter greater than 20 mm, absence of visible fimbriae, dense pelvic adhesions, ovarian adhesions, advanced age of the female partner, and duration of the infertility problem[120] (Fig. 20–12). Infertile women with bilateral proximal and distal tubal disease have low chances of conceiving after surgical treatment.[121] Treatment with IVF is much more successful than surgical treatment in this group of women.

A major advance in the treatment of proximal tubal occlusion associated with infertility is the development of flexible-tip guide wire techniques to restore patency to the proximal portion of the fallopian tube[122] (Figs. 20–13 and 20–14). In one study of transcervical fluoroscopic catheter recanalization of the fallopian tube, successful recanalization was achieved in 47 of 65 tubes treated (72 percent). Of the 40 women with open tubes after the procedure, 9 achieved livebirths (23 percent), 4 had ectopic pregnancies (10 percent), and 1 woman became pregnant but had an

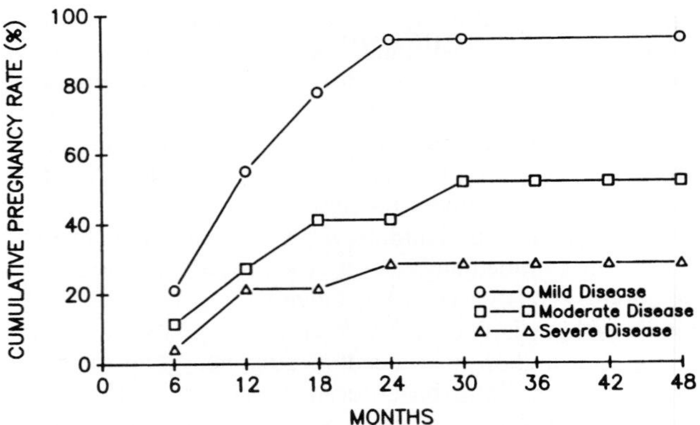

Figure 20–12 ■ Life table analysis of pregnancy outcome after neosalpingostomy by extent of disease. (From Schlaff WE, Hassiakos D, Damewood MD, Rock JA. Neosalpingostomy for distal tubal obstruction: Prognostic factors and impact of surgical technique. Fertil Steril 54:984–990, 1990. Reproduced with permission of the American Society for Reproductive Medicine.)

early abortion. In the 11 women in whom tubal recanalization was not successful, there were no pregnancies.[123]

One of the most successful surgical procedures for infertility is the microsurgical reanastomosis of fallopian tubes that were subjected to surgical sterilization procedures. The clinical characteristics associated with a high success rate for surgical reanastomosis include female partner younger than 40 years; tubal length greater than 4 cm; previous Falope ring, clip, or Pomeroy tubal ligation; and absence of associated pelvic disease.[124] Cumulative pregnancy rates in the year after the procedure are in the range of 50 to 80 percent. Laparoscopic surgical reanastomosis has recently been proposed as an alternative to traditional laparotomy approaches to tubal reanastomosis.[125]

Cervical Factor Infertility

The cervix is an active participant in shepherding sperm from the vagina to the upper reproductive tract. In the normal cervix, the secreted cervical mucus has physicochemical properties that facilitate the transport of sperm. Congenital malformation and trauma to the cervix may impair the ability of the cervix to produce normal mucus.

The postcoital test is the procedure most frequently used to examine the adequacy of the cervical mucus and the sperm-mucus interaction. Late in the follicular phase, the infertile couple is instructed to have sexual intercourse. The female partner is seen after intercourse, and a small amount of cervical mucus is obtained by use of oval forceps with a hollow aperture. The glycoproteins in the mucus support the property of spinnbarkeit or stretchability of the mucus. By allowing the prongs of the forceps to separate, the spinnbarkeit of the mucus can be tested. A separate aliquot is dried on a glass slide. Because of the high concentration of salts in the normal mucus in the late follicular phase, the dried mucus will crystallize in a "fern" pattern. A third aliquot is placed on a glass slide overlaid with a coverslip and examined under the high-power microscope objective for the presence of sperm.

Two major problems with the postcoital test are that there is little consensus on the "normal range" and that the test has poor predictive value for pregnancy. For example, some authorities suggest that a normal test result requires more than 20 sperm per high-power field.[126] Other authorities conclude that the presence of a single sperm indicates a normal test result.[127] In one study of the relationship between the postcoital test and fecundability, 20 percent of fertile women were observed to have 1 sperm or less per high-power field.[126] In another study, fecundability did not seem to be altered by the presence of between 0 and 11 sperm per high-power field.[128] Further reducing the potential validity of the postcoital test is the observation that the interobserver and intraobserver reproducibility is poor.[129]

Endometriosis

Endometriosis is the presence of tissue that resembles endometrial glands or stroma outside the uterus. The most common sites of endometriosis lesions are the peritoneal surfaces of the cul-de-sac of Douglas, the peritoneum cov-

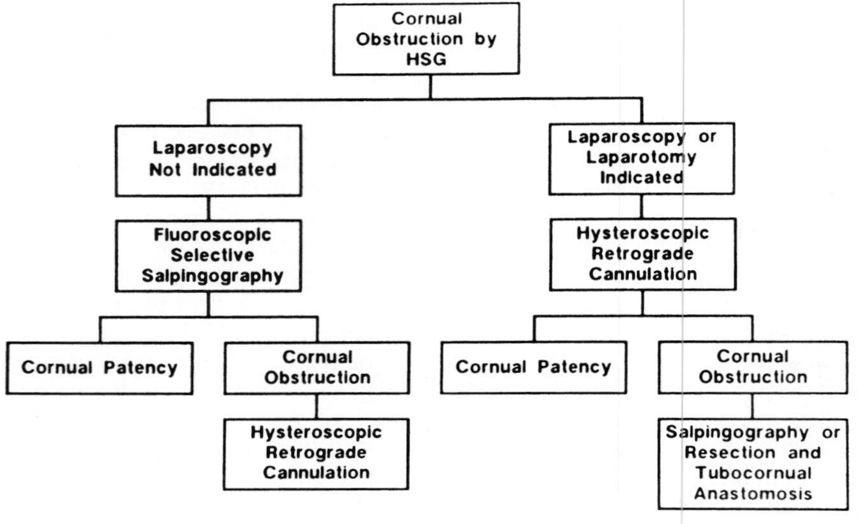

Figure 20–13 ■ Schematic algorithm for treatment of women with proximal tubal obstruction. If laparoscopy or laparotomy is planned because of known major pelvic disease, proximal obstruction can be evaluated and treated by a hysteroscopic procedure performed at the same operation. If the patient is not thought to require a surgical procedure for pelvic disease, proximal tubal obstruction can be evaluated and treated by fluoroscopic selective salpingography and catheter treatment. HSG, hysterosalpingography. (From Novy MJ, Thurmond AS, Patton P, et al. Diagnosis of cornual obstruction by transcervical fallopian tube cannulation. Fertil Steril 50:434–440, 1988. Reproduced with permission of the American Society for Reproductive Medicine.)

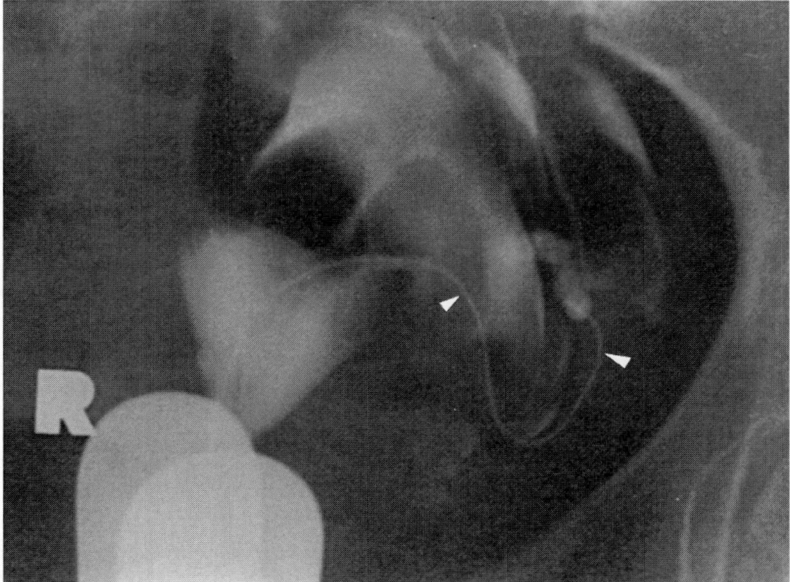

Figure 20–14 ■ Transcervical bougie dilatation recanalizes an obstructed right tube. Note residual strictures around arrowheads at the isthmic segment of the tube, suggesting the presence of salpingitis isthmica nodosa. (From Lang EK, Dunaway HH. Recanalization of obstructed fallopian tube by selective salpingography and transvaginal bougie dilatation: Outcome and cost analysis. Fertil Steril 66:210–215, 1996. Reproduced with permission of the American Society for Reproductive Medicine.)

ering the bladder, the ovarian surfaces, the stroma of the ovary, the bowel serosa, the fallopian tubes, the uterine surfaces, and the appendix. Women with endometriosis usually present for treatment of pelvic pain, infertility, or an adnexal mass (an ovarian endometrioma). Women with large adnexal masses that might be an endometrioma should have a surgical procedure to remove the mass.[130] Women with endometriosis and pelvic pain are typically treated with surgical ablation of the lesions or with hormone therapy that suppresses estrogen production and menstrual cyclicity. The treatment of women with endometriosis and infertility is complex, and clinical recommendations are limited because of the lack of sufficient clinical trials.[131] The fecundability of women with endometriosis is probably related to the disease stage.

The American Society for Reproductive Medicine has advocated the use of a surgical staging system for endometriosis that divides the disease into four stages (Fig. 20–15). Women with stage III and stage IV endometriosis often have major pelvic adhesions that involve the ovarian surface and distort the fallopian tube. In women with stage III and stage IV endometriosis, both anatomic defects and functional defects probably contribute to the infertility experienced by these women. Women with stage I and stage II endometriosis often have no significant anatomic distortion of the pelvic organs. In stage I and stage II endometriosis, small implants of endometriosis affect the surface structures of the pelvis. In women with infertility and stage I and stage II endometriosis, functional abnormalities in peritoneal, tubal, and endometrial function probably contribute to the subfertility experienced by these women.

Infertility in Women with Stage III and Stage IV Endometriosis

The hypothesis that advanced endometriosis (stage III and stage IV disease) causes a decrease in fecundability in women has not been tested by use of a rigorous scientific design in humans. However, studies in rabbits, rats, and monkeys suggest that experimentally induced advanced endometriosis causes a decrease in fecundability in all three of these species. Endometriosis is experimentally induced in laboratory animals by suturing small squares of endometrium on pelvic peritoneal surfaces or bowel mesentery. In experiments in rabbits, Schenken and Asch[132] removed the right uterine horn from New Zealand white rabbits and sutured endometrial squares of 25 mm^2 onto pelvic peritoneal surfaces. Control animals had adipose tissue sutured onto their peritoneal surfaces. Twenty-five days after the initial surgery, a surgical staging procedure was performed. In the group that received the endometrial implants, the majority of animals were observed to have significant adhesions from bowel and pelvic organs to the implants. Only 13 percent of the animals in the control group developed major adhesions. Fourteen days after the surgical staging procedure, the animals received a dose of chorionic gonadotropin and were inseminated with sperm from bucks with proven fertility. In the control group, 75 percent of the animals became pregnant. In the experimental group, only 25 percent of the animals became pregnant. Hahn and coworkers[133] have reported similar results.

Similar results have been reported in rats[134] and monkeys. Schenken and colleagues[135] studied the effects of experimentally induced endometriosis on fertility in monkeys. Animals with surgically induced endometriosis and control animals with adipose tissue autografts were mated. In control animals and animals with minimal endometriosis, the cycle pregnancy rates were similar, 42 percent and 35 percent, respectively. However, in the animals with advanced endometriosis, the cycle pregnancy rate was reduced to 12 percent. The presence of ovarian adhesions was associated with a 0 percent pregnancy rate. These studies support the hypothesis that advanced endometriosis is associated with a reduction in fecundability in laboratory animals. The major pelvic adhesions associated with advanced endometriosis may contribute to reduced fecundability by impairing egg release from the ovary, blocking

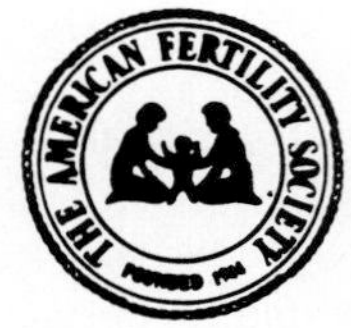

THE AMERICAN FERTILITY SOCIETY
REVISED CLASSIFICATION OF ENDOMETRIOSIS

Patient's Name ______________________ Date ______________

Stage I (Minimal) - 1-5
Stage II (Mild) - 6-15
Stage III (Moderate) - 16-40
Stage IV (Severe) - >40
Total ______________

Laparoscopy ________ Laparotomy ________ Photography ________
Recommended Treatment ______________________
Prognosis ______________

	ENDOMETRIOSIS	<1cm	1-3cm	>3cm
PERITONEUM	Superficial	1	2	4
	Deep	2	4	6
OVARY	R Superficial	1	2	4
	Deep	4	16	20
	L Superficial	1	2	4
	Deep	4	16	20

POSTERIOR CULDESAC OBLITERATION	Partial	Complete
	4	40

	ADHESIONS	<1/3 Enclosure	1/3-2/3 Enclosure	>2/3 Enclosure
OVARY	R Filmy	1	2	4
	Dense	4	8	16
	L Filmy	1	2	4
	Dense	4	8	16
TUBE	R Filmy	1	2	4
	Dense	4*	8*	16
	L Filmy	1	2	4
	Dense	4*	8*	16

*If the fimbriated end of the fallopian tube is completely enclosed, change the point assignment to 16.

Additional Endometriosis: ______________________

Associated Pathology: ______________________

To Be Used with Normal Tubes and Ovaries

L R

To Be Used with Abnormal Tubes and/or Ovaries

L R

Figure 20–15 ■ Revised American Fertility Society classification for endometriosis. Scoring system and patient information. (Reproduced with permission of the American Society for Reproductive Medicine [formerly the American Fertility Society].)

sperm entry into the peritoneal cavity, and inhibiting tubal pickup of the oocyte.

In women with infertility and advanced endometriosis, surgical treatment of the pelvic adhesions and resection of the endometriosis implants (conservative surgery) may improve fecundability. Olive and Lee[136] retrospectively analyzed 130 infertile women treated with expectant management, surgery, or both. In women with mild or moderate endometriosis,[137] expectant management and surgical treatment were associated with similar fecundability. In women with severe (advanced) endometriosis, surgical treatment resulted in an increase in fecundability. In 32 women with advanced endometriosis observed with expectant management, none became pregnant with 231 months of cumulative follow-up. In 34 women with advanced endometriosis treated with conservative surgery, 10 became pregnant during 702 months of follow-up. Garcia and David[138] have reported similar findings. Telimaa[139] reported that in women with infertility and advanced endometriosis due to the presence of deep endometriomas, surgical treatment of the endometriomas resulted in improved pregnancy rates. These studies suggest that expectant management is not warranted in the treatment of infertility associated with advanced endometriosis.

In women with infertility and stage III and stage IV endometriosis, surgical treatment to excise or ablate endometriosis lesions, resect adhesions, and restore pelvic anatomy to normal is warranted. Fecundability is highest in the 6 to 12 months after the surgical procedure. If pregnancy does not occur after the first surgery, additional surgical procedures have not been demonstrated to be effective in increasing fecundability. In couples who do not become pregnant after a surgical procedure, empirical treatment with ovarian stimulation with or without intrauterine insemination (IUI) can be used if the fallopian tubes are patent. IVF and gamete intrafallopian tube transfer are alternative choices for treatment of infertile women with advanced endometriosis (Table 20–5).

There are no large randomized controlled clinical trials that definitively demonstrate that IVF or gamete intrafallopian tube transfer increases fecundability in women with advanced endometriosis. In one small randomized study, 21 women with endometriosis and infertility were randomized to receive either IVF (N = 15) or expectant management (N = 6).[140] None of the women in the expectant management group became pregnant. Five of the 15 women who were treated with IVF became pregnant (not statistically significant). Because of the small sample size, this study did not have sufficient statistical power to detect true differences between the two groups.

In women with advanced endometriosis, a history of previous bilateral ovarian surgery may influence the success of IVF. Women with advanced endometriosis and a previous oophorectomy and a contralateral ovarian cystectomy appear to have poor responses to ovarian stimulation and a low pregnancy rate.[141] Matson and Yovich[142] analyzed the relationship between the stage of endometriosis and parameters of response to IVF including the number of oocytes recovered and fertilization and pregnancy rates. Women with tubal infertility served as a control group. The number of oocytes recovered was similar in all groups: tubal factor, 4.3 oocytes; stage I endometriosis, 4.2 oocytes; stage II endometriosis, 3.8 oocytes; stage III endometriosis, 3.2 oocytes; and stage IV endometriosis, 3.1 oocytes. The fertilization rate was similar in all groups. The per cycle pregnancy rate was reduced in the women with advanced endometriosis. The per cycle pregnancy rates were tubal factor, 18 percent; stage I endometriosis, 13 percent; stage II endometriosis, 8 percent; stage III endometriosis, 6 percent; and stage IV endometriosis, 2 percent. Other investigators have also reported that advanced endometriosis may reduce the success of IVF.

■ TABLE 20–5

Treatment of Infertility in Women with Advanced Endometriosis

Step 1	Identify and treat all reversible causes of infertility.
Step 2	If an endometrioma is diagnosed, consider surgical resection.
Step 3	If major pelvic adhesions are present and the patient has had no previous fertility surgery, consider a conservative surgical procedure to resect adhesions and endometriosis implants and to restore pelvic anatomy to normal.
Step 4	Consider empirical clomiphene treatment with or without intrauterine insemination.
Step 5	Consider empirical gonadotropin treatment with or without intrauterine insemination.
Step 6	Consider in vitro fertilization.

Infertility in Women with Stage I and Stage II Endometriosis

Women with infertility and stage I or stage II endometriosis have decreased fecundability. However, it is not clear whether the endometriosis is causally linked to the decreased fecundability. The mechanisms that link infertility and minimal or mild endometriosis have not been definitively identified, but functional abnormalities in peritoneal, tubal, and endometrial function are likely culprits.

Most women with stage I or stage II endometriosis do not have major pelvic adhesions. If endometriosis causes a decrease in fecundability in these women, it is probably due to functional factors. Many functional abnormalities of reproduction have been described in women with minimal and mild endometriosis and infertility. Numerous investigators have reported that women with endometriosis have an increased volume of peritoneal fluid[143]; increased peritoneal concentrations of activated macrophages[144]; and increased peritoneal fluid concentration of prostaglandin, interleukin-1, tumor necrosis factor, and proteases.[145] These functional alterations in the peritoneal environment may impair gamete, embryo, and fallopian tube function.

Some investigators have reported that antiendometrial antibodies are increased in women with endometriosis and that these antibodies may impair endometrial function.[146, 147] Some women with early-stage endometriosis have luteal-phase dysfunction,[148] abnormal follicle growth,[149] multiple and premature LH surges,[150] and luteinized unruptured follicle syndrome.[151]

A recently evolving concept is that the eutopic endometrium may be abnormal in women with endometriosis. This suggests that a müllerian tract "field defect" may be present in women with endometriosis. Lessey and colleagues[12] reported that the endometrial expression of the intercellular ligand protein β_3 integrin is significantly suppressed in women with stage I and stage II endometriosis. It is possible that the decrease in β_3 integrin expression is associated with an impaired interaction of the embryo with the endometrium.

As noted before, it is unclear whether stage I and stage II endometriosis causes infertility. However, women with infertility and stage I or stage II endometriosis clearly have reduced fecundability. Most studies suggest that the fecundability of infertile women with stage I or stage II endometriosis is in the range of 0.04 to 0.05 if no treatment is provided. Four major treatment regimens have been used to treat the infertility associated with early-stage endometriosis: (1) hormone suppression of ovarian function to suppress endometriosis implants with use of drugs such as leuprolide, buserelin, or danazol; (2) surgical treatment of endometriosis lesions; (3) empirical ovarian hyperstimulation (with clomiphene or gonadotropins) with or without IUI; and (4) assisted reproductive technologies.

Most clinical trials report that hormone therapy of endometriosis lesions does not improve fecundability in infertile women with early-stage endometriosis.[152] Seibel and colleagues[153] reported the first prospective randomized trial of hormone treatment of endometriosis lesions for the treatment of infertility. Couples with 1 year of failure to conceive, a normal basic infertility examination, and a laparoscopy that demonstrated minimal endometriosis (Kistner stage I) were randomized to receive either danazol (N = 37) or no treatment (N = 36). The couples were observed for 1 year beginning immediately after laparoscopy in the no-treatment group or for 1 year after the completion of the danazol therapy. During the 1-year follow-up, 35 percent of the danazol-treated women and 47 percent of the untreated women became pregnant (Fig. 20–16). The per cycle pregnancy rates were 0.035 and 0.051 in the danazol-treated and the control groups, respectively. This study demonstrated that danazol treatment of endometriosis lesions did not improve fecundability in women with infertility and early-stage endometriosis.

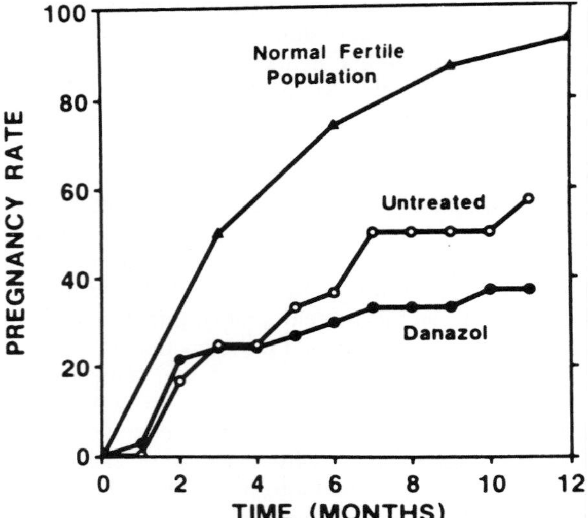

Figure 20–16 ■ Cumulative pregnancy rates in danazol-treated and untreated patients with minimal endometriosis. The cumulative pregnancy rate in an ideal fertile population is also shown for comparison. (From Bayer SR, Seibel MM, Saffan DS, et al. The efficacy of danazol treatment for minimal endometriosis in infertile women: A prospective randomized study. J Reprod Med 33:179–183, 1988.)

Similar findings have been reported by Fedele and colleagues.[154] Women with revised American Society for Reproductive Medicine stage I or stage II endometriosis were randomized to receive hormone treatment with the GnRH agonist analogue buserelin for 6 months or to a no-treatment group. Median follow-up was approximately 18 months in both groups. The 1-year actuarial pregnancy rate was 30 percent in the group treated with buserelin and 37 percent in the group that received no treatment. The 2-year actuarial pregnancy rate was 61 percent in the buserelin group and 60 percent in the control group. By use of the 2-year actuarial cumulative pregnancy rates (60 to 61 percent), the per cycle fecundability in each group was approximately 0.04. These data demonstrate that in women with infertility and American Society for Reproductive Medicine stage I or stage II endometriosis, treatment with buserelin does not improve fecundability.

The effect of surgical treatment on fecundability in women with infertility and early-stage endometriosis is controversial. Small randomized prospective clinical trials have demonstrated that surgical ablation or excision of endometriosis implants does not improve fecundability in women with infertility and early-stage endometriosis.[155, 156] In retrospective and prospective nonrandomized studies, laparoscopic treatment of early-stage endometriosis in women with infertility is associated with a fecundability in the range of 0.03 to 0.05.[157–159] Numerous studies suggest that a fecundability of 0.03 to 0.05 can be achieved in this population of patients with expectant management. Recently, Marcoux and colleagues[159a] have reported that surgical treatment of stage I and stage II endometriosis improves fecundability in infertile women. The investigators randomized 341 women with stage I or stage II endometriosis to a diagnostic laparoscopy only or a diagnostic laparoscopy combined with surgical resection or ablation of endometriosis lesions. During 36 weeks of postoperative follow-up, the fecundability was 0.024 in the group that underwent diagnostic laparoscopy and 0.047 in the group that had surgical resection or ablation of the endometriosis lesions ($P < 0.006$). This report is the first, large-scale clinical trial that documents an increase in fecundability after surgical treatment of early-stage endometriosis. Additional prospective randomized studies are needed to compare the efficacy of surgical treatment with that of empirical ovarian stimulation with clomiphene or gonadotropins in the treatment of infertility associated with early-stage endometriosis.

Two studies suggest that treatment of infertility with empirical, controlled ovarian stimulation may increase fecundability in women with minimal or mild endometriosis. Fedele and colleagues[160] randomized 40 women with stage I or stage II endometriosis to three cycles of hMG ovarian stimulation plus IUI or no treatment. The per cycle pregnancy rate was 0.045 in the no-treatment group. This per cycle pregnancy rate is similar to that observed in the control group of many other studies of infertility in early-stage endometriosis. In the women who received hMG-IUI, the per cycle pregnancy rate was 0.15 ($P < .05$).

This study indicates that fecundability can be increased in women with infertility and early-stage endometriosis by hMG-IUI treatment. The separate roles of the hMG ovarian stimulation and the IUI treatment are not yet clearly resolved. In a similar study, Kemmann and colleagues[161] randomized women with infertility and early-stage endometriosis to one of four treatment groups: (1) no treatment, (2) clomiphene ovarian stimulation, (3) clomiphene plus hMG, or (4) IVF. Women who received no treatment had a per cycle pregnancy rate of 0.028. Women who received clomiphene ovarian stimulation had a pregnancy rate of 0.066, a fecundability not significantly different from that of the no-treatment group. The women who received clomiphene plus hMG ovarian stimulation had a per cycle pregnancy rate of 0.114 ($P < .05$ compared with the control group). This suggests that the stimulation of the ovary to produce multiple oocytes may increase the per cycle pregnancy rate in these women. Alternatively, the ovarian stimulation may better prepare the endometrium for embryo implantation. The women treated with IVF had a per cycle pregnancy rate of 0.22 ($P < .05$). This suggests that the highest fecundability is achieved with IVF treatment.

Given these observations, a stepwise approach to the treatment of infertility in women with early-stage endometriosis is warranted (Table 20–6). Step 1 is the identification and treatment of all reversible causes of infertility in the couple. Step 2 is the use of timed cycles (measurement of urine LH or use of basal body temperature recordings). Step 3 is empirical clomiphene treatment, with or without IUI. Step 4 is empirical gonadotropin ovarian stimulation with or without IUI. Step 5 is the use of assisted reproductive technologies such as IVF or gamete intrafallopian tube transfer. Although the available data suggest that IVF and gamete intrafallopian tube transfer are the most effective methods for achieving pregnancy in couples with early-stage endometriosis, the cost of these procedures precludes their use as first-step treatments in most clinical situations. The stepwise approach attempts to balance the two variables of effectiveness and cost in a rational clinical pathway.

Uterine Leiomyomas

Uterine leiomyomas, also known as fibroids or uterine myomas, are benign smooth muscle tumors of the uterus.

■ TABLE 20–6

Treatment of Infertility in Women with Early-Stage Endometriosis

Step 1	Identify and treat all reversible causes of infertility in the couple.
Step 2	If the woman is younger than 32 years, consider expectant management or timed intercourse by monitoring of urine luteinizing hormone or use of basal body temperature charts. If the woman is older than 32 years, consider expectant management, timed intercourse, or immediate progression to step 3.
Step 3	Consider empirical treatment with clomiphene with or without intrauterine insemination.
Step 4	Consider empirical treatment with gonadotropins with or without intrauterine insemination.
Step 5	Consider in vitro fertilization or gamete intrafallopian tube transfer.

Myomas are the most common pelvic tumors of women. Uterine leiomyomas are monoclonal tumors that demonstrate nonrandom cytogenetic mutations. The most frequently reported cytogenetic abnormalities in myomas are t(12;14)(q13–15,q23–24), del(7)(q21), and t(1;2)(p36,p24).[162] A gene at 12q15 encoding high-mobility group protein HMGI-C was discovered to be mutated in many cases of uterine myomata.[163] HMGI-C is an architectural factor that binds to the minor groove of DNA and may play a role in organizing satellite chromatin. HMGI-C is a phosphoprotein that is a substrate for cell-regulatory kinases such as casein kinase and p34/cdc2. One current working hypothesis is that somatic mutations in genes, such as HMGI-C, in uterine myocytes result in dysregulated growth that produces a myoma.[164] In addition, the high-mobility group mutation appears to increase the sensitivity of the mutated smooth muscle cells to the effects of estradiol.[165] The mechanisms that cause a high rate of mutations in the HMGI-C gene in uterine myocytes are unknown, but estradiol and progesterone probably play a role in regulating the rate of mitosis and mutation in the uterine myocyte.

There are few well-designed clinical studies that analyze the effect of uterine leiomyomas on fecundability. Farhi and colleagues[166] reported the effect of uterine leiomyomas on the results of IVF treatment. The investigators reported that among 46 women with uterine myomas treated with IVF, the pregnancy rate per transfer was 22 percent and the abortion rate was 36 percent. In a control group of women with mechanical causes of infertility, the pregnancy rate per transfer was 25 percent and the abortion rate was 25 percent. There were no statistically significant differences between the two groups. A further analysis divided the women with uterine myomas into two groups, those with a normal uterine cavity and those with an abnormal uterine cavity as assessed by HSG. In the 28 women with uterine myomas and a normal uterine cavity, there was a 30 percent pregnancy rate per transfer. In the 18 women with uterine myomas and an abnormal uterine cavity, there was a 9 percent pregnancy rate per embryo transfer. This study suggests that uterine leiomyomas that distort the uterine cavity may be associated with a decrease in fecundability.

DISORDERS OF SPERM PRODUCTION: THE "MALE FACTOR"

The process of spermatogenesis and sperm transport and maturation through the male reproductive tract is complex and reviewed in Chapter 23. For the fertility specialist, the initial approach to the evaluation of sperm production is the semen analysis. The semen analysis is noninvasive and requires modest laboratory resources to complete. There are problems inherent to the semen analysis. Variability can be introduced by laboratory technicians or by the large variation between ejaculates in the same man. Some of the variation between ejaculates in the same man may be due to environmental exposures (season, illness, stress).[167] It is widely believed that low sperm concentration is associated with decreased fecundability (Table 20–7). However, not all studies have consistently reported a relationship between abnormal semen parameters and low fecundability.

■ TABLE 20–7
Relative Risk of Infertility Stratified by Sperm Count

SPERM CONCENTRATION (million/ml)	RELATIVE RISK OF INFERTILITY	STATISTICAL SIGNIFICANCE COMPARED WITH UNIT RISK (*P* value)
<10	10.3	$P < .000000001$
10 up to 20	5.2	$P < .00001$
20 up to 40	3.1	$P < .001$
40 up to 60	1.7	$P < .02$
60 up to 160	1.0	Unit risk
160 up to 200	1.3	Not significant
>200	1.5	Not significant

Data from Nelson CMK, Bunge R. Fertil Steril 4:10, 1953; and DeCherney AH. *In* Kase NG, Weingold AB (eds). Principles and Practice of Clinical Gynecology. New York, Churchill Livingstone, 1983.

For example, in one study, the semen measures of volume, sperm concentration, motility, and morphology did not independently predict fecundability. However, a combination of sperm concentration and motility, the "motile sperm density," was a predictor of fecundability. A motile sperm density below 5 million motile sperm per milliliter was associated with a decrease in fecundability.[168] Another study that used receiver operator characteristics curve analysis to evaluate the predictive utility of semen parameters also observed that a sperm density of less that 5 million motile sperm per milliliter was a predictor of low fecundability.[169] In addition, total motile sperm in the ejaculate (volume × sperm concentration × motility) of less than 5 million was also associated with low fecundability.[169]

The basic semen analysis measures semen volume, sperm concentration, and sperm motility and morphology. Many laboratories recommend collection of the semen specimen by masturbation after 2 to 3 days of abstinence from ejaculation. The specimen is collected into a clean container that does not have any spermicidal agents. The specimen is typically analyzed within 2 hours of collection. The volume is measured by graduated cylinder or pipette and is typically between 2 and 6 ml. The sperm count is performed after complete liquefaction of the seminal fluid. Two techniques used to count sperm are specially designed hemocytometers and automated cell-counting systems. The sperm concentration is normally greater than 20 million sperm per milliliter of semen. Motility should ideally be analyzed immediately on liquefaction of the semen sample and is normally greater than 50 percent. The analysis of sperm morphology continues to evolve. Light microscopy is less sensitive than electron microscopy for identification and classification of sperm morphology. By use of standard analysis of morphology, normal semen has greater than 40 percent normal forms. By use of the "strict" criteria of Kruger and colleagues,[170] semen with greater than 14 percent normal forms is considered to be normal. If the semen has greater than 14 percent normal forms, then the sperm demonstrates normal fertilization when it is used for IVF. Semen with less than 4 percent normal forms is associated with low fertilization when it is used for IVF.[170]

In addition to basic semen testing, numerous advanced tests of semen quality and sperm characteristics have been developed. In many semen specimens, round cells are identified by microscopy. These round cells are usually either immature germ cells or leukocytes. The origin of the round cells can be distinguished on the basis of specific staining techniques such as the Endtz test.[171] In one study, the presence of immature germ cells in the ejaculate (possibly reflecting a disorder of spermatogenesis) but not the presence of leukocytes was associated with reduced fertilizing capacity.[172]

The hamster egg penetration test is one of the most commonly used tests of sperm function.[173] In this test, human sperm, preincubated in a medium that promotes capacitation, is exposed to zona pellucida–free hamster eggs. The percentage of oocytes penetrated by a sperm and the number of sperm penetrating each oocyte are measured. It is unlikely that this test provides a definitive analysis of the fertilizing capacity of sperm with human oocytes.[174]

Other advanced tests of sperm characteristics include the human zona-binding assay, the hypo-osmotic swelling test, and the measurement of adenosine triphosphate in the semen. The clinical utility of these tests remains to be determined.

The biologic processes that control male gamete production are incompletely characterized. It is likely that there are dozens of diseases of sperm production that remain to be discovered. Consequently, a listing of the common causes of male factor infertility is in part a reflection of our lack of understanding of the male reproductive process. In one study of male partners of infertile couples presenting to a urologist's practice, the most commonly identified conditions causing or associated with male factor infertility were varicocele (37 percent), idiopathic (26 percent), testicular failure (9 percent), obstruction (6 percent), cryptorchidism (6 percent), low semen volume (5 percent), sperm agglutination (3 percent), excessive semen viscosity (2 percent), and other causes (6 percent).

Varicocele

A varicocele is a dilatation of the pampiniform plexus of the scrotal veins. Approximately 11 percent of men with a normal semen analysis have a clinically detected varicocele. Approximately 25 percent of men with an abnormal semen analysis have a varicocele.[175] Varicoceles are believed to influence semen quality by increasing testicular temperature or by exposing the testis to abnormally high levels of an inhibitor of sperm function through alterations in venous efflux from the testis.

The clinical effect of the surgical treatment of varicoceles is controversial. Most authorities believe that treatment of subclinical varicoceles (varicoceles detected only by an imaging procedure such as ultrasonography or venography) does not improve fecundability.[176] Most studies suggest that treatment of clinically evident varicoceles improves semen parameters. For example, Madgar and colleagues[177] demonstrated that high spermatic vein ligation of clinically detected varicoceles resulted in an increase in sperm concentration from approximately 15 million/ml before surgery to approximately 35 million/ml after surgery. Men with varicoceles randomized to no surgical treatment did not demonstrate an increase in sperm concentration. Motility also increased after varicocelectomy.

Numerous other investigators have reported that semen parameters improve in men with varicocele after high spermatic vein ligation.[178] The effect of varicocele surgery on fecundability is controversial. Madgar and colleagues[177] reported that in men with varicoceles, high spermatic vein ligation improved fecundability. In this study, in the 12 months after randomization, fecundability in the men who did not have surgery was approximately 0.01. Fecundability was approximately 0.04 in the men who had high spermatic vein ligation. Other investigators have not confirmed these findings. For example, Breznik and coworkers[178] reported that management of varicocele by surgery or no treatment resulted in similar fecundability.

Idiopathic Oligospermia and Asthenospermia

Even with extensive evaluation, infertile men with abnormal semen characteristics often have no identified cause for their problem. These cases of idiopathic oligospermia or asthenospermia have been treated with many hormone regimens, most of which do not appear to be effective. Treatment with testosterone rebound therapy, hCG injections, clomiphene, or testolactone (an inhibitor of aromatase) has not been proved to be effective.[179]

Gonadal Failure

The most common cause of gonadal failure in the male is Klinefelter's syndrome (47,XXY). There is no known treatment for the sterility associated with Klinefelter's syndrome. This condition is discussed in more detail in Chapter 23. Mumps orchitis and severe cryptorchidism can be associated with gonadal failure.

Hypogonadotropic Hypogonadism

Men with anosmia and low concentrations of LH, FSH, and testosterone, in the absence of a primary pituitary disorder, have Kallmann's syndrome, which is due to the lack of adequate GnRH production by the hypothalamus. This disease and other causes of hypogonadotropic hypogonadism can be treated with gonadotropin therapy. One regimen is to use hCG 2000 IU intramuscularly three times weekly for 6 months followed by the addition of 37.5 IU of hMG or FSH intramuscularly three times weekly.[180] Another approach to treatment is to replace the missing hormone, GnRH, by pulsatile administration of approxmately 4 μg every 3 hours by a portable infusion pump.[181] Treatment of these men is often associated with successful pregnancy at sperm concentrations less than 5 million/ml. This suggests that in men with pure endocrine causes of infertility, the production of only a few good sperm is adequate to achieve fertility.

Obstructive Abnormalities of Vas Deferens or Epididymis

Congenital absence of the vas deferens can be diagnosed by the absence of fructose in the semen and confirmed by vasography. Recent data suggest that many men with congenital absence of the vas deferens are carriers of mutations in the cystic fibrosis transmembrane regulator gene *(CFTR)*. In one study of 102 men with congenital absence of the vas deferens, 19 of the 102 men had mutations in both copies of the *CFTR* gene.[182] Fifty-four men had a mutation in one copy of *CFTR* and 34 also had a mutation in the noncoding region of *CFTR* (5T allele) in the other *CFTR* gene. Seven men had a mutation in the noncoding region of *CFTR*. Twenty-two men had no identifiable mutation. In most men with congenital absence of the vas deferens, pulmonary function and gastrointestinal function are normal.[183]

The most common cause of blockage of the vas deferens is previous vasectomy or accidental ligation during inguinal surgery. Treatment of infertility in these cases may require microsurgical correction. Vasovasostomy is typically performed by use of microsurgical techniques. After vasovasostomy, patency rates are in the range of 70 to 97 percent. The pregnancy rate is high in reversals performed within 3 years of vasectomy (crude pregnancy rate, 70 percent) and significantly lower 15 years after vasectomy (crude pregnancy rate, 30 percent).[184]

Retrograde Ejaculation

Retrograde ejaculation is caused by injury to the lumbar sympathetic nerves or damage to the bladder neck. The diagnosis is made by demonstrating a high number of sperm in the urine after ejaculation. Medical treatment with phenylproprolamide (75 mg twice daily) or ephedrine sulfate (25 mg four times daily) can be effective by stimulating closure of the bladder neck. Alternatively, the urine can be collected and sperm harvested from the urine by centrifugation for insemination.

Spinal Cord Injury

Men with spinal cord injury often have failure of ejaculation. Electroejaculation can be used to obtain semen, but the semen often demonstrates abnormalities of sperm motility.[185]

Environmental Exposures

Alkylating chemotherapeutic agents are associated with a high rate of gonadal failure. For example, in men treated with chemotherapy for Hodgkin's disease, complete gonadal failure is common.[186] The relationship between other exposures, such as cigarette smoking, and decreased fecundability is more difficult to demonstrate, suggesting only a modest effect.

Donor Insemination

For men with azoospermia and for couples with significantly abnormal semen parameters who do not want gamete micromanipulation or IVF, donor insemination is effective treatment. Recent advances in methods for harvesting sperm from testis biopsies in azoospermic men increase the options for these couples. Donor insemination raises the possibility of transmitting infectious agents in the donor sperm or semen. This requires that semen donors submit specimens that are frozen and quarantined for 6 months until follow-up testing can be done on the donor to minimize the risk of transmitting known infectious agents. Current protocols test donors for human immunodeficiency virus (HIV) infection, hepatitis B and C, syphilis, gonorrhea, chlamydial infection, and cytomegalovirus infection. Donors are also screened for a family history of genetic disease. In many centers, the infertile couple is also screened for sexually transmitted infectious disease to reduce the likelihood of the male partner's transmitting a disease such as HIV infection to the female partner during the course of donor insemination. In 12 cycles of donor insemination, the cumulative pregnancy rate in women younger than 30 years is approximately 75 percent.

Donor insemination is associated with many complex psychosocial and legal issues. In many programs, all couples treated with donor insemination receive counseling by psychologists or social workers with a special interest in fertility issues. In many states, the male partner is the legal father of offspring conceived through donor insemination.

Odem and colleagues[187] studied the clinical utility of timing donor insemination by measurement of urine LH or by the physician's interpretation of the basal body temperature record. Interestingly, the physician-interpreted basal body temperature was associated with better fecundability and lower costs than was home measurement of urine LH.

DISORDERS OF IMPLANTATION

Implantation is one of the least understood processes in human reproduction. Findings in laboratory models offer the best hope of furthering our understanding of the process of implantation. The process of implantation and fertility disorders associated with implantation defects are reviewed in Chapters 8 and 21.

OTHER DISORDERS ASSOCIATED WITH INFERTILITY

Immunologic Factors

Antisperm Antibodies

Antigenic determinants on spermatozoa are capable of eliciting an immune response.[188] In women, antisperm antibodies can be detected in the serum and cervical mucus. It is conceivable that agglutinating antibodies in the cervical mucus could interfere with sperm function. In men, antisperm antibodies can be detected in the semen and serum.

The relationship between antisperm antibodies and infertility is controversial. A prospective study was unable to demonstrate differences in fecundability in couples with and without antisperm antibodies.[189]

Antiphospholipid Antibodies

Antiphospholipid antibodies refer to a heterogeneous group of autoantibodies that bind to negatively charged phospholipids. The lupus anticoagulant antibodies and the anticardiolipin antibodies are types of antiphospholipid antibodies. The antiphospholipid antibody syndrome refers to the association of antiphospholipid antibodies with clinical problems such as arterial or venous thrombosis, thrombocytopenia, or recurrent spontaneous abortion. Other pregnancy complications associated with antiphospholipid antibodies include intrauterine growth restriction, preeclampsia, placental abruption, and intrauterine fetal demise.[190]

The type of phospholipid antibody and the antibody titer are probably important predictors of the impact of the antibodies on pregnancy outcome. For example, one prospective study reported an increase in the risk of fetal loss for those women with lupus anticoagulant but not for women with anticardiolipin antibodies.[191] In another study, women with anticardiolipin immunoglobulin G titers of more than 20 binding units were more likely than women with low titers or no titers of antiphospholipid antibodies to develop an antiphospholipid disorder.[192]

Treatment of pregnant women with antiphospholipid antibodies and a history of fetal loss is empirical. Heparin plus low-dose aspirin appears to be superior to prednisone plus low-dose aspirin because of a lower risk of both preterm delivery and other detrimental side effects associated with prednisone treatment.[193] A commonly used regimen includes aspirin 80 mg daily plus heparin 5000 to 10,000 units every 12 hours. Long-term therapy with unfractionated heparin can be associated with thrombocytopenia, osteopenia, and bleeding.

Recurrent Abortion

Recurrent abortion is defined as the occurrence of two consecutive spontaneous abortions. The most common causes of recurrent abortion include genetic factors (major chromosome abnormalities), 5 percent; anatomic factors, including uterine anomalies, 10 percent; endocrine factors, including luteal-phase deficiency, 10 percent; infectious factors, less than 5 percent; immunologic factors, 5 percent; and unidentified factors, 65 percent[194, 195] (Table 20–8).

In chromosomally abnormal fetuses, the most commonly identified abnormalities are trisomy, monosomy X, triploidy, tetraploidy, and rearrangements. The most common uterine abnormalities associated with recurrent abortion are the müllerian anomalies including the septate uterus, diethylstilbestrol-related changes,[196] incompetent cervix, and Asherman's syndrome. Of the major uterine anomalies, septate uterus is associated with the highest rate of spontaneous abortion (more than 50 percent), and the didelphic uterus is associated with the lowest rate of spontaneous abortion (approximately 30 percent) (Table 20–9). For infertile women with recurrent abortion and a septate uterus, hysteroscopic resection of the septum appears to significantly reduce the risk of a spontaneous abortion in a subsequent pregnancy.[197] No surgical treatment is recommended for an infertile woman with recurrent abortion and a didel-

■ TABLE 20–8

Laboratory Tests Commonly Employed in the Evaluation of Recurrent Abortion

Hysterosalpingography
Endometrial biopsy in midluteal or late luteal phase
Karyotype on peripheral white blood cells in male and female partner
Lupus anticoagulant and anticardiolipin antibody screen
Thyroid-stimulating hormone measurement, and prolactin if indicated

■ TABLE 20–9

Spontaneous Abortion Rate Associated with Different Types of Uterine Anomalies

UTERINE ANOMALY	NUMBER OF WOMEN STUDIED	RATE OF SPONTANEOUS ABORTION (%)
Septate	113	53
Unicornuate	220	35
Bicornuate	154	33
Didelphic	31	29
In utero diethylstilbestrol exposure	472	28

From Patton P, Novy MJ. Reproductive potential of the anomalous uterus. Semin Reprod Endocrinol 6:217–233, 1988. Reprinted by permission of Thieme Medical Publishers.

phic uterus, and no surgical procedure has been described that can enlarge a unicornuate uterus.

The most common endocrine factors associated with abortion are luteal-phase deficiency, uncontrolled diabetes, hypothyroidism, and hyperandrogenism. As noted before, the relationship between luteal-phase deficiency and pregnancy outcome is controversial. There are clearly isolated cases in which endocrine abnormalities such as a modest degree of hyperprolactinemia produce poor follicular development and result in reduced progesterone production in the luteal phase. These endocrine abnormalities might result in a pregnancy at high risk for spontaneous abortion.

Genetic Causes of Infertility

For many decades, it has been known that major chromosome abnormalities are often associated with infertility. For example, women with 45,X (Turner's syndrome) have premature depletion of the oocyte pool and are typically sterile. Men with 47,XXY (Klinefelter's syndrome) typically have azoospermia and are sterile.[198] A major goal of reproductive scientists is to identify individual genes that are associated with infertility. Most genes that participate in the process of conception remain to be identified. A few genes in men and women that influence fecundability have recently been identified.

Galactose 1-phosphate uridyltransferase (GALT) is a crucial enzyme in the pathway subserving the metabolism of galactose to glucose. At least three major alleles have been identified for GALT. The wild-type allele is associated with normal enzyme activity. The galactosemia allele is associated with nearly complete suppression of enzyme production. Women with two copies of the galactosemia allele have the inborn error of metabolism galactosemia and develop liver failure, cataracts, mental retardation, and ovarian failure unless they are treated with severe restriction of dietary galactose. The Duarte allele is associated with an approximately 50 percent reduction in enzyme activity. Women with galactosemia usually develop ovarian failure during their early teens.[199] Cramer and associates[97, 200] reported that women with one copy of the Duarte or galactosemia allele have a partially reduced level of GALT and develop elevated FSH levels during their late 30s. One explanation for these observations is that nearly complete loss of the enzyme GALT results in the accumulation of toxic metabolites that causes a greatly accelerated loss of oocytes, whereas a partial reduction in the GALT enzyme results in only a minor increase in toxic metabolites that is associated with a slightly accelerated loss of oocytes. The effect on FSH of carrying a single allele for galactosemia appears to be similar to the effect of cigarette smoking.[97] Interestingly, women who carry one copy of the Duarte or galactosemia allele also have an increased rate of infertility compared with women with two copies of the wild-type allele.[200]

In 1976, Tiepolo and Zuffardi[201] observed that in some men with azoospermia, there was a deletion of a portion of the Y chromosome. Reijo and colleagues[202] reported that approximately 13 percent of azoospermic men have new mutations (not carried by their fathers) in a small region of the Y chromosome that includes the newly described *DAZ* gene. In follow-up of these findings, Reijo and colleagues[203] reported that approximately 10 percent of men with severe oligospermia have a de novo deletion of a small portion of the Y chromosome that includes the *DAZ* gene. The *DAZ* gene appears to be expressed in the gonocytes and spermatogonia of rodents and is a ribonucleic acid–binding protein that may help regulate gene expression in the gonad.

Deficiencies in the *GALT* gene in women and deficiencies in the *DAZ* gene in men provide examples of the families of genes that are likely to be involved in the process of conception. Identification of the genes most likely to be causally related to infertility will significantly advance our understanding of the causes of decreased fecundability.

EMPIRICAL THERAPY FOR INFERTILITY

For many infertile couples, the cause of the fertility problem cannot be identified. For example, in couples with unexplained infertility, approximately 5 to 15 percent of the infertile population, a complete fertility evaluation fails to identify a specific cause of the fertility problem.[7, 8] Because no fertility problem was identified, the proper course of treatment is often unclear. In addition to unexplained infertility, other diseases associated with infertility may not have a clear cause-effect relationship with the fertility problem. For example, for infertile women with early-stage endometriosis or infertile men with borderline abnormal semen parameters, it is not clear whether these abnormal findings cause the reduced fecundability. In all of these clinical situations, a staircase approach to empirical infertility treatment has gained in popularity because of its efficacy (Fig. 20–17).

In the staircase approach to empirical infertility treatment, the progression of therapy is from IUI or clomiphene with or without IUI to gonadotropin induction of ovulation with or without IUI to IVF. The rationale for this staircase approach is that treatment is initiated with low-cost and low-risk interventions; with each step in the program, interventions that use greater resources and carry more risk are initiated. An important feature of the staircase approach to empirical treatment of infertility is that the interventions

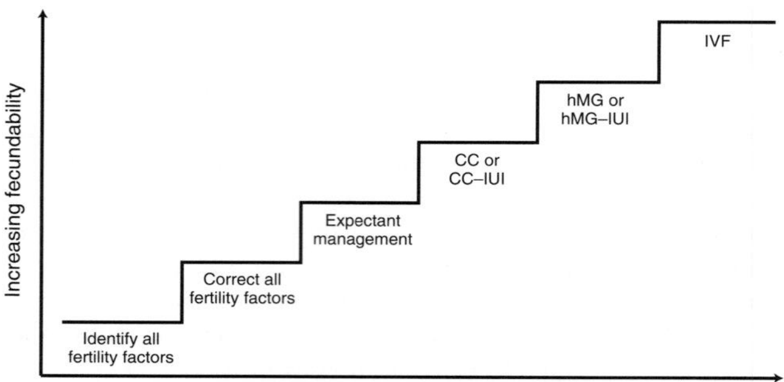

Figure 20–17 ■ Staircase approach to empirical infertility treatment. For women older than 35 years, the first three steps in the algorithm should be rapidly completed. In women younger than 30 years, more time can be spent on the first three steps in the staircase. CC, clomiphene citrate; IUI, intrauterine insemination; hMG, human menopausal gonadotropin; IVF, in vitro fertilization.

with progressively greater pregnancy rates are applied sequentially (see Fig. 20–17).

Serhal and colleagues[204] were among the first investigators to report the efficacy of empirical treatment of unexplained infertility. They randomized couples with unexplained infertility to receive IUI, ovarian stimulation with Pergonal, or ovarian stimulation with Pergonal plus IUI. The per cycle pregnancy rates in these three treatment groups were 0.022, 0.061, and 0.264, respectively. Similar results have been reported by other investigators.[205, 206]

Empirical induction of ovulation with clomiphene with or without IUI also appears to increase fecundability in couples with unexplained infertility, early-stage endometriosis, or borderline normal semen factors (Fig. 20–18). For example, Glazener and coworkers[207] randomized 118 women with unexplained infertility to receive either placebo or clomiphene. The per cycle pregnancy rates were approximately 0.05 in the placebo group and 0.07 in the group treated with clomiphene. This resulted in a statistically significant difference in cumulative pregnancy rates after three cycles (0.15 versus 0.22, $P < .05$). In another randomized study, Deaton and colleagues[208] randomized 67 couples with unexplained infertility or endometriosis to either clomiphene-IUI or observation only. In the observation-only group, the fecundability was 0.033. In the group randomized to clomiphene-IUI, the fecundability was 0.095. Similar results have been reported by Dickey and colleagues,[209] who treated 849 women with 1974 cycles of clomiphene-IUI treatment. The crude per cycle pregnancy rate was 0.072. The presence of endometriosis, tubal adhesions, low sperm motility (<20 percent), and low sperm concentration (<5 million/ml) each reduced the fecundability of the couples. These studies suggest that empirical treatment with clomiphene is more effective than empirical treatment with IUI for unexplained infertility.

The precise efficacy of IUI in programs of empirical infertility treatment remains to be established. Reports on the efficacy of IUI are contradictory. For example, Arcaini and colleagues[210] reported that IUI increased fecundability in women undergoing empirical ovulation induction. Arcaini and colleagues[210] randomized 68 couples with unexplained infertility to treatment with ovarian stimulation with clomiphene and gonadotropins versus ovarian stimulation with clomiphene and gonadotropins plus IUI. The age of the female partner, duration of infertility, and response to ovarian stimulation were similar in both groups. The initial per cycle pregnancy rate (0.19 versus 0.10) and the cumulative pregnancy rate in five cycles (0.63 versus 0.38) were better in the group that received ovarian stimulation plus IUI than in the group that received ovarian stimulation without IUI. This study supports the liberal use of IUI in programs of empirical infertility treatment.

Numerous other investigators have reported that ovarian stimulation plus IUI is associated with a per cycle pregnancy rate in the range of 0.10 to 0.20 in couples with unexplained infertility, early-stage endometriosis, or borderline abnormal semen parameters.[211] In contrast, Melis and associates[212] reported that IUI did not increase fecundability in couples receiving gonadotropin induction of ovulation for unexplained or male factor infertility. Melis and

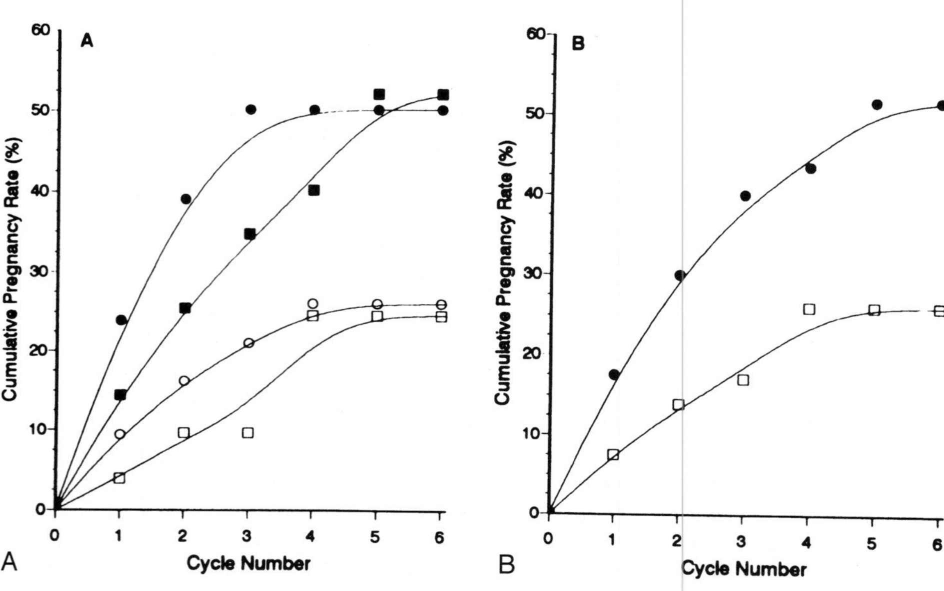

Figure 20–18 ■ Cumulative pregnancy rates by Kaplan-Meier life table analysis for 290 infertile couples undergoing clomiphene-IUI therapy stratified by the age of the female partner. *A,* Ages of women: closed circles, younger than 30 years; closed squares, 31 to 35 years; open circles, 36 to 40 years; open squares, 41 years or older. *B,* Ages of women: closed circles, younger than 35 years; open squares, older than 35 years. (From Agarwal SK, Buyalos RP. Clomiphene citrate with intrauterine insemination: Is it effective therapy in women above the age of 35 years? Fertil Steril 65:759–763, 1996. Reproduced with permission of the American Society for Reproductive Medicine.)

associates[212] randomized 200 couples with unexplained or mild male factor infertility to receive gonadotropin treatment with or without IUI. Each couple was treated for three cycles. IUI treatment did not increase the fecundability in the couples. For the couples with unexplained infertility, the per cycle pregnancy rate was 0.18 with gonadotropin treatment and 0.18 with gonadotropin plus IUI treatment. For the couples with mild male factor infertility, the per cycle pregnancy rate was 0.11 with gonadotropin treatment and 0.11 with gonadotropin plus IUI treatment. Karlstrom and colleagues[213] studied the relative efficacy of intercourse versus IUI in 157 couples with unexplained infertility or early-stage endometriosis. The fecundability was 0.149 in the couples randomized to ovulation induction plus vaginal intercourse versus 0.125 in the group randomized to ovulation induction and IUI. The investigators concluded that IUI did not significantly increase the fecundability in this population. Arici and coworkers[214] have reported that IUI alone was less effective than IUI plus clomiphene in the treatment of unexplained infertility. The per cycle pregnancy rate with IUI alone was 0.05. The per cycle pregnancy rate with clomiphene plus IUI was 0.26. A problem with this study is that the reported pregnancy rate with clomiphene plus IUI is considerably higher than that observed by other investigators. Similarly, Nulsen and colleagues[215] reported that IUI alone was much less effective than hMG plus IUI in increasing fecundability in couples with unexplained infertility, endometriosis, and male factor infertility (Fig. 20–19).

The efficacy of IUI may be easier to demonstrate in couples with male factor infertility. Ho and coworkers[216] randomized couples with abnormal semen factors as the only identifiable cause of the decreased fertility to gonadotropin alone or gonadotropin plus IUI. The gonadotropin-only treatment resulted in no pregnancies in 42 cycles. The gonadotropin plus IUI resulted in six pregnancies in 42 cycles (0.143).

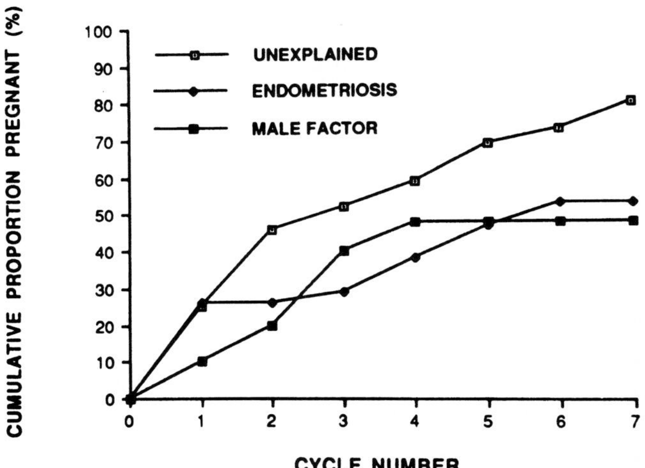

Figure 20–19 ■ Cumulative pregnancy rate for gonadotropin-IUI treatment of various fertility conditions: unexplained, early-stage endometriosis, and male factor. (From Nulsen JC, Walsh S, Dumex S, Metzger DA. A randomized and longitudinal study of human menopausal gonadotropin with intrauterine insemination in the treatment of infertility. Obstet Gynecol 82:780–786, 1993. Reproduced with permission of The American College of Obstetricians and Gynecologists.)

Although IUI appears to increase fecundability in some infertile couples, direct placement of sperm in the fallopian tube does not appear to increase fecundability over that observed with IUI treatment. Karande and associates[217] randomized infertile couples to receive either ovarian stimulation with fallopian tube sperm perfusion or ovarian stimulation with IUI. The per cycle pregnancy rate in each group was 0.11. The investigators concluded that fallopian sperm perfusion is more resource intensive than is IUI and offered no therapeutic benefit in the population studied. Similarly, Gregoriou and colleagues[218] reported that direct placement of the sperm in the peritoneal cavity did not increase fecundability over that observed with IUI.

In the empirical treatment of infertility, the combination of GnRH agonist analogues plus gonadotropin does not appear to increase fecundability over that observed with gonadotropin alone. Sengoku and colleagues[219] randomized 91 couples with unexplained infertility to receive hMG alone or hMG plus GnRH agonist. The per cycle pregnancy rates in the two groups were 0.11 and 0.13, respectively. These rates were not statistically different.

In summary, most studies suggest that the relative rank order of efficacy for the treatment of unexplained infertility, early-stage endometriosis, or mild male factor infertility is IVF > gonadotropin-IUI > gonadotropin > clomiphene-IUI or clomiphene alone > IUI alone or observation alone (Figs. 20–20 and 20–21).

ADOPTION

The most difficult decision in fertility treatments is deciding when to cease active interventions designed to increase fecundability. Throughout the process of fertility treatment, it is prudent to raise the issue of when to cease active intervention and to offer adoption as a method of building a family. It may be useful for couples to explore the option of adoption at the same time that they are undergoing fertility therapy. If the fertility therapy fails, adoption may help couples cope with the loss caused by their infertility.

PSYCHOSOCIAL ASPECTS OF INFERTILITY

Infertility and the associated diagnostic and therapeutic procedures can produce significant stress for each partner in the couple and their relationship. Each diagnostic and therapeutic procedure offers hope for an imminent successful conception, but each subsequent menstrual cycle rekindles the feeling of loss. The repetitive cycles of hope and loss can be stressful for couples with infertility.[220] Infertility can be perceived by the couple as a loss that is often difficult to grieve for because the absence of fertility is somewhat intangible. Infertility may be especially stressful for those couples when the cause of the infertility is difficult to identify.[221] The classic progression of emotions related to a loss is often expressed by the infertile couple.[222] These emotions include the feelings of disbelief and surprise, denial, anger, isolation, guilt, grief, and resolution. For many couples, the female partner bears a disproportionate degree of responsibility for the loss that infertility

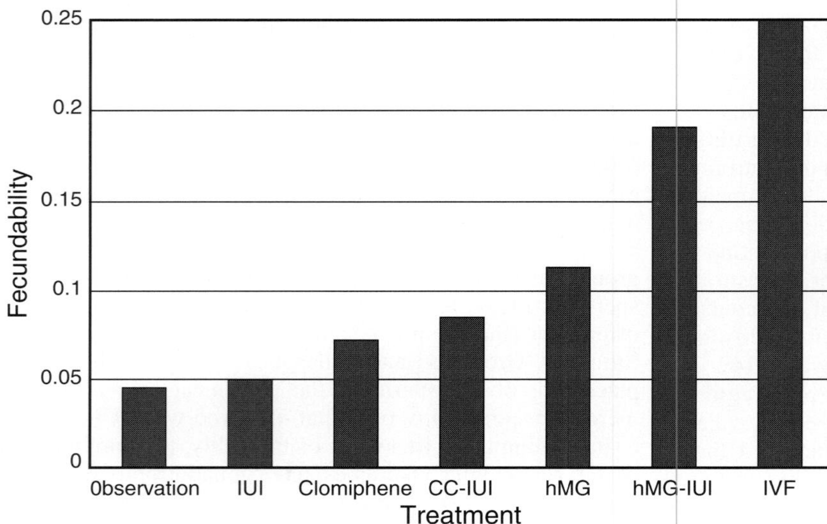

Figure 20–20 ■ Fecundability associated with empirical treatment of unexplained infertility. IUI, intrauterine insemination; CC, clomiphene citrate; hMG, human menopausal gonadotropin; IVF, in vitro fertilization.

represents. Although infertility treatment is often perceived as extremely stressful, infertility treatment does not appear to be associated with long-term emotional distress, dysfunction, or de novo psychiatric conditions.[223] Recent preliminary findings suggest that effective management of the stress and psychosocial sequelae of infertility might decrease the cost of fertility treatments and increase the fecundability of the couple.

INFERTILITY: SOCIAL AND ETHICAL ISSUES

Medicine is an ethical profession that has long adhered to basic principles of human rights: respect for the dignity of human life, the right of an individual to participate in decisions that affect his or her health, an unwavering dedication to seek good and to avoid unnecessary harm, and a commitment to treat the patient fairly. Fertility practitioners also have an ethical obligation to protect the security of the genetic human material in their custody.

Most ethicists are in agreement that the inviolability of each human precludes any medical intervention without the individual's consent. Free and informed consent is the cornerstone of ethical medical practice. Practices that are deceptive or could have the appearance of being deceptive undermine the credibility of clinicians in the fertility profession.

Embryonic development is a continuous biologic process. Current law tends to assign gradually increasing rights to the developing life. A human does not acquire full legal identity until birth but is offered some legal protections in utero (e.g., restrictions on legal abortion in the third trimester). Modern society is not unified on the point in the developmental process at which the developing life becomes a unique individual with full rights to inviolability and inalienability. This disagreement, which is most obvious in the debate over abortion, will make it difficult to reach consensus on the ethics of certain types of fertility research, such as research on discarded embryos. However, most practitioners and ethicists are in agreement that clon-

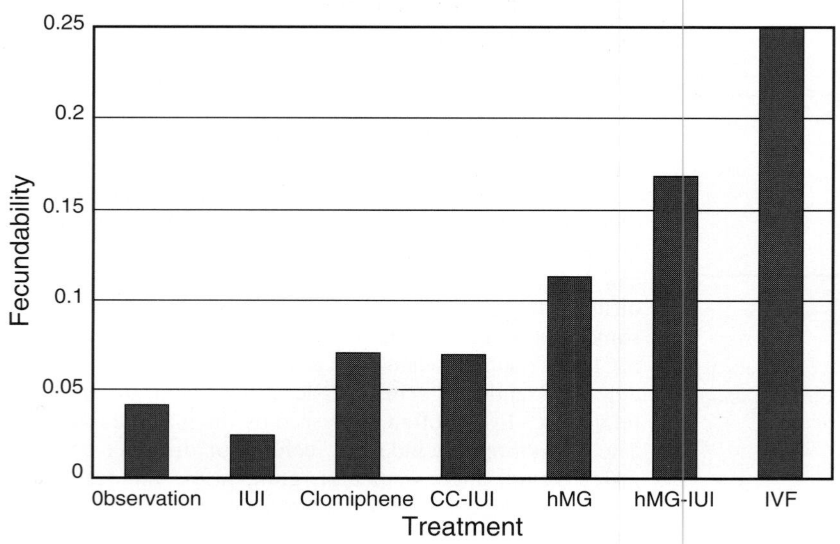

Figure 20–21 ■ Fecundability associated with empirical treatment of early-stage endometriosis. IUI, intrauterine insemination; CC, clomiphene citrate; hMG, human menopausal gonadotropin; IVF, in vitro fertilization.

ing of humans, interspecies fertilization, and the creation of chimeras are not ethical.

References

1. Mosher WD. Infertility: Why business is booming. Am Demograph 9:42–43, 1987.
2. Cramer DW, Walker AM, Schiff I. Statistical methods in evaluating the outcome of infertility therapy. Fertil Steril 32:80–86, 1979.
3. Guttmacher AF. Factors affecting normal expectancy of conception. JAMA 161:855–860, 1956.
4. Zinaman MJ, Clegg ED, Brown CC, et al. Estimates of human fertility and pregnancy loss. Fertil Steril 65:503–509, 1996.
5. Wilcox AJ, Weinburg CR, O'Connor J, et al. Incidence of early loss of pregnancy. N Engl J Med 319:189–194, 1988.
6. Bloch SK. Occult pregnancy: A pilot study. Obstet Gynecol 48:365–368, 1976.
7. WHO Scientific Group Report. Recent Advances in Medically Assisted Conception. WHO Technical Report Series 820. Geneva, World Health Organization, 1992.
8. Collins JA. Unexplained infertility. *In* Keye WR, Chang RJ, Rebar RW, Soules MR (eds). Infertility: Evaluation and Treatment. Philadelphia, WB Saunders, 1995, pp 249–262.
9. Wilcox AJ, Weinberg CR, Baird DD. Timing of sexual intercourse in relation to ovulation. N Engl J Med 333:1517–1521, 1995.
10. Filicori M, Butler JP, Crowley WF Jr. Neuroendocrine regulation of the corpus luteum in the human. Evidence for pulsatile progesterone secretion. J Clin Invest 73:1638–1647, 1984.
11. Hull MG, Savage PE, Bromham DR, et al. The value of a single serum progesterone measurement in the midluteal phase as a criterion of a potentially fertile cycle derived from treated and untreated conception cycles. Fertil Steril 37:355–360, 1982.
12. Lessey BA, Castlebaum AJ, Sawin SW, et al. Aberrant integrin expression in the endometrium of women with endometriosis. J Clin Endocrinol Metab 79:643–649, 1994.
13. Hamilton CJ, Wetzels LC, Evers JL, et al. Follicle growth curves and hormonal patterns in patients with the luteinized unruptured follicle syndrome. Fertil Steril 43:541–548, 1985.
14. Kerin JF, Kirby C, Morris D, et al. Incidence of the luteinized unruptured follicle phenomenon in cycling women. Fertil Steril 40:620–626, 1983.
15. Scheenjes E, te Velde ER, Kremer J. Inspection of the ovaries and steroids in serum and peritoneal fluid at various time intervals after ovulation in fertile women: Implications for the luteinized unruptured follicle syndrome. Fertil Steril 54:38–41, 1990.
16. Reindollar RH, Novak M, Tho SPT, McDonough PG. Adult onset amenorrhea: A study of 262 patients. Am J Obstet Gynecol 155:531–543, 1986.
17. Laufer MR, Floor AE, Parsons KE, et al. Hormone testing in women with adult onset amenorrhea. Gynecol Obstet Invest 40:200–203, 1995.
18. Barbieri RL, Ryan KJ. The menstrual cycle. *In* Ryan KJ, Berkowitz RS, Barbieri RL (eds). Kistner's Gynecology: Principles and Practice, 6th ed. St. Louis, Mosby, 1995, pp 11–49.
19. Collins JA, Wrixon W, Janes LB, Wilson EH. Treatment of independent pregnancy among infertile couples. N Engl J Med 309:1202–1206, 1983.
20. Frisch RE. The right weight: Body fat, menarche and ovulation. Baillieres Clin Obstet Gynecol 4:419–439, 1990.
21. Grodstein F, Goldman MB, Cramer DW. Body mass index and ovulatory infertility. Epidemiology 5:247–250, 1994.
22. Pasquali R, Antenucci D, Casimirri F. Clinical and hormonal characteristics of obese and amenorrheic hyperandrogenic women before and after weight loss. J Clin Endocrinol Metab 68:173–178, 1989.
23. Clark AM, Ledger W, Galletly C, et al. Weight loss results in significant improvement in pregnancy and ovulation rates in anovulatory obese women. Hum Reprod 10:2705–2712, 1995.
24. Schneider JS, Snow RC, Barbieri RL. High dietary fiber and low saturated fat intake among oligomenorrheic undergraduates. Fertil Steril 54:632–637, 1990.
25. Snow R, Barbieri RL, Frisch RA. Estrogen 2-hydroxylase activity and menstrual function in elite oarsmen. J Clin Endocrinol Metab 69:369–376, 1989.
26. Abraham S, Mira M, Llewellyn-Jones D. Should ovulation be induced in women recovering from an eating disorder or who are compulsive exercisers? Fertil Steril 53:566–568, 1990.
27. Greenblatt RB, Barfield WE, Jungck EC, Ray AW. Induction of ovulation with MRL-41. JAMA 178:101–106, 1961.
28. Adashi EY. Clomiphene citrate initiated ovulation: A clinical update. Semin Reprod Endocrinol 4:255–272, 1986.
29. Young RL, Goldzieher JW, Elkind-Hirsch K, et al. A short-term comparison of the effects of clomiphene citrate and conjugated equine estrogen in menopausal/castrate women. Int J Fertil 36:167–171, 1991.
30. Jones GS, Moraes-Ruehsen M. Induction of ovulation with human gonadotropins and with clomiphene. Fertil Steril 16:461–484, 1965.
31. Kerin JF, Liu JH, Phillipou G, Yen SSC. Evidence for a hypothalamic site of action of clomiphene citrate in women. J Clin Endocrinol Metab 61:265–268, 1985.
32. Vaitukaitis JL, Bermudez JA, Cargille CM, et al. New evidence for an antiestrogenic action of clomiphene citrate in women. J Clin Endocrinol Metab 32:503–508, 1971.
33. Tobias A, Carr LA, Voogt JL. Effects of estradiol benzoate and clomiphene on tyrosine hydroxylase activity and on luteinizing hormone and prolactin levels in ovariectomized rat. Life Sci 29:711–715, 1981.
34. Miyake A, Tasaka K, Sakumoto T, et al. Clomiphene citrate induces luteinizing hormone release through hypothalamic luteinizing hormone releasing hormone in vitro. Acta Endocrinol (Copenh) 103:289–293, 1983.
35. Adashi EY, Hsueh AJ, Bambino TH, Yen SSC. Disparate effect of clomiphene and tamoxifen on pituitary gonadotropin release in vitro. Am J Physiol 240:E125–E130, 1981.
36. Zhuang L, Adashi EY, Hsueh AJ. Direct enhancement of gonadotropin-stimulated ovarian estrogen biosynthesis by estrogen and clomiphene citrate. Endocrinology 110:2219–2225, 1982.
37. Pildes RB. Induction of ovulation with clomiphene. Am J Obstet Gynecol 91:466–473, 1965.
38. Van Campenhout J, Simard R, Leduc B. Antiestrogenic effect of clomiphene in the human being. Fertil Steril 19:700–706, 1968.
39. WHO Scientific Group Report. Consultation on the Diagnosis and Treatment of Endocrine Forms of Female Infertility. WHO Technical Report Series 514. Geneva, World Health Organization, 1976.
40. Hull MG, Knuth UA, Murray MA, Jacobs HS. The practical value of the progestogen challenge test, serum estradiol estimation or clinical examination in assessment of the estrogen state and response to clomiphene in amenorrhea. Br J Obstet Gynecol 86:799–805, 1979.
41. Turksoy RN, Biller BJ, Farber M, et al. Ovulatory response to clomiphene citrate during bromocriptine failed ovulation in amenorrhea-galactorrhea and hyperprolactinemia. Fertil Steril 37:441–444, 1982.
42. Wu CH, Winkel CA. The effect of therapy initiation day on clomiphene citrate therapy. Fertil Steril 52:564–568, 1989.
43. Gysler M, March CM, Mishell DR, Bailey EJ. A decade's experience with an individualized clomiphene treatment regimen including its effect on the postcoital test. Fertil Steril 37:161–167, 1982.
44. O'Herlihy C, Pepperell RJ, Brown JB, et al. Incremental clomiphene therapy; a new method for treating persistent anovulation. Obstet Gynecol 58:535–539, 1981.
45. Hammond MG, Halme JK, Talbert LM. Factors affecting the pregnancy rate in clomiphene citrate induction in ovulation. Obstet Gynecol 62:196–202, 1983.
46. Rossing MA, Daling JR, Weiss NS, et al. Ovarian tumors in a cohort of infertile women. N Engl J Med 331:771–776, 1994.
47. Whittemore AS, Harris P, Itnyre J. The Collaborative Ovarian Cancer Group: Collaborative analysis of twelve U.S. case control studies. II. Invasive epithelial cancer in white women. Am J Epidemiol 136:1184–1189, 1992.
48. Cramer DW, Hutchinson GB, Welch WR, et al. Determinants of ovarian cancer risk. I. Reproductive experiences and family history. J Natl Cancer Inst 71:711–716, 1983.
49. Swyer GI, Radwanska E, McGarrigle HH. Plasma estradiol and progesterone estimation for the monitoring of induction of ovulation with clomiphene and chorionic gonadotropin. Br J Obstet Gynecol 82:794–799, 1975.

50. O'Herlihy C, Pepperell RJ, Robinson HP. Ultrasound timing of human chorionic gonadotropin administration in clomiphene-stimulated cycles. Obstet Gynecol 59:40–46, 1982.
51. Palopoli FP, Feil VJ, Allen RE, et al. Substituted aminoalkoxytriarylhaloethylenes. J Med Chem 10:84–86, 1967.
52. Merrell Dow Pharmaceuticals. Product Information Bulletin. Cincinnati, OH, National Laboratories, 1972.
53. Rein M, Barbieri RL, Greene M. High order multiple gestation associated with the use of clomiphene and human menopausal gonadotropin. Int J Fertil 35:154–156, 1990.
54. Jansen RP. Spontaneous abortion incidence in the treatment of infertility. Am J Obstet Gynecol 143:451–456, 1982.
55. Daly DC, Walters CA, Soto-Albors CE, et al. A randomized study of dexamethasone in ovulation induction with clomiphene citrate. Fertil Steril 41:844–848, 1984.
56. Maruo T, Katayama K, Barnea ER, Mochizuki M. A role for thyroid hormone in the induction of ovulation and corpus luteum function. Horm Res 37(suppl 1):12–18, 1992.
57. Laohaprasitiporn C, Barbieri RL, Yeh J. Induction of ovulation with the sole use of clomiphene citrate in late onset 21-hydroxylase deficiency. Gynecol Obstet Invest 41:224–226, 1996.
58. Birnbaum MD, Rose LI. Late onset adrenocortical hydroxylase deficiencies associated with menstrual dysfunction. Obstet Gynecol 63:445–451, 1984.
59. Kistner RW. Sequential use of clomiphene citrate and human menopausal gonadotropin in ovulation induction. Fertil Steril 27:72–82, 1976.
60. Jarrell J, McInnes R, Crooke R. Observations on the combination of clomiphene citrate–hMG–hCG in the management of anovulation. Fertil Steril 35:634–639, 1981.
61. Gemzell CA, Diczfalusy E, Tillinger KG. Clinical effect of human pituitary follicle stimulating hormone. J Clin Endocrinol Metab 18:1333–1339, 1958.
62. Lunenfeld B, Sulimovici S, Rabau E, Eshkol A. L'induction de l'ovulation dans les amenorrhea hypophysaires par un traitement combaine de gonadotropine urinaires menopausiques et de gonadotropines chorionique. C R Soc Fr Gynecol 35:346–351, 1962.
63. Karnitis VJ, Townson DH, Friedman CI, Danforth DR. Recombinant human follicle stimulating hormone stimulates multiple follicular growth, but minimal estrogen production in gonadotropin releasing hormone antagonist treated monkeys: Examining the role of luteinizing hormone in follicular development and steroidogenesis. J Clin Endocrinol Metab 79:91–97, 1994.
64. Lunenfeld B, Eshkol A. Induction of ovulation with gonadotropin. *In* Rolland R, van Hall EV, Hillier SG (eds). Follicular Maturation and Ovulation. Amsterdam, Excerpta Medica, 1982, p 361.
65. Gemzell CA. Experience with the induction of ovulation. J Reprod Med 21:205–207, 1978.
66. Schwartz M, Jewelewicz R, Dyrenfurth I, et al. Use of hMG/hCG for induction of ovulation: Sixteen years experience at Sloan Hospital for Women. Am J Obstet Gynecol 138:801–807, 1980.
67. Grazi RV, Taney FH, Gagliardi LL. The luteal phase during gonadotropin therapy: Effect of two human chorionic gonadotropin regimens. Fertil Steril 55:1088–1092, 1991.
68. Messinis IE, Bergh T, Wide L. The importance of human chorionic gonadotropin support of the corpus luteum during human gonadotropin therapy in women with anovulatory infertility. Fertil Steril 50:31–36, 1988.
69. Homburg R, Levy T, Ben Rafael Z. A comparative study of conventional regimen with low dose FSH for ovulation in PCOS. Fertil Steril 63:729–733, 1995.
70. Buyalos RP, Lee CT. Polycystic ovary syndrome: Pathophysiology and outcome with in vitro fertilization. Fertil Steril 65:1–10, 1996.
71. Wada I, Matson PL, Troup SA, Lieberman BA. Assisted conception using buserelin and human menopausal gonadotropins in women with polycystic ovary syndrome. Br J Obstet Gynecol 100:3665–3669, 1993.
72. Urman B, Fluker MR, Yuen BH, et al. The outcome of in vitro fertilization and embryo transfer in women with polycystic ovary syndrome failing to conceive after ovulation induction with exogenous gonadotropins. Fertil Steril 57:1269–1273, 1992.
73. Schenker JG, Weinstein D. Ovarian hyperstimulation syndrome: A current survey. Fertil Steril 30:255–259, 1978.
74. Lanzone A, Fulghesu AM, Spina MA, et al. Successful induction of ovulation and conception with combined gonadotropin releasing hormone agonist plus highly purified follicle stimulating hormone in patients with polycystic ovarian disease. J Clin Endocrinol Metab 65:1253–1258, 1987.
75. Dodson WC, Hughes CL, Whiteside DB, Haney AF. The effect of leuprolide acetate on ovulation induction with human menopausal gonadotropins in polycystic ovary syndrome. J Clin Endocrinol Metab 65:95–100, 1987.
76. Homburg R, Levy T, Berkovitz D, et al. Gonadotropin releasing hormone agonist reduces the miscarriage rate for pregnancies achieved in women with polycystic ovarian syndrome. Fertil Steril 59:527–531, 1993.
77. Homburg R, West C, Torresani T, Jacobs HS. Cotreatment with human growth hormone and gonadotropins for induction of ovulation: A controlled clinical trial. Fertil Steril 53:254–260, 1990.
78. Santoro N, Wierman ME, Filicori M, et al. Intravenous administration of pulsatile gonadotropin releasing hormone in hypothalamic amenorrhea. Effects of dosage. J Clin Endocrinol Metab 62:109–116, 1986.
79. Crowley WF, McArthur JW. Stimulation of the normal menstrual cycle in Kallmann's syndrome by pulsatile administration of luteinizing hormone releasing hormone. J Clin Endocrinol Metab 51:173–179, 1980.
80. Seibel MM, Kamrava M, McArdle C, Taymor ML. Ovulation induction and conception using subcutaneous pulsatile luteinizing hormone releasing hormone. Obstet Gynecol 61:292–297, 1983.
81. Martin KA, Hall JE, Adams JM, Crowley WF. Comparison of exogenous gonadotropins and pulsatile gonadotropin releasing hormone for induction of ovulation in hypogonadotropic amenorrhea. J Clin Endocrinol Metab 77:125–129, 1993.
82. Barbieri RL, Ryan KJ. Bromocriptine: Endocrine pharmacology and therapeutic applications. Fertil Steril 39:727–741, 1983.
83. Soules MR, McLachlan RI, Ek M, et al. Luteal phase deficiency: Characterization of reproductive hormones over the menstrual cycle. J Clin Endocrinol Metab 69:804–812, 1989.
84. Chrousos GP, MacLusky NJ, Brandon DD, et al. Progesterone resistance. Adv Exp Med Biol 196:317–328, 1986.
85. Tredway DR, Mishell DR, Moyer DL. Correlation of endometrial dating with luteinizing hormone peak. Am J Obstet Gynecol 117:1030–1036, 1973.
86. Davis OK, Berkley AS, Naus GJ, et al. The incidence of luteal phase defect in normal fertile women determined by serial endometrial biopsies. Fertil Steril 51:582–586, 1989.
87. Shoupe D, Mishell DR, Lacarra M, et al. Correlation of endometrial maturation with four methods of estimating day of ovulation. Obstet Gynecol 73:88–92, 1989.
88. Nakajima ST, Gibson M. Pathophysiology of luteal-phase deficiency in human reproduction. Clin Obstet Gynecol 34:167–179, 1991.
89. Jones GS, Aksel S, Wentz AC. Serum progesterone values in the luteal phase defects. Obstet Gynecol 44:26–31, 1974.
90. Baker TG. Radiosensitivity of mammalian oocytes with particular reference to the human female. Am J Obstet Gynecol 110:746–761, 1971.
91. Schwartz D, Mayaux MJ. Female fecundity as a function of age: Results of artificial insemination in 2193 nulliparous women with azoospermic husbands. Federation CECOS. N Engl J Med 306:404–406, 1982.
92. Toner JP, Philput CB, Jones GS, Muasher SJ. Basal follicle-stimulating hormone level is a better predictor of in vitro fertilization performance than age. Fertil Steril 55:784–791, 1991.
93. Reame NE, Kelch RP, Beitins IZ, et al. Age effects of follicle stimulating hormone and pulsatile luteinizing hormone secretion across the menstrual cycle of premenopausal women. J Clin Endocrinol Metab 81:1512–1518, 1996.
94. Scott RT, Hormann GE. Prognostic assessment of ovarian reserve. Fertil Steril 63:1–11, 1995.
95. Scott RT, Toner JP, Muasher SH, et al. Follicle stimulating hormone levels on cycle day 3 are predictive of in vitro fertilization outcome. Fertil Steril 51:651–654, 1989.
96. Jick H, Porter J, Morrison AS. Relation between smoking and age of natural menopause. Lancet 1:1354–1355, 1972.
97. Cramer DW, Barbieri RL, Xu H, Reichart JKV. Determinants of

basal follicle stimulating hormone levels in premenopausal women. J Clin Endocrinol Metab 79:1105–1109, 1994.
98. Clark ST, Radford JA, Crowther D, et al. Gonadal function following chemotherapy for Hodgkin's disease: A comparative study of MVPP and a seven-drug hybrid regimen. J Clin Oncol 13:134–139, 1995.
99. Scott RT, Leonardi MR, Hofmann GE, et al. A prospective evaluation of clomiphene citrate challenge test screening in the general infertility population. Obstet Gynecol 82:539–545, 1993.
100. Sharara FI, Beaste SN, Leonardi MR, et al. Cigarette smoking accelerates the development of diminished ovarian reserve as evidenced by the clomiphene citrate challenge test. Fertil Steril 62:257–262, 1994.
101. Agarwal SK, Buyalos RP. Clomiphene citrate with intrauterine insemination: Is it effective therapy in women above the age of 35 years? Fertil Steril 65:759–763, 1996.
102. Warburton D. Reproductive loss: How much is preventable? N Engl J Med 316:158–160, 1987.
103. Society for Assisted Reproductive Technology. Assisted reproductive technology in the United States and Canada: 1993 results generated from the American Society for Reproductive Medicine/Society for Assisted Reproductive Technology Registry. Fertil Steril 64:13–21, 1995.
104. Westrom L. Incidence, prevalence and trends of acute pelvic inflammatory disease and its consequences in industrialized countries. Am J Obstet Gynecol 138:880–892, 1980.
105. Patton DL, Askienazy-Elbhar M, Henry-Suchet J, et al. Detection of *Chlamydia trachomatis* in fallopian tube tissue in women with postinfectious tubal infertility. Am J Obstet Gynecol 171:95–101, 1994.
106. Mueller BA, Daling JR, Moore DE, et al. Appendectomy and the risk of tubal infertility. N Engl J Med 315:1506–1508, 1986.
107. DeCherney AH, Mezer HC. The nature of post tuboplasty pelvic adhesions as determined by early and late laparoscopy. Fertil Steril 41:643–649, 1984.
108. Diamond MP, DeCherney AH. Pathogenesis of adhesion formation/reformation: Application to reproductive pelvic surgery. Microsurgery 8:103–107, 1987.
109. Diamond MP, Linsky CB, Cunningham T, et al. Synergistic effects of Interceed (TC7) and heparin in reducing adhesion formation in the rabbit uterine horn model. Fertil Steril 55:389–394, 1991.
110. Boyers SP, Diamond MP, DeCherney AH. Reduction of postoperative pelvic adhesions in the rabbit with Gore-Tex surgical membrane. Fertil Steril 49:1066–1070, 1988.
111. Diamond MP, Cunningham T, Linsky CB, et al. Interceed (TC7) as an adjuvant for adhesion prevention: Animal studies. Prog Clin Biol Res 358:131–143, 1990.
112. Nordic Adhesion Prevention Group. The efficacy of Interceed for prevention of reformation of postoperative adhesions on ovaries, fallopian tubes and fimbriae in microsurgical operations for fertility: A multi center study. Fertil Steril 63:709–714, 1995.
113. Franklin RR. Reduction of ovarian adhesions by the use of Interceed. Ovarian Adhesions Study Group. Obstet Gynecol 86:335–340, 1995.
114. Stumpf PG, March CM. Febrile morbidity following hysterosalpingography: Identification of risk factors and recommendations for prophylaxis. Fertil Steril 33:487–492, 1980.
115. Watson A, Vanderkerckhove P, Lilford R, et al. A meta analysis of the therapeutic role of oil-soluble contrast media at hysterosalpingography: A surprising result? Fertil Steril 61:470–477, 1994.
116. Alper MM, Garner PR, Spence JEH, Quarrington AM. Pregnancy rates after hysterosalpingography with oil and water soluble contrast media. Obstet Gynecol 68:6–11, 1986.
117. de Boer AD, Vemer HM, Willemsen WN, Sanders FB. Oil or aqueous contrast media for hysterosalpingography: A prospective randomized clinical study. Eur J Obstet Gynecol Reprod Biol 28:65–68, 1988.
118. Dlugi AM, Reddy S, Saleh WA, et al. Pregnancy rates after operative endoscopic treatment of total or near total distal tubal occlusion. Fertil Steril 62:913–920, 1994.
119. Canis M, Mage G, Pouly JL, et al. Laparoscopic distal tuboplasty: Report of 87 cases and a 4-year experience. Fertil Steril 56:616–621, 1991.
120. Schlaff WD, Hassiakos DK, Damewood MD, Rock JA. Neosalpingostomy for distal tubal obstruction: Prognostic factors and impact of surgical technique. Fertil Steril 54:984–989, 1990.
121. Singhal V, Li TC, Cooke ID. An analysis of factors influencing the outcome of 232 consecutive tubal microsurgery cases. Br J Obstet Gynecol 98:628–636, 1991.
122. Sulak PJ, Letterie GS, Hayslip CC, et al. Hysteroscopic cannulation and lavage in the treatment of proximal tubal occlusion. Fertil Steril 48:493–494, 1987.
123. Thurmond AS, Burry KA, Novy MJ. Salpingitis isthmica nodosa: Results of transcervical fluoroscopic catheter recanalization. Fertil Steril 63:715–722, 1995.
124. Silber SH, Cohen R. Microsurgical reversal of female sterilization; the role of tubal length. Fertil Steril 33:598–601, 1980.
125. Istre O, Olsboe F, Trolle B. Laparoscopic tubal anastomosis: Reversal of sterilization. Acta Obstet Gynecol Scand 72:680–681, 1993.
126. Jette NT, Glass RH. Prognostic value of the postcoital test. Fertil Steril 23:29–32, 1972.
127. Kovacs GT, Newman GB, Henson GL. The postcoital test: What is normal? BMJ 23:29–32, 1978.
128. Collins JA, So Y, Wilson EH, et al. The postcoital test as a predictor of pregnancy among 355 infertile couples. Fertil Steril 41:703–708, 1984.
129. Glatstein IZ, Best CL, Palumbo A, et al. The reproducibility of the postcoital test: A prospective study. Obstet Gynecol 85:396–400, 1995.
130. Hornstein MD, Barbieri RL. Endometriosis. *In* Ryan KJ, Berkowitz RS, Barbieri RL (eds). Kistner's Gynecology: Principles and Practice, 5th ed. Chicago, Year Book Medical Publishers, 1990, p 320.
131. Barbieri RL. Infertility aspects of endometriosis. *In* Sciarra JJ. Gynecology and Obstetrics. Philadelphia, Lippincott-Raven, 1996, pp 1–17.
132. Schenken RS, Asch RH. Surgical induction of endometriosis in the rabbit; effect on fertility and concentration of peritoneal fluid prostaglandins. Fertil Steril 34:581–587, 1980.
133. Hahn DW, Carraher R, Foldesy R. Studies on the mechanism of infertility associated with endometriosis and the effect of an LHRH agonist in an animal model for endometriosis. *In* Labrie F, Belanger A, Dupont A (eds). LHRH and its Analogues. New York, Elsevier, 1984, p 203.
134. Vernon MW, Wilson EA. Studies on the surgical induction of endometriosis in the rat. Fertil Steril 44:684–689, 1985.
135. Schenken RS, Asch RH, Williams RF. Etiology of infertility in monkeys with endometriosis: Luteinized unruptured follicles, luteal phase defects, pelvic adhesions and spontaneous abortions. Fertil Steril 41:122–127, 1984.
136. Olive DL, Lee KL. Analysis of sequential treatment protocols for endometriosis-associated infertility. Am J Obstet Gynecol 154:613–619, 1986.
137. Acosta AA, Buttram VC, Besch PK. A proposed classification of pelvic endometriosis. J Reprod Med 3:757–761, 1988.
138. Garcia CR, David SS. Pelvic endometriosis: Infertility and pelvic pain. Am J Obstet Gynecol 129:740–746, 1977.
139. Telimaa S. Danazol and medroxyprogesterone acetate is efficacious in the treatment of infertility in endometriosis. Fertil Steril 50:872–878, 1988.
140. Soliman S, Daya S, Collins J. A randomized trial of in vitro fertilization versus conventional treatment for infertility. Fertil Steril 59:1239–1245, 1993.
141. Hornstein MH, Barbieri RL, McShane PM. The effects of previous ovarian surgery on the follicular response to ovulation induction in an in vitro fertilization program. J Reprod Med 134:277–281, 1989.
142. Matson PL, Yovich JL. The treatment of infertility associated with endometriosis by in vitro fertilization. Fertil Steril 56:432–437, 1986.
143. Haney AF, Muscato JJ, Weinberg JB. Peritoneal fluid cell populations in infertility patients. Fertil Steril 41:122–128, 1984.
144. Halme J, Becker S, Haskill S. Altered maturation and function of peritoneal macrophages: Possible role in pathogenesis of endometriosis. Am J Obstet Gynecol 156:783–789, 1987.
145. Fakih H, Baggett B, Holtz G. Interleukin-1: A possible role in the infertility associated with endometriosis. Fertil Steril 47:213–218, 1987.

146. Badawy SZ, Cuenca V, Stitzel A. Autoimmune phenomena in infertile patients with endometriosis. Obstet Gynecol 63:271–276, 1984.
147. Weed JC, Aquembourg PC. Endometriosis: Can it produce an autoimmune response resulting in infertility? Clin Obstet Gynecol 23:885–891, 1980.
148. Cheesman KL, Cheesman SD, Chatterton RT. Alterations in progesterone metabolism and luteal function in infertile women with endometriosis. Fertil Steril 29:270–275, 1978.
149. Wardle PG, McLaughlin EA, McDermott A. Endometriosis and ovulatory disorder: Reduced fertilization in vitro compared with tubal and unexplained infertility. Lancet 2:236–242, 1985.
150. Polan ML, Totora M, Caldwell BV, et al. Abnormal ovarian cycles as diagnosed by ultrasound and serum estradiol levels. Fertil Steril 37:342–347, 1982.
151. Marik J, Hulka J. Luteinized unruptured follicle syndrome: A subtle cause of infertility. Fertil Steril 29:270–275, 1978.
152. Barbieri RL. Medical treatment of infertility associated with minimal to mild endometriosis. Int J Fertil 41:276–278, 1996.
153. Seibel MM, Berger MJ, Weinstein FG. The effectiveness of danazol on subsequent fertility in minimal endometriosis. Fertil Steril 38:534–539, 1982.
154. Fedele L, Parazzini F, Radici E. Buserelin acetate versus expectant management in the treatment of infertility associated with minimal or mild endometriosis; a randomized clinical trial. Am J Obstet Gynecol 166:1345–1350, 1992.
155. Hughes EG, Fedorkow DM, Collins JA. A quantitative overview of controlled trials in endometriosis-associated infertility. Fertil Steril 59:963–970, 1993.
156. Gant NF. Infertility and endometriosis: Comparison of pregnancy outcomes with laparotomy versus laparoscopy techniques. Am J Obstet Gynecol 166:1072–1081, 1992.
157. Adamson GD. Laparoscopic treatment is better than medical treatment for minimal or mild endometriosis. Int J Fertil 41:396–399, 1996.
158. Adamson GD, Hurd SJ, Pasta DJ. Laparoscopic endometriosis treatment: Is it better? Fertil Steril 59:35–44, 1993.
159. Chong AP, Keene ME, Thornton NL. Comparison of pregnancy outcomes with three modes of treatment for infertility patients with minimal pelvic endometriosis. Fertil Steril 53:407–410, 1990.
159a. Marcoux S, Maheux R, Berube S, The Canadian Collaborative Group on Endometriosis. Laparoscopic surgery in infertile women with minimal or mild endometriosis. N Engl J Med 1997;337:217–222.
160. Fedele L, Bianchi S, Marchini M, et al. Superovulation with human menopausal gonadotropins in the treatment of infertility associated with minimal or mild endometriosis. Fertil Steril 58:28–31, 1992.
161. Kemmann E, Chazi D, Corsan G. Does ovulation stimulation improve fertility in women with minimal/mild endometriosis after laser laparoscopy? Int J Fertil 38:16–21, 1993.
162. Rein MS, Freidman AJ, Barbieri RL, et al. Heterogenous cytogenetic abnormalities are associated with uterine leiomyomata. Obstet Gynecol 77:923–926, 1991.
163. Schoenmakers EF, Wanschura S, Mols R, et al. Recurrent rearrangements in the high mobility group protein gene, HMGI-C, in benign mesenchymal tumours. Nat Genet 10:436–441, 1995.
164. Barbieri RL, Andersen J. Uterine leiomyomata: The somatic mutation theory. Semin Reprod Endocrinol 10:301–309, 1992.
165. Andersen J, DyReyes V, Barbieri RL, et al. Leiomyoma primary cultures have elevated transcriptional response to estrogen compared to autologous myometrial cultures. J Soc Gynecol Invest 2:542–551, 1995.
166. Farhi J, Ashkenazi J, Feldberg D, et al. Effect of uterine leiomyomata on results of IVF treatment. Hum Reprod 10:2576–2578, 1995.
167. Jequier AM, Ukombe EB. Errors inherent in the performance of a routine semen analysis. Br J Urol 55:434–436, 1983.
168. Dunphy BC, Neal LM, Cooke ID. The clinical value of conventional semen analysis. Fertil Steril 51:324–329, 1989.
169. Peng HQ, Collins JA, Wilson EH, Wrixon W. Receiver operating characteristics curves for semen analysis variables: Methods for evaluating diagnostic tests of male gamete function. Gamete Res 17:229–236, 1987.
170. Kruger TF, Acosta AA, Simmons KF, et al. Predictive value of abnormal sperm morphology in in vitro fertilization. Fertil Steril 49:112–117, 1988.
171. Wolff H, Anderson DJ. Immunohistologic characterization and quantitation of leukocyte subpopulations in human semen. Fertil Steril 49:497–504, 1988.
172. Tomlinson MJ, Barratt CLR, Bolton AE, et al. Round cells and sperm fertilizing capacity: The presence of immature germ cells but not seminal leukocytes is associated with reduced success of in vitro fertilization. Fertil Steril 58:1257–1259, 1992.
173. Yanagimachi R, Yanagimachi H, Rogers BJ. The use of zona-free animal ova as a test for assessment of fertilizing capacity of human spermatozoa. Biol Reprod 15:471–476, 1976.
174. Mao C, Grimes DA. The sperm penetration assay: Can it discriminate between fertile and infertile men? Am J Obstet Gynecol 159:279–286, 1988.
175. World Health Organization. The influence of varicocele on parameters of fertility in a large group of men presenting to infertility clinics. Fertil Steril 57:1289–1293, 1992.
176. Yamamoto M, Hibi H, Hirata Y, et al. Effect of varicocelectomy on sperm parameters and pregnancy rate in patients with subclinical varicocele: A randomized prospective controlled study. J Urol 155:1636–1638, 1996.
177. Madgar I, Weissenberg R, Lunenfeld B, et al. Controlled trial of high spermatic vein ligation for varicocele in infertile men. Fertil Steril 63:120–124, 1995.
178. Breznik R, Vlaisavljevic V, Borko E. Treatment of varicocele and male fertility. Arch Androl 30:157–160, 1993.
179. Howards SS. Treatment of male infertility. N Engl J Med 332:312–317, 1995.
180. Finkel DM, Phillips JL, Snyder PJ. Stimulation of spermatogenesis by gonadotropins in men with hypogonadotropic hypogonadism. N Engl J Med 313:651–655, 1985.
181. Schopohl J, Mehltretter G, von Zumbusch R, et al. Comparison of gonadotropin releasing hormone and gonadotropin therapy in male patients with idiopathic hypothalamic hypogonadism. Fertil Steril 56:1143–1170, 1991.
182. Chillon M, Casals T, Mercier B, et al. Mutations in the cystic fibrosis gene in patients with congenital absence of the vas deferens. N Engl J Med 332:1475–1480, 1995.
183. Colin AA, Sawyer SM, Mickle JE, et al. Pulmonary function and clinical observations in men with congenital bilateral absence of the vas deferens. Chest 110:440–445, 1996.
184. Belker AM, Thomas AJ, Fuchs EF, et al. Results of 1469 microsurgical vasectomy reversals by the Vasovasostomy Study Group. J Urol 145:505–511, 1991.
185. Denil J, Ohl DA, McGuire EJ, Jonas U. Treatment of anejaculation with electroejaculation. Acta Urol Belg 60:15–25, 1992.
186. Bokemeyer C, Schmoll HJ, van Rhee J, et al. Long term gonadal toxicity after therapy for Hodgkin's and non-Hodgkin's lymphoma. Ann Hematol 68:105–110, 1994.
187. Odem RR, Durso NM, Long CA, et al. Therapeutic donor insemination: A prospective randomized study of scheduling methods. Fertil Steril 55:976–982, 1991.
188. Bronson R, Cooper G, Rosenfeld DL. Sperm antibodies: Their role in infertility. Fertil Steril 42:171–183, 1984.
189. Collins JA, Burrows EA, Yeo J, Young Lai EV. Frequency and predictive value of antisperm antibodies among infertile couples. Hum Reprod 8:592–598, 1993.
190. Yasuda M, Takakuwa K, Tokunaga A, Tanaka K. Prospective studies of the association between anticardiolipin antibody and outcome of pregnancy. Obstet Gynecol 86:555–559, 1995.
191. Out HJ, Bruinse HW, Christaens GC, et al. A prospective controlled multicenter study on the obstetrics risk of pregnant women with antiphospholipid antibodies. Am J Obstet Gynecol 167:26–32, 1992.
192. Silver RM, Porter TF, van Leeuween I, et al. Anticardiolipin antibodies: Clinical consequences of low titers. Obstet Gynecol 87:494–500, 1996.
193. Cowchuck FS, Reece EA, Balaban D, et al. Repeated fetal losses associated with antiphospholipid antibodies: A collaborative randomized trial comparing prednisone with low dose heparin treatment. Am J Obstet Gynecol 166:1318–1323, 1992.
194. Scott JR, Branch DW. Evaluation and treatment of recurrent miscarriages. *In* Keye WR, Chang RJ, Rebar RW, Soules MR (eds). Infertility: Evaluation and Treatment. Philadelphia, WB Saunders, 1995, pp 230–248.

195. Hill JA. Immunological mechanisms of pregnancy maintenance and failure: A critique of theories and therapy. Am J Reprod Immunol 22:33–42, 1990.
196. Patton P, Novy MJ. Reproductive potential of the anomalous uterus. Semin Reprod Endocrinol 6:217–233, 1988.
197. Fayez JA. Comparison between abdominal and hysteroscopic metroplasty. Obstet Gynecol 68:399–432, 1986.
198. Check JH, Caro JF, Criden L, et al. Leydig cell responsiveness with germinal cell resistance to gonadotropin therapy in Kallmann's syndrome. Am J Med 67:495–497, 1979.
199. Kaufman FR, Reichardt JK, Ng WG, et al. Correlation of cognitive, neurologic and ovarian outcome with the Q188R mutation of the galactose-1-phosphate uridyl transferase gene. J Pediatr 125:225–227, 1994.
200. Cramer DW, Harlow BL, Barbieri RL, Ng WG. Galactose-1-phosphate uridyl transferase activity associated with age at menopause and reproductive history. Fertil Steril 51:609–615, 1989.
201. Tiepolo L, Zuffardi O. Localization of factors controlling spermatogenesis in the non-fluorescent portion of the human Y chromosome long arm. Hum Genet 34:119–124, 1976.
202. Reijo R, Lee TY, Salo P, et al. Diverse spermatogenetic defects in humans caused by Y chromosome deletions encompassing a novel RNA binding protein gene. Nat Genet 10:383–393, 1995.
203. Reijo R, Alagappan RK, Patrizio P, Page DC. Severe oligozoospermia resulting from deletions of azoospermia factor gene on Y chromosome. Lancet 347:1290–1293, 1996.
204. Serhal PF, Katz M, Little V, Woronowski H. Unexplained infertility: The value of Pergonal superovulation combined with intrauterine insemination. Fertil Steril 49:602–608, 1988.
205. Sher G, Knutzen VK, Stratton CJ, et al. In vitro sperm capacitation and transcervical intrauterine insemination for the treatment of refractory infertility. Fertil Steril 41:260–264, 1984.
206. Dodson WC, Whiteside DB, Hughes CL, et al. Superovulation with intrauterine insemination in the treatment of infertility: A possible alternative to gamete intrafallopian transfer and in vitro fertilization. Fertil Steril 48:441–445, 1987.
207. Glazener CM, Coulson C, Lambert PA, et al. Clomiphene treatment for women with unexplained infertility: Placebo-controlled study of hormonal responses and conception rates. Gynecol Endocrinol 4:75–83, 1990.
208. Deaton JL, Gibson M, Blackmer KM, et al. A randomized controlled trial of clomiphene citrate and intrauterine insemination in couples with unexplained infertility or surgically corrected endometriosis. Fertil Steril 54:1083–1088, 1990.
209. Dickey RP, Olar TT, Taylor SN, et al. Relationship of follicle number and other factors to fecundability and multiple pregnancy in clomiphene citrate–intrauterine insemination cycles. Fertil Steril 57:613–619, 1992.
210. Arcaini L, Bianchi S, Baglioni A, et al. Superovulation and intrauterine insemination vs superovulation alone in the treatment of unexplained infertility. J Reprod Med 41:614–618, 1996.
211. Karacan M, Shelden R, Corsan GH. Controlled ovarian hyperstimulation–intrauterine insemination cycles in subfertile couples. J Reprod Med 41:767–771, 1996.
212. Melis GB, Paoletti AM, Ajossa S, et al. Ovulation induction with gonadotropins as sole treatment in infertile couples with open tubes: A randomized prospective comparison between intrauterine insemination and timed vaginal intercourse. Fertil Steril 64:1088–1093, 1995.
213. Karlstrom PO, Bergh T, Lundkvist O. A prospective randomized trial of artificial insemination versus intercourse in cycles stimulated with human menopausal gonadotropin or clomiphene citrate. Fertil Steril 59:554–559, 1993.
214. Arici A, Byrd W, Bradshaw K, et al. Evaluation of clomiphene citrate and human chorionic gonadotropin treatment: A prospective randomized crossover study during intrauterine insemination cycles. Fertil Steril 61:314–318, 1994.
215. Nulsen JC, Walsh S, Dumez S, Metzger DA. A randomized and longitudinal study of human menopausal gonadotropin with intrauterine insemination in the treatment of infertility. Obstet Gynecol 82:780–786, 1993.
216. Ho PC, So WK, Chan YF, Yeung WS. Intrauterine insemination after ovarian stimulation as a treatment for subfertility because of subnormal semen: A prospective randomized controlled trial. Fertil Steril 58:995–999, 1992.
217. Karande VC, Rao R, Pratt DE, et al. A randomized prospective comparison between intrauterine insemination and fallopian sperm perfusion for the treatment of infertility. Fertil Steril 64:638–640, 1995.
218. Gregoriou O, Papadias C, Konidaris S, et al. A randomized comparison of intrauterine and intraperitoneal insemination in the treatment of infertility. Int J Gynecol Obstet 42:33–36, 1993.
219. Sengoku K, Tamate K, Takaoka Y, et al. A randomized prospective study of gonadotropin with or without gonadotropin releasing hormone agonist for treatment of unexplained infertility. Hum Reprod 9:1043–1047, 1994.
220. Seibel MM, Levin S. A new era in reproduction technologies; the emotional stages of in vitro fertilization. J In Vitro Fertil Embryo Transf 4:135–140, 1987.
221. Wasser SK, Sewall G, Soules MR. Psychosocial stress as a cause of infertility. Fertil Steril 59:685–689, 1993.
222. Menning BE. The emotional needs of infertile couples. Fertil Steril 34:313–319, 1980.
223. Freeman WE, Rickels K, Tausig J, et al. Emotional and psychosocial factors in follow-up of women after IVF-ET treatment. A pilot investigation. Acta Obstet Gynecol Scand 66:517–521, 1987.

Chapter 21

ASSISTED REPRODUCTION

Robert L. Barbieri

■ CHAPTER OUTLINE

KEY POINTS

- Assisted reproductive technologies are those infertility treatment procedures that involve the manipulation of oocytes, sperm, or embryos in vitro.
- In vitro fertilization (IVF) is indicated for the treatment of most causes of infertility that have not responded to less resource intensive treatments.
- Success rates with IVF are dependent on the clinical characteristics of the couple, including age of the female partner and cause of the infertility.
- Pregnancy occurring after IVF treatment can be associated with multiple gestations. In 1994, of the pregnancies resulting from IVF, approximately 29 percent were twins, 7 percent were triplet gestations, and 0.6 percent were higher order multiple gestations.
- Intracytoplasmic sperm injection is an evolving and effective treatment for male factor infertility.
- As the cost of treatment by assisted reproductive techniques decreases and the success increases, assisted reproductive technologies will increase in importance in the treatment of infertility.

The essence of mammalian reproduction is the fusion of a sperm and egg resulting in a conceptus, which can grow and differentiate into a new organism. Mammalian reproduction is an efficient process that typically occurs entirely within the bodies of the male and female partners and requires no intervention or assistance from a third party to achieve success. The essence of *assisted reproduction* is that a third party, the reproductive biologist, directly handles the oocyte and sperm to enhance the probability of achieving a pregnancy. In general, at least part of the manipulation of the sperm and oocyte occurs outside of the body of the male and female partners. Assisted reproductive technologies refer to a large number of techniques including in vitro fertilization and embryo transfer (IVF-ET), gamete intrafallopian tube transfer (GIFT), zygote intrafallopian tube transfer (ZIFT), intracytoplasmic sperm injection (ICSI), and cryopreservation of embryos.

The history of assisted reproduction is more than 100 years old, beginning with the attempts of Schenck to achieve fertilization in vitro and the successful transfer of embryos from a donor to a recipient rabbit by Heape.[1] In 1959, Chang[2] successfully fertilized a rabbit oocyte in vitro. In the human, successful capacitation of sperm in vitro and the fertilization of human oocytes matured in vitro[3] were followed by the insight that preovulatory oocytes provided optimal performance for in vitro fertilization.[4] These exploratory steps culminated in 1978 with a term birth resulting from the in vitro fertilization of a single preovulatory human oocyte obtained from a natural menstrual cycle.[5]

Assisted reproduction is the jewel in the crown of reproductive medicine. It is one of the best examples in reproductive medicine of the transfer of knowledge gained by laboratory scientists to an application that treats human disease. Assisted reproduction is a vast field encompassing both the sublime secrets of how two haploid cells combine to create a zygote that contains all the information necessary to grow and develop into a complex mammal and the pragmatically empirical application of the technology to treatment of infertility. As assisted reproduction becomes the standard treatment for the disease of infertility, the pace of the transfer of knowledge from bench to bedside is increasing, challenging our concepts of self, family, and society.

THE GAMETES

Sex is not necessary for successful reproduction. Single-cell organisms propagate directly by mitotic division. Some reptiles are all female and reproduce without mating. However, the majority of fish, birds, reptiles, and mammals reproduce sexually. The key feature of sexual reproduction is that unique haploid cells fuse at fertilization to form diploid cells that can grow and develop into an entire organism. In turn, some diploid cells divide by the process of meiosis to produce unique haploid cells that can fuse to yield a new, totally unique diploid organism.

Sexual reproduction has two critical features. One crucial feature of sexual reproduction is that diploid cells give rise to unique haploid cells because of genetic recombination between homologous chromosomes, a process that occurs during meiosis (see Chapter 12). Exchange of genetic material between maternally and paternally derived chromosomes markedly increases the genetic diversity of the resultant haploid cells (Figs. 21–1 and 21–2). One theoretical advantage of sexual reproduction is that the process of meiosis permits the random recombination of genetic material. The recombination of genetic material increases the range of traits displayed by members of the species. The diversity generated by genetic recombination increases the success of the species in adapting to an ever-changing environment. A second unique feature of sexual reproduction is that the haploid cells fuse in the process of fertilization to form a new diploid cell. The single-cell diploid zygote has all the information necessary to grow and develop into an adult organism.

The generation of both oocytes and sperm begins with the process of meiosis (see Figs. 21–1 and 21–2). During meiosis, duplication of diploid deoxyribonucleic acid (DNA) in the progenitor cell is followed by two successive cell divisions, which results in derivative packets of haploid DNA. In the meiotic process, the majority of time is spent in prophase of the first meiotic division. As the progenitor cell enters prophase I, each chromosome consists of two joined sister chromatids. During prophase I, homologous chromosomes are aligned in bivalents and genetic recombination occurs. In the first meiotic division, one chromosome pair (consisting of linked sister chromatids) is distributed to each daughter cell (see Fig. 21–1). In the second meiotic division, no DNA replication occurs, and the strands of the sister chromatids are separated to the derivative haploid cells (see Fig. 21–2).

In most species that reproduce by sexual reproduction, two types of gametes are produced. The egg or ovum is large and nonmotile. The developing egg or ovum is referred to as an oocyte. The sperm or spermatozoa are small and motile. In many species, the oocyte is totipotent; once stimulated, it can give rise to an entire adult organism. The stimulus can occur through the process of fertilization by a sperm or other mechanisms, such as by mechanical activation (parthenogenesis).

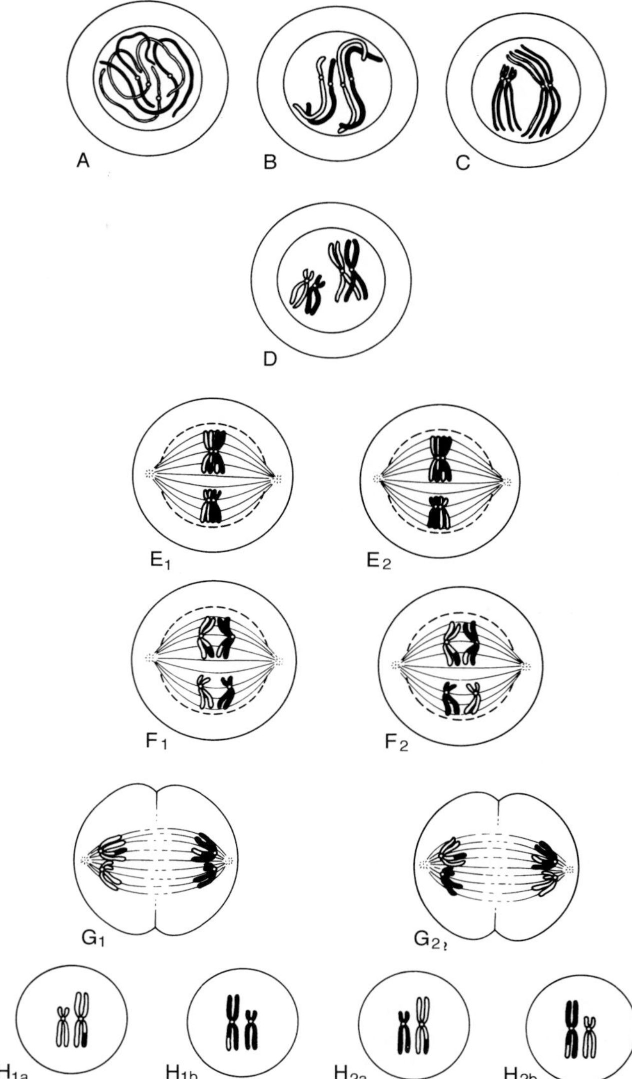

Figure 21–1 ■ The first meiotic division. Two of the 23 chromosome pairs are shown to simplify the presentation. Chromosomes from the maternal source are shown in outline, chromosomes from the paternal source are shown in black. A, leptotene; B, zygotene; C, pachytene; D, diplotene; E_1 and E_2, metaphase; F_1 and F_2, early anaphase; G_1 and G_2, late anaphase; H_1 and H_2, telophase. One set of distributions of chromosome pairs is delineated in E_1 through H_1, an alternative combination in E_2 through H_2. Homologous recombination and random segregation increase the diversity of genetic material passed to the gametes. (From Thompson JS, Thompson MW. Genetics in Medicine. Philadelphia, WB Saunders, 1986, p 19.)

The process of oogenesis begins when the primordial germ cells migrate into the embryonic gonad and become oogonia. The oogonia proliferate by mitotic division, become invested with a single layer of granulosa cells, and differentiate into primary oocytes. The primary oocyte en-

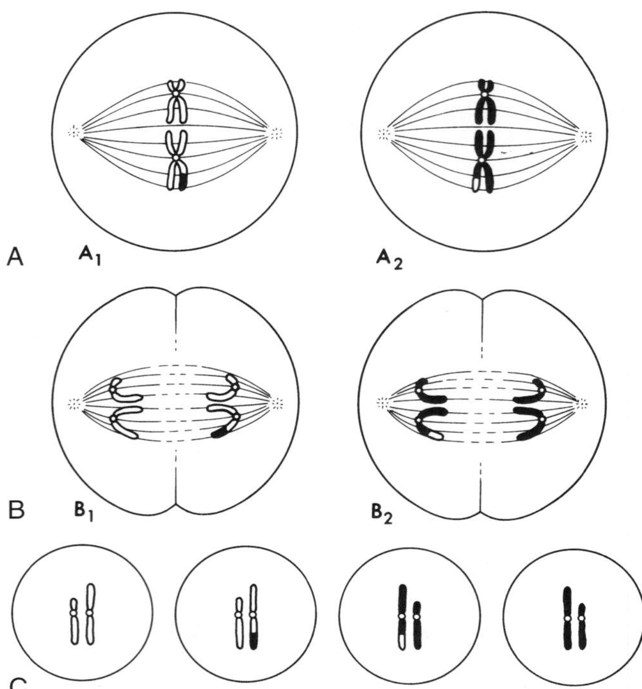

Figure 21–2 ■ The second meiotic division. A, metaphase; B, anaphase; C, telophase; A_1 and A_2 represent H_{1a} and H_{1b} from Figure 21–1. (From Thompson JS, Thompson MW. Genetics in Medicine. Philadelphia, WB Saunders, 1986, p 20.)

ters the meiotic process, duplicates its complement of DNA, reaches prophase I of meiosis, and then enters a state of prolonged "hibernation." The primary oocyte synthesizes a coat of glycoproteins, the zona pellucida. The mechanisms used by the oocyte to become one of the largest cells in the body are not fully characterized. However, one possible mechanism is that the extra copies of genes that are present in prophase I (diploid chromosome complement in duplicate) allow the oocyte to increase the rate of ribonucleic acid and protein synthesis. The primary oocyte remains arrested in this state until it is recruited into a pool of developing follicles. Under the influence of the luteinizing hormone (LH) surge, the oocyte completes meiosis I, extrudes a polar body, and becomes a secondary oocyte. The secondary oocyte proceeds to metaphase II of meiosis and awaits fertilization (Fig. 21–3).

In contrast to the egg, sperm are among the smallest cells in mammals. Sperm are highly specialized for the sole purpose of transporting DNA to an oocyte. Sperm consist of four key functional components: (1) the acrosomal vesicle; (2) the nucleus containing highly compacted DNA; (3) a midpiece enriched in mitochondria; and (4) the tail, which contains the axoneme and the dynein motor proteins. To maximize transport efficiency, the sperm has no ribosomes, endoplasmic reticulum, or Golgi apparatus.

Spermatogenesis differs significantly from oogenesis (Fig. 21–4). In the embryo, primordial germ cells migrate to the testis and enter a state of hibernation until puberty. Under the influence of testosterone and other hormones, the spermatogonia divide mitotically and generate two pools of derivative cells. The cells of one pool continue to divide mitotically and serve as the spermatogonial stem cells. The second pool of cells will enter meiosis and become primary spermatocytes (46 duplicated chromosomes). The primary spermatocytes proceed through the first meiotic division and then become secondary spermatocytes (22 duplicated autosomal chromosomes plus a duplicated X chromosome or a duplicated Y chromosome). After the second meiotic division, the secondary spermatocytes become spermatids (haploid number of single chromosomes), which then differentiate into mature sperm. The process of meiotic maturation of the spermatogonia occurs inside the seminiferous tubule, with the precursor cells located at the outer border of the tubule and the mature sperm in the lumen of the tubule. The developing sperm cells undergo nuclear division but do not complete cytoplasmic division until near the end of sperm differentiation (see Fig. 21–4). Consequently, the developing germ cells are connected by cytoplasmic bridges in a syncytium. The syncytium arrangement allows the diploid spermatogonium to produce proteins and cellular materials for the haploid sperm.

The sperm then enters the epididymis, where its surface is reorganized both by absorbing secretions from the epididymis and by internal processes.[6] When the sperm enters the female reproductive tract, it undergoes the process of capacitation. During capacitation, the proteins and lipids of the sperm membrane change in preparation for interaction with the oocyte.[7] At the end of the process of capacitation, the sperm is prepared to undergo the acrosome reaction and fertilize an egg. The acrosome is a large secretory granule that contains proteases and hyaluronidases. In the acrosome reaction, the outer acrosome membrane fuses with the plasma membrane of the sperm, and the contents of the acrosome are emptied. In many species, the acrosome reaction is initiated by the proteins of the zona pellucida and can be accelerated by progesterone.[8]

FERTILIZATION

The process of fertilization involves at least two key initial steps: interaction and penetration of the zona pellucida by the sperm, and fusion of the sperm and oocyte membranes

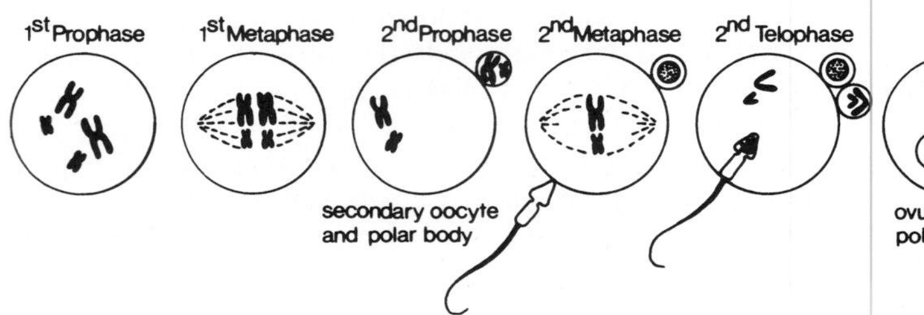

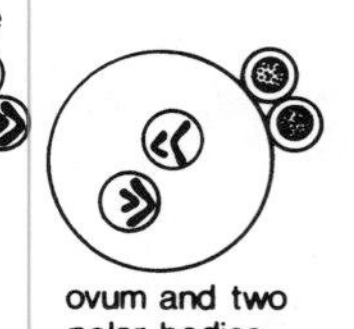

Figure 21–3 ■ Illustration of the stages of human oogenesis and fertilization. The primary oocytes remain in suspended prophase (dictyotene) until the follicle begins to grow. (From Thompson JS, Thompson MW. Genetics in Medicine. Philadelphia, WB Saunders, 1986, p 23.)

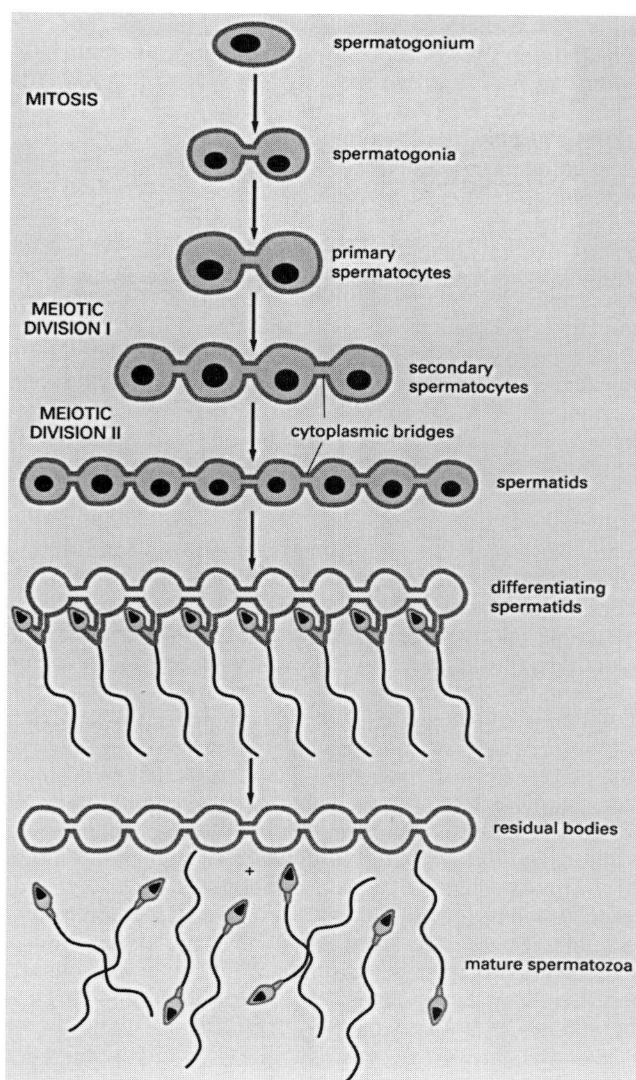

Figure 21–4 ■ The progeny of a single maturing spermatogonium remain connected to each other by cytoplasmic bridges. The cytoplasmic bridges allow the spermatids to receive proteins from the parent cell apparatus without bearing the burden of protein machinery (e.g., endoplasmic reticulum). (Redrawn from Alberts B, Bray D, Lewis J, et al. Molecular Biology of the Cell. New York, Garland Publishing, 1994, p 1031.)

(Fig. 21–5). Although the mechanisms that allow the human sperm and zona pellucida of the oocyte to interact are not fully characterized, most data suggest that a complex glycoprotein on the zona pellucida interacts with a sperm surface carbohydrate-binding protein.[9] In the mouse, the zona pellucida contains three glycoproteins, ZP1, ZP2, and ZP3. ZP2 and ZP3 have a filament structure, and ZP1 appears to link ZP2 and ZP3 in a complex three-dimensional array. Purified ZP3 blocks, in a dose-dependent manner, the ability of sperm to bind to the oocyte zona pellucida. This implies that ZP3 is the zona pellucida sperm receptor.[10] It appears that an O-linked oligosaccharide in ZP3 subserves the interaction of ZP3 and the sperm receptor.[11] The interaction of the sperm with ZP3 induces the acrosome reaction. ZP3 cross-links the sperm receptors on the sperm membrane, inducing an influx of calcium that causes the exocytotic release of proteases and hyaluronidases from the acrosome. Induction of the acrosome reaction can be inhibited by pertussis toxin, implying that a G protein complex is necessary for the acrosome reaction.[12]

After completion of the acrosome reaction, the sperm lose their affinity for ZP3.[13] After the acrosome reaction, the continued attachment of the sperm to the oocyte appears to be dependent on ZP2.[14] The sperm penetrates the zona pellucida, in part, by the forward mechanical thrust provided by the flagellum and by the hydrolytic enzymes secreted by the acrosome that cause disruption of the continuity of the zona pellucida.

A small number of proteins on the sperm surface appear to be responsible for the interaction with ZP3. For example, β1,4-galactosyltransferase on the sperm surface appears to bind with high affinity to ZP3.[15] Other putative sperm receptors for ZP3 are sp56[16] and a cell surface tyrosine kinase.[17] The role of ZP3 in fertilization in the human is not fully characterized. Studies suggest that some metaphase II oocytes that fail to fertilize demonstrate reduced ZP3 levels in the zona pellucida as determined by immunohistochemistry.[18]

In the hamster, the interaction and fusion of the sperm and oocyte plasma membranes probably involve the interaction of the sperm protein fertilin (PH-30) and an integrin receptor on the egg membrane.[19, 20] PH-30 is composed of two glycosylated transmembrane subunits, α and β. The

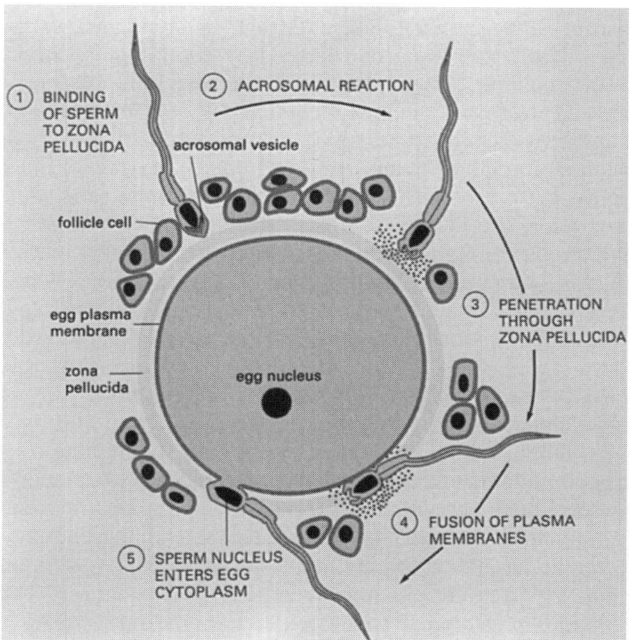

Figure 21–5 ■ Key steps in the process of fertilization. Step 1, Binding of sperm to zona pellucida involves zona protein ZP3 and a sperm protein, probably a carbohydrate-binding protein such as β1,4-galactosidase. Step 2, Acrosome reaction. Step 3, Penetration of sperm through zona pellucida. Step 4, Fusion of plasma membranes of sperm and oocyte. Depolarization of oocyte membrane and secretion of cortical granules—the primary and secondary blocks to polyspermy. Step 5, Sperm nucleus enters egg cytoplasm. (Redrawn from Alberts B, Bray D, Lewis J, et al. Molecular Biology of the Cell. New York, Garland Publishing, 1994, p 1031.)

β-subunit contains an integrin binding domain that interacts with the oocyte membrane. The α-subunit contains a fusigenic region that has high homology to viral fusion proteins. The β-subunit may serve to allow high-affinity sperm-oocyte interaction; the α-subunit subserves the process of sperm-oocyte membrane fusion.

Once the sperm and oocyte membranes fuse, a depolarization of the egg plasma membrane occurs that acts as the primary block to polyspermy. Shortly thereafter, the inositol phospholipid cell-signaling pathway is activated, resulting in an increase in cytosolic calcium, which induces the submembrane cortical granules to release their contents. The contents of the cortical granules change the glycoprotein coat of the zona pellucida, preventing sperm binding by hydrolyzing the oligosaccharides of ZP3 and by the proteolytic cleavage of ZP2. This process creates a secondary block to polyspermy.

THE EARLY CONCEPTUS AND IMPLANTATION

The prezygote is formed once the sperm penetrates the oocyte. The prezygote is characterized by the presence of two pronuclei and two polar bodies. Pronuclear membrane breakdown will then occur and a zygote will form. During this process, the maternal and paternal chromosomes reorganize and pair on the first cleavage spindle. The pre-embryo then proceeds through an exceptionally complex series of early events. In mammalian pre-embryos, up to the 8-cell stage, the blastomeres are totipotent. Up to the 8-cell stage, removal of blastomeres does not necessarily disrupt embryo development. After the 8-cell stage, the cells in the pre-embryo clearly differentiate; the surface cells become the trophoblast (and give rise to the extraembryonic structures, such as the placenta), and the inner cell mass gives rise to the embryo. The blastocyst is the stage of the pre-embryo when it develops a fluid-filled inner cavity. With use of strict terminology, the embryonic stage consists of the period from the development of the primitive streak through the initial steps in the development of all the major organs. In the human, the embryonic stage begins approximately 14 days after fertilization. In assisted reproduction, most authorities use the term embryo to describe the conceptus from the first cleavage through the initial stages of organ development. In the remainder of this chapter, I follow this convention.

In humans, the molecular biology of implantation is not well characterized (see Chapter 8). The trophectoderm nearest the inner cell mass probably plays an important role in the interaction of the blastocyst and the endometrium.[21] The interaction of the blastocyst with the endometrium involves an attachment and an invasion phase. The blastocyst can attach to the endometrium only during a critical window of implantation corresponding to menstrual cycle days 19 to 23. Although the molecules that control the attachment of the blastocyst and endometrium are not well characterized, integrins, fibronectin, and laminin have been proposed as playing a role. After attachment, the conceptus enters the endometrium and by 12 days after fertilization is completely embedded in the endometrial stroma. At the same time, the trophoblast invades the maternal endothelium, establishing a hemochorial placentation. Once this contact is established, human chorionic gonadotropin (hCG) can be measured in the maternal circulation.

ASSISTED REPRODUCTIVE TECHNOLOGIES

A large number of techniques have been described that involve manipulation of oocytes, sperm, and conceptuses to improve fecundability or enhance pregnancy outcome. In this chapter, the focus is on the most commonly performed procedures including IVF-ET, GIFT, ZIFT, ICSI, and blastomere biopsy. IVF-ET (in vitro fertilization and embryo transfer) is the laboratory culture of aspirated oocytes and spermatozoa in vitro, followed by the transcervical replacement of the embryo into the uterine cavity. GIFT (gamete intrafallopian tube transfer) is the direct placement of aspirated oocytes and spermatozoa into the fallopian tube. ZIFT (zygote intrafallopian tube transfer) is the laboratory culture of aspirated oocytes with spermatozoa followed by the direct placement of fertilized zygotes into the fallopian tubes. ICSI (intracytoplasmic sperm injection) is a technique that involves the injection of a single sperm into the cytoplasm of the oocyte, with transcervical transfer of the conceptus to the uterus.

A major deficiency in the field of assisted reproduction is that there are few randomized studies demonstrating the superior efficacy of assisted reproductive techniques versus other forms of fertility treatment. Consequently, much of the discussion of clinical assisted reproductive technologies is limited to data reported in descriptive studies that often do not have adequate control groups for comparison. Another deficiency is that many new assisted reproductive technologies are introduced into clinical practice without a clinical trial to demonstrate their utility over "standard" methods of treatment. Notwithstanding these deficiencies, there has been a consistent improvement in the success of IVF during the past decade (Table 21–1). IVF is the core

■ TABLE 21–1

In Vitro Fertilization Outcomes as Reported by Those Programs Participating in the Society for Assisted Reproductive Technology/American Society for Reproductive Medicine Registry, 1986 and 1994

	1986	1994
Cycles initiated	4,867	26,555
Cycle cancellations per cycle initiated	28%	13.2%
Oocyte retrievals	3,504	23,050
Embryo transfer per retrievals	85%	90.3%
Clinical pregnancies	485	6,089
Deliveries	NR	4,896
Deliveries per cycle initiated	<9%*	18.4%

NR, not reported.

*Assumes an abortion and ectopic rate of at least 10 percent.

Adapted from Medical Research International, The American Fertility Society Special Interest Group. In vitro fertilization/embryo transfer in the United States: 1985 and 1986 results from the National IVF/ET Registry. Fertil Steril 49:212–215, 1988; and Society for Assisted Reproductive Technology and the American Society for Reproductive Medicine. Assisted reproductive technology in the United States and Canada: 1994 results generated from the American Society for Reproductive Medicine/Society for Assisted Reproductive Technology Registry. Fertil Steril 66:697–705, 1996. Reprinted with permission of the American Society for Reproductive Medicine.

procedure in assisted reproduction, and this chapter focuses on its indications, implementation, and outcomes.

IN VITRO FERTILIZATION

Indications for In Vitro Fertilization

In current clinical practice, the standard indications for IVF are tubal factor infertility, endometriosis, male factor infertility, and idiopathic or unexplained infertility. However, as techniques improve, IVF is being recommended for essentially all infertility conditions that have not been successfully treated by other modalities. For example, IVF has recently been advocated for the treatment of polycystic ovary syndrome (PCOS) and immunologic infertility.

Tubal Factor Infertility

As noted before, a major deficiency in the assisted reproductive technologies literature is that few clinical trials are available that address key issues in the application of the technique. Few randomized trials are available comparing assisted reproductive techniques with other fertility treatments such as pelvic reconstructive surgery or empirical ovarian stimulation with gonadotropins. For example, for women with infertility and complete distal fallopian tube occlusion, expectant management is unlikely to be successful. For treatment of infertility due to distal tubal occlusion, both surgical treatment and IVF are possible therapeutic options. Unfortunately, a prospective randomized controlled trial comparing pelvic reconstructive surgery versus IVF for the treatment of infertility due to tubal occlusion has not been reported. One randomized study did demonstrate that IVF was more effective than expectant management for infertility due to tubal disease.[22] In a retrospective study reporting the results of IVF for the treatment of tubal factor infertility, the investigators reported a 70 percent cumulative livebirth rate after up to four cycles of IVF.[23] This cumulative success compared favorably with surgical treatment of infertility due to tubal disease. Notwithstanding the absence of clinical trials, as IVF success increases and the cost of IVF decreases, IVF is likely to become the preferred treatment of tubal factor infertility.

Endometriosis

For indications such as infertility in women with early-stage endometriosis, IVF has not been documented by a randomized clinical trial to be superior to other available treatments such as expectant management, human menopausal gonadotropin (hMG) with intrauterine insemination (IUI), or surgical treatment (see Chapter 20). However, some studies suggest that IVF treatment results in a higher pregnancy rate per cycle than that observed after surgical treatment, hMG-IUI, clomiphene treatment with IUI, or expectant management. For example, in one retrospective study of infertile women with advanced endometriosis, surgical treatment was associated with a cumulative pregnancy rate of 24 percent at 9 months after surgery. In a similar group of infertile women with advanced endometriosis, two cycles of IVF treatment were associated with a 70 percent pregnancy rate.[24] This study demonstrates the "time"-effectiveness of IVF treatment. For infertile couples, the older the female partner, the greater the importance of the time-effectiveness of IVF. For example, Kodama and associates[25] demonstrated that in women older than 31 years with endometriosis, treatment with IVF resulted in a significantly higher pregnancy rate than that observed in the control group (Fig. 21–6). In the women older than 31, the cumulative pregnancy rate was 59 percent in those women treated with IVF and 29 percent in women treated with expectant management. In contrast, in women younger than 32 years, the cumulative pregnancy rate during 3 years was 64 percent in the women treated with IVF and 53 percent in the control group. Because IVF is often more expensive per cycle than other treatments, such as hMG-IUI, it is usually reserved for couples who have failed to conceive after trials of these other forms of treatment.

IVF was originally developed as a method to treat tubal factor infertility. Retrospective analyses from many IVF centers indicate that IVF treatment of infertility associated with endometriosis is associated with a pregnancy rate similar to that observed with IVF treatment of tubal factor infertility. For example, Olivennes and colleagues[26] reported that IVF treatment resulted in a livebirth rate per cycle of 31 percent for women with endometriosis and 32 percent for women with tubal factor infertility. When the results were analyzed by surgical stage of the endometriosis (revised American Society for Reproductive Medicine classification), the livebirth rate per cycle was stage I, 27 percent; stage II, 31 percent; stage III, 36 percent; and stage IV, 33 percent.

Male Factor

Male factor is a broad category that ranges from men with minimally abnormal semen parameters to men with total

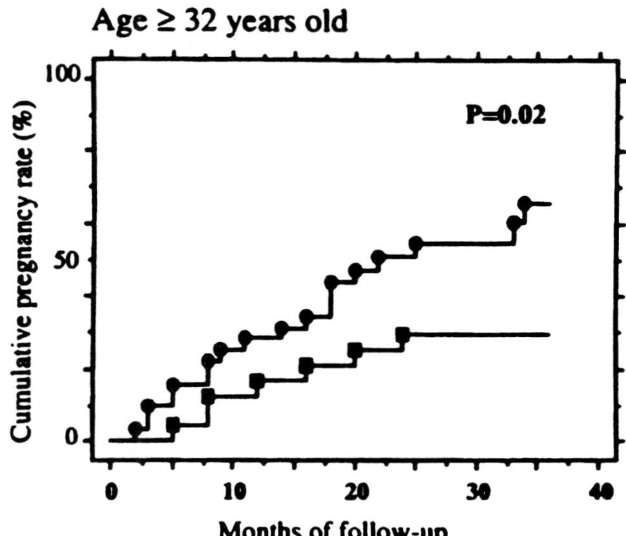

Figure 21–6 ■ Cumulative conception rate curves during 36 months for women older than 32 years with infertility and endometriosis. *Top curve,* Cumulative conception rate after IVF treatment. *Bottom curve,* Cumulative conception rate with expectant management after laparoscopy. (From Kodama H, Fukuda J, Karube H, et al. Benefit of in vitro fertilization treatment for endometriosis associated infertility. Fertil Steril 66:974–979, 1996. Reproduced with permission of the American Society for Reproductive Medicine.)

sperm counts less than 5 million per ejaculate. In general, men with severe semen abnormalities are probably best treated with ICSI (see later). Men with minimally to moderately abnormal semen parameters who have no reversible cause of the abnormality are good candidates for IVF. Male factor infertility is associated with reduced fertilization rates in IVF. Severe decreases in the number of motile sperm per ejaculate (<1.5 million) and decreases in the number of sperm with normal morphology are associated with poor pregnancy rates in standard IVF.[27]

Idiopathic Infertility

Approximately 10 to 17 percent of infertile couples have no identifiable cause of infertility after a thorough evaluation. Unexplained infertility refers to those couples who have completed a thorough infertility evaluation that includes laparoscopy. For the purposes of this chapter, idiopathic infertility refers to those couples who have completed the basic steps of the infertility evaluation but who may not have had laparoscopy as a component of their evaluation.

Many couples with idiopathic infertility achieve successful pregnancies after a stepwise empirical treatment approach (see Chapter 20), which includes empirical clomiphene treatment followed by empirical gonadotropin ovarian stimulation, with or without IUI treatment.[28] If the couple fails to conceive after treatment with empirical gonadotropin ovarian stimulation with IUI, IVF treatment often results in a successful pregnancy. In one study of 117 couples with idiopathic infertility, the clinical pregnancy rate per cycle of IVF treatment was similar to that observed for couples with tubal factor infertility (21 percent and 22 percent). However, there was a lower fertilization rate in the couples with idiopathic infertility compared with the couples with tubal factor infertility (44 percent versus 56 percent, $P < .005$), and there was a higher frequency of complete fertilization failure in the group with idiopathic infertility (20 percent versus 8 percent, $P < .001$). The cumulative pregnancy rate after three cycles of IVF was similar in both groups (45 percent versus 44 percent). These results indicate that IVF can be effective for the treatment of unexplained infertility after ovarian stimulation with gonadotropins has failed.[29]

Polycystic Ovary Syndrome

Women with PCOS are often infertile because of anovulation. Ovulation induction with clomiphene results in a high rate of ovulation (>80 percent), but cumulative pregnancy rates after clomiphene are in the range of 50 percent. For women with PCOS who do not achieve a pregnancy with clomiphene, gonadotropin treatment is often successful. Until recently, infertile women with PCOS in whom both clomiphene and gonadotropin ovulation induction failed had no remaining treatment option except ovarian wedge resection or related surgical procedures. Evidence is accumulating that IVF can be effective for the treatment of PCOS. In one study, the effects of IVF were compared between 68 infertile women with PCOS who did not become pregnant after six ovulatory cycles of gonadotropin treatment and 68 age-matched women with tubal factor infertility. Comparison of the outcome in the two groups showed that the women with PCOS had more oocytes retrieved (14 versus 11) but a lower fertilization rate (57 percent versus 66 percent) than the women with tubal factor infertility. The clinical pregnancy rate per embryo transfer (23 percent versus 26 percent) and the multiple gestation rate (19 percent versus 16 percent) were similar for the PCOS and the tubal factor infertility groups.[30] Similar results have been reported by other investigators with a clinical pregnancy rate per embryo transfer of 27 percent in the PCOS women and 22 percent in the control group.[31] It is likely that IVF will become an accepted treatment for infertility caused by PCOS after attempts at ovulation induction have not resulted in a pregnancy.

Immunologic Infertility

In some infertile couples, abnormal sperm function appears to be due to coating of the sperm with antibodies. Both IVF and ICSI have been used to treat couples with dysfunctional sperm caused by antisperm antibodies. In one study, IVF treatment of male immunologic infertility was associated with a 32 percent clinical pregnancy rate per cycle. Treatment of the male with prednisolone before IVF did not improve the pregnancy rate.[32] In some cases, when the density of antibodies on the surface of the sperm is high, ICSI but not IVF may result in a successful pregnancy.[33, 34]

Multiple Infertility Factors

Many couples have multiple factors contributing to their low fecundability. In general, the greater the number of infertility factors, the lower the success with IVF treatment. For example, in one study of the impact of IVF on infertile women with endometriosis, the livebirth rate per cycle was 31 percent in women with endometriosis as the only infertility factor. In women with endometriosis and a male partner with an abnormal semen analysis, the livebirth rate per cycle was 16 percent. For women with both endometriosis and tubal disease, the livebirth rate per cycle was 8 percent.[26] Similarly, in one study of the impact of IVF on women with tubal disease, the livebirth rate per transfer was 30 percent in women with tubal disease alone. The livebirth rate per transfer was lower when tubal factor occurred in combination with male factor (25 percent), previous diethylstilbestrol exposure (20 percent), or immunologic infertility (19 percent).[23]

Overview of In Vitro Fertilization Statistics

As IVF evolves as a scientific and clinical field, the reporting of outcomes associated with IVF procedures has continued to improve. Currently, most authorities recognize that the live delivery (birth) rate per cycle initiated provides the most realistic estimate of the likely outcome of an IVF cycle. For the calculation of the delivery rate, multiple gestations are counted as one delivery (birth), not two deliveries in the case of twins or three deliveries in the case of triplets. Unfortunately, many investigators use other numerators (clinical pregnancy, ongoing pregnancy) and denominators (transfer cycles, retrieval cycles) in calculating IVF success rates. These rates may be overly optimistic

■ TABLE 21–2

Deliveries Per Retrieval for In Vitro Fertilization Cycles as Influenced by the Age of the Female Partner and Status of Semen Factors*

	FEMALE PARTNER <40 yr	FEMALE PARTNER >40 yr
No male factor	24.5% (3671/14,990)	9% (243/2709)
Male factor	20.2% (908/4485)	8.5% (74/866)

*Parentheses reflect number of pregnancy cycles divided by number of cycles initiated.

From Society for Assisted Reproductive Technology and the American Society for Reproductive Medicine. Assisted reproductive technology in the United States and Canada: 1994 results generated from the American Society for Reproductive Medicine/Society for Assisted Reproductive Technology Registry. Fertil Steril 66:697–705, 1996. Reprinted with permission of the American Society for Reproductive Medicine.

in the evaluation of IVF success. From 1986 to 1994, there was a significant increase in the livebirths per cycle initiated from less than 9 percent to more than 18 percent[35, 36] (see Table 21–1).

Clinical characteristics of the male and female partners play a major role in determining the success rate of IVF treatment (Table 21–2). For example, in 1994, the highest success was reported for couples in which the female partner was younger than 40 years and the male had a normal semen analysis (24.5 percent deliveries per retrieval). The lowest success was reported for women older than 40 years with a male partner with a normal (9 percent deliveries per retrieval) or abnormal (8.5 percent deliveries per retrieval) semen analysis. As data sets for IVF treatment become larger and more complete, it should be possible to develop a statistical model that will predict the IVF success rate for each couple on the basis of epidemiologic and biochemical characteristics, such as age of the female partner, cycle day 3 follicle-stimulating hormone (FSH) level, and semen characteristics.

Table 21–3 presents the deliveries per cycle initiated for IVF, GIFT, ZIFT, IVF with donor oocytes, and embryo transfers using cryopreserved embryos from IVF cycles. The descriptive statistics reported for these different procedures of assisted reproduction are problematic because the clinical characteristics of the patients are not described in sufficient detail to determine whether the observed differences are due to the procedures themselves or to factors in the selection of patients. It is likely that variations in characteristics of patients are a major factor determining the differences observed among the assisted reproductive procedures.

■ TABLE 21–3

Deliveries Per Cycle Initiated for Various Assisted Reproductive Technology Procedures in the United States and Canada in 1994

	CYCLES INITIATED	DELIVERIES PER CYCLE INITIATED (%)
IVF	26,961	18.2
GIFT	4,214	25
ZIFT	962	24
IVF with donor oocyte	3,119	30
ET with cryopreserved embryos from IVF	7,193	15

IVF, in vitro fertilization; GIFT, gamete intrafallopian tube transfer; ZIFT, zygote intrafallopian tube transfer; ET, embryo transfer.

From Society for Assisted Reproductive Technology and the American Society for Reproductive Medicine. Assisted reproductive technology in the United States and Canada: 1994 results generated from the American Society for Reproductive Medicine/Society for Assisted Reproductive Technology Registry. Fertil Steril 66:697–705, 1996. Reprinted with permission of the American Society for Reproductive Medicine.

Selection of Patients

As IVF-ET results continue to improve, it has become increasingly clear that IVF-ET is most successful for couples in which the woman has an adequate ovarian follicular pool and the male partner has a normal semen analysis. As a woman ages, the ovarian follicular pool declines. Some reports suggest that the decline in the oocyte pool accelerates after 37 years of age (Fig. 21–7). Interestingly, age alone is not as accurate a predictor of the oocyte reserve as is measurement of a follicular-phase cycle day 3 FSH concentration[37] or the FSH response to clomiphene citrate.

In one study of the relationship between cycle day 3 FSH concentration and IVF pregnancy and delivery rates, the investigators observed that a cycle day 3 FSH level greater than 25 mIU/ml was associated with a clinical pregnancy rate in the range of 5 percent per cycle, and the delivery rate was in the range of 2 percent per cycle (Fig. 21–8). In contrast, for a cycle day 3 FSH level less than 15 mIU/ml, the clinical pregnancy rate was approximately 23 percent per cycle, and the delivery rate was approximately 16 percent per cycle.[38] When the interaction of age and the results of a clomiphene challenge test were examined, the investigators observed that for women with a normal clomiphene challenge test response (suggesting the presence of an adequate follicular pool), age of the female partner remained an important prognostic variable.[38] Similar results have been observed in a general infertility population (Fig. 21–9). Many authorities advise that both women with a depleted oocyte pool and women older than 40 years with a poor response to gonadotropin stimulation should consider treatment with donor oocytes.

For men with severely abnormal semen parameters, standard IVF therapy is associated with low success rates. Many authorities suggest that these men consider treatment with ICSI rather than standard IVF. For men with less than 5 million sperm per ejaculate, ICSI may be indicated as primary treatment.

One review of more than 80,000 follicle aspirations provides a concise overview of the characteristics of IVF cycles, including indications, ovulation induction methods, aspiration methods, embryos generated, luteal-phase support used, gestational rank, and pregnancy loss (Fig. 21–10). The next portion of this chapter focuses on these key components of IVF.

Ovarian Stimulation

Many techniques for preparing the ovary for oocyte retrieval have been developed. Techniques that have been

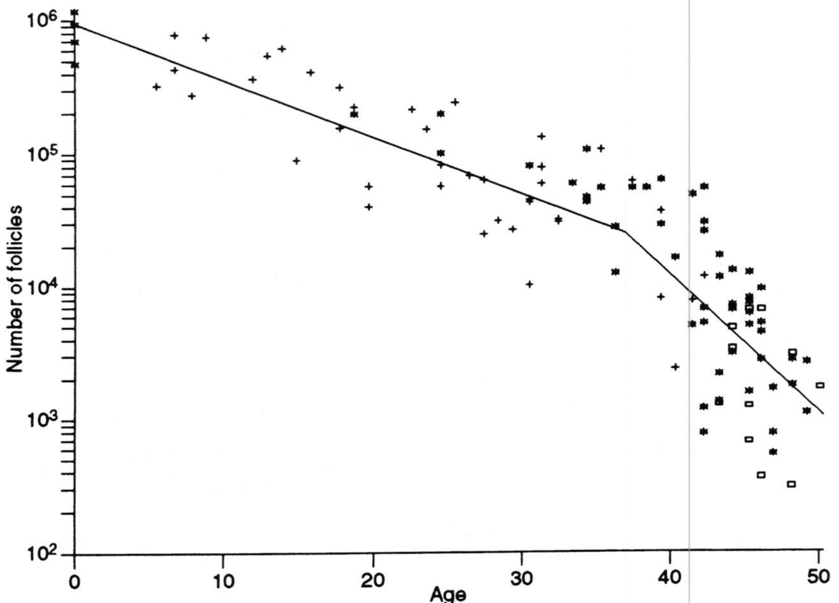

Figure 21–7 ■ Biexponential model of declining follicle numbers in women up to 51 years of age. Accelerated rate of follicle loss appears to occur after age 37 years. (From Faddy MI, Gosden R, Gougeon A, et al. Accelerated disappearance of ovarian follicles in mid-life: Implications for forecasting menopause. Hum Reprod 7:1342–1346, 1992.)

used to prepare the ovary for oocyte retrieval include monitoring the natural cycle; clomiphene treatment; clomiphene-hMG; hMG alone; highly purified human FSH (hFSH) alone; recombinant human FSH (rhFSH) alone; combinations of hMG, hFSH, and rhFSH; and pulsatile gonadotropin-releasing hormone (GnRH) (Fig. 21–11). Most programs currently use a combination of a GnRH agonist plus gonadotropin treatment to stimulate the ovary for IVF-ET cycles (Fig. 21–12).

Careful monitoring of the menstrual cycle with serum hormones and pelvic sonography can identify the time in the "natural" cycle when the dominant follicle can be aspirated to yield a fertilizable oocyte. Although conceptually appealing, natural cycle IVF is associated with low pregnancy rates. In one study of 74 natural cycle IVF procedures, oocytes were harvested in approximately 50 percent of the cycles, and the per cycle pregnancy rate was 3 percent on the basis of the number of cycles initiated.[39]

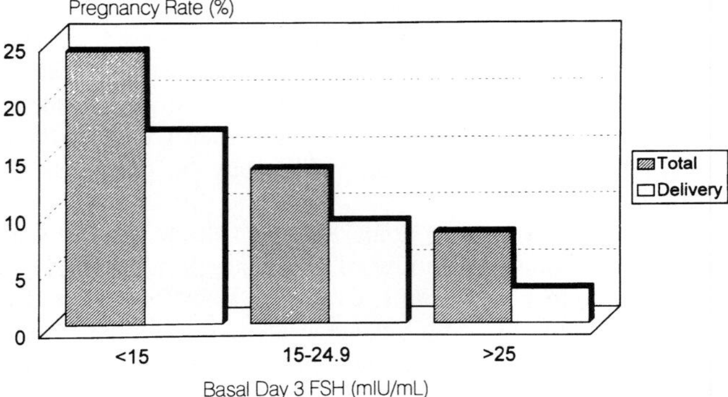

Figure 21–8 ■ Clinical pregnancy and delivery rates after IVF treatment as a function of the cycle day 3 FSH concentration of the female partner. Note the decrease in livebirth rates with day 3 FSH levels greater than 25 mIU/ml. Data based on 758 couples. (From Scott RT, Hofmann GE. Prognostic assessment of ovarian reserve. Fertil Steril 63:1–11, 1995. Reproduced with permission of the American Society for Reproductive Medicine.)

Clomiphene citrate, at doses of 100 mg daily for 5 days, induces one to three follicles in normally cycling women. In IVF cycles in which clomiphene stimulation is used, one or two oocytes are retrieved and the pregnancy rate per cycle initiated is in the range of 10 percent. For example, in one randomized study comparing IVF using a natural cycle versus clomiphene stimulation, the mean number of oocytes retrieved was 1.8 in the clomiphene group and 0.3 in the natural cycle group. The clinical pregnancy rate per cycle initiated was 12 percent in the clomiphene group and 0 percent in the natural cycle group.[40] In IVF cycles in which clomiphene is used for ovarian stimulation, support of the luteal phase with both estradiol and progesterone may improve the clinical pregnancy rate.[41]

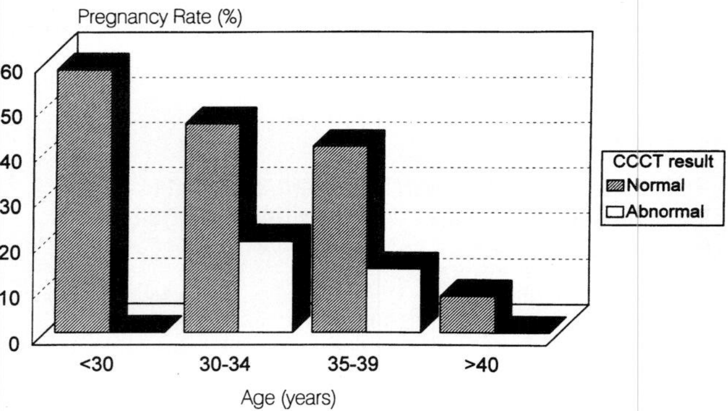

Figure 21–9 ■ Clinical pregnancy rates as a function of both age and the response to a clomiphene citrate challenge test (CCCT) in a general infertility population observed prospectively. The illustration is based on data from 236 couples. In women with an abnormal CCCT result (suggestive of a depleted oocyte pool), pregnancy rates are low regardless of the age of the female partner. In women older than 40 years, pregnancy rates are low with IVF even if the CCCT result is normal. (From Scott RT, Hofmann GE. Prognostic assessment of ovarian reserve. Fertil Steril 63:1–11, 1995. Reproduced with permission of the American Society for Reproductive Medicine.)

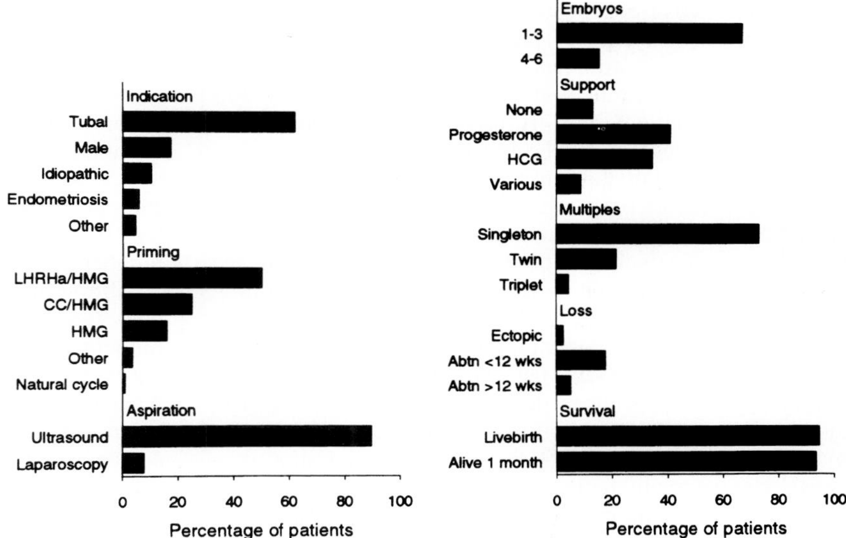

Figure 21–10 ■ Characteristics of IVF treatment in 80,000 cycles based on practices at more than 500 clinics, including indication for IVF, ovarian stimulation regimens used, aspiration techniques, embryos obtained, luteal-phase support, gestational rank, and pregnancy outcomes. (From Edwards RG, Brody SA. Principles and Practice of Assisted Human Reproduction. Philadelphia, WB Saunders, 1995, p 659. Data from Testart J. World collaborative report on IVF-ET and GIFT: 1989 results. Hum Reprod 7:362–369, 1992. Reproduced by permission of the Oxford University Press.)

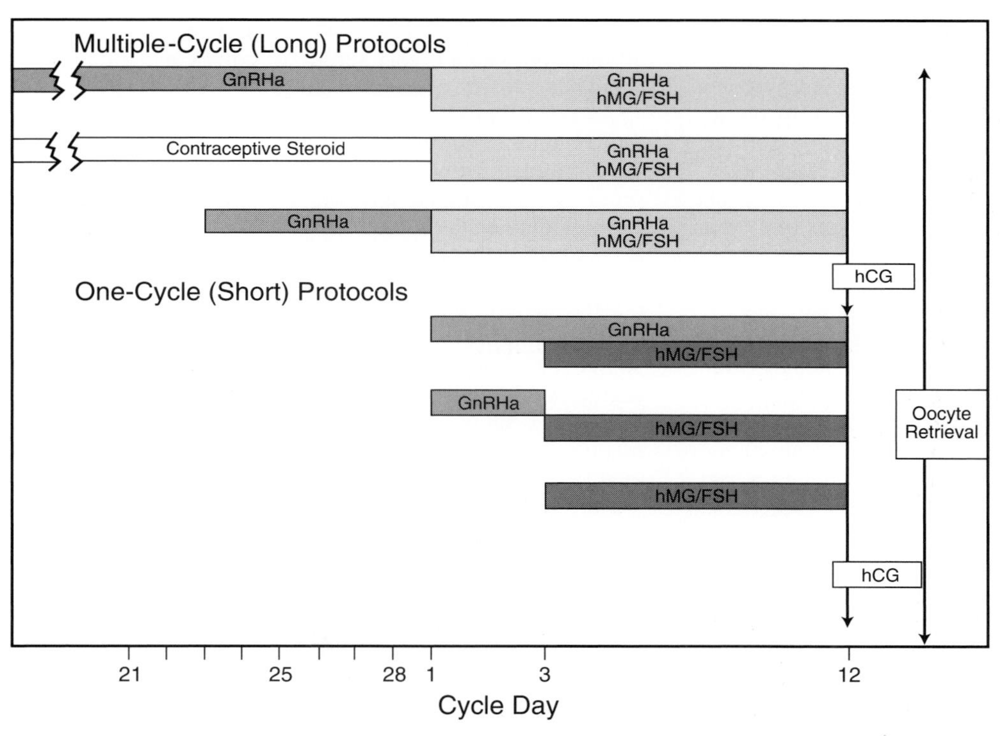

Figure 21–11 ■ Schematic representation of the different approaches to ovarian stimulation that have been used in IVF programs. GnRHa, gonadotropin releasing hormone agonist analogues; hMG, human menopausal gonadotropin; FSH, follicle stimulating hormone; hCG, human chorionic gonadotropin.

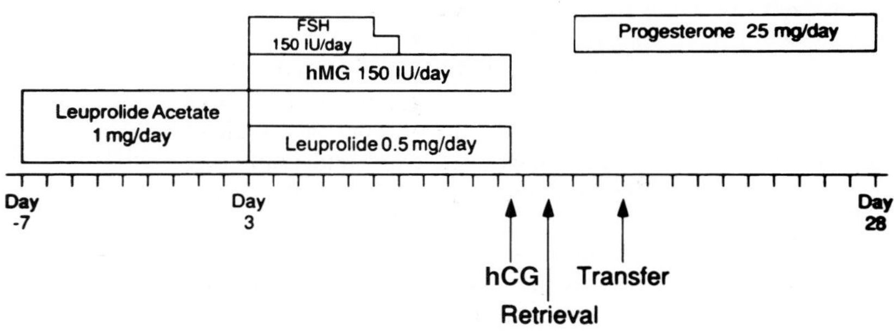

Figure 21–12 ■ Schematic representation of the long gonadotropin-releasing hormone agonist analogue protocol with step-down gonadotropin stimulation. (From Davis OK, Rosenwaks Z. In Vitro Fertilization. *In* Keye WR, Chang RJ, Rebar RW, Soules MR [eds]. Infertility: Evaluation and Treatment. Philadelphia, WB Saunders, 1995, p 763.)

Pulsatile, native decapeptide GnRH, at the proper doses (approximately 14 μg per pulse every 90 minutes), can induce one to three follicles in normally cycling women. When sequential stimulation with clomiphene citrate followed by pulsatile GnRH is used, up to seven mature follicles can be obtained.[42] Use of pulsatile GnRH requires a programmable infusion pump and chronic parenteral access. These factors have limited its application in IVF.

The use of exogenous gonadotropins permits the overriding of the mechanisms that produce mono-ovulation. At the proper doses, clomiphene-hMG, hMG, and hFSH ovarian stimulation regimens will produce numerous follicles capable of being fertilized and a pregnancy rate in the range of 10 to 20 percent, or more, per cycle initiated. However, a number of studies suggest that the combination of GnRH agonist plus gonadotropin stimulation is more effective for ovarian stimulation in IVF-ET cycles.[43] The addition of a GnRH agonist analogue to a gonadotropin stimulation regimen appears to suppress premature LH surges, reduces the chance of premature luteinization of granulosa cells, and reduces cycle cancellation due to premature luteinization or ovulation.

GnRH agonist analogues differ from native decapeptide GnRH in amino acid positions 6 and 10 and are resistant to degradation, giving them long half-lives. The initial administration of GnRH agonist analogues is associated with an increase in LH and FSH secretion (agonist phase). Long-term administration causes down-regulation and partial desensitization of the pituitary GnRH receptor, resulting in the suppression of LH and FSH secretion. The addition of GnRH agonist analogues to regimens of ovarian hyperstimulation for IVF-ET appears to be associated with an increase in the number of oocytes retrieved, the number of embryos transferred, and the clinical pregnancy rate.[44, 45]

For example, one study demonstrated that treatment with a GnRH agonist (buserelin) plus hMG resulted in more oocytes retrieved (9.3 versus 6.2), more embryos (4.3 versus 2.8), and a higher clinical pregnancy rate (20 percent versus 14 percent) than did stimulation with clomiphene-hMG.[46] In another study, comparison of a stimulation regimen using the same medications also demonstrated that buserelin-hMG stimulation resulted in a higher pregnancy rate than that observed with clomiphene-hMG (36 percent versus 18 percent).[47] The type of GnRH agonist analogue used appears not to be crucial to obtaining the improved outcomes. Studies with D-Trp^6 GnRH agonist analogue also demonstrate improved pregnancy rates (21 percent versus 12 percent) compared with ovarian stimulation regimens that do not use GnRH agonists for IVF-ET.[48]

GnRH agonist analogues are typically started in the luteal phase preceding the IVF-ET cycle (long protocol) or in the early follicular phase of the IVF-ET cycle (short or flare protocol) (see Fig. 21–11). A meta-analysis of the two protocols did not demonstrate significant differences in pregnancy rates.[44] In most cases, the long protocol requires a higher dose of gonadotropins, but the number of follicles stimulated, the number of oocytes retrieved and embryos obtained, and the pregnancy rate are similar in the long and short protocols.[49]

One problem with luteal-phase initiation of GnRH agonist analogues before IVF is that it is difficult to determine whether the woman is pregnant at the time of agonist initiation. Some authorities recommend that when the long protocol is used, the GnRH agonist should be started in the follicular phase, approximately 4 weeks before the start of gonadotropin stimulation, and that a barrier contraceptive be prescribed. The follicular-phase long protocol has the advantage of reducing the likelihood that an early pregnancy is present at the time of medication initiation. The follicular-phase long protocol has the disadvantage that the GnRH agonist will need to be administered for a greater number of days.[50]

Although GnRH agonist–gonadotropin protocols are now the standard in IVF-ET (see Fig. 21–12), further refinements in stimulation protocols are likely. The current doses of GnRH agonist used in IVF-ET do not fully suppress pituitary secretion of LH, and small LH surges may occur after each dose of GnRH agonist. This phenomenon can be used to augment ovarian stimulation, either by using a flare protocol or by administering microdoses of GnRH agonist analogue in combination with gonadotropin. In one study, women with a poor response to standard long-protocol GnRH agonist down-regulation plus gonadotropin stimulation were treated with microdose leuprolide acetate (20 μg every 12 hours) plus gonadotropin. The treatment with the microdose GnRH agonist resulted in greater ovarian stimulation with a higher serum estradiol concentration and a greater number of follicles and retrieved oocytes.[51]

As noted before, recent evidence suggests that doses of GnRH agonist currently used in IVF produce partial pituitary desensitization but not complete suppression of the pituitary. A potential advance in ovarian stimulation for IVF-ET may be the use of GnRH antagonists. At the proper dose, GnRH antagonists can produce complete suppression of LH secretion. Unlike the GnRH agonist analogues, GnRH antagonists do not cause LH stimulation. In one study comparing the effects of a GnRH antagonist (Nal-Glu antagonist, 5 mg daily) versus a GnRH agonist (leuprolide acetate, 0.25 mg daily) for ovarian stimulation for IVF-ET, the GnRH antagonist resulted in lower LH levels, more mature oocytes retrieved, and a higher proportion of high-quality embryos.[52]

Current regimens of ovarian stimulation for IVF produce major increases in circulating estradiol. Estradiol concentrations in the range of 1200 pg/ml are routinely reached during ovarian stimulation for IVF. Interestingly, studies demonstrate that circulating androgen levels also increase significantly in women undergoing ovarian stimulation for IVF[53] (Fig. 21–13). The impact of the elevated circulating androgens on the ovary and endometrium remains to be fully characterized.

Although GnRH agonist analogues have few side effects when they are used in ovarian stimulation protocols for IVF-ET, a few cases of ovarian hyperstimulation caused by the administration of the GnRH agonist alone have been reported.[54]

Oocyte Retrieval

Oocyte retrieval is typically performed approximately 36 hours after hCG administration by a transvaginal sonography-guided technique. Descriptive studies of the appearance of oocytes in the human fallopian tube after hCG administration suggest that a time interval between hCG

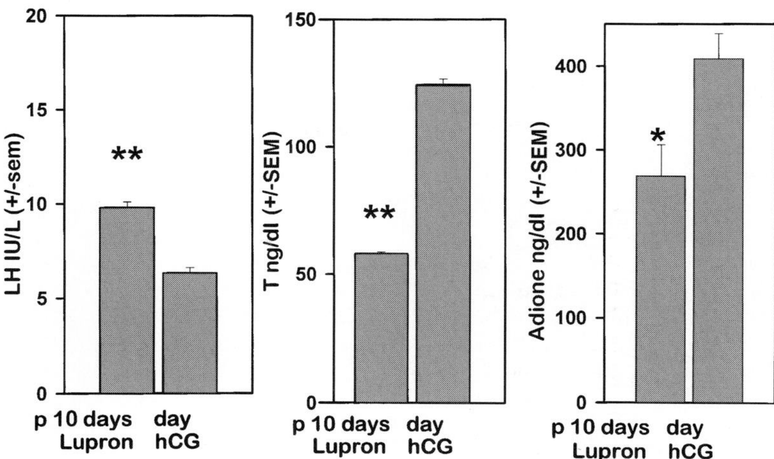

Figure 21–13 ■ Androgen levels in normal ovulatory infertile women undergoing IVF and receiving leuprolide and hMG for ovarian stimulation in preparation for oocyte retrieval. LH, testosterone (T), and androstenedione (Adione) were measured after 10 days of leuprolide acetate treatment, 1 mg daily by subcutaneous injection, and then again after leuprolide plus hMG stimulation, just before the administration of hCG. After 10 days of leuprolide treatment, LH concentrations were in the normal follicular-phase range. Testosterone and androstenedione concentrations increase significantly with ovarian stimulation. Mean (SEM), $^{**}P < .001$, $^{*}P < .05$. (From Martin KA, Hornstein MD, Taylor AE, et al. Exogenous gonadotropin stimulation is associated with increases in serum androgens in IVF-ET cycles. Fertil Steril 68:1011–1016, 1997. Reproduced with permission of the American Society for Reproductive Medicine.)

administration and oocyte retrieval of about 36 hours maximizes oocyte maturation and minimizes the chance of spontaneous ovulation (Fig. 21–14). Before 30 hours, oocyte maturation may not be fully developed, and ovulation begins to occur after 36 hours.[4] Lewin and colleagues[55] randomized 120 women undergoing oocyte retrieval for IVF to either laparoscopic oocyte retrieval under general anesthesia or transvaginal sonography-guided oocyte retrieval with local anesthesia. The number of oocytes recovered (5.3 versus 4.0), the number of embryos transferred (3.0 versus 2.3), and the clinical pregnancy rate (13 percent versus 15 percent) were similar in both the laparoscopy and transvaginal oocyte retrieval groups. The number of oocytes retrieved is largely dependent on the number of large follicles present at the time of retrieval. In general, oocytes can be harvested with a high rate of success from follicles with a mean diameter greater than 12 mm (Fig. 21–15).[56]

Evaluating Oocyte Quality and Meiotic Stage

The science of evaluating the quality of oocytes obtained by ovarian follicle aspiration is at a primitive stage. Currently, embryos are evaluated on the basis of their morphologic appearance with use of a light microscope (Fig. 21–16). According to the criteria established by the Brigham and Women's Hospital Assisted Reproductive Technology Laboratory, oocytes are scored from 0 to 5 on the basis of their morphologic characteristics. Grade 0 oocytes have a microscopic appearance suggesting the degeneration of the oocyte. Grade 1 oocytes have virtually no cumulus cells, and the oocyte is in meiotic prophase (Fig. 21–17). Grade 2 oocytes have an adequate cumulus of granulosa cells, and the oocyte has not completed metaphase I. Grade 3 oocytes have a normal cumulus, and the oocyte has completed metaphase I (Fig. 21–18). Grade 4 oocytes are "post mature" with no visible distinct corona and a zona that refracts light. Most retrieved oocytes are grade 2 or grade 3. These oocytes have a fertilization rate in the range of 50 to 65 percent. Oocytes are fully prepared for fertilization when they reach metaphase II (Fig. 21–19).

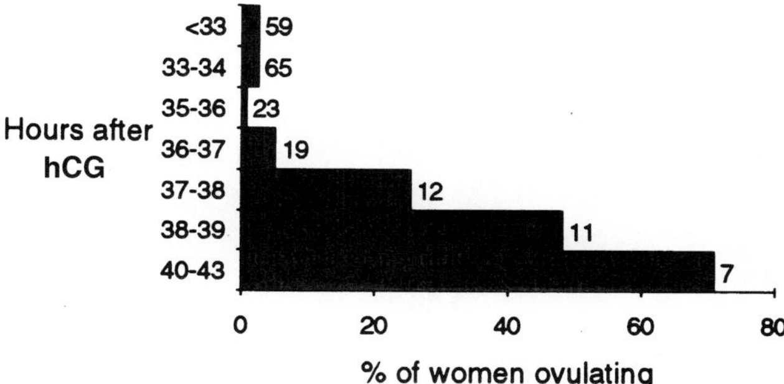

Figure 21–14 ■ Interval between an injection of hCG and the percentage of women in whom follicular rupture has occurred. The number of women studied is indicated to the right of the bar. (From Edwards RG. Physiological aspects of human ovulation. J Reprod Fertil 18[suppl]:87–101, 1973.)

Incubation of Oocytes and Sperm

For IVF procedures, semen is collected by masturbation or occasionally by sexual intercourse with use of a condom.

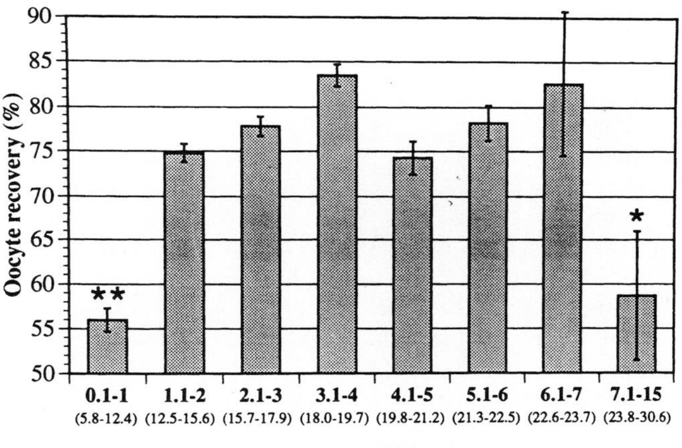

Figure 21–15 ■ Percentage of follicles from which an oocyte was obtained at the time of retrieval as a function of follicle size. Mean (SEM), $^{*}P < .01$, $^{**}P < .001$. Numbers in parentheses represent corresponding follicular diameter in millimeters as determined by sonography. (From Wittmaack FM, Kreger DO, Blasco L, et al. Effect of follicular size on oocyte retrieval, fertilization, cleavage, and embryo quality in in vitro fertilization cycles: A 6-year data collection. Fertil Steril 62:1205–1210, 1994. Reproduced with permission of the American Society for Reproductive Medicine.)

OOCYTE CLASSIFICATION

SCORE	APPEARANCE	NUCLEAR MATURITY (Theoretical)	% of POP	%FERT
0	Egg; Zona; Corona Cells; Cumulus	Degenerating	2%	0%
1	Zona; Egg; Corona Cells (tightly associated w/egg); Germinal Vesicle stg nucleus (w/prominent nucleolus)	Germinal Vesicle Stage Meiotic Prophase (4N)	5%	0%
2	Egg; Zona; Corona Cells (< 1/2 the diameter of the egg); Cumulus	Metaphase I Incomplete (4N)	48%	50%
3	!st polar body; Metaphase II plate; Egg; Zona; Corona Cells (≥ the diameter of the egg); Cumulus	Metaphase I Complete Arrested @ Metaphase II (2N)	42%	65%
4	1st polar body; Metaphase II plate; Egg; Zona (no corona cells visable, light refracts off zona); Cumulus	(Post Mature) Metaphase I Complete Arrested @ Metaphase II (2N)	<1%	60%
5	Zona; Corona Cells; Cumulus	No egg, just a corona with a broken zona inside	3%	

Figure 21–16 ■ Oocyte classification based on morphologic appearance. (From the Brigham and Women's Hospital Assisted Reproductive Technology Laboratory Manual, 1993.)

The semen specimens are processed for sperm collection by a variety of techniques including swim-up and Percoll gradient centrifugation techniques. For normal semen specimens, both techniques generate high-motility sperm for oocyte insemination.[57] However, most studies demonstrate that for semen with abnormal sperm characteristics (e.g., low sperm concentration), sperm prepared by the Percoll gradient centrifugation technique have a greater fertilization capacity than sperm prepared by the swim-up technique. For example, in one study on semen with sperm concentration less than 15 million/ml, the swim-up technique resulted in the collection of more sperm with higher motility, but the Percoll gradient centrifugation sperm were associated with a higher fertilization rate.[58] The superiority of the Percoll gradient centrifugation technique when semen characteristics are abnormal has been reported by other investigators.[59] The FDA regulatory process has led many laboratories to perform gradient centrifugation with other preparations, such as isolate.

Sperm prepared by either the swim-up or gradient centrifugation technique are then incubated in a protein-sup-

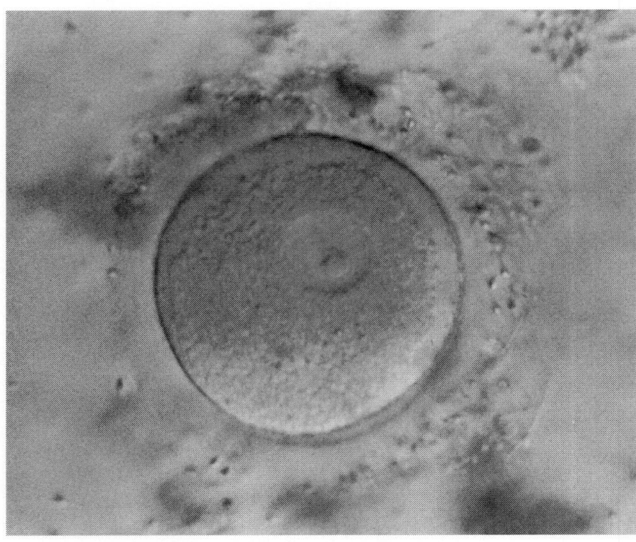

Figure 21–17 ■ Oocyte at prophase I. Note the germinal vesicle and the dark ooplasm. (Courtesy of Aida Nureddin, PhD, Brigham and Women's Hospital ART Embryology Laboratory, Boston, MA.)

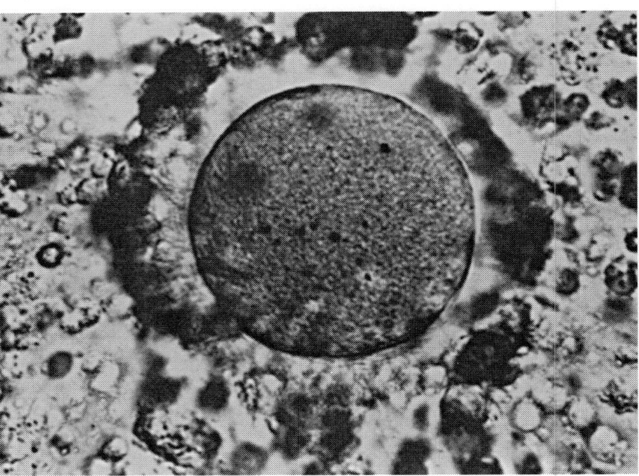

Figure 21–18 ■ Oocyte at metaphase I. Note the absence of both a germinal vesicle and a polar body. The cytoplasm is clearer than that observed with the prophase I oocyte. (From Veeck LL. The gamete laboratory design, management and techniques. *In* Keye WK, Chang RJ, Regar RW, Soules MR [eds]. Infertility: Evaluation and Treatment. Philadelphia, WB Saunders, 1995, p 808.)

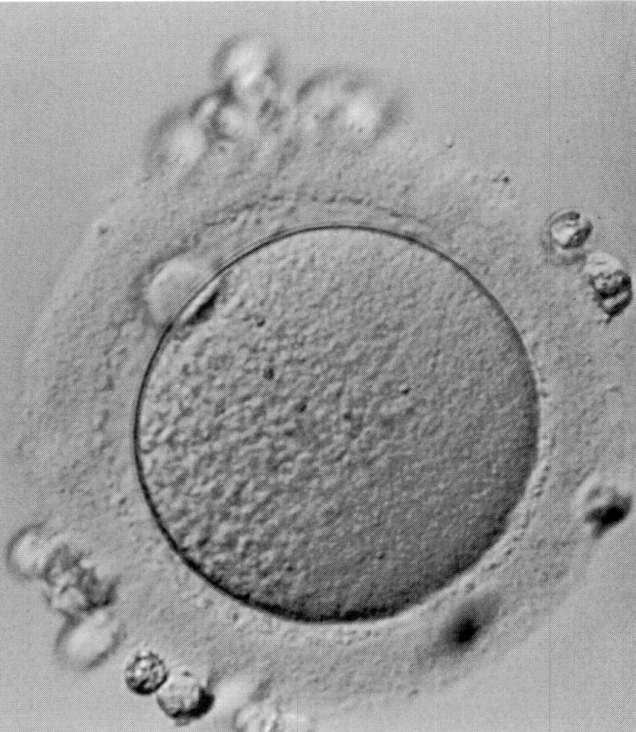

Figure 21–19 ■ Oocyte at metaphase II. The first polar body can be seen at the 10 o'clock position. (Courtesy of David Travassos, BS, Brigham and Women's Hospital ART Embryology Laboratory, Boston, MA.)

plemented media for up to 4 hours, to initiate the process of capacitation, before their coincubation with the oocytes. For standard IVF, approximately 50,000 to 100,000 capacitated sperm are incubated with a single oocyte. Preliminary studies suggest that for men with normal semen parameters, higher concentrations of sperm (250,000 to 500,000 per oocyte) do not significantly improve the fertilization rate. For mature oocytes, insemination is performed approximately 4 hours after oocyte retrieval. Approximately 18 hours later, the oocytes are examined for fertilization. A zygote with two pronuclei and two polar bodies is morphologic evidence of fertilization (Fig. 21–20).

Embryo Transfer

Embryo transfer is commonly performed 72 hours after oocyte retrieval. Before 1990, most programs transferred embryos 48 hours after oocyte retrieval. Recent trends indicate that most programs transfer embryos 72 hours (or more) after oocyte retrieval. Embryos are often at the 4- to 8-cell stage at the time of transfer. Two important goals of IVF treatment are to maximize the livebirth rate per cycle initiated and to minimize the number of multiple gestations. Unfortunately, both the livebirth rate and the rate of multiple gestations are positively correlated with the number of embryos transferred and the quality of the embryos transferred. For example, in one study of women younger than 35 years, the pregnancy rate increased as the number of embryos transferred increased from one to four. However, the multiple gestation rate also increased as the number of embryos transferred increased[60] (Table 21–4). The quality of the embryos transferred is an important determinant of both pregnancy and multiple gestation rates. Some centers take advantage of this relationship by calculating a cumulative embryo score.[61] This score is determined for each embryo on the day of transfer by multiplying the number of blastomeres in the embryo by the score for each embryo. The embryo score is determined by morphologic assessment of the embryo with a light microscope based on variables such as fragmentation and granulation. The score is summed for the embryos. In general, an attempt is made to transfer embryos with a cumulative score up to a threshold that maximizes the pregnancy rate but minimizes the multiple gestation rate. The remaining embryos are then cryopreserved. The pregnancy and multiple gestation rates are also dependent on the age of the female partner. For women older than 36 years, increasing numbers of embryos must be transferred to achieve the pregnancy rates observed in younger women[62, 63] (Fig. 21–21). At many centers, an additional embryo (or two) is transferred for women over age 36.

■ TABLE 21–4

Rate of Singleton and Multiple Gestations (Reaching >20 Weeks of Gestation) in Women Younger Than 35 Years as a Function of the Number of Embryos Transferred

	RATE (%) PER NUMBER OF EMBRYOS			
	1	2	3	4
Singleton	8.7	12.8	15.8	17.2
Twin	—	1.3	4.2	7.4
Triplet	—	—	0.3	2.4
Quadruplet	—	—	—	0.3
Cumulative pregnancy rate	8.7	14	15	27

From Svendsen TO, Jones D, Butler L, Muasher SJ. The incidence of multiple gestations after in vitro fertilization is dependent on the number of embryos transferred and maternal age. Fertil Steril 65:561–565, 1996. Reprinted with permission of the American Society for Reproductive Medicine.

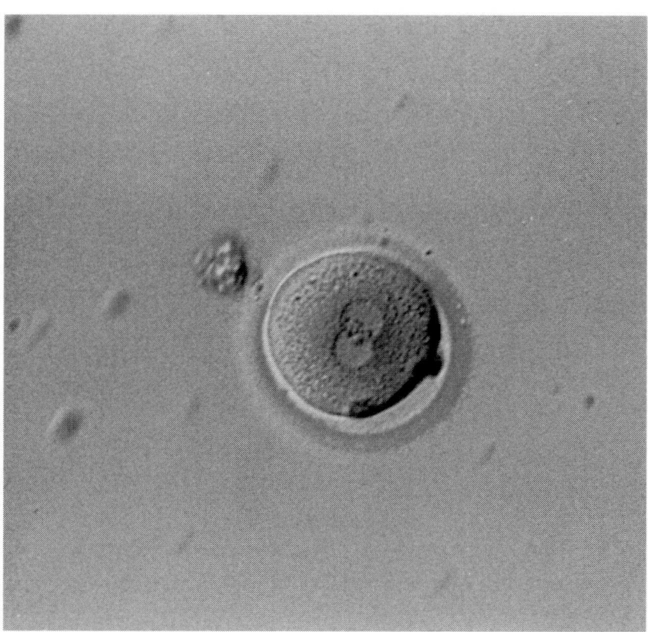

Figure 21–20 ■ Zygote with two pronuclei in the center of the figure and two polar bodies in the perivitelline space. (Courtesy of Glen Adaniya, PhD, Brigham and Women's Hospital ART Embryology Laboratory, Boston, MA.)

At some centers, the goal of preventing multiple gestations is assigned a high priority. In these centers, only two embryos are transferred in most cycles with the intent of reducing the rate of triplet pregnancy. It is likely that the cumulative pregnancy rate achieved by these centers is lower than at those centers where there is flexibility in the number of embryos transferred.[64] Many groups are now performing transfers 120 hours after oocyte retrieval. Transfer of 2 blastocysts markedly reduces triplet pregnancy incidence without a decrease in pregnancy rate.

Luteal-Phase Support

In IVF cycles, the ovary and endometrium are buffeted by numerous countervailing forces that are not controlled by normal feedback mechanisms. For example, the endometrium is exposed to extremely high levels of estradiol and abnormally high levels of androgen. These exposures may result in abnormal endometrial maturation, especially if luteal progesterone does not adequately balance the estrogen effect. Because oocyte retrieval is associated with the removal of a large number of granulosa cells, the adequacy of ovarian progesterone production after oocyte retrieval has been a major concern since the inception of IVF. Reviews of the literature suggest that luteal-phase support using either hCG or progesterone improves the pregnancy rate in IVF.[65]

The two major methods of luteal-phase support that have

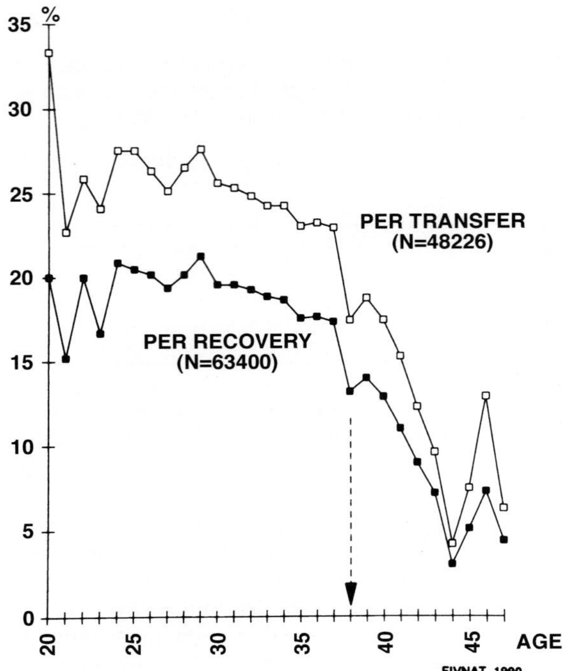

Figure 21–21 ■ Relationship between the age of the female partner and pregnancy rate per oocyte retrieval *(lower line)* and pregnancy rate per transfer *(upper line)*. (From French In Vitro National. French National IVF Registry: Analysis of 1986 to 1990 data. Fertil Steril 59:587–595, 1993. Reproduced with permission of the American Society for Reproductive Medicine.)

been used in IVF cycles are progesterone supplementation, usually given by injection at doses of 25 to 50 mg daily,[66] and hCG at doses ranging from 1500 to 10,000 IU given intramuscularly once or more during the luteal phase.[67] Both hCG and progesterone appear to be associated with an increased pregnancy rate compared with no luteal support.[65] In general, hCG appears to be associated with a slightly higher pregnancy rate than progesterone, but hCG also appears to cause a higher rate of ovarian hyperstimulation syndrome.[65]

Repeated In Vitro Fertilization Cycles

The majority of couples completing a single IVF cycle do not become pregnant. Many couples will request a repeated IVF cycle. In some cases, a specific cause of the IVF cycle failure can be identified (elevated cycle day 3 FSH concentrations). In most cases, a specific cause of the IVF failure cannot be identified. At many centers, repeated IVF cycles appear to have a per cycle pregnancy rate similar to that observed for the first cycle[68] (Fig. 21–22). At some centers, repeated IVF cycles are associated with decreased per cycle pregnancy rates compared with the results from the first treatment cycle. At these centers, the decrease in per cycle pregnancy rate appears to be particularly significant after cycle number four[69] (Fig. 21–23).

Risks of In Vitro Fertilization

Ovarian stimulation with gonadotropin is associated with an approximately 1 percent risk of ovarian hyperstimulation syndrome. In IVF cycles, risk factors for ovarian hyperstimulation syndrome appear to be peak estradiol concentrations greater than 2000 pg/ml, more than 15 follicles greater than 12 mm in diameter, and the establishment of a successful pregnancy.[70] Ovarian hyperstimulation syndrome that develops during IVF cycles typically resolves with conservative management (see Chapter 20). Harvesting of granulosa cells at the time of oocyte retrieval may reduce the chance for development of severe ovarian hyperstimulation syndrome in an IVF cycle.[71]

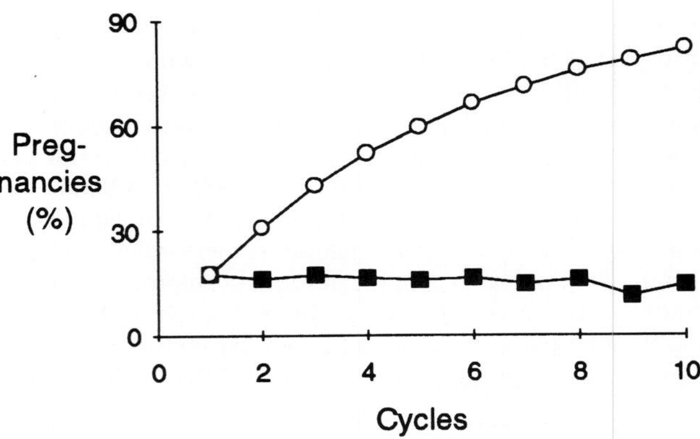

Figure 21–22 ■ Relationship between the number of in vitro fertilization–embryo transfer cycles and the cumulative clinical pregnancy rate *(circles)* and the clinical pregnancy rate per cycle *(squares)*. (From Cohen J. The efficiency and efficacy of IVF and GIFT. Hum Reprod 6:613–618, 1991. Reproduced by permission of the Oxford University Press.)

Some epidemiologists have suggested that drugs used to induce ovulation may be associated with an increased risk of ovarian cancer. The data suggesting this association are weak. A reasonably strong association appears to exist between ovarian cancer and having no children, whether because of infertility or by choice. Oocyte retrieval can be

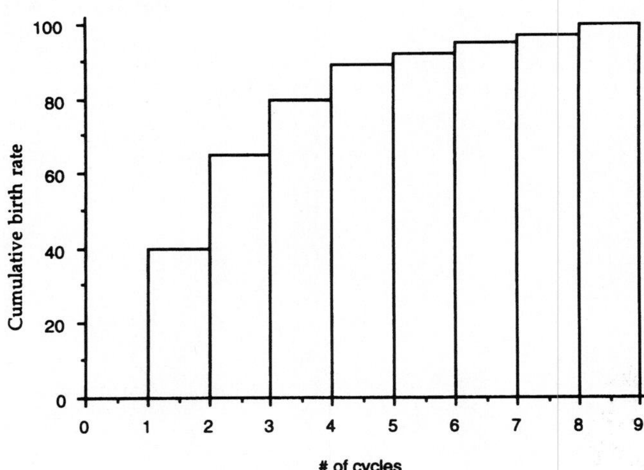

Figure 21–23 ■ Plot of the number of in vitro fertilization–embryo transfer cycles and the cumulative clinical livebirth rate. (From Cooperman AB, Selick CE, Grunfeld, et al. Cumulative number and morphological score of embryos resulting in success: Realistic expectations from in vitro fertilization embryo transfer. Fertil Steril 64:88–92, 1995. Reproduced with permission of the American Society for Reproductive Medicine.)

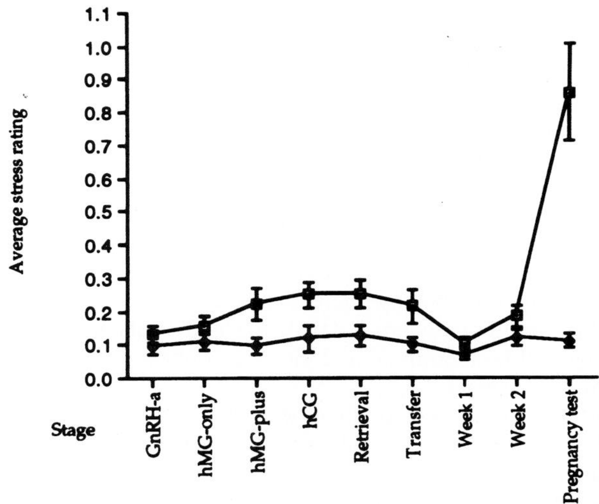

Figure 21–24 ■ Stress ratings throughout an IVF cycle. The upper line represents self-reported scores from women who did not become pregnant. The lower line represents self-reported scores from women who did become pregnant. Note the large increase in stress rating at the time the woman learns that her pregnancy test result is negative. (From Boivin J, Takefman JE. Stress level across stages of in vitro fertilization in subsequently pregnant and nonpregnant women. Fertil Steril 64:802–810, 1995. Reproduced with permission of the American Society for Reproductive Medicine.)

associated with pelvic bleeding, requiring transfusion or surgical exploration, or pelvic infection. Both complications are rare, less than 1 per 500 cases.

Many couples in IVF cycles experience significant stress. In one study, stress scores were reported by the female partner of the couple across an entire IVF cycle[72] (Fig. 21–24). Ovarian stimulation was associated with an increase in self-reported stress. Stress levels increased markedly at the time that couples were informed that the result of a pregnancy test obtained 2 weeks after embryo transfer was negative. When couples were told that the pregnancy test result was positive, there was no significant increase in the self-report of stress. This observation supports the theory that failure to conceive in an IVF cycle is similar to a significant loss and that the couple must grieve for that loss. Support, counseling, and relaxation techniques can all help reduce the stress associated with IVF. The major medical risk associated with IVF is the potential for high-order multiple gestations.

Pregnancy Outcome

For women who achieve pregnancy after treatment with IVF, approximately 20 percent will experience a spontaneous abortion and up to 5 percent will have an ectopic pregnancy. Early pregnancy can be monitored both by transvaginal sonography and by serial hCG levels (Figs. 21–25 and 21–26). For livebirths after IVF treatment, the rate of congenital malformations is somewhat higher (3.5 percent) than that observed after natural conception (2.1 percent). The rate of minor congenital malformations after IVF treatment (3.1 percent) is also somewhat higher than that observed with natural conception. Many of the malformations occurred in pregnancies with multiple gestations.[73, 74]

The outcome of pregnancies produced by IVF treatment is probably directly related to the number of gestations established. In 1994, of the pregnancies resulting from IVF, approximately 29 percent were twins, 7 percent were triplet gestations, and 0.6 percent were higher order gestations. Singleton pregnancies produced by IVF treatment appear to have an outcome that is similar to spontaneous singleton pregnancy, if factors such as maternal age are appropriately controlled.[75] Compared with naturally occurring twin gestations, twin gestations produced from IVF treatment appear to have a similar prematurity rate (39 percent), low birth weight (18 percent), and perinatal mortality (35 per 1000).[76] Triplet and other high-order multiple gestations are associated with increased prematurity, low birth weight, and increased perinatal mortality.

Triplet pregnancies occur in approximately 7 percent of IVF pregnancies. Triplet pregnancies are associated with a high perinatal mortality rate, as high as 100 to 200 per 1000. Average gestational age at delivery is 37 weeks for twin pregnancy and 34 weeks for triplets.[77]

During the past decade, the number of multiple gestation pregnancies has increased, owing in part to the multiple gestations resulting from IVF treatment (Table 21–5). Approximately 22 percent of all triplet pregnancies are produced by IVF treatment. The remainder of triplet pregnancies are due to use of ovulation-inducing drugs or are spontaneous.[78]

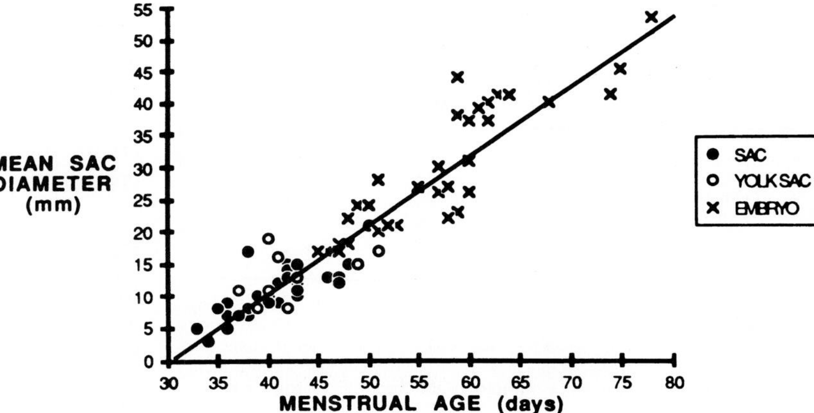

Figure 21–25 ■ Relationship between pregnancy dating as determined by menstrual age and gestational sac size as measured by the mean sac diameter. (From Nyberg DA, Mack LA, Liang FC, Patten RM. Distinguishing normal from abnormal gestational sac growth in early pregnancy. J Ultrasound Med 6:23–27, 1987.)

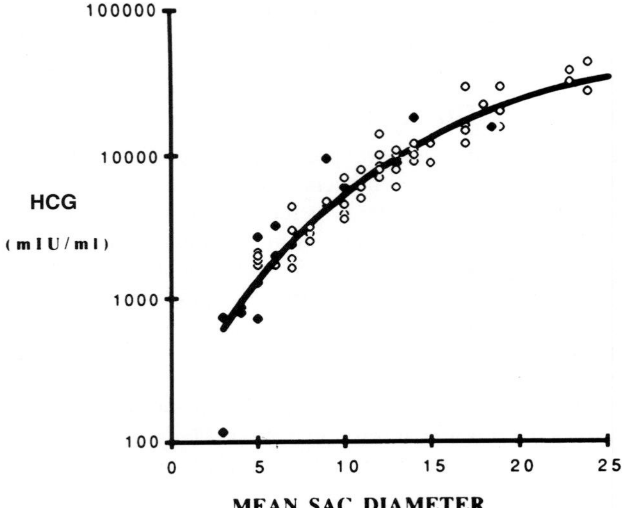

Figure 21–26 ■ Relationship between mean gestational sac diameter as measured by the mean sac diameter and the serum hCG concentration. (From Nyberg DA, Mack LA, Liang FC, Jeffrey RB. Early pregnancy complications: Endovaginal sonographic findings correlated with human chorionic gonadotropin levels. Radiology 167:619–622, 1988.)

Couples who achieve triplet pregnancy are faced with two major options: expectant management or reduction of the triplet pregnancy to a twin or singleton gestation. The two most widely used methods of pregnancy reduction are the transvaginal approach and the transabdominal approach for the injection of potassium chloride into the fetal heart. The transabdominal approach is usually performed at 10 to 13 weeks of gestation. The transvaginal approach is typically performed earlier in gestation. For couples choosing expectant management, approximately 15 percent will spontaneously lose one embryo-fetus, resulting in a twin pregnancy.[79] Of couples who are offered selective reduction, approximately 20 percent choose to undergo the procedure.[80] The complete pregnancy loss after reduction of a multifetal pregnancy is approximately 10 percent.[81] Some studies demonstrate that the reduction of a triplet gestation to a twin gestation may decrease the risk of preeclampsia, increase the gestational age at birth, and increase the mean birth weights.[82, 83]

An alternative to embryo reduction for triplet pregnancy due to IVF is to reduce the number of embryos transferred to the woman. It is likely that reducing the number of transferred embryos will reduce the overall pregnancy rate per cycle initiated, but the decrease in the number of triplets produced by IVF will improve the overall perinatal outcome of the resulting pregnancies.[84] Some investigators have proposed that by increasing the number of days of embryo culture (up to 5 days), the truly outstanding embryos will be identified, and then two outstanding embryos could be transferred.[85]

Many authorities conclude that it is "fairly well established" that multifetal reduction for quadruplet pregnancy results in improved pregnancy outcomes.[86] Although no randomized studies have been reported, some series observe a 4-week increase in the length of gestation, from 31 weeks to 35 weeks, in quadruplet pregnancies that have been successfully reduced to twins. Reduction in the number of quadruplet pregnancies after IVF treatment is probably best achieved by transferring no more than three high-quality embryos in those women at highest risk for multifetal pregnancy.

■ TABLE 21–5

Distribution of Multiple Gestations in Women Pregnant after In Vitro Fertilization Treatment in 1991 and 1994

	PERCENTAGE OF ALL DELIVERIES	
	1991	**1994**
Singleton	70	64
Twin	25	29
Triplet	4.8	6.5
Quadruplet or quintuplet	0.2	0.6
Total deliveries	3215	4912

From Society for Assisted Reproductive Technology and the American Society for Reproductive Medicine. Assisted reproductive technology in the United States and Canada: 1994 results generated from the American Society for Reproductive Medicine/Society for Assisted Reproductive Technology Registry. Fertil Steril 66:697–705, 1996. Reprinted with permission of the American Society for Reproductive Medicine.

Embryo Cryopreservation

IVF often generates substantial numbers of excess embryos that cannot be safely transferred in the cycle of oocyte retrieval because of the risk of high-order multiple gestation. The development of successful embryo cryopreservation techniques allows multiple transfer cycles after just one ovarian stimulation and oocyte retrieval.[87] Embryo cryopreservation increases the cumulative pregnancy rate per oocyte retrieval and helps to diminish the multiple gestation rate. An important issue in embryo cryopreservation is the optimal cryoprotectant. In one randomized prospective study, dimethyl sulfoxide (DMSO) was observed to be a better cryoprotectant for multicellular human embryos than 1,2-propanediol.[88] Embryos were randomized to freezing with DMSO (N = 232) or 1,2-propanediol (N = 250). The livebirth rates per embryo thawed were 3.5 percent for DMSO and 0.8 percent for 1,2-propanediol. Preliminary results suggest that embryos can be successfully frozen for at least 7 years[89] (Fig. 21–27). Interestingly, embryos that were cryopreserved for only 2 to 10 months did not result in as many pregnancies as did embryos cryopreserved for more than 12 months. This is probably due to the observation that women who became pregnant with the initial embryo transfer (suggesting that many high-quality embryos were present) did not need to access their cryopreserved embryos until after they completed their first pregnancy.

Cost-Benefits of In Vitro Fertilization

In a medical care environment where resource constraints assume greater importance in medical decision making, the cost-benefit of IVF has been keenly debated. Some authorities suggest that the cost of an IVF livebirth is in the range of $44,000 to $211,940 (U.S. dollars).[90] This

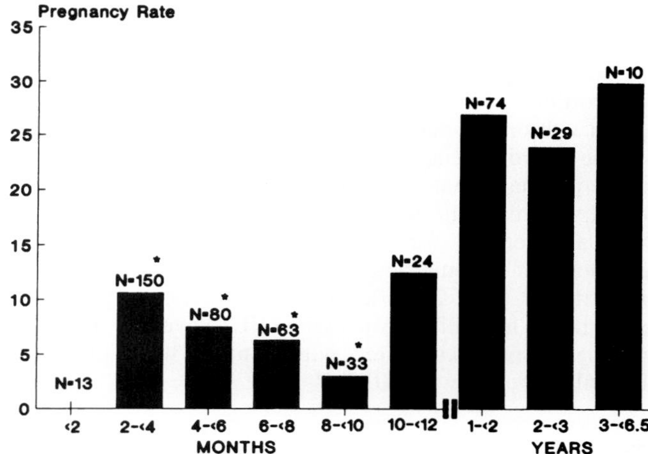

Figure 21–27 ■ Relationship between the length of time that embryos were preserved in cryostorage and the clinical pregnancy rate resulting from the thawing and transfer of the cryopreserved embryos. The embryos that were stored for 1 to 6.5 years had a high rate of establishing pregnancy when they were thawed and transferred. One explanation of this result is that women who became pregnant on the initial in vitro fertilization–embryo transfer cycle kept their embryos cryopreserved for a long time before accessing them. (From Lin YP, Cassidenti DL, Chacon RR, et al. Successful implantation of frozen sibling embryos is influenced by the outcome of the cycle from which they were derived. Fertil Steril 63:262–267, 1995. Reproduced with permission of the American Society for Reproductive Medicine.)

analysis assumed a livebirth rate in the range of 10 percent per cycle, far below what is actually achieved at most centers. In a report from the Brigham and Women's Hospital IVF program, actual charges and livebirths for calendar year 1993 were analyzed.[91] Couples were assigned to one of three groups on the basis of their clinical characteristics. Group A consisted of couples in which the woman was younger than 32 years and the male partner had a normal semen analysis. Group B consisted of women younger than 40 years with a male partner with an abnormal semen analysis. Group C consisted of women 40 to 42 years of age with a male partner with a normal semen analysis. The livebirth rates in the three groups were 35 percent, 24 percent, and 19 percent. For group A, the cost of a livebirth was $23,000. For group B, the cost of a livebirth was $34,000. For group C, in the first cycle of IVF, the cost of a livebirth was $43,000. Because the livebirth rate was "low" in group C, many of these couples had multiple cycles of IVF. When the analysis was restricted to couples in group C who completed three cycles of IVF, the cost of a livebirth was $75,000.

These studies demonstrate that the cost of a livebirth from IVF is directly related to the clinical characteristics of the couples. Currently, the cost of adoption in the United States is in the range of $12,000 to $30,000. The cost of detecting one abnormal fetus by α-fetoprotein screening is in the range of $40,000. These comparisons support the use of IVF for the treatment of infertility that has not responded to less intensive treatments.

As the cost of IVF decreases and the success of IVF increases, there will continue to be an increase in the utilization of this technique. If the cost of IVF decreases to $2000 per cycle and the success rate increases to 50 percent per cycle, the evaluation of the infertile couple might be limited to those tests that will not cost far more than $2000. Non-IVF treatment would be limited to those interventions for which the total cost of the treatment was less than approximately $4000 per livebirth. This trend might reduce the use of classic surgical interventions for the diagnosis and treatment of infertility.

In Vitro Fertilization with Oocyte Donation

A venerable question in reproduction is, Which factor has a greater impact on fecundability, oocyte age or uterine age? On the basis of results from IVF with oocyte donation, both oocyte age and uterine age have an impact on fecundability, but oocyte age appears to have a far greater impact on fecundability than uterine age. Early studies of IVF with oocyte donation clearly established the feasibility of the technique and reported pregnancy rates in the range of 25 percent per cycle.[92, 93] Studies suggest that oocyte age and uterine age both influence pregnancy rates in programs of IVF with oocyte donation. For example, one study of 114 women undergoing IVF with oocyte donation examined implantation and pregnancy rates for women younger than 40 years and women between 40 and 49 years of age.[94] The clinical pregnancy rates per embryo transfer were 47 percent and 25 percent for the women younger than 40 years and 40 to 49 years of age, respectively. In another study of IVF with oocyte donation, the pregnancy losses were significantly higher in the women older than 40 years compared with women younger than 40 years.[95]

The reproductive options for women with ovarian failure are limited. For women with depletion of the oocyte pool, IVF with donor oocytes is the only current method that can allow these women to be the gestational carrier of a pregnancy. The initial applications of IVF with oocyte donation were to women with premature ovarian failure. As the technique developed, it has been applied more frequently to women older than 40 years.[96] An important ethical issue is at what age women should be advised not to pursue IVF with oocyte donation. Some centers have treated women older than 60 years. Other centers restrict the application of this technique to women younger than 50 years.

The technique of IVF with oocyte donation requires the coordination of the reproductive tracts of both the donor and recipient (Fig. 21–28). An important insight provided by this technique is that for women with ovarian failure, steroid replacement with estradiol and progesterone is adequate to prepare the endometrium for successful pregnancy. No other ovarian hormone is required to achieve a successful pregnancy. Most oocyte donation programs use "fresh" oocytes, and the problem of possible transmission of infection from oocyte donor to recipient has not been fully solved. At the current time, cryopreservation of oocytes has many technical limitations, but advances are being made.[97, 97a] Gook and colleagues[97b] have reported that the use of intracytoplasmic sperm injection (ICSI) may partially overcome the damage to oocytes caused by cryopreservation. They observed that cryopreserved-thawed oocytes failed to demonstrate normal embryo development after

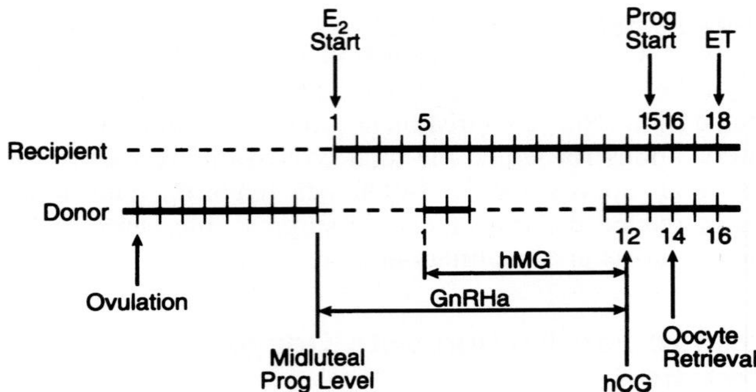

Figure 21–28 ■ Schematic of the synchronization of oocyte donor and embryo recipient on a gonadotropin-releasing hormone agonist analogue (GnRHa) with exogenous estrogen (E_2) and progesterone (Prog) protocol. hMG, human menopausal gonadotropin; hCG, human chorionic gonadotropin; ET, embryo transfer. (From Schmidt-Sarosi CL. In vitro fertilization with donor oocytes. *In* Keye WR, Chang RJ, Rebar RW, Soules MR [eds]. Infertility: Evaluation and Treatment. Philadelphia, WB Saunders, 1995, p 781.)

being fertilized with standard insemination-incubation techniques. In contrast, some of the cryopreserved-thawed oocytes demonstrated normal embryo development up to the blastocyst stage after being fertilized by ICSI. Preliminary reports suggest that pregnancy can be achieved with cryopreserved-thawed oocytes fertilized by ICSI. However, the efficiency of the approach is poor. In preliminary reports, approximately 100 cryopreserved-thawed oocytes need to be used to achieve one pregnancy. It is hoped that advances in oocyte cryopreservation will lead to the development of anonymous oocyte donor banks, in which the donors have been screened for infectious diseases at an appropriate time after the oocyte donation.

GAMETE INTRAFALLOPIAN TUBE TRANSFER

Infertile women with dysfunctional fallopian tubes are ideal candidates for IVF. Infertile women with functional fallopian tubes are often ideal candidates for GIFT. The core concept that supports the use of GIFT is that the fallopian tube may be a better site for nurturing the interaction of oocyte and sperm than a synthetic media in a plastic dish kept in an incubator. Unfortunately, there are no contemporary, large-scale randomized studies that directly assess the effectiveness of IVF versus GIFT in the treatment of infertility of various causes. One small study that compared the effectiveness of IVF versus GIFT for the treatment of idiopathic or male factor infertility reported similar pregnancy rates with the two procedures.[98]

One important issue regarding GIFT is whether it offers a higher per cycle pregnancy rate than ovarian stimulation with gonadotropin alone (with or without IUI). A requirement for GIFT is that the fallopian tubes be patent. Consequently, it is possible that much of the success of GIFT could be due to the ovarian stimulation and multiple follicular development achieved with gonadotropin administration. In one randomized trial, couples with unexplained infertility or failed donor insemination were randomized to either GIFT or ovarian stimulation with gonadotropins. The per cycle clinical pregnancy rate was similar in the group treated with GIFT (13 percent) and the group treated with ovarian stimulation alone (9 percent).[99] This suggests that before being treated with GIFT, couples should consider one to three cycles of ovarian stimulation with gonadotropins (with or without IUI).

The infertility diagnosis of the couple may affect the per cycle pregnancy rate associated with GIFT treatment. For example, treatment with GIFT appears to be associated with a lower per cycle pregnancy rate in women with a diagnosis of endometriosis than in women with idiopathic infertility[100] (Fig. 21–29). In some centers, couples with male factor infertility treated with GIFT have low per cycle pregnancy rates compared with couples with idiopathic infertility treated with GIFT.[101]

Transcervical Gamete Intrafallopian Tube Transfer

One major problem with standard GIFT is that anesthesia (usually general anesthesia) and laparoscopy, a major surgical procedure, are key features of the treatment. An alternative method of accomplishing GIFT is to retrieve the oocytes by a transvaginal sonography-guided technique and transfer the sperm and oocytes to the fallopian tube by a hysteroscopic technique. In a prospective randomized study comparing standard GIFT with hysteroscopic GIFT, the pregnancy rate was similar.[102]

Zygote Intrafallopian Tube Transfer

ZIFT combines features of IVF (transvaginal oocyte retrieval, fertilization in vitro) and GIFT (transfer of conceptuses to fallopian tube). ZIFT has the theoretical advantage of providing a direct observation of the success of the

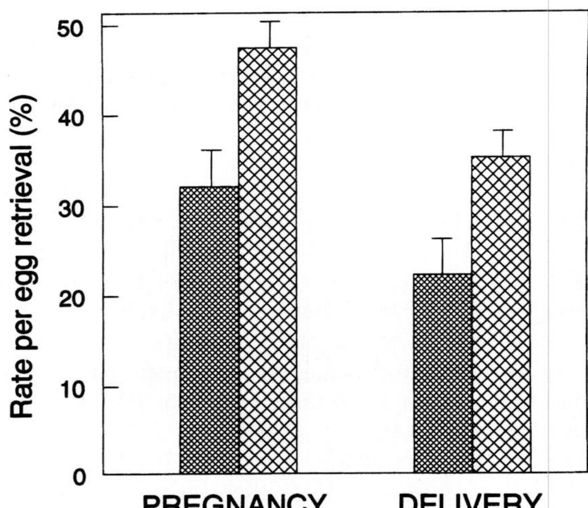

Figure 21–29 ■ Comparison of the clinical pregnancy and delivery rates between couples with endometriosis (dense hatching) and couples without endometriosis (less dense hatching) during a cycle of gamete intrafallopian tube transfer. The women with endometriosis had lower pregnancy and delivery rates per GIFT cycle than did the women without endometriosis. (From Guzick DS, Yao YAS, Berga SL, et al. Endometriosis impairs the efficacy of gamete intrafallopian transfer: Results of a case-control study. Fertil Steril 62:1186–1191, 1994. Reproduced with permission of the American Society for Reproductive Medicine.)

fertilization process in vitro (not possible with GIFT) and the incubation of the conceptus in the fallopian tube, potentially a better incubator than a plastic dish and laboratory incubator. Most clinical trials have reported that ZIFT is not superior to IVF. For example, in one randomized prospective trial comparing IVF and ZIFT for the treatment of male factor infertility, the embryo implantation and clinical pregnancy rate was similar with both treatments.[103] Similar results have been reported in other clinical trials.[104, 105] ZIFT is more complex than IVF. Unless future trials establish superior outcomes for ZIFT over IVF, the use of ZIFT should be limited.

Fallopian Tube Transfer of Cryopreserved Embryos

A potential application of fallopian tube placement of embryos is in programs of embryo cryopreservation. Van Voorhis and coworkers[106] have reported a randomized trial of intrauterine versus laparoscopic tubal placement of thawed, previously cryopreserved embryos. The ongoing pregnancy rate was significantly higher when the embryos were placed in the fallopian tube by laparoscopy than when the embryos were placed directly in the uterus (58 percent versus 19 percent).

CIGARETTE SMOKING AND ASSISTED REPRODUCTION TECHNIQUES

Assisted reproduction procedures provide a unique opportunity to explore the effects of environmental exposures on fecundability. The effect of cigarette smoking has been studied for both IVF and GIFT cycles. In IVF cycles, cigarette smoking is associated with no major change in peak estradiol concentration or number of oocytes retrieved. However, cigarette smoking appears to decrease the pregnancy and livebirth rates in IVF cycles if the female partner smokes but not if the male partner smokes[107] (Fig. 21–30). The effect of smoking on IVF outcome may be dose dependent. The largest effects of smoking on IVF outcome are observed when the female partner smokes more than 20 cigarettes daily[108] (Fig. 21–31). Similarly, cigarette smoking also appears to decrease pregnancy and livebirth rates in infertile couples treated with GIFT.[109]

A mechanism that may link cigarette smoking and reduced pregnancy rates in IVF and GIFT is the observation that smoking accelerates the rate of oocyte loss. Smoking appears to prematurely increase cycle day 3 FSH concentration in women who smoke.[110] In addition, women between 35 and 39 years of age who smoke achieve a post clomiphene FSH level more than twice as high as that of women who do not smoke.[111] Both the elevated cycle day 3 FSH concentration and the elevated FSH level in response to clomiphene suggest that women who smoke have a depleted oocyte pool and may have prematurely aged follicles. Components of smoking may increase the rate of oocyte loss. Although the effects of smoking on ovarian function may be irreversible, women who smoke cigarettes should consider discontinuing smoking before undergoing an IVF or GIFT cycle.

MICROMANIPULATION OF GAMETES

Male factor infertility is due to many different types of semen abnormalities including low sperm production (oligospermia), poor sperm motility (asthenospermia), and abnormal sperm morphology (teratospermia). Until recently, the treatment of severe male factor infertility has been associated with relatively low success rates compared with the treatment of anovulatory or tubal factor infertility.[112] For example, in most IVF programs, the livebirth rate for couples with male factor infertility is approximately 50 percent lower than the livebirth rate for couples with tubal factor or endometriosis. Male partners with semen abnormalities that resulted in less than 500,000 motile high-quality sperm being harvested per ejaculate have low fertilization and pregnancy rates in IVF[113] (Table 21–6). Gamete micromanipulation techniques, especially ICSI, offer important advantages for couples with severe male factor infertility. Gamete micromanipulation techniques include

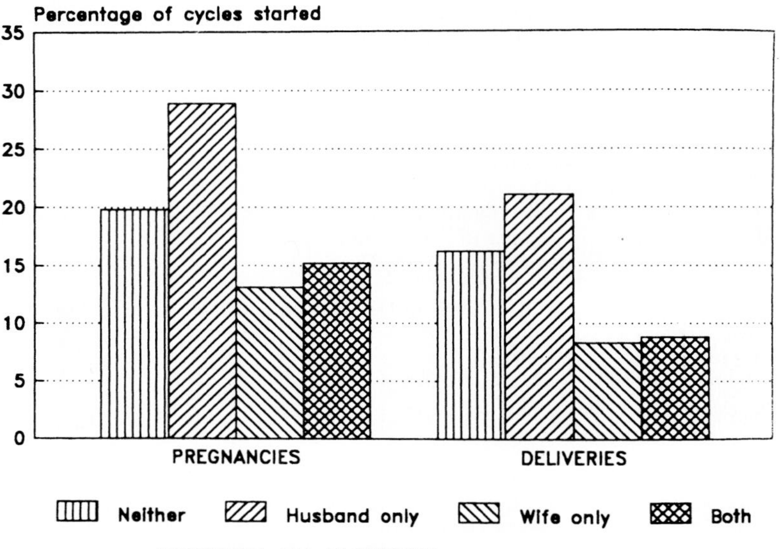

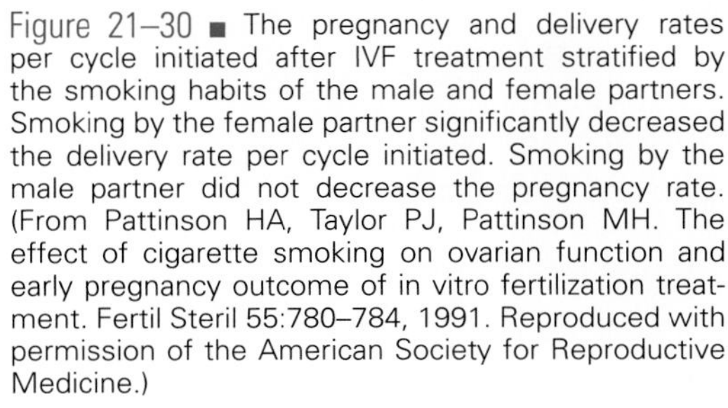
Figure 21–30 ■ The pregnancy and delivery rates per cycle initiated after IVF treatment stratified by the smoking habits of the male and female partners. Smoking by the female partner significantly decreased the delivery rate per cycle initiated. Smoking by the male partner did not decrease the pregnancy rate. (From Pattinson HA, Taylor PJ, Pattinson MH. The effect of cigarette smoking on ovarian function and early pregnancy outcome of in vitro fertilization treatment. Fertil Steril 55:780–784, 1991. Reproduced with permission of the American Society for Reproductive Medicine.)

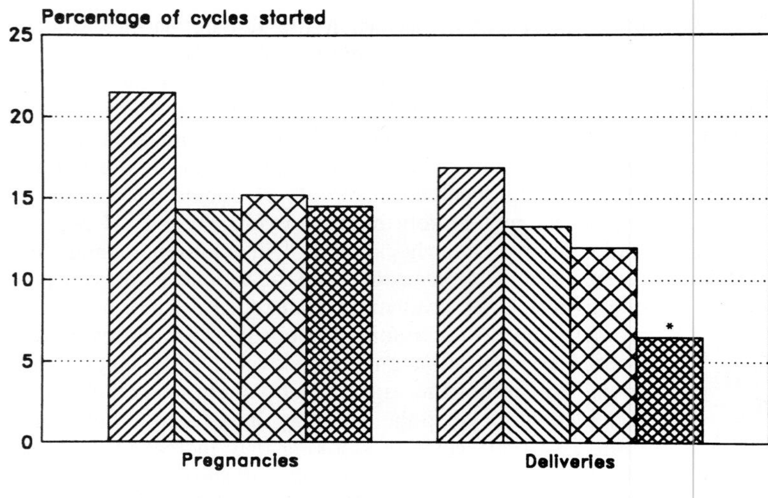

Figure 21–31 ■ The IVF pregnancy and delivery rates per cycle initiated stratified by the magnitude of the exposure of the female partner to cigarette smoke. When the female partner smoked more than 20 cigarettes per day, there was a significant decrease in the delivery rate per cycle initiated. (From Pattinson HA, Taylor PJ, Pattinson MH. The effect of cigarette smoking on ovarian function and early pregnancy outcome of in vitro fertilization treatment. Fertil Steril 55:780–784, 1991. Reproduced with permission of the American Society for Reproductive Medicine.)

partial zona drilling (PZD), subzonal sperm injection (SUZI), and ICSI[114] (Fig. 21–32).

PZD can be performed by applying a solution of acid Tyrode's to the oocyte or by mechanical disruption of the zona with a sharp instrument (partial zona dissection).[115] Zona drilling of oocytes with acid Tyrode's solution can be successfully accomplished with mouse oocytes, but human oocytes are often damaged by the acid Tyrode's solution. Partial zona dissection is performed by creating a slit in the zona with a glass microneedle. Partial zona dissection appears to result in a higher fertilization rate in couples in which the male partner has an abnormal semen analysis. In one study of male factor infertility, the fertilization rate was 26 percent after PZD and 9 percent after standard IVF.[116] However, these results are not consistently obtained by all gametologists. In addition, incubation of oocytes in a high concentration of sperm appears to achieve a fertilization rate similar to that observed with partial zona dissection.[117]

SUZI involves the direct placement of 5 to 30 sperm into the perivitelline space between the zona pellucida and the oocyte cell membrane.[118] SUZI appears to increase the fertilization rate compared with standard IVF in couples with male factor infertility. For example, in one study of male factor infertility, the oocyte fertilization rate was 39 percent after SUZI compared with 6 percent after standard IVF.[119] Problems associated with SUZI include increased polyploidy and a high rate of fertilization failure with all the oocytes obtained from a single woman.

■ TABLE 21–6

Results of In Vitro Fertilization in Couples with Severe Male Factor, Analyzed by Number of Total Motile Sperm Harvested After Semen Preparation by Swim-Up

Total motile sperm after swim-up ($\times 10^6$)	<0.50	0.51 to 1.00	1.01 to 1.50	>1.50
Fertilization rate (%)	22 ± 5	40 ± 4	60 ± 5	64 ± 1
Clinical pregnancy rate per oocyte retrieval (%)	8	15	21	22

From Ben-Chetrit A, Senoz S, Greenblatt EM, Casper RM. In vitro fertilization outcome in the presence of severe male factor infertility. Fertil Steril 63:1032–1037, 1995. Reprinted with permission of the American Society for Reproductive Medicine.

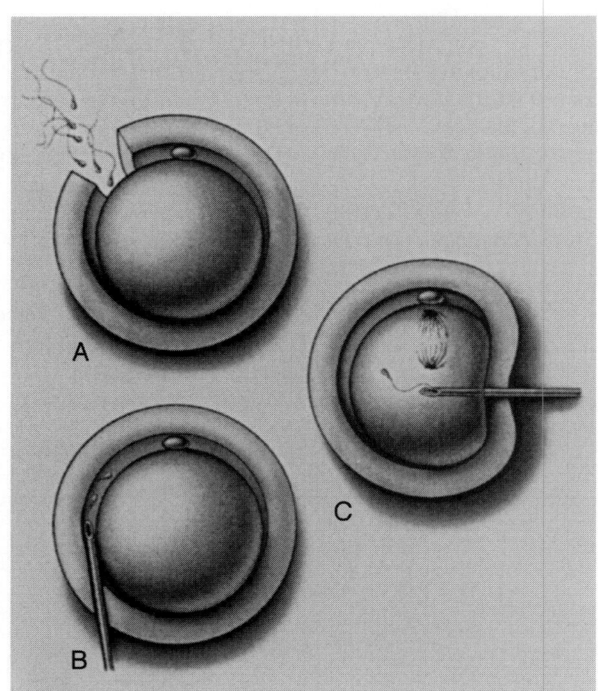

Figure 21–32 ■ Schematic of three types of gamete micromanipulation. *A,* Partial zona dissection (PZD). *B,* Subzonal sperm injection (SUZI). *C,* Intracytoplasmic sperm injection (ICSI). In couples with severe male factor infertility, ICSI is associated with higher pregnancy rates than either SUZI or PZD. (From Schlegel PN, Girardi S. In vitro fertilization for male factor infertility. J Clin Endocrinol Metab 82:709–716, 1997. © The Endocrine Society.)

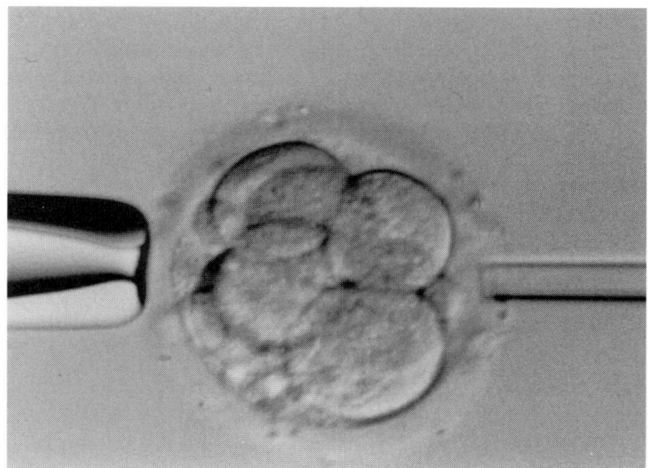

Figure 21–33 ■ Zona drilling for assisted hatching of human embryo with acid Tyrode's solution. (Courtesy of Katharine Jackson, BS, Brigham and Women's Hospital ART Embryology Laboratory, Boston, MA.)

ICSI is the direct injection of a single sperm into the cytoplasm of the oocyte[120] (Fig. 21–34). Most authorities believe that ICSI is more effective than PZD or SUZI for the treatment of male factor infertility. In general, most studies suggest that ICSI results in higher rates of both fertilization and embryo development and a higher pregnancy rate than SUZI or PZD. For example, in one randomized study of the treatment of severe male factor infertility, greater fertilization was achieved by ICSI than by SUZI (33 percent versus 16 percent).[121] Similar results have been reported by Catt and associates,[122] who prepared sperm for injection by using both polyvinylpyrrolidone to immobilize the sperm and incision of the sperm tail before injection. Fertilization rates for ICSI (42 percent) were greater than the fertilization rates observed with SUZI (21 percent). In one review of these three techniques, the author reported that the pregnancy rate per oocyte retrieval was 25 percent, 10 percent, and 4 percent for ICSI, SUZI, and PZD, respectively.[123] ICSI is now the state-of-the-art technique for the treatment of severe male factor infertility.

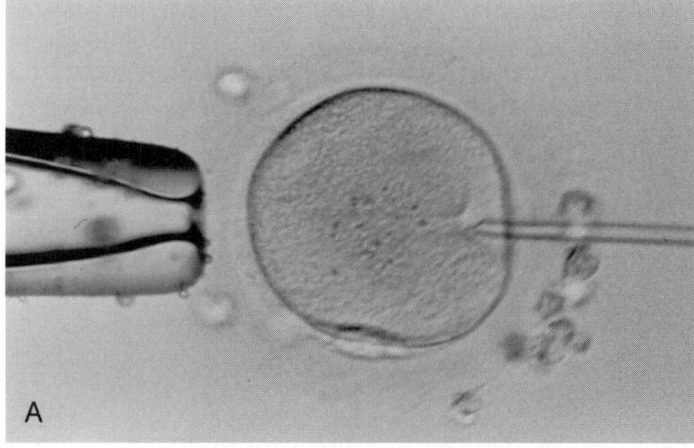

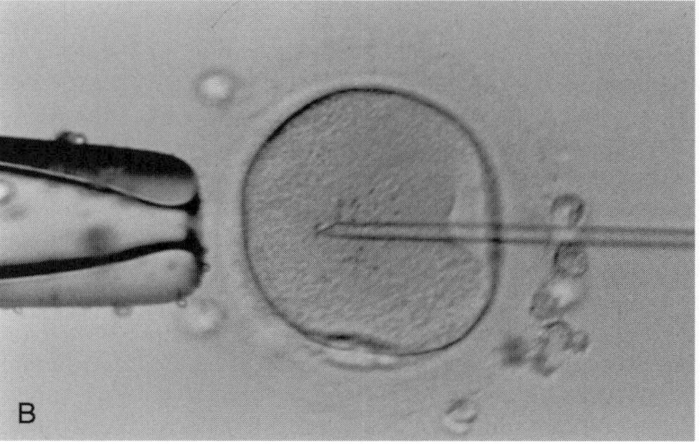

Figure 21–34 ■ *A* and *B*, Intracytoplasmic sperm injection. (*A* and *B* courtesy of Katharine Jackson, BS, Brigham and Women's Hospital ART Embryology Laboratory, Boston, MA.)

The indications for ICSI continue to evolve. Currently, the best established indication for ICSI is the treatment of severe male factor infertility. With ICSI, there is little relationship between sperm concentration in the semen, sperm motility, or sperm morphology and the pregnancy rate.[124] If a single live sperm can be identified, success with ICSI is possible. ICSI may simplify the approach to the treatment of male factor infertility. If severe male factor is present, extensive diagnostic and therapeutic interventions may not be indicated if ICSI is available and appropriate.

A remarkable paradox of the success of ICSI in the treatment of male factor infertility is that success in ICSI cycles is highly dependent on the number and quality of the oocytes retrieved. The major predictors of ICSI success are likely to be age of the female partner, early follicular-phase FSH level, and FSH response to a clomiphene challenge.[125]

For ICSI, sperm can be prepared by high-speed centrifugation (1800 g). The collected motile sperm are then "immobilized" in a drop of polyvinylpyrrolidone under oil. Many gametologists nick, roll, or cut the sperm tail before drawing the sperm into the microinjection pipette. Before sperm injection, the oocyte is prepared by removing the cumulus mass with hyaluronidase. The oocyte is fixed in place with the polar body at the 6 or 12 o'clock position with suction applied by a micropipette in a drop of medium under oil. The pipette containing the sperm is inserted into the oocyte at the 3 o'clock position followed by injection of the sperm. Injection of the sperm near the meiotic spindle appears to modestly increase the number of high-quality embryos obtained with ICSI.[126] Immobilization of the sperm may increase sperm membrane permeability, which increases the success of mechanisms of zygote formation.[127]

In one large series reported by Van Steirteghem and colleagues,[128] 18,778 oocytes were injected in 1816 separate treatment cycles. The fertilization rate was 62 percent, and the ongoing pregnancy rate was 37 percent. In a follow-up of 424 pregnancies that occurred after ICSI, approximately 25 percent of the pregnancies aborted. Thirty percent of the pregnancies were twins, and 2 percent were triplets. The perinatal mortality rate was 19 per 1000 births.[129] In one follow-up study of 432 children born after ICSI, there was a 3.3 percent rate of major malformations and a 1 percent rate of chromosome abnormalities. Neurologic and developmental problems at 2 months of age were observed in 14 children.[130] Long-term follow-up of large numbers of births from ICSI will be needed to fully evaluate the effects of the procedure on the offspring.

An important refinement of ICSI is to combine surgical harvesting of epididymal or testicular sperm with ICSI in men with no sperm in the ejaculate. Testicular biopsy specimens are minced and subjected to Percoll gradient centrifugation. The sperm obtained are then used for ICSI.[131] Epididymal sperm is typically obtained by microsurgical epididymal sperm aspiration in men with congenital absence of the vas deferens or for irreparable obstructive azoospermia. Surgical harvesting of sperm from the epididymis or testis followed by ICSI produces embryos for transfer in up to 90 percent of cases with livebirth rates per cycle in the range of 30 percent.[132] In contrast, use of sperm obtained by microsurgical epididymal aspiration with IVF results in a livebirth rate per cycle less than 5 percent.[133]

As ICSI develops, clinicians are attempting more daring treatments for previously "untreatable" disorders. For example, Bourne and colleagues[134] reported that ICSI can be used to successfully fertilize oocytes with round-headed sperm missing the acrosome.

ICSI may completely transform the diagnostic and treatment approach to male factor infertility. With ICSI, the important operative question is, Can one live sperm be obtained from the infertile male? If the answer is yes, then the couple is eligible for treatment with ICSI. If the answer is no, the only available effective fertility treatment is the use of donor sperm.

ICSI does not appear to improve pregnancy rates in IVF when it is applied to infertile couples with a normal semen analysis. In one trial, couples with tubal factor and a normal semen analysis were randomized to receive either standard IVF or ICSI. The clinical pregnancy rate was similar in both groups (31 percent and 33 percent).[135] Given the greater resources used with ICSI, it is probably not warranted to apply this technique for tubal factor infertility treated with IVF.

GENETIC DISEASES CAUSING MALE INFERTILITY: TRANSMISSION TO A NEW GENERATION WITH MICROMANIPULATION TECHNIQUES

Many human diseases are due to genetic abnormalities that have not been fully characterized. It is likely that many cases of male factor infertility are due to genetic abnormalities. In the natural state, many of these genetic abnormalities cause infertility and would not be transmitted to male offspring. With the use of gamete micromanipulation techniques, especially ICSI, the possibility that these abnormalities will be transmitted to male progeny is substantial. Approximately 15 percent of men with azoospermia have chromosome abnormalities, such as 47,XXY, Klinefelter's syndrome.[136] Studies demonstrate that men with oligospermia, like those with azoospermia, have an increased frequency of chromosome abnormalities. In two studies of more than 700 men with oligospermia (semen concentrations of sperm less than 20 million/ml), aneuploidy was detected in approximately 3 percent of the men.[137, 138] Among men with semen concentrations of sperm less than 10 million/ml, chromosome abnormalities were detected in approximately 6 percent of the men. Most of the abnormalities seen in oligospermic men involve autosomal abnormalities including reciprocal and Robertsonian translocations. Theoretically, up to two thirds of sperm from a balanced translocation carrier contain an abnormal complement of chromosome material. However, most of the conceptions resulting from fertilization with chromosomally abnormal sperm will result in pregnancy loss. In large populations of men with a reciprocal translocation, the risk of transmission to a child ranges from approximately 1 to 25 percent and depends on the size of the chromosome abnormality, the specific chromosome involved, and the type of translocation.[139]

In addition to chromosome abnormalities, oligospermic men also have genetic abnormalities that cannot be detected by karyotype analysis.[140] For example, the *DAZ* gene (deleted in azoospermia) is deleted in approximately 2 to 13 percent of men with azoospermia and less than 1 percent of men with severe oligospermia. In one study of the *DAZ* gene in infertile men consulting an infertility clinic, 5 of 168 azoospermic or severely oligospermic men were noted to have deletions in sY254 or sY255 (markers for the *DAZ* gene). Four of these men had elevated FSH levels, and all five had abnormally low testicular volume by physical examination. None of the men with semen concentrations of sperm greater than 1 million/ml had a deletion of the *DAZ* gene.[141] Recent clinical reports suggest that with use of ICSI, sperm from men with the *DAZ* deletion can fertilize oocytes and produce liveborn children.

In the next decade, many genes will be identified that are associated with oligospermia. With use of assisted reproduction techniques, such as ICSI, men with severe oligospermia will father male offspring who are at risk for having oligospermia. Until more is known concerning these risks, couples should be counseled and karyotype analysis should be offered when severe oligospermia or azoospermia is present and the couple plans to use ICSI. The probability of detecting a chromosome abnormality in couples in which the male partner has severe oligospermia or azoospermia is similar to that reported for couples with recurrent abortion.[142]

EMBRYO MICROMANIPULATION

One technique that has been proposed to improve embryo implantation is assisted hatching. Assisted hatching involves the deliberate thinning or disruption of the zona of a conceptus by enzymatic or mechanical techniques (Figs. 21–33 and 21–35). The goal of assisted hatching is to allow the conceptus that reaches the blastocyst stage to expand through the zona and thereby facilitate the interaction of the conceptus with the endometrium (Fig. 21–35). Assisted hatching can be performed by the mechanical technique of partial zona dissection or by the chemical technique of zona drilling using acid Tyrode's solution. Zona drilling for assisted hatching is often performed on day 3 of embryonic development, after interblastomere adhesion has increased.[143]

Preliminary data suggest that embryos derived from women older than 37 years[144] (Fig. 21–36) or from women with elevated early follicular-phase FSH concentrations have a decreased implantation rate per embryo. One poten-

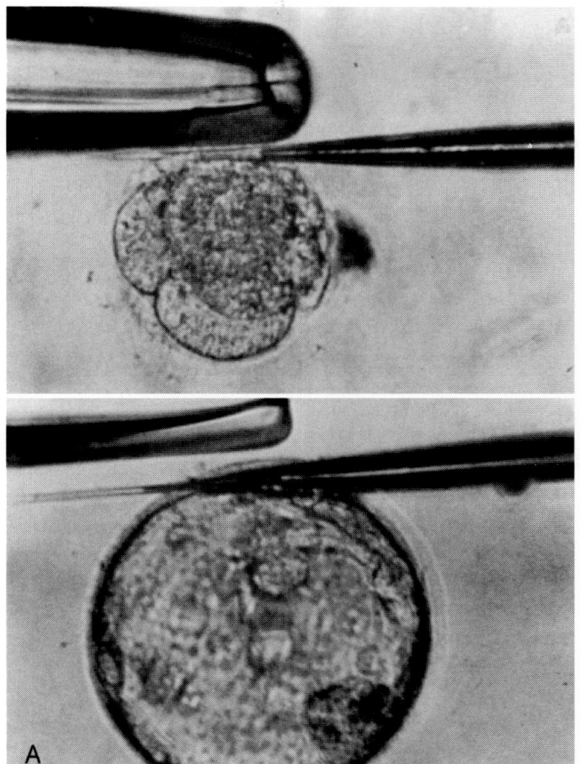

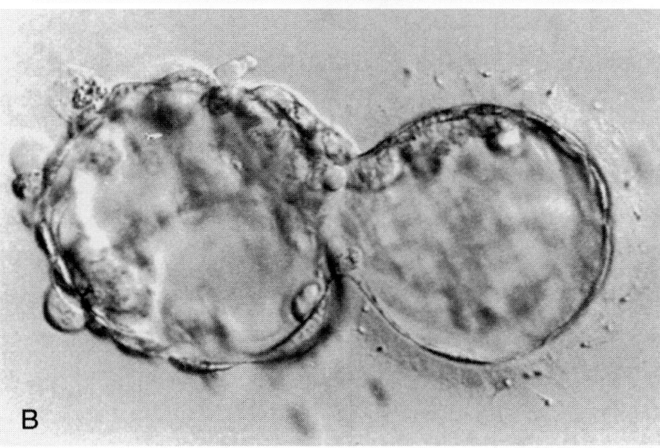

Figure 21–35 ■ *A,* Micromanipulation of a human embryo on day 2 to make a mechanical slit in the zona pellucida. *B,* Hatching blastocyst after assisted hatching procedure. (*A* and *B* from Dokras A, Ross C, Gosden B, et al. Micromanipulation of human embryos to assist hatching. Fertil Steril 61:514–520, 1994. Reproduced with permission of the American Society for Reproductive Medicine.)

tial application of assisted hatching is to try to improve the implantation rate in these women. In one study examining the effects of zona drilling using acid Tyrode's solution on pregnancy in women with elevated FSH, an increase in clinical pregnancy was observed.[145] In a refinement of the technique, only those embryos with a zona thicker than 15 μm were treated with zona drilling. The implantation rate per embryo increased from 18 percent in the control embryos to 25 percent in the zona-drilled embryos. When zona drilling is applied to embryos with a zona less than 12 μm in diameter, or when embryos from young women with low basal FSH concentrations are subjected to drilling, there is no improvement in pregnancy rate.[145] Additional clinical trials are needed to better define the indications and effectiveness of zona drilling.

PREIMPLANTATION GENETIC DIAGNOSIS: BLASTOMERE BIOPSY

An important potential advantage of assisted reproductive technology is that both the gametes and embryos can be directly examined, tested, and manipulated. In the future, assisted reproductive techniques may be widely used for genetic diagnosis and gene therapy. Gene therapy on human gametes and embryos is not yet practical, but preimplantation genetic diagnosis can currently be performed for a significant number of genetic diseases (Table 21–7). Conceptuses from many species implant normally and result in liveborn infants after blastomere biopsy. In the human, removal of one blastomere from 6- to 8-cell conceptuses is technically feasible and appears to be compatible with implantation and pregnancy.[146, 147] Blastomere preimplantation genetic diagnosis is performed by removing a blastomere from an embryo generated by IVF or, less commonly, by uterine flushing. Blastomere biopsy for the preimplantation diagnosis of genetic disorders requires a reliable method for genetic diagnosis on single blastomeres. Techniques such as fluorescence in situ hybridization and polymerase chain reaction are suitable for such analyses because results can be obtained within 12 hours (see Chapter 12).

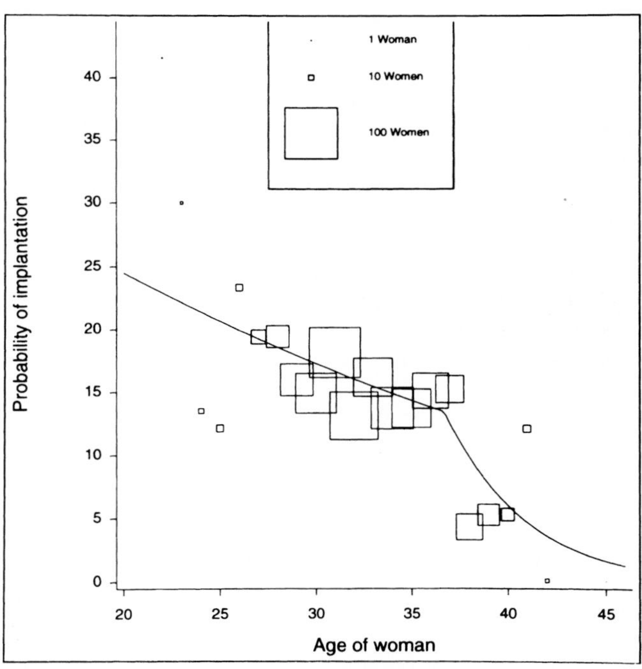

Figure 21–36 ■ Relationship between the age of the female partner and the estimated probability of embryo implantation resulting from IVF treatment. The implantation rate per age group is represented by the blocks. The size of the block is proportional to the number of data points for the observation. The calculated solid line shows a decrease in implantation rate after age 37 years. (From van Kooij RJ, Looman CWN, Habbema JDF, et al. Age-dependent decrease in embryo implantation rate after in vitro fertilization. Fertil Steril 66:769–775, 1996. Reproduced with permission of the American Society for Reproductive Medicine.)

■ TABLE 21–7
Genetic Disorders That Can Be Diagnosed by Blastomere Biopsy

α_1-Antitrypsin deficiency
Cystic fibrosis
Tay-Sachs disease
Duchenne's muscular dystrophy
Turner's syndrome
Down syndrome
Hemophilia A
Fragile X syndrome
X-linked disorders

NUCLEAR CLONING

The genomic DNA and its linear sequence of A, G, C, and T nucleotides contains all the information that is necessary to produce an organism. The diploid cells in the body inherit the same DNA that was present in the fertilized egg. It is theoretically possible to harvest the DNA from a diploid adult cell, inject it into an oocyte that has had its DNA removed, and stimulate the development of the oocyte into an adult organism. Successful nuclear transplantation of DNA from an adult cell into an oocyte was first accomplished in the amphibian. In the frog, cloning can be accomplished by first destroying the DNA in an oocyte by ultraviolet radiation and then injecting a nucleus from an adult skin cell or an erythrocyte into the oocyte. The trauma of the injection activates the egg, and a swimming tadpole is the product.[148–150]

Similar techniques have recently been used to clone mammals.[151, 152] Oocytes were recovered from Scottish Blackface ewes 28 to 33 hours after the injection of GnRH. The oocytes were enucleated and then fused with donor cells by use of electrical pulses. Before fusion with the enucleated oocyte, the donor cells were forced into quiescence (G_0 stage of the cell cycle) by culturing in media with low serum concentration. By this technique, liveborn sheep were obtained with the use of donor cells derived from adult mammary tissue, fetal tissue, and an embryonic cell line. These results demonstrate that it is possible to reproduce some mammalian species without the use of sperm.

The aspect of these experiments that drew the attention of the public was the possibility of generating a large number of genetically identical clones. The investigators suggest that nuclear transfer from the cells of elite animals to recipient oocytes may enhance the replication of animals with enhanced performance characteristics. Although nuclear cloning may be supported by some experts in animal husbandry, many scientists are concerned about the potential misuse of cloning technology. Ironically, one major advantage of sexual reproduction is to increase the genetic diversity of the species. Excessive use of cloning would have exactly the opposite result. Public awareness of the technical advances achieved with nuclear cloning resulted in a call for either a moratorium or ban on all cloning work with humans. The potential of this technology may be too threatening to our societal concepts of self, family, and society to ever allow widespread application of these techniques to humans.

References

1. Heape W. Preliminary note on the transplantation and growth of mammalian ova within a uterine foster mother. Proc R Soc 48:457–458, 1891.
2. Iwamatsu T, Chang MC. In vitro fertilization of mouse eggs in the presence of bovine follicular fluid. Nature 224:919–920, 1969.
3. Edwards RG, Bavister BD, Steptoe PC. Early stages of fertilization in vitro of human oocytes matured in vitro. Nature 221:632–635, 1969.
4. Edwards RG. Physiological aspects of human ovulation, fertilization and cleavage. J Reprod Fertil 18(suppl):87–101, 1973.
5. Steptoe PC, Edwards RG, Purdy JM. Clinical aspects of pregnancies established with cleaving embryos grown in vitro. Br J Obstet Gynaecol 87:757–768, 1980.
6. Millete CF. Cell surface antigens during mammalian spermatogenesis. Curr Top Dev Biol 13:1–30, 1979.
7. Langlais J, Zollinger M, Plante L, et al. Localization of cholesteryl sulfate in human spermatozoa in support of a hypothesis for the mechanism of capacitation. Proc Natl Acad Sci USA 78:7266–7270, 1981.
8. Kopf GS, Gerton GL. The mammalian sperm acrosome and the acrosome reaction. *In* Wassarman PM (ed). Elements of Mammalian Fertilization. Boston, CRC Press, 1991, pp 153–203.
9. Macek MB, Shur BD. Protein-carbohydrate complementarity in mammalian gamete recognition. Gamete Res 20:93–109, 1988.
10. Bleil JD, Wassarman PM. Mammalian sperm-egg interaction: Identification of a glycoprotein in mouse egg zonae pellucidae possessing receptor activity for sperm. Cell 20:873–882, 1980.
11. Florman HM, Wassarman PM. O-linked oligosaccharides of mouse egg ZP3 account for its sperm receptor activity. Cell 41:313–324, 1985.
12. Ward CR, Kopf GS. Molecular events mediating sperm activation. Dev Biol 158:9–34, 1993.
13. Mortillo S, Wassarman PM. Differential binding of gold labeled zona pellucida glycoproteins mZP2 and mZP3 to mouse sperm membrane compartments. Development 113:141–149, 1991.
14. Bleil JD, Greve JM, Wassarman PM. Identification of a secondary sperm receptor in the mouse egg zona pellucida: Role in maintenance of binding of acrosome reacted sperm to eggs. Dev Biol 128:376–385, 1988.
15. Miller DJ, Macek MB, Shur BD. Complementarity between sperm surface β1,4-galactosyltransferase and egg-coat ZP3 mediates sperm-egg binding. Nature 357:589–593, 1992.
16. Bookbinder LH, Cheng A, Bleil JD. Tissue and species specific expression of sp56, a mouse sperm fertilization protein. Science 269:86–89, 1995.
17. Leyton L, Saling P. 95 kd sperm proteins bind ZP3 and serve as tyrosine kinase substrates in response to zona binding. Cell 57:1123–1130, 1989.
18. Oehninger S, Hinsch E, Pfisterer S, et al. Use of specific zona pellucida protein 3 antiserum as a clinical marker for human ZP integrity and function. Fertil Steril 65:139–145, 1996.
19. Blobel VP, Wolfsberg TG, Turck CW, et al. A potential fusion peptide and an integrin ligand domain in a protein, active in sperm egg fusion. Nature 356:248–252, 1992.
20. Myles DG, Kimmel LH, Blobel CP, et al. Identification of a binding site in the disintegrin domain of fertilin required for sperm-egg fusion. Proc Natl Acad Sci USA 91:4195–4198, 1994.
21. Lindenberg S, Hyttel P, Lenz S, Holmes PV. Ultrastructure of the early human implantation in vitro. Hum Reprod 1:533–538, 1986.
22. Soliman S, Daya S, Collins J, Jarrell J. A randomized trial of in vitro fertilization versus conventional treatment for infertility. Fertil Steril 59:1239–1244, 1993.
23. Benadiva CA, Kligman I, Davis O, Rosenwaks Z. In vitro fertilization versus tubal surgery: Is pelvic reconstructive surgery obsolete? Fertil Steril 64:1051–1061, 1995.
24. Pagidas K, Falcone T, Hemmings R, Miron P. Comparison of reoperation for moderate and severe endometriosis-related infertility with in vitro fertilization embryo transfer. Fertil Steril 65:791–795, 1996.
25. Kodama H, Fukuda J, Karube H, et al. Benefit of in vitro fertilization treatment for endometriosis associated infertility. Fertil Steril 66:974–979, 1996.
26. Olivennes F, Feldberg D, Liu HC, et al. Endometriosis: A stage by

stage analysis—role of in vitro fertilization. Fertil Steril 64:392–398, 1995.
27. van Uem JFHM, Acosta AA, Swanson RG, et al. Male factor evaluation in in vitro fertilization. Fertil Steril 44:375–383, 1985.
28. Dodson WC, Whitesides DB, Hughes CL, et al. Superovulation with intrauterine insemination in the treatment of infertility: A possible alternative to gamete intrafallopian transfer and in vitro fertilization. Fertil Steril 48:441–445, 1987.
29. Gurgan T, Urman B, Yarali H, Kisnisci HA. The results of in vitro fertilization embryo transfer in couples with unexplained infertility failing to conceive with superovulation and intrauterine insemination. Fertil Steril 64:93–97, 1995.
30. Homburg R, Berkowitz D, Levy T, et al. In vitro fertilization and embryo transfer for the treatment of infertility associated with polycystic ovary syndrome. Fertil Steril 60:858–863, 1993.
31. Wada I, Matson PL, Troup SA, Lieberman BA. Assisted conception using buserelin and human menopausal gonadotropins in women with polycystic ovary syndrome. Br J Obstet Gynaecol 100:365–369, 1993.
32. Lahteenmaki A, Rasanen M, Hovatta O. Low-dose prednisolone does not improve the outcome of in vitro fertilization in male immunologic infertility. Hum Reprod 10:3124–3129, 1995.
33. Nagy ZP, Verheyen G, Liu J, et al. Results of 55 intracytoplasmic sperm injection cycles in the treatment of male-immunological infertility. Hum Reprod 10:1775–1780, 1995.
34. Lahteenmaki A, Reima I, Hovatta O. Treatment of severe male immunological infertility by intracytoplasmic sperm injection. Hum Reprod 10:2824–2828, 1995.
35. Society for Assisted Reproductive Technology and The American Society for Reproductive Medicine. Assisted reproductive technology in the United States and Canada: 1994 results generated from the American Society for Reproductive Medicine/ Society for Assisted Reproductive Technology Registry. Fertil Steril 66:697–705, 1996.
36. Medical Research International, The American Fertility Society Special Interest Group. In vitro fertilization/embryo transfer in the United States: 1985 and 1986 results from the National IVF/ET Registry. Fertil Steril 49:212–215, 1988.
37. Toner JP, Philput CB, Jones GS, Muasher SJ. Basal follicle stimulating hormone level is a better predictor of in vitro fertilization performance than age. Fertil Steril 55:784–791, 1991.
38. Scott RT, Hofmann GE. Prognostic assessment of ovarian reserve. Fertil Steril 63:1–11, 1995.
39. Claman P, Domingo M, Garner P, et al. Natural cycle in vitro fertilization embryo transfer at the University of Ottawa: An inefficient therapy for tubal infertility. Fertil Steril 60:298–302, 1993.
40. MacDougall MJ, Tan SL, Hall V, et al. Comparison of natural with clomiphene citrate stimulated cycles in in vitro fertilization: A prospective randomized trial. Fertil Steril 61:1052–1057, 1994.
41. Hurd WW, Randolph JF, Christman GM, et al. Luteal support with both estradiol and progesterone after clomiphene citrate stimulation for in vitro fertilization. Fertil Steril 66:587–592, 1996.
42. Shaw RW, Ndukwe G, Imoedemhe D, et al. Stimulation of multiple follicular growth for in vitro fertilization by administration of pulsatile luteinizing hormone releasing hormone. Fertil Steril 46:135–137, 1986.
43. Porter RN, Smith W, Craft IL, et al. Induction of ovulation for in vitro fertilization using buserelin and gonadotropins. Lancet 2:1284–1285, 1984.
44. Hughes EG, Fedorkow DM, Daya S, et al. The routine use of gonadotropin releasing hormone agonists prior to in vitro fertilization and gamete intrafallopian tube transfer: A meta-analysis of randomized controlled trials. Fertil Steril 58:888–896, 1992.
45. Liu HC, Lai YM, Davis O, et al. Improved pregnancy outcome with gonadotropin releasing hormone agonist stimulation is due to the improvement in oocyte quantity rather than quality. J Assist Reprod Genet 9:338–344, 1992.
46. Lejune B, Barlow P, Puissant F, et al. Use of buserelin acetate in an in vitro fertilization program: A comparison with classical clomiphene citrate–human menopausal gonadotropin treatment. Fertil Steril 54:475–481, 1990.
47. MacNamee MC, Howles CM, Edwards RG, et al. Short term luteinizing hormone agonist treatment prospective trial of a novel ovarian stimulation regimen for in vitro fertilization. Fertil Steril 52:264–269, 1989.
48. Antoine JM, Salat-Baroux J, Alvarez S, et al. Ovarian stimulation using human menopausal gonadotropins with or without LHRH analogues in a long protocol for in vitro fertilization: A prospective randomized comparison. Hum Reprod 5:565–569, 1990.
49. Garcia JE, Padilla SL, Bayati J, Baramki TA. Follicular phase gonadotropin releasing hormone agonist and human gonadotropins: A better alternative for ovulation induction in in vitro fertilization. Fertil Steril 53:302–305, 1990.
50. Kondaveeti-Gordon U, Harrison RF, Barry-Kinsella C, et al. A randomized prospective study of early follicular or midluteal initiation of long protocol gonadotropin releasing hormone in an in vitro fertilization program. Fertil Steril 66:582–586, 1996.
51. Scott RT, Navot D. Enhancement of ovarian responsiveness with microdoses of gonadotropin releasing hormone agonist during ovulation induction for in vitro fertilization. Fertil Steril 61:880–885, 1994.
52. Minaretzis D, Alper MM, Oskowitz SP, et al. Gonadotropin releasing hormone antagonist versus agonist administration in women undergoing controlled ovarian hyperstimulation: Cycle performance and in vitro steroidogenesis of granulosa cells. Fertil Steril 172:1518–1525, 1995.
53. Martin KA, Hornstein MD, Taylor AE, et al. Exogenous gonadotropin stimulation is associated with increases in serum androgens in IVF-ET cycles. Fertil Steril 68:1011–1016, 1997.
54. Yeh J, Ravnikar V, Barbieri RL. Ovarian hyperstimulation syndrome associated with leuprolide suppression: A case report. J In Vitro Fertil 6:261–263, 1989.
55. Lewin A, Laufer N, Rabinowitz R, et al. Ultrasonically guided oocyte collection under local anesthesia: The first choice method for in vitro fertilization—a comparative study with laparoscopy. Fertil Steril 46:257–261, 1986.
56. Wittmaack FM, Kreger DO, Blasco L, et al. Effect of follicular size on oocyte retrieval, fertilization, cleavage and embryo quality in in vitro fertilization cycles: A 6-year data collection. Fertil Steril 62:1205–1210, 1994.
57. Chan SY, Chan YM, Tucker MJ. Comparison of characteristics of human spermatozoa selected by the multiple tube swim up and simple discontinuous Percoll gradient centrifugation. Andrologia 23:213–218, 1991.
58. Sapienza F, Verheyen G, Tournaye H, et al. An auto-controlled study in in vitro fertilization reveals the benefit of Percoll centrifugation to swim up in the preparation of poor quality semen. Hum Reprod 8:1856–1862, 1993.
59. van der Zwalmen P, Bertin-Segal G, Geerts L, et al. Sperm morphology and IVF pregnancy rate: Comparison between Percoll gradient centrifugation and swim up procedures. Hum Reprod 6:581–588, 1991.
60. Svendsen TO, Jones D, Butler L, Muasher SJ. The incidence of multiple gestations after in vitro fertilization is dependent on the number of embryos transferred and maternal age. Fertil Steril 65:561–565, 1996.
61. Steer CV, Mills CL, Tan SL, et al. The cumulative embryo score: A predictive embryo scoring technique to select the optimal number of embryos to transfer in an in vitro fertilization and embryo transfer programme. Hum Reprod 7:117–119, 1992.
62. Roseboom TJ, Vermeiden JP, Schoute E, et al. The probability of pregnancy after embryo transfer is affected by the age of the patient, cause of infertility, number of embryos transferred and the average morphology score, as revealed by multiple logistic regression analysis. Hum Reprod 10:3035–3041, 1995.
63. French In Vitro National. French National IVF Registry: Analysis of 1986 to 1990 data. Fertil Steril 59:587–595, 1993.
64. Preutthipan S, Amso N, Curtis P, Shaw RW. The influence of number of embryos transferred on pregnancy outcome in women undergoing in vitro fertilization and embryo transfer. J Med Assoc Thai 79:613–617, 1996.
65. Soliman S, Daya S, Collins J, Hughes EG. The role of luteal phase support in infertility treatment: A meta analysis of randomized trials. Fertil Steril 61:1068–1076, 1994.
66. Van Steirteghem AC, Smitz J, Camus M, et al. The luteal phase after in vitro fertilization and related procedures. Hum Reprod 3:161–164, 1988.

67. Hutchinson-Williams KA, DeCherney AH, Lavy G, et al. Luteal rescue in in vitro fertilization embryo transfer. Fertil Steril 53:459–501, 1990.
68. Cohen J. The efficiency and efficacy of IVF and GIFT. Hum Reprod 6:613–618, 1991.
69. Cooperman AB, Selick CE, Grunfeld, et al. Cumulative number and morphological score of embryos resulting in success: Realistic expectations from in vitro fertilization embryo transfer. Fertil Steril 64:88–92, 1995.
70. Forman RG, Frydman R, Egan D, et al. Severe ovarian hyperstimulation syndrome using agonists of gonadotropin releasing hormone for in vitro fertilization: A European series and a proposal for prevention. Fertil Steril 53:502–509, 1990.
71. Gonen Y, Powell WA, Casper RF. Effect of follicular aspiration on hormonal parameters in patients undergoing ovarian stimulation. Hum Reprod 6:356–358, 1991.
72. Boivin J, Takefman JE. Stress level across stages of in vitro fertilization in subsequently pregnant and nonpregnant women. Fertil Steril 64:802–810, 1995.
73. Palermo GD, Colombero LT, Schattman GL, et al. Evolution of pregnancies and initial follow-up of newborns delivered after intracytoplasmic sperm injection. JAMA 276:1893–1897, 1996.
74. Cohen J, Mayaux MJ, Guihard-Moscato ML. Pregnancy outcomes after in vitro fertilization. Ann N Y Acad Sci 541:1–6, 1988.
75. Olivennes F, Kerbrat V, Rufat P, et al. Follow-up of a cohort of 422 children ages 6 to 13 years conceived by in vitro fertilization. Fertil Steril 67:284–289, 1997.
76. Olivennes F, Kadhel P, Rufat P, et al. Perinatal outcome of twin pregnancies obtained after in vitro fertilization: Comparison with twin pregnancies obtained spontaneously or after ovarian stimulation. Fertil Steril 66:105–109, 1996.
77. Roest J, van Heusden AM, Verhoeff A, et al. A triplet pregnancy after in vitro fertilization is a procedure related complication that should be prevented by the replacement of two embryos only. Fertil Steril 67:290–295, 1997.
78. Wilcox LS, Kiely JL, Melvin CL, Martin MC. Assisted reproductive technologies: Estimates of their contribution to multiple births and newborn hospital days in the United States. Fertil Steril 65:361–366, 1996.
79. Bollen N, Camus M, Tournaye H, et al. Embryo reduction in triplet pregnancies after assisted procreation: A comparative study. Fertil Steril 60:504–509, 1993.
80. Radestad A, Bui TH, Nygren KG. Multifetal pregnancy reduction in Sweden. Utilization rate and pregnancy outcome. Acta Obstet Gynecol Scand 73:403–406, 1994.
81. Evans MI, Dommergues M, Timor-Tritsch I, et al. Transabdominal versus transcervical and transvaginal multifetal pregnancy reduction: International collaborative experience of more than 1000 cases. Am J Obstet Gynecol 170:902–909, 1994.
82. Smith Levitan M, Kowalik A, Birnholz J, et al. Selective reduction of multifetal pregnancies to twins improves outcome over non-reduced triplet gestations. Am J Obstet Gynecol 175:878–883, 1996.
83. Bollen N, Camus M, Tournaye H, et al. Embryo reduction in triplet pregnancies after assisted procreation: A comparative study. Fertil Steril 60:504–509, 1993.
84. Staessen C, Janssenswillen C, Van den Abbeel E, et al. Avoidance of triplet pregnancies by elective transfer of two good quality embryos. Hum Reprod 8:1650–1653, 1993.
85. Scholtes MCW, Zeilmaker GH. A prospective randomized study of embryo transfer results after 3 or 5 days of embryo culture in in vitro fertilization. Fertil Steril 65:1245–1248, 1996.
86. Berkowitz RL, Lynch L, Stone J, Alvarez M. The current status of multifetal pregnancy reduction. Am J Obstet Gynecol 174:1265–1272, 1996.
87. Zeilmaker GH, Alberda AT, van Gent I, et al. Two pregnancies following transfer of intact frozen thawed embryos. Fertil Steril 42:293–296, 1984.
88. Van der Elst J, Camus M, Van den Abbeel E, et al. Prospective randomized study on the cryopreservation of human embryos with dimethylsulfoxide or 1,2-propanediol protocols. Fertil Steril 63:92–100, 1995.
89. Lin YP, Cassidenti DL, Chacon RR, et al. Successful implantation of frozen sibling embryos is influenced by the outcome of the cycle from which they were derived. Fertil Steril 63:262–267, 1995.
90. Neumann PJ, Gharib SD, Weinstein MC. The cost of a successful delivery with in vitro fertilization. N Engl J Med 331:239–243, 1994.
91. Trad FS, Hornstein MD, Barbieri RL. In vitro fertilization: A cost effective alternative for infertile couples? J Assist Reprod Genet 12:418–421, 1995.
92. Lutjen P, Trounson A, Leeton J, et al. The establishment and maintenance of pregnancy using in vitro fertilization and embryo donation in a patient with primary ovarian failure. Nature 307:174–175, 1984.
93. Sauer MV, Paulson RJ. Human oocyte and pre-embryo donation: An evolving method for the treatment of female infertility. Am J Obstet Gynecol 163:1421–1424, 1990.
94. Borini A, Bianchi L, Violini F, et al. Oocyte donation program: Pregnancy and implantation rates in women of different ages sharing oocytes from single donor. Fertil Steril 65:94–97, 1996.
95. Cano F, Simon C, Remohi J, Pellecier A. Effect of aging on the female reproductive system: Evidence for a role of uterine senescence in the decline in female fecundity. Fertil Steril 64:584–589, 1995.
96. Morris RS, Sauer MV. Oocyte donation in 1990s and beyond. Assist Reprod Rev 3:211–217, 1993.
97. Veeck LL, Mundson CH, Brothman LJ, et al. Significantly enhanced pregnancy rates per cycle through cryopreservation and thaw of pronuclear stage oocytes. Fertil Steril 59:1202–1207, 1993.
97a. Gook DA, Schiewe MC, Osborn SM, et al. Intracytoplasmic sperm injection and embryo development of human oocytes cryopreserved using 1,2-propanediol. Hum Reprod 10:2637–2641, 1995.
98. Leeton J, Rogers P, Caro C, et al. A controlled study between the use of gamete intrafallopian transfer and in vitro fertilization and embryo transfer in the management of idiopathic and male infertility. Fertil Steril 48:605–607, 1987.
99. Hogerzeil HV, Spiekerman JC, de Vries JW, de Schepper G. A randomized trial between GIFT and ovarian stimulation for the treatment of unexplained infertility and failed artificial insemination by donor. Hum Reprod 7:1235–1239, 1992.
100. Guzick DS, Yao YAS, Berga SL, et al. Endometriosis impairs the efficacy of gamete intrafallopian transfer: Results of a case control study. Fertil Steril 62:1186–1191, 1994.
101. Seracchioli R, Maccolini A, Porcu E, et al. The role of gamete intrafallopian transfer (GIFT) and tubal embryo transfer (TET) in the treatment of patients with patent tubes associated with male infertility factor. J Assist Reprod Genet 10:266–270, 1993.
102. Seracchioli R, Porcu E, Ciotti P, et al. Gamete intrafallopian transfer: Prospective randomized comparison between hysteroscopic and laparoscopic transfer techniques. Fertil Steril 64:355–359, 1995.
103. Tournaye H, Devroey P, Camus M, et al. Zygote intrafallopian transfer or in vitro fertilization and embryo transfer for the treatment of male-factor infertility: A prospective randomized trial. Fertil Steril 58:344–350, 1992.
104. Fluker MR, Zouves CG, Bebbington MW. A prospective randomized comparison of zygote intrafallopian transfer and in vitro fertilization–embryo transfer for non-tubal factor infertility. Fertil Steril 60:515–519, 1993.
105. Preutthipan S, Amso N, Curtis P, Shaw RW. A prospective randomized cross over comparison of zygote intrafallopian tube transfer and in vitro fertilization embryo transfer in unexplained infertility. J Med Assoc Thai 77:599–604, 1994.
106. Van Voorhis BJ, Syrop CH, Vincent RD, et al. Tubal versus uterine transfer of cryopreserved embryos: A prospective randomized trial. Fertil Steril 63:578–583, 1995.
107. Rowlands DJ, McDermott A, Hull MGR. Smoking and decreased fertilization rates in vitro. Lancet 340:1409–1410, 1992.
108. Pattinson HA, Taylor PJ, Pattinson MH. The effect of cigarette smoking on ovarian function and early pregnancy outcome of in vitro fertilization treatment. Fertil Steril 55:780–783, 1991.
109. Chung PH, Yeko TR, Mayer JC, et al. Gamete intrafallopian transfer: Does smoking play a role? J Reprod Med 42:65–70, 1997.
110. Cramer DC, Barbieri RL, Xu H, Reichardt JKV. Determinants of basal follicle stimulating hormone levels in premenopausal women. J Clin Endocrinol Metab 79:1105–1109, 1994.
111. Sharara FI, Beatse SN, Leonardi MR, et al. Cigarette smoking

accelerates the development of diminished ovarian reserve as evidenced by the clomiphene citrate challenge test. Fertil Steril 62:257–262, 1994.
112. O'Donovan PA, Vandekerckhove P, Lilford RJ, Hughes E. Treatment of male infertility: Is it effective? Hum Reprod 8:1209–1222, 1993.
113. Ben-Chetrit A, Senoz S, Greenblatt EM, Casper RF. In vitro fertilization outcome in the presence of severe male factor infertility. Fertil Steril 63:1032–1037, 1995.
114. Schlegel PN, Girardi S. In vitro fertilization for male factor infertility. J Clin Endocrinol Metab 82:709–716, 1997.
115. Cohen J, Malter H, Wright G, et al. Partial zona dissection of human oocytes when failure of zona pellucida penetration is anticipated. Hum Reprod 4:435–442, 1989.
116. Tummon IS, Gore-Langton RE, Daniel SA, et al. Randomized trial of partial zona dissection for male infertility. Fertil Steril 63:842–848, 1995.
117. Hammitt DG. Treatment of male factor infertility by in vitro insemination with HCI of motile sperm. Semin Reprod Endocrinol 11:72–78, 1993.
118. Cohen J, Alikani M, Malter HE, et al. Partial zona dissection or subzonal sperm insertion: Microsurgical fertilization alternatives based on evaluation of sperm and embryo morphology. Fertil Steril 56:696–706, 1991.
119. Fishel S, Timson J, Lisi F, Rinaldi L. Evaluation of 225 patients undergoing subzonal insemination for the procurement of fertilization in vitro. Fertil Steril 57:840–849, 1992.
120. Palermo G, Joris H, Devroey P, et al. Pregnancies after intracytoplasmic injection of single spermatozoon into an oocyte. Lancet 340:17–18, 1992.
121. Levran D, Bider D, Yonesh M, et al. A randomized study of intracytoplasmic sperm injection (ICSI) versus subzonal insemination (SUZI) for the management of severe male factor infertility. J Assist Reprod Genet 12:319–321, 1995.
122. Catt J, Ryan J, Pike I, O'Neill C. Fertilization rates using intracytoplasmic sperm injection are greater than subzonal insemination but are dependent on prior treatment of sperm. Fertil Steril 64:764–769, 1995.
123. Tarin JJ. Subzonal insemination, partial zona dissection or intracytoplasmic sperm injection. Hum Reprod 10:165–170, 1995.
124. Nagy ZP, Liu J, Joris H, et al. The result of intracytoplasmic sperm injection is not related to any of the three basic sperm parameters. Hum Reprod 10:1123–1129, 1995.
125. Sherins RJ, Thorsell LP, Dorfmann A, et al. Intracytoplasmic sperm injection facilitates fertilization even in the most severe forms of male infertility: Pregnancy outcome correlates with maternal age and number of eggs available. Fertil Steril 64:369–375, 1995.
126. Nagy ZP, Liu J, Joris H, et al. The influence of the site of sperm deposition and mode of oolema breakage at intracytoplasmic sperm injection on fertilization and embryo development rates. Hum Reprod 10:3171–3177, 1995.
127. Parrington J, Swann K, Shevchenko VI, et al. Calcium oscillations in mammalian eggs triggered by a soluble sperm protein. Nature 379:364–368, 1996.
128. Van Steirteghem AC, Joris H, Liu J, et al. Evolution of intracytoplasmic results. Fertil Steril 63:S83, 1994.
129. Wisanto A, Magnus M, Bonduelle M, et al. Obstetric outcome of 424 pregnancies after intracytoplasmic sperm injection. Hum Reprod 10:2713–2718, 1995.
130. Bonduelle M, Legein J, Buyusse A, et al. Prospective follow-up study of 423 children born after intracytoplasmic sperm injection. Hum Reprod 11:1558–1564, 1996.
131. Verheyen G, De Croo I, Tournaye H, et al. Comparison of four mechanical methods to retrieve spermatozoa from testicular tissue. Hum Reprod 10:2965–2969, 1995.
132. Silber SJ, Nagy Z, Liu J, et al. The use of epididymal and testicular spermatozoa for intracytoplasmic sperm injection: The genetic implications for male infertility. Hum Reprod 10:2031–2043, 1995.
133. Silber SJ, Devroey P, Tournaye H, Van Steirteghem AC. Fertilizing capacity of epididymal and testicular sperm using intracytoplasmic sperm injection (ICSI). Reprod Fertil Dev 7:281–292, 1995.
134. Bourne H, Liu DY, Clarke GN, Baker HW. Normal fertilization and embryo development by ICSI of round headed acrosomeless sperm. Fertil Steril 63:1329–1332, 1995.
135. Aboulghar MA, Mansour RT, Serour GI, et al. Prospective controlled randomized study of in vitro fertilization versus intracytoplasmic sperm injection in the treatment of tubal factor infertility with normal semen parameters. Fertil Steril 66:753–756, 1996.
136. Chandley AC. The chromosomal basis of human infertility. Br Med Bull 35:181–186, 1979.
137. Matsuda T, Horii Y, Nomomura M, et al. Chromosomal survey of 1001 subfertile males: Incidence and clinical features of males with chromosomal anomalies. Hinyokika Kiyo 38:803–809, 1992.
138. Abyholm T, Stray-Pedersen S. Hypospermiogenesis and chromosomal aberrations. A clinical study of azoospermia and oligospermic men with normal and abnormal karyotype. Int J Androl 4:546–558, 1981.
139. Daniel A, Hook EB, Wulf G. Risks of unbalanced progeny at amniocentesis to carriers of chromosome rearrangements: Data from United States and Canadian laboratories. Am J Med Genet 31:14–53, 1989.
140. Reijo R, Alagappan RK, Patrizio P, Page DC. Severe oligospermia resulting from deletions of azoospermia factor gene on Y chromosome. Lancet 347:1290–1293, 1996.
141. Simoni M, Gromoll J, Dworniczak B, et al. Screening for deletions of the Y chromosome involving the *DAZ* gene in azoospermia and severe oligospermia. Fertil Steril 67:542–547, 1997.
142. Portnoi M, Joye N, den Akker J, et al. Karyotypes of 1142 couples with recurrent abortion. Obstet Gynecol 72:31–34, 1988.
143. Cohen J. Assisted hatching of human embryos. J In Vitro Fertil Embryo Transf 8:179–190, 1991.
144. van Kooij RJ, Looman CWN, Habbema JDF, et al. Age-dependent decrease in embryo implantation rate after in vitro fertilization. Fertil Steril 66:769–775, 1996.
145. Cohen J, Alikani M, Trowbridge J, Rosenwaks Z. Implantation enhancement by selective assisted hatching using zona drilling of embryos with poor prognosis. Hum Reprod 7:685–691, 1992.
146. Handyside AH, Kontogianni EH, Hardy K, Winston RM. Pregnancies from biopsied human preimplantation embryos sexed by Y-specific DNA amplification. Nature 344:768–770, 1990.
147. Grifo JA, Tang YX, Cohen J, et al. Pregnancy after embryo biopsy and coamplification of DNA from X and Y chromosomes. JAMA 268:727–729, 1992.
148. DeBerardino MA, Orr NH, McKinnell RG. Feeding tadpoles cloned from *Rana* erythrocyte nuclei. Proc Natl Acad Sci USA 83:8231–8234, 1986.
149. Gurdon JB. Transplanted nuclei and cell differentiation. Sci Am 219:24–35, 1968.
150. Gurdon JB, Laskey RA, Reeves OR. The developmental capacity of nuclei transplanted from keratinized skin cells of adult frogs. J Embryol Exp Morphol 34:93–112, 1975.
151. Campbell KHS, McWhir J, Ritchie WA, Wilmut I. Sheep cloned by nuclear transfer from cultured cell line. Nature 380:64–66, 1996.
152. Wilmut I, Schnieke AE, McWhir J, et al. Viable offspring derived from fetal and adult mammalian cells. Nature 385:810–813, 1997.

Chapter 22

MALE HYPOTHALAMIC-PITUITARY-GONADAL AXIS

Johannes D. Veldhuis

CHAPTER OUTLINE

KEY POINTS

- The male hypothalamic-pituitary-gonadal axis is a multicomponent but integrated feedback system with intraglandular (paracrine and autocrine) control at each major level of the axis and interglandular communication between major control loci (i.e., the pituitary gland signals the testis, and the testis signals the hypothalamic-pituitary unit).
- Steroidal (testosterone and estrogen) and nonsteroidal (GnRH, opiate peptides, inhibin, activin, follistatin) regulators act within the male reproductive axis as local or systemic first messengers to direct moment-to-moment responses as well as long-term adaptations in target organs.
- New cellular, biochemical, biomathematical, and molecular methodologies to investigate mechanisms of regulated hormone action are likely to yield exciting insights in the next decade.

The healthy male hypothalamic-pituitary-gonadal axis orchestrates two principal functions that are essential to reproductive performance in the male, namely, the production of physiologic quantities of appropriate sex steroid hormones, including androgens, and the generation of healthy spermatogenic cells that become mature male gametes capable of fertilizing the oocyte. These reproductively crucial activities must be conducted under diverse and potentially unfavorable genetic and environmental conditions.

The hypothalamus and the anterior pituitary gland participate jointly in regulating the steroidogenic and spermatogenic functions of the testis. The testis also receives critical instruction from cells contained within it through paracrine and autocrine regulation. Overall function of the male reproductive system requires physiologic integration among individual neuroglandular elements (hypothalamus, pituitary gland, and testis), each of which is inherently complex. This concept of a so-called feedback and feedforward control system is illustrated in Figure 22–1.

HYPOTHALAMIC AND PITUITARY CONTROL MECHANISMS

GnRH Pulse Generator

Direct monitoring of hypothalamic-pituitary venous blood in animals indicates that gonadotropin-releasing hormone (GnRH) pulses appear to drive most luteinizing hormone (LH) release episodes.[1] The concept of a hypothalamic GnRH pulse generator has emerged as a multineuronal ensemble capable of episodic release of bursts of GnRH.[2] Immortalized GnRH neurons produced by targeted oncogenesis in the mouse also show in vitro pulsatility of GnRH release, suggesting intrinsic hypothalamic neuronal rhythmicity.[3] Whereas multiple neuroregulatory molecules

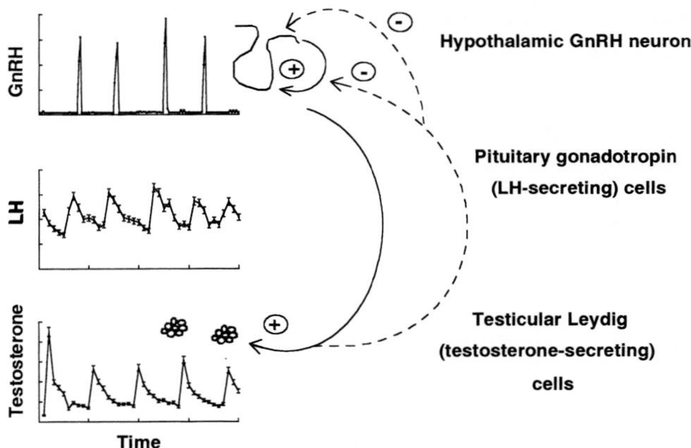

Figure 22–1 ■ Schematic depiction of the feedback and feedforward relationships operating within the hypothalamic (GnRH)–pituitary (LH)–testicular (testosterone) axis. Episodic GnRH release drives pulsatile LH and in turn testosterone release (feedforward), whereas testosterone negatively regulates both GnRH and LH secretion (feedback action). The feedback relationships maintain normal blood LH and testosterone concentrations throughout the day and night.

modulate GnRH secretion, including GnRH itself, their exact roles in the human are not known (e.g., somatostatin, galanin, norepinephrine, neuropeptide Y, neurotensin, β-endorphin, dopamine).

Since the identification of GnRH in the early 1970s,[4] this decapeptide has been found widely distributed within the central nervous system. Central nervous system GnRH appears to influence sexual behavior, at least in the rodent. Recent cloning of the GnRH receptor in the rat, mouse, and human has shown its widespread brain distribution, including in limbic regions that are concerned with behavior.[5]

Embryologic studies in the mouse have evinced the extrahypothalamic origin of brain GnRH neurons. Fetal GnRH neurons arise at the base of the nose in the olfactory placode and then migrate into the forebrain and hypothalamus along the terminal nerve, septum, and preoptic area. This embryonic itinerary is interrupted in the syndrome of isolated hypogonadotropic hypogonadism, or Kallmann syndrome (see Chapter 23), in which mutations in one or more adhesion molecules are postulated to impede the migration of GnRH neurons prenatally.[6]

Endogenous Opioid Peptides

Men who abuse potent opiates commonly exhibit decreased libido and potentia and reduced serum concentrations of LH and testosterone.[7] This is accounted for predominantly by inhibition of the GnRH pulse generator. Conversely, treatment with mu opioid receptor antagonists amplifies the pulsatile release of LH in normal men[8] but not in boys before puberty.[9] A similar response in the male rat is dependent on testosterone and abolished by castration.[10] The inhibitory feedback actions of androgen on GnRH secretion in the human may be mediated in part by opiatergic neurons.[11] Pathophysiologic states of presumptive opiate-mediated suppression of the GnRH pulse generator include administration of opioid drugs, stress, marked physical overexertion, severe anxiety, and depression. However, few clinical studies have directly tested this important hypothesis.

Inhibition of the Hypothalamic-Pituitary Unit by Androgens

Large doses of testosterone or anabolic steroids will suppress pulsatile LH and presumptively GnRH release[11–14] or inhibit the ability of GnRH to stimulate LH secretion.[11, 15, 16] Androgen's negative feedback is exerted in part through aromatization of testosterone to estradiol (as based on experiments with pulsatile GnRH treatment in Kallmann's patients)[15–17] and also through the androgen receptor (as suggested from studies with nonsteroidal androgenic and antiandrogen drugs in normal men).[14, 18, 19]

Effects of Estrogen on Pulsatile LH Release

Men with estrogen overproduction manifest feminization (gynecomastia, redistribution of fat) and androgen deficiency (decreased libido, potency, and prostate size).[20] Mechanistic studies indicate that excess estrogen suppresses the amplitude, but not so evidently the frequency, of pulsatile LH release.[11, 12, 21] On the other hand, antiestrogen drugs increase the amplitude and frequency of LH secretory bursts in normal men,[21, 22] suggesting tonic negative feedback actions of endogenous estrogen on the male hypothalamic-pituitary unit.

α-Adrenergic Pathways

Infusion of α-adrenergic receptor antagonists rapidly suppresses GnRH pulse generator activity in the rhesus monkey[23] but not in the human.[24] Clinically, adrenergic inhibitors used in treating hypertension often impair sexual function in men, primarily by suppressing neuronal mechanisms involved in erection or ejaculation.[7]

Serotoninergic or GABAergic Neurons

Facilitative and suppressive effects of serotoninergic pathways have been inferred in the rat[13] but not yet in the human.[25] However, a selective serotonin reuptake inhibitor, fluoxetine hydrochloride, enhances the amplitude of pulsatile prolactin release in the human.[26] Whereas the γ-aminobutyric acid (GABA) agonists modulate LH secretion in the rat,[27] similar actions of GABA in men are not yet defined.

Dopaminergic Pathways

In healthy men, infusion of dopamine suppresses exogenous GnRH-stimulated LH release and also attenuates the expected stimulatory effect of opioid receptor blockade on LH secretion.[28] Although "stress-associated" (hypothalamic/functional) hypogonadotropism in some women can be reversed by acute administration of a dopamine receptor antagonist,[29] the relevance of this response to the pathophysiology of various male hypogonadotropic states will require further study.

Effect of Aging in Healthy Men

Healthy aging affects the male reproductive axis.[30–33] Most studies indicate that serum total, free, and especially bioavailable testosterone concentrations decline with age.[31, 34] Although daily LH production in older men is normal or slightly increased, high-amplitude bioactive LH pulses are lost,[35–37] and administration of naloxone or tamoxifen fails to stimulate endogenous LH release maximally.[35, 38] On the other hand, older men can increase bioactive LH secretion in response to antiandrogen treatment, indicating preservation of testosterone's negative feedback actions.[18, 19, 39] Because older individuals can respond with normal or heightened LH release to low doses of GnRH,[40] hypothalamic GnRH-deficient hypogonadotropism has been suggested in older men.[36] Loss of diurnal testosterone rhythmicity[41] as well as possibly increased sensitivity to suppressive (negative feedback) effects of androgen on the LH axis[42] also develops with aging.

Healthy aging also affects the testis. In older men, injected human chorionic gonadotropin (hCG) is less effective in stimulating testosterone secretion, testicular volume and spermatogenesis decrease, and serum α-inhibin concentrations fall (intact inhibin levels have not yet been reported).[7, 31, 32]

Other dynamic abnormalities of LH neuroregulation are evident in healthy older men, namely, a greater irregularity (or approximate entropy) of the LH release process with high-frequency but low-amplitude LH excursions and reduced synchrony of LH-testosterone secretion, which probably reflects loss of network coordination within the reproductive axis.[43] These changes may be more specific to the aging process than to the reproductive axis, because a similar phenomenon is observed for growth hormone release in older individuals.[44]

Factors Inducing the Dissociated Release of LH and FSH

Although GnRH can stimulate the release of both LH and FSH in vitro and in vivo, discrepant release of LH and FSH also occurs. For example, GnRH antagonists rapidly suppress LH secretion by 50 to 70 percent in 2 to 6 hours but reduce immunoreactive FSH release by only 10 to 15 percent even after 24 hours,[45] although FSH bioactivity may decrease.[46] In addition, slower GnRH pulse frequencies favor FSH synthesis and secretion.[47, 48] This may explain the selective increases in serum FSH concentration in idiopathic oligospermic men, who exhibit reduced LH pulse frequency in some[49, 50] but not all studies. FSH is also differentially controlled by feedback actions of sex steroid hormones and possibly by intrapituitary autocrine and paracrine factors (e.g., by locally produced activin, inhibin, and follistatin).[51, 52] For example, in the rat in vivo, estradiol suppresses but testosterone (paradoxically) increases FSH β-subunit messenger ribonucleic acid (mRNA) expression in the absence of GnRH. In vitro, activin predominantly evokes FSH secretion, which can be inhibited by follistatin or inhibin,[7, 53–56] thus controlling low rates of basal (nonpulsatile) FSH release.[51, 57]

GONADOTROPIN-RELEASING HORMONE ACTIONS

GnRH stimulates gonadotropin biosynthesis and secretion through receptor-specific calcium-dependent mechanisms.[58] GnRH receptor expression is regulated by GnRH itself and sex steroid feedback, even as early as in utero.[7] In the decade before puberty, GnRH preferentially releases FSH; but after puberty, when testosterone concentrations rise, GnRH triggers predominantly LH secretion.[13] The dose-response curve for GnRH has been studied in men with Kallmann's syndrome (isolated GnRH deficiency) after GnRH priming. The half-maximally effective dose of GnRH is 25 to 100 ng/kg. In a 50- to 70-kg adult, the injected dose is thus several micrograms (1 to 5 μg),[59] which is much less than the amount (50 or 200 μg) usually injected in clinical tests of gonadotroph function. Not only the *amount* but also the *waveform* or *time course* of GnRH delivery influences LH secretion.[60, 61] Indeed, continuous GnRH delivery markedly down-regulates gonadotroph cell output (see later).

GnRH Analogues

Potent GnRH peptide agonists and antagonists have been evaluated. GnRH agonists (e.g., leuprolide) have the clinically important property of selectively *down-regulating* GnRH receptors and gonadotroph cell secretory mechanisms.[58] An agonist initially stimulates LH release (in 1 to 4 days) and then suppresses LH secretion (after 10 to 21 days). FSH secretion is less markedly suppressed, and serum free α-subunit concentrations may actually increase, reflecting differential sensitivities of gonadotropin subunit genes to constant versus pulsatile GnRH drive. Other novel GnRH analogues are pure *antagonists,* such as Nal-Glu or Nal-Lys GnRH.[45, 62] These experimental agents reduce LH and testosterone secretion within 1 to 3 hours without initial stimulation but have limited solubility and cause local histamine release.[45]

GnRH and Testis

GnRH receptors exist in the rodent testis, where GnRH exerts direct effects.[63] Similar gonadal actions of GnRH have not been demonstrated unequivocally in the human.

THE ROLE OF LUTEINIZING HORMONE

LH Structure

Biochemically, LH (like FSH, thyroid-stimulating hormone, and hCG) consists of two polypeptide chains, termed α and β. β-Subunits are hormone specific. Recent crystallization of hCG has unraveled some of its three-dimensional structure.[64] Although small amounts of hCG are produced within the testis, pituitary gland, and other nonplacental tissues, their role is not known. LH is post-translationally modified by addition of various oligosaccharides, sialic acid and sulfate moieties, which profoundly affect its charge, biochemical isoform, in vivo half-life, and biologic activity.[65] Rare mutations of the β-subunit of LH or FSH glycoproteins may reduce bioactivity, but not necessarily immunoreactivity, and cause hypogonadism.[66, 67] Allelic variants of LH structure (polymorphisms) can occur in as many as 10 to 25 percent of some healthy populations and may falsely lower LH immunoradiometric activity.[68, 69]

LH Kinetics

Human LH injected into hypopituitary men has an average half-life of 47 ± 7 minutes by radioimmunoassay and 65 ± 5 minutes by Leydig cell in vitro bioassay. The metabolic clearance rate approximates 26 (±3) ml/m²/min for bioactive LH and 34 (±3) ml/m²/min for immunoreactive hormone.[70] In functionally anephric rats or humans, the half-life of LH in blood increases twofold to threefold.[71–73]

LH Action on the Testis

LH stimulates Leydig cell production of androgens and nonsteroidal regulatory factors. Synthesis of adult quantities (3 to 7 mg/daily) of testosterone to maintain masculinization requires multiple enzymatic steps in LH-responsive Leydig cells, available lipoprotein receptors to provide sterol substrate for the cholesterol side-chain cleavage reaction, free cholesterol delivery to mitochondrial enzymes, and functional androgen receptors in target tissues.[7, 74–78] Inborn biochemical defects exist at almost all of these steps, including LH-driven cholesterol transport into mitochondria, which occurs through a steroidogenic acute regulatory (StAR) protein recently cloned from mouse Leydig tumor cells.[79]

Secretion of testosterone, estradiol, and inhibin into the human spermatic vein is distinctly pulsatile, with approximately hourly pulses[80, 81] like LH.[13, 19, 36, 82–84] Minute to minute testosterone secretion in men depends on immediately (0.5 to 2 hours) prior LH release, because a GnRH antagonist rapidly lowers secretion of both LH and testosterone.[45]

LH and FSH Receptor Mutations

Mutations of the LH receptor that result in its constitutive (unregulated) activation cause "testotoxicosis," that is, gonadotropin-independent testosterone overproduction in familial male sexual precocity.[85] Conversely, LH receptor mutations that abolish its function result in male pseudohermaphroditism, characterized by feminized external genitalia in the genetic male. Loss-of-function mutations of the FSH receptor in women produce primary ovarian failure.[86] The consequences in men are less well defined to date.

PREPUBERTAL PULSATILE LUTEINIZING HORMONE RELEASE

In the male neonatal monkey and human, a marked surge of LH and testosterone secretion occurs transiently, lasting 3 to 4 months,[7] before declining to prepubertal levels.[87] Prepubertal LH pulsatility is evident in high-sensitivity immunofluorometric assays and bioassays.[88–90] An ultrasensitive immunofluorometric assay recently disclosed a 30-fold increase in LH secretory burst amplitude (and mass) versus a 1.5-fold or lesser rise in LH secretory burst frequency in late pubertal boys.[90] This remarkable pubertal activation of LH release is illustrated in Figure 22–2. Such increases are presaged by augmented nighttime LH and testosterone secretion.[91] Adult LH and testosterone release show 24-hour variations of lesser magnitude (10 to 30 percent).[82, 92, 93] Both non–rapid eye movement sleep and circadian variations modulate nighttime LH and testosterone secretion.[94] Hypothalamic GnRH pulsatility and true circadian rhythms are linked in male rodents, because a dominant mutation affecting the circadian clock in the hamster also alters pulsatile (ultradian) LH release.[95]

REGULATION OF PULSATILE FOLLICLE-STIMULATING HORMONE RELEASE

Little is known about the regulation of pulsatile FSH secretion in boys and men, although immunofluorometric assays indicate a 3-fold to 30-fold increase in mean serum FSH concentrations across puberty.[96] The physiologic significance of the multiple (up to 15 different) biochemical isoforms of FSH is also not yet apparent,[97] although in vivo half-lives and biopotencies of these isoforms vary. Sex steroids differentially modulate pulsatile FSH secretion, because estradiol infusion in young men decreases the calculated *half-life* of endogenous FSH,[98] whereas pure androgen treatment reduces the *mass* of FSH secreted per burst. Conversely, tamoxifen and flutamide, which respectively inhibit estrogen and androgen receptor activity, augment FSH secretory burst amplitude and mass, with no evident change in FSH pulse frequency.[99]

FSH Kinetics

The metabolic clearance rate of purified urinary FSH in men is 4 to 12 ml/min,[100] and FSH half-lives average 5.8 hours (monoexponential) or 1.7 hours (biexponential fast component) and 8.3 hours (slow component). *Bioactive* FSH kinetics are comparable.[100] Recombinant human FSH may have a longer slow-phase half-life approaching 18 to 24 hours.[101]

Concordance of Pulsatile FSH and LH Release

There is a statistically significant (35 to 50 percent) concordance between individual FSH and LH release episodes in normal young men.[45, 102, 103] Imperfect concordance suggests that LH and FSH pulse detection methods have unequal sensitivities or specificities[104, 105] or that distinct mechanisms regulate pulsatile secretion of these two glycoproteins (see earlier).

Role of Testicular Factors in the Regulation of FSH Release

Serum FSH concentrations rise in response to diffuse testicular disease involving the seminiferous tubules.[7, 84, 106, 107] However, the roles of circulating or intrapituitary inhibin, activin, and follistatin in FSH pathophysiology remain unknown. Testosterone is a major feedback signal; in functionally agonadal men, testosterone treatment reduces elevated LH pulse frequency and amplitude toward normal values[108] and suppresses elevations in FSH secretory burst

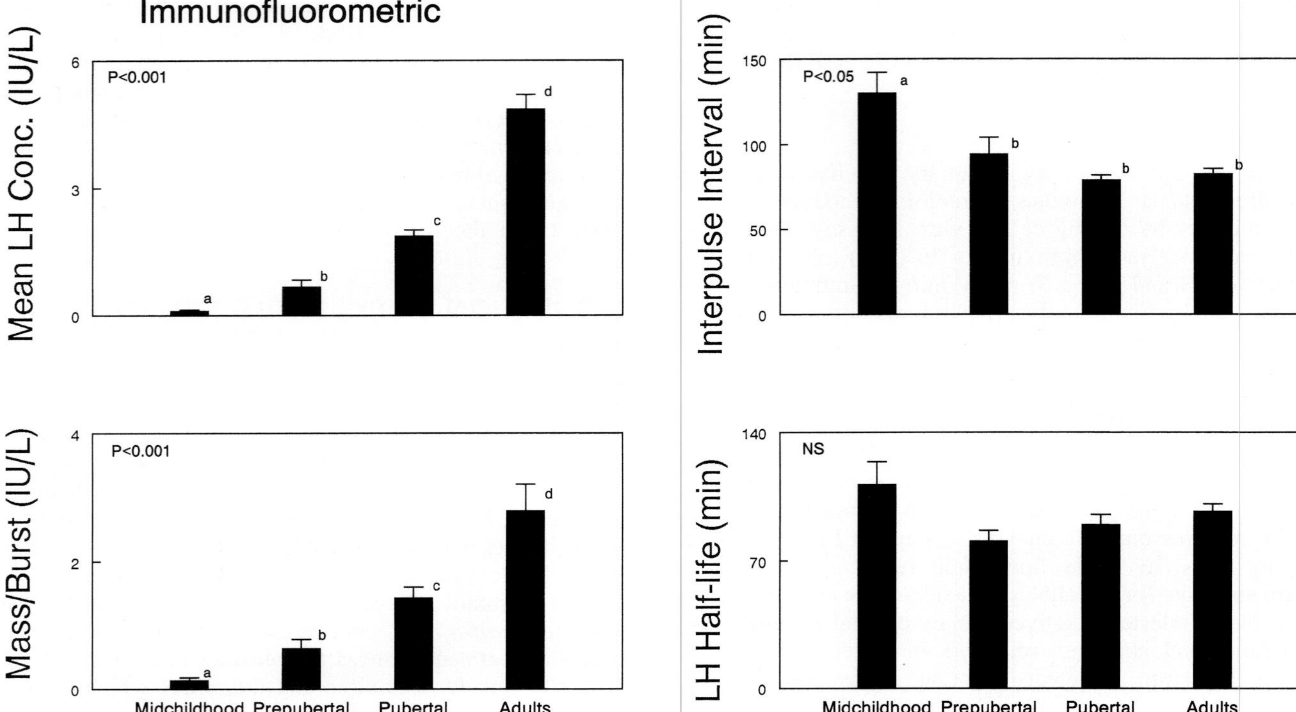

Figure 22–2 ■ Neuroendocrine mechanisms of human pubertal activation of the male gonadotropic axis, as reflected by amplified pulsatile LH secretion across puberty in boys. A high-sensitivity immunofluorometric LH assay and deconvolution analysis were used to evaluate the changing amplitude and frequency of pulsatile LH release in prepubertal (midchildhood) and pubertal boys and young men. The calculated mass of LH secreted per burst increased 30-fold in midpuberty, whereas the frequency of detectable LH pluses rose less than 2-fold, and the estimated LH half-life did not change. (Adapted from Wu FCW, Butler GE, Kelnar CJH, et al. Patterns of pulsatile luteinizing hormone secretion from childhood to adulthood in the human male: A study using deconvolution analysis and an ultrasensitive immunofluorometric assay. J Clin Endocrinol Metab 81:1798–1805, 1996. © The Endocrine Society.)

mass or basal FSH release.[109] FSH pulse frequency, unlike that of LH, does not appear to rise with gonadal ablation.[109]

STATES OF REVERSIBLE AND ACQUIRED HYPOGONADOTROPIC HYPOGONADISM

Acquired conditions of relative LH and FSH deficiency in the male include obesity, healthy aging, stress, nutritional deprivation, uremia, hyperprolactinemia, treatment with opiates or narcotic agonists, sex steroid hormone excess (aromatizable or nonaromatizable androgen or estrogen administration, or tumoral overproduction), uncontrolled diabetes mellitus, and other catabolic states. These conditions are contrasted with structural hypothalamic-pituitary disease (Table 22–1), as discussed in greater detail elsewhere.[7, 84, 86]

Stress of various types (e.g., psychologic, physical [heat, burns, exertion, trauma], metabolic [diabetes mellitus, fasting]) can disturb reproductive function.[7, 13, 84, 86, 110–112] Stress may disrupt the male gonadal axis in part at the level of the testes, because stress-released mediators such as adrenocorticotropic hormone (ACTH), corticotropin-releasing hormone (CRH [ACTH-releasing hormone]), tumor necrosis factor-α, catecholamines, vasopressin, interleukins, and glucocorticoids can exert in vitro actions on gonadal cells (see Chapter 23).[113] Second, LH secretion and pituitary responsiveness to GnRH can be reduced by large amounts of glucocorticoids.[114] Third, and most plausibly, inhibition of hypothalamic GnRH synthesis or release, such as by central CRH (ACTH-releasing hormone) and opiatergic pathways, may mediate stress-induced hypogonadotropism. Thus, pharmacologic inhibitors of CRH and opiate receptors attenuate some but not all stress-induced decreases in LH release in the male rat and rhesus monkey, suggesting a role also for non–CRH-dependent and non–opiate-dependent central nervous system and intrapituitary mechanisms.[84, 115]

Nutrient deprivation suppresses the male reproductive axis.[116] Thus, short-term (1 to 5 days) voluntary starvation of healthy young men reduces LH and testosterone concentrations.[117] Although increased gonadotropinuria occurs in fasted subjects,[118] this route of gonadotropin removal remains quantitatively minor. Rather, calculated LH secretion rates fall about 50 percent in fasted young men.[117] Hypogonadotropism probably reflects decreased GnRH release from the median eminence, because there is preserved gonadotroph cell responsiveness to exogenous GnRH,[117] and pulsatile GnRH treatment will reverse LH deficiency in fasting men.[119] Experiments in the castrated male rodent also suggest increased negative feedback potency of androgen in the fasted animal.[120] Testosterone secretion in response to hCG treatment is also not diminished in acutely underfed animals, suggesting preserved gonadal function.[116] In chronic malnutrition, diminished Leydig cell function and increased serum FSH concentration may occur; the

■ TABLE 22–1
Mechanisms of Altered GnRH-LH Secretion

Fixed Deficiency of GnRH

Congenital: Kallmann's syndrome (anosmia)
Hypothalamic lesions
  Tumors: craniopharyngioma, hamartoma, glioma
  Vascular: contusion, infarction, vasculitis
  Infiltrative: granulomatous disease (histoplasmosis, sarcoidosis)
  Others: metastatic lesions, arachnoid cysts

Reversible GnRH Deficiency

Weight loss, starvation, type I diabetes mellitus
Stress (physical, psychologic, metabolic)
Opiates (e.g., heroin, methadone)
Exercise (nearly exhaustive levels)
Exogenous (anabolic) steroids
Others

Intrapituitary Disease

Parasellar or intrasellar mass (e.g., meningioma, aneurysms)
Adenomas (e.g., prolactinoma, acromegaly)
Ischemic infarction (e.g., pituitary apoplexy)
Metastatic carcinoma (e.g., adenocarcinoma, melanoma)
Abscess (e.g., tuberculosis)

Adapted from Reyes-Fuentes A, Veldhuis JD. Neuroendocrine physiology of the normal male gonadal axis. Endocrinol Metab Clin North Am 22:93–124, 1993.

latter is consistent with seminiferous tubule or Sertoli cell dysfunction. Accompanying nutrient deficiencies (e.g., vitamin A, trace minerals like zinc) can also have negative influences on the reproductive axis.[7]

THE INHIBIN AND ACTIVIN FAMILY

The existence of inhibin as a nonsteroidal inhibitor of FSH release was postulated six decades ago.[86] Only recently have reliable bioassays allowed cloning of inhibin in the pig, human, cow, sheep, and rat. Two forms of inhibin are identified, both of which are heterodimers consisting of a common α-subunit and one of two distinct β-subunits, termed β_A or β_B. The resultant dimer is referred to as either inhibin A or inhibin B; they are equipotent in inhibiting FSH secretion. In contrast, heterodimers and homodimers of the *two β-subunits* are called *activins,* which *stimulate* FSH secretion.[53, 86] This is a slow-onset effect, unlike that of GnRH, and is possibly mediated by stabilization of FSH-β mRNA turnover. Activins are designated as activin AB (β_A and β_B heterodimer)[121] and activin A or B (a homodimer of β_A or β_B).[122]

Inhibin and activin are part of a larger "superfamily" of glycoproteins characterized by structural homology with each other and with transforming growth factor-β, a mitogenic protein, and müllerian-inhibiting substance, a Sertoli cell glycoprotein causing regression of internal müllerian duct (female anlage) structures in the developing male fetus.[123] Production of müllerian-inhibiting substance by the male gonad is not androgen dependent, because in utero regression of the uterus, fallopian tubes, and distal vagina occurs even in androgen receptor–defective patients.[86]

Passive immunoneutralization and inhibin infusion studies have suggested that inhibin acting alone is not a dominant inhibitor of basal FSH secretion in the intact adult male rat, but it may be more important prepubertally in the rodent[124] as well as in the adult rhesus monkey.[56, 125] The role of inhibin in the human is largely unknown.

The mRNAs encoding α and β inhibin subunits are detected in rodent *brain* tissue.[126] *Intrapituitary* activin and inhibin production also occurs, which may coregulate FSH synthesis and secretion at least in the rat.[51, 52, 57, 126, 127]

Inhibin subunits are identified in Sertoli cells in the testis. Thus, intragonadal actions of inhibin on both the steroidogenic and gametogenic compartments are also possible.[113, 128–131] Unexpectedly, α-inhibin "knockout" mice manifest a high incidence of adrenal and gonadal tumors, thus suggesting an important tumor suppressor role for this subunit.[130] Inhibin biosynthesis is stimulated in the gonad by FSH, growth factors, and some sex steroids.

Follistatin, a single-chain polypeptide structurally distinct from the inhibins and activins,[132] also inhibits FSH secretion. Follistatin is produced in the gonad and anterior pituitary gland and possibly functions primarily as a high-affinity activin-binding and inhibiting protein to regulate local actions of activin.[51] The recent cloning of several activin receptors, such as type I (a serine phosphorylating protein) and type II (a ligand-specific activin-binding moiety), should stimulate additional insights into the mechanisms of activin action on target cells within the male reproductive axis.[133–136]

ANDROGEN RECEPTOR PATHWAY

Androgen acts through its cognate receptor not only on peripheral "androgenized" target tissues but also as a negative feedback steroid physiologically, because patients with complete and partial androgen resistance (testicular feminization) due to receptor defects have significantly elevated serum LH levels[86] despite adult concentrations of testosterone and estradiol. Multiple molecular defects associated with androgen resistance have now been defined after cloning of the classical androgen receptor gene (see Chapter 4). Because treatment with estrogen will suppress LH in such patients,[137] LH secretion must be modulated by both androgens and estrogens (see earlier). Whereas relative resistance to steroid feedback occurs in long-standing hypergonadotropic hypogonadism (e.g., Klinefelter's syndrome),[138] the basis for this phenomenon is not known. Importantly, intratesticular androgen action is required for fertility,[76] which suggests that subfertility in some men may be due to otherwise inapparent androgen receptor defects.

Acknowledgments

We thank Patsy Craig for her skillful preparation of the manuscript and Paula P. Azimi for the artwork. This work was supported in part by NIH Grant RR 00847 to the Clinical Research Center of the University of Virginia, RCDA 1 KO4 HD00634, the Diabetes and Endocrinology Research Center Grant NIH DK-38942, the NIH-supported Clinfo Data Reduction Systems, the Baxter Healthcare Corporation (Round Lake, IL), the University of Virginia Academic Enhancement Fund, the NSF Science Center for Biological Timing, and an NIH P-30 Center for Reproductive Research Grant (NICHD) HD28934.

References

1. Clarke IJ, Cummins JT. The temporal relationship between gonadotropin-releasing hormone (GnRH) and luteinizing hormone (LH) secretion in ovariectomized ewes. Endocrinology 111:1737–1739, 1982.
2. Knobil E. The electrophysiology of the GnRH pulse generator in the rhesus monkey. J Steroid Biochem 33:669–671, 1989.
3. Krsmanovic LZ, Stojilkovic SS, Merelli F, et al. Calcium signaling and episodic secretion of gonadotropin-releasing hormone in hypothalamic neurons. Proc Natl Acad Sci USA 89:8462–8466, 1992.
4. Amoss M, Burgus R, Blackwell R, et al. Purification, amino acid composition and N-terminus of the hypothalamic luteinizing hormone releasing factor (LRF) of ovine origin. Biochem Biophys Res Commun 44:205–210, 1971.
5. Eidne KA, Sellar RE, Couper G, et al. Molecular cloning and characterisation of the rat pituitary gonadotropin-releasing hormone (GnRH) receptor. Mol Cell Endocrinol 90:R5–R9, 1992.
6. Schwanzel-Fukuda M, Bick D, Pfaff DW. Luteinizing hormone–releasing hormone (LHRH)–expressing cells do not migrate normally in an inherited hypogonadal (Kallmann) syndrome. Brain Res Mol Brain Res 6:311–326, 1989.
7. Veldhuis JD. The hypothalamic-pituitary-testicular axis. *In* Yen SSC, Jaffe RB (eds). Reproductive Endocrinology, 3rd ed. Philadelphia, WB Saunders, 1991, pp 409–459.
8. Veldhuis JD, Rogol AD, Johnson ML, et al. Endogenous opiates modulate the pulsatile secretion of biologically active luteinizing hormone in man. J Clin Invest 72:2031–2040, 1983.
9. Veldhuis JD, Kulin HE, Warner BA, et al. Responsiveness of gonadotropin secretion to infusion of an opiate-receptor antagonist in hypogonadotropic individuals. J Clin Endocrinol Metab 55:649–653, 1982.
10. Cicero TJ, Wilcox CE, Meyer ER. Naloxone-induced increases in serum luteinizing hormone in the male: Mechanisms of action. J Pharmacol Exp Ther 212:573–578, 1980.
11. Veldhuis JD, Rogol AD, Samojlik E, et al. Role of endogenous opiates in the expression of negative feedback actions of estrogen and androgen on pulsatile properties of luteinizing hormone secretion in man. J Clin Invest 74:47–55, 1984.
12. Santen RJ. Is aromatization of testosterone to estradiol required for inhibition of luteinizing hormone secretion in man? J Clin Invest 56:1555–1563, 1975.
13. Urban RJ, Evans WS, Rogol AD, et al. Contemporary aspects of discrete peak detection algorithms: I. The paradigm of the luteinizing hormone pulse signal in men. Endocr Rev 9:3–37, 1988.
14. Marynick SP, Loriaux DL, Sherins RJ, et al. Evidence that testosterone can suppress pituitary gonadotropin secretion independently of peripheral aromatization. J Clin Endocrinol Metab 49:396–398, 1979.
15. Shecker CB, Matsumoto AM, Bremner WJ. Testosterone administration inhibits gonadotropin secretion by an effect directly on the human pituitary. J Clin Endocrinol Metab 68:397–401, 1989.
16. Finkelstein JS, Whitcomb R, O'Dea L, et al. Sex steroid control of gonadotropin secretion in the human male. I. Effects of testosterone administration in normal and gonadotropin-releasing hormone–deficient men. J Clin Endocrinol Metab 73:609–620, 1991.
17. Finkelstein JS, O'Dea LSL, Whitcomb RW, et al. Sex steroid control of gonadotropin secretion in the human male. II. Effects of estradiol administration in normal and gonadotropin-releasing hormone–deficient men. J Clin Endocrinol Metab 73:621–628, 1991.
18. Veldhuis JD, Urban RJ, Dufau ML. Differential responses of biologically active LH secretion in older versus young men to interruption of androgen negative feedback. J Clin Endocrinol Metab 79:1763–1770, 1994.
19. Urban RJ, Davis MR, Rogol AD, et al. Acute androgen receptor blockade increases luteinizing-hormone secretory activity in men. J Clin Endocrinol Metab 67:1149–1155, 1988.
20. Veldhuis JD, Sowers JR, Rogol AD, et al. Pathophysiology of male hypogonadism associated with endogenous hyperestrogenism: Evidence for dual defects in the gonadal axis. N Engl J Med 312:1371–1375, 1985.
21. Veldhuis JD, Dufau ML. Estradiol modulates the pulsatile secretion of biologically active luteinizing hormone in man. J Clin Invest 80:631–638, 1987.
22. Winters SJ, Troen P. Evidence for a role of endogenous estrogen in the hypothalamic control of gonadotropin secretion in men. J Clin Endocrinol Metab 61:842–845, 1985.
23. Bhattacharya AN, Dierschke DJ, Yamaji T, et al. The pharmacological blockade of the circhoral mode of LH secretion in the ovariectomized rhesus monkey. Endocrinology 90:778–786, 1972.
24. Veldhuis JD, Rogol AD, Williams FA, et al. Do alpha-adrenergic mechanisms regulate spontaneous or opiate-modulated pulsatile LH secretion in man? J Clin Endocrinol Metab 57:1292–1296, 1983.
25. Urban RJ, Veldhuis JD. Effects of short-term stimulation of serotoninergic pathways on the pulsatile secretion of luteinizing hormone in the absence and presence of acute opiate-receptor blockade. J Androl 11:227–232, 1990.
26. Urban RJ, Veldhuis JD. A selective serotonin re-uptake inhibitor, fluoxetine HCl, modulates the pulsatile release of prolactin in postmenopausal women. Am J Obstet Gynecol 164:147–152, 1991.
27. Wuttke W, Jarry H, Demling J, et al. Involvement of GABA in the neuroendocrinology of reproduction. *In* Leung PCK, Armstrong DT, Ruf KB, et al. Endocrinology and Physiology of Reproduction. New York, Plenum Press, 1987, pp 65–69.
28. Delitala G, Devilla L, Musso NR. On the role of dopamine receptors in the naloxone-induced hormonal changes in man. J Clin Endocrinol Metab 55:181–184, 1983.
29. Quigley ME, Sheehan KL, Casper RF, et al. Evidence for increased dopaminergic and opioid activity in patients with hypothalamic hypogonadotropic amenorrhea. J Clin Endocrinol Metab 50:949–954, 1980.
30. Winters SJ, Troen P. Episodic luteinizing hormone (LH) secretion and the response of LH and follicle-stimulating hormone to LH-releasing hormone in aged men: Evidence for coexistent primary testicular insufficiency and an impairment in gonadotropin secretion. J Clin Endocrinol Metab 55:560–565, 1982.
31. Urban RJ, Veldhuis JD. Hypothalamo-pituitary concomitants of aging. *In* Sowers JR, Felicetta JV (eds). The Endocrinology of Aging. New York, Raven Press, 1988, pp 41–74.
32. Tenover JS, McLachlan RI, Dahl KD, et al. Decreased serum inhibin levels in normal elderly men: Evidence for a decline in Sertoli cell function with aging. J Clin Endocrinol Metab 67:455–461, 1988.
33. Blackman MR, Weintraub BD, Rosen SW, et al. Comparison of the effects of lung cancer, benign lung disease, and normal aging on pituitary-gonadal function in men. J Clin Endocrinol Metab 66:88–95, 1988.
34. Tenover JS, Matsumoto AM, Plymate SR, et al. The effects of aging in normal men on bioavailable testosterone and luteinizing hormone secretion: Response to clomiphene citrate. J Clin Endocrinol Metab 65:1118–1125, 1987.
35. Urban RJ, Veldhuis JD, Blizzard RM, et al. Attenuated release of biologically active luteinizing hormone in healthy aging men. J Clin Invest 81:1020–1029, 1988.
36. Veldhuis JD, Urban RJ, Lizarralde G, et al. Attenuation of luteinizing hormone secretory burst amplitude is a proximate basis for the hypoandrogenism of healthy aging in men. J Clin Endocrinol Metab 75:707–713, 1992.
37. Mitchell R, Hollis S, Rothwell C, et al. Age related changes in the pituitary-testicular axis in normal men; lower serum testosterone results from decreased bioactive LH drive. Clin Endocrinol (Oxf) 42:501–507, 1995.
38. Vermeulen A, Deslypere JP, Kaufman JJ. Influence of antiopioids on luteinizing hormone pulsatility in aging men. J Clin Endocrinol Metab 68:68–72, 1989.
39. Veldhuis JD, Urban RJ, Dufau ML. Evidence that androgen negative-feedback regulates hypothalamic GnRH impulse strength and the burst-like secretion of biologically active luteinizing hormone in men. J Clin Endocrinol Metab 74:1227–1235, 1992.
40. Zwart AD, Urban RJ, Odell WD, Veldhuis JD. Contrasts in the GnRH dose-response relationships for LH, FSH, and alpha subunit release in young versus older men: Appraisal with high-specificity immunoradiometric assay and deconvolution analysis. Eur J Endocrinol 135:399–406, 1996.
41. Bremner WJ, Vitiello MV, Prinz PN. Loss of circadian rhythmicity

in blood testosterone levels with aging in normal men. J Clin Endocrinol Metab 56:1278–1281, 1983.
42. Winters SJ, Sherins RJ, Troen P. The gonadotropin suppressive activity of androgen is increased in elderly men. Metabolism 33:1052–1060, 1984.
43. Pincus SM, Mulligan T, Iranmanesh A, et al. Older males secrete luteinizing hormone and testosterone more irregularly, and jointly more asynchronously, than younger males: Dual novel facets. Proc Natl Acad Sci USA 93:14100–14105, 1996.
44. Veldhuis JD, Liem AY, South S, et al. Differential impact of age, sex-steroid hormones, and obesity on basal versus pulsatile growth hormone secretion in men as assessed in an ultrasensitive chemiluminescence assay. J Clin Endocrinol Metab 80:3209–3222, 1995.
45. Pavlou SN, Veldhuis JD, Lindner J, et al. Persistence of concordant LH, testosterone and alpha subunit pulses following LHRH antagonist administration in normal men. J Clin Endocrinol Metab 70:1472–1478, 1990.
46. Dahl KD, Pavlou SN, Kovacs WJ, et al. The changing ratio of serum bioactive to immunoreactive follicle-stimulating hormone in normal men following treatment with a potent gonadotropin releasing hormone antagonist. J Clin Endocrinol Metab 63:792–794, 1986.
47. Wildt L, Hausler A, Marshall G, et al. Frequency and amplitude of gonadotropin releasing hormone stimulation and gonadotropin secretion in the rhesus monkey. Endocrinology 109:373–385, 1981.
48. Haisenleder DJ, Dalkin AC, Ortolano GA, et al. A pulsatile GnRH stimulus is required to increase transcription of the gonadotropin subunit genes: Evidence for differential regulation of transcription by pulse frequency in vivo. Endocrinology 128:509–517, 1991.
49. Reyes-Fuentes A, Chavarria ME, Carrera A, et al. Combined alterations in pulsatile LH and FSH secretion in idiopathic oligospermic men: Assessment by deconvolution analysis. J Clin Endocrinol Metab 81:524–529, 1996.
50. Gross KM, Matsumoto AM, Southworth MB, et al. Evidence for decreased luteinizing hormone–releasing hormone pulse frequency in men with selective elevations of follicle-stimulating hormone. J Clin Endocrinol Metab 60:197–203, 1985.
51. Corrigan AZ, Bilezikjian LM, Carroll RS, et al. Evidence for an autocrine role of activin B within rat anterior pituitary cultures. Endocrinology 128:1682–1684, 1991.
52. Roberts V, Meunier H, Vaughan J, et al. Production and regulation of inhibin subunits in pituitary gonadotropes. Endocrinology 124:552–554, 1989.
53. McLachlan RI, Dahl KD, Bremner WJ, et al. Recombinant human activin-A stimulates basal FSH and GnRH-stimulated FSH and LH release in the adult male macaque, *Macaca fascicularis*. Endocrinology 125:2787–2789, 1989.
54. Paul SJ, Ortolano GA, Haisenleder DJ, et al. Gonadotropin subunit mRNA concentrations after blockade of GnRH action: Testosterone selectively increases FSH beta subunit mRNA by posttranscriptional mechanisms. Mol Endocrinol 4:1943–1955, 1990.
55. Shupnik MA, Gharib SD, Chin WW. Estrogen suppresses rat gonadotropin gene transcription in vivo. Endocrinology 122:1842–1846, 1988.
56. Medhamurthy R, Culler MD, Gay VL, et al. Evidence that inhibin plays a major role in the regulation of follicle-stimulating hormone secretion in the fully adult male rhesus monkey *(Macaca mulatta)*. Endocrinology 129:389–395, 1991.
57. Kirk SE, Dalkin AC, Yasin M, et al. GnRH pulse frequency regulates expression of pituitary follistatin mRNA: A mechanism for differential gonadotrope function. Endocrinology 135:876–880, 1994.
58. Conn PM, Crowley WF. Gonadotropin-releasing hormone and its analogs. N Engl J Med 324:93–103, 1991.
59. Veldhuis JD, O'Dea LS, Johnson ML. The nature of the gonadotropin-releasing hormone stimulus–luteinizing hormone secretory response of human gonadotrophs in vivo. J Clin Endocrinol Metab 68:661–670, 1989.
60. Handelsman DJ, Cummins JT, Clarke IJ. Pharmacodynamics of gonadotropin-releasing hormone. I. Effects of gonadotropin-releasing hormone pulse contour on pituitary luteinizing hormone secretion in vivo in sheep. Neuroendocrinology 48:432–438, 1988.
61. Spratt DI, Crowley WF, Butler JP, et al. Pituitary luteinizing hormone responses to intravenous and subcutaneous administration of gonadotropin-releasing hormone in men. J Clin Endocrinol Metab 61:890–895, 1985.
62. Pavlou SN, Debold CR, Island DP, et al. Single subcutaneous doses of a luteinizing hormone–releasing hormone antagonist suppress serum gonadotropin and testosterone levels in normal men. J Clin Endocrinol Metab 63:303–308, 1986.
63. Hsueh AJW, Erickson GF. Extrapituitary inhibition of testicular function by luteinizing hormone releasing hormone. Nature 281:66–67, 1979.
64. Lapthorn AJ, Harris DC, Littlejohn A, et al. Crystal structure of human chorionic gonadotropin. Nature 369:455–461, 1994.
65. Dufau ML, Veldhuis JD. Pathophysiological relationships between the biological and immunological activities of luteinizing hormone. Baillieres Clin Endocrinol Metab 1:153–176, 1987.
66. Matthews CH, Borgato S, Beck-Peccoz P. Primary amenorrhea and infertility due to a mutation in the beta-subunit of follicle-stimulating hormone. Nat Genet 5:83–86, 1993.
67. Weiss J, Axelrod L, Whitcomb RW. Hypogonadism caused by a single amino acid substitution in the beta-subunit of luteinizing hormone. N Engl J Med 326:179–183, 1992.
68. Pettersson K, Ding Y-Q, Huhtaniemi I. An immunologically anomalous luteinizing hormone variant in a healthy woman. J Clin Endocrinol Metab 74:164–171, 1992.
69. Furui K, Suganuma N, Tsukahara S-I. Identification of two point mutations in the gene coding luteinizing hormone (LH) beta-subunit, associated with immunologically anomalous LH variants. J Clin Endocrinol Metab 78:107–113, 1994.
70. Veldhuis JD, Fraioli F, Rogol AD, et al. Metabolic clearance of biologically active luteinizing hormone in man. J Clin Invest 77:1122–1128, 1986.
71. de Kretser DM, Atkins RC, Paulsen CA. Role of the kidney in the metabolism of luteinizing hormone. J Endocrinol 58:425–434, 1973.
72. Veldhuis JD, Wilkowski MJ, Urban RJ, et al. Evidence for attenuation of hypothalamic GnRH impulse strength with preservation of gonadotropin-releasing hormone (GnRH) pulse frequency in men with chronic renal failure. J Clin Endocrinol Metab 76:648–654, 1993.
73. Schaefer F, Veldhuis JD, Robertson WR, et al. Immunoreactive and bioactive luteinizing hormone in pubertal patients with chronic renal failure. Kidney Int 45:1465–1476, 1995.
74. Tilley WD, Marcelli M, Wilson JD, et al. Characterization and expression of a cDNA encoding the human androgen receptor. Proc Natl Acad Sci USA 76:327–331, 1989.
75. Imperato-McGinley J, Guerrero L, Gautier T, et al. Steroid 5-alpha-reductase deficiency in man: An inherited form of male pseudohermaphroditism. Science 186:1213–1215, 1974.
76. Aiman J, Griffin JE, Gazak JM, et al. Androgen insensitivity as a cause of infertility in otherwise normal men. N Engl J Med 300:223–227, 1979.
77. Miller WL. Molecular biology of steroid hormone synthesis. Endocr Rev 9:295–318, 1988.
78. Gwynne JT, Strauss JF III. The role of lipoproteins in steroidogenesis and cholesterol metabolism in steroidogenic cells. Endocr Rev 3:299–321, 1982.
79. Clark BJ, Wells J, King SR, et al. The purification, cloning, and expression of a novel luteinizing hormone–induced mitochondrial protein in MA-10 mouse Leydig tumor cells. J Biol Chem 269:28314–28322, 1994.
80. Winters SJ, Troen PE. Testosterone and estradiol are co-secreted episodically by the human testis. J Clin Invest 78:870–872, 1986.
81. Winters SJ. Inhibin is released together with testosterone by the human testis. J Clin Endocrinol Metab 70:548–550, 1990.
82. Veldhuis JD, King JC, Urban RJ, et al. Operating characteristics of the male hypothalamo-pituitary-gonadal axis: Pulsatile release of testosterone and follicle-stimulating hormone and their temporal coupling with luteinizing hormone. J Clin Endocrinol Metab 65:929–941, 1987.
83. Veldhuis JD, Johnson ML, Dufau ML. Physiological attributes of endogenous bioactive luteinizing hormone secretory bursts in man: Assessment by deconvolution analysis and in vitro bioassay of LH. Am J Physiol 256:E199–E207, 1989.
84. Reyes-Fuentes A, Veldhuis JD. Neuroendocrine physiology of the normal male gonadal axis. Endocrinol Metab Clin North Am 22:93–124, 1993.

85. Shenker A, Laue L, Kosugi S, et al. A constitutively activating mutation of the luteinizing hormone receptor in familial male precocious puberty. Nature 365:652–654, 1993.
86. Veldhuis JD. Male hypothalamic-pituitary-gonadal axis. *In* Lipshultz LI, Howards SS (eds). Infertility in the Male. Philadelphia, Mosby–Year Book, 1996, pp 23–58.
87. Waldhauser F, Weissenbacher G, Frisch H, et al. Pulsatile secretion of gonadotropins in early infancy. Eur J Pediatr 137:71–76, 1981.
88. Mauras N, Veldhuis JD, Rogol AD. Role of endogenous opiates in pubertal maturation: Opposing actions of naltrexone in prepubertal and late pubertal boys. J Clin Endocrinol Metab 62:1256–1263, 1986.
89. Veldhuis JD, Weiss J, Mauras N, et al. Appraising endocrine pulse signals at low circulating hormone concentrations: Use of regional coefficients of variation in the experimental series to analyze pulsatile luteinizing hormone release. Pediatr Res 20:632–637, 1986.
90. Wu FCW, Butler GE, Kelnar CJH, et al. Patterns of pulsatile luteinizing hormone secretion from childhood to adulthood in the human male: A study using deconvolution analysis and an ultrasensitive immunofluorometric assay. J Clin Endocrinol Metab 81:1798–1805, 1996.
91. Reiter EO, Dufau ML, Root AW. Bioactive and immunoreactive serum LH in normal prepubertal and pubertal boys. Pediatr Res 12:330–336, 1978.
92. Veldhuis JD, Johnson ML. Operating characteristics of the human male hypothalamo-pituitary-gonadal axis: Circadian, ultradian and pulsatile release of prolactin, and its temporal coupling with luteinizing hormone. J Clin Endocrinol Metab 67:116–123, 1988.
93. Mauras N, Rogol AD, Veldhuis JD. Appraising the instantaneous secretory rates of luteinizing hormone and testosterone in response to selective mu opiate receptor blockade in late pubertal boys. J Androl 8:201–207, 1987.
94. Kapen S, Boyar RM, Finkelstein JW, et al. Effect of sleep-wake cycle reversal on luteinizing hormone secretory pattern in puberty. J Clin Endocrinol Metab 39:293–299, 1974.
95. Loudon ASI, Wayne NL, Kreig R, et al. Ultradian endocrine rhythms are altered by a circadian mutation in the Syrian hamster. Endocrinology 135:712–718, 1994.
96. Dunkel L, Alfthan H, Stenman UH, et al. Pulsatile secretion of LH and FSH in prepubertal and early pubertal boys revealed by ultrasensitive time-resolved immunofluorometric assay. Pediatr Res 27:215–219, 1990.
97. Stanton PG, Robertson DM, Burgon PG, et al. Isolation and physicochemical characterization of human follicle-stimulating hormone isoforms. Endocrinology 130:2820–2832, 1992.
98. Urban RJ, Dahl KD, Padmanabhan V, et al. Specific regulatory actions of dihydrotestosterone and estradiol on the dynamics of FSH secretion and clearance in man. J Androl 12:27–35, 1991.
99. Urban RJ, Dahl KD, Lippert MC, et al. Endogenous androgen and estrogen modulate immunoradiometric and bioactive FSH secretion and clearance in young and elderly men. J Androl 13:579–586, 1992.
100. Urban RJ, Padmanabhan V, Beitins I, et al. Metabolic clearance of human follicle-stimulating hormone assessed by radioimmunoassay, immunoradiometric assay, and in vitro Sertoli cell bioassay. J Clin Endocrinol Metab 73:818–823, 1991.
101. le Cotonnec Y-Y, Porchet HC, Beltrami V, et al. Clinical pharmacology of recombinant human follicle-stimulating hormone. II. Single doses and steady state pharmacokinetics. Fertil Steril 61:679–686, 1994.
102. Veldhuis JD, Iranmanesh A, Clarke I, et al. Random and non-random coincidence between luteinizing hormone peaks and follicle-stimulating hormone, alpha subunit, prolactin, and gonadotropin-releasing hormone pulsations. J Neuroendocrinol 1:185–194, 1989.
103. Veldhuis JD, Johnson ML, Seneta E. Analysis of the co-pulsatility of anterior pituitary hormones. J Clin Endocrinol Metab 73:569–576, 1991.
104. Urban RJ, Johnson ML, Veldhuis JD. In vivo biological validation and biophysical modeling of the sensitivity and positive accuracy of endocrine peak detection: I. The LH pulse signal. Endocrinology 124:2541–2547, 1989.
105. Urban RJ, Johnson ML, Veldhuis JD. In vivo biological validation and biophysical modeling of the sensitivity and positive accuracy of endocrine peak detection: II. The FSH pulse signal. Endocrinology 128:2008–2014, 1991.
106. Franchimont P, Chari S, Hazee-Hajelstin MT, et al. Evidence for the existence of inhibin. *In* Troen P, Nankin H (eds). The Testis in Normal and Infertile Men. New York, Raven Press, 1977, p 253.
107. Ho KY, Veldhuis JD, Johnson ML, et al. Fasting enhances growth hormone secretion and amplifies the complex rhythms of growth hormone secretion in man. J Clin Invest 81:968–975, 1988.
108. Winters SJ, Troen P. A reexamination of pulsatile luteinizing hormone secretion in primary testicular failure. J Clin Endocrinol Metab 57:432–435, 1983.
109. Veldhuis JD, Iranmanesh A, Urban RJ. Primary gonadal failure in men selectively increases the mass of follicle stimulating hormone (FSH) secreted per burst and increases the disorderliness of FSH release: reversibility with testosterone replacement. Int J Androl 20:297–305, 1997.
110. Veldhuis JD, Evans WS, Demers LM, et al. Altered neuroendocrine regulation of gonadotropin secretion in women distance runners. J Clin Endocrinol Metab 61:557–563, 1985.
111. MacConnie SE, Barkan A, Lampman RM, et al. Decreased hypothalamic gonadotropin-releasing hormone secretion in male marathon runners. N Engl J Med 315:411–417, 1986.
112. Vogel AV, Peake GT, Rada RT. Pituitary-testicular axis dysfunction in burned men. J Clin Endocrinol Metab 60:658–665, 1985.
113. Shikone T, Matzuk MM, Perlas E. Characterization of gonadal sex cord–stromal tumor cell lines from inhibin-alpha and p53-deficient mice: The role of activin as an autocrine growth factor. Mol Endocrinol 8:983–995, 1994.
114. Veldhuis JD, Lizarralde G, Iranmanesh A. Divergent effects of short-term glucocorticoid excess on the gonadotropic and somatotropic axes in normal men. J Clin Endocrinol Metab 74:96–102, 1992.
115. Briski KP, Quigley K, Meites J. Endogenous opiate involvement in acute and chronic stress-induced changes in plasma LH concentrations in the male rat. Life Sci 34:2485–2493, 1984.
116. Bergendahl M, Veldhuis JD. Altered pulsatile gonadotropin signaling in nutritional deficiency in the male. Trends Endocrinol Metab 6:145–159, 1995.
117. Veldhuis JD, Iranmanesh A, Evans WS, et al. Amplitude suppression of the pulsatile mode of immunoradiometric LH release in fasting-induced hypoandrogenemia in normal men. J Clin Endocrinol Metab 76:587–593, 1993.
118. Beitins IZ, Barkan A, Klibanski A, et al. Hormonal responses to short term fasting in postmenopausal women. J Clin Endocrinol Metab 60:1120–1126, 1985.
119. Aloi JA, Bergendahl M, Iranmanesh A, Veldhuis JD. Pulsatile intravenous gonadotropin-releasing hormone administration averts fasting-induced hypogonadotropism and hypoandrogenemia in healthy, normal-weight men. J Clin Endocrinol Metab 82:1543–1548, 1997.
120. Pirke KM, Spyra B. Influence of starvation on testosterone–luteinizing hormone feedback in the rat. Acta Endocrinol (Copenh) 96:413–421, 1981.
121. Vale W, Rivier J, Vaughan J, et al. Purification and characterization of an FSH releasing protein from porcine ovarian follicular fluid. Nature 321:776–779, 1986.
122. Ling N, Ying SY, Ueno N, et al. Pituitary FSH is released by a heterodimer of the beta-subunits from the two forms of inhibin. Nature 321:779–782, 1986.
123. Cate RL, Mattaliano RJ, Hession C. Isolation of the bovine and human genes for müllerian inhibiting substance and expression of the human gene in animal cells. Cell 45:685–698, 1986.
124. Culler MD, Negro-Vilar A. Passive immunoneutralization of endogenous inhibin: Sex-related differences in the role of inhibin during development. Mol Cell Endocrinol 58:263–273, 1988.
125. Medhamurthy R, Abeyawardene SA, Culler MD, et al. Immunoneutralization of circulating inhibin in the hypophysiotropically clamped male rhesus monkey *(Macaca mulatta)* results in a selective hypersecretion of follicle-stimulating hormone. Endocrinology 126:2116–2124, 1990.
126. Meunier H, Rivier C, Evans RM, et al. Gonadal and extragonadal expression of inhibin A, BA, and BB subunits in various tissues predicts diverse functions. Proc Natl Acad Sci USA 85:247–251, 1988.

127. Roberts VJ, Peto CA, Vale W, et al. Inhibin/activin subunits are costored with FSH and LH in secretory granules of the rat anterior pituitary gland. Neuroendocrinology 56:214–224, 1992.
128. Mather JP, Attie KS, Woodruff TK, et al. Activin stimulates spermatogonial proliferation in germ-Sertoli cell cocultures from immature rat testis. Endocrinology 127:3206–3214, 1990.
129. Griswold MD. Interactions between germ cells and Sertoli cells in the testis. Biol Reprod 52:211–216, 1995.
130. Matzuk MM, Finegold MJ, Su J-GJ, et al. Alpha-inhibin is a tumour suppressor gene with gonadal specificity in mice. Nature 360:313–319, 1992.
131. Vassalli A, Matzuk MM, Gardner HAR, et al. Activin/inhibin beta B subunit gene disruption leads to defects in eyelid development and female reproduction. Genes Dev 8:414–427, 1994.
132. Ueno N, Ling N, Ying S-Y, et al. Isolation and partial characterization of follistatin: A single-chain Mr 35,000 monomeric protein that inhibits the release of follicle-stimulating hormone. Proc Natl Acad Sci USA 84:8282–8288, 1987.
133. Cameron VA, Nishimura E, Mathews LS, et al. Hybridization histochemical localization of activin receptor subtypes in rat brain, pituitary, ovary, and testes. Endocrinology 134:799–808, 1994.
134. Mathews LS. Activin receptors and cellular signaling by the receptor serine kinase family. Endocr Rev 15:310–325, 1994.
135. Gonzalez-Manchon C, Bilezikjian LM, Corrigan AZ, et al. Activin-A modulates gonadotropin-releasing hormone secretion from a gonadotropin-releasing hormone–secreting neuronal cell line. Neuroendocrinology 54:373–377, 1991.
136. Matzuk MM, Finegold MJ, Mather JP, et al. Development of cancer cachexia syndrome and adrenal tumors in inhibin-deficient mice. Proc Natl Acad Sci USA 91:8817–8821, 1994.
137. Veldhuis JD, Rogol AD, Perez-Palacios G, et al. Endogenous opiates participate in the regulation of pulsatile LH release in an unopposed estrogen milieu: Studies in estrogen-replaced, gonadectomized patients with testicular feminization. J Clin Endocrinol Metab 61:790–793, 1985.
138. Winters SJ, Sherins RJ, Loriaux DL. Studies on the role of sex steroids in the feedback control of gonadotropin concentrations in men. III. Androgen resistance in primary gonadal failure. J Clin Endocrinol Metab 48:553–558, 1979.

Chapter 23

THE TESTIS: Function and Dysfunction

Richard J. Santen

■ CHAPTER OUTLINE

KEY POINTS

- The human testes secrete androgenic hormones and excrete mature spermatozoa. A useful classification scheme divides disorders involving these two processes into hypogonadotropic, hypergonadotropic, and eugonadotropic subtypes.
- Appropriate assessment of patients requires an understanding of the normal actions of androgens in utero, during puberty, and in adulthood. Evaluation includes measurement of basal and stimulated hormone levels, genetic testing, and delineation of anatomic features.
- Hypogonadotropic disorders may be characterized by isolated deficiency of LH or FSH or may involve multiple trophic hormone deficiencies or hyperprolactinemia. Physiologic delayed puberty may present as a hypogonadotropic syndrome that resolves in a period of months to a few years.
- Hypergonadotropic syndromes commonly result from Klinefelter's syndrome but may also reflect manifestations of myotonic dystrophy and other genetic disorders, gonadal toxins, enzyme defects, mumps orchitis, diabetes mellitus, aging, or hormone resistance.
- Treatment of androgen deficiency involves use of injectable androgens or transdermal delivery devices. Careful attention focuses on dosage, duration of action, metabolism of testosterone to dihydrotestosterone and estradiol, and nadir and peak androgen levels in blood.
- Stimulation of spermatogenesis in hypogonadotropic patients involves injection of gonadotropins or administration of GnRH in a pulsatile mode.
- Germinal cell dysfunction affects 3 to 5 percent of men. Hypergonadotropic causes include the Sertoli cell–only syndrome as well as idiopathic seminiferous tubule failure with hyalinization.
- A new technique, intracytoplasmic sperm injection, appears highly promising as a means of using sperm with severe degrees of dysfunction to fertilize ova.
- Gynecomastia results from an imbalance of androgens and estrogens, often associated with drugs or with obesity. A directed work-up seeks to exclude serious underlying causes and to identify medications that are associated with this condition.
- Erectile dysfunction results from vascular, neurologic, endocrine, or psychogenic causes, and multifactorial abnormalities often coincide to exacerbate the problem.

The human testis serves two separate functions: secretion of androgenic hormones and excretion of mature spermatozoa. Although the anatomic basis and physiologic control of these two processes are highly interrelated, androgen secretion and germinal cell maturation are best considered separately. Clinical disorders may involve the androgen secretory component, the germinal cell axis, or both functional compartments simultaneously. A useful classification scheme, providing a frame of reference to evaluate and treat patients, divides disorders into hypogonadotropic, hypergonadotropic, and eugonadotropic subtypes.

EVALUATION OF THE HYPOTHALAMIC-PITUITARY-TESTICULAR AXIS

Clinical Evaluation

Appropriate assessment of patients requires an understanding of the normal actions of androgens in utero, during puberty, and in adulthood (Table 23–1). Patients with congenital hypogonadism present with sexual infantilism and retarded growth for age. The history and physical examination should focus on external genitalia, hair growth, linear growth, accessory sex organs, voice, psyche, and muscle mass. Acquired hypogonadism results in a loss of androgen-mediated effects (see Table 23–1) and directs attention toward patterns of hair growth, testis size, libido and sexual potentia, behavioral patterns, maintenance of bone density, spermatogenesis, and hematopoiesis.

Assessment of Hormonal Status

Basal Hormone Level

Recent technologic developments have substantially improved the sensitivity and specificity of gonadotropin immunoassays. Antibodies directed at two sites on the gonadotropin molecule improve specificity, and fluorometric or chemoluminescent detection markedly enhances assay sensitivity.[1] When values are substantially above or below the normal range, gonadotropin measurements in single serum samples can identify patients with hypergonadotropic and hypogonadotropic conditions. When values border the normal range, interpretation of results is confounded by pulsatile gonadotropin secretion, which introduces errors in estimates from single samples of ±60 percent for luteinizing hormone (LH) and ±20 percent for follicle-stimulating hormone (FSH).[2] On the basis of considerations of cost and precision, a practical recommendation for gonadotropin assessment includes obtaining a single measurement of LH and FSH in serum and confirming by repeated measurements in a pool of four samples taken at 20-minute intervals if the initial level is borderline high or low. Single samples are usually adequate for clinical assessment of testosterone, dihydrotestosterone (DHT), or estradiol levels.[3]

Several factors may confound interpretation of gonadotropin and testosterone levels[4] (Fig. 23–1). Aging influences normative values, and use of age-related normal ranges is advisable. The diurnal rhythm of testosterone necessitates obtaining early morning (i.e., 8 AM to 10 AM) samples. When abnormal values for total testosterone are detected, the possibility of sex hormone–binding globulin (SHBG) abnormalities should be considered and measurements of free or non–SHBG-bound testosterone obtained (Fig. 23–2).

Immunoassays for LH and FSH may be influenced by aberrant antigenic determinants on the gonadotropin molecule. Under these circumstances, alterations of the biologic to immunologic (B:I) ratios for LH and FSH may occur. Research methods are now available to measure the biologic activity of plasma LH and FSH.[5, 6] These techniques are highly sensitive and detect properties of the gonadotropin molecule that differ from antigenic recognition sites reacting with antibodies used in immunologic systems. Most bioassays detect a greater amount of gonadotropin than do immunoassays, and B:I ratios are usually greater than unity.[5–9] Controversy regarding the interpretation of B:I ratios exists because assay conditions, gonadotropin standards, species used for Leydig cell harvest, and physiologic circumstances can alter results.[8] These considerations suggest that much of the prior data regarding B:I ratio changes with puberty and chronic illness are of questionable value. On the other hand, several precisely definable conditions can alter the B:I ratio. Genetic mutations of the LH gene result in molecules that are biologically active but lack appropriate antigenic recognition sites.[10] One such mutation occurs in 28 percent of the Finnish population.[11] Variations in the carbohydrate content of the LH and FSH molecules occur during basal and gonadotropin-releasing hormone (GnRH)–stimulated secretion.[12, 13] The practical conclusion from these data is that gonadotropin assay results that are not congruent with the clinical situation may be explained by genetic or carbohydrate alterations of the gonadotropin molecule. When this occurs, use of research bioassay measurements may prove useful.

Measurements of inhibin provide an emerging means of assessing Sertoli cell function. The α-subunit of inhibin

■ TABLE 23–1
Effects of Androgens

In utero

External genitalia development
Wolffian duct development

Prepubertal

Possible male behavioral effects

Pubertal

External genitalia: penis and scrotum increase in size and become pigmented, and rugal folds appear in scrotal skin
Hair growth: mustache and beard develop and scalp line undergoes recession; pubic hair develops; axillary, body, extremity, and perianal hair grows
Linear growth: pubertal growth spurt appears; androgens interact with growth hormone to increase insulin-like growth factor I levels
Accessory sex organs: prostate and seminal vesicles enlarge and secretion begins
Voice: pitch is lowered because of enlargement of larnyx and thickening of vocal cords
Psyche: more aggressive attitudes are manifest and sexual potentia develops
Muscle mass: muscle bulk increases and positive nitrogen balance is demonstrable

Adult

Hair growth: androgenic patterns are maintained; male baldness may be initiated
Psyche: behavioral attitudes and sexual potency are maintained
Bone: bone loss and osteoporosis are prevented
Spermatogenesis: interaction with follicle-stimulating hormone to modulate Sertoli cell function and to stimulate spermatogenesis occurs
Hematopoiesis: stimulation of erythropoietin and direct marrow effect on erythropoiesis are present

Adapted from Bardin CW, Paulsen CA. The testes. *In* Williams RD (ed). Textbook of Endocrinology, 6th ed. Philadelphia, WB Saunders, 1981, p. 303.

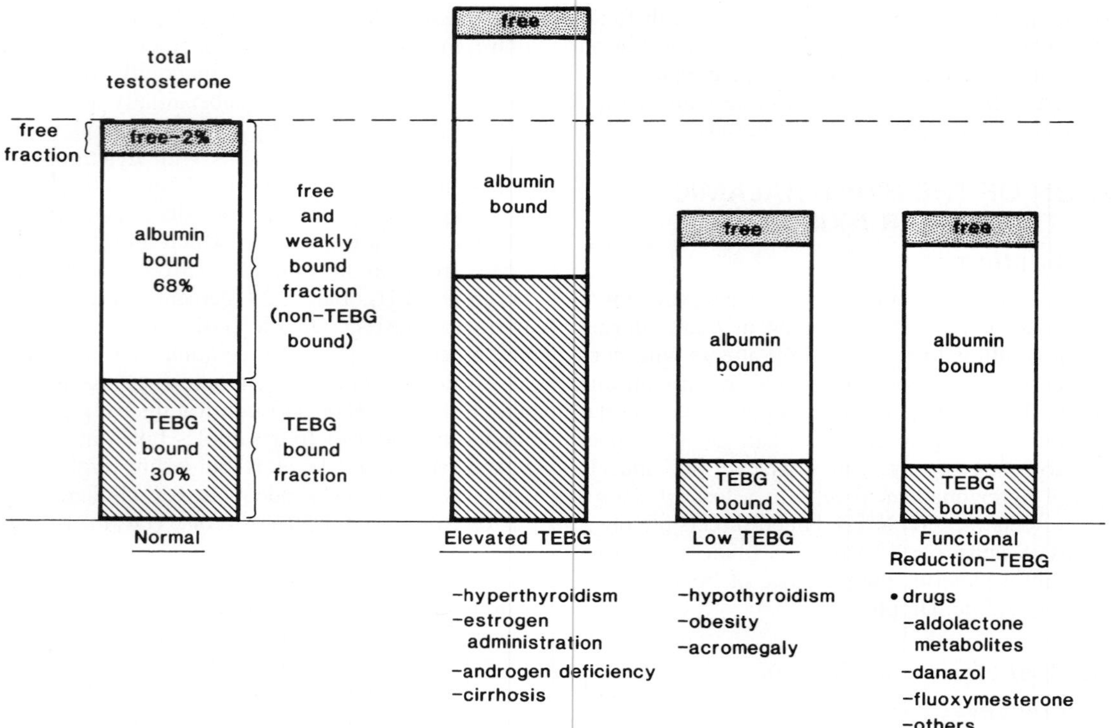

Figure 23–1 ■ Fractions of bound, weakly bound, and free testosterone in normal men and in men with disorders producing high or low levels of testosterone-estradiol–binding globulin (TEBG).

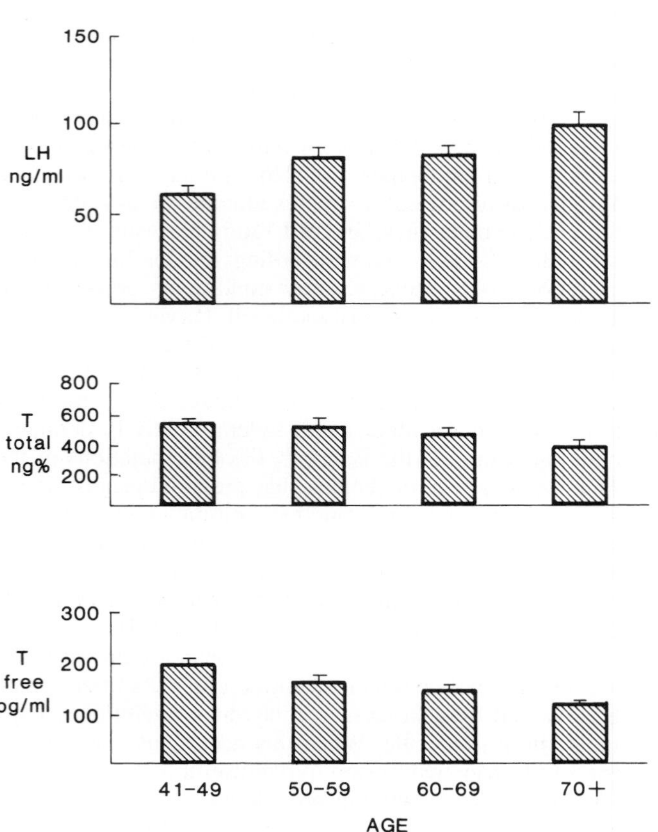

Figure 23–2 ■ Age-related changes in LH and total free testosterone (T) concentrations in normal men. (Adapted from data of Davidson JM, Chen JJ, Crapo L, et al. Hormonal changes and sexual function in aging men. J Clin Endocrinol Metab 57:71–77, 1983. © The Endocrine Society.)

forms a disulfide link with either β-subunit A or β-subunit B to form inhibin A and inhibin B. Secretion is stimulated by FSH and to a lesser extent by LH.[14–17] Currently used two-site immunoassays demonstrate that the circulating form of inhibin is predominantly inhibin B. The levels of inhibin B correlate well with FSH levels in semen donors, infertile men, and men with elevated FSH levels but not in normal men.[14–19] These data suggest that inhibin measurements might ultimately be useful as a means to assess testicular function, but they are presently a research tool.[17–19]

Dynamic Tests

Interruption of the estrogen negative feedback axis with clomiphene citrate (Clomid) (Figs. 23–3 to 23–5) stimulates release of LH and FSH and, secondarily, testosterone and estradiol. Clomiphene is a potent estrogen antagonist (and weak agonist) that exerts antiestrogenic effects predominantly at the hypothalamic level. In men, administration of 100 mg daily for 7 days can be used as a provocative test to evaluate the entire hypothalamic-pituitary axis

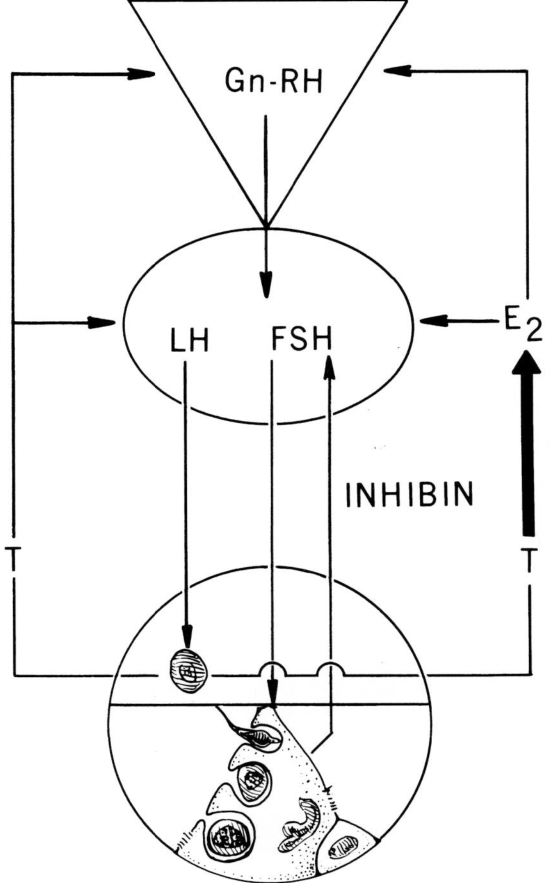

Figure 23–3 ■ Integrated control of LH and FSH secretion involving both the Leydig cell and Sertoli cell compartments of the testis. The hypothalamus *(inverted triangle)*, pituitary *(oval)*, and testis *(circle)* with its Leydig cell compartment *(upper)* and Sertoli and germinal cell compartments *(lower)* are shown. The feedback relationship of testosterone (T), estradiol (E_2), and LH and FSH is indicated. The specific interaction of the Sertoli cell compartment of the testis, inhibin, and pituitary FSH secretion is indicated.

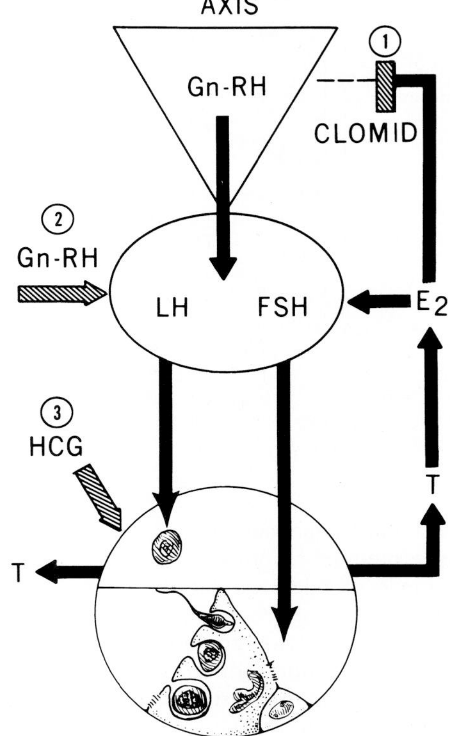

Figure 23–4 ■ The sites of action of stimulation tests of the testis: 1, clomiphene citrate (Clomid); 2, gonadotropin-releasing hormone; 3, human chorionic gonadotropin. Inverted triangle, hypothalamus; oval, pituitary; circle, Leydig and germ cell compartments of the testis; E_2, estradiol; T, testosterone.

(see Fig. 23–5). A 100 percent rise in LH and a 50 percent rise in FSH concentrations represent mean normal increments observed with this test. When clomiphene is given for a 6-week period, LH concentration increases further by 200 to 700 percent and FSH by 70 to 360 percent, reaching a plateau at approximately 1 month.

The GnRH test evaluates the functional capacity of the gonadotrophs to release LH and FSH (see Fig. 23–5). Two factors influence this response: the number of gonadotrophs present and the priming of these cells by prior exposure to endogenous GnRH secretion. If the gonadotrophs are not primed, the response to a single bolus of GnRH is limited. For this reason, use of the GnRH test to distinguish between hypothalamic and pituitary causes of reduced gonadotropin secretion is problematic. Operationally, the test consists of administration of 25 μg of GnRH as a single bolus with a measurement of plasma LH before and three to six times after the injection during a 3-hour period. No standard means of interpreting results has been agreed upon. As a general guideline, a doubling of LH and a 50 percent increase in FSH concentrations represent minimally normal results (Table 23–2).

Several reports describe refinements of the GnRH test.[20–22] One method infuses 0.25 μg of GnRH per minute during a 4-hour period. This method is based on physiologic data indicating that polypeptide hormones are se-

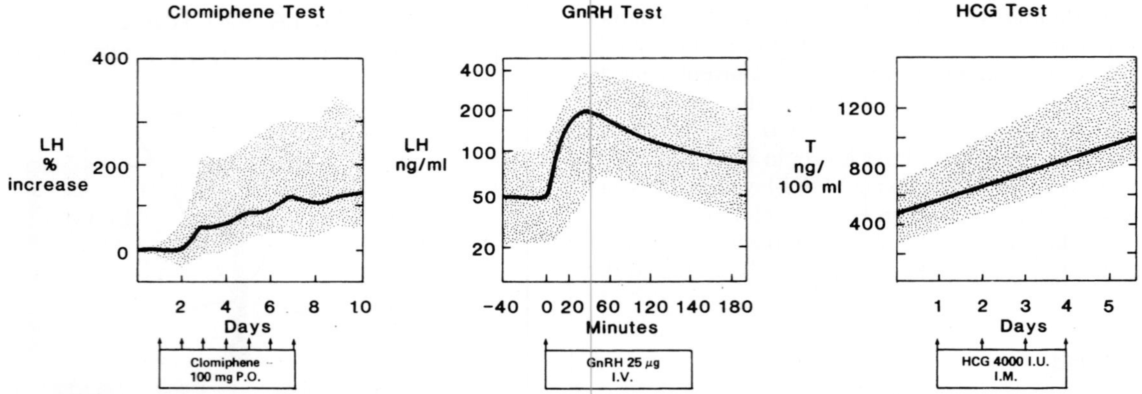

Figure 23–5 ■ Mean *(solid lines)* and ranges *(shaded areas)* of LH and testosterone (T) concentration increments during clomiphene, GnRH, and hCG stimulation tests. (Data from Santen RJ, Kulin HE. Evaluation of gonadotropins in man. *In* Hafez ESE [ed]. Techniques of Human Andrology. Amsterdam, Elsevier North Holland, 1977; Santen RJ, Leonard JM, Sherins RJ, et al. Short- and long-term effects of clomiphene citrate on the pituitary-testicular axis. J Clin Endocrinol Metab 33:970–979, 1971; Santen RJ, Paulsen CA. Hypogonadotropic eunuchoidism. II. Gonadal responsiveness to exogenous gonadotropins. J Clin Endocrinol Metab 36:55–63, 1973; and Santen RJ. Is aromatization of testosterone to estradiol required for inhibition of LH secretion in men? J Clin Invest 56:1555–1563, 1975.)

creted in a bimodal manner. Initially, presynthesized hormone is secreted in response to the stimulus; later, a secondary mode of release of newly synthesized or processed material occurs. A second iteration uses a long-acting GnRH analogue to provide continuous stimulation during a 24-hour period. A third administers GnRH pulses in a 36-hour period. All require further validation under a wide variety of clinical circumstances before general acceptance for clinical use.

Direct provocative testing of the testes requires administration of human chorionic gonadotropin (hCG) and assessment of plasma testosterone increments at various time intervals (see Figs. 23–4 and 23–5). Traditional test procedures use multiple injections on a daily basis; however, one injection of 1500 to 4000 IU intramuscularly is a sufficient stimulus.[23] Plasma testosterone is measured before and 5 days after hCG injections. Normal responses vary from a doubling of the initial testosterone level in adult patients to a rise greater than 150 ng/dl in prepubertal subjects (see Table 23–2). Alternatively, in prepubertal boys a longer protocol can be used, during which testosterone reaches the adult male range after 16 days of stimulation.

Genetic Tests

Buccal smears can be used to detect Barr bodies, the condensed second X chromosome in a male. Karyotype analysis of blood lymphocytes, skin fibroblasts, or gonadal tissues provides more definitive information regarding the presence of supernumerary X chromosomes. Special fluorescent stains are available that can identify the Y chromosomes in cells from buccal smears, from metaphase plates, or from meiotic spreads of gonadal tissue. A deoxyribonucleic acid (DNA) segment, *SRY*, has been shown to be necessary and sufficient to initiate testis determination.[24] Complementary DNA (cDNA) probes are now available to demonstrate the presence of this portion of the Y chromosome.

Structural and Functional Assessment

Testis and Surrounding Structure

Testis size is assessed by simple measurement of longitudinal and horizontal axes or by comparison with a series of ellipsoids of increasing volume (Table 23–3) using an apparatus called a Prader orchidometer. This technique

■ TABLE 23–2
Normal Basal and Stimulated Hormone Levels

		STIMULATED		
		Mean Percentage Increase (Range)		
	BASAL	***Clomiphene***	***GnRH***	***hCG***
Plasma				
LH	4–20 mIU/ml	100 (30–400)	450 (50–1200)	—
FSH	4–20 mIU/ml	50 (20–200)	70 (9–176)	—
Testosterone	300–1200 ng/dl	25 (0–65)	No rise	100 (50–200)

Test Protocols

Clomiphene test: 100 mg clomiphene citrate (Clomid) daily by mouth for 7 days; draw blood sample before and on day 8.
GnRH test: 25 μg intravenously with collection of blood before and at 30, 60, 90, and 120 minutes after administration.
hCG test: 4000 IU hCG on day 1; draw blood sample before and on day 5.

■ TABLE 23–3
Assessment of Testicular Size

METHOD	TESTICULAR SIZE Prepubertal	Pubertal	Adult
Orchidometer (ml)	1–6	8–15	20–30*
Ruler measurement (cm)			
Length	1.6–2.9	3.1–4.0	4.1–5.5
Width	1.0–1.8	2.0–2.5	2.7–3.2

*24 ± 4 ml (SD); N = 44.

Adapted from Sherins RJ, Howards SS. Male infertility. *In* Walsh PC, Gittes RF, Perlmutter AD, Stamey TA (eds). Campbell's Urology, 5th ed, Vol 1. Philadelphia, WB Saunders, 1986, p 640.

correlates precisely with objective measurements obtained by testicular ultrasound examination.[25] Special techniques of testicular examination must be used under certain circumstances. In boys with pseudocryptorchidism or retractile testes, the gonads may be palpated only when the patient exits from a warm bath or assumes a squatting position. Dilatation of veins in the scrotum, a condition called varicocele, may be detected only when the patient is upright and performing a Valsalva maneuver.

Special diagnostic tools are available to provide further anatomic information.[26] Pelvic ultrasonography can be of assistance in locating intra-abdominal testicular structures in older boys or adults and to identify occult testicular tumors.[27] Testicular vein venography delineates the location of cryptorchid testes and identifies the presence of a varicocele. Laparoscopy allows visualization of intra-abdominal testicular structures. The vas deferens may be cannulated during surgery and injected with dye (operative vasogram) to establish patency of the epididymis and vas deferens.

Before the availability of plasma FSH assays, testicular biopsy provided the only information regarding the degree of functional impairment of the spermatogenic process. Currently, plasma FSH measurements are also used to assess the amount of testicular damage, because FSH concentration rises with increasing testicular destruction.[28] For this reason, testicular biopsy is now used less commonly. However, this procedure may be helpful in distinguishing obstructive azoospermia from idiopathic azoospermia with peritubular hyalinization. With obstruction of the excurrent duct system, normal spermatogenesis is found on biopsy specimens; with idiopathic azoospermia, severe tubular sclerosis and peritubular hyalinization are observed. FSH determination also distinguishes these two groups of patients because those with obstruction exhibit normal FSH levels whereas those with hyalinization have high titers.[28] Testicular biopsy causes a transient but reversible reduction in sperm count.[29]

Seminal fluid analysis provides information regarding the production of sperm by the testes and the patency of the excurrent duct system. Standardized collection involves abstinence from ejaculation for 3 days or longer; submission of the specimen by masturbation into a clean, dry, wide-mouth container; and completion of sperm counting and other analyses within 2 hours of collection. Computerized video analytic techniques allow precise quantitation of several sperm variables. The presence of fructose indicates patency of the excurrent duct system from the seminal vesicles to the urethra.

The sperm count in multiple specimens from the same subject usually varies by an average of 75 percent but may undergo even more extreme fluctuations.[30] For example, counts in samples from normal volunteers ranged from 5 $\times$ 10^6/ml to 200 $\times$ 10^6/ml in the same individuals during a 2- to 3-year period. Some of the variability may be seasonal and related to the summer climate.[31] For these reasons, only general ranges describing relative normal values can be given (Table 23–4). Several authors have reported reductions in mean sperm concentrations observed in normal men during the past two decades. This finding, attributed by some to environmental estrogen exposure, has been a controversial issue.[32–34]

A minimum of three samples should be collected in a 3-month period. The variability in single samples can be minimized by averaging the results from these separate collections. Independently assessed variables, such as total sperm count, sperm concentration, percentage of motility, and percentage of normal forms, covary in the same individual.[35] Under some circumstances, however, specimens with low counts (as low as 5 $\times$ 10^6/ml) can be normal with respect to motility and morphologic features and, consequently, have high fertilization potential.

The capability of sperm to fertilize can be assessed with several in vitro functional tests including the zona-free hamster oocyte penetration test, the hypo-osmotic swelling test, analysis of sperm–zona pellucida binding, acrosome reactability, and oolemma binding capability. These assays add information independent from that gained from analysis of semen volumes, sperm count, percentage of sperm motility, and percentage of normal spermatozoa. Overall prediction of fertility increases only from 70 to 78 percent when the zona-free hamster oocyte penetration test and hypo-osmotic swelling test are added to the routine semen measurements.[35] Emerging data suggest that sperm zona binding properties, acrosome reactability, and oolemma binding ability might be better predictors of fertilization potential.[36, 37] Further data are required before these become proven and established methods.

HYPOGONADOTROPIC HYPOGONADISM

See Table 23–5 for the classification of hypogonadotropic hypogonadism.

■ TABLE 23–4
Normal Values for Semen Analysis

PARAMETER	NORMAL VALUE
Sperm concentration	>20 $\times$ 10^6/ml
Total sperm in ejaculate	>50 $\times$ 10^6
Semen volume	>1 ml
Percentage motile	>60

Summarized from MacLeod J, Gold RZ. The male factor in fertility and infertility: II. Spermatozoon counts in 1000 men of known fertility and in 1000 cases of infertile marriage. J Urol 66:436, 1951; Naghma-E-Rehan, Sobrero AJ, Fertig JW. The semen of fertile men: Statistical analysis of 1300 men. Fertil Steril 26:492–502, 1975; Nelson CMK, Bunge RG. Semen analysis: Evidence for changing parameters of male fertility potential. Fertil Steril 25:503–507, 1974; and Smith KD, Steinberger E. What is oligospermia? *In* Troen P, Nankin HR (eds). The Testis in Normal and Infertile Men. New York, Raven Press, 1977, p 489.

■ TABLE 23–5
Classfication of Hypogonadotropic Hypogonadism

Organic Causes

Multiple trophic hormone deficiencies
- Idiopathic
- Secondary to tumor
- Miscellaneous causes
  - Histiocytosis X
  - Tuberculosis
  - Sarcoidosis
  - Collagen-vascular diseases
  - Hypophysitis
  - Sequela of pituitary irradiation

Secondary to hyperprolactinemia

Isolated gonadotropin deficiency
- Hypogonadotropic eunuchoidism (Kallmann's syndrome)
  - Complete
  - Partial (predominant luteinizing hormone deficiency—fertile eunuch syndrome)
  - Variant form (isolated follicle-stimulating hormone deficiency)
- Specific genetic syndromes
  - Prader-Labhart-Willi
  - Laurence-Moon
  - Bardet-Biedl
  - Möbius'
  - Other rarer disorders

Acute and chronic illness
- Acute illness
- Chronic illnesses
- Emotional disorders
- Acquired immunodeficiency syndrome (AIDS)
- Obesity
- Drugs
- Liver disease—one subgroup
- Renal disease—one component
- Hemochromatosis
- Spinal cord damage
- Hypophysitis

Glucocorticoids

Functional Causes

Physiologic delayed puberty (constitutional delay)

Organic Causes

Multiple Trophic Hormone Deficiencies

Prepubertal patients with multiple trophic hormone deficiencies (hypopituitarism) commonly experience severe growth retardation, whereas older boys exhibit delayed adolescence. Adults seek medical attention because of erectile dysfunction, headaches, or visual disturbance. Symptoms may be present that suggest deficient secretion of thyroid-stimulating hormone, adrenocorticotropic hormone, or antidiuretic hormone. The patient may complain of progressive headache or visual disturbance caused by the pituitary tumor.

Idiopathic hypopituitarism is the most common cause of multiple pituitary hormone deficiencies in early childhood or early adolescence. Pituitary tumors are common in the adult patient. Nonfunctioning macroadenomas are most likely to induce panhypopituitarism, whereas growth hormone–producing macroadenomas are associated with relative sparing of anterior pituitary function.[38] Gonadotropin-producing tumors secrete FSH but relatively little LH, and consequently patients present with symptoms of androgen deficiency.[39] Other causes include craniopharyngioma, pinealoma, dysgerminoma, glial tumors, and autoimmune or necrotizing hypophysitis.[40] Disorders recognizable by their extrapituitary manifestations but causing hypogonadotropism (see Table 23–5) include histiocytosis X, tuberculosis, sarcoidosis, and certain collagen-vascular diseases with central nervous system vasculitis. Gonadotropin deficiency may result several years after pituitary irradiation for nasopharyngeal carcinoma or other disorders.[41]

LH, FSH, and testosterone concentrations are low in patients with each of these conditions; release of these hormones in response to clomiphene is blunted or absent. GnRH produces release of LH and FSH variably, depending on the degree of pituitary gonadotropin reserve and pre-exposure to endogenous GnRH from the hypothalamus. Elevated lipid levels and decreased bone density are observed as a reflection of long-standing androgen deficiency.[42–44]

Hyperprolactinemia

Serum prolactin elevations result in hypogonadism through both direct and indirect mechanisms. Prolactin acts directly on the hypothalamus to alter aminergic function, lower GnRH messenger ribonucleic acid (mRNA) levels,[45] and diminish GnRH, gonadotropin, and testosterone secretion.[46] Prolactin also reduces the concentration of 5α-reductase in androgen-dependent tissues[47] and may cause a disproportionate reduction in DHT as opposed to testosterone levels.[48] A direct antagonistic effect of prolactin on the testes has been suggested[49] but is probably not functionally important because testosterone responses to hCG are normal in hyperprolactinemia from a variety of drug-induced or organic causes.[50]

Prolactin elevations result from prolactinomas and from functional causes. With small prolactinomas, the major clinical manifestations are delayed puberty in children[51] and hypogonadism in adults.[52] Erectile dysfunction resulting from androgen deficiency or perhaps from direct effects of elevated prolactin levels on erectile function is nearly always present in adult men. With large prolactinomas, symptoms related to growing tumor mass predominate, such as headache, visual field abnormalities, and functional hypopituitarism. Notably, most men with prolactinomas are found to have large lesions.[52] Functional causes of hyperprolactinemia usually result from centrally acting pharmacologic agents such as the phenothiazines and antihypertensive medications with α-adrenergic or dopamine-blocking properties.

Treatment when tumor is present consists of dopaminergic agonist therapy with bromocriptine, pergolide or cabergoline either alone or in combination with surgery. Testosterone levels rise slowly for a period of 1 year and usually return toward, but not into, the normal range. Exogenous testosterone administration may be necessary, but caution is advised because tumor stimulation resulting from increased aromatization of testosterone to estradiol has been observed, albeit rarely.[53] Correction of androgen deficiency alone is not usually sufficient to relieve symptoms of erectile dysfunction, and reduction of prolactin concentration is also necessary. This observation, which suggests that prolactin has a direct role in the erectile process, remains to be explained by rigorous physiologic studies.

Isolated Gonadotropin Deficiency

HYPOGONADOTROPIC EUNUCHOIDISM (KALLMANN'S SYNDROME)

Hypogonadotropic eunuchoidism, or Kallmann's syndrome, although the most common cause of isolated gonadotropin deficiency, occurs in less than 1 in 10,000 live male births. Probably representing several specific diseases, Kallmann's syndrome may exhibit autosomal dominant inheritance with relative sex limitation to males[54] or an autosomal recessive or X-linked pattern.[55, 56]

In the X-linked form, the KAL1 gene, localized at Xp22.3 (Fig. 23–6), is defective. An adhesion molecule coded for by KAL1 mediates the early embryonic migration of GnRH neurons from the nasal anlage to the hypothalamus. Genetic defects in this molecule prevent migration and result in absence of GnRH neurons in the hypothalamus (Fig. 23–7). Depending on the relative degree of reduction of these hypothalamic neurons, GnRH secretion can be absent or blunted. The KAL1 gene is flanked by genes coding for X-linked ichthyosis, mental retardation, and short stature (see Fig. 23–6). Consequently, patients with Kallmann's syndrome may present with complex phenotypes characterized by a combination of hypogonadotropic hypogonadism and X-linked ichthyosis due to steroid sulfatase deficiency, chrondroplasia punctata, short stature, and mental retardation.[56, 57] Other abnormalities observed include hyposmia or anosmia, cryptorchidism, cleft lip or cleft palate, and congenital deafness in addition to the hypogonadism.[54, 55] Mirror movements, eye movement abnormalities, cerebellar dysfunction, pes cavus deformity of feet, and café au lait macules occur in a substantial fraction of additional patients.[58] No pathophysiologic distinction can be made at present between subjects with a familial pattern of gonadotropin deficiency and sporadic or nonfamilial forms.

The degree of gonadotropin deficiency in patients with Kallmann's syndrome ranges from partial to complete.

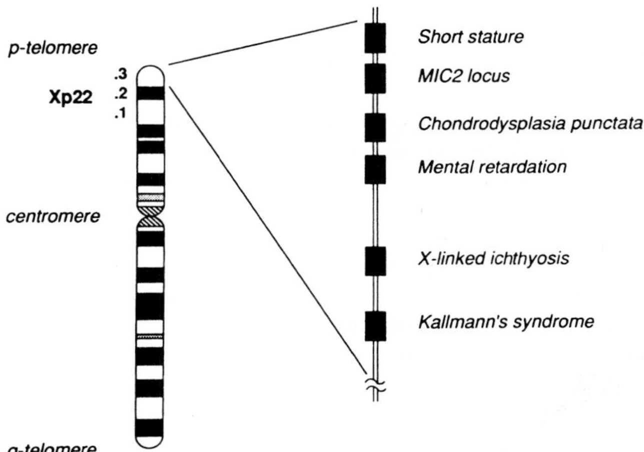

Figure 23–6 ■ Schematic representation of the X chromosome with the relative locations of the major identified genes in the Xp22.3 region. (From X-chromosome–linked Kallmann's syndrome: Pathology at the molecular level [Editorial]. J Clin Endocrinol Metab 76:824–826, 1993. © The Endocrine Society.)

With a highly sensitive urinary concentration assay, basal urinary FSH excretion ranged from 10 to 500 mIU/hr (a 50-fold variation), whereas LH excretion varied from 10 to 700 mIU/hr in a group of 16 subjects with this disorder (Fig. 23–8). Plasma testosterone concentration was as low as 5 ng/dl and as high as 60 ng/dl.[59]

The amplitude and frequency of spontaneous LH pulses also vary substantially from a complete absence of pulses to those with normal amplitude but decreased frequency[60] (Fig. 23–9). Subjects with infrequent pulses could be returned to normal testicular function by administration of GnRH episodically at a frequency comparable with that in normal individuals. Surprisingly, a few of these patients (approximately 5 percent) maintained normal function even after cessation of GnRH therapy, perhaps as a result of pituitary priming or further hypothalamic maturation.[61]

The degree of gonadotropin deficiency influences the clinical presentation. In the complete form, both FSH and LH levels are low, and no evidence of sexual maturation is apparent. With partial deficits, FSH secretion predominates, and germinal cell maturation of the testis proceeds even to late spermatid or spermatozoa formation whereas sexual development is incomplete. These patients have been referred to as fertile eunuchs because spermatozoa may be present in testicular biopsy specimens or in the ejaculate,[62] but few are actually fertile. On clinical examination, the presence of gynecomastia is more frequent in patients with partial than with complete gonadotropin deficiency. The fertile eunuch syndrome is considered a variation of hypogonadotropic eunuchoidism because anosmia and other anomalies of the genetic disorder may be present. Another variant, isolated FSH deficiency, has been described.[63]

The severity of the gonadotropin secretory defect may have practical significance regarding therapy. Subjects with relative preservation of FSH may respond with normal spermatogenesis to treatment with hCG alone.[64] Testis size before treatment is a good predictor of response to hCG alone. Presumably, a sufficient amount of FSH is present to initiate and complete normal spermatogenesis after intratesticular testosterone levels are normalized by the effects of exogenous LH or hCG. Rowe and colleagues[65] reported that two subjects with incomplete gonadotropin deficiency developed normal spermatogenesis with testosterone treatment alone, but this phenomenon is probably uncommon.

The major problem in diagnosis of isolated gonadotropin deficiency is to differentiate patients with an organic defect from those with physiologic delayed puberty. A positive family history or presence of nongonadal abnormalities associated with hypogonadotropic eunuchoidism (e.g., anosmia and cleft lip) provides the best means of confirming the diagnosis of Kallmann's syndrome.[54, 55] Because approximately 80 percent of boys with hypogonadotropic hypogonadism exhibit either anosmia or hyposmia, this clinical finding is useful.[54] A scratch, sniff, and smell test developed by Doty and associates[66] has been clinically useful to detect patients with hyposmia.

If no associated congenital abnormalities are present, other diagnostic measures are needed. It was originally thought that the gonadotropin responses to GnRH might

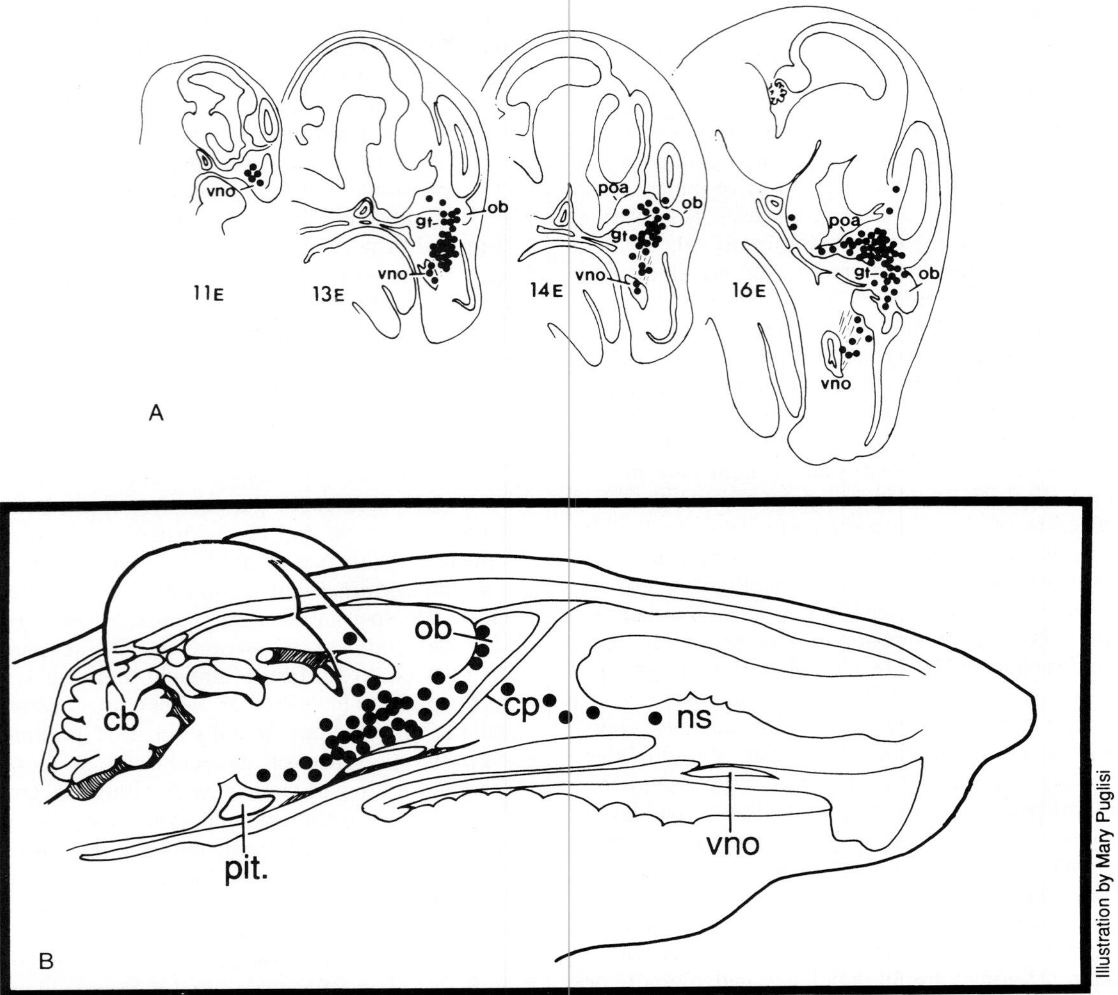

Figure 23–7 ■ Migration of GnRH cells from the olfactory pit to the brain begins about 11.5 days after conception in the mouse.
A, Most cells are still close to the vomeronasal organ (vno) at embryonic day 11 to 11.5. By 13 days, the number of GnRH neurons has increased and the first cells are crossing into the brain near the olfactory bulb (ob). By 14 days, GnRH neurons have begun to arc back through the forebrain to the preoptic area (poa). Migration is largely complete by 15 to 16.5 days after conception. ctx, cerebral cortex; gt, ganglion terminale. (Adapted from Schwanzel-Fukada M, Pfaff DW. Origin of luteinizing hormone releasing hormone neurons. Nature 338:161–164, 1989. Copyright © 1989 Macmillan Magazines Ltd.)
B, Distribution of GnRH neurons in the brain of the adult rat. Cerebellum (cb), pituitary gland (pit), olfactory bulb (ob), cribriform plate (cp), nasal septum (ns), and vomeronasal organ (vno) are indicated.

allow earlier differentiation between subjects with physiologic delay of puberty and those with isolated gonadotropin deficiency. However, variable increments in LH and FSH concentrations have been observed after single injections of GnRH in patients with hypogonadotropic eunuchoidism, particularly in those with the incomplete forms. Patients with physiologic delayed puberty, on the other hand, may exhibit diminished responses to GnRH before the onset of testicular enlargement. When sexual maturation has progressed, as reflected by testicular enlargement, the LH concentration increments after GnRH stimulation may become normal.

With use of highly sensitive immunoassays, most patients with hypogonadotropic hypogonadism have lower basal and post-GnRH gonadotropin levels than do patients with constitutional delay.[1] Stimulation tests using a long-acting GnRH agonist in conjunction with sensitive immunoassays may also suggest gonadotropin deficiency if basal and stimulated values are low.[67] Nonetheless, these methods do not provide complete discrimination because of the overlap[68, 69] in the amount of gonadotropin secretion between patients with constitutional delay and those with hypogonadotropic hypogonadism. A more precise method is to obtain serial measurements of LH and FSH concentrations during a period of several months. Progressive increments in the levels of these hormones strongly suggest physiologic delayed puberty[69] (Fig. 23–10). However, it may be necessary to wait until the patient is older than 18 to 20 years to be certain about permanent hypogonadotropism because most boys with a physiologic delay will have undergone pubertal changes by that time. However, some patients undergo spontaneous puberty even after age 20 years.[70, 71]

Clinical observations suggest that certain patients with

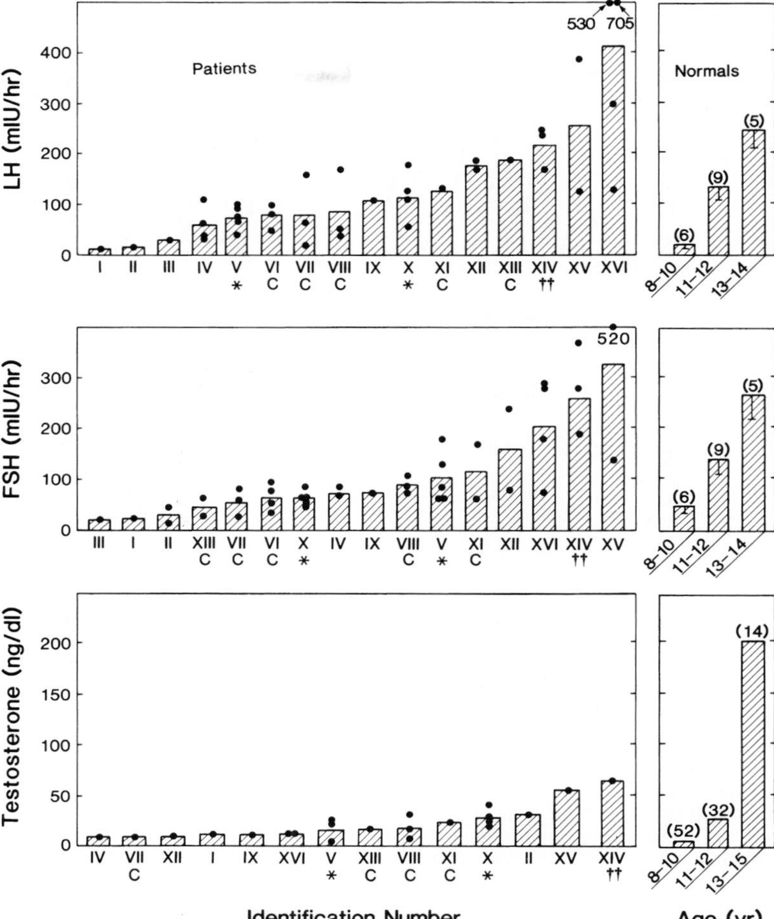

Figure 23–8 ■ Heterogeneity of gonadotropin deficiency in hypogonadotropic hypogonadism. Levels of urinary LH were ranked according to increased concentration in 16 patients with hypogonadotropic hypogonadism *(top).* Circles represent separate determinations; height of bar indicates mean level. For comparison *(middle, bottom),* levels of urinary FSH and plasma testosterone are shown. *Testis size, 2.0 to 2.5 cm on the long axis, all others less than 2.0 cm; C, unilateral cryptorchidism; †† bilateral cryptorchidism. Normal ranges and number of individuals in normal range are shown on the right panels for comparison. (From Santen RJ, Kulin HE. Evaluation of delayed puberty and hypogonadotropism. *In* Santen RJ, Swerdloff RS [eds]. Male Reproductive Dysfunction: Diagnosis and Management of Hypogonadism, Infertility, and Impotence. New York, Marcel Dekker, 1986, pp 145–190. Reproduced by courtesy of Marcel Dekker, Inc.)

hypogonadotropic eunuchoidism may have Leydig cells that are relatively unresponsive to hCG[72] or to GnRH-induced LH increments. The associated Leydig cell defect may be limited to patients with bilateral cryptorchidism[73] or to subjects with more severe intrauterine GnRH deficiency and lack of full testicular development.

Evaluation of patients with isolated gonadotropin deficiency requires a careful family history to identify other affected family members, many of whom may have hyposmia or anosmia without reproductive dysfunction. Quantitative estimation of olfactory threshold or absence of olfactory bulbs or tracts on magnetic resonance imaging can identify 80 percent of subjects with this disorder. Measurements of LH, FSH, and testosterone concentrations define the degree of deficit. Additional evaluation includes demonstration of normal growth hormone and thyroid function and exclusion of hyperprolactinemia and sellar or parasellar mass lesions. Assay of dehydroepiandrosterone sulfate (DHEA-S) level, as an indicator of adrenal adrenarche, is useful in patients with Kallmann's syndrome. Gonadarche and adrenarche reflect two separate physiologic processes that can be dissociated clinically. Adrenarche, as reflected by DHEA-S levels, is normal for age in Kallmann's syndrome. Delayed adrenarche with low DHEA-S levels is found with physiologic delayed puberty or organic lesions of the pituitary.

SPECIFIC GENETIC SYNDROMES WITH PREDOMINANT HYPOGONADOTROPISM

Prader-Labhart-Willi Syndrome. This syndrome[74] is an inherited disorder causing hypogonadism (Table 23–6). Boys with this disorder may have hypotonia (especially in infancy), obesity, mental retardation, short stature, and adult-onset diabetes mellitus. The mnemonic HHHO syndrome (hypomentia, hypotonia, hypogonadism, obesity) has been applied to this disorder. Other distinguishing features often present include acromicria, micrognathia, strabismus, fish-like or Cupid's bow mouth, clinodactylism, and absence of auricular cartilage. The degree of hypogonadotropism in this disorder is variable but ranges from partial to severe. Paradoxically, some cases with hypergonadotropic hypogonadism or diminished responsiveness to hCG have been recognized.[74] The diagnosis is made by identifying the clinical stigmata of this syndrome and documenting the presence of reduced LH and FSH levels. A karyotype analysis of peripheral blood lymphocytes may also be helpful. A defect in chromosome 15 arising from the paternal chromosome has been described in approximately half of the cases.[74, 75] A few older subjects with this disorder have responded to clomiphene citrate with reversal of hypogonadotropism and spontaneous onset of puberty.[76]

Laurence-Moon and Bardet-Biedl Syndromes. Hypogonadism in association with retinitis pigmentosa, obesity,

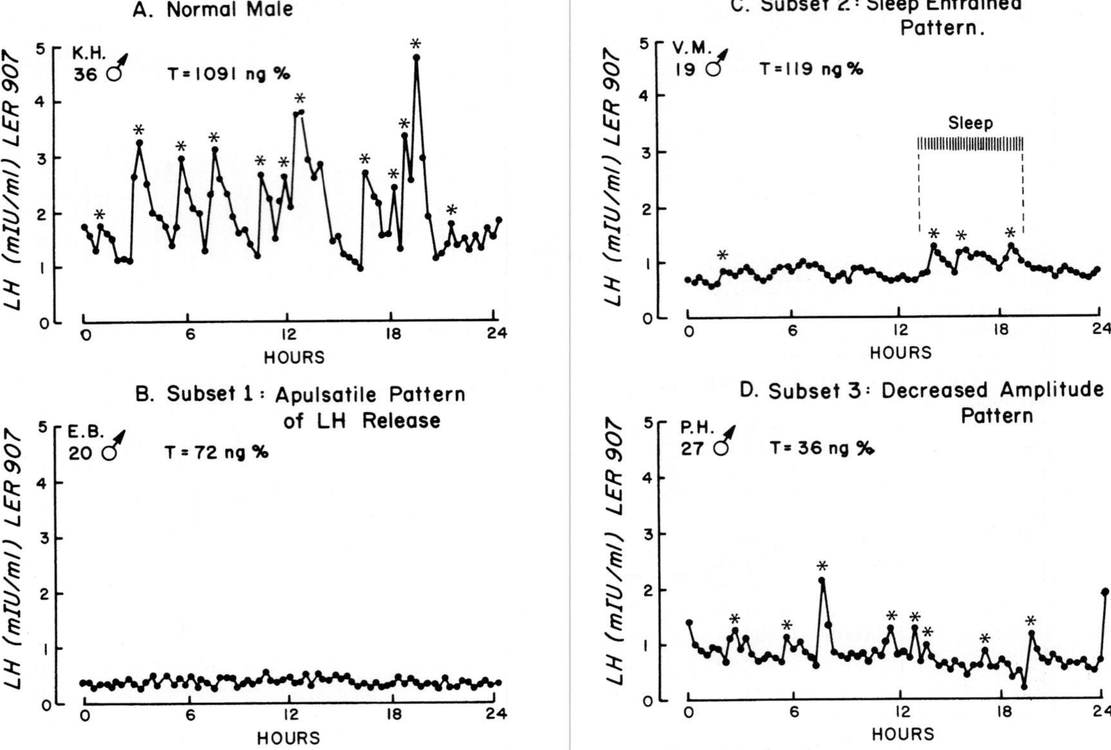

Figure 23–9 ■ Patterns of endogenous LH secretion in idiopathic hypogonadotropic hypogonadal (IHH) men.

A, LH values determined every 20 minutes for 24 hours in a normal man displaying discrete LH pulsations occurring about every 2 hours and resulting in a normal plasma testosterone (T) concentration.

B, LH determinations in a man with IHH displaying no detectable LH pulsations and a prepubertal testosterone level.

C, Sleep-entrained LH pulsations of decreased amplitude associated with prepubertal testosterone levels in an 18-year-old IHH man.

D, LH pulsations of decreased amplitude occurring during sleep and wake periods in a 27-year-old IHH man. (*A* to *D* from Spratt DI, Hoffman AR, Crowley WF Jr. Hypogonadotropic hypogonadism and its treatment. *In* Santen RJ, Swerdloff RS [eds]. Male Reproductive Dysfunction: Diagnosis and Management of Hypogonadism, Infertility, and Impotence. New York, Marcel Dekker, 1986, p 227. Reproduced by courtesy of Marcel Dekker, Inc.)

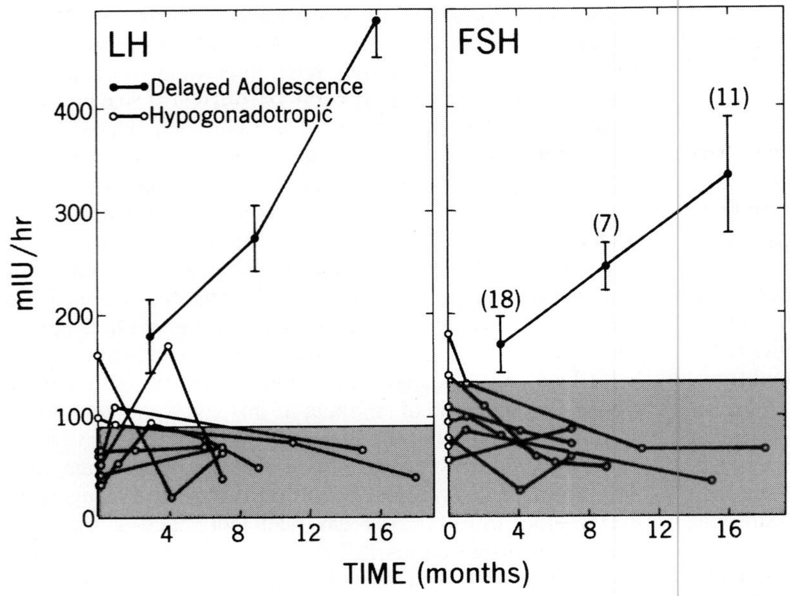

Figure 23–10 ■ Sequential gonadotropin changes in 10 boys with constitutionally delayed adolescence and in 7 patients with hypogonadotropic hypogonadism observed for 6 to 28 months. Shaded areas indicate normal prepubertal male ranges. (From Kulin HE, Santen RJ. Normal and aberrant pubertal development in man. *In* Vaitukaitis JL [ed]. Current Endocrinology: Comprehensive Reproductive Neuroendocrinology. New York, Elsevier Biomedical, 1982, p 19.)

■ TABLE 23–6
Clinical Features of Common* Genetic Hypogonadotropic Hypogonadal Syndromes

PRADER-LABHART-WILLI	LAWRENCE-MOON	BARDET-BIEDL	RUD'S	HYPOGONADOTROPISM/ATAXIA	MÖBIUS'	MULTIPLE LENTIGENES
Hypomentia Hypotonia Short stature Cupid's-bow mouth Diabetes mellitus Hypogonadism† Obesity	Hypogonadism† Mental retardation Ataxia Nystagmus Pigmentary retinopathy Spastic paraplegia Obesity Short stature	Hypogonadism† Dysmorphic extremities, (polydactyly, syndactyly, or bradydactyly) Retinal dystrophy Renal disease Obesity	Mental retardation Epilepsy Congenital ichthyosis	Cerebellar ataxia Pes cavus Spina bifida	Multiple cranial nerve abnormalities Anosmia Mental retardation	Multiple lentigenes Cardiac defects, hypertelorism Short stature Deafness Delayed or no puberty Genital and urologic defects

*For rare disorders, consult Rimoin DL, Schimke RN. The gonads. *In* Rimoin DL, Schimke RN (eds). Genetic Disorders of the Endocrine Glands. St. Louis, CV Mosby, 1971.
†Hypergonadotropic types have also been described.

mental retardation, and polydactyly has commonly been termed the Laurence-Moon-Biedl syndrome.[77] Hypogonadism occurs in 50 percent of affected patients and delayed adolescence in another 30 percent. Some authorities distinguish two distinct entities, the Laurence-Moon and Bardet-Biedl syndromes[77] (see Table 23–6).

Most studies of endocrine function have not distinguished these two syndromes and describe abnormalities in groups of patients with both entities. Early reports suggested that hypogonadism occurs in 80 percent of boys with Laurence-Moon-Biedl syndrome. However, more than half of these patients were younger than 15 years at diagnosis; examination of older boys revealed only a 50 percent prevalence of hypogonadism.[78] This finding suggests that delayed adolescence is a common feature of this syndrome. In prepubertal boys, microphallus, hypospadias, and undescended testes are common. The major manifestations of this syndrome are apparent early in life. Retinal degeneration occurs between ages 4 and 10 and obesity begins somewhat earlier. Many reports attribute the hypogonadism to a hypothalamic-pituitary disorder. Other studies identified patients with hypergonadotropic hypogonadism. A family study of eight males with the Bardet-Biedl syndrome identified seven with small testes and genitalia and two with low serum testosterone levels.[77] These two subjects had low to normal LH levels and an exaggerated response to GnRH. Although interpreted differently,[77] these findings suggest an incomplete form of hypogonadotropic hypogonadism. Thus, both hypogonadotropic and hypergonadotropic forms of these syndromes probably exist.

Other Syndromes. Hypogonadotropic hypogonadism may also be associated with several other syndromes with characteristic congenital anomalies (see Table 23–6).

Acute Illness. Studies in hospitalized men with acute illness demonstrate a pattern of falling LH, FSH, and testosterone levels (Fig. 23–11). Disorders examined included severe burns, head injury, septic shock, cardiac surgery, myocardial infarction, and a variety of other conditions.[79] Increasing severity of illness as assessed by the Acute Physiology and Chronic Health Evaluation (APACHE) score correlates with degree of testosterone and FSH but not LH reductions.[79] The time course of suppression and recovery parallels that observed in the euthyroid sick syndrome and also occurs under similar circumstances.

The pathophysiology of the hypogonadotropic syndrome associated with acute illness is multifactorial. A stress response can reduce LH and testicular androgen levels.[79–81] Drugs such as dopamine, exogenous glucocorticoids,[81] and opioids, which are frequently being administered, can suppress LH or testosterone directly. Head injury can interdict pituitary LH release through mechanical stalk section or through metabolic mechanisms. Complete fasting or diminished nutritional intake lowers LH by diminishing the amplitude of LH pulses.[82] Interestingly, acute regulation of estrogen production by the enzyme aromatase occurs as well. As shown in men undergoing cardiac surgery or in groups with septic shock, the rate of aromatization of androgens to estrogens increases by up to sixfold.[83] The mechanism for this acute regulation is unexplained but could reflect a rise in cortisol or certain cytokines that are known enhancers of aromatase transcription. These observations support the clinical caveat that evaluation of the hypothalamic-pituitary-testicular axis to assess permanent defects should not be undertaken in hospitalized patients with acute illness.

Chronic Illnesses. Systemic illness of sufficient severity may cause hypogonadism in the adult.[84] Malnutrition is a factor in some instances.[85] Studies in male primates suggest that there is a defect in GnRH release at the level of the hypothalamic pulse generator during restricted food intake.[86] Intestinal disease that produces weight loss or frank malabsorption may be associated with hypogonadotropic hypogonadism. Adolescents are particularly sensitive to the gonadotropin-suppressing effects of systemic illness and weight loss.

Relative hypogonadotropism is also observed in a group of patients presenting with erectile dysfunction and low testosterone levels. These men frequently take multiple medications and have a variety of underlying medical conditions. Normal responses to clomiphene suggest that the problem is functional and may be related to chronic illness.[87]

Strenuous Exercise. Military endurance training for a 5-day period causes a profound reduction of testosterone and LH levels.[88] Chronic long-distance running may also reduce testosterone and LH levels although the results reported have varied, perhaps as a reflection of the degree of exercise intensity or associated stress.[89] Only anecdotal reports suggest the presence of diminished libido. No systematic studies have shed light on the presence, degree, or

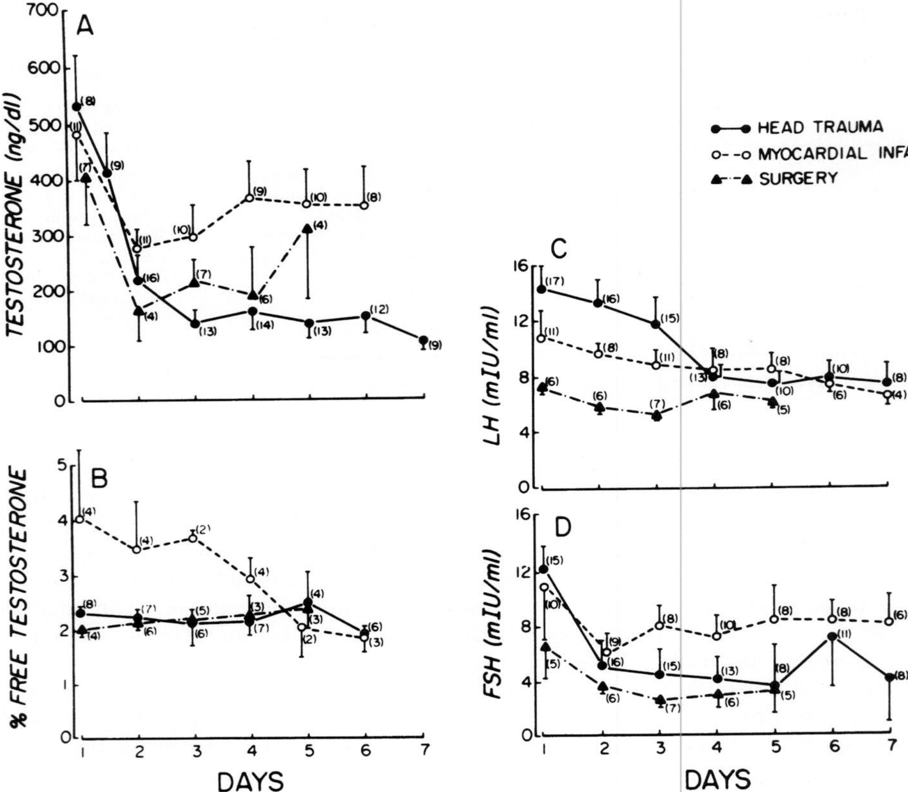

Figure 23–11 ■ Daily plasma total and percentage of ultrafilterable testosterone, LH, and FSH levels in 17 men with traumatic brain injury, 11 men with myocardial infarction, and 7 men undergoing elective surgery. (*A* to *D* from Wolff PD, Hamill RW, McDonald JV, et al. Transient hypogonadotropic hypogonadism caused by critical illness. J Clin Endocrinol Metab 60:444–450, 1985. © The Endocrine Society.)

severity of hypogonadal symptoms that may occur as a result of prolonged strenuous activity.[90] Acute marathon running is paradoxically associated with an increase in testosterone levels as a result of hemoconcentration and perhaps also of reduced testosterone clearance.[91]

Emotional Disorders. Adult men with anorexia nervosa have gonadotropin deficiency and hypogonadism in association with weight loss. In adolescents, psychiatric illness or emotional stress may cause inhibition of gonadotropin secretion or delay the pubertal process. In children, severe psychiatric illness as a cause of delayed puberty is usually not difficult to diagnose. Milder forms of psychologic problems, however, may be confirmed only by excluding the presence of organic disease. One variant of this condition appears to be a fear of becoming obese.[92]

A unifying pathophysiologic mechanism for hypogonadotropic hypogonadism in these disorders may relate to the effects of stress.[88] Corticotropin-releasing factor (CRF) levels increase in response to stress. CRF, in turn, stimulates β-endorphin levels, which then directly inhibit release of GnRH. Administration of opiate antagonists to experimentally stressed primates reversed the inhibition of stress-induced gonadotropin secretion.[93] These observations suggest that various systemic illnesses induce stress, which in turn produces increased CRF levels, increased endogenous opiate secretion, and decreased GnRH release. Hypogonadotropic hypogonadism would then occur as a result.

Acquired Immunodeficiency Syndrome (AIDS). Histopathologic changes in the testes of men dying of AIDS are common and include decreased spermatogenesis, thickened basement membranes, and interstitial infiltrates.[94] With polymerase chain reaction methodology, human immunodeficiency virus DNA can be shown to selectively infect the spermatogonia.[95] *Mycobacterium avium-intracellulare*, toxoplasma, or cytomegalovirus is present in the testes of 39 percent of patients with disseminated AIDS.[96] Low testosterone levels occur in approximately half of men with AIDS and AIDS-related complex.[94, 97, 98] Impotence is common. Several studies that measured LH levels indicated hypogonadotropism as the cause of androgen deficiency.[94] Adequate responses to GnRH suggested lack of involvement of the pituitary itself. The mechanism for low androgen levels is controversial, however, because other investigators detected primarily hypergonadotropic hypogonadism.[99] Medications can also be associated with lowered testosterone levels and particularly ketoconazole and megestrol acetate, drugs frequently given to men with AIDS.[94]

Obesity. Massive obesity is associated with low testosterone levels, low to low-normal LH levels, and reduced LH pulse amplitude.[100] Reductions in levels of SHBG (see Fig. 23–1) are partially responsible for the lowering of total testosterone levels, but free or weakly bound testosterone levels are low as well. Leydig cell function, as assessed by responsiveness to exogenous hCG, is normal. Increased aromatization of testosterone to estradiol is present, but the testosterone levels can be returned to normal with weight loss of insufficient degree to lower estradiol levels. Consequently, aromatization of testosterone to estradiol is not the only factor involved in diminished gonadotropin secretion.[101]

Drugs. Narcotic analgesics reduce the secretion of LH

and testosterone, resulting in hypogonadotropic hypogonadism of reversible type. Men who abuse narcotics often develop symptoms of erectile dysfunction.

Liver Disease. Hypogonadism, gynecomastia, and testicular atrophy are commonly observed in men with hepatic cirrhosis.[102] The extent of reduction in testosterone correlates with the severity of liver disease. One of several different mechanisms may be responsible for these findings. Men with hypogonadotropic and hypergonadotropic subtypes of hypogonadism are encountered. In the hypogonadotropic subgroup, LH and FSH levels may be suppressed because of associated malnutrition or because of enhanced aromatization of testosterone to estradiol and increased estrogen negative feedback.[102] The hypergonadotropic group has a form of primary gonadal disease characterized by high LH levels and diminished testosterone response to exogenous hCG. The direct inhibiting effects of alcohol on testicular steroidogenesis may partially explain this abnormality. Additional effects of alcohol on the liver, which increase testosterone metabolic clearance rate, may also lower circulating androgen concentrations.

Renal Disease. Chronic renal failure is associated with hypogonadism and hyperprolactinemia.[103] Erectile dysfunction, related partially to the low androgen levels and partially to associated neuropathy and vascular disease, is a common complaint. The pathophysiology of the hypogonadism is complex. A reduced metabolic clearance rate of LH leads to an increased plasma LH concentration in patients with a marked reduction in renal function. A component of primary testicular failure leads to an increase in LH production rate in approximately 20 percent of men. However, the major defect involves hypothalamic dysfunction, which results in relative hypogonadotropism. Administration of the antiestrogen clomiphene citrate stimulates return of gonadotropin and testosterone secretion to normal in these patients, suggesting that an abnormality of negative feedback set-point exists.[103] Analysis of pulsatile LH secretion suggests that impaired release of GnRH results in a reduction of the mass of LH released per pulse. This compromises the ability to increase LH secretion sufficiently to overcome the primary testicular defect.[104]

Hemochromatosis. Hemochromatosis of both primary and secondary (e.g., β-thalassemia with transfusion-induced iron overload) origin involves the pituitary, and iron can be demonstrated there by magnetic resonance imaging. Gonadotropin deficiency and hypogonadism are commonly present. Impotence usually precedes the diagnosis of hemochromatosis. Symptoms are exacerbated in the presence of cirrhosis and diabetes. Although primary testicular involvement may also occur, the pituitary defect appears to predominate. Marked iron deposition in the pituitary leads to functional impairment of the gonadotrophs. Some but not all patients experience improved gonadal function after prolonged therapy with phlebotomy.[105]

Spinal Cord Damage. Injury to the spinal cord induces a variable reduction in testosterone production, resulting in erectile dysfunction and hypospermatogenesis in more than half of such patients.[106]

Hypophysitis. Lymphocytic hypophysitis causes isolated gonadotropin deficiency and fractional panhypopituitarism. This rare disorder occurs predominantly in women and is associated with autoantibodies to multiple endocrine organs but particularly the thyroid.[40, 107] Granulomatous and necrotizing forms occur less commonly.[40]

Glucocorticoids. Cushing's syndrome and glucocorticoid administration are associated with reduced testosterone levels. Both central and direct gonadal effects of glucocorticoids are involved.[108]

Functional Causes: Physiologic Delayed Puberty (Constitutional Delay)

Physiologic delayed puberty is a common disorder that often appears to be familial but may occur sporadically.[109] From an early age, boys with this disorder lag 1 to 3 years behind their peers in linear growth and in bone age; they may fall as low as the first percentile on growth charts. Puberty is usually initiated between ages 14 and 18 years but may be delayed to age 20 to 24 years in rare instances. The diagnosis is suspected in a short adolescent boy with no significant testicular enlargement whose father, brothers, or cousins initiated puberty between the ages of 14 and 18 years. In some instances, no family history can be elicited. The absence of hyposmia, anosmia, cryptorchidism, and other congenital anomalies supports the diagnosis of physiologic delay. Retardation in bone age or height to more than 3.5 SD below the mean raises the possibility that there is an organic cause of delayed puberty. In addition, clinical evidence of growth hormone, thyroxine, or cortisol deficiency by history or physical examination points to organic rather than physiologic causes of delayed sexual maturation.

The major problem in diagnosis is the differentiation of boys with physiologic delayed puberty from those with complete or incomplete forms of hypogonadotropic eunuchoidism. Because it is inappropriate to withhold treatment until late in the teenage period in patients with organic hypogonadotropic hypogonadism, efforts have been made to develop functional tests to identify patients who will ultimately undergo spontaneous sexual development. No definitive methods to make this distinction currently exist (see Kallmann's syndrome earlier). Progressive increments in gonadotropin titers during a period of months point to physiologic delayed adolescence rather than to organic hypogonadotropic hypogonadism (see Fig. 23–10). A clearly pubertal response to a single bolus of GnRH, GnRH infusions, or long-acting GnRH favors physiologic delay, although caution must be advised in drawing definitive conclusions from these tests.

HYPERGONADOTROPIC HYPOGONADISM

See Table 23–7 for the classification of hypergonadotropic hypogonadism.

Gonadal Defects

Genetic Disorders

KLINEFELTER'S SYNDROME

Klinefelter's syndrome, the most common disorder causing male hypogonadism, is defined as a type of testicular dysgenesis characterized by the presence of one or more super-

■ TABLE 23–7
Classification of Hypergonadotropic Hypogonadism

Gonadal Defects

Genetic
- Klinefelter's syndrome
- Myotonic dystrophy
- Webbed neck, ptosis
- XYY syndrome
- Down syndrome
- Miscellaneous

Anatomic
- Functional prepubertal castrate

Gonadal toxin–induced
- Drugs
- Ionizing radiation

Enzymatic
- 17α-hydroxylase/17,20-lyase deficiency
- 17-ketoreductase deficiency
- 5 α-reductase deficiency

Viral
- Mumps orchitis

Diabetes mellitus

Gerontologic
- Male climacteric

Hormone Resistance

Androgen insensitivity
Luteinizing hormone resistance

numerary X chromosomes (Table 23–8). The classic (XXY) form occurs in approximately 1 in 500 males (0.21 percent of infants, 0.15 to 0.24 percent of adults).[110] In boys, the defect in testosterone secretion is often partial; androgen-related somatic changes occur at puberty but are incomplete. In adults, this disorder is suspected in men with firm testes less than 2.0 cm in length who have clinical signs of androgen deficiency of variable degree. Gynecomastia occurs in 85 percent of patients. The arm span is usually more than 2 cm longer than the patient's height, and the floor to pubis length is usually 2 cm greater than the distance from the pubis to the crown of the head. These disproportionate body measurements are called eunuchoidal proportions. Patients with this syndrome are of normal stature or are tall.

Large prospective surveys show that mean intelligence test scores and educational levels achieved are lower in men with Klinefelter's syndrome compared with those of control subjects of similar age.[110] A slightly increased proportion of patients with Klinefelter's syndrome may have frankly subnormal intelligence; however, case selection methods may bias these results toward identification of a greater number of patients of subnormal intelligence than occurs among the general population. Personality disorders are reported to occur more commonly in men with Klinefelter's syndrome than in the general population. This finding could be ascribed to the problems encountered in adjusting to androgen deficiency and altered physical habitus or could occur as a primary manifestation of the genetic process.

Patients with this disorder are most commonly detected on routine physical examination on the basis of small testes. Additional cases are discovered among patients with azoospermia (i.e., complete lack of spermatozoa) at infertility clinics. Patients with Klinefelter's syndrome usually do not seek medical attention because of signs or symptoms of androgen deficiency, even though these features are commonly present. For this reason, the majority of patients with this common syndrome escape diagnosis.

The testes of pubertal boys with Klinefelter's syndrome

■ TABLE 23–8
Clinical Features of Klinefelter's Syndrome

	CLASSIC FORM		VARIANT FORM	
VARIABLE	**XXY**	**XX**	**Mosaic Forms***	**Poly X + Y***
Incidence	1:500	1:9000	Unknown	Unknown
Clinical features	Testes <2 cm and firm Eunuchoid proportions Gynecomastia Personality disorder Androgen deficiency of variable degree	Shorter in stature Hypospadias	Testes may be normal size	Increased incidence of cryptorchidism and radioulnar synostosis
Laboratory findings	Luteinizing hormone increased Follicle-stimulating hormone increased Testosterone decreased in 50% Barr body (+) 47,XXY karyotype Azoospermia	46,XX karyotype	XXY/XY, XXY/XX Spermatogenesis variably present	XXXY, XXXXY, XXXXXY
Testis biopsy	Hyalinized tubules Relative Leydig cell hyperplasia		Less severe damage	

*Divergent features only are listed.
Adapted from Bardin CW, Paulsen CA. The testes. *In* Williams RD (ed). Textbook of Endocrinology, 6th ed. Phiadelphia, WB Saunders, 1981, p 293.

are smaller than normal. By adulthood, nearly all patients with classic Klinefelter's syndrome have lost their total complement of germinal cells in the testes. As a consequence, their testes remain small, and their semen contains no spermatozoa. The exact mechanisms responsible for the testicular dysfunction are inferred from observations in animals. The presence of an extra X chromosome commits the germ cells to a shortened life span. In a variety of animal species as well as in humans, a normal complement of primordial germ cells is present in the fetal testis of XXY males, but these die at an accelerated rate during the patient's childhood.

The degree of Leydig cell dysfunction in Klinefelter's syndrome is variable. Mean testosterone concentrations in patients as a group are approximately half those in normal men (i.e., 300 ng/dl compared with 600 ng/dl). However, 43 percent of men in one series had total testosterone levels in the normal (albeit low-normal) range.[111] Plasma estradiol concentration, on the other hand, was twofold higher in patients than in control subjects (30 versus 15 pg/ml).[111] This results from an increased fraction of testosterone converted to estradiol in peripheral tissues (0.60 percent in Klinefelter's syndrome versus 0.38 percent in normal men).[111] In response to elevated estradiol concentration, plasma SHBG level increases and the fraction of non–SHBG-bound testosterone is reduced. Consequently, some patients with normal total testosterone levels exhibit low free and weakly bound testosterone concentrations.

A common variant form of Klinefelter's syndrome is the XX subtype (the "sex reversal syndrome"), which occurs in 1 in 9000 men and mimics the XXY variety in most respects (see Table 23–8). However, XX individuals are shorter (168 ± 0.77 cm) and have a 9 percent incidence of hypospadias.[112] The testis-determining factor *(SRY)* gene, present in normal males on the Y chromosome, is uniformly present on the X chromosome in such patients, as shown by DNA hybridization testing.

Patients with mosaic forms of Klinefelter's syndrome exhibit variable cytogenetic findings. Mosaicism may be present in cell lines from all tissues. Supernumerary X cell lines may also exist exclusively in testicular tissue. Testicular biopsy with karyotyping of testicular fibroblasts is required to diagnose such mosaicism. Variable degrees of spermatogenesis and, occasionally, normal-sized testes may be present in some of these individuals; fertility is possible. Such individuals usually undergo a progressive loss of spermatogenesis, Leydig cell function, and testicular size if they are observed over time. In the poly X plus Y variant of Klinefelter's syndrome, the incidence of cryptorchidism is increased, severe deficits in intellectual function occur, and radioulnar synostosis is found.

The diagnosis of Klinefelter's syndrome of any type is presumed when buccal smear analysis reveals Barr bodies in a phenotypic male. Confirmation requires karyotype analysis of blood lymphocytes or of testis tissue in rare instances when mosaicism is limited to the testis. Elevation of plasma FSH concentration is uniformly present and LH nearly so. Response to exogenous hCG is blunted, indicating that testicular reserve function is decreased.

Testicular biopsy reveals peritubular hyalinization, tubular sclerosis, and adenomatous hyperplasia of Leydig cells. The hyperplastic appearance of the Leydig cells is deceiving; it reflects the marked reduction in seminiferous tubule mass with relative preservation of interstitial tissue. In actuality, quantitative morphometric studies reveal a reduced number of Leydig cells.

Treatment consists of counseling regarding the presence of infertility and provision of androgen replacement therapy if clinical circumstances warrant. Individuals with testosterone levels in the low-normal range in the face of high LH levels deserve a therapeutic trial of androgen replacement, even though they may not complain of androgen deficiency symptoms. Many of these individuals improve their sense of well-being and sexual potency during such therapy.

MYOTONIC DYSTROPHY

Myotonic dystrophy is a familial disorder characterized by cataracts, baldness, muscle weakness, and hypogonadism in 80 percent of affected males. The testes are small and soft, resulting from partial to complete germinal cell destruction. Leydig cell morphologic features appear normal, but function is compromised and maintained only by secretion of high levels of LH. Testosterone concentration ranges from moderately reduced to low-normal. Clinical signs of androgen deficiency vary and correlate with the level of plasma testosterone. FSH concentration is uniformly increased.[113] Definitive diagnosis is possible with DNA analysis.

SYNDROME OF WEBBED NECK, PTOSIS, HYPOGONADISM, CONGENITAL HEART DISEASE, AND SHORT STATURE (NOONAN'S SYNDROME, MALE TURNER'S SYNDROME)

The clinical association of diminished testicular function and phenotypic stigmata of Turner's syndrome was once classified as the male Turner's syndrome. Clinical findings in these patients may include facies typical of Turner's syndrome in girls, a webbed neck, short stature, low-set ears, ptosis, shield-like chest, cryptorchidism, diminished spermatogenesis, decreased Leydig cell function, cubitus valgus, and cardiovascular anomalies (especially pulmonic stenosis).[114] Also present may be mental retardation, low hairline, small penis, and lymphedema of the hands and feet, particularly at birth.

The diagnosis is limited to patients with four or more cardinal features of the syndrome and a normal chromosomal constitution. Use of the term *male Turner's syndrome* has been discouraged because more than 95 percent of patients with the cardinal features of this syndrome have a normal karyotype.[114] Gonadotropin levels may be elevated, reflective of a reduction in germ cell or Leydig cell function. Sterility and cryptorchidism are common.

XYY SYNDROME

This disorder has been identified with higher frequency among men with tall stature and severe nodular cystic acne. The condition is common and affects 0.1 to 0.2 percent of live male newborns.[110] Mean intelligence and educational level achieved by these patients are lower than those for normal control subjects of the same age.[110] These individuals have a high incidence of convictions for criminal behavior (i.e., 45 percent) compared with 9.3 percent in a control group in one study.[110] However, the criminal behavior appears to relate more to the diminished intellectual function and its concomitant adjustment patterns than to aggressive behavior imparted by the extra Y chromosome.

Endocrine studies reveal normal LH, FSH, and testosterone levels in the majority of these patients and elevated gonadotropin titers in the minority.[115, 116] Numerous case reports of patients with an XYY karyotype with defective sperm production or Leydig cell function have appeared. The actual frequency of these abnormalities among all patients with this karyotype is unknown. The significance of an XYY karyotype in an otherwise normal patient is unclear, and caution is advised so as to avoid alarming the patient or his parents if the diagnosis is made fortuitously on the basis of routine screening.

DOWN SYNDROME

A mild degree of testicular dysfunction occurs in patients with the Down syndrome. LH levels are elevated, even though Leydig cells appear normal on testicular biopsy. A moderate to severe reduction in all germ cell types, germ cell arrest, and Sertoli cell–only patterns can be seen. Levels of FSH may be normal or elevated.

MISCELLANEOUS GENETIC DISORDERS

A variety of clinical syndromes identified on the basis of their specific nontesticular features involve testicular dysfunction. Sickle cell disease is associated with low testosterone levels in conjunction with high LH and FSH concentrations and a reduced response to exogenous GnRH.[117] Certain autoimmune disorders are associated with testicular failure and other endocrine deficiency states.[118]

Functional Prepubertal Castrate Syndrome (Anorchia)

Individuals with functional prepubertal castrate syndrome[119] manifest signs and symptoms of severe androgen deficiency and lack anatomically demonstrable or functioning testes. The appearance of the external genitalia is normal, with the exception of an empty scrotum. Bilateral testicular torsion probably explains the loss of testes in most of these patients. This disorder may be partial, resulting from incomplete interference with the vascular supply to the testes, occurring on occasion during bilateral hernia repair or performance of bilateral orchidopexy.

Patients with complete anorchia present with suspected bilateral cryptorchidism before puberty or sexual infantilism in the teenage or adult years. Palpation of the scrotum reveals the vas deferens or small masses of tissue consisting of wolffian duct remnants. Elevated gonadotropin levels for age may be documented even in childhood. In the pubertal years, the levels of LH and FSH increase and ultimately reach adult castrate levels in patients with anorchia. The finding of normal gonadotropin levels in a pubertal or adult patient suspected of having anorchia excludes this condition and prompts a search for cryptorchid testes. Alternatively, levels of LH and FSH in the castrate (high) range, in conjunction with very low testosterone levels, strongly suggest anorchia.

The differential diagnosis between bilateral cryptorchidism and anorchia can usually be made at any age by employing the hCG test. After 2 weeks of administration of 1000 to 2000 IU of hCG three times per week, patients with functioning testes generally attain adult male testosterone levels, whereas those without testes exhibit no increase in testosterone concentration. Cryptorchid testes often descend during this regimen.

Gonadal Toxins

Cytotoxic drugs used as treatment of the nephrotic syndrome or of neoplastic diseases commonly produce testicular damage.[120] The alkylating agents are particularly common offenders. Nearly 100 percent of patients receiving MOPP (mechlorethamine, vincristine, procarbazine, prednisone) chemotherapy develop azoospermia and compromised androgen production. Dactinomycin, vincristine, and vinblastine appear not to affect spermatogenesis regardless of dose, whereas agents such as cisplatin produce intermediate effects. For Hodgkin's disease, ABVD (doxorubicin, bleomycin, vinblastine, and dacarbazine) produces azoospermia in only 35 percent of patients, whereas an equally efficacious regimen such as MOPP produces azoospermia in 100 percent of subjects. Other drugs may also cause testicular dysfunction. Amiodarone is associated with increases in LH and FSH levels and sexual dysfunction in aging men that exceed those in men not taking this drug.

Radiation therapy that includes the gonads results in testicular failure.[121] Damage occurs in prepubertal and adult men and may be potentiated by cytotoxic chemotherapy.[122–126] Damage is dependent on the dose and the duration of therapy.[126] Spermatogenic elements are more sensitive than Leydig cells to radiation therapy or radiomimetic drugs. Consequently, each of these agents may compromise spermatogenesis to a greater extent than androgen production, and monotropic FSH rises may be observed. Radiation doses as low as 15 rad transiently compromise the pool of spermatogonial cells, and 600 rad permanently destroys germinal elements.[127] Permanent Leydig cell dysfunction occurs with doses of 2000 to 3000 rad, as in treatment of lymphoblastic leukemia with testicular involvement. Subtle defects in LH secretion occur in patients receiving chemotherapeutic agents as well.[128] Various regimens designed to induce protection of the testes during chemotherapy have been attempted, but results are generally disappointing.[129]

When potential fertility is discussed with patients about to undergo cytotoxic therapy, the possibility of banking of sperm requires exploration. However, studies have revealed a high incidence of hypogonadism before initiation of therapy in groups of patients with malignant disorders.[130] Defects in both pituitary and gonadal function are encountered, which explains the reduction in testosterone levels.

Environmental toxins or habitually abused agents that adversely affect Leydig cell function or spermatogenesis have been insufficiently investigated. Under experimental conditions, marijuana causes a reduction in sperm count and motility[131]; the frequency and the severity of the abnormalities produced under noncontrolled conditions are currently unknown. Alcohol also exerts a direct effect on testicular steroidogenesis and may contribute to testicular dysfunction.[132] Industrial hydrocarbon exposure, particularly to polychlorinated insecticides and dibromochloropropane, has been associated with a reduction in sperm count.[133]

Enzyme Defects

Several defects in steroidogenic enzymes result in deficient testosterone production and reflex elevations in gonadotropin production (see Chapters 14 and 15). Three involve cortisol secretion and can be life threatening. Signs and symptoms of adrenal insufficiency bring these patients to clinical attention, and a diagnosis is made after exploring causes of cortisol deficiency. Three other defects involve androgen but not cortisol secretion.[134–137] These include 17α-hydroxylase/17,20-lyase, 17-ketosteroid reductase, and 5α-reductase deficiencies.[136, 137] (17α-hydroxylase deficiency causes decreased cortisol levels, but not clinical cortisol deficiency.) Patients with these defects present as phenotypic females with partial virilization at puberty. However, incomplete defects may result in androgenized males with hypospadias, gynecomastia, and lack of full pubertal development. In the 17α-hydroxylase defect, hypertension and hypokalemia are present because of increased adrenal mineralocorticoid production. The 5α-reductase deficiency syndrome is described later. Definitive diagnosis is made by demonstration of elevated levels of precursor steroids in the presence of low testosterone or DHT levels.

Mumps Orchitis

In 15 to 25 percent of pubertal or postpubertal subjects, mumps involves the testes and produces a highly painful, inflammatory disorder. After the acute illness subsides, the germ cells gradually degenerate during a period of several years, and Leydig cell dysfunction develops. Gynecomastia and testicular atrophy may be present as well as clinical evidence of androgen deficiency. Evaluation reveals low testosterone levels, low sperm counts, and high serum or urine LH and FSH concentrations. The diagnosis is made in a patient with a clinical picture suggesting Klinefelter's syndrome but with a history of mumps and a normal blood cell karyotype.

Diabetes Mellitus

Erectile dysfunction occurs in 50 percent of diabetic men[138] and may reflect neurologic, vascular, psychologic, or endocrine causes. The possibility that primary gonadal failure may explain erectile dysfunction in a subset of diabetic patients has been generally controversial. Conflicting reports indicate normal or low serum testosterone[138–147] and variable gonadotropin concentrations in these patients.[138] One study separated diabetic patients into those with psychogenic impotence and those with organic impotence on the basis of nocturnal penile tumescence testing.[138] In the organic impotence group, extensive evaluation revealed convincing evidence of gonadal dysfunction. Specifically, free testosterone concentrations were low and urinary and integrated plasma LH levels were high compared with those in control subjects and diabetic men with psychogenic impotence. Androgen replacement in the group with organic impotence without vascular disease improved nocturnal penile tumescence testing results, and symptoms of impotence improved.[138]

Male Climacteric

Clinical, histopathologic, and hormonal studies indicate that gonadal function declines gradually as a function of age in men. The defect exists both at the level of the testes and in the hypothalamic-pituitary axis. Clinical observations include a gradual reduction in total, free, and bioavailable testosterone (see Fig. 23–2); increases in the levels of LH and FSH measured by some but not all assays; and blunted testosterone responses to hCG.[148–153] Inhibin levels[154] are lower in elderly than in young men as a reflection of reduced Sertoli cell function. Histologic studies reveal an age-related decline in Leydig[149] as well as in Sertoli cells,[150] and sperm production diminishes.[151] Symptoms of decreased sexual function may correlate with these changes.[148] Subsets of healthy men exhibit lesser degrees of these abnormalities,[155] suggesting that an age-related increase in chronic illness may contribute to the observed gonadal dysfunction.[156]

Although a primary testicular defect is present, careful assessment of LH pulsatility in aging men revealed an increase in frequency but reduction in pulse amplitude and mass of LH secreted per pulse.[157, 158] Other studies using less stringent methodology have found divergent effects.[159, 160] Additional abnormalities include loss of the diurnal pattern of testosterone secretion[161] and alterations of opiate tone[160] and androgen negative feedback.[162]

Hormone Resistance

Androgen Insensitivity

The genetic male with complete insensitivity to androgens presents as a phenotypic female with primary amenorrhea and breast development, the so-called testicular feminization syndrome. As a manifestation of androgen resistance, these individuals lack facial, axillary, and pubic hair and have female external genitalia. The distal two thirds of the vagina is well developed, but the proximal third and the uterus and fallopian tubes are absent. Testosterone, estradiol, and LH levels are high, whereas FSH levels are normal. Testicular biopsy reveals immature germ cells because of the insensitivity to androgen. The Leydig cells are hyperplastic as a result of the elevated LH levels, and adenomatous clumps may be observed. The androgen resistance may be due to a complete lack of androgen receptors, a defect in receptor function, or postreceptor defects.[163] Most commonly, point mutations of the androgen receptor occur[164–166] (Fig. 23–12). These mutations can result in premature termination of transcription of the androgen receptor mRNA, derangements of splicing of the mRNA sequences, or synthesis of androgen receptors with reduced affinity for androgen. Less commonly, whole exons are deleted and the androgen receptor mRNA is markedly truncated.[167] Each of these mutations produces androgen receptors with reduced or absent capacity to mediate androgenic effects.[165–168] It is of interest that all mutations have involved the DNA- or hormone-binding regions of the receptor but not the N-terminal portion that is involved in

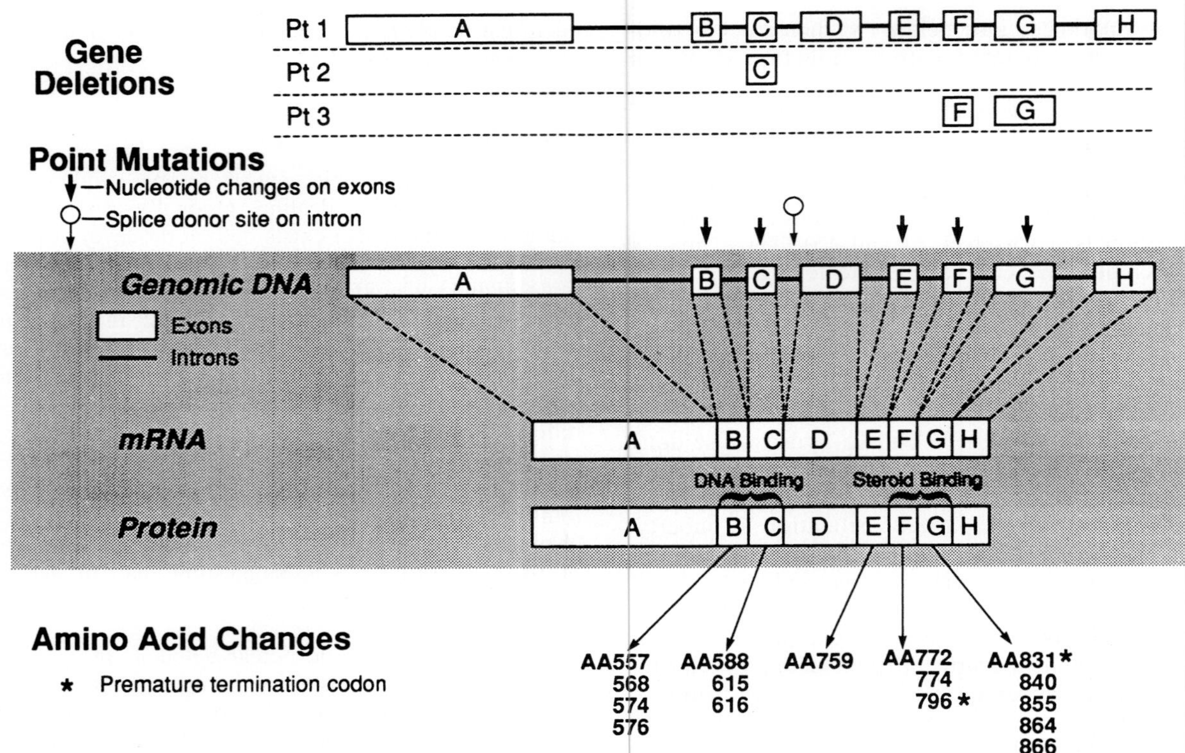

Figure 23–12 ■ Diagrammatic representation of recently described genetic mutations associated with androgen insensitivity. Gene deletions, sites of point mutations, and locations of amino acid changes are indicated. (From Santen RJ. The testis. *In* Felig P, Baxter JD, Frohman LA [eds]. Endocrinology and Metabolism, 3rd ed. New York, McGraw-Hill, 1995, p 934.)

the AF-1 mediation of receptor-induced transcription. Some individuals have receptor defects that reduce the affinity of androgen for the receptor. These individuals can be treated with high doses of androgen to overcome the reduced affinity state.

Increases in the number of glutamine repeats in exon 1 result in androgen insensitivity associated with spinal and bulbar muscular atrophy (Kennedy's syndrome).[169] Although incompletely understood, the neurologic deficit may relate to the known presence of androgen receptors in the spinal and bulbar motor neurons.

Incomplete insensitivity to androgens produces a clinical spectrum ranging from features of severe undervirilization to normally virilized men with infertility or even fertile men with minimal undervirilization. These patients experience pubertal onset at an appropriate age but usually fail to androgenize completely. Gynecomastia, hypospadias, bifid scrotum, and cryptorchidism are common. LH levels are usually elevated, reflecting resistance to androgens at the hypothalamic-pituitary level.[170] FSH levels are usually normal.

Diagnosis requires demonstration of quantitative or qualitative abnormalities of the androgen receptor[171] and demonstration of the genetic aberration. Lack of suppression of SHBG levels with the anabolic androgen stanozolol may provide a screening method to identify patients for definitive receptor measurements,[172] but its use requires wider confirmation. Treatment with high-dose androgen therapy in postpubertal patients produced limited results, whereas encouraging beneficial effects were observed in one prepubertal patient.[171]

Partial androgen resistance may represent a common cause of oligospermia or azoospermia in patients with infertility. Clinically, these men exhibit minimal evidence of undervirilization and normal levels of LH and testosterone. The reported frequency of this disorder in men with azoospermia ranges from rare to as high as 40 percent.[173–177]

Another type of partial androgen resistance results from the loss-of-function mutation of 5α-reductase, the enzyme that converts testosterone to DHT.[178, 179] Patients with this defect exhibit a characteristic form of male pseudohermaphroditism, originally termed pseudovaginal perineoscrotal hypospadias. They are usually raised as females. Their excretory duct system, including epididymides, vasa deferentia, seminal vesicles, and ejaculatory ducts, are normal male in type, but the ejaculatory ducts terminate in a vagina and the external genitalia are ambiguous. At puberty, partial virilization with penile growth and increase in muscle mass ensue. Facial hair, acne, and frontal balding are lacking. In primitive cultures, these individuals take on a male role at puberty. Spermatogenesis is usually impaired, either as a result of 5α-reductase deficiency and subsequent reduction of testicular DHT levels or as a consequence of the cryptorchid position of the testes.[179] Semen volume, as a reflection of low DHT levels, is significantly reduced.[180]

Luteinizing Hormone Resistance

LH resistance is associated with sexual immaturity, elevated LH and low testosterone concentrations, and unstimulated testes.[181] Two novel homozygous, inactivating, missense mutations of the LH receptor gene (Arg 554→stop codon 554(TGA) and Ser 616→Tyr 616) are responsible for LH resistance in one reported series. Secretion of an immunologically recognizable but biologically inactive LH molecule exactly mimics this syndrome; measurement of LH concentration by bioassay as well as by radioimmunoassay is required to identify this disorder.[182]

Estradiol Resistance and Aromatase Deficiency

A defect in the estrogen receptor causing complete estradiol resistance results in elevated LH, FSH, and testosterone levels as well as delayed or absent closure of the epiphyses. A defect in estrogen production due to a mutation in the aromatase gene causes an identical phenotype. These syndromes, supported by observations in an estrogen receptor knockout experiment in mice, indicate that estradiol is required for epiphyseal closure whereas testosterone stimulates long bone growth.[183–185]

TREATMENT OF HYPOGONADISM

(Table 23–9)

Delayed Adolescence

Major psychologic effects may result from a delay in adolescent sexual development. Patients with untreated delayed puberty exhibit continued diminution of the bone mineral density of the femoral neck, radius, and spine on evaluation several years after they have completed puberty.[186] Precise differentiation of physiologically delayed adolescence from isolated gonadotropin deficiency may not always be possible in boys of pubertal age. These considerations favor treatment empirically in patients older than 14 years when clinical circumstances, and specifically the psychologic needs of the patient, warrant. The usual strategy is to initiate androgenic effects with intermittent subreplacement doses of testosterone (i.e., maintenance of testosterone levels of 100 to 300 ng/dl) and then interrupt therapy periodically to observe for spontaneous maturational changes.[187] Two therapeutic modalities, administration of hCG and testosterone, are available. Testosterone is preferred because of ease of administration, cost, and predictability of response. The administration of hCG is efficacious in hypogonadotropic syndromes when Leydig cell responsiveness is adequate. A dosage of 1500 IU once or twice weekly stimulates testosterone to levels between 100 and 300 ng/dl.[188] This regimen is expensive and requires frequent injections. Its only advantage over replacement testosterone is its effect to stimulate testis size. Consequently, hCG is infrequently used as a long-term treatment modality.

Injectable esters such as testosterone enanthate or testosterone cypionate provide sustained blood levels of testosterone for 1 to 2 weeks. To initiate pubertal changes, 25 mg is administered every 2 weeks intramuscularly for 3 months followed by cessation for an equal time period. Similar intermittent courses of 50 and 100 mg intramuscularly are then administered.[187] The goal is to promote the development of secondary sexual characteristics and normal linear growth. Evidence of spontaneous pubertal development, such as testicular enlargement and spontaneous

■ TABLE 23–9
Treatment of Testis Disorders

GROUP	GOAL OF TREATMENT	TREATMENT MODALITY	DOSAGE
Delayed adolescence	Initiate androgenic effects with subreplacement doses of testosterone to maintain plasma levels of 100–300 ng/dl Promote secondary sex characteristics and normal linear growth Observe for spontaneous maturational changes during periods off medication	Testosterone enanthate or cypionate	25–100 mg q* 3–4 weeks IM† Treat for 3-month periods alternating with no therapy for 3 months for a 1- to 2-year period if physiologically delayed puberty is suspected After 2 years, if there is no spontaneous pubertal rise in testosterone, increase to adult replacement levels of testosterone
Adult hypogonadotropic hypogonadism	Long-term maintenance of testosterone levels at 300–1200 ng/dl	Transdermal patch	One scrotal patch per day *or* one 5.0 mg patch on back per day
		Testosterone enanthate or cypionate	100 mg q 7 days IM *or* 200 mg q 10–14 days *or* 300 mg q 21 days IM
		hCG	1000–4000 IU 2–3 times per week
		GnRH	2–20 μg SC‡ 2–3 times per hour
		Testosterone undecanoate	200 mg PO 4 times daily (not available in the United States)
Adult hypergonadotropic hypogonadism	Long-term maintenance of testosterone levels at 300–1200 ng/dl	Transdermal patch	One scrotal patch per day *or* one 5.0 mg patch on back per day
		Testosterone enanthate or cypionate	100 mg q 7 days IM *or* 200 mg q 10–14 days IM *or* 300 mg q 21 days IM
		Testosterone undecanoate	200 mg PO 4 times daily (not available in the United States)
	Provide subreplacement doses of androgen	Fluoxymesterone	5–10 mg PO daily
		Methyltestosterone	25 mg daily by linguet

*q = every; †IM = intramuscular; ‡SC = subcutaneous.

increments of gonadotropins and testosterone levels, should be sought during the 3 months without therapy. If no significant progression is noted, intermittent courses of low-dose testosterone at increasing increments can be administered until spontaneous puberty is initiated or the need for long-term exogenous therapy is confirmed. If the doses are kept small, this regimen has no harmful effect on potential for full somatic growth[189] or subsequent testicular function. Patients with isolated gonadotropin deficiency, when left untreated for periods of 6 years or more, experience a modest increase in adult height (approximately 5 cm) above that normally expected when androgen therapy is initiated. This information should not impede initiation of androgen therapy because final height with treatment is not reduced to below-normal levels.[190] Although not studied extensively in the setting of delayed puberty, testosterone patches may also be used provided that plasma testosterone levels are carefully monitored.

Hypergonadotropic Hypogonadism

Exogenous testosterone administration provides the only effective therapy in adults with hypergonadotropic hypogonadism and can be used as well in hypogonadotropic patients not immediately desiring to father children.[191] The goal of therapy is to maintain plasma testosterone concentration in the range of 300 to 1200 ng/dl. After elapse of sufficient time, full secondary sexual characteristics and sexual potency are attained. Testicular enlargement, an effect observed only with hCG therapy, does not occur. Oral androgens are not adequate to induce full androgen maintenance. Consequently, injectable testosterone or transdermal patches must be used.

Pharmacologic studies have fully characterized the dose-response profiles over time for the available agents[191] (Fig. 23–13). Higher doses produce more prolonged effects at the expense of higher peak levels. Because toxic effects of pharmacologic plasma concentrations of testosterone are rare, higher doses are usually chosen to prolong the effect. Suggested regimens include 300 mg of testosterone enanthate or testosterone 17β-cypionate intramuscularly every 14 to 21 days, 200 mg every 10 to 14 days, or 100 mg every 5 to 10 days. Measurement of plasma testosterone concentration at the nadir, just before the next injection, allows empirical adjustment of dosage. Levels of testosterone below 250 ng/dl during therapy can often be perceived by patients as causing impaired sexual potency or reduced endurance during physical activity.

Transdermal patches containing testosterone provide another effective means of maintaining plasma testosterone levels between 300 and 1200 ng/dl. Two delivery systems, one applied to scrotal skin and the other to the back, have recently been approved by the U.S. Food and Drug Administration (FDA).[192, 193] The concentrations of testosterone and estradiol produced with both patches mimic the diurnal levels observed in normal men (Fig. 23–14). The scrotal patch increases plasma DHT levels because of the presence of the 5α-reductase enzyme in scrotal skin. The nonscrotal patch increases DHT to normal levels. It is not known whether elevated DHT levels may produce adverse effects during long-term use of scrotal patches. Both systems are better accepted by patients than testosterone injections, predominantly because of the lack of fluctuations in hormone level that occur uniformly after injections. Cost is greater with the patches and rash occurs in up to 10 percent of subjects, particularly with the nonscrotal patches.[194] Testosterone microcapsules[195] and long-acting analogues are also undergoing development as approved means of maintaining stable testosterone levels during replacement therapy.[196, 197]

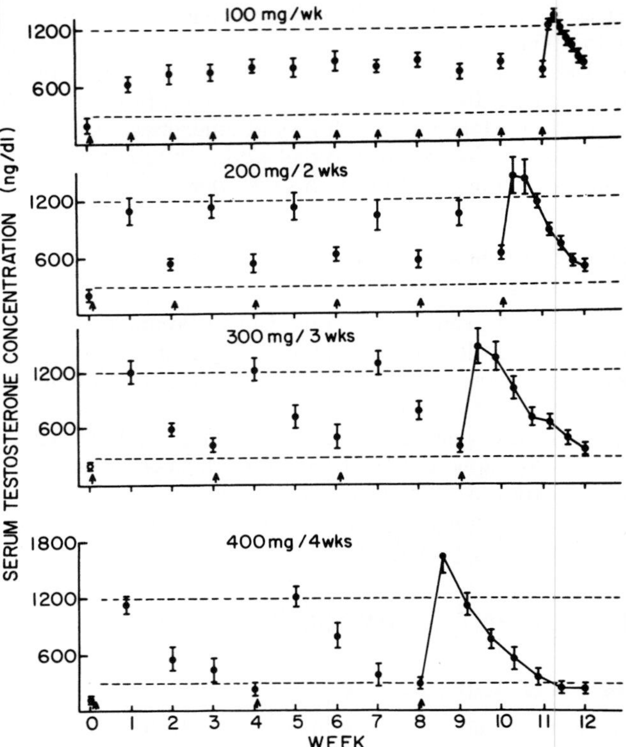

Figure 23–13 ■ Serum testosterone levels in hypogonadal men receiving androgen replacement therapy with intramuscular testosterone enanthate injections for 12 weeks in four dosage regimens: 100 mg weekly; 200 mg every 2 weeks; 300 mg every 3 weeks; and 400 mg every 4 weeks. Blood was sampled weekly until the last dose and then less frequently. Serum testosterone concentrations exhibit large fluctuations but are maintained above the lower limit of the normal range *(dashed lines)* except for the dosage regimen of 400 mg every 4 weeks, in which testosterone levels fall below the normal range after 3 weeks. (From Snyder PJ. Clinical use of androgens. Annu Rev Med 35:207–217, 1984.)

Side effects and toxicity due to testosterone replacement are uncommon. However, an increased hematocrit due to bone marrow stimulation, acne, sleep apnea syndrome, gynecomastia as a result of aromatization of testosterone to estradiol, and prostatic hypertrophy in the elderly are physiologic consequences of this therapeutic approach. Rarely, hepatic tumors have occurred in patients receiving pharmacologic levels of androgen. Only anecdotal reports have associated androgen therapy with prostatic carcinoma, and systematic data regarding this association are required to determine causative associations.[198, 199] Nonaromatizable androgens (anabolic steroids) increase low-density lipoprotein and decrease high-density lipoprotein cholesterol levels, particularly when they are given orally to exert a first-pass effect on the liver. These agents could potentially increase the risk for development of cardiovascular disease.

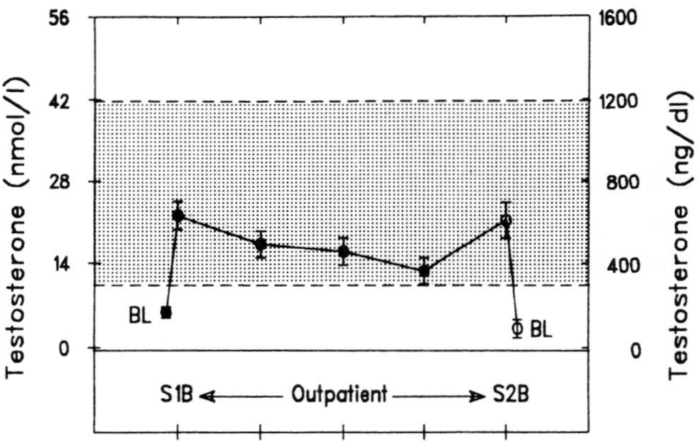

Figure 23–14 ■ Plasma testosterone levels resulting from wearing two enhanced transdermal patches on the back. The patches were applied at 2200 hours, and the plasma testosterone levels were measured in samples collected at 1000 hours. The morning testosterone levels are shown by the lines and the normal ranges by the shaded area. Testosterone levels denoted BL represent baseline levels before and after wearing the patch. The time points on the abscissa represent days 0, 7, 14, 21, and 28. (From Meikle AW, Arver S, Dobs AS, et al. Pharmacokinetics and metabolism of a permeation-enhanced testosterone transdermal system in hypogonadal men: Influence of application site—a clinical research center study. J Clin Endocrinol Metab 81:1832–1840, 1996. © The Endocrine Society.)

With aromatizable androgens (e.g., testosterone), these effects are offset by the concomitant increase in estrogen levels.[200]

Oral androgens available in the United States such as fluoxymesterone and methyltestosterone are insufficiently potent for full androgen replacement. Testosterone undecanoate, another orally absorbable androgen ester, is not available for use in the United States but is sufficiently potent for full androgen replacement.

Adult Hypogonadotropic Hypogonadism

Treatment goals in patients with adult hypogonadotropic hypogonadism include (1) maintenance of androgen levels in the normal adult male range (i.e., 300 to 1200 ng/dl) to allow full virilization and maintenance of normal bone density and (2) stimulation of spermatogenesis to allow fertility. Studies have demonstrated an improvement in mood and in muscle mass in hypogonadal men receiving testosterone.[201, 202] Therapy with exogenous testosterone is usually chosen to induce virilization, because this approach requires less frequent injections and is less costly than hCG administration. Exogenous androgen administration does not compromise later potential for fertility.[203] The approach is identical to that used in patients with hypergonadotropic hypogonadism.

Administration of hCG provides another means of maintaining normal adult male androgen levels (Fig. 23–15). A dosage of 1000 to 4000 IU intramuscularly is given two or three times per week. The exact dosage is established empirically in individual patients by measuring plasma testosterone concentrations. Testicular enlargement can be achieved, but the testes seldom exceed 3.5 cm in length in response to hCG alone. This approach is expensive, requires frequent injections, and has no advantage over direct androgen replacement therapy unless fertility is an immediate goal.

Unproven Indications for Treatment

Reductions of testosterone levels occur with aging and associated illness. No clear indications have as yet emerged

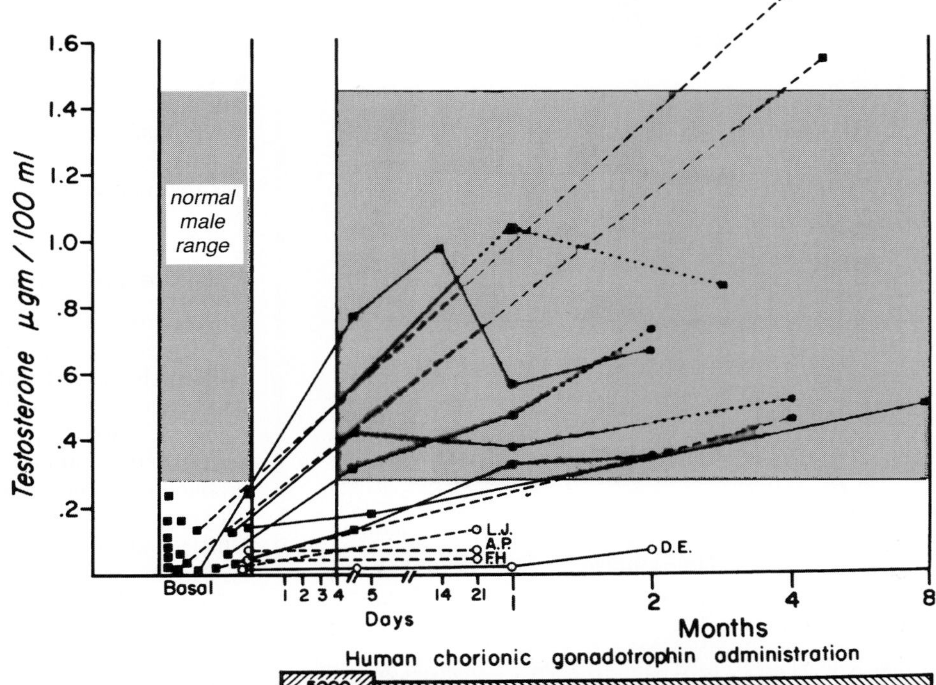

Figure 23–15 ■ Basal and stimulated levels of serum testosterone concentration in men with hypogonadotropic hypogonadism. Open circles refer to men with bilateral cryptorchidism. Dashed lines refer to patients not studied with 4-day hCG stimulation. Dotted lines refer to nonconsecutive observations of serum testosterone concentratoin. Black squares represent data points in patients with hypogonadotropic hypogonadism. (Adapted from Santen RJ, Paulsen CA. Hypogonadotropic eunuchoidism. II. Gonadal responsiveness to exogenous gonadotropins. J Clin Endocrinol Metab 36:55–63, 1973. © The Endocrine Society.)

regarding which individuals to treat. Short-term studies during androgen administration demonstrated an increase in lean body mass, a reduction in urinary hydroxyproline, an increase in hematocrit, a decline in total and low-density lipoprotein cholesterol, and a sustained increase in prostate-specific antigen levels in older men selected because of slightly reduced testosterone levels.[204, 205] Long-term studies are not yet available. Evidence of primary gonadal failure in an older man with symptoms of erectile dysfunction warrants consideration of testosterone replacement. This therapeutic option must be weighed against the possibility of adversely affecting prostate size and uroflow dynamics. At present, treatment of aging men with testosterone is considered experimental.[206] Further study is required for demonstration of efficacy and development of clear guidelines regarding evaluation and treatment of such patients.

More than two decades ago, physicians prescribed androgen to debilitated patients. A study substantiates the effects of pharmacologic doses of testosterone to increase strength, reduce lean body mass, and add bulk to muscle groups[207, 208] (Fig. 23–16). Interestingly, these doses did not increase expression of anger as assessed by objective psychologic inventory testing.[209] There is now renewed enthusiasm for use of androgens for men with chronic debilitating illness with muscle wasting and other manifestations of a catabolic state. Use of androgens in the catabolic stages of AIDS has been reported and could be beneficial. Further studies are required to establish that the benefits of this approach outweigh the risks.

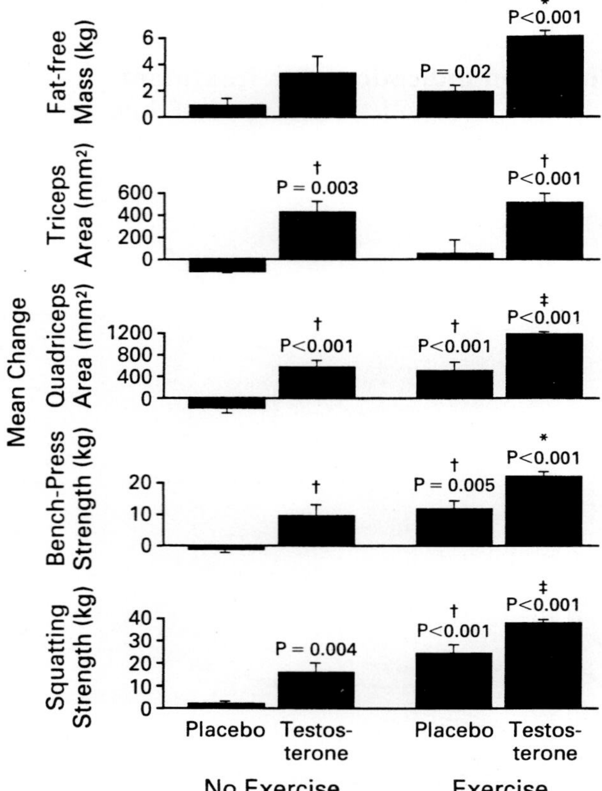

Figure 23–16 ■ Effects of high-dose testosterone in normal men. (From Bhasin S, Storer TW, Berman N, et al. The effects of supraphysiologic doses of testosterone on muscle size and strength in normal men. N Engl J Med 335:1–7, 1996. Reproduced by permission of The New England Journal of Medicine. © 1996, Massachusetts Medical Society.)

Stimulation of Spermatogenesis

Human Chorionic Gonadotropin and Human Menopausal Gonadotropin

In this method exogenous LH-like material in the form of hCG initially is administered followed by coadministration of FSH (in the form of human menopausal gonadotropin [hMG]) if necessary. Patients with adult-onset (acquired) hypogonadotropinism and incomplete forms of gonadotropin deficiency frequently achieve normal spermatogenesis when they are given 1000 to 4000 IU of hCG alone, two or three times per week for a period of 1 to 2 years. Response to monotherapy is predicted by the presence of testes that exceed prepubertal size before therapy is initiated.[210] Other patients require the addition of 75 to 150 IU of menotropins (Pergonal) three times weekly for 1 to 2 years. Administration of menotropins is started after testosterone levels have been normalized in response to hCG for at least 6 months. On average, sperm appear in the ejaculate after 18 months, and maximal sperm counts are observed after approximately 2 years of therapy. Even though quantitatively normal spermatogenesis is not achieved, more than half of the patients are successful in impregnating their sexual partners.[210] After full stimulation of spermatogenesis with hCG and hMG, maintenance of sperm production is often possible with hCG administration alone. Antibodies to hCG occasionally develop but rarely present a clinical problem.

Approximately 10 percent of patients do not achieve sperm in the ejaculate even after prolonged gonadotropin administration. It is not clear what distinguishes these patients from others. Pharmacokinetic studies indicated that standard FSH regimens produce only low-normal plasma levels of FSH. The authors suggested that use of subcutaneous injections to prolong the duration of effect and daily rather than three-times-weekly injections would increase plasma FSH levels. However, no data on the efficacy of this regimen to increase sperm counts are available.[211]

Pulsatile GnRH Therapy

On theoretical grounds, it was predicted that pulsatile GnRH treatment might provide the most physiologic means of normalizing LH and FSH levels in patients with GnRH deficiency (Kallmann's syndrome). In initial trials, patients received 5 to 30 μg of GnRH subcutaneously every 2 hours by programmed pump for 2 years or longer. Sperm production occurred, and patients were often able to impregnate their sexual partners. Direct comparisons of GnRH and hCG/hMG regimens in both randomized and crossover designs revealed that larger testis size was achieved during the GnRH treatment, but no significantly greater sperm concentrations.[212, 213] Because pulsatile GnRH therapy by pump is more difficult for the patient to tolerate, I prefer to use hCG/hMG until more data on the use of GnRH are available.

GERMINAL CELL FAILURE

Infertility, defined as a lack of conception for more than 1 year of adequate, unprotected intercourse, occurs in 10 percent of marriages. A male factor of oligospermia or azoospermia is present in 30 to 50 percent of cases. Appropriate calculations from these data indicate that the prevalence of germinal cell dysfunction in men approaches 3 to 5 percent. Disorders of germinal cell function can be classified as hypogonadotropic, hypergonadotropic, and eugonadotropic in type. The hypogonadotropic forms produce a clinical picture of Leydig cell dysfunction as well as germinal cell failure and are best considered with hypogonadotropic syndromes as discussed before. In contrast, germinal cell failure of the hypergonadotropic and eugonadotropic types produces only subclinical Leydig cell dysfunction and is generally recognized clinically because of infertility rather than testosterone deficiency.

Hypergonadotropic Syndromes

When germinal cell mass or Sertoli cell function is sufficiently reduced, plasma or urine FSH levels increase, often without a concomitant rise in LH concentration. Most but not all studies demonstrate a similar increase in FSH levels with in vitro bioassays and with immunoassays.[214–216] Detailed clinical observations demonstrate an inverse relationship between the remaining germinal cell mass and the level of circulating FSH. An exact relationship between FSH secretion and the presence of a specific germinal cell type is not found. Several lines of evidence suggest that FSH secretion may directly correlate with Sertoli cell function and only indirectly with germinal cell maturation. Regardless of the exact relationships, the degree of elevation of FSH concentration in plasma can be used as an index of the severity of germinal cell dysfunction.[28] An exaggerated release of FSH in response to GnRH appears to uncover lesser degrees of germinal cell failure.[217] Several specific disorders produce monotropic FSH elevation or disproportionate FSH to LH ratios in association with germinal cell failure.[218]

Sertoli Cell–Only Syndrome

The Sertoli cell–only syndrome is a disorder diagnosed by testicular biopsy and characterized by azoospermia, elevated FSH, and absence of germinal cells on testicular biopsy. Clinical examination reveals normal pubic and axillary hair but small, soft testes averaging 2 to 4 cm in their long axes (volume, 10 to 20 ml). Half of the patients exhibit subclinical Leydig cell dysfunction, characterized by elevated LH concentration with normal or slightly reduced testosterone concentration and blunted response to hCG.[217] The seminiferous tubules are slightly reduced in diameter, contain only Sertoli cells, and are not sclerotic in appearance. The Sertoli and Leydig cells appear normal by light microscopy but on electron microscopy contain minor abnormalities.[219] Normal seminiferous tubules with full germinal cell maturation are occasionally seen, but the majority are completely depleted of germinal elements. A definitive diagnosis requires a testicular biopsy and demonstration of markedly depleted germinal cells.

Idiopathic Seminiferous Tubule Failure with Hyalinization

In a major subgroup of men with oligospermia or azoospermia, no specific cause is found but FSH concentrations are elevated. Testicular biopsies reveal hyalinization of the peritubular elements in conjunction with variable degrees of germinal cell loss. Testis size may be reduced to below adult normal limits of 4.0 cm in the long axis or 20 ml.

Eugonadotropic Syndromes

Idiopathic Germinal Cell Failure

Oligospermia or azoospermia of unknown cause may be less severe and may be associated with normal basal FSH levels. Two subtypes have been described: arrest of germinal cell maturation at a specific step or generalized hypospermatogenesis affecting all germinal cell elements (Table 23–10). Clinical examination reveals no abnormality, and testis size is usually normal. Subclinical hypergonadotropism can be uncovered in approximately 30 percent of these patients by the demonstration of exaggerated FSH (and often LH) increments after administration of exogenous GnRH.[217] Prolactin levels are elevated in 5 percent of oligospermic patients, but the pathophysiologic significance of this is unclear.[220]

Numerous treatments for patients with germinal cell failure,[221] and particularly the eugonadotropic subgroup, have been proposed, including (1) induction of rebound from testosterone- or anabolic androgen–induced azoospermia; (2) administration of exogenous gonadotropins or gonadotropin-releasing factors; (3) use of clomiphene citrate or tamoxifen to stimulate endogenous gonadotropin secretion; (4) administration of low doses of mesterolone, an oral synthetic androgen; and (5) use of an aromatase inhibitor, such as testolactone. A general review of available data reveals that sperm count increases in 20 to 40 percent of

■ TABLE 23–10

Relative Frequency of Causes and Histologic Findings in Infertile Men

CAUSES	%	HISTOLOGIC FINDINGS	%
Idiopathic	33	Hypospermatogenesis	61
Varicocele	25	Maturation arrest	15
Undescended testes (surgically corrected or uncorrected)	7	Sertoli cell–only	13
		Normal appearance	8
		Hyalinized tubules	2
Excurrent duct obstruction	4.8	Immature testis	1
Mumps orchitis	3.3		
Hypogonadotropinism	2.3		
Klinefelter's syndrome	1.9		
Miscellaneous	23		

Data from Baker HWG, Burger HG, de Kretser DM, Hudson B. Relative incidence of etiologic disorders in male infertility. *In* Santen SJ, Swerdloff RS (eds). Male Reproductive Dysfunction: Diagnosis and Management of Hypogonadism, Infertility, and Impotence. New York, Marcel Dekker, 1986, p 341; Tyler ET, Singher HO. Male infertility—status of treatment, prevention, and current research. JAMA 160:91, 1956; Dubin L, Amelar RD. Etiologic factors in 1294 consecutive cases of male infertility. Fertil Steril 22:469–474, 1971; Greenberg SH, Lipshultz LI, Wein AJ. Experience with 425 subfertile male patients. J Urol 119:507–510, 1978; and Abyholm T. Azoospermia and oligozoospermia etiology and clinical findings. Arch Androl 10:57–65, 1983.

these patients in association with each of these treatments. Baker[222] suggested that these increments represent merely regression to the mean in men selected on the basis of a limited number of sperm counts. Increased sperm counts in men receiving a placebo in one study supported this conclusion.[223] Few controlled randomized trials using a placebo have been conducted, and no study has conclusively established the benefit of these treatments.[224] Strictly controlled studies of extensively characterized patients are required to establish that any of the currently available treatment modalities has a role in reversing the spermatogenic deficiency.

Given the lack of effective therapies, clinical investigators have applied in vitro fertilization (IVF) techniques to enhance the fertilizing capacity of a limited number of sperm in men with oligospermia.[37] For men with mild to moderate degrees of sperm impairment, standard IVF offers a means to improve rates of conception. Selection techniques are used to enhance the quality of sperm used. These include swim-up, migration gravity, and sedimentation methods. More complex procedures include use of albumin or Percoll gradients. Other approaches attempt to increase sperm-egg interactions and include motility enhancers such as caffeine and its derivatives, reduction of volume of insemination medium through use of microdrops, and removal of the cumulus cells surrounding the oocyte. These methods appear to be effective in cases of moderate oligospermia and asthenospermia. However, in couples in whom sperm function is severely impaired, the fertilization rate is minimal or at best less than 20 percent with standard IVF techniques.[225] The success of the procedure is related to the degree of severity of the defect in sperm function. Thus, the rate of spontaneous conceptions in the most favorable groups compared with the rate obtained with IVF has not been determined in a rigorous manner. Insemination improves only minimally with use of higher sperm concentrations or micromanipulation of eggs by partial zona dissection.

A recently described technique, intracytoplasmic sperm injection (ICSI), holds substantial promise as an effective new method for treatment of severe oligospermia or qualitative sperm dysfunction.[226, 227] This involves the isolation of an egg from the female partner by use of standard techniques for IVF. A single mobile sperm is then microinjected into the cytoplasm of the egg with the assistance of a mechanical micromanipulator and micropipette. This technique is available at specialized centers. A large study of 190 couples, including a majority in whom standard IVF failed, reported 52 pregnancies.[226] Surprisingly, the severity of semen abnormalities had only a small effect on fertilization rate. This method appears to be a potentially powerful new tool for the treatment of severe male infertility. On the basis of preliminary results of this technique, it has been suggested that the main determinants of success in treating male infertility are the egg number and quality obtained from the female partner.

The process of selection of patients for ICSI is now undergoing critical analysis, and guidelines proposed are only provisional. This technique is clearly appropriate for men with profound oligospermia and counts less than 2 million/ml and for those with zero motility. Additional recommended criteria for selection are based on pathophysiologic principles but not data from controlled trials. One proposed criterion is to use the acrosome reaction or proportion of sperm binding to the zona pellucida as algorithmic branch points. Men with failure of the acrosome reaction or zona binding are selected for the ICSI technique because their sperm cannot adequately penetrate eggs during standard IVF techniques. Those with an acrosome reaction may be candidates for observation or for standard IVF procedures based on these parameters. However, the validity of IVF with or without partial zona dissection or subzonal microinjection in men with acrosome reactions and zona pellucida binding remains to be fully established by further controlled studies. In the meantime, ICSI appears to represent a major advance, not on the basis of controlled trials but on the basis of its efficacy in patients in whom standard IVF procedure fail.[226]

Varicocele

Incompetence of the left or, less commonly, the right testicular vein results in the formation of dilated veins in the scrotum, a condition called varicocele.[228, 229] Detection of varicocele clinically requires examination of a standing patient during the Valsalva maneuver. Subclinical varicocele is suggested by thermography and confirmed by retrograde testicular vein venography, but the significance of this finding remains controversial.[228]

A series of observations suggest an etiologic association between varicocele and infertility. Varicoceles can be palpated in approximately 40 percent of men with oligospermia or azoospermia and 23 percent of normal men.[230, 231] Sperm motility is often reduced, and a "stress" pattern of sperm morphologic features, with increased numbers of immature or tapered forms, is commonly found.[229] The stress pattern, however, is not specific to oligospermic patients with varicocele and can be found in other oligospermic patients as well. Sperm from men with varicocele penetrate into denuded ova from hamsters, as a test of sperm function, less well than do normal sperm.[232]

High venous ligation of the testicular veins in the inguinal canal is the standard treatment of varicocele.[228, 229] Venous occlusion can also be induced by the injection of thrombogenic agents through a venous catheter.[228] The clinician should be aware that 10 percent of varicoceles recur after surgery and can be detected on careful repeated examination. The majority of reports indicate a pregnancy rate of approximately 30 percent compared with 15 percent in control patients receiving either medical treatment or no therapy.[229] Because the mechanism of induction of oligospermia is unknown and prospective controlled trials of therapy have not been completed, some investigators question the etiologic association of varicocele with infertility and the efficacy of surgical therapy.[233] Data for and against this conclusion have been presented.[233–235] Until a definitive answer is obtained from controlled studies, the question of the efficacy of varicocele repair will remain open.

No clearly defined criteria allow a prediction of responders to corrective surgery. Carefully conducted studies suggest that patients with subclinical Leydig cell dysfunction, as detected by exaggerated LH and FSH responses to GnRH infusion, may be more likely to respond to varicocele repair.[236, 237] Azoospermic patients are unlikely to benefit from this procedure.

Varicoceles occur in approximately 15 percent of adolescent boys.[231] Progressive testicular atrophy has been observed in some of these subjects.[238] An increase in the volume of the affected testis follows varicocele repair in the majority of patients with an ipsilateral testis smaller than the contralateral one.[239] These findings raise questions about the management of adolescent patients with varicocele.[240] Many investigators advocate varicocele repair for patients with large varicoceles and progressive atrophy of the ipsilateral testis.[239] An operation for oligospermia is generally not performed because systematic collection of prospective data based on semen analyses is not practical. Adolescents with varicocele should probably be observed with a physical examination every 6 months, and an attempt should be made to obtain a baseline semen analysis. Growth failure of the testis ipsilateral to the varicocele is an indication for varicocele ligation.

Ductal Obstruction

Nearly 40 percent of patients with azoospermia are found to have ductal obstruction. Inflammatory, iatrogenic, or congenital defects of the vas deferens or epididymis are the most common causes. These patients have normal FSH levels and testis size and are diagnosed by demonstration of normal spermatogenesis on testicular biopsy and obstructed ducts on vasographic study. An algorithm for the evaluation of azoospermic patients recommends testicular biopsy only for those with normal testes and vas deferens on physical examination and normal FSH levels.[241]

Congenital Adrenal Hyperplasia

Elevated adrenal androgen levels suppress the production of LH and FSH in men with congenital adrenal hyperplasia. The majority of these patients have normal spermatogenesis.[242, 243] Some, particularly those with adrenal rest tumors in the testes, exhibit oligospermia. Treatment with exogenous glucocorticoids reverses the oligospermia and reduces the size of testicular masses in such patients.[243]

Heat

Exposure to heat reproducibly reduces sperm production temporarily in a number of animal species. Although this effect has been incompletely documented in men, studies suggest that the heat encountered in a sauna may be sufficient to temporarily reduce sperm production.[244]

Infections

In the majority of patients with eugonadotropic seminiferous tubule failure, no cause can be identified. A thorough search for infectious agents has identified a variety of organisms in the seminal fluid of men with oligospermia or with decreased sperm motility.[245] Mycoplasmal infection, particularly by *Ureaplasma urealyticum,* has been suggested as a causative factor in infertility, but this conclusion remains controversial.[245] *U. urealyticum* was found in 26 percent of 100 infertile men compared with 13 percent of 30 fertile men in one study. *Escherichia coli* has been implicated in other studies. No characteristic features are apparent by history or physical examination in these men. The presence of an excessive number of leukocytes in the seminal fluid suggests the possibility of infection. A cause-effect relationship between the documented infection and the associated infertility has not yet been established. However, most large infertility clinics routinely treat with antibiotics such as doxycycline when infection is suspected on the basis of the presence of pus cells on several seminal fluid examinations or positive cultures.[245]

Sinopulmonary-Infertility Syndrome

In a number of disorders, a correlation between infertility and recurrent sinopulmonary infections is apparent[246] (Table 23–11). In the immotile cilia syndrome, sperm motility and ciliary function in the respiratory tract are defective because of abnormal flagellar function. One subtype of this syndrome is identified by electron microscopic study. It consists of absence of dynein arms on the sperm tail and respiratory cilia. Partial deletions of the dynein arms may also exist but are difficult to detect because of considerable variability in the appearance of normal sperm tails on electron microscopy. Deficiency of protein carboxymethylase, an enzyme required for motility,[247] has been demonstrated in the sperm of patients with necrospermia.

Cystic fibrosis is characterized by congenital malformation of the vas deferens with azoospermia and tenacious bronchopulmonary secretions. Young's syndrome, on the other hand, is associated with inspissated secretions in the

■ TABLE 23–11
Clinical Features of the Sinopulmonary-Infertility Syndrome

SYNDROME	SINOPULMONARY INFECTION	SPERM AND CILIA ULTRASTRUCTURE	VAS AND EPIDIDYMIS	SPERM ANALYSIS	PANCREATIC FUNCTION	SWEAT TEST
Immotile cilia syndrome	Present	Abnormal*	Normal sperm	Immotile	Normal	Normal
Cystic fibrosis	Present	Normal	Malformation†	Azoospermia	Abnormal	Abnormal
Young's syndrome	Present	Normal	Obstruction by inspissated secretions	Azoospermia	Normal	Normal

*Biochemical variants with enzymatic defects may also exist.
†Rare cases with intact vas and epididymides and fertility have been reported.
Adapted from Handelsman DE, Conway AJ, Boylan LM, Turtle JK. Young's syndrome: Obstructive azoospermia and chronic sinopulmonary infections. N Engl J Med 310:3–9, 1984.

vas deferens in association with azoospermia. Both disorders produce recurrent respiratory tract infections; the infections are severe in the case of cystic fibrosis and mild in those with Young's syndrome.[246]

Genetic Syndromes

Surveys of karyotype analyses or of meiotic chromosomes in men with infertility document the frequency of genetic disorders.[248] Prior studies showed that 15 percent of men with azoospermia were found to have various genetic abnormalities including XXY and XYY karyotypes, reciprocal autosomal and Robertsonian translocations, and a variety of other abnormalities. The frequency of these disorders in oligospermic men with sperm counts of 1 to 20 $\times$ 10^6/ml was 1.65 percent. In 2372 infertile men screened by Chandley,[248] 24 had an XXY karyotype, 10 had reciprocal autosomal translocations, 5 were of XYY karyotype, 4 had Robertsonian translocations, and 8 had miscellaneous abnormalities on somatic karyotype analysis.

More recent studies detect DNA microdeletions on the long arm of the Y chromosome in a substantial number (18 percent) of men with either azoospermia or severe oligospermia. There is increasing evidence that genes on the long arm of the Y chromosome and especially within deletion interval 6 are important for mammalian spermatogenesis.[249–252] Studies in men with Y/autosome translocations or large deletions of portion of the Y chromosome suggest that all of the euchromatic portion of Y must be present to achieve normal germ cell development. If macroscopic portions in interval 6 are missing, men are azoospermic. Polymerase chain reaction techniques are used to identify microdeletions or macrodeletions in this region.[253] Two closely related Y-specific genes have been proposed as the putative azoospermia factor.[254]

Autoimmunity

Infertility and oligospermia occur in association with certain autoimmune disorders such as Addison's disease and the familial autoimmune endocrine deficiency syndrome.[255] The presence of autoantibodies against the testis has been demonstrated in these subjects. Autoantibodies directed against either the testes or sperm occur in other patients with oligospermia or azoospermia as well. Indirect quantitative radioimmunoassay detects antisperm antibodies on spermatozoa in seminal plasma and in the sera of men with oligospermia with greater frequency than in the normal population. Both continuous and intermittent prednisolone therapy have been shown to be effective in some placebo-controlled trials in patients with autoantibodies but not in others.[37, 256, 257]

Approach to the Diagnosis of the Infertile Male

Initial evaluation of the infertile male involves documentation of low sperm counts with at least three semen analyses at monthly intervals. Specimens are obtained after 3 days of abstinence from intercourse. If counts are consistently below 20 $\times$ 10^6/ml or 50 $\times$ 10^6 total, germinal cell dysfunction should be highly suspected. A work-up should then be started to identify possible causes (see Table 23–10). A carefully directed history should initially be obtained. A decrease in libido and potency, energy, and shaving frequency and a loss of body hair are consistent with hypogonadism. Retrograde ejaculation with spermaturia is suggested if patients void cloudy urine after intercourse. A history of testicular maldescent or trauma, prior genitourinary or hernia surgery, a past history of genitourinary infection, and a history of pain or swelling of the testes should be elicited. Systemic illnesses such as recent febrile episodes, renal disease, and inflammatory bowel disease can impair fertility. A history of recurrent respiratory illnesses is associated with Young's syndrome and obstructive azoospermia. Because in utero exposure to diethylstilbestrol may be associated with infertility in males, information regarding this risk factor should be obtained.[258] Medications and drugs can affect germ cell function as well.

Physical examination requires an overall assessment of the patient's degree of virilization, body proportions, musculature, and hair distribution. Examination of the scrotal veins during a Valsalva maneuver is required to exclude a minimal varicocele. Examination of the genitourinary system should include accurate measurement of testicular volume (using a ruler, an orchidometer, or ultrasound examination) and palpation of the epididymis, checking specifically for tenderness (infection) and fullness (obstruction). Necessary laboratory data include measurements of LH, FSH, testosterone, and prolactin concentrations. Seminal fluid should be cultured if pus cells are detected on semen analysis or if excurrent duct infection is apparent. Examination of urine voided after intercourse allows documentation of retrograde ejaculation.[259] Testicular biopsy may be requested in subjects with normal FSH levels, normal testicular size, and a palpable vas deferens on physical examination. This procedure is now less commonly performed but is useful in identifying patients who are likely to have ductal obstruction. Measurement of antisperm antibodies is available only to certain investigative groups but may be useful under certain circumstances. Testing to determine candidates for ICSI now becomes an important practical issue.[225–227] Whereas no agreement exists, some investigators suggest that ICSI should be the initial treatment in men with sperm counts less than 5 million/ml, with 0 percent sperm motility, and with sperm that lack the acrosome reaction.[37, 226, 227] The female partner of an oligospermic male requires complete evaluation as well. Reproductive abnormalities commonly exist in both partners.

The clinician should keep in mind the relative prevalence of different etiologic disorders in infertile men. Five series involving 3478 men[260] revealed the following frequencies of etiologic factors: idiopathic, 33 percent; varicocele, 25 percent; undescended testes, 7 percent; excurrent duct obstruction, 4.8 percent; hypogonadotropic hypogonadism, 2.3 percent; and Klinefelter's syndrome, 1.9 percent. A large category of miscellaneous causes remains. In another series of 280 men, testicular biopsy revealed hypospermatogenesis in 61 percent, maturation arrest in 15 percent, Sertoli cell–only syndrome in 13 percent, normal appearance in 8 percent, hyalinized tubules in 2 percent, and immature testes in 1 percent[260] (see Table 23–10).

GYNECOMASTIA

A disordered balance between the stimulatory effects of estradiol and the inhibitory actions of testosterone on the male breast underlies the development of the pathologic forms of gynecomastia in men. Gynecomastia may also occur as a normal physiologic process at various stages of life as a reflection of hormonal changes. Major emphasis is placed on the balance between estradiol, the major facilitative hormone, and testosterone, as an inhibitor, in both physiologic and pathologic types.

Physiologic Forms

Pubertal Gynecomastia

Beginning at age 11 years, approximately 30 percent of boys develop detectable gynecomastia (i.e., glandular tissue greater than 0.5 cm in diameter); by age 14 years, gynecomastia is detectable in 65 percent. Surprisingly, unilateral gynecomastia is common, occurring on the left in 19 percent and on the right in 26 percent; gynecomastia occurs bilaterally in 55 percent of those with palpable breast tissue.[261] Gynecomastia resolves spontaneously in the majority 1 year after it is detected by a physician.

Adult Gynecomastia

Four studies found that gynecomastia was present in hospitalized adults with high prevalence. Thirty-three percent of men in their mid-20s and 57 percent between ages 45 and 59 years had palpable breast tissue exceeding 2 cm in diameter. In 83 percent of hospitalized men with gynecomastia, the diameter of breast tissue was 5 cm or less.[262] Autopsy confirmed the physical findings in 60 consecutive cases in one study and independently detected gynecomastia in another.[262] Two subtypes of gynecomastia can be distinguished histologically. Glandular predominance occurs in 5 to 9 percent of patients and presumably represents active hormonal stimulation of ductal elements. Stromal tissue predominates in 8 percent and probably reflects the aftermath of a process that becomes quiescent.[263, 264]

Pathologic Forms

In adolescence, a group of boys develop an exaggerated form of gynecomastia with breast development to Tanner stage 3 (greater than 4 cm of glandular breast tissue), stage 4 (near-adult female), or stage 5 (normal adult female). This condition, called persistent pubertal macromastia, is not associated with specific endocrine disorders or with recognized hormonal or receptor abnormalities.[265] Tumors of the testis or adrenal and exogenous sources of estrogen are rare causes of gynecomastia in prepubertal or pubertal boys.

Causes of the pathologic forms of gynecomastia in adults are multiple, but the physiologic variety is common, particularly in men with obesity (Fig. 23–17). Consequently, the clinician must be concerned only when there is breast tenderness, a progressive increase in breast size, or enlargement beyond the physiologic range (2 to 5 cm). A distinction must also be made between pseudogynecomastia (fat tissue present underneath the nipple) and true gynecomastia. Mammography may be helpful in making this distinction.[266] Ultrasonography can also be used, but it is not considered as sensitive as mammography.[267]

The differential diagnosis of gynecomastia is extensive and difficult to remember because of the variety of causes. Two approaches are useful for the clinician: consideration of the various disorders on a pathophysiologic basis (Table 23–12) and practical attention to the most frequent causes of this condition (Fig. 23–18).

Evaluation

The clinician must decide when to evaluate men with gynecomastia, a condition found in approximately 50 percent of hospitalized men.[268] Clear indications for evaluation include breast tenderness, rapid enlargement, and eccentric or hard irregular masses and lesions greater than 5 cm. Asymptomatic stable gynecomastia less than 5 cm in diameter, particularly in obese patients, probably requires only a careful history and physical examination for evaluation. In lean subjects, gynecomastia with a breast diameter of 2 to 5 cm should probably be evaluated more extensively.

The appropriate technique for physical examination to detect gynecomastia is pinching the tissue between thumb and forefinger lateral to the nipple. Ability to "flip an edge" of tissue at the interface of normal and glandular tissue confirms the presence of gynecomastia. Comparison of consistency with that of the fat tissue over the abdomen

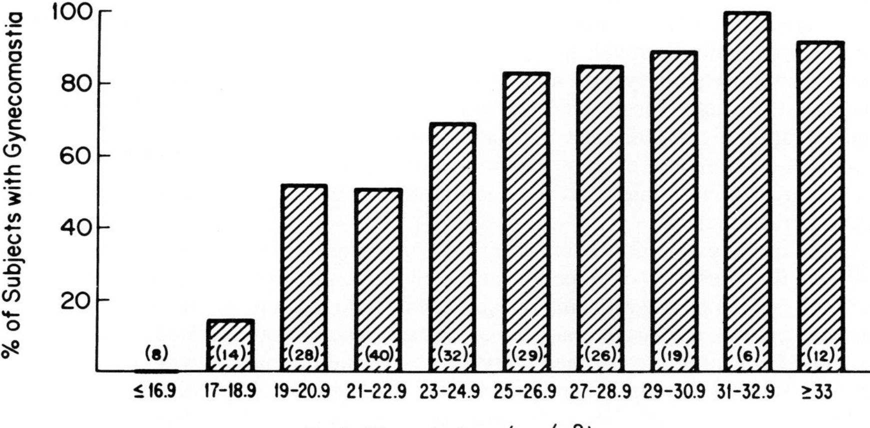

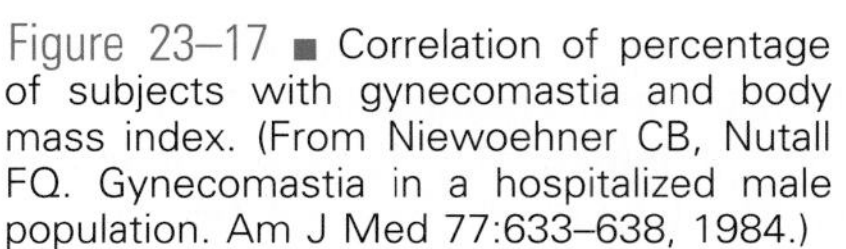
Figure 23–17 ■ Correlation of percentage of subjects with gynecomastia and body mass index. (From Niewoehner CB, Nutall FQ. Gynecomastia in a hospitalized male population. Am J Med 77:633–638, 1984.)

■ TABLE 23–12
Causes of Gynecomastia

Stimulatory Hormone Excess

- Estradiol
  - Adrenal or testicular tumors
  - Drug therapy with
    - Estrogens
    - Estrogen creams
    - Embalming cream
    - Delousing powder
    - Hair oil
    - Estrogen analogues; *digitoxin**
    - Estrogen precursors: aromatizable androgens
      - *Testosterone enanthate*
      - *Testosterone propionate*
  - Increased peripheral aromatase activity due to
    - Heredity
    - Obesity
- Prolactin
  - Pituitary tumor
  - Drug therapy with catecholamine antagonists or depleters
    - *Sulpiride* — *Phenothiazines*
    - *Metoclopramide* — *Reserpine*
    - *Domperidone* — *Tricyclic antidepressants*
    - *Methyldopa*
  - Hypothyroidism

Inhibitory Hormone Deficiency

- Androgen resistance
  - Complete testicular feminization
  - Partial: Reifenstein, Lubbs, Rosewater, and Dreyfus syndromes
- Androgen antagonist drugs
  - *Spironolactone* — *Progestagens*
  - *Cimetidine* — *Flutamide*
  - *Marijuana* — *Finasteride*

Stimulatory-Inhibitory Hormone Imbalance

- Hypergonadotropic syndromes
  - Primary gonadal diseases
  - Cytotoxic drug–induced hypogonadism from
    - *Busulfan* — *Nitrosourea*
    - *Vincristine* — Combination chemotherapy
  - Steroid synthesis inhibitory drugs
    - *Ketoconazole*
    - *Metronidazole*
  - Tumor-related hCG-producing tumors (testis, lung, gastrointestinal tract)
    - Hepatic tumor with aromatase
  - hCG administration
- Hypogonadotropic syndromes
  - Isolated gonadotropin deficiency, particularly fertile eunuch syndrome
  - Panhypopituitarism
- Systemic illnesses
  - Renal disease
  - Severe liver disease

Miscellaneous Endocrine Causes

- Hyperthyroidism
- Acromegaly
- Cushing's syndrome

Local Trauma

- Hip spica cast
- Chest injury
- Herpes zoster of chest wall
- Post thoracotomy

Primary Breast Tumor

Uncertain Causes

- Refeeding
- Other chronic illnesses
  - Pulmonary tuberculosis
  - Diabetes mellitus
  - Leprosy
- Persistent pubertal macromastia
- Idiopathic
  - Familial

*Drugs are listed in italics.

or along the axillary line is useful. Palpation of tissue with the fingers by pressing over the nipple or lateral to it is an insensitive technique.

After the decision has been made that it is warranted, a directed evaluation (see algorithm, Fig. 23–19) should be initiated, including in all patients (1) a careful drug and environmental exposure history; (2) identification of the presence of systemic renal, hepatic, cardiac, or pulmonary disease and, particularly, previous malnutrition due to these disorders; (3) detection of obvious signs and symptoms of underlying malignant disease, especially testicular; and (4) detection of clinically evident syndromes of estradiol, prolactin, growth hormone, cortisol, or thyroxine excess or androgen deficiency.

If the initial evaluation is unrevealing, screening tests to exclude the presence of a neoplasm, including measurement of hCG-β as a tumor marker and chest radiograph to rule out pulmonary carcinoma, should be performed on all patients. Clinical judgment then dictates whether additional studies, such as thyroxine, prolactin, LH, FSH, estradiol, testosterone, and DHEA-S concentrations, should be obtained. Most commonly, these measurements are ordered to exclude hypogonadism, thyroid dysfunction, and adrenal and testicular tumors. Frequently the only abnormality is a mild elevation of plasma estradiol. Testicular ultrasound examination in such patients is useful, because testicular tumors may not be large enough to palpate but can be detected by ultrasonography. Adrenal computed tomography or magnetic resonance imaging is obtained only if DHEA-S levels are concomitantly elevated or other reasons for suspicion of adrenal disease exist.

Treatment

Specific therapy for treatable diseases should be used if it is feasible, and the use of offending drugs should be discontinued. Reduction mammaplasty is required under certain circumstances. Persistent pubertal macromastia is resistant to medical therapy and requires surgical excision. Reduction mammaplasty is occasionally necessary in men with painful or cosmetically disabling lesions. A highly experienced surgeon should be asked to perform this procedure because of the precise sculpturing necessary to produce an excellent cosmetic effect. Boys with pubertal gyne-

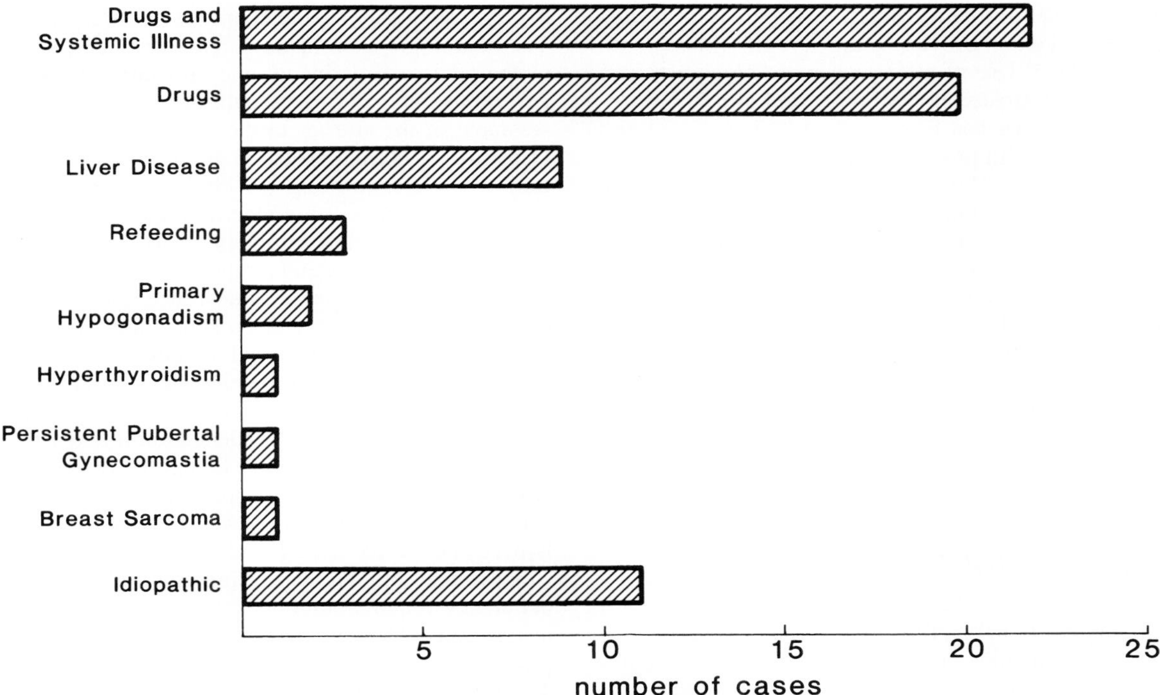

Figure 23–18 ■ Frequency of causes of gynecomastia in men hospitalized at a Veterans Administration hospital. The "drugs and systemic illness" category includes male climacteric, cirrhosis, hepatitis, hyperthyroidism, refeeding syndrome, and primary hypogonadism. The "drugs" category includes methyldopa, phenothiazines, amitriptyline, imipramine, spironolactone, isoniazid, testosterone, narcotics, estradiol, amphetamines, and reserpine. (Adapted from information appearing in Carlson HE. Current concepts: Gynecomastia. N Engl J Med 303:795–799, 1980.)

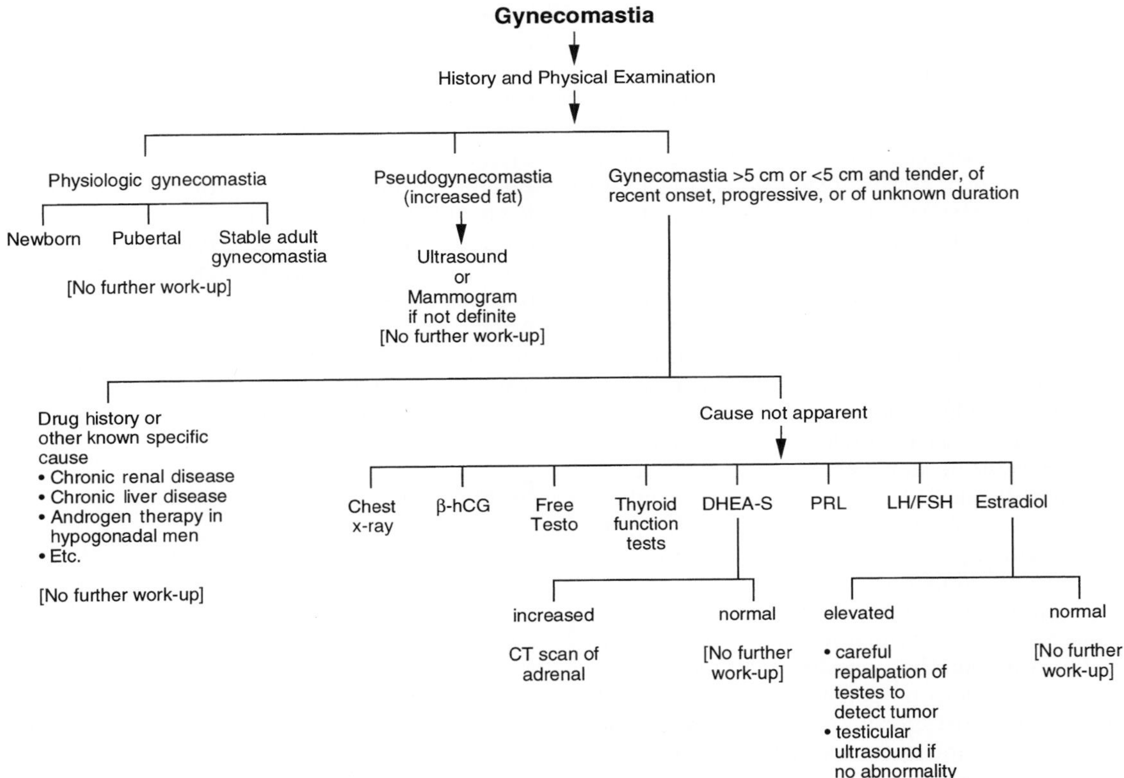

Figure 23–19 ■ Algorithm depicting evaluation of the patient with gynecomastia.

comastia can generally be reassured that regression occurs after 2 to 3 years in the majority of those with gynecomastia.[261, 269] Use of antiestrogens to block estrogen action, stimulate testosterone secretion, and alter the estrogen-androgen balance has been evaluated in pubertal and adult gynecomastia; improvement has been seen in some but not all patients.[270] The aromatase inhibitor testolactone has also been used to suppress estradiol but not androgen levels. Each of these agents can be considered when pubertal gynecomastia is severe and psychologically debilitating. However, surgical therapy with reduction mammaplasty is usually required for more severe gynecomastia. The pharmacologic agents mentioned can be used in adult patients with idiopathic gynecomastia, but experience with these drugs is limited. No comparative trials among medical agents are available, and choices of therapy are based on drug availability, experience of the physician, and cost factors.

ERECTILE DYSFUNCTION

The term impotence has been replaced by consensus with the less pejorative term erectile dysfunction. This condition is defined as the inability to achieve or sustain an erection for a sufficient duration to have coitus. Disorders of libido or orgasmic potential should be distinguished from erectile dysfunction. The frequency of erectile dysfunction increases with age such that 1.9 percent of men at age 40 years and 25 percent of men at age 65 experience this symptom.[271] The causes of erectile dysfunction can be divided into five general categories: psychogenic, vascular, neuropathic, endocrinologic, and drug related.[272] In patients presenting to urologists for treatment, the relative frequencies of these causes approximate 15 percent for psychogenic, 50 percent for vascular, 15 percent for neurogenic, and 20 percent for mixed.[272]

The erectile dysfunction of vascular insufficiency is often associated with symptoms of intermittent claudication, angina, or transient ischemic attacks of the anterior or posterior cerebral circulation. Historical features suggesting neuropathic impotence include stocking-glove paresthesias, symptoms of autonomic insufficiency, and a history of diabetes mellitus or renal disease. Endocrine-related erectile dysfunction causes decreased libido as well as decreased potency, loss of morning erections, inability to masturbate, and loss of secondary sexual characteristics after a prolonged period. Drug-related dysfunction is obvious, provided that the physician considers the diagnosis.[272] Endocrine causes are considered relatively uncommon.

Psychogenic erectile dysfunction was once considered the most common diagnosis but is made less frequently as more sensitive techniques are available to detect organic causes. Patients with a psychogenic etiology often recount alternating periods of normal potency and impotence. Suggestive historical features include premature ejaculation or stress-related premature detumescence, abrupt onset of impotence after heavy alcohol ingestion, and maintenance of normal libido but loss of potency. Characteristically, physiologic control of the erectile process remains intact; these individuals continue to experience morning and sleep-related erections and retain their ability to masturbate.

Physical examination is directed toward careful assessment of secondary sexual characteristics and testicular size. The neurologic examination should include sensory testing of the penis and perineum and an evaluation of the bulbocavernous reflex. The vascular examination involves assessment of the arteries in the penis and lower extremities. Detection of normal prolactin and free testosterone concentrations in the morning (to eliminate diurnal variability) practically excludes an endocrinologic cause.

The major clinical problem is to distinguish between organic and psychogenic impotence. Quantitative assessment of nocturnal penile tumescence and correlation with electroencephalographic sleep stages are the best available methods to assess nocturnal erections. The snap gauge band provides a home screening device, and the Rigiscan provides a more quantitative instrument for home detection of nocturnal erections.[273, 274] Detection of a low testosterone concentration in the morning favors the diagnosis of endocrine-related impotence. A specific cause should then be sought from the various causes of hypogonadotropic and hypergonadotropic hypogonadism described in this chapter.

Treatment of erectile dysfunction related to androgen deficiency requires administration of adequate amounts of testosterone. Objective measures of erectile function improve in hypogonadal men who receive this therapy.[275] Testosterone enanthate, 200 mg every 2 weeks, can be given as a therapeutic trial. As confirmation of a physiologic rather than a placebo response, the physician can substitute a sterile vehicle for 1-month periods with 1-month androgen replacement therapy interspersed.

Treatment of erectile dysfunction related to prolactin excess requires identification and treatment of the specific cause of hyperprolactinemia. If no specific cause is found, prolactin levels should then be lowered with bromocriptine. Androgen therapy is initiated only after reduction of prolactin levels. As emphasized before, erectile dysfunction often persists when prolactin levels are elevated, even if the testosterone deficiency is corrected.

Vascular, psychogenic, and neurogenic forms of erectile dysfunction can be effectively treated by the use of intracavernosal injections of alprostadil, a prostaglandin analogue (FDA approved). It can also be administered by a urethral delivery device. Urologists frequently combine agents such as papaverine, phentolamine, and alprostadil to lower doses of individual agents and reduce side effects. Approaches to the diagnosis of and therapy for impotence of nonendocrine nature entail extensive laboratory and clinical support. A recent review provides an excellent overview from a practical and treatment-oriented perspective.[276]

References

1. Haavisto A-M, Dunkel L, Pettersson K, Huhtaniemi I. LH measurements by in vitro bioassay and a highly sensitive immunofluorometric assay improve the distinction between boys with constitutional delay of puberty and hypogonadotropic hypogonadism. Pediatr Res 27:211, 1990.
2. Santen RJ, Bardin CW. Episodic luteinizing hormone secretion in man: Pulse analysis, clinical interpretation, physiologic mechanisms. J Clin Invest 52:2617, 1973.
3. Vermeulen A, Verdonck G. Representativeness of a single point plasma testosterone level for the long term hormonal milieu in men. J Clin Endocrinol Metab 74:939, 1992.
4. Field AE, Colditz GA, Willett WC, et al. The relation of smoking, age, relative weight, and dietary intake to serum adrenal steroids,

sex hormones, and sex hormone–binding globulin in middle-aged men. J Clin Endocrinol Metab 79:1310, 1994.

5. Veldhuis JD, Urban RJ, Dufau ML. Differential responses of biologically active luteinizing hormone secretion in older versus young men to interruption of androgen negative feedback. J Clin Endocrinol Metab 79:1763, 1994.
6. Jia X-C, Kessel B, Yen SSC, et al. Serum bioactive follicle-stimulating hormone during the human menstrual cycle in hyper- and hypogonadotropic states: Application of a sensitive granulosa cell aromatase bioassay. J Clin Endocrinol Metab 62:1243, 1986.
7. Warner BA, Dufau ML, Santen RL. Effects of aging and illness on the pituitary testicular axis in men: Qualitative as well as quantitative changes in luteinizing hormone. J Clin Endocrinol Metab 60:263, 1985.
8. Burstein S, Schaff-Blass E, Blass J, Rosenfield RL. The changing ratio of bioactive to immunoreactive luteinizing hormone (LH) through puberty principally reflects changing LH radioimmunoassay dose-response characteristics. J Clin Endocrinol Metab 61:508, 1985.
9. Kletter GB, Padmanabhan V, Brown MB, et al. Serum bioactive gonadotropins during male puberty: A longitudinal study. J Clin Endocrinol Metab 76:432, 1993.
10. Furui K, Suganuma N, Tsukahara S-I, et al. Identification of two point mutations in the gene coding luteinizing hormone (LH) β-subunit, associated with immunologically anomalous LH variants. J Clin Endocrinol Metab 78:107, 1994.
11. Haavisto A-M, Pettersson K, Bergendahl M, et al. Occurrence and biological properties of a common genetic variant of luteinizing hormone. J Clin Endocrinol Metab 80:1257, 1995.
12. Papandreou M-J, Asteria C, Pettersson K, et al. Concanavalin A affinity chromatography of human serum gonadotropins: Evidence for changes of carbohydrate structure in different clinical conditions. J Clin Endocrinol Metab 76:1008, 1993.
13. Phillips DJ, Wide L. Serum gonadotropin isoforms become more basic after an exogenous challenge of gonadotropin-releasing hormone in children undergoing pubertal development. J Clin Endocrinol Metab 79:814, 1994.
14. Seminara SB, Boepple PA, Nachtigall LB, et al. Inhibin B in males with gonadotropin-releasing hormone (GnRH) deficiency: Changes in serum concentration after short term physiologic GnRH replacement—a clinical research center study. J Clin Endocrinol Metab 81:3692, 1996.
15. Illingworth PJ, Groome NP, Byrd W, et al. Inhibin-B: A likely candidate for the physiologically important form of inhibin in men. J Clin Endocrinol Metab 81:1321, 1996.
16. Robertson D, Burger HG, Sullivan J, et al. Biological and immunological characterization of inhibin forms in human plasma. J Clin Endocrinol Metab 81:669, 1996.
17. De Kretser DM, McFarlane JR. Inhibin in the male. J Androl 17:179, 1996.
18. Nachtigall LB, Boepple PA, Seminara SB, et al. Inhibin B secretion in males with gonadotropin-releasing hormone (GnRH) deficiency before and during long-term GnRH replacement: Relationship to spontaneous puberty, testicular volume, and prior treatment—a clinical research center study. J Clin Endocrinol Metab 81:3520, 1996.
19. Anwalt BD, Bebb RA, Matsumoto AM, et al. Serum inhibin B levels reflect Sertoli cell function in normal men and men with testicular dysfunction. J Clin Endocrinol Metab 81:3341, 1996.
20. Bremner WJ, Paulsen CA. Two pools of luteinizing hormone in the human pituitary: Evidence from constant administration of luteinizing hormone–releasing hormone. J Clin Endocrinol Metab 39:811, 1974.
21. Ghai K, Rosenfield RL. Maturation of the normal pituitary-testicular axis, as assessed by gonadotropin-releasing hormone agonist challenge. J Clin Endocrinol Metab 78:1336, 1994.
22. Smals AGH, Hermus ARM, Boers GHJ, et al. Predictive value of luteinizing hormone releasing hormone (LHRH) bolus testing before and after 36-hour pulsatile LHRH administration in the differential diagnosis of constitutional delay of puberty and male hypogonadotropic hypogonadism. J Clin Endocrinol Metab 78:602, 1994.
23. Forest MG. How should we perform the human chorionic gonadotrophin (hCG) stimulation test? Int J Androl 6:1, 1983.
24. McElreavey K, Barbaux S, Ion A, Fellous M. The genetic basis of murine and human sex determination: A review. Heredity 75:599, 1995.
25. Behre HM, Nashan D, Nieschlag E. Objective measurement of testicular volume by ultrasonography: Evaluation of the technique and comparison with orchidometer estimates. Int J Androl 12:395, 1989.
26. Lowe DH, Brock WA, Kaplan GW. Laparoscopy for localization of nonpalpable testes. J Urol 131:728, 1984.
27. Coen P, Kulin H, Ballantine T, et al. An aromatase-producing sex-cord tumor resulting in prepubertal gynecomastia. N Engl J Med 324:317, 1991.
28. de Kretser DM, Burger HG, Fortune D, et al. Hormonal, histological and chromosomal studies in adult males with testicular disorders. J Clin Endocrinol Metab 35:392, 1972.
29. Gordon DL, Barr AB, Heerigel JE, Paulsen CA. Testicular biopsy in man: Effect on sperm concentration. Fertil Steril 16:522, 1965.
30. Berman NG, Wang C, Paulsen CA. Methodological issues in the analysis of human sperm concentration data. J Androl 17:68, 1996.
31. Levine RJ, Mathew RM, Chenault CB, et al. Differences in the quality of semen in outdoor workers during summer and winter. N Engl J Med 323:12, 1990.
32. Sherins RJ. Ar semen quality and male fertility changing? N Engl J Med 332:327, 1995.
33. Keiding N, Skakkebaek NE. Sperm decline—real or artifact? Fertil Steril 65:450, 1996.
34. Olsen GW, Bodner KM, Ramlow JM, et al. Have sperm counts been reduced 50 percent in 50 years? A statistical model revisited. Fertil Steril 63:887, 1995.
35. Wang C, Chan SYW, Ng M, et al. Diagnostic value of sperm function tests and routine semen analyses in fertile and infertile men. J Androl 9:384, 1988.
36. Liu DY, Baker HWG. Tests of human sperm function and fertilization in vitro. Fertil Steril 58:465, 1992.
37. Baker HWG. Male infertility. *In* DeGroot LJ (ed). Endocrinology, 3rd ed, Vol 3. Philadelphia, WB Saunders, 1995, pp 2404–2433.
38. Greenman T, Tordjman K, Eisch E, et al. Relative sparing of anterior pituitary function in patients with growth hormone–secreting macroadenomas: Comparison with nonfunctioning macroadenomas. J Clin Endocrinol Metab 80:1577, 1995.
39. Penabad JL, Bashey HM, Asa SL, et al. Decreased follistatin gene expression in gonadotroph adenomas. J Clin Endocrinol Metab 81:3397, 1996.
40. Ahmed SR, Aiello DP, Page R, et al. Necrotizing infundibulohypophysitis: A new syndrome of diabetes insipidus and hypopituitarism. J Clin Endocrinol Metab 76:1499, 1993.
41. Rappaport R, Brauner R, Czernichow P, et al. Effect of hypothalamic and pituitary irradiation on puberty development in children with cranial tumours. J Clin Endocrinol Metab 54:1164, 1982.
42. Stepan JJ, Lachman M, Zverina J, et al. Castrated men exhibit bone loss: Effect of calcitonin treatment on biochemical indices of bone remodeling. J Clin Endocrinol Metab 69:523, 1989.
43. Finkelstein JS, Klibanski A, Neer RM, et al. Osteoporosis in men with idiopathic hypogonadotropic hypogonadism. Ann Intern Med 106:354, 1987.
44. Oppenheim DS, Greenspan SL, Zervas NT, et al. Elevated serum lipids in hypogonadal men with and without hyperprolactinemia. Ann Intern Med 111:288, 1989.
45. Selmanoff M, Shu C, Petersen SL, et al. Single cell levels of hypothalamic messenger ribonucleic acid encoding luteinizing hormone–releasing hormone in intact, castrated, and hyperprolactinemic male rats. Endocrinology 128:459, 1991.
46. Thorner MO, Evans WS, MacLeod RM, et al. Hyperprolactinemia: Current concepts of management including medical therapy with bromocriptine. *In* Goldstein M, Calne DB, Lieberman A, Thorner MO (eds). Ergot Compounds and Brain Function: Neuroendocrine and Neuropsychiatric Aspects. New York, Raven Press, 1980, p 165.
47. Magrini G, Pellaton M, Felber JP. Prolactin induced modifications of testosterone metabolism in man. Acta Endocrinol Suppl 212:143, 1977.
48. Magrini G, Ebiner JR, Burckhardt P, Felber JP. Study on the relationship between plasma prolactin levels and androgen metabolism in man. J Clin Endocrinol Metab 43:944, 1976.

49. Fung MC, Wah GC, Odell WD. Effects of prolactin on luteinizing hormone–stimulated testosterone secretion in isolated perfused rat testis. J Androl 10:37, 1989.
50. Martikainen H, Vihko R. hCG-stimulation of testicular steroidogenesis during induced hyper- and hypoprolactinaemia in man. Clin Endocrinol (Oxf) 16:227, 1982.
51. Patton ML, Woolf PD. Hyperprolactinemia and delayed puberty: A report of three cases and their response to therapy. Pediatrics 71:572, 1983.
52. Carter JN, Tyson JE, Tolis G, et al. Prolactin-secreting tumors and hypogonadism in 22 men. N Engl J Med 299:847, 1978.
53. Prior JC, Cox TA, Fairholm D, et al. Testosterone-related exacerbation of a prolactin producing macroadenoma: Possible role for estrogen. J Clin Endocrinol Metab 64:391, 1987.
54. Santen RJ, Paulsen CA. Hypogonadotropic eunuchoidism: 1. Clinical study of the mode of inheritance. J Clin Endocrinol Metab 36:47, 1973.
55. Lieblich JM, Rogol AD, White BJ, Rosen SW. Syndrome of anosmia with hypogonadotropic hypogonadism (Kallmann syndrome). Clinical and laboratory studies in 23 cases. Am J Med 73:506, 1982.
56. Hardelin JP, Levilliers J, Young J, et al. X-22.3 deletions in isolated familial Kallmann's syndrome. J Clin Endocrinol Metab 76:827, 1993.
57. X-chromosome–linked Kallmann's syndrome: Pathology at the molecular level (Editorial). J Clin Endocrinol Metab 76:824, 1993.
58. Schwankhaus JD, Currie J, Jaffe MJ, et al. Neurologic findings in men with isolated hypogonadotropic hypogonadism. Neurology 39:223, 1989.
59. Santen RJ. The testis. *In* Felig P, Baxter JD, Frohman LA (eds). Endocrinology and Metabolism, 3rd ed. New York, McGraw-Hill, 1995, pp 885–972.
60. Spratt DI, Carr DB, Merriam GR, et al. The spectrum of abnormal patterns of gonadotropin-releasing hormone secretion in men with idiopathic hypogonadotropic hypogonadism: Clinical and laboratory correlations. J Clin Endocrinol Metab 64:283, 1987.
61. Finkelstein JS, Spratt DI, O'Dea LSL, et al. Pulsatile gonadotropin secretion after discontinuation of long term gonadotropin-releasing hormone (GnRH) administration in a subset of GnRH-deficient men. J Clin Endocrinol Metab 69:377, 1989.
62. Santen RJ, Leonard JM, Sherins RJ, et al. Short- and long-term effects of clomiphene citrate on the pituitary-testicular axis. J Clin Endocrinol Metab 33:970, 1971.
63. Mozaffarian GA, Higley M, Paulsen CA. Clinical studies in adult male patient with "isolated follicle stimulating hormone (FSH) deficiency." J Androl 4:393, 1983.
64. Finkel DM, Phillips JL, Snyder PJ. Stimulation of spermatogenesis by gonadotropins in men with hypogonadotropic hypogonadism. N Engl J Med 313:651, 1985.
65. Rowe RC, Schroeder ML, Faiman C. Testosterone induced fertility in a patient with previously untreated Kallmann's syndrome. Fertil Steril 40:400, 1983.
66. Doty RL, Shaman P, Dann M. Development of the University of Pennsylvania smell identification test: A standardized microencapsulated test of olfactory function. Physiol Behav 32:489, 1984.
67. Ehrmann DA, Rosenfield RL, Cuttler L, et al. A new test of combined pituitary-testicular function using the gonadotropin-releasing hormone agonist nafarelin in the differentiation of gonadotropin deficiency from delayed puberty: Pilot studies. J Clin Endocrinol Metab 69:963, 1989.
68. Yeh J, Rebar RW, Liu JH, Yen SSC. Pituitary function in isolated gonadotrophin deficiency. Clin Endocrinol 31:375, 1989.
69. Kulin HE, Santen RJ. Normal and aberrant pubertal development in man. *In* Vaitukaitis JL (ed). Current Endocrinology: Clinical Reproductive Neuroendocrinology. New York, Elsevier Biomedical, 1982, p 19.
70. Bauman A. Markedly delayed puberty or Kallmann's syndrome variant. J Androl 7:224, 1986.
71. Santen RJ, Kulin HE. Evaluation of delayed puberty and hypogonadism. *In* Santen RJ, Swerdloff RS (eds). Male Reproductive Dysfunction: Diagnosis and Management of Hypogonadism, Infertility, and Impotence. New York, Marcel Dekker, 1986, pp 145–189.
72. Bardin CW, Ross GT, Rifkind AB, et al. Studies of the pituitary–Leydig cell axis in young men with hypogonadotropic hypogonadism and hyposmia: Comparison with normal men, prepubertal boys, and hypopituitary patients. J Clin Invest 48:2046, 1969.
73. Santen RJ, Kulin HE. Hypogonadotropic hypogonadism and delayed puberty. *In* Burger H, de Kretser D (eds). The Testis. New York, Raven Press, 1981, p 329.
74. Jeffcoate WJ, Laurence BM, Edwards CRW, Besser GM. Endocrine function in the Prader-Willi syndrome. Clin Endocrinol (Oxf) 12:81, 1980.
75. Pauli RM, Meisner LF, Szmanda RJ. Expanded Prader-Willi syndrome in a boy with an unusual 15q chromosome deletion. Am J Dis Child 137:1087, 1983.
76. Hamilton CR Jr, Scully RE, Kliman B. Hypogonadotropism in Prader-Willi syndrome. Am J Med 52:322, 1972.
77. Green JS, Parfrey PS, Harnett JD, et al. The cardinal manifestations of Bardet-Biedl syndrome, a form of Laurence-Moon-Biedl syndrome. N Engl J Med 321:1002, 1989.
78. Dekaban NS, Parks JS, Ross GT. Laurence-Moon syndrome: Evaluation of endocrinological function and phenotypic concordance and report of cases. Med Ann DC 41:687, 1972.
79. Spratt DI, Cox P, Orav J, et al. Reproductive axis suppression in acute illness is related to disease severity. J Clin Endocrinol Metab 76:1548, 1993.
80. Barbarino A, DeMarinis L, Tofani A, et al. Corticotropin-releasing hormone inhibition of gonadotropin release and the effect of opioid blockade. J Clin Endocrinol Metab 68:523, 1989.
81. Veldhuis JD, Lizarralde G, German L, Iranmanesh A. Divergent effects of short term glucocorticoid excess on the gonadotropic and somatotropic axes in normal men. J Clin Endocrinol Metab 74:96, 1992.
82. Veldhuis JD, Iranmanesh A, Evans WS, et al. Amplitude suppression of the pulsatile mode of immunoradiometric luteinizing hormone release in fasting-induced hypoandrogenemia in normal men. J Clin Endocrinol Metab 75:587, 1993.
83. Spratt DI, Lapp PR, Nye L, Longcope C. Peripheral aromatization is markedly increased during critical illness. Free Communications, IV International Aromatase Conference; June 1996; Tahoe City, CA, p 26.
84. Woolf PD, Hamill RW, McDonald JV, et al. Transient hypogonadotropic hypogonadism caused by critical illness. J Clin Endocrinol Metab 60:444, 1985.
85. Hoffer LJ, Beitins IZ, Kyung N-H, Bistrian BR. Effects of severe dietary restriction on male reproductive hormones. J Clin Endocrinol Metab 62:288, 1986.
86. Dubey AK, Cameron JL, Steiner RA, Plant TM. Inhibition of gonadotropin secretion in castrated male rhesus monkeys *(Macaca mulatta)* induced by dietary restriction: Analogy with the prepubertal hiatus of gonadotropin release. Endocrinology 118:518, 1986.
87. Glass AR. Pituitary-testicular reserve in men with low serum testosterone and normal serum luteinizing hormone. J Androl 9:224, 1988.
88. Opstad PK. Androgenic hormones during prolonged stress, sleep, and energy deficiency. J Clin Endocrinol Metab 74:1176, 1992.
89. MacDougall JD, Webber CE, Martin J, et al. Relationship among running mileage, bone density, and serum testosterone in male runners. J Appl Physiol 73:1165, 1992.
90. Howlett TA. Hormonal responses to exercise and training: A short review. Clin Endocrinol (Oxf) 26:723, 1987.
91. Demers LM, Harrison TS, Halbert DR, Santen RJ. Effect of prolonged exercise on plasma prostaglandin levels. Prostaglandins Med 6:413, 1981.
92. Pugliese MT, Lifshitz F, Grad G, et al. Fear of obesity. A cause of short stature and delayed puberty. N Engl J Med 309:513, 1983.
93. Sapolsky RM, Krey LC. Stress-induced suppression of luteinizing hormone concentrations in wild baboons: Role of opiates. J Clin Endocrinol Metab 66:722, 1988.
94. Sellmeyer DE, Grunfeld C. Endocrine and metabolic disturbances in human immunodeficiency virus infection and the acquired immune deficiency syndrome. Endocr Rev 17:518, 1996.
95. De Paepe ME, Waxman M. Testicular atrophy in AIDS: A study of 57 autopsy cases. Hum Pathol 20:210, 1989.
96. De Paepe ME, Guerri C, Waxman M. Opportunistic infections of the testis in the acquired immune deficiency syndrome. Mt Sinai J Med 57:25, 1990.

97. Grinspoon S, Corcoran C, Lee K, et al. Loss of lean body and muscle mass correlates with androgen levels in hypogonadal men with acquired immunodeficiency syndrome and wasting. J Clin Endocrinol Metab 81:4051, 1996.
98. Dobs AS, Few WL III, Blackman MR, et al. Serum hormones in men with human immunodeficiency virus–associated wasting. J Clin Endocrinol Metab 81:4108, 1996.
99. Croxson TS, Chapman WE, Miller LK, et al. Changes in the hypothalamic-pituitary-gonadal axis in human immunodeficiency virus–infected homosexual men. J Clin Endocrinol Metab 68:317, 1989.
100. Vermeulen A, Kaufman JM, Deslypere JP, Thomas G. Attenuated luteinizing hormone (LH) pulse amplitude but normal LH pulse frequency, and its relation to plasma androgens in hypogonadism of obese men. J Clin Endocrinol Metab 76:1140, 1993.
101. Strain GW, Zumoff B, Miller LK, et al. Effect of massive weight loss on hypothalamic-pituitary-gonadal function in obese men. J Clin Endocrinol Metab 66:1019, 1988.
102. Baker HWG, Burger HG, de Kretser DM, et al. A study of the endocrine manifestations of hepatic cirrhosis. Q J Med 45:145, 1976.
103. Emmanouel DS, Lindheimer MD, Katz AI. Pathogenesis of endocrine abnormalities in uremia. Endocr Rev 1:28, 1980.
104. Veldhuis JD, Wilkowski MJ, Zwart AD, et al. Evidence for attenuation of hypothalamic gonadotropin-releasing hormone (GnRH) impulse strength with preservation of GnRH pulse frequency in men with chronic renal failure. J Clin Endocrinol Metab 76:648, 1993.
105. Wang C, Tso SC, Todd D. Hypogonadotropic hypogonadism in severe β-thalassemia: Effect of chelation and pulsatile gonadotropin-releasing hormone therapy. J Clin Endocrinol Metab 68:511, 1989.
106. Claus-Walker J, Scurry M, Carter RE, Campos RJ. Steady state hormonal secretion in traumatic quadriplegia. J Clin Endocrinol Metab 44:530, 1977.
107. Jenkins PJ, Chew SL, Lowe DG, et al. Lymphocytic hypophysitis: Unusual features of a rare disorder. Clin Endocrinol (Oxf) 42:529, 1995.
108. MacAdams MR, White RH, Chipps BE. Reduction of serum testosterone levels during chronic glucocorticoid therapy. Ann Intern Med 104:648, 1986.
109. Rosenfield RL. Diagnosis and management of delayed puberty. J Clin Endocrinol Metab 70:559, 1990.
110. Philip J, Lundsteen C, Owen D. The frequency of chromosome aberrations in tall men with special reference to 47,XYY and 47,XXY. Am J Hum Genet 28:404, 1976.
111. Wang C, Baker HWG, Burger HG, et al. Hormonal studies in Klinefelter's syndrome. Clin Endocrinol (Oxf) 4:399, 1975.
112. de la Chappelle A. Analytic review: Nature and origin of males with XX sex chromosomes. Am J Hum Genet 24:71, 1972.
113. Harper P, Penny R, Foley TP Jr, et al. Gonadal function in males with myotonic dystrophy. J Clin Endocrinol Metab 35:852, 1972.
114. Grumbach MM, Conte FA. Disorders of sexual differentiation. *In* Wilson JD, Foster DW (eds). Textbook of Endocrinology, 7th ed. Philadelphia, WB Saunders, 1985, p 312.
115. Santen RJ, de Kretser DM, Paulsen CA, Vorhees J. Gonadotropins and testosterone in the XYY syndrome. Lancet 2:371, 1970.
116. Schiavi RC, Owen D, Fogel M, et al. Pituitary-gonadal function in XYY and XXY men identified in a population survey. Clin Endocrinol (Oxf) 9:233, 1978.
117. Abbasi AA, Prasad AS, Ortega J, et al. Gonadal function abnormalities in sickle cell anemia. Studies in adult male patients. Ann Intern Med 85:601, 1976.
118. Elder M, Maclaren N, Riley W. Gonadal autoantibodies in patients with hypogonadism and/or Addison's disease. J Clin Endocrinol Metab 52:1137, 1981.
119. Aynsley-Green A, Zachmann M, Illig R, et al. Congenital bilateral anorchia in childhood: A clinical, endocrine and therapeutic evaluation of twenty-one cases. Clin Endocrinol (Oxf) 5:381, 1976.
120. da Cunha MF, Meistrich ML, Fuller LM, et al. Recovery of spermatogenesis after treatment for Hodgkin's disease: Limiting dose of MOPP chemotherapy. J Clin Oncol 2:571, 1984.
121. Bauner R, Czernichow P, Cramer P, et al. Leydig-cell function in children after direct testicular irradiation for acute lymphoblastic leukemia. N Engl J Med 309:25, 1983.
122. Tsatsoulis A, Shalet SM, Robertson WR, et al. Plasma inhibin levels in men with chemotherapy-induced severe damage to the seminiferous epithelium. Clin Endocrinol (Oxf) 29:659, 1988.
123. Quigley C, Cowell LC, Jimenez M, et al. Normal or early development of puberty despite gonadal damage in children treated for acute lymphoblastic leukemia. N Engl J Med 321:143, 1989.
124. Aubier F, Flamant F, Brauner R, et al. Male gonadal function after chemotherapy for solid tumors in childhood. J Clin Oncol 7:304, 1989.
125. Schilsky RL. Male fertility following cancer chemotherapy. J Clin Oncol 7:295, 1989.
126. Meirow D, Schenker JG. Cancer and male infertility. Hum Reprod 10:2017, 1995.
127. Ash P. The influence of radiation on fertility in man. Br J Radiol 53:271, 1980.
128. Talbot JA, Shalet SM, Tsatsoulis A, et al. Luteinizing hormone pulsatility in men with damage to the germinal epithelium. Int J Androl 13:223, 1990.
129. Morris ID, Shalet SM. Endocrine-mediated protection from cytotoxic-induced testicular damage. J Endocrinol 120:7, 1989.
130. Chlebowski RT, Heber D. Hypogonadism in male patients with metastatic cancer prior to chemotherapy. Cancer Res 42:2495, 1982.
131. Hembree WC III, Nahas GG, Zeidenberg P, Huang HFS. Changes in human spermatozoa associated with high dose marihuana smoking. *In* Nahas GG, Paton WDM (eds). Marihuana: Biological Effects. New York, Pergamon Press, 1979, p 429.
132. Adler RA. Clinically important effects of alcohol on endocrine function. J Clin Endocrinol Metab 74:957, 1992.
133. Lantz GD, Cunningham GR, Huckins C, Lipshultz LL. Recovery from severe oligospermia after exposure to dibromochloropropane (DBCP). Fertil Steril 35:46, 1981.
134. Imperato-McGinley J, Akgun S, Ertel NH, et al. The coexistence of male pseudohermaphrodites with 17-ketosteroid reductase deficiency and 5α-reductase deficiency within a Turkish kindred. Clin Endocrinol (Oxf) 27:135, 1987.
135. Wilson SC, Hodgins MB, Scott JS. Incomplete masculinization due to a deficiency of 17β-hydroxysteroid dehydrogenase: Comparison of prepubertal and peripubertal siblings. Clin Endocrinol (Oxf) 26:459, 1987.
136. Eckstein B, Cohen S, Farkas A, Rosler A. The nature of the defect in familial male pseudohermaphroditism in Arabs of Gaza. J Clin Endocrinol Metab 68:477, 1989.
137. Rösler A, Silverstein S, Abeliovich D. A (R80Q) mutation in 17β-hydroxysteroid dehydrogenase type 3 gene among Arabs of Israel is associated with pseudohermaphroditism in males and normal asymptomatic females. J Clin Endocrinol Metab 81:1827, 1996.
138. Murray FT, Wyss HU, Thomas RG, et al. Gonadal dysfunction in diabetic men with organic impotence. J Clin Endocrinol Metab 65:127, 1987.
139. Ellenberg M. Impotence in diabetes: The neurological factor. Ann Intern Med 75:213, 1971.
140. Geisthovel W, Niedergerke U, Morgner KD, et al. Androgenstatus bei mannlichen Diabetikern. Med Klin 70:1417, 1975.
141. McCulloch DK, Campbell IW, Wu FC, et al. The prevalence of diabetic impotence. Diabetologia 18:279, 1980.
142. Clarke BF, Ewing DJ, Campbell IW. Diabetic autonomic neuropathy. Diabetologia 17:195, 1979.
143. Buck AC, Reed PL, Siddiq YK, et al. Bladder dysfunction and neuropathy in diabetics. Diabetologia 12:258, 1976.
144. Melman A, Henry DP, Felten DL, O'Connor BL. Alteration of the penile corpora in patients with erectile impotence. Invest Urol 17:474, 1980.
145. Barrett-Conner E. Lower endogenous androgen levels and dyslipidemia in men with non–insulin dependent diabetes mellitus. Ann Intern Med 117:807, 1992.
146. Berchtold P, Berger M, Cuppers HJ, et al. Non-glucoregulatory hormones during physical exercise in juvenile-type diabetics. Horm Metab Res 6:335, 1974.
147. Gattucio F, Porcelli P, Morici V, et al. The hypothalamic-pituitary-testicular axis in diabetic subjects. *In* Fabrini A, Steinberger E (eds). Recent Progress in Andrology. New York, Academic Press, 1979, p 351.
148. Davidson JM, Chen JJ, Crapo L, et al. Hormonal changes and sexual function in aging men. J Clin Endocrinol Metab 57:71, 1983.

149. Kaler LW, Neaves WB. Attrition of the human Leydig cell population with advancing age. Anat Rec 192:513, 1978.
150. Johnson L, Zane RS, Petty CS, Neaves WB. Quantification of the human Sertoli cell population: Its distribution, relation to germ cell numbers, and age-related decline. Biol Reprod 31:785, 1984.
151. Johnson L, Petty CS, Neaves WB. Influence of age on sperm production and testicular weights in men. J Reprod Fertil 70:211, 1984.
152. Paniagua R, Martin A, Nistal M, Amat P. Testicular involution in elderly men: Comparison of histologic quantitative studies with hormone patterns. Fertil Steril 47:671, 1987.
153. Pincus SM, Mulligan T, Iranmanesh A, et al. Older males secrete luteinizing hormone and testosterone more irregularly, and jointly more asynchronously, than younger males. Proc Natl Acad Sci USA 93:14100, 1996.
154. Tenover JS, McLachlan RI, Dahl KD, et al. Decreased serum inhibin levels in normal elderly men: Evidence for a decline in Sertoli cell function with aging. J Clin Endocrinol Metab 67:455, 1988.
155. Tsitouras PD, Martin CE, Harman SM. Relationship of serum testosterone to sexual activity in healthy elderly men. J Gerontol 37:288, 1982.
156. Vermeulen A, Kaufman JM, Giagulli VA. Influence of some biological indexes on sex hormone–binding globulin and androgen levels in aging or obese males. J Clin Endocrinol Metab 81:1821, 1996.
157. Role of the hypothalamo-pituitary function in the hypoandrogenism of healthy aging (Editorial). J Clin Endocrinol Metab 75:704, 1992.
158. Mulligan T, Iranmanesh A, Gheorghiu S, et al. Amplified nocturnal luteinizing hormone (LH) secretory burst frequency with selective attenuation of pulsatile (but not basal) testosterone secretion in healthy aged men: Possible Leydig cell desensitization to endogenous LH signaling—a clinical research center study. J Clin Endocrinol Metab 80:3025, 1995.
159. Deslypere JP, Kaufman JM, Vermeulen T, et al. Influence of age on pulsatile luteinizing hormone release and responsiveness of the gonadotrophs to sex hormone feedback in men. J Clin Endocrinol Metab 64:68, 1987.
160. Vermeulen A, Deslypere JP, Kaufman JM. Influence of antiopioids on luteinizing hormone pulsatility in aging men. J Clin Endocrinol Metab 68:68, 1989.
161. Plymate SR, Tenover JS, Bremner WJ. Circadian variation in testosterone, sex hormone–binding globulin, and calculated non–sex hormone–binding globulin bound testosterone in healthy young and elderly men. J Androl 10:366, 1989.
162. Winters S, Shawns R, Troen P. The gonadotropin suppressive activity of androgens is increased in elderly men. Metabolism 33:1052, 1984.
163. Grino PB, Griffin JE, Wilson JD. Androgen resistance due to decreased amounts of androgen receptor: A reinvestigation. J Steroid Biochem 35:647, 1990.
164. Rodien P, Mebarki F, Mowszowicz I, et al. Different phenotypes in a family with androgen insensitivity caused by the same M780I point mutation in the androgen receptor gene. J Clin Endocrinol Metab 81:2994, 1996.
165. Lumbroso S, Lobaccaro JM, Georget V, et al. A novel substitution (Leu707Arg) in exon 4 of the androgen receptor gene causes complete androgen resistance. J Clin Endocrinol Metab 81:1984, 1996.
166. Choong CS, Sturm MJ, Strophair JA, et al. Partial androgen insensitivity caused by an androgen receptor mutation at amino acid 907 (Gly→Arg) that results in decreased ligand binding affinity and reduced androgen receptor messenger ribonucleic acid levels. J Clin Endocrinol Metab 81:236, 1996.
167. Di Lauro SL, Behzadian A, Tho SPT, McDonough PG. Probing genomic deoxyribonucleic acid for gene rearrangement in 14 patients with androgen insensitivity syndrome. Fertil Steril 55:481, 1991.
168. French FS, Lubahn DB, Brown TR, et al. Molecular basis of androgen insensitivity. Recent Prog Horm Res 46:1, 1990.
169. MacLean HE, Choi W-T, Rekaris G, et al. Abnormal androgen receptor binding affinity in subjects with Kennedy's disease (spinal and bulbar muscular atrophy). J Clin Endocrinol Metab 80:508, 1995.
170. Faiman C, Winter JSD. The control of gonadotropin secretion in complete testicular feminization. J Clin Endocrinol Metab 39:631, 1974.
171. Grino PB, Isidro-Gutierrez RF, Griffin JE, Wilson JD. Androgen resistance associated with a qualitative abnormality of the androgen receptor and responsive to high dose androgen therapy. J Clin Endocrinol Metab 68:578, 1989.
172. Sinnecker G, Kohler S. Sex hormone–binding globulin response to the anabolic steroid stanozolol: Evidence for its suitability as a biological androgen sensitivity test. J Clin Endocrinol Metab 68:1195, 1989.
173. Aiman J, Griffin JE. The frequency of androgen receptor deficiency in infertile men. J Clin Endocrinol Metab 54:725, 1982.
174. Morrow AF, Gyorki S, Warne GL, et al. Variable androgen receptor levels in infertile men. J Clin Endocrinol Metab 64:1115, 1987.
175. Bouchard P, Wright F, Portois MC, et al. Androgen insensitivity in oligospermic men: A reappraisal. J Clin Endocrinol Metab 63:1242, 1986.
176. Migeon CJ, Brown TR, Lanes R, et al. A clinical syndrome of mild androgen insensitivity. J Clin Endocrinol Metab 59:672, 1984.
177. Eil C, Gamblin GT, Hodge JW, et al. Whole cell and nuclear androgen uptake in skin fibroblasts from infertile men. J Androl 6:365, 1985.
178. Boudon C, Lumbroso S, Lobaccaro JM, et al. Molecular study of the 5α-reductase type 2 gene in three European families with 5α-reductase deficiency. J Clin Endocrinol Metab 80:2149, 1995.
179. Johnson L, George FW, Neaves WB, et al. Characterization of the testicular abnormality in a 5α-reductase deficiency. J Clin Endocrinol Metab 63:1091, 1986.
180. Cia L-Q, Fratianni CM, Gautier T, Imperato-McGinley J. Dihydrotestosterone regulation of semen in male pseudohermaphrodites with 5α-reductase-2 deficiency. J Clin Endocrinol Metab 79:409, 1994.
181. Latronico AC, Anasti J, Arnhold IJP, et al. Brief report: Testicular and ovarian resistance to luteinizing hormone caused by inactivating mutations of the luteinizing hormone–receptor gene. N Engl J Med 334:507, 1996.
182. Beitins IZ, Axelrod L, Ostrea T, et al. Hypogonadism in a male with an immunologically active, biologically inactive luteinizing hormone. J Clin Endocrinol Metab 52:1143, 1981.
183. Morishima A, Grumbach MM, Simpson ER, et al. Aromatase deficiency in male and female siblings caused by a novel mutation and the physiological role of estrogens. J Clin Endocrinol Metab 80:3689, 1995.
184. Smith EP, Boyd J, Frank GR, et al. Estrogen resistance caused by a mutation in the estrogen-receptor gene in a man. N Engl J Med 331:1056, 1994.
185. Korach KS, Couse JF, Curtis SW, et al. Estrogen receptor gene disruption: Molecular characterization and experimental and clinical phenotypes. Recent Prog Horm Res 51:159, 1996.
186. Finkelstein JS, Klibanski A, Neer RM. A longitudinal evaluation of bone mineral density in adult men with histories of delayed puberty. J Clin Endocrinol Metab 81:1152, 1996.
187. Kulin HE. Extensive personal experience—delayed puberty. J Clin Endocrinol Metab 81:3460, 1996.
188. Balducci R, Toscano V, Casilli D, et al. Testicular responsiveness following chronic administration of hCG (1500 IU every six days) in untreated hypogonadotropic hypogonadism. Horm Metab Res 19:216, 1987.
189. Adan L, Souberbielle JC, Brauner R. Management of the short stature due to pubertal delay in boys. J Clin Endocrinol Metab 78:478, 1994.
190. Uriarte MM, Baron J, Garcia HB, et al. The effect of pubertal delay on adult height in men with isolated hypogonadotropic hypogonadism. J Clin Endocrinol Metab 74:436, 1992.
191. Snyder PJ. Clinical use of androgens. Annu Rev Med 35:207, 1984.
192. Cofrancesco J Jr, Dobs AS. Transdermal testosterone delivery systems. Endocrinologist 6:207, 1996.
193. Meikle AW, Arver S, Dobs AS, et al. Pharmacokinetics and metabolism of a permeation-enhanced testosterone transdermal system in hypogonadal men: Influence of application site—a clinical research center study. J Clin Endocrinol Metab 81:1832, 1996.

194. Testosterone patches for hypogonadism. Med Lett 38:49, 1996.
195. Bhasin S, Swerdloff RS, Steiner B, et al. A biodegradable testosterone microcapsule formulation provides uniform eugonadal levels of testosterone for 10–11 weeks in hypogonadal men. J Clin Endocrinol Metab 74:75, 1992.
196. Burris AS, Ewing LL, Sherins RL. Initial trial of slow-release testosterone microspheres in hypogonadal men. Fertil Steril 50:493, 1988.
197. Handelsman DJ, Conway AJ, Boylan LM. Pharmacokinetics and pharmacodynamics of testosterone pellets in man. J Clin Endocrinol Metab 70:216, 1990.
198. Jackson JA, Waxman J, Spiekerman M. Prostatic complications of testosterone replacement therapy. Arch Intern Med 149:2365, 1989.
199. Bardin CW, Swerdloff RS, Santen RJ. Androgens: Risk and benefits. J Clin Endocrinol Metab 73:4, 1991.
200. Friedl KE, Hannan CJ, Jones RE, Plymate SR. High density lipoprotein cholesterol is not decreased if an aromatizable androgen is administered. Metabolism 39:69, 1990.
201. Brodsky IG, Balagopal P, Nair KS. Effects of testosterone replacement on muscle mass and muscle protein synthesis in hypogonadal men—a clinical research center study. J Clin Endocrinol Metab 81:3469, 1996.
202. Wang C, Alexander G, Berman N, et al. Testosterone replacement therapy improves mood in hypogonadal men—a clinical research study. J Clin Endocrinol Metab 81:3578, 1996.
203. Ley SB, Leonard JM. Male hypogonadotropic hypogonadism: Factors influencing response to human chorionic gonadotropin and human menopausal gonadotropin, including prior exogenous androgens. J Clin Endocrinol Metab 61:746, 1985.
204. Tenover JS. Effects of testosterone supplementation in the aging male. J Clin Endocrinol Metab 75:1092, 1992.
205. Morley JE, Perry HM III, Kaiser FE, et al. Effects of testosterone replacement therapy in old hypogonadal males: A preliminary study. J Am Geriatr Soc 41:149, 1993.
206. Bagatell CJ, Bremner WJ. Androgens in men—uses and abuses. N Engl J Med 334:707, 1996.
207. Bardin CW. The anabolic action of testosterone. N Engl J Med 335:52, 1996.
208. Bhasin S, Storer TW, Berman N, et al. The effects of supraphysiologic doses of testosterone on muscle size and strength in normal men. N Engl J Med 335:1, 1996.
209. Tricker R, Casaburi R, Storer TW, et al. The effects of supraphysiologic doses of testosterone on angry behavior in healthy eugonadal men—a clinical research center study. J Clin Endocrinol Metab 81:3754, 1996.
210. Burris AS, Rodbard HW, Winters SJ, Sherins RJ. Gonadotropin therapy in men with isolated hypogonadotropic hypogonadism: The response to human chorionic gonadotropin is predicted by initial testicular size. J Clin Endocrinol Metab 66:1144, 1988.
211. Handelsman DJ, Turner L, Boylan LM, Conway AJ. Pharmacokinetics of human follicle-stimulating hormone in gonadotropin-deficient men. J Clin Endocrinol Metab 80:1657, 1995.
212. Liu L, Banks SM, Barnes KM, Sherins RJ. Two-year comparison of testicular responses to pulsatile gonadotropin-releasing hormone and exogenous gonadotropins from the inception of therapy in men with isolated hypogonadotropic hypogonadism. J Clin Endocrinol Metab 67:1140, 1988.
213. Liu L, Chaudhari N, Corle D, Sherins RJ. Comparison of pulsatile subcutaneous gonadotropin-releasing hormone and exogenous gonadotropins in the treatment of men with isolated hypogonadotropic hypogonadism. Fertil Steril 49:302, 1988.
214. Jockenhovel F, Khan SA, Nieschlag E. Diagnostic value of bioactive FSH in male infertility. Acta Endocrinol (Copenh) 121:802, 1989.
215. Fauser BCJM, Bogers JW, Hop WCJ, De Jong FH. Bioactive and immunoreactive FSH in serum of normal and oligospermic men. Clin Endocrinol (Oxf) 32:433, 1990.
216. Wang C, Dahl KD, Leung A, et al. Serum bioactive follicle-stimulating hormone in men with idiopathic azoospermia and oligospermia. J Clin Endocrinol Metab 65:629, 1987.
217. Bain J, Moskowitz JP, Clapp JJ. LH and FSH response to gonadotropin releasing hormone (GnRH) in normospermic, oligospermic and azoospermic men. Arch Androl 1:147, 1978.
218. Wu FCW, Edmond P, Raab G, Hunter WM. Endocrine assessment of the subfertile male. Clin Endocrinol (Oxf) 14:493, 1981.
219. Chemes HE, Dym M, Fawcett DW, et al. Pathophysiological observations of Sertoli cells in patients with germinal aplasia or severe germ cell depletion. Biol Reprod 17:108, 1977.
220. Rjosk HK, Schill WB. Serum prolactin in male infertility. Andrologia 11:297, 1979.
221. Howards SS. Treatment of male infertility. N Engl J Med 332:312, 1995.
222. Baker HWG. Development of clinical trials in male infertility research. *In* Serio M (ed). Perspectives in Andrology, Vol 53. New York, Raven Press, 1989, p 307.
223. World Health Organization Task Force on the Diagnosis and Treatment of Infertility. Mesterolone and idiopathic male infertility: A double-blinded study. Int J Androl 12:254, 1989.
224. Sokol RZ. The diagnosis and treatment of male infertility. Curr Opin Obstet Gynecol 7:177, 1995.
225. Palermo GD, Cohen J, Rosenwaks Z. Intracytoplasmic sperm injection: A powerful tool to overcome fertilization failure. Fertil Steril 65:899, 1996.
226. Sherins RJ, Thorsell LP, Dorfmann A, et al. Intracytoplasmic sperm injection facilitates fertilization even in the most severe forms of male infertility: Pregnancy outcome correlates with maternal age and number of eggs available. Fertil Steril 64:3699, 1995.
227. Van Steirteghem AC, Liu J, Joris H, et al. Higher success rate by intracytoplasmic sperm injection than by subzonal insemination. A report of a second series of 300 consecutive treatment cycles. Hum Reprod 8:1055, 1993.
228. Comhaire FH. Evaluation and treatment of varicocele. *In* Santen RJ, Swerdloff RS (eds). Male Reproductive Dysfunction: Diagnosis and Management of Hypogonadism, Infertility, and Impotence. New York, Marcel Dekker, 1986, pp 387–406.
229. Pryor JL, Howards SS. Varicocele. Urol Clin North Am 14:499, 1987.
230. Kursh ED. What is the incidence of varicocele in a fertile population? Fertil Steril 48:510, 1987.
231. Steeno O, Knops J, Declerck L, et al. Prevention of fertility disorders by detection and treatment of varicocele at school and college age. Andrologia 8:47, 1971.
232. Plymate SR, Nagao RR, Muller CH, Paulsen CA. The use of sperm penetration assay in evaluation of men with varicocele. Fertil Steril 47:680, 1987.
233. Baker HWG, Burger HG, de Kretser DM, et al. Testicular vein ligation and fertility in men with varicoceles. Br Med J 291:1678, 1985.
234. Vermeulen A, Vandeweghe M. Improved fertility after varicocele correction: Fact or fiction? Fertil Steril 42:249, 1984.
235. Okuyama A, Fujisue H, Doi MY, et al. Surgical repair of varicocele: Effective treatment from subfertile men in a controlled study. Eur Urol 14:298, 1988.
236. Hudson RW. The endocrinology of varicoceles. Fertil Steril 49:199, 1988.
237. Bickel A, Dickstein G. Factors predicting the outcome of varicocele repair for subfertility: The value of the luteinizing hormone–releasing hormone test. J Urol 142:1230, 1989.
238. Lipshultz LL, Corriere JN Jr. Progressive testicular atrophy in the varicocele patient. J Urol 117:175, 1977.
239. Kass EJ, Belman AB. Reversal of testicular growth failure by varicocele ligation. J Urol 137:475, 1987.
240. Lyon RP, Marshall S, Scott MP. Varicocele in childhood and adolescence: Implication in adulthood infertility? Urology 19:641, 1982.
241. Jarow JP, Espeland MA, Lipshultz LI. Evaluation of the azoospermic patient. J Urol 142:62, 1989.
242. Urban MD, Lee PA, Migeon CJ. Adult height and fertility in men with congenital virilizing adrenal hyperplasia. N Engl J Med 299:1392, 1978.
243. Bonaccorsi AC, Adler I, Figuieredo JG. Male infertility due to congenital adrenal hyperplasia: Testicular biopsy findings, hormonal evaluation, and therapeutic results in three patients. Fertil Steril 47:664, 1987.
244. Brown-Woodman PDC, Post EJ, Gass GC, White IG. The effect of a single sauna exposure on spermatozoa. Arch Androl 12:9, 1984.
245. Berger RE, Holmes KK. Infection and male infertility. *In* Santen RJ, Swerdloff RS (eds). Male Reproductive Dysfunction: Diagnosis and Management of Hypogonadism, Infertility, and Impotence. New York, Marcel Dekker, 1986, p 407.

246. Handelsman DJ, Conway AJ, Boylan LM, Turtle JR. Young's syndrome: Obstructive azoospermia and chronic sinopulmonary infections. N Engl J Med 310:3, 1984.
247. Gagnon C, Sherins RJ, Phillips DM, Bardin CW. Deficiency of protein–carboxyl methylase in immobile spermatozoa of infertile men. N Engl J Med 306:821, 1982.
248. Chandley AC. Assessment of blood karyotypes and germinal cell meiosis in the evaluation of male infertility. *In* Santen RJ, Swerdloff RS (eds). Male Reproductive Dysfunction: Diagnosis and Management of Hypogonadism, Infertility, and Impotence. New York, Marcel Dekker, 1986, p 457.
249. Kotecki M, Jaruzelska J, Skowronska M, Fichna P. Deletion mapping of interval 6 of the human Y chromosome. Hum Genet 87:234, 1994.
250. Vogt P, Chandley AC, Hargreave TV, et al. Microdeletions in interval 6 of the Y-chromosome of males with idiopathic sterility point disruption of *AZF,* a human spermatogenesis gene. Hum Genet 89:491, 1992.
251. Nagafuchi S, Namiki M, Nakahor Y, et al. A minute deletion of the Y-chromosome in men with azoospermia. J Urol 150:1155, 1993.
252. Ma K, Sharkey A, Kirsh S, et al. Towards the molecular localization of the *AZF* locus: Mapping of microdeletions in azoospermic men within fourteen subintervals of interval 6 of the human Y-chromosome. Hum Mol Genet 1:29, 1992.
253. Najmabadi H, Huang V, Yen P, et al. Substantial prevalence of microdeletions of the Y-chromosome in infertile men with idiopathic azoospermia and oligozoospermia detected using a sequence-tagged site-based mapping strategy. J Clin Endocrinol Metab 81:1347, 1996.
254. Ma K, Inglis JD, Sharkey A, et al. A Y chromosome gene family with RNA-binding protein homology: Candidates for the azoospermia factor *AZF* controlling human spermatogenesis. Cell 75:1287, 1993.
255. Smith BR, Furmaniak J. Adrenal gonadal autoimmune diseases (Editorial). J Clin Endocrinol Metab 80:1502, 1995.
256. Hendry WF, Hughes L, Scammell G, et al. Comparison of prednisolone and placebo in subfertile men with antibodies to spermatozoa. Lancet 335:85, 1990.
257. Bals-Pratsch M, Doren M, Karbowski B, et al. Cyclic corticosteroid immunosuppression is unsuccessful in the treatment of sperm antibody related male infertility: A controlled study. Hum Reprod 7:99, 1992.
258. Stenchever MA, Williamson RA, Leonard J, et al. Possible relationship between in utero diethylstilbestrol exposure and male fertility. Am J Obstet Gynecol 140:186, 1981.
259. Shangold GA, Cantor B, Schreiber JR. Treatment of infertility due to retrograde ejaculation: A simple, cost-effective method. Fertil Steril 54:175, 1990.
260. Baker HWG, Burger HG, de Kretser DM, Hudson B. Relative incidence of etiologic disorders in male infertility. *In* Santen RJ, Swerdloff RS (eds). Male Reproductive Dysfunction: Diagnosis and Management of Hypogonadism, Infertility, and Impotence. New York, Marcel Dekker, 1986, pp 341–372.
261. Biro FM, Lucky AW, Huster GA, Morrison JA. Hormonal studies and physical maturation in adolescent gynecomastia. J Pediatr 116:450, 1990.
262. Niewoehner CB, Nuttal FQ. Gynecomastia in a hospitalized male population. Am J Med 77:633, 1984.
263. Andersen JA, Gram JB. Male breast at autopsy. Acta Pathol Microbiol Immunol Scand A 90:191, 1982.
264. Sandison AT. An autopsy study of the adult human breast. Natl Cancer Inst Monogr 8:77, 80, 1962.
265. Eil C, Lippman ME, de Moss EKY, Loriaux DL. Androgen receptor characteristics in skin fibroblasts from men with pubertal macromastia. Clin Endocrinol (Oxf) 19:223, 1983.
266. Dershaw DD. Male mammography. AJR 146:127, 1986.
267. Jackson VP, Gilmore RL. Male breast carcinoma and gynecomastia: Comparison of mammography with sonography. Radiology 149:533, 1986.
268. Ley SR, Mozaffarian GA, Leonard JM, et al. Palpable breast tissue versus gynecomastia as a normal physical finding. Clin Res 28:24A, 1980.
269. Nydick M, Bustos J, Dale JH Jr, Rawson RW. Gynecomastia in adolescent boys. JAMA 178:449, 1961.
270. Santen RJ. Gynecomastia. *In* DeGroot LJ, Besser M, Burger HG, et al (eds). Endocrinology, 3rd ed, Vol 3. Philadelphia, WB Saunders, 1995, pp 2474–2484.
271. Krane RJ, Goldstein I, De Tejada IS. Impotence. N Engl J Med 321:1648, 1989.
272. Linet OI, Ogrinc FG, for the Alprostadil Study Group. Efficacy and safety of intracavernosal alprostadil in men with erectile dysfunction. N Engl J Med 334:873, 1996.
273. Burris AS, Banks SM, Sherins RJ. Quantitative assessment of nocturnal penile tumescence and rigidity in normal men using a home monitor. J Androl 10:492, 1989.
274. Fabbri A, Jannini EA, Ulisse S, et al. Low serum bioactive luteinizing hormone in nonorganic male impotence: Possible relationship with altered gonadotropin-releasing hormone pulsatility. J Clin Endocrinol Metab 67:867, 1988.
275. Cunningham GR, Hirshkowitz M, Korenman SG, Karacan I. Testosterone replacement therapy and sleep-related erections in hypogonadal men. J Clin Endocrinol Metab 70:792, 1990.
276. Korenman SG. Advances in the understanding and management of erectile dysfunction. J Clin Endocrinol Metab 80:1985, 1995.

Chapter 24

INHIBIN, ACTIVIN, AND NEOPLASIA

Henry G. Burger

CHAPTER OUTLINE

KEY POINTS

- The inhibins are a family of dimeric proteins made up of an α-subunit linked to one of two β-subunits, β_A or β_B, to give the major species, inhibins A and B.
- Inhibins A and B are products of the ovarian granulosa cell and the testicular Sertoli cell and are differentially regulated throughout the menstrual cycle. Only inhibin B is found in significant amounts in adult men.
- There is substantial evidence that the inhibins exert negative feedback effects on pituitary FSH secretion.
- The activins are dimers of the β-subunits that stimulate FSH and have a diverse range of nonreproductive effects.
- The follistatins are activin-binding proteins.
- Evidence has been obtained experimentally that the inhibin α-subunit may be a tumor suppressor gene. In contrast, the inhibins and activins and their subunits are demonstrable in various ovarian cancer types by immunohistochemistry.
- Circulating inhibin levels are elevated in postmenopausal women with granulosa cell and mucinous epithelial cancers and in a proportion of those with serous epithelial cancers.
- Serum inhibin levels are useful markers of disease progression, particularly in granulosa cell tumors.
- Current studies suggest a role for the inhibin/activin family in prostate cancer.
- Assays for inhibin represent an important advance, aiding in the management of certain types of ovarian malignant disease in particular, and their roles in other malignant neoplasms are the subject of current research.

The postulate that a nonsteroidal gonadal factor exerts feedback effects on pituitary gonadotropin secretion was confirmed by the successful isolation and characterization of inhibin, a hormone identified by its ability to selectively suppress the synthesis and secretion of follicle-stimulating hormone (FSH). The subsequent cloning of inhibin established it to be a heterodimeric protein consisting of an α-subunit linked to one of two structurally similar but nonidentical β-subunits to give inhibin A ($\alpha\beta_A$) and inhibin B ($\alpha\beta_B$). Soon afterward, the intriguing observation was made that homodimers of the β-subunits had an action on FSH opposite to that of inhibin; that is, they stimulated rather than suppressed FSH secretion, and they were called activins. The β-subunits were recognized to belong, on the basis of structural homologies, to the larger family of peptides generally called the transforming growth factor-β family.[1, 2] Additional β-subunits have recently been identified (e.g., β_C, β_D), but their roles and significance await elucidation.

Within 2 years of the initial isolation of inhibin, another single-chain peptide, structurally unrelated to the inhibins, was identified on the basis of its shared property of suppressing FSH and was called follistatin. Its FSH-suppressing action appears to result primarily from its ability to bind activin and hence to negate its FSH-stimulating activity.[3] The establishment of a radioimmunoassay for inhibin and its application to the sera of patients with ovarian granulosa cell tumors[4] led to the current interest in the role of the inhibin/activin family in neoplasia, particularly in ovarian cancer. In this chapter, a general description of the inhibins, activins, and follistatins is followed by a consideration of their roles in the pathogenesis, diagnosis, and monitoring of reproductive tract and other malignant neoplasms.

THE INHIBINS

Inhibin was originally isolated from ovarian follicular fluid, in which it was shown that FSH-suppressing activity was present in a range of molecular weight species. Inhibin in serum also exists in a variety of molecular weights; Figure 24–1 shows in diagrammatic form the structures of the inhibin subunits, their precursors, and the various inhibin dimers that have been isolated.[5] The precise contribution of each molecular weight form to the biologic activity present in serum has not been determined, but it is clear that several forms (e.g., the 55-kDa and the 32-kDa forms) are biologically active.[6] The higher molecular weight forms represent various combinations of subunit precursors, and present evidence indicates that biologic activity depends on at least one of the two subunits being in its mature rather than its precursor form. It is likely that the lowest biologically active molecular weight form, 32 kDa, represents the ultimate product of proteolytic cleavage of larger molecular weight precursors. In addition to the presence of various dimeric forms in the circulation, free α-subunit–derived peptides also circulate and have complicated the interpretation of the originally developed radioimmunoassays.[7] The origins and functions of the free α-subunits are unclear.

Dimeric inhibins are products of the ovarian granulosa cell and the testicular Sertoli cell; inhibin subunit messenger ribonucleic acids (mRNAs) have been identified in a number of other organs and tissues, including the adrenal.[1, 2] Because dimeric inhibin forms are not detectable in plasma in either sex after castration, it appears that at least from the point of view of circulating hormone, the only significant sources are the gonads.

The isolation of inhibin was initially facilitated by the development of bioassays in which the suppression of FSH content or secretion by cultured pituitary cells was the assay endpoint.[1, 2] Radioimmunoassays were developed that are now recognized to have been of rather broad specificity, in that they recognize both inhibin A and B in addition to the subunit precursors.[7] Specific assays have recently been developed that recognize only dimeric inhibin A or B or the α-subunit precursor pro-αC (see Fig. 24–1). Studies of the secretion of the specific dimeric inhibins during the human menstrual cycle have indicated that their secretion is differentially regulated.[8] Inhibin A is secreted at relatively low levels for most of the follicular phase of the cycle, rises in association with the midcycle gonadotropin surge, and reaches its highest levels in the luteal phase, in parallel with the secretion of progesterone. It is a product of follicular granulosa cells and of the corpus luteum. The levels fall rapidly in parallel with those of luteal progesterone and estradiol toward the end of the cycle and may contribute to the FSH increase that occurs at the time of the luteal-follicular transition.

On the other hand, inhibin B rises subsequent to the

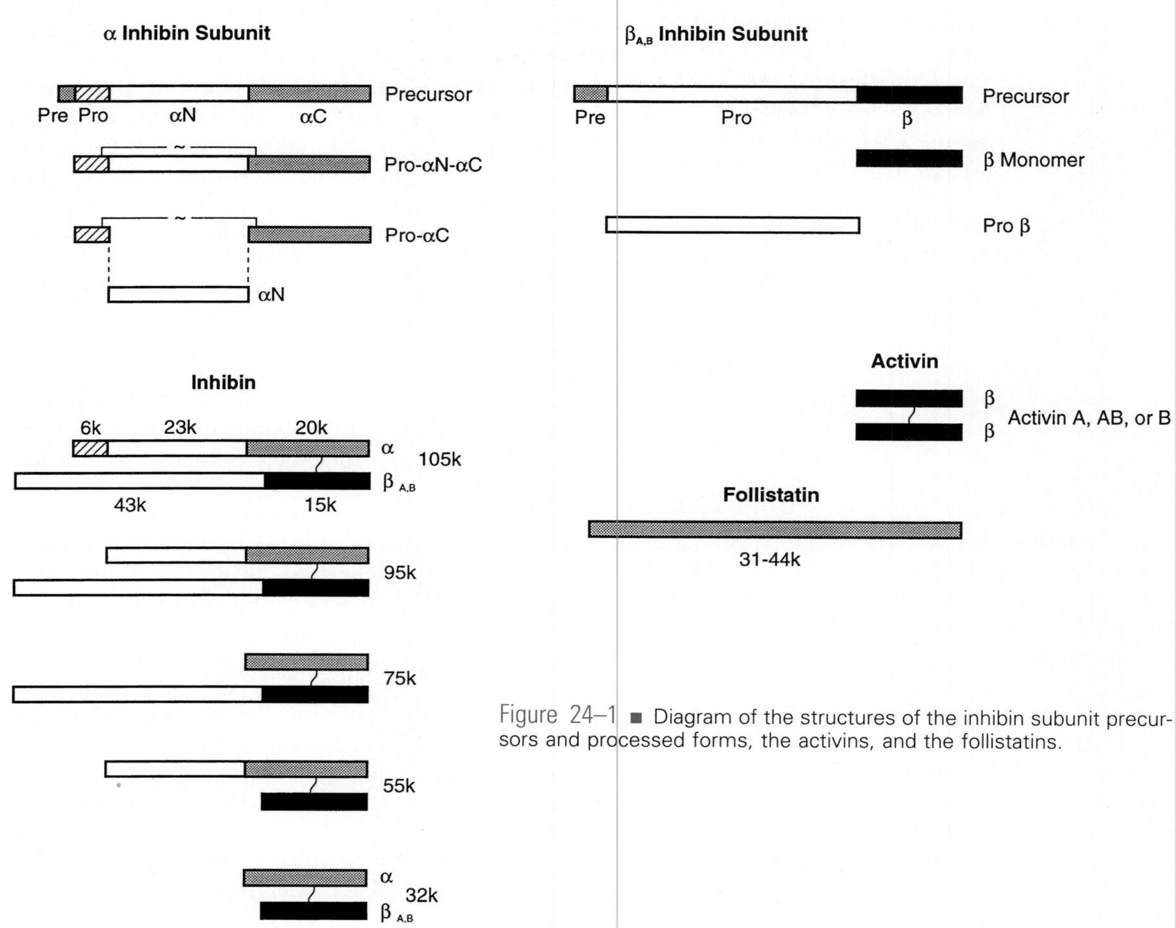

Figure 24–1 ■ Diagram of the structures of the inhibin subunit precursors and processed forms, the activins, and the follistatins.

early follicular FSH peak and reaches its maximal levels in the midfollicular phase. A small peak occurs around midcycle, but levels subsequently fall throughout the luteal phase. Inhibin B may thus be a product of the cohort of developing follicles from which the dominant follicle is selected and may be involved in the feedback regulation of FSH during the follicular phase, whereas inhibin A may exert its major effects during the luteal phase, acting in concert with estradiol and progesterone to suppress FSH to its lowest cycle levels.

In contrast to the situation in the female, the human male appears to secrete only inhibin B. Evidence for a likely physiologic role for inhibin B in the control of FSH secretion in the male has been obtained.[9]

In the human female, there is a considerable body of evidence that is compatible with a physiologic role for the inhibins in the regulation of FSH, although much of this has used the less specific radioimmunoassay in which α-subunit cross-reactivity has been demonstrated.[10] Nevertheless, there may be a role for inhibin in the feedback regulation of FSH throughout the menstrual cycle, and declining inhibin secretion appears to contribute significantly to the rising FSH levels observed during the menopausal transition and after the menopause.[11] Inhibin levels are normally low or undetectable postmenopausally, and this has made the postmenopausal period, in particular, a time when inhibin measurements may contribute to the diagnosis and monitoring of ovarian malignant disease.

Although inhibin was initially isolated on the basis of its postulated role as a feedback regulator of pituitary FSH, it has been demonstrated that local pituitary production of the inhibin family of peptides occurs, and thus local autocrine and paracrine mechanisms are also operative.

Major and unresolved issues with regard to the inhibins are the identification of the inhibin receptor or receptors and an elucidation of their mechanism of action, particularly at the receptor and signal transduction level. A number of groups have attempted to isolate and characterize the inhibin receptor, but none has so far reported success.

THE ACTIVINS

As predicted from the existence of two forms of the inhibin subunit, there are three forms of activin, activin A ($\beta_A\beta_A$), activin B ($\beta_B\beta_B$), and activin AB ($\beta_A\beta_B$), with the possibility that further members of this group may be developed (e.g., $\beta_C\beta_C$ or $\beta_D\beta_D$). High-molecular-weight forms of activin occur in vivo. Whereas the inhibins appear to have been involved primarily in the regulation of FSH secretion, the activins have been shown to have much wider biologic roles. These include erythropoiesis, mesodermal differentiation, neurotransmitter function, regulation of secretion of other pituitary and pancreatic hormones, and various aspects of placental function.[2] The development of assays for circulating activins has proved to be more difficult than has the development of inhibin assays, primarily because of the presence of activin-binding proteins in the circulation, particularly the follistatins. However, several activin assays have been reported, and unlike the situation with inhibin, activin does not appear to be involved primarily as a feedback regulator of gonadotropin secretion. If anything, activin levels rise progressively with increasing age and show little fluctuation throughout the menstrual cycle.[12] Activin A levels rise throughout pregnancy, particularly in the third trimester. Because of the wide variety of activin biologic activities, there may be an important role for the activins in the pathogenesis of a number of malignant neoplasms.

In contrast to the situation with the inhibins, a variety of activin receptors have been characterized. There are two main activin receptor subtypes, Act-RI and Act-RII, with several isoforms of the Act-RII receptor.[13] The mechanism of activin action involves the binding of the hormone to the RII receptor with subsequent complex formation with the RI receptor, which in turn leads to signal transduction through a serine-threonine kinase mechanism (Fig. 24–2). The identification of the activin receptors has led to a number of publications in which both activin and activin receptor levels have been characterized in various tissues.

THE FOLLISTATINS

The follistatins are a family of single-chain polypeptides with two major molecular weight forms resulting from the differential splicing of follistatin mRNA, follistatin 288 and follistatin 315.[3] Both are glycosylated to varying degrees, giving rise to a total of nine different forms of the

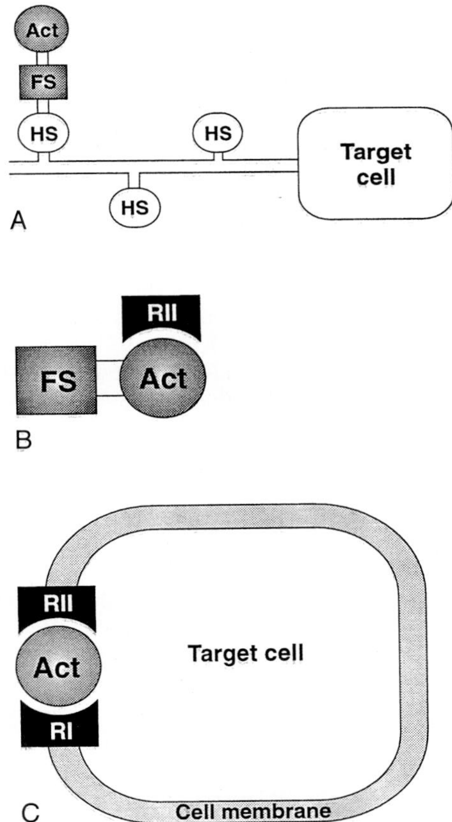

Figure 24–2 ■ Follistatin (FS) can bind to cell surface heparan sulfate (HS) proteoglycans *(A)* and also bind activin (Act). The follistatin-activin complex may be a mechanism for presentation of activin to the Act-RII receptor *(B)*. The Act-RII–activin complex then dimerizes with Act-RI, resulting in intracellular signal transduction *(C)*.

mature molecule. The major role of the follistatins appears to be to act as activin-binding proteins. They also show the property of binding to cell surface glycoproteins and may thus participate in the process of presenting activin to its receptors as illustrated in Figure 24–2. Follistatins appear to be produced locally in tissues that also produce the activins and therefore seem likely to exhibit crucial modulatory roles in the actions of the activins.

THE GONADAL PEPTIDES AND NEOPLASIA

To date, in the field of oncology, the most widely characterized role of the inhibin-related family of peptides has been in ovarian malignant neoplasms of various types. A potential role in placental neoplasms has also been postulated, and limited studies of the inhibin-related family in testicular and prostatic tumors have been published. The possibility that the inhibin α-subunit is a tumor suppressor has been raised as a result of studies in mice transgenic for deletion of the subunit, and this animal model has also suggested the possibility of an involvement of the inhibin family in the pathogenesis of adrenal tumors. Finally, the application of an assay specific for activin A to the sera of patients with various solid tumors has indicated that some such tumors are characterized by elevated activin levels.[12]

Ovarian Cancer

Types of Ovarian Cancer

The most common form of ovarian malignant disease is epithelial ovarian cancer, constituting approximately two thirds of all ovarian tumors. Among these, the predominant variety is the serous cystadenocarcinoma; other less frequent forms include mucinous cystadenocarcinoma, endometrioid carcinoma, and clear cell carcinoma. About one quarter of ovarian tumors are of the germ cell type, including teratomas, dysgerminomas, and yolk sac tumors; the minority (approximately 10 percent) are made up of sex cord stromal tumors, including granulosa cell tumors, thecomas, and luteomas. Deaths from ovarian cancer outnumber those from other forms of gynecologic cancer combined, and in Western societies, the lifetime risk for the development of ovarian cancer is estimated to be in the range 1:80 to 1:100. There is currently substantial interest in the possibility that ovarian cancer may have increased as the result of the development of assisted reproductive technologies, particularly those involving ovarian hyperstimulation. Regrettably, most patients with ovarian cancer present at an advanced stage, with a resulting poor 5-year survival. The inhibin-related family may be involved in the pathogenesis of ovarian tumors, but currently their most practical role is as markers in the monitoring of patients with granulosa cell tumors, with the potential to be of value in other types of ovarian malignant disease.

The Inhibin Family and Ovarian Tumor Pathogenesis

That the inhibin family might be involved in the pathogenesis of certain types of ovarian tumor was strongly suggested by the finding that mice transgenic for deletion of the inhibin α-subunit gene developed mixed or incompletely differentiated gonadal stromal tumors in the females and Sertoli-Leydig cell tumors in the males.[14] If the gonads were removed, the surviving animals went on to develop adrenal tumors, suggesting a tumor-suppressing role for the α-subunit in both ovarian and adrenal neoplasia.

The precise mechanism for tumor production in such transgenic mice is as yet unclear. Deletion of the inhibin α-subunit gene will clearly abolish inhibin secretion, leading to partially unregulated secretion of FSH. Because FSH is mitogenic for granulosa cells and is known to stimulate the synthesis and secretion of inhibin and its subunits, the stromal tumors might result from unregulated FSH secretion. On the other hand, the actions of α-subunit could lead to the unregulated expression of β-subunit dimers. Because activin is known to influence adrenal cortical, ovarian, and testicular cell proliferation, it could be the unregulated secretion of activin that leads to the development of ovarian and subsequently adrenocortical neoplasia. Further, the development of tumors in the transgenic mice was rapidly followed by a cachexia-like syndrome, which appears to result from an Act-RII receptor–mediated effect of activin.[15] When mice transgenic for the α-subunit deletion were crossed with mice in which the Act-RII receptor had been deleted, the resulting offspring did not develop cachexia and hepatic necrosis, but gonadal tumors were still observed. This suggested either that activin was not involved in the pathogenesis of the tumors or that its action might involve a different receptor.

The development of tumor-derived cell lines from such transgenic mice is facilitated by crossing them with mice in which the *P53* gene has also been deleted, suggesting that the development of the full malignant phenotype may require a "second hit." Studies of a variety of ovarian cancer–derived cell lines have also shown differential expression and production of inhibin/activin subunits, follistatin, and Act-RII receptors. Activin stimulated proliferation of cell lines that did not produce follistatin. These studies provide further evidence of potential roles for this group of hormones in ovarian neoplasia.[15–17] The pathogenesis of ovarian tumors and the potential role of the inhibin family in this process have been reviewed.[18]

The Localization of Inhibin and Activin in Ovarian Tumors

Several reports have indicated the presence of inhibin or activin in ovarian malignant neoplasms. Biologically and immunologically active inhibin was extracted from a granulosa cell tumor[19]; the ovarian vein draining the tumor was shown to have levels of immunoreactive inhibin higher than those in peripheral blood, whereas the contralateral ovarian vein had levels not statistically different from those in the periphery. An immunohistochemical investigation, using antibodies for the inhibin/activin subunits as well as intact inhibin A and activins A and B, demonstrated the presence of inhibin, activin, and their subunits in several mucinous cystadenocarcinomas of the ovary and in one granulosa cell tumor. Several serous cystadenocarcinomas, a clear cell tumor, and control endocervical tissues showed no staining. The mucinous tumors showed that the peptides were present in the epithelial cells and not in the stroma.[20] The demonstration of activin in several ovarian tumors raises the possibility that circulating activin levels might be raised, but no studies of such levels have yet been published. The demonstration of α-subunit in ovarian tumors seems to contradict the potential role of the α-subunit as a tumor suppressor. It could be, however, that the α-subunit is a tumor suppressor in some circumstances but that in others, when the α-subunit is present, a defect in the FSH-stimulated signal transduction pathway preceding α-subunit synthesis may be responsible for tumor pathogenesis. Whereas Lyons and colleagues[21] reported that 30 percent of sex cord tumors contained activating mutations of the $G\alpha_{i\text{-}2}$ subunit gene, this has not been confirmed in a subsequent study.[22]

Inhibins as Markers of Ovarian Tumors

The first report that the circulating immunoreactive inhibin levels might be useful as markers of ovarian tumors was the description by Lappohn and colleagues[4] of elevated inhibin concentrations in sera from patients with granulosa cell tumors. These samples were drawn from a tissue bank and were obtained at various stages of the evolution of the disease. The authors noted that elevations in serum immunoreactive inhibin could be present as long as 2 years before the development of clinically recurrent disease. Kauppila and associates[23] reported the use of immunoreactive inhibin as a marker of response or lack of response of a small group of patients treated with a gonadotropin-releasing hormone agonist. The immunoreactive inhibin levels broadly paralleled the clinical evolution of the disease in these patients. The most extensive study of the use of immunoreactive inhibin as a marker of granulosa cell tumors was that of Jobling and coworkers,[24] which confirmed the useful role of the assay in the monitoring of disease progression in patients with granulosa cell tumors. A major portion of the inhibin immunoreactivity that circulates in patients with granulosa cell tumors is biologically active dimeric inhibin A.[25, 26] In such patients, an inverse relationship between inhibin A and FSH concentrations has been demonstrated.[27] It is of interest that levels of a related gonadal peptide, müllerian-inhibiting substance, have also been reported as being elevated in patients with sex cord tumors, including granulosa cell tumors.[28]

Serum immunoreactive inhibin levels in patients with granulosa cell tumors are usually markedly in excess of those found during the menstrual cycle. Thus, inhibin measurements can be useful in patients with granulosa cell tumor both during the reproductive age and postmenopausally. However, if a granulosa cell tumor is removed unilaterally, with preservation of the contralateral ovary, the measurement of inhibin as a marker of tumor recurrence is unlikely to be helpful, unless levels again rise well above those found during the cycle. In contrast, in women who have had both ovaries removed or who are spontaneously postmenopausal, inhibin levels are of value in the monitoring of granulosa cell tumor progression.

Immunoreactive inhibin levels are elevated in the majority of patients with mucinous cystadenocarcinomas, both of clear-cut malignant potential and of borderline malignancy.[27] Because inhibin levels in mucinous cystadenocarcinoma are not nearly as elevated as those in granulosa cell tumor, the practical application of the assay in this situation is limited to postmenopausal or oophorectomized women. The most extensive report to date indicated elevated inhibin concentrations in 16 of 18 postmenopausal women with mucinous cystadenocarcinomas. Levels were shown to fall into the normal range within a week of surgery. There was no correlation between immunoreactive inhibin and serum CA125 levels. Specific inhibin A assay has also shown elevated levels in some patients with mucinous tumors,[25] but there was no correlation between immunoreactive inhibin and inhibin A in these tumors. Furthermore, in contrast to the situation with granulosa cell tumors, there was no relationship between circulating FSH and immunoreactive inhibin levels in patients with mucinous tumors,[27] suggesting that these secrete members of the inhibin family other than biologically active dimeric inhibin A or alternatively that they could secrete varying levels of activin, thus perturbing any relationship between inhibin and FSH. Because of these findings, the less specific assays that recognize a variety of inhibin-related family members appear to be those most likely to contribute significantly to the clinical diagnosis and monitoring of patients with ovarian malignant disease.

It can be suggested that postmenopausal women in particular suspected of having an ovarian malignant neoplasm should have preoperative serum taken for subsequent inhibin assay. If an ovarian malignant neoplasm is identified, postoperative serum should be obtained and both preoperative and postoperative samples subjected to assay by use of one of the less specific inhibin assays. The finding of elevated preoperative levels would suggest that monitoring with use of the inhibin assay may be of practical value. Because CA125, widely used in the monitoring particularly of serous epithelial tumors, is not consistently elevated in mucinous or granulosa cell tumors, the inhibin assay may have an important role complementary to that of CA125 and other ovarian tumor markers in the clinical management of patients with this disease.

Hydatidiform Mole and Choriocarcinoma

An early report[29] in which the relatively nonspecific inhibin immunoassay was applied suggested that inhibin measurement might be a useful marker of the presence and progress of hydatidiform mole and choriocarcinoma. Circulating inhibin levels were reported to fall more rapidly than those of the more classic human chorionic gonadotropin (hCG)–related tumor markers. A subsequent study[30] has not confirmed this observation and has in fact suggested that the hCG assay is a more useful tumor marker than is inhibin. Further studies using both a nonspecific inhibin assay and the more specific inhibin A assay in particular are needed to establish whether the inhibin-related family of peptides has a role in the monitoring of placental tumors.

Testicular Tumors

Limited reports have been published of inhibin measurements in men with testicular tumor.[31] The precise nature of circulating inhibin immunoreactivity in males has been clarified only recently with the recognition that the physiologically active peptide is inhibin B.[9] The sera of males contain relatively large quantities of inhibin α-subunit–related material, the origin of which is unclear.[6] Limited observations suggest that exogenous sex steroid administration results in suppression of these levels, consistent with their being gonadotropin dependent and perhaps of Leydig cell origin. Levels have in particular been noted to be elevated in men with Klinefelter's syndrome. The fact that only unilateral orchiectomy is carried out in most men with testicular tumor has made the interpretation of postoperative inhibin measurements unreliable and difficult. Whereas the remaining testis is capable of secreting inhibin, the peptide is unlikely to be useful as a tumor marker.

The possible role of the inhibin-related family in the pathogenesis of the rare Sertoli-Leydig cell tumors has been described before. Of interest are experimental studies of testicular tumorigenesis in transgenic mice that express the 6-kilobase mouse inhibin α-subunit promoter/simian virus 40 T-antigen (SV40 Tag) fusion gene, in which the tumors are confined to the Leydig cells.[32]

Prostate Cancer

Inhibin-related proteins have been demonstrated in the rat prostate,[33] and mRNAs for activin β_A and β_B subunits have been found in the human prostate.[34] In addition, the capacity to synthesize activins and follistatins has been supported by the localization of immunoreactivity for β_A and β_B subunit proteins, activin A, and follistatin to the epithelial cells of men with advanced stage carcinoma of the prostate.[34] Collectively, these data show that inhibin-related proteins (particularly activins) are present in the prostate, but their role in the progression to prostate cancer remains to be determined.

Other Malignant Neoplasms

Although no diagnostic monitoring role has been described for the inhibin-related family of peptides in other malignant neoplasms, the potential that they may be involved is clear. Thus, the expression of inhibin subunit mRNAs in pituitary adenomas has been described,[35] and the possible role of the α-subunit peptide in the pathogenesis of adrenal tumors has been noted. A publication in which an assay specific for activin A was applied to patients with a variety of diseases showed elevated activin A levels in some patients with solid tumors.[12] It seems likely that the wider application of immunoassays for specific types of inhibin-related family members may increase the scope and application of such assays in the diagnosis and monitoring of various neoplasms.

CONCLUSION

A growing body of evidence has implicated the inhibin-related family of peptides, including the activins, in the pathogenesis of various neoplasms, particularly those of the ovary. In addition, the measurement of circulating levels of immunoreactive inhibin has been shown to be of value in the monitoring of patients with ovarian granulosa cell tumors and may prove valuable also in other epithelial ovarian cancers such as mucinous cystadenocarcinoma. With the recent availability of assays for serum activin, the potential role of this peptide as a diagnostic marker for various malignant neoplasms can now be evaluated.

References

1. Burger HG. Inhibin. Reprod Med Rev 1:1, 1992.
2. Vale W, Rivier C, Hsueh A, et al. Chemical and biological characterization of the inhibin family of protein hormones. Recent Prog Horm Res 44:1, 1988.
3. Michel U, Farnworth P, Findlay JK. Follistatins: More than follicle-stimulating hormone suppressing proteins (Review). Mol Cell Endocrinol 91:1, 1993.
4. Lappohn RE, Burger HG, Bouma J, et al. Inhibin as a marker for granulosa-cell tumors. N Engl J Med 321:790, 1989.
5. Robertson DM, Sullivan J, Cahir N. Inhibin forms in human plasma. J Endocrinol 144:261, 1995.
6. Robertson DM, Burger HG, Sullivan J, et al. Biological and immunological characterization of inhibin forms in human plasma. J Clin Endocrinol Metab 81:669, 1996.
7. Burger HG. Clinical review: Clinical utility of inhibin measurements. J Clin Endocrinol Metab 76:1391, 1993.
8. Groome NP, Illingworth PJ, O'Brien M, et al. Measurement of dimeric inhibin B throughout the human menstrual cycle. J Clin Endocrinol Metab 81:1401, 1996.
9. Illingworth PJ, Groome NP, Byrd W, et al. Inhibin-B: A likely candidate for the physiologically important form of inhibin in men. J Clin Endocrinol Metab 81:1321, 1996.
10. Burger HG. Evidence for a negative feedback role of inhibin in FSH regulation in women. Hum Reprod 8:129, 1993.
11. Burger HG, Dudley EC, Hopper JL, et al. The endocrinology of the menopausal transition: A cross-sectional study of a population-based sample. J Clin Endocrinol Metab 80:3537, 1995.
12. Harada K, Shintani Y, Sakamoto Y, et al. Serum immunoreactive activin A levels in normal subjects and patients with various diseases. J Clin Endocrinol Metab 81:2125, 1996.
13. Mathews LS. Activin receptors and cellular signaling by the receptor serine kinase family. Endocr Rev 15:310, 1994.
14. Matzuk MM, Finegold MJ, Su JG, et al. Alpha-inhibin is a tumour-suppressor gene with gonadal specificity in mice. Nature 360:313, 1992.
15. Coerver KA, Woodruff TK, Finegold MJ, et al. Activin signaling through activin receptor type II causes the cachexia-like symptoms in inhibin-deficient mice. Mol Endocrinol 10:534, 1996.
16. Di Simone N, Crowley WF Jr, Wang Q-F, et al. Characterization of inhibin/activin subunit, follistatin, and activin type II receptors in human ovarian cancer cell lines: A potential role in autocrine growth regulation. Endocrinology 137:486, 1996.
17. Shikone T, Matzuk MM, Perlas E, et al. Characterization of gonadal sex cord–stromal tumor cell lines from inhibin- and p53-deficient mice: The role of activin as an autocrine growth factor. Mol Endocrinol 8:983, 1994.
18. Burger HG, Fuller PJ. The inhibin/activin family and ovarian cancer. Trends Endocrinol Metab 7:197, 1996.
19. Sluijmer AV, Heineman MJ, Evers JLH, et al. Peripheral vein, ovarian vein and ovarian tissue levels of inhibin in a postmenopausal patient with a granulosa cell tumour. Acta Endocrinol (Copenh) 12:311, 1993.
20. Gurusinghe CJ, Healy DL, Jobling T, et al. Inhibin and activin are demonstrable by immunohistochemistry in ovarian tumor tissue. Gynecol Oncol 57:27, 1995.
21. Lyons J, Landis CA, Harsh G, et al. Two G protein oncogenes in human endocrine tumors. Science 249:655, 1990.
22. Shen Y, Mamers P, Jobling T, et al. Absence of the previously reported G-protein oncogene (*gip2*) in ovarian granulosa cell tumors. J Clin Endocrinol Metab 81:4159, 1996.
23. Kauppila A, Bangah M, Burger HG, et al. GnRH agonist therapy in advanced/recurrent granulosa cell tumors: Further evidence of a role of inhibin in monitoring response to treatment. Gynecol Endocrinol 6:271, 1992.
24. Jobling T, Mamers P, Healy DL, et al. A prospective study of inhibin in granulosa cell tumors of the ovary. Gynecol Oncol 55:285, 1994.
25. Burger HG, Robertson DM, Cahir N, et al. Characterisation of

inhibin immunoreactivity in post-menopausal women with ovarian tumours. Clin Endocrinol (Oxf) 44:413, 1996.
26. Cooke I, O'Brien M, Charnock FM, et al. Inhibin as a marker for ovarian cancer. Br J Cancer 71:1046, 1995.
27. Healy DL, Burger HG, Mamers P, et al. Inhibin: A serum marker for mucinous ovarian cancers. N Engl J Med 329:1539, 1993.
28. Gustafson ML, Lee MM, Scully RE, et al. Müllerian inhibiting substance as a marker for ovarian sex-cord tumor. N Engl J Med 326:466, 1992.
29. Yohkaichiya T, Fukaya T, Hoshiai H, et al. Inhibin: A new circulating marker of hydatidiform mole? Br Med J 298:1684, 1989.
30. Badonnel Y, Barbé F, Legagneur H, et al. Inhibin as a marker for hydatidiform mole: A comparative study with the determinations of intact human chorionic gonadotrophin and its free β-subunit. Clin Endocrinol (Oxf) 41:155, 1994.
31. Brennerman W, Stoffel-Wagner B, Bidlingmaier F, et al. Immunoreactive plasma inhibin levels in men after polyvalent chemotherapy of germinal cell cancer. Acta Endocrinol (Copenh) 126:224, 1992.
32. Kananen K, Markkula M, el-Hafnawy T, et al. The mouse inhibin α-subunit promoter directs SV40 T-antigen to Leydig cells in transgenic mice. Mol Cell Endocrinol 119:135, 1996.
33. Risbridger G, Thomas T, Gurusinghe CJ, et al. Inhibin-related proteins in rat prostate. J Endocrinol 149:93, 1996.
34. Thomas T, Wang H, Niclasen P, et al. Expression and localization of activin subunits and follistatins in tissues from men with high grade prostate cancer. J Clin Endocrinol Metab 82:3851, 1997.
35. Alexander JM, Swearingen B, Tindall GT, et al. Human pituitary adenomas express endogenous inhibin subunit and follistatin messenger ribonucleic acids. J Clin Endocrinol Metab 80:147, 1995.

Chapter 25

CONTRACEPTION

Daniel R. Mishell, Jr.

CHAPTER OUTLINE

KEY POINTS

- The effectiveness and incidence of use in the United States of the various types of contraceptives currently available are discussed.
- Information about spermicidal and barrier contraception is presented.
- The effectiveness, mechanisms of action, pharmacodynamics, and endocrinologic effects of the various types of steroid contraceptives currently available are reviewed.
- Information about the most commonly used steroid contraceptive, the oral combination formulations, is presented.
- Progestins given by injection as well as in subdermal capsules are described.
- For use of these agents, data are summarized regarding their adverse clinical and metabolic effects as well as their neoplastic effects and effects on future reproduction after use is discontinued.
- Information about the various types of postcoital contraceptive agents is presented as well as the data involving use of the progesterone receptor agonist mifepristone as an oral agent to induce abortion in early gestation.
- The types of intrauterine devices and their mechanisms of action as well as the adverse effects of these contraceptive agents are summarized.

Reversible contraception is defined as the temporary prevention of fertility and includes all the currently available contraceptive methods except sterilization. Sterilization should be considered a permanent prevention of fertility even though both vasectomy and tubal interruption can usually be reversed by a meticulous surgical procedure. The reversible methods are also called active methods; sterilization is also called a terminal method. A perfect method of contraception for all individuals is not currently available and probably will never be developed. Each of the various methods of contraception currently available has certain advantages and disadvantages. Therefore, when giving advice about contraception, the clinician should explain to the couple the advantages and disadvantages of each method so that they will be fully informed and can rationally choose the method most suitable for them.

CONTRACEPTIVE USE IN THE UNITED STATES

In 1995, it was estimated that there were 69.5 million women between the ages of 15 and 50 years in the United States, and 53 percent of them were married.[1] Of the nearly 70 million women in the reproductive age group in the United States in 1995, slightly more than half used a reversible method of contraception, about one fourth had one member of the couple sterilized by tubal ligation or vasectomy, and about one fifth used no method. Among the group using no method of contraception, about half had

■ TABLE 25–1
Contraceptive Methods Used by U.S. Women Aged 15 to 50 Years

	1993 (%)	1994 (%)	1995 (%)
Oral contraceptives	25	24	26
Sterilization	27	26	24
Tubal ligation	15	15	15
Vasectomy	13	12	10
Condom	19	19	19
Withdrawal	6	5	6
Rhythm	3	3	3
Diaphragm	2	2	2
Sponge	2	1	1
Vaginal suppository	2	1	1
Douche	1	1	1
Foam	1	1	1
IUD	1	1	1
Cream/jelly alone	1	1	1
Progestin implant	1	1	1
Progestin injection	*	1	1
Cervical cap	*	*	*
Female condom/pouch	*	*	*
No method	19	19	20
Hysterectomy/menopause	8	9	6
Pregnant	2	2	3
Trying to conceive	2	2	2

*Less than 1 percent.
From 1995 Ortho Birth Control Survey. Raritan, NJ, Ortho Pharmaceutical, 1996.

a prior hysterectomy or were pregnant, infertile, or trying to conceive. The other half either were not sexually active or were having infrequent episodes of coitus or otherwise did not believe there was a need for contraception. Thus, about 56 million women, approximately 80 percent of those in the reproductive age group in the United States, used some method of contraception in 1995[1] (Table 25–1).

Of the nonsurgical, reversible methods of contraception, oral contraceptives (OCs) were most popular, used by 26 percent of all women in this age group. OCs were followed in frequency of use by the condom, withdrawal, progestin injection, periodic abstinence, diaphragm, and spermicides alone. The intrauterine device (IUD) and progestin implants, the two most effective methods of reversible contraception, were each used by less than 1 million women.

Of women who initiated contraception in 1995, about one third selected OCs. Of all women currently in the reproductive age group in the United States, more than three fourths, 77 percent, have taken OCs at some time in their life. The average length of time of OC use by an individual woman is 5.8 years. Condom use has increased in the United States in the past two decades and is the third most popular method of contraception used by about one fifth of reproductive age women.

CONTRACEPTIVE EFFECTIVENESS

It is difficult to determine the actual effectiveness of a contraceptive method because of the many factors that affect contraceptive failure. The terms method effectiveness and use effectiveness (or method failure and patient failure) were previously used to describe conception occurring while the contraceptive method was being used correctly or incorrectly. These have now been replaced by the terms typical use and perfect use.

The percentage of failure rates with the first year of use for the various methods of contraception available in the United States is shown in Table 25–2. In this table is an estimate of the percentage of women continuing to use the method after 1 year has elapsed since starting to use the method.[2] The actual use failure rates for durations more than 1 year are available for certain methods of long-acting contraceptives. The failure rate for 5 years of use of the six progestin implants, Norplant, in clinical trials is 1.1 percent.[3] The cumulative failure rate of the copper T380 IUD was 1.0, 1.4, and 1.6 per 100 women after 3, 5, and 7 years of use in a large World Health Organization (WHO) study.[4] The failure rate of all types of tubal sterilization is 1.31 after 5 years and 1.85 per 100 women after 10 years, being highest for tubal fulguration and lowest for segmental resection in the 10 years after the procedure.[5] In counseling women about long-term failure rates, they should be in-

■ TABLE 25–2
Failure Rates of Various Contraceptive Methods

METHOD	PERCENTAGE OF WOMEN EXPERIENCING AN ACCIDENTAL PREGNANCY WITHIN THE FIRST YEAR OF USE		PERCENTAGE OF WOMEN CONTINUING USE AT 1 YEAR
	Typical Use	**Perfect Use**	
Chance	85	85	
Spermicides	21	6	43
Periodic abstinence	20		67
Calendar		9	
Ovulation method		3	
Symptothermal		2	
Post ovulation		1	
Withdrawal	19	4	
Cap			
Parous women	36	26	45
Nulliparous women	18	9	58
Sponge			
Parous women	36	20	45
Nulliparous women	18	9	58
Diaphragm	18	6	58
Condom			
Female (Reality)	21	5	56
Male	12	3	63
Pill	3		72
Progestin-only		0.5	
Combined		0.1	
IUD			
Progesterone T	2.0	1.5	81
Copper T380A	0.8	0.6	78
LNg20	0.1	0.1	81
Depo-Provera	0.3	0.3	70
Norplant (six capsules)	0.09	0.09	85
Female sterilization	0.4	0.4	100
Male sterilization	0.15	0.10	100

Emergency contraceptive pills treatment initiated within 72 hours after unprotected intercourse reduces the risk of pregnancy by at least 75%.
Lactational amonorrhea methods a highly effective, *temporary* method of contraception.

From Contraceptive Technology update. Monthly newsletter from Health Professionals, American Health Consultants. Don't neglect perfect-use failure rates when talking to patients. Contraceptive Technology, Feb. 1996, Vol. 17, No. 1, pp 13–24.

formed about the high incidence of ectopic pregnancies that occur in women who conceive using progestin-only methods, the IUD, and female sterilization. Ectopic pregnancy rates for women conceiving while they are using these methods range from about 30 percent with tubal sterilization failure, 25 percent with implant failure, and 5 percent with copper IUD failure.[5, 6]

SPERMICIDES: FOAMS, CREAMS, AND SUPPOSITORIES

All spermicidal agents contain a surfactant, usually nonoxynol 9, that immobilizes or kills sperm on contact. They also provide a mechanical barrier and need to be placed into the vagina before each coital act. The effectiveness of these agents increases with increasing age of the woman and is similar to that of the diaphragm in all age and income groups. Although a few early studies linked the use of a spermicide at the time of conception with an increased risk of some congenital malformations, several well-performed studies have shown no increased risk of congenital malformation in the newborns[7–9] or karyotypic abnormalities in the spontaneous abortuses[10] of women who conceived while using spermicides.

BARRIER TECHNIQUES

Diaphragm

A diaphragm must be carefully fitted by the health care provider. The largest size that does not cause discomfort or undue pressure on the vaginal epithelium should be used. After the fitting, the woman should remove the diaphragm and reinsert it herself. She should then be examined to make sure the diaphragm is covering the cervix. The diaphragm should be used with a spermicide and be left in place for at least 8 hours after the last coital act. If repeated intercourse takes place or coitus occurs more than 8 hours after insertion of the diaphragm, additional spermicide should be used.

Although it is advisable to use a spermicide with the diaphragm, it may not be necessary because it has not been conclusively demonstrated that pregnancy rates are lower when a spermicide is used with a diaphragm than when the diaphragm is used alone.[11] The number of urinary tract infections in women who use diaphragms is significantly higher than in nonusers, probably because of the mechanical obstruction of the outflow of urine by the diaphragm.[12] Diaphragm users should also be cautioned not to leave the device in place for more than 24 hours, because ulceration of the vaginal epithelium may occur with prolonged usage.

Cervical Cap

The cervical cap, a cup-shaped plastic or rubber device that fits around the cervix, has been used as a barrier contraceptive for decades, mainly in Britain and other parts of Europe.

There has been a recent resurgence of interest in the use of this older method because the cervical cap can be left in place longer than the diaphragm and is more comfortable. The various types of caps are manufactured in different sizes and should be fitted to the cervix by a clinician. The Prentif cavity-rim cervical cap was approved for general use in the United States in 1988. The product labeling stipulates that the cap should be left on the cervix for no more than 48 hours and that a spermicide should always be placed inside the cap before use.[13] The cap is manufactured in four sizes and requires more training than the diaphragm, both for the provider to fit it and for the user to place it correctly. Failure rates with the cervical cap are similar to those observed with the diaphragm. Because of concern about a possible adverse effect of the cap on cervical tissue, the cervical cap should be used only by women with normal cervical cytology, and it is recommended that users have another cervical cytologic examination 3 months after starting to use this method.

Male Condom

Use of the male condom by individuals with multiple sex partners should be encouraged. The male condom is the most effective method of contraception to prevent transmission of sexually transmitted diseases. The male condom should not be applied tightly. The tip should extend beyond the end of the penis by about ½ inch to collect the ejaculate. Care must be taken on withdrawal not to spill the ejaculate. When used by strongly motivated couples, the male condom is highly effective.

Female Condom

A female condom was approved for marketing in the United States in 1994. It consists of a soft, loose-fitting sheath and two flexible polyurethane rings. One ring lies inside the vagina at the closed end of the sheath and serves as an insertion mechanism and internal anchor. The outer ring forms the external edge of the device and remains outside the vagina after insertion, thus providing protection to the labia and the base of the penis during intercourse. The condom is prelubricated and is intended for one-time use only. Fitting by a health professional is not required.[14]

In comparison to the male condom, the female condom has the advantage of being able to be inserted before beginning sexual activity and to be left in place for a longer time after ejaculation occurs. Because the female condom also covers the external genitalia, it should offer greater protection against the transfer of certain sexually transmitted organisms, particularly genital herpes. Because polyurethane is stronger than the latex used in male condoms, the female condom is less likely to rupture. In a multicenter clinical trial, the cumulative pregnancy rate in U.S. centers at 6 months was 12.4 percent. The 6-month pregnancy rate with perfect use was 2.6 percent, indicating that the probable 1-year pregnancy rate with perfect use would be slightly more than 5 percent.[15] At the end of 6 months in the U.S. study, about one third of the women had discontinued use of this method. Because clinical trials with use of the female condom have not compared its use with other barrier techniques, an exact comparison with other contraceptive methods cannot be made. Trussel and colleagues,[15] using the data of other studies, concluded that the efficacy rate of the female condom with perfect use would be similar to that of the diaphragm and cervical cap, but the failure rate of the female condom with typical use would be higher than that of the diaphragm. Because of the lack of prospective clinical trials with the male condom, no statistical comparison of the effectiveness of the two types of condoms can be made. No data exist in which the effectiveness of the female condom for reducing sexual disease transmission is analyzed. Because polyurethane does not allow virus transmission, it should reduce the risk of a woman's acquiring human immunodeficiency virus infection.

ORAL STEROID CONTRACEPTIVES

Oral steroid contraceptives (OCs) were initially marketed in the United States in 1960. Because contraceptive steroid formulations with more than 50 μg of estrogen were associated with a greater incidence of adverse effects without greater efficacy, they are no longer marketed for contraceptive use in the United States, Canada, and Great Britain. Indications for prescribing formulations with 50 μg of estrogen are uncommon. In 1996, only about 2.5 percent of all OC prescriptions in the United States were for formulations with 50 μg of estrogen. OC formulations currently marketed in the United States, excluding generic brands, are listed in Table 25–3.

Pharmacology

There are three major types of OC formulations: fixed-dose combination, combination phasic, and daily progestin. The combination formulations are the most widely used and most effective. They consist of tablets containing both an estrogen and progestin given continuously for 3 weeks. No steroids are given for the next 7 days, after which time the active combination is given for an additional 3 weeks. Uterine bleeding usually occurs in the week when no steroid is ingested. Without estrogenic stimulation, the endometrium usually begins to slough 1 to 3 days after steroid ingestion is stopped. Withdrawal bleeding usually lasts 3 to 4 days and uterine blood loss averages about 25 ml, less than the mean of about 35 ml that occurs during menses in a normal ovulatory cycle.

All currently marketed formulations are made from synthetic steroids and contain no natural estrogens or progestins. There are two major types of synthetic progestins: derivatives of 19-nortestosterone and derivatives of 17α-acetoxyprogesterone. The latter group are C_{21} progestins, called pregnanes, and are structurally related to progesterone. Medroxyprogesterone acetate and megestrol acetate are C_{21} progestins marketed as tablets for noncontraceptive usage. In contrast to the 19-nortestosterone derivatives, when high dosages of the C_{21} progestins were given to female beagle dogs (an animal previously used for OC toxicology testing), the animals developed an increased incidence of mammary cancer. Because of this carcinogenic effect, oral contraceptives containing these progestins are no longer marketed despite the fact that the beagle, unlike the human, metabolizes C_{21} progestins to estrogen, which then stimulates mammary nodules that can become carcinogenic in this animal.

The steroid structure of the 19-nortestosterone progestins more closely resembles testosterone than the C_{21} acetoxyprogestins. Therefore, all progestational agents currently used in OCs have some degree of androgenic activity. The 19-nortestosterone progestins used in OCs are of two major types, called estranes and gonanes. Although the original estrane, norethynodrel, is no longer used in currently marketed OCs, other estranes, norethindrone and its derivatives with one or two acetates, norethindrone acetate and ethynodiol diacetate, are used in several marketed formulations (Fig. 25–1). Gonanes have greater progestational activity per unit weight than estranes do, and thus a smaller amount of the gonane type of progestin is used in OC formulations. The parent compound of the gonanes is *dl*-norgestrel, which consists of two isomers, dextro and levo. Only the levo form is biologically active. Both *dl*-norgestrel and its active isomer levonorgestrel are present in several OC formulations. Three less androgenic derivatives of levonorgestrel, namely, desogestrel, norgestimate, and gestodene, have also been synthesized (Fig. 25–2). Formulations with each of these three progestins have been marketed in Europe for many years, and formulations with desogestrel and norgestimate, but not gestodene, have been marketed in the United States since 1992.

With the exception of two daily progestin-only formulations, the progestins are combined with varying dosages of two estrogens, ethinyl estradiol and ethinyl estradiol 3-methyl ether, also known as mestranol (Fig. 25–3). All the older, higher dosage OC formulations contained mestranol, and this steroid is still present in some 50-μg formulations. All formulations with less than 50 μg of estrogen contain only the parent compound ethinyl estradiol. In common

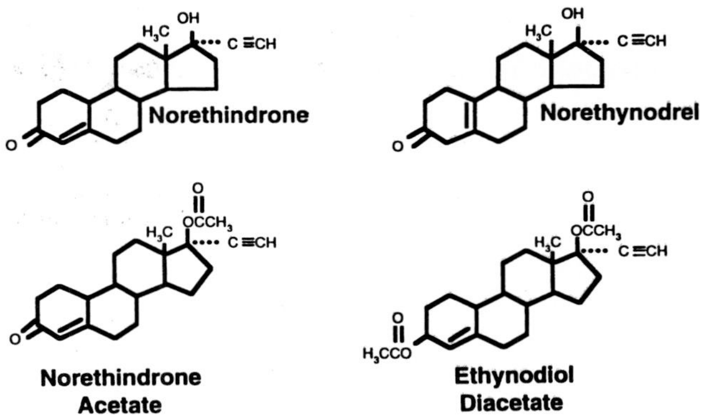

Norethindrone
Norethynodrel
Norethindrone Acetate
Ethynodiol Diacetate

Figure 25–1 ■ Chemical structures of the estrane progestins used in oral contraceptives.

Levonorgestrel
Gestodene
Norgestimate
Desogestrel

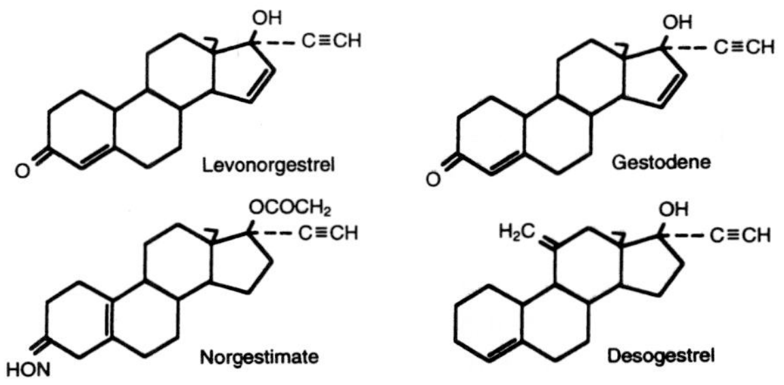

Figure 25–2 ■ Chemical structure of the gonane progestins used in oral contraceptives.

■ TABLE 25–3

Estrogen and Progestin Components of Oral Contraceptives

MANUFACTURER	PRODUCT TYPE	PROGESTIN	ESTROGEN*
Berlex			
Levlen	Combination	0.15 mg levonorgestrel	30 μg
Tri-Levlen 6/	Combination, triphasic	0.05 mg levonorgestrel	30 μg
5/		0.075 mg levonorgestrel	40 μg
10/		0.125 mg levonorgestrel	30 μg
Bristol-Myers Squibb			
Ovcon 35	Combination	0.4 mg norethindrone	35 μg
Ovcon 50	Combination	1.0 mg norethindrone	50 μg
Organon			
Desogen	Combination	0.15 mg desogestrel	35 μg
Ortho-MacNeil Pharmaceutical			
Micronor	Progestin-only	0.35 mg norethindrone	
Modicon	Combination	0.5 mg norethindrone	35 μg
Ortho-Cept	Combination	0.15 mg desogestrel	30 μg
Ortho-Cyclen	Combination	0.25 mg norgestimate	35 μg
Ortho-Novum 1/35	Combination	1.0 mg norethindrone	35 μg
Ortho-Novum 1/50	Combination	1.0 mg norethindrone	50 μg†
Ortho-Novum 7/	Combination, triphasic	0.5 mg norethindrone	35 μg
7/		0.75 mg norethindrone	35 μg
7/		1.0 mg norethindrone	35 μg
Ortho-Novum 10/	Combination, biphasic	0.5 mg norethindrone	35 μg
11/		1.0 mg norethindrone	35 μg
Ortho-Tricyclin	Combination, triphasic	0.18 mg norgestimate	35 μg
		0.215 mg norgestimate	35 μg
		0.25 mg norgestimate	35 μg
Parke-Davis			
Estrostep	Combination	1.0 mg norethindrone acetate	20 μg
		1.0 mg norethindrone acetate	30 μg
		1.0 mg norethindrone acetate	35 U
Loestrin 1/20	Combination	1.0 mg norethindrone acetate	20 μg
Loestrin 1.5/30	Combination	1.5 mg norethindrone acetate	30 μg
Norlestrin 1/50	Combination	1.0 mg norethindrone acetate	50 μg†
Norlestrin 2.5/50	Combination	2.5 mg norethindrone acetate	50 μg†
Roche Laboratories			
Brevicon	Combination	0.5 mg norethindrone	35 μg
Norinyl 1 + 35	Combination	1.0 mg norethindrone	35 μg
Norinyl 1 + 50	Combination	1.0 mg norethindrone	50 μg
Nor-QD	Progestin-only	0.35 mg norethindrone	
Tri-Norinyl 7/	Combination, triphasic	0.5 mg norethindrone	35 μg
9/		1 mg norethindrone	35 μg
5/		0.5 mg norethindrone	35 μg
Searle			
Demulen 1/35	Combination	1.0 mg ethynodiol diacetate	35 μg
Demulen 1/50	Combination	1.0 mg ethynodiol diacetate	50 μg
Wyeth-Ayerst			
Alesse	Combination	0.1 mg levonorgestrel	20 μg
Lo/Ovral	Combination	3.0 mg norethindrone	30 μg
Nordette	Combination	0.15 mg norethindrone	30 μg
Ovral	Combination	0.5 mg norgestrel	50 μg
Ovrette	Progestin-only	0.075 μg norgestrel	30 μg
Triphasil 6/	Combination, triphasic	0.05 μg levonorgestrel	30 μg
5/		0.75 μg levonorgestrel	40 μg
10/		1.25 μg levonorgestrel	30 μg

*Ethinyl estradiol unless noted.
†Mestranol.

usage, formulations with 50 μg or more of estrogen (ethinyl estradiol or mestranol) have been termed first-generation OCs. Those with less than 50 μg of estrogen, 20 to 35 μg of ethinyl estradiol, are called second-generation products if they contain any progestin except the three newest levonorgestrel derivatives. Those formulations with desogestrel, norgestimate, and gestodene are called third-generation formulations. All the synthetic estrogens and progestins in OCs have an ethinyl group at position 17. The presence of this ethinyl group enhances the oral activity of these agents, because their essential functional groups are not as rapidly metabolized as they pass through the intestinal mucosa and the liver through the portal system, in contrast to what occurs when natural sex steroids are ingested orally. The synthetic steroids thus have greater oral potency per unit of weight than the natural steroids. It has been estimated that ethinyl estradiol has about 100 times the potency of an equivalent weight of conjugated equine

Mestranol Ethinylestradiol

Figure 25–3 ■ Structures of the two estrogens used in combination oral contraceptives.

estrogen or estrone sulfate for stimulating synthesis of various hepatic globulins.

The various modifications in chemical structure of the different synthetic progestins and estrogens also affect their biologic activity. Thus, one cannot define the pharmacologic activity of the progestin or estrogen in a particular contraceptive steroid formulation on the basis of only the amount of steroid present. The biologic activity of each steroid also has to be considered. By use of established tests for progestational activity in animals, it has been found that a given weight of norgestrel is several times more potent than the same weight of norethindrone. Studies in humans, using delay of menses[16] or endometrial histologic alterations such as subnuclear vacuolization[17, 18] as endpoints, also determined that norgestrel is about 10 times more potent than the same weight of norethindrone. Norethindrone acetate and ethynodiol diacetate are metabolized in the body to norethindrone. Studies in humans, measuring progestational activity as described before, as well as other studies comparing the effects of serum lipids in humans indicate that each of these three progestins has approximately equal potency per unit of weight, whereas levonorgestrel is 10 to 20 times as potent.[19] Each of the three most recently developed levonorgestrel derivatives has been shown in animal but not human studies to have similar or greater progestogenic potency than an equivalent weight of levonorgestrel, with less androgenic activity.[20] The magnitude of difference in androgenic and progestational effects produced by each progestin is called selectivity.

The two estrogenic compounds used in OCs, ethinyl estradiol and its 3-methyl ether, mestranol, also have different biologic activity in women. To become biologically effective, mestranol must be demethylated to ethinyl estradiol, because mestranol does not bind to the estrogen cytosol receptor. The degree of conversion of mestranol to ethinyl estradiol varies among individuals; some are able to convert it completely, whereas others convert only a portion of it. Thus, in some women, a given weight of mestranol is as potent as the same weight of ethinyl estradiol; in other women, it is only about half as potent. Overall, it has been estimated, by use of human endometrial response and effect on liver corticosteroid-binding globulin production as endpoints, that ethinyl estradiol is about 1.7 times as potent as the same weight of mestranol.[21] The biologic activity as well as the quantity of both steroid components needs to be evaluated in comparing potency of the various formulations.

Radioimmunoassay methods have been developed to measure blood levels of these synthetic estrogens and progestins. Peak plasma levels of ethinyl estradiol are lower and occur about 2 to 4 hours later after ingestion of mestranol than after ingestion of ethinyl estradiol.[22] The delay is due to the time necessary for mestranol to be demethylated to ethinyl estradiol in the liver.

When different doses of *dl*-norgestrel were administered to women, it was found that the serum levels of levonorgestrel were related to the dosage.[23] Peak serum levels were found 0.5 to 3 hours after oral administration, followed by a rapid, sharp decline (Fig. 25–4). However, 24 hours after ingestion, 20 to 25 percent of the peak level of levonorgestrel was still present in the serum. After 5 days of norgestrel administration, measurable amounts of levonorgestrel were present for at least the following 5 days.

Brenner and coworkers[24] measured serum levels of levonorgestrel, follicle-stimulating hormone (FSH), luteinizing hormone (LH), estradiol, and progesterone 3 hours after ingestion of a combination OC containing 0.5 mg of *dl*-norgestrel and 50 μg of ethinyl estradiol in three women during two consecutive cycles as well as during the intervening pill-free interval. Daily levels of levonorgestrel rose during the first few days of ingestion, reached a plateau thereafter, and declined after ingestion of the last pill (Fig. 25–5). Nevertheless, substantial amounts of levonorgestrel remained in the serum for at least the first 3 to 4 days after the last pill was ingested. These steroid levels were sufficient to suppress gonadotropin release during the 1-week interval when no steroid was administered. Thus, follicle maturation, as evidenced by rising estradiol levels,

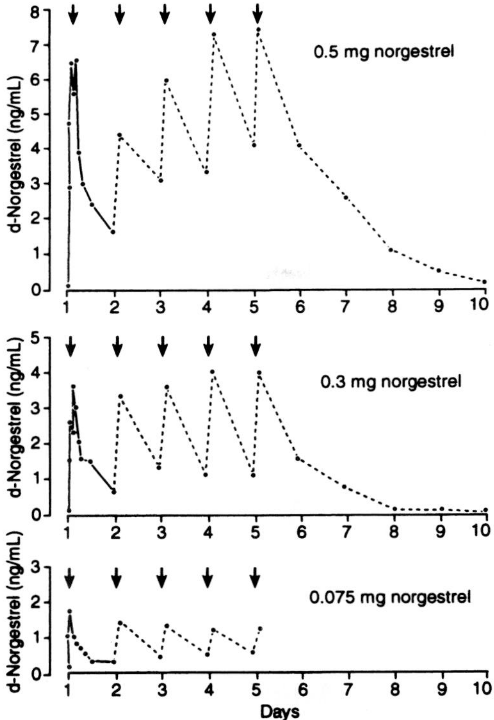

Figure 25–4 ■ Serum *d*-norgestrel levels in three subjects receiving 500 μg of *dl*-norgestrel and 50 μg of ethinyl estradiol (Ovral). Arrows indicate time of ingestion. (From Brenner PF, Mishell DR Jr, Stanczyk FZ, Goebelsmann U. Serum levels of *d*-norgestrel, luteinizing hormone, follicle-stimulating hormone, estradiol, and progesterone in women during and following ingestion of combination oral contraceptives containing *dl*-norgestrel. Am J Obstet Gynecol 129:133–140, 1977.)

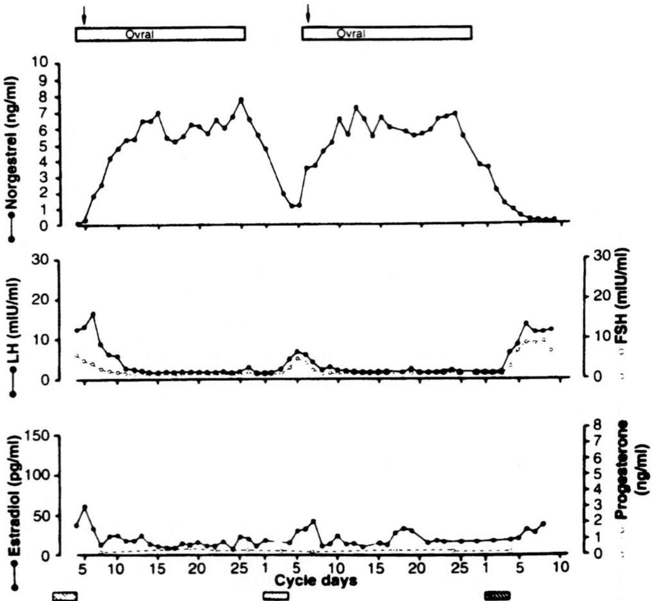

Figure 25–5 ■ Serum *d*-norgestrel, FSH, LH, estradiol, and progesterone levels in patients during and after oral administration of 500 μg of *dl*-norgestrel and 50 μg of ethinyl estradiol (Ovral) for two subsequent 21-day periods interrupted by a pill-free interval of 6 days. (From Brenner PF, Mishell DR Jr, Stanczyk FZ, Goebelsmann U. Serum levels of *d*-norgestrel, luteinizing hormone, follicle-stimulating hormone, estradiol, and progesterone in women during and following ingestion of combination oral contraceptives containing *dl*-norgestrel. Am J Obstet Gynecol 129:133–140, 1977.)

did not occur during the 1 week when no steroid was being ingested. When lower doses of steroids are administered, follicular growth but not ovulation may occur because of initiation of growth of the dominant follicle during the time that no steroid is being ingested.

From these data, it seems reasonable to conclude that accidental pregnancies during OC use probably occur not because of failure to ingest one or two pills more than a few days after a treatment cycle is initiated but rather because initiation of the next cycle of medication is delayed for a few days. Therefore, it is important that the pill-free interval is not extended more than 7 days. This is best accomplished by ingesting either a placebo or iron tablet daily during the steroid-free interval (the so-called 28-day package). If a 3-week pill package is used, treatment is best started on the first Sunday after menses begins instead of the first or fifth day of the cycle. It is easier to remember to start the new package on a Sunday. Women should be advised that the most important pill to remember to take is the first one of each cycle.

Mechanisms of Action

The estrogen-progestin combination is the most effective type of OC formulation, because these preparations consistently inhibit the midcycle gonadotropin surge and thus prevent ovulation. The progestin-only formulations have a lower dose of progestin than the combined agents and do not consistently inhibit ovulation. Both types of formulations also act on other aspects of the reproductive process: (1) they alter the cervical mucus, making it thick, viscid, and scanty, which retards sperm penetration; (2) they alter motility of the uterus and oviduct, thus impairing transport of both ova and sperm; (3) they alter the endometrium so that its glandular production of glycogen is diminished and less energy is available for the blastocyst to survive in the uterine cavity; and (4) they may alter ovarian responsiveness to gonadotropin stimulation. With both types of formulations, neither gonadotropin production nor ovarian steroidogenesis is completely abolished. Levels of endogenous estradiol in the peripheral blood during ingestion of high-dose combination OCs are similar to those found in the early follicular phase of the normal cycle.[25]

Contraceptive steroids prevent ovulation both by interfering with release of gonadotropin-releasing hormone (GnRH) from the hypothalamus and by suppressing pituitary release of LH and FSH. Several studies in humans showed most women who had been ingesting combination OCs had suppression of the release of LH and FSH after infusion of GnRH, indicating that the steroids had a direct inhibitory effect on the pituitary as well as on the hypothalamus.[26]

Direct pituitary inhibition occurs in about 80 percent of women ingesting high-dose combination OCs. Pituitary suppression is unrelated to the age of the woman or the duration of steroid use but is related to the potency of the formulation. The effect is more pronounced with formulations containing a more potent progestin[27] and with those containing 50 μg or more of estrogen than with 30- to 35-μg estrogen-containing formulations.[28] It has not been demonstrated that the degree of pituitary suppression is related to the occurrence of amenorrhea after OC use is stopped. There are data showing that the mean time to conception after discontinuation of OC use is shorter in women ingesting preparations with less than 50 μg of estrogen (4.01 cycles) than in those ingesting formulations with 50 μg of estrogen or more (4.79 cycles).[29]

The daily progestin-only preparations do not consistently inhibit ovulation. They exert their contraceptive action by the other mechanisms listed before, but because of the inconsistent ovulation inhibition, their effectiveness is significantly less than that of the combination types of OCs.[2] Because a lower dose of progestin is used in these formulations than in the combination tablets, it is important that these preparations be consistently taken at the same time of day to ensure that blood levels do not fall below the effective contraceptive level.

No significant difference in clinical effectiveness has been demonstrated among the various combination formulations currently available in the United States. As long as no tablets are omitted (perfect use), the pregnancy rate is less than 0.2 percent at the end of 1 year with all marketed combination formulations.

Metabolic Effects

The synthetic steroids in OC formulations have many metabolic effects in addition to their contraceptive actions (Table 25–4). These metabolic effects can produce both the more common, less serious side effects as well as the rare, potentially serious complications. The magnitude of these effects is directly related to the dosage and potency of the

■ TABLE 25–4
Metabolic Effect of Contraceptive Steroids

	CHEMICAL EFFECTS	CLINICAL EFFECTS
Estrogen: Ethinyl estradiol		
Proteins		
Albumin	↓	None
Amino acids	↓	None
Globulins	↑	
Angiotensinogen		↑ Blood pressure
Clotting factors		Hypercoagulability
Carrier proteins (CBG, TBG, transferrin, ceruloplasmin)		None
Carbohydrate		
Plasma insulin	None	None
Glucose tolerance	None	None
Lipids		
Cholesterol	↑	None
Triglyceride	↑	None
HDL cholesterol	↑	? ↓ Cardiovascular disease
LDL cholesterol	↓	? ↓ Cardiovascular disease
Electrolytes		
Sodium excretion	↓	Fluid retention Edema
Vitamins		
B-complex	↓	None
Ascorbic acid	↓	None
Vitamin A	↑	None
Other		
Breast	↑	Breast tenderness
Endometrial steroid receptors	↑	Endometrial hyperplasia
Skin	↓	↓ Sebum production ↑ Facial pigmentation
Progestins: 19-Nortestosterone derivatives		
Proteins	None	None
Carbohydrate		
Plasma insulin	↑	None
Glucose tolerance	↓	None
Lipids		
Cholesterol	↓	None
Triglyceride	↓	None
HDL cholesterol	↓	? ↑ Cardiovascular disease
LDL cholesterol	↑	? ↑ Cardiovascular disease
Other		
Nitrogen retention	↑	↑ Body weight
Skin—sebum production	↑	↑ Acne
CNS effects	↑	Nervousness, fatigue, depression
Endometrial steroid receptors	↓	No withdrawal bleeding

CBG, corticosteroid-binding globulin; TBG, thyroid-binding globulin; HDL, high-density lipoprotein; LDL, low-density lipoprotein; CNS, central nervous system.

steroids in the formulations. Fortunately, in most instances, the more common adverse effects are relatively mild.

The most frequent symptoms produced by the estrogen component include nausea (a central nervous system effect), breast tenderness, and fluid retention (which usually does not exceed 3 to 4 pounds of body weight) because of decreased sodium excretion. Minor, clinically insignificant changes in circulating vitamin levels also occurred after ingestion of the higher dosage OCs. These changes included a decrease in levels of the B-complex vitamins and ascorbic acid and increases in levels of vitamin A. Even with use of the agents containing a high steroid dose, dietary vitamin supplementation was not necessary, because the changes in circulating vitamin levels were small and clinically insignificant. Estrogen can also cause melasma, pigmentation of the malar eminences, to develop. Melasma is accentuated by sunlight and usually takes a long time to disappear after OCs are discontinued. The incidence of all these estrogenic side effects is much less with use of formulations of lower estrogen dose than with those of high estrogen dose.

With high doses of estrogen, OC usage was found to accelerate the development of the symptoms of gallbladder disease in young women but did not increase the overall incidence of cholelithiasis. The results of the large British Family Planning Association study[30] and a case-control study[31] indicate that the use of high-dose OCs does not increase the incidence of gallbladder disease in women. When the data were stratified among women of different body weight or different age, no increased risk of gallbladder disease was found in any subgroup. These results indicate that development of gallbladder disease is not a risk factor associated with OC use, even if these agents contain high doses of steroids and are used for more than 8 years.[32]

Mood and Depression

It was previously postulated that high dosages of the synthetic estrogens could also produce changes in mood and depression brought about by diversion of tryptophan metabolism from its minor pathway in the brain to its major pathway in the liver. The end product of tryptophan metabolism, serotonin, is thus decreased in the central nervous system, and it was postulated that the resultant lowering of serotonin could produce depression in some women and sleepiness and mood changes in others.

Analysis of the data from the Royal College of General Practitioners (RCGP) cohort study indicated that OC use was positively correlated with the incidence of depression, which in turn was directly related to the dose of estrogen in the formulation.[33] In this study, an increased incidence of depression was not found to occur among users of OCs containing less than 50 μg of estrogen. Data from postmenopausal women receiving estrogen therapy alone as well as estrogen-progestin sequential therapy indicate that administration of physiologic doses of estrogen alone, which is less potent than the pharmacologic dose used in OCs, improves the mood of women, whereas the addition of a progestin increases the amount of depression, irritability, tension, and fatigue.[34] These studies indicate that the progestin component of the agents may be the major cause of the adverse mood changes and tiredness observed in some women after ingestion of OCs, but it has not been definitely established which of the steroid components is the major factor in producing adverse mood changes. Possibly, both are involved.

Androgenic Effects

The progestins, because they are structurally related to testosterone, also produce certain adverse androgenic effects. These include weight gain, acne, and a symptom perceived by some women as nervousness. Some women gain a considerable amount of weight when they take OCs, and this weight gain is believed to be produced by the anabolic effect of the progestin component. Although estrogens decrease sebum production, progestins increase it and can cause acne to develop or worsen. Thus, women who have acne should be given a formulation with a low progestin-estrogen ratio.

The final symptom produced by the progestin component is failure of withdrawal bleeding or amenorrhea. Because the progestins decrease the synthesis of estrogen receptors in the endometrium, endometrial growth is decreased, and some women have failure of withdrawal bleeding. This symptom is not important medically, but because bleeding serves as a signal that the woman is not pregnant, it is desirable to have some amount of periodic withdrawal bleeding during the days she is not taking these steroids. The two steroid components can act together to produce irregular bleeding. Unscheduled (breakthrough) bleeding (which is usually produced by insufficient estrogen, too much progestin, or a combination of both) as well as failure of withdrawal bleeding can be alleviated by increasing the amount of estrogen in the formulation or by switching to a more estrogenic formulation.

Hepatic Proteins

The synthetic estrogens used in OCs cause an increase in the hepatic production of several globulins. Progesterone and androgenic progestins do not affect the synthesis of globulins except that of sex hormone–binding globulin (SHBG). Synthesis of SHBG is reduced by androgens, including the androgenic progestins. Some of the globulins that are increased by ethinyl estradiol ingestion, such as factors V, VIII, and X and fibrinogen, enhance thrombosis,[35] whereas another globulin, angiotensinogen, may be converted to angiotensin and increase blood pressure in some users.[36] The circulating levels of each of these globulins are directly correlated with the amount of estrogen in the OC formulation. Epidemiologic studies have shown that the incidence of both venous and arterial thrombosis is also directly related to the dose of estrogen.[35, 37, 38]

Although angiotensinogen levels are lower in women who ingest formulations with 30 to 35 μg of ethinyl estradiol than in those who ingest formulations of higher estrogen dosage, a slight but significant increase in mean blood pressure still occurs in women who ingest the lower dosage formulations.[36, 39] Thus, blood pressure should be monitored in all users of OCs. There is some indirect evidence that the progestin component may also raise blood pressure. However, women who receive progestins without estrogen do not have an increase in blood pressure over time,[36] indicating that the estrogen component is the major cause of elevated blood pressure in a few users of OCs.

Another globulin, SHBG, binds circulating levels of estrogens and androgens. Progesterone is bound to corticosteroid-binding globulin, but because the progestins used in oral contraceptives are 19-nortestosterone derivatives, they are bound to SHBG. Estrogens increase SHBG levels, whereas androgens, including 19-nortestosterone derivatives, decrease SHBG levels. Thus, measurement of SHBG is one way to determine the relative estrogenic/androgenic balance of different OC formulations. Van der Vange and associates[40] measured SHBG levels before and 6 months after ingestion of several OC formulations containing about the same amount of ethinyl estradiol. The greatest increase occurred with formulations containing cyproterone acetate (not used in OC formulations in the United States), desogestrel, and gestodene. SHBG increases of lesser magnitude occurred after ingestion of formulations containing low doses of norethindrone and levonorgestrel. Because SHBG binds endogenous testosterone and prevents it from acting on the target tissue, formulations causing the greatest increase in SHBG should be associated with the least amount of androgenic effects. These formulations are particularly useful for treating women with symptoms of hyperandrogenism such as polycystic ovary syndrome.

Carbohydrate Metabolism

The effect of OCs on glucose metabolism is mainly related to the dose, potency, and chemical structure of the progestin. Conflicting data exist as to whether the estrogen component affects carbohydrate metabolism. The estrogen may act synergistically with the progestin to impair glucose tolerance. In general, the higher the dose and potency of the progestin, the greater the magnitude of impaired glucose metabolism. The degree of alteration appears to be greater with gonanes than with estranes. Several studies have shown that formulations with a low dose of progestin, including one containing levonorgestrel, do not significantly alter levels of glucose, insulin, or glucagon after a glucose load in healthy women[41, 42] or in those with a history of gestational diabetes.[43] However, other studies indicate that the multiphasic formulations with norgestrel, but not those with norethindrone, produce some deterioration of glucose tolerance in normal women[44] as well as in those with a history of gestational diabetes.[45] Some studies have shown increased levels of both glucose and insulin when glucose tolerance tests were administered to women ingesting desogestrel-containing OCs.[46–48]

Data from 20 years of experience using mainly high-dose formulations in the large RCGP cohort study indicated that there was no increased risk for development of diabetes mellitus among current OC users (relative risk [RR], 0.80) or former OC users (RR, 0.82) even among women who had used OCs for 10 years or more.[49] More than 1 million person-years of follow-up of OC users in the large Nurses' Health Study cohort were analyzed in 1992. Although type II diabetes mellitus developed in more than 2000 women, the risk was not increased among current OC users (RR, 0.71) and only marginally increased in past OC users (RR, 1.11),[50] only among women who had used high-dose formulations many years previously, not for those who had used lower dose formulations.

Kjos and colleagues[51] observed a group of women with a history of gestational diabetes mellitus for several years after the end of the pregnancy. In the first year, women ingesting a low-dose levonorgestrel formulation had a greater risk of developing diabetes mellitus than did a control group not taking OCs. On the other hand, women ingesting a low-dose norethindrone formulation did not have a greater risk of developing diabetes mellitus than control subjects did. After the first year following delivery, women ingesting both types of OCs had no greater risks of developing diabetes mellitus than did the control group. When OCs are prescribed for women with a history of glucose intolerance, formulations with a low dose of a norethindrone-type progestin are probably preferable to levonorgestrel preparations. In addition, glucose tolerance should be monitored periodically.

Lipids

The estrogen component of OCs causes an increase in high-density lipoprotein (HDL) cholesterol, a decrease in low-density lipoprotein (LDL) cholesterol, and an increase in total cholesterol and triglyceride levels. The progestin component causes a decrease in HDL, an increase in LDL, and a decrease in total cholesterol and triglyceride levels.

The older formulations with high doses of progestin had adverse effects on the lipid profile although they also contained high doses of the synthetic estrogen. These progestin-dominant formulations produced a decrease in HDL cholesterol levels and an increase in LDL cholesterol levels.[52] They also caused an increase in serum triglyceride levels because the estrogen has a greater effect on triglyceride synthesis than does the progestin. Short-term longitudinal studies of several phasic formulations containing levonorgestrel and norethindrone found that a significant increase in triglyceride levels still occurred but there was little change in either HDL cholesterol or LDL cholesterol levels as well as in total cholesterol levels because the effects of each steroid on lipid synthesis were offset by the other.[53, 54]

In a cross-sectional study in which lipid levels were measured in a large number of women ingesting several OC formulations and compared with those of nonusers, Godsland and colleagues[47] reported that there were insignificant differences in HDL and LDL cholesterol levels compared with those of nonusers when low-dose monophasic and triphasic levonorgestrel and norethindrone formulations were ingested. The women ingesting formulations with only 0.5 mg of norethindrone or 150 μg of desogestrel had a significant increase in HDL cholesterol levels and a significant decrease in LDL cholesterol levels.[46] The three most recently developed progestins have less androgenic activity than the older progestins and as such, when combined with an estrogen, would be expected to have less adverse effect on lipid metabolism than the older formulations. Speroff and associates,[20] in 1993, reviewed data from the published studies in which lipid levels were measured in women ingesting formulations with the three less androgenic progestins. They reported that with use of these formulations, there was a significant increase in HDL cholesterol levels, a significant decrease in LDL cholesterol levels, little change in total cholesterol levels, and a substantial increase in triglyceride levels (Table 25–5). The long-term effect, if any, of these changes in lipid parameters remains to be determined.

Coagulation Parameters

As previously mentioned, the estrogen component of OCs increases the synthesis of several coagulation factors, including fibrinogen, which enhances thrombosis in a dose-dependent manner. The effect of OCs on parameters that inhibit coagulation, such as protein C, protein S, and antithrombin III, is less clear because of the diversity of techniques used to measure these parameters in different laboratories. A similar lack of consistency occurs when parameters that enhance fibrinolysis (such as plasminogen) or inhibit fibrinolysis (such as plasminogen activator inhibitor 1) are measured in OC users.

Changes in most of these coagulation parameters in OC users are small, if they occur at all, and there is no evidence that these minor alterations in levels of coagulation parameters measured in the laboratory have any effect on the clinical risk of developing venous or arterial thrombosis. Nevertheless, if the woman has an inherited coagulation disorder that increases her risk of developing thrombosis, such as protein C, protein S, or antithrombin III deficiency or the more common activated protein C resistance, her risk of developing thrombosis is increased several-fold if she ingests estrogen-containing OCs.[55] Vandenbroucke and coworkers[56] reported that the relative risk of developing deep venous thrombosis among women with activated protein C resistance with OC use was increased 30-fold compared with that of nonusers without the mutation. They estimated that the annual incidence of deep venous thrombosis in a woman of reproductive age with this genetic mutation was about 6 per 10,000 women if she did not take OCs and about 30 per 10,000 women if she took them. At present, it is not recommended that screening for these coagulation deficiencies be undertaken before OC use

■ TABLE 25–5
Lipid Changes With Oral Contraceptives Containing New Progestins

		PERCENTAGE CHANGE FROM BASELINE					
PROGESTIN	N	TG	C	LDL-C	HDL-C	Apo B	Apo A-I
Desogestrel	608	29.3	2.8	−2.1	12.9	10.5	11.3
Gestodene	296	38.3	3.8	−2.5	8.1	16.0	7.1
Norgestimate	>2550	14.8	4.3	−0.2	9.9	5.3	7.3

TG, triglyceride; C, total cholesterol; LDL-C, low-density lipoprotein cholesterol; HDL-C, high-density lipoprotein cholesterol; apo, apoprotein.
From Speroff L, DeCherney A, and the Advisory Board for the New Progestins.
Evaluation of a new generation of oral contraceptives. Obstet Gynecol 81:1034–1047, 1993.

is started unless the woman has a personal or family history of thrombotic events.

Cardiovascular Events

The cause of the increased incidence of both venous and arterial cardiovascular disease, including myocardial infarction (MI), in users of OCs appears to be thrombosis and not atherosclerosis.

Venous Thromboembolism

Gerstman and colleagues[38] analyzed the effect of OCs with different doses of estrogen on the incidence of venous thromboembolism (VTE) in a historical cohort study of more than 230,000 women aged 15 to 44 years. Among users of OC formulations with less than 50 μg of estrogen, the rate of VTE per 10,000 woman-years was 4.2; with use of the 50-μg estrogen formulation, the rate was 7.0; and in users of formulations with more than 50 μg of estrogen, the rate increased to 10.0 per 10,000 woman-years (Table 25–6). These data confirm earlier findings indicating that the risk of VTE is directly related to the dose of estrogen in the formulation. The background rate of VTE in women of reproductive age is about 0.8 per 10,000 woman-years. A large observational study found that the incidence of venous thromboembolic events among users of OCs with 20 to 50 μg of ethinyl estradiol was 3 per 10,000 woman-years, about four times the background rate of women of reproductive age but half the rate of 6 per 10,000 woman-years associated with pregnancy.[57]

Three population-based studies have been performed to determine the risk of VTE in users of OCs containing mainly less than 50 μg of estrogen.[58–60] These studies were consistent and showed that the risk of deep venous thrombosis was increased approximately fourfold among women using OCs compared with women not using OCs. Thus, use of OCs with less than 50 μg of estrogen is associated with about a threefold to fourfold increased risk of VTE compared with a nonpregnant population not taking OCs but about a 50 percent reduction in risk of VTE compared with a pregnant or recently postpartum population.

In late 1995 and early 1996, results of four observational studies showed that the risk of VTE among women ingesting low-estrogen formulations containing desogestrel or gestodene was increased about 1.5 to 2.5 times that of women ingesting formulations containing less than 50 μg of estrogen and levonorgestrel.[58, 60–62] Because these studies were not prospective comparative trials, controversy exists as to whether the increased risk of VTE was causally related to formulations containing these progestins or whether the increased risk was due to certain types of bias. Selection bias, diagnostic bias, and referral bias could have accounted for the differences, but a causal relation cannot be disproved.[63] Few data have been published to date regarding the risk of VTE with norgestimate-containing compounds, so it remains uncertain whether formulations containing this progestin are associated with an increased risk of VTE compared with use of low-estrogen levonorgestrel compounds.

■ TABLE 25–6

Rates of Deep Venous Thromboembolic Disease in Oral Contraceptive Estrogen Dose–Refined Cohorts

ESTROGEN-DEFINED COHORTS (μg)	NUMBER OF CASES	PERSON-YEARS (×10,000)	RATES/10,000 PERSON-YEARS
<50	53	12.7	4.2
50	69	9.8	7.0
>50	20	2.0	10.0
All	142	24.5	5.8

From Gerstman BB, Piper JM, Tomita DK, et al. Oral contraceptive estrogen dose and the risk of deep venous thromboembolic disease. Am J Epidemiol 133:32–37, 1991.

Myocardial Infarction

Neither epidemiologic studies of humans nor experimental studies with subhuman primates have observed an acceleration of atherosclerosis with the ingestion of OCs. Nearly all the published epidemiologic studies indicate that there is no increased risk of MI among former users of OCs.[64–66] The incidence of cardiovascular disease is also not correlated with the duration of OC use.[67] Further data indicating that the increased risk of MI in OC users is due to thrombosis, not atherosclerosis, are provided by an angiographic study of young women who had an MI performed in 1983 by Engel and associates.[68] In this study, only 36 percent of users of OCs containing 50 μg of ethinyl estradiol had evidence of coronary atherosclerosis compared with 79 percent of nonusers.

A study with cynomolgus macaque monkeys found that the ingestion of an OC containing high doses of norgestrel and ethinyl estradiol lowered HDL cholesterol levels significantly.[69] However, after 2 years of ingesting this formulation and being fed an atherogenic diet, these animals had a significantly smaller area of coronary artery atherosclerosis than did a control group of female monkeys not ingesting OCs but fed the same diet. Another group of monkeys that received levonorgestrel without estrogen also had lowered HDL cholesterol levels. In this group, the extent of coronary atherosclerosis was significantly increased compared with that of the control group. The results of this study have since been confirmed in a larger study with two high-dose estrogen-progestin formulations.[70] Both of these compounds lowered the HDL cholesterol levels by half and tripled the ratio of cholesterol to HDL cholesterol. In this study, the mean extent of coronary artery plaque formation in the high-risk control group of female animals was more than 3 times greater than that found in animals ingesting a high-dose norgestrel compound and more than 10 times greater than that found in animals ingesting a high-dose ethynodiol diacetate compound. These studies suggest that the estrogen component of OCs has a direct protective effect on the coronary arteries, reducing the extent of atherosclerosis that would otherwise be accelerated by decreased levels of HDL cholesterol.

The epidemiologic studies that reported an increased incidence of MI in older users of OCs were published in the late 1970s and thus used as a database women who ingested only formulations with 50 μg or more of estrogen.

In these case-control and cohort studies, a significantly increased incidence of MI was found mainly among older users who had risk factors that caused arterial narrowing, such as pre-existing hypercholesterolemia, hypertension, diabetes mellitus, or smoking more than 15 cigarettes a day.[71]

Data accumulated during the first 10 years of the RCGP study (1968 to 1978), in which the majority of users ingested formulations with more than 50 μg of estrogen and high doses of progestin, showed that a significantly increased relative risk of death from circulatory disease occurred only among women older than 35 years who also smoked.[67] A more recent analysis of data obtained during the first 20 years of this study (1968 through 1987) revealed that there was no significant increased relative risk of acute MI among current or former users of OCs who did not smoke any cigarettes[72] (Table 25–7). Women who smoked and did not use OCs had a greater risk of MI than did nonsmokers whether or not they used OCs. Even though most of the women in this study used high-dose formulations, a significantly increased risk of MI with OC use compared with that of smokers not using OCs occurred only among both light (fewer than 15 cigarettes per day) and heavy cigarette smokers. OC users who were heavy smokers had a greater relative risk than did light smokers. A case-control study analyzed the relation between OC use and the risk of MI among women admitted to a group of New England hospitals between 1985 and 1988. The relative risk of MI among current OC users was not significantly increased (RR, 1.1; confidence interval [CI], 0.4 to 3.1).[66] Among women who smoked at least 25 cigarettes a day, current OC use increased the risk of MI 30-fold. Smoking alone, without use of OCs, increased the risk of MI about ninefold. These data indicate that cigarette smoking is an independent risk factor for MI, but the use of high-dose OCs by cigarette smokers significantly enhances their risk of experiencing an MI, the two factors acting synergistically. Current or prior OC use is not associated with an increased risk of MI in nonsmokers.

Stroke

Although epidemiologic data from studies performed in the 1970s indicated that there was possibly a causal relation between ingestion of high-dose OC formulations and stroke, the data were conflicting; some studies showed a significantly increased risk of thrombotic stroke, others an increased risk of hemorrhagic stroke, and still others no significantly increased risk of either entity.[73] Furthermore, as occurred with MI, the studies that did show a significantly increased risk of stroke in OC users indicated that the increased risk was mainly limited to older women who also smoked or were hypertensive.[74]

Data from the epidemiologic studies of OC use and cardiovascular disease performed in the 1960s and 1970s are not relevant to their current use, because the dose of both steroid components in the formulations now being marketed is markedly less, and women with cardiovascular risk factors such as uncontrolled hypertension are no longer receiving these agents. Furthermore, it is strongly recommended not to prescribe OCs to women older than 35 years who also smoke.

A nested case-control analysis by Hannaford and colleagues[75] examined the data obtained between 1968 and 1990 during the RCGP's Oral Contraception Study to determine the relationship between OC use and the risk of first-ever stroke including the diagnosis of subarachnoid hemorrhage, cerebral hemorrhage, or thromboembolic stroke. Women using OCs containing a high estrogen dose, more than 50 μg, had nearly a sixfold increase in the risk of stroke; women ingesting OC formulations containing 30 to 35 μg of estrogen did not have an increased risk. An analysis of strokes occurring in a large health maintenance organization in California during the years 1991 to 1994 indicated that the users had no significant increase of either thromboembolic or hemorrhagic stroke with OC use. In this study, the relative risk of thromboembolic stroke was 0.65 and of hemorrhagic stroke 1.01 for OC users compared with women who never used OCs and 1.18 and 1.13 compared with never users and past users.[76]

The results of these recent epidemiologic studies indicate that use of low-dose estrogen-progestin OC formulations by nonsmoking women without risk factors for cardiovascular disease is not associated with an increased incidence of either MI or stroke. Smoking is a risk factor for arterial but not venous thrombosis. Combination OCs should not be prescribed to women older than 35 years who smoke cigarettes or use alternative forms of nicotine.

Reproductive Effects

In an attempt to determine whether the reproductive endocrine system recovers normally after cessation of OC therapy, Klein and Mishell[77] measured serum levels of FSH, LH, estradiol, progesterone, and prolactin in six women every day for 2 months after they discontinued use of high-dose OCs. Except for a variable prolongation of the follicular phase of the first postcontraceptive cycle, the

■ TABLE 25–7
Relative Risk of Myocardial Infarction in Relation to Smoking and Oral Contraceptive Use*

SMOKING	ORAL CONTRACEPTIVE USE		
	Never (CL)	Previously (CL)	Current (CL)
Never	1.0	1.1 (0.6–2.2)	0.9 (0.3–2.7)
<15 cig/day	2.0 (1.0–3.9)	1.3 (0.6–2.8)	3.5 (1.3–9.5)
≥15 cig/day	3.3 (1.6–6.7)	4.3 (2.3–8.0)	20.8 (5.2–83.1)

*Royal College of General Practitioners study, 1968–1987. N = 158. CL, confidence limits.
Modified from Croft P, Hannaford PC. Risk factors for acute myocardial infarction in women. Br Med J 298:1245, 1991.

patterns and levels of all of these hormones were indistinguishable from those found in normal ovulating subjects. In these six women, the initial LH peak occurred from 21 to 28 days after ingestion of the last tablet. These results indicate that after a variable but usually short interval after the cessation of oral steroids, their suppressive effect on the hypothalamic-pituitary-ovarian axis disappears. After the initial recovery, completely normal endocrine function occurs.

As previously mentioned, the delay in the return of fertility is greater for women discontinuing use of OCs with 50 μg of estrogen or more than with those containing lower doses of estrogen.[29] However, use of the low-dose formulations still causes a significant reduction in time to conception rates, with a mean of 5.88 cycles for OC users compared with 3.18 cycles for women discontinuing other contraceptive methods. Among women stopping use of OCs to conceive, the reduced probability of conception compared with that of women stopping use of other methods is greatest in the first month after their use is stopped and decreases steadily thereafter. There is little if any effect of duration of OC use on the length of delay of subsequent conception, but the magnitude of the delay to return of conception after OC use is greater among older primiparous women than among others.

Thus, for about 2 years after the discontinuation of contraceptives to conceive, the rate of return of fertility is lower for users of OCs than for women who have used barrier methods, but eventually the percentage of women who conceive after ceasing to use each of these contraceptive methods becomes the same.[78] Thus, the use of OCs does not cause permanent infertility.

Neither the rate of spontaneous abortion nor the incidence of chromosome abnormalities[79] in abortuses is increased in women who conceive in the first or subsequent months after they cease to use OCs. Several cohort and case-control studies of large numbers of babies born to women who stopped using OCs have been undertaken. These studies indicate that these infants have no greater chance of being born with any type of birth defect than do infants born to women in the general population, even if conception occurred in the first month after the medication was discontinued.[80–82] If OCs are accidentally ingested during the first few months of pregnancy, a large cohort study reported that there is no significantly increased risk of congenital malformations among the offspring of users overall or among those of nonsmoking users.[82]

Neoplastic Effects

OCs have been extensively used for more than 35 years, and numerous epidemiologic studies of both cohort and case-control design have been performed to determine the relation between use of these agents and the development of various types of neoplasms. Because as yet no elderly women have used OCs during their early reproductive years, the studies thus far published usually restrict the analysis to women younger than 60 years. Because hormones are mainly considered to be promoters, not initiators, of cancers, any adverse oncologic effects of these steroids should show a dose response, as demonstrated by an increased risk occurring with increased duration of use. In 1995, Schlesselman[83] addressed this issue by performing a meta-analysis of the epidemiologic studies reported between 1980 and 1994 that analyzed the effect of OCs according to their duration of use on cancer of the breast, organs of the female reproductive tract, and liver.[83]

Breast Cancer

Because estrogen stimulates the growth of breast tissue, there have been concerns that the high dose of exogenous estrogen in OCs could either initiate or promote breast cancer in humans. Accordingly, numerous epidemiologic studies have been published in which breast cancer risk among OC users has been determined. In 1991, Thomas[84] published a comprehensive review of the results of all previously published epidemiologic studies of breast cancer risk in relation to use of combined OCs. Both case-control and cohort studies were analyzed, and the summary relative risk was determined by meta-analysis. There were 15 case-control studies conducted in developed countries that included women of all ages at risk for having used OCs. These papers were published between 1974 and 1990, and the relative risk of breast cancer with OC use ranged from 0.7 to 1.6 in the individual studies. Only one of these studies reported a significant increase in breast cancer risk, and the summary relative risk obtained by combining data for all the studies was 1.0 (CI, 1.0 to 1.1).[84]

Eight case-control and one cohort study investigated the relative risk of breast cancer in OC users who did and did not have a family history of breast cancer. None of the studies showed a significant difference in risk of breast cancer among OC users who did and did not have a family history of breast cancer.

In 1996, a large international collaborative group reanalyzed the entire worldwide epidemiologic data that had investigated the relation between risk of breast cancer and use of OCs. Analysis was done of data from 54 studies performed in 25 countries, involving more than 53,000 women with breast cancer and more than 100,000 control subjects. The analysis indicated that while women took OCs, they had a slightly increased risk of having breast cancer diagnosed (RR, 1.24; CI, 1.15 to 1.30)[85] (Fig. 25–6). The magnitude of risk of having breast cancer diagnosed declined steadily after stopping OCs, so there was no longer a significantly increased risk 10 years or more after stopping their use (RR, 1.01; CI, 0.96 to 1.05).[85] It is of interest that the cancers diagnosed in women taking OCs were less advanced clinically than those that occurred in the nonusers. The risk of having breast cancer that had spread beyond the breast compared with a localized tumor was significantly reduced (RR, 0.88; CI, 0.81 to 0.95) in OC users compared with nonusers. The group concluded that these results could be explained by the fact that breast cancer is diagnosed earlier in OC users than in nonusers or could be due to biologic effects of the OCs.[86]

The clinical meaning of this vast amount of epidemiologic data with small changes in relative risk is difficult to interpret. It appears that the dose or type of either steroid as well as duration of OC use is not related to breast cancer risk. Because there is no relation between dose or duration of use of estrogen, it is unlikely that OCs initiate breast cancer. Furthermore, the collaborative analysis found that

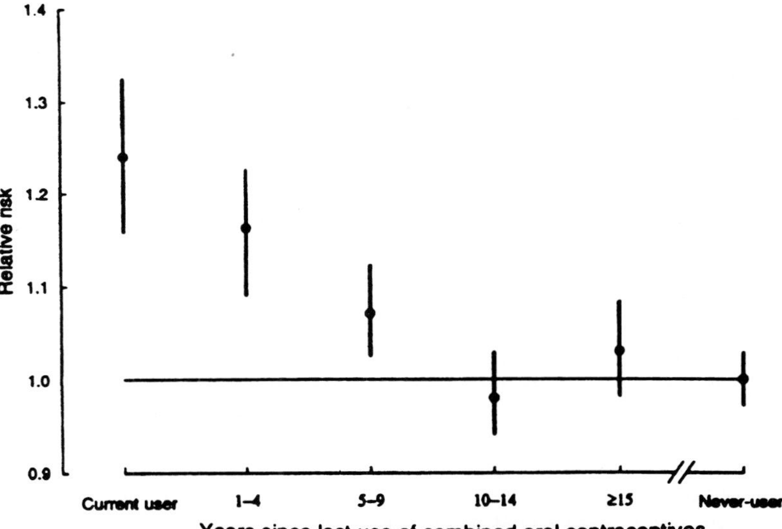

Figure 25–6 ■ Relative risk of breast cancer by time since last use of combined oral contraceptives. Dots are point estimates. Vertical line indicates 95 percent confidence intervals. (From Collaborative Group on Hormonal Factors in Breast Cancer. Breast cancer and hormonal contraceptives: Collaborative reanalysis of individual data on 53,297 women with breast cancer and 100,239 women without breast cancer from 54 epidemiological studies. Lancet 347:1713–1727, 1996. © by The Lancet Ltd.)

there was no significant increase in risk of breast cancer with OC use at very young ages, use before a first birth, or use by women with a family history of breast cancer. Two findings are important. One is that with current OC use or use within 5 years, the risk of breast cancer diagnosis is increased by about 25 percent. The second is that the increased risk of breast cancer in current OC users is limited to localized disease, and OC users have a significantly reduced incidence of disease that has spread beyond the breast. A decreased risk of advanced disease is also found in more older former OC users than nonusers who have breast cancer. Because the increased risk of breast cancer with OC use is confined to current and recent users, if there is an excess in incidence, the magnitude of increased incidence is small because breast cancer is uncommon before the age of 45 years. Furthermore, the contraceptive steroids probably act to promote the growth or increase the chance of diagnosis of existing cancers because breast cancer has been thought to usually take many years to become clinically evident after the cancer is initiated. Overall, the large body of data regarding OC use and breast cancer risk is reassuring.

Cervical Cancer

The epidemiologic data regarding the risk of invasive cervical cancer as well as cervical intraepithelial neoplasia and OC use are conflicting. Confounding factors such as the woman's age at first sexual intercourse, number of sexual partners, exposure to human papillomavirus (possibly greater among OC users), cytologic screening (probably more frequent among OC users), and use of barrier contraceptives or spermicides (primarily by women in the control group) as well as cigarette smoking (an independent risk factor for this disease) could account for the different results in different studies. In most of these studies, statistical corrections were made for these confounding factors, and the control group did not use barrier methods of contraception in many of them.

As reported by Schlesselman's review of 14 studies of more than 3800 women with invasive cervical cancer, there is a significant trend of increased risk of this disease with increased duration of OC use. The relative risk of disease with 4, 8, and 12 years of OC use increased from 1.37 to 1.60 to 1.77, respectively.[83]

Two of three case-control studies also reported that the risk of invasive cervical cancer was significantly increased with long-term OC use, with a relative risk between 1.5 and 2.5.[87–89] Three case-control studies have reported that the risk of adenocarcinoma of the cervix was significantly increased about twofold among OC users compared with nonusers.[87, 90, 91] In two of these studies, the risk of this type of tumor increased with increasing duration of use; in one study, a fourfold increased risk was reached with more than 12 years of OC use. Adenocarcinoma of the cervix is uncommon before the age of 55 years, with an incidence of about 1 per 1000 women. In contrast to these findings, the majority of well-controlled studies indicate that there is no significant change in risk of cervical intraepithelial neoplasia with OC use.[88] Because invasive epithelial cervical cancer is usually preceded by dysplasia, the relation between OC use and increased risk of epithelial cervical cancer is unlikely to be causal. However, it is possible that a causal relation exists between OC use and an increased risk of cervical adenocarcinoma.

Endometrial Cancer

Twelve case-control studies and three cohort studies have examined the relation between OCs and endometrial cancer, and all but two of these studies have indicated that the use of these agents has a protective effect against endometrial cancer, the third most common cancer among United States women.[83, 92] Women who use OCs for at least 1 year have an age-adjusted relative risk of 0.5 for diagnosis of endometrial cancer between the ages of 40 and 55 years compared with nonusers. This protective effect is related to duration of use, increasing from a 20 percent reduction risk with 1 year of use to a 40 percent reduction with 2 years of use to about a 60 percent reduction with 4 years of use. Voigt and colleagues[93] reported that the protective effect of OCs on endometrial cancer occurred with use of combination formulations with both high and low doses of progestin.

Ovarian Cancer

As summarized by Hankinson and coworkers[94] in 1992, there were 20 published reports examining the use of OCs with subsequent development of ovarian cancer, and 18 of these found a reduction in risk specifically of the most common type—epithelial ovarian cancers (Fig. 25–7). The summary relative risk of ovarian cancer among ever-users of OCs was 0.64, a 36 percent reduction. OCs reduce the risk of the four main histologic types of epithelial ovarian cancer (serous, mucinous, endometrioid, and clear cell), and the risk of invasive ovarian cancers as well as of those with low malignant potential is reduced. The magnitude of the decrease in risk is directly related to the duration of OC use, increasing from about a 40 percent reduction with 4 years of use to a 53 percent reduction with 8 years of use and a 60 percent reduction with 12 years of use. Beyond 1 year, there is about an 11 percent reduction in ovarian cancer risk for each of the first 5 years of use. The protective effect begins within 10 years of first use and continues for at least 20 years after the use of OCs ends. A study by Rosenberg and associates[95] found a similar level of protection with low-dose monophasic formulations as well as with higher dose agents. Insufficient data on ovarian cancer risk with use of phasic formulations are currently available. As with endometrial cancer, the protective effect occurs only in women of low parity (≤4), who are at greatest risk for this type of cancer.

Liver Adenoma and Cancer

The development of a benign hepatocellular adenoma is a rare occurrence in long-term users of OCs, and the increased risk of this tumor was associated with prolonged use of high-dose formulations, particularly those containing mestranol. Although two British studies reported an increased risk of liver cancer among users of OCs, the number of patients was small and the results could have been influenced by confounding factors.[96, 97] The rate of death from the disease has remained unchanged in the United States during the past 25 years, a period when millions of women have used these agents. Data from a large multicenter epidemiologic study coordinated by the WHO found no increased risk of liver cancer associated with OC users in countries with a high prevalence rate of this neoplasm.[98] This study found no change in risk with increasing duration of use or time since first or last use.

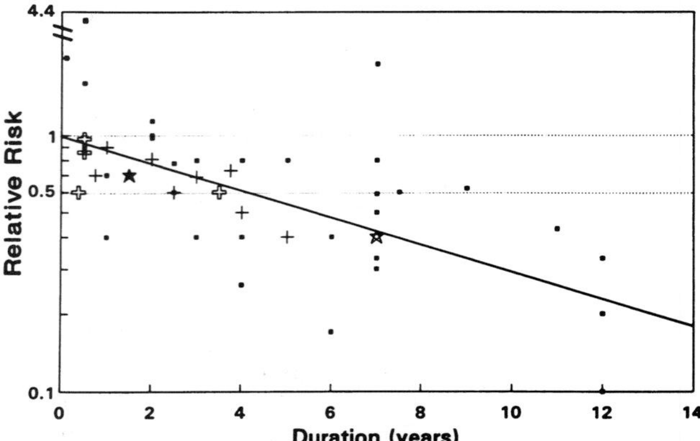

Figure 25–7 ■ Relative risk of ovarian cancer associated with different durations of oral contraceptive use: findings of 15 studies. Study categories, indicating category weights ranging from smallest (weight in bottom 25 percent of range) to largest (weight in top 25 percent of range): squares = 1 (smallest); pluses = 2; open crosses = 3; stars = 4 (largest). (From Hankinson SE, Colditz GA, Hunter DJ, et al. A quantitative assessment of oral contraceptive use and risk of ovarian cancer. Obstet Gynecol 80:708–714, 1992.)

Pituitary Adenoma

OCs mask the predominant symptoms produced by prolactinoma—amenorrhea and galactorrhea. When OC use is discontinued, these symptoms occur, suggesting a causal relation. However, data from three studies indicate that the incidence of pituitary adenoma among users of OCs is not higher than that among matched control subjects.[99]

Malignant Melanoma

Several epidemiologic studies have been undertaken to assess the relation of OC use and malignant melanoma. The results are ambiguous, because an increased risk, a decreased risk, and no effect have all been reported. In a review by Prentice and Thomas[73] in 1987, the summary relative risk for eight case-control studies was 1.0 and for three cohort studies 1.4, an insignificant increase. A more recent analysis of the two large British cohort studies that were initiated in 1968, involving more than 40,000 women, reported that the adjusted relative risk of malignant melanoma in OC users was 0.92 and 0.85.[100] The results of these large studies of long duration indicate that OC use does not increase the risk of malignant melanoma.

Contraindications to Use

OCs can be prescribed for the majority of women of reproductive age, because these women are young and generally healthy. However, there are certain absolute contraindications: a history of vascular disease (including thromboembolism, thrombophlebitis, atherosclerosis, and stroke) and systemic disease that has altered the vascular system, such as lupus erythematosus or diabetes with retinopathy or nephropathy. Cigarette smoking by OC users older than 35 and uncontrolled hypertension are also contraindications. One of the contraindications listed in the product labeling is cancer of the breast or endometrium, although there are no data indicating that OCs are harmful to women with these diseases. Pregnant women should not take OCs, because it has been theorized that there may be masculinizing effect of the 19-nonprogestins on the external genitalia of female fetuses.

Women with functional heart diseases should not use OCs, because the fluid retention they produce could result in congestive heart failure. There is no evidence, however, that individuals with asymptomatic mitral valve prolapse should not use OCs. Women with active liver disease should not take OCs. However, women who have recovered from liver disease, such as viral hepatitis, and whose liver function test results have returned to normal can safely take OCs.

Relative contraindications to OC use include heavy cigarette smoking by women younger than age 35, migraine headaches, undiagnosed causes of amenorrhea, and depression. About 20 percent of women have migraine headaches, and their frequency and severity can be worsened by OC use. There is currently no evidence that the risk of stroke is significantly increased in women with migraine headaches who use OCs compared with nonusers. Unless the women have peripheral neurologic symptoms with the migraine headaches, OCs can be used. If fainting, temporary loss of vision or speech, or paresthesias develop in an OC user, the use of OCs should be stopped because of their thrombophilic effect.

Because OC use may mask the symptoms produced by a prolactin-secreting adenoma (amenorrhea and galactorrhea), amenorrheic women should not receive OCs until the diagnosis for this symptom is established. If galactorrhea develops during OC use, OCs should be discontinued, and after 2 weeks a serum prolactin level should be measured. If it is elevated, further diagnostic evaluations are indicated. The presence of a prolactin-secreting macroadenoma but not a microadenoma is a contraindication for OC use. Use of OCs does not cause enlargement of prolactin-secreting pituitary microadenomas or worsen functional prolactinoma as was previously believed. Women with gestational diabetes can take low-dose OC formulations, because these agents do not affect glucose tolerance or accelerate the development of diabetes mellitus.[101] Insulin-dependent diabetes without vascular disease is also not a contraindication for low-dose OC use.

Contraceptive Use

Initiation

ADOLESCENTS

In deciding whether a sexually active pubertal girl should use OCs for contraception, the clinician should be more concerned about compliance with the regimen than about possible physiologic harm. As long as she has demonstrated maturity of the hypothalamic-pituitary-ovarian axis with at least three regular, presumably ovulatory, menstrual cycles, it is safe to prescribe OCs without concern that their use will permanently alter future reproductive endocrinologic function. It is not necessary to be concerned about accelerating epiphyseal closure in the postmenarcheal female. Endogenous estrogens have already initiated the process a few years before menarche, and use of contraceptive steroids will not hasten it.

AFTER PREGNANCY

There is a difference in the relationship of the return of ovulation and bleeding between the postabortal woman and one who has had a term delivery. The first episode of menstrual bleeding in the postabortal woman is usually preceded by ovulation. After a term delivery, the first episode of bleeding is usually but not always anovulatory. Ovulation occurs sooner after an abortion, usually between 2 and 4 weeks, than after a term delivery, when ovulation is usually delayed beyond 6 weeks but may occur as early as 4 weeks in a woman who is not breast feeding.

Thus, after spontaneous or induced abortion of a fetus of less than 12 weeks' gestation, OCs should be started immediately to prevent conception after the first ovulation. For women who deliver after 28 weeks and are not nursing, the combination pills should be initiated 2 to 3 weeks after delivery. If the termination of pregnancy occurs between 21 and 28 weeks, contraceptive steroids should be started 1 week later; the reason for delay in this instance is that the normally increased risk of thromboembolism occurring post partum may be further enhanced by the thrombophilic effects of combination OCs. Because the first ovulation is delayed for at least 4 weeks after a term delivery, there is no need to expose the woman to this increased risk.

Estrogen inhibits the action of prolactin in breast tissue receptors; therefore, the use of combination OCs (those containing both estrogen and progestin) diminishes the amount of milk produced by OC users who breast feed their babies. Although the diminution of milk production is directly related to the amount of estrogen in the contraceptive formulation, only one study has been published in which the amount of breast milk was measured by breast pump in women using formulations with less than 50 μg of estrogen. In this study, the use of this low dose of estrogen reduced the amount of breast milk.[102] Thus, it is probably best for women who are nursing not to use combination OCs unless supplemental feeding is given to the infant.

Women who are breast feeding every 4 hours, including during the night, will not ovulate until at least 10 weeks after delivery and thus do not need contraception before that time. Because only a small percentage of breast feeding women will ovulate as long as they continue full nursing and remain amenorrheic, either a barrier method or a progestin-only OC can be used until menses resume. Progestins do not diminish the amount of breast milk, and progestin-only OCs are effective in this group of women. Once supplemental feeding is introduced, ovulation can resume promptly, and more effective contraception is then needed. Combination OCs should be used once supplemental feeding is initiated.

CYCLING WOMEN

At the initial visit, after a history and physical examination have determined that there are no medical contraindications for OCs, the woman should be informed about the benefits and risks. For medicolegal reasons, it is best to note on the patient's medical record that the benefits and risks have been explained to her.

Type of Formulation

In determining which formulation to use, it is best initially to prescribe a formulation with less than 50 μg of ethinyl estradiol, because these agents are associated with less cardiovascular risk as well as fewer estrogenic side effects than formulations with 50 μg of estrogen. It would also appear reasonable to use formulations with the lowest androgenic potency of progestin, because there would be less androgenic, metabolic, and clinical adverse effects associated with their use. The development of multiphasic formulations has allowed the total dose of progestin to be reduced compared with some monophasic formulations, without increasing the incidence of breakthrough bleeding. However, several monophasic formulations have a lower total dose of progestin per cycle than the multiphasic formulations, and the incidence of follicular enlargement is more frequent with multiphasic than with monophasic formulations.[103]

The U.S. Food and Drug Administration (FDA) has stated that the product prescribed should be one that contains the least amount of estrogen and progestin that is compatible with a low failure rate and the needs of the individual woman. Because few randomized studies have been performed comparing the different marketed formulations, until large-scale comparative studies are performed, the clinician must decide on the formulation to use on the basis of which have the least adverse effects among women in his or her practice. If estrogenic or progestogenic side effects occur with one formulation, a different agent with less estrogenic or progestogenic activity can be given.

The contraceptive formulations containing progestins and no estrogen have a lower incidence of adverse metabolic effects than do the combination formulations. Because the factors that predispose to thromboembolism are caused by the estrogen component, the incidence of thromboembolism in women ingesting these compounds is not increased. Furthermore, blood pressure is not affected, nausea and breast tenderness are eliminated, and milk production and quality are unchanged. Despite these advantages, these agents have the disadvantages of a high frequency of intermenstrual and other abnormal bleeding patterns (including amenorrhea) and a lower rate of effectiveness than the combined formulations. The failure rate of these preparations is higher than with the combined formulations, and a relatively high percentage of the pregnancies that do occur are ectopic. Because nursing mothers have reduced fertility and are amenorrheic, the major disadvantages of these preparations are minimized for these individuals. Furthermore, because milk production and quality are unaffected in contrast to the changes produced by combination pills, the formulations with only a progestin may be offered to these women while they are nursing. However, a small portion of these synthetic steroids have been detected in breast milk. The long-term effects (if any) of these progestins on the infant are not known, but none has been detected to date. A long-term follow-up study of breast fed children whose mothers ingested combined OCs containing 50 μg of estrogen while they were lactating revealed no difference in mean body weight or height up to 8 years of age compared with breast fed children whose mothers did not ingest OCs.[104] There was also no difference of occurrence of disease or in intellectual or psychologic behavior between the two groups.

Follow-up

If a healthy woman has no contraindications to OC use, it is unnecessary to perform any laboratory tests including cervical cytology unless these are necessary for routine health maintenance. At the end of 3 months, the woman should be seen again; at this time, a nondirected history should be obtained and the blood pressure measured. After this visit, the woman should be seen annually, at which time a nondirected history should again be taken, blood pressure and body weight measured, and a physical examination (including breast, abdominal, and pelvic examination with cervical cytology) performed. It is important to perform annual cervical cytologic screening of OC users, because they are a group at relatively high risk for development of cervical neoplasia. The routine use of other laboratory tests is not indicated unless the woman has a family history of diabetes or vascular disease at a young age. Routine use of these tests in women is not indicated, because the incidence of positive results is extremely low. However, if the woman has a family history of vascular disease, such as MI occurring in family members younger than 50, it would be advisable to obtain a lipid panel before OC use is started; hypertriglyceridemia may be present, and OC use will further raise triglyceride levels. Because the low-dose formulations do not adversely alter the lipid profile except for triglycerides, it is not necessary to measure lipids, other than the routine cholesterol screening every 5 years, in women with no cardiovascular risk factors, even if they are older than 35. If the woman has a family history of diabetes or evidence of diabetes during pregnancy, a 2-hour postprandial blood glucose test should be performed before OCs are started, and if the blood glucose level is elevated, a glucose tolerance test should be performed. If the woman has history of liver disease, a liver panel should be obtained to make certain that liver function is normal before OCs are started.

Drug Interactions

Although synthetic sex steroids can retard the biotransformation of certain drugs (e.g., phenazone and meperidone) as a result of substrate competition, such interference is not important clinically. OC use has not been shown to inhibit the action of other drugs. However, some drugs can interfere clinically with the action of OCs by inducing liver enzymes that convert the steroids to more polar and less biologically active metabolites.

Certain drugs have been shown to accelerate the biotransformation of steroids in humans. These include barbiturates, sulfonamides, cyclophosphamide, and rifampin. Several investigators have reported a relatively high incidence of OC failure in women ingesting rifampin, and these two agents should not be given concurrently.[105] The clinical data concerning OC failure in users of other antibiotics (e.g., penicillin, ampicillin, and sulfonamides), analgesics (e.g., phenytoin), and barbiturates are less clear. A few anecdotal studies have appeared in the literature, but reliable evidence for a clinical inhibitory effect of these drugs on OC effectiveness, such as occurs with rifampin, is not available. One study by Murphy and colleagues[106] showed that when 2 gm of tetracycline was given daily in divided doses, the levels of both ethinyl estradiol and norethindrone in OC users were similar to those before antibiotic use. Women with epilepsy requiring medication should probably be treated with formulations containing 50 μg of estrogen; a higher incidence of abnormal bleeding has been reported in these women with the use of lower dose estrogen formulations owing to lower circulating levels of ethinyl estradiol brought about by the action of most antiepileptic medications.[107]

Noncontraceptive Health Benefits

In addition to being the most effective method of contraception, OCs provide many other health benefits.[108] Some are due to the fact that the combination OCs contain a potent, orally active progestin as well as an orally active estrogen, and there is no time when the estrogenic target tissues are stimulated by estrogens without a progestin (unopposed estrogen).

Both natural progesterone and the synthetic progestins inhibit the proliferative effect of estrogen, the so-called antiestrogenic effect. Estrogens increase the synthesis of both estrogen and progesterone receptors, whereas progesterone decreases their synthesis. Thus, one mechanism whereby progesterone exerts its antiestrogenic effects is by decreasing the synthesis of estrogen receptors. Relatively little progestin is needed to exert this action, and the amount present in OCs is sufficient. Another way progesterone produces its antiestrogenic action is by stimulating the activity of the enzyme estradiol-17β-dehydrogenase within the endometrial cell. This enzyme converts the more potent estradiol to the less potent estrone, reducing estrogenic action within the cell.

As a result of the antiestrogenic action of the progestins in OCs, the height of the endometrium is less than in an ovulatory cycle, and there is less proliferation of the endometrial glands. These changes produce several substantial benefits for the OC user. One is a reduction in the amount of blood loss at the time of endometrial shedding. In an ovulatory cycle, the mean blood loss during menstruation is about 35 ml, compared with 20 ml for women ingesting OCs. This decreased blood loss makes the development of iron deficiency anemia less likely in OC users than in nonusers.

Because OCs produce regular withdrawal bleeding, it would be expected that OC users would have fewer menstrual disorders than do control subjects. The results of the RCGP study confirmed the fact that OC users were significantly less likely to have menorrhagia, irregular menstruation, or intermenstrual bleeding develop.[109] Because these disorders are frequently treated by curettage or hysterectomy, OC users require these procedures less frequently than do nonusers.

Estrogen exerts a proliferative effect on breast tissue, which also contains estrogen receptors. Progestins may also inhibit the synthesis of estrogen receptors in this organ. Several studies have shown that OCs reduce the incidence of benign breast disease, and two prospective studies have indicated that this reduction is directly related to the amount of progestin in the compounds.[110, 111]

Benefits from Inhibition of Ovulation

Other noncontraceptive medical benefits of OCs result from their main action—inhibition of ovulation. Some disorders, such as dysmenorrhea and premenstrual tension, occur much more frequently in ovulatory than in anovulatory cycles.

Lanes and coworkers[103] studied the rate of functional cysts more than 2 cm in diameter, which required either hospitalization or outpatient surgery, by ultrasonography. They found that low-dose monophasic formulations resulted in about a 50 percent reduction in functional cysts, lower than the 75 percent reduction with high-dose formulations, whereas use of multiphasic formulations had only a slight reduction of ovarian cyst development.

Other Benefits

Several European studies, including the RCGP study, showed that the risk of development of rheumatoid arthritis in OC users was only about half that in control subjects.[112, 113] Another benefit is protection against salpingitis, commonly referred to as pelvic inflammatory disease (PID). The relative risk of PID developing among OC users in most studies is about 0.5, a 50 percent reduction.[114] OCs reduce the clinical development of salpingitis in women infected with gonorrhea. OCs reduce the risk of ectopic pregnancy by more than 90 percent in current users and may reduce the incidence in former users by decreasing their chance of development of salpingitis.

Limited epidemiologic data indicate that OCs may reduce bone loss in perimenopausal women, particularly those with oligomenorrhea.[115] There are noncontraceptive health benefits associated with continuing OC use beyond the age of 40 years into the perimenopausal years. Because the estrogen given for hormone replacement is not as thrombophilic as the estrogen dose currently used in OCs, it is best to switch from OCs to estrogen replacement at about the age of 50 years. To avoid discontinuing OC use when the woman is still ovulating, measurement of the FSH and estradiol levels on the last day of the pill-free interval provides information about ovarian follicular activity. When the FSH level is elevated and the estradiol level is low, OCs should be discontinued and estrogen hormonal replacement begun.[116]

LONG-ACTING CONTRACEPTIVE STEROIDS

To avoid contraceptive failure associated with the need to remember to take OC daily, methods of administering contraceptive steroid formulations at infrequent intervals have been developed. To date, two types of long-acting steroids, injectable suspensions and subdermal implant formulations, have been developed and are being used by women in the United States and elsewhere. Because most of the long-acting steroid formulations contain only a progestin, without an estrogen, endometrial integrity is not maintained and uterine bleeding occurs at irregular and unpredictable intervals. Therefore, women wishing to use these methods need to be counseled about the development of irregular bleeding before their use to enhance continuity of use.

Injectable Suspensions

Three types of injectable steroid formulations are currently in use for contraception throughout the world. These include depot medroxyprogesterone acetate (DMPA), given in a dose of 150 mg every 3 months; norethindrone enanthate, given in a dose of 200 mg every 2 months; and several once-a-month injections of combinations of different progestins and estrogens. Only the first of these three types is currently available in the United States. Injectable contraceptives are a popular method of contraception worldwide. In the United States, they are used by about 3 percent of women of reproductive age.

Medroxyprogesterone acetate (MPA) is a 17-acetoxyprogesterone compound and is the only progestin used for contraception that is not a 19-nortestosterone derivative. In all currently marketed oral contraceptives, the progestins are all 19-nortestosterone compounds, either estranes or gonanes, and as such have varying degrees of androgenic activity.

The 17-acetoxyprogestins, which do not have androgenic activity and are structurally related to progesterone instead of testosterone, were used in OC formulations about 30 years ago. Although they were approved for contraception in many Western countries in the 1960s, regulatory approval for these agents in the United States was stopped when tests on beagle dogs showed that ingestion of OCs with 17-acetoxyprogestins was associated with an increased risk of mammary cancer. It was discovered later that, unlike humans and other animals, the beagle uniquely metabolizes 17-acetoxyprogestins to estrogen, which causes mammary hyperplasia. Thus, when MPA is ingested by the beagle, this substance behaves differently than it does in the human, in whom it is not metabolized to estrogen. After epidemiologic studies showed that DMPA does not increase the risk of breast cancer in humans, regulatory approval for marketing this agent as a contraceptive was obtained in the United States in 1992.

Depot Formulation of Medroxyprogesterone Acetate

MPA is a 17-acetoxy-6-methyl progestin that has progestogenic activity in the human[117] (Fig. 25–8). Because MPA is not metabolized as rapidly as the parent compound, progesterone, it can be given in smaller amounts than progesterone, with an equivalent amount of progestational activity. DMPA, the long-acting injectable formulation of MPA, consists of a crystalline suspension of this progestational hormone. The effective contraceptive dosage is 150 mg DMPA, which is given by injection deep into the gluteal or deltoid muscle, after which the progestin is released slowly into the systemic circulation. The area should not be massaged, so that the drug is released slowly into the circulation and maintains its contraceptive effectiveness for at least 4 months.

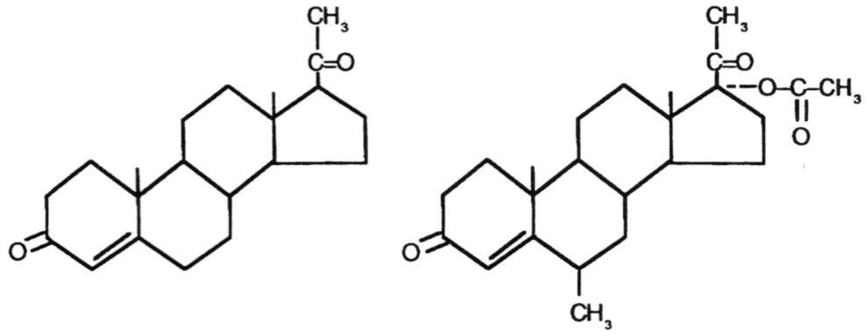

Progesterone

Medroxyprogesterone Acetate (MPA)

Figure 25–8 ■ Comparative structures of progesterone and MPA. (From Mishell DR Jr. Pharmacokinetics of depot medroxyprogesterone acetate contraception. J Reprod Med 41[suppl]:381–390, 1996.)

DMPA is an extremely effective contraceptive. In a large WHO clinical trial studying use of DMPA, the pregnancy rate at 1 year was only 0.1 percent; at 2 years, the cumulative rate was 0.4 percent.[118] Three mechanisms of action are involved. The major effect is inhibition of ovulation. Second, the endometrium becomes thin and does not secrete sufficient glycogen to provide nutrition for a blastocyst entering the endometrial cavity. Third, DMPA keeps the cervical mucus thick and viscous, so sperm are unlikely to reach the oviduct and fertilize an egg. With these multiple mechanisms of action, DMPA is one of the most effective reversible methods of contraception currently available.

PHARMACOKINETICS

MPA can be detected in the systemic circulation within 30 minutes after its intramuscular injection.[119] Although serum MPA levels vary among individuals, they rise steadily to contraceptively effective blood levels (>0.5 ng/ml) within 24 hours after the injection.

The pattern of MPA clearance from the circulation varies among different studies according to the type of assay used. After DMPA was administered to three subjects, Ortiz and coworkers[119] assayed blood MPA levels daily for 2 weeks, then three times a week for the next 3 months, and then weekly until MPA was undetectable. In two subjects, MPA levels initially plateaued at 1.0 to 1.5 ng/ml for about 3 months, after which they declined slowly to about 0.2 ng/ml during the fifth month (Fig. 25–9). In a third subject, the blood levels were higher during the first month, then ranged between 1.0 and 1.5 ng/ml for the next 2 months, after which there was a further decline. MPA levels remained detectable in the circulation (>0.2 ng/ml) for 7 to 9 months in all three subjects, after which it was not detectable. Estradiol levels were found to be in the range of the early follicular to midfollicular phase, but consistently below 100 pg/ml during the first 4 months after injection. After 4 to 6 months, when MPA levels decreased to less than 0.5 ng/ml, estradiol concentrations rose to preovulatory levels, indicating follicular activity, but ovulation did not occur, as evidenced by persistently low progesterone levels. Return of follicular activity preceded the return of luteal activity by 2 to 3 months. This delay in resumption of luteal activity is probably due to the fact that the circulating MPA levels inhibit the positive feedback effect of the rise of estradiol on the hypothalamic-pituitary axis, which in the absence of MPA would stimulate the midcycle release of LH. The return of luteal activity in this study, indicated by a rise in serum progesterone levels, did not occur until 7 to 9 months after the injection, when the MPA levels were below 0.1 ng/ml.

In another study, performed by Kirton and Cornette[120] using a different assay, MPA levels were much higher, although the pattern was similar to that found in the study by Ortiz,[119] and luteal activity also did not occur until about 7 months after the injection.

A third study of DMPA pharmacokinetics was reported

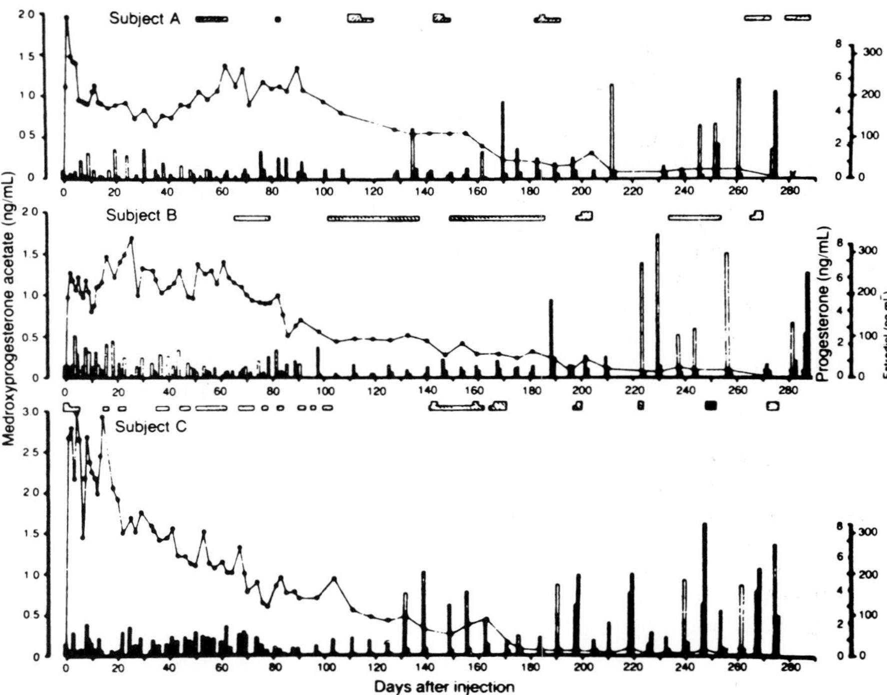

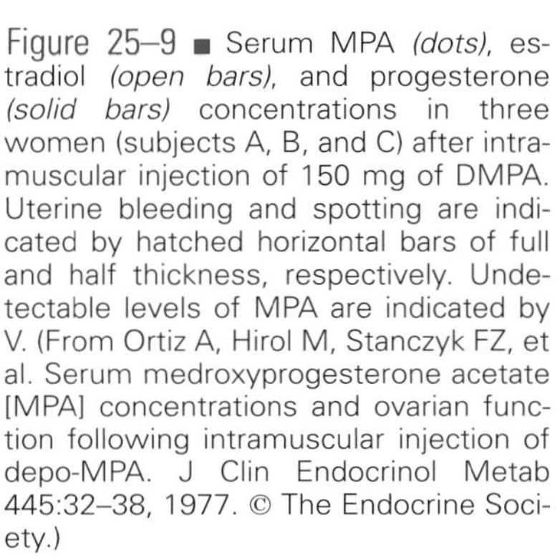
Figure 25–9 ■ Serum MPA *(dots)*, estradiol *(open bars)*, and progesterone *(solid bars)* concentrations in three women (subjects A, B, and C) after intramuscular injection of 150 mg of DMPA. Uterine bleeding and spotting are indicated by hatched horizontal bars of full and half thickness, respectively. Undetectable levels of MPA are indicated by V. (From Ortiz A, Hirol M, Stanczyk FZ, et al. Serum medroxyprogesterone acetate [MPA] concentrations and ovarian function following intramuscular injection of depo-MPA. J Clin Endocrinol Metab 445:32–38, 1977. © The Endocrine Society.)

by Fotherby and colleagues[121] and showed an entirely different pattern of MPA clearance after the injection. In this study, the MPA levels fell more rapidly than in the other two studies, and the progesterone levels initially rose about 3.5 months after the injection. On the basis of this study, the product labeling states that if the time interval after the last injection is more than 13 weeks, the provider should determine that the woman is not pregnant before administering the drug. Additional studies are needed to determine more precisely the pharmacodynamics of MPA clearance and time of initial resumption of ovulation because of the differences observed in previous studies.

OVULATORY SUPPRESSION

To determine the effect of DMPA on the hypothalamic-pituitary axis, Mishell and colleagues[122] measured serum LH and FSH levels daily during a control cycle and then for 2 months after a single injection was given. Although the midcycle LH peak was suppressed after the injection, tonic LH was still being secreted in a pulsatile manner, and serum tonic levels were about the same as those found in the follicular phase of the control cycle. The normally occurring peak level of FSH at midcycle was also suppressed after the injection, but tonic FSH levels were in the range of those found in the luteal phase of the control cycle, indicating a lack of complete suppression of the hypothalamic-pituitary axis.

Mishell and colleagues[122] reported that daily progesterone levels were consistently in the follicular-phase range during the first 2 months after the initial injection of DMPA. To obtain suppression of ovulation in the initial injection cycle, DMPA has to be administered within several days after the onset of menses. Siriwongse and associates[123] reported that when the drug was initially given on day 5 or 7 of the cycle, none of the women ovulated, but when it was given on day 9, 2 of 13 subjects had presumptive evidence of ovulation. The results of this study indicated that DMPA should be given no later than 7 days after the onset of menses to be effective in the first ovulatory cycle. The product labeling states that to ensure the woman is not pregnant at the time of the first injection, it must be given during the first 5 days of the cycle.

Mishell and colleagues[122] reported that circulating estradiol levels during the first 2 months after the initial 150-mg injection of DMPA were similar to the levels found in the follicular phase of the control cycle. Therefore, there is incomplete suppression of follicular activity in the first two cycles after an injection of DMPA.

A cross-sectional study was performed by Mishell and colleagues[122] of 121 women who received 150 mg of DMPA every 3 months for more than 1 year. An assay performed on a serum sample obtained on the day of the next scheduled injection showed marked differences in the estradiol levels, which varied from approximately 15 pg/ml to nearly 100 pg/ml (mean, approximately 42 pg/ml). A similar range and mean value were also found among women who had been receiving DMPA for 1 to 2 years and those who had used it for 4 to 5 years. All these women had moist, well-rugated vaginas, and none stated that her breast size had decreased. None of the women complained of hot flashes. This use of contraceptive doses of DMPA does not decrease endogenous estradiol levels to the postmenopausal range and does not cause symptoms of estrogen deficiency.

RETURN OF FERTILITY

Because of the lag time in clearing DMPA from the circulation, resumption of ovulation is delayed for a variable time, which may last as long as 1 year after the last injection. Women who wish to become pregnant and stop using

DMPA should be informed that there will be a delay in the resumption of fertility until the drug is cleared from the circulation. After this initial delay, fecundability resumes at a rate similar to that found after discontinuation of a barrier contraceptive[124] (Fig. 25–10). Thus, use of DMPA does not prevent return of fertility; it only delays the time at which conception will occur. Because of its long and unpredictable duration of release from the injection site, the time until resumption of fertility may be delayed for 1 year or more after the last injection. Information about the possibility of a long duration of DMPA action needs to be given to women who are considering this method of contraception.

ENDOMETRIAL CHANGES

The histology of the endometrium at various intervals after starting DMPA was examined by Mishell and associates.[125] Histologic examination of endometrial biopsy specimens revealed three types of patterns: proliferative, quiescent, and atrophic. Secretory endometrium was not seen. Most of the women had a quiescent pattern, characterized by narrow, widely spaced glands and decidualization of the stroma.

ADVERSE EFFECTS

Clinical Effects

Bleeding Irregularities. The major side effect of DMPA is complete disruption of the menstrual cycle. In the first 3 months after the first injection, about 30 percent of women are amenorrheic and another 30 percent have irregular bleeding and spotting occurring more than 11 days per month.[126] The bleeding is usually small in amount and does not cause anemia to occur. As duration of therapy increases, the incidence of frequent bleeding steadily declines and the incidence of amenorrhea steadily increases, so that at the end of 2 years about 70 percent of the women treated with DMPA are amenorrheic[126] (Fig. 25–11). Women who use this method of contraception should be counseled that, with time, the irregular bleeding episodes will cease and amenorrhea will most likely occur.

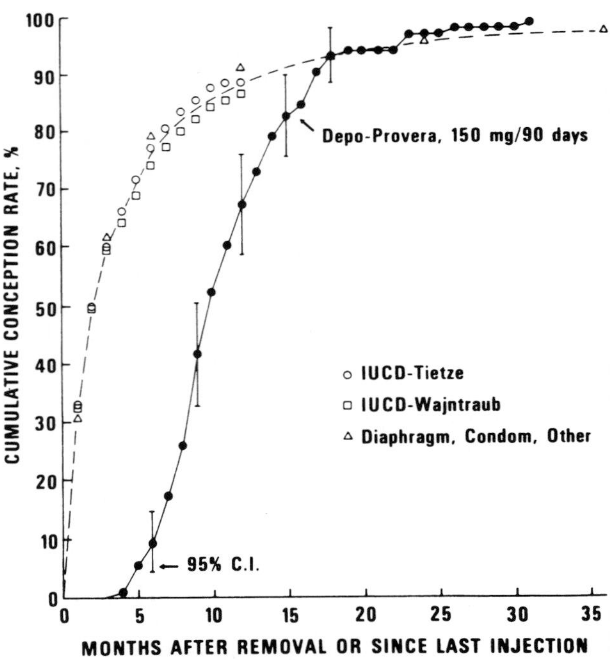

Figure 25–10 ■ Cumulative conception rates of women who discontinued a contraceptive method to become pregnant. (From Schwallie PC, Assenzo JR. The effect of depo-medroxyprogesterone acetate on pituitary and ovarian function, and the return of fertility following its discontinuation: A review. Contraception 10:181–202, 1974.)

Weight Changes. In five cross-sectional studies, users of DMPA weighed more than a comparison group not using hormonal contraceptives.[127] Several longitudinal studies have indicated that DMPA users gain between 1.5 and 4 kg in their first year of use and continue to gain weight thereafter. None of these studies included a control group, so the weight could be due to factors other than DMPA use. In one retrospective comparative longitudinal study, Moore and coworkers[128] found no significant change in mean weight of DMPA, progestin implant, and OC users. Thus, the effect among DMPA on body weight remains unclear. If DMPA users gain weight, they should be counseled to decrease calorie intake and increase their expenditure of energy.

Mood Changes. The product labeling lists depression and mood changes as side effects of DMPA. Several studies, however, indicate that the incidence of depression and mood change in women using this method of contraception is less than 5 percent.[127] No clinical trials with a comparison group not using DMPA have been performed to determine whether a causal relation between use of DMPA and development of depression exists.

Headache. Although development of headaches is the most frequent medical event reported by DMPA users[129] and a common reason for discontinuation of its use, there are no comparative studies to indicate that use of DMPA increases the incidence or severity of tension or migraine headaches. Therefore, the presence of migraine headaches is not an absolute contraindication for use of DMPA. However, women should be counseled that if the frequency or severity of headaches increases after the injection is given, it may be several months before the drug is cleared from the circulation. For this reason, the presence of migraine headaches may be considered to be a relative contraindication for use of DMPA.

Metabolic Effects

Protein. Because DMPA does not increase liver globulin production as does the estrogen component of OC (ethinyl estradiol), no alteration in blood clotting factors or angiotensinogen levels is associated with its use. Thus, unlike OCs, DMPA has not been associated with an increased incidence of hypertension or thromboembolism.[36] A WHO study reported that mean blood pressure measurements were unchanged in DMPA users after 2 years of injections.[118]

Carbohydrate. There have been two studies in which oral glucose tolerance tests have been performed on long-term DMPA users and matched control subjects not using hormonal contraceptives.[130, 131] The mean glucose levels were slightly greater among the DMPA users than among the control subjects in one but not the other study. Mean insulin levels were also higher. The slight deterioration

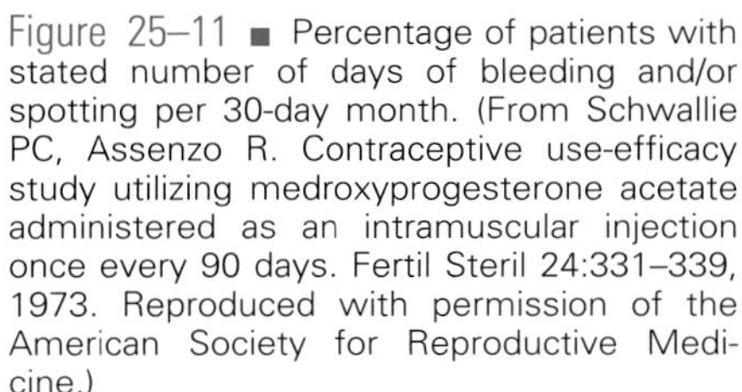

Figure 25–11 ■ Percentage of patients with stated number of days of bleeding and/or spotting per 30-day month. (From Schwallie PC, Assenzo R. Contraceptive use-efficacy study utilizing medroxyprogesterone acetate administered as an intramuscular injection once every 90 days. Fertil Steril 24:331–339, 1973. Reproduced with permission of the American Society for Reproductive Medicine.)

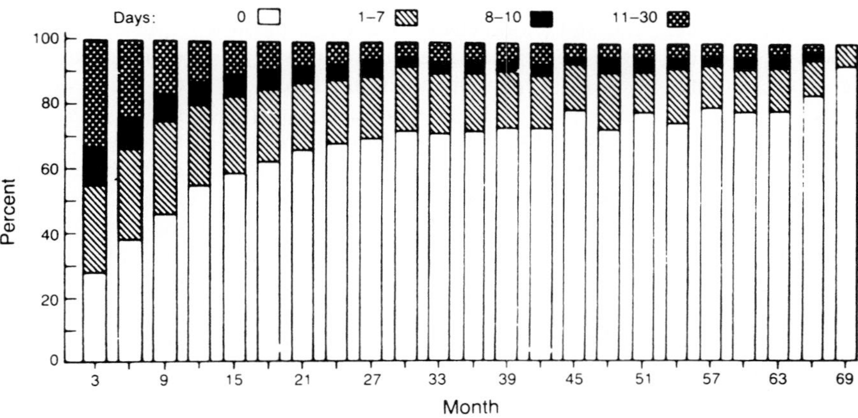

in glucose tolerance among DMPA users is probably not clinically significant and returns to normal after use of DMPA is stopped.

Lipids. Westhoff[127] reviewed the findings of 11 studies that evaluated plasma lipids among groups of women using DMPA. Most of the studies were cross-sectional and compared lipid levels among DMPA users with those of women not using hormonal methods of contraception. There was little or no change in mean triglyceride and total cholesterol levels; however, in all seven studies in which mean HDL cholesterol levels were measured, the levels were lower among the DMPA users. Of the five studies in which LDL cholesterol was measured, three noted an increase among the DMPA users. There are no studies in which the incidence of cardiovascular events among current or former long-term DMPA users was compared with that among control subjects. Therefore, although the lipid changes with DMPA use are not beneficial, there is no evidence to date that they are associated with an acceleration of atherosclerosis.

Bone Loss. One cross-sectional study of 30 long-term DMPA users indicated that they had a reduction in lumbar spine and femoral bone density compared with 30 premenopausal control subjects that was of lesser magnitude than occurred in 30 postmenopausal women whose bone density was also measured concurrently with dual-energy x-ray absorption.[132] A subsequent report by the same group of investigators indicated that after use of DMPA was stopped, there was an increase in bone mineral density of the lumbar spine.[133] Other longitudinal studies have not shown a decrease in bone density in DMPA users.[134–136] The reported effect of DMPA on bone density remains to be clarified with ongoing long-term longitudinal studies. To date, no studies have reported a change in incidence of fractures in current or former long-term DMPA users.

NEOPLASTIC EFFECTS

Breast Cancer. Two large case-control studies, the WHO study[137] and a New Zealand study,[138] indicated that the relative risk of diagnosis of breast cancer among all DMPA users was not significantly changed (RR of 1.2 and CI of 0.96 to 1.15,[137] and RR of 1.0 and CI of 0.8 to 1.3,[138] respectively). When the data from these studies were pooled, the overall breast cancer diagnosis risk among DMPA users was 1.1 (CI, 0.97 to 1.4).[139] In long-term users, those who had used the drug more than 5 years and those who had started use more than 14 years earlier, the risk of diagnosis of breast cancer was also not increased (RR of 1.0 and CI of 0.70 to 1.5, and RR of 0.89 and CI of 0.6 to 1.3, respectively). However, among those women who had started use within the past 5 years and were mainly younger than 35, there was a significant increased risk of diagnosis of breast cancer (RR, 2.0; CI, 1.5 to 2.8), similar to that found with use of OCs and women with first term pregnancy at an early age. Thus, like other contraceptive steroids, DMPA does not appear to change the overall incidence of diagnosis of breast cancer, and women should be counseled accordingly.

Endometrial Cancer. A WHO case-control study found the risk of endometrial cancer to be significantly reduced among DMPA users (RR, 0.21; CI, 0.06 to 0.79).[140] This reduction in risk persisted for at least 8 years after use was stopped and was similar in magnitude to the protective effect observed with combination OCs.

Ovarian Cancer. In a WHO case-control study, the risk of ovarian cancer among DMPA users was unchanged (RR, 1.07; CI, 0.6 to 1.8).[141] These findings do not demonstrate a protective effect similar to that observed with OCs despite inhibition of ovulation with both agents. The lack of a protective effect observed with DMPA was probably due to the fact that in the countries studied, DMPA was given only to multiparous women, women at low risk of developing epithelial ovarian cancer, who differ from the higher risk women taking OCs.

Cervical Cancer. In a large WHO case-control study, the risk of invasive cancer of the cervix was not increased (RR, 1.1; CI, 0.96 to 1.29),[142] similar to findings observed in a large case-control study in Costa Rica.[143] Long-term use and long time since first use were also not associated with a significant increase in risk of cervical cancer in these studies. The risk of cancer in situ was slightly increased in the WHO study (RR, 1.4; CI, 1.2 to 1.7) but not in the Costa Rica study (RR, 1.1; CI, 0.6 to 1.8) or two New Zealand studies investigating the risk of cancer dysplasia.[144, 145] Thus, the reports in which the neoplastic effects of DMPA on breast and reproductive tract have been investigated are reassuring.

NONCONTRACEPTIVE HEALTH BENEFITS

In a summarization by Cullins,[146] there is good epidemiologic evidence that use of DMPA reduces the risk of iron deficiency anemia, PID, and endometrial cancer and has a beneficial effect on hematologic parameters in women with sickle cell disease as well as reducing their incidence of clinical problems. DMPA also reduces seizure frequency in women with epilepsy[147] and probably should reduce the incidence of primary dysmenorrhea, ovulation pain, and functional ovarian cyst because it inhibits ovulation. DMPA also reduces the symptoms of endometriosis and in two small studies reduced the incidence of vaginal candidiasis.[148, 149]

CLINICAL RECOMMENDATIONS

Women should be thoroughly counseled about the occurrence of abnormal bleeding and development of amenorrhea with use of DMPA before receiving the first injection. It has been shown that pretreatment counseling improves continuation rates.[150] In addition, women should be counseled that the duration of action may last as long as 1 year after the last injection if they decide to discontinue use to become pregnant or if they experience side effects.

In cycling women, the initial injection should be given no later than day 5 of the cycle to be certain to inhibit ovulation in the initial treatment cycle.[151] Because of an absence of thrombophilic effects, the first injection should be given within 5 days post partum in nonlactating women; but, in women who exclusively breast feed their infants, the product labeling states that the first injection should not be given until at least 6 weeks post partum.[151] DMPA does not affect the quantity or quality of breast milk or the health of children who breast feed during its use.[152] If a woman with lactational amenorrhea wishes to institute DMPA use, it is unlikely that she is pregnant if a qualitative test response for human chorionic gonadotropin (hCG) is negative; therefore, she can receive the injection at that time. If concern about pregnancy exists, use of a barrier contraceptive should be advised for an additional 2 weeks, at which time the assay for hCG should be repeated. If the response is still negative, the injection can be given. A similar protocol can be used for the woman who has received DMPA in the past but is delayed beyond 13 weeks in returning for her next injection and is still amenorrheic. If accidental pregnancy does occur in a DMPA user, there is no evidence that the agent is teratogenic or has an adverse effect on the outcome of the pregnancy.[153]

Subdermal Implants

Subdermal implants of capsules made of polydimethylsiloxane (Silastic) containing levonorgestrel for use as contraceptives have been developed and patented by The Population Council as Norplant. It was approved by the U.S. FDA in 1990, and marketing in this country began in 1991. As with all steroid-containing Silastic devices, the rate of steroid delivery is directly proportional to the surface area of the capsules, whereas duration of action depends on the amount of steroid within the capsules. To produce effective blood levels of norgestrel, it was found necessary to use six capsules filled with crystalline levonorgestrel. The cylindrical capsules are 3.4 cm long and 2.4 mm in outer diameter, with the ends sealed with Silastic medical adhesive. Each capsule contains 36 mg of crystalline levonorgestrel for a total amount of 215 mg in each six-capsule set.

Insertion is performed in an outpatient setting, and the entire procedure takes about 5 minutes. After infiltration of the skin with local anesthetic, a small (3-mm) incision is made with a scalpel, usually in the upper arm, although the lower arm and the inguinal, scapular, and gluteal regions have also been used. When the capsules are inserted in any area of subcutaneous tissue, the steroid diffuses into the circulation at a relatively constant rate. The capsules are implanted into the subcutaneous tissue in a radial pattern through a large (10- to 12-gauge) trocar, and the incision is closed with adhesive. Sutures are not necessary. Because polydimethylsiloxane is not biodegradable, the capsules have to be removed through another incision when desired by the user or at the end of 5 years, which is the duration of maximal contraceptive effectiveness.

After insertion, blood levels of levonorgestrel rise rapidly to reach levels between 1000 and 2000 pg/ml in 24 hours.[154] These levels fall markedly in the first week and then gradually in the first month and then remain relatively constant during the first year of use with the mean level ranging between 250 and 600 pg/ml, which is usually sufficient to inhibit ovulation[155] (Fig. 25–12). At the end of 5 years, mean levonorgestrel levels range between 170 and 350 pg/ml.[156] Blood levels vary considerably among women, mainly because of differences in body weight. Heavier women have lower circulating levonorgestrel levels than thin women do. When the amount of steroid was measured in capsules removed from women after various times, it was found that the rate of release was fairly constant during the first year of use, averaging about 50 μg of levonorgestrel per day from the six-capsule set. From about the end of the first year of use until 8 years of use, daily release rates declined to about 30 μg/day but remained constant during each day.[154]

With this low level of levonorgestrel, gonadotropin levels are not completely suppressed, and ovarian follicular activity results in periodic peaks of estradiol. Because the level of circulating levonorgestrel is usually sufficient to inhibit the positive feedback effect of these estradiol peaks on LH release, LH levels are lower than normal, even in Norplant users with regular cycles, and ovulation during the first 2 years of use occurs infrequently.[157]

Thus, inhibition of ovulation is one of the major mechanisms of action of this method of contraception. The consistently elevated circulating levels of norgestrel also prevent the normal midcycle thinning of the cervical mucus from occurring. The cervical mucus remains scanty and viscid, and normal sperm penetration does not take place, as demonstrated by both in vivo and in vitro studies.[158, 159] These two mechanisms of action result in a high level of contraceptive effectiveness.

With the less dense tubing currently used, annual pregnancy rates for the first 5 years of use are about 0.2 per 100 women of all body weights, yielding a cumulative 5-year pregnancy rate of 1.1 percent.[154] As with all progestin-only methods of contraception, when pregnancies occur with Norplant, a high percentage, about 20 percent, are ectopic. However, because of its high rate of effectiveness, the overall rate of ectopic pregnancies in Norplant users, 0.28 per 1000 woman-years of use, is reduced compared with ectopic pregnancy rates in the entire United States

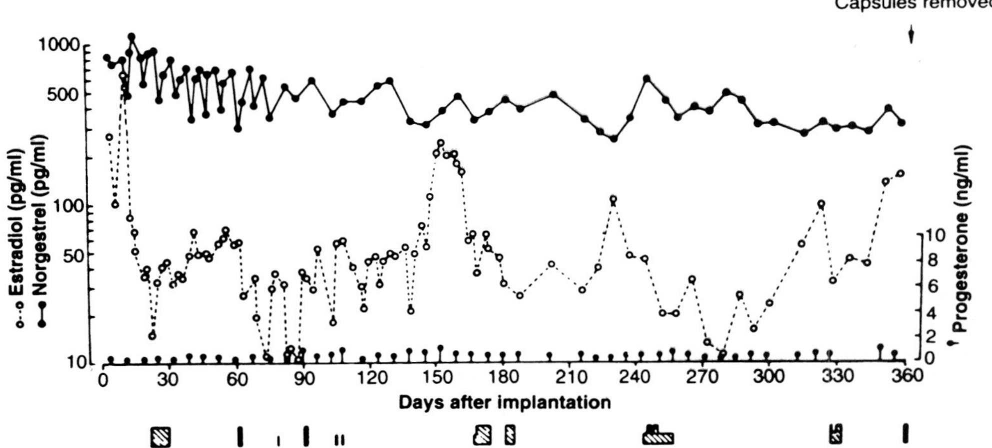

Figure 25–12 ■ Serum levels of estradiol, progesterone, and *d*-norgestrel in a subject with six polysiloxane capsules, each containing 33.9 mg of *d*-norgestrel, implanted on day 0. Hatched bars represent uterine bleeding. (From Moore LL, Valuck R, McDougall C, et al. A comparative study of one-year weight gain among users of medroxyprogesterone acetate, levonorgestrel implants, and oral contraceptives. Contraception 52:215–220, 1995.)

population of women of reproductive age, 1.5 per 1000 women annually.[160]

Mean estradiol levels in Norplant users, whether they are ovulatory or anovulatory, are about the same as in women with regular ovulatory cycles who used IUDs,[161] and three patterns of estradiol activity have been observed. About half of Norplant users have periodic, irregular peaks of estradiol within the normal range (up to 400 pg/ml), 30 percent have fluctuating estradiol levels with high broad peaks above 400 pg/ml, and about 10 percent have consistently low estradiol levels below 75 pg/ml.[161] After a fall in estradiol level, endometrial sloughing and uterine bleeding or spotting usually occur. Because the peaks and declines in estradiol levels occur at irregular intervals, uterine bleeding also occurs at irregular intervals in the majority of Norplant users.

The major side effect of Norplant use is the irregular pattern of uterine bleeding. Other alterations in uterine blood flow involve changes in duration and volume, with most bleeding episodes being scanty in amount. About half the bleeding episodes can be characterized as fairly regular, with the interval between bleeding episodes ranging between 21 and 35 days; about 40 percent as irregular, with intervals outside this range; and about 10 percent as amenorrheic, with no bleeding for more than a 13-month interval.[162] Bleeding episodes tend to be more prolonged and irregular during the first year of use, after which there is greater frequency of a more regular pattern. Shoupe and colleagues[163] reported that during the first year of use, about one fourth of the cycles were regular, two thirds irregular, and 7 percent amenorrheic. By the fifth year, about two thirds of the cycles were regular and one third irregular, and none was amenorrheic (Fig. 25–13). The mean number of days of bleeding also declines steadily with use.[160] Mean total blood loss in Norplant users is about 25 ml per month.[164] Several clinical studies have shown that the mean hemoglobin concentration in the first 3 years of Norplant use tends to rise slightly. When pregnancies occur in Norplant users, they almost always occur in women with a recent history of regular cyclic uterine bleeding.

Other problems associated with this method of contraception include infection, local irritation, and painful reaction at the insertion site. Expulsion of a capsule, usually in association with infection, occurs occasionally. The incidence of insertion site infection is less than 1 percent. Headache is the single most frequent medical problem causing removal of the implants, accounting for about 30 percent of the medical reasons for removal.[160] Weight gain was a common reason for medical removal in U.S. studies, whereas weight loss was more common in the Dominican Republic. Other medical problems among Norplant users include acne, mastalgia, and mood changes, including anxiety, depression, and nervousness. Because ovarian follicular

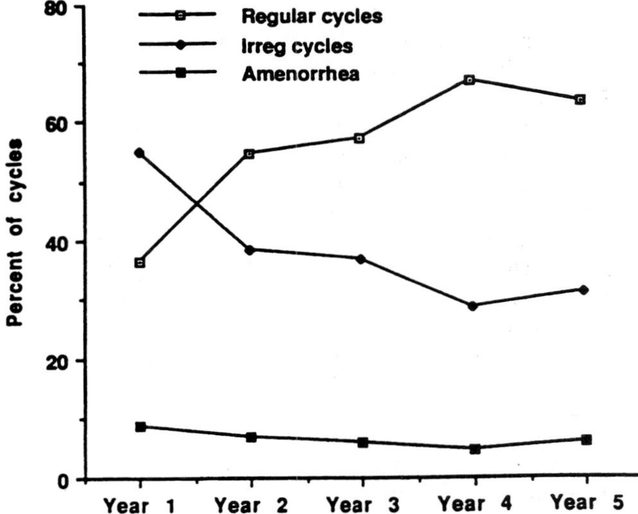

Figure 25–13 ■ Bleeding patterns calculated on a monthly basis in implant users during 5 years of use. (From Shoupe D, Mishell DR Jr, Bopp BL, Fielding M. The significance of bleeding patterns in Norplant implant users. Obstet Gynecol 77:256–260, 1991.)

development without subsequent ovulation is common among Norplant users, adnexal enlargement due to persistent unruptured follicles has been noted during routine bimanual pelvic examination in many Norplant users. These enlarged follicles, which may reach 5 to 7 cm in diameter, usually spontaneously regress in 1 to 2 months without therapy.

A great number of metabolic studies have been performed among Norplant users in various population groups. Studies of carbohydrate metabolism, serum chemistries, liver function, serum cortisol levels, thyroid function, and blood coagulation have revealed only minimal changes, which remain within the normal range.[162] Several studies have been performed in different countries in which lipoproteins were measured before and after Norplant insertion. In most of these studies, levels of triglycerides, total cholesterol, and LDL cholesterol declined, whereas HDL cholesterol declined slightly or increased.[162] There was little change in the ratio of cholesterol to HDL cholesterol, indicating that Norplant should not enhance the development of atherosclerosis.

The removal process, like the insertion procedure, is performed in the clinic area with use of local anesthesia and a small skin incision. Removal of Norplant is a more difficult process than insertion, because fibrous tissue develops around the capsule and must be cut before removal of the capsules. It is important to insert the capsules superficially to enhance the ease of removal; deeply implanted capsules are more difficult to remove.

After removal, the incision is closed without sutures, and a pressure dressing is applied for about 24 hours. If the woman wishes to continue use, another set can be inserted through the same incision or in the opposite arm. If another set of Norplant is not inserted after removal, the steroid is rapidly cleared from the circulation and serum levels of norgestrel fall rapidly, reaching nearly undetectable levels in 96 hours.[165] If pregnancy is desired, return to ovulation is prompt and is similar to that in women discontinuing nonhormonal methods of reversible contraception, reaching 50 percent at 3 months and 86 percent at 1 year.[160] Continuation rates with Norplant method of contraception are high, ranging from 76 to 99 percent at 1 year in different countries and from 33 to 78 percent at 4 years.[160]

Manufacture of the capsules is complicated, and placing or removing six capsules creates some difficulties; therefore, norgestrel has been fabricated into solid rods that are a homologous mixture of Silastic and crystalline levonorgestrel covered with Silastic tubing. The rods are easier to manufacture, insert, and remove than the capsules. Because of different properties of diffusion, higher blood levels of norgestrel are achieved with a smaller total surface area of the rods. Thus, with two 4-cm covered rods with the same diameter as the capsules, the same release rate for norgestrel, about 50 μg/day, can be achieved as with placement of six 3-cm capsules. During a 3-year clinical study comparing rods and capsules, the serum norgestrel levels, bleeding patterns, and incidence of elevated progesterone levels were similar.[166] A multicenter clinical study has confirmed these findings, and use of the two covered rods has recently been approved by the U.S. FDA for clinical use. Single implants with other progestins such as desogestrel have been manufactured and studied in clinical trials. These implants have a probable duration of action of 2 years and are much easier to insert and remove than the multiple levonorgestrel-releasing implants.

EMERGENCY CONTRACEPTION

Various estrogenic compounds have been used for emergency contraception. The estrogen compounds that have been used for this purpose include diethylstilbestrol, 25 to 50 mg/day; ethinyl estradiol, 5 mg/day; and conjugated estrogen, 30 mg/day. Treatment is continued for 5 days. If treatment is begun within 72 hours after an isolated midcycle act of coitus, its effectiveness is good. If more than one episode of coitus has occurred, or if treatment is initiated later than 72 hours after coitus, the method is less effective.

Pregnancy rates among women treated with ethinyl estradiol were 0.6 percent; with diethylstilbestrol, 0.7 percent; and with conjugated estrogen, 1.6 percent.[167] It has been estimated that the clinical pregnancy rate for a single act of midcycle coitus without use of a contraceptive is about 7 percent. Thus, high-dose estrogen is an effective method of postcoital contraception. Side effects associated with this high-dose estrogen therapy are common and severe. They include nausea, vomiting, breast soreness, and menstrual irregularities, which tend to reduce compliance.

Because the side effects of high-dose estrogens cause many women to fail to complete the 5-day treatment course, a regimen of four tablets of an ethinyl estradiol, 0.05 mg, and *dl*-norgestrel, 0.5 mg, combination OC (Ovral), given in doses of two tablets 12 hours apart, was initially tested in Canada. This regimen was found to have a similar degree of effectiveness with a shorter duration of adverse symptoms than with 5 days of estrogen.

Fasoli and colleagues[167] summarized the results of 11 studies with this treatment regimen involving 3802 women. Failure rates varied widely, from a low of 0.2 percent in a Canadian study to a high of 7.4 percent in an Italian study. The total pregnancy rate in the 11 studies was 1.8 percent, similar to the individual failure rate in the largest studies in this review. Trussell and associates[168] pooled the data from studies that were published between 1977 and 1993 involving 5226 women treated with this regimen. They calculated that the failure rate was 1.5 percent and use of this regimen prevented about 75 percent of the expected pregnancies. Trussell and colleagues also analyzed results of nine published studies in which the effectiveness of this regimen was determined when treatment was initiated 1, 2, or 3 days after midcycle unprotected intercourse. Using logistic regimen analysis, they found that there was no significant difference in failure rates when the first pill was taken on the first, second, or third day after unprotected intercourse.

Ho and Kwan[169] reported results of a randomized trial comparing the use of four tablets of ethinyl estradiol and levonorgestrel taken in divided doses 12 hours apart with a single tablet of 0.75 mg levonorgestrel taken initially and another one 12 hours later. Both regimens were ingested within 48 hours of unprotected intercourse. Failure rates of both regimens, about 2 percent, were similar, but there was significantly less nausea and vomiting with the progestin alone than with the one combined with estrogen. A strip of four tablets of the combination steroid pills is marketed in several countries under a variety of brand names.

Several authors have advocated that intrauterine insertion of a copper IUD within 5 to 10 days of midcycle coitus is an effective method to prevent continuation of the pregnancy. Fasoli and coworkers[167] summarized the results of four published studies in nine countries involving 875 women. Only one pregnancy occurred after a copper IUD was inserted in these women. Insertion of a copper IUD and ingestion of high-dose estrogens are the most effective methods of emergency contraception, but side effects limit acceptance of the latter, and cost and concern about introducing pathogens into the upper genital tract with IUD insertion limit its widespread use. Because no manufacturer has applied for U.S. FDA approval to market an emergency method of contraception, it is infrequently prescribed by clinicians, and few women in the United States are aware that it is effective, accessible, and safe.

PROGESTERONE ANTAGONISTS

A few years ago Healy and colleagues[170] synthesized a progestogenic steroid compound that had weak progestational activity but marked affinity for progesterone receptors in the endometrium. This compound, called RU 486 or mifepristone (Fig. 25–14), because of its high receptor affinity prevents progesterone from binding to its receptors and thus inhibits the action of circulating progesterone on its target tissue. In clinical trials, it was found that if a single 600-mg dose of RU 486 was administered orally in early pregnancy, before 7 weeks after the onset of the last menses, about 85 percent of the pregnancies spontaneously terminated.[171] When this treatment was combined with administration of a prostaglandin 36 to 48 hours later, the efficacy increased to 96 percent.[172] However, side effects include nausea, vomiting, and abdominal pain. Two prostaglandin analogues, intramuscular sulprostone and vaginal gemeprost, were the agents initially used after mifepristone. Sulprostone is no longer marketed for this purpose, because three women who received this agent with mifepristone suffered an MI. Gemeprost is much more expensive than misoprostol, a prostaglandin analogue widely used to prevent peptic ulcer disease. Therefore, oral administration of misoprostol is now being used more extensively than gemeprost after mifepristone.

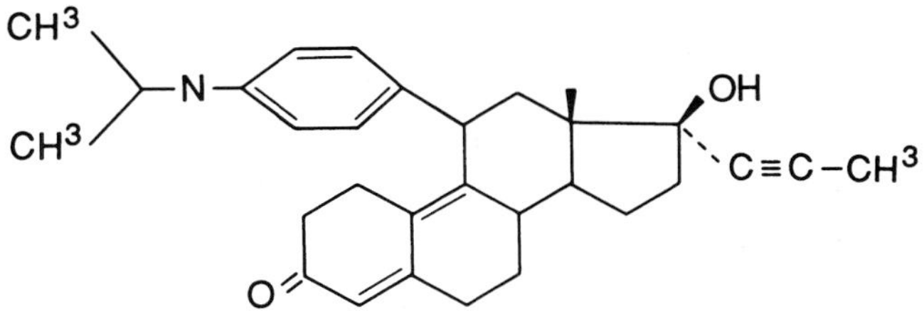

Figure 25–14 ■ Molecular structure of RU 486. Molecular weight is 430, and empirical formula is $C_{29}H_{35}NO_2$. (From Healy DL, Baulieu EE, Hodgen GD. Induction of menstruation by an antiprogesterone steroid [RU 486] in primates: Site of action, dose-response relationships, and hormonal effects. Fertil Steril 40:253–257, 1983. Reproduced with permission of the American Society for Reproductive Medicine.)

The results of a randomized trial with misoprostol given vaginally or orally suggest that when misoprostol is given vaginally instead of orally, it is more effective and has fewer side effects.[173] A large, multicenter clinical trial with mifepristone followed by oral misoprostol was recently performed in the United States. Therefore, when this drug combination does become available for use in this country, the oral administration of misoprostol will most likely be recommended, even though vaginal administration is probably preferable. The main disadvantage of this medical abortifacient method is prolonged and sometimes heavy uterine bleeding that on occasion can cause anemia, necessitating a blood transfusion and possibly curettage. The mean duration of bleeding after administration of this drug is about 12 days when it is administered alone and 9 days when it is used with a prostaglandin. Distribution of mifepristone is currently limited to a few European countries and China, but compounds with similar activity or steroid enzymatic inhibitors that prevent progesterone synthesis are also being studied.[174]

INTRAUTERINE DEVICES

The main benefits of IUDs are (1) a high level of effectiveness, (2) a lack of associated systemic metabolic effects, and (3) the need for only a single act of motivation for long-term use. Despite these advantages, less than 1 percent of married women of reproductive age use the IUD for contraception in the United States compared with 15 to 30 percent in most European countries and Canada.

Types

In the past 35 years, many types of IUDs have been designed and used clinically. The devices developed and initially used in the 1960s were made of a plastic, polyethylene, impregnated with barium sulfate to make them radiographic. In the 1970s, to diminish the frequency of the side effects of increased uterine bleeding and pain, smaller plastic devices covered with copper were developed and widely used. In the 1980s, devices were developed bearing a larger amount of copper, including sleeves on the horizontal arm, such as the copper T380A and the copper T220C, as well as the Multiload Cu250 and Cu375. These devices have a longer duration of high effectiveness and thus need to be reinserted at less frequent intervals than the devices bearing a smaller amount of copper. The copper T380A IUD is the only copper-bearing IUD currently marketed in the United States, but the Multiload Cu375 is widely used in Europe (Fig. 25–15).

Because of the constant dissolution of copper, which amounts daily to less than that ingested in the normal diet, all copper IUDs have to be replaced periodically. The copper T380A is currently approved for use in the United States for 10 years and may maintain its effectiveness for a longer time. At the scheduled time of removal, the device can be removed and another inserted during the same office visit.

Adding a reservoir of progesterone to the vertical arm also increases the effectiveness of the T-shaped devices. The currently marketed progesterone-releasing IUD allows 65 mg of progesterone to diffuse into the endometrial

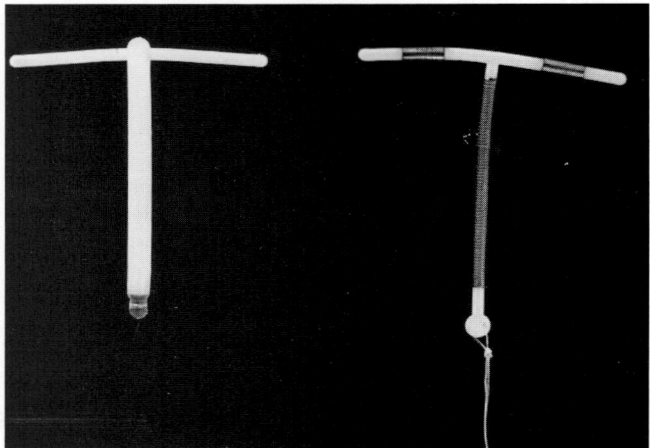

Figure 25–15 ■ Intrauterine devices currently being marketed in the United States: *left,* progesterone-releasing IUD; *right,* copper T380A.

cavity each day. This amount is sufficient to prevent pregnancy by local action within the endometrial cavity but is not enough to cause a measurable increase in peripheral serum progesterone levels. Because of the progestational effect on the endometrium, the amount of uterine bleeding is reduced with use of this device, and it has been used therapeutically to treat menorrhagia. The currently approved progesterone-releasing IUD needs to be replaced annually, because the reservoir of progesterone becomes depleted after about 18 months of use and the surface area of plastic in this small device is insufficient to produce a sufficiently large leukocytic response to yield a high level of contraceptive effectiveness.

A T-shaped device containing a reservoir of levonorgestrel on the vertical arm has been developed and undergone extensive clinical testing. A large comparative trial of the copper T380A and the levonorgestrel-releasing IUD found that the effectiveness and continuation rates of both devices were similar.[175] Because of the slower rate of release of levonorgestrel than progesterone, the levonorgestrel-releasing IUD has an estimated duration of use of at least 5 years. The levonorgestrel-releasing IUD also reduces menstrual blood loss and has been used therapeutically to treat abnormal uterine bleeding. This device is currently marketed in only a few European countries.

Mechanisms of Action

The main mechanism of contraceptive action of copper-bearing IUDs in the human is a spermicidal effect. This effect is caused by a local sterile inflammatory reaction produced by the presence of the foreign body in the uterine cavity. There is about 1000 percent increase in the number of leukocytes in washings of the human endometrial cavity 18 weeks after the insertion of an IUD, compared with washings obtained before insertion. In addition to causing phagocytosis of spermatozoa, tissue breakdown products of these leukocytes are toxic to all cells, including spermatozoa and the blastocyst. The amount of inflammatory reaction, and thus contraceptive effectiveness, is directly related to the size of the intrauterine foreign body. Copper markedly increases the extent of the inflammatory reaction, so this metal has been added to the small-sized frame of T-shaped devices.[176] In addition, copper impedes sperm transport and viability in the cervical mucus.[177] Because the copper T380 has about twice as much copper surface area as the previously marketed copper 7 IUD, the former has a lower failure rate than the latter IUD. Sperm transport from the cervix to the oviduct in the first 24 hours after coitus is markedly impaired in women wearing IUDs.[178] Because of the spermicidal action of IUDs, few if any sperm reach the oviducts, and the ovum usually does not become fertilized.[179] Thus, the principal mechanism of action of the copper T380A IUD is as a spermicide, preventing fertilization of the ovum. The progesterone-releasing IUD has a much higher ectopic pregnancy rate than the copper IUD[180] and probably acts mainly by slowing tubal transport of the embryo as well as by preventing implantation of the blastocyst owing to the presence of a high level of progesterone in the uterine cavity.

On removal of the IUD, the inflammatory reaction rapidly disappears. Resumption of fertility after IUD removal is prompt and occurs at the same rate as resumption of fertility after discontinuation of the barrier methods of contraception.[181] The incidence of term deliveries, spontaneous abortion, and ectopic pregnancies in conceptions occurring after IUD removal is the same as in the general noncontracepting population.

Time of Insertion

Although it is widely believed that the optimal time for insertion of an IUD is during the menses, there are data indicating that the IUD can be safely inserted on any day of the cycle provided that the woman is not pregnant.

Adverse Effects

Incidence

In general, in the first year of use, copper IUDs have less than a 1 percent pregnancy rate, a 10 percent expulsion rate, and a 15 percent rate of removal for medical reasons, mainly bleeding and pain. The incidence of each of these events, especially expulsion, diminishes steadily in subsequent years.

In an ongoing WHO study of the copper T380A, termination rates for adverse effects continued to decline annually after the first year following insertion for each of the 7 years in which sufficient data had been accumulated.[4] In this study, the cumulative percentage discontinuation rate for pregnancy, bleeding and pain, and expulsion at the end of 7 years was 1.6, 22.7, and 8.6, respectively.

Uterine Bleeding

The majority of women discontinuing this method of contraception do so for medical reasons. Nearly all the medical reasons accounting for removal of copper-bearing or inert IUDs involve one or more types of abnormal bleeding: heavy or prolonged menses or intermenstrual bleeding.

The copper T380A IUD is associated with about a 55 percent increase in menstrual blood loss.[182] In contrast, with the progesterone-releasing IUD, the amount of blood loss is significantly reduced to about 25 ml per cycle.[183] There is also reduced blood loss with the levonorgestrel-releasing IUD.

Excessive bleeding in the first few months after IUD insertion should be treated with reassurance and supplemental oral iron as well as systemic administration of one of the prostaglandin synthetase inhibitors during menses. The bleeding usually diminishes with time, as the uterus adjusts to the presence of the foreign body.

Mefenamic acid ingested in a dosage of 500 mg three times a day during the days of menstruation has been shown to reduce menstrual blood loss significantly in IUD users.[184] If excessive bleeding continues despite this treatment, the device should be removed. After a 1-month interval, another type of device may be inserted if the woman still wishes to use an IUD for contraception. Consideration should be given to using a progestin-releasing IUD, because this device is associated with less blood loss than the copper-bearing IUDs.

Perforation

Although uncommon, one of the potentially serious complications associated with use of the IUD is perforation of the uterine fundus. Perforation always occurs at the time of insertion.

In large multiclinic studies, perforation rates for the copper 7 were about 1 per 1000 insertions, but in contrast, perforation rates for the copper T380A were only about 1 in 3000 insertions.[185] Any type of IUD found to be outside the uterus, even if it is asymptomatic, should be removed from the peritoneal cavity because complications such as severe adhesions and bowel obstruction have been reported with intraperitoneal IUDs. Therefore, it is best to remove intraperitoneal IUDs shortly after the diagnosis of perforation is made. Unless severe adhesions have developed, most intraperitoneal IUDs can be removed by means of laparoscopy.

Complications Related to Pregnancy

CONGENITAL ANOMALIES

There is no evidence of an increased incidence of congenital anomalies in infants born with a plastic, copper-bearing, or progesterone-releasing IUD in utero.

SPONTANEOUS ABORTION

In all reported series of pregnancies with any type of IUD in situ, the incidence of fetal death was not significantly increased; however, a significant increase in spontaneous abortion has been consistently observed. If a woman conceives while wearing an IUD that is not subsequently removed, the incidence of spontaneous abortion is about 55 percent, approximately three times greater than would occur in pregnancies without an IUD.[186, 187]

After conception, if the IUD is spontaneously expelled, or if the appendage is visible and the IUD is removed by traction, the incidence of spontaneous abortion is significantly reduced. In one study of women who conceived with copper T devices in place, the incidence of spontaneous abortion was only 20 percent if the device was removed or spontaneously expelled.[186] This figure is similar to the normal incidence of spontaneous abortion and significantly less than the 54 percent incidence of abortion reported in the same study among women retaining the devices in utero. Thus, if a woman conceived with an IUD in place and wishes to continue the pregnancy, the IUD should be removed if the appendage is visible to significantly reduce the chance of spontaneous abortion. If the appendage is not visible, blind probing of the uterine cavity may increase the chance of abortion as well as sepsis. However, several reports indicate that with sonographic guidance, it is possible during early gestation to remove intrauterine IUDs in the lower uterine cavity without a visible appendage and not adversely affect the outcome of the pregnancy.[188, 189]

There was an increased risk of septic abortion if a patient conceived with a shield IUD in place, because of the structure of the multifilament appendage of the shield. However, there is no conclusive evidence that IUDs with monofilament tail strings cause sepsis during pregnancy.

ECTOPIC PREGNANCY

There is about a threefold increase in the risk of the pregnancy's being ectopic if a woman becomes pregnant with a copper IUD in place than if she is using no contraception method. However, because the copper T380 IUD so effectively prevents all pregnancies, with a total pregnancy rate of about 3.4 per 1000 women per year, the estimated ectopic pregnancy rate is only 0.2 to 0.4 per 1000 women per year in women using the IUD.[180] The estimated ectopic pregnancy rate among sexually active U.S. women using no method of contraception has been estimated to be between 3.25 and 4.5 per 1000 woman-years. Thus, the relative risk of ectopic pregnancy with the copper T380A is 0.1.[180]

The total number of pregnancies in women using the progesterone-releasing IUD is approximately 230, and about one in four pregnancies occurring in women using the device will be ectopic. The rate of ectopic pregnancies of 6.8 per 1000 woman-years in women using this device is higher than the 3.25 to 4.5 rate of ectopic pregnancy per 1000 noncontracepting women per year.[180]

The action of progesterone on oviductal motility increases the relative risk of having an ectopic pregnancy with this IUD 1.5 to 1.8 times compared with women using no method of contraception. Thus, the two types of IUDs currently marketed in the United States have differing effects on the risk of ectopic pregnancy. The copper T380 IUD lowers the risk and the progesterone IUD increases the risk compared with use of no contraception. Because a woman's risk of ectopic pregnancy is increased if she becomes pregnant with either IUD in place compared with the overall population of pregnant women, appropriate diagnostic studies should take place early in gestation to establish the diagnosis before tubal rupture occurs.

The increased risk of ectopic pregnancy for a woman who conceives while wearing an IUD is temporary and does not persist after removal of the IUD.[190]

PREMATURITY

In the previously cited study of conceptions occurring in the presence of copper T devices, the rate of prematurity among livebirths was four times greater when the copper T was left in place than when it was removed.[186]

INFECTION IN THE NONPREGNANT IUD USER

In 1966, a study was performed in which aerobic and anaerobic cultures were made of homogenates of endometrial tissue obtained transfundally from uteri removed by vaginal hysterectomy at various intervals after insertion of the loop IUD.[191] During the first 24 hours after IUD insertion, the normally sterile endometrial cavity was consistently infected with bacteria. Nevertheless, in 80 percent of uteri removed during the following 24 hours, the women's natural defenses had destroyed these bacteria and the endometrial cavities were sterile. In this study, when transfundal cultures were obtained more than 30 days after IUD insertion, the endometrial cavity, the IUD, and the portion of the thread within the cavity were always found to be sterile (Fig. 25–16). These findings indicate that development of PID more than a month after insertion of the IUD is due to infection with a sexually transmitted pathogen and is unrelated to the presence of the device.

Results of a large multicenter study coordinated by the WHO revealed similar findings. In this study of 22,908 women inserted with IUDs, the PID rate was highest in the first 3 weeks after insertion but remained lower and constant during the 8 years thereafter at 0.5 per 1000 woman-years (Fig. 25–17).[192] The results of both of these studies indicate that an IUD should not be inserted into a woman who may have been recently infected with gonococci or chlamydiae. Insertion of the device will transport these pathogens from the cervix into the upper genital tract where the large number of organisms may overcome the host defense and cause salpingitis. If there is clinical suspicion of infectious endocervicitis, cultures should be obtained and the IUD insertion delayed until the results reveal that no pathogenic organisms are present. It does not appear to be cost-effective to administer systemic antibiotics routinely with every IUD insertion, but the insertion procedure should be as aseptic as possible.

There is evidence that IUD users may have an increased

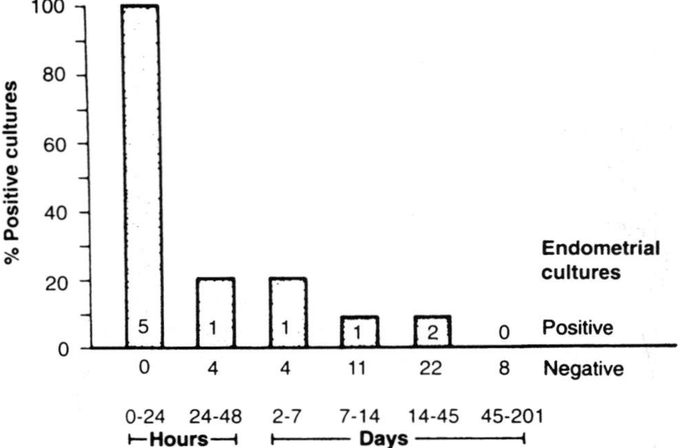

Figure 25–16 ■ Relationship between incidence of positive endometrial cultures and duration of IUD use before hysterectomy. (From Mishell DR Jr, Bell JH, Good RG, et al. The intrauterine device: A bacteriologic study of the endometrial cavity. Am J Obstet Gynecol 96:119–126, 1966.)

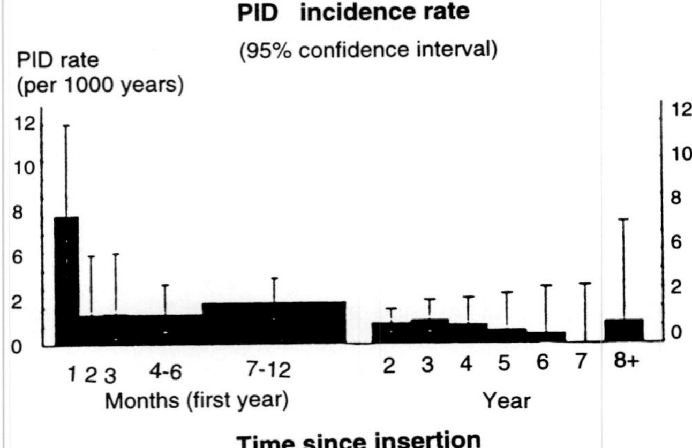

Figure 25–17 ■ Pelvic inflammatory disease (PID) incidence by time since insertion. Incidence rate estimated by the number of PID cases and years of exposure in each time interval; 95 percent confidence intervals were calculated from the Poisson distribution. (From Farley TM, Rosenberg MJ, Rowe PJ, et al. Intrauterine devices and pelvic inflammatory disease: An international perspective. Lancet 339:785–788, 1992. © by The Lancet Ltd.)

risk for colonizing actinomycosis organisms in the upper genital tract. The relationship of actinomycosis to PID is unclear because many women without IUDs have actinomycosis in their vagina and are asymptomatic.[193] If actinomycosis organisms are identified on the routine examination of cervical cytology and the woman is asymptomatic, she may be treated with appropriate antimicrobal therapy to erradicate the organisms or observed without therapy. The IUD should not be removed from an asymptomatic woman who is colonized but not infected with actinomycosis.

Overall Safety

Several long-term studies have indicated that the IUD is not associated with an increased incidence of endometrial or cervical carcinoma and may actually be associated with a reduction in risk of developing these neoplasms during and after its insertion.[194, 195] The IUD is a particularly useful method of contraception for women who have completed their families and do not wish permanent sterilization and have contraindications to, or do not wish to use, other effective methods of reversible contraception. An analysis reported that after 5 years of use, the IUD was the most cost-effective method of all methods of contraception including sterilization.[196] Women in the United States who use an IUD have a higher level of satisfaction with their method of contraception than do women using any of the other methods of reversible contraception.

References

1. 1995 Ortho Birth Control Survey. Raritan, NJ, Ortho Pharmaceutical, 1996.
2. Contraceptive Technology update. Monthly newsletter from Health Professionals, American Health Consultants. Don't neglect perfect-use failure rates when talking to patients. Contraceptive Technology 17(1):13, 1996.
3. Sivin I. Contraception with Norplant implant. J Reprod Med 9:1818, 1994.

4. World Health Organization. The TCu220C, multiload 250 and Nova T IUDs at 3.5 and 7 years of use. Results from three randomized multicentre trials. Contraception 42:141, 1990.
5. Peterson HB, Xia Z, Hughes JM, et al. The risk of pregnancy after tubal sterilization: Findings from the U.S. Collaborative Review of Sterilization. Am J Obstet Gynecol 174:1161, 1996.
6. Sivin I. Dose- and age-dependent ectopic pregnancy risks with intrauterine contraception. Obstet Gynecol 78:291, 1991.
7. Linn S, Schoenbaum SC, Monson RR, et al. Lack of association between contraceptive usage and congenital malformations in offspring. Am J Obstet Gynecol 147:923, 1983.
8. Bracken MB, Vita K. Frequency of non-hormonal contraception around conception and association with congenital malformations in offspring. Am J Epidemiol 117:281, 1983.
9. Louik C, Mitchell AA, Werler MM, et al. Maternal exposure to spermicides in relation to certain birth defects. N Engl J Med 317:474, 1987.
10. Strobino B, Kline J, Lai A, et al. Vaginal spermicides and spontaneous abortion of known karyotype. Am J Epidemiol 123:432, 1986.
11. Craig S, Hepburn S. The effectiveness of barrier methods of contraception with and without spermicide. Contraception 26:347, 1982.
12. Fihn SD, Latham RH, Roberts P, et al. Association between diaphragm use and urinary tract infection. JAMA 254:240, 1986.
13. Klitsch M. FDA approval ends cervical cap's marathon. Fam Plann Perspect 20:137, 1988.
14. Farr G, Gabelnlick H, Sturgen-K, Dorflinger L. Contraceptive efficacy and acceptability of the female condom. Am J Public Health 84:1960, 1994.
15. Trussel J, Sturgen K, Strickler J, Dominik R. Comparative contraceptive efficacy of the female condom and other barrier methods. Fam Plann Perspect 26:66, 1994.
16. Swyer GIM. Potency of progestogens in oral contraceptives—further delay of menses data. Contraception 26:23, 1982.
17. Ferin J. Orally active progestational compounds. Human studies: Effects on the utero-vaginal tract. *In* International Encyclopedia of Pharmacology and Therapeutics, Vol 2. Oxford, UK, Pergamon Press, 1972.
18. Grant ECG. Hormone balance of oral contraceptives. J Obstet Gynaecol Br Commonw 74:908, 1967.
19. Dorflinger L. Relative potency of progestins used in oral contraceptives. Contraception 557:31, 1985.
20. Speroff L, DeCherney A, and the Advisory Board for the New Progestins. Evaluation of a new generation of oral contraceptives. Obstet Gynecol 81:1034, 1993.
21. Goldzieher JW, Dozier TS, de la Pena A. Plasma levels and pharmacokinetics of ethynyl estrogens in various populations. Contraception 21:17, 1980.
22. Brenner PF, Goebelsmann U, Stanczyk FZ, Mishell DR Jr. Serum levels of ethinylestradiol following its ingestion alone or in oral contraceptive formulations. Contraception 22:85, 1980.
23. Mishell DR Jr, Stanczyk FZ, Hiroi M, et al. Steroid contraception. *In* Crosignani PG, Mishell DR Jr (eds). Ovulation in the Human. London, Academic Press, 1976, pp 141–151.
24. Brenner PF, Mishell DR Jr, Stanczyk FZ, Goebelsmann U. Serum levels of *d*-norgestrel, luteinizing hormone, follicle-stimulating hormone, estradiol, and progesterone in women during and following ingestion of combination oral contraceptives containing *dl*-norgestrel. Am J Obstet Gynecol 129:133, 1977.
25. Mishell DR Jr, Thorneycroft IH, Nakamura RM, et al. Serum estradiol in women ingesting combination oral contraceptive steroids. Am J Obstet Gynecol 114:923, 1972.
26. Mishell DR Jr, Kletzky OA, Brenner PF, et al. The effect of contraceptive steroids on hypothalamic-pituitary function. Am J Obstet Gynecol 130:817, 1978.
27. Scott JA, Brenner PF, Kletzky OA, et al. Factors affecting pituitary gonadotropin function in users of oral contraceptive steroids. Am J Obstet Gynecol 130:8817, 1978.
28. Scott JA, Kletzky OA, Brenner PF, et al. Comparison of the effects of contraceptive steroid formulations containing two doses of estrogen on pituitary function. Fertil Steril 30:141, 1978.
29. Bracken MB, Hellenbrand KG, Holford TR. Conception delay after oral contraceptive use: The effect of estrogen dose. Fertil Steril 53:21, 1990.
30. Vessey M, Painter R. Oral contraceptive use and benign gallbladder disease; revisited. Contraception 50:167, 1994.
31. La Vecchcia C, Negri E, D'Avanzo B, et al. Oral contraceptives and noncontraceptive oestrogens in the risk of gallstone disease requiring surgery. J Epidemiol Community Health 46:234, 1992.
32. Strom BL, Tamragouri RN, Morse ML, et al. Oral contraceptives and other risk factors for gallbladder disease. Clin Pharmacol Ther 39:335, 1986.
33. Kay CR. The Royal College of General Practitioners' Oral Contraception Study: Some recent observations. Clin Obstet Gynaecol 11:759, 1984.
34. Holst J, Backstrom T, Hammarback S, von Schoultz B. Progestogen addition during oestrogen replacement therapy—effects on vasomotor symptoms and mood. Maturitas 11:13, 1989.
35. Meade TW. Oral contraceptives, clotting factors, and thrombosis. Am J Obstet Gynecol 142:758, 1982.
36. Wilson ES, Cruickshank J, McMaster M, et al. A prospective controlled study of the effect on blood pressure of contraceptive preparations containing different types and dosages and progestogen. Br J Obstet Gynaecol 91:1254, 1984.
37. Mann JI. Progestogens in cardiovascular disease: An introduction to the epidemiologic data. Am J Obstet Gynecol 142:752, 1982.
38. Gerstman BB, Piper JM, Tomita DK, et al. Oral contraceptive estrogen dose and the risk of deep venous thromboembolic disease. Am J Epidemiol 133:32, 1991.
39. Khaw K-T, Peart WS. Blood pressure and contraceptive use. Br Med J 285:403, 1982.
40. Van der Vange N, Blankenstein MA, Kloosterboer HJ, et al. Effects of seven low-dose combined oral contraceptives on sex hormone binding globulin, corticosteroid binding globulin, total and free testosterone. Contraception 41:345, 1990.
41. Van der Vange N, Kloosterboer HG, Haspels AA. Effect of seven low-dose combined oral contraceptive preparations on carbohydrate metabolism. Am J Obstet Gynecol 156:918, 1987.
42. Bowes WA, Katta LR, Droegemueller W, et al. Triphasic randomized clinical trial: Comparison of effects on carbohydrate metabolism. Am J Obstet Gynecol 161:1402, 1989.
43. Kung AW, Ma JT, Wong VC, et al. Glucose and lipid metabolism with triphasic oral contraceptives in women with history of gestational diabetes. Contraception 35:257, 1987.
44. Luyckx AS, Gaspard UJ, Romus MA, et al. Carbohydrate metabolism in women who used oral contraceptives containing levonorgestrel or desogestrel: A 6-month prospective study. Fertil Steril 45:635, 1986.
45. Skouby SO, Kuhl C, Molsted-Pedersen L, et al. Triphasic oral contraception: Metabolic effects in normal women and those with previous gestational diabetes. Am J Obstet Gynecol 153:495, 1985.
46. Petersen KR, Skouby SO, Pedersen RG. Desogestrel and gestodene in oral contraceptives: 12 months' assessment of carbohydrate and lipoprotein metabolism. Obstet Gynecol 78:666, 1991.
47. Godsland IF, Crook D, Simpson R, et al. The effects of different formulations of oral contraceptive agents on lipid and carbohydrate metabolism. N Engl J Med 323:1375, 1990.
48. Godsland IF, Crook D, Worthington M, et al. Effects of a low-estrogen, desogestrel-containing oral contraceptive on lipid and carbohydrate metabolism. Contraception 48:217, 1993.
49. Hannaford PC, Kay CR. Oral contraceptives and diabetes mellitus. Br Med J 299:315, 1989.
50. Rimm EB, Manson JE, Stampfer MJ, et al. Oral contraceptive use and the risk of type 2 (non–insulin-dependent) diabetes mellitus in a large prospective study of women. Diabetologia 35:9967, 1992.
51. Kjos SL, Xiang A, Schafer U, et al. Hormonal contraception in the development of type II diabetes mellitus in high risk women. Unpublished data.
52. Wahl IP, Walden C, Knopp R, et al. Effect of estrogen/progestin potency on lipid/lipoprotein cholesterol. N Engl J Med 308:862, 1981.
53. Patsch W, Brown SA, Gotto AM, et al. The effect of triphasic oral contraceptives on plasma lipids and lipoproteins. Am J Obstet 161:1396, 1989.
54. Notelovitz M, Feldman EB, Gillespy M, et al. Lipid and lipoprotein changes in women taking low-dose, triphasic oral contraceptives: A controlled, comparative, 12-month clinical trial. Am J Obstet Gynecol 160:1269, 1989.

55. Pabinger I, Schneider B. Thrombotic risk of women with hereditary antithrombin III-, protein C- and protein S–deficiency taking oral contraceptive medication. The GTH Study Group on Natural Inhibitors. Thromb Haemost 71:548, 1994.
56. Vandenbroucke JP, Koster T, Briet E, et al. Increased risk of venous thrombosis in oral-contraceptive users who are carriers of factor V Leiden Mutation. Lancet 344:1453, 1994.
57. Farmer RDT, Preston NTD. The risk of venous thrombosis associated with low oestrogen oral contraceptives. J Obstet Gynaecol 15:195, 1995.
58. Jick H, Jick SS, Gurewich V, et al. Risk of idiopathic cardiovascular death and nonfatal venous thromboembolism in women using oral contraceptives with differing progestagen components. Lancet 346:1589, 1994.
59. World Health Organization Collaborative Study of Cardiovascular Disease and Steroid Hormone Contraception. Venous thromboembolic disease and combined oral contraceptives: Results of international multicenter case-control study. Lancet 346:1575, 1995.
60. Spitzer WO, Lewis MA, Heinemann LAJ, et al. Third generation oral contraceptives and risk of venous thromboembolic disorders: An international case-control study. Br Med J 312:83, 1996.
61. World Health Organization Collaborative Study of Cardiovascular Disease and Steroid Hormone Contraception. Effect of different progestagens in low-oestrogen oral contraceptives on venous thromboembolic disease. Lancet 346:1582, 1995.
62. Bloemenkamp KWM, Rosendaal FR, Helmerhorst FM, et al. Enhancement of factor V Leiden mutation of risk of deep-vein thrombosis associated with oral contraceptives containing a third-generation progestagen. Lancet 346:1593, 1995.
63. Lidegaard O, Milsom I. Oral contraceptives and thrombotic diseases: Impact of new epidemiological studies. Contraception 53:135, 1996.
64. Layde PM, Ory HW, Schlesselman JJ. The risk of myocardial infarction in former users of oral contraceptives. Fam Plann Perspect 14:78, 1982.
65. Stampfer MJ, Willett WC, Colditz GA, et al. A prospective study of past use of oral contraceptive agents and risk of cardiovascular diseases. N Engl J Med 319:1313, 1988.
66. Rosenberg L, Palmer JR, Zauber AG. A case-control study of oral contraceptive use and invasive epithelial ovarian cancer. Am J Epidemiol 139:654, 1994.
67. Royal College of General Practitioners' Oral Contraception Study. Further analyses of mortality in oral contraceptive users. Lancet 1:541, 1981.
68. Engel H-J, Engel E, Lichtlen PR. Coronary atherosclerosis and myocardial infarction in young women—role of oral contraceptives. Eur Heart J 4:1, 1983.
69. Adams MR, Clarkson TB, Kortinik DR, et al. Contraceptive steroids and coronary artery atherosclerosis in cynomolgus macaques. Fertil Steril 47:1010, 1987.
70. Clarkson TB, Shively CA, Morgan TM, et al. Oral contraceptives and coronary artery atherosclerosis of cynomolgus monkeys. Obstet Gynecol 75:217, 1990.
71. Mann JI, Doll R, Thorogood M, et al. Risk factors for myocardial infarction in young women. Br J Prev Soc Med 30:94, 1986.
72. Croft P, Hannaford PC. Risk factors for acute myocardial infarction in women. Br Med J 298:165, 1989.
73. Prentice RL, Thomas DB. On the epidemiology of oral contraceptives and disease. Adv Cancer Res 49:285, 1987.
74. Ramcharan S, Pelligrin FA, Ray R, et al. The Walnut Creek Contraceptive Drug Study: A Prospective Study of the Side Effects of Oral Contraceptives III. Washington, DC, U.S. Government Printing Office, 1981. NIH publication 81–564.
75. Hannaford PC, Croft PR, Kay CR. Oral contraception and stroke: Evidence from the Royal College of General Practitioners' Oral Contraception Study. Stroke 25:935, 1993.
76. Pettiti DB, Sidney S, Bernstein A, et al. Stroke in users of low-dose oral contraceptives. N Engl J Med 335:18, 1996.
77. Klein TA, Mishell DR Jr. Gonadotropin, prolactin and steroid hormone levels after discontinuation of oral contraceptives. Am J Obstet Gynecol 127:585, 1977.
78. Vessey MP, Wright NH, McPherson K, et al. Fertility after stopping different methods of contraception. Br Med J 1:265, 1978.
79. Jacobsen C. Cytogenic Study of Immediate Post Contraceptive Abortion. Washington, DC, U.S. Government Printing Office, 1974.
80. Rothman KJ, Louik C. Oral contraceptives and birth defects. N Engl J Med 299:522, 1978.
81. Janerich DT, Piper JM, Glebatis DM. Oral contraceptives and birth defects. Am J Epidemiol 112:73, 1980.
82. Harlap S, Shiono PH, Ramcharan S. Congenital abnormalities in the offspring of women who used oral and other contraceptives around the time of conception. Int J Fertil 30:39, 1985.
83. Schlesselman JJ. Net effect of oral contraceptive use on the risk of cancer in women in the United States. Obstet Gynecol 85:793, 1995.
84. Thomas DB. Oral contraceptives and breast cancer: Review of the epidemiologic literature. Contraception 43:597, 1991.
85. Collaborative Group on Hormonal Factors in Breast Cancer. Breast cancer and hormonal contraceptives: Collaborative reanalysis of individual data on 53,297 women with breast cancer and 100,239 women without breast cancer from 54 epidemiological studies. Lancet 347:1713, 1996.
86. Collaborative Group on Hormonal Factors in Breast Cancer. Breast cancer and hormonal contraceptives: Further results. Contraception 54:1S, 1996.
87. Brinton LA, Reeves WC, Brenes MM, et al. Oral contraceptive use and risk of invasive cervical cancer. Int J Epidemiol 19:4, 1990.
88. Kjaer SK, Engholm G, Dahl C, et al. Case-control study of risk factors for cervical squamous-cell neoplasia in Denmark. III. Role of oral contraceptive use. Cancer Causes Control 4:513, 1993.
89. Parazzini F, La Vecchia C, Negri E, Maggi R. Oral contraceptive use and invasive cervical cancer. Int J Epidemiol 19:259, 1990.
90. Ursin G, Peters RK, Henderson BE, et al. Oral contraceptive use and adenocarcinoma of cervix. Lancet 344:1390, 1994.
91. Thomas DB, Ray RM and the World Health Organization Collaborative Study of Neoplasia and Steroid Contraceptives and invasive adenocarcinomas and adenosquamous carcinomas of the uterine cervix. Am J Epidemiol 144:281, 1996.
92. Centers for Disease Control. Combination oral contraceptives use and risk of endometrial cancer. JAMA 257:976, 1987.
93. Voigt LF, Deng Q, Weiss NS. Recency, duration, and progestin content of oral contraceptives in relation to the incidence of endometrial cancer. Cancer Causes Control 5:227, 1994.
94. Hankinson SE, Colditz GA, Hunter DJ, et al. A quantitative assessment of oral contraceptive use and risk of ovarian cancer. Obstet Gynecol 80:708, 1992.
95. Rosenberg L, Palmer JR, Lesko SM, et al. Oral contraceptive use and the risk of myocardial infarction. Am J Epidemiol 131:1009, 1990.
96. Forman D, Vincent TJ, Doll R. Cancer of the liver and the use of oral contraceptives. Br Med J 292:1357, 1986.
97. Neuberger J, Forman D, Doll R, Williams R. Oral contraceptives and hepatocellular carcinoma. Br Med J 292:1355, 1986.
98. World Health Organization. Combined oral contraceptives and liver cancer. Int J Cancer 43:254, 1989.
99. Pituitary Adenoma Study Group. Pituitary adenomas and oral contraceptives: A multicenter case-control study. Fertil Steril 39:753, 1983.
100. Hannaford PC, Villard-Mackintosh L, Vessey MP, Kay CR. Oral contraceptives and malignant melanoma. Br J Cancer 63:430, 1991.
101. Kjos SL, Shoupe D, Douhan S, et al. Effect of low-dose oral contraceptives on carbohydrate and lipid metabolism in women with recurrent gestational diabetes: Results of a controlled randomized prospective study. Am J Obstet Gynecol 163:1822, 1990.
102. Lonnerdel IB, Forsum E, Hambraeus L. Effect of oral contraceptives on composition and volume of breast milk. Am J Clin Nutr 33:816, 1980.
103. Lanes AF, Birmann B, Walter AM, Singer S. Oral contraceptive type and functional ovarian cysts. Am J Obstet Gynecol 166:956, 1992.
104. Nilsson S, Mellbin T, Hofvander Y, et al. Long-term follow-up of children breast fed by mothers using oral contraceptives. Contraception 34:443, 1986.
105. Back DJ, Breckenridge AM, Crawford FE, et al. The effects of

rifampicin on the pharmacokinetics of ethinylestradiol in women. Contraception 21:135, 1980.
106. Murphy AA, Zacur HA, Charache P, Burkmand RT. The effect of tetracycline on levels of oral contraceptives. Am J Obstet Gynecol 164:28, 1991.
107. Mattson RH, Rebar RW. Contraceptive methods for women with neurologic disorders. Am J Obstet Gynecol 168:2027, 1993.
108. Mishell DR Jr. Noncontraceptive health benefits of oral steroidal contraceptives. Am J Obstet Gynecol 142:809, 1981.
109. Royal College of General Practitioners. Oral Contraceptives and Health: An Interim Report from The Oral Contraceptive Study of the Royal College of General Practitioners. New York, Pitman Medical Publishing, 1974.
110. Ory H, Cole IP, MacMahon B, et al. Oral contraceptives and reduced incidence of benign breast disease. N Engl J Med 294:419, 1976.
111. Brinton LA, Vessy MP, Flavell R, et al. Risk factors for benign breast disease. Am J Epidemiol 113:203, 1981.
112. Spector TD, Romas E, Silman AJ. The pill, parity, and rheumatoid arthritis. Arthritis Rheum 33:782, 1990.
113. Hazes JMW, Dijkmans BAC, Vanderbroucke JP, et al. Reduction of the risk of rheumatoid arthritis among women who take oral contraceptives. Arthritis Rheum 33:173, 1990.
114. Senanayake P, Kramer DG. Contraception and the etiology of pelvic inflammatory disease: New perspectives. Am J Obstet Gynecol 138:852, 1980.
115. Gambacciani M, Spinetti A, Toponeco F, et al. Longitudinal evaluation of perimenopausal vertebral bone loss: Effects of a low-dose oral contraceptive preparation on bone mineral density and metabolism. Obstet Gynecol 83:392, 1993.
116. Castracane VD, Gimpel T, Goldzieher JW. When is it safe to switch from oral contraceptives to hormonal replacement therapy? Contraception 52:371, 1995.
117. Mishell DR Jr. Pharmacokinetics of depot medroxyprogesterone acetate contraception. J Reprod Med 41:381, 1996.
118. World Health Organization Expanded Programme of Research, Development and Research Training in Human Reproduction Task Force on Long-Acting Systemic Agents for the Regulation of Fertility. Multinational comparative clinical evaluation of two long-acting injectable contraceptive steroids: Norethisterone enanthate and medroxyprogesterone acetate. Final report. Contraception 18:1, 1983.
119. Ortiz A, Hirol M, Stanczyk FZ, et al. Serum medroxyprogesterone acetate (MPA) concentrations and ovarian function following intramuscular injection of depo-MPA. J Clin Endocrinol Metab 44:32, 1977.
120. Kirton KT, Cornette JC. Return of ovulatory cyclicity following an intramuscular injection of medroxyprogesterone acetate (Provera). Contraception 10:39, 1974.
121. Fotherby K, Kowetsawang S, Mathrubutham M. A pharmacokinetic study of different doses of Depo-Provera. Contraception 22:527, 1980.
122. Mishell DR Jr, Kharma KM, Thorneycroft IH, et al. Estrogenic activity in women receiving an injectable progestogen for contraception. Am J Obstet Gynecol 113:372, 1972.
123. Siriwongse T, Snidvongs W, Tantayaporn P, et al. Effect of depo-medroxyprogesterone acetate on serum progesterone levels when administered on various cycle days. Contraception 26:487, 1982.
124. Schwallie PC, Assenzo JR. The effect of depo-medroxyprogesterone acetate on pituitary and ovarian function, and the return of fertility following its discontinuation: A review. Contraception 10:181, 1974.
125. Mishell DR Jr, el-Habashy MA, Good RG, et al. Contraception with an injectable progestin: A study of its use in postpartum women. Am J Obstet Gynecol 101:1046, 1968.
126. Schwallie PC, Assenzo JR. Contraceptive use—efficacy study utilizing medroxyprogesterone acetate administered as an intramuscular injection once every 90 days. Fertil Steril 24:331, 1973.
127. Westhoff C. Depot medroxyprogesterone acetate contraception. Metabolic parameters and mood changes. J Reprod Med 41(suppl):401, 1996.
128. Moore LL, Valuck R, McDougall C, et al. A comparative study of one-year weight gain among users of medroxyprogesterone acetate, levonorgestrel implants, and oral contraceptives. Contraception 52:215, 1995.
129. Food and Drug Administration, Fertility and Maternal Health Drugs Advisory Committee. Meeting Transcript. Washington, DC, U.S. Department of Health and Human Services, 1992.
130. Lieu DFM, Ng CSA, Yong YM, et al. Long-term effects of Depo-Provera on carbohydrate and lipid metabolism. Contraception 31:51, 1985.
131. Virutamasen P, Wongsrichanalai C, Tangkeo P, et al. Metabolic effects of depot medroxyprogesterone acetate in long-term users: A cross-sectional study. Int J Gynaecol Obstet 24:291, 1986.
132. Cundy T, Evans M, Roberts H, et al. Bone density in women receiving depot medroxyprogesterone acetate for contraception. Br Med J 303:13, 1991.
133. Cundy T, Cornish J, Evans MC, et al. Recovery of bone density in women who stop using medroxyprogesterone acetate. Br Med J 308:247, 1994.
134. Mark S. Premenopausal bone loss and depot medroxyprogesterone acetate administration. Int J Gynaecol Obstet 47:269, 1994.
135. Virutamasen P, Wangsuphachart S, Reinproayoon D, et al. Trabecular bone in long-term depot medroxyprogesterone acetate users. Asia Oceania J Obstet Gynaecol 20:269, 1994.
136. Naessen T, Olsson S-E, Gudmundson J. Differential effects on bone density of progestogen-only methods for contraception in premenopausal women. Contraception 52:35, 1995.
137. World Health Organization Collaborative Study of Neoplasia and Steroid Contraceptives. Breast cancer and depot medroxyprogesterone acetate: A multinational study. Lancet 338:833, 1991.
138. Paul C, Skegg DCG, Spears GFS. Depot medroxyprogesterone (Depo-Provera) and risk of breast cancer. Br Med J 299:759, 1989.
139. Skegg DC, Noonan EA, Paul C, et al. Depot medroxyprogesterone acetate and breast cancer: A pooled analysis of the World Health Organization and New Zealand studies. JAMA 273:799, 1995.
140. World Health Organization Collaborative Study of Neoplasia and Steroid Contraceptives. Depot medroxyprogesterone acetate (DMPA) and risk of endometrial cancer. Int J Cancer 49:186, 1991.
141. World Health Organization Collaborative Study of Neoplasia and Steroid Contraceptives. Depot medroxyprogesterone acetate (DMPA) and risk of epithelial ovarian cancer. Int J Cancer 49:191, 1991.
142. World Health Organization Collaborative Study of Neoplasia and Steroid Contraceptives. Depot medroxyprogesterone acetate (DMPA) and risk of squamous cell cervical cancer. Contraception 45:299, 1992.
143. Oberle MW, Rosero-Bixiby L, Irwin KL, et al. Cervical cancer risk and use of depot medroxyprogesterone acetate in Costa Rica. Int J Epidemiol 17:718, 1988.
144. The New Zealand Contraception and Health Study Group. Risk of cervical dysplasia in users of oral contraceptives, intrauterine devices or depot medroxyprogesterone acetate. Contraception 50:431, 1994.
145. The New Zealand Contraception and Health Study Group. History of long-term use of depot medroxyprogesterone acetate in patients with cervical dysplasia: Case-control analysis nested in a cohort study. Contraception 50:443, 1994.
146. Cullins VE. Noncontraceptive benefits and therapeutic uses of depot medroxyprogesterone acetate. J Reprod Med 41(suppl):428, 1996.
147. Mattson RH, Cramer JA, Caldwell BVD, et al. Treatment of seizures with medroxyprogesterone acetate. Preliminary report. Neurology 34:1255, 1984.
148. Dennerstein GJ: Depo-Provera in the treatment of recurrent vulvovaginal candidiasis. J Reprod Med 31:801, 1986.
149. Tooppozada M, Onsy FA, Fares E, et al. The protective influence of progesterone-only contraception against vaginal moniliasis. Contraception 20:99, 1979.
150. Lei Z-W, Wu SC, Garceau RJ, et al. Effect of pretreatment counseling on discontinuation rates in Chinese women given depo-medroxyprogesterone acetate for contraception. Contraception 53:357, 1996.
151. Patient labeling information. Physicians' Desk Reference, 50th ed. Montvale, NJ, Medical Economics, 1996.
152. Koetsawang S. The effects of contraceptive methods on the quality and quantity of breast milk. Int J Gynaecol Obstet Suppl 25:115, 1987.

153. Gray RH, Pardthaisong T. In utero exposure to steroid contraceptives and survival during infancy. Am J Epidemiol 134:804, 1991.
154. Sivin I. Contraception with Norplant implants. Hum Reprod 9:1818, 1974.
155. Moore DE, Roy S, Stanczyk FZ, et al. Bleeding and serum d-norgestrel, estradiol, and progesterone patterns in women using d-norgestrel subdermal polysiloxane capsules for contraception. Contraception 17:315, 1978.
156. Diaz S, Pavez M, Miranda P, et al. Long-term follow-up of women treated with Norplant implants. Contraception 35:551, 1987.
157. Alvarez F, Brache V, Tejada AS, et al. Abnormal endocrine profile among women with confirmed or presumed ovulation during long-term Norplant use. Contraception 33:111, 1986.
158. Croxatto HB, Diaz S, Salvatierra AM, et al. Treatment with Norplant subdermal implants inhibits penetration through cervical mucus in vitro. Contraception 36:193, 1987.
159. Brache V, Faundes A, Johansson E, et al. Anovulation, inadequate luteal phase and poor sperm penetration in cervical mucus during prolonged use of Norplant implants. Contraception 31:261, 1985.
160. Sivin I. International experience with Norplant and Norplant 2. Stud Fam Plann 38:465, 1988.
161. Croxatto HB, Diaz S, Pavez M, et al. Estradiol plasma levels during long term treatment with Norplant subdermal implants. Contraception 38:465, 1988.
162. Darney PD, Klaisle CM, Tanner S, et al. Sustained-release contraceptives. Curr Probl Obstet Gynecol Fertil 13:87, 1990.
163. Shoupe D, Mishell DR Jr, Bopp BL, Fielding M. The significance of bleeding patterns in Norplant implant users. Obstet Gynecol 77:256, 1991.
164. Nilsson CG, Holma P. Menstrual blood loss with contraceptive subdermal levonorgestrel implants. Fertil Steril 35:304, 1981.
165. Croxatto HB, Diaz S, Pavez M, et al. Clearance of levonorgestrel from the circulation following removal of Norplant subdermal implants. Contraception 38:509, 1988.
166. Koopersmith TB, Lacarra M, Mishell DR Jr. Equal efficacy and acceptability of the Norplant 2 and Norplant implant systems. Submitted for publication.
167. Fasoli M, Parazzini F, Cecchetti G, et al. Post-coital contraception: An overview of published studies. Contraception 39:459, 1989.
168. Trussell J, Ellertson C, Stewart F. The effectiveness of the Yuzpe regimen of emergency contraception. Fam Plann Perspect 28:58, 1996.
169. Ho PC, Kwan MSW. A prospective randomized comparison of levonorgestrel with the Yuzpe regimen in post-coital contraception. Hum Reprod 8:389, 1993.
170. Healy DL, Baulieu EE, Hodgen GD. Induction of menstruation by an antiprogesterone steroid (RU 486) in primates: Site of action, dose-response relationships, and hormonal effects. Fertil Steril 40:253, 1983.
171. Couzinet B, LeStrat N, Ulmann A, et al. Termination of early pregnancy by the progesterone antagonist RU 486 (mifepristone). N Engl J Med 315:1565, 1986.
172. Silvestre L, Dubois C, Renault M, et al. Voluntary interruption of pregnancy with mifepristone (RU 486) and a prostaglandin analogue. N Engl J Med 322:6455, 1990.
173. El-Rafaey H, Rajasekar D, Abdalla M, et al. Induction of abortion with mifepristone (RU 486) and oral or vaginal misoprostol. N Engl J Med 332:983, 1995.
174. Crooij MJ, de Nooyer CCA, Rao BR, et al. Termination of early pregnancy by the 3β-hydroxysteroid dehydrogenase inhibitor epostane. N Engl J Med 319:813, 1988.
175. Sivin I, Stern J. Long-acting, more effective copper T IUDs: A summary of U.S. experience, 1970–75. Stud Fam Plann 10:276, 1979.
176. Cuadros A, Hirsch J. Copper on intrauterine devices stimulates leukocyte exudation. Science 175:175, 1972.
177. Hefnawi F, Handil O, Askalani A, et al. Mode of action of the copper IUD: Effect on endometrial copper and cervical mucus sperm migration. Proceedings of the Third International Symposium on IUDs; December 1973; Cairo, Egypt, p 456.
178. El-Habashi M, el-Sahwi S, Gawish S, Osman M. Effect of Lippes loop on sperm recovery from human fallopian tubes. Contraception 22:549, 1980.
179. Alvarez F, Guiloff E, Brache V, et al. New insights on the mode of action of intrauterine contraceptive devices in women. Fertil Steril 49:768, 1988.
180. Sivin I. Dose- and age-dependent ectopic pregnancy risks with intrauterine contraception. Obstet Gynecol 78:291, 1991.
181. Vessey MP, Lawless M, McPherson K, et al. Fertility after stopping use of intrauterine contraceptive device. Br Med J 286:106, 1983.
182. Milson I, Anderson K, Jonasson K, et al. The influence of the Gyne-T 380A IUD on menstrual blood loss and iron status. Contraception 52:175, 1995.
183. Rybo G. The IUD and endometrial bleeding. J Reprod Med 20:715, 1978.
184. Anderson ABM, Haynes PJ, Guillebaud J, et al. Reduction of menstrual blood loss by prostaglandin synthetase inhibitors. Lancet 1:774, 1976.
185. Sivin I, Stern J. Long-acting, more effective copper T IUDs: A summary of U.S. experience, 1970–75. Stud Fam Plann 10:276, 1979.
186. Tatum HJ, Schmidt FH, Jain AK. Management and outcome of pregnancies associated with the copper T intrauterine contraceptive device. Am J Obstet Gynecol 126:869, 1976.
187. Vessey MP, Johnson B, Doll R, et al. Outcome of pregnancy in women using an intrauterine device. Lancet 1:495, 1974.
188. Shalev E, Edelstein S, Engelhard J, et al. Ultrasonically controlled retrieval of an intrauterine contraceptive device (IUCD) in early pregnancy. J Clin Ultrasound 15:525, 1987.
189. Stubblefield PG, Fuller AF Jr, Foster SC. Ultrasound-guided intrauterine removal of intrauterine contraceptive devices in pregnancy. Obstet Gynecol 72:961, 1988.
190. Chow W-H, Daling JR, Weiss NS, et al. IUD use and subsequent tubal pregnancy. Am J Public Health 66:131, 1986.
191. Mishell DR Jr, Bell JH, Good RG, et al. The intrauterine device: A bacteriologic study of the endometrial cavity. Am J Obstet Gynecol 96:119, 1966.
192. Farley TM, Rosenberg MJ, Rowe PJ, et al. Intrauterine devices and pelvic inflammatory disease: An international perspective. Lancet 339:785, 1992.
193. Persson E, Holmberg K, Dahlgren S, et al. *Actinomyces israelii* in genital tract of women with and without intrauterine contraceptive devices. Acta Obstet Gynecol Scand 62:563, 1983.
194. Castellsagué X, Thompson WD, Dubrow R. Intra-uterine contraception and the risk of endometrial cancer. Int J Cancer 54:911, 1993.
195. Lassise D, Savitz D, Hamman R, et al. Invasive cervical cancer and intrauterine device use. Int J Epidemiol 20:865, 1991.
196. Trussell J, Keveque JA, Koenig JD, et al. The economic value of contraception: A comparison of 15 methods. Am J Public Health 85:494, 1995.

Chapter 26

PRACTICAL EVALUATION OF HORMONAL STATUS

Robert W. Rebar

■ CHAPTER OUTLINE

KEY POINTS

- The female patient with a disorder of reproductive function serves as her own bioassay.
- The history and physical examination are most important in evaluating any patient with reproductive dysfunction.
- Evaluating the individual clinically with normal pubertal development as a reference is often useful in determining the cause of the reproductive dysfunction.
- Laboratory tests are generally used only to confirm what is suspected on the basis of the initial evaluation.
- Measurements of basal FSH, prolactin, and TSH in the circulation appear warranted in all amenorrheic women once pregnancy has been excluded.
- Radiographic studies of the sella turcica are indicated in amenorrheic women with low levels of circulating LH and FSH, whether prolactin is elevated or not.
- Individuals with large hypothalamic or pituitary tumors and those with presumptive hypopituitarism should undergo dynamic testing of pituitary function.
- Individuals with hirsutism should have a serious etiologic factor eliminated by appropriate laboratory testing.

CLINICAL ASPECTS: THE PATIENT AS A BIOASSAY SUBJECT

Clinical assessment of the woman with possible endocrine dysfunction is aided by the fact that the patient serves as her own bioassay. In general, the expression of abnormal endocrine function depends on the age of the individual at the onset of the disorder. Whereas hormonal abnormalities beginning in adulthood are characterized largely by metabolic and physiologic disturbances, such imbalances in young children and adolescents may produce marked deviations from the usual patterns of growth and development. These maturational events may be altered by several groups of hormones. Acceleration may be seen in response to increased secretion of growth hormone, the thyroid hormones, and androgens and estrogens from whatever source. The glucocorticoids, if secreted in excessive quantities by the adrenal cortex or when administered therapeutically, inhibit growth. Diminished growth hormone or thyroid hormone secretion also results in growth retardation.

Disordered sexual development can be of several types. The time of onset or the progression of development of secondary sex characteristics at puberty may be altered as a result of modified steroid secretion or of resistance to steroids at the end organ. In addition, altered hormonal milieu in utero may lead to ambiguous genitalia. Endocrine dysfunction after completion of somatic growth and sexual development will produce completely different biologic effects, although the resultant clinical changes may still be apparent.

It is important to evaluate the clinical signs and symptoms in relation to puberty and to the influence of altered hormonal secretion on the pubertal process. In general terms, puberty is associated with (1) an increase in growth of the skeleton, the skeletal muscles, and the viscera, more commonly known as the adolescent growth spurt; (2) sexual dimorphism with sex-specific changes in growth, such as increased shoulder width in males and increased hip width in females; (3) changes in body composition, exemplified by increased muscle and bone and decreased fat; and (4) development of the reproductive system and secondary sex characteristics.

Longitudinal studies such as those of Marshall and Tanner[1] have documented the relationships among the different events occurring at puberty and have noted the probabilities of the various events occurring concomitantly. As suggested by these workers and described in more detail in Chapter 15 and illustrated in Figure 26–1, puberty in females can be divided into specific developmental stages on the basis of somatic signs, including the amount of pubic hair and the degree of breast development. The time of menarche, the age of achievement of maximal velocity in linear growth, and the skeletal or bone age are also important. In assessing puberty, it is essential to establish whether a patient's development is or was within normal limits for her age and whether the breasts and the pubic hair have developed at a normal rate, in unison, and in proper relation to the growth spurt and to menarche.

Clinical History: Elucidation of Hormonal Effects

Within this framework, the clinician should obtain the history from the individual with the aim of assessing the biologic effects of each of the various hormones. The history should be constructed around the chief complaint (Table 26–1). It is apparent that the patient will present most commonly with altered sexual development or sexual or reproductive dysfunction.

Altered sexual development will take the form of sexual precocity, complaints of heterosexual signs or development, delayed puberty, or what can be termed asynchronous pubertal development (Table 26–2). Sexual precocity can result from several disorders, but invariably the manifestations of sexual precocity are secondary to the biologic effects of increased production of the sex steroids, caused by increased gonadotropin secretion from either pituitary or extrapituitary sources or by intrinsic adrenal or ovarian disease.[2] Pubertal changes probably should not be considered precocious unless they begin before the individual has reached the age of 8 years. In females, increased estrogen secretion for age results in isosexual precocity (consistent with the sex of the individual), whereas increased androgen production for age leads to heterosexual precocity (development of secondary sex characteristics of the opposite sex).

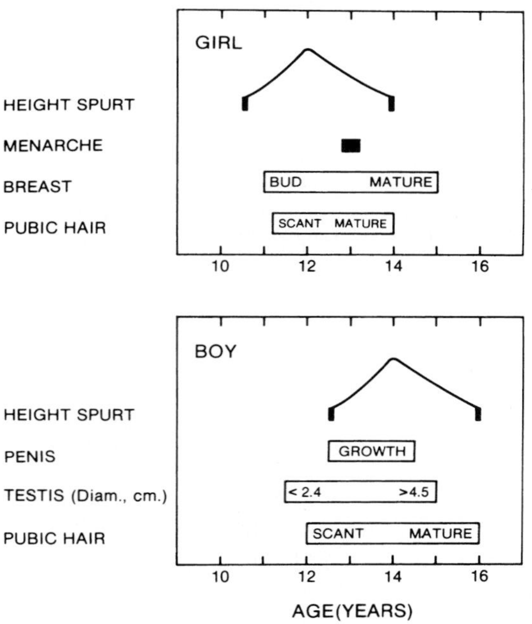

Figure 26–1 ■ Schematic sequence of events at puberty. An average girl *(upper panel)* and an average boy *(lower panel)* are represented. There is a wide range of ages over which these changes can occur in normal children. (Adapted from Tanner, J. M., Sequence and tempo in the somatic changes in puberty. *In* Grumbach MM, Grave GD and Mayer FE [eds]. The Control of the Onset of Puberty. New York, John Wiley & Sons, 1974.)

■ TABLE 26–1

Important Historical Features in Evaluating the Amenorrheic Woman

Pubertal milestones
Abnormalities of growth and development
Diet
Exercise
Weight change
Lifestyle: environmental and psychologic stresses
Drug use
Systemic diseases
Evidence of increased androgen
Galactorrhea
Past gynecologic problems and procedures
Past reproductive and sexual history
Family history of genetic anomalies
Evidence of other endocrinopathies

With regard to isosexual precocity, true precocious puberty in females must be distinguished from precocious thelarche, which is characterized only by breast enlargement and possibly results from transient elevation of plasma estradiol concentrations,[2, 3] and precocious adrenarche, which is typified by the isolated development of sexual hair, most commonly pubic, and increased (adrenal) production of weakly androgenic steroids.[2, 3] In both of these disorders, pubertal maturation occurs at the expected age. However, premature pubic hair growth may in fact be the earliest sign of isosexual or heterosexual precocity as well as an isolated finding in premature adrenarche. Although most isosexual precocity in girls is idiopathic, the clinician must determine whether a neoplasm involving the central nervous system, the ovary, or the adrenal is present or whether ectopic production of chorionic gonadotropin exists (see Chapter 23). A careful history may provide the clues. Behavioral changes or symptoms suggestive of psychomotor epilepsy may be the only evidence of central nervous system disease in the child. The well-documented association of hypothyroidism and sexual precocity[4] demands careful questioning for symptoms of thyroid hormone deficiency. Furthermore, the availability of oral contraceptive preparations requires searching for a history of drug ingestion; estrogens may be present in some skin creams, vitamins, and other health food store products as well.

Heterosexual changes, regardless of the age at which they become apparent, must be considered evidence of increased production of biologically active androgens in the genetic female or, more rarely, signs of fetal errors in gonadal development or gonaductal or genital differentiation. The special considerations of abnormal genitalia and virilization observed in the neonatal period are beyond the scope of this chapter but suggest the need for chromosomal

■ TABLE 26–2
Possible Abnormalities in Pubertal Development in Girls

ABNORMALITY	DEFINITION	EXAMPLES
Precocious puberty	Pubertal development beginning before age 8 years	
Isosexual precocity	Development consistent with the sex of the individual	Idiopathic; central nervous system, ovarian, or adrenal neoplasm
Heterosexual precocity	Development characteristic of the opposite sex	Congenital adrenal hyperplasia; androgen-producing neoplasm
Heterosexual puberty	Development characteristic of the opposite sex at the expected age of puberty	Polycystic ovary syndrome; congenital adrenal hyperplasia (rarely)
Delayed puberty	Absence of any secondary sexual characteristics by age 13, absence of menarche by age 16, or passage of 5 years or more from breast budding to menarche	Gonadal dysgenesis; isolated gonadotropin deficiency; panhypopituitarism
Asynchronous puberty	Deviation from the normal pattern of puberty	Androgen insensitivity syndrome

evaluation. Regardless of the age of the patient, the existence of signs and symptoms of androgen excess should be ascertained, including acne, hirsutism, temporal balding, alterations in body contour and muscle mass, and voice change.

Hirsutism alone frequently begins during the pubertal years and, in this context, is most often associated with polycystic ovary syndrome (PCOS) or is possibly "idiopathic" (see Chapter 18). The onset of hirsutism or virilization at any other time should alert the clinician to the possibility of Cushing's syndrome or adrenal or ovarian neoplasms. Even though hirsutism, as a manifestation of adrenal disease, is infrequently accompanied by amenorrhea in comparison with the incidence of amenorrhea in ovarian disease, both should be considered. Congenital adrenal hyperplasia, characterized by only partial 11β- or 21-hydroxylase deficiency, is occasionally not recognized until the signs and symptoms of heterosexual precocity become evident. (PCOS and congenital adrenal hyperplasia can almost always be easily distinguished on physical examination, because girls with PCOS feminize as well as masculinize, whereas those with classic congenital adrenal hyperplasia generally only masculinize.) On the other hand, some women with presumed PCOS really have nonclassic "adult-onset," or "cryptic," congenital adrenal hyperplasia.[5] Virilization at puberty may suggest incomplete androgen insensitivity or other forms of male pseudohermaphroditism[6]; in such patients, a family history of sexual immaturity and infertility may be elicited. Chromosomal evaluation is obviously indicated in cases of suspected pseudohermaphroditism.

Puberty should be considered delayed in girls who have not developed any secondary sex characteristics by age 13 years, who have the absence of menarche by age 16 or if more than 5 years pass between the onset of breast development and menarche. In general, such patients present with primary amenorrhea (see Chapters 14 and 15). Errors in gender assignment may not be recognized until the expected age of puberty, when such patients fail to attain puberty or have primary amenorrhea; therefore, chromosomal evaluation often plays a prominent role in the diagnosis.

When obtaining the history, the clinician should phrase the questions to elicit evidence of the existence of any biologic effect of sex steroids. A history of interruption of the orderly progression of pubertal changes is suggestive of neoplasms of the pituitary region or of idiopathic panhypopituitarism and is also being increasingly observed in patients receiving chemotherapy.[7] In individuals treated with chemotherapeutic (especially alkylating) agents, permanent or transitory gonadal failure is the cause of disrupted pubertal development. Asynchronous pubertal progression, with breast development in the absence of pubic and axillary hair, is characteristic of complete androgen insensitivity (i.e., testicular feminization)[6] and suggests the need for chromosomal evaluation. Normal onset and progression of pubertal changes in the absence of menses are associated with aplasia or dysplasia of müllerian duct derivatives.

Among patients with the syndrome of "pure gonadal dysgenesis" without the stigmata of Turner's syndrome, who may be chromatin-positive, a familial history of sexual immaturity and infertility may exist.[6] In the more common forms of gonadal dysgenesis with the stigmata of Turner's syndrome, there may be a history of pedal edema during the neonatal period as well as of cardiac and renal abnormalities and short stature.[6] Patients with Kallmann's syndrome (i.e., isolated gonadotropin deficiency) may give a history of hyposmia, color blindness, congenital deafness, or cleft lip or palate in themselves or in family members.[3] Although the condition is relatively common, the diagnosis of constitutionally delayed puberty should always be one of exclusion. This disorder is frequently familial. It is likely that this disorder forms a structural continuum with other midline defects, with septo-optic dysplasia representing the most severe disorder.

With regard to altered reproductive function, it is most often menstrual dysfunction that initially brings the patient to the clinician. A woman may be so concerned with her menstrual symptoms that she may fail to note other obvious symptoms of endocrine disorder. In any amenorrheic woman, pregnancy and even gestational trophoblastic disease must be excluded at the onset. Careful evaluation of any past reproductive history, as well as of the patient's sexual activity and contraceptive practices, can provide useful indications of the likelihood of pregnancy. Furthermore, the reproductive history may suggest the possibility of Sheehan's syndrome of postpartum pituitary necrosis[8] if menses did not resume after a delivery complicated by significant hemorrhage. In such instances, evidence of adrenal and thyroid insufficiency should be sought. Classically, women with Sheehan's syndrome are unable to breast feed and note that their pubic and axillary hair does not grow after delivery.

In secondary amenorrhea, any association with other events should be established. Strenuous exercise is not infrequently associated with amenorrhea.[9, 10] Weight loss often precedes or accompanies secondary amenorrhea and has been suggested as evidence of hypothalamic dysfunction. A bizarre dietary history may be suggestive of bulimia or of anorexia nervosa.[11] A history of dilatation and curettage, postpartum endometritis, or disseminated tuberculosis with absent to scanty menses should suggest the possibility of Asherman's syndrome of intrauterine synechiae.[12] The presence of any signs or symptoms of estrogen deficiency, including dyspareunia, atrophic vaginitis, emotional lability, and vasomotor instability, should suggest amenorrhea of a central nature with low concentrations of circulating gonadotropins (see Chapter 19) or ovarian failure with elevated gonadotropins.[13, 14]

A history of galactorrhea in patients presenting with amenorrhea is often elicited if it is sought. Nonpuerperal galactorrhea suggests a host of diagnostic possibilities and is frequently a manifestation of excessive prolactin secretion, although it may be a result of increased sensitivity of breast tissue to the hormones necessary for milk production.[15] The history will frequently reveal drug ingestion as the cause. Various drugs (including several of the psychotropic agents, which may cause amenorrhea alone, and antihypertensive agents as well as oral contraceptive preparations) have been implicated. Primary hypothyroidism may be associated with precocious puberty with galactorrhea in the child[4] and with amenorrhea, galactorrhea, or both in the adult woman. Any history of excessive nipple manipulation or chest wall disease should be elicited and may well be the etiologic factor. A prolactin-secreting pituitary tumor is also a possibility.

Careful delineation of the family history may be revealing, because several endocrine disorders have pronounced hereditary tendencies. Among other important examples, the familial nature of thyroid disorders is well recognized. Also of particular note is the background of patients with multiple endocrine dysfunction characterized by hypoparathyroidism, Addison's disease, mucocutaneous candidiasis, and ovarian failure; numerous relatives may be found with one or more of the disorders present in the propositus.[14]

The clinician should not conclude the history taking without questioning the patient about symptoms pertaining to general endocrinopathies. Questions should be asked concerning headaches, fatigue, palpitations, nervousness, altered libido, polyphagia or anorexia, polydipsia, and polyuria. Sexual dysfunction is frequently only one manifestation of panhypopituitarism; when questioned closely, the patient may describe symptoms characteristic of thyroid or adrenal insufficiency, of growth hormone excess, or even of diabetes insipidus.

The General Physical Examination: Manifestations of Endocrine Disorders and Hormonal Action

In an even more dramatic manner than the history, the physical examination reveals to the observant clinician the manifestations of the biologic effects of the several hormones. Detailed clinical assessment will often make the diagnosis apparent and will obviate the need for prolonged and complicated testing. In evaluating a female patient with a potential reproductive abnormality, the clinician should direct special attention toward assessing those items cited in Figure 26–2.

In the evaluation of any patient with a suspected endocrine disorder, height and weight should be carefully determined and, especially in children, should be plotted on any of several available charts relating height and weight to age and comparing these with normal findings. Because the rate of growth is important in establishing the etiology in several endocrinopathies, the examiner should attempt to obtain historical data from physicians who have previously cared for the patient. Because sexual precocity, with its increased estrogen or androgen production, induces marked acceleration of both growth and epiphyseal development, children with this disorder will be tall for their age initially. However, early epiphyseal fusion brings growth to an end, often before normal adult height is reached. In general, the earlier sexual precocity begins, the greater the stunting. Short stature is also common in hypopituitarism characterized by growth hormone deficiency, whereas unusual height may be seen in growth hormone excess. Patients with Turner's syndrome are typically below 5 feet in height.

Skeletal proportions are also of diagnostic significance. The lower segment can easily be measured with the patient in the standing position and is the distance from the top of the symphysis pubis to the floor. One can then obtain the upper segment length by subtracting the lower segment length from the total height. The ratio of the upper segment to the lower segment is approximately 1.7:1 at birth. Because the legs grow more rapidly than the trunk, the ratio rapidly decreases until the individual is approximately 10 years of age, when the segments are of equal length; they remain so thereafter. Measurement of the arm span is also of aid. In normal adults, the span is similar to the height (i.e., within 5 cm of each other), whereas in eunuchoid individuals, both the span and the lower segment are increased because of delayed epiphyseal fusion in the absence of sex steroids. Also, for example, hypothyroid dwarfs frequently retain infantile body proportions. Similarly, infantile upper to lower segment ratios are observed in most chondrodystrophies. In hypopituitary and other types of dwarfs, the skeletal proportions become more mature and are commensurate with the chronologic age.

Even the vital signs may provide useful clues. Decreased or absent pulses in the lower extremities may suggest coarctation of the aorta, which is frequently found in patients with gonadal dysgenesis. Also common in such patients is aortic stenosis, characterized by an anacrotic pulse, with its slow rise and delayed peak. A bounding pulse is characteristic of thyrotoxicosis. Hypertension occurs in patients with congenital adrenal hyperplasia and 17α-hydroxylase deficiency, resulting from increased mineralocorticoid production; essential hypertension is common in Turner's syndrome.

If possible, initial inspection should be carried out with the patient fully undressed. A good policy, if practical, is to obtain photographs of the unclothed patient before a height grid at the time of this examination. The general

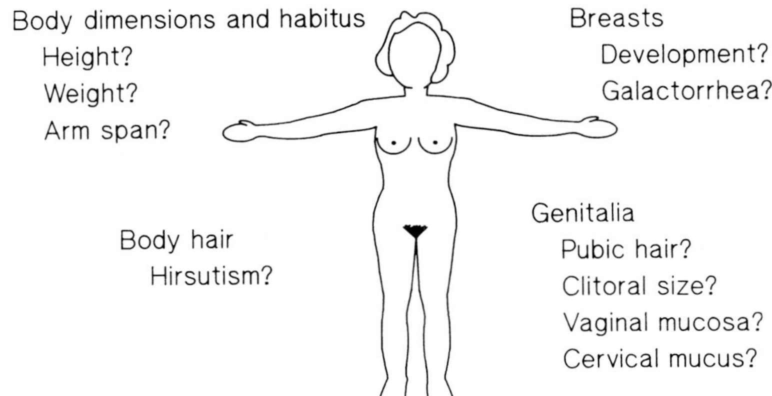

Figure 26–2 ■ Features of special importance in examining the female patient with reproductive dysfunction.

habitus, nutritional status, and distribution of fat should be noted.

The biologic effects of glucocorticoid excess in Cushing's syndrome are generally evident and include centripetal obesity, a plethoric and rounded "moon facies," and a "buffalo hump." There may be some virilization as well. Glucocorticoid deficiency (Addison's disease) is characterized by increased brown pigmentation of the skin and the mucous membranes, particularly over pressure points, in scars, in body folds, on the areolae and the nipples, and in the creases of the palms. Body hair may be decreased, and the patient may appear asthenic.

Likewise, excessive growth hormone production in the adult, with generalized overgrowth of bony cartilaginous and soft tissue, is usually apparent; the coarseness of the facial features, the frontal and mandibular prominence, and the enlarged and broadened hands and feet are seen at first glance. Early changes may be difficult to detect in the absence of photographs of the patient taken before the onset of the disease. Growth hormone excess in childhood, with open epiphyseal plates, is characterized by proportionate increased growth with or without signs of other pituitary hormone dysfunction. In the young adult, features of both acromegaly and gigantism may be observed. With respect to disorders of thyroid hormone secretion, the infantile appearance of children with hypothyroidism is characteristic. In the adult, myxedema results in a puffy face and thickened lips and tongue, and the skin appears thick, rough, and scaly. The thyrotoxic individual appears nervous and tremulous with a fine, moist skin. The eyes may be protuberant in Graves' disease. Thyroid enlargement or nodules may be apparent on inspection or may require more careful examination for detection.

The combined effect of decreased production of thyroid, adrenal, and gonadal hormones in hypopituitary patients results in skin that is pallid, hairless, smooth, and dry—the so-called alabaster skin. If hypopituitarism with growth hormone deficiency begins in childhood, short stature will result, and axillary and pubic hair and other secondary sex characteristics will fail to develop in the absence of adrenal and gonadal steroids.

The quality of the skin should be appraised in detail for excessive dryness or oiliness, pigmentary changes, striae, evidence of easy bruisability, and other characteristics of thyroid and adrenocortical dysfunction. Black freckles and café au lait spots are seen in gonadal dysgenesis. Patchy brown irregular skin pigmentation is seen in the McCune-Albright syndrome (with fibrous dysplasia of bone); café au lait spots and neurofibromas are found in von Recklinghausen's disease; and shagreen spots, café au lait spots, depigmented areas, and fibroadenomas of facial sebaceous glands are present in tuberous sclerosis. These last three diseases are found in association with sexual precocity.[2, 3]

The distribution and quantity of hair should be considered in light of the familial history. Hypertrichosis—the excessive growth of hair on the extremities, the head, and the back—must be distinguished from true hirsutism, which is the development of facial hair, chest hair, and a male escutcheon with or without signs of overt virilization in response to increased production of biologically active androgens. Some degree of hypertrichosis is not uncommon in women of Mediterranean descent, whereas the occurrence of any facial hirsutism in the relatively hairless and androgen-insensitive Asian woman may require thorough investigation.

Although complex and detailed methods of assessing hirsutism clinically have been proposed and are useful in clinical studies,[16] the most practical method may well be that of Bardin and Lipsett.[17] Facial hirsutism only may be graded, giving a rating of 1+ each for excess chin, upper lip, or sideburn hair and 4+ for a full beard. No method is an adequate replacement for photographs. Acne is frequently the earliest and most sensitive indicator of excessive androgen production. Other signs of virilization should be carefully sought.

Meticulous inspection of the breasts is of paramount importance in all women. These end organs are extremely sensitive to a wide variety of reproductive hormones. Classification of the stage of breast development according to the method of Marshall and Tanner[1] is a convenient and valuable adjunct (see Chapter 15 and Fig. 26–1). Whether the breasts appear to have decreased in size recently, whether the areolae are well formed and pigmented (as they are in pregnancy), and whether Montgomery glands are obvious should be assessed. The syndrome of complete androgen insensitivity is characterized by sparse to absent axillary hair (due to androgen resistance) with breasts that, although they are relatively well developed (because of adequate estrogen), may have immature nipples and hypopigmented areolae (Tanner stage 3).[6]

Cardiac and abdominal examinations are also important. As stated previously, cardiac abnormalities are commonly found in association with gonadal dysgenesis. Furthermore, a hyperdynamic heart, as expected, is seen in thyrotoxicosis, often in association with arrhythmias. Careful abdominal and rectal palpation for adrenal or ovarian neoplasms, particularly in patients with sexual precocity or signs of virilization, is essential. Inguinal masses and hernias are not uncommon in several forms of male pseudohermaphroditism.[6]

Musculoskeletal abnormalities are typical of several syndromes with endocrine manifestations. Congenital asymmetry is found in the Silver-Russell syndrome with its characteristic dwarfism and occasional sexual precocity.[18] Polydactyly may be the clue to the diagnosis of the Laurence-Moon-Bardet-Biedl syndrome with its obesity, hypogonadism, mental retardation, and retinitis pigmentosa, which is so characteristic that ophthalmoscopic examination should confirm this diagnosis.[19] The features suggestive of gonadal dysgenesis include short metacarpals or metatarsals, cubitus valgus, and hypoplasia and aplasia of various muscle groups.[6] Inverted nipples are almost invariably present in untreated girls with a 45,X karyotype. Association of musculoskeletal malformations with anomalies of müllerian duct derivatives is common.[6] Skeletal defects in association with short stature and a history of recurrent otitis media, polydipsia, and polyuria should suggest Langerhans cell–type histiocytosis (Hand-Schüller-Christian disease) involving the pituitary region.[20]

The female genitalia also provide a sensitive indicator of the hormonal milieu. Because sensitivity of the genitalia to androgens decreases in time from the early stages of fetal development to adulthood, the extent of any virilization can be helpful in suggesting the etiology. The most pronounced changes—labial fusion or marked clitoral enlargement with or without formation of a penile urethra—are generally observed in those patients exposed to androgens during the first 3 months of fetal development. Such findings have been described in patients with congenital adrenal hyperplasia, hermaphroditism, and drug-induced virilization (see Chapter 14). Significant postnatal clitoromegaly, on the other hand, requires marked hormonal stimulation and, in the absence of significant exogenous steroids, strongly implicates an androgen-secreting tumor. However, it is always important to exclude excessive masturbation as the cause of clitoromegaly. The glans clitoris is enlarged when it measures 1 cm or more in diameter. A clitoral index, defined as the product of the sagittal and transverse diameters of the glans at the base, greater than 35 mm^2 falls outside the 95 percent confidence interval.[21] Estrogen-induced change is also apparent in the development of the labia minora at puberty.

After careful inspection of the external genitalia and grading of stage according to the method of Marshall and Tanner[1] (see Chapter 15 and Fig. 26–1), the remainder of the pelvic examination should be conducted with care. Overt anomalies of müllerian duct derivatives, including imperforate hymen, vaginal and uterine aplasia, and vaginal septa, should be sought.[6] Visual inspection of the quality of the vaginal mucosa and the cervical mucus is important. Under the influence of estrogen, the vaginal mucosa progresses during sexual maturation from a tissue with a shiny, bright red appearance with sparse, thin secretions to a dull, gray-pink rugated surface with copious, thick secretions. Well-estrogenized vaginal mucosa with moderate quantities of cervical mucus may be indicative of Asherman's syndrome in the proper historical setting. In such patients, absence of progestin-induced withdrawal bleeding warrants radiographic or hysteroscopic examination of the uterine cavity to establish the diagnosis. Bimanual palpation can document the existence of pelvic disease, including tumors.

The hormone-induced changes in vaginal cytology and cervical mucus can be particularly useful to the clinician in the assessment of biologic estrogenic activity and therefore merit further comment.

Internal Genitalia: Steroid Hormone Action at the End Organ

Vaginal Epithelium

The extreme sensitivity of the epithelium of the vagina to various hormonal agents has long been recognized.[22] Although all epithelial tissues respond similarly to changes in their endocrine milieu, none is as sensitive an indicator as the epithelium of the vaginal vault in quality, quantity, and rapidity of response. The stratified squamous epithelium lining the vagina consists of superficial, intermediate, parabasal, and basal layers, and the cells of these layers are commonly shed in the vaginal secretions as they are replaced. Consequently, cytohormonal evaluation of a polychrome stain of a lateral vaginal wall scraping, obtained at the time of initial examination, can be a valuable adjunct to the total evaluation of hormonal status.

With certain limitations, evaluation of vaginal cytology can be carried out on a temporary wet mount at the time of examination in the physician's office or after routine fixation and staining by the Papanicolaou method as a part of every "Pap smear" in any pathology laboratory. Only specimens from the lateral wall of the posterior third of the vagina and vaginal pools should be evaluated. An aspirate obtained through a glass pipette, a scraping obtained by use of a wooden spatula, and a specimen collected on a cotton-tipped applicator stick all yield satisfactory results.

Although the vaginal mucosa responds to various hormones, it is much more sensitive to estrogen than to any other substance. In the absence of any interfering factors, such as inflammation and local disease, and when no progesterone is present and other steroids are found only in physiologic quantities, the vaginal smear becomes essentially an index of estrogenic activity.

By far the major effect of estrogen on the vagina is promotion of growth of the epithelium and maturation of the lining cells. The most mature of the desquamated cells seen in the vaginal smear, the superficial cells, can be further categorized on the basis of the morphologic appearance of their nuclei and the staining reactions of their cytoplasm. In the presence of marked estrogenic stimulation, the nuclei become pyknotic, that is, condensed by degenerative change to a dense, structureless mass of chromatin, and the cytoplasm becomes eosinophilic; these cells are often termed cornified. In contrast, precornified cells have vesicular nuclei and basophilic cytoplasm.

On the basis of such changes, a plethora of indices has been developed in an attempt to quantify the estrogenic stimulation of the vaginal epithelium. The two most commonly used are the maturation index and the maturation value,[23] as shown in Figure 26–3. The isolated index in one smear often has little diagnostic significance; serial patterns are important and must be compared with well-established norms.

The vaginal cytology in the normal female is characteristic of the hormonal milieu of each period of life.[24] During the first few days of life, clusters of desquamating superficial cells reflect the large quantities of placental estrogen and progesterone present in utero. Within a few weeks of birth, the vaginal smear becomes atrophic and remains so until just before puberty, when slight proliferative changes that progress through puberty begin. Just before menarche, the vaginal smear generally consists mainly of superficial cells as estrogen production increases. During pregnancy, the vaginal smear reflects the progressively rising levels of estrogen and progesterone, and the smear during the postpartum period is also characteristic.[23] With the approach of menopause, the pattern becomes atrophic, although the majority of women continue to show some estrogenic effect during the postmenopausal years, as characterized by an intermediate type of smear, probably reflecting adrenal secretion of androgen and peripheral conversion of androgens to estrogens.

Characteristic changes also occur during the normal menstrual cycle. Immediately after menses, the smear consists chiefly of precornified cells with vesicular nuclei and basophilic cytoplasm. As the circulating estrogen concentration rises before ovulation, there is a corresponding progressive increase in the number of cornified, eosinophilic cells. After ovulation, there is progressive desquamation, clustering, and folding of cells, so noticeable that with serial samples, possibly obtained by the patient herself, it is possible to determine the day of ovulation, although more reliable methods clearly exist (see Chapter 7). The effects in the luteal phase of the menstrual cycle induced by progesterone are nonspecific and may be imitated by high concentrations of androgens and adrenal steroids.[24] Marked degenerative changes are noted immediately before menses.

In general, the usefulness of the vaginal smear in amenorrheic patients is primarily as an indication of the degree of ovarian function present. The smear patterns observed may range from the highly proliferative to the completely atrophic. Atrophic smears suggest that the ovaries are producing little if any estrogen, whereas highly estrogenic smears are suggestive of estrogen-producing tumors in the appropriate clinical setting.

Of use in the pediatric population is the observation that smears from the lateral vaginal wall and urinary sediment from the first morning urine sample demonstrate parallel changes.[25] This is not surprising in view of the fact that the cells in the urinary sediment originate from the lower part of the urethra and appear similar but not identical to cells of the vaginal epithelium.

Cervical Mucus

Cervical mucus is another easily examined physical characteristic that is a direct expression of hormonal activity. The mucus is a heterogeneous secretion regulated by steroid hormones normally produced by the ovary that changes in concert with the hormonal alterations observed during the normal menstrual cycle. In general, estrogen stimulates the secretion of copious amounts of watery mucus, and progesterone inhibits the secretory activity of the cervical glands.[26] Certain physical properties and chemical constituents also show cyclic variation.

Although the observed changes occur gradually and pro-

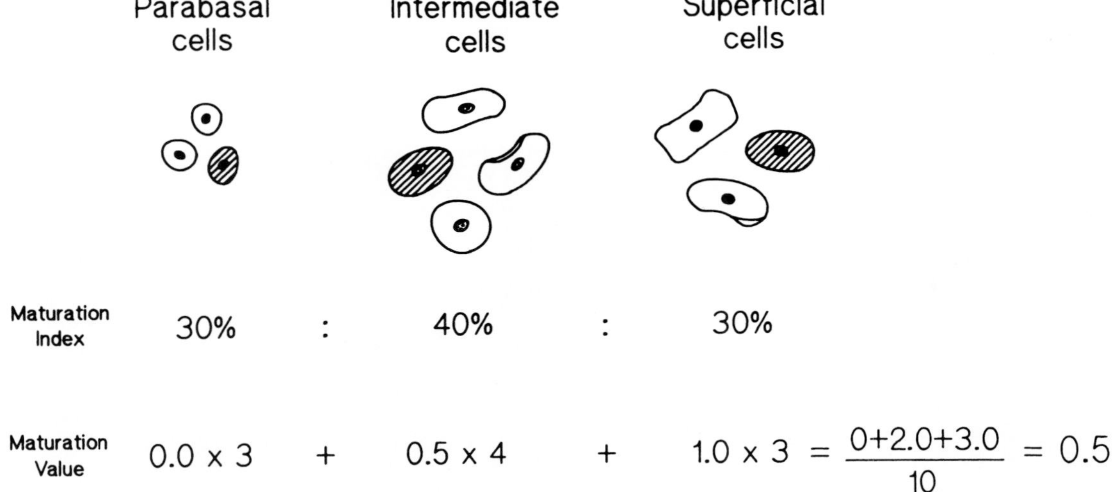

Figure 26–3 ■ Commonly used indices of vaginal cytology. In this idealized representation the smallest cells are parabasal. The cross-hatched cells stain eosinophilic, and the clear cells stain cyanophilic. The Maturation Index *(MI)* represents the relation between parabasal, intermediate, and superficial cells expressed as percentages. The Maturation Value *(MV)* assigns certain values to each cell type. Thus, a specimen consisting of parabasal cells only would have a MV of zero. To calculate this value, 100 cells are typically counted. The number of parabasal cells are multiplied by 0.0, the number of intermediate cells by 0.5, and the number of superficial cells by 1.0. This total number is then divided by the number of cells counted: the higher the value, the greater the effect of estrogen (maximum of 1.0). (Adapted from Wied GL, Boschann HW, Ferin J, et al. Symposium on hormonal cytology. Acta Cytol 12:87, 1968.)

gressively, it is convenient to think of the menstrual cycle as divided into three phases. During the first phase (days 1 through 7), little cervical mucus is produced, and that which is present is viscous and sticky. If a sample of mucus is left to dry on a glass slide, an abundance of vaginal and cervical epithelial cells, leukocytes, and mucous masses can be seen under the microscope. This cellular pattern without arborization (ferning) is diagnostic of little estrogenic activity or suppression of this activity by progesterone (Fig. 26–4*A*).

The second phase extends from approximately day 8 through day 21 of the cycle. During this period, the cervical os opens from approximately 1 to 3 mm in diameter. The secretion of mucus increases 10-fold, from 20 to 60 mg/day to 200 to 700 mg/day at the time of ovulation. The viscosity decreases considerably, and the water content and the concentration of sodium chloride rise. The mucus becomes glassy, transparent, and highly elastic; it can be drawn into a long thread (spinnbarkeit), and when it is ejected onto a slide, bubbles (like soap) may appear. In dried mucus, ferning is a prominent feature until ovulation (Fig. 26–4*B*). This pattern is the result of crystallization of sodium chloride from dilute solutions of proteins; it is always indicative of estrogenic stimulation when it is observed in secretions of endocervical glands. During this period, the mucus is permeable to spermatozoa.

After ovulation, the mucus remains transparent and elastic until approximately the beginning of the third week, although many of the other properties begin to change immediately after ovulation. From the third week until the onset of menses, there is a progressive decrease in cervical mucus production as the cervical os closes. Ferning disappears coincidentally with the maximal production of progesterone, and a cellular pattern once more predominates. The mucus is thready with little elasticity.

During pregnancy, cervical secretions form a thick and turbid mucous plug that serves as an effective barrier against invasion of the uterine cavity by bacteria and spermatozoa. The mucus is highly cellular and elastic and has a great deal of plasticity and tack; it has little spinnbarkeit. The chemical properties of the mucus are also different from those of the mucus of nonpregnant women.[26]

Elasticity (spinnbarkeit) and arborization can be used as aids in determining the timing of ovulation,[26, 27] as can other properties of the mucus, including glucose content and pH (Fig. 26–5). In general, 13 mm or more of spinnbarkeit is noted just before ovulation. Ferning can be graded on a scale from 0 to 3+; 3+ indicates the presence of arborization in most places under low power through the microscope, 2+ indicates ferning in several places, and 1+ indicates ferning in a few places. At midcycle, just before ovulation, 3+ ferning is noted; if subsequently there is no arborization premenstrually, then there is evidence of corpus luteum function. The addition of semen to cervical mucus inhibits ferning. It is important that the sample of mucus to be assessed for ferning is collected from an external cervical os that has been swabbed clean and that the sample is spread thickly on a glass slide and allowed to dry completely before inspection.

The value of the inspection of cervical mucus lies in the fact that clinicians can assess the mucus for themselves without reference to any specialized laboratory and can form a definite opinion about hormonal status. Careful naked-eye inspection alone may be sufficient, supplemented at times by microscopic examination. For example, if moderate secretion of clear ferning mucus is observed in patients with primary amenorrhea, then normal menses may still occur because of estrogenic stimulation of the genital tract. In patients with postmenopausal bleeding who are not receiving hormonal medication, the presence alone of a moderate quantity of mucus is evidence of estrogenic activity and should alert the physician to the possibility of an estrogen-producing tumor. Persistent ferning through the second half of the menstrual cycle suggests failure to ovulate or defective corpus luteum function. The use of the characteristic appearance of cervical mucus as a bioassay can easily be expanded.

Indirect Tests

Assessment of Target Organ Response

Progestin-Induced Withdrawal Bleeding. A progestational agent can be administered to the amenorrheic patient to test for the presence of intact pelvic organs with an

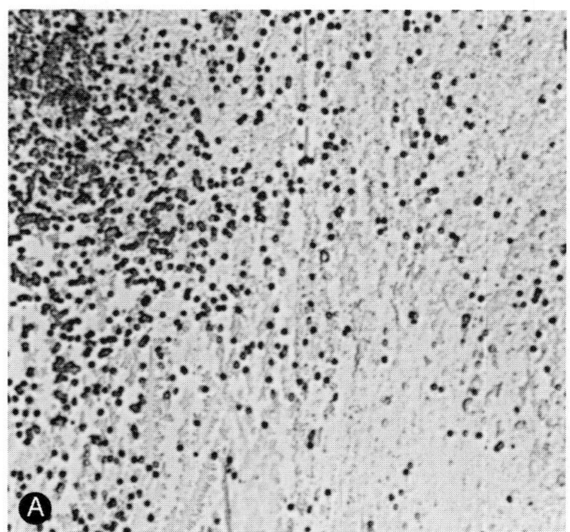

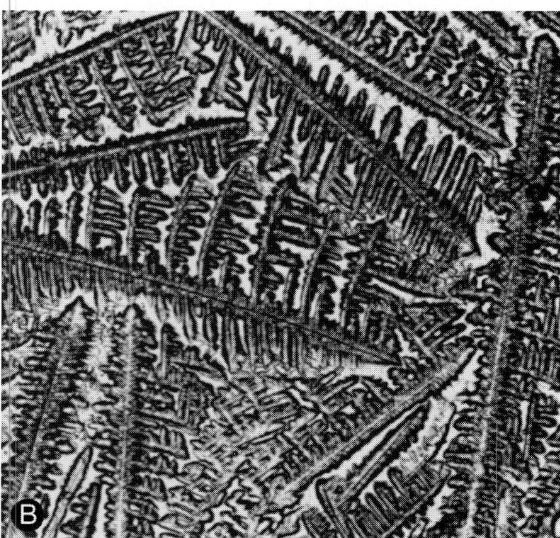

Figure 26–4 ■ *A*, The absence of arborization (ferning) in a vaginal smear obtained during the immediate postmenstrual period (day 5) from a normally cycling woman (x88). *B*, Ferning in a vaginal smear obtained just prior to ovulation (x88).

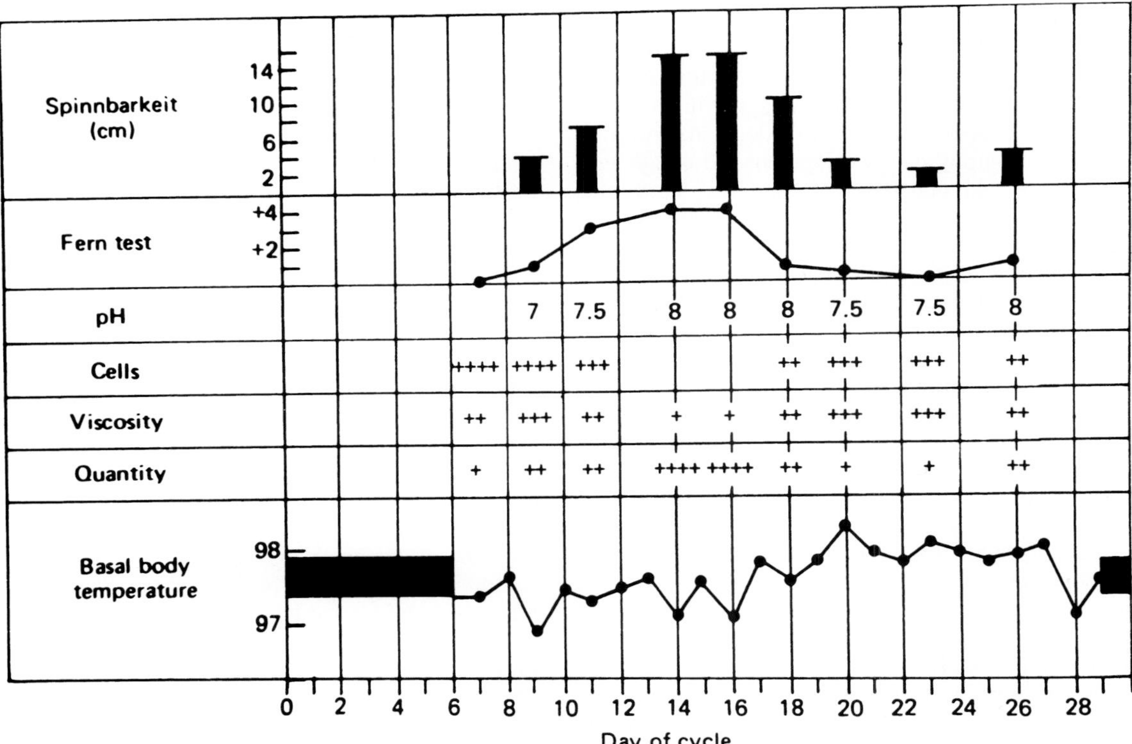

Figure 26–5 ■ Changes in the composition and properties of cervical mucus during the menstrual cycle. (From Goldfien A, Monroe SE. The ovaries. *In* Greenspan FS, Forsham PH [eds]. Basic and Clinical Endocrinology, 2nd ed. Los Altos, CA, Lange Medical Publications, 1986, p 400.)

estrogen-primed endometrium. Either an orally active (medroxyprogesterone acetate, 5 to 20 mg/day for 5 days) or an intramuscularly administered (progesterone in oil, 50 to 100 mg) agent is suitable, and each has its advantages. Compliance of patients is always uncertain with oral preparations that must be ingested at specified intervals. Variable absorption of any injected preparation is always a possibility.

In either case, any quantity of uterine bleeding within 10 days of the final time of administration demonstrates at least minimal functioning of the hypothalamic-pituitary-ovarian axis. The careful examiner can almost always accurately predict if bleeding will result; as a consequence, the use of progestin as a diagnostic test in evaluating amenorrheic women is not great. Moreover, data indicate that almost half the women with presumptive ovarian failure withdraw to progestin, diminishing the value of this clinical test.[13] Because almost all such hypergonadotropic women do not ovulate in response to clomiphene citrate, progestin-induced withdrawal bleeding cannot be used to identify patients who will respond to clomiphene.

Despite the limited value of progestin administration as a diagnostic tool, it seems reasonable to conclude that in amenorrheic patients with progesterone-induced uterine bleeding, (1) the pituitary gland is capable of secreting gonadotropins, (2) in response to gonadotropin stimulation, the ovary secretes sufficient estrogen for endometrial proliferation, and (3) the endometrium is capable of responding to progesterone as well as to estrogen. However, a negative test response does not necessarily imply that the axis is nonfunctional. Absorption of progesterone after intramuscular injection in obese individuals may be slow and incomplete. Moreover, an appropriate ratio of estrogen to progestin at the level of endometrial receptors may not be achieved, resulting in no endometrial response.

In the event that withdrawal bleeding fails to occur and if müllerian dysgenesis has been excluded by appropriate examination, further studies are warranted to fix the locus of the abnormality. Administration of estrogen and progestin together for 3 weeks, most conveniently in the form of combined oral contraceptive pills, should identify women with functional endometrium. Failure to withdraw may suggest either Asherman's syndrome or pelvic tuberculosis. It is also true that some bleeding may occur in both of these disorders.

Determination of Bone Maturation. As an adjunct to measurements recorded during the examination, radiographs of the epiphyseal centers should be obtained in patients with disorders of growth and sexual development. Classically, "bone age" is determined by comparing x-ray films of the hand and wrist of the patient with films from normal children at different ages as shown in the Greulich and Pyle atlas.[28] X-ray films of other sites, such as the knee, may also be used, although the bone age of the wrist is the most thoroughly documented. In general, a skeletal age more than 2 standard deviations from the mean makes it highly probable that the child is abnormally advanced or retarded.

Several endocrinopathies affect the degree of bone maturation. Hypothyroidism, in which the bone age is more retarded than the height age, is not an uncommon cause of short stature. Cushing's syndrome in children is characteristically accompanied by growth retardation, with skeletal maturation affected as well. Hypopituitarism with its onset before puberty, regardless of the etiology, leads to progressive retardation of epiphyseal development. Although the bone age in patients with gonadal dysgenesis may be within normal limits, there is wide variation, with retardation occurring during the teenage years in the absence of hormonal therapy; characteristic skeletal abnormalities, including a short fourth metacarpal and depressed medial tibial plateaus, may be present as well. Congenital adrenal hyperplasia and sexual precocity are also commonly associated with ultimate short stature, although increased linear growth and skeletal maturation customarily occur in these patients during the prepubertal years. An increased growth rate associated with advanced bone age is typically seen in hyperthyroid children as well. Hypogonadism from any cause can lead to increased linear growth with delayed fusion of the epiphyses (eunuchoidism), assuming that growth hormone function is intact.

It becomes especially important to determine the bone (or skeletal) age in girls with altered pubertal development to predict final adult height by use of the Bayley-Pinneau tables.[29] This can also be estimated by plotting the bone age on a standard growth chart. Individuals with delayed puberty and retarded bone age can be advised that further growth will occur with therapy to induce development of secondary sex characteristics. The efficacy of therapy can be determined in individuals with precocious puberty and accelerated bone age. Discussing ultimate height with adolescent patients is a most important part of any therapy.

Evaluation of Bone Density. It is now clear that estrogen deficiency results in accelerated bone loss in menopausal, oophorectomized, and hyperprolactinemic individuals and in women with premature ovarian failure and hypothalamic and exercise-associated amenorrhea. Moreover, accelerated bone loss occurs during therapy with gonadotropin-releasing hormone agonists. These findings have led to intense interest in evaluating bone density in women at risk of developing osteoporosis and bone fractures. Several noninvasive methods are available to assess bone mass with reasonable accuracy and precision. Moreover, prospective studies have shown that there is a progressive increase in the risk of future fracture as bone mass decreases. For each standard deviation below age-predicted mean values, there is a twofold to threefold increase in prospective future risk.[30] Because the type of bone and the rate and magnitude of bone loss vary throughout the body, estimates of bone density at one or two sites may not reflect the propensity of a patient to develop an osteoporotic fracture at an unexamined site. The selection of the site at which bone density is measured and its composition are important in interpreting bone mineral results.

The most commonly employed methods for assessing bone mineral content are the transmission densitometric techniques (single- and dual-photon absorptiometry and dual-energy x-ray absorptiometry) as well as quantitative computed tomography (QCT) (Table 26–3). Dual-energy x-ray absorptiometry has become the preferred technique for most purposes because of its superior precision and lower radiation dose.[30, 31] X-ray absorptiometry and ultrasound densitometry of the calcaneus also are being suggested as screening tools.

Single-Energy Photon Absorptiometry. Single-energy photon absorptiometry measures bone mineral content in the appendicular skeleton, usually the radius. The technique is simple, rapid, noninvasive, and relatively inexpensive and involves only a small amount of radiation. Rectilinear scanning allows measurement of the density of the calcaneus as well. A monoenergetic photon source, typically ^{146}I, is coupled with a sodium iodide scintillation counter/detector. The site for measurement is placed between the photon source and the detector, and the direct mineral content is computed from the amount of gamma radiation that is blocked. The bone mineral content is then expressed

■ TABLE 26–3

Comparison of Approximate Worldwide Distribution and of Precision Error, Accuracy Error, and Radiation Dose of Techniques for Bone Mineral Measurement

TECHNIQUE (WORLD DISTRIBUTION)	SITE	PRECISION (%)	ACCURACY (%)	EFFECTIVE DOSE EQUIVALENT* (μSv)
RA (500)	Phalanx/metacarpal	1–2	5	~5
SXA/DXA (3000)	Radius/calcaneus	1–2	4–6	<1
DXA (6000)	PA spine	1–1.5	4–10	~1
	Lat spine	2–3	5–15	~3
	Proximal femur	1.5–3	6	~1
	Forearm	~1	5	~1
	Whole body	~1	3	~3
QCT (4000)	Spine trabecular	2–4	5–15	~50
	Spine integral	2–4	4–8	~50
pQCT (1000)	Radius trabecular	1–2	?	~1
	Radius total	1–2	2–8	~1
QUS (2000)	SOS calcaneus/tibia	0.3–1.2	?	0
	BUA calcaneus	1.3–3.8	?	0

Modified from Genant HK, Ingelke K, Fuerst T, et al. Noninvasive assessment of bone mineralization and structure: state of the art. J Bone Miner Res 11(6):697, 1996.

*Dose for annual background ~2000 μSv, for abdominal radiograph ~500 μSv, and for abdominal CT ~4000 μSv.

The numbers given for precision errors and accuracy errors are from various publications. Because these numbers were obtained using different methods and sometimes distinct statistical approaches, they should be seen as a guideline for clinical practice.

as bone mineral per square centimeter scanned. This method is dependent on careful positioning of the bone site examined during sequential testing, and instruments manufactured by various companies attempt to standardize the site in different ways. In addition, numerous studies have indicated that mineral measurements of the radius do not correlate well with measurements of the axial skeleton (where most osteoporotic fractures occur).[30, 31] This technique may have a role in screening large populations of women to identify those who merit further investigation.

Dual-Energy Photon Absorptiometry. Dual-energy photon absorptiometry, a modification of the single-energy technique, uses a radioisotope, typically ^{175}Gd, that emits photons at two different energy levels. Dual-photon absorption measurement eliminates the need for constant soft tissue thickness across the path scanned and thus permits measurement of spinal mineral content. Routine spinal films for localizations do increase the radiation exposure associated with the technique. Dual-energy photon absorption does not provide absolute bone mineral content because the amount of bone scanned differs with skeletal size and thus must be normalized. Measurements of the spine become inaccurate in the presence of the "spurring" that occurs with osteoarthritis.

Dual-Energy X-ray Absorptiometry. Dual-energy x-ray absorptiometry uses the higher radiation flux and finer spatial resolution of x-rays to produce results similar to dual-energy photon absorptiometry.

Computed Tomography. Computed tomography (CT) can also be used to measure bone mineral content, and advanced software and hardware capabilities have improved results. Typically, mineral content is measured in the midportion of the first and second lumbar vertebrae, and the results are referenced to a mineral-equivalent calibration standard scanned with the patient. Either single- or dual-energy techniques may be used. Dual-energy CT has less precision, but it allows more reliable determination of bone mineral content independent of marrow fat.

Results obtained by use of dual-photon absorptiometry and QCT of the spine frequently differ.[30, 31] If the measurement of purely trabecular bone provides a better method of quantifying bone loss, QCT is preferred. Both, however, appear to be reasonably precise, although photon absorptiometry correlates better with results from neutron activation analysis.[32]

Total Body Neutron Activation Analysis. Total body neutron activation analysis can be used to measure the calcium content of the skeleton. A source of high-energy neutrons is used to activate body ^{48}Ca to ^{49}Ca. The subsequent decay back to ^{48}Ca is then measured with a gamma radiation counter to provide a measure of total body calcium. Because greater than 98 percent of total body calcium is skeletal, this method determines total bone calcium content. Modifications of the technique can allow the assessment of regional calcium stores. Although neutron activation analysis provides the most accurate measurement of total skeletal calcium, the distribution of calcium within bone may be more important than the amount of calcium present. In addition, radiation exposure from this procedure varies from 300 to 5000 mrad (compared with 20 to 40 mrad for a routine chest film).[32]

Markers of Bone Formation and Resorption

The rates of bone formation and resorption can be assessed indirectly by measuring some enzymatic activity of osteoblasts and osteoclasts or by measuring bone matrix components released into the circulation during formation or resorption[33] (Table 26–4). Unfortunately, none of the markers is disease specific.

Markers of bone formation include osteocalcin, a secretory product of osteoblasts also known as bone Gla protein; total and bone alkaline phosphatase; and a type I procollagen extension peptide. The first two are available for clinical use and appear to correlate reasonably well with bone formation rates.

Markers of bone resorption include urinary hydroxyproline and the pyridinolines, both of which reflect collagen breakdown. Hydroxyproline is an amino acid almost entirely confined to collagen that is not catabolized in the body. In the absence of major muscle loss, urinary hydroxyproline reflects bone turnover. Because dietary collagen also gives rise to urinary hydroxyproline, the diet must be free of meat and gelatin before and during urine collection. Because not all of the covalent bonds that cross-link the strands of collagen are destroyed when collagen is degraded, collagen cross-links, termed pyridinoline and deoxypyridinoline moieties, are released into the circulation and excreted as well. Fasting urinary calcium measured in a timed morning sample and corrected by creatinine excretion is the least expensive assay of bone resorption but lacks sensitivity. Other potential markers of bone resorption include plasma tartrate-resistant acid phosphatase and hydroxylysine that is excreted in glycosylated form.

The use of these bone markers is controversial. Some experts believe that some combination of bone mass measurement and assessment of bone turnover by a battery of specific markers will be helpful in the future in screening women at risk of osteoporosis. Others believe that the primary value of these markers is in following the response to therapy in women with documented osteoporosis.

Evaluation of Follicular Development

Follicular development can be monitored during normal menstrual cycles and in anovulatory women undergoing ovulation induction by serially measuring estradiol concentrations in the serum or urine and by pelvic ultrasonography

■ TABLE 26–4
Biochemical Markers of Bone Turnover

FORMATION	RESORPTION
Serum	**Plasma**
Osteocalcin (bone Gla protein)	Tartrate-resistant acid phosphatase
Total and bone alkaline phosphatase	Pyridinoline and pyridinoline-containing peptides
Procollagen I extension peptide (C-terminal)	**Urine**
	Pyridinoline and deoxypyridinoline (collagen cross-links)
	Fasting calcium
	Hydroxyproline
	Hydroxylysine glycosides

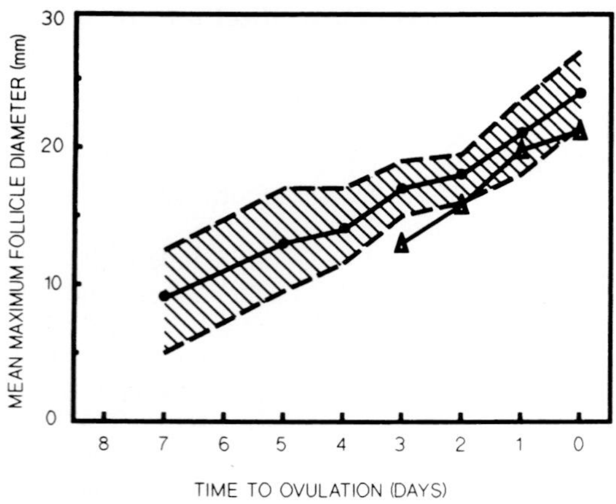

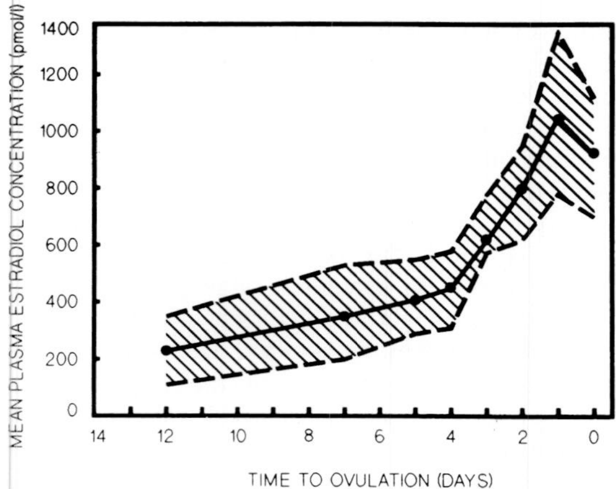

Figure 26–6 ■ Ovulatory cycles. *Left panel*: The relationship of follicle diameter on ultrasound to time to ovulation during the menstrual cycle (in days). Ovulation was determined by use of ultrasonic criteria. Mean values for maximum follicular diameter (in mm) are shown by the solid circles with the 95% confidence intervals shown by the shaded areas. The open triangles show the mean maximum follicular diameters in clomiphene-stimulated cycles. *Right panel*: The relationship of plasma estradiol to time to ovulation during the menstrual cycle (in days). Mean values for mean estradiol are shown by the solid circles with the 95% confidence intervals shown by the shaded areas. (Data from Bryce RL, Shuter B, Sinosich MJ, Stiel JN, Picker RH, and Saunders DM. The value of ultrasound, gonadotropin, and estradiol measurements for precise ovulation prediction. Fertil Steril 37:42, 1982, and O'Herlihy C, Pepperell RJ, and Robinson HP. Ultrasound timing of human chorionic gonadotropin administration in clomiphene-stimulated cycles, Obstet Gynecol 59:40, 1982.)

(Fig. 26–6). However, both estradiol levels and measurements of follicular diameter vary, depending on the methodology (vaginal versus abdominal scans) and the type of stimulation of follicular development (clomiphene citrate versus exogenous gonadotropins versus spontaneous). Estradiol concentrations are much higher in stimulated than in spontaneous cycles, largely because of multiple follicular development in the former. The use of rapid methods to measure estradiol also makes values less accurate and precise. Still, concentrations of estradiol in the serum just

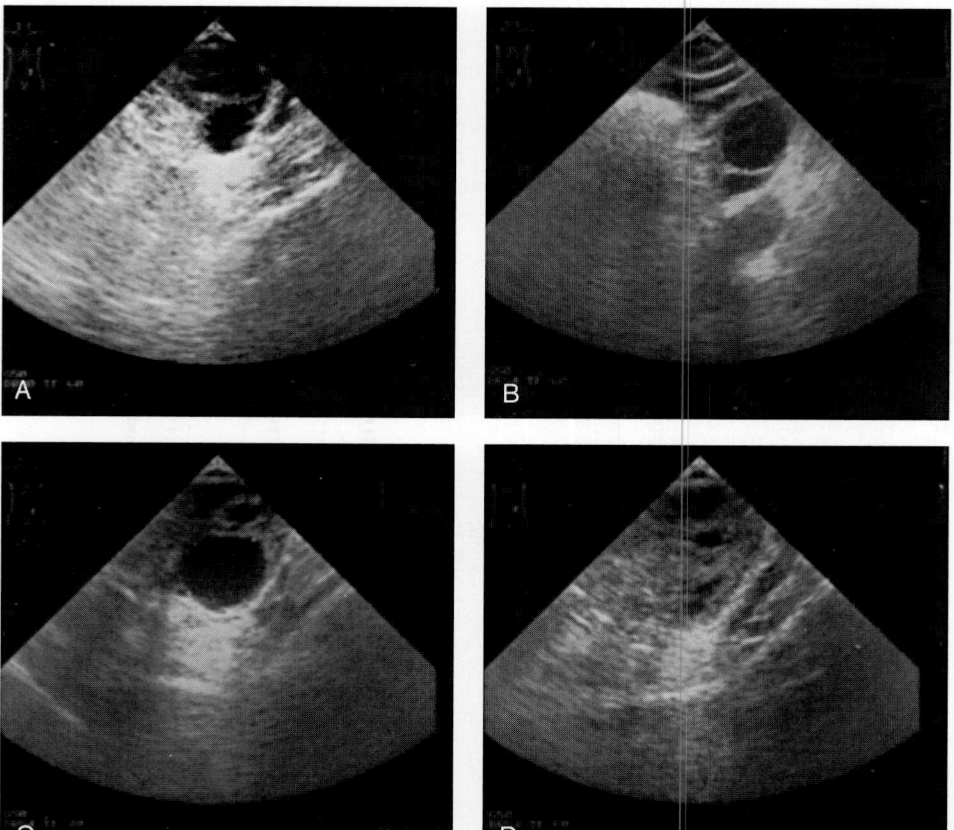

Figure 26–7 ■ Sequential views obtained by vaginal ultrasound of a follicle's development and collapse following ovulation in the left ovary during a normal menstrual cycle. *A*, Six days before ovulation: follicle measured 14 × 16 mm in diameter. *B*, Three days before ovulation, 18 × 21 mm. *C*, One day before ovulation, 21 × 23 mm. *D*, Follicular collapse indicating ovulation (day 0).

before ovulation do provide evidence of the number of mature follicles: each mature follicle secretes approximately 200 to 350 pg/ml.

Pelvic ultrasonography can also be used to confirm ovulation by observing the appearance of a significant amount of fluid in the cul-de-sac, a decrease in follicular diameter, or the development of the hypoechoic areas within the follicle that represent hemorrhage and the formation of a corpus luteum (Fig. 26–7).

Evaluation of the Endometrium by Ultrasonography

Transvaginal sonography is assuming increasing importance as a method of evaluating the endometrium.[34] In the absence of estrogenic stimulation, the total thickness of atrophic endometrium is normally less than 5 mm on transvaginal sonography regardless of the instrument used (Fig. 26–8*A*). Estrogenic stimulation of the endometrium invariably results in a trilaminar appearance to the full thickness of the endometrium on ultrasound examination (Fig. 26–8*B*). It is also clear that sonography can be used to screen for endometrial hyperplasia, cancer, and other lesions. The predictive value is greatest in postmenopausal women not taking exogenous estrogen. Many clinicians biopsy only the endometrium in women with a total endometrial thickness of 5 mm or greater so long as the entire uterus is normal and not distorted by any lesions. Extrapolation of these findings to estrogen-stimulated women is inappropriate, and sonography is clearly of less value in evaluating abnormal bleeding in estrogen-stimulated women. Transvaginal sonography and sonohysterography can be of great value, however, in identifying intrauterine lesions such as submucous myomas and endometrial polyps in such instances. Some clinicians are also attempting to correlate endometrial thickness with the chances of pregnancy in women undergoing ovulation induction and in vitro fertilization, but results to date are confusing and not definitive.

Consideration of Possible Causative Factors

Diagnostic Imaging of the Sellar Region. Radiographic imaging of the sella turcica and the hypothalamic region is important in evaluating many women with endocrine disorders[35] (Figs. 26–9 to 26–13). Just how extensive imaging should be is controversial. Traditionally, the first imaging examination in the evaluation of the sellar region consisted of lateral and anteroposterior screening views of the sella turcica. However, microadenomas of the pituitary gland clearly can exist in patients with normal screening views of the sella turcica. Thus, one approach is to obtain more detailed studies in any patient with amenorrhea and persistent hyperprolactinemia, whether or not galactorrhea is present (see Fig. 26–9). Because the probability of a pituitary tumor increases as the basal concentration of prolactin rises, some clinicians use screening views of the sella unless prolactin levels are greater than 100 ng/ml. Screening views of the sella can also be obtained in patients in whom gonadotropin levels are low and prolactin concentrations are normal to rule out large hypothalamic or pituitary lesions (see Fig. 26–9). In women with a history consistent with hypothalamic chronic anovulation (as discussed in Chapter 19), the likelihood of a lesion in the hypothalamic or pituitary area is extremely small. However, neoplasms can exist in individuals who do not have hyperprolactinemia.

Two different types of radiographic studies are commonly obtained today to assess the sellar region in detail: CT and magnetic resonance imaging (MRI). In CT scanning, coronal images that are perpendicular to the sellar floor are best for identifying normal and abnormal structures in the region of the sella.[36] The intravenous injection of contrast medium opacifies the intrasellar and parasellar structures, with pituitary adenomas enhancing less densely than normal glandular tissue. However, soft tissue characterization is less than ideal, but this modality identifies calcified lesions effectively (see Fig. 26–11). Dynamic

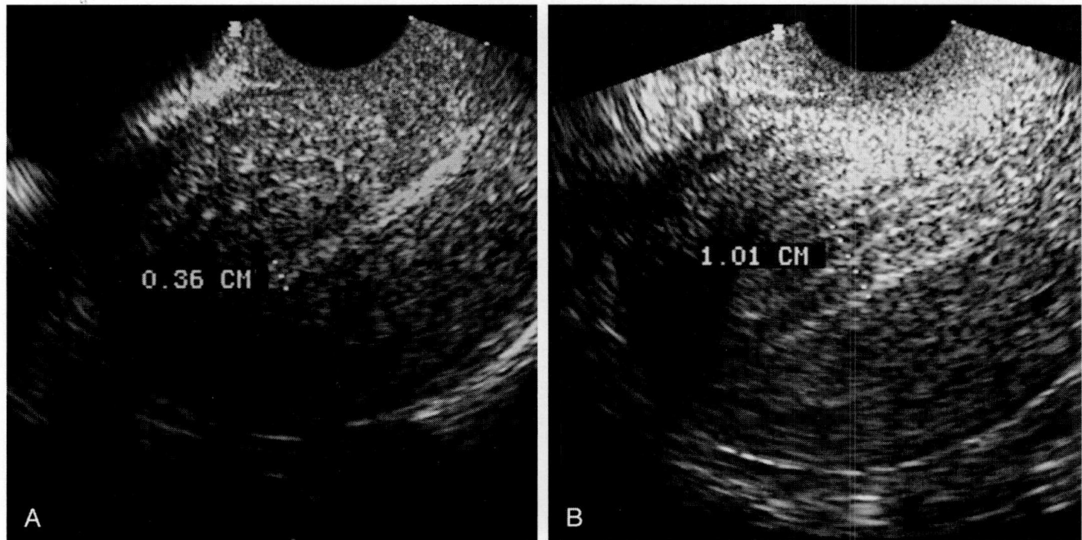

Figure 26–8 ■ *A*, The simple structure of the postmenopausal uterus on transvaginal sonography. Any stimulation or lesion of the atrophic endometrium, which measures 0.3 mm here, will thicken the endometrium. *B*, The typical "three-layered" appearance of estrogen-stimulated endometrium in a 32-year-old woman with idiopathic secondary infertility treated with human menopausal gonadotropin with a serum estradiol of 1460 pg/ml cyclic estrogen and progestogen. (Courtesy of M. Scheiber, Cincinnati, Ohio.)

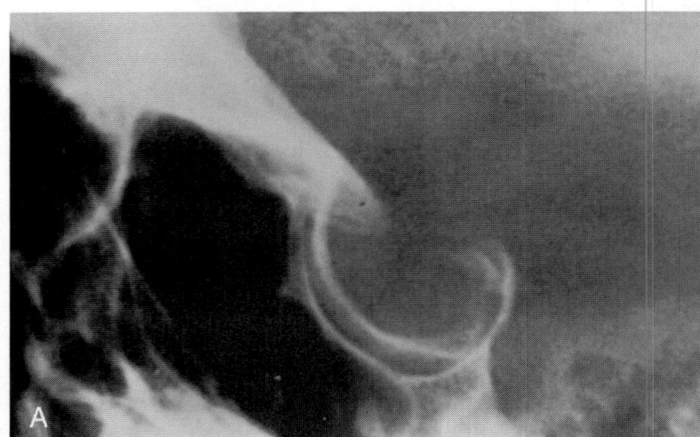

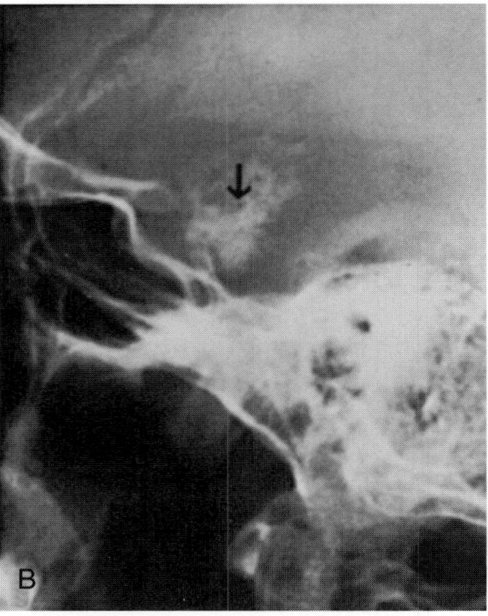

Figure 26–9 ■ Assessment of the sella turcica. *A*, Cone down view of the sella turcica showing ballooning, a double floor, and mild erosion of the posterior clinoid processes in a 38-year-old woman with amenorrhea-galactorrhea. Further evaluation of such a patient with a large tumor is warranted. *B*, Calcification in the hypothalamic area visible on a lateral cone down view of the sellar area in a 20-year-old woman with primary amenorrhea, LH of 8.0 mIU/ml, FSH of 5.0 mIU/ml and prolactin of 19 ng/ml. Her history revealed no features characteristic of hypothalamic amenorrhea. Subsequent MRI was consistent with craniopharyngioma.

scanning helps in evaluating vascular and neoplastic tissues in the pituitary fossa because the carotid arteries, pituitary gland, and cavernous sinuses are opacified successively. Intrathecal injection of a contrast agent may be used as an adjunct to diagnose an empty sella or to define a suspected suprasellar cystic mass.

MRI is more effective than CT in visualizing pituitary lesions and does not use ionizing radiation. Except when cost is a consideration, MRI is probably the method of choice for evaluating the sellar and juxtasellar structures. The pituitary stalk, tuber cinereum, and optic chiasm are well visualized in MRI, especially in the sagittal and coronal planes.[37] Contrast material may be injected during MRI to further increase detail.

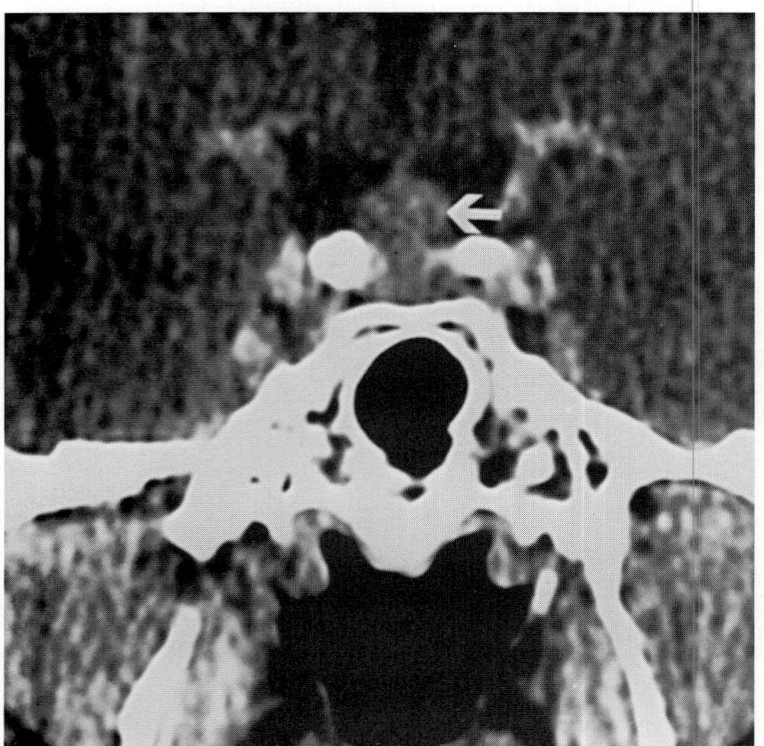

Figure 26–10 ■ A typical close-up coronal view of a pituitary microadenoma by CT scan. The neoplasm cannot be distinguished from normal pituitary. Thus, the arrow indicates an enlarged abnormal pituitary bulging superiorly. The stalk is seen superior to the gland in the midline. The bone appears white on CT scan. MRI may allow better resolution of neoplasm from normal pituitary.

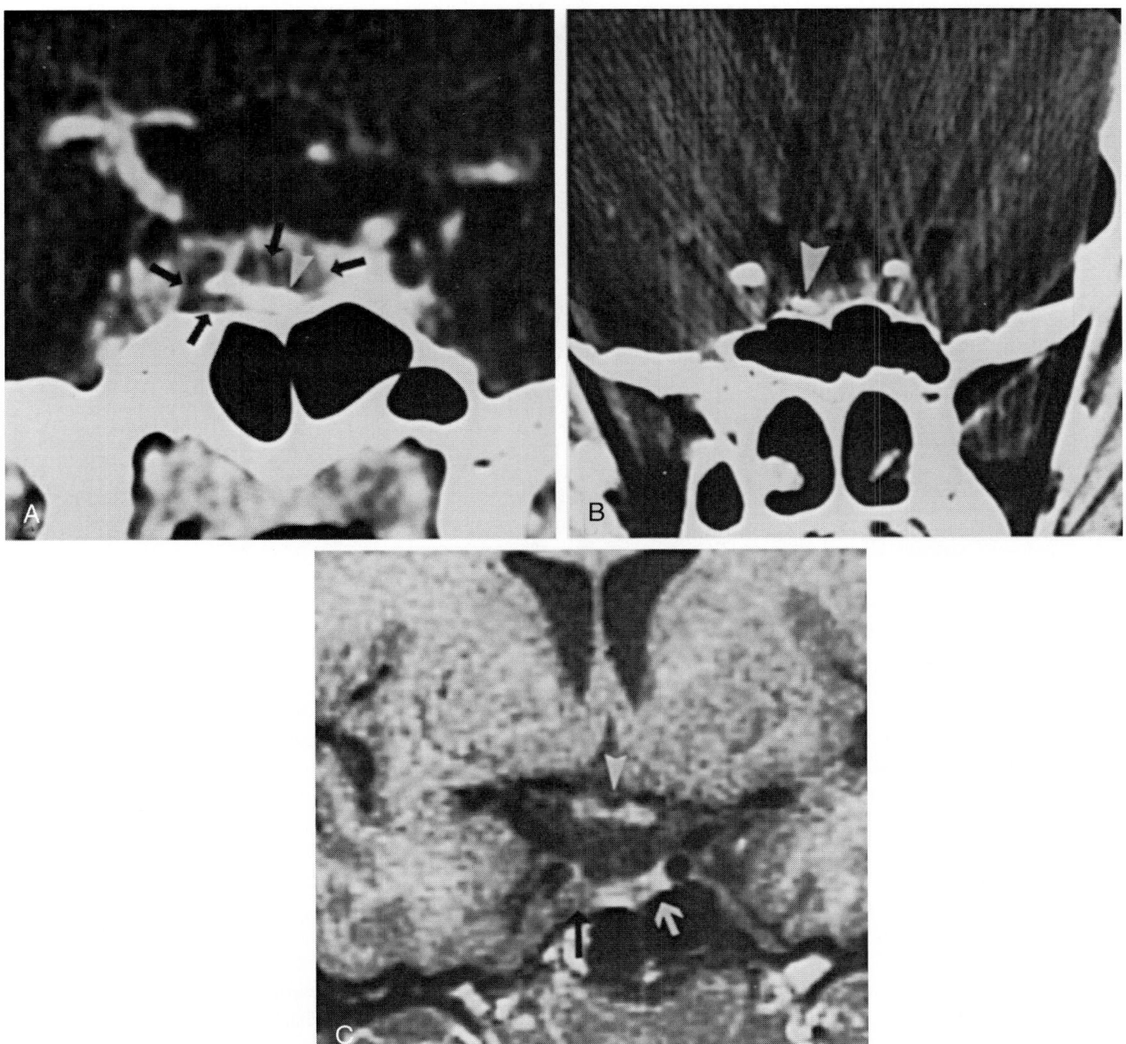

Figure 26–11 ■ Selected close-up coronal views of sequential studies in a 32-year-old woman with amenorrhea-galactorrhea and basal prolactin concentration of 160 ng/ml. *A*, Initial CT scan shows the enlarged, irregular pituitary gland *(black arrows)*, containing a calcified mass *(white arrowhead)*. Such calcification is rare in prolactinomas. *B*, The patient was treated with bromocriptine and a subsequent CT scan was obtained 1 year later. The pituitary and the calcified mass *(arrowhead)* have decreased in size. *C*, Simultaneous MRI suggests the continued presence of a neoplasm because of the sloping floor of the diaphragm sella *(white arrow)* and an area of decreased attenuation *(black arrow)* at the lateral margin of the pituitary. Note that the calcification seen on CT does not appear on the MRI. The optic chiasm is indicated by the white arrowhead.

Normal anatomic variability (particularly on screening radiographs) may suggest the possibility of a pituitary neoplasm even in individuals without a tumor. Therefore, the radiographic findings must always be interpreted in light of the patient's clinical presentation. The views of the sella may reveal a double floor, erosion of the posterior clinoid processes, enlargement, ballooning, or suprasellar extension. Calcification may be seen in the region, most often as a result of a craniopharyngioma and less frequently due to tuberculous meningitis or some other cause.

It is controversial as to how frequently individuals treated or monitored for hypothalamic-pituitary lesions should be evaluated radiographically. The slow growth of pituitary tumors has been well documented.[38, 39] The availability of MRI permits visualization of the sella as frequently as is necessary, but there is probably little need to evaluate the sellar region more often than yearly. Moreover, endocrine aberrations may well be more sensitive than radiographic tools in evaluating hypothalamic-pituitary function.

Evaluation for Genetic Disorders. When apparent disorders of sexual differentiation (see Chapter 14) are present or amenorrhea occurs with elevated gonadotropin levels in young women,[13, 14] chromosomal evaluation is required as an adjunct to clinical assessment and other laboratory studies. In many cases, such evaluation will merely serve to confirm the clinical impression and will aid in the planning of treatment.

The human karyotype may now be obtained from almost any tissue grown in culture, although leukocytes are most commonly used. Techniques have been developed to stain the bands of the chromosomes using both fluorescent meth-

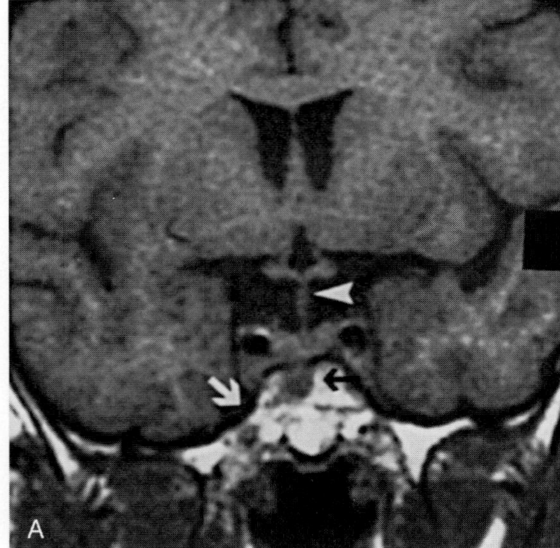

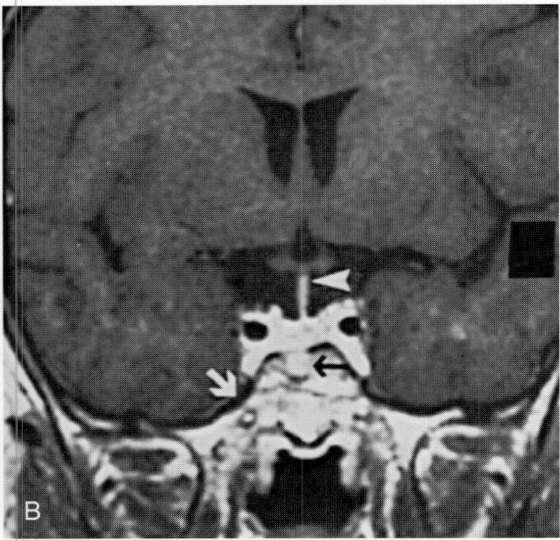

Figure 26–12 ■ Selected close-up views of coronal sections of an MRI *(A)* without and *(B)* with contrast material (gadolinium) in a 35-year-old with amenorrhea-galactorrhea. The neoplasm *(black arrow)* can be seen eroding the floor of the diaphragm sella seen as a black line *(white arrow)*. The pituitary stalk is also visible *(white arrowhead)*.

ods, with such substances as quinacrine mustard and specific staining methods, such as Giemsa staining (see Chapter 12). In this way, even small abnormalities may be detected. Because the heterochromatin in the long arm of the Y chromosome has an affinity for fluorescent stains, it is possible to visualize the Y chromosome throughout the cell cycle and in the resting nucleus. Although much heterochromatin fluoresces, the Y chromosome is generally more conspicuous because of its larger size. In individuals suspected of genetic mosaicism, karyotypes should be determined in two cell lines, typically leukocytes cultured from blood and fibroblasts from connective tissue obtained at skin biopsy. The use of fibroblasts from skin biopsy should generally obviate the need for gonadal biopsy solely for karyotype.

The use of molecular probes to evaluate individuals for specific gene mutations is increasing (see Chapter 12). Possible uses of these techniques are detailed in Chapters 1 and 12.

LABORATORY ASPECTS: EVALUATION OF HORMONAL SECRETION

Today it is possible to measure the minute quantities of hormones present in the circulation with relative ease, and specific tests of endocrine function are numerous and relatively straightforward. However, clinical testing and laboratory measurement must always serve as adjuncts to clinical evaluation of the patient. In this respect, it is essential for clinicians to be acutely aware of the tools at their disposal, so that they may proceed with testing in the simplest, most logical, and most informative manner.

The Principle of Competitive Binding Assays

With Berson and Yalow's report of a radioimmunoassay for insulin in plasma,[40] clinical endocrinology entered a new era. During the next several years, by use of the same principle, in vitro assays were developed for dozens of body substances, predominantly hormones. For the first time, hundreds of samples could be processed in a single day by one individual, and minute quantities (in the picogram range) of substances in the blood could be quantified.

Numerous terms have been used to describe "binding assays" using similar principles, including saturation analysis, radioimmunoassay, immunoradiometric assay, radioligand assay, displacement analysis, radiostereoassay, radioenzymatic assay, competitive protein-binding assay, and radioreceptor assay. More recently, a number of immunoassays employing enzymes, such as enzyme-multiplied immune technique assays and enzyme-linked immunosorbent assays, and assays employing fluoresceinated compounds rather than radioisotopes have been developed. All are based on the principle of competitive binding, following the law of mass action.

Required for such assays is a suitable binding protein, antibody, or receptor (P) to which a known substance (S) binds specifically. The pure substance S must be available so that it can be "labeled" to contain, for example, a radioisotope or fluorescein, thus allowing quantitation. Simply stated, P is then mixed with the substance S to form a complex, PS (Fig. 26–14). A known quantity of the labeled form of the substance (S*) is added and can also form a complex, PS*. Because the quantity of the binding protein P is held constant, the unlabeled S and the labeled S* compete for the limited binding sites in proportion to their concentration. Increasing the unknown substance S results in progressively less binding of S* to form PS*. In some way, the complexed bound substance is separated from the unbound (free), and plotting the change in either the bound or the free labeled substance, S*, against the equivalent unlabeled compound S results in a standard curve. The amount of bound or free S* in the presence of an unknown quantity of S reveals the concentration of S compared with the standard curve.

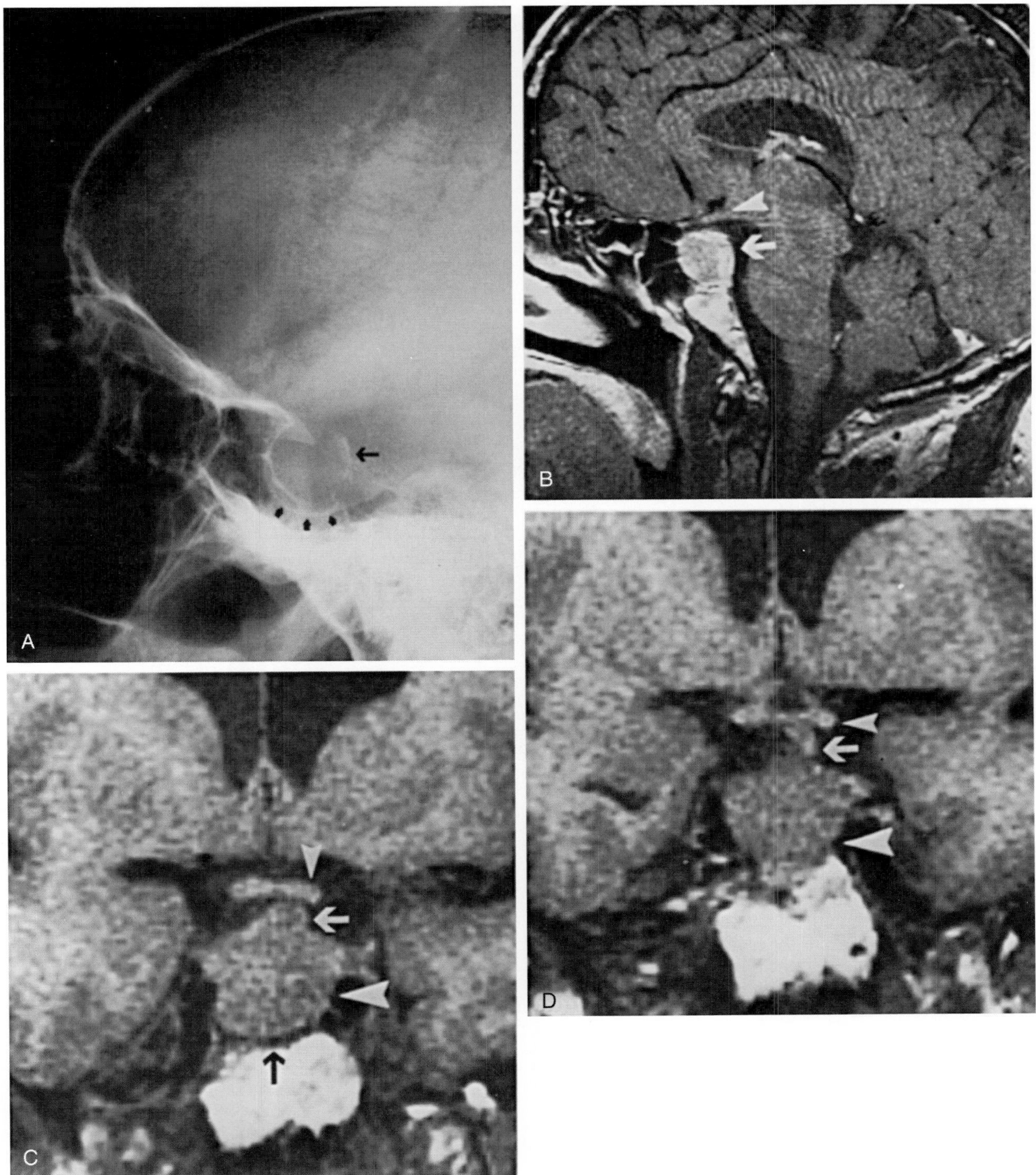

Figure 26–13 ■ Selected views in a 39-year-old woman with a probable nonsecreting neoplasm who presented with amenorrhea-galactorrhea and had prolactin levels of approximately 50 ng/ml. The x-rays suggest the mild hyperprolactinemia is due to stalk compression. *A*, Lateral skull film showing ballooning of the sella turcica with a thin double floor *(small black arrows)* and erosion of the clinoid processes posteriorly *(large black arrow)*. *B*, Sagittal view of MRI with contrast material showing the large pituitary tumor *(white arrow)* and normally positioned optic chiasm *(white arrowhead)*. *C*, Coronal view showing the large neoplasm *(large white arrowhead)* bulging superiorly *(white arrow)* toward the optic chiasm *(small white arrowhead)*. The black arrow notes the diaphragm sella in black. *D*, Another view of the neoplasm shows displacement of the optic chiasm *(white arrow)* below the optic nerves and chiasm *(small white arrowhead)*. The diaphragm is indistinct and there is the suggestion here of bony erosion.

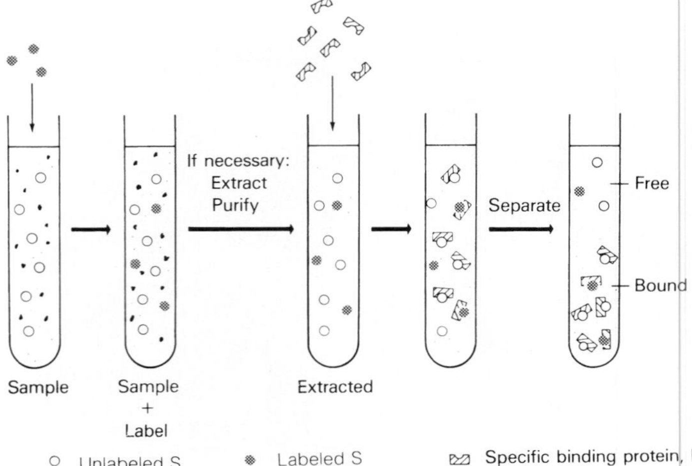

Figure 26–14 ■ The principle of competitive binding assays. Such assays are based on the binding of any substance, S (which is generally a hormone), with some protein, P, to which it will bind specifically. In a typical assay, a known quantity of the labeled substance, S*, is added to the sample containing an unknown quantity of S, and this mixture is then exposed to a known quantity of the binding protein, P. The amount of S* appearing both in the free form and in the bound form after separation is dependent on how much unknown S competed with it. Either the bound or the free S* may be counted, and, by comparison with a standard curve, S may be quantitated.

Antibodies for use in such assays have been produced for substances such as steroids, which are not normally antigenic (haptens). This has been accomplished by coupling the haptens chemically with antigenic proteins, such as albumin, and injecting these substances into animals for production of antibody. With this principle of competitive binding, estradiol, for example, can be measured by use of a receptor (from the uterus), a plasma protein (estrogen-binding globulin of rat pregnancy plasma), or an antibody (produced against an estradiol-bovine serum albumin complex).

Obviously required for assays involving antibodies is antibody specificity. Yet antibodies to cortisol, for example, commonly also bind to a number of endogenous and exogenous glucocorticoids. Thus, if the antibody is not highly specific, some means of separating the substance to be measured from other similar substances in the plasma or urine, such as chromatography, must be used before assay.

Until recently, most antibodies were prepared by immunizing animals and were polyclonal, implying that several antigenic sites on the immunogenic hormone were recognized. Antibodies prepared in different animals are each unique and react differently when used in assays. This problem is particularly acute for peptide hormones, which are generally large molecules with many possible antigenic determinants. Thus, different antibodies yield different results quantitatively.

Monoclonal antibodies, which react against one highly specific antigenic determinant of a given hormone, can be produced in unlimited quantities and can help alleviate interlaboratory differences in results. Unfortunately, the avidity of such antibodies has not been as great as anticipated. By combining monoclonal antibodies to different antigenic sites on the same molecule, avidity is increased. Consequently, assays using combinations of monoclonal antibodies are becoming more common.

For a competitive binding assay system to be employed with confidence, it is essential that its reliability in each particular laboratory be established and that strict quality-control measures be taken. Utmost precision and care are required. Guidelines for assessing the reliability of such assays have been established.[41, 42]

Antibodies detect the presence of an antigen. Antibodies do not provide any information about the biologic activity of the antigenic hormone being measured. This fact is important in measuring peptide hormones that may circulate as inactive large-molecular-weight prohormones and as smaller metabolites with little or no bioactivity in addition to circulating in several active forms. Thus, the aim in developing any hormone immunoassay is to develop a test that correlates well with bioactivity. Unfortunately, this ideal relationship, with immunoactivity equating with bioactivity, does not always hold.

Steroid Hormone Determinations

Clinically relevant determinations of steroid hormone levels can be made in either the serum or the urine. Today, serum concentrations are measured almost exclusively by competitive binding assays. The pattern of relevant gonadal steroid levels in the serum through the normal menstrual cycle is illustrated in Figure 26–15. Measurement of steroid levels in 24-hour urine specimens is still sometimes employed, invariably by immunoassay. First morning void and timed urinary measurements of estradiol or estrone glucuronide and pregnanediol glucuronide have been used to describe the normal menstrual cycle.

The most closely corresponding plasma and urinary tests of steroid determinations are listed in Table 26–5. Special note should be made of the normal ranges of pregnanetriol glucuronide in the urine and of 17-hydroxyprogesterone in the serum in any particular laboratory. Elevated levels are found in congenital adrenal hyperplasia and are almost diagnostic. Elevations may also be seen in patients with adrenal or ovarian neoplasma. Mild elevation in comparison with the levels found in normal women may also occasionally be observed in hirsute women with PCOS. However, the unique historical and clinical bioassay findings in congenital adrenal hyperplasia should normally pose little problem to the clinician when this diagnosis is made. Serum 17-hydroxyprogesterone levels are almost invariably less than 200 ng/dl in normal women.

Collection of 24-hour specimens requires the complete cooperation of the patient as well as an understanding of what is required. The patient should be instructed to void, preferably between 7:00 and 9:00 AM, and to discard this specimen. All successive voidings, including the one at the end of the period that will complete the 24-hour cycle, are pooled in a container that is kept refrigerated. After collection, total volume should be measured. Urinary creatinine concentration should always be obtained in an additional effort to ensure that the specimen does indeed represent a complete 24-hour collection, and appropriate steroid determinations should be made. Day-to-day variation often mandates at least 3 consecutive days of collection for the purpose of a reliable diagnosis.

The total urinary 17-ketosteroids (17-KS) consist of many of the major androgenic metabolites of both the adrenal gland and the ovary; all those included have a ketone group at the 17-position and, in addition, are "neutral." Consequently, testosterone itself is not included, even though many of the metabolites of dehydroepiandrosterone, Δ^4-androstenedione, testosterone, and 11β-hydroxyandrostenedione are. In fact, only a small fraction of the 17-KS excretion results from testosterone secretion in the normal woman (see Chapter 4).

Obviously, no conclusion about the amount of any particular precursor can be based on such studies, even though such information would be valuable because of marked differences in biologic activity among the various androgens. Although fractionation of the 17-KS can be accomplished, even this does not identify the precursors or indicate their biologic activity. Interference in measurement of 17-KS occurs as a result of "nonspecific chromogens," which are either present in the urine or formed during hydrolysis.

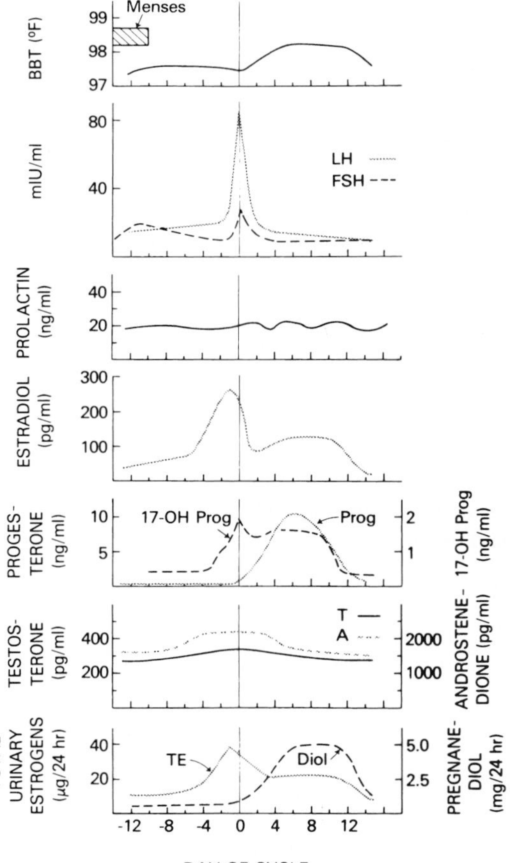

Figure 26–15 ■ Schematic representation of serum gonadotropin, prolactin, and steroid hormone profiles during the normal menstrual cycle as determined by radioimmunoassay. The 24-hr urinary excretion pattern of total estrogens and pregnanediol is included *(lowest panel)* as well as serum steroid concentration profiles. The well-known thermogenic properties of progesterone account for the characteristic shift of basal body temperature (BBT) in ovulatory cycles.

■ TABLE 26–5

Corresponding Urinary and Serum Steroid Measurements

URINE	SERUM
Total urinary estrogens	Estradiol-17β
Estradiol or estrone glucuronide	Estradiol-17β
Pregnanediol glucuronide	Progesterone
Pregnanetriol glucuronide	17-Hydroxyprogesterone
17-Hydroxycorticosteroids (Porter-Silber)	Cortisol
17-Ketosteroids	Dehydroepiandrosterone sulfate (major steroid)
17-Ketogenic steroids	No corresponding test available: best estimation a combination of cortisol and 17-hydroxyprogesterone

When interpreting values for any individual, one must consider age and total body surface. In women of reproductive years, 17-KS excretion, as measured by the Zimmermann reaction, is approximately 10 mg/24 hr.[43] However, a tall, heavy patient will generally excrete amounts greater than the mean for a normal population. Furthermore, 17-KS excretion is much reduced in the prepubertal girl (2 to 5 mg/24 hr). It increases rapidly to adult levels during adolescence and then decreases again with increasing age. 17-KS excretion is also dependent on nutritional state, gonadal status, and sex.

Although such difficulties and the resultant variability detract from the diagnostic value of urinary 17-KS, the results can be of use when they are considered in the context of the clinical presentation. Significant androgenic manifestations in association with normal or only slightly elevated 17-KS excretion are probably caused by testosterone, the most biologically potent androgen, and are typical of disorders with an ovarian etiology. Almost all disorders associated with hirsutism and virilization and attributable to adrenocortical dysfunction are associated with a marked increase in 17-KS excretion, largely because of the great quantities of dehydroepiandrosterone and its sulfate that are produced. Total 17-KS of greater than 20 mg/24 hr probably suggests adrenal disease.

Measurements of testosterone in the blood by radioimmunoassay and its glucuronide in the urine have generally added little to attempts to localize the site of excess androgen production. Testosterone production tends to be increased in both adrenal and ovarian disorders producing hirsutism,[44] because testosterone is formed not only in secretory organs but also from its precursors in other body locations (i.e., liver and skin). Furthermore, serum testosterone levels may be normal in such circumstances, possibly because of increased end organ sensitivity, because of other active androgens produced in excess, or even because of formation of testosterone from precursors in the hair follicle itself. Serum measurements more than twice normal (greater than 200 ng/100 ml), however, should alert the clinician to the real possibility of an androgen-producing tumor.

The fact that testosterone may be synthesized from its biologically inactive precursors in the liver and immediately conjugated to glucuronide means that large proportions of testosterone glucuronide measured in the urine may never have had biologic activity.[45] Furthermore, only 1 percent of plasma testosterone is excreted in the urine as its glucuronide.[46] Such data imply that measurements of testosterone glucuronide in the urine of the female are of little significance.

Both 17-hydroxycorticosteroid (17-OHCS) and 17-ketogenic (17-KG) steroid determinations measure urinary metabolites of glucocorticoids. Because both assays require the presence of a 17α-hydroxyl group and the mineralocorticoids do not have a C-17 hydroxyl group, they are not included in measurements of 17-OHCS and 17-KG steroids. The 17-KG steroid measurement is obtained as follows: compounds are oxidized to give 17-KS and are measured by the Zimmermann reaction; the 17-KS are then subtracted, and the difference represents the 17-KG steroids.[43] The 17-OHCS, on the other hand, as measured by the Porter-Silber reaction, include urinary metabolites that have a hydroxyl group present at C-21 and a ketone group present at C-20, in addition to the C-17 hydroxyl group. Consequently, 17-KG steroid measurements include more glucocorticoid metabolites than do 17-OHCS measurements. In fact, all the C_{21} steroids are ketogenic and are estimated by the various urinary 17-KG steroid assays. Thus, the urinary 17-KG steroid method assays slightly more than half of the total daily production of cortisol, and the Porter-Silber reaction (17-OHCS) measures approximately one third of the total cortisol production.[47]

The 17-KG steroids include cortisol and cortisone and their tetrahydro-derivatives as well as further reduction products of tetrahydrocortisol and cortisone; they are almost always of adrenocortical origin. Because pregnanetriol is also included among the 17-KG steroids, this assay is increased in congenital adrenal hyperplasia. Pregnanetriol is not among the metabolites included in measurement of 17-OHCS.

As with the 17-KS, normal ranges of 17-KG steroids and 17-OHCS vary with age and sex. In addition, numerous drugs interfere with the assay. In measurement of 17-KG steroids, nonspecific interfering chromogens pose less of a problem than they do with 17-KS determinations. In females of reproductive age, 17-KG steroids generally range from 6 to 14 mg/24 hr. Normal 17-OHCS levels are approximately 4.4 ± 1.7 mg per gram of creatinine per 24 hours, regardless of age.[48]

Clinical conditions in which hepatic conjugation of steroids is impaired or in which steroid excretion is elevated may warrant determination of free corticosteroids for diagnostic purposes. Increased quantities of free urinary cortisol are found in early and mild Cushing's syndrome.

Assessment of the Hypothalamic–Pituitary–End Organ Axis

Assessment of endocrine function begins with the measurement of hormone concentrations in the circulation or urine in the basal state. However, the values obtained must be interpreted with full knowledge of the clinical presentation of the patient. In addition, virtually all hormones are secreted in a pulsatile manner, and many vary throughout the day and the night in response to various endogenous and exogenous stimuli. Despite these limitations, the value of basal concentrations in single serum samples should not be forgotten in the rush to proceed to more sophisticated testing with various provocative stimuli.

Individuals suspected of having partial or complete hypopituitarism will often require dynamic testing of pituitary reserve. However, the diagnosis of a pituitary tumor cannot be established on the basis of such testing alone. Many patients with hypopituitarism continue to respond normally to several provocative stimuli; others present with symptoms related only to the mass effects of the tumor (e.g., headaches and visual field defects).

Testing with agents that provoke or inhibit secretion of various pituitary hormones is expensive and time-consuming. The tests to be conducted, therefore, should be chosen with care. It has become clear that administration of synthetic hypothalamic releasing hormones is of great value in assessing pituitary reserve. To this end, several groups have documented the efficacy of administering several such provocative stimuli together or sequentially on the same day as a combined anterior pituitary function test.[49–51]

In patients in whom the diagnosis of a pituitary lesion has been established, it is imperative to determine the status of the thyroid and adrenal axes and to institute replacement when appropriate. The institution of replacement therapy in the absence of definite and documented hormonal deficits, even after therapy by surgery or irradiation, seems unjustified. After treatment of a pituitary tumor, evaluation of hormonal status should be undertaken at frequent intervals, preferably at 3 and 6 months post therapy and at yearly intervals thereafter. How complete such evaluation should be is open to question. However, some assessment of thyroid and adrenal function, as well as radiographic evaluation of the sella and a visual field examination, must be included.

Evaluation of the Hypothalamic-Pituitary-Ovarian Axis

Measurement of Gonadotropins. Gonadotropins can now be measured by immunoassay, radioreceptor assay, or biologic assay in the serum and in the urine. Although immunoassay determinations are generally used for diagnostic purposes, bioassay measurements are important because of the realization that immunologically active hormone need not be biologically active. The bioassay most frequently employed for measurement of luteinizing hormone (LH) and human chorionic gonadotropin (hCG) is the sensitive and precise in vitro assay using preparations of dispersed Leydig cells.[52] The responses of rat granulosa or Sertoli cells in culture to follicle-stimulating hormone (FSH) form the basis for its bioassay[53]; these assays, however, are difficult and expensive with marked variation from day to day. Receptor assays do not appear to have any advantage over more convenient immunoassays. The mouse uterine weight assay fails to discriminate among LH, FSH, and hCG and is no longer commonly used.[54]

However, it still remains the standard with which other assays must be compared.

Immunologic Measurements of hCG. Measurement of hCG is commonly done by immunoassay today, with enzyme-linked immunoassays forming the basis for almost all of the available sensitive pregnancy tests. Almost all of the assays available today are so-called β-subunit assays and measure either the intact or whole hCG molecule only or intact plus any circulating free β-subunit.[55]

Because hCG is structurally similar to LH, antibodies to one will bind to both hormones. Even antibodies directed to the C-terminal peptide unique to the β-subunit of hCG show a small degree of cross-reactivity with LH.

The β-subunit of hCG can be detected in the circulation by immunoassays currently available before the date of expected menses and approximately 9 to 11 days after the LH surge. Levels of hCG generally approach 100 mIU/ml by the date of expected menses.

Serial measurements of hCG in early pregnancy are helpful in distinguishing viable normal from abnormal pregnancies.[56] Early in pregnancy, hCG values double approximately every 48 hours until levels of 1000 to 1500 mIU/ml are attained; from then until levels of approximately 6000 mIU/ml, values double at about 72-hour intervals. It is rare for an extrauterine pregnancy to have hCG levels above 6000 mIU/ml. By use of vaginal ultrasonography, gestational sacs can be identified with hCG concentrations even below 1000 mIU/ml in some cases. However, because different hCG reference preparations are used in different assays, values differ considerably among assays and laboratories. Appropriate values must be developed for every medical center.

Immunologic Measurements of LH and FSH. The immunoassay of serum gonadotropins secreted by the pituitary gland has been hampered even more profoundly by the use of different standard preparations by different laboratories. At present, most gonadotropin results in the United States are presented in terms of the Second International Reference Preparation of Human Urinary Menopausal Gonadotropin (2nd IRP-hMG) or in terms of a purified pituitary preparation, LER-907. This is true despite the fact that the 2nd IRP-hMG is no longer available for use as a reference preparation. Other reference preparations are compared with this previous standard. In addition, the World Health Organization's International Laboratory for Biological Standards is now providing qualified investigators with an International Reference Preparation of Human Pituitary Luteinizing Hormone for Immunoassay (coded 68/40) and an International Reference Preparation of Human Pituitary Gonadotrophins (FSH and LH) for Bioassay (coded 69/104). Of note is that data compared with these last two standard preparations can be reported in terms of international units; yet these units differ from those obtained with use of the 2nd IRP-hMG. Thus, the importance of knowing the standard preparation that is used and the "normal range" for any given laboratory is obvious. Also important is that commercially available assays may use different standards, and some of the kits do not even state what reference preparation is provided. Because it is clear that biochemically different gonadotropins exist in blood and urine,[57] the difficulties involved in using one reference preparation to compare blood and urine are immediately evident. Coupled with the number of different antisera now in use, it becomes apparent that results may, and often do, differ significantly among laboratories. Despite such difficulties, however, the pattern of gonadotropin concentrations observed in the blood during the normal menstrual cycle is remarkably constant. Typical concentrations are depicted in Figure 26–15.

In general, the immunoassays now available for LH and FSH in blood and urine correlate well with bioassay results. However, existing immunoassays have demonstrated little ability to discriminate among low values in serum, particularly in the prepubertal years. The ability of immunoassays to measure integrated gonadotropin content in timed urinary specimens has allowed differences in the prepubertal years to be documented.[58]

Despite the pulsatile release of gonadotropins, single determinations of serum levels made at the time of the initial office visit can be of diagnostic aid to the clinician. Elevated levels of serum FSH generally indicate ovarian failure, although it is clear that elevated immunoassayable FSH levels may be found in patients with viable ovarian follicles.[13, 14] An elevated LH level and a normal FSH concentration in an amenorrheic patient suggest PCOS[59] or, less commonly and if the clinical picture warrants, complete androgen insensitivity.[60] Serum LH levels appear greater than 25 mIU/ml in more than 80 percent of patients with PCOS at the time of the first office visit.[61] However, the ratio of LH to FSH can be normal in women with PCOS. Low serum gonadotropin levels in the amenorrheic woman suggest hypothalamic or pituitary dysfunction and occur together with low peripheral estradiol concentrations. Radiographic evaluation of the sella turcica should be conducted to rule out a pituitary tumor whenever gonadotropin output is decreased (both LH and FSH levels less than 10 mIU/ml) in the amenorrheic woman or if galactorrhea or hyperprolactinemia is present. Although rare, elevated gonadotropin levels may result from pituitary gonadotropin-producing tumors[62] or ectopic gonadotropin-producing neoplasms. Figure 26–16 shows ranges of serum gonadotropins observed in various clinical states.

GnRH Testing. All subjects respond to a dose of 10 μg of synthetic gonadotropin-releasing hormone (GnRH), and a maximal response can be elicited by 100 μg or more injected intravenously as a bolus with a release of both LH and FSH.[63] Except in patients receiving chronic estrogen therapy,[64] the maximal response is generally observed at 15 to 30 minutes after injection for LH and 30 to 45 minutes for FSH.[63–65] Marked variation in responsiveness to GnRH has been noted during the menstrual cycle, with the greatest responses observed just before the LH surge.[65] The responses of both LH and FSH are diminished in prepubertal children, with the FSH response greater than the LH response; significant changes in the patterns of response occur during puberty.[66]

In general, the magnitudes of the responses for both LH and FSH are directly proportional to the basal level of each gonadotropin just before the test. Only patients with a presumed central "hypothalamic" etiology to their amenorrhea, with low to normal basal levels of gonadotropins and no evidence of pulsatile gonadotropin secretion, sometimes show increased responsiveness to GnRH in comparison with the low basal levels.[67] Patients with documented pitu-

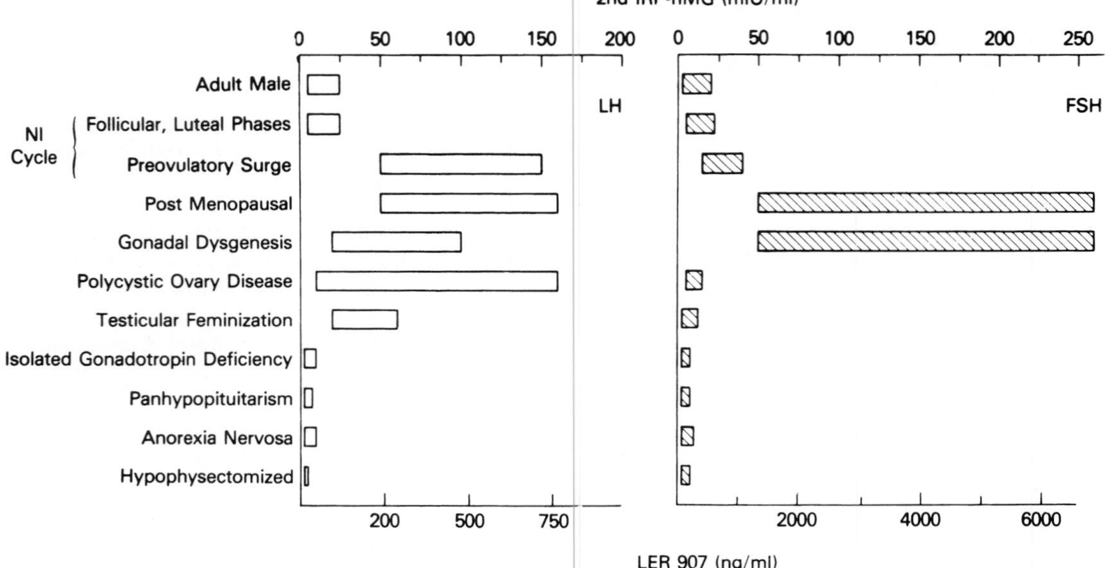

Figure 26–16 ■ Schematic representation of the range of basal serum gonadotropin concentrations observed in various clinical states. The ranges seen will differ from laboratory to laboratory, but concentrations less than 2 mIU/ml are generally undetectable.

itary tumors or with hypothalamic lesions cannot be distinguished with certainty on the basis of their responses to GnRH.[50, 64] Typical responses are illustrated in Figure 26–17*A* and *B*. The individual variability of the responses to GnRH[63, 64] decreases its utility as a clinical test capable of differentiating among various pathologic states. The GnRH test can demonstrate only that the pituitary gland can release gonadotropin in response to GnRH; for this purpose, the 100-μg dose is recommended. It is now apparent that GnRH can be used as a clinical tool to induce pubertal development in children with Kallmann's syndrome and to induce ovulation in a variety of situations if it is administered in a pulsatile manner.[68] Agonists and antagonists of GnRH are also useful in several clinical situations in which "functional castration" is deemed advisable.

Evaluation of the Hypothalamic-Pituitary-Thyroid Axis

Thyrotropin-releasing hormone (TRH) has not proved to be clinically useful except in specially selected cases. Administration of synthetic TRH to normal human subjects causes a prompt release of thyroid-stimulating hormone (TSH), which can be detected readily by conventional immunoassay, whether the TRH is administered intravenously, intramuscularly, or in much larger doses orally.[69, 70] When TRH is given intravenously as a bolus, the serum TSH concentration reaches a peak 15 to 30 minutes after administration, followed by a decline to basal levels within 4 hours[69, 70] (see Fig. 26–17*C*). In euthyroid individuals, the increase in TSH concentration is proportional to the dose of TRH, up to a maximal dose of 100 to 400 μg, depending on the study,[69, 70] and there is considerable variability among individuals.[69, 70] Consequently, a 500-μg dose is recommended here as providing a maximal stimulus to TSH release.

Transient side effects, generally appearing within 1 minute of intravenous administration of TRH and disappearing within 5 minutes, have been observed in approximately 70 percent of patients.[69] These include nausea (41 percent), a flushed feeling (24 percent), urinary urgency (19 percent), a peculiar taste in the mouth (18 percent), lightheadedness (8 percent), headache (6 percent), and, less frequently, an urge to defecate and a dry mouth. No serious or long-lasting toxicity has been reported.

The levels of serum TSH in patients with hyperthyroidism are generally the only values that are undetectable in the ultrasensitive TSH assays, which can measure as little as 0.1 to 0.3 μU/ml (Fig. 26–18). There are also a few well-documented cases of TSH-dependent hyperthyroidism in which TSH levels are elevated.[71] In hyperthyroidism, TSH secretion is suppressed by the high circulating concentrations of thyroid hormones (i.e., thyroxine and triiodothyronine). Almost all hyperthyroid patients fail to show a response to TRH, although in some patients there is a small, blunted response[69, 70]; the sensitive TSH assays, however, eliminate the need to administer TRH to document hyperthyroidism. It remains possible that all hyperthyroid patients respond to TRH with increased TSH secretion but that available radioimmunoassays still are not sufficiently sensitive to record these small changes. The response to TRH can be blunted by even a slight excess of thyroxine or triiodothyronine, demonstrating a sensitive pituitary "set-point," with diminished responses occurring even when thyroid hormones are in the normal range.[72]

Euthyroid Graves' disease may provide a diagnostic use for TRH. In this disorder, patients have infiltrative ocular findings characteristic of Graves' disease but no evidence of clinical or chemical hyperthyroidism. Routinely, the diagnosis has been based on abnormal thyroid suppressibility: thyroid uptake of radioiodine does not fall markedly after administration of triiodothyronine (100 μg/day for 1 week) in quantities sufficient to suppress pituitary TSH secretion in normal individuals. However, only approxi-

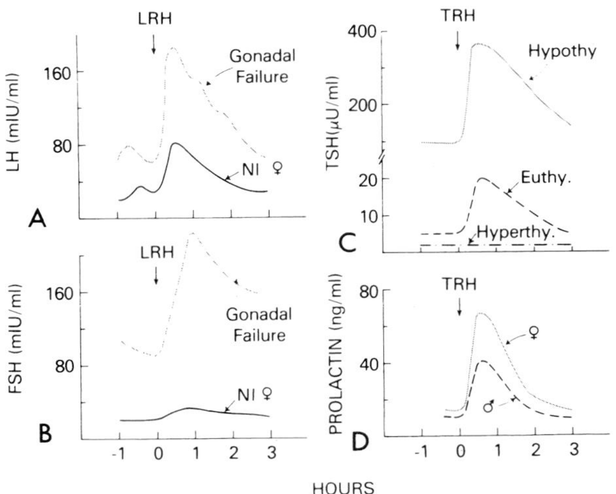

Figure 26–17 ■ Schematic representations of the responses of the various pituitary hormones to gonadotropin-releasing hormone (GnRH; also known as luteinizing hormone-releasing hormone, LRH) and thyrotropin-releasing hormone (TRH). Typical patterns of release of luteinizing hormone (LH-β) and follicle-stimulating hormone (FSH-β) in a normal female during the early follicular phase of the menstrual cycle and in a patient with gonadal failure who is not receiving estrogen therapy following a bolus of GnRH of 100 μg or greater are depicted in the left hand panels (A and B). The pulsatile pattern of LH release is shown in panel A. The release of FSH is markedly accentuated in the absence of functioning gonads (panel B). In panel C are illustrated typical TSH responses of hypothyroid, euthyroid, and hyperthyroid individuals to a supramaximal bolus of intravenous TRH (500 μg). Hyper-responsiveness from elevated basal levels is typical of hypothyroidism, whereas no response or only a blunted response is commonly seen in hyperthyroidism. In panel D are illustrated the typical prolactin responses of normal males and females to the same supramaximal bolus of TRH (500 μg). The responses of females are generally greater than the responses of males. In general, in individuals responding to releasing factors, the response is rapid, with the peak observed 15 to 45 minutes following intravenous administration. Abnormal responses may be observed in some, but not all, patients with hypothalamic or pituitary dysfunction.

mately two thirds of patients with euthyroid Graves' disease do not suppress normally. Most fail to respond to TRH because they are chemically hyperthyroid. Thus, the sensitive TSH assay may also assist in making this diagnosis. Still, a few patients may respond normally to TRH, and others may even have the elevated basal TSH levels characteristic of primary hypothyroidism; this could well be a result of coexisting thyroid disease other than Graves' disease.[73] In any event, the TRH test is far simpler to perform than the thyroid suppression test; those who fail to respond to TRH are likely to have nonsuppressible thyroid function, hence Graves' disease.

In most patients with primary hypothyroidism, basal levels of TSH are markedly elevated (see Fig. 26–18), and the response to TRH is also elevated, indicating increased thyrotropin reserve (see Fig. 26–17*C*). When the basal serum TSH concentration is elevated, testing with TRH is unnecessary to establish the diagnosis of primary hypothyroidism. Levels of thyroid hormones are rarely near the lower limits of the normal ranges and TSH levels are borderline elevated. Hyperresponsiveness to TRH will establish the diagnosis of borderline hypothyroidism. If TSH levels are low or undetectable in the presence of hypothyroidism, the diagnosis of secondary hypothyroidism is established.

Either hypothalamic or pituitary disease may have an absent, normal, or delayed and exaggerated response to TRH. Thus, TRH cannot be used to localize the site of central disease.

The interaction of the thyroid and adrenal axes has long been recognized and must be remembered when the thyroid axis is tested. Steroids reduce the basal secretion of TSH, and patients with Cushing's disease may have no TSH response to TRH.

A more complete treatment of thyroid pathophysiology is found in Chapter 16.

Evaluation of Prolactin Secretion

Fetal prolactin is only slightly elevated in comparison with normal adult levels (generally less than 20 ng/ml in most assay systems), but the concentration of prolactin in amniotic fluid is extremely high and may be as much as 1.0 μg/ml at term.[74] In the neonate, too, prolactin levels are elevated (up to 500 ng/ml), although they fall rapidly after birth.[74] Prolactin levels remain elevated longer in premature infants—up to 3 to 6 months.[75] Levels of prolactin in males and females are uniformly low until puberty, when the increased estrogen in females leads to slightly increased prolactin levels in women.[75]

Although basal levels do not appear to vary markedly during the menstrual cycle, there is more variation in prolactin during the secretory phase compared with the follicular phase of the cycle.[75] Diurnal variation is present, with the highest levels observed 2 to 3 hours after the onset of sleep.[76] Prolactin is released in response to the noon meal as well.[77] In pregnancy, elevated levels are first seen at approximately 8 weeks' gestation, with levels rising to about 200 ng/ml at term.[78] If the woman does not breast feed, prolactin levels return to normal in 2 to 3 weeks. Prolactin levels increase with each episode of suckling.[78] With menopause, there is no marked change in prolactin levels, although there is a suggestion of an increase after the age of 75 years.[75] Surgical and psychologic stress are known to be potent stimuli to release of prolactin.[74]

Data combined from several studies indicate that about 75 percent of women with amenorrhea and galactorrhea have hyperprolactinemia.[15] Because about 15 percent of amenorrheic women are also hyperprolactinemic, prolactin concentrations should be evaluated in all anovulatory women. In addition, although galactorrhea may be present in about 5 to 10 percent of normal menstruating women, basal prolactin concentrations are normal in more than 90 percent of these individuals. A few normoprolactinemic anovulatory women apparently have exaggerated prolactin responses to provocative stimuli.[79]

Efforts to determine the incidence of abnormal prolactin secretion in women with unexplained infertility have yielded conflicting results. It has been suggested that mild nocturnal hyperprolactinemia may be present in some women with regular menses and unexplained infertility.[80] Also suggested is that galactorrhea in some women with unexplained infertility may reflect increased bioavailable prolactin.[81]

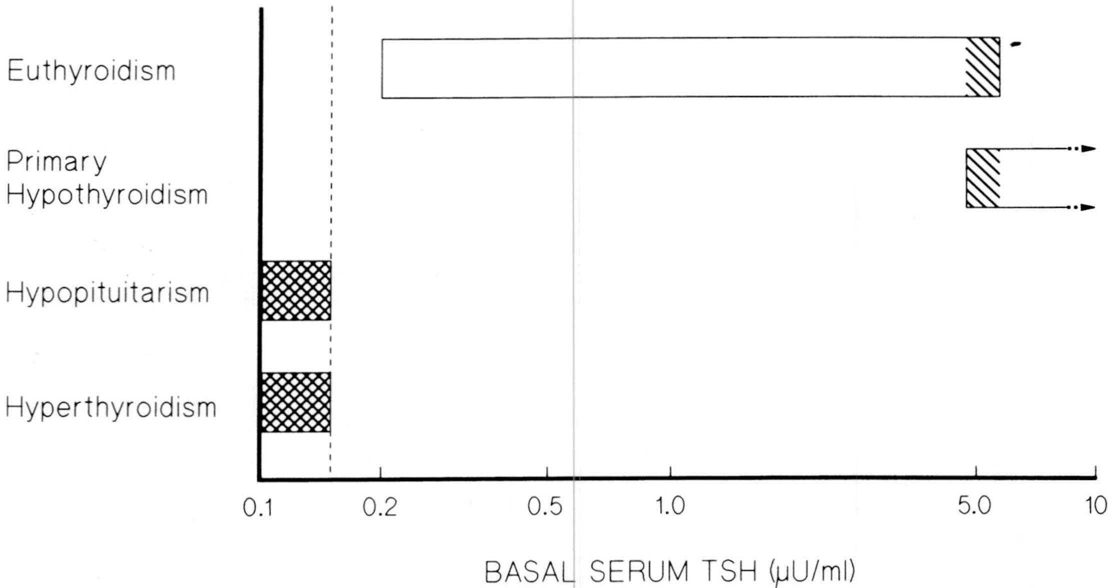

Figure 26–18 ■ The range of basal serum thyroid-stimulating hormone (TSH) concentrations observed in various clinical states. The range of values is plotted on a logarithmic scale. The dotted line represents the limit of assay sensitivity. The shaded areas indicate that values in both hypopituitarism and hyperthyroidism are generally undetectable. Note the overlap between euthyroidism and primary hypothyroidism, sometimes resolved only by TRH testing. In primary hypothyroidism, basal TSH concentrations may be greater than 100 μU/ml in some individuals, as suggested by the arrows indicating that the upper limit of the range is not shown.

In patients with persistent hyperprolactinemia, the normal diurnal variation with augmentation during sleep is frequently lost, even though secretion of prolactin remains episodic.[82] In other studies, increased secretion of prolactin has been demonstrated in patients receiving various medications, including phenothiazines, tricyclic antidepressants, oral contraceptives, reserpine, and methyldopa, to name a few[15] (see Chapter 9).

Also complicating the understanding of the secretion of prolactin in pathophysiologic states is the observation that several molecular forms of prolactin, some glycosylated, are present in the circulation.[83] These different molecular forms apparently also have different biologic activity but are measured by radioimmunoassay. They are found in different proportions under various physiologic and pathologic states.

It is important to collect blood samples for measurement of prolactin in a true basal state in the awake, unstressed patient who is not receiving interfering medication. Many endocrinologists recommend obtaining several serial samples through an indwelling cannula or obtaining several samples on various occasions for estimation of basal prolactin concentration.

The response of serum prolactin to TRH, however, is distinctly different from that of TSH. Some response can be elicited with as little as 4 μg, and a maximal response is observed when 100 μg or more of TRH are administered as an intravenous bolus[15] (see Fig. 26–17*D*). Consequently, if the test is used, serum prolactin can be measured in the same samples as serum TSH levels after the 500-μg dose of TRH recommended for assessing TSH function. Again, the peak response is noted within 15 to 30 minutes. Numerous other stimulatory (chlorpromazine, metoclopramide) and inhibitory (L-dopa, dopamine, dopamine agonists) tests of prolactin secretion have been developed.

Using the various provocative tests of prolactin secretion, numerous studies have attempted to distinguish prolactin-secreting pituitary tumors from abnormal hypothalamic control.[15] Unfortunately, to date no single test or combination of tests has proved of discriminatory value in a single given patient. It appears that basal serum prolactin concentrations are as useful as provocative testing in this regard.[15] Elevated levels of prolactin should alert the clinician to the possibility of a pituitary neoplasm; indeed, there should be a high index of suspicion in any patient with nonpuerperal galactorrhea in whom other causes have been eliminated. The patient should be screened for other possible pituitary hormone disorders, even in the absence of radiographic changes or visual field abnormalities. The suspicion of a pituitary tumor will obviously be increased by the demonstration of other endocrine abnormalities.

Before extensive pituitary investigation is undertaken, a true elevation in basal prolactin levels should be documented. If basal prolactin concentrations are elevated on a single occasion, at least one additional sample collected in the basal state should be measured before further evaluation. Hypothyroidism as a cause for hyperprolactinemia should be excluded as well. Similarly, radiographic assessment of the sella turcica is warranted only after persistent hyperprolactinemia is documented and primary hypothyroidism is excluded. It is well known that the pituitary gland is increased in size by thyrotroph hyperplasia in primary hypothyroidism.[84]

The one fact that has been noted is that the mean basal serum prolactin concentration in patients with prolactin-secreting pituitary tumors is often significantly higher compared with the means of other groups with galactorrhea; however, individually there is much overlap.[15, 75] Examples of the range of basal serum prolactin levels observed in various states are illustrated in Figure 26–19.

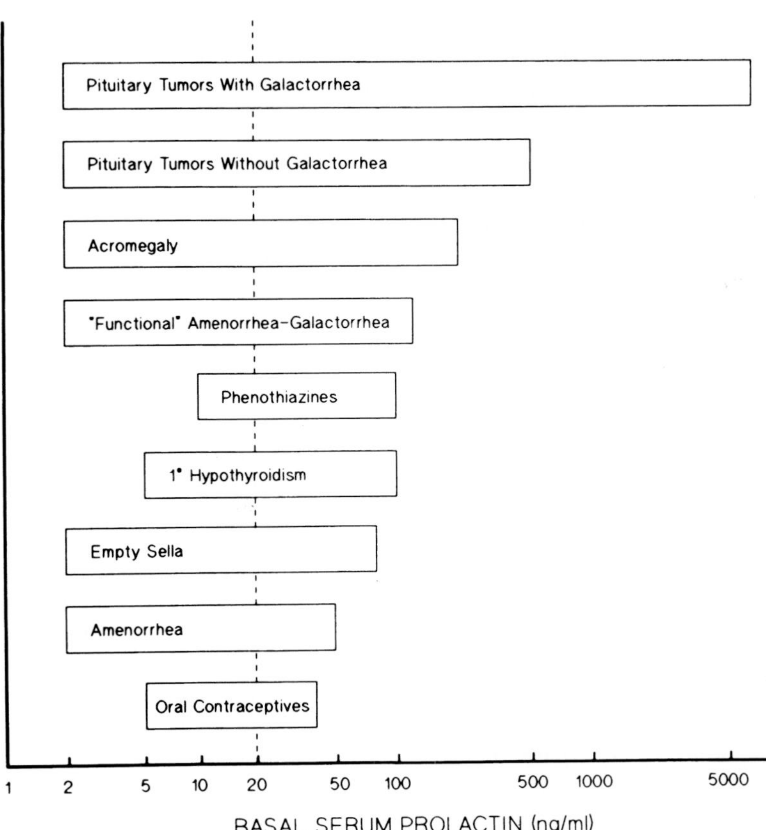

Figure 26–19 ■ Schematic representation of the range of basal serum prolactin levels observed in various pathologic and pharmacologic states. The range of values is plotted on a logarithmic scale, and the dotted line at 20 ng/ml signifies the upper limit of the normal range in many laboratories. Values less than 2 ng/ml are generally undetectable. Measured values may differ significantly, depending on the laboratory and immunoassay system employed.

How intensive follow-up should be in women with apparent idiopathic hyperprolactinemia is unresolved at present. At least yearly physical examinations and determination of the basal serum prolactin level would seem warranted for such patients. Radiographic evaluation of the sella turcica should be obtained if there is any significant increase in basal prolactin concentrations or any change in the patient's presentation.

Evaluation of Growth Hormone Secretion

Evaluation of human growth hormone secretion by the pituitary gland can be important in the patient with suspected hypothalamic-pituitary axis dysfunction. Idiopathic hypopituitarism is frequently associated with diminished growth hormone secretion, and pituitary tumors may exist that produce either increased quantities (as in acromegaly and gigantism) or that are associated with markedly decreased secretion of growth hormone. Manifestations of both mild overproduction and underproduction of growth hormone can indeed be so subtle that only laboratory estimations of the hormone after provocative stimuli can firmly establish the disorder. Growth hormone is among those hormones decreased early by "nonsecretory" tumors of the pituitary gland.

A variety of tests have been developed to assess the adequacy of growth hormone function. It is generally agreed that a single fasting blood sample is not sufficient for screening for growth hormone deficiency. In fact, many clinicians believe that inadequate growth hormone secretion is not established until absence of significant release is documented after several provocative stimuli. Because growth hormone release is decreased in the presence of abnormal thyroid function,[85, 86] thyroid status must be evaluated first, and replacement therapy, if necessary, must be instituted several weeks before testing of growth hormone.

Two simple screening tests for growth hormone deficiency are useful. Obtaining a blood sample 60 to 120 minutes after the onset of sleep for measurement of growth hormone serves as one effective screening test because growth hormone release is associated with the onset of deep sleep.[87, 88] Strenuous exercise has also been recognized as a potent physiologic stimulus to growth hormone secretion.[89] Obtaining a blood sample after approximately 20 minutes of vigorous exercise, such as running up and down stairs, is effective in documenting growth hormone release, particularly in children.

Serum insulin-like growth factor I (IGF-I; also known as somatomedin C) measurements may also be helpful in diagnosing growth hormone deficiency.[90] Low serum concentrations of IGF-I are found in patients with growth hormone deficiency. Unfortunately, the usefulness of this measurement is diminished by the wide range of values observed in normal individuals, especially children. Serum IGF-I levels in normal children younger than 9 years may be so low as to be indistinguishable from those seen in hypopituitarism. Serum IGF-I levels increase during puberty, only to decrease again with aging. IGF-I levels are also reduced in starvation, protein deficiency, and anorexia nervosa (leading to increased secretion of growth hormone in these conditions). Thus, low levels of IGF-I may indicate growth hormone deficiency, be normal for that individual, or indicate the presence of other nonendocrine conditions.

If a clinical diagnosis of growth hormone deficiency is strongly suspected or if the screening tests fail to elicit significant release of growth hormone, or both, then further studies of growth hormone secretion are necessary. Perhaps the most thoroughly substantiated and effective test is that of insulin-induced hypoglycemia.[91] Unfortunately, it is uncomfortable and potentially hazardous, although it is almost always well tolerated (Table 26–6). When combined with arginine, as in the arginine-insulin tolerance test,[92] the test appears to be approximately 95 percent effective in detecting patients with growth hormone deficiency. The use of insulin has another advantage in that adrenal function may be tested simultaneously. Clonidine hydrochloride is being used increasingly to stimulate growth hormone release because the test has few side effects. Synthetic growth hormone–releasing hormone (GHRH) appears no more useful than any of the other provocative stimuli.[93] It is not uncommon for individuals with hereditary growth hormone deficiency to have significant increases in serum growth hormone levels after a single intravenous bolus of GHRH, indicating a hypothalamic defect as the cause of the growth hormone deficiency. Thus, GHRH cannot be used to document growth hormone deficiency from any cause. In addition, with chronic GHRH deficiency, the content of growth hormone within the pituitary is diminished, leading to decreased or absent responses to GHRH in individuals with no intrinsic pituitary disease. Last, as with other stimuli to growth hormone release, responses of growth hormone to GHRH are variable. Despite these limitations, responses to GHRH in patients with documented pituitary neoplasms eliminate the diagnosis of growth hormone deficiency. Of course, the same conclusion can be reached if any stimulus results in growth hormone release.

A number of conditions inhibit growth hormone release. These include obesity, Cushing's syndrome, and administration of corticosteroids and tranquilizers. Growth hormone responses to insulin may be inadequate unless adequate hypoglycemia is induced (see Table 26–6). Particularly in males, responses to arginine are increased by pretreatment with an estrogen.

In general, any growth hormone determination greater than 10 ng/ml or any response of greater than 5 ng/ml after a stimulus is sufficient to rule out growth hormone deficiency. However, rare abnormalities in somatomedins in the presence of normal and elevated growth hormone secretion have been demonstrated in some individuals with short stature.[94, 95]

The diagnosis of excess growth hormone secretion as manifested by acromegaly and gigantism is obvious in many instances; in others, it may be surprisingly difficult to diagnose on appearance alone without old photographs. Serial photographs of the patient, a history of increasing shoe and glove or ring size, and the patient's overall appearance may make laboratory tests merely confirmatory. An elevated fasting growth hormone level obtained with the patient awake and in the basal state is diagnostic when it is greater than 10 ng/ml (in most assay systems).[96] IGF-I levels are also markedly elevated in individuals with acromegaly.[97] These growth hormone levels are generally nonsuppressible in response to an oral glucose tolerance test, whereas the growth hormone levels in normal individuals generally decrease to less than 5 ng/ml during the test.[98] On occasion, individuals with true acromegaly are found who do not have elevated growth hormone levels in the basal state but who do fail to suppress in response to glucose.[99]

Evaluation of Adrenocortical Function

Establishment of normal adrenocortical function is a problem with which clinicians are being confronted increasingly. The diagnosis of Cushing's syndrome, of no difficulty in patients with obvious clinical signs, is often painstaking when the disease is subtle in its manifestations (see Chapter 18). Similarly, signs and symptoms of adrenocortical insufficiency may appear abruptly with potentially life-threatening collapse or may develop so slowly and insidiously that the deficiency may be unrecognized. Although inadequate secretion of adrenocorticosteroids may be the result of either diminished adrenocorticotropic hormone (ACTH) secretion or primary partial or complete destruction of the adrenal glands, the clinician will generally be faced with determining whether adrenal function is sufficient in patients with suspected or proven pituitary tumor.

Once the diagnosis of either hyperfunction or hypofunction of the adrenal glands is suspected, the diagnosis must be established by careful laboratory investigation. Because of the profound effect of abnormal thyroid function on urinary steroid excretion,[100, 101] it is essential that thyroid status be evaluated first and that the patient be euthyroid at the time of adrenal testing.

ADRENOCORTICAL HYPERFUNCTION

Studies should be directed toward establishing overproduction of cortisol and determining the etiology of the disorder. Either urinary or serum screening tests may be employed. Elevated urinary 17-OHCS excretion or, better still, elevated urinary free cortisol[102] in at least three successive 24-hour periods will establish absolute cortisol secretory excess. However, 17-OHCS excretion may not be elevated early in the disease process. Furthermore, because of the sometimes fluctuating course of the disease, urinary steroids may be normal on some days and elevated on others in patients with documented Cushing's syndrome; consequently, the need for several 24-hour urine specimens is apparent. Because urinary 17-KS may be low, normal, or most commonly elevated, depending on the cause of the disorder, their determination is generally of little value. Elevated values are occasionally found in otherwise normal obese individuals, and elevated values are found in pregnancy because of pregnanediol and pregnanetriol excretion. Because of possible drug interference, the patient should not be receiving any medication during the collection period.

The most useful test for evaluating cortisol secretion is the 24-hour urinary free cortisol excretion. Typically, the normal basal excretion of urinary free cortisol is less than 100 μg/day. Values consistently greater than 250 μg/day are virtually diagnostic of Cushing's syndrome. However,

Text continued on page 739

■ TABLE 26–6

Specific Provocative Tests of Hormonal Function

TEST	DRUG AND DOSE	PURPOSE	HORMONES MEASURED AND MINIMAL SAMPLING TIMES	NORMAL RESPONSE	SPECIAL CONSIDERATIONS	SIDE EFFECTS
GnRH[63, 64]	Synthetic GnRH, 100 μg IV bolus for maximal responses 10 μg IV bolus deemed more discriminatory by some	Assessment of gonadotropin secretion by the pituitary gland	LH, FSH at 0, 30, 60 min	2- to 3-fold increase above basal LH Smaller increase in FSH	Little response before puberty, with responses increasing during puberty. Gonadal steroids greatly modify responses. The test has great variability and little reproducibility. Responses are increased by renal failure.	None reported
TRH[69, 70]	Synthetic TRH, 500 μg IV bolus for maximal responses	Assessment of status of TSH and PRL secretion by the pituitary gland	TSH, PRL at 0, 30, 60 min	2- to 4-fold increase in TSH 4- to 8-fold increase of PRL in women	For TSH, exaggerated and prolonged responses from elevated baseline in primary hypothyroidism; blunted or absent responses in hyperthyroidism. For PRL, the response in females is greater than the response in males. For both, normal or blunted responses may be observed in patients with documented central nervous system lesions.	Transient side effects in approximately 70% of subjects. Nausea, facial flushing, urge to urinate, and strange taste in the mouth are most common. Lightheadedness, transient headache, dry mouth, urge to defecate, and chest tightness are also reported.
GHRH[93]	Synthetic GHRH-40 or GHRH-44, 1.0 μg/kg or 100 μg IV bolus for maximal response	Assessment of the ability of the pituitary gland to secrete GH	GH at 0, 30, 60 min	Up to a 10-fold increase above basal levels	Not yet approved for use in the United States. Responses vary widely, and normal individuals rarely may fail to have any increase in GH.	Occasional facial flushing
CRH[109, 110, 116, 132]	Synthetic ovine CRH 1.0 μg/kg or 100 μg IV bolus for maximal response	Assessment of ACTH secretion by the pituitary gland	ACTH at 0, 30, 60 min Cortisol at 0, 60, 90 min	2- to 4-fold increase in ACTH Increase in cortisol to >20 μg/dl or of >7 μg/dl	Not yet approved for use in the United States. Synthetic ovine CRH is used because of prolonged responses due to lower metabolic clearance rate than of human CRH. Blunted responses are seen in forms of Cushing's syndrome other than Cushing's disease.	Perhaps one third experience warmth and flushing of face.
L-Dopa[91]	500 ng PO for adults 10 mg/kg body weight PO for children	Assessment of GH secretion and suppressibility of PRL	GH, PRL at 0, 60, 90, 120 min	Increase in GH to >10 ng/ml or of >5 ng/ml Decrease in PRL of 50% or more	Normal response of GH does not always occur in normal individuals; release of GH may be augmented by pretreatment with diethylstilbestrol (5 mg PO bid × 3 days).[133] Suppression of PRL is not a reliable test for distinguishing neoplasms from "idiopathic" hyperprolactinemia.	Nausea and vomiting occur in up to 40% of subjects.

Table continued on following page

■ TABLE 26–6

Specific Provocative Tests of Hormonal Function *Continued*

TEST	DRUG AND DOSE	PURPOSE	HORMONES MEASURED AND MINIMAL SAMPLING TIMES	NORMAL RESPONSE	SPECIAL CONSIDERATIONS	SIDE EFFECTS
Clonidine	Clonidine hydrochloride 0.15 mg/m² PO (maximum, 0.2 mg)	Assessment of GH secretion	GH at 0, 60, 90, 120 min	Increase in GH to >10 ng/ml or of >5 ng/ml	Normal response of GH does not always occur in normal individuals.	Mild somnolence and hypotension
Insulin tolerance test[92, 118]	Regular insulin 0.05–0.15 unit/kg body weight (Dosage 0.1 unit/kg indicated in most; 0.05 if adrenal insufficiency strongly suspected and 0.15–0.20 if obese)	Assessment of GH status and the integrity of the hypothalamic-pituitary-adrenal axis	GH, cortisol, and glucose at 0, 20, 30, 45, 60, 90 min	Increase in GH to >10 ng/ml or of >5 ng/ml Increase in cortisol of >7 µg/dl or to >20/dl Decrease in glucose of >50% to <40 mg/dl	The test is safe as long as a medical attendant is present. Test results cannot be interpreted in the absence of the normal expected fall in glucose. Absence of any symptoms may suggest that adequate hypoglycemia did not occur. The patient should be fasted from midnight before the morning of the test.	Usually only transient perspiration, tachycardia, and nervousness. Palpitations, loss of consciousness, or a seizure should lead to prompt termination of the test by administration of 50% glucose IV.
Arginine tolerance test[92, 134, 135]	12.5% solution of arginine hydrochloride in sterile water at a dose of 500 mg/kg body weight (maximum, 30 gm) infused IV during 30 min	Assessment of GH secretion	GH at 0, 30, 60, 90 min	Increase in GH to >10 ng/ml or of >5 ng/ml	The test may be most effective when it is immediately followed by the insulin tolerance test.	May exacerbate acidosis in patients with renal failure and may be hazardous in those with liver disease.
Rapid screening dexamethasone[103, 106]	Dexamethasone 1 mg PO at 11:00 PM	Screening for nonsuppressible ACTH or cortisol production	Cortisol at 8:00 AM after dexamethasone	Cortisol <5 µg/dl	Abnormal suppression may be observed in some normal individuals and particularly in obesity and in psychiatric and other chronic and acute illnesses and during administration of an estrogen preparation.	None reported
Dexamethasone suppression[107]	Low dose: dexamethasone 0.5 mg q 6 hr × 48 hr beginning at 8:00 AM followed immediately by high dose: dexamethasone 2.0 mg q 6 hr × 48 hr	Evaluate the suppressibility of the pituitary-adrenal axis Specifically, the test is used to diagnose Cushing's syndrome and to attempt to determine its cause	24-hr urine samples for 17-OHCS, 17-KS, and creatinine or free cortisol and creatinine for at least 2 days before and each day of dexamethasone beginning at 8:00 AM Plasma cortisol may be measured each morning	**Low dose:** Decrease in 17-OHCS to <3 mg or to <50% of basal levels; plasma cortisol to <6 µg/dl; decrease in free cortisol to <20 µg/dl or to <50% of basal levels. **High dose:** Most patients with Cushing's disease (ACTH-dependent adrenocortical hyperplasia) suppress <50%. Failure to suppress is common in adrenal tumors, whereas patients with ectopic ACTH-producing tumors respond unpredictably.	Severely stressed individuals without endocrine disease may fail to respond to low-dose suppression. Paradoxical responses have been noted in patients with hypothalamic-pituitary axis dysfunction. This test may be useful in establishing congenital adrenal hyperplasia in patients with hirsutism when other test results are confusing. Prompt suppression should occur with low-dose dexamethasone.	None reported

Rapid ACTH (Cortrosyn)[106, 126]	ACTH 25 USP units or α^{1-24}-corticotropin 250 μg IV bolus	Screening test of adrenocortical function Also used to identify individuals with 21-hydroxylase deficiency	Cortisol at 0, 60, 120 min to assess adrenocortical function 17-Hydroxyprogesterone at 30 min to determine if 21-hydroxylase deficiency exists	Increase in cortisol of >7 μg/dl or to >20 μg/dl excludes adrenal insufficiency. In women who do not have 21-hydroxylase deficiency, values of 17-hydroxyprogesterone are typically <400 ng/dl. With classical deficiency, ≥3000 ng/dl; with nonclassic, ≥1500 ng/dl; heterozygote carriers achieve levels of about 1000 ng/dl.	In hirsute individuals who appear to have 21-hydroxylase deficiency, it is important to document that 17-hydroxyprogesterone is suppressed by dexamethasone (0.5 mg q 6 hr × 3 days).	None reported
ACTH infusion, 48 hr[117]	ACTH 40 USP units in 500 ml normal saline q 12 hr × 4 doses beginning at 8:00 AM	Assessment of adrenocortical function Identification of patients with primary and secondary adrenocortical insufficiency	Plasma cortisol at 8:00 AM and 8:00 PM until infusion completed 24-hr urine samples for 17-OHCS and creatinine for 1 day before test, during the 48-hr infusion, and for 1 day after infusion	Plasma cortisol >20 μg/dl and increase >7 μg/dl. Normal subjects increase 17-OHCS to >27 mg on day 1 and >47 mg on day 2. Patients with secondary adrenocortical insufficiency have 17-OHCS >4 mg on day 1 and >10 mg on day 2. With primary adrenocortical insufficiency, 17-OHCS are <3 mg on day 1 and <4 mg on day 2.	If a 10% overlap between primary and secondary adrenal insufficiency can be tolerated, the test can be shortened to 24 hr.	Some fluid retention occurs in most patients and is thought to be caused by trace contamination of the ACTH with ADH. Occasional hyperexcitation in some normal subjects is believed to be due to high levels of glucocorticoids.
Metyrapone[115, 119]	Metyrapone 750 mg PO every 4 hr × 6 doses beginning at 8:00 AM In children, 300 mg/m² body surface area PO q 4 hr × 6 doses Some give metyrapone 35 mg/kg body weight (to a maximum of 1 gm) IV in 250–500 ml saline during 4 hr with measurement of plasma 11-deoxycortisol to children[136]	Assessment of ACTH reserve Differential diagnosis of Cushing's syndrome	24-hr urine samples for 17-OHCS and creatinine basal and day of test and day after test Plasma cortisol at 8:00 AM before first dose and at 8:00 AM the following day	Increase in 17-OHCS by 2-fold or ≥10 mg/24 hr on day of or day after metyrapone. Those with "limited reserve" excrete ≥3 mg/24 hr in the basal state and ≥15 gm/24 hr in response to ACTH infusion. In the differential diagnosis of Cushing's syndrome, patients with Cushing's disease have an exaggerated response to metyrapone. Impaired or absent responses are seen in patients with adenoma or carcinoma of the adrenal. Plasma cortisol should fall to low levels to document 11β-hydroxylase blockade.	ACTH 50 USP units in 500 ml normal saline can be administered during 8 hr on the third day after metyrapone.[119] Plasma cortisol may be measured at 0, 4, and 8 hr. Numerous patients with Cushing's syndrome fail to show the "typical" responses.	Dizziness and nausea are frequent. Bed rest is of aid in alleviating these symptoms.

Table continued on following page

■ TABLE 26–6

Specific Provocative Tests of Hormonal Function *Continued*

TEST	DRUG AND DOSE	PURPOSE	HORMONES MEASURED AND MINIMAL SAMPLING TIMES	NORMAL RESPONSE	SPECIAL CONSIDERATIONS	SIDE EFFECTS
Dehydration[128]	Patients with mild polyuria or those who are normal are deprived of fluids from 6:00 PM before the test; those with marked polyuria are deprived from 7:00 AM. Patients are weighed at the start of dehydration and at least every 4 hr thereafter. Aqueous vasopressin (Pitressin) 5 units SC is injected when there is a change of <30 mOsm/kg between 2 consecutive collection periods	Assessment of posterior pituitary function by evaluation for vasopressin deficiency (diabetes insipidus)	Aliquots of urine for osmolality are collected at start of dehydration and hourly from 7:00 AM until 60 min after aqueous vasopressin Serum for electrolytes and osmolality at start of dehydration, at 7:00 AM day of testing, and just before vasopressin is given	A normal response is defined as a maximal urine osmolality that exceeds plasma osmolality after dehydration and does not increase ≥5% after vasopressin. Patients with diabetes insipidus cannot concentrate urine and increase urine osmolality >50% after vasopressin. Patients with partial diabetes insipidus may concentrate urine osmolality above plasma but have an increase >9% after vasopressin.	If there is any question about the patient's reliability, he or she should be observed throughout the test. The period required to establish constant urine osmolality in normal individuals is generally 16–18 hr and 4–18 hr in polyuric patients. The test is far safer than a saline load.	Severe dehydration is possible if the patient is not observed closely.
Clomiphene citrate challenge[137–139]	Clomiphene citrate 100 mg PO daily on days 5–9 of menstrual cycle If amenorrheic, menses can be induced with medroxyprogesterone acetate 5–10 mg PO × 5 days before testing	Assessment of ovarian reserve and probability of pregnancy in women ≥35 years	Serum FSH measured in morning on cycle days 3 and 10	The threshold value for FSH must be determined for each laboratory. Any value for FSH >95% confidence interval for premenopausal women is considered abnormal and has varied from 10–26 mIU/ml.	An abnormal test response does not preclude pregnancy. The test has only limited sensitivity because of age-related reduction in fertility independent of the test, but it appears specific. Some do not believe that the test is justified because it is so often in error.[140]	Ovarian hyperstimulation is exceedingly rare but possible.

even normal values may be observed in Cushing's syndrome, and values greater than 100 μg/day are common in obesity, depression, alcoholism, hypoglycemia, and chronic stress.

Determination of plasma cortisol levels in the basal state has been advocated as a method of establishing increased cortisol secretion. Absence of the normal diurnal variation in plasma cortisol levels often occurs before overt elevation of these levels.[103] Blood specimens should optimally be obtained at 8:00 AM and 12:00 midnight. Some clinicians suggest collecting blood samples at 30-minute intervals between 6:00 AM and 8:00 AM and between 10:00 PM and 12:00 midnight for the measurement of cortisol. Assuming a normal sleep-wake cycle, the mean evening value should be less than half the mean morning value. This is true because the plasma cortisol level varies widely in normal individuals from approximately 5 to 30 μg/100 ml at 8:00 AM and is generally reduced by more than 50 percent at midnight. Patients with Cushing's syndrome generally do not demonstrate the evening reduction in plasma cortisol. Cortisol levels are lower at midnight than they are earlier in the day.[104]

That the diurnal rhythm of plasma cortisol values may be "normal" in Cushing's syndrome has also been suggested by studies indicating that the normal episodic pulsatile secretion of cortisol is exaggerated in patients with the disease[105]; thus, an 8:00 AM sample obtained from a patient with Cushing's syndrome during a secretory burst of cortisol and a midnight sample obtained between secretory episodes might well show the "diurnal variation" characteristic of the normal subject. Despite such variations, a midnight sample of greater than 5 μg/100 ml is probably abnormal.

Elevated values are observed during pregnancy, during estrogen administration, and often during acute illness; the normal diurnal variation as determined by only two samples per day may be absent in some normal subjects, some obese individuals, and patients with severe acute and chronic disease. However, despite such limitations, the collection of such specimens in resting, pain-free patients is a valuable screening test.[103]

A simple screening suppression test may also be conducted on an outpatient basis.[103, 106] A specimen for plasma cortisol determination is obtained at 8:00 AM. The patient is then instructed to take 1 mg of dexamethasone by mouth between 11:00 PM and midnight. A second specimen for plasma cortisol is obtained the next morning at 8:00 AM. In normal individuals, the plasma cortisol levels generally fall to below 5 μg/100 ml after the dexamethasone, whereas they remain above 10 μg/100 ml in patients with Cushing's syndrome. Once again, abnormal values can be found in psychiatric (especially depression) and other chronic and acute illnesses and during the administration of estrogens or oral contraceptives.[103]

If the screening tests either confirm or strongly suggest the diagnosis of Cushing's syndrome, thorough evaluation is indicated to verify the diagnosis and to determine the etiology of the disorder. The dexamethasone suppression test as standardized by Liddle[107] is most commonly used to verify the diagnosis. Normal individuals, as opposed to those with Cushing's syndrome, will suppress adrenocorticosteroid production when they are given 2 mg of dexamethasone (0.5 mg four times per day) daily for 2 days ("low-dose" test). Conveniently, dexamethasone does not interfere with the estimation of corticosteroids, and normal subjects show falls of urinary 17-OHCS to values less than 3 mg/day or to less than 50 percent of basal levels to values approaching zero. Although this test can be performed on an outpatient basis in reliable patients, this cannot be recommended, because complete urine collections are difficult to obtain even from hospitalized patients. Therefore, it is best to decrease stress by requiring bed rest for the patient.

The availability of reliable corticotropin (ACTH) measurements by immunoassay and of corticotropin-releasing hormone (CRH) has led to a new approach to the differential diagnosis of Cushing's syndrome. Measurement of plasma ACTH concentrations offers the most reliable means of making the differential diagnosis and is the next logical step in the assessment of hypercortisolism. Studies indicate that values are high in patients without adrenal tumors, undetectable in patients with adrenal tumors, and normal or elevated in patients with pituitary neoplasms and the ectopic ACTH syndrome.[108] Thus, low values of ACTH point to adrenal disease, whereas normal or elevated values indicate that the hypercortisolism is ACTH dependent. If plasma ACTH levels are low or undetectable, primary adrenal disease should be sought by CT scanning of the adrenals. A factitious cause of Cushing's syndrome must also be considered.

If ACTH dependency is documented by the finding of normal or elevated ACTH levels, CRH (1 μg/kg intravenously during 1 minute) can be administered. Approximately 90 percent of ACTH-secreting pituitary tumors release increased quantities of ACTH in response to CRH. In contrast, individuals with extrapituitary ACTH-secreting neoplasms only rarely respond to CRH.[109, 110] Patients with normal or increased levels of ACTH who do not respond to CRH are still just as likely to have a pituitary adenoma as an ectopic ACTH-producing tumor as the cause of the Cushing's syndrome because Cushing's disease is far more common than ectopic ACTH-producing neoplasms. In patients not responding to CRH, inferior petrosal sinus sampling for ACTH can localize the site of ACTH production if radiographic studies of the sella turcica fail to reveal an adenoma and radiographic studies of the chest also fail to demonstrate any tumor.

Blood sampling of the right and left inferior petrosal sinuses permits measurement of ACTH concentrations in blood immediately draining from the pituitary gland.[111] A marked gradient or "step-up" from concentrations in the peripheral blood stream is seen in patients with pituitary ACTH excess, whereas the maximal gradient seen in patients with a paraneoplastic source of ACTH is close to 1.0. The test also allows lateralization of any pituitary microadenoma before surgery in the absence of radiographic evidence of a neoplasm. This procedure is not readily available, however, and it should be performed only by individuals experienced in the technique.

Most ectopic ACTH-producing neoplasms are localized to the chest. Simple radiographs may fail to detect a small neoplasm, and consequently CT or MRI scanning should be used.

If reliable measurements of plasma ACTH cannot be

obtained, the "high-dose" dexamethasone suppression test (2 mg four times per day for 2 days immediately after low-dose suppression) should be used in an attempt to differentiate among the various causes of the disease.[107] Most patients with Cushing's disease (pituitary-dependent adrenocortical hyperplasia) will show at least 50 percent suppression of plasma or urinary corticosteroids, or both. Patients with adrenal tumors do not suppress adequately even with this high dose, and patients with ACTH-producing tumors of nonendocrine organs have unpredictable responses to ACTH. However, no suppression, or even a paradoxical increase in corticosteroids, has also been observed in patients with hypothalamic-pituitary-adrenal axis dysfunction; consequently, as in all the commonly employed tests, the reliability of high-dose dexamethasone is not great.[112, 113]

Stimulation with ACTH[114] and stimulation with metyrapone[115] have also been extensively used as discriminatory tests, with widely varying success. In brief, most patients with Cushing's disease without adrenal tumor show exaggerated responses of plasma cortisol to intravenous ACTH, and metyrapone administration often provokes an excessive rise in urinary 17-OHCS in individuals with "bilateral adrenal hyperplasia" with little or no rise in patients with adrenocortical tumors. The metyrapone test, however, is more useful as a test of pituitary ACTH reserve than it is as an aid in the differential diagnosis of Cushing's syndrome.

ADRENOCORTICAL HYPOFUNCTION

Adrenocortical insufficiency may be primary, resulting from destruction of the adrenal glands themselves (Addison's disease), or secondary, resulting from impaired hypothalamic or pituitary function with consequent diminished ACTH secretion and adrenocortical atrophy. Although hypoadrenalism may be partial or complete, or acute or chronic, the reproductive endocrinologist almost always will be concerned with detecting subtle abnormalities in patients with a proven or suspected pituitary tumor. Two practical screening tests exist. The simpler and more convenient procedure involves the rapid intravenous injection of ACTH (25 USP units) or α^{1-24}-corticotropin (250 μg). α^{1-24}-Corticotropin is a synthetic subunit of ACTH with complete biologic and steroidogenic activity. Blood samples for cortisol are obtained before ACTH injection and 60 and 120 minutes after injection. Although results vary among laboratories, if the plasma corticosteroids rise by more than 7 μg/100 ml or to a level above 20 μg/100 ml, a diagnosis of Addison's disease can be excluded.[106] The second screening procedure involves the serial collection of 24-hour urine specimens for 17-OHCS and creatinine. Values of 2.0 mg 17-OHCS per gram of creatinine per 24 hours or less strongly suggest adrenocortical hypofunction.

Numerous other tests assessing the adequacy of adrenocortical reserve have been used. Those tests that are described here appear to be of most value. The use of synthetic CRH, which is discussed in further detail in Table 26–6, has not proved to be of great value in discriminating between secondary adrenocortical insufficiency of hypothalamic and of pituitary origin.[116]

Rose and colleagues[117] suggested the use of a continuous 48-hour infusion of ACTH (40 units every 12 hours) to distinguish among normal adrenocortical function and primary and secondary adrenocortical insufficiency. Although the investigators initially also determined plasma cortisol and urinary 17-KS values, they concluded that urinary 17-OHCS values were the most discriminating. Details of the test may be found in Table 26–6.

The accurate measurement of basal ACTH concentrations may be the most accurate method of determining the cause of adrenal insufficiency. High concentrations of ACTH localize the problem to the adrenal gland, whereas normal or low concentrations of ACTH imply a hypothalamic or pituitary defect.[117]

Insulin-induced hypoglycemia, which generally results in a detectable rise in plasma corticosteroids 40 to 60 minutes after intravenous injection of 0.1 unit per kilogram body weight of regular insulin, is thought by many to be the most reliable of the various tests aimed at assessing the integrity of the hypothalamic-pituitary-adrenal axis.[118] The normal response is regarded as a minimal rise in plasma cortisol of 7 μg/100 ml, or to a value of greater than 20 μg/100 ml, provided that blood glucose has been suppressed by 50 percent or more. Hypoglycemic side effects are common, however, and the test is not entirely safe in a variety of clinical states (see Table 26–6).

Metyrapone, a drug that prevents 11β-hydroxylation, can be used to block cortisol and corticosterone synthesis. In normal individuals, this blockade prevents feedback inhibition of ACTH by cortisol, resulting in increased release of ACTH and additional stimulation of the adrenal gland. Because cortisol cannot be produced in the presence of metyrapone, 11-deoxycortisol secretion is increased. The excessive production of this compound can be followed in the plasma or, more easily, in the urine by measurement of 17-OHCS, because the metabolites of 11-deoxycortisol are included among such substances.[115] Several variations have been proposed, but oral administration for 24 hours remains the preferred method for producing maximal, although incomplete, inhibition of 11β-hydroxylation.[115] Metyrapone tests only the steroid-suppressible control mechanism, and thus stressful situations may cause release of ACTH even in patients failing to respond.[115] As proposed by Liddle,[119] an ACTH stimulation test is generally performed on the last day of the test to distinguish adrenal from hypothalamic-pituitary insufficiency. However, the response is reduced below normal levels or absent in patients with hypoadrenalism or hypopituitarism. Diminished responses to metyrapone are often observed in cases of pregnancy, hyperthyroidism, myxedema, and pseudotumor cerebri and in patients taking oral contraceptives and phenytoin.[120]

Some additional comments are warranted. Cortisol response to stress can be evaluated in patients taking dexamethasone; thus, the insulin tolerance test can be used to evaluate adrenocortical function in patients receiving steroids for questionable reasons. In patients with documented tumors involving the sellar region who are undergoing CT scanning with contrast injection, blood samples for plasma cortisol obtained before and during the procedure can provide an excellent test of the adrenal axis.[121] Coverage of the patient with dexamethasone during the test will not interfere with this test of pituitary-adrenal function.

In the event that a patient is acutely ill with hypotension, anorexia, weight loss, and weakness, it may be most desirable to proceed with therapy for Addison's disease immediately, rather than to institute a battery of diagnostic tests. In such cases, a sample of venous blood for determination of serum cortisol should be obtained, and a 24-hour collection of 17-OHCS and creatinine should be instituted. The patient should then be given 4 mg of dexamethasone immediately and should be maintained with that steroid while a 48-hour ACTH infusion test is conducted (see Table 26–6). Additional intravenous fluids should be given as indicated for management of shock and dehydration. No cortisone or hydrocortisone should be given, because these compounds are included in measurements of serum cortisol and urinary 17-OHCS.

Evaluation of Hirsutism

Numerous suppression and stimulation tests have been proposed as means of identifying the adrenal gland or the ovary as the site of excess androgen production in masculinizing syndromes and attempting to predict the outcome of long-term therapy. Virtually all tests that have been used to date fail to discriminate reliably between the adrenal gland and the ovary in virilized individuals. For example, ACTH and hCG may stimulate and dexamethasone may suppress steroid production by both glands. In addition, measurement of androgenic steroids in either serum or urine also fails as a method of determining the etiology of the disorder. Even pathologic documentation of the existence of polycystic ovaries fails to prove a primary ovarian etiology, because the ovaries respond to any excess androgen in this characteristic manner. However, it has been claimed that agonists of luteinizing hormone–releasing hormone (GnRH) will suppress only ovarian androgen production.[122]

The most logical approach for the clinician evaluating the hirsute woman is to attempt to formulate a presumptive diagnosis on the basis of the clinical findings and then to document the correctness of this diagnosis with the aid of laboratory tests. The history and clinical findings, especially concerning the progression of the disease, are most important in this regard. Measurement of the appropriate steroid hormone concentrations can then aid in confirming one's suspicions.

In women with hirsutism, it is essential that Cushing's syndrome, congenital adrenal hyperplasia, and adrenal and ovarian neoplasms be excluded. In most cases, this can easily be done at the bedside alone. A random sample for measurement of serum testosterone and dehydroepiandrosterone sulfate (DHEA-S) concentrations should be obtained from all women with hirsutism. If the serum testosterone level is greater than 200 ng/100 ml, then the possibility of an ovarian androgen-producing neoplasm should be considered. Values of testosterone greater than 80 ng/100 ml but less than 200 ng/100 ml are commonly associated with benign processes, but at least periodic reassessment at 3- to 6-month intervals is warranted to identify those few patients with progressive disorders. If the serum DHEA-S level is more than twice normal, then the possibility of an adrenal neoplasm must be entertained. CT scanning or MRI will diagnose an adrenal tumor in almost all cases. Pelvic ultrasonography will visualize most virilizing ovarian tumors because these tend to be large. Percutaneous venous catheterization of the ovarian and adrenal vessels with measurement of androgenic steroids from each site is now rarely needed to localize a neoplasm before surgery and should be carried out only by experienced radiologists.

Because the reason for measuring testosterone and DHEA-S is to rule out any serious cause for hirsutism, there is no need for extensive testing if neither testosterone nor DHEA-S is elevated markedly. In addition, because the patient serves as her own bioassay, the fact that the patient is hirsute makes the measurement of biologically active free testosterone unnecessary. Yet some clinicians measure free rather than total testosterone levels because free testosterone levels are more sensitive indicators of increased androgen secretion and action. Some clinicians have also suggested measuring 3α-androstanediol glucuronide levels as a marker of androgen action in peripheral tissues such as skin.[123] Again, there seems little need to measure this hormone in hirsute women. It is clear that androgen action in the periphery must be increased in women with idiopathic hirsutism who do not have increased secretion of androgens. It has become clear that idiopathic hirsutism represents enhanced androgen action and metabolism at the hair follicle.[123]

Because Cushing's syndrome and congenital adrenal hyperplasia can generally be eliminated at the bedside on the basis of the physical findings, estimates of cortisol secretion need be obtained only if Cushing's syndrome is suspected clinically.

Some clinicians also advocate measurement of 17-hydroxyprogesterone in all women with hirsutism. There is no doubt that this hormone is the single best test for diagnosing congenital adrenal hyperplasia due to 21-hydroxylase deficiency. Routine measurement of this hormone may be of value in populations at high risk of nonclassic adult-onset 21-hydroxylase deficiency (see Chapter 18). However, because of the low incidence of this disorder in most populations (perhaps 1 to 5 percent of hirsute women),[124, 125] 17-hydroxyprogesterone need be measured in most populations only in women with features characteristic of nonclassic congenital adrenal hyperplasia, including severe hirsutism beginning at puberty, height shorter than other family members, flattening of the breasts on physical examination (i.e., defeminization), and increased DHEA-S levels of between 5.0 and 7.0 μg/ml, or in those with a strong family history of hirsutism (Fig. 26–20).

In women with regular cyclic menses, it is important to measure 17-hydroxyprogesterone only in the follicular phase because levels normally increase at midcycle and in the luteal phase (see Chapter 7). Circulating 17-hydroxyprogesterone levels vary throughout the day and are highest in the morning. Plasma levels should be less than 200 ng/dl in normal women. Most patients with 21-hydroxylase deficiency have levels of at least 1000 ng/dl. Even if basal 17-hydroxyprogesterone levels are normal, ACTH testing is indicated in individuals suspected of having this enzyme deficiency.

Determination of 17-hydroxyprogesterone 30 minutes after intravenous injection of 250 μg of synthetic $^{1-24}$ACTH is the most commonly used diagnostic test[126] (Fig. 26–21; see Table 26–6). Because 17-hydroxyprogesterone may be secreted in excess by virilizing ovarian and adrenal neo-

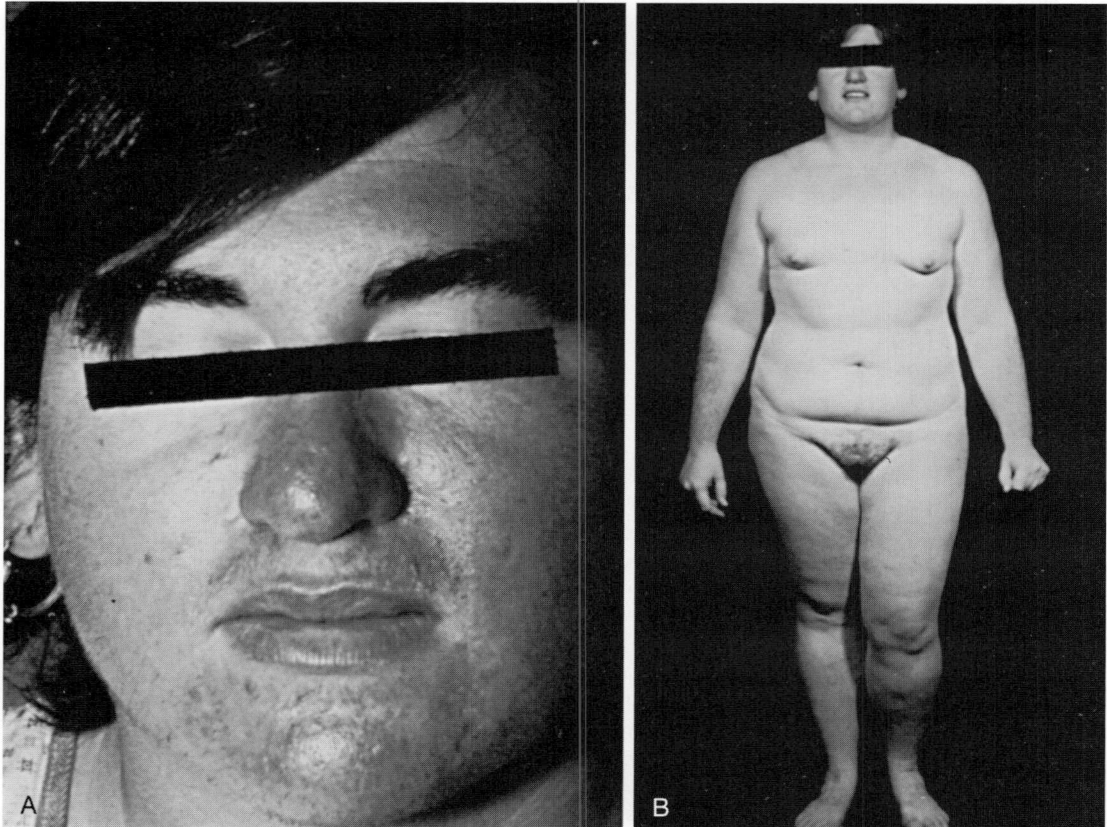

Figure 26–20 ■ A 19-year-old woman with secondary amenorrhea and hirsutism with "nonclassic" adult-onset 21-hydroxylase deficiency. Note the oiliness of her skin, the acne, hirsutism, and plethora *(A)* as well as the flattening of the breasts and unusual habitus *(B)*.

plasms, it is important to show that plasma levels of 17-hydroxyprogesterone are suppressed by dexamethasone (0.5 mg four times per day for 3 days).

The diagnosis of nonclassic congenital adrenal hyperplasia can be confirmed by human leukocyte antigen (HLA) studies.[126] Family studies of patients with symptomatic nonclassic 21-hydroxylase deficiency have documented that this disorder is HLA-linked and is in strong genetic disequilibrium with HLA-B14 sometimes together with disequilibrium in HLA-Bw47.

Similarly, the diagnosis of the much less common 11-hydroxylase deficiency is made by documenting increased circulating concentrations of 11-deoxycortisol. Because this steroid may be secreted in excess by some adrenal neoplasms, it is necessary to distinguish the 11-hydroxylase form of congenital adrenal hyperplasia from tumors by documenting that suppression with dexamethasone lowers 11-deoxycortisol levels into the normal range.

Once serious causes of hirsutism have been eliminated, the clinician has performed only the first of two difficult tasks. The second involves treating the hirsutism, which is difficult at best. What is true is that the site of androgen excess and the response to various dynamic tests do not seem to influence the success of the various treatment modalities.

Evaluation of Posterior Pituitary Function

Although the neurohypophysis is known to secrete two cyclic octapeptides, vasopressin (or antidiuretic hormone [ADH]) and oxytocin, no disease process has yet been associated with oxytocin excess or deficiency. In contrast, diabetes insipidus (vasopressin deficiency) and inappropriate secretion of ADH (vasopressin excess) are well-established disorders.

Diabetes insipidus is characterized by polyuria (of 2.5 L or more per 24 hours) and polydipsia, with as much as 20 to 25 L of urine excreted daily. Fluid restriction leads to insatiable thirst and dehydration. Because normal glucocorticoid function is required to excrete a water load, it is necessary to evaluate adrenocortical function and institute replacement therapy, if necessary, before testing for the possible existence of diabetes insipidus.

Although diabetes insipidus of central origin must be distinguished from nephrogenic diabetes insipidus, and although a large proportion of all cases are idiopathic, the majority of cases are associated with primary or metastatic tumors of the neurohypophyseal area or with a variety of lesions, including trauma, sarcoidosis, meningitis, and Langerhans cell–type histiocytosis, or occur after intracranial surgery. In addition, partial diabetes insipidus may be associated with anorexia nervosa.[11]

After high pituitary stalk section in humans (as may occur at hypophysectomy), a triphasic response is frequently observed in patients developing diabetes insipidus.[127] First, polyuria and polydipsia commence, generally lasting 4 to 5 days. This is followed by a period of intense antidiuresis of approximately 1 week's duration. Finally, a permanent diabetes insipidus may or may not result, de-

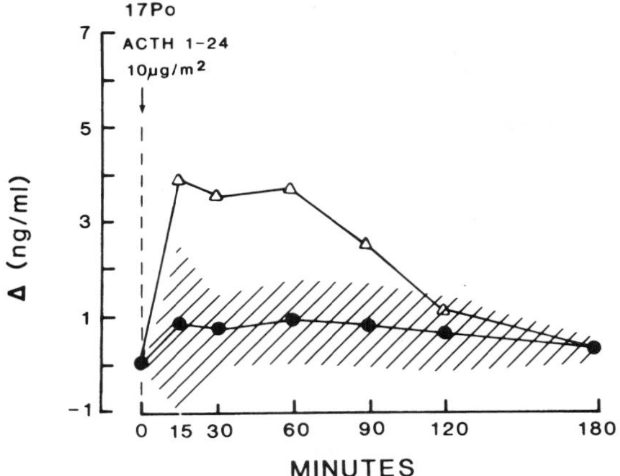

Figure 26–21 ■ Testing with corticotropin (ACTH$^{1-24}$) in the patient depicted in Figure 26–20. In this case a very small dose of corticotropin was given as an intravenous bolus of 10 μg/m^2 following dexamethasone suppression. The increase (Δ) in 17-hydroxyprogesterone (17 Po) in ng/ml was greater than two standard deviations *(shaded area)* of the increase observed in normal women in the early follicular phase of the menstrual cycle. The patient's responses are indicated by open triangles and the mean of responses in normal women by the closed circles. The ACTH$^{1-24}$ was administered at time 0.

pending on the extent of permanent damage. It is generally agreed that the initial diuretic phase results from acute damage to hypothalamic function, so that stored hormone is not released. The second antidiuretic phase is thought to result from degeneration of neurohypophyseal cells containing vasopressin, with release of the contained hormone.

The majority of cases seen by the reproductive endocrinologist will have concurrent evidence of hypothalamic or anterior pituitary dysfunction or will occur after hypophysectomy. In such cases, the diagnosis is frequently obvious by history alone. If diabetes insipidus exists, failure to treat with available preparations of vasopressin can lead to permanent renal damage. Recognition of partial defects and confirmation of cases of complete diabetes insipidus can still be best established by the dehydration test.[128] Details of this procedure are given in Table 26–6. Infusion of hypertonic saline can also be used to document diabetes insipidus, but this test is more dangerous than is dehydration.[129]

The increasing availability and use of sensitive and specific immunoassays capable of detecting physiologically low circulating concentrations of ADH simplify the diagnosis of diabetes insipidus. It appears that the measurement of plasma ADH in the basal state is of little diagnostic value, but measurement after osmotic stimulation by fluid deprivation or infusion of hypertonic saline may be of diagnostic value.[130] After dehydration or hypertonic saline infusion, individuals with compulsive psychogenic water drinking (sometimes termed primary polydipsia) and nephrogenic diabetes insipidus have plasma ADH and plasma osmolality values that fall within (or even above) the normal range. In contrast, individuals with central diabetes fail to have any appreciable increase in ADH levels with osmotic stimulation.

Vasopressin excess resulting in a state of hyponatremia with normal blood urea nitrogen, a competent circulatory system, considerable quantities of sodium in the urine, and no edema was first noted in patients with bronchogenic carcinoma.[131] This syndrome of inappropriate ADH secretion has since been observed in several clinical conditions, most of which involve pulmonary or intracranial lesions. Although rare, it has been observed in patients with tumors in the hypothalamic or pituitary area and must be distinguished from acute adrenocortical insufficiency. Although strict limitation of fluid intake will correct all the physiologic disturbances of this syndrome despite persistent excess antidiuretic activity, glucocorticoids are essential for treatment of adrenal failure.

SUMMARY: THE APPROACH TO THE AMENORRHEIC WOMAN

As described here, a detailed history and a thorough physical examination are of paramount importance in the evaluation of any amenorrheic patient. Diagnostic tests should be used to confirm the suspected diagnosis or to differentiate among likely possibilities. It is useful to think of the patient as a bioassay subject in whom even subtle hormonal alterations may be manifested by obvious signs and symptoms. Central to the consideration of the patient as a bioassay subject is an evaluation of the individual with regard to puberty and to the influence of altered hormonal secretion on the pubertal process. The simple classification of Marshall and Tanner[1] thus provides a framework for the initial examination. The use of progestational (and estrogenic) agents to induce withdrawal bleeding is of diagnostic use only in women in whom uterine end organ failure is a possibility.

One approach to the laboratory evaluation of amenorrheic and anovulatory woman is outlined in Figure 26–22. Measurements of basal concentrations of FSH, prolactin, and TSH in the circulation appear indicated in all amenorrheic individuals. Clearly, it is important to exclude pregnancy at the outset in any amenorrheic woman. If the physical findings are not conclusive, the sensitive pregnancy tests available today should provide a definitive answer. The fact that hCG cross-reacts with LH in all LH immunoassays also means immunoassayable LH levels will be markedly elevated in all but the earliest pregnancies.

Increased TSH concentrations (generally greater than 5 μU/ml) with or without increased levels of prolactin indicate primary hypothyroidism. The increased secretion of TRH present in this disorder stimulates increased secretion of prolactin as well as of TSH in many affected women.

If thyroid function is normal and basal prolactin levels are *persistently* elevated, then further evaluation is warranted to rule out a pituitary adenoma.

Increased FSH concentrations (generally greater than 30 mIU/ml) imply ovarian "failure." Chromosomal evaluation is warranted in young women (certainly younger than 30 years) with this disorder to rule out a chromosome abnormality. Gonadectomy is warranted in individuals with a Y chromosome complement because of the malignant potential of abnormal gonads endowed with a portion of a Y chromosome (see Chapter 14).

If prolactin, TSH, and FSH levels are either within the normal range or low, then further evaluation should be based on the clinical presentation. Here one is attempting

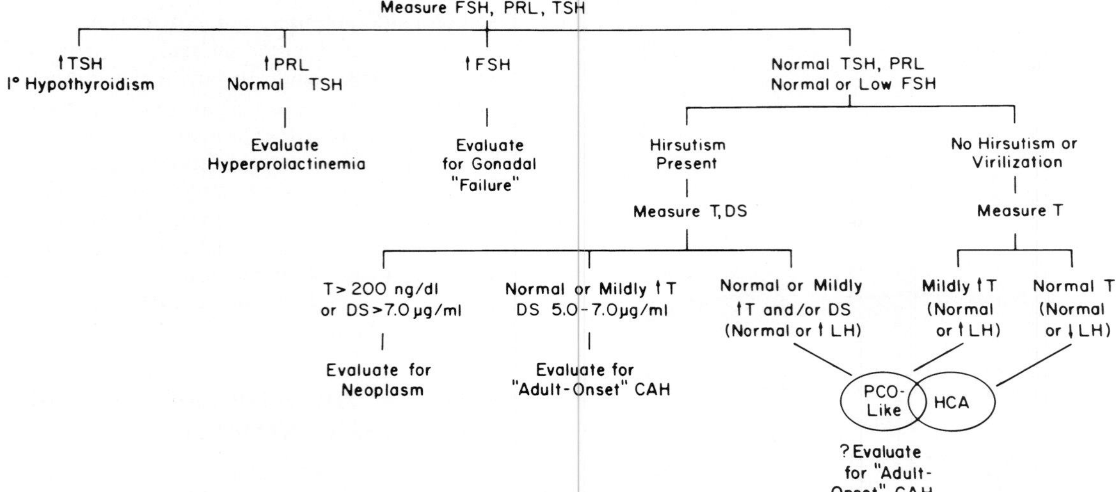

Figure 26–22 ■ Flow diagram for the laboratory evaluation of amenorrhea. Such a scheme must be considered as an adjunct to the clinical evaluation of the patient (see text). FSH, follicle-stimulating hormone; PRL, prolactin; TSH, thyroid-stimulating hormone; CAH, congenital adrenal hyperplasia; PCO, polycystic ovary syndrome; LH, luteinizing hormone; HCA, hypothalamic chronic anovulation; DS, dehydroepiandrosterone sulfate; T, testosterone. (From Rebar RW. The ovaries. *In* Wyngaarden JB, Smith LH Jr, Bennett JC [eds]. Cecil Textbook of Medicine, 19th ed. Philadelphia, WB Saunders, 1992, p 1367.)

to distinguish between PCOS-like disorders and hypothalamic-pituitary dysfunction. Circulating thyroid hormone levels should be determined if there is evidence of hyperthyroidism because of low TSH levels. One can argue for the measurement of total testosterone in women who are not hirsute but who have a history and clinical picture otherwise compatible with PCOS (see Chapter 17). Not all hyperandrogenic women are hirsute owing to relative insensitivity of the hair follicles to androgen in some women. Moreover, alterations in the metabolic clearance rates of androgens and in the concentrations of sex hormone–binding globulin in PCOS probably reduce the chances of hirsutism in individuals with decreased sensitivity to androgen. Circulating concentrations of LH may also aid in distinguishing PCOS from hypothalamic-pituitary dysfunction or failure. LH levels are frequently, but not always, increased in PCOS such that the ratio of LH to FSH is also increased.[63] In contrast, levels of LH and FSH tend to be normal or slightly reduced in women with hypothalamic-pituitary dysfunction. Thus, as shown in Figure 26–16, there is some overlap in laboratory values between women with PCOS-like disorders and those with hypothalamic-pituitary dysfunction, most commonly hypothalamic chronic anovulation.

As noted previously, radiographic studies of the sella turcica are indicated in all amenorrheic women in whom both LH and FSH levels are low (generally less than 10 mIU/ml) to exclude a pituitary or a hypothalamic lesion, regardless of whether or not prolactin levels are increased. Obviously, pituitary testing, especially of adrenal and thyroid function, is warranted whenever panhypopituitarism is suspected. The evaluation of hirsute women should proceed as delineated previously.

More detailed diagnostic studies are based on the results of the initial investigations. The determination of the etiology of the amenorrhea should always begin with the patient and not in the laboratory and should facilitate rational treatment.

References

1. Marshall WA, Tanner JM. Variations in patterns of pubertal changes in girls. Arch Dis Child 44:291, 1969.
2. Kaplan SL, Grumbach MM. Pathogenesis of sexual precocity. *In* Grumbach MM, Sizonenko PC, Aubert ML (eds). Control of the Onset of Puberty. Baltimore, Williams & Wilkins, 1990, p 620.
3. Rosen D, Kelch RP. Precocious and delayed puberty. *In* Becker KL, et al (eds). Principles and Practice of Endocrinology and Metabolism, 2nd ed. Philadelphia, JB Lippincott, 1995, p 830.
4. VanWyk JJ, Grumbach MM. Syndrome of precocious menstruation and galactorrhea in juvenile hypothyroidism: An example of hormonal overlap in pituitary feedback. J Pediatr 57:416, 1960.
5. Speiser PW. Congenital adrenal hyperplasia. *In* Becker KL, et al (eds). Principles and Practice of Endocrinology and Metabolism, 2nd ed. Philadelphia, JB Lippincott, 1995, p 686.
6. Simpson JL, Rebar RW. Normal and abnormal sexual differentiation and development. *In* Becker KL, et al (eds). Principles and Practice of Endocrinology and Metabolism, 2nd ed. Philadelphia, JB Lippincott, 1995, p 788.
7. Damewood MD, Grochow LB. Prospects for fertility after chemotherapy or radiation for neoplastic disease. Fertil Steril 45:443, 1986.
8. Sheehan HL, Davis JC. Pituitary necrosis. Br Med Bull 24:59, 1968.
9. Feicht CB, Johnson TS, Martin BJ, et al. Secondary amenorrhea in athletes. Lancet 2:1145, 1978.
10. Schwartz B, Cumming DC, Riordan E, et al. Exercise-associated amenorrhea: A distinct entity? Am J Obstet Gynecol 141:662, 1981.
11. Mecklenburg RJ, Loriaux DL, Thompson RH, et al. Hypothalamic dysfunction in patients with anorexia nervosa. Medicine (Baltimore) 53:147, 1974.
12. Asherman JG. Amenorrhea traumatica (atretica). J Obstet Gynecol Br Emp 55:23, 1948.
13. Rebar RW, Connolly HV. Clinical features of young women with hypergonadotropic amenorrhea. Fertil Steril 53:804, 1990.
14. Rebar RW, Cedars MI. Hypergonadotropic forms of amenorrhea in young women. Endocrinol Metab Clin North Am 21:173, 1992.
15. Molitch ME, Reichlin S. Hyperprolactinemic disorders. Dis Mon 28:1, 1982.
16. Ferriman D, Gallwey JD. Clinical assessment of body hair growth in women. J Clin Endocrinol Metab 21:1440, 1961.
17. Bardin CW, Lipsett MB. Testosterone and androstenedione blood production rates in normal women and women with idiopathic hirsutism or polycystic ovaries. J Clin Invest 46:891, 1967.

18. Silver HK. Asymmetry, short stature, and variations in sexual development. Am J Dis Child 107:495, 1964.
19. Klein D, Ammann F. The syndrome of Laurence-Moon-Bardet-Biedl and allied diseases in Switzerland: Clinical, genetic and epidemiological studies. J Neurol Sci 9:479, 1969.
20. Braunstein GD, Whitaker JN, Kohler PO. Cerebellar dysfunction in Hand-Schüller-Christian disease. Arch Intern Med 132:387, 1973.
21. Tagatz GE, Kopher RA, Nagel TC, Okagaki T. The clitoral index: A bioassay of androgenic stimulation. Obstet Gynecol 54:562, 1979.
22. Papanicolaou GN. The sexual cycle in the human female as revealed by vaginal smears. Am J Anat 52:519, 1933.
23. Weid GL, Boschann H-W, Ferin J, et al. Symposium on hormonal cytology. Acta Cytol 12:87, 1968.
24. Rakoff AE. Hormonal cytology in gynecology. Clin Obstet Gynecol 4:1045, 1961.
25. Collett-Solberg PR, Grumbach MM. A simplified procedure for evaluating estrogenic effects and the sex chromatin pattern in exfoliated cells in urine. Studies in premature thelarche and gynecomastia of adolescence. J Pediatr 66:883, 1965.
26. Boyers SP. Evaluation and treatment of disorders of the cervix. *In* Keye WR Jr, Chang JR, Rebar RW, Soules MR (eds). Infertility. Evaluation and Treatment. Philadelphia, WB Saunders, 1995, pp 195–229.
27. Moghissi KS, Syner FN, Evans TN. A composite picture of the menstrual cycle. Am J Obstet Gynecol 114:405, 1972.
28. Greulich WW, Pyle SI. Radiographic Atlas of Skeletal Development of the Hand and Wrist, 2nd ed. London, Oxford University Press, 1959.
29. Bayley N, Pinneau SR. Tables for predicting adult height from skeletal age: Revised for use with the Greulich-Pyle hand standards. J Pediatr 40:423, 1952.
30. Johnston CC Jr, Melton LJ III. Bone density measurement and the management of osteoporosis. *In* Favus MJ (ed). Primer on the Metabolic Bone Diseases and Disorders of Mineral Metabolism, 2nd ed. New York, Raven Press, 1993, p 137.
31. Genant HK, Block JE, Steiger P, et al. Appropriate use of bone densitometry. Radiology 170:817, 1989.
32. Health and Public Policy Committee of the American College of Physicians. Radiologic methods to evaluate bone mineral content. Ann Intern Med 100:908, 1984.
33. Delmas PD. Markers of bone formation and resorption. *In* Favus MJ (ed). Primer on the Metabolic Bone Diseases and Disorders of Mineral Metabolism, 2nd ed. New York, Raven Press, 1993, p 108.
34. Parsons AK. Detection and surveillance of endometrial hyperplasia/carcinoma. *In* Lobo RA (ed). Treatment of the Postmenopausal Woman: Basic and Clinical Aspects. New York, Raven Press, 1994, p 385.
35. Oehler M, Chakeres D. Diagnostic imaging of the sellar region. *In* Becker KL, et al (eds). Principles and Practice of Endocrinology and Metabolism, 2nd ed. Philadelphia, JB Lippincott, 1995, p 207.
36. Taylor S. High resolution computed tomography of the sella. Radiol Clin North Am 20:207, 1982.
37. Daniels DL, Haughton VM, Naidich T (eds). Cranial and Spinal Magnetic Resonance Imaging: Atlas and Guide. St. Louis, CV Mosby, 1988.
38. Sheline GE. Untreated and recurrent chromaphobe adenomas of the pituitary. Radiology 12:768, 1971.
39. Weisberg LA. Asymptomatic enlargement of the sella turcica. Arch Neurol 32:483, 1975.
40. Yalow RS, Berson SA. Immunoassay of endogenous plasma insulin in man. J Clin Invest 39:1157, 1960.
41. Midgley AR Jr, Niswender GD, Rebar RW. Principles for the assessment of the reliability of radioimmunoassay methods (precision, accuracy, sensitivity, specificity). Acta Endocrinol Suppl 142:163, 1969.
42. Rodbard D. Statistical quality control and routine data processing for radioimmunoassays (RIA) and immunoradiometric assays (IRMA). Clin Chem 20:1255, 1974.
43. Kane KK, Kelly WG. Chemical measurements of 17-ketosteroids and 17-ketogenic steroids. *In* Sunderman FW, Sunderman FW Jr (eds). Laboratory Diagnosis of Endocrine Disease. St. Louis, Warren H. Green, 1971, p 510.
44. Korenman SG, Kirschner MA, Lipsett MB. Testosterone production in normal and virilized women and in women with the Stein-Leventhal syndrome or idiopathic hirsutism. J Clin Endocrinol Metab 25:798, 1965.
45. Lipsett MB, Wilson H, Kirschner MA, et al. Studies on Leydig cell physiology and pathology: Secretion and metabolism of testosterone. Recent Prog Horm Res 22:245, 1966.
46. Bardin CW, Kirschner MA. The clinical usefulness of testosterone measurements in virilizing syndromes in women. *In* Sunderman FW, Sunderman FW Jr (eds). Laboratory Diagnosis of Endocrine Disease. St. Louis, Warren H. Green, 171, p 559.
47. Peterson RE. The miscible pool and turnover rate of adrenocortical steroids in man. Recent Prog Horm Res 15:23, 1959.
48. Franks RC. Urinary 17-hydroxycorticosteroid and cortisol excretion in childhood. J Clin Endocrinol Metab 36:702, 1973.
49. Harsoulis P, Marshall JC, Kuku SF, et al. Combined test for assessment of anterior pituitary function. Br Med J 4:326, 1973.
50. Rakoff J, VandenBerg G, Siler TM, Yen SSC. An integrated direct functional test of the adenohypophysis. Am J Obstet Gynecol 119:358, 1974.
51. Sheldon WR Jr, DeBold CR, Evans WS, et al. Rapid sequential intravenous administration of four hypothalamic releasing hormones as a combined anterior pituitary function test in normal subjects. J Clin Endocrinol Metab 60:623, 1985.
52. Dufau ML, Mendelson CR, Catt KJ. A highly sensitive in vitro bioassay for luteinizing hormone and chorionic gonadotropin: Testosterone production by dispersed Leydig cells. J Clin Endocrinol Metab 39:610, 1974.
53. Jia XC, Hsueh AJ. Granulosa cell aromatase bioassay for follicle-stimulating hormone: Validation and application of the method. Endocrinology 199:1570, 1986.
54. Ross GT. Biological methods for the measurement of gonadotropin in man and their clinical application. *In* Sunderman FW, Sunderman FW Jr (eds). Laboratory Diagnosis of Endocrine Disease. St. Louis, Warren H. Green, 1971, p 138.
55. Vaitukaitis JL, Braunstein GD, Ross GT. A radioimmunoassay which specifically measures human chorionic gonadotropin in the presence of human luteinizing hormone. Am J Obstet Gynecol 113:751, 1972.
56. Kadar N, DeCherney AH, Romero R. Receiver operating serial chorionic gonadotropin determinations in the early diagnosis of ectopic pregnancy. Fertil Steril 37:542, 1982.
57. Ryan RY. A comparison of biologic and immunologic potency estimates of human luteinizing (LH) and follicle stimulating (FSH) hormones. Acta Endocrinol Suppl 142:300, 1969.
58. Hansen JW, Hoffman PG, Ross GT. Monthly gonadotropin cycles in premenarcheal girls. Science 190:161, 1975.
59. Yen SSC, Vela P, Rankin J. Inappropriate secretion of follicle-stimulating hormone and luteinizing hormone in polycystic ovarian disease. J Clin Endocrinol Metab 30:435, 1970.
60. Judd HL, Hamilton CR, Barlow JJ, et al. Androgen and gonadotropin dynamics in testicular feminization syndrome. J Clin Endocrinol Metab 34:229, 1972.
61. Rebar R, Judd HL, Yen SSC, et al. Characterization of the inappropriate gonadotropin secretion in polycystic ovary syndrome. J Clin Invest 57:1320, 1976.
62. Snyder PJ, Sterling FH. Hypersecretion of LH and FSH by a pituitary adenoma. J Clin Endocrinol Metab 42:544, 1976.
63. Rebar RW, Yen SSC, VandenBerg G, et al. Gonadotropin responses to synthetic LRF: Dose-response relationship in men. J Clin Endocrinol Metab 36:10, 1973.
64. Yen SSC, Rebar R, VandenBerg G, et al. Pituitary gonadotropin responsiveness to synthetic LRF in subjects with normal and abnormal hypothalamic-pituitary-gonadal axis. J Reprod Fertil 20:137, 1973.
65. Yen SSC, VandenBerg G, Rebar R, Ehara Y. Variation of pituitary responsiveness to synthetic LRF during different phases of the menstrual cycle. J Clin Endocrinol Metab 35:931, 1972.
66. Job JC, Garnier PE, Chaussain JL, Milhaud G. Elevation of serum gonadotropins (LH and FSH) after releasing hormone (LH-RH) injection in normal children and in patients with disorders of puberty. J Clin Endocrinol Metab 35:475, 1972.
67. Yen SSC, Rebar R, VandenBerg G, Judd H. Hypothalamic amenorrhea and hypogonadotropinism: Responses to LRF. J Clin Endocrinol Metab 36:811, 1973.

68. Reid RL, Leopold GR, Yen SSC. Induction of ovulation and pregnancy with pulsatile luteinizing hormone–releasing factor: Dosage and mode of delivery. Fertil Steril 36:553, 1981.
69. Anderson MS, Bowers CY, Kastin AJ, et al. Synthetic thyrotropin-releasing hormone: A potent stimulator of thyrotropin secretion in man. N Engl J Med 285:1279, 1971.
70. Snyder PJ, Utiger RD. Response to thyrotropin releasing hormone (TRH) in man. J Clin Endocrinol Metab 34:380, 1972.
71. Gershengorn MC, Weintraub BD. Thyrotropin-induced hyperthyroidism caused by selective pituitary resistance to thyroid hormone: A new syndrome of "inappropriate secretion of TSH." J Clin Invest 56:633, 1975.
72. Snyder PJ, Utiger RD. Inhibition of thyrotropin response to thyrotropin-releasing hormone by small quantities of thyroid hormones. J Clin Invest 51:2077, 1972.
73. Franco PS, Hershman JM, Haigler ED Jr, Pittman JA Jr. Response to thyrotropin-releasing hormone compared with thyroid suppression tests in euthyroid Graves' disease. Metabolism 22:1357, 1973.
74. Friesen HG. Human prolactin in clinical endocrinology: The impact of radioimmunoassays. Metabolism 22:1039, 1973.
75. Fournier PJR, Desjardins PD, Friesen HG. Current understanding of human prolactin physiology and its diagnostic and therapeutic applications. A review. Am J Obstet Gynecol 118:337, 1974.
76. Sassin JF, Frantz AG, Weitzman ED, Kapen S. Human prolactin: 24-hour pattern with increased release during sleep. Science 177:1205, 1972.
77. Quigley ME, Ropert JF, Yen SSC. Acute prolactin release triggered by feeding. J Clin Endocrinol Metab 52:1043, 1981.
78. Tyson JE, Hwang P, Guyda H, Friesen HG. Studies of prolactin secretion in human pregnancy. Am J Obstet Gynecol 113:14, 1972.
79. Suginami H, Katsuyuki H, Yano K, et al. Ovulation induction with bromocriptine in normoprolactinemic anovulatory women. J Clin Endocrinol Metab 62:899, 1986.
80. Board JA, Storlazzi E, Schneider V. Nocturnal prolactin levels in infertility. Fertil Steril 36:720, 1983.
81. DeVane GW, Gusick DS. Bromocriptine therapy in normoprolactinemic women with unexplained infertility and galactorrhea. Fertil Steril 46:1026, 1986.
82. Boyar RM, Kapen S, Finkelstein JW, et al. Hypothalamic-pituitary function in diverse hyperprolactinemic states. J Clin Invest 53:1588, 1974.
83. Markoff E, Lee DW. Glycosylated prolactin is a major circulating variant in human serum. J Clin Endocrinol Metab 65:1102, 1987.
84. Yamada T, Tsukui T, Ikejiri K, et al. Volume of the sella turcica in normal subjects and in patients with primary hypothyroidism and hyperthyroidism. J Clin Endocrinol Metab 42:817, 1976.
85. MacGillivray MH, Aceto T Jr, Frohman LA. Plasma growth hormone responses and growth retardation of hypothyroidism. Am J Dis Child 115:273, 1968.
86. Burgess JA, Smith BR, Merimee TJ. Growth hormone in thyrotoxicosis: Effect of insulin-induced hypoglycemia. J Clin Endocrinol Metab 26:1257, 1966.
87. Mace JW, Gotlin RW, Sassin JF, et al. Usefulness of post-sleep human growth hormone release as a test of physiologic growth hormone secretion. J Clin Endocrinol Metab 31:225, 1970.
88. Underwood JE, Azumi K, Voina SJ, Van Wyk JJ. Growth hormone levels during sleep in normal and growth hormone deficient children. Pediatrics 48:946, 1971.
89. Buckler JMH. Exercise as a screening test for growth hormone release. Acta Endocrinol (Copenh) 69:219, 1972.
90. Underwood LE, Clemmons DR, Van Wyk JJ. Plasma immunoreactive somatomedin C/IGF I in the evaluation of short stature. *In* Martin Spenser E (ed). Insulin-Like Growth Factors/Somatomedins. New York, Walter de Gruyter, 1983, p 235.
91. Frasier SD. A review of growth hormone stimulation tests in children. Pediatrics 53:6, 1974.
92. Penny R, Blizzard RM, Davis WT. Sequential arginine and insulin tolerance tests on the same day. J Clin Endocrinol Metab 29:1499, 1969.
93. Rosenthal SM, Schriock EA, Kaplan SL, et al. Synthetic human pancreas growth hormone releasing factor (hpgrf [1-44]-NH_2) stimulates growth secretion in normal men. J Clin Endocrinol Metab 57:677, 1983.
94. Laron Z, Pertzelan A, Karp M. Pituitary dwarfism with high serum levels of growth hormone. Isr J Med Sci 4:883, 1968.
95. Daughaday WH, Laron Z, Pertzelan A, Heins JH. Defective sulfation factor generation: A possible etiological link in dwarfism. Trans Assoc Am Physicians 82:129, 1969.
96. Daughaday WH. The diagnosis of hypersomatotropism in man. Med Clin North Am 52:371, 1968.
97. Clemmons DR, Van Wyk JJ, Ridgway EC, et al. Evaluation of acromegaly by radioimmunoassay of somatomedin-C. N Engl J Med 301:1138, 1979.
98. Earill JM, Sparks LL, Forsham PH. Glucose suppression of serum growth hormone in the diagnosis of acromegaly. JAMA 201:628, 1967.
99. Mims RB, Bethune JE. Acromegaly with normal fasting growth hormone concentrations but abnormal growth hormone regulation. Ann Intern Med 81:781, 1974.
100. Hellman L, Bradlow HL, Zumoff B, Gallagher TF. The influence of thyroid hormone on hydrocortisone production and metabolism. J Clin Endocrinol Metab 21:1231, 1961.
101. Gallagher TF, Hellman L, Finkelstein J, et al. Hyperthyroidism and cortisol secretion in man. J Clin Endocrinol Metab 34:919, 1972.
102. Mattingly D, Tyler C. Simple screening test for Cushing's syndrome. Br Med J 4:394, 1967.
103. Sawin CT. Measurement of plasma cortisol in the diagnosis of Cushing's syndrome. Ann Intern Med 68:624, 1968.
104. Hellman L, Nakada F, Curti J, et al. Cortisol is secreted episodically by normal men. J Clin Endocrinol Metab 30:411, 1970.
105. Hellman L, Weitzman ED, Roffwarg H, et al. Cortisol is secreted episodically in Cushing's syndrome. J Clin Endocrinol Metab 30:686, 1970.
106. Melby JC. Assessment of adrenocortical function. N Engl J Med 285:735, 1971.
107. Liddle GW. Tests of pituitary adrenal suppressibility in the diagnosis of Cushing's syndrome. J Clin Endocrinol Metab 20:1539, 1960.
108. Ney RL, Shimizu N, Nicholson WE, et al. Correlation of plasma ACTH concentration with adrenocortical response in normal human subjects, surgical patients, and patients with Cushing's syndrome. J Clin Invest 42:1669, 1963.
109. Nahara M, Shibasaki T, Shizume K, et al. Corticotropin-releasing factor test in normal subjects and patients with hypothalamic-pituitary-adrenal disorders. J Clin Endocrinol Metab 57:963, 1983.
110. Chrousos GP, Schulte HM, Oldfield EH, et al. The corticotropin-releasing factor stimulation test: An aid in the evaluation of patients with Cushing's syndrome. N Engl J Med 310:622, 1984.
111. Oldfield EH, Chrousos GP, Schulte HM, et al. Preoperative lateralization of ACTH-secreting pituitary microadenomas by bilateral and simultaneous inferior petrosal venous sinus sampling. N Engl J Med 312:100, 1985.
112. Silverman SR, Marnell RT, Sholiton LJ, Werk EE Jr. Failure of dexamethasone suppression test to indicate bilateral adrenocortical hyperplasia in Cushing's syndrome. J Clin Endocrinol Metab 23:167, 1963.
113. Cassidy CE, Rosenfeld PS, Bokat MA. Suppression of activity of the adrenal cortex by dexamethasone in Cushing's syndrome. J Clin Endocrinol Metab 26:1181, 1966.
114. Nichols J, Nugent CA, Tyler FH. Steroid laboratory tests in the diagnosis of Cushing's syndrome. Am J Med 45:116, 1968.
115. Liddle GW, Estep HL, Kendall JW Jr, et al. Clinical application of a new test of pituitary reserve. J Clin Endocrinol Metab 19:875, 1959.
116. Schulte HM, Chrousos GP, Avgerinos P, et al. The corticotropin-releasing hormone stimulation test: A possible aid in the evaluation of adrenal insufficiency. J Clin Endocrinol Metab 58:1064, 1984.
117. Rose LI, Williams GH, Jagger PI, Lauler DP. The 48-hour adrenocorticotrophin infusion test for adrenocortical insufficiency. Ann Intern Med 73:49, 1970.
118. Landon J, Greenwood FC, Stamp TCB, Wynn V. The plasma sugar, free fatty acid, cortisol, and growth hormone response to insulin, and the comparison of this procedure with other tests of pituitary and adrenal function. II. In patients with hypothalamic or pituitary dysfunction or anorexia nervosa. J Clin Invest 43:437, 1966.
119. Liddle GW, Island D, Meador CK. Normal and abnormal regulation of corticotropin secretion in man. Recent Prog Horm Res 18:125, 1962.

120. Loriaux DL. Tests of adrenocortical function. *In* Becker KL, et al (eds). Principles and Practice of Endocrinology and Metabolism, 2nd ed. Philadelphia, JB Lippincott, 1995, p 662.
121. Allen JP, Kendall JW, McGilvra R, et al. Adrenocorticotrophic and growth hormone secretion: Studies during pneumoencephalography. Arch Neurol 31:325, 1974.
122. Chang J, Laufer L, Meldrum D, et al. Sex steroid secretion in polycystic ovarian disease (PCO) following ovarian suppression by a long-acting GnRh agonist (Abstract 642). Program and Abstracts of the 64th Annual Meeting of the Endocrine Society. Bethesda, MD, The Society, 1982, p 240.
123. Horton R, Hawks D, Lobo R. 3α,17β-Androstanediol glucuronide in plasma: A marker of androgen action in idiopathic hirsutism. J Clin Invest 69:1203, 1982.
124. Lobo RA, Goebelsmann U. Adult manifestation of congenital hyperplasia due to incomplete 21-hydroxylase deficiency mimicking polycystic ovarian disease. Am J Obstet Gynecol 138:720, 1980.
125. Chrousos GP, Loriaux DL, Mann DL, Cutler GB. Late-onset 21-hydroxylase deficiency mimicking idiopathic hirsutism or polycystic ovarian disease. Ann Intern Med 96:143, 1982.
126. New MI, Lorenzen F, Lerner AJ, et al. Genotyping steroid 21-hydroxylase deficiency: Hormonal reference data. J Clin Endocrinol Metab 57:320, 1983.
127. Randall RV, Clark EC, Dodge HW Jr, Love JG. Polyuria after operation for tumors in the region of the hypophysis and hypothalamus. J Clin Endocrinol Metab 20:1614, 1960.
128. Miller M, Dalakos T, Moses AM, et al. Recognition of partial defects in antidiuretic hormone secretion. Ann Intern Med 73:721, 1970.
129. Moses A, Streeten D. Differentiation of polyuric states by measurement of responses to changes in plasma osmolality induced by hypertonic saline infusions. Am J Med 42:368, 1967.
130. Baylis PH, Thompson CJ. Diabetes insipidus and hyperosmolar syndromes. *In* Becker KL, et al (eds). Principles and Practice of Endocrinology and Metabolism, 2nd ed. Philadelphia, JB Lippincott, 1995, p 257.
131. Goldberg M. Hyponatremia and the inappropriate secretion of antidiuretic hormone. Am J Med 35:293, 1963.
132. Orth DN, Jackson RV, DeCherney GS, et al. Effect of synthetic ovine corticotropin-releasing factor. J Clin Invest 71:587, 1983.
133. Lippe B, Wong S-LR, Kaplan SA. Simultaneous assessment of growth hormone and ACTH reserve in children pretreated with diethylstilbestrol. J Clin Endocrinol Metab 33:949, 1971.
134. Merimee TJ, Rabinowitz D, Fineberg SE. Arginine-initiated release of human growth hormone: Factors modifying the response in normal man. N Engl J Med 280:1434, 1969.
135. Parker ML, Hammond JM, Daughaday WH. The arginine provocative test: An aid in the diagnosis of hyposomatotropism. J Clin Endocrinol Metab 27:1129, 1967.
136. Keenan BS, Beitins IZ, Lee PA, et al. Estimation of ACTH reserve on normal and hypopituitary subjects: Comparison of oral and intravenous metyrapone with insulin hypoglycemia. J Clin Endocrinol Metab 37:540, 1973.
137. Nanot D, Rosenwaks Z, Margalioth EJ. Prognostic assessment of female fecundity. Lancet 2:647, 1987.
138. Scott RT, Leonardi MR, Hoffman GE, et al. A prospective evaluation of clomiphene citrate challenge test screening of the general infertility population. Obstet Gynecol 82:539, 1993.
139. Scott RT Jr, Hoffman GE. Prognostic assessment of ovarian reserve. Fertil Steril 63:1, 1995.
140. Wallach EE. Pitfalls in evaluating ovarian reserve. Fertil Steril 63:12, 1995.

Part III

Endocrinology of Pregnancy

Chapter 27

NEUROENDOCRINE-METABOLIC REGULATION OF PREGNANCY

Robert B. Jaffe

■ CHAPTER OUTLINE

KEY POINTS

- Implantation requires a coordinated sequence of events involving trophoblast, embryo, and maternal uterus.
- The fetal endocrine system is established early in intrauterine life.
- The fetal hypothalamic-pituitary-adrenal axis maintains intrauterine homeostasis, prepares the fetus for independent extrauterine existence, and may play a role in the initiation of parturition.
- The fetal hypothalamic-pituitary-gonadal axis is functional during intrauterine life, and the testis secretes testosterone and müllerian-inhibiting substance essential for the development of the derivatives of the wolffian ducts and inhibition of müllerian ductal development, respectively.
- Progesterone and estrogen production requires the interplay of fetus, placenta, and mother, the *fetoplacental unit.*
- The placenta synthesizes a wide array of hypothalamic-like and pituitary-like hormones, growth factors, and neurotransmitters and many of their receptors.

The endocrine system is one of the first—if not the first—of the homeostatic systems to develop during fetal life. The neuroendocrine axis appears early in fetal development, and the full repertoire of neurotransmitter, neuropeptide, and hormonal factors is available to regulate pituitary function. Further, the pituitary gland can respond to hypophysiotropic substances in early fetal life.[1] The interplay among fetus, placenta, and mother represents an intriguing, unique feature of human endocrine biology.

In this chapter, after describing the process of implantation, I trace the neuroanatomical and neuroendocrinologic development of the fetus and placenta, their interdependence in steroid hormone formation, and the role of placental peptides, proteins, and growth factors in intrauterine biology and in the timing of parturition and preparation for extrauterine existence.

IMPLANTATION AND EARLY PREGNANCY

Implantation

Appropriate implantation of the embryo is essential for survival and a normal pregnancy. The rate of spontaneous abortions is high (about one third of human pregnancies end in spontaneous abortion, and 22 percent of these occur before pregnancy is detected clinically).[2] The placenta develops through the formation of the trophoblast cells and the development of the endodermal and mesodermal components of the placenta that arise from a portion of the inner cell mass. After the placenta has formed, cells from the inner cell mass give rise to the embryo proper.

A major unanswered question is why trophoblasts, which express paternal proteins and interact directly with maternal immune cells, avoid rejection as an allograft. A key may lie in the elucidation of a unique HLA antigen, HLA-G.[3–5] HLA-G is a novel class Ib human major histocompatibility complex antigen. Unlike its class Ia counterparts (HLA-A, B, and C), HLA-G is smaller (37 to 39 kDa versus 41 to 42 kDa), exhibits reduced polymorphism, and is expressed by differentiated cytotrophoblasts that lie at the maternal-fetal interface. Because of its reduced polymorphism, HLA-G is less immunogenic and could prevent immunologic recognition by cytotoxic T cells. In addition, there is recent evidence that HLA-G can inhibit natural killer cell activity, suggesting that HLA-G could be playing a crucial role in maternal immune tolerance of the fetal-placental unit.

Implantation occurs soon after the blastocyst hatches from the zona pellucida. Many of the molecules involved in the implantation process in mammals, including humans, have been elucidated and are described in an excellent review.[6]

Within a few hours of implantation, the endometrium is modified to form the decidua. In addition, inflammatory and endothelial cells are recruited, and there is transepithelial invasion of trophoblasts into the endometrium, coupled with apoptosis (programmed cell death) of the uterine epithelium.

Although the preimplantation embryo is able to develop without maternal signals, effective intercommunication between the maternal compartment and the blastocyst is essential. Close synchronization between the development of the uterus and blastocyst must occur for successful implantation to be accomplished. Lack of this synchronization is probably responsible for the high failure rate of embryo transfer in advanced reproductive technology programs.

Another crucial aspect of successful implantation is the establishment of a vasculature. Advances in the understanding of new blood vessel formation[7] are shedding light on the mechanisms by which this occurs. Human placentation represents a balance between the concurrent degradation of the maternal decidual vasculature and the highly coordinated angiogenesis directed by the developing embryo. The maternal effects are regulated by the invading cytotrophoblasts, whereas the villous mesenchyme gives rise to the fetal vessels under the regulation of local macrophages (Hofbauer cells).

During the preimplantation period, the uterus undergoes striking developmental changes under the influence of ovarian estrogen and progesterone. These ovarian sex steroids prepare the uterus for implantation.

Estrogen elicits several events that permit the initiation of implantation. It induces the secretion of cytokines, including members of the epidermal growth factor (EGF) family[8] and leukemia inhibitory factor,[9–11] at least in rodents. During the peri-implantation period in the rodent, four members of the EGF family, EGF, transforming growth factor (TGF)–α, heparin-binding EGF, and amphiregulin, are produced in the uterus. Although TGF-α is produced in large amounts in the mouse uterus, it does not appear to be essential, because implantation occurs normally in mice lacking a functional TGF-α gene.[12] Comparable studies in humans or subhuman primates have not been published as of this writing.

In addition to changes in the maternal uterus, there are events elicited by the blastocyst itself. Again, most studies to date have been performed in rodents, although there are some reports in humans. Interleukin-1β is made by mouse trophoblast beginning at the blastocyst stage, and the type I interleukin-1 receptor is expressed on trophoblasts, uterine epithelium, and endometrial stroma.[13] Interleukin-1β is also produced by human trophoblasts[14] and induces markers of trophoblast differentiation, including aromatase activity,[15] and production of corticotropin-releasing hormone (CRH), adrenocorticotropic hormone (ACTH), human chorionic gonadotropin (hCG),[16, 17] and gelatinase B.[18]

At implantation, the nonadhesive surface of the trophectoderm becomes adhesive. The molecules concerned with this event are not well defined; the known aspects of the process are well described in reference 6.

At the initiation of pregnancy, the secretory endometrium undergoes decidualization accompanied by widespread vascular expansion and reorganization as well as by an increase in focal vascular permeability at the implantation site.[19] Angiogenesis at the implantation site may actually occur before the physical apposition of the blastocyst.[20] After implantation, cytotrophoblasts invade and migrate through the endometrium, forming physical connections to the uterus and villous networks where future fetal neovascularization will occur.[21] The cytotrophoblasts reach the inner third of the myometrium, initially plugging the maternal spiral arterioles and then replacing the maternal endothelial cells and musculoelastic tissue.[22] A low-resistance arteriolar system is thus created in the absence of maternal vasomotor control. The lack of autoregulation of placental blood flow allows the dramatic increase in blood supply necessary to serve the growing demands of the fetus.[23] Despite a 15-fold increase in uterine volume and weight, 85 percent of the uterine blood flow is directed to fetoplacental tissues.[24] Limitation of this blood supply may have adverse clinical effects. For example, in preeclampsia, cytotrophoblast invasion is restricted to the superficial decidual segments, leaving the myometrial spiral arterioles undisturbed and responsive to vasomotor influences.[25] These pathologic changes result in an impaired blood supply to the fetoplacental unit.[26, 27]

Angiogenesis and the Placenta. The presence of angiogenic activity within the placenta has long been recognized. Several known angiogenic factors have been localized to the placenta. Basic fibroblast growth factor has been immunolocalized in trophoblast and endothelial cells throughout gestation.[28] Platelet-derived endothelial cell growth factor has been isolated from both human placenta[29] and choriocarcinoma cell lines.[30] Similarly, vascular endothelial growth factor is expressed in several components of the human placenta, including maternal glandular epithelium, fetal and maternal macrophages, and cytotrophoblasts.[31] Although the vascular endothelial growth factor receptor is limited to vascular endothelium in other tissues, its expression by cytotrophoblasts[32] suggests that this growth factor may regulate other processes besides angiogenesis. These may include the regulation of amniotic fluid dynamics through the modulation of vascular permeability.[33] In addition to these angiogenic factors, two potent inhibitors of angiogenesis have been isolated from mouse placenta.[34] The specific interplay between angiogenic factors and their inhibitors in the placenta is not well understood.

The Corpus Luteum of Pregnancy and Luteal-Placental Transition

Almost immediately after implantation, hCG (discussed in detail subsequently) is secreted by the trophoblast. The hCG is luteotropic and maintains the function of the corpus luteum. In response to hCG, the corpus luteum secretes increasing concentrations of progesterone, 17α-hydroxyprogesterone, estradiol, and estrone, as well as stimulates the secretion of relaxin. Aspects of progesterone, estrogen, and relaxin biology in pregnancy are detailed subsequently in this chapter.

Relaxin is in the insulin/insulin-like growth factor (IGF) family, with which it shares extensive structural homologies. The rise of relaxin in early pregnancy parallels that of hCG. It may synergize with progesterone in maintaining myometrial quiescence in early pregnancy.[35, 36] The corpus luteum retains the capacity to synthesize progesterone throughout most of pregnancy. However, its functional activity decreases markedly after the seventh week. At this time, the luteal-placental transition occurs, and the placenta and decidua subsume the production of progesterone throughout the remainder of pregnancy. Removal of the ovary or corpus luteum before the eighth week of pregnancy results in abortion, whereas after the ninth week it does not.[37]

FETOPLACENTAL ENDOCRINE DEVELOPMENT, REGULATION, AND FUNCTION

Fetal Neuroendocrinologic Development

The earliest events in primate organogenesis include development of the brain. The classic view of pituitary organogenesis, described in the 1950s for the human, held that the pituitary primordium appears as the epithelial evagination of Rathke's pouch arising from a diverticulum of the stomodeum. The forebrain appears by 3 weeks' gestation, and the telencephalon and diencephalon can be distinguished by 5 weeks. The evaginated pituitary primordium appears at 4 weeks and has separated from the stomodeum by 5 weeks. The floor of the sella turcica is in place by 7 weeks and separates the pituitary from its epithelial origins.[38] Subsequently, the classic view of pituitary organogenesis was questioned. The emergence of the amine precursor uptake and decarboxylation concept as signifying a common origin of certain peptide-secreting cells[39] suggests that the progenitors of hormone-secreting cells originate in the ventral neural ridges of the primitive neural tube. This region also gives rise to the diencephalon, which further suggests that the hypothalamus and anterior pituitary share a common embryonic origin.[40] The pituitary increases in size and cell number through proliferation of cell cords into mesenchyme from week 6.[41] Capillaries interdigitate among the mesenchymal tissue about Rathke's pouch and the diencephalon at 8 weeks,[42, 43] and the median eminence is distinguishable by 9 weeks.[44] Vascular casts have demonstrated the presence of an intact hypothalamic-hypophyseal vascular system in fetuses of 11.5 to 16.8 weeks' fetal age.[45] In addition to the neurovascular link between the developing hypothalamus and pituitary, it is possible that hypophysiotropic factors reach the pituitary by local diffusion from the hypothalamus.[46]

Ontogeny of Fetal Hypothalamic Hormones. The hypothalamic nuclei and fiber tracts can be distinguished at 14 to 16 weeks,[47] and the hypophysiotropic hormones—gonadotropin-releasing hormone (GnRH),[46] thyrotropin-releasing hormone (TRH),[46, 48] and somatostatin (somatotropin release–inhibiting hormone)[46]—appear in the fetal hypothalamus by this period (Table 27–1). Catecholamine fluorescence in cells projecting from the arcuate nuclei to the internal and external layers of the median eminence appears during the interval from 12 to 16 weeks.[49] Dopamine is present in the fetal hypothalamus at weeks 11 to 15 at a concentration twice that of the adult.[45] Consistent with the effects of dopamine functioning as the prolactin release–inhibiting factor, fetal hypothalami taken within this interval display a prolactin release–inhibiting activity when tested with adult rat anterior pituitary cells.[50] Immunocytochemical studies of growth hormone–releasing hormone (GHRH) have indicated the appearance of this peptide at 18 weeks' fetal age, with increasing levels found up to 30 weeks.[51] Interestingly, a paucity of GHRH in the neonate was observed, with the peptide reappearing at 2 months. CRH nerve terminals in the fetal median eminence are seen at 16 weeks' fetal age, neurohemal connections at 17 weeks, and CRH-immunopositive cell bodies at 19 weeks.[52]

Ontogeny of Fetal Pituitary Hormones. The anterior pituitary ultimately differentiates into five types of specialized epithelium-derived secretory cells, producing and secreting six hormones (see Table 27–1). Classically, these are lactotropes producing prolactin (PRL), somatotropes producing growth hormone (GH), corticotropes producing ACTH, thyrotropes producing thyroid-stimulating hormone (TSH), and gonadotropes producing luteinizing hormone (LH) and follicle-stimulating hormone (FSH). The first three are proteins or peptides; the last three are glycoproteins consisting of a common α-subunit and a unique β-subunit. As discussed in Chapter 9, transcriptional regulation of lactotrope, somatotrope, and thyrotrope differentiation and development is effected by Pit-1. Within the pituitary, ACTH-containing cells have been detected immunocytochemically at 7 weeks,[53, 54] β-lipotropin and β-endorphin at 8 weeks,[54, 55] GH-containing and LH-containing cells both at 10.5 weeks,[53] and TSH-containing cells at 13 weeks.[53] Melanocyte-stimulating hormone (MSH)–containing cells, which probably contain β-lipotropin, have

■ TABLE 27–1

Ontogeny of Human Fetal Hypothalamic and Pituitary Hormones

HORMONE	AGE DETECTED (weeks)
Hypothalamic	
Gonadotropin-releasing hormone	14
Thyrotropin-releasing hormone	10
Somatostatin	14
Dopamine	11
Growth hormone–releasing hormone	18
Corticotropin-releasing hormone	16
Pituitary	
Prolactin	16.5
Growth hormone	10.5
Corticotropin (ACTH)	7
Thyroid-stimulating hormone (thyrotropin)	13
Luteinizing hormone	10.5
Follicle-stimulating hormone	10.5

also been reported to appear at 14 weeks,[53] and PRL-containing cells appear at 16.5 weeks' fetal age.[53] About the time of detection in the fetal pituitary by immunocytochemistry, GH can be detected by immunoassay of pituitary tissue at 10 weeks,[56] PRL at 17 weeks,[57, 58] TSH at 12 weeks, LH and FSH at 10 weeks,[45] ACTH at 9 weeks,[59] and MSH (again probably β-lipotropin) at 10 weeks' fetal age.[46] Thus, many of the components required for the normal regulated function of the anterior pituitary, that is, the secretory cells of the anterior pituitary, the hypophysiotropic factors elaborated by the hypothalamus, and the neurohemal link connecting the hypothalamus and pituitary, are present in the fetus well before the end of the first half of pregnancy.

The functional relationship between these components is not clearly established. The primate fetal pituitary is competent to respond in vitro to virtually all of the known hypophysiotropic factors by midgestation. Whether it does indeed respond to these compounds in vivo remains to be demonstrated directly, although studies in the catheterized rhesus fetus in utero suggest that responses to at least one of the hypophysiotropic factors, GnRH, can occur.[60]

The role of the fetal hypothalamus in the differentiation of the anterior pituitary is uncertain. In studies of anencephalic fetuses, only quantitative reductions in pituitary hormone content have been reported compared with normal fetuses. Therefore, these studies are interpreted as supporting an intrinsic mechanism for the expression of the anterior pituitary cell types. The vestigial secretion of a hypothalamic hormone may be sufficient for the appearance of a particular cell type, although the secretion may be insufficient to develop normal hormone content and secretion. Organ cultures of fetal pituitaries originating as early as 5 weeks' gestation will also secrete GH, PRL, LH, FSH, TSH, and ACTH.[61] Thus, the fetal pituitary appears to have at least a limited potential for differentiation in the absence of hypothalamic input.

Fetal Hypothalamic Hormones

GONADOTROPIN-RELEASING HORMONE

The hypothalamus of the fetus produces the decapeptide GnRH during intrauterine life.[48] In both the human[62] and the monkey[60] fetus, GnRH has the capacity to stimulate gonadotropin production, although the magnitude of the response increases after birth. Immunoreactive GnRH is present in the human fetal hypothalamus in significant amounts by 10 weeks of gestation (0.54 pg/mg). There was no significant correlation between the concentration of GnRH in the fetal hypothalamus and either sex or gestational age during the 10- to 22-week gestational age interval studied. During this period, the content varied from 208 to 4300 pg and the concentration from 0.27 to 13.1 pg/mg.

Rasmussen and colleagues[63] demonstrated the pulsatile release of GnRH from the human fetal hypothalamus in vitro. In vivo, with use of a monkey preparation in which indwelling catheters were placed in the vascular system of the male fetus in utero, the fetus was challenged with GnRH and demonstrated an increase in both LH and testosterone.[60] Thus, at least by the last third of gestation, the pituitary-gonadal axis of the male monkey fetus responds to GnRH stimulation. It is likely that a similar situation exists in the human fetus.

THYROTROPIN-RELEASING HORMONE

As with GnRH, significant levels of immunoreactive TRH are found in the human fetal hypothalamus early in gestation.[46] By 10 weeks, the hypothalamic content is 1500 pg. In fetuses of 10 to 22 weeks' gestation, the concentration varies from 0.2 to 218 pg/mg; the content ranges from 0.64 to 184 ng. As is also true with GnRH, there is no significant correlation with sex or gestational age. The presence of TRH in the fetal hypothalamus in early gestation and midgestation suggests its possible role in the regulation of secretion of TSH and possibly PRL.

GROWTH HORMONE RELEASE–INHIBITING HORMONE (SOMATOSTATIN)

Immunoreactive somatostatin, like GnRH and TRH, was demonstrated in the hypothalamus of human fetuses from 10 to 22 weeks' gestational age.[46] At 10 weeks, the concentration was 7.3 pg/ml. In contrast to GnRH and TRH, concentrations of somatostatin increased with advancing gestational age; the mean level at 10 to 15 weeks of gestation was 10.2 pg/mg, with significantly higher levels (28.5 pg/mg) at midgestation. The hypothalamic content of somatostatin rose from 7 to 8 ng early in gestation to 36.6 ng by midgestation. These findings suggest that the pattern of GH secretion in the fetus may reflect maturational changes in the secretion of GHRH and somatostatin.

CORTICOTROPIN-RELEASING HORMONE

The chemical structure of CRH, which can stimulate the secretion of ACTH, has been elucidated and the gene that encodes it has been cloned.[64] It is a 41–amino acid peptide with a molecular mass of approximately 4.7 kDa. CRH is a potent secretagogue for ACTH and β-endorphin release in the human fetal pituitary gland.[65] Further, arginine vasopressin can also release ACTH from the fetal pituitary, and CRH and arginine vasopressin can synergize in stimulating ACTH release.[65] Large quantities of CRH are also produced by the placenta, particularly toward the end of pregnancy, as detailed subsequently. Therefore, the extent to which fetal hypothalamic CRH and arginine vasopressin and placental CRH interact in regulating fetal ACTH release remains to be elucidated.

Fetal Pituitary-Adrenal Functions and Interactions

Steroid hormones produced by the fetal adrenal cortex regulate intrauterine homeostasis, the maturation of fetal organ systems necessary for extrauterine life, and, in some species, the timing of parturition.[66, 67] Appropriate development and function of the fetal adrenal cortex, therefore, are crucial for fetal maturation and perinatal survival. Moreover, the fetal adrenal cortex must itself undergo maturational changes in preparation for its essential role postnatally (i.e., production of glucocorticoids and mineralocorticoids) and to ensure adrenal cortical autonomy once the placenta has separated.

Development and function of the primate fetal adrenal

cortex are distinct from those in other species. During the last two thirds of gestation in humans and higher primates, the fetal adrenal glands are disproportionately enlarged and exhibit extraordinary growth and steroidogenic activity in a specialized inner cortical compartment known as the fetal zone[68, 69] (Fig. 27–1). The fetal zone exists only during fetal life; it involutes or undergoes remodeling soon after birth. During midgestation, the fetal zone occupies 80 to 90 percent of the cortical volume and produces 100 to 200 mg/day of the androgenic C_{19} steroid dehydroepiandrosterone sulfate (DHEA-S), which is quantitatively the principal steroid product of the primate fetal adrenal gland throughout gestation. The primate fetal adrenal cortex also produces cortisol, which promotes the maturation of fetal organ systems needed for extrauterine life, including the lungs, liver, thyroid, and gut.[66] In some species (e.g., sheep, goats, and rabbits), cortisol produced by the fetal adrenals also regulates the timing of parturition[67]; however, the mechanism in primates is incompletely understood.

Experiments of nature in humans (e.g., anencephaly)[70, 71] and studies in pregnant rhesus monkeys[72] indicate that ACTH secreted from the fetal pituitary is the principal trophic regulator of the fetal adrenal cortex. However, several observations indicate that ACTH may not be acting directly. During the last two thirds of gestation, the fetal zone grows rapidly and produces large amounts of steroids even though circulating ACTH concentrations in one study did not rise.[73] Furthermore, soon after birth, the fetal zone rapidly involutes although exposure to ACTH continues, albeit at lower concentrations. This may reflect ACTH secretion by the placenta. Thus, other factors, possibly specific to the intrauterine environment, appear to play a role in the regulation of fetal adrenal cortical growth and function. Substances produced by the placenta (e.g., chorionic gonadotropin, hCG) have been implicated,[71, 74] and peptide growth factors produced locally within the fetal adrenal[75] appear to influence fetal adrenal cortical growth and function by mediating or modulating the trophic actions of ACTH. Specific nuclear receptor transcription factors, discussed subsequently, also appear to be important regulators of adrenal cortical development by influencing early embryonic differentiation of adrenal cortical progenitors and the maintenance of steroidogenic function.[76, 77] Thus, regulation of the primate fetal adrenal cortex is a complex process involving the net effect of a cohort of factors that modulate or mediate the trophic actions of ACTH.

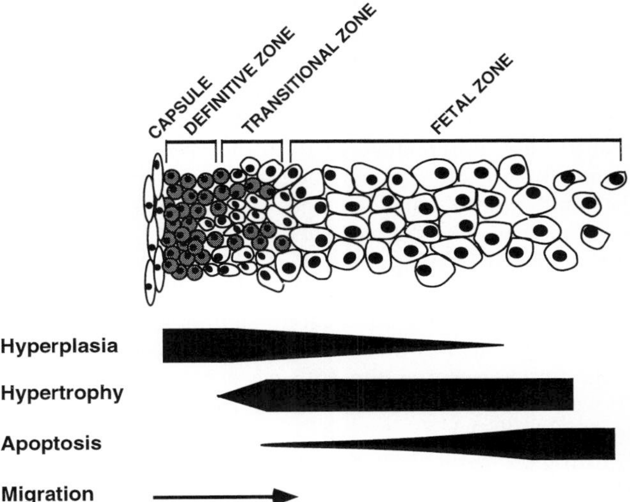

Figure 27–1 ■ Schematic structure of the midgestation human fetal adrenal gland and proposed primary modes of growth in each cortical zone and cell migration. Hyperplasia occurs mainly in the definitive zone; hypertrophy occurs mainly in the fetal zone; apoptosis occurs mainly in the central areas of the fetal zone; and cells migrate from the periphery to the center of the gland. (From Mesiano S, Jaffe RB. Developmental and functional biology of the primate fetal adrenal cortex. Endocr Rev 18:378–403, 1997. © The Endocrine Society.)

FETAL ADRENAL DEVELOPMENT

Development of the primate fetal and neonatal adrenal cortex differs qualitatively and quantitatively from that of other species and is characterized by extraordinarily rapid growth, high steroidogenic activity, and a unique morphologic appearance. For much of gestation, the human fetal adrenal cortex is composed of two morphologically distinct zones, the fetal zone and the definitive zone (see Fig. 27–1). The fetal zone accounts for the bulk (80 to 90 percent) of the cortex and is the primary site of growth and steroidogenesis. The definitive zone (also referred to as the adult cortex, neocortex, or permanent zone) occupies the remainder of the cortex and comprises a narrow band of tightly packed cells surrounding the fetal zone (for reviews, see references 78 and 79).

Ontogeny of the Fetal Adrenal Cortex. The anlage of the human adrenal cortex is first identified at about the fourth week of gestation as a thickening of the coelomic epithelium in the notch between the primitive urogenital ridge and the dorsal mesentery. By the fifth week, these primitive cells begin to migrate, forming cords that stream medially and cranially, eventually accumulating at the cranial end of the mesonephros where they condense to form the earliest recognizable manifestation of the adrenal gland. Cells destined to become the steroidogenic cells of the adrenal and gonad appear to be derived from neighboring areas of the coelomic epithelium and are morphologically identical.[78] In general, the portion medial to the mesonephros produces cells destined for the adrenal cortex, whereas the portion ventral to the mesonephros produces cells destined for the gonad.

By the eighth week of gestation, the mass of cells migrating into the adrenal blastema organize into anastomosing cords and exhibit ultrastructural characteristics consistent with steroidogenic capability. These cells eventually differentiate into large polyhedral cells and become the primordium of the fetal zone. The definitive zone is derived at approximately the same time when a separate population of cells in the same area of coelomic epithelium migrates to the adrenal blastema and surrounds the primordial fetal zone. By the eighth week of human pregnancy, the fetus acquires a rudimentary but distinct adrenal cortex made up of two zonal compartments. Whether there is a common progenitor cell type or two separate populations[78] of cells make up the two zones is debated.

At around the ninth week of gestation, the adrenal blastema is completely enclosed by the adrenal capsule, which is composed of specialized mesenchymal cells migrating from the area of Bowman's capsule. At the same time, an extensive network of sinusoidal capillaries develops between the cords of the fetal zone. This vasculature predominates in the central portion of the fetal zone and persists throughout fetal life.[80] Consequently, the adrenal cortex is one of the most highly vascularized organs in the primate fetus. Abundant vascularization is probably required to facilitate access of hormonal products to the circulation.

After 10 to 12 weeks of gestation, the morphology of the adrenal cortex remains relatively constant. By midgestation (16 to 20 weeks), the fetal zone clearly dominates and is composed of large eosinophilic cells that exhibit ultrastructural characteristics typical of steroid-secreting cells. In the outer regions of the fetal zone, the cells are arranged in tightly packed cords. However, the cells in the central portion are more widely spaced in a reticular pattern and separated by many vascular sinusoids. Clusters of immature neuroblasts that will aggregate eventually into a functional medulla are also present between the innermost fetal zone cells.[80, 81]

The definitive zone is composed of a narrow band of small, tightly packed basophilic cells that exhibit structural characteristics typical of cells in a proliferative state. Its inner layers form arched cords that send finger-like columns of cells into the outer rim of the fetal zone. Although definitive zone cells are lipid poor during midgestation, they accumulate some cytoplasmic lipid and begin to resemble steroidogenically active cells in late pregnancy. By late gestation, the definitive zone cells are similar to cells of the adult zona glomerulosa.[80]

Ultrastructural studies have also demonstrated a third zone between the fetal and definitive zones, the cells of which have intermediate characteristics,[82] referred to as the transitional zone[83] (see Fig. 27–1). After midgestation, transitional zone cells have the capacity to synthesize cortisol and thus may be analogous to cells of the zona fasciculata of the adult adrenal. By the 30th week of gestation, the definitive zone and transitional zone begin to take on the appearance of the zona glomerulosa and the zona fasciculata, respectively.[84] Thus, by late gestation, the fetal adrenal cortex resembles a rudimentary form of the adult adrenal cortex.

Soon after birth, the primate adrenal cortex undergoes dramatic remodeling. The postnatal remodeling of the primate adrenal cortex involves a complex wave of differentiation such that the inner portion of the fetal zone atrophies and the zonae glomerulosa and fasciculata develop.[84] Studies indicate that fetal zone remodeling in the human is an apoptotic process.[85, 88]

It has generally been thought that the adult cortical zones develop from the persistent definitive zone. However, there is no evidence of adrenal cortical insufficiency during the perinatal period and the postnatal remodeling process. Thus, it is likely that the nascent adult cortical zones are present and functional before birth. Indeed, morphologic studies have identified rudimentary zonae glomerulosa and fasciculata during late gestation.[84] This lends support to the notion that the postnatal remodeling of the primate adrenal cortex involves apoptosis of a portion of the fetal zone and the simultaneous expansion of pre-existing zonae glomerulosa and fasciculata.

FETAL ADRENAL GROWTH

Rapid growth of the human fetal adrenal cortex begins at approximately the 10th week of gestation and continues to term (see Fig. 27–1). The growth is almost entirely due to enlargement of the fetal zone. Between the 10th and 15th weeks, the fetal zone begins to enlarge; as a consequence, the gland becomes as large as the fetal kidney by 20 weeks, and its weight increases 20-fold. During the next 10 weeks, the fetal adrenal gland doubles in size and weight, achieving a relative size 10- to 20-fold that of the adult adrenal. A further doubling occurs after 30 weeks of gestation, and by term the gland weighs approximately 3 to 4 gm. The dynamics of primate fetal adrenal cortical growth involve cellular hyperplasia, hypertrophy, migration, and senescence. Growth of the embryonic adrenal cortex probably occurs by hyperplasia, because mitotic activity can be observed throughout the adrenal blastema. However, after 8 weeks, when the definitive and fetal zones can be delineated, mitotic activity is limited to the definitive zone.[86] The cells of the fetal zone are not necessarily more numerous but are much larger than those of the definitive zone. In the fetal rhesus monkey, growth of the fetal zone in response to increased endogenous ACTH secretion occurs primarily by hypertrophy,[87] at least initially. Taken together, these data suggest that the fetal zone enlarges by hypertrophy and limited proliferation, whereas definitive zone growth occurs mainly by hyperplasia.

Centripetal migration of lipid-containing cells from the definitive to the fetal zone occurs.[88] The disparate level of proliferation between the definitive and fetal zones and evidence of centripetal migration lend support to the migration theory of adrenal cortical cytogenesis and suggest that the definitive zone is the germinal/stem cell compartment from which the inner cortical zones are derived. Thus, cells proliferate in the definitive zone and then migrate inward to form the fetal zone. The adrenal cortical zones therefore appear to be interdependent and derived from a common pool of cells in the periphery.

Thus, the primate fetal adrenal cortex is a dynamic organ in which cells proliferate in the periphery, migrate centripetally, differentiate to form the specialized cortical compartments (and possibly continue to proliferate within the compartments), and then undergo senescence when they reach the center of the cortex (see Fig. 27–1).

Functional Development. Fetal adrenal steroidogenesis is first seen at 6 to 8 weeks when the cells in the adrenal blastema differentiate and acquire steroidogenic characteristics. The fetus has the capacity to produce cortisol from progestins as early as the 16th week of gestation.[89–91] At 20 weeks, low levels of aldosterone can be produced from corticosterone.[92]

Estrogens, particularly estriol, in the maternal circulation are indicative of fetal adrenal steroidogenic activity. The placenta, which is the principal source of estrogens during pregnancy, uses exogenous androgens supplied to an increasing extent by the fetal adrenal cortex and to a decreasing extent by the maternal adrenal cortex as gestation proceeds[93] as precursors for estrogen synthesis (see later). Low levels of estriol can first be detected in the maternal circulation at the eighth week of gestation, indicating that DHEA-S is being produced by the fetus. At around the 12th week of gestation, estriol concentrations in the maternal circulation rapidly increase approximately 100-fold. This increase coincides with the initiation of fetal zone enlargement and ACTH secretion by the fetal pituitary gland.[53] In contrast, estriol levels are markedly decreased and sometimes undetectable in women bearing anencephalic fetuses,[93, 94] if fetal death occurs,[93] or in placental sulfatase deficiency.[95] These observations indicate that the human fetal adrenal cortex produces DHEA-S beginning at around 8 to 10 weeks of gestation in sufficient quantities to effect increases in maternal estrogen levels. Production of DHEA-S by the fetal adrenal cortex continues for the remainder of pregnancy and during the second and third trimesters increases considerably such that by term the human fetal adrenal produces around 200 mg/day.[93]

A major unanswered question is when in gestation the fetal adrenal cortex begins producing cortisol. Observations of infants with congenital adrenal hyperplasia, in whom excess ACTH is produced as a result of loss of negative feedback, suggest that the fetal adrenal cortex produces cortisol early in gestation. These observations imply that under normal circumstances the fetal adrenal produces cortisol early in pregnancy, which exerts negative feedback control on fetal pituitary ACTH secretion. These observations also suggest that the human fetal pituitary produces ACTH before 10 weeks of gestation, which regulates fetal adrenal steroidogenesis. The presence of corticotropes in the human fetal pituitary can be seen at about this time.[53]

Although the human fetal adrenal cortex is responsive to ACTH and can produce corticoids and DHEA-S as early as the 10th week of gestation, the pattern of glucocorticoid production by the primate fetal adrenal cortex during the rest of pregnancy is not clear. Expression of key steroid-metabolizing enzymes suggests that the human fetal adrenal cortex does not produce cortisol de novo from cholesterol until around week 30 of gestation (see later). However, this does not preclude the possibility that cortisol is produced by use of progesterone as a precursor early in gestation.[91]

Mineralocorticoid production by the primate fetal adrenal cortex is low early in gestation but increases during the third trimester. At term, 80 percent of the aldosterone in human and rhesus monkey fetal blood appears to originate from the fetal adrenal.[92] In 18- to 21-week human fetal adrenals, the mineralocorticoid metabolic pathway is localized to the definitive zone, although its activity is low and unresponsive to secretagogues.[97, 98] The angiotensin II receptors AT_1 and AT_2 are present on human fetal adrenal cortical cells after 16 weeks of gestation.[99] The AT_2 receptor is localized mainly on definitive zone cells, whereas the AT_1 receptor is detectable to a lesser extent in cells from both fetal and definitive zones. Thus, during the first and second trimesters, the ability of the human fetal adrenal cortex to synthesize mineralocorticoids is minimal even though the cells express angiotensin II receptors.

Functional Zonation and Ontogeny of Steroidogenic Enzyme Expression. Earlier studies[96] indicated that in response to ACTH, fetal zone cells produce mainly DHEA-S and little corticoid, whereas definitive zone cells produce mainly corticoids and little DHEA-S. It was concluded that during midgestation the fetal zone is the site of DHEA-S synthesis and the definitive zone is the site of corticoid synthesis.[96] Another approach to assessing the steroidogenic potential of adrenal cortical zones has been to determine which steroidogenic enzymes are expressed by the cells of each zone. Because the fate of pregnenolone metabolism is determined by the branch point enzymes cytochrome P450 17α-hydroxylase/17,20-lyase (P450c17) and 3β-hydroxysteroid dehydrogenase/Δ^{4-5}-isomerase (3βHSD), the steroidogenic potential of cells may be inferred by the pattern of expression of these two enzymes. Expression of 3βHSD by the primate fetal adrenal cortex appears to be the critical step in the metabolism of pregnenolone, because it confers on cells the ability to convert Δ^5–3β-hydroxysteroids to Δ^{4-3}-ketosteroids essential for mineralocorticoid and glucocorticoid production (Fig. 27–2). At no time in gestation is 3βHSD expression detected in the fetal zone. This ontogenetic pattern suggests that the human fetal adrenal cortex cannot synthesize cortisol de novo between 16 and 22 weeks because it cannot convert pregnenolone to progesterone owing to the lack of 3βHSD.

Expression of P450c17, although highly abundant in the transitional and fetal zones, is lacking in the definitive zone at all gestational ages.[83, 100] The lack of P450c17 in the definitive zone implies that these cells cannot synthesize cortisol in vivo either de novo or from progesterone. Expression of P450c17 is highest in the transitional zone cells, which late in gestation also express 3βHSD. Therefore, the

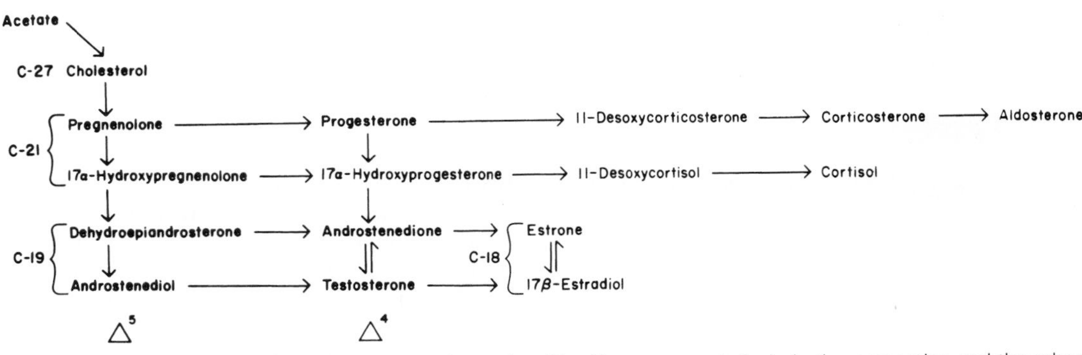

Figure 27–2 ■ Biosynthetic pathways in steroid hormone formation. The C_{21} compounds include the progestins and the adrenal corticosteroids. The C_{19} compounds include the androgens, and the C_{18} compounds include the estrogens. Steroids with a double bond between the 5 and 6 positions in the steroid nucleus (Δ^5-steroids) are shown on the left, and those with a double bond between the 4 and 5 positions (Δ^4-steroids) are depicted on the right.

transitional zone may be the site of de novo glucocorticoid production and may acquire this capability later in gestation when its cells begin to express 3βHSD.

Thus, each fetal adrenal cortical zone has a different rate of functional maturation depending on the ontogeny of expression of specific steroidogenic enzymes. Furthermore, the human fetal adrenal cortex appears to be composed of three functionally distinct zones: (1) the definitive zone, which late in gestation is the likely site of mineralocorticoid synthesis; (2) the transitional zone, which appears to be the site of glucocorticoid synthesis because it expresses the necessary biosynthetic enzymes; and (3) the fetal zone, which is the site of Δ^5-steroid production, particularly DHEA-S (Fig. 27–3).

Responsiveness to ACTH. The rapid growth and abundant steroid production by the human fetal adrenal cortex are not paralleled by increases in plasma ACTH. Instead, mean circulating ACTH levels in the human fetus were reported to decrease by almost 50 percent during this period in one study.[73] One possible explanation is that placental ACTH, discussed subsequently, plays a role in fetal adrenal growth and function. Another explanation for this paradox is that responsiveness of the fetal adrenals to ACTH increases during the second and third trimesters. Responsiveness to ACTH by human fetal adrenal cortical cells is augmented by ACTH itself[101–103] and other factors, particularly IGF-I and IGF-II.[104] Exposure of fetal zone and definitive zone cells to ACTH increases the subsequent acute response to further ACTH stimulation.[101, 102] This increased responsiveness is due to increased ACTH binding capacity[102] as a result of increased expression of the ACTH receptor.[103]

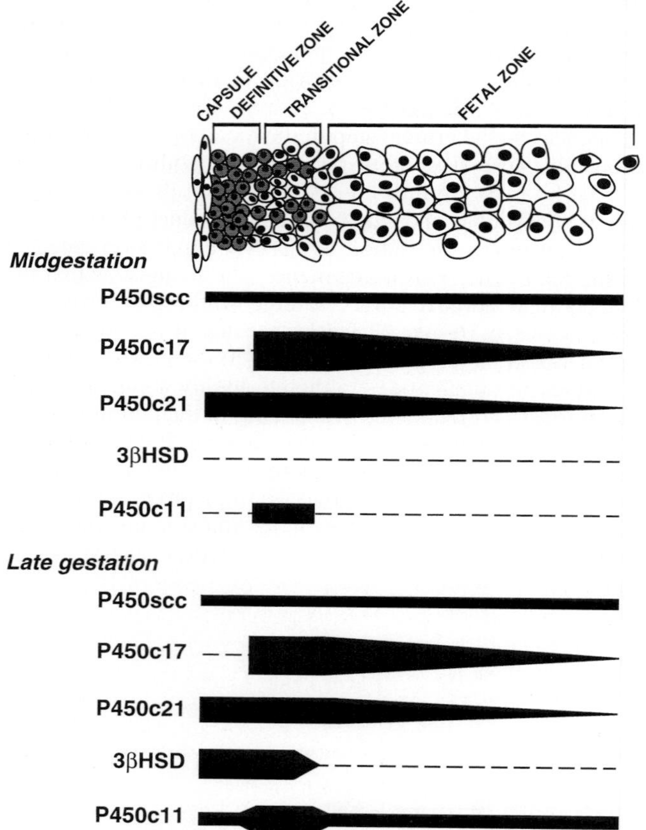

Figure 27–3 ■ Schematic representation of the localization of expression of P450scc, P450c21, 3βHSD, and P450c11 in the primate fetal adrenal cortex during midgestation and late gestation. Thickness of the line indicates relative abundance of expression. Dashed line indicates lack of expression. Note the lack of P450c17 expression in the definitive zone at all stages of gestation and the ontogenetic expression of 3βHSD only in the definitive and transitional zones late in gestation. (From Mesiano S, Jaffe RB. Developmental and functional biology of the primate fetal adrenal cortex. Endocr Rev 18:378–403, 1997. © The Endocrine Society.)

Ligand-induced up-regulation of ACTH receptor expression may be an important adaptive process directed toward optimizing adrenal responsiveness to ACTH in concert with physiologic requirements for hypothalamic-pituitary-adrenal activity. This is particularly important for the physiologic response to stress and the maintenance of metabolic homeostasis, in which the adrenals play a pivotal role. Inhibition, by ligand-induced receptor down-regulation, of mechanisms involved in the response to stress would be detrimental, whereas enhancement by ligand-induced up-regulation would be advantageous by permitting a more efficient and rapid response. Whether such a process is advantageous for fetal development is not clear. It is possible that this up-regulation is part of the process by which the fetus prepares for responding to the stresses of delivery and the perinatal period.

THE FETAL PITUITARY AND ACTH

It is not unexpected that the extraordinary growth and steroidogenic activity of the primate fetal adrenal cortex are dependent on an intact fetal pituitary gland, because it produces ACTH, the primary trophic regulator of the adrenal cortex postnatally.

The mechanism by which ACTH regulates fetal adrenal cortical growth and function is not clearly understood. The actions of ACTH are mediated through its interaction with specific receptors on the cell surface of adrenal cortical cells. A human ACTH receptor has been cloned and characterized.[105]

Although the principal regulator of fetal adrenal cortical development appears to be ACTH, several observations support the concept that human fetal adrenal growth and function are also influenced by factors that act independently from, or in conjunction with, ACTH.[79] Specific growth factors, acting in an autocrine or paracrine manner, are likely candidates as mediators or modulators of the trophic actions of ACTH on the primate fetal adrenal cortex. Studies of growth factor involvement in the regulation of fetal adrenal development have addressed (1) the effects of growth factors on proliferation and function of cultured fetal adrenal cortical cells, (2) growth factor expression by the fetal adrenals, and (3) the regulation of this growth factor expression.

Basic Fibroblast Growth Factor. Basic fibroblast growth factor (bFGF) is a peptide mitogen that stimulates the proliferation of mesoderm- and neurectoderm-derived cells and is also a potent angiogenic and neurotrophic agent. Proliferation of both fetal and definitive zone cells from midgestation human adrenals is stimulated by bFGF.[106, 107] Basic FGF elicits a greater proliferative response in definitive zone cells than in fetal zone cells. This suggests that the definitive zone may be more sensitive than the fetal zone to the mitogenic actions of bFGF and that bFGF may preferentially influence definitive zone development in vivo.

Basic FGF bioactivity and messenger ribonucleic acid (mRNA) were detected in midgestation human fetal adrenals[75]; mRNA encoding bFGF was also detected in cultured human fetal adrenal cortical cells, and its abundance was increased twofold to threefold by ACTH. Thus, bFGF, a potent mitogen for human fetal adrenal cortical cells, is expressed by these cells and regulated by ACTH and may be an important mediator of ACTH action in human fetal adrenal development.

Epidermal Growth Factor and Transforming Growth Factor-α. EGF is also a potent mitogen for cultured fetal and definitive zone cells from midgestation human fetal adrenals.[106, 107] As with their response to bFGF, definitive zone cells were more responsive to the proliferative action of EGF than were fetal zone cells, suggesting that EGF (like bFGF) preferentially regulates definitive zone growth. High-affinity surface binding sites, characteristic of EGF receptors, were detected in both cell types.[106] These findings imply that the human fetal adrenal cortex is a target for EGF or, more likely, TGF-α, which binds to the EGF receptor and is present in fetal adrenal glands whereas EGF is not (Smikle CB, Kim HS, Mesiano S, Jaffe RB. Unpublished data).

In the rhesus monkey fetus in utero, EGF stimulated hypertrophy and not hyperplasia of definitive zone cells, an unexpected effect given the potent mitogenic action of EGF on definitive zone cells in vitro.[108] Thus, in vivo, TGF-α may not be a direct mitogen for definitive zone cells but instead may affect its growth by modulating the hypothalamic-pituitary axis and possibly increasing ACTH secretion or ACTH responsiveness.

Insulin-Like Growth Factors I and II. IGF-I and IGF-II affect growth and function in a wide variety of cell types and can act as autocrine, paracrine, or endocrine factors. IGF-I (formerly known as somatomedin C) mediates many of the somatotropic actions of growth hormone. Although the role of IGF-II is less defined, it is thought to be involved in the regulation of fetal development because its circulating and tissue levels are highest during fetal life and fall postnatally.[109] Two IGF receptors, designated type I and type II, have been identified.[110] The type I receptor is structurally related to the insulin receptor and binds both IGF-I and IGF-II with high affinity and insulin with lower affinity. Most of the known actions of IGF-I and IGF-II appear to be mediated by activation of the type I receptor. The IGF system is made more complex by the presence of six high-affinity IGF-binding proteins, which associate with the IGF peptides and modulate their biologic activity.[111]

Studies of IGFs in human fetal adrenal development indicate that IGF-II is quantitatively the predominant IGF expressed during fetal life. In the fetal adrenals, abundance of mRNA encoding IGF-II was high (second only to the liver), whereas mRNA encoding IGF-I was low.[112, 113] All of the components of the IGF system (i.e., IGFs, receptors, and binding proteins) are expressed by human fetal adrenals.[114]

A high level of IGF-II expression is present both in vivo[112] and in vitro and can be stimulated by ACTH and factors that increase intracellular cyclic adenosine monophosphate (cAMP).[115, 116] IGF-II is expressed by all ACTH-responsive cortical cells in high abundance, whereas IGF-I is detectable only in the adrenal capsule. Similarly, in cultured human fetal adrenal cortical cells, mRNA encoding IGF-II is highly abundant, and its abundance is markedly up-regulated by ACTH. In contrast, IGF-I mRNA is not detected in cultured fetal adrenal cortical cells and cannot be stimulated with ACTH. These findings were confirmed in the fetal rhesus monkey in vivo in which endogenous ACTH secretion was increased by administration of metyrapone.[87] Adrenals of metyrapone-treated fetuses were larger than those of control fetuses and expressed higher levels of IGF-II but not of IGF-I. Taken together, these data strongly implicate IGF-II as an important local regulator of fetal adrenal development and a possible mediator of at least some of the trophic actions of ACTH. Adrenal cortical cells from a 6-week human neonate responded to ACTH with increased cortisol production but failed to express IGF-II,[117] suggesting that expression of IGF-II by the human adrenal cortex and its regulation by ACTH are unique to fetal life.

In cultured human fetal adrenal cortical cells, IGF-II is a specific mitogen.[116] The IGFs act cooperatively with bFGF and presumably TGF-α, other known mitogens for human fetal adrenal cortical cells (see earlier), resulting in an additive effect on cell proliferation.

In conjunction with its mitogenic activity, IGF-II also affects the differentiated function of human fetal adrenal cortical cells. IGF-II augments ACTH-stimulated cortisol and DHEA-S production in human fetal adrenal cortical cells and ACTH-stimulated expression of the steroidogenic enzymes P450scc, P450c17, and 3βHSD.[104, 118] Whereas IGF-II directly up-regulates basal expression of P450c17, it does not enhance basal expression of P450scc or 3βHSD. The increased P450c17 activity suggests that IGF-II may be an important regulator of adrenal androgen production. Activation of the type I IGF receptor by either IGF-I (postnatally) or IGF-II (prenatally) may directly augment adrenal androgen synthetic capacity by augmenting P450c17 expression and activity. This may be an important mechanism by which adrenal androgen production is regulated during fetal and postnatal life.

Activin/Inhibin. Activin and inhibin are homodimeric ($\beta_A\beta_A$, $\beta_B\beta_B$, or $\beta_A\beta_B$) and heterodimeric ($\alpha\beta_A$ or $\alpha\beta_B$) glycoproteins, respectively, that are structurally related to other members of the TGF-β family of peptides. Both inhibin and activin originally were isolated from follicular fluid. It is now apparent that activin's actions extend beyond the pituitary-gonadal axis to affect many key biologic functions. The amino acid sequence of activin is strongly conserved between species. Activin appears to play a role in the regulation of adrenal cortical development and function. This is not unexpected because activin has profound effects on the growth and function of granulosa cells,[119] which originate from the same germ layer as adrenal cortical cells. Each of the activin/inhibin subunit proteins and their mRNAs were detected in human fetal and adult adrenals.[120, 121] In cultured fetal adrenal cortical cells, ACTH stimulated secretion of immunoreactive α-subunit. This suggests that ACTH stimulates inhibin production by fetal adrenal cortical cells, because the α-subunit is present only in the inhibin molecule. ACTH enhances the abundance of mRNAs encoding the α-subunit and β_A-subunit, but not the β_B-subunit, in cultured fetal adrenal cortical cells. Thus, during midgestation, the human fetal adrenals express each of the activin/inhibin subunits and appear to produce immunoreactive activin A in the definitive and transitional zones (see Fig. 27–1). ACTH stimulates expression of the α-subunit and β_A-subunit, suggesting that fetal adrenal production of activin and inhibin is under trophic hormone regulation.

Recombinant human activin A inhibits proliferation of fetal zone cells and increases ACTH-stimulated cortisol production.[120, 121] Activin has no effect on DHEA-S production by fetal zone cells or growth and steroidogenesis in definitive zone or adult adrenal cortical cells. Recombinant human inhibin has no effect on proliferation or function of any of the adrenal cortical cell types. Thus, activin acts directly and specifically on fetal zone cells to inhibit their rate of growth and enhance their capacity for cortisol production in response to ACTH. Activin appears to inhibit fetal zone cell growth by stimulating cellular apoptosis and therefore may be involved in the postnatal demise of the fetal zone, a process involving apoptosis.[88, 99] In addition, activin may coordinately stimulate the differentiation of other fetal zone cells into a cortisol-producing phenotype.

Transforming Growth Factor-β. TGF-β is the prototypical peptide of a large family of growth factor proteins including activin, inhibin, müllerian-inhibiting substance, bone morphogenic protein, and several closely related proteins. Specific receptors for TGF-β have been identified on almost all mammalian cells. The effect of TGF-β is variable and appears to be dependent on the cell type. In general, TGF-β stimulates proliferation of cells of mesenchymal origin and inhibits proliferation of cells of epithelial or neurectodermal origin.[122] TGF-β also modulates the differentiated function of cells and in particular has marked effects on the function of steroid-producing cells.

Both basal and ACTH-stimulated DHEA-S and cortisol production and expression of P450c17 by fetal and definitive zone cells are inhibited by TGF-β.[123] TGF-β binds to specific sites on human fetal adrenal cortical cells, and these binding sites are regulated by ACTH.[124] Whether TGF-β is expressed by human fetal adrenal cortical cells is unknown. Taken together, these data indicate that TGF-β–related peptides (particularly TGF-β and activin) are significant negative regulators of human fetal adrenal growth and may play an important role in balancing the positive effects of other growth factors during adrenal development.

Nuclear Receptors/Transcription Factors. Nuclear receptors are essential elements in cellular regulation because they mediate the link between an extracellular signal and the transcriptional response. Many transcription factors have been identified that share sequence homology (especially in the DNA and ligand binding domains) with classical nuclear receptors, but their ligands have not been identified. These are referred to as "orphan" nuclear receptors. Two of these, steroidogenic factor 1 (SF-1) and DAX-1, appear to play major roles in adrenal development and function.

SF-1 regulates the expression of genes encoding steroidogenic enzymes.[125, 126] Consensus binding sites for SF-1 have been identified in the promoter regions of genes for most steroidogenic enzymes. Interestingly, in the mouse, SF-1 is also expressed in the embryonic anlage of steroidogenic cells before their acquisition of a steroidogenic phenotype, suggesting that it is involved in the early embryonic development of steroidogenic tissues. Mice deprived of SF-1 had normal survival in utero but died by postnatal day 8 because of severe adrenal insufficiency. These animals lacked adrenal glands and gonads, and all animals (male and female) had female internal reproductive organs, demonstrating the essential role of SF-1 in the embryonic differentiation of steroidogenic tissues, in particular the embryonic development of the adrenal cortex. A similar role of SF-1 in the regulation of adrenal development in humans is likely but presently unproved. Several studies have demonstrated SF-1 expression in human steroidogenic tissues, and a growing body of literature demonstrates a role for SF-1 in the regulation of the genes for human steroidogenic enzymes.[126]

Another transcription factor that appears to be an important regulator of adrenal development is DAX-1. Mutations in the gene encoding DAX-1 are responsible for X-linked adrenal hypoplasia congenita (AHC), an inherited disorder in humans that is characterized by hypoplasia of the fetal adrenal glands with absence of the definitive zone and the structural disorganization of the fetal zone[127, 128] (see reference 84 for review). The *DAX-1* gene derives its name from its proximity to the dosage-sensitive sex reversal locus and the *AHC* locus on the X chromosome.[128] Like SF-1, DAX-1 is also a member of the nuclear receptor superfamily, and because its ligand is not yet known, it is considered an orphan nuclear receptor. DAX-1 is expressed in the human adrenal gland and testis and, to a lesser extent, in the ovary. Abundance of mRNA encoding DAX-1 is much lower in the adult adrenal than in the fetal adrenal,[128] possibly reflecting its more important role in fetal adrenal development. The tissue distribution of DAX-1 expression is similar to that for SF-1,[129] suggesting that these two factors may be coregulators of steroidogenic tissue development and function. Putative SF-1 response elements have been identified in the 5′ flanking region of the human *DAX-1* gene,[130, 131] suggesting that SF-1 is involved in the regulation of DAX-1 expression and that SF-1 is proximal to DAX-1 in the regulatory cascade. The complete absence of adrenals and gonads associated with SF-1 deficiency but not with DAX-1 deficiency suggests that SF-1 is obligatory for adrenal and gonadal development, whereas the requirement for DAX-1 is partial; DAX-1 appears to be required for the development of the definitive zone but not the fetal zone. The molecular mechanism underlying the actions of DAX-1 is not yet fully characterized.

Fetal Pituitary-Gonadal Functions and Interactions

The foundation for normal puberty and adult reproductive function is established during fetal life. On the basis of studies of primate fetal endocrine physiology, it is apparent that the endocrine system is one of the earliest, if not the earliest, systems to develop. This is true particularly for intrauterine gonadal development, which is essential for normal sexual development. The consequence of impairment of this system can be irreparable loss of germ cells, endocrine function, and reproductive potential.

TESTIS

The development of the fetal testis is described in Chapter 14 and that of the fetal ovary in Chapters 6 and 14. Therefore, their development is only encapsulated here from a slightly different perspective. Sexual development in humans, as in most mammals, can be divided into four stages: (1) pregonadal, (2) indifferent, (3) primary sex differentiation, and (4) secondary sex differentiation.[132] The first three stages and part of the fourth occur in the embryo in the human (first 8 weeks after conception). These facets of embryonic development are pivotal to understanding the subsequent events occurring during human fetal life.

The pregonadal stage begins with the differentiation of primordial germ cells in 4.5-day-old blastocysts,[133] a time when there are no specific gonadal structures. The indifferent stage is initiated with the development of the gonadal or genital ridges and lasts about 7 to 10 days in the human embryo.[134] The indifferent gonad forms as a result of proliferation and thickening of the genital ridge and its coelomic epithelium on the medioventral surface of the mesonephric fold to the root of the dorsal mesentery. The epithelium lies directly on the underlying tissue without an intervening basement membrane.[134]

Simultaneously, the primordial germ cells begin ameboid migration from the yolk sac endoderm into the mesoderm of the coelomic epithelium and the urogenital ridge. By 5 to 6 weeks' gestation, the indifferent gonad is composed of primordial germ cells, supporting cells of the coelomic epithelium, and gonadal ridge mesenchyme. The first sign of primary sex differentiation is the appearance of Sertoli cells,[135] which aggregate to form testicular cords at about 43 to 50 days, which subsequently enclose the germ cells. This is followed by differentiation of mesenchymal somatic cells into Leydig cells.

During secondary sex differentiation, androgen and müllerian-inhibiting substance (see Chapter 14) production by the male testis causes müllerian duct regression and stabilization of the wolffian duct and its derivatives. In the absence of these testicular products, the müllerian duct and female genitalia form. As described in Chapter 14 and illustrated in Figure 14–4, the development of a male gonad is directed by the sex-determining region of the Y chromosome (*SRY*). The appearance and morphologic differentiation of Sertoli cells are followed by development of adherent junctions between adjacent Sertoli cells and formation of a basement membrane along the base of the tubules.[136] This is followed by secretion of müllerian-inhibiting substance and later differentiation of interstitial or Leydig cells.[137] Important paracrine (müllerian-inhibiting substance) and endocrine (inhibin/activin)[138] Sertoli cell functions continue throughout embryonic and fetal development. The testicular cords that do not have a lumen grow, become circular, and anastomose during the fetal period. They are enveloped by a basal lamina that is detectable in the human fetus by 44 to 48 days.[139]

The fetal spermatogonia are found in the cords surrounded by Sertoli cells; germ cells not enclosed by testicular cords degenerate rapidly. In contrast to those of the female, male germ cells do not start meiotic division before puberty. The spermatogonia in the periphery of the testicular tubules cease mitotic division at 18 to 20 weeks.[140]

Androgen-secreting Leydig cells are seen in the testis at 8 weeks.[141] Concentrations of androgens in testicular tissue, blood, and amniotic fluid reach a maximum at 15 to 18 weeks,[142, 143] paralleled by an increase in Leydig cell number. Their numbers subsequently decrease, and only a few Leydig cells are seen at term.[141]

OVARY

In the human fetal ovary, meiosis begins shortly after ovarian differentiation. Although the capacity for limited steroidogenesis exists, few if any steroids are produced de novo in the ovary at this time. During female fetal and neonatal development, there is no apparent need for ovarian function. In contrast, adequate fetal and prepubertal ovarian development is necessary for normal puberty and reproductive life.

Between 7 and 9 weeks, large ameboid-appearing cells, the majority of which are oogonia, are scattered throughout the ovarian parenchyma.[144] Intraovarian mesonephric cell cords occupy the medulla before meiosis begins.[145] Meiotic prophase begins at around 11 to 12 weeks. With increasing gestational age, more germ cells enter meiosis and go through leptotene, zygotene, and pachytene stages.[146] The diplotene stage of prophase is completed shortly after birth, and oocytes enter a resting stage until reproductive life. The peak number of germ cells is reached at 16 to 20 weeks,[147] at which time their number increases to about 6 million, with subsequent progressive reduction to about 2 million at term (for a more detailed discussion of this process, see reference 148).

At 13.5 to 14 weeks, diplotene oocytes begin to be surrounded by an incomplete layer of flattened follicular cells. After 16 weeks, follicular development intensifies, and shortly thereafter all diplotene oocytes are in primordial follicles[149] (oocytes surrounded by a single layer of flat granulosa cells and a basement membrane without a defined theca cell layer). Further development of the follicle and the development of the zona pellucida surrounding the oocyte are discussed in Chapter 6 and reference 148.

Interstitial cells possessing ultrastructural characteristics of steroid-producing cells can be seen after 12 weeks,[150] perhaps accounting for the steroidogenic capacity of the early fetal ovary. During the last trimester, theca cells with steroidogenic capacity surround the developing follicles.[146] Despite this steroidogenic capacity, it is unlikely that significant secretion of fetal ovarian steroids occurs during most of pregnancy.

REGULATION OF GONADAL GROWTH AND DIFFERENTIATION

The control of fetal gonadal function by fetal pituitary or placental gonadotropins is not fully understood. As discussed subsequently in other contexts, hCG has close biologic, structural, and immunologic similarities to LH. Maternal levels of hCG are detectable shortly after implantation of the blastocyst about 9 to 13 days after conception.[151, 152] Levels of hCG in the maternal circulation peak at about 10 weeks and subsequently decline to a nadir at 20 weeks.[153, 154] Fetal levels parallel those of the mother but are about 5 percent of those in maternal serum. Circulating levels of fetal FSH peak at 28 weeks and are higher in female fetuses than in males until the last 6 weeks of pregnancy.[154, 155]

Studies of anencephalic fetuses indicate that embryonic sexual differentiation and early gonadal development do not depend on fetal pituitary gonadotropes. In anencephalics, there is a reduction in Leydig cell number, whereas a reduction in the number of spermatogonia is uncommon.[156] There is also a similar time of appearance of seminiferous tubules in anencephalic and normal fetuses.[156] In female anencephalics, the ovary appears to develop normally until 32 weeks; testicular development is impaired earlier.[156] At term, ovaries of anencephalic fetuses are smaller than normal, and central follicles are absent.[156] In anencephalics, proliferation of oogonia with progression through meiosis until development of primordial follicles is not initiated.[156] Thus, pituitary gonadotropins are necessary for granulosa cell/follicular proliferation near term and, to a lesser extent, through granulosa cell regulation, for oocyte survival. In at least some mammalian species, Kit ligand (stem cell factor), produced locally by the granulosa cell, influences oocyte development. The receptor for Kit ligand, c-*kit*, is located on the oocyte.[157] On the basis of studies in fetal rhesus monkeys, fetal pituitary gonadotropins appear necessary for granulosa cell proliferation and follicular fluid formation during the latter part of pregnancy.[158]

Placental hCG has long been regarded as the gonadotropic stimulus to steroidogenesis in early pregnancy on the basis of the observations that (1) fetal circulating hCG concentrations reach a peak at 12 weeks, a time when testicular Leydig cell content is highest[141]; (2) when hCG and fetal testosterone levels fall in the second half of pregnancy, there is a parallel regression in Leydig cells in the testis[159]; and (3) fetal testes contain binding sites for hCG.[160, 161] However, one group failed to show hCG-dependent testosterone secretion in 10- to 18-week testes,[162] perhaps because the high endogenous hCG in the freshly excised testes had fully occupied the hCG receptors, precluding exogenous hCG from eliciting an additional response.

Gonadotropic regulation differs for males and females in human and monkey (a model for late gestation) fetal gonads. FSH receptors are present in the second-trimester human and late gestational rhesus monkey fetal testes.[163] Specific FSH binding is not found in human second-trimester ovaries but is present in near-term monkey fetal ovaries.[163] Thus, the ovary develops gonadotropin receptors only at a later stage of pregnancy.

GONADAL STEROIDOGENESIS AND ITS REGULATION

In contrast to the ovary, fetal testes can synthesize testosterone de novo.[164, 165] Testosterone secretion by Leydig cells is necessary at different stages of pregnancy for adequate growth of internal and external genitalia. In the human fetal testis, the Δ^5-pathway appears to be of greater significance than the Δ^4-pathway in testosterone biosynthesis (see Fig. 27–2). A temporal relationship exists between the rise and fall of testicular and serum testosterone levels and the pattern of serum gonadotropin concentrations[159] (Fig. 27–4). In the fetal rhesus monkey in utero, testosterone production can be elicited by hCG injection and by stimulating the fetal pituitary-testicular axis with GnRH.[60, 166] Low-density lipoprotein cholesterol can serve as a precursor for steroid synthesis in the fetal testes[167] and may function as an inducer of testicular steroidogenesis as well.[167]

The gradual decline of Leydig cells in the fetus is accompanied by the decline of the mRNA levels for the steroidogenic enzymes P450scc and P450c17.[168] Levels of aromatase activity, necessary for estrogen formation, are low in the fetal testis.[169]

In contrast to the male, ovarian steroid production is not essential for female phenotypic development. Furthermore, meiosis in the ovary begins relatively early, but significant estrogen production does not occur until late in fetal life, although the capacity for aromatization exists by the eighth week.[170] The preponderance of data indicates that although certain enzymatic activity can be demonstrated in the fetal ovary,[171] it cannot form estrogen de novo and is probably steroidogenically quiescent through most of pregnancy. It is possible that locally produced growth factors, acting in

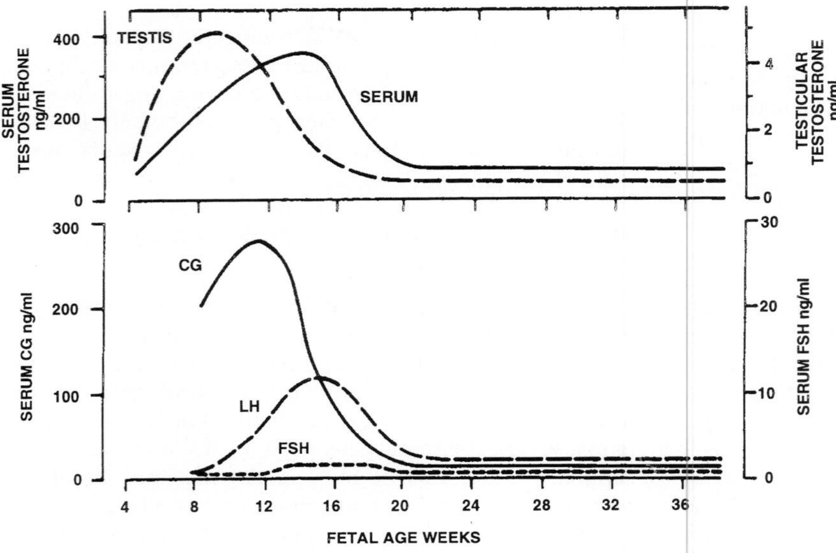

Figure 27–4 ■ Schematic depiction of serum chorionic gonadotropin (CG) and pituitary gonadotropin levels in the human male fetus and their temporal relationship to mean testicular and circulating testosterone levels. (From Wartenberg H. Differentiation and development of the testes. *In* Burger H, DeKretzer D [eds]. The Testis. New York, Raven Press, 1989, p 41.)

an autocrine/paracrine manner, play a role in growth and development of the fetal gonads, but this has not been studied extensively to date in the human (see reference 172 for discussion). The mRNA for one of these growth factors, IGF-II, has been demonstrated in the midtrimester human fetal testis and ovary.[172]

Fetal Pituitary-Thyroid Functions and Interactions

In the human fetus, the thyroid gland has acquired its characteristic morphologic appearance and the capacity to concentrate radioiodine and to synthesize iodothyronines by 10 to 12 weeks of gestation.[173] In addition, by this stage, thyrotropes can be detected in the fetal pituitary[53] and radioimmunoassayable TSH can be found in the fetal pituitary and serum. Thyroxine (T_4) has also been found in the fetal circulation.[173]

Hypothalamic TRH is detectable at 10 to 12 weeks. The maturation of the fetal hypothalamus is accompanied by maturation of the hypothalamic-pituitary portal system.

Thyroid function remains in a basal state until midgestation. At this time, secretory activity of the thyroid gland and serum T_4 concentrations begin to increase (Fig. 27–5). It is likely that this rise is related to the establishment of continuity between the hypothalamic and pituitary portions of the portal vascular system.[173, 174] Pituitary and serum TSH concentrations begin to rise shortly before the rise in T_4 levels. Maximal TSH concentrations are reached early in the third trimester and do not increase further until term. In the rhesus monkey, a TSH response to TRH administration is present early in the third trimester[175] and may well be present much earlier. In contrast with the adult, triiodothyronine (T_3) administration to the fetus does not suppress the pituitary TSH response to TRH in primates.[175] The human infant born after 26 to 28 weeks of gestation responds to exogenous administration of TRH with an increase of circulating TSH levels similar to those seen in adults.[173, 176]

At term, TSH secretion by the human fetus can be inhibited by the administration of T_4. Intra-amniotic injection of T_4 24 hours before elective cesarean section almost doubles cord T_4 concentrations, with only a minimal increase in the mean cord serum T_3.[174, 176] In addition, the elevated cord T_4 is associated with marked suppression of the neonatal TSH surge.[174] This inhibitory effect of T_4 is presumably mediated through pituitary conversion of T_4 to T_3.[173] Human fetal serum T_4 and free T_4 levels increase progressively during the last trimester, although serum TSH levels do not[174] (see Fig. 27–5).

Serum T_3 concentrations are usually unmeasurable in the human fetus until approximately 30 weeks' gestation.[174] Thereafter, concentrations rise to a mean level of approximately 50 ng/dl at term. The prenatal increase in serum T_3 concentrations occurs during several weeks and may be related to increased cortisol concentrations.[177] Immediately after birth (during the first 4 to 6 hours), circulating T_3 levels increase still further to concentrations three to six times those occurring in utero.[177, 178] The interesting substance reverse T_3 (3, 3′, 5′-triiodothyronine) reaches concentrations in the human fetus greater than 250 ng/dl early in the last trimester; these decrease progressively until term.[174, 178, 179] In contrast with T_3 levels, serum reverse T_3 concentrations remain virtually unchanged during early neonatal life in term infants.

An acute increase in pituitary TSH levels occurs when the term fetus is exposed to the extrauterine environment. This, in turn, stimulates thyroidal iodine uptake and evokes release of thyroid hormones.[174, 180] The maximal TSH concentrations are attained 30 minutes after birth. Thereafter, there is a rapid decrease in serum TSH during the first day of extrauterine life and a slower decrease during the succeeding 2 days. Serum T_4 and free T_4 levels reach a peak at 24 hours and then decrease slowly during the first weeks of life.[181]

Binding of iodothyronine and maturation of thyroid hormone receptors have not been reported in the human fetus. In the rat, hepatic nuclear T_3 receptors mature during the

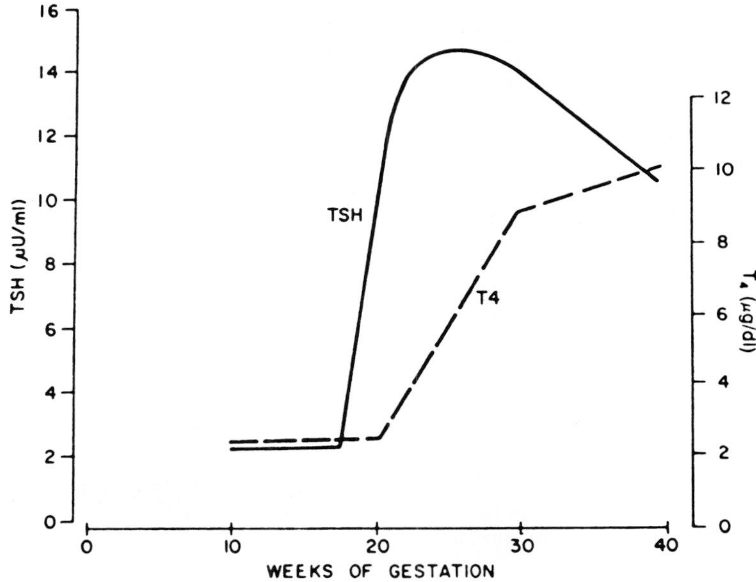

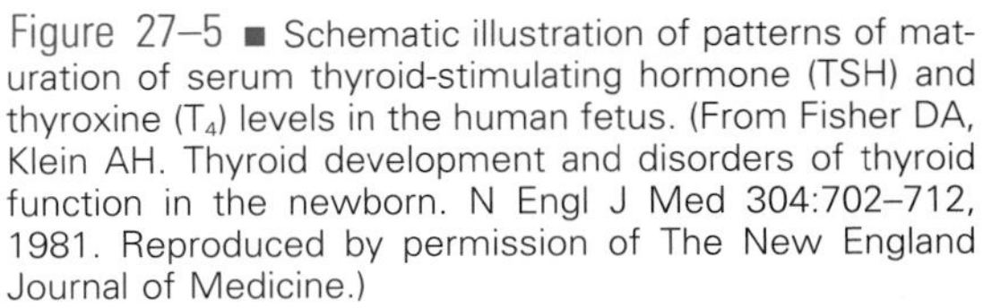

Figure 27–5 ■ Schematic illustration of patterns of maturation of serum thyroid-stimulating hormone (TSH) and thyroxine (T_4) levels in the human fetus. (From Fisher DA, Klein AH. Thyroid development and disorders of thyroid function in the newborn. N Engl J Med 304:702–712, 1981. Reproduced by permission of The New England Journal of Medicine.)

first few weeks after birth.[182] T_3 receptor capacity, and possibly affinity, increases during the first 3 to 4 weeks. In the brain, in contrast with the liver, T_3 nuclear receptor binding develops early.[183] Binding to T_3 by fetal brain cells is comparable with that in the adult and increases still further in the first 3 days of neonatal life.[183] However, there appears to be a discrepancy between T_3 nuclear receptor binding and brain tissue responsiveness in both the neonate and the adult. Neither appears to respond to exogenous T_3 administration with an increase in oxygen consumption.[183] Other enzyme markers of brain activity, such as α-glycerophosphate dehydrogenase and malic enzyme, also fail to respond to T_3 stimulation.[183] Of interest is the observation that thyroid hormones increase nerve growth factor concentrations in adult and newborn mouse brain[184]; it has been postulated that this nerve growth factor may modulate the effects of thyroid hormones on brain development.[183]

Steroidogenesis and the Fetoplacental Unit

In large measure, the integrated *fetoplacental unit* must control its destiny—its growth, development, and function as well as the subsequent expulsion of the fetus and senescence of the placenta and even its ability to survive in an alien environment.

From the endocrinologic point of view, these functions are subsumed by steroid hormone production by the fetal adrenal, gonad, and placenta; by neuropeptide and polypeptide hormone production by the fetal hypothalamic-pituitary unit and placenta; and by hormonal production by the fetal thyroid and pancreas. Contributing to this fetal and placental activity are the changes in maternal endocrine economy and the influence these have on the function of fetus and placenta.

Steroid Formation

In regard to steroid hormone formation in pregnancy, two aspects must be considered: (1) the integrated role and constant interaction of fetus, placenta, and mother in the formation of the large quantities of the sex steroids—estrogens and progesterone—extant during pregnancy; and (2) steroid hormone formation and regulation within the fetus itself. The latter has been discussed in the preceding section.

The concept has evolved that the placenta is an incomplete steroid-producing organ—unlike the adult adrenal, testis, and ovary—and must rely on precursors reaching it from the fetal and maternal circulations. From the unique interdependence of fetus, placenta, and mother arose the concept of an integrated *fetoplacental-maternal unit.* To understand this concept, the reader will find it useful to review the general biosynthetic pathways in steroid hormone formation (see Figs. 27–2 and 14–9).

The individual adult steroid-producing glands are capable of the formation of progestins, androgens, and estrogens, but this is not true of the placenta. There is a constant interplay of fetus, placenta, and mother to form the bulk of the sex steroids in pregnancy. For estrogen formation by the placenta to occur, precursors must reach it from both the fetal and maternal compartments, whereas placental progesterone formation is accomplished in large part from circulating maternal low-density lipoprotein cholesterol.[185, 186] In the placenta, the cholesterol is converted first to pregnenolone and then rapidly and efficiently to progesterone.[187] Production of progesterone approximates 250 mg/day by the end of pregnancy, at which time circulating levels are on the order of 130 ng/ml[188] (Fig. 27–6). To form estrogens, the placenta, which has an active aromatizing capacity, uses circulating androgens, primarily from the fetus but also from the mother. The major androgenic precursor in placental estrogen formation is DHEA-S, mainly from the fetal adrenal gland. Because the placenta has an abundance of the sulfatase (sulfate-cleaving) enzyme, DHEA-S is converted to free (unconjugated) DHEA when it reaches the placenta, then to androstenedione, thereafter to testosterone, and finally to estrone and 17β-estradiol.

In human pregnancy, however, by far the major estrogen formed is neither estrone nor estradiol but another estrogen, estriol. Estriol is not secreted by the ovary of nonpregnant women. It has an additional hydroxyl group in the 16 position and constitutes more than 90 percent of the known estrogen in pregnancy urine, into which it is excreted as sulfate and glucuronide conjugates. Concentrations increase with advancing gestation and range from approximately 2 mg/24 hr at 26 weeks to 35 to 45 mg/24 hr at term.[189] Estriol is also found in high concentrations in amniotic fluid[190] and in the maternal circulation. At term, the concentration of estriol in the maternal circulation is between approximately 8 and 13 ng/dl.[191]

Estriol is formed by a unique biosynthetic process during pregnancy, which demonstrates the interdependence of fe-

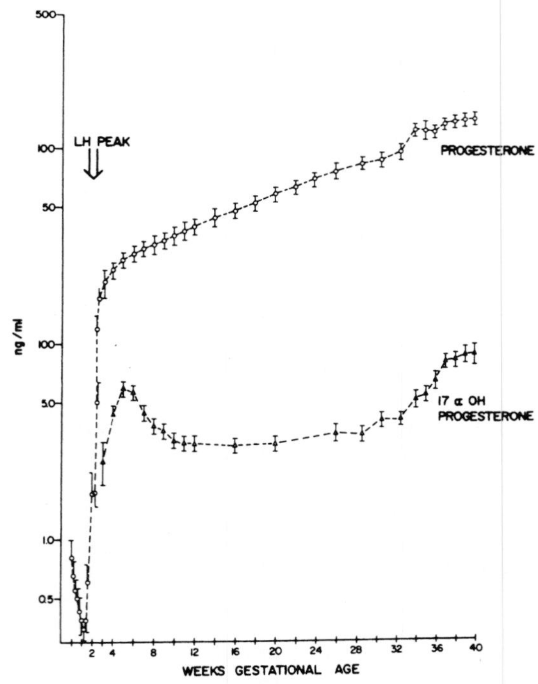

Figure 27–6 ■ Relative increments of circulating concentrations (mean ± SE) of progesterone and 17α-hydroxyprogesterone during the course of human pregnancy. The data are values before and after the LH peak at midcycle.

tus, placenta, and mother (Fig. 27–7). Quantitatively, DHEA-S is the major steroid produced by the fetal adrenal gland; almost all of it is produced in the fetal zone, as discussed previously.[96] When DHEA-S of either fetal or maternal origin reaches the placenta, estrone and estradiol are formed. However, little of either is converted to estriol by the placenta. Instead, some of the DHEA-S undergoes 16α-hydroxylation, primarily in the fetal liver and, to a limited extent, in the fetal adrenal itself.[192] When the 16α-hydroxydehydroepiandrosterone sulfate (16α-OH-DHEA-S) so formed reaches the placenta, the placental sulfatase enzyme cleaves the sulfate side chain, and the unconjugated 16α-OH-DHEA, after further metabolism, is aromatized to form estriol. The estriol is then secreted into the maternal circulation. When it reaches the maternal liver, it is conjugated to form estriol sulfate, estriol glucosiduronate, and a mixed conjugate, estriol sulfoglucosiduronate, in which forms it is excreted by way of the maternal urine.[193]

Another placental estrogen derived from a fetal precursor is estetrol, formed after 15-hydroxylation of 16α-OH-DHEA-S. Its function is not known.

With such relatively copious amounts of progesterone and estriol produced each day, the question of the function of these two steroids during pregnancy must be addressed. In the case of progesterone, attention has focused on its effect in maintaining the uterine myometrium in a state of relative quiescence during much of the pregnancy.

Putative Functional Roles of Progesterone and Estrogen. Siiteri and colleagues[194] proposed that progesterone produced by the placenta, the ovaries, or both is the essential hormone of mammalian pregnancy because of its ability to inhibit T lymphocyte cell–mediated responses involved in tissue rejection. On the basis of their experiments demonstrating the role of progesterone in prolonging xenogeneic grafts, preventing inflammation, and promoting the survival of human trophoblastic tissue in rodents, they suggested that a high local (intrauterine) concentration of progesterone can effectively block cellular immune responses to foreign antigens. They pointed out that progesterone has been aptly called the "hormone of pregnancy" because it appears to be essential for maintenance of pregnancy in all mammals examined, and its presence has been detected in species representing all classes of vertebrates and lower forms, such as mollusks. The essential nature of progesterone for pregnancy maintenance has been demonstrated by experiments in which abortion was induced after the administration of drugs that either inhibit progesterone synthesis or compete with progesterone for binding sites or the administration of progesterone antibodies. The specificity of the abortifacient effect was demonstrated by the concurrent administration of progesterone in some of these experiments.

The functional role of estriol in pregnancy has caused a great deal of speculation. In many biologic systems, estriol is a weak estrogen, with approximately 0.01 times the

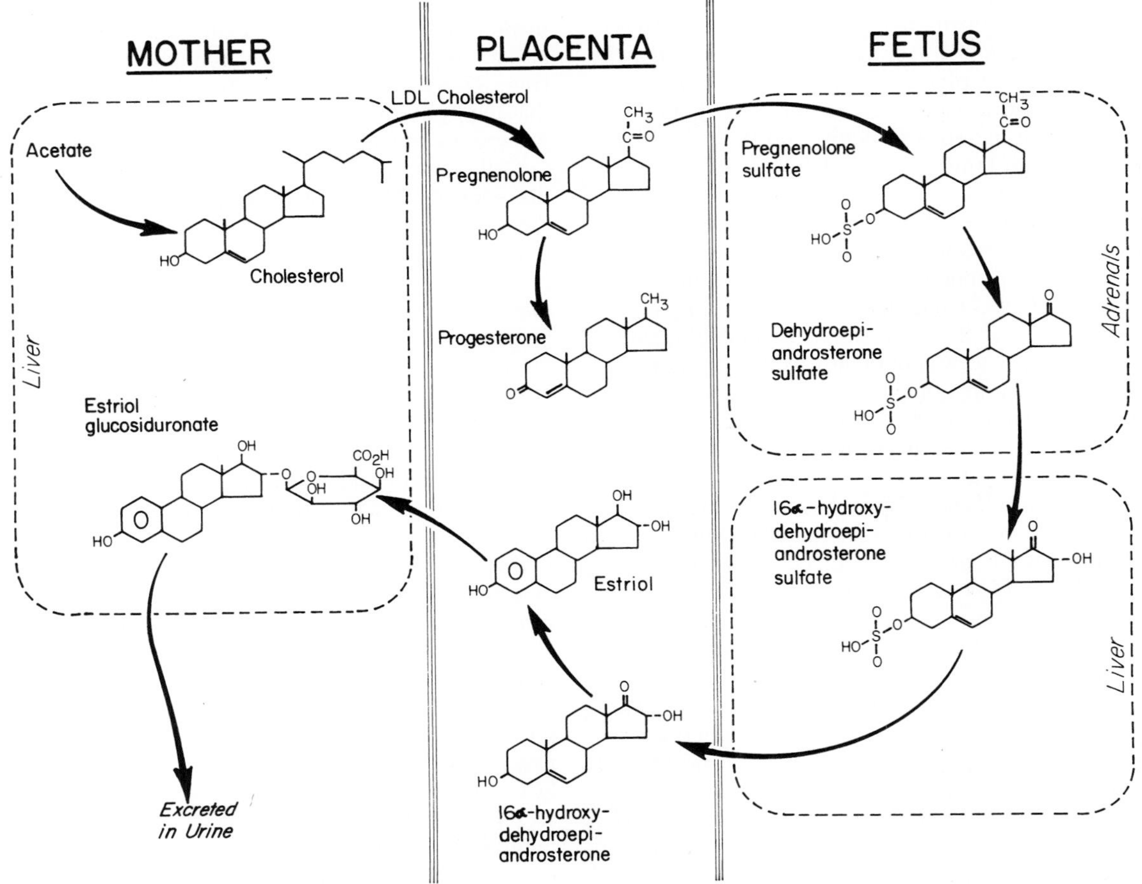

Figure 27–7 ■ Overall pathway of estriol biosynthesis in late pregnancy.

potency of estradiol and 0.1 times the potency of estrone on a weight basis. However, there is one function for which estriol appears to be as effective as the other estrogens: its ability to increase uteroplacental blood flow. Therefore, this may be a primary function of the large amounts of estriol produced each day.[195] Its relatively weak estrogenic effects on other organ systems may make it an ideal candidate for this purpose. Estrogens exert their effect on blood flow by prostaglandin stimulation.[196] Although acute administration of estriol is ineffective as an estrogen and does not demonstrate extensive binding to estrogen receptors, prolonged exposure to estriol does produce estrogen effects and binding occurs.[197, 198]

Placental Proteins, Peptides, and Growth Factors and Their Interactions

The placenta serves to transmit nutrients to the fetus and waste products from the fetus to the maternal circulation. The placenta also exerts hormonal modulation of maternal metabolism at different stages of gestation. The functional unit of the placenta is the chorionic villus, which has a central core of loose connective tissue with an extensive capillary network linking it with the fetal circulation. Surrounding the core are the inner syncytiotrophoblast and outer cytotrophoblast.

A plethora of data indicate that in addition to the pituitary trophic hormone–like proteins of the placenta—hCG, human chorionic somatomammotropin (hCS), and human chorionic corticotropin (hCC)—hypothalamic peptides, including GnRH, corticotropin-releasing hormone (CRH), and somatostatin, are also synthesized by trophoblastic cells. Not only has the placental synthesis of an array of hypothalamic-like hormones been demonstrated, but the presence of many of the growth factors and their receptors, as well as the inhibin family of gonadal peptides, has been as well.

Intriguingly, production of placental protein hormones is no longer seen as autonomous; an increasing number of in vitro studies point to endogenous placental regulation of its hormonal products, simulating a miniature hypothalamic–pituitary–target hormone unit. In addition, substances reaching the placental circulation may also regulate placental hormone production. If these in vitro studies are confirmed in vivo, the concept of autoregulation within the placenta will replace that of autonomous hormone production and constitute a new chapter in our understanding of placental biology. This subject has been extensively reviewed.[199, 200] The sites of origin and putative interactions of these placental hormones are presented schematically in Figure 27–8. In addition to their actions within the placenta, a number of these placental hormones may exert effects on the fetus or the mother and thus participate in fetal and maternal homeostasis during pregnancy and perhaps the timing of parturition. Hormonal regulation within the placenta may be paracrine, autocrine, or endocrine.

Many of the analogues of the hypothalamic hormones are produced primarily in the cytotrophoblastic layer of the placenta. These include GnRH and its precursor GnRH-associated peptide, somatostatin, TRH, and the family of opioid peptides. CRH, originally thought to be produced in the cytotrophoblast, is now thought to be primarily produced in the syncytiotrophoblast. GHRH has been found in the rat placenta but has not yet been identified in the human.

Gonadotropin-Releasing Hormone or Luteinizing Hormone–Releasing Factor

GnRH was first demonstrated in the human placenta in 1975.[201] It is synthesized by the placenta and can stimulate LH/hCG in vitro and in vivo.[202] Further, GnRH antagonists prevent the GnRH-induced increase in hCG release as well as decrease basal hCG production.[203] Subsequently, cloned genomic and complementary deoxyribonucleic acid (cDNA) sequences encoding the precursor form of GnRH in the human placenta were described,[204] further supporting its local synthesis. The GnRH-like material was localized immunocytochemically principally in the cytotrophoblastic layer of the placental villus as well as in syncytiotrophoblast of hydatidiform moles, choriocarcinoma, and trophoblasts from early placentas.[205] Whereas GnRH mRNA levels remain constant during pregnancy,[206] immunocytochemically assessed GnRH content is highest during the second trimester and remains constant thereafter[207]; quantitative immunocytochemistry showed the most intense staining in 8-week-gestation placentas with a subsequent decrease in immunostaining during the rest of pregnancy.[208]

Placental GnRH stimulates the production of both the α-subunit and β-subunit of hCG in placental explants. Intriguingly, GnRH-binding sites have been demonstrated in the human placenta,[209] raising the possibility that there is "autoregulation" of hCG production within the placenta (Fig. 27–9). As discussed subsequently, it is also possible that the hCG influences placental steroidogenesis, thus suggesting a complete placental internal regulatory system.

Cell membrane depolarization results in the release of placental GnRH by promoting the influx of calcium into the cells.[210] This is the same mechanism involved in the release of hypothalamic GnRH. Prostaglandins (PGE_2 and PGF_2) and epinephrine increase the release of GnRH from placental cells, probably acting through cAMP. Because propranolol (a β-adrenergic receptor antagonist) reverses the release of GnRH effected by epinephrine, and because isoproterenol (a β-adrenergic receptor agonist) mimics the effect of epinephrine on GnRH, it is possible that adrenergic receptors play a role in modulating placental GnRH release. Insulin and vasoactive intestinal peptide can also stimulate placental GnRH in a dose-dependent manner[211] (Fig. 27–9), as can EGF.[212]

Because inhibin and activin are also synthesized in the cytotrophoblast,[213] they may be involved in regulating placental hCG production by regulating GnRH activity (Fig. 27–9). The addition of inhibin antiserum to placental cell cultures caused an increase in GnRH release and a parallel rise in hCG secretion. Further, addition of a GnRH antagonist reduced the effect of inhibin antiserum on hCG secretion, pointing to the interaction of inhibin and GnRH on hCG secretion. The suppressive effect of inhibin on hCG secretion could be demonstrated only in the latter part of pregnancy.[214] Addition of purified inhibin had no effect on hCG or GnRH production but reversed GnRH-induced hCG release from cultured placenta cells[213] (Fig. 27–9).

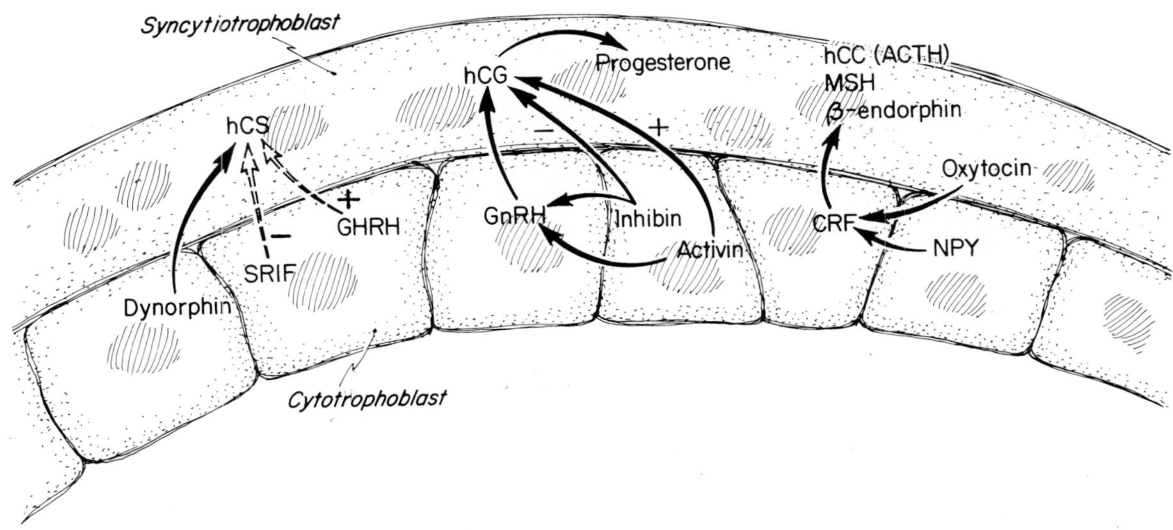

Figure 27–8 ■ Schematic representation of neurohormones and their potential interactions in the placenta. CRF, corticotropin-releasing factor (corticotropin-releasing hormone, CRH); hCS, human chorionic somatomammotropin; hCC, human chorionic corticotropin; hCG, human chorionic gonadotropin; NPY, neuropeptide Y; ACTH, adrenocorticotropic hormone; GHRH, growth hormone–releasing hormone; SRIF, somatostatin (somatotropin release–inhibiting factor); GnRH, gonadotropin-releasing hormone; MSH, melanocyte-stimulating hormone. (Modified from Petraglia FA, Volpe AO, Genazzani AR, et al. Neuroendocrinology of the human placenta. Front Neuroendocrinol 11:6, 1990.)

Therefore, it is possible that inhibin exerts an autocrine or paracrine effect on hCG secretion acting through GnRH.

In contrast, activin augments the GnRH-induced release of hCG in cultured trophoblast cells, an effect that can be reduced by the addition of inhibin.[213] Therefore, at least in vitro, GnRH can play a role in the regulation of hCG secretion, and this action of GnRH can be modulated by inhibin (inhibitory) and activin (stimulatory), acting in a paracrine manner (Fig. 27–9).

Another peptide family that can modulate (inhibit) placental GnRH release is the opioid peptides, as they do in

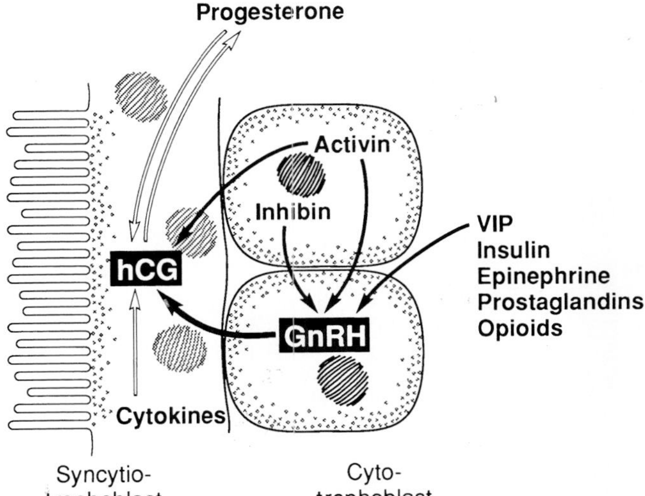

Figure 27–9 ■ The regulatory system of gonadotropin-releasing hormone (GnRH) and human chorionic gonadotropin (hCG) between cytotrophoblasts and syncytiotrophoblasts. The autocrine and paracrine modes of regulation of GnRH by inhibin (inhibitory) and activin (stimulatory) as well as a variety of modulating factors are depicted. The microvilli of the syncytiotrophoblast are depicted by the zigzag lines. VIP, vasoactive intestinal peptide.

hypothalamic GnRH neurons. Because there are opioid receptors on placental membranes,[216] this is a plausible regulatory mechanism.

In addition to the peptides discussed before, steroid hormones can also modulate GnRH release in placental cultures.[215] Both estradiol and estriol potentiate, and progesterone inhibits, the action of 8-bromo-cAMP on GnRH release from cultured placental cells. These observations are consistent with previous studies of estrogen's increasing and progesterone's decreasing basal and GnRH-stimulated hCG release and hCG mRNA levels.[217–219] The presence of estrogen and progesterone receptors in the placenta is also consistent with this concept.[220]

GnRH has been measured in the circulation of pregnant women.[221] Its concentration parallels that of placental GnRH, being highest in the first trimester. That there is a correlation between circulating GnRH and hCG[221] again suggests a possible role of GnRH in regulating hCG production.

Somatostatin

Immunoreactive somatostatin-like material has been demonstrated in human placental villi in early pregnancy.[222] Immunocytochemical localization studies have demonstrated the presence of somatostatin in the cytotrophoblast but not in the syncytiotrophoblast.[222, 223] With advancing gestational age, the amount of immunoreactive somatostatin decreases.[223] Because hCS increases as pregnancy progresses, the suggestion has been made that the placenta-derived somatostatin may exert an inhibitory influence on hCS,[223] and the diminution in somatostatin production by the cytotrophoblast may permit the progressive increase in hCS secretion by the syncytiotrophoblast. This, then, would be the parallel (albeit inhibitory rather than stimulatory) to the regulation of hCG production by placental GnRH. A receptor for somatostatin in the human placenta was recently described.[224]

Corticotropin-Releasing Hormone

In the pituitary gland, CRH of hypothalamic origin stimulates the release of the derivatives of pro-opiomelanocortin. These include ACTH, β-endorphin, β-lipotropin, and α-MSH. The human placenta synthesizes and secretes CRH, which is immunologically and biologically similar to hypothalamic CRH.[225, 226] The CRH extracted from human placenta can stimulate the release of ACTH and β-endorphin from rat pituitary cells as well as the ACTH-like material in the placenta.[227, 228]

There is a remarkable increase in the mRNA for CRH of more than 20-fold in the last 5 weeks of pregnancy[229] (Fig. 27–10). This parallels the increase in circulating maternal CRH levels and placental CRH content. The mRNA for CRH can be detected by the seventh week of human gestation. Interestingly, in contrast to the negative feedback effect of cortisol on hypothalamic CRH, glucocorticoids enhance CRH mRNA expression in the placenta.[230] CRH mRNA can be found in both the cytotrophoblast and syncytiotrophoblast.[230] Studies by Riley and colleagues[231] indicate that the syncytiotrophoblast is the major site of placental CRH production, with some also noted in the intermediate trophoblast. It was also found in amnion, chorion, and decidua.

There is a binding protein for CRH, a 37-kDa protein that binds CRH and reduces its biologic action.[232, 233] Although CRH-binding protein is present in the circulation in pregnancy, its levels are similar to those of nonpregnant women and men. There is a significant decrease of CRH-binding protein during the last 4 weeks of pregnancy.[234]

Prostaglandins, neurotransmitters, and peptides can stimulate placental CRH release in vitro[235]; prostaglandins F_2 and E_2, norepinephrine, and acetylcholine all stimulate CRH release from cultured placental cells. In addition, the neuropeptides arginine vasopressin and angiotensin II, along with oxytocin, can stimulate CRH from placental cells as they can from adult hypothalami. Further, the cytokine interleukin-1 can stimulate the release of CRH from cultured placental cells, whereas interleukin-2 does not.

The marked increase in CRH expression at the end of gestation and the capacity of glucocorticoids to enhance this expression led Robinson and colleagues[230] to propose a biologic role for CRH in the fetoplacental unit and in parturition. They suggested that the marked rise in placental CRH that precedes parturition could result from the rise in fetal glucocorticoids that occurs at this time. They suggested additionally that the increase in placental CRH may stimulate, through fetal ACTH, a further rise in fetal glucocorticoids, "completing a positive feedback loop that would be terminated by delivery." Because CRH of fetal hypothalamic origin may also stimulate fetal pituitary ACTH,[65, 236, 237] they postulate that environmental stresses may stimulate fetal hypothalamic as well as placental CRH production, leading to increases in fetal ACTH production. In addition, placental ACTH may stimulate the fetal adrenal directly.[238] Although these observations and hypotheses remain to be substantiated in vivo, they raise intriguing possibilities regarding the maintenance of fetal homeostasis and the initiation of parturition (see subsequent section on timing of parturition).

Thyrotropin-Releasing Hormone

A substance similar to the hypothalamic tripeptide TRH has been found in the human placenta.[201, 239] It can stimulate pituitary thyrotropin (TSH) release in the rat both in vitro and in vivo.[201, 239] Youngblood and colleagues[240] have concluded that the material found in the placenta is not identical to hypothalamic TRH, although it has TSH-stimulating capacity. To date, a placental TSH has not been identified. Whether placental TRH plays a role in stimulating fetal or maternal pituitary TSH remains to be ascertained. As discussed subsequently, the thyroid-stimulating activity of the placenta has been ascribed to hCG.

Human Chorionic Gonadotropin

Human chorionic gonadotropin was the first placental protein hormone to be described. In 1927, Ascheim and Zon-

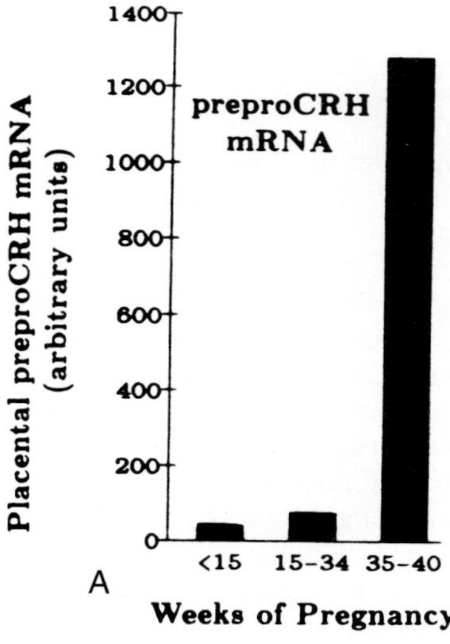

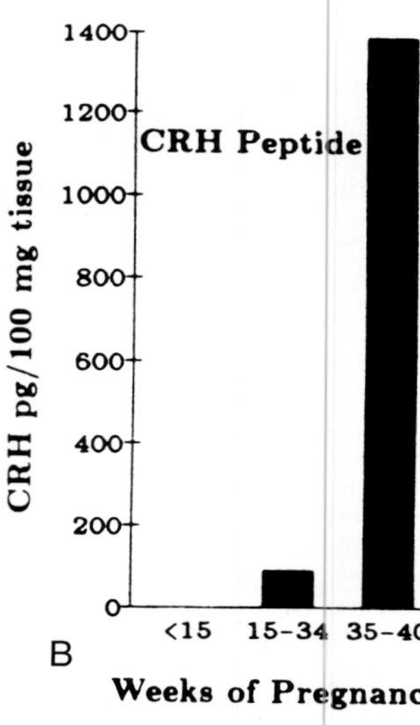

Figure 27–10 ■ Changes in placental corticotropin-releasing hormone (hCRH) mRNA *(A)* and hCRH peptide *(B)* during gestation. *A*, Derived from densitometric scanning of autoradiograms from Northern blot analysis of total RNA from placentas of gestational ages varying between 7 and 40 weeks. *B*, Radioimmunoassays of placental hCRH peptide extracted from the same placentas from which the values of RNA in *A* were derived. (From Frim DM, Emanuel RL, Robinson BG, et al. Characterization and gestational regulation of corticotropin-releasing hormone messenger RNA in human placenta. J Clin Invest 82:287–292, 1988. © American Society of Clinical Investigation.)

dek[241] found a substance in the urine of pregnant women that they initially thought was produced by the anterior pituitary gland of the mother. Later studies indicated its production by the placenta.

Human chorionic gonadotropin, which has a molecular weight of 36,000 to 40,000, is a glycoprotein hormone that is biologically and immunologically similar to pituitary LH. Details of its purification and chemical properties have been elucidated in studies by Bahl.[242, 243] The site of origin of hCG has been the subject of controversy; immunocytochemical localization studies suggest that it is produced by the syncytiotrophoblastic layer of the placenta[244] rather than the cytotrophoblast, as first believed. It is elaborated by all types of trophoblastic tissue, including that from hydatidiform mole, chorioadenoma destruens, and choriocarcinoma. It is also produced by choriocarcinoma not following a pregnancy as well as in the testes of men and the ovaries of women.

Like all glycoprotein hormones (LH, FSH, TSH), hCG is composed of two subunits, α and β. With minor modifications, the α-subunit is common to all of the glycoprotein hormones and the β-subunit confers unique specificity to the hormone. The subunits can be recombined, and the α-subunits are interchangeable to a large degree. Several of the subunits have been characterized chemically. Antibodies have been developed to the β-subunits of several of the hormones. By use of an antibody to the β-subunit of hCG, a specific radioimmunoassay was developed.[245] This assay can distinguish hCG from pituitary LH, which most radioimmunoassays for the intact hormone are incapable of doing because of immunologic cross-reaction. The β-subunit hCG radioimmunoassay is useful clinically to follow the progress of trophoblastic disease, because LH will not interfere. Conventional immunologic pregnancy tests can be employed until titers become too low. The β-subunit assay can then be used to assess whether hCG titers disappear entirely.

In normal pregnancy, the primitive trophoblast produces hCG early. In a spontaneous pregnancy, hCG was detectable 9 days after the midcycle LH peak, which is 8 days after ovulation and only 1 day after implantation[151] (Fig. 27–11). Therefore, pregnancy can be detected before the first missed menstrual period. This has clinical utility when it is important to determine the presence of pregnancy at an early stage. Radioreceptor assays have been developed that can also detect the presence of early pregnancies. These tests can be performed in several hours and may be of value in ectopic pregnancies. Home pregnancy test kits are also available and widely used.

Concentrations of hCG rise to peak values by 60 to 90 days of gestation. In early pregnancy, there is an approximate doubling of hCG levels every 2 to 3 days. Thereafter, there is a decrement in hCG levels to a plateau that is maintained during the remainder of the pregnancy (Fig. 27–12). Maternal immunoassayable LH and FSH levels are virtually undetectable throughout pregnancy.[246, 247] Bioactive FSH-like material has been found in the maternal circulation,[248] perhaps secreted by the placenta. The half-life of hCG is approximately 32 to 37 hours,[249] appreciably longer than most other protein and steroid hormones, the half-lives of which are often measured in minutes.

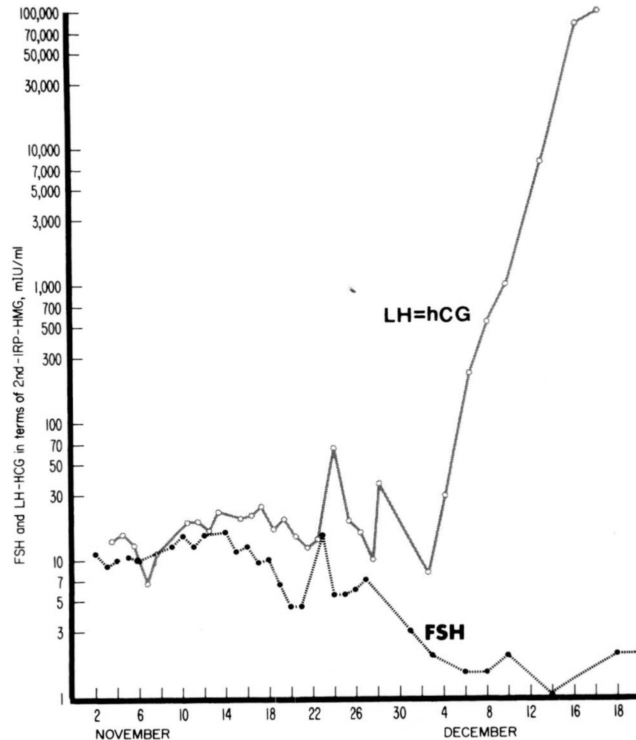

Figure 27–11 ■ Serum gonadotropin concentrations (log scale) during the normal menstrual cycle and the early period of an ensuing pregnancy. (From Jaffe RB, Lee PA, Midgley AR Jr. Serum gonadotropins before, at the inception of, and following human pregnancy. J Clin Endocrinol Metab 29:1281–1283, 1969. © The Endocrine Society.)

Although much has been learned about the chemical nature, concentration, and site of production of hCG, information is still accumulating concerning its functional roles in pregnancy. It is known to play a luteotropic role in early pregnancy; it maintains the corpus luteum of the menstrual cycle, permitting its conversion to the corpus luteum of pregnancy, thus allowing the continued production of progesterone necessary for decidual development until the placenta takes over progesterone production. In addition, hCG may regulate steroid production in the fetus—both DHEA-S by the fetal zone of the adrenal gland and testosterone by the testis[250–252] (see previous sections). The hCG content is high not only in the fetal testis, in which there is specific hCG binding and testosterone stimulation,[252, 253] but also in other fetal tissues, including kidney, ovary, and thymus. These observations led to an investigation of the source of the hCG in these fetal tissues.[254] It was speculated that hCG was being actively synthesized by these tissues rather than just being taken up from the fetal circulation. Therefore, human fetal kidney, liver, and lung were compared with placenta in a tissue explant system, studying incorporation of ^{35}S-methionine (Fig. 27–13). The tissue homogenates were immunoprecipitated with specific hCG-β antiserum. Figure 27–13 depicts the amount of labeled protein reactive with β-subunit antiserum, expressed per milligram of protein. These data suggest that not only does the placenta produce hCG, but the human fetal kidney actively synthesizes and secretes hCG as well. Subsequently, synthesis of α-subunit was demonstrated, and it

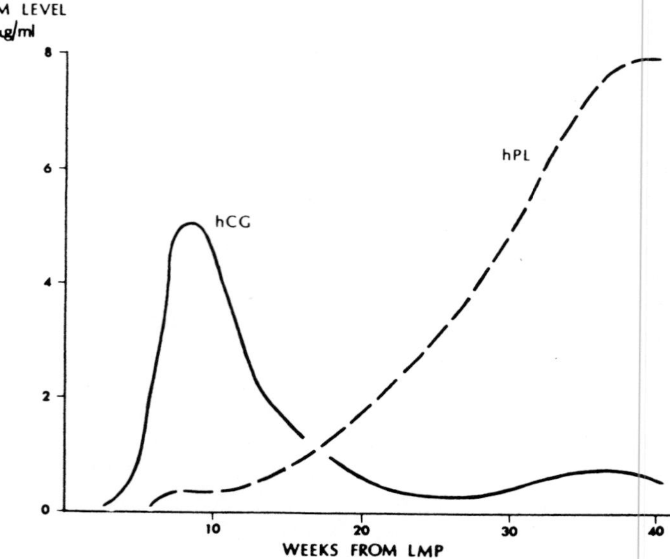

Figure 27–12 ■ Schematic representation of concentrations of human chorionic gonadotropin (hCG) and human chorionic somatomammotropin (here called human placental lactogen, hPL) throughout gestation. Note differences in the magnitude of the concentrations of the two hormones in early and late pregnancy.

was determined that the newly synthesized hCG was biologically active.[255] Immunocytochemical staining lent further support to these observations.[256] The fetal pituitary gland also has the capacity to synthesize hCG. It is possible that the finding of chorionic gonadotropin in some adult nontrophoblastic tumors represents an atavistic reversion to a fetal form of hormone synthesis. This also represented the first evidence that the genome of a human fetal tissue directs synthesis of what has been considered a placental hormone.

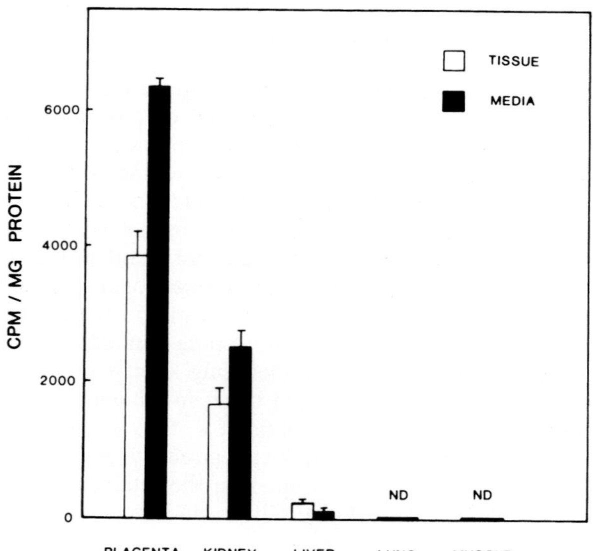

Figure 27–13 ■ Incorporation of radiolabeled amino acid (^{35}S-methionine) into immunoprecipitable hCG-β. Placental and fetal tissue samples were incubated in buffer containing ^{35}S-methionine. Tissue homogenates and media were analyzed for immunoreactive hCG-β. CPM, counts per minute. (From McGregor WG, Raymoure WJ, Kuhn RW, Jaffe RB. Fetal tissue can synthesize a placental hormone: Evidence for chorionic gonadotropin β-subunit synthesis by human fetal kidney. J Clin Invest 68:306–309, 1981. © American Society of Clinical Investigation.)

Two groups have shown that hCG has thyroid-stimulating activity and that much of the increased thyroid activity that occurs in pregnancy is a result of hCG.[257, 258] The hCG molecule contains the structural characteristics required for interaction with the human TSH receptor and activation of the membrane adenylate cyclase that regulates thyroid cell function. Highly purified hCG exhibits specific binding to human thyroid gland membranes.[259] In addition, hCG inhibits the binding of TSH,[259, 260] and highly purified hCG stimulates adenylate cyclase in human thyroid gland membranes.[259] Furthermore, partial digestion of the hCG molecule with carboxypeptidase results in an increase in human thyroid adenylate cyclase–stimulating activity while retaining the ability to stimulate rat testicular adenylate cyclase activity.[261]

Finally, it is important to speculate whether hCG may have steroid-regulatory effects within the placenta. Because hCG is produced in the syncytiotrophoblast and because steroids are also produced within this cell layer, the intriguing possibility of "autoregulation" within the cell exists. The finding of hCG-specific adenylate cyclase stimulation in the placenta lends credence to this possibility.[262]

Human Chorionic Somatomammotropin

Another protein hormone, hCS, with immunologic and certain biologic similarities to pituitary growth hormone (hGH), was isolated from the human placenta by several groups of investigators in the early 1960s. Both hCS and hGH genes cluster on the long arm of chromosome 17.[263] Josimovich and MacLaren,[264] who found this material in peripheral maternal and retroplacental serum as well as in the placenta, designated it human placental lactogen because it was lactogenic in the pigeon crop sac assay and promoted milk production by the mammary gland of the pseudopregnant rabbit.[264] However, whether it has lactogenic properties in women remains to be established. The hormone has luteotropic properties in the pseudopregnant, hypophysectomized rat.[264] Grumbach and associates[265] suggested that this hormone, because of its similarity to GH and its possible metabolic effects on the mother, may have important anabolic effects in pregnancy, particularly during the second half of gestation by mobilizing maternal metabolic fuels for transport to the fetus.

The syncytiotrophoblastic layer of the placenta synthesizes hCS. It is present in the serum and urine in both normal and molar pregnancies, and it disappears rapidly from the serum and urine after delivery of the placenta or evacuation of the uterus. After normal delivery, serum hCS cannot be detected after the first postpartum day. In addition to being found in normal and molar pregnancies, hCS has been found in the urine of patients harboring trophoblastic tumors and in men with choriocarcinoma of the testis.

In vitro biosynthesis of hCS has been accomplished.[266] Seeburg and coworkers[267] established the nucleotide sequence of part of the gene encoding hCS. The hCS molecule is a single-chain polypeptide of 191 amino acids with two disulfide bridges and has a 96 percent homology with GH.[268, 269] When circular dichroism is used, a marked similarity in secondary structure is also demonstrated.[270]

The somatotropic activity of hCS is 3 percent or less that of hGH, although the PRL-like activity of the two hormones in animals is similar. Further, hCS does have GH-like effects on tibial epiphyseal growth, body weight gain, and sulfate uptake by costal cartilage in the hypophysectomized rat, although the effective dose required is 100 to 200 times that of GH.[271] In vitro, hCS stimulates thymidine incorporation into DNA and enhances the action of hGH and insulin.

In patients with idiopathic hypopituitarism, hCS has growth-promoting activity, as suggested by significant nitrogen and potassium retention and a decrease in blood urea nitrogen.[265] To demonstrate these changes, amounts of hCS were administered that achieved blood levels of 1 to 3 μg/ml, slightly below those of pregnant women in late gestation.

The effects of hCS on fat and carbohydrate metabolism are similar to those after treatment with hGH, including inhibition of peripheral glucose uptake and stimulation of insulin release. An increase in plasma free fatty acids occurs after administration of hCS or hGH to patients with hypopituitarism.[272]

Both radioimmunoassays and hemagglutination inhibition tests have been developed to quantify hCS. It is present in microgram per milliliter quantities in early pregnancy. Its concentration increases as pregnancy progresses, with peak levels being reached during the last 4 weeks (Fig. 27–14). There may be a 10-fold or greater increase in circulating levels of hCS from the first to the third trimester. Low levels of hCS (7 to 10 ng/ml) are present in the maternal circulation by 20 to 40 days of gestation. By the last 4 weeks of pregnancy, levels of 5.4 μg/ml are achieved.[265] Some investigators have found a significant relationship between placental weight and circulating hCS concentrations, as can be seen in Figure 27–14, although this has not been observed consistently. Cellular hCS mRNA levels remain fairly constant during pregnancy, supporting the concept that the content of hCS mRNA per unit of syncytial mass remains constant during gestation.[273] The concentration of hCS in maternal peripheral blood is about 300 times that in umbilical vein blood. Further, the concentration of hCS in the blood leaving the gravid uterus is markedly greater than that in the peripheral circulation. The concentration of hCS is less in amniotic fluid than in maternal plasma but greater than in fetal plasma.

As noted, there is a rapid disappearance of circulating hCS after removal of the placenta. Kaplan and colleagues[274] found multiexponential disappearance curves, with the half-life of the major component being 9 to 15 minutes. To maintain circulating concentrations, this would imply placental production of between 1 and 4 gm of the hormone per day at term. Production of this hormone, therefore, must represent one of the major metabolic and biosynthetic activities of the syncytiotrophoblast.

A number of factors known to alter pituitary GH secretion are ineffective in altering hCS concentrations. Prolonged fasting at midgestation[275] and insulin-induced hypoglycemia, however, were reported to raise hCS concentrations, and intra-amniotic instillation of prostaglandin $F_{2\alpha}$ causes a marked reduction in hCS levels.

Grumbach and coworkers[271] proposed that hCS exerts its major metabolic effect on the mother to ensure the nutritional demands of the fetus. As pregnancy progresses, the fetus increases its substrate requirements, which leads to an increased functional role for this hormone in the second and third trimesters. Kaplan[276] suggested that hCS is the "growth hormone" of pregnancy. She noted that during pregnancy, blood glucose is decreased and insulin secretion is increased, with resistance to endogenous insulin. In addi-

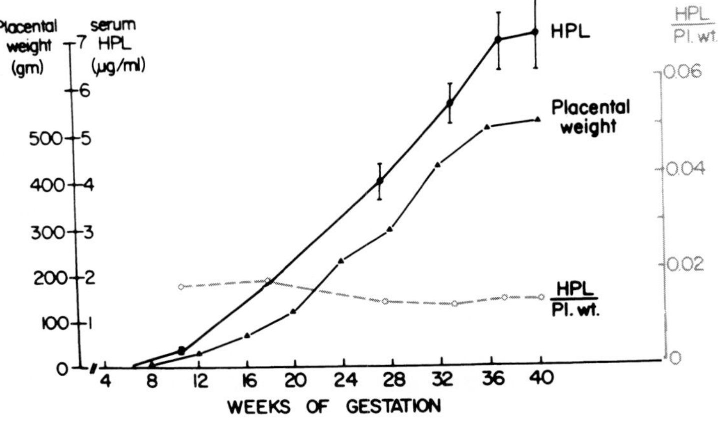

Figure 27–14 ■ Concentrations of human chorionic somatomammotropin (here called human placental lactogen, HPL) during normal pregnancy. (From Selenkow HA, Saxena BM, Dana CL, Emerson K Jr. Measurements and pathologic significance of human placental lactogen. *In* Pecile A, Fenzi C [eds]. The Foeto-Placental Unit. Amsterdam, Excerpta Medica, 1969, pp 340–362. Courtesy of Elsevier Science Publishers.)

tion, elevations in plasma free fatty acids occur. These GH-like and contra-insulin effects of hCS would lead to impaired glucose uptake and stimulation of free fatty acid release, with resultant decreased effective insulin.

Kaplan pointed out that although free fatty acids cross the placenta, the increased ketones induced by their metabolism are a more important energy source for the fetus. As a consequence of decreased effective insulin, muscle proteolysis and the formation of ketones may be enhanced. The decreased glucose use induced by hCS would ensure a steady supply of glucose for the fetus. In midgestation, hypoglycemia, which occurs with fasting, is related to fetal glucose consumption and not to an overall decrease in gluconeogenesis. In contrast, in the fed state, Kaplan suggests that the plasma insulin response to glucose would overcome the contrainsulin effects of hCS. This would allow restoration of hepatic glycogen and lipid stores. The increased insulin, acting in concert with hCS, would result in increased protein synthesis.

Kaplan also postulated that in the late postprandial or fasted state, hCS may be predominantly a catabolic hormone. This would be consistent with the observation that fasting is a stimulus to hCS during pregnancy. Increased hCS concentration and decreased insulin levels in this situation would enhance lipolysis, with the release of free fatty acids and glycerol, resultant ketosis, and decreased glucose use. These effects have been observed during periods of fasting in pregnant women.

In this manner, maternal metabolism would be directed toward mobilization of maternal sources to furnish substrate for the fetus. There would be a steady source of various fuels for the fetus, of which glucose would predominate. Insulin is seen as a fluctuating modifier of the effects of hCS on the mother. Feasting increases effective insulin and restores maternal substrates, whereas fasting results in decreased effective insulin and primary catabolic effects of hCS to ensure an adequate supply of metabolic nutrients for the fetus.

Human Chorionic Corticotropin

The placenta is likely to be the source of another pituitary-like hormone, hCC.[277] Both immunoassayable and bioassayable ACTH activity in extracts of extensively washed human placental tissue and dispersed viable trophoblasts have been demonstrated. When trophoblasts were incubated in tissue culture medium, the ACTH content of both the cells and medium was significantly greater than during the preincubation level, suggesting its synthesis by trophoblastic cells. The physiologic role, if any, of hCC and its regulation remain to be elucidated. It may be responsible for the relative resistance to negative feedback suppression of pituitary ACTH by glucocorticoids during pregnancy.[278] As noted earlier, however, because glucocorticoids stimulate expression of placental CRH, placental CRH may play a role in hCC production.

Other ACTH-Related Peptides

As detailed in Chapter 1, there is a common precursor glycoprotein in the pituitary gland, with a molecular weight of approximately 31,000, that gives rise to ACTH and a group of peptides, including β-lipotrophic hormone (β-LPH, β-lipotropin), β-endorphin, and α-MSH. These substances are post-translationally derived from the parent hormone, variously referred to as pro-opiomelanocortin or 31K ACTH/endorphin.

Both ACTH and β-endorphin–like peptides have been demonstrated in human placental extracts by a variety of assay techniques.[277–280] Thus, the synthesis of both the 31K parent molecule and β-endorphin by the placenta furnishes yet another example of some of the similar biosynthetic capacities of placenta and pituitary. The biologic role, if any, of placenta-derived β-endorphin awaits further study.

Immunoreactive β-endorphin in the maternal circulation remains relatively low throughout pregnancy, with mean levels of approximately 15 pg/ml.[281] Mean levels rise to approximately 70 pg/ml during late labor and rise further (mean, 113 pg/ml) at delivery.[281] Similar concentrations of β-endorphin (mean, 105 pg/ml) are also seen in cord plasma at term, suggesting secretion by the placenta or fetal pituitary. Many factors that cause an increase in pituitary ACTH also result in an increase in β-endorphin. Hypoxia and acidosis may cause an increase in β-endorphin (and β-LPH) as well as ACTH.[282]

In addition to β-endorphin and β-LPH, which are derived from the parent pro-opiomelanocortin molecule, there are two other families of endogenous opioids—enkephalins and dynorphins. Immunoreactive methionine-enkephalin has been found in the human placenta and is chemically identical to the native molecule.[283] Circulating levels of metenkephalin do not change appreciably throughout pregnancy.[283]

Three forms of dynorphin have been found in the human placenta.[284, 285] Dynorphin binds to kappa opiate receptors; these are abundant in human placenta,[286] and receptor number increases at term.[287] The placental content of dynorphin at term is of similar magnitude to that found in the pituitary gland and brain.[285] Relatively high concentrations of dynorphin have been found in amniotic fluid and umbilical venous plasma, and maternal plasma levels in the third trimester and at delivery are higher than in nonpregnant women.[285] Because kappa receptor agonists stimulate the release of hCS,[288] it is possible that dynorphin exerts local regulatory effects on hCS production.

Neuropeptide Y

Neuropeptide Y (NPY) is a 36–amino acid substance that is found in the central and peripheral nervous systems and can exert effects centrally on such behavioral events as eating and satiety as well as on neuroendocrine function.[289, 290] Immunoreactive NPY has been found in extracts of term placenta, and its elution profile is similar to that of synthetic NPY.[291] In the placenta, NPY is found principally in the cytotrophoblast and intermediate trophoblast layers.[291] In addition, binding sites for NPY have been found in the placenta.[291]

Maternal NPY levels are increased above those of nonpregnant women beginning early in gestation. They remain elevated until term and rise still further during labor, reaching their acme with cervical dilatation and parturition.[292] There is no significant change in NPY concentrations in the circulation of women undergoing cesarean section who are not in labor.[292] The levels of NPY fall rapidly after delivery, again suggesting a placental source of this neuropeptide. Elevated concentrations of NPY are also found in the amniotic fluid.[292]

Because NPY can stimulate CRH release from cultured placental cells, but not the release of GnRH, hCG, or hCS, it may play a role in the regulation of placental CRH release (Fig. 27–15).

Growth Factor–Related Placental Peptides

THE INHIBIN FAMILY OF PEPTIDES

As noted (see earlier discussion of inhibin/activin regulation of placental GnRH), inhibin, which preferentially inhibits pituitary FSH, is a heterodimer composed of an α-subunit and one of two β-subunits, β_A or β_B. The major known sites of production of inhibin are the testis and ovary. As also indicated previously, in the human midtrimester fetus, the interstitial (Leydig) cells produce the α-subunit and both β-subunits.

In addition to inhibin, which is a heterodimer, the homodimers β_{AA} and β_{BB} stimulate FSH production. These compounds have been termed *activins*. The inhibin subunits have been found in the placenta with the use of both immunocytochemical and in situ hybridization techniques.[293, 294] Placental inhibin has biologic activity,[293] and inhibin antibodies can block this activity. By use of immunocytochemistry, immunoreactive cells in the cytotrophoblastic layer of human placental villi were found,[293] and all three subunits were found in the syncytiotrophoblast.[294] There were no observable changes in localization with advancing gestation.

Analogues of cAMP and adenylate cyclase activators increase inhibin release from placental cells in culture, suggesting that cAMP may be the second messenger involved in the release of placental inhibin. This may also explain the increase in inhibin effected by hCG in placental cell cultures.[293] Further, the neuropeptides vasoactive intestinal peptide and NPY also increase inhibin release from the placenta in a dose-related manner.[211]

Patients with premature ovarian failure, who had demonstrated undetectable circulating inhibin levels before becoming pregnant, had high levels after in vitro fertilization and embryo transfer with use of donor ova[295]; this again points to a placental source for the inhibin present in the maternal circulation. Levels of inhibin are high in both the maternal circulation and cord blood. Although it was thought initially that inhibin is secreted by the corpus luteum of pregnancy, a study indicates that inhibin A is a product of the fetoplacental unit and not of the corpus luteum.[296] Activin A appears to be produced by both the corpus luteum and placenta.[296]

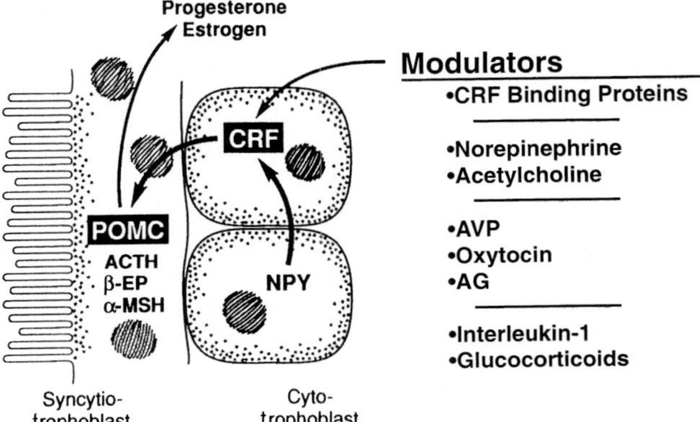

Figure 27–15 ■ Diagrammatic depiction of the potential placental CRF-POMC system and its modulators. CRF, corticotropin-releasing factor; NPY, neuropeptide Y; POMC, pro-opiomelanocortin; ACTH, adrenocorticotropic hormone; EP, endorphin; MSH, melanocyte-stimulating hormone; AVP, arginine vasopressin; AG, angiotensin.

OTHER GROWTH FACTORS IN THE PLACENTA

Inhibin is in the family of growth factors that includes TGF-β. Not only TGF-β[297] but also many other growth factors and their receptors have been found in the human placenta. These include insulin-like growth factors,[298] epidermal growth factor,[299, 300] platelet-derived growth factor,[301] and fibroblast growth factor.[302] Some or all of these may play a role in growth, development, and differentiated function of the placenta, a fascinating biochemical factory, as well as subserving these roles in the fetus.

Steroid Sulfates and Placental Sulfatase Deficiency

An interesting facet of steroid hormone metabolism in the human fetus is the formation of sulfate conjugates of the steroid hormones. The process of sulfoconjugation of hydroxylated steroids is a ubiquitous one in the fetus, occurring in a variety of sites—the lung, the gut, and the liver as well as the adrenal gland. In the adrenal, sulfurylation leads to the formation of a variety of steroid sulfates, including pregnenolone sulfate, 17α-hydroxypregnenolone sulfate, and DHEA-S, quantitatively the most significant androgen. The DHEA-S can be formed de novo in the fetal adrenal gland from acetate by the following metabolic chain[303]: acetate→cholesterol→cholesterol sulfate→pregnenolone sulfate→17α-hydroxypregnenolone sulfate→DHEA-S. This is a pathway of "direct" steroid sulfate to steroid sulfate metabolism without loss of the sulfate side chain. Steroid sulfates can also be formed from the corresponding free (unconjugated) steroid. It is interesting that although the capacity for direct steroid sulfate metabolism is possessed by adult hyperplastic and neoplastic adrenal tissue, this has not been demonstrated in the normal adult adrenal gland.[304] Thus, it appears that the neoplastic tissue reverts to a fetal mode of metabolism.

The role of steroid sulfates in the endocrine economy of pregnancy has not been defined completely. These agents can serve as precursors of placental estrogens. In addition, they may serve as reservoirs of available substrates for active hormones, or conversely, the sulfurylation of a steroid may be a mechanism by which it is rendered inactive.

Whereas the fetal adrenal gland rapidly sulfurylates several unconjugated steroids, the fetal testis does this to a far lesser degree.[305] When presented with testosterone, the adrenal forms significant amounts of testosterone sulfate, whereas the testis does not demonstrate this conversion. Furthermore, although there is de novo synthesis of steroid sulfates from acetate in the adrenal,[303] there is no demonstrable de novo steroid sulfate formation in the fetal testis. However, there is de novo formation of testosterone in the fetal testis in similar experiments.[306] It appears, therefore, that the major biosynthetic activity of the fetal testis is directed toward active androgen (testosterone) formation and that the testosterone, once formed, is not inactivated by sulfate conjugation but is kept in an active form so that its role in secondary sexual development can be maintained.

Placental Sulfatase Deficiency

As noted, the human fetus has the capacity to sulfurylate steroids extensively in a variety of tissues, including the adrenal gland. In a complementary manner, the placenta possesses extensive sulfatase activity (i.e., the ability to cleave steroid sulfates, liberating the "free," or unconjugated, steroid) in normal pregnancy. Thus, when steroid sulfates reach the placenta, the sulfate side chain—when it is in the 3 position—is rapidly and efficiently cleaved by placental sulfatase. Sulfurylated steroids serve as the principal precursors of placental estrogens. Enzymatic cleavage of sulfate conjugates is essential for estrogen formation by the placenta. That this is indeed the case was supported by the observation that urinary estrogen excretion was low throughout the pregnancy of women whose placentas had a deficiency of sulfatase activity.[307] In a case studied by France and colleagues,[95] urinary excretion of estriol was approximately 5 percent of that found in normal pregnancy, and excretion of estrone and estradiol was approximately 15 percent of the level in normal pregnancy. In contrast, urinary pregnanediol excretion was in the range of normal pregnancy. No significant increase in estrogen excretion was noted when the patient was given a load of DHEA-S. In contrast, when unconjugated DHEA was given, increases in estrogens were similar to those seen in normal pregnancies. Thus, the placenta could metabolize the DHEA but not the DHEA-S. Incubation studies with the placenta from this patient indicated that the other enzymes involved in estrogen formation (3β-hydroxysteroid dehydrogenase/Δ^{4-5}-isomerase and aromatase) were not affected. Others have confirmed these observations.[308]

If the disorder is suspected during pregnancy, DHEA-S (50 mg intravenously) can be administered to the mother.[309] Plasma and urinary estrogen concentrations can then be measured and compared with those values obtained before DHEA-S administration. If placental sulfatase deficiency exists, plasma and urinary estrogen levels will not rise after DHEA-S administration, whereas they will be elevated in normal pregnancies. In normal pregnancy, at least 10 percent of the injected DHEA-S is recovered as estrogens in maternal urine during the first 24 hours.[309] In maternal plasma, DHEA-S administration results in an increase in concentration of various estrogens. This increase is more marked and rapid for estradiol and is usually more than 200 percent after 30 minutes. Values then reach a plateau that lasts approximately 180 minutes, returning to control values within 12 to 24 hours. If no significant rise in estrogen concentration follows the administration of DHEA-S, one can confirm the diagnosis by administering free DHEA to the mother a few days later, following the same procedure. When urinary estrogens and plasma estradiol increase after the administration of DHEA, the location of the block has been identified.

The disorder occurs in male offspring. This observation, coupled with the finding of the disorder in the fetuses of two sisters who were pregnant at the same time,[310] suggests that placental sulfatase deficiency is an X-linked recessive characteristic. Furthermore, ichthyosis of an X-linked nature is commonly found in offspring of women with placental sulfatase deficiency and has been found in two sons of one of the sisters mentioned previously.[310] The offspring usually do well otherwise after delivery. Thus, the disorder does not seem a threat to the later health of the infant. There remains some controversy regarding the frequency of the delay in the onset of spontaneous labor in these cases and the problem of complicated deliveries.

Decidua and Fetal Membranes as Endocrine Tissues

Although the decidua and fetal membranes formerly were not thought of as endocrine-active tissues, there is strong evidence that these structures not only are capable of hormone production and metabolism but also contain hormonal receptors, suggesting their susceptibility to endocrine effects.

The uterine decidua, composed of glycogen-containing cells of stromal origin, can be seen during the late luteal phase of the menstrual cycle and increases markedly in size if pregnancy ensues. The decidua of pregnancy is composed of three portions, depending on anatomic location: (1) the decidua basalis, which underlies the site of implantation and forms the maternal component of the placenta; (2) the decidua capsularis, which overlies the gestational sac (this portion disappears in the later stages of pregnancy); and (3) the decidua vera, which lines the remainder of the uterine cavity (and becomes intimately approximated to the chorion). Thus, the decidua can communicate both with the fetus through the amniotic fluid and with the adjacent uterine myometrium.

Two groups[311, 312] demonstrated the synthesis of PRL by human decidual tissue. Both groups suggested that this may be the source of the high concentrations of PRL found in amniotic fluid.[312, 313] Although the amnion does not produce PRL, it does selectively localize PRL and thus is a potential target for it.[314]

It has been suggested that PRL produced by the decidua increases myometrial contractility and that this activity can be antagonized by relaxin.[315, 316] The location of the decidua, with its immediate proximity to the myometrium, would seem ideal in this regard.

Relaxin is also produced by the decidua.[317] Its concentrations in pregnancy are depicted in Figure 27–16. In contrast to PRL, relaxin can inhibit uterine contractility.[316] These two decidual hormones, therefore, may exert counteractive forces on the myometrium, with various factors governing the predominance of one or the other. In addition to inhibiting uterine contractility, relaxin increases distensibility of the cervix and induces interpubic ligament formation.[317] The actual biologic role of relaxin in human pregnancy remains to be ascertained definitively. Porcine relaxin causes dilatation and effacement of the human cervix in late gestation.[318]

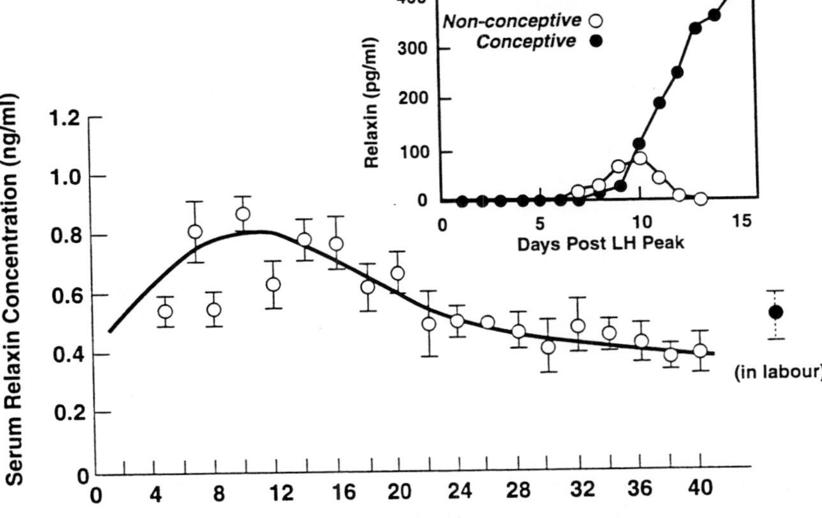

Figure 27–16 ■ Serum relaxin concentrations throughout pregnancy. (From Bryant-Greenwood GD, Schwabe C. Human relaxins: Chemistry and biology. Endocr Rev 15:5–26, 1994. © The Endocrine Society.)

That the decidua may also serve as a target of hormone action is suggested by the studies of Fuchs and associates.[319] They demonstrated that oxytocin receptors increased progressively with advancing gestation and reached peak levels in early labor in decidua and myometrium in a parallel manner. They also demonstrated that oxytocin can induce the production of prostaglandin by the decidua but not by the myometrium. Thus, oxytocin can stimulate uterine contractions both by acting directly on the myometrium and by stimulating prostaglandin synthesis by the decidua. Of interest were the earlier increases in concentration of oxytocin receptors in decidua and myometrium in cases of premature labor. The striking increase in oxytocin receptors may reflect one of the initial steps in the initiation of labor, even though maternal oxytocin concentrations were not found to increase during labor.[320]

CRH can also stimulate secretion of prostaglandins by placental, decidual, and amnion cells.[321, 322]

Finally, the decidua has the capacity to effect 1α-hydroxylation of the biologic precursor 25-hydroxyvitamin D_3 to the biologically active 1,25-dihydroxyvitamin D_3.[323] It is possible that this may play a role in modulating calcium activity in the myometrium or in providing a source of vitamin D_3 to the fetus through the amniotic fluid. The extent to which this occurs awaits further exploration.

Fetal Maturation and Timing of Parturition

The pioneering work of Liggins[66] in sheep first demonstrated that increased activity of the fetal hypothalamic-pituitary-adrenal axis triggers the initiation of parturition and stimulates the maturation of the fetal organ systems essential for extrauterine life. In this species, increased secretion of cortisol from the fetal adrenal glands during the final week of pregnancy initiates a cascade of events that culminates in the birth of a viable neonate. In most mammalian species, including humans, cortisol also stimulates events associated with preparation for extrauterine life (e.g., surfactant production by the fetal lungs; activity of enzyme systems in the fetal gut, retina, pancreas, thyroid, and brain; and deposition of glycogen in the fetal liver).[66] As in the sheep, the primate fetal adrenal cortex must produce cortisol de novo toward the end of gestation to ensure fetal maturation and neonatal competence. Perinatal survival is dependent on the timely initiation of labor when organ systems necessary for extrauterine life are sufficiently mature to allow the newborn to live outside of the uterus and independently of the placenta. Thus, in some species, regulation of fetal maturation and the timing of parturition are controlled by a single hormone, cortisol, produced by the fetal adrenals, which appears to coordinate these processes so that fetal maturation proceeds appropriately before parturition.

In anencephalics and infants with congenital abnormalities that prevent glucocorticoid synthesis, pregnancy is not significantly prolonged, on average, although labor occurs during a wider time interval.[324] Similarly, adrenalectomy[325] or experimental anencephaly[326] in fetal rhesus monkeys does not prevent parturition but increases the window of time in gestation during which birth occurs. Treatment of rhesus monkey fetuses with dexamethasone does not lead to premature induction of parturition, as it does in sheep, but instead results in prolonged pregnancy.[327] Because glucocorticoid treatment inhibits ACTH production by the fetal pituitary leading to a decrease in DHEA-S production and suppression of the fetoplacental unit, these findings implicate the fetoplacental unit in the regulation of primate parturition. Infusion of androstenedione, which is readily aromatized by the placenta to estrogen, into pregnant rhesus monkeys late in gestation increased maternal estrogen and nocturnal oxytocin concentrations and induced cervical dilatation and normal parturition.[328] Thus, in primates, androgen produced by the fetal adrenals as a source of aromatizable substrate for estrogen synthesis by the placenta can be a link between the fetus and mother in the initiation of parturition.

Studies of CRH production by the primate placenta have led to novel theories regarding the mechanism by which the fetoplacental unit is involved in the regulation of parturition. Majzoub and colleagues[230, 329] found that unlike its effects on hypothalamic CRH production, glucocorticoid increases CRH expression by the human placenta. The marked increase of CRH expression and maternal circulating concentrations at the end of gestation, and the capacity of glucocorticoids to enhance placental CRH expression, led these investigators to propose a biologic role for CRH in the fetoplacental unit and parturition. They suggested that the rise in placental CRH that precedes parturition could result from the rise in fetal glucocorticoids that occurs at this time. The increase in placental CRH may stimulate, by stimulation of fetal pituitary ACTH,[65] a further rise in fetal glucocorticoids, completing a positive feedback loop that would be terminated by delivery. Because CRH of fetal hypothalamic origin may also stimulate fetal pituitary ACTH, they postulated that environmental stresses may stimulate fetal hypothalamic as well as placental CRH production, leading to increases in fetal ACTH production and activation of the positive feedback loop (Fig. 27–17). Subsequent studies showed that CRH receptors are present in the myometrium and fetal membranes[330] and that CRH stimulates the release of prostaglandins from human decidua and amnion in vitro[321] and can potentiate the action of oxytocin and prostaglandin $F_{2\alpha}$ in vitro[331, 332] and in vivo.[333] These observations provide further circumstantial evidence that placental CRH may be directly involved in the regulation of human parturition by increasing myometrial contractility associated with labor. In addition, placental ACTH may stimulate the fetal adrenal directly.[200]

More recently, Majzoub and colleagues[329] investigated the mechanism by which glucocorticoid increases CRH expression in the human placenta. Their data indicate that cortisol may compete with progesterone for binding to the glucocorticoid receptor late in gestation and that because progesterone, by interacting with this receptor, inhibits placental CRH expression, its displacement would result in increased CRH expression. They proposed that the increased fetal cortisol, which stimulates increased placental CRH, competes with the action of progesterone in regulating the placental CRH gene.[329] They suggested that placental CRH stimulates fetal ACTH, which in turn stimulates fetal zone DHEA, the precursor of placental estrogen. The increased fetal ACTH might also stimulate increased fetal adrenal cortisol production. They postulated that the positive feedback loop between placental CRH and cortisol, which is suggested by the exponential increase in fetal cortisol, CRH, and DHEA seen at the end of gestation, might be the "motor" of a biologic clock that drives the mediators of labor. The antagonism of progesterone's binding to placental glucocorticoid receptors by cortisol could further stimulate placental CRH expression. In their theoretical model (see Fig. 27–17), concomitant stimulation of fetal cortisol and DHEA by placental CRH would couple the glucocorticoid effects on fetal organ maturation with

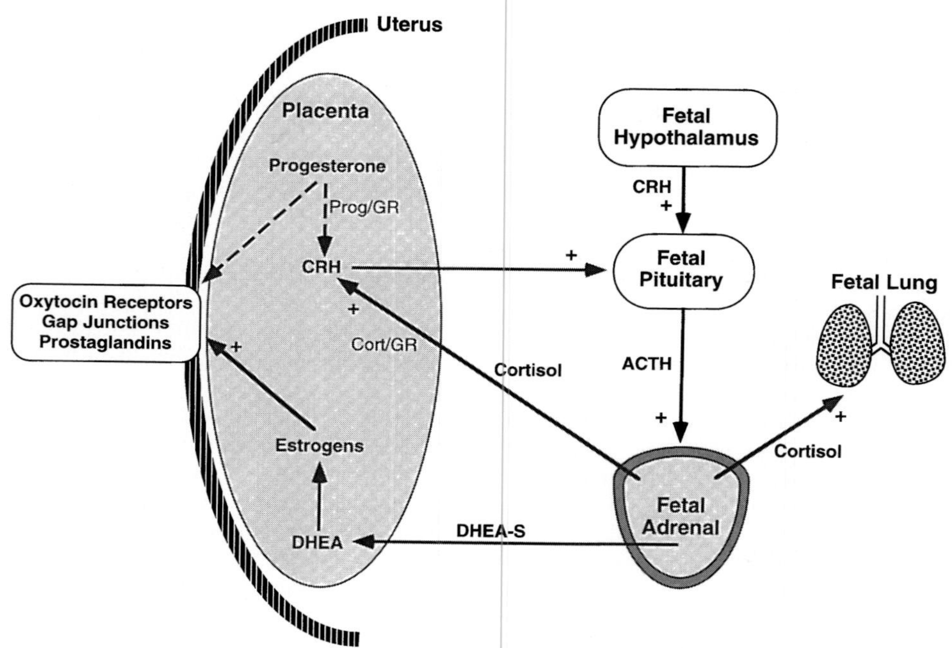

Figure 27–17 ■ Schematic depiction of the theoretical model proposed by Karalis and coworkers describing the endocrine interaction between the fetal hypothalamic-pituitary-adrenal axis and the placenta in the regulation of human parturition. Late in gestation, cortisol produced by the fetal adrenal cortex blocks the inhibitory effects of progesterone on placental CRH production by competing with progesterone for the glucocorticoid receptor (GR). As a consequence, CRH secretion by the placenta into the fetal compartment increases, providing further stimulation to fetal pituitary ACTH production, which in turn stimulates cortisol and DHEA-S production by the fetal adrenal cortex. Cortisol promotes maturation of fetal organ systems, such as the lungs, in preparation for extrauterine life and, by further enhancing placental CRH production, completes a positive feedback loop. DHEA-S is converted to estrogens by the placenta, which stimulates gap junction formation and oxytocin receptor expression by the myometrium and prostaglandin production by the amnion and decidua, events necessary to facilitate uterine contraction and labor. CRH may also directly enhance prostaglandin production and myometrial responsiveness to oxytocin. These events are inhibited by progesterone. (Adapted from Karalis K, Goodwin G, Majzoub JA. Cortisol blockade of progesterone: A possible molecular mechanism involved in the initiation of human labor. Nat Med 2:556–560, 1996.)

the timing of parturition, which, as they note, is of obvious benefit for postnatal survival. A similar model involving the stimulation of prostaglandin production in human fetal membranes by CRH has been proposed by Jones and Challis.[321, 322]

McLean and colleagues[334] proposed that placental CRH is associated with a "placental clock," which is active beginning at least by the 16th week of pregnancy and participates in the determination of the length of pregnancy and the timing of parturition. They found that concentrations of CRH in the maternal circulation, presumably secreted by the placenta, are predictive of the subsequent length of gestation. Maternal plasma CRH concentrations were predictive of those women who were destined to have normal term, preterm, or post-term delivery. The CRH curve in women who delivered before term was shifted to the left by a magnitude of 6 weeks, which was equivalent to the degree of prematurity later observed at delivery in this group. Conversely, in women who delivered post term, the CRH curve was shifted to the right by a magnitude of 2 weeks, which corresponded to the extent of postmaturity that was observed subsequently.

As noted previously, the exponential rise in maternal plasma CRH concentrations with advancing pregnancy is associated with a concomitant fall in the concentrations of the CRH-binding protein in late pregnancy. The implication of these reciprocal concentration curves is that there is a rapid increase in circulating levels of bioavailable CRH concurrent with the onset of parturition. The causal relationship between the increase in unbound CRH and the timing of parturition remains to be elucidated. Because CRH receptors are present in the myometrium and fetal membranes[335, 336] and CRH stimulates the release of prostaglandins from human decidua and amnion in vitro, and can potentiate the action of oxytocin and prostaglandin $F_{2\alpha}$ in vitro and in vivo, this relationship may be involved in the increased myometrial contractility associated with labor. In addition, CRH is present in amniotic fluid and the fetal circulation where it has the ability to stimulate the fetal pituitary-adrenal axis to increase fetal adrenal glucocorticoid secretion, which can stimulate further placental CRH secretion as indicated before.

Recently, a receptor for CRH was found in the human fetal adrenal gland.[337] When CRH was incubated with human fetal adrenal cells, DHEA-S was preferentially stimulated, compared to stimulation of cortisol. The magnitude of CRH stimulation of DHEA-S was similar to that of ACTH stimulation of fetal adrenal DHEA-S. Interestingly, the mechanism by which CRH stimulates steroidogenesis in the fetal adrenal gland is via the inositol phosphate-phosphokinase C pathway,[338] rather than the cyclic AMP-phosphokinase A pathway utilized by CRH in stimulating the human fetal pituitary gland.[65] This raises the possibility that the increasing concentrations of placental CRH that occur toward the end of gestation directly stimulate fetal adrenal DHEA-S production (perhaps also stimulating fetal pituitary ACTH secretion). The increased DHEA-S might lead to increased production of placental estrogen via aromatization. The increased estrogen could then function in a paracrine manner to evoke uterine contractions, a phenomenon demonstrated in the pregnant rhesus monkey in vivo.[339] Therefore, it is possible that increasing placental CRH may orchestrate a series of events in the fetal pituitary, adrenal, placenta, and membranes, culminating in the initiation of parturition.

Thus, the role of the fetal-placental-adrenal axis in the regulation of parturition in primates is highly complex and different from that in other species. In addition, the primate may have several redundant mechanisms that may regulate parturition. This is not surprising given the critical nature of the timing and occurrence of this event.

References

1. Mulchahey JJ, DiBlasio AM, Martin MC, et al. Hormone production and peptide regulation in the human fetal pituitary gland. Endocr Rev 8:406, 1987.
2. Wilcox AJ, Weinberg CR, O'Connor JF, et al. Incidence of early loss of pregnancy. N Engl J Med 319:187, 1988.
3. Schmidt CM, Orr HT. Maternal/fetal interactions: The role of the MHC class 1 molecule HLA-G. Crit Rev Immunol 13:207, 1993.
4. Rouas-Freiss N, Marchal RE, Kirszenbaum M, et al. The alpha 1 domain of HLA-G1 and HLA-G2 inhibits cytotoxicity induced by natural killer cells: Is HLA-G the public ligand for natural killer cell inhibitory receptors? Proc Natl Acad Sci USA, 94:5249, 1997.
5. Munz C, Holmes N, King A, et al. Human histocompatibility leukocyte antigen (HLA-G) molecules inhibit NKAT3 expressing natural killer cells. Exp Med 185:385, 1997.
6. Cross JC, Werb Z, Fisher SJ. Implantation and the placenta: Key pieces of the development puzzle. Science 266:1508, 1994.
7. Gordon JD, Shifren JL, Foulk RA, et al. Angiogenesis in the human female reproductive tract. Obstet Gynecol Surv 50:693, 1995.
8. Das SK, Wang X-N, Parin BC, et al. Heparin-binding EGF-like growth factor gene is induced in the mouse uterus temporally by the blastocyst solely at the site of apposition: A possible ligand for interaction with blastocyst EGF receptor in implantation. Development 120:1071, 1994.
9. Shen MM, Leder P. Leukemia inhibitory factor is expressed by the preimplantation uterus and selectively blocks primitive ectoderm formation in vitro. Proc Natl Acad Sci USA 89:8240, 1992.
10. Bhatt H, Brunet LJ, Stewart CL. Uterine expression of leukemia inhibitory factor coincides with the onset of blastocyst implantation. Proc Natl Acad Sci USA 88:11408, 1991.
11. Stewart CL, Kaspar P, Brunet LJ, et al. Blastocyst implantation depends on maternal expression of leukemia inhibitory factor. Nature 359:76, 1992.
12. Luetteke NC, Qiu TH, Peiffer RL, et al. TGFα deficiency results in hair follicle and eye abnormalities in targeted and waved-1 mice. Cell 73:263, 1993.
13. Simon C, Frances A, Piquette GN, et al. Embryonic implantation in mice is blocked by interleukin-1 receptor antagonist. Endocrinology 134:521, 1994.
14. Hu XL, Yang J, Hunt JS. Differential distribution of interleukin-1β proteins in human placentas. J Reprod Immunol 22:257, 1992.
15. Nestler JE. Interleukin-1 stimulates the aromatase activity of human placental cytotrophoblasts. Endocrinology 132:566, 1993.
16. Yagel S, Lala PK, Powell WA, Casper RF. Interleukin-1 stimulates human chorionic gonadotropin secretion by first trimester human trophoblast. J Clin Endocrinol Metab 68:992, 1989.
17. Masuhiro K, Matsuzaki N, Nishino E, et al. Trophoblast-derived interleukin-1 (IL-1) stimulates the release of human chorionic gonadotropin by activating IL-6 and IL-6 receptor system in first trimester human trophoblasts. J Clin Endocrinol Metab 72:594, 1991.
18. Librach CL, Feigenbaum SL, Bass KE, et al. Interleukin-1β regulates human cytotrophoblast metalloproteinase activity and invasion in vitro. J Biol Chem 269:17125, 1994.
19. O'Shea J, Kleinfeld R, Morrow H. Ultrastructure of decidualization in the pseudopregnant rat. Am J Anat 166:271, 1983.
20. Goodger AM, Rogers PA. Uterine endothelial cell proliferation before and after embryo implantation in rats. J Reprod Fertil 99:451, 1993.

21. Fisher SJ, Damsky CH. Human cytotrophoblast invasion. Semin Cell Biol 4:183, 1993.
22. Pijnenborg R. Trophoblast invasion and placentation in the human: Morphological aspects. Trophoblast Res 4:33, 1990.
23. Greiss FJ, Anderson SG, Still JG. Uterine pressure-flow relationships during early gestation. Am J Obstet Gynecol 126:799, 1976.
24. Makowski EL, Meschia G, Droegemueller W, et al. Distribution of uterine blood flow in the pregnant sheep. Am J Obstet Gynecol 101:409, 1968.
25. Khong TY, De WF, Robertson WB, et al. Inadequate maternal vascular response to placentation in pregnancies complicated by preeclampsia and by small-for-gestation age infants. Br J Obstet Gynaecol 93:1049, 1986.
26. Trudinger BJ, Giles WB, Cook CM, et al. Fetal umbilical artery flow velocity waveforms and placental resistance: Clinical significance. Br J Obstet Gynaecol 92:23, 1985.
27. Frusca T, Morassi L, Pecorelli S, et al. Histological features of uteroplacental vessels in normal and hypertensive patients in relation to birthweight. Br J Obstet Gynaecol 96:835, 1989.
28. Carney E, Lye S, Peek W, et al. Cellular localization of basic fibroblast growth factor within human placenta throughout gestation (Abstract 533). 39th Annual Meeting of the Society for Gynecologic Investigation; March 18–21, 1992; San Antonio, TX.
29. Usuki K, Norberg L, Larsson E, et al. Localization of platelet-derived endothelial cell growth factor in human placenta and purification of an alternatively processed form. Cell Regul 1:677, 1990.
30. Ishikawa F, Miyazono K, Hellman U, et al. Identification of angiogenic activity and the cloning and expression of platelet-derived endothelial cell growth factor. Nature 338:567, 1989.
31. Sharkey AM, Charnock JD, Boocock CA, et al. Expression of mRNA for vascular endothelial growth factor in human placenta. J Reprod Fertil 99:609, 1993.
32. Charnock JD, Sharkey AM, Boocock CA, et al. Vascular endothelial growth factor receptor localization and activation in human trophoblast and choriocarcinoma cells. Biol Reprod 51:524, 1994.
33. Cheung C, Singh M, Brace R. Expression of vascular endothelial growth factor and its ribonucleic acid in ovine placenta and fetal membranes (Abstract p393). 42nd Annual Meeting of the Society for Gynecologic Investigation; March 15–18, 1995; Chicago, IL.
34. Jackson D, Volpert OV, Bouck N, et al. Stimulation and inhibition of angiogenesis by placental proliferin and proliferin-related protein. Science 266:1581, 1994.
35. Szlachter N, O'Byrne EM, Goldsmith L, et al. Myometrial inhibiting activity of relaxin containing extracts of human corpora lutea of pregnancy. Am J Obstet Gynecol 136:594, 1980.
36. Bigazzi M, Nardi E. Prolactin and relaxin: Antagonism on the spontaneous motility of the uterus. J Clin Endocrinol Metab 53:665, 1981.
37. Csapo AL, Pulkkinen MO, Weist WG. Effects of lutectomy and progesterone replacement in early pregnant patients. Am J Obstet Gynecol 115:759, 1973.
38. Daikoku S. Studies on the human foetal pituitary: 2. On the form and histological development, especially that of the anterior pituitary. Tokushima J Exp Med 5:214, 1958.
39. Pearse AGE, Takor TT. Neuroendocrine embryology and the APUD concept. Clin Endocrinol 5:229, 1976.
40. Takor TT, Pearse AGE. Neuroectodermal origin of avian hypothalamo-hypophyseal complex: The role of the ventral neural ridge. J Embryol Exp Morphol 34:311, 1975.
41. Conklin JL. The development of the human fetal adenohypophysis. Anat Rec 160:79, 1968.
42. Anderson H, von Bulow FA, Mollgard K. The early development of the pars distalis of the human foetal pituitary gland. Z Anat Entwicklungsgesh 135:117, 1971.
43. Failin LI. The development of human hypophysis and differentiation of cells of its anterior lobe during embryonic life. Acta Anat 44:188, 1961.
44. Hyyppa M. Hypothalamic monoamines in human fetuses. Neuroendocrinology 9:257, 1972.
45. Thiveris JA, Currie RW. Observations on the hypophyseal portal vasculature in the developing human fetus. Am J Anat 157:441, 1980.
46. Kaplan SL, Grumbach MM, Aubert ML. The ontogenesis of pituitary hormones and hypothalamic factors in the human fetus: Maturation of central nervous system regulation of anterior pituitary function. Recent Prog Horm Res 32:161, 1976.
47. Raiha N, Hjelt L. The correlation between the development of the hypophysial portal system and the onset of neurosecretory activity in the human fetus and infant. Acta Paediatr Scand 46:610, 1957.
48. Winters AJ, Eskay RL, Porter JC. Concentration and distribution of TRH and LRH in the human fetal brain. J Clin Endocrinol Metab 39:269, 1974.
49. Nobin A, Bjorkland A. Topography of the monoamine neuron systems in the human brain as revealed in fetuses. Acta Physiol Scand 388:1, 1973.
50. McNeilly AS, Gilmore D, Dobbie G, Chard T. Prolactin releasing activity in the early human foetal hypothalamus. J Endocrinol 73:533, 1977.
51. Bresson JL, Clavequin M-C, Fellman D, Bugnon C. Ontogeny of the neuroglandular system revealed with HPGRF44 antibodies in human hypothalamus. Neuroendocrinology 39:68, 1984.
52. Bugnon C, Fellman D, Gouget A, et al. Corticoliberin neurons: Cytophysiology, phylogeny and ontogeny. J Steroid Biochem 20:183, 1984.
53. Baker BL, Jaffe RB. The genesis of cell types in the adenohypophysis of the human fetus as observed with immunocytochemistry. Am J Anat 143:137, 1975.
54. Begeot M, Dubois MP, Dubois PM. Mise en evidence par immunocytochemie de la β-lipotropine (β-LPH) des α- et β-endorphines dans l'anterhypophysyse de foetus humains normaux et anencephales. Ann Endocrinol (Paris) 39:235, 1978.
55. Begeot M, Dubois MP, Dubois PM. Immunologic localization of α- and β-endorphins and β-lipotropin in corticotrophic cells of the normal and anencephalic fetal pituitaries. Cell Tissue Res 193:413, 1978.
56. Kaplan SL, Grumbach MM. Immunologic assay and characterization of growth hormone in the pituitary gland of the human fetus. Am J Dis Child 104:528, 1973.
57. Grumbach MM, Kaplan SL. Ontogenesis of growth hormone, insulin, PRL, and gonadotropin secretion in the human fetus. *In* Cross KW, Nathanielsz P (eds). Foetal and Neonatal Physiology. New York, Cambridge University Press, 1973, p 462.
58. Aubert ML, Grumbach MM, Kaplan SL. The ontogenesis of human fetal hormones: III. Prolactin. J Clin Invest 56:155, 1975.
59. Allen JP, Cook DM, Kendall JW, McGilvra R. Maternal-fetal ACTH relationships in man. J Clin Endocrinol Metab 37:320, 1973.
60. Huhtaniemi IT, Koritnik DR, Korenbrot CC, et al. Stimulation of pituitary-testicular function with gonadotropin-releasing hormone in fetal and infant monkeys. Endocrinology 105:109, 1979.
61. Siler-Khodr TM, Morganstern LL, Greenwood FC. Hormone synthesis and release from human fetal adenohypophyses in vitro. J Clin Endocrinol Metab 39:960, 1974.
62. Groom GV, Boyns AR. Gonadotropin release from human foetal pituitary cultures induced by fragments of the luteinizing hormone–releasing hormone. J Endocrinol 59:511, 1973.
63. Rasmussen DD, Liu JH, Wolf PL, Yen SSC. Endogenous opioid regulation of gonadotropin-releasing hormone release from the human fetal hypothalamus in vitro. J Clin Endocrinol Metab 57:881, 1983.
64. Arbiser JL, Morton CC, Bruns GA, Majzoub JA. Human corticotropin releasing hormone gene is located on the long arm of chromosome 8. Cytogenet Cell Genet 47:113, 1988.
65. Blumenfeld Z, Jaffe RB. Hypophysiotropic and neuromodulatory regulation of ACTH in the human fetal pituitary gland. J Clin Invest 78:288, 1986.
66. Liggins GC. Adrenocortical-related maturational events in the fetus. Am J Obstet Gynecol 126:931, 1976.
67. Liggins GC. Endocrinology of parturition. *In* Novy MJ, Resko JA (eds). Fetal Endocrinology. New York, Academic Press, 1981, pp 211–237.
68. Hornsby PJ. The regulation of adrenocortical function by control of growth and structure. *In* Anderson DC, Winter JSD (eds). Adrenal Cortex. London, Butterworth, 1985, pp 1–31.
69. Jaffe RB, Serón-Ferré M, Crickard K, et al. Regulation and function of the primate fetal adrenal gland and gonad. Recent Prog Horm Res 37:41, 1981.

70. Gray ES, Abramovich DR. Morphologic features of the anencephalic adrenal gland in early pregnancy. Am J Obstet Gynecol 137:491, 1980.
71. Benirschke K. Adrenals in anencephaly and hydrocephaly. Obstet Gynecol 8:412, 1956.
72. Walsh SW, Norman RL, Novy MJ. In utero regulation of rhesus monkey fetal adrenals: Effects of dexamethasone, adrenocorticotropin, thyrotropin-releasing hormone, prolactin, human chorionic gonadotropin, and alpha-melanocyte–stimulating hormone on fetal and maternal plasma steroids. Endocrinology 104:1805, 1979.
73. Winters AJ, Oliver C, Colston C, et al. Plasma ACTH levels in the human fetus and neonate as related to age and parturition. J Clin Endocrinol Metab 39:269, 1974.
74. Serón-Ferré M, Lawrence CC, Jaffe RB. Role of hCG in regulation of the fetal zone of the human fetal adrenal gland. J Clin Endocrinol Metab 46:834, 1978.
75. Mesiano S, Mellon SH, Gospodarowicz D, et al. Basic fibroblast growth factor expression is regulated by ACTH in the human fetal adrenal: A model for adrenal growth regulation. Proc Natl Acad Sci USA 88:5428, 1991.
76. Burris TP, Guo W, McCabe ER. The gene responsible for adrenal hypoplasia congenita, *DAX-1*, encodes a nuclear hormone receptor that defines a new class within the superfamily. Recent Prog Horm Res 51:241, 1996.
77. Luo X, Ikeda Y, Parker KL. A cell-specific nuclear receptor is essential for adrenal and gonadal development and sexual differentiation. Cell 77:481, 1994.
78. Hatano O. Takakusi A, Nomura M, Morohashi KI. Identical origin of adrenal cortex and gonad revealed by expression profiles of Ad4BP/SF-1. Genes Cells 1:663, 1996.
79. Mesiano S, Jaffe RB. Developmental and functional biology of the primate fetal adrenal cortex. Endocr Rev 18:378, 1997.
80. McClellan M, Brenner RM. Development of the fetal adrenals in nonhuman primates: Electron microscopy. *In* Novy MJ, Resko JA (eds). Fetal Endocrinology New York, Academic Press, 1981, pp 383–403.
81. Wilburn LA, Goldsmith PC, Chang K-J, Jaffe RB. Ontogeny of enkephalin and catecholamine synthesizing enzymes in the primate fetal adrenal medulla. J Clin Endocrinol Metab 63:974, 1986.
82. McNutt NS, Jones AL. Observations of the ultrastructure of cytodifferentiation in the human fetal adrenal cortex. Lab Invest 11:513, 1970.
83. Mesiano S, Coulter CL, Jaffe RB. Localization of cytochrome P450 cholesterol side chain cleavage, cytochrome P450 17α-hydroxylase/17,20-lyase, and 3β-hydroxysteroid dehydrogenase-isomerase steroidogenic enzymes in the human and rhesus fetal adrenal gland: Reappraisal of functional zonation. J Clin Endocrinol Metab 77:1184, 1992.
84. Sucheston ME, Cannon MS. Development of zonular patterns in the human adrenal gland. J Morphol 126:477, 1968.
85. Spencer SJ, Mesiano S, Jaffe RB. Programmed cell death in remodelling of the human fetal adrenal cortex: Possible role of activin-A (Abstract 027). 42nd Annual Meeting of the Society for Gynecologic Investigation; March 15–18, 1995; Chicago, IL.
86. Johannisson E. The foetal adrenal cortex in the human. Its ultrastructure at different stages of development and in different functional states. Acta Endocrinol (Copenh) 130(Suppl):1, 1968.
87. Coulter CL, Goldsmith PC, Mesiano S, et al. Functional maturation of the primate fetal adrenal in vivo: 1. Role of insulin-like growth factors, IGF-I receptor and IGF binding proteins in growth regulation. Endocrinology 137:4487, 1996.
88. Spencer SJ, Mesiano S, Lee JY, Jaffe RB. Unpublished data.
89. Pasqualini JR, Lowy J, Wiqvist N, Diczfalusy E. Biosynthesis of cortisol from 3β,17α,21-trihydroxypregnenolone by the intact human foetus at midpregnancy. Biochim Biophys Acta 152:648, 1968.
90. Solomon S, Bird CE, Ling W, et al. Formation and metabolism of steroids in the fetus and placenta. Recent Prog Horm Res 23:297, 1967.
91. MacNaughton MC, Taylor T, McNally EM, Coutts JRT. The effect of synthetic ACTH on the metabolism of [4-^{14}C]-progesterone by the previable human fetus. J Steroid Biochem 8:499, 1977.
92. Bayard F, Ances IG, Tapper AJ, et al. Transplacental passage and fetal secretion of aldosterone. J Clin Invest 49:1389, 1970.
93. Siiteri PK, MacDonald PC. The utilization of circulating dehydroepiandrosterone sulfate for estrogen synthesis during human pregnancy. Steroids 2:713, 1963.
94. Fransden VA, Stakeman G. The site of production of oestrogenic hormones in human pregnancy. Hormone excretion in pregnancy with anencephalic foetus. Acta Endocrinol (Copenh) 38:383, 1961.
95. France JT, Seddon RJ, Liggins GC. A study of pregnancy with low estrogen production due to placental sulfatase deficiency. J Clin Endocrinol Metab 36:1, 1973.
96. Serón-Ferré M, Lawrence CC, Siiteri PK, Jaffe RB. Steroid production by definitive and fetal zones of the human fetal adrenal gland. J Clin Endocrinol Metab 47:603, 1978.
97. Nelson HP, Kuhn RW, Deyman ME, Jaffe RB. Human fetal adrenal definitive and fetal zone metabolism of pregnenolone and corticosterone: Alternate biosynthetic pathways and absence of detectable aldosterone synthesis. J Clin Endocrinol Metab 70:693, 1990.
98. Serón-Ferré M, Biglieri EG, Jaffe RB. Regulation of mineralocorticoid secretion by the superfused fetal monkey adrenal gland: Lack of stimulation of aldosterone by ACTH. J Dev Physiol 13:33, 1990.
99. Breault L, Lehoux JG, Gallo-Payet N. The angiotensin AT_2 receptor is present in the human fetal adrenal gland throughout the second trimester of gestation. J Clin Endocrinol Metab 81:3914, 1996.
100. Doody KM, Carr BR, Rainey WE, et al. 3β-Hydroxysteroid dehydrogenase/isomerase in the fetal zone and neocortex of the human fetal adrenal gland. Endocrinology 126:2487, 1990.
101. DiBlasio AM, Jaffe RB. Adrenocorticotropic hormone does not induce desensitization in human adrenal cells during fetal life. Biol Reprod 39:617, 1988.
102. Rainey WE, McAllister JM, Byrd EW, et al. Regulation of corticotropin responsiveness in human fetal adrenal cells. Am J Obstet Gynecol 165:1649, 1991.
103. Mesiano S, Fujimoto VY, Nelson LR, et al. Localization and regulation of corticotropin receptor expression in the midgestation human fetal adrenal cortex: Implications for in utero homeostasis. J Clin Endocrinol Metab 81:340, 1996.
104. Mesiano S, Katz SL, Lee JY, Jaffe RB. Insulin-like growth factors augment steroid production and expression of steroidogenic enzymes in human fetal adrenal cortical cells: Implications for adrenal androgen regulation. J Clin Endocrinol Metab 82:1390, 1997.
105. Mountjoy KG, Robbins LS, Mortrud MT, Cone RD. The cloning of a family of genes that encode the melanocortin receptors. Science 257:1248, 1992.
106. Crickard K, Ill CR, Jaffe RB. Control of proliferation of human fetal adrenal cells in vitro. J Clin Endocrinol Metab 53:790, 1981.
107. Hornsby PJ, Sturek M, Harris SE, Simonian MH. Serum and growth factor requirements for proliferation of human adrenocortical cells in culture: Comparison with bovine adrenocortical cells. In Vitro 19:863, 1983.
108. Coulter CL, Read LC, Carr BR, et al. A role for epidermal growth factor in the morphological and functional maturation of the adrenal gland in the fetal rhesus monkey in vivo. J Clin Endocrinol Metab 81:1254, 1996.
109. D'Ercole AJ. The insulin-like growth factors and fetal growth. *In* Spencer E (ed). Modern Concepts of Insulin-Like Growth Factors. New York, Elsevier, 1991, p 9.
110. Rosenfeld RG, Hintz RL. Somatomedin receptors; structure, function and regulation. *In* Conn P (ed). The Receptors. New York, Academic Press, 1986, p 281.
111. Baxter RC. Physiological roles of IGF binding proteins. *In* Spencer E (ed). Modern Concepts of Insulin-Like Growth Factors. New York, Elsevier, 1991, p 371.
112. Han VKM, D'Ercole AJ, Lund PK. Cellular localization of somatomedin (insulin-like growth factor) messenger RNA in the human fetus. Science 236:193, 1987.
113. Han VKM, Lund PK, Lee DC, D'Ercole AJ. Expression of somatomedin/insulin-like growth factor messenger ribonucleic acids in the human fetus: Identification, characterization, and tissue distribution. J Clin Endocrinol Metab 66:422, 1988.
114. Ilvesmaki V, Blum WF, Voutilainen R. Insulin-like growth factor binding proteins in the human adrenal gland. Mol Cell Endocrinol 97:71, 1993.

115. Voutilainen R, Miller WL. Coordinate tropic hormone regulation of mRNAs for insulin-like growth factor II and cholesterol side-chain-cleavage enzyme, P450ssc, in steroidogenic tissues. Proc Natl Acad Sci USA 84:1590, 1987.
116. Mesiano S, Mellon SH, Jaffe RB. Mitogenic action, regulation and localization of insulin-like growth factors in the human fetal adrenal gland. J Clin Endocrinol Metab 76:968, 1992.
117. Mesiano S, Jaffe RB. Regulation of growth and function of the human fetal adrenal. *In* Saez JM, Brownie AC, Capponi A, et al. (eds). Cellular and Molecular Biology of the Adrenal Cortex. London, John Libby and Company, 1992, pp 235–245.
118. Mesiano S, Jaffe RB. Interaction of insulin-like growth factor-II and estradiol directs steroidogenesis in the human fetal adrenal toward dehydroepiandrosterone sulfate production. J Clin Endocrinol Metab 77:754, 1993.
119. Rabinovici J, Spencer SJ, Doldi N, et al. Activin-A as an intraovarian modulator: Actions, localization, and regulation of the intact dimer in human ovarian cells. J Clin Invest 89:1528, 1992.
120. Spencer SJ, Rabinovici J, Jaffe RB. Human recombinant activin-A inhibits proliferation of human fetal adrenal cells in vitro. J Clin Endocrinol Metab 71:1678, 1990.
121. Spencer SJ, Rabinovici J, Mesiano S, et al. Activin and inhibin in the human adrenal gland: Regulation and differential effects in fetal and adult cells. J Clin Invest 90:142, 1992.
122. Roberts AB, Flanders KC, Kondalah P, et al. Transforming growth factor beta: Biochemistry and roles in embryogenesis, tissue repair and remodeling and carcinogenesis. Recent Prog Horm Res 44:157, 1990.
123. Stankovic AK, Dion LD, Parker CR Jr. Effects of transforming growth factor-beta by human fetal adrenal steroid production. Mol Cell Endocrinol 99:145, 1994.
124. Stankovic AK, Parker CR Jr. Receptor binding of transforming growth factor-beta by human fetal adrenal cells. Mol Cell Endocrinol 109:159, 1995.
125. Ikeda Y, Lala DS, Luo X, et al. Characterization of the mouse FTZ-F1 gene, which encodes a key regulator of steroid hydroxylase gene expression. Mol Endocrinol 7:852, 1992.
126. Parker KL, Schimmer BP. Steroidogenic factor I: A key determinant of endocrine development and function. Endocr Rev 18:361, 1997.
127. Muscatelli F, Strom TM, Walker AP, et al. Mutations in the DAX-1 gene give rise to both X-linked adrenal hypoplasia congenita and hypogonadotropic hyogonadism. Nature 372:672, 1994.
128. Zanaria E, Muscatelli F, Bardoni B, et al. An unusual member of the nuclear hormone receptor superfamily responsible for X-linked adrenal hypoplasia congenita. Nature 372:635, 1994.
129. Ikeda Y, Shen WH, Ingraham HA, Parker KL. Developmental expression of mouse steroidogenic factor-1, an essential regulator of the steroid hydroxylases. Mol Endocrinol 8:654, 1994.
130. Guo W, Burris TP, Zhang YH, et al. Genomic sequence of the *DAX1* gene: An orphan nuclear receptor responsible for X-linked adrenal hypoplasia congenita and hypogonadotropic hypogonadism. J Clin Endocrinol Metab 81:2481, 1996.
131. Burris TP, Guo W, Le T, McCabe ER. Identification of a putative steroidogenic factor-1 response element in the *DAX-1* promoter. Biochem Biophys Res Commun 214:576, 1995.
132. Mittwoch U. Sex differentiation in mammals and tempo of growth: Probabilities. J Theor Biol 137:445, 1989.
133. Hertig AT, Adams EC, McKay DC, et al. A description of 34 human ova within the first 17 days of development. Am J Anat 98:435, 1956.
134. Jirasek JE. Development of the genital system in human embryos and fetuses. *In* Cohen MM Jr (ed). Development of the Genital System and Male Pseudohermaphroditism. Baltimore, Johns Hopkins Press, 1971, p 3.
135. Jost A. Initial stages of gonadal development. Theories and methods. Arch Anat Microsc Morphol Exp 74:39, 1985.
136. Pelliniemi LJ. Development of sexual dimorphism of the embryonic gonad. Hum Genet 58:64, 1981.
137. Jost A. Organogenesis and endocrine cytodifferentiation of the testis. Arch Anat Microsc Morphol Exp 74:101, 1985.
138. Rabinovici J, Goldsmith PC, Roberts VJ, et al. Localization and secretion of inhibin/activin subunits in the human and subhuman primate fetal gonads. J Clin Endocrinol Metab 73:1141, 1991.
139. Van Wagenen G, Simpson ME. Embryology of the Ovary and Testis in *Homo sapiens and Macaca mulatta*. New Haven, CT, Yale University Press, 1965.
140. Gondos B, Hobel C. Ultrastructure of germ cell development in the human fetal testis. Z Zellforsch Mikrosk Anat 119:1, 1971.
141. Pelliniemi LJ, Niei M. Fine structure of the human foetal testis. I. The interstitial tissue. Z Zellforsch Mikrosk Anat 99:507, 1969.
142. Reyes FI, Boroditsky RS, Winter JS, Faiman C. Studies on human sexual development. II. Fetal and maternal serum gonadotropin and sex steroid concentration. J Clin Endocrinol Metab 38:612, 1974.
143. Siiteri PK, Wilson JD. Testosterone formation and metabolism during male sexual differentiation in the human embryo. J Clin Endocrinol Metab 38:113, 1974.
144. Kurilo LF. Oogenesis in antenatal development in man. Hum Genet 57:86, 1981.
145. Byskov AG, Hoyer PE. Embryology of mammalian gonads and ducts. *In* Knobil E, Neill J (eds). The Physiology of Reproduction. New York, Raven Press, 1988, p 265.
146. Gondos B, Westergaard L, Byskov A. Initiation of oogenesis in the human fetal ovary: Ultrastructural and squash preparation study. Am J Obstet Gynecol 155:189, 1986.
147. Gondos B, Bhiraleus P, Hobel CJ. Ultrastructural observations on germ cells in human fetal ovaries. Am J Obstet Gynecol 110:644, 1971.
148. Rabinovici J, Jaffe RB. Development and regulation of growth and differentiated function in human and subhuman primate fetal gonads. Endocr Rev 11:532, 1990.
149. Konishi I, Fujii S, Okamura H, et al. Development of interstitial cells and ovigerous cords in the human fetal ovary: An ultrastructural study. J Anat 148:121, 1986.
150. Gondos B, Hobel CJ. Interstitial cells in the human fetal ovary. Endocrinology 93:736, 1973.
151. Jaffe RB, Lee PA, Midgley AR Jr. Serum gonadotropins before, at the inception of, and following human pregnancy. J Clin Endocrinol Metab 29:1281, 1969.
152. Catt KJ, Dufau ML, Vaitukaitis JL. Appearance of hCG in pregnancy plasma following the initiation of implantation of the blastocyst. J Clin Endocrinol Metab 40:537, 1975.
153. Marshall JR, Hammond CB, Ross GT, et al. Plasma and urinary chorionic gonadotropin during early human pregnancy. Obstet Gynecol 32:760, 1968.
154. Clements JA, Reyes FI, Winter JSD, Faiman C. Studies on human sexual development. III. Fetal pituitary and serum and amniotic fluid concentrations of LH, CG and FSH. J Clin Endocrinol Metab 42:9, 1976.
155. Kaplan SL, Grumbach MM. The ontogenesis of human foetal hormones. II. Luteinizing hormone (LH) and follicle stimulating hormone (FSH). Acta Endocrinol (Copenh) 81:808, 1976.
156. Baker TG, Scrimogeour JB. Development of the gonad in normal and anencephalic human fetuses. J Reprod Fertil 60:193, 1980.
157. Lammie A, Drobnjak M, Gerald W, et al. Expression of c-*kit* and kit ligand proteins in normal human tissues. J Histochem Cytochem 42:1417, 1994.
158. Gulyas B, Hodgen G, Tullner W, Ross G. Effects of fetal and maternal hypophysectomy on endocrine organs and body weight in infant rhesus monkeys (*Macaca mulatta*) with particular reference to oogenesis. Biol Reprod 16:216, 1977.
159. Wartenberg H. Differentiation and development of the testes. *In* Burger H, DeKretzer D (eds). The Testis. New York, Raven Press, 1989, p 67.
160. Molsberry RL, Carr BR, Mendelson CR, Simpson ER. Human chorionic gonadotropin binding to human fetal testes as a function of gestational age. J Clin Endocrinol Metab 55:791, 1982.
161. Huhtaniemi I, Korenbrot C, Jaffe R. hCG binding and stimulation of testosterone biosynthesis in the human fetal testis. J Clin Endocrinol Metab 44:963, 1977.
162. Word RA, George FW, Wilson JD, Carr BR. Testosterone synthesis and adenylate cyclase activity in the early human fetal testis appear to be independent of human chorionic gonadotropin control. J Clin Endocrinol Metab 69:204, 1989.
163. Huhtaniemi IL, Yamamoto M, Ranta T, et al. Follicle-stimulating hormone receptors appear earlier in the primate fetal testis than in the ovary. J Clin Endocrinol Metab 65:1210, 1987.
164. Serra GB, Perez PG, Jaffe RB. De novo testosterone biosynthesis in the human fetal testis. J Clin Endocrinol Metab 30:141, 1970.
165. Rice BF, Johanson CA, Sternberg WH. Formation of steroid

hormones from acetate-1-^{14}C by a human fetal testis preparation grown in organ culture. Steroids 7:79, 1966.
166. Huhtaniemi I, Korenbrot C, Séron-Ferré M, et al. Stimulation of testosterone production in vivo and in vitro in the male rhesus monkey fetus in late gestation. Endocrinology 100:839, 1977.
167. Carr BR, Parker CRJ, Ohashi M, et al. Regulation of human fetal testicular secretion of testosterone: Low-density lipoprotein-cholesterol and cholesterol synthesized de novo as steroid precursor. Am J Obstet Gynecol 146:241, 1983.
168. Voutilainen R, Miller WL. Developmental expression of genes for the steroidogenic enzymes P450scc (20,22-desmolase), P450c17 (17 α-hydroxylase/17,20-lyase) and P450c21 (21-hydroxylase) in the human fetus. J Clin Endocrinol Metab 63:1145, 1986.
169. Tapanainen J, Voutilainen R, Jaffe RB. Low aromatase activity and gene expression in human fetal testes. J Steroid Biochem 33:7, 1989.
170. George FW, Wilson JD. Conversion of androgen to estrogen by the human fetal ovary. J Clin Endocrinol Metab 47:550, 1978.
171. Payne AH, Jaffe RB. Androgen formation from pregnenolone sulfate by the human fetal ovary. J Clin Endocrinol Metab 39:300, 1974.
172. Voutilainen R, Miller WL. Developmental and hormonal regulation of mRNAs for insulin-like growth factor II and steroidogenic enzymes in human fetal adrenals and gonads. DNA 7:9, 1989.
173. Fisher DA, Klein AH. Thyroid development and disorders of thyroid function in the newborn. N Engl J Med 304:702, 1981.
174. Fisher DA, Dussault JH, Sack J, Chopra IJ. Ontogenesis of hypothalamic-pituitary-thyroid function and metabolism in man, sheep, and rat. Recent Prog Horm Res 33:59, 1977.
175. Melmed S, Harad A, Murata Y, et al. Fetal response to the thyrotropin-releasing hormone after thyroid hormone administration to the rhesus monkey: Lack of pituitary suppression. Endocrinology 150:334, 1979.
176. Jacobsen BB, Andersen H, Dige-Petersen H, Hummer L. Thyrotropin response to thyrotropin-releasing hormone in fullterm, euthyroid and hypothyroid newborns. Acta Paediatr Scand 65:438, 1975.
177. Osathanondh R, Chopra IJ, Tulchinksy D. Effects of dexamethasone on fetal and maternal thyroxine, triiodothyronine, reverse triiodothyronine, and thyrotropin levels. J Clin Endocrinol Metab 47:1236, 1978.
178. Isaac RM, Hayek A, Standefer JC, Eaton RP. Reverse triiodothyronine to triiodothyronine ratio and gestational age. J Pediatr 94:477, 1979.
179. Chopra IJ, Sack J, Fisher DA. Circulating 3,3′,5′-triiodothyronine (reverse T_3) in the human newborn. J Clin Invest 55:1137, 1975.
180. Fisher DA, Odell WD. Acute release of thyrotropin in the newborn. J Clin Invest 48:1670, 1969.
181. Abuid J, Stinson DA, Larsen PR. Serum triiodothyronine and thyroxine in the neonate and acute increases in these hormones following delivery. J Clin Invest 52:1195, 1973.
182. DeGroot IJ, Robertson M, Rue PA. Triiodothyronine receptors during maturation. Endocrinology 100:1511, 1977.
183. Schwartz HL, Oppenheimer JH. Ontogenesis of 3,5,3′-triiodothyronine receptors in neonatal rat brain: Dissociation between receptor concentration and stimulation of oxygen consumption by 3,5,3′-triiodothyronine. Endocrinology 103:943, 1978.
184. Walker P, Weichsel ME Jr, Fisher DA, Gris SM. Thyroxine increases nerve growth factor concentration in adult mouse brain. Science 204:427, 1979.
185. Hellig HD, Gattereau D, Lefevbre Y, Bolte E. Steroid production from plasma cholesterol: I. Conversion of plasma cholesterol to placental progesterone in humans. J Clin Endocrinol Metab 30:624, 1970.
186. Carr BR, Simpson ER. Cholesterol synthesis in human fetal tissues. J Clin Endocrinol Metab 55:447, 1982.
187. Pion R, Jaffe RB, Erickson G, et al. Studies on the metabolism of C-21 steroids in the human foeto-placental unit: 1. Formation of α,β-unsaturated 3-ketones in mid-term placentas perfused in situ with pregnenolone and 17α-hydroxypregnenolone. Acta Endocrinol (Copenh) 48:234, 1965.
188. Johansson ENB. Plasma levels of progesterone in pregnancy measured by a rapid competitive protein binding technique. Acta Endocrinol (Copenh) 61:607, 1979.
189. Frandsen VA, Stakeman G. The clinical significance of oestriol estimators in late pregnancy. Acta Endocrinol (Copenh) 44:183, 1963.
190. Schindler AE, Siiteri PK. Isolation and quantitation of steroids from normal human amniotic fluid. J Clin Endocrinol Metab 28:1189, 1968.
191. Goebelsmann U, Chen LC, Saga M, et al. Plasma concentration and protein binding of oestriol and its conjugates in pregnancy. Acta Endocrinol (Copenh) 74:592, 1973.
192. Peréz-Palaciós G, Peréz AE, Jaffe RB. Conversion of pregnenolone 7α-^{3}H-sulfate to other Δ^5-3β-hydroxysteroid sulfates by the human fetal adrenal in vitro. J Clin Endocrinol Metab 28:19, 1968.
193. Goebelsmann U, Jaffe RB. Oestriol metabolism in pregnant women. Acta Endocrinol (Copenh) 66:679, 1971.
194. Siiteri PK, Febres F, Clemens LE, et al. Progesterone and maintenance of pregnancy: Is progesterone nature's immunosuppressant? Ann N Y Acad Sci 286:384, 1977.
195. Resnik R, Killam AP, Battaglia FC, et al. The stimulation of uterine blood flow by various estrogens. Endocrinology 94:1192, 1974.
196. Resnik R, Brink GW. Modulating effects of prostaglandins on the uterine vascular bed. Gynecol Invest 8:10, 1977.
197. Martucci C, Fishman J. Direction of estradiol metabolism as a control of its hormonal action—uterotrophic activity of estradiol metabolites. Endocrinology 101:1709, 1977.
198. Clark JH, Paszko Z, Peck EJ Jr. Nuclear binding and retention of the receptor estrogen complex: Relation to the agonistic and antagonistic properties of estriol. Endocrinology 100:91, 1977.
199. Petraglia F, Florio P, Nappi C, Genazzani AR. Peptide signaling in human placenta and membranes: Autocrine, paracrine and endocrine mechanisms. Endocr Rev 178:156, 1991.
200. Waddell BJ. The placenta as hypothalamus and pituitary: Possible impact on maternal and fetal adrenal function. Reprod Fertil Dev 5:47, 1996.
201. Gibbons JM, Mitnick M, Chieffo V. In vitro biosynthesis of TSH- and LH-releasing factors by the human placenta. Am J Obstet Gynecol 121:127, 1975.
202. Khodr GS, Siler-Khodr TM. Placental luteinizing hormone–releasing factor and its synthesis. Science 207:315, 1980.
203. Siler-Khodr TM, Khodr GS, Vickery BH, Nestor JJ. Inhibition of hCG, α-hCG and progesterone release from human placental tissue in vitro by a GnRH antagonist. Life Sci 32:2741, 1983.
204. Seeburg PH, Adelman JP. Characterization of cDNA for precursor of human luteinizing hormone releasing hormone. Nature 311:666, 1984.
205. Lehtovin P, Lee JN, Leppalautin J. Immunohistochemical demonstration of luteinizing hormone–releasing factor–like material in human syncytiotrophoblast and trophoblastic tumors. Clin Endocrinol (Oxf) 12:441, 1980.
206. Kelly AC, Rodgers A, Dong KW, et al. Gonadotropin-releasing hormone and chorionic gonadotropin gene expression in human placental development. DNA Cell Biol 10:411, 1991.
207. Siler-Khodr TM, Khodr GS. Luteinizing hormone releasing factor content of the human placenta. Am J Obstet Gynecol 130:216, 1978.
208. Miyake A, Sakumoto T, Aono T, et al. Changes in luteinizing-hormone-releasing hormone in human placenta throughout pregnancy. Obstet Gynecol 60:444, 1987.
209. Currie AJ, Fraser HM, Sharpe RM. Human placental receptors for luteinizing hormone releasing hormone. Biochem Biophys Res Commun 99:332, 1981.
210. Petraglia F, Lim ATW, Vale W. Adenosine 3′,5′-monophosphate, prostaglandins, and epinephrine stimulate the secretion of immunoreactive gonadotropin-releasing hormone from cultured human placental cells. J Clin Endocrinol Metab 65:1020, 1987.
211. Petraglia F, Volpe AO, Genazzani AR, et al. Neuroendocrinology of the human placenta. Front Neuroendocrinol 11:6, 1990.
212. Barnea ER, Feldman D, Kaplan M, Morrish DW. The dual effect of epidermal growth factor upon human chorionic gonadotropin secretion by the first trimester placenta in vitro. J Clin Endocrinol Metab 71:923, 1990.
213. Petraglia F, Vaughan J, Vale W. Inhibin and activin modulate the release of GnRH, hCG and progesterone from cultured human placental cells. Proc Natl Acad Sci USA 86:5114, 1989.

214. Mersol-Barg MS, Miller KF, Choi CM, et al. Inhibin suppresses human chorionic gonadotropin secretion in term, but not first trimester, placenta. J Clin Endocrinol Metab 71:1294, 1990.
215. Petraglia F, Vaughan J, Vale W. Steroid hormones modulate the release of immunoreactive gonadotropin-releasing hormone from cultured human placental cells. J Clin Endocrinol Metab 70:1173, 1990.
216. Belisle S, Petit A, Gallo-Payet N, et al. Functional opioid receptor sites in human placenta. J Clin Endocrinol Metab 66:283, 1988.
217. Ringler GE, Kao L-C, Miller WL, Strauss JF III. Effects of 8-bromo-cAMP on expression of endocrine functions by cultured human trophoblast cells. Regulation of specific mRNAs. Mol Cell Endocrinol 61:13, 1989.
218. Wilson EEA, Jawad MJ, Powell DE. Effect of estradiol and progesterone on human chorionic gonadotropin secretion in vitro. Am J Obstet Gynecol 149:143, 1984.
219. Maruo T, Matsuo H, Ohtani T, et al. Differential modulation of chorionic gonadotropin (CG) subunit messenger ribonucleic acid level and CG secretion by progesterone in normal placenta and choriocarcinoma cultured in vitro. Endocrinology 119:858, 1986.
220. Younes MA, Besch NF, Besch PK. Estradiol and progesterone binding in human term placental cytosol. Am J Obstet Gynecol 141:170, 1981.
221. Siler-Khodr TM, Khodr GS, Valenzuela G. Immunoreactive GnRH levels in maternal circulation throughout pregnancy. Am J Obstet Gynecol 150:376, 1984.
222. Kumasaka T, Nishi N, Jai Y, et al. Demonstration of immunoreactive somatostatin-like substance in villi and decidua in early pregnancy. Am J Obstet Gynecol 134:39, 1979.
223. Watkins WB, Yen SSC. Somatostatin in cytotrophoblast of the immature human placenta: Localization by immunoperoxidase cytochemistry. J Clin Endocrinol Metab 50:969, 1980.
224. Caron P, Buscail L, Esteve JP, Susini C. Expression of somatostatin receptor SST 4 in human placenta (Abstract OR-35). Annual Meeting of the Endocrine Society; June 11–14, 1997; Minneapolis, MN, p 115.
225. Campbell EA, Linton EA, Wolfe CDA, et al. Plasma corticotropin releasing hormone concentrations during pregnancy and parturition. J Clin Endocrinol Metab 64:1054, 1987.
226. Sasaki A, Tempst P, Liotta AS, et al. Isolation and characterization of a corticotropin-releasing hormone–like peptide from human placenta. J Clin Endocrinol Metab 67:768, 1988.
227. Margioris AN, Grino M, Protos P, et al. Corticotropin-releasing hormone and oxytocin stimulate the release of placental proopiomelanocortin peptides. J Clin Endocrinol Metab 66:922, 1988.
228. Petraglia F, Sawchenko P, Rivier J, Vale W. Evidence for local stimulation of ACTH secretion by corticotropin-releasing factor in human placenta. Nature 328:717, 1987.
229. Frim DM, Emanuel RL, Robinson BG, et al. Characterization and gestational regulation of corticotropin-releasing hormone messenger RNA in human placenta. J Clin Invest 82:287, 1988.
230. Robinson BG, Emanuel RL, Frim DM, Majzoub JA. Glucocorticoid stimulates expression of corticotropin-releasing hormone gene in human placenta. Proc Natl Acad Sci USA 85:5244, 1988.
231. Riley SC, Walton JC, Herlick JM, Challis JRG. The localization and distribution of corticotrophin-releasing hormone in the human placenta and fetal membranes throughout gestation. J Clin Endocrinol Metab 72:1001, 1991.
232. Linton EA, Wolfe CDA, Behan DP, Lowry PJ. A specific carrier substance for human corticotropin releasing factor in late gestational maternal plasma which could mask the ACTH-releasing activity. Clin Endocrinol 28:315, 1988.
233. Potter E, Behan DP, Fisher WH, et al. Cloning and characterization of the cDNAs for human and rat corticotropin-releasing factor binding proteins. Nature 349:429, 1991.
234. Perkins AV, Eben F, Wolfe CAD, et al. Plasma measurements of corticotropin-releasing hormone–binding protein in normal and abnormal human pregnancy. J Endocrinol 138:149, 1993.
235. Petraglia F, Sutton S, Vale W. Neurotransmitters and peptides modulate the release of immunoreactive corticotropin-releasing factor from human cultured placental cells. Am J Obstet Gynecol 160:247, 1989.
236. Gibbs DM, Stewart RD, Vale W, et al. Synthetic corticotropin-releasing factor stimulates secretion of immunoreactive β-endorphin/β-lipotropin and ACTH by human fetal pituitaries in vitro. Life Sci 32:547, 1983.
237. Jaffe RB, Mulchahey JJ, DiBlasio AM, et al. Peptide regulation of pituitary and target tissue function and growth in the primate fetus. Recent Prog Horm Res 44:431, 1988.
238. Liotta A, Osathanondh R, Ryan KJ, Krieger DK. Presence of corticotropin in human placenta: Demonstration of in vitro synthesis. Endocrinology 101:1552, 1977.
239. Shambaugh G, Kubek M, Wilson JF. Thyrotropin-releasing hormone activity in the human placenta. J Clin Endocrinol Metab 48:483, 1979.
240. Youngblood WW, Humm J, Lipton MA, Kizer JS. Thyrotropin-releasing hormone–like bioactivity in placenta: Evidence for the existence of substances other than pyro-glu-his-pro-NH_2 (TRH) capable of stimulating pituitary-thyrotropin release. Endocrinology 106:541, 1980.
241. Ascheim S, Zondek B. Anterior pituitary hormone and ovarian hormone in the urine of pregnant women. Klin Wochenschr 6:1322, 1927.
242. Bahl OP. Human chorionic gonadotropin: I. Purification and physiochemical properties: II. Nature of the carbohydrate units. J Biol Chem 244:575, 1969.
243. Carlsen RB, Bahl OP, Swaminathan N. Human chorionic gonadotropin: Linear amino acid sequence of the α subunit. J Biol Chem 248:6810, 1973.
244. Midgley AR Jr, Pierce GB Jr. Immunohistochemical localization of human chorionic gonadotropin. J Exp Med 115:289, 1962.
245. Vaitukaitis JL, Braunstein GD, Ross GT. A radioimmunoassay which specifically measures human chorionic gonadotropin in the presence of human luteinizing hormone. Am J Obstet Gynecol 113:751, 1972.
246. Talas M, Midgley AR Jr, Jaffe RB. Regulation of human gonadotropins: XIV. Gel filtration and electrophoretic analysis of endogenous and extracted immunoreactive human follicle-stimulating hormone of pituitary, serum and urinary origin. J Clin Endocrinol Metab 36:817, 1973.
247. Reyes FL, Winter JSD, Faiman C. Pituitary gonadotropin function during human pregnancy: Serum FSH and LH levels before and after LHRH administration. J Clin Endocrinol Metab 42:590, 1976.
248. Padmanebhen V, Sonstein J, Olton PL, et al. Serum bioactive follicle-stimulating hormone–like activity increases during pregnancy. J Clin Endocrinol Metab 69:986, 1968.
249. Midgely AR Jr, Jaffe RB. Regulation of human gonadotropins: II. Disappearance of human chorionic gonadotropin following delivery. J Clin Endocrinol Metab 28:1712, 1968.
250. Serón-Ferré M, Lawrence CC, Jaffe RB. Role of hCG in the regulation of the fetal zone of the human fetal adrenal gland. J Clin Endocrinol Metab 46:834, 1978.
251. Jaffe RB, Serón-Ferré M, Huhtaniemi I, Korenbrot C. Regulation of the primate fetal adrenal gland and testes in vitro and in vivo. J Steroid Biochem 8:479, 1977.
252. Huhtaniemi IT, Korenbrot CC, Jaffe RB. HCG binding and stimulation of testosterone biosynthesis in the human fetal testis. J Clin Endocrinol Metab 44:963, 1977.
253. Huhtaniemi IT, Korenbrot CC, Jaffe RB. Content of chorionic gonadotropin in human fetal tissues. J Clin Endocrinol Metab 46:994, 1978.
254. McGregor WG, Raymoure WJ, Kuhn RW, Jaffe RB. Fetal tissue can synthesize a placental hormone: Evidence for chorionic gonadotropin β-subunit synthesis by human fetal kidney. J Clin Invest 68:306, 1981.
255. McGregor WG, Kuhn RW, Jaffe RB. Biologically active chorionic gonadotropin: Synthesis by the human fetus. Science 220:306, 1983.
256. Goldsmith PC, McGregor WG, Raymoure WJ, et al. Identification of cellular sites of chorionic gonadotropin synthesis in human fetal kidney and liver. J Clin Endocrinol Metab 57:654, 1983.
257. Nisula BC, Kettslergers JM. Thyroid-stimulating activity and chorionic gonadotropin. J Clin Invest 54:494, 1974.
258. Kenimer JG, Hershman JM, Higgins HP. The thyrotropin in hydatidiform moles is human chorionic gonadotropin. J Clin Endocrinol Metab 40:482, 1975.
259. Carayon P, Lefort G, Nisula B. Interaction of human chorionic gonadotropin and human luteinizing hormone with human thyroid membranes. Endocrinology 106:1907, 1980.

260. Pekonen F, Weintraub BD. Interaction of crude and pure chorionic gonadotropin with the thyrotropin receptor. J Clin Endocrinol Metab 50:280, 1980.
261. Carayon P, Amir S, Nisula B, Lissitzky S. Effect of carboxypeptidase digestion of the human choriogonadotropin molecule on its thyrotropic activity. Endocrinology 108:1891, 1981.
262. Menon KMJ, Jaffe RB. Chorionic gonadotropin–sensitive adenyl cyclase in human term placenta. J Clin Endocrinol Metab 36:1104, 1973.
263. Barsh GS, Seeburg PH, Gelinas RE. The human growth hormone gene family: Structure and evolution of the chromosomal locus. Nucleic Acids Res 11:3939, 1983.
264. Josimovich JB, MacLaren JA. Presence in human placenta and term serum of highly lactogenic substance immunologically related to pituitary growth hormone. Endocrinology 71:209, 1962.
265. Grumbach MM, Kaplan SL, Sciarra JJ, Burr IM. Chorionic growth hormone–prolactin (CGP): Secretion, disposition, biologic activity in man, and postulated function as the "growth hormone" of the second half of pregnancy. Ann N Y Acad Sci 148:501, 1968.
266. Suwa S, Friesen H. Biosynthesis of human placental proteins and human placental lactogen (HPL) in vitro: I. Identification of ^{3}H-labeled HPL. Endocrinology 85:1028, 1969.
267. Seeburg PH, Shine J, Martial J, et al. Nucleotide sequence of part of the gene for human chorionic somatomammotropin: Purification of DNA complementary to predominant mRNA species. Cell 12:157, 1977.
268. Li CH, Dixon JS, Chung D. Primary structure of the human chorionic somatomammotropin (HCS) molecule. Science 173:56, 1971.
269. Niall HD, Hogan ML, Sauer R, et al. Sequences of pituitary and placental lactogenic and growth hormones. Evolution from a primordial peptide by gene reduplication. Proc Natl Acad Sci USA 68:866, 1971.
270. Bewley TA, Li CH. Circular dichroism studies on human pituitary growth hormone and ovine pituitary lactogenic hormone. Biochemistry 11:884, 1972.
271. Grumbach MM, Kaplan SL, Vinek A. Human chorionic somatomammotropin (HCS). *In* Berson SA, Yalow RS (eds). Methods in Investigative and Diagnostic Endocrinology. Amsterdam, Elsevier North Holland, 1973.
272. Grumbach MM, Kaplan SL, Abrams CL, et al. Plasma free fatty acid response to the administration of chorionic "growth hormone–prolactin." J Clin Endocrinol Metab 26:476, 1966.
273. Hoshina M, Boothby M, Boime I. Cytological localization of chorionic gonadotropin α and placental lactogen mRNAs during development of the human placenta. J Cell Biol 93:190, 1982.
274. Kaplan SL, Gurpide E, Sciarra JJ, Grumbach MM. Metabolic clearance rate and production rate of chorionic growth hormone–prolactin in late pregnancy. J Clin Endocrinol Metab 28:1450, 1968.
275. Kim YJ, Felig P. Plasma chorionic somatomammotropin levels during starvation in midpregnancy. J Clin Endocrinol Metab 32:864, 1971.
276. Kaplan S. *In* Jaffe RB (ed). The Endocrine Milieu of Pregnancy, Puerperium and Childhood: Report of the Third Ross Conference on Obstetric Research. Human Chorionic Somatomammotropin: Secretion, Biologic Effects, and Physiologic Significance, Columbus, OH, Ross Laboratories, 1974, p 75.
277. Liotta A, Osathanondh R, Ryan KJ, Kreiger DT. Presence of corticotropin in human placenta: Demonstration of in vitro synthesis. Endocrinology 101:1551, 1977.
278. Reese LH, Burke CW, Chard T, et al. Possible placental origin of ACTH in normal human pregnancy. Nature 154:620, 1975.
279. Odagiri ED, Sherrell BJ, Mount CD, et al. Human placental immunoreactive corticotropin, lipotropin, and β-endorphin: Evidence for a common precursor. Proc Natl Acad Sci USA 76:2027, 1971.
280. Liotta AS, Houghten R, Krieger DT. Identification of a β-endorphin–like peptide in cultured human placental cells. Nature 295:593, 1982.
281. Golund RS, Wardlaw SL, Stark RI, Frantz AG. Human plasma β-endorphin during pregnancy, labor and delivery. J Clin Endocrinol Metab 52:74, 1981.
282. Wardlaw SL, Stark RI, Baxi L, Frantz AG. Plasma β-endorphin and β-lipoprotein in the human fetus at delivery: Correlation with arterial pH and pO_2. J Clin Endocrinol Metab 79:888, 1979.
283. Rama Sastry BV, Barnwell LS, Tayeb OS, et al. Occurrence of methionine enkephalin in human placental villus. Biochem Pharmacol 29:475, 1980.
284. Lemaire S, Valette A, Chouinard L, et al. Purification and identification of multiple forms of dynorphin in human placenta. Neuropeptides 3:181, 1983.
285. Valette A, Desprat R, Cros J, et al. Immunoreactive dynorphin in maternal blood, umbilical vein and amniotic fluid. Neuropeptides 7:145, 1986.
286. Belisle S, Petit A, Gallo-Payet N, et al. Functional opioid receptor sites in human placentas. J Clin Endocrinol Metab 66:283, 1988.
287. Ahmed MS, Randall LW, Cavinato AG, et al. Human placental opioid peptides: Correlation to the route of delivery. Am J Obstet Gynecol 155:703, 1986.
288. Ahmed MS, Horst MA. Opioid receptors of human placental villi modulate acetylcholine release. Life Sci 39:535, 1986.
289. O'Donahue TL, Chronwell BM, Pruss RM, et al. Neuropeptide Y and peptide YY neuronal and endocrine systems. Peptides 6:755, 1985.
290. Tatemoto K. Neuropeptide Y: Complete amino acid sequence of the brain peptide. Proc Natl Acad Sci USA 79:5485, 1982.
291. Petraglia F, Calza L, Giardino L, et al. Identification of immunoreactive neuropeptide-Y in human placenta: Localization, secretion, and binding sites. Endocrinology 124:2016, 1989.
292. Petraglia F, Coukos G, Battaglia C, et al. Plasma and amniotic fluid immunoreactive neuropeptide-Y levels change during pregnancy, labor and at parturition. J Clin Endocrinol Metab 69:324, 1989.
293. Petraglia F, Sawchenko PA, Lim ATW, et al. Localization, secretion, and action of inhibin in human placenta. Science 237:187, 1987.
294. Rabinovici J, Goldsmith P, Librach C, Jaffe RB. Localization and regulation of the activin-A dimer in human placental cells. J Clin Endocrinol Metab 75:571, 1992.
295. McLachlan RI, Healy DL, Lutjen PF, et al. The maternal ovary is not the source of circulating inhibin levels during human pregnancy. Clin Endocrinol (Oxf) 27:663, 1987.
296. Muttrishna S, Child TJ, Groone NP, Ledger WL. Source of circulating levels of inhibin A, pro alpha C–containing inhibins and activin A in early pregnancy. Hum Reprod 12:1089, 1997.
297. Frolik CA, Dart LL, Meyers CA, et al. Purification and initial characterization of type β transforming growth factor from human placenta. Biochemistry 80:3676, 1983.
298. Fant M, Munro H, Moses AC. An autocrine/paracrine role for insulin-like growth factors in the regulation of human placental growth. J Clin Endocrinol Metab 63:499, 1986.
299. Lai W, Guyda HJ. Characterization and regulation of epidermal growth factor receptors in human placental cell cultures. J Clin Endocrinol Metab 58:344, 1984.
300. Maruo T, Matsuo H, Oishi T, et al. Induction of differentiated trophoblast function by epidermal growth factor: Relation of immunohistochemically detected cellular epidermal growth factor levels. J Clin Endocrinol Metab 64:744, 1987.
301. Goustin AS, Betsholtz C, Pfeifer-Ohlsson S, et al. Coexpression of the *sis* and *myc* proto-oncogenes in developing human placenta suggests autocrine control of trophoblast growth. Cell 41:301, 1985.
302. Gospodarowicz D, Cheng J, Lui GM, et al. Fibroblast growth factor in the human placenta. Biochem Biophys 128:554, 1985.
303. Jaffe RB, Peréz-Palaciós G, Lamont KG, Givner ML. De novo steroid sulfate biosynthesis. J Clin Endocrinol Metab 16:71, 1968.
304. Killinger DW, Solomon S. Synthesis of pregnenolone sulfate, dehydroisoandrosterone sulfate, 17α-hydroxypregnenolone sulfate, and Δ^5-pregnanetriol sulfate by the normal human adrenal gland. J Clin Endocrinol Metab 25:290, 1965.
305. Jaffe RB, Payne AH. Gonadal steroid sulfates and sulfatase: IV. Comparative studies on steroid sulfokinase in the human fetal testis and adrenal. J Clin Endocrinol Metab 33:592, 1971.
306. Serra GB, Peréz-Palaciós G, Jaffe RB. De novo testosterone biosynthesis in the human fetal testis. J Clin Endocrinol Metab 30:128, 1970.
307. France JT, Seddon RJ, Liggins GC. Placental sulfatase deficiency. J Clin Endocrinol Metab 29:138, 1969.

308. Oakey RE, Cawoods M, MacDonald RR. Biochemical and clinical observations in a pregnancy with placental sulphatase and other enzyme deficiencies. J Clin Endocrinol Metab 3:131, 1974.
309. Lauritzen C. Conversion of DHA-sulfate to estrogens as a test of placental function. Horm Metab Res 1:96, 1969.
310. Bedin M, Tanguy G, Cedard L, et al. Deficit en sulfatase placentaire et icthyose recessive liée au sexe. Deux cas observés chez deux soeurs. J Gynecol Obstet Biol Reprod 8:533, 1979.
311. Riddick DH, Luciano AA, Kusnik WF, Maslar IA. De novo synthesis of prolactin by human decidua. Life Sci 23:1913, 1978.
312. Golanden A, Hurley T, Barrett J, et al. Prolactin synthesis by human-chorion-decidual tissue: A possible source of prolactin in the amniotic fluid. Science 202:311, 1978.
313. Riddick DH, Kusnik WF. Decidua: A possible source of amniotic fluid PRL. Am J Obstet Gynecol 127:187, 1977.
314. McCoshen JA, Tomita K, Fernandez C, Tyson JE. Specific cells of human amnion selectively localize prolactin. J Clin Endocrinol Metab 55:166, 1982.
315. Bigazzi M, Pollicino G, Nardi E. Is human decidua a specialized endocrine organ? J Clin Endocrinol Metab 49:847, 1979.
316. Bigazzi M, Nardi E. Prolactin and relaxin: Antagonism on the spontaneous motility of the uterus. J Clin Endocrinol Metab 53:665, 1981.
317. Bryant-Greenwood GD. Relaxin as a new hormone. Endocr Rev 3:62, 1982.
318. Evans MI, Dougan MB, Moawad AH, et al. Ripening of the human cervix with porcine ovarian relaxin. Am J Obstet Gynecol 147:410, 1983.
319. Fuchs AR, Fuchs F, Husslein P. Oxytocin receptors and human parturition: A dual role for oxytocin in the initiation of labor. Science 215:1396, 1982.
320. Leake RD, Weitzman RE, Glatz TH, Fisher DA. Plasma oxytocin concentrations in men, nonpregnant women, and pregnant women before and during spontaneous labor. J Clin Endocrinol Metab 53:730, 1981.
321. Jones SA, Challis JRG. Local stimulation of prostaglandin production by corticotropin-releasing hormone in human fetal membranes and placenta. Biochem Biophys Res Commun 159:192, 1989.
322. Jones SA, Challis JRG. Steroid corticotropin-releasing hormone, ACTH and prostaglandin, interactions in the amnion and placenta of early pregnancy in man. J Endocrinol 125:159, 1990.
323. Gray TK, Lowe W, Lester GE. Vitamin D and pregnancy: The maternal-fetal metabolism of vitamin D. Endocr Rev 2:264, 1981.
324. Honnebier WJ, Jobis AC, Swaab DF. The effect of hypophyseal hormones and human chorionic gonadotropin (HCG) on the anencephalic fetal adrenal cortex and parturition in the human. J Obstet Gynaecol Br Commonu 81:423, 1974.
325. Mueller-Heubach E, Myers RE, Adamsons K. Effects of adrenalectomy on pregnancy length in the rhesus monkey. Am J Obstet Gynecol 112:221, 1972.
326. Novy MJ, Walsh SW, Kittinger GW. Experimental fetal anencephaly in the rhesus monkey: Effect on gestational length and fetal and maternal plasma steroids. J Clin Endocrinol Metab 45:1031, 1977.
327. Novy MJ, Walsh SW. Dexamethasone and estradiol treatment in pregnant rhesus macaques: Effects of gestational length, maternal plasma hormones, and fetal growth. Am J Obstet Gynecol 145:920, 1983.
328. Mecenas CA, Giussani DA, Owiny JR, et al. Production of premature delivery in pregnant rhesus monkeys by androstenedione infusion. Nat Med 2:443, 1996.
329. Karalis K, Goodwin G, Majzoub JA. Cortisol blockade of progesterone: A possible molecular mechanism involved in the initiation of human labor. Nat Med 2:556, 1996.
330. Hillhouse EW, Grammatopoulos D, Milton NG, Quartero HW. The identification of a human myometrial corticotropin-releasing hormone receptor that increases in affinity during pregnancy. J Clin Endocrinol Metab 76:736, 1993.
331. Benedetto C, Petraglia F, Marozio L, et al. Corticotropin-releasing hormone increases prostaglandin $F_{2\alpha}$ activity on human myometrium in vitro. Am J Obstet Gynecol 171:126, 1994.
332. Quartero HWP, Fry CH. Placental corticotropin releasing factor may modulate human parturition. Placenta 10:439, 1989.
333. McLean M, Thompson D, Zhang HP, et al. Corticotrophin-releasing hormone and beta-endorphin in labour. Eur J Endocrinol 131:167, 1994.
334. McLean M, Bisits A, Davies J, et al. A placental clock controlling the length of human pregnancy. Nat Med 1:460, 1995.
335. Sasaki A, Shinkawa O, Margioris AN, et al. Immunoreactive corticotropin-releasing hormone concentrations during pregnancy and parturition. J Clin Endocrinol Metab 64:1054, 1987.
336. Sasaki A, Liotta AS, Luckey MM, et al. Immunoreactive corticotropin-releasing factor is present in human plasma during the third trimester of pregnancy. J Clin Endocrinol Metab 59:812, 1984.
337. Smith R, Mesiano S, Chan EC, et al. Corticotropin-releasing hormone directly and preferentially stimulates dehydroepiandrosterone sulfate secretion by human fetal adrenal cortical cells. J Clin Endocrinol Metab 83:2916, 1998.
338. Chakravorty A, Mesiano S, Jaffe RB. Corticotropin releasing hormone (CRH) stimulates phosphatidylinositol metabolism in human fetal adrenal cells: evidence for a novel signaling pathway (Abstract OR30-5). Annual Meeting of the Endocrine Society; June 24–27, 1998; New Orleans, LA, p 92.
339. Nathanielsz PW, Jenkins SL, Tame JD, et al. Local paracrine effects of estradiol are central to parturition in the rhesus monkey. Nature Med 4:456, 1998.

Chapter 28

ENDOCRINE DISORDERS IN PREGNANCY

Robert L. Barbieri

CHAPTER OUTLINE

KEY POINTS

- Four placental genes, placental growth hormone (GH-V) and the three chorionic somatomammotropin genes (hCS-A, hCS-B, hCS-L), are responsible for many of the changes in central metabolism that occur in pregnancy. The most important of these alterations is a marked increase in insulin resistance.
- The metabolic changes of pregnancy allow the fetus to use maternal glucose and amino acids as fuel sources and provide extra free fatty acids, ketones, and glycerol as maternal fuel sources.
- The insulin resistance of pregnancy can cause the onset of gestational diabetes, one of the most common endocrine disorders of pregnancy.
- During pregnancy, pituitary production of LH, FSH, and growth hormone is markedly suppressed, and the production of prolactin and ACTH is increased. The placenta produces hCG and placental growth hormone as "replacements" for the suppressed pituitary hormones.
- The placenta produces many hypothalamic and pituitary hormones, governed by regulatory systems that mimic those observed in the hypothalamic-pituitary unit. This is the basis for Yen's hypothesis that the placenta is a "third brain."
- In pregnancy, the most common cause of Cushing's syndrome is an adrenal adenoma secreting cortisol.
- For women with a history of delivering a child with classic adrenal hyperplasia, prenatal counseling and glucocorticoid treatment may reduce the risk of delivering a daughter with classic adrenal hyperplasia in a subsequent pregnancy.
- Preterm labor may be due to a placental clock that is set to run too fast. Placental secretion of corticotropin-releasing hormone may play a major role in timing the onset of human labor.

For most women, pregnancy and birth are seminal events, treasured among the most rewarding of all life experiences. The majority of pregnant women are healthy and have no endocrine disorders during their pregnancy. For a few women, pre-existing endocrine abnormalities complicate their pregnancy. The most common pre-existing endocrine disorders that can complicate pregnancy are obesity, thyroid dysfunction (reviewed in Chapter 16), and diabetes mellitus. Less common pre-existing endocrine disorders that can complicate pregnancy include pituitary tumors, diabetes insipidus, and hyperparathyroidism. In some women, pregnancy *causes* the onset of a newly diagnosed endocrine disorder, the most common of which are gestational diabetes and disorders of the endocrine and sympathetic nervous system associated with preeclampsia.

DIABETES MELLITUS

Alterations in Central Metabolism During Pregnancy

In pregnancy, control of central metabolism is significantly altered by the action of placental hormones including placental growth hormone (GH-V), placental chorionic somatomammotropins (hCS, placental lactogens), placental corticotropin-releasing hormone (CRH), cortisol, and progesterone. In many respects, during late pregnancy, control of maternal central metabolism shifts to the fetal-placental unit.

Insulin Resistance

In pregnancy, major functional changes occur in insulin production and action. Insulin levels increase during pregnancy.[1–3] In early pregnancy, insulin responsiveness to nutrients, especially glucose, appears to be enhanced. In later pregnancy, insulin resistance appears to predominate.[4–6] Insulin resistance is characterized by a marked decrease in the ability of a fixed amount, or concentration, of insulin to stimulate glucose uptake in muscle and adipocytes. In response to insulin resistance, the pancreas with adequate beta cell reserve will increase insulin secretion in an attempt to overcome the peripheral insulin resistance. This compensatory response tends to return glucose levels to normal at the cost of chronically elevated insulin levels both in the fasting and in the fed state.

Insulin resistance in pregnancy can be demonstrated by the insulin tolerance test and by glucose loading tests. During pregnancy, the injection of a standard dose of insulin does not result in a normal decrease in circulating insulin[7] (Fig. 28–1). In pregnancy, intravenous administration of glucose results in significant hyperinsulinemia compared with the nonpregnant state[6] (Fig. 28–2). The result of these changes is marked hyperinsulinemia after meals (Fig. 28–3). In pregnancy, the peripheral resistance to insulin is accompanied by a decrease in the maternal circulating glucose pool, suggesting that increases in maternal plasma volume and extraction of glucose by the fetal-placental unit are dominant features. The increase in insulin concentration observed in pregnancy is not due to changes in the half-life of insulin, which is approximately 7 minutes both before and during pregnancy[7] (see Fig. 28–1). The increase in insulin levels during pregnancy is paralleled by islet cell hyperplasia, which has been demonstrated in all mammalian species studied to date.

The mechanisms that cause insulin resistance in pregnancy are not fully delineated. A study compared insulin receptor function in abdominal adipocytes obtained from pregnant and nonpregnant women.[8] High-affinity insulin receptors were significantly reduced in cells from pregnant women compared with those from nonpregnant women (20,000 versus 58,000 receptors per cell) (Fig. 28–4). Insulin receptor kinase activity was similar in adipocytes obtained from pregnant and nonpregnant women. However, pregnant women had a threefold decrease in insulin-stimulated glucose transport (Fig. 28–5). These results suggest that both decreased insulin receptor number and a "postreceptor" defect in insulin action are the key causes of pregnancy-induced insulin resistance.[9, 10]

Insulin resistance in pregnancy may also be caused by perturbations in the glucose transport system. Glucose transport into adipocytes and skeletal muscle is mediated by the glucose transport proteins GLUT-1 and GLUT-4. GLUT-1 is responsible for basal glucose transport and is not responsive to insulin. GLUT-4 is an insulin-responsive transporter that translocates to the cell surface after stimulation by insulin.[11] In gestational diabetes, glucose transport is reduced in both the basal and insulin-stimulated states. GLUT-4 appears to be markedly reduced in some gestational diabetics and fails to translocate to the cell surface with insulin stimulation.[12] The mechanisms that cause the dysregulation in GLUT-4 function in gestational diabetes are unclear.

Regardless of the cellular mechanisms of pregnancy-induced insulin resistance, it is clear that pregnancy tissues cause the insulin resistance. In most women, after delivery, insulin-glucose dynamics rapidly return to normal.[5] In

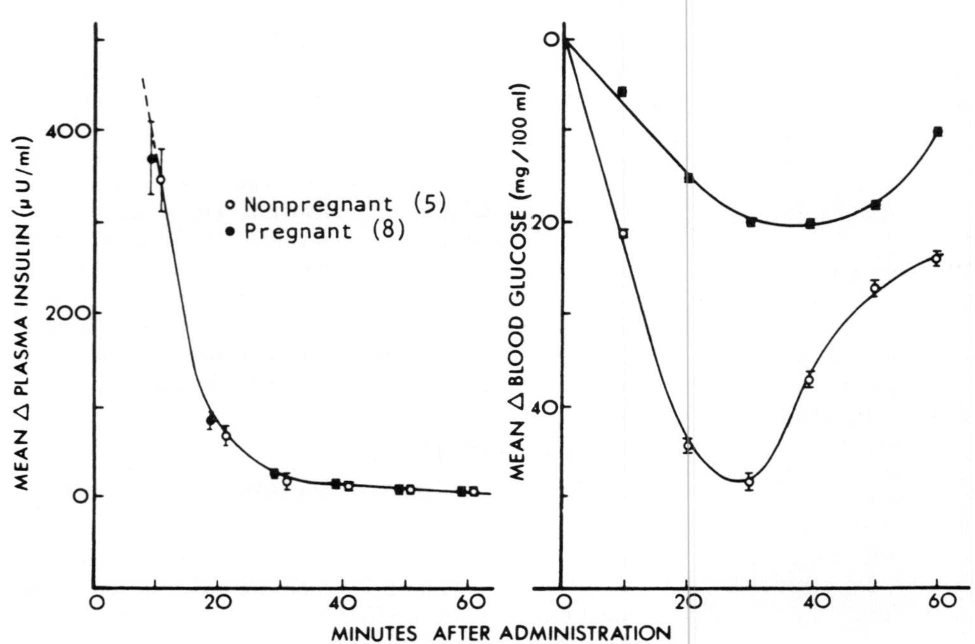

Figure 28–1 ■ *Left,* Intravenous injection of insulin (0.1 unit/kg) results in identical disappearance curves for circulating insulin in nonpregnant *(open circles)* and pregnant *(closed circles)* subjects. *Right,* In pregnant subjects *(closed circles),* the intravenous injection of insulin results in a smaller decline in circulating glucose than that seen in nonpregnant subjects. The blunted biologic effect of insulin in pregnancy suggests that pregnancy is an "insulin-resistant" state. (From Burt RL, Davidson WF. Insulin half-life and utilization in normal pregnancy. Obstet Gynecol 43: 161–170, 1974. Reprinted with permission from The American College of Obstetricians and Gynecologists.)

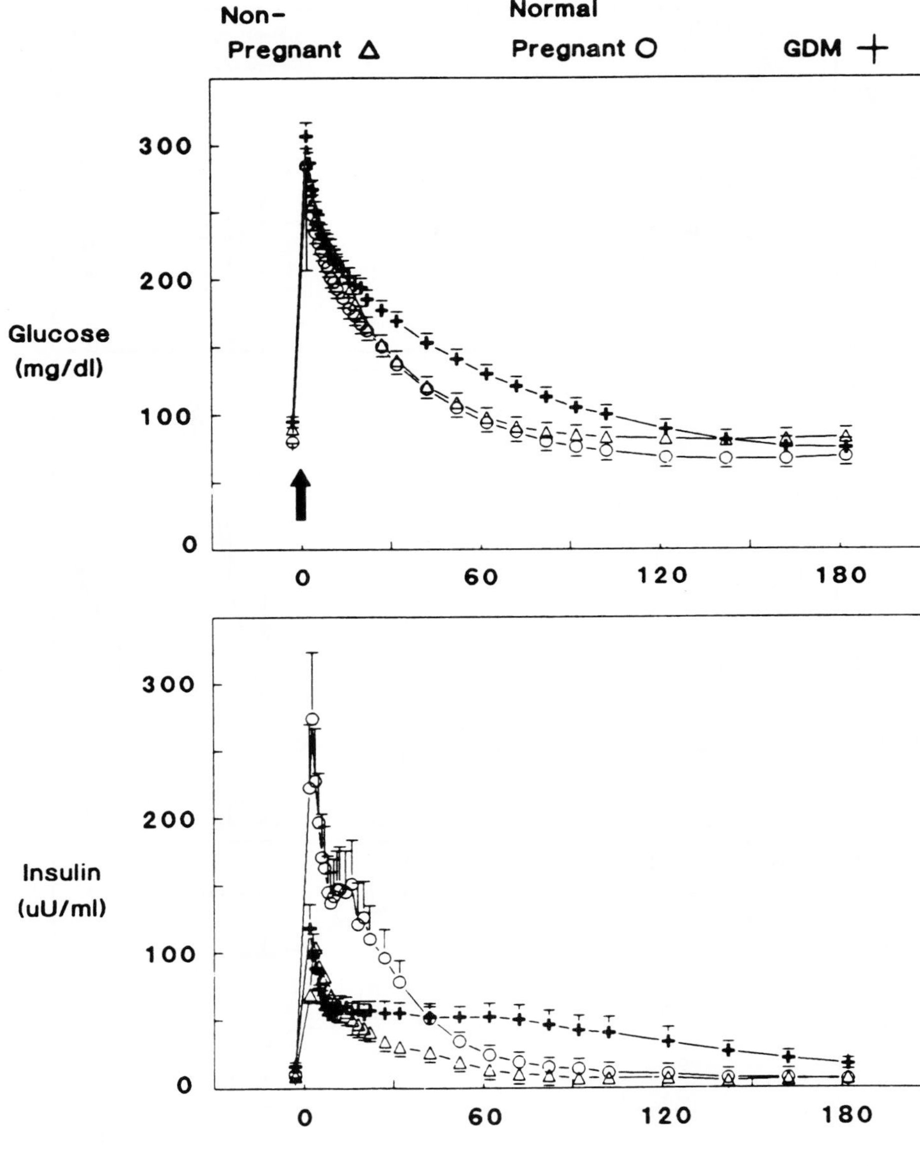

Figure 28–2 ■ Comparison of insulin and glucose responses to the rapid intravenous glucose tolerance test (300 mg/kg) in nonpregnant women, pregnant women, and pregnant women with gestational diabetes (GDM). In gestational diabetes, there are both elevated glucose and insulin concentrations, suggesting that gestational diabetes is an insulin-resistant state. The arrow indicates injection of glucose. (From Buchanan TA, Metzger BE, Freinkel N, Bergman B. Insulin sensitivity and beta-cell responsiveness to glucose during late pregnancy in lean and moderately obese women with normal glucose tolerance or mild gestational diabetes. Am J Obstet Gynecol 162:1008–1014, 1990.)

pregnancy, postreceptor insulin resistance is probably due to the production of placental counterregulatory hormones including GH-V, hCS, CRH, cortisol, and progesterone.

PLACENTAL COUNTERREGULATORY HORMONES

Insulin promotes glucose uptake in muscle and adipose tissue. Counterregulatory hormones such as growth hormone, hCS, cortisol, and progesterone inhibit insulin-mediated glucose uptake into muscle and adipose tissue, acting, in part, at a post–insulin receptor site. During pregnancy, there is a major transition in the locus of control of the growth hormone axis from the maternal hypothalamic-pituitary unit to the placenta.

Placental Growth Hormone and Chorionic Somatomammotropins. The human genes coding for growth hormone and chorionic somatomammotropins (hCS) are clustered on chromosome 17 in the following order: 5′ hGH-N (the pituitary growth hormone gene), hCS-L, hCS-A, hGH-V (the placental growth hormone gene), and hCS-B 3′.[13] The placenta does not express the hGH-N gene (pituitary growth hormone). At 8 weeks of pregnancy, hCS-A and hCS-B are expressed equally, but by term, hCS-A is expressed fivefold more abundantly than hCS-B; hCS-L generates two distinct messenger ribonucleic acids (mRNAs) on the basis of alternative splice-acceptor sites; hGH-V generates two distinct transcripts on the basis of generation of a minor mRNA (hGH-V2) that retains intron 4.[14] Multiple genes, multiple mRNA species, and heterogeneity in post-translational processing result in many isoforms of these key placental growth hormones. The teleologic purpose of having multiple placental growth hormone–like genes in tandem is to ensure that the placenta

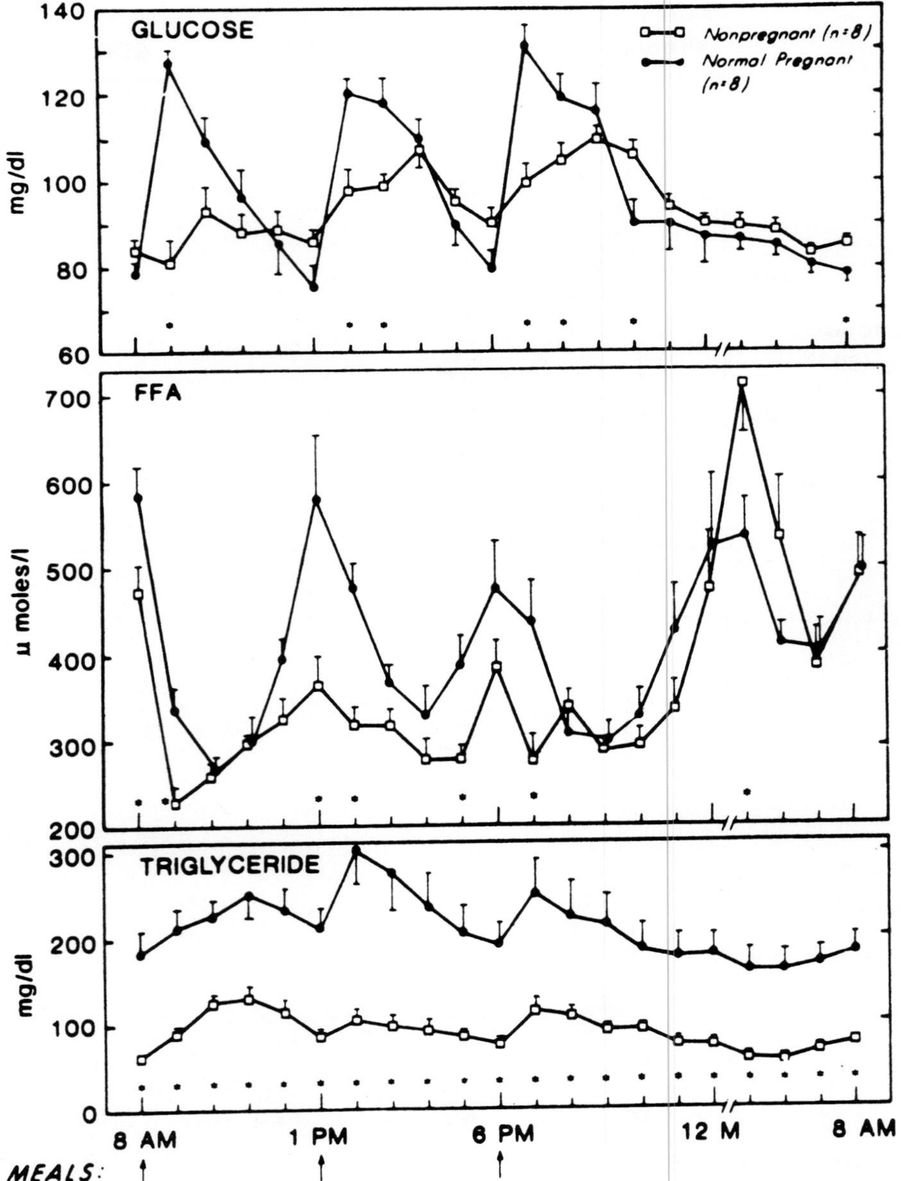

Figure 28–3 ■ Glucose and insulin response to 24 hours of feeding and fasting in the third trimester of pregnancy *(closed circles)* and the nonpregnant state *(open squares)*. In the fed state (asterisk), pregnancy is associated with elevated levels of both circulating glucose and insulin. In the fasting state, pregnancy is associated with decreases in glucose below those that are seen in the nonpregnant state. FFA, free fatty acids. (From Phelps RL, Metzger BE, Freinkel N. Carbohydrate metabolism in pregnancy. Am J Obstet Gynecol 140:730–736, 1981.)

can generate sufficient quantities of growth hormones to regulate maternal and fetal metabolism. "Knockout" of a single gene has a low likelihood of disrupting pregnancy outcome.

Human placental growth hormone circulates in at least three forms, with molecular masses of 22, 25, and 26 kDa. Placental growth hormone differs from pituitary growth hormone by 13 amino acid substitutions (of 191 residues).[15] The 25-kDa form is glycosylated, and the 26-kDa isoform results from alternative splicing of mRNA.[16] During the first trimester of pregnancy, pituitary growth hormone is detectable in maternal serum and is secreted in a pulsatile manner.[17] During the second and third trimesters of pregnancy, pituitary growth hormone secretion progressively declines. During the third trimester of pregnancy, pituitary growth hormone secretion is largely suppressed and minimally responsive to normal stimulation by hypoglycemia or amino acid infusions (see later).[18, 19] During the second and third trimesters of pregnancy, there is a progressive increase in the circulating concentration of placental growth hormone. The physiologic impact of the increase in placental growth hormone is discussed later.

The human chorionic somatomammotropins are single-chain proteins produced largely by the syncytiotrophoblast with high homology to growth hormone and prolactin. In primates, hCS genes appear to have evolved from a precursor growth hormone gene. In nonprimate species, the placental lactogens appear to have evolved from a precursor prolactin gene. Because of these differences in evolution, we have chosen to use "human chorionic somatomammotropins" to refer to these genes.[20] A dominant form of hCS is 191 amino acids with a molecular mass of 23 kDa.[15, 21] The factors that control hCS synthesis and secretion are not fully delineated, but somatostatin and growth hormone–

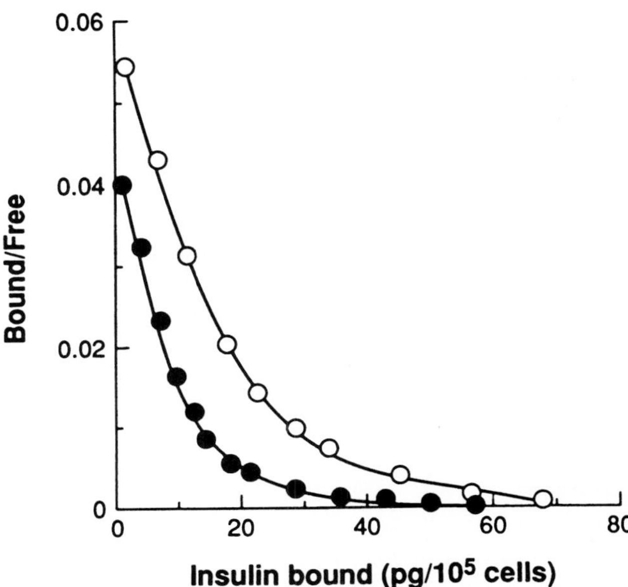

Figure 28–4 ■ Composite Scatchard curves of insulin binding to isolated adipocytes from control nonpregnant subjects *(open circles)* and pregnant subjects *(closed circles)*. Specific binding of insulin to freshly isolated cells was measured at 37°C. (From Ciaraldi TP, Kettel M, el-Roeiy A, et al. Mechanism of cellular insulin resistance in human pregnancy. Am J Obstet Gynecol 170:635–641, 1994.)

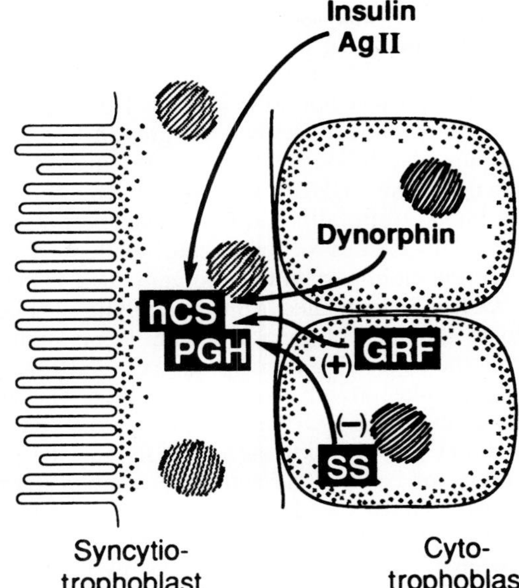

Figure 28–6 ■ Diagrammatic depiction of a potential placental regulatory system involving growth hormone–releasing hormone (GRF), somatostatin (SS), human chorionic somatomammotropin (hCS), and placental growth hormone (PGH). The modulating roles of dynorphin, insulin, and angiotensin II (AgII) are also shown. The placenta has endocrine regulatory systems that parallel those in the maternal and fetal hypothalamic-pituitary units. Yen has proposed that the placenta is a "third brain."

releasing hormone produced by the cytotrophoblast may respectively play inhibitory and stimulatory roles[22–24] (Fig. 28–6). This intraplacental regulatory system would partially parallel that observed in the hypothalamic-pituitary unit. Yen has proposed that the placenta is a "third brain," which has endocrine regulatory systems similar to those

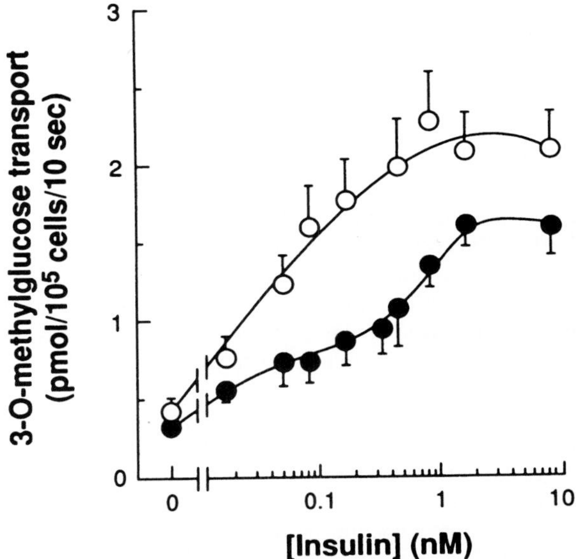

Figure 28–5 ■ Concentration dependence of insulin stimulation of glucose transport in isolated adipocytes from control nonpregnant *(open circles)* and pregnant *(closed circles)* subjects. Results are rates of glucose transport, mean (SEM). (From Ciaraldi TP, Kettel M, el-Roeiy A, et al. Mechanism of cellular insulin resistance in human pregnancy. Am J Obstet Gynecol 170:635–641, 1994.)

observed in the hypothalamic-pituitary unit of the mother and fetus. Additional regulation of hCS is provided by insulin and angiotensin II, which stimulate hCS release.[25, 26] Dynorphin may also regulate hCS secretion.[27]

Both GH-V and hCS increase throughout pregnancy. Acting through growth hormone receptors (growth hormone and prolactin receptors belong to a superfamily of cytokine receptors that share homology),[20] these proteins stimulate the production of insulin-like growth factor I (IGF-I). IGF-I increases throughout pregnancy, reaching a peak near term.[28, 29] The increase in IGF-I with pregnancy is also observed in dwarfs with complete pituitary growth hormone deficiency, suggesting that placental hormones modulate this effect.[19] IGF-binding protein 1 (IGFBP-1) rises in the first trimester, peaks at about 12 to 14 weeks of gestation, and then remains relatively stable throughout the remainder of gestation.[30] During pregnancy, the high bioavailable IGF-I concentration probably contributes to the suppression of pituitary GH-N secretion (see below). At term, estimates of growth hormone activity based on radioreceptor assays suggest that the relative contributions to circulating growth hormone activity are 85 percent from placental GH-V, 12 percent from hCS, and less than 3 percent from pituitary GH-N.[31] GH-V and the hCS are primary metabolic regulators of pregnancy.

In the circulation, growth hormone can exist in a free or bound form. In humans, growth hormone–binding protein (GHBP) is an ectodomain of the cellular growth hormone receptor, which enters the circulation through proteolytic cleavage of the cellular growth hormone receptor. GHBP appears to have both inhibitory and potentiating effects on growth hormone action. Approximately 30 percent of growth hormone circulates bound to GHBP.[32] The 30 percent of growth hormone bound to GHBP is probably not bioavailable, indicating that GHBP can have inhibitory actions on the growth hormone system. However, GHBP can also have potentiating effects on growth hormone action. Veldhuis and colleagues[33] concluded that at physiologic concentrations, GHBP acts as a buffer to prevent growth hormone from falling to low values between secretory pulses. This creates a "feminizing" pattern of growth hormone action on important target organs such as the liver. Because GHBP is generated from proteolytic cleavage of the cellular growth hormone receptor, some authorities believe that the circulating concentration of GHBP parallels that of the cellular growth hormone receptor. The greater the levels of circulating GHBP, the greater the concentration of cellular growth hormone receptors and the greater the sensitivity of cells to the actions of growth hormone. In pregnancy, GHBP tends to decline as gestation advances.[34] The physiologic meaning of this change is unclear. In women with gestational diabetes, two independent groups have reported that GHBP levels are elevated compared with those in nondiabetic pregnant women. This suggests that in gestational diabetes, at the tissue level, there may be an increased concentration of growth hormone receptors and a degree of sensitization to the effects of GH-V, hCS, and GH-N.[35] Increasing cellular sensitivity to the effects of growth hormone should result in increased insulin resistance and higher glucose levels and may be a risk factor for fetal macrosomia. Normal pregnancy is possible in Laron dwarfism, in which both the growth hormone receptor and GHBP are absent.[36]

GH-V, IGF-I, and the IGFBPs appear to correlate with birth weight. In a series of studies, a decrease in both placental GH-V and IGF-I has been reported to be associated with growth-restricted newborns.[37] The decrease in GH-V production appears to be due to both a decrease in placental mass and a decrease in the density of GH-V–secreting cells normalized for a given placental area.[38] There is a strong negative correlation between maternal IGFBP-1 concentrations and birth weight in term and preterm pregnancies.[39, 40] The higher the maternal IGFBP-1 levels, the lower the bioavailable IGF-I and the lower the birth weight. Many investigators have reported a positive correlation between fetal circulating concentrations of IGF-I and birth weight.[41, 42] Reece and colleagues[41] reported that in neonates below mean birth weight for gestational age, IGF-I concentration was lower than in neonates above the mean for birth weight (mean [SEM], 40 [11] ng/ml versus 86 [6] ng/ml, $P < .02$). In these two groups of neonates, there were no differences in IGF-II concentrations. Similar findings were reported by Lassarre and colleagues.[42] These findings suggest that maternal, fetal, and placental regulation of growth hormone, GH-V, hCS, GHBP, and the IGFBPs may play an important role in governing fetal growth and pregnancy outcome.

Cortisol. Cortisol is a potent diabetogenic hormone. Cortisol promotes lipolysis in adipocytes and protein breakdown in muscle. This results in an increase in circulating free fatty acids and amino acids.[43] During pregnancy, both adrenocorticotropic hormone (ACTH) and cortisol concentrations increase.[44] The increase in ACTH concentration is probably due, in part, to increases in placental production of CRH (see later). Much of the increase in total cortisol concentration is due to an increase in corticosteroid-binding globulin. The production of corticosteroid-binding globulin is stimulated by estrogen. However, there is also a significant increase in urinary free cortisol excretion during pregnancy, suggesting that free cortisol may be increased.[45] The physiologic contribution of an increase in free cortisol to the insulin resistance of pregnancy is unclear.

Progesterone. In both isolated cell systems and laboratory animals, high concentrations of progesterone cause insulin resistance.[46–48] The insulin resistance caused by progesterone appears to be due to both a decrease in insulin receptor number and postreceptor defects in insulin action. In pregnancy, the high concentration of progesterone may contribute to the insulin resistance.

Fed State

Many of the pregnancy-associated adaptations in central metabolism are meant to provide a preferential and uninterrupted supply of metabolic fuel from mother to fetus as dictated by the progressively increasing metabolic needs of a growing fetus. Placental hormones help promote lipolysis during fasting and hypertriglyceridemia in the fed state. These changes allow the mother to use fats for fuel and preserve glucose and amino acids for fetal use (Fig. 28–7).

In pregnancy, a glucose load is associated with a greater increase in glucose concentration than that seen in the nonpregnant state[49] (see Fig. 28–3). In pregnancy, a glucose load produces a smaller decline in free fatty acids and a larger increase in triglycerides than are seen in the nonpregnant state (see Fig. 28–7). The relatively high levels of free fatty acids, ketone bodies, and triglycerides are probably due to the lipolytic action of the counterregulatory hormones GH-V, hCS, progesterone, and cortisol.

The placenta is relatively impermeable to fat but readily transports glucose, amino acids, and ketone bodies. The mother uses the available triglycerides, glycerol, and free fatty acids for fuel and allows the fetus to draw preferentially from the glucose and amino acid pools.

Fasted State

In normal nonpregnant women, an overnight fast is associated with a need to preserve glucose production for use by the brain. Glucose is released from the liver with contributions from glycogenolysis (75 percent) and gluconeogenesis (25 percent). The precursors for gluconeogenesis include pyruvate, lactate, alanine (from muscle), and glycerol (from the breakdown of triglycerides to glycerol in adipose tissue).

In pregnancy, there is an increase in glucose and alanine use due to the uptake of glucose and alanine by the conceptus. Consequently, in pregnancy, the fasted state is marked by exaggerated and accelerated hypoglycemia and a decrease in alanine concentration. To preserve glucose and alanine for fetal use, maternal metabolism shifts to the preferential use of free fatty acids (derived from triglyceride breakdown in adipose cells) and ketone bodies. In pregnancy, fasting is associated with hyperketonemia and an increase in free fatty acids[50, 51] (Table 28–1). The enhanced lipolysis of late pregnancy is probably due in part

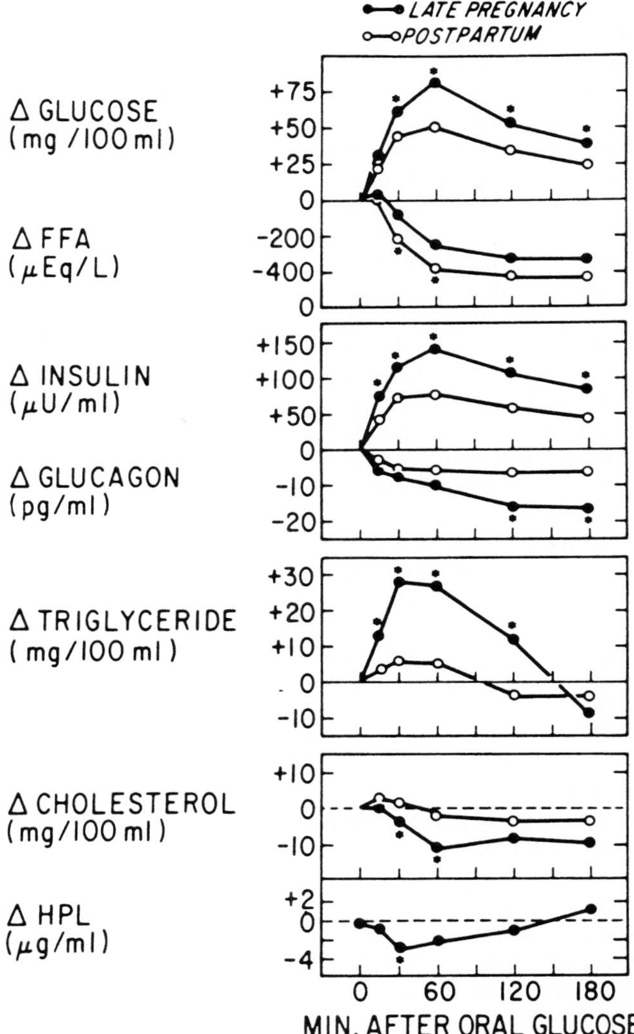

Figure 28–7 ■ Differences in the central metabolic response to an oral glucose load (100 gm) in pregnant *(closed circles)* and nonpregnant *(open circles)* subjects. FFA, free fatty acids; HPL, human placental lactogen (chorionic somatomammotropin). (From Freinkel N, Metzger BE, Nitzan M, et al. Facilitated anabolism in late pregnancy: Some novel maternal compensations for accelerated starvation. *In* Malaisse WJ, Pirart J [eds]. Diabetes International Series 312. Amsterdam, Excerpta Medica, 1973, p 474. Courtesy of Elsevier Science Publishers.)

to insulin resistance in adipose cells caused by counterregulatory hormones secreted by the placenta (GH-V, hCS). The enhanced lipolysis of late pregnancy results in hyperketonemia. In pregnancy, the acceleration of lipid catabolism during fasting helps the mother to rely on fat as a major energy source, minimizing protein catabolism and freeing both glucose and amino acids for fetal use (Fig. 28–8). These adaptations have been termed accelerated starvation by Freinkel.[52] In some respects, this characterization of pregnancy may be inaccurate in that fat mass significantly increases in pregnancy.[53]

Hyperlipemia

Pregnancy is associated with hyperlipemia. Total plasma lipid concentrations increase progressively after 24 weeks

■ TABLE 28–1

Fasting Maternal Glucose, Insulin, Glucagon, Amino Acid, Alanine, Free Fatty Acid, and Cholesterol Concentrations in Late Pregnancy and the Nonpregnant State

	MEAN (SEM) CONCENTRATION	
MEASUREMENT	Nonpregnant	Late Pregnancy
Glucose (mg/dl)	79 (2.4)	68 (1.5)*
Insulin (μU/ml)	9.8 (1.1)	16.2 (2.0)*
Glucagon (pg/ml)	126 (6.1)	130 (5.2), NS
Amino acids (μM)	3.82 (0.13)	3.18 (0.11)*
Alanine (μM)	286 (15)	225 (9)*
Free fatty acids (mg/dl)	76 (7)	181 (10)*
Cholesterol (mg/dl)	163 (8.7)	205 (5.7)*

*$P < .05$. NS, not significantly different.

From Freinkel N, Metzger BE, Nitzan M, et al. Facilitated anabolism in late pregnancy: Some novel maternal compensations for accelerated starvation. *In* Malaisse WJ, Pirart J (eds). Diabetes International Series 312. Amsterdam, Excerpta Medica, 1973, p 474.

of gestation. Increases in triglycerides, cholesterol, and free fatty acids are significant (Fig. 28–9 and Table 28–2). High-density lipoprotein cholesterol levels rise during early pregnancy, and low-density lipoprotein cholesterol concentrations increase in later pregnancy.[54, 55]

Definition of Diabetes

The American Diabetes Association recognizes four types of diabetes: type I diabetes (beta cell dysfunction usually leading to absolute insulin deficiency); type II diabetes (typically associated with insulin resistance and varying degrees of insulin secretory defect); gestational diabetes; and other types, including genetic defects and drug-induced diabetes. The fasting glucose cutoff for diagnosing nongestational diabetes was recently reduced from 140 to 126 mg/dl.[56] On the basis of this change in the diagnosis of

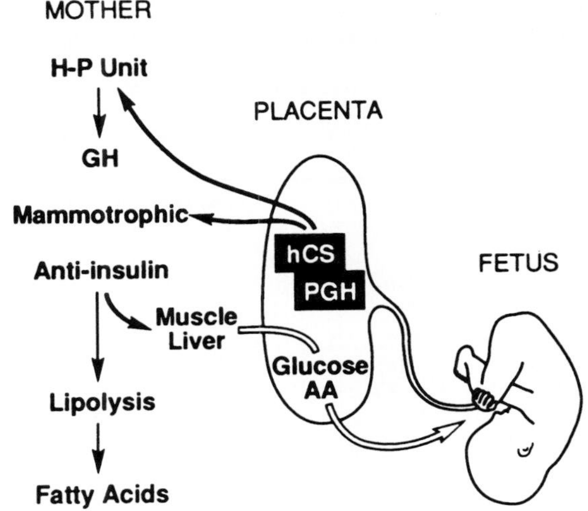

Figure 28–8 ■ The proposed functional role of human chorionic somatomammotropin (hCS) and placental growth hormone (PGH) in the adjustment of maternal metabolic homeostasis with preferential transfer of amino acid (AA) and glucose to the fetus. Maternal metabolism relies on triglycerides and fatty acids.

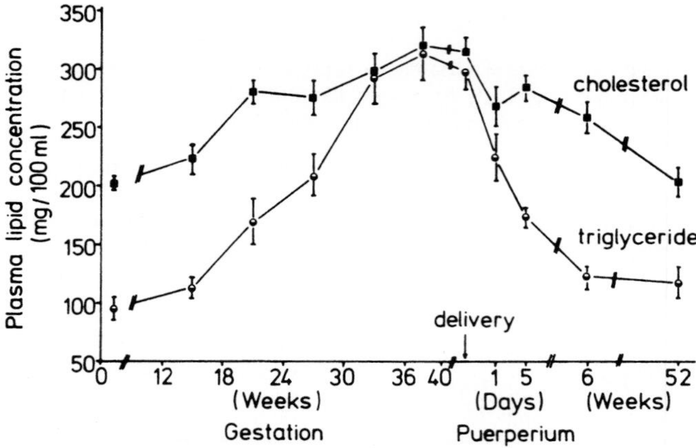

Figure 28–9 ■ Changes in plasma cholesterol and triglyceride concentrations during pregnancy and in the puerperium. Fasting lipid concentrations were measured serially throughout pregnancy, at delivery, in the puerperium, and at 12 months. The results are the mean (SEM). (From Potter JM, Nestel PJ. The hyperlipidemia of pregnancy in normal and complicated pregnancies. Am J Obstet Gynecol 133:165–170, 1979.)

nongestational diabetes, as many as 16 million citizens of the United States are diabetic.

Gestational Diabetes

Gestational diabetes is defined as any degree of glucose intolerance with the onset of pregnancy or first recognized during pregnancy.[57] Gestational diabetes complicates approximately 4 percent of all pregnancies in the United States, resulting in 140,000 cases annually.[58] Women with gestational diabetes far exceed the number of pregnant women with pre-existing diabetes, the ratio being approximately 10 to 1. Gestational diabetes may include a small group of women with previously unrecognized overt type I or type II diabetes. "True" gestational diabetes is associated with a normal glycosylated hemoglobin level and a normal glucose tolerance test after delivery.

Clinical recognition of gestational diabetes is important because it can be associated with increased perinatal mortality, increased birth trauma, and maternal hypertension.[59] In the past, some expert panels have recommended screening all pregnant women for gestational diabetes. However, there is a group of women at extremely low risk for gestational diabetes for which universal screening is probably not cost-effective. The women at low risk are younger than 25 years, are of normal body mass index, have no family history of diabetes (first-degree relatives), and are not members of ethnic or racial groups with a high prevalence of diabetes (e.g., Hispanic, Native American, Asian, African-American). For women who fulfill all of these criteria, screening during pregnancy is not necessary.

The most commonly used screening test for gestational diabetes is a 50-gm oral glucose challenge, followed by a plasma glucose measurement at 1 hour.[57] Screening is most commonly performed during 24 to 28 weeks of gestation. If the screening test reveals a 1-hour glucose level greater than 140 mg/dl, a full diagnostic 100-gm, 3-hour oral glucose tolerance test should be performed in the fasting state.

There is little consensus about the glucose values that define the upper range of normal for a full diagnostic 3-hour oral glucose tolerance test. The recommendations of the American Diabetes Association and those proposed by other authorities are presented in Table 28–3.[60–62]

For the gestational diabetic, increased perinatal mortality and fetal and maternal problems associated with fetal macrosomia are the two most common complications of diabetes.[63] Treatment of gestational diabetes includes blood glucose monitoring, dietary counseling, fetal surveillance near term, and insulin therapy if it is needed. The gestational diabetic should be observed with fasting and postprandial glucose determinations. If the fasting glucose level is greater than 100 mg/dl or if the postprandial level is greater than 120 mg/dl, consideration should be given to instituting insulin therapy.[64] Oral hypoglycemic agents are not used

■ TABLE 28–2

Comparison of Lipoprotein and Apoprotein Concentrations at 36 Weeks' Gestation Versus Nonpregnant Control Subjects

	MEAN (SD) CONCENTRATION (mg/dl)		
	36-Week Gestation	**Control, Nonpregnant**	**Percentage Change**
Total triglyceride	222 (60)	59 (19)	+376
Total cholesterol	251 (32)	171 (26)	+176
VLDL			
Triglyceride	107 (41)	33 (14)	+324
LDL			
Triglyceride	72 (21)	14 (10)	+514
Cholesterol	161 (39)	104 (23)	+154
Apo A-I	84 (23)	61 (10)	+138
HDL			
Triglyceride	29 (9)	2 (6)	+1450
Cholesterol	64 (9)	56 (12)	+114
Apo A-I	164 (16)	128 (23)	+128

VLDL, very low density lipoprotein; LDL, low-density lipoprotein; HDL, high-density lipoprotein; Apo A-I, apolipoprotein A-I.

From Knopp RH, Warth MR, Charles D, et al. Lipoprotein metabolism in pregnancy, fat transport to the fetus and the effects of diabetes. Biol Neonate 50:297–317, 1986. Reproduced with permission of S. Karger AG, Basel.

■ TABLE 28–3

Diagnostic Thresholds for Gestational Diabetes During 100-gm Glucose Tolerance Test

	PLASMA GLUCOSE VALUES, mg/dl (mmol)		
	National Diabetes Data Group	**Sacks et al**	**Carpenter and Coustan**
Fasting	105 (5.8)	96 (5.3)	95
1-hour	190 (10.6)	172 (9.4)	180
2-hour	165 (9.2)	152 (8.3)	155
3-hour	145 (8.1)	131 (7.2)	140

From National Diabetes Data Group. Classification and diagnosis of diabetes and other categories of glucose intolerance. Diabetes 28:1039–1057, 1979; Sacks DA, Abu-Fadil S, Greenspoon JS, Fotheringham N. Do the current standards for glucose tolerance testing in pregnancy represent a valid conversion of O'Sullivan's original criteria? Am J Obstet Gynecol 161:638–641, 1989; Carpenter MW, Coustan DR. Criteria for screening tests for gestational diabetes. Am J Obstet Gynecol 144:768–773, 1982.

during pregnancy because if they cross the placenta, they can produce hypoglycemia in the fetal compartment. The Third International Workshop on Gestational Diabetes recommended exercise as a mainstay to the treatment of gestational diabetes.[65] However, some randomized studies have demonstrated no beneficial effect of exercise on glucose control in women with gestational diabetes.[66]

Many of the complications of gestational diabetes are due to macrosomia. Increased birth weight is associated with increased delivery trauma to both the mother (vaginal, perineal, and rectal trauma) and fetus (brachial plexus nerve injury and fractured clavicle). Macrosomia is also associated with increased rates of operative delivery. Shoulder dystocia and brachial plexus nerve injury are serious consequences of fetal macrosomia, especially because the macrosomia of diabetes is associated with increased diameters in the upper thorax. Interventions that definitively decrease the risk of macrosomia have not been identified. Prophylactic insulin therapy has been proposed as one method for decreasing the risk of macrosomia.[64]

The risk of stillbirth is increased in women with gestational diabetes. Many centers recommend weekly fetal biophysical profiles that begin at 32 weeks' gestation if a pregnancy complication is identified (fetal macrosomia, polyhydramnios, hypertension, or insulin therapy); otherwise, biophysical profiles are often instituted at 38 weeks' gestation. Delivery is recommended by many authorities before 40 weeks if insulin therapy has been instituted or before 42 weeks if the diabetes is diet controlled. If estimated fetal weight is greater than 4500 gm, elective cesarean section is often recommended to reduce the risk of birth trauma and shoulder dystocia.

Women with gestational diabetes are at increased risk for developing diabetes later in life.[67] These women should consider interventions that include weight reduction, increased exercise, and prospective screening for diabetes.

Pregnancy in Women with Type I or Type II Diabetes

For women with type I or type II diabetes diagnosed before conception, the most important risk is congenital malformations associated with hyperglycemia during fertilization and embryo development. As many as 30 to 50 percent of the perinatal mortality in diabetic pregnancy is due to fetal malformations.[68] The congenital defects that are most characteristic of diabetic embryopathy are sacral agenesis and caudal dysplasia. These anomalies are 400 times more common in offspring of women with diabetes than in women with normal glucose metabolism.[69] Other anomalies associated with diabetes include anencephaly, open spina bifida, renal agenesis, ventricular septal defects, and transposition of the great vessels. Glucose[70] and ketone bodies such as β-hydroxybutyrate[71] may be teratogens that are capable of altering embryogenesis. High glucose concentration may perturb intracellular protein phosphorylation and decrease the production of heparan sulfate proteoglycan (perlecan), a modulator of cell-cell interaction. Perlecan modulates epithelial-mesenchymal interactions, which may be important in embryogenesis. Perturbations in perlecan synthesis may lead to dysmorphogenesis in many different organ systems.[72]

Prospective randomized studies suggest that tight control of glucose before conception is effective in reducing the risk of congenital malformations in women with established diabetes.[73] In one trial, intensive preconception treatment of diabetic women with vascular disease reduced the malformation rate from 19 percent to 8.5 percent.[74] Unfortunately, the minority of diabetic women receive intensive preconceptional treatment.[75] Elevated glycosylated hemoglobin levels at the time of conception are associated with a marked increase in congenital malformations.[76] Maternal α-fetoprotein testing and sonography at approximately 18 weeks' gestation can be useful in screening for fetal malformations.

The goal of treatment is to measure blood glucose regularly and to adjust diet, exercise, and insulin to achieve tight glucose control. Blood glucose goals should be fasting values less than 105 mg/dl and postprandial values less than 120 mg/dl.

Hypertension, prematurity, and late fetal demise are the most common complications of pregnancy in diabetic women. In diabetic women, approximately 30 percent will develop hypertension in the third trimester. Pregnancy-induced hypertension often results in induced delivery and is a major contributor to prematurity in diabetic women. Late fetal demise is probably due to abnormalities in oxygen delivery to the fetus. Maternal hyperglycemia results in fetal hyperglycemia, which causes fetal hyperinsulinemia. Fetal hyperglycemia and hyperinsulinemia increase fetal oxygen demand, which may exceed oxygen delivery capabilities, resulting in asphyxia.[77] For pregnant women with diabetes, weekly fetal testing usually starts at 32 weeks with fetal heart rate testing. After 36 weeks, testing is usually performed twice weekly. If the fetal heart rate is abnormal, oxytocin challenge testing or fetal biophysical profile should be used.

A common problem for pregnant diabetic women is the proper timing of delivery. In pregnant diabetic women, most late fetal demises occur after 36 weeks' gestation. No pregnant diabetic woman should be delivered after 40 weeks because of the increased risk of late fetal demise. Delivery before 37 weeks is associated with an increased risk of fetal respiratory distress syndrome. Fetal lung maturation is enhanced by cortisol, thyroxine, prolactin, and estradiol. Fetal lung maturation is inhibited by insulin and testosterone. In infants of diabetic mothers, hyperinsulinemia and hyperandrogenemia are common findings and may contribute to the delay in lung maturation observed in diabetic pregnancies.[78–80] The increased testosterone observed in male infants of diabetic mothers may be due to elevated concentrations of human chorionic gonadotropin (hCG) that stimulate fetal Leydig cell testosterone synthesis.

Women with poorly controlled diabetes should probably be delivered at 37 to 38 weeks after testing for fetal lung maturity. Women with well-controlled diabetes can be delivered at 38 to 40 weeks. As many as 25 percent of infants of diabetic mothers are macrosomic. If the estimated fetal weight is greater than 4500 gm, many authorities recommend cesarean delivery to reduce the risk of birth trauma, such as shoulder dystocia.

During labor, maternal glucose levels should be in the range of 100 mg/dl to reduce fetal hyperglycemia. Fetal hyperglycemia increases oxygen demand and increases the risk of neonatal hypoglycemia by causing excessive fetal insulin secretion. Before an elective induction, the morning insulin dose is withheld, and an infusion of insulin (approximately 1 unit/hour) and glucose is initiated. An insulin infusion rate of 1 unit/hour often results in a glucose level between 70 and 120 mg/dl. Glucose concentration is measured hourly and the insulin infusion adjusted. Post partum, the need for tight control is reduced, and glucose values up to 200 mg/dl are acceptable pending discharge from the hospital and regulation of glucose levels in the home environment.

OBESITY AND PREGNANCY

There is a strong relationship between obesity and reproductive function. Leptin is a protein secreted by adipocytes that may help integrate central metabolism and reproductive processes. Leptin suppresses appetite and increases energy expenditure, thereby regulating body weight. In the obese/obese mouse, the absence of a functional leptin gene results in obesity and anovulation. Administration of human leptin to the *ob/ob* mouse increases energy expenditure, reduces weight and fat mass, and restores ovulation and fertility.[81]

At delivery, leptin levels are increased in maternal serum (term, 20 ng/ml; pre-pregnancy, 5.5 ng/ml) and lower in cord blood (arterial 9.7 and venous 8.9 ng/ml) and amniotic fluid (3.6 ng/ml). Cord leptin levels correlate positively with birth weight (r = 0.5') and placental weight (r = 0.50).[82] Maternal serum leptin levels are correlated with maternal body mass, both at 36 weeks' gestation and 3 and 6 months post partum.[83] It is conceivable that manipulations of leptin or its receptor system will be the basis for safe and effective treatments of obesity.

Obesity is a complex central nervous system–endocrine disorder that is associated with a large number of adverse pregnancy outcomes. Obesity is associated with an increased risk of congenital malformations, preeclampsia, gestational diabetes, insulin treatment, macrosomia, cesarean sections, and urinary tract infections.[84] The preferred method of weight assessment is the body mass index. Body mass index is calculated as the body weight in kilograms divided by the square of the height in meters. Obesity is defined as a body mass index greater than 25 kg/m^2 before age 34 years and a body mass index greater than 27 kg/m^2 after age 34 years. An advantage of using body mass index for defining obesity is that no adjustments need to be made for gender, and no tables are required for determining the normal range. The waist to hip ratio is an independent risk for adverse outcomes in obese women. This measurement is made by taking the minimum circumference at the waist and dividing by the maximum circumference taken at the hip-buttocks. A waist to hip ratio greater than 0.8 is an independent risk factor for adverse medical outcomes in obese women independent of body mass index.[85, 86]

Obesity is associated with a significant increase in the risk of congenital malformations including neural tube defects, ventral wall defects, and abnormalities of the great vessels.[87–89] In one study, relative to a control population weighing 50 to 59 kg, obese women weighing more than 110 kg had a fourfold (95 percent confidence interval, 1.6 to 9.9) increased risk of having a fetus with a neural tube defect. For women weighing between 80 and 89 kg, the risk was 1.9 (5 percent confidence interval, 1.2 to 2.9). Interestingly, folic acid replacement at recommended levels (0.4 mg daily) did not appear to reduce the risk of neural tube defects in the obese women.[87] Similar results have been reported by other investigators, who reported that a body mass index greater than 29 kg/m^2 was associated with a 1.9-fold increase in the risk for neural tube defects.[88] Obesity appears to be one of the most important human teratogens. It is conceivable that in obese women, subtle abnormalities in the metabolism of glucose and insulin contribute to the increased risk of congenital malformations.

Obesity, like gestational diabetes, is associated with a significant increase in the risk of developing preeclampsia. In one prospective study of 2947 pregnant women, 5.3 percent developed preeclampsia. Four risk factors were identified that increased the risk of developing preeclampsia: (1) increased systolic blood pressure at first prenatal visit, (2) obesity, (3) previous spontaneous or therapeutic abortions, and (4) cigarette smoking.[90] In another study, obesity was associated with a 3.5-fold increased risk of developing severe preeclampsia (95 percent confidence interval, 1.68 to 7.46).[91]

Obesity, like gestational diabetes, is associated with an increased risk of fetal macrosomia, birth trauma, and an increased risk of cesarean section. In a study of 20,130 births, a body mass index greater than 39 kg/m^2 was associated with a 46 percent cesarean section rate, compared with a 20 percent cesarean section rate for women with a body mass index less than 29 kg/m^2.[92] In obese women, limiting total pregnancy weight gain to no more than 15 to 25 pounds appears to decrease the risk of fetal macrosomia but does not increase the risk of low birth weight.[93] During the next decade, one of the greatest challenges for endocrinologists is to develop effective treatments for obesity. For women in developed countries, obesity is the most important "endocrine" disease contributing to excess morbidity and mortality.

HYPOTHALAMIC-PITUITARY DISEASES

Pregnancy-Associated Changes in Pituitary Structure and Function

The pituitary gland is composed of three major parts: the anterior lobe (adenohypophysis), the intermediate lobe (prominent in the fetus but attenuated in the adult), and a posterior lobe (the neurohypophysis). During pregnancy, the structure and function of the anterior lobe of the pituitary gland are significantly altered. These changes have been reviewed in detail in a previous publication.[94] In the nonpregnant state, the pituitary gland is approximately 15 mm across, 10 mm long, and 5 mm deep and weighs between 0.5 and 1.0 gm. During pregnancy, the volume of the pituitary increases significantly and the shape of the gland changes. One autopsy study of 118 pregnant women demonstrated a 30 percent increase in the weight of the gland (term, 1070 mg; nonpregnant, 820 mg).[95] With use of magnetic resonance imaging, a 136 percent increase in pituitary gland volume during pregnancy has been reported[96] (Table 28–4). In pregnancy, the pituitary gland develops a convex, dome-shaped superior surface.[97] This upward bulging of the pituitary may account, in part, for the bitemporal hemianopia observed in some apparently healthy pregnant women.[98, 99]

The adenohypophysis is composed of at least six distinct cell types: lactotroph, corticotroph, somatotroph, gonadotroph, thyrotroph, and other. During gestation, the number of these cell types and their function change significantly.

The greatest changes occur in the lactotrophs. On the basis of immunohistochemistry, approximately 20 percent of the pituitary cells are lactotrophs in the nonpregnant state.[100, 101] In the third trimester, approximately 60 percent of the pituitary cells are lactotrophs. The increase in lactotrophs is most pronounced in the lateral portions of the adenohypophysis. By 1 month post partum, the number of lactotrophs decreases in nonlactating women. Postpartum resolution of lactotroph hyperplasia is incomplete, and nonpregnant multiparas have more lactotrophs than nulligravid women do. During pregnancy, the number of gonadotrophs and α-subunit–secreting cells decreases markedly. The number of somatotrophs decreases significantly, and minimal changes occur in the number of thyrotrophs.

Prolactin

During pregnancy, there are three major sources of prolactin production: maternal pituitary, fetal pituitary, and uterine decidua. Most prolactin in the maternal circulation is derived from the maternal pituitary. Prolactin levels rise throughout pregnancy, reaching concentrations of approximately 140 ng/ml at term[102] (Fig. 28–10). Estradiol is believed to be a major factor accounting for the hyperprolactinemia of pregnancy. The decidua is a major site of prolactin production during pregnancy, and decidual production of prolactin accounts for the elevated amniotic fluid prolactin levels (6000 ng/ml at the end of the second trimester).[103] Evidence to support the hypothesis that significant quantities of decidual prolactin do not enter the maternal circulation is provided by the observation that in pregnant women with pre-existing hypopituitarism, prolactin in the maternal circulation is low throughout pregnancy.[104, 105]

The control of pituitary prolactin secretion during pregnancy appears to be preserved except for the presence of a higher set-point to basal secretion. In pregnant women, prolactin secretion is stimulated by thyrotropin-releasing

■ TABLE 28–4

Volume of the Pituitary Gland Throughout Pregnancy as Determined by Magnetic Resonance Imaging

GESTATIONAL AGE (weeks)	SUBJECT NUMBER	PITUITARY VOLUME (mm³), Mean (SEM)
Nonpregnant	20	300 (60)
9	10	437 (90)
21	11	534 (124)
37	11	708 (123)

From Gonzalez JG, Elizondo G, Saldivar D, et al. Pituitary gland growth during normal pregnancy: An in vivo study using magnetic resonance imaging. Am J Med 85:217–220, 1988. Elsevier Science Inc.

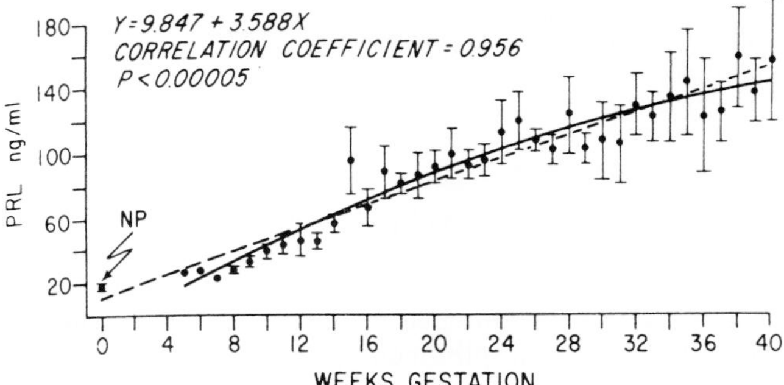

Figure 28–10 ■ Prolactin concentration in maternal circulation throughout gestation. (From Rigg LA, Lein A, Yen SSC. Pattern of increase in circulating prolactin levels during human gestation. Am J Obstet Gynecol 129:454–456, 1977.)

hormone (TRH),[106] arginine,[107] meals,[107] and sleep[108] in a manner similar to that seen in nonpregnant women. After delivery, maternal prolactin concentrations decrease to prepregnancy levels within 3 months in women who are not nursing.[109] In nursing women, baseline serum prolactin levels slowly decline to nonpregnant levels with intermittent episodes of "hyperprolactinemia" occurring in conjunction with nursing.

During gestation, there is a shift in the circulating isoforms of prolactin. In the nonpregnant state, most circulating prolactin is an *N*-linked glycosylated form (G-PRL). As pregnancy progresses, increasing amounts of nonglycosylated prolactin appear in the circulation.[110] In the third trimester, the concentration of circulating nonglycosylated prolactin exceeds that of G-PRL. In some bioassay systems, nonglycosylated prolactin is more biologically active than G-PRL.[111] The high levels of nonglycosylated prolactin in pregnancy may help prepare the breast for lactation.[110]

Adrenocorticotropin

Pregnancy is marked by an increase in the concentration of ACTH in the maternal circulation. Carr and colleagues[44] reported an increase in ACTH in the maternal circulation from 10 pg/ml in the nonpregnant state to 50 pg/ml at term (Fig. 28–11). Further increases in ACTH in the maternal circulation (300 pg/ml) were observed in labor.[44] Although the placenta can produce ACTH,[112] the majority of the ACTH in the maternal circulation is probably derived from the maternal pituitary.[113]

The increase in maternal circulating ACTH is associated with an increase in serum free cortisol,[114, 115] salivary free cortisol,[116] and urinary free cortisol.[114, 115, 117] Maternal hypercortisolemia is also observed in complete molar pregnancy, implying that the increased cortisol is not derived from a fetal source. Placental production of CRH may be a cause of the elevated ACTH observed during pregnancy.[118–120] In nonpregnant women, circulating CRH is in the range of 10 to 100 pg/ml. In the third trimester of pregnancy, maternal CRH concentrations are 500 to 3000 pg/ml, and levels drop precipitously after delivery.[120] Elevated placental CRH may alter the maternal ACTH-cortisol set-point, resulting in reduced suppressibility of the maternal ACTH-cortisol axis with exogenous glucocorticoids,[114,

[115, 121] enhanced response to ACTH stimulation by vasopressin,[118, 119] and decreased ACTH response to exogenous CRH.[118, 119]

Growth Hormone

During pregnancy, maternal pituitary secretion of somatotropin (GH-N) is markedly suppressed, and placental production of growth hormone (GH-V) replaces pituitary production of growth hormone (GH-N).[31] Blunted maternal GH-N response to insulin-induced hypoglycemia[18] and arginine stimulation[122] suggests that maternal pituitary growth hormone secretory reserve is markedly diminished in pregnancy (Figs. 28–12 and 28–13).

Gonadotropins

During pregnancy, maternal serum luteinizing hormone (LH) and follicle-stimulating hormone (FSH) are decreased by 6 to 7 weeks of pregnancy and are below the detection limits of many radioimmunoassays by the second trimester.[123–125] Immunohistochemical and immunochemical analysis of pituitary glands from pregnant women demonstrate a decrease in pituitary LH and FSH concentration.[126, 127] In pregnancy, LH and FSH response to exogenous gonadotropin-releasing hormone (GnRH) stimulation is markedly diminished[123–125] (Fig. 28–14). It is likely that the high pregnancy concentrations of estradiol and progesterone and possibly inhibins cause the suppression of LH and FSH.

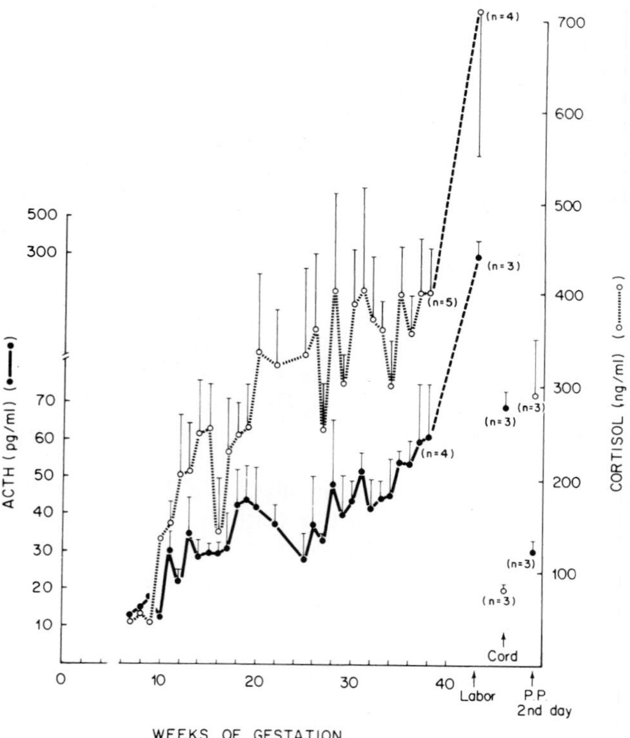

Figure 28–11 ■ ACTH and total cortisol concentration in the maternal circulation throughout gestation. (From Carr BR, Parker CR, Madden JD, et al. Maternal plasma adrenocorticotropin and cortisol relationships throughout human pregnancy. Am J Obstet Gynecol 139:416–422, 1981.)

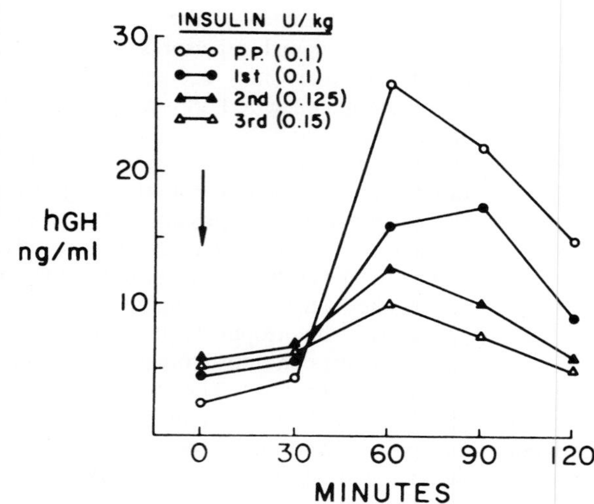

Figure 28–12 ■ Human pituitary growth hormone response to insulin-induced hypoglycemia throughout pregnancy. In the third trimester of pregnancy, pituitary growth hormone response to hypoglycemia is blunted. (From Yen SSC, Vela P, Tsai CC. Impairment of growth hormone secretion in response to hypoglycemia during early and late pregnancy. J Clin Endocrinol Metab 31:29–32, 1970. © The Endocrine Society.)

Thyrotropin

Maternal concentration of thyrotropin (thyroid-stimulating hormone [TSH]) is within the normal range throughout pregnancy.[128, 129] TSH response to TRH stimulation is normal throughout pregnancy.[128, 129] At 9 to 13 weeks of gestation, there is a modest decline in maternal circulating TSH[130, 131] (Fig. 28–15). This decrease coincides with peak placental production of hCG. The decrease in TSH may be due to the weak thyrotropic properties of hCG.[132, 133] An alternative hypothesis is that the placenta secretes a chorionic TSH or TRH, but this hypothesis is not supported by most data.[134]

Imprinting of the Pituitary During Pregnancy

Pregnancy produces changes in prolactin secretion that persist long after delivery. In a study of 24 women before and after delivery and 40 nulliparous control subjects, Musey and colleagues[135] observed that basal serum prolactin concentration and prolactin response to perphenazine were lower after pregnancy than before pregnancy. In a cross-sectional study of 19 nulliparous women and 29 parous women, serum prolactin concentration was found to be lower in the parous women (4.8 ng/ml) than in the nulliparous women (8.9 ng/ml, $P < .01$).[135] These findings and others[136, 137] suggest that pregnancy permanently lowers the secretion of prolactin.

Pituitary Tumors in Pregnancy

Many pituitary tumors are monoclonal, indicating that a somatic mutation in a single progenitor cell is the cause of the tumor formation. In one study, 100 percent of growth hormone–producing tumors and 75 percent of ACTH-producing tumors were demonstrated to be monoclonal.[138] In

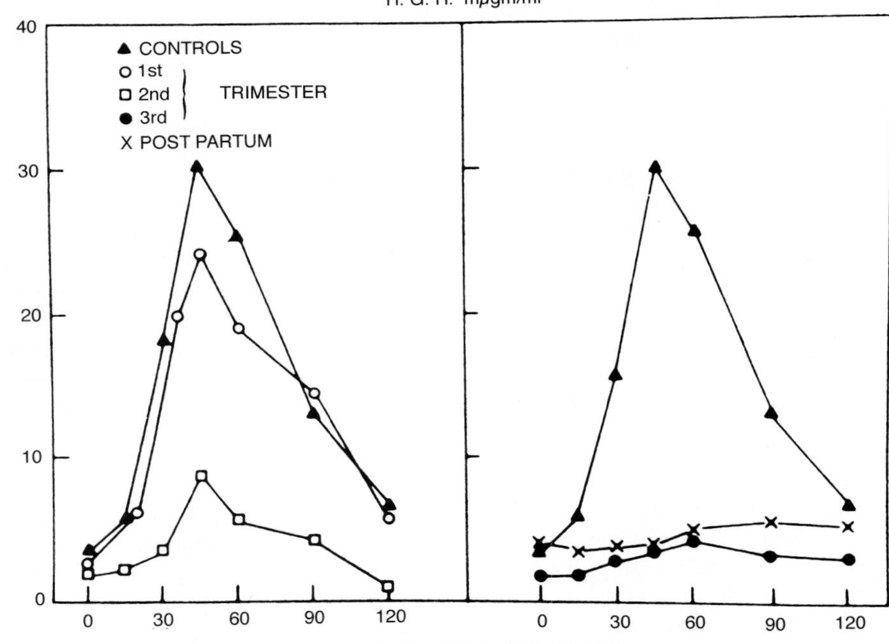

Figure 28–13 ■ Human pituitary growth hormone response to arginine throughout pregnancy. In the second and third trimesters of pregnancy, there is markedly suppressed pituitary growth hormone response to arginine infusion. (From Samaan NA, Goplerud CP, Bradbury JT. Effect of arginine infusion on plasma levels of growth hormone, insulin and glucose during pregnancy and the puerperium. Am J Obstet Gynecol 107:1002–1007, 1970.)

growth hormone–secreting tumors, mutations in the gene that codes for the G_s protein have been reported in 10 of 25 tumors. The mutations result in the production of a mutant G_s protein that is constitutively activated.[139] Genetic mutations are the primary cause of pituitary tumor growth.

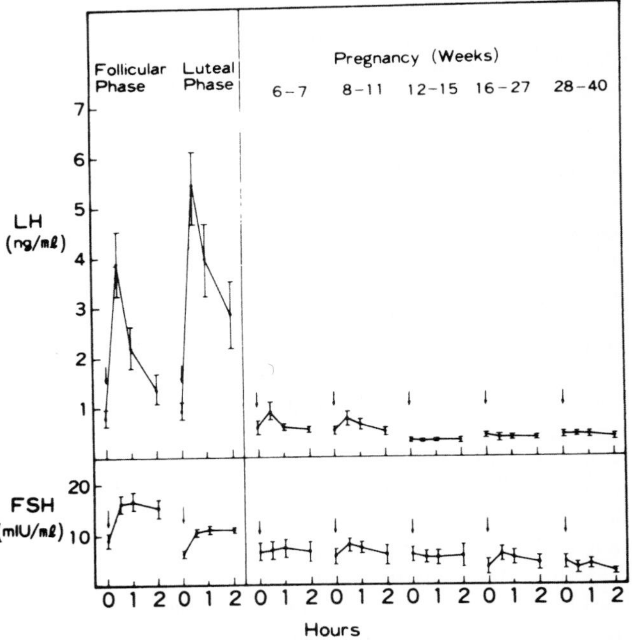

Figure 28–14 ■ Serum levels of LH and FSH before and after a 100-μg bolus of GnRH in pregnant women and normal menstruating women. During pregnancy, LH and FSH levels are markedly suppressed. (From Miyake A, Tanizawa O, Aono T, Kurachi K. Pituitary responses in LH secretion to LHRH during pregnancy. Obstet Gynecol 49:549–551, 1977. Reprinted with permission from The American College of Obstetricians and Gynecologists.)

Factors that change during pregnancy (estradiol, progesterone, dopamine) are secondary modulators of tumor phenotype. In general, pituitary tumors are benign and grow slowly.

Prolactinomas

In the initial evaluation of a suspected prolactinoma, it is important to measure circulating prolactin, thyroxine, thyroid hormone–binding globulin uptake, thyrotropin (TSH), and serum IGF-I. A structural study of the hypothalamus and pituitary is useful, and computerized evaluation of the

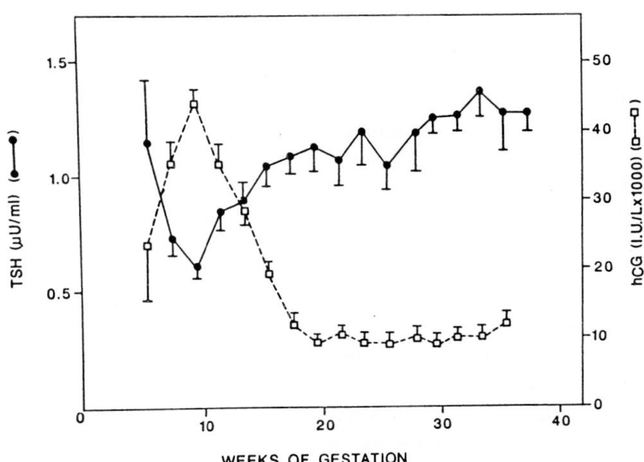

Figure 28–15 ■ Maternal concentration of serum TSH and hCG as a function of gestational age. The decrease in serum TSH at approximately 10 weeks' gestation may be due to thyrotropic effects of hCG. (From Glinoer D, de Nayer P, Bourdoux P, et al. Regulation of maternal thyroid during pregnancy. J Clin Endocrinol Metab 71:276–287, 1990. © The Endocrine Society.)

visual fields is necessary if compression of the optic chiasm is suspected. This evaluation will exclude both occult hypothyroidism (thyroxine, TSH) and acromegaly (IGF-I) as causes of the hyperprolactinemia.

Women with significant hyperprolactinemia are usually anovulatory and require treatment to ovulate and achieve a pregnancy. If a woman with hyperprolactinemia does not desire pregnancy, treatment with estrogen-progestin combinations will reduce the risk of osteoporosis and regulate the menstrual cycle. In women with microprolactinomas, treatment with estrogen-progestin combinations appears to be safe and is associated with few tumor complications such as tumor growth.[140]

For infertile women with significant hyperprolactinemia, treatment is usually required to induce ovulation and achieve a pregnancy. Controversy continues as to whether surgery or dopamine agonist treatment represents the best first-line therapy for the infertile woman with hyperprolactinemia. Many authorities support the concept that dopamine agonist therapy is the best first-line treatment for infertile women with hyperprolactinemia.[141, 142]

The four goals for the treatment of a prolactinoma are to (1) suppress prolactin and induce ovulation, (2) decrease tumor size, (3) preserve pituitary reserve, and (4) prevent recurrence. Treatment with a dopamine agonist is effective in achieving the first three of these goals. For example, bromocriptine can normalize prolactin levels, establish regular ovulation, decrease tumor size, and preserve pituitary reserve.[143, 144] A disadvantage of dopamine agonist treatment is that it is not effective in preventing tumor recurrence once treatment is discontinued. Four dopamine agonists have been demonstrated to be effective in the treatment of hyperprolactinemia: bromocriptine, pergolide, quinagolide, and cabergoline. Cabergoline is administered once weekly and may be more efficacious than bromocriptine in the treatment of microadenomas.[145] However, little information is available concerning the effects of pergolide, quinagolide, and cabergoline on pregnancy. In contrast, substantial experience has accumulated that bromocriptine can be safely administered during pregnancy, with no significant increase in recognizable malformations. In women who have conceived using bromocriptine, the rate of congenital abnormalities is no higher than in a control group.[146] The most common problems with bromocriptine therapy are the side effects of nausea, vomiting, and postural hypotension. These side effects can be minimized by starting treatment at 0.625 mg daily and increasing to the target dose during a few weeks. In some patients, doses as low as 2.5 mg daily are effective. During initiation of treatment, prolactin levels can be checked every month for 3 months, then every 3 months until the prolactin level is returned to normal.

Pituitary tumors are commonly classified by size as microadenomas ($<$10 mm in diameter) or macroadenomas ($>$10 mm in diameter). Macroadenomas can be associated with extrasellar extension, local invasion, or compression of the optic chiasm. During pregnancy, the clinical behavior of microadenomas and macroadenomas is significantly different. In general, in pregnant women, microadenomas tend to behave in a benign manner with no evidence of loss of pituitary secretory function and a low risk of neurologic complications. For example, of 215 women with microprolactinomas who became pregnant, less than 1 percent had changes in visual fields, polytomograms, or neurologic signs. Approximately 5 percent developed headaches.[94]

For women with microprolactinomas, the majority will have no neurosurgical complications during pregnancy. For those women who do develop neurologic symptoms such as headache or cranial nerve dysfunction, bromocriptine therapy can be reinstituted during the pregnancy. An occasional woman will need neurosurgical intervention during the pregnancy for marked enlargement of the tumor with neurologic sequelae.

In contrast, in pregnant women with macroadenomas, pituitary insufficiency and neurosurgical complications are common. In women with a macroprolactinoma, testing for panhypopituitarism should be completed before dopamine agonist treatment is initiated. Of 60 women with macroadenomas who became pregnant, approximately 20 percent developed changes in visual fields, polytomograms, or neurologic signs.[94] For women with macroprolactinomas, one approach to treatment is to discontinue bromocriptine once pregnancy is established and reinstitute bromocriptine therapy if symptoms or signs of increasing tumor volume occur.[147] An alternative plan is to continue bromocriptine treatment throughout pregnancy.[148, 149]

For infertile women with prolactinomas, some authorities recommend surgical treatment before attempts at pregnancy both to reduce the need for dopamine agonist treatment and to decrease the incidence of neurologic complications during pregnancy.[150] However, microsurgical resection of a prolactinoma can result in death (0.3 percent of cases) or serious morbidity, such as a cerebrospinal fluid leak (0.4 percent). In addition, surgery is successful in producing a long-term cure in only approximately 60 percent of cases.[151]

Post partum, lactation does not appear to worsen the clinical course of prolactinomas, and nursing can be encouraged.[152]

Cushing's Disease and Acromegaly

As noted before, the majority of ACTH- and growth hormone–secreting pituitary tumors are monoclonal and arise from a somatic mutation in a progenitor cell. The somatic mutation is the cause of the tumor. Changes in estradiol, progesterone, and other hormones during pregnancy can only modulate the tumor phenotype.

Cushing's disease is typically associated with depressed gonadotropin secretion, and pregnancy rarely occurs in women with established Cushing's disease unless the tumor is treated. Most cases of Cushing's disease are due to microadenomas, and therefore neurosurgical problems seldom occur during pregnancy. However, the metabolic derangements associated with Cushing's disease can increase maternal and fetal mortality. In pregnant women with Cushing's disease, premature labor, pregnancy-induced hypertension, and gestational diabetes are common (see discussion later).

Acromegaly is often associated with anovulation, but pregnancy occasionally occurs.[153, 154] In general, except for complications associated with pituitary enlargement, acromegaly does not have a marked detrimental effect on pregnancy outcome. In most women, definitive treatment for acromegaly can be deferred until after delivery. Bromocriptine and transsphenoidal surgery have been successfully used to treat acromegaly during pregnancy.

Pituitary Insufficiency

Sheehan's Syndrome

Sheehan's syndrome is the onset of hypothalamic and pituitary dysfunction after severe obstetric hemorrhage and maternal hypotension at delivery. During pregnancy, the pituitary volume increases by approximately 100 percent. The increase in pituitary size and the low-flow, low-pressure nature of the portal circulation may make the pituitary, and parts of the hypothalamus, susceptible to ischemia caused by obstetric hemorrhage and hypotension. In developing countries, the risk of obstetric hemorrhage resulting in significant hypotension is much greater than in the developed world. Consequently, the majority of cases of Sheehan's syndrome occur in developing countries. Worldwide, Sheehan's syndrome is the most common cause of hypopituitarism.

In Sheehan's syndrome, every imaginable pattern of pituitary hormone deficiency can be observed. Growth hormone and prolactin deficiency are the most common abnormalities in women with Sheehan's syndrome. In a study of 10 African women with Sheehan's syndrome, Jialal and coworkers[155] reported the pituitary hormone response to a combined intravenous insulin (0.1 unit/kg), TRH (200 μg), and GnRH (100 μg) challenge test. The pattern of pituitary hormone response revealed the following loss of secretory reserve: 100 percent of these women had both prolactin and growth hormone deficiency, 90 percent had cortisol deficiency, 80 percent had TSH deficiency, 70 percent had LH deficiency, and 40 percent had FSH deficiency. These pituitary abnormalities cause failure of lactation, failure of hair growth over areas shaved for delivery, poor wound healing after cesarean section, and weakness.

The best single test to diagnose Sheehan's syndrome is to administer TRH 100 μg intravenously with prolactin measurements at 0 and 30 minutes. The ratio of prolactin at 30 minutes to prolactin before the TRH injection (time 0) should be greater than 3.[156] If the ratio is subnormal, the woman should have a complete evaluation for panhypopituitarism.

Loss of anterior pituitary hormone reserve is the most common presentation of Sheehan's syndrome. Mild hypothalamic and posterior pituitary dysfunction occur frequently in women with Sheehan's syndrome. Sheehan and Whitehead[157] reported that at autopsy, 90 percent of women with postpartum hypopituitarism demonstrated "atrophy and scarring" of the neurohypophysis on neuropathologic examination. Whitehead[158] performed detailed pathologic studies on the hypothalamus of 13 patients and observed atrophy of the supraoptic and paraventricular nuclei. Clinical studies demonstrate that most women with Sheehan's syndrome have mild defects in both vasopressin secretion and maximal urinary concentrating capability.[159, 160]

Lymphocytic Hypophysitis

Lymphocytic hypophysitis is a rare disorder caused by infiltration of the adenohypophysis with lymphocytes and plasma cells. Most cases of lymphocytic hypophysitis occur in women in the third trimester of pregnancy or immediately post partum.[161] Circulating antipituitary, antinuclear, and antimitochondrial antibodies are detected in some cases. Pituitary enlargement can result in neurologic complications requiring surgical intervention.[162] Bromocriptine and high-dose glucocorticoids may be effective in managing some cases of lymphocytic hypophysitis when headache, visual field defects, and cranial nerve palsy are present.

Diabetes Insipidus

In early pregnancy, plasma osmolality decreases by 9 to 10 mOsm/kg and remains at these low levels throughout gestation. Arginine vasopressin levels do not change.[163] This suggests that there is a modest resetting of the osmostat with a decrease in the osmotic threshold for vasopressin release of 9 to 10 mOsm/kg.

Diabetes insipidus in pregnancy is a rare disease characterized by polyuria (more than 3 L of urine in 24 hours), polydipsia, and plasma hyperosmolarity. Diabetes insipidus can be caused by diseases of the hypothalamus-pituitary (central) or kidney (peripheral resistance). The differential diagnosis of central diabetes insipidus is extensive and includes idiopathic causes, pituitary surgery or trauma, and infiltration of the neurohypophysis by tumors or inflammatory cells and infectious agents. Central diabetes insipidus usually presents acutely with urine output in the range of 4 to 15 L daily. Transient nephrogenic forms of diabetes insipidus can occur in pregnancy, usually associated with preeclampsia, the HELLP syndrome, or acute fatty liver of pregnancy.[164] High levels of placental vasopressinase may contribute to pregnancy-associated nephrogenic forms of diabetes insipidus by destroying endogenous vasopressin. During pregnancy, D-arginine vasopressin (DDAVP), which is resistant to degradation by vasopressinase, may be somewhat more effective in treatment than native vasopressin. The increase in vasopressinase may also cause women with partial central vasopressin deficiency to develop diabetes insipidus during pregnancy. In many cases, the diabetes insipidus improves after delivery.[165]

The diagnosis of diabetes insipidus is confirmed by a water deprivation test, which should probably be performed only by an endocrinologist owing to risks associated with dehydration. The test starts in the early morning after an overnight fast. The patient is denied water until 3 percent of body weight is lost or urine osmolarity shows no increment in three successive specimens. At the end of the test, serum osmolarity and vasopressin concentrations are measured. In women with diabetes insipidus, urine osmolarity will remain low, but plasma osmolarity will increase significantly. Plasma vasopressin levels are low in central diabetes insipidus and elevated in nephrogenic diabetes insipidus. To help separate the two main causes of diabetes insipidus, 10 μg of D-arginine vasopressin (DDAVP) can be administered immediately after the completion of the water deprivation test. In women with central diabetes insipidus, there will be a decrease in urine output and an increase in urine osmolarity. In women with nephrogenic diabetes insipidus, only minimal changes are observed in urine output and osmolarity.[166]

DISORDERS OF CALCIUM METABOLISM

The key features of calcium metabolism are a large skeletal pool of "inert" calcium (1 kg) and a small extracellular pool of bioavailable calcium that are in a dynamic equilibrium controlled by parathyroid hormone (PTH), which stimulates release of calcium from the bone, and calcitonin, which suppresses calcium release from bone surfaces. Calcium enters the system from the gastrointestinal tract, regulated by vitamin D metabolites. Calcium leaves the system through urinary excretion and by loss of calcium in the skeleton of a fetus.

During pregnancy, there is a net accumulation of 25 to 30 gm of calcium at term, largely in the fetal skeleton. Increased calcium absorption from the gastrointestinal tract is probably facilitated by increases in intestinal calcium-binding protein and increases in 1,25-dihydroxyvitamin D.[167] The pregnancy-associated increase in 1,25-hydroxyvitamin D appears to be greater than the rise in the vitamin D–binding protein.[168] Free 1,25-hydroxyvitamin D levels appear to be increased in pregnancy.[169] These findings suggest that pregnancy is a state of physiologic hyperabsorption of calcium from the gastrointestinal tract. The decidua may be one source of the elevated 1,25-hydroxyvitamin D levels in pregnancy.[170]

During pregnancy, there is a major decrease in the circulating concentration of albumin (Fig. 28–16). This causes a decrease in the concentration of total calcium. The upper limit of normal for total serum calcium during pregnancy is approximately 9.5 mg/dl. Ionized calcium changes little during pregnancy.[171] Calcitonin levels remain relatively constant throughout gestation. Using early radioimmunoassays for PTH, some investigators reported that PTH levels rise during pregnancy.[172] Studies with dual antibody assays that have high specificity for intact PTH suggest that PTH levels tend to be constant during pregnancy.[171]

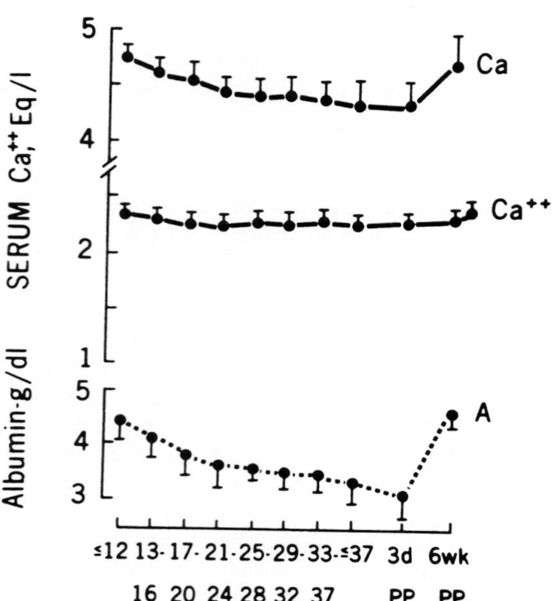

Figure 28–16 ■ Serum calcium, ionized calcium, and albumin concentrations during pregnancy. During pregnancy, there is a marked decrease in circulating albumin concentration; this results in a decrease in total calcium. There is no change in ionized calcium. (From Pitkin RM, Reynolds WA, Williams GA, Hargis GK. Calcium metabolism in normal pregnancy: A longitudinal study. Am J Obstet Gynecol 133:781–790, 1979.)

Calcium from the maternal compartment is actively transported across the placenta up a concentration gradient to the fetal compartment. This process appears to be regulated in part by the production of PTH-related protein by the fetal parathyroid gland.[173] In mice with a knockout of the gene encoding PTH-related protein, calcium transport from the maternal to fetal compartment is markedly impaired and can be returned to normal by the injection of PTH-related protein.[174] The fetus is relatively hypercalcemic compared with the mother; cord calcium levels exceed maternal levels by 1 mEq/L. At birth, the fetus is relatively hypercalcemic, hypercalcitonemic, and hypoparathyroid. A fall in serum calcium at birth due to the loss of the maternal source of calcium is accompanied by a rise in serum PTH and a fall in calcitonin. Although urinary excretion of calcium tends to rise during pregnancy,[175] the ratio of urinary calcium to creatinine tends to fall,[176] suggesting an attempt to conserve calcium even though renal glomerular filtration is increasing. In general, bone density during pregnancy is relatively stable; some investigators report a slight decrease in bone density in the third trimester.[177]

Hyperparathyroidism

Primary hyperparathyroidism in pregnancy is unusual with only a few hundred reported cases. The causes of hyperparathyroidism are a solitary parathyroid adenoma (80 percent of cases), four-gland hyperplasia (15 percent of cases), multiple adenomas (3 percent of cases), and carcinoma (less than 2 percent of cases). The maternal complications of hyperparathyroidism include hyperemesis, weakness, headache, confusion, emotional lability, nephrolithiasis, pancreatitis, and hypertension.[178] Fetal death and spontaneous abortion rates are increased in pregnancies complicated by hyperparathyroidism,[179] but in recent series, with better management, the fetal death rate appears to be decreasing.[180] At birth, neonatal hypocalcemic tetany is common and typically occurs in the first 2 weeks of life.[181] Most authorities recommend surgical excision of the adenoma in symptomatic women.[178] Controversy persists as to the optimal management for asymptomatic women or women with mild hyperparathyroidism.

Unusual causes of hypercalcemia in pregnancy include familial hypocalciuric hypercalcemia (FHH) and rare cases of inappropriate secretion of the PTH-related protein.[182] In FHH, women present with mild hypercalcemia, mild elevations in PTH, and low urinary calcium. Because of the autosomal dominant nature of the disease and the high penetrance, infants can present with either hypercalcemia (neonate affected with FHH) or hypocalcemia (neonate not affected with FHH, neonate responding to the maternal hypercalcemia).[183]

Hypoparathyroidism

The most common cause of maternal hypoparathyroidism is incidental resection of the parathyroid glands at the time of thyroidectomy. This complication occurs in approximately 1 percent of thyroidectomy cases. Symptoms of hypocalcemia include numbness and tingling of the fingers and orofacial area. Chvostek's sign (twitching of the facial muscles when the facial nerve is tapped) and Trousseau's sign (induction of carpopedal spasm by applying pressure to the upper arm with a blood pressure cuff) are often present. In pregnancies complicated by hypoparathyroidism, the fetus demonstrates a compensatory hyperparathyroidism with bone demineralization. The treatment of maternal hypoparathyroidism is calcium (1.2 gm daily) and vitamin D (50,000 to 150,000 IU daily). If calcium levels can be maintained near the normal range, pregnancy outcome is excellent.[184] During labor, tetany is common in women with hypocalcemia, possibly exacerbated by respiratory alkalosis. Calcium for intravenous administration should be available. Lactation may not be advisable in women with hypoparathyroidism taking vitamin D. Vitamin D is present in breast milk and may pose a risk for hypercalcemia in the newborn.[185]

ADRENAL DISEASES

Adrenal Insufficiency

Adrenal insufficiency is caused by destruction of the adrenal cortex (primary adrenal insufficiency, Addison's disease) or adrenocortical atrophy due to ACTH deficiency (secondary adrenal insufficiency) from pituitary or hypothalamic disease. In secondary adrenal insufficiency, the zona glomerulosa and mineralocorticoid production are preserved because they are under the control of the renin-angiotensin system.[186] Most cases of Addison's disease are caused by autoimmune destruction of the adrenal, which can occur in isolation or in association with the destruction of other endocrine organs (autoimmune polyglandular diseases type I and type II)[187] (Table 28–5). In the autoimmune adrenal insufficiency cases, antibodies against cytochrome P450 monooxygenases involved in steroidogenesis are common.[188] Other causes of Addison's disease include human immunodeficiency virus disease, tuberculosis, sarcoidosis, and adrenal leukodystrophy.

■ TABLE 28–5
Autoimmune Polyglandular Syndromes*

TYPE I	TYPE II
Common	**Common**
Addison's disease	Addison's disease
Hypoparathyroidism	Thyroid dysfunction
Mucocutaneous candidiasis	Type I diabetes
Less Common	**Less Common**
Hypogonadism	Hypogonadism
Malabsorption	Myasthenia gravis
Vitiligo	Vitiligo
Pernicious anemia	Pernicious anemia
Alopecia	Alopecia
Hypothyroidism	

*Autoimmune polyglandular syndromes are important becuase given the presence of one disease, certain other endocrinopathies are more likely both in the patient and in relatives. Type I is also named autoimmune polyendocrinopathy–candidiasis–ectodermal dystrophy syndrome.

From Neufeld M, MacLaren NK, Blizzard RM. Two types of autoimmune Addison's disease associated with different polyglandular autoimmune syndromes. Medicine (Baltimore) 60:355–362, 1981.

The most common symptoms of adrenal insufficiency are weakness, fatigue, nausea, anorexia, diarrhea, and weight loss. Pigmentation in the creases of the palms of the hands, knuckles, and knees may be seen in some patients with Addison's disease. Vitiligo is present in about 10 percent of patients. Laboratory features of Addison's disease include hyponatremia, hyperkalemia, and an increase in blood urea nitrogen. Addison's disease can be diagnosed by administering synthetic $^{1-24}$ACTH (cosyntropin) 0.25 mg by intravenous bolus and measuring cortisol 60 minutes after the injection. The stimulated cortisol concentration should be greater than 18 μg/dl.[189] If secondary adrenal insufficiency is a consideration, an aldosterone measurement can be obtained. In secondary adrenal insufficiency, there will be a subnormal rise in cortisol, but the aldosterone concentration will be normal.[190]

Therapy for Addison's disease consists of the physiologic replacement of cortisol and mineralocorticoid, if necessary. Normal cortisol production rates are in the range of 20 to 30 mg daily. Hydrocortisone (cortisol) at doses of 20 to 30 mg daily is prescribed; two thirds of the dose is administered in the morning and one third in the late afternoon or early evening. Fluorohydrocortisone (Florinef) at doses in the range of 0.1 mg daily will treat mineralocorticoid deficiency. In pregnancy, the kidney synthesizes large amounts of deoxycorticosterone from progesterone.[191] Deoxycorticosterone is a weak glucocorticoid and mineralocorticoid. The renal production of deoxycorticosterone during pregnancy may account for the observation that adrenal crises during pregnancy are unusual, but they frequently occur in the immediate postpartum interval.[192]

Adrenal crisis requires treatment with normal saline, glucose, and high doses of cortisol. Many clinicians give both intramuscular and intravenous injections of glucocorticoid to reduce the risk that loss of intravenous access might prevent the patient from receiving the full dose of glucocorticoid. The maximal adrenal cortisol production is approximately 300 mg daily. Many clinicians give a 100-mg bolus of cortisol at the initiation of treatment and then give a constant infusion of cortisol, 300 mg daily.

For women undergoing elective surgery, stress doses of cortisol should be administered. On the day of surgery, 300 mg of cortisol can be administered, and this dose can be reduced by 50 mg daily until oral glucocorticoid replacement is reinitiated. For pregnant women, cortisol requirements appear not to be increased during pregnancy, but labor may be managed with stress doses of glucocorticoids. The fetus is highly resistant to suppression of the fetal adrenals by maternal ingestion of glucocorticoids.[193]

Cushing's Syndrome

Cushing's syndrome can be due to ACTH-dependent causes (ACTH-secreting pituitary adenoma [Cushing's disease], ACTH- or CRH-secreting tumors such as bronchial carcinoids) and ACTH-independent causes (administration of glucocorticoids, adrenal adenoma, or carcinoma). In nonpregnant women, Cushing's disease is three times more common than an adrenal adenoma as the cause of Cushing's syndrome. In pregnant women, adrenal adenomas are the most common cause of Cushing's syndrome[194] (Table 28–6). Cushing's syndrome can be difficult to recognize and diagnose during pregnancy because of the physiologic "hypercortisolism" of pregnancy.

The most common symptoms and signs of Cushing's disease are muscle weakness, personality changes, centripetal obesity ("potato stick" person: thick trunk, thin arms and legs), facial plethora, supraclavicular and dorsal (buffalo hump) fat pads, violaceous striae, hirsutism, and hypokalemia. The most specific signs of Cushing's disease are spontaneous hypokalemia, violaceous striae greater than 2 cm in width, and proximal muscle weakness. It is often helpful to obtain a photograph of the patient from many years in the past to compare facial changes.

In pregnant women, Cushing's syndrome is associated with an increased risk of hypertension (65 percent), diabetes (32 percent), preeclampsia (10 percent), congestive heart failure, and death. Congestive heart failure and death often occurred in association with severe hypertension or preeclampsia. Perinatal morbidity and mortality are high in pregnancies complicated by Cushing's disease. Prematurity (65 percent), intrauterine growth restriction (26 percent), and perinatal death (16 percent) were the major adverse pregnancy outcomes.

During pregnancy, establishing the diagnosis of Cushing's syndrome and identifying the cause can be difficult. In nonpregnant women, significant and persistent elevation in urinary free cortisol excretion (>200 μg/day) is the single best laboratory marker for Cushing's syndrome. In normal pregnancy, urinary free cortisol excretion increases, with mean levels as high as 130 μg/day (60 to 250 μg/day) being reported.[195] However, these assays may have been performed with anticortisol antibodies that lacked specificity. With use of more specific testing techniques, which include sample extraction and high-performance liquid chromatography, normal subjects have 24-hour urinary free cortisol excretion in the range of 23 μg; the urinary cortisol excretion in Cushing's disease is in the range of 165 to 3360 μg daily.[196] Urinary free cortisone and cortisol as determined by high-performance chromatography may have greater sensitivity and specificity in the diagnosis of Cushing's syndrome than does the measurement of urinary free cortisol by standard assay techniques.[197]

Given the high rate of adrenal adenomas in pregnant women with Cushing's syndrome, one approach to the differential diagnosis might be to first perform a high-resolution imaging study on the adrenal glands (computed tomography or magnetic resonance imaging). This test would identify adrenal adenomas and adrenal carcinomas. If these two causes of Cushing's syndrome are excluded, then a test to identify an ACTH-secreting pituitary tumor (CRH stimulation followed by petrosal sinus sampling for ACTH) or an extrapituitary source of ACTH or CRH (computed tomography of the chest) could be performed.[198]

Because of the relatively few cases of Cushing's syndrome complicating pregnancy, no clinical trials have been performed to identify an optimal treatment strategy. Owing to the high maternal and perinatal morbidity associated with Cushing's syndrome during pregnancy, it is warranted to treat the cause of the problem as soon as it is identified. In the case of an adrenal adenoma, a unilateral adrenalectomy can be performed. Alternatively, experimental therapy with antiglucocorticoids or inhibitors of adrenal steroidogenesis could be used. Metyrapone,[199, 200] aminoglutethimide,[201] and ketoconazole[202, 203] have been used to treat Cushing's syndrome in pregnancy. However, no studies have established the efficacy or safety of these agents. In the case of an ACTH-secreting pituitary tumor, transsphenoidal resection during pregnancy can be successful.[204]

■ TABLE 28–6

Comparision of the Etiology of Cushing's Syndrome in Nonpregnant Versus Pregnant Populations

ETIOLOGY	NONPREGNANT	PREGNANT
Number of subjects	108	58
ACTH-secreting pituitary tumor–bilateral adrenal hyperplasia	64 (59%)	19 (33%)
Adrenal adenoma	17 (16%)	29 (50%)
Adrenal carcinoma	10 (9%)	6 (10%)
Ectopic ACTH	17 (16%)	1 (2%)
Unknown	0	3 (5%)

From Buescher MA, McClamrock HD, Adashi EY. Cushing's syndrome in pregnancy. Obstet Gynecol 79:130–137, 1992. Reprinted with permission from The American College of Obstetricians and Gynecologists.

Adrenal Hyperplasia

Classic (congenital) adrenal hyperplasia (CAH) occurs in approximately 1 in 14,000 livebirths. In select populations, the risk is much higher. In the Yupik Eskimos, CAH occurs at a frequency of 1 in 300 livebirths.[205] In CAH, the loss of 21-hydroxylase activity results in a decrease in cortisol production, which results in a compensatory increase of ACTH and increase in the flux of steroid precursors through the adrenal, causing adrenal androgen overproduction. The exposure of the female fetus to high levels of androgen during early development can lead to clitorimegaly, labioscrotal fusion, abnormal course of the urethra, and virilization. In severe forms of 21-hydroxylase deficiency, the conversion of progesterone to the mineralocorticoids deoxycorticosterone, corticosterone, and aldosterone is reduced, resulting in "salt wasting." The salt-wasting form of the disease is associated with hyponatremia, hyperkalemia, and death in the perinatal period if it is undetected and untreated. In CAH due to 21-hydroxylase deficiency, 75 percent of cases are associated with salt wasting and 25 percent present with virilization but no salt wasting. For the obstetrician evaluating a newborn with ambiguous genitalia, the most important disease to exclude is 21-hydroxylase deficiency associated with salt wasting. Failure to recognize this condition can result in discharge of the newborn, dehydration, and death.

Women with 21-hydroxylase deficiency may inquire about the risk that their daughters will be affected by the disease. Women with nonclassic 21-hydroxylase deficiency who have not delivered a child with CAH do not require prenatal intervention. The likelihood that a mother with nonclassic adrenal hyperplasia will have a child who is more severely affected than the mother is low, less than 1 percent in most cases. However, if the mother has delivered one child with CAH, or if the mother or father has CAH, then the parents can consider prenatal counseling, prenatal glucocorticoid treatment, and genetic testing.

Speiser and colleagues[206] have reported a protocol that may be effective in the prenatal treatment of families with one child affected by CAH (Fig. 28–17). The mother is treated with dexamethasone (20 μg/kg) as soon as pregnancy is diagnosed. Chorionic villus sampling is performed between 8 and 10 weeks of gestation. If a male fetus is identified, therapy is discontinued. Chromosomal deoxyribonucleic acid is analyzed for defects in the 21-hydroxylase gene by use of restriction fragment length polymorphisms. If an affected female fetus is identified, glucocorticoid treatment is continued for the entire pregnancy. Clitorimegaly and labioscrotal fusion may be prevented by this approach. Maternal estriol, which is derived from fetal adrenal precursors, can be used to monitor the effectiveness of maternal glucocorticoid therapy to suppress fetal adrenal steroidogenesis. Maternal circulating estriol concentration less than 0.2 nM is associated with marked suppression of the fetal adrenal. Maternal circulating estriol greater than 10 nM is associated with minimal suppression of the fetal adrenal.[207]

Application of this protocol to 14 fetuses at risk resulted in the treatment of two affected female fetuses with success in one of the affected female fetuses. A follow-up report reviewed the effects of prenatal glucocorticoid treatment on 15 female fetuses diagnosed as being affected with CAH on the basis of genetic testing in utero. Of the 15 female infants, 5 responded completely and 10 responded partially.[208] A major problem with this protocol is the development of iatrogenic Cushing's syndrome in the mothers receiving dexamethasone at a dose of 20 μg/kg daily.[207]

OVARIAN ENDOCRINE TUMORS

During normal pregnancy, maternal circulating testosterone[209] and androstenedione[210] increase, peaking in the third trimester. Before 28 weeks' gestation, although total testosterone increases, no significant change occurs in free testos-

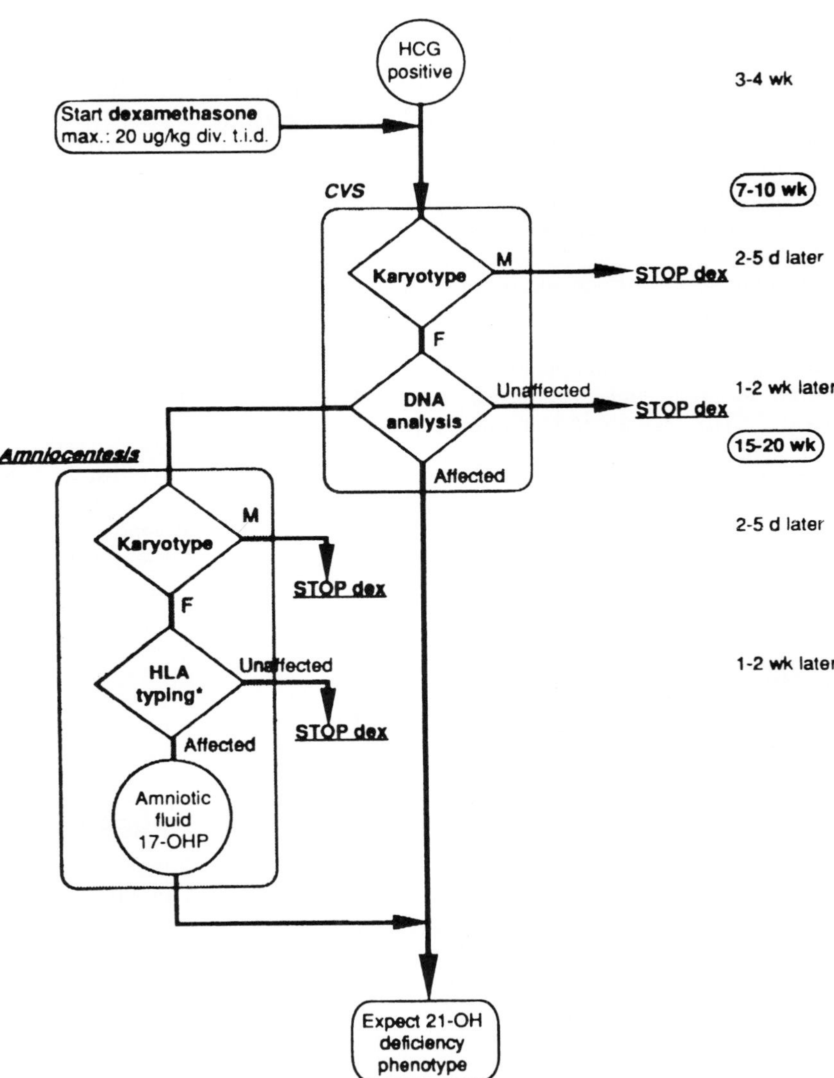

Figure 28–17 ■ Proposed protocol for the management of pregnant women at risk for congenital adrenal hyperplasia. CVS, chorionic villus sampling. (From Speiser PW, Laforgia N, Kato K, et al. First trimester prenatal treatment and molecular genetic diagnosis of congenital adrenal hyperplasia [21-hydroxylase deficiency]. J Clin Endocrinol Metab 70:838–848, 1990. © The Endocrine Society.)

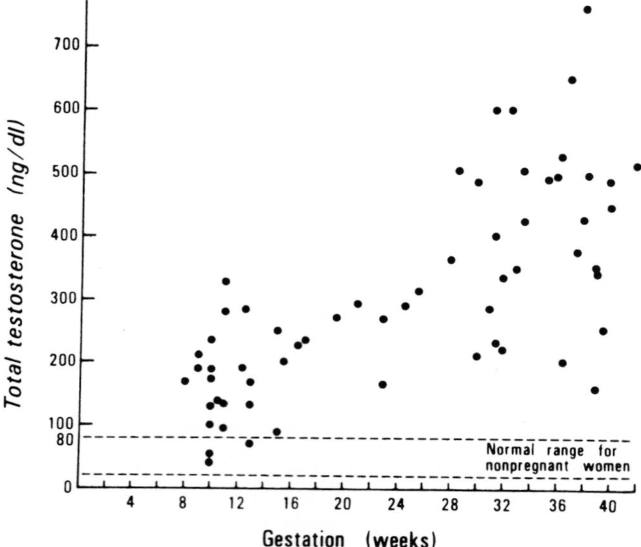

Figure 28–18 ■ Maternal circulating total testosterone levels throughout normal pregnancy. (From Bammann BL, Coulam CB, Jiang NS. Total and free testosterone during pregnancy. Am J Obstet Gynecol 137:293–298, 1980.)

terone, suggesting that much of the increase in total testosterone is due to increases in sex hormone–binding globulin.[211] This is consistent with the observation that the metabolic clearance rate of testosterone decreases during pregnancy.[212] After 28 weeks, an increase in both total and free testosterone has been reported (Figs. 28–18 and 28–19).

In contrast, dehydroepiandrosterone and dehydroepiandrosterone sulfate (DHEA-S) concentrations decrease during pregnancy.[213] DHEA-S levels fall to half of the concentration in the nonpregnant state. This decrease occurs even though the maternal production rate of DHEA-S increases.[214] The decrease in maternal DHEA-S concentration is probably due to increased placental clearance of this estrogen precursor.[213, 214]

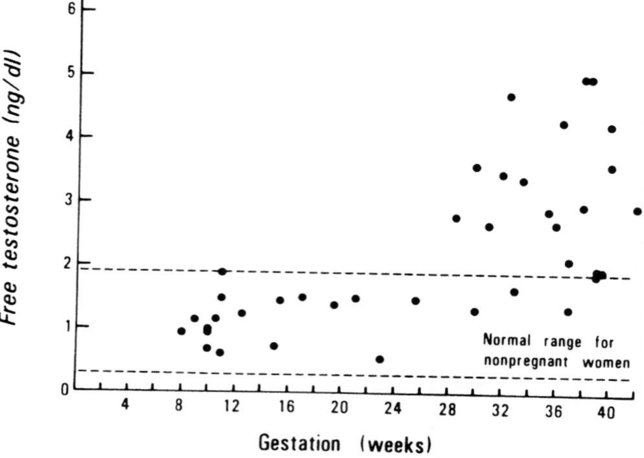

Figure 28–19 ■ Maternal circulating free testosterone levels throughout normal pregnancy. (From Bammann BL, Coulam CB, Jiang NS. Total and free testosterone during pregnancy. Am J Obstet Gynecol 137:293–298, 1980.)

Most cases of virilization in pregnancy are due to either ovarian endocrine "tumors" or exogenous androgen administration. Three distinct endocrine disorders of the ovary can cause maternal virilization: luteomas, hyperreactio luteinalis (gestational theca-lutein cysts), and Sertoli-Leydig cell tumors (arrhenoblastomas).[215] All three tumor types can be associated with markedly elevated levels of testosterone, dihydrotestosterone, and androstenedione.

The luteoma appears to be derived from luteinization and hyperplasia of theca interna or stromal cells.[216, 217] Luteomas are bilateral in approximately 45 percent of cases.[215] Maternal virilization or severe hirsutism occurs in approximately 35 percent of cases, and the risk of virilization of a female fetus is high. In contrast, hyperreactio luteinalis is associated with a lower risk of virilization of a female fetus. Maternal diseases associated with hyperreactio luteinalis include gestational trophoblastic tumors, diabetes, and Rh isoimmunization. In all three diseases associated with hyperreactio luteinalis, elevated hCG production has been reported; hCG appears to be the cause of the development of the theca-lutein cysts and a major stimulator of the steroid production from cysts. In the majority of cases, the cysts are bilateral. The risk of maternal and fetal virilization is highest with the Sertoli-Leydig cell tumor. These tumors are usually unilateral. Fortunately, Sertoli-Leydig cell tumors are typically associated with anovulation, so few cases occurring in pregnancy have been reported.

The female fetus is partially protected from developing virilization by at least three mechanisms. The high sex hormone–binding globulin concentration during pregnancy tends to dampen the amount of free testosterone available to cross the placenta as the amount of total testosterone rises.[211] A second mechanism is that the placenta has a high capacity to aromatize androgens such as testosterone and androstenedione to the estrogens estradiol and estrone.[218] By aromatizing androgens, the placenta acts as a protective barrier to prevent the female fetus from being exposed to excessive concentrations of testosterone and androstenedione. Dihydrotestosterone is not a substrate for aromatization. The placenta may be less effective in preventing this steroid from crossing into the fetal compartment and causing virilization. Finally, some female fetuses appear to be somewhat resistant to virilizing effects of androgens. Cases have been reported in which high cord concentrations of androgens have been present at birth but fetal virilization did not occur.[219] The female fetus may be especially sensitive to becoming virilized in the first trimester of pregnancy and may become less sensitive to the virilizing effects of androgens in the third trimester.

PREECLAMPSIA

Preeclampsia is a uniquely human disorder, most commonly characterized by both hypertension and proteinuria during the second or third trimester of pregnancy. Both the hypertension and proteinuria resolve after delivery of the placenta. Investigators have proposed many markers for preeclampsia including autocoids, lipids, oxidant activity, markers of neutrophil activation, adhesion molecules, cytokines, albumin isoforms, urinary calcium excretion, and many others.[220] Increase in responsiveness to angiotensin

II has been repetitively demonstrated to be a marker of preeclampsia.[221] The increase in responsiveness to angiotensin II demonstrated by women with preeclampsia is thought to be due to changes in endothelial function associated with preeclampsia.

Inhibin A and activin A have recently been reported to be markedly elevated in the circulation of women with pregnancies complicated by preeclampsia[222] (Fig. 28–20). In one study of 20 women with preeclampsia, the maternal circulating concentrations of inhibin A and activin A were approximately 10-fold higher in the women with preeclampsia than in the control subjects. The women with preeclampsia and the control subjects were matched for gestational age (29 weeks), but little information was provided concerning the clinical characteristics of the women with preeclampsia. It is likely that the elevated inhibin A and activin A concentrations in preeclampsia were caused by a combination of placental dysfunction resulting in overproduction of the proteins and decreased metabolic clearance of the proteins due to renal dysfunction. The biologic function of the inhibins and activins in the placenta is yet to be determined.

In preeclampsia, there are both perturbations in the control of the endocrine system and abnormalities in the nervous system. Schobel and colleagues[223] demonstrated that postganglionic sympathetic nerve activity was increased more than twofold in women with preeclampsia compared with pregnant women without hypertension. Using intraneural microelectrodes to measure sympathetic nerve activity in the blood vessels of skeletal muscle, the investigators demonstrated that the firing rate was 10 bursts per minute in normotensive pregnant women, 12 bursts per minute in normotensive nonpregnant women, and 15 bursts per minute in hypertensive nonpregnant women. In women with preeclampsia, 33 bursts per minute ($P < .05$) were recorded. These data suggest that the increases in peripheral vascular resistance and blood pressure that characterize preeclampsia may be due, in part, to increased firing of sympathetic neurons. Interestingly, heart rate was not increased in the women with preeclampsia, implying either that increased vagal tone suppressed sympathetic activity in the heart or that the increase in peripheral sympathetic activity is a secondary compensation to plasma volume contraction.

PRETERM AND POST-DATES LABOR

Human gestation averages approximately 40 weeks, but many pregnancies are complicated by preterm or post-dates delivery. Just before the onset of labor, numerous biochemical and structural changes occur in the myometrium that prepare the uterus for labor. For example, the membrane concentration of connexin-43, the myocyte gap junction protein, increases markedly just before labor. The high membrane concentration of connexin-43 permits the individual myocytes to efficiently transmit chemical signals to neighboring cells, allowing the myocytes to act in unison as a syncytium.[224] The mechanism that determines the onset

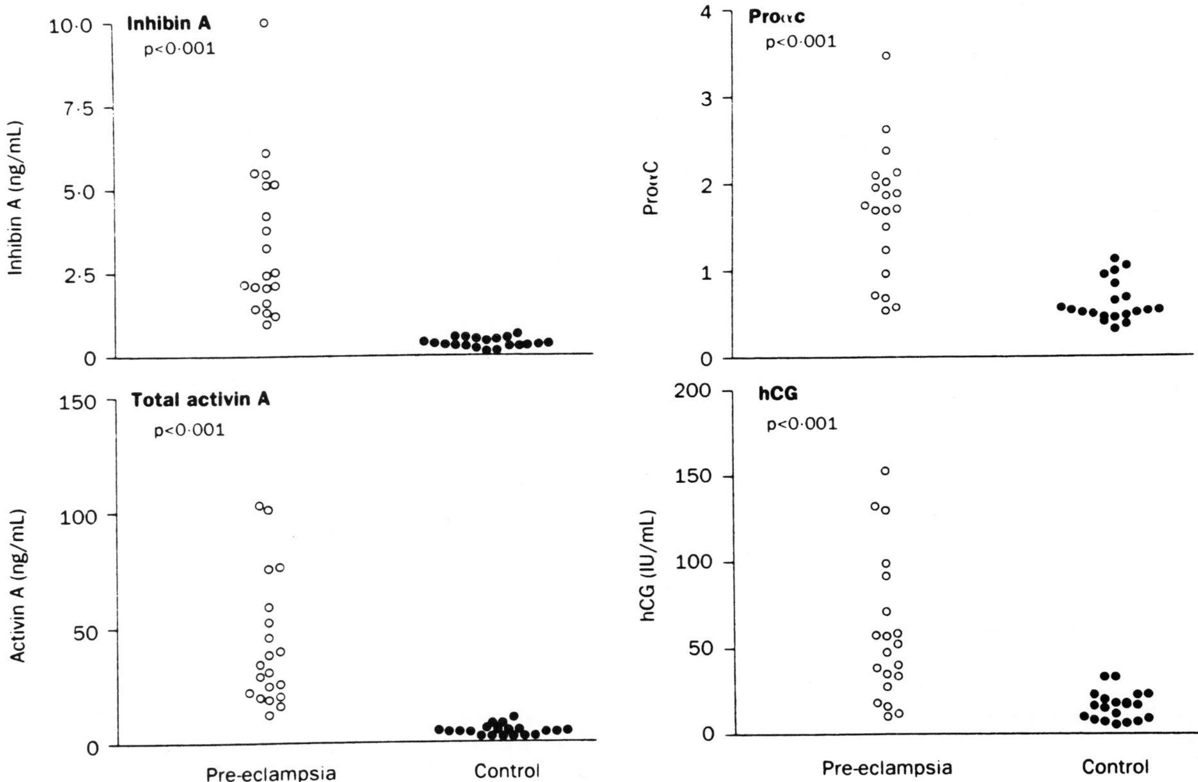

Figure 28–20 ■ Concentrations of inhibin A, total activin A, pro-αC, and hCG in preeclampsia and control women. (From Muttukrishna S, Knight PG, Groome NP, et al. Activin A and inhibin A as possible endocrine markers for preeclampsia. Lancet 349:1285–1288, 1997. © by The Lancet Ltd.)

of labor in humans is not well characterized, but evidence is accumulating that placental CRH may play an important role in the timing of labor in humans.[225] Maternal plasma CRH rises throughout pregnancy (Fig. 28–21). During the first two trimesters of pregnancy, CRH bioactivity is probably blocked by the presence of high circulating concentrations of CRH-binding protein. Just before the onset of labor, plasma CRH concentrations increase significantly and CRH-binding protein concentrations decrease. The net effect of these two changes is a marked increase in bioactive CRH. CRH receptors are present in the myometrium[226] and the fetal membranes.[227] CRH can stimulate secretion of prostaglandins from the decidua and amnion[228] and can potentiate the myometrial effects of oxytocin and prostaglandin.[229] Placental CRH enters the fetal circulation, where it can increase pituitary ACTH secretion and adrenal cortisol secretion. Fetal secretion of cortisol in the third trimester may control the final maturation of the fetal lung, gut, and cerebral vasculature.[230] Interestingly, in preterm labor, placental CRH production is abnormally increased and advanced for gestational age. In post-dates labor, placental CRH production is abnormally decreased and delayed for gestational age. These observations support the hypothesis that the rate of maturation and the onset of the prelabor placental CRH production control the timing of labor. In pregnancies in which the placental clock is "running fast," placental CRH secretion increases markedly before term, causing the onset of preterm labor. In pregnancies in which the placental clock is "running slow," the prelabor increase in placental secretion of CRH is delayed, resulting in post-dates pregnancy.[225] Measurement of CRH through all three trimesters of pregnancy suggests that the placental clock may be set to run fast or slow as early as the first or second trimester of pregnancy.[225] Once the speed of the placental clock is set, the timing of delivery may be predetermined.

As our understanding of placental physiology expands, it is clear that the placenta is an exceptionally complex endocrine organ. Many neuroendocrine-pituitary factors are secreted and regulated in the placenta in a way paralleling that observed in the hypothalamic-pituitary unit. During pregnancy, the placenta acts as a "third brain" playing

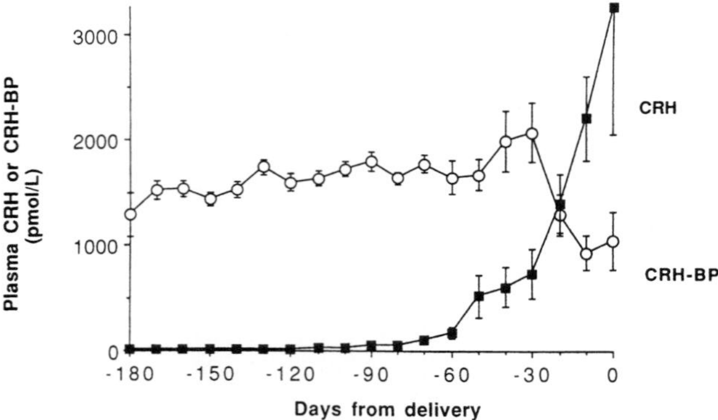

Figure 28–21 ■ Comparison of the molar concentration of corticotropin-releasing hormone *(closed squares)* and CRH-binding protein *(open circles)* in maternal plasma during the final 180 days of pregnancies resulting in the normal timing of delivery (37 to 42 weeks' gestation). (From McLean M, Bisits A, Davies J, et al. A placental clock controlling the length of human pregnancy. Nat Med 1:460–463, 1995.)

important roles in the regulation of metabolism, fetal growth, and the timing of the onset of labor.

References

1. Spellacy WN, Goetz FE. Plasma insulin in normal late pregnancy. N Engl J Med 268:988, 1963.
2. Kalkhoff RK, Schalch DS, Walker JW, et al. Diabetogenic factors associated with pregnancy. Trans Assoc Am Physicians 77:270, 1964.
3. Bleicher SJ, O'Sullivan JB, Freinkel N. Carbohydrate metabolism in pregnancy. V. The interrelations of glucose, insulin and free fatty acids in late pregnancy and post-partum. N Engl J Med 271:866, 1964.
4. Yen SSC, Tsai CC, Vela P. Gestational diabetogenesis: Quantitative analyses of glucose insulin interrelationship between normal pregnancy and pregnancy with gestational diabetes. Am J Obstet Gynecol 11:792, 1971.
5. Yen SSC. Endocrine regulation of metabolic homeostasis during pregnancy. Clin Obstet Gynecol 16:130, 1973.
6. Buchanan TA, Metzger BE, Freinkel N, Bergman RN. Insulin sensitivity and beta-cell responsiveness to glucose during late pregnancy in lean and moderately obese women with normal glucose tolerance or mild gestational diabetes. Am J Obstet Gynecol 162:1008, 1990.
7. Burt RL, Davidson WF. Insulin half life and utilization during pregnancy. Obstet Gynecol 43:161, 1974.
8. Ciaraldi TP, Kettel M, el-Roeiy A, et al. Mechanism of cellular insulin resistance in human pregnancy. Am J Obstet Gynecol 170:635, 1994.
9. Moore P, Kolterman O, Weyant J, Olefsky JM. Insulin binding in human pregnancy: Comparisons to the postpartum, luteal and follicular states. J Clin Endocrinol Metab 52:937, 1981.
10. Puavilai G, Drobny EC, Domont LA, Baumann G. Insulin receptors and insulin resistance in human pregnancy. Evidence for a post-receptor defect in insulin action. J Clin Endocrinol Metab 54:247, 1982.
11. Thorens B, Charron MJ, Lodish HF. Molecular physiology of glucose transporters. Diabetes Care 13:209, 1990.
12. Garvey WT, Maianu L, Zhu JH, et al. Multiple defects in the adipocyte glucose transport system cause cellular insulin resistance in gestational diabetes. Heterogeneity in the number and novel abnormality in subcellular localization of GLUT4 glucose transporters. Diabetes 42:1773, 1993.
13. Jacquemin P, Oury C, Peers B, et al. Characterization of a single strong tissue specific enhancer downstream from the three human genes encoding placental lactogen. Mol Cell Biol 14:93, 1994.
14. MacLeod JN, Lee AK, Liebhaber SA, Cooke NE. Developmental control and alternative splicing of the placentally expressed transcripts from the human growth hormone gene cluster. J Biol Chem 267:14219, 1992.
15. Barsh GS, Seeburg PH, Gelinas RE. The human growth hormone gene family: Structure and evolution of the chromosomal locus. Nucleic Acids Res 11:3939, 1983.
16. Igout A, Frankenne F, L'Hermite-Baleriaux M, et al. Somatogenic and lactogenic activity of the recombinant 22 kDa isoform of human placental growth hormone. Growth Regul 5:60, 1995.
17. Eriksson L, Frankenne F, Eden S, et al. Growth hormone 24 hour serum profiles during pregnancy: Lack of pulsatility for the secretion of the placental variant. Br J Obstet Gynecol 96:949, 1989.
18. Yen SSC, Vela P, Tsai CC. Impairment of growth hormone secretion in response to hypoglycemia during early and late pregnancy. J Clin Endocrinol Metab 31:29, 1970.
19. Merimee TJ, Zapt J, Foresch ER. Insulin-like growth factor in pregnancy: Studies in a growth hormone deficient dwarf. J Clin Endocrinol Metab 54:1101, 1982.
20. Goffin V, Shiverick KT, Kelly PA, Martial JA. Sequence-function relationships within the expanding family of prolactin, growth hormone, placental lactogen and related proteins in mammals. Endocr Rev 17:385, 1996.
21. Berrera-Saldana HA, Seeburg PH, Saunders GF. Two structurally different genes produce the same human placental lactogen hormone. J Biol Chem 258:3787, 1983.

22. Watkins WB, Yen SSC. Somatostatin in cytotrophoblast of the immature human placenta. J Clin Endocrinol Metab 50:969, 1980.
23. Kumasaka T, Nishi N, Yaoi Y. Demonstration of immunoreactive somatostatin-like substance in villi and decidua in early pregnancy. Am J Obstet Gynecol 134:39, 1979.
24. Hochberg Z, Bick T, Perlman R. Two pathways of placental lactogen secretion by cultured human trophoblast. Biochem Med Metabol Biol 39:111, 1988.
25. Hochberg Z, Perlman R, Brandes JM, Benderly A. Insulin regulates placental lactogen and estradiol secretion by cultured human term trophoblast. J Clin Endocrinol Metab 57:1311, 1983.
26. Petit A, Guillon G, Tence M, et al. Angiotensin II stimulates both inositol phosphate production and human placental lactogen release from human trophoblast cells. J Clin Endocrinol Metab 69:280, 1989.
27. Ahmed MS, Horst MA. Opioid receptors of human placental villi modulate acetylcholine release. Life Sci 39:535, 1986.
28. Wilson DM, Bennett A, Adamson GD. Somatomedin in pregnancy: A cross sectional study of IGF-I and -II and somatomedin peptide content in normal human pregnancy. J Clin Endocrinol Metab 55:858, 1982.
29. Hall K, Enberg G, Hellem E, et al. Somatomedin levels in pregnancy: Longitudinal study in healthy subjects and patients with GH deficiency. J Clin Endocrinol Metab 59:587, 1984.
30. Wang HS, Perry LA, Kanisius J, et al. Purification and assay of insulin like growth factor binding protein 1: Measurement of circulating levels throughout pregnancy. J Endocrinol 128:161, 1991.
31. Daughaday WH, Rivedi B, Winn HN, Yan H. Hypersomatotropism in pregnant women as measured by a human liver radioreceptor assay. J Clin Endocrinol Metab 70:215, 1990.
32. Baumann G, Amburn K, Shaw MA. The circulating growth hormone binding protein complex: A major constituent of plasma GH in man. Endocrinology 122:976, 1988.
33. Veldhuis JD, Johnson ML, Fant LM, et al. Influence of the high affinity GHBP on plasma profiles of free and bound GH and on the apparent half life of GH. J Clin Invest 91:629, 1993.
34. Barnard R, Chan FY, Mulchay J, et al. The Australian fetal growth study. I. Investigations of GH and GHBP throughout normal and pathologic gestation. Proceedings of the 10th International Congress of Endocrinology; June 1996; San Francisco, CA, p 480.
35. Luthman M, Stock S, Werner S, Bremme K. Growth hormone binding protein in plasma is inversely correlated to placental lactogen and augmented with increasing body mass index in healthy pregnant women and women with gestational diabetes mellitus. Gynecol Obstet Invest 38:145, 1994.
36. Pertzelan A, Lazar L, Klinger B, Laron Z. Puberty in fifteen patients with Laron syndrome: A longitudinal study. Pediatr Adolesc Endocrinol 24:27, 1993.
37. Evain-Brion D. Hormonal regulation of fetal growth. Horm Res 42:207, 1994.
38. Chowen JA, Evain-Brion D, Pozo J, et al. Decreased expression of placental growth hormone in intrauterine growth retardation. Pediatr Res 39:736, 1996.
39. Baldwin S, Chung T, Rogers M, et al. Insulin like growth factor binding protein-1, glucose tolerance and fetal growth in human pregnancy. J Endocrinol 136:319, 1993.
40. Wang HS, Lee CL, Chard T. Levels of insulin-like growth factor I and IGFBP-1 in pregnancy with pre-term delivery. Br J Obstet Gynaecol 100:472, 1993.
41. Reece EA, Wiznitzer A, Le E, et al. The relation between human fetal growth and fetal blood levels of insulin-like growth factors I and II, their binding proteins and receptors. Obstet Gynecol 84:88, 1994.
42. Lassarre C, Hardouin S, Daffos F, et al. Serum insulin like growth factors and insulin like growth factor binding proteins in human fetus. Relationships with growth in normal subjects and subjects with intrauterine growth retardation. Pediatr Res 29:219, 1991.
43. Perley M, Kipnis DM. Effect of glucocorticoids on plasma insulin. N Engl J Med 274:1237, 1966.
44. Carr BR, Parker CR, Madden JD, et al. Maternal plasma adrenocorticotropin and cortisol relationships throughout human pregnancy. Am J Obstet Gynecol 139:416, 1981.
45. Cousins L, Rigg L, Hollingsworth D, et al. Qualitative and quantitative assessment of the circadian rhythm of cortisol in pregnancy. Am J Obstet Gynecol 145:411, 1983.
46. Ryan EA, Enns L. Role of gestational hormones in the induction of insulin resistance. J Clin Endocrinol Metab 67:341, 1988.
47. Kumagai S, Homang A, Bjorntorp P. The effects of estrogens and progesterone on insulin sensitivity in female rats. Acta Physiol Scand 149:91, 1993.
48. Sutter-Dub MT, Kaaya A, Sfaxi A, et al. Progesterone and synthetic steroids produce insulin resistance at the post-receptor level in adipocytes of female rats. Steroids 52:583, 1988.
49. Phelps RL, Metzger BE, Freinkel N. Carbohydrate metabolism in pregnancy. Am J Obstet Gynecol 140:730, 1981.
50. Felig P, Kim YJ, Lynch V, Hendler R. Amino acid metabolism during starvation in human pregnancy. J Clin Invest 51:1195, 1972.
51. Freinkel N, Metzger BE, Nitzan M, et al. Facilitated anabolism in late pregnancy: Some novel maternal compensations for accelerated starvation. *In* Malaisse WJ, Pirart J (eds). Diabetes International Series 312. Amsterdam, Excerpta Medica, 1973, p 474.
52. Freinkel N. Effects of the conceptus on maternal metabolism during pregnancy. *In* Leibel BS, Wrenshall GA (eds). On the Nature and Treatment of Diabetes. Amsterdam, Excerpta Medica, 1965, p 679.
53. Hopkinson JM, Butte NF, Ellis KJ, et al. Body fat estimation in late pregnancy and early post-partum: Comparison of two-, three-, and four component models. Am J Clin Nutr 65:432, 1997.
54. Knopp RH, Warth MR, Charles D, et al. Lipoprotein metabolism in pregnancy, fat transport to the fetus and the effects of diabetes. Biol Neonate 50:297, 1986.
55. Potter JM, Nestel PJ. The hyperlipidemia of pregnancy in normal and complicated pregnancies. Am J Obstet Gynecol 133:165, 1979.
56. The Expert Committee on the Diagnosis and Classification of Diabetes Mellitus. Report of the Expert Committee on the Diagnosis and Classification of Diabetes Mellitus. Diabetes Care 20:1183, 1997.
57. Metzger GE. Organizing Committee: Summary and recommendations of the Third International Workshop-Conference on Gestational Diabetes Mellitus. Diabetes 40:197, 1991.
58. Engelgau MM, Herman WH, Smith PJ, et al. The epidemiology of diabetes and pregnancy in the U.S., 1988. Diabetes Care 18:1029, 1995.
59. Magee MS, Walden CE, Benedetti TJ. Influence of diagnostic criteria on the incidence of gestational diabetes and perinatal morbidity. JAMA 269:609, 1993.
60. National Diabetes Data Group. Classification and diagnosis of diabetes mellitus and other categories of glucose intolerance. Diabetes 28:1039, 1979.
61. Sacks DA, Abu-Fadil S, Greenspoon JS, Fotheringham N. Do the current standards for glucose tolerance testing in pregnancy represent a valid conversion of O'Sullivan's original criteria? Am J Obstet Gynecol 161:638, 1989.
62. Carpenter MW, Coustan DR. Criteria for screening tests for gestational diabetes. Am J Obstet Gynecol 144:768, 1982.
63. Widness JA, Cowett RM, Coustan DR, et al. Neonatal morbidities in infants of mothers with glucose intolerance in pregnancy. Diabetes 34(suppl 2):61, 1985.
64. Coustan DR, Imarah J. Prophylactic insulin treatment of gestational diabetes reduces the incidence of macrosomatia, operative delivery and birth trauma. Am J Obstet Gynecol 150:836, 1984.
65. Jovanovic-Peterson L, Durak E, Peterson C. Randomized trial of diet versus diet plus cardiovascular conditioning on glucose levels in gestational diabetes. Am J Obstet Gynecol 161:415, 1989.
66. Avery MD, Leon AS, Kopher RA. Effects of a partially home-based exercise program for women with gestational diabetes. Obstet Gynecol 89:10, 1997.
67. O'Sullivan J. Diabetes mellitus after GDM. Diabetes 40:131, 1991.
68. Simpson JL, Elias S, Martin AO, et al. Diabetes in pregnancy, Northwestern University series (1977–1981). Prospective study of anomalies in offspring of mothers with diabetes mellitus. Am J Obstet Gynecol 146:263, 1983.
69. Kucera J. Rate and type of congenital anomalies among offspring of diabetic women. J Reprod Med 7:61, 1971.
70. Freinkel N, Cockroft DL, Lewis NJ, et al. The 1986 McCollom award lecture. Fuel mediated teratogenesis during early organogenesis: The effects of increased concentrations of glucose, ketones or somatomedin inhibitor during rat embryo culture. Am J Clin Nutr 44:986, 1986.

71. Horton WE, Sadler TW. Effects of maternal diabetes on early embryogenesis: Alterations in morphogenesis produced by the ketone body beta-hydroxybutyrate. Diabetes 32:610, 1983.
72. Kanwar YS, Liu ZZ, Kumar A, et al. D-Glucose induced dysmorphogenesis of embryonic kidney. J Clin Invest 98:2478, 1996.
73. Fuhrmann K, Reiher H, Semmler K, Glockner E. The effect of intensified conventional insulin therapy before and during pregnancy on the malformation rate in offspring of diabetic mothers. Exp Clin Endocrinol 83:173, 1984.
74. Molsted-Pedersen L. Pregnancy and diabetes, a survey. Acta Endocrinol (Copenh) 94(suppl 238):13, 1980.
75. Landon MB, Gabbe SG, Sachs L. Management of diabetes mellitus and pregnancy: A survey of obstetricians and maternal fetal specialists. Obstet Gynecol 75:635, 1990.
76. Miller E, Hare JW, Cloherty JP, et al. Elevated maternal HbA_1 in early pregnancy and major congenital anomalies in infants of diabetic mothers. N Engl J Med 304:1331, 1981.
77. Carsons BS, Phillips AF, Simmons MA, et al. Effects of a sustained insulin infusion upon glucose uptake and oxygenation of the ovine fetus. Pediatr Res 14:147, 1980.
78. Barbieri RL, Saltzman D, Phillippe M, et al. Elevated beta-human chorionic gonadotropin and testosterone in cord serum of male infants of diabetic mothers. J Clin Endocrinol Metab 61:976, 1985.
79. Barbieri RL, Saltzman DH, Torday JS, et al. Elevated concentrations of the beta-subunit of human chorionic gonadotropin and testosterone in the amniotic fluid of infants of diabetic mothers. Am J Obstet Gynecol 154:1039, 1986.
80. Saltzman DH, Barbieri RL, Frigoletto FD. Decreased fetal cord prolactin concentration in diabetic pregnancies. Am J Obstet Gynecol 154:1035, 1986.
81. Chehab FF, Lim ME, Lu R. Correction of the sterility defect in homozygous obese female mice by treatment with the human recombinant leptin. Nat Genet 12:318, 1996.
82. Schubring C, Kiess W, Englaro P, et al. Levels of leptin in maternal serum, amniotic fluid and arterial and venous cord blood: Relation to neonatal and placental weight. J Clin Endocrinol Metab 82:1480, 1997.
83. Butte NF, Hopkinson JM, Nicolson MA. Leptin in human reproduction: Serum leptin levels in pregnant and lactating women. J Clin Endocrinol Metab 82:585, 1997.
84. Calandra C, Abell DA, Beischer NA. Maternal obesity in pregnancy. Obstet Gynecol 57:8, 1981.
85. Egger G. The case for using waist to hip ratio measurements in routine medical checks. Med J Aust 156:280, 1992.
86. Morris RD, Rimm AA. Association of waist to hip ratio and family history with the prevalence of NIDDM among 25,272 adult white females. Am J Public Health 81:507, 1991.
87. Werler MM, Louik C, Shapiro S, Mitchell AA. Prepregnant weight in relation to risk of neural tube defects. JAMA 275:1089, 1996.
88. Shaw GM, Velie EM, Schaffer D. Risk of neural tube defect–affected pregnancies among obese women. JAMA 275:1093, 1996.
89. Waller DK, Mills JL, Simpson JL, et al. Are obese women at higher risk for producing malformed offspring? Am J Obstet Gynecol 170:541, 1994.
90. Sibai BM, Gordon T, Thom E, et al. Risk factors for preeclampsia in healthy nulliparous women: A prospective multicenter study. Am J Obstet Gynecol 172:642, 1995.
91. Stone JL, Lockwood CJ, Berkowitz GS, et al. Risk factors for severe preeclampsia. Obstet Gynecol 83:357, 1994.
92. Crane SS, Wojtowycz MA, Dye TD, et al. Association between pre-pregnancy obesity and the risk of cesarean delivery. Am J Obstet Gynecol 89:213, 1997.
93. Edwards LE, Hellerstedt WL, Alton IR, et al. Pregnancy complications and birth outcomes in obese and normal weight women: Effects of gestational weight change. Obstet Gynecol 87:389, 1996.
94. Barbieri RL. The maternal adenohypophysis. *In* Tulchinsky D, Little BA (eds). Maternal-Fetal Endocrinology. Philadelphia, WB Saunders, 1994, pp 119–131.
95. Erdheim J, Stumme E. Über die Schwangerschaftsveranderung der Hypophyse. Beitr Pathol Anat 46:1, 1909.
96. Gonzalez JG, Elizondo G, Saldivar D, et al. Pituitary gland growth during normal pregnancy: An in vivo study using magnetic resonance imaging. Am J Med 85:217, 1988.
97. Hinshaw DB, Hasso AN, Thompson JR, Davidson BJ. High resolution computed tomography of the post partum pituitary gland. Neuroradiology 26:299, 1984.
98. Carvill M. Bitemporal contractions of the visual fields during pregnancy. Am J Ophthalmol 6:885, 1923.
99. Finlay CE. Visual field defects in pregnancy. Arch Ophthalmol 12:207, 1934.
100. Scheithauer BW, Sano T, Kovacs ST, et al. The pituitary gland in pregnancy: A clinicopathologic and immunohistochemical study of 69 cases. Mayo Clin Proc 65:461, 1990.
101. Asa SI, Penz G, Kovacs K, Ezrin C. Prolactin cells in the human pituitary: A quantitative immunocytochemistry analysis. Arch Pathol Lab Med 106:360, 1982.
102. Rigg LA, Lein A, Yen SSC. Pattern of increase in circulating prolactin levels during human gestation. Am J Obstet Gynecol 129:454, 1977.
103. Fang VS, Kim MH. Study on maternal, fetal and amniotic human prolactin at term. J Clin Endocrinol Metab 41:1030, 1975.
104. Kauppila A, Chatelain P, Kirkinen P, et al. Isolated prolactin deficiency in a woman with puerperal lactogenesis. J Clin Endocrinol Metab 64:309, 1987.
105. Riddick DH, Luciano AA, Kusmick WF, Maslar IA. Evidence for a nonpituitary source of amniotic fluid prolactin. Fertil Steril 31:35, 1979.
106. Hershman JM, Burrow GN. Lack of release of human chorionic gonadotropin by thyrotropin releasing hormone. J Clin Endocrinol Metab 42:970, 1976.
107. Quigley ME, Ishizuka B, Ropert JF, Yen SSC. The food entrained prolactin and cortisol release in late pregnancy and prolactinemia patients. J Clin Endocrinol Metab 54:1109, 1982.
108. Boyar RM, Finkelstein JW, Kapen S, Hellman L. Twenty four hour prolactin secretory patterns during pregnancy. J Clin Endocrinol Metab 40:1117, 1975.
109. Bonnar J, Franklin M, Nott PN, McNeilly AS. Effect of breast feeding on pituitary ovarian function after childbirth. BMJ 4:82, 1975.
110. Markoff E, Lee DW, Hollingsworth DR. Glycosylated and nonglycosylated prolactin in serum during pregnancy. J Clin Endocrinol Metab 67:519, 1988.
111. Pellegrini I, Gunz G, Ronin C, et al. Polymorphism of prolactin secreted by human prolactinoma cells: Immunological, receptor binding, and biological properties of the glycosylated and nonglycosylated forms. Endocrinology 122:2667, 1988.
112. Genazzani AR, Fraioli F, Hurlimann J, et al. Immunoreactive ACTH and cortisol plasma levels during pregnancy. Detection and partial purification of corticotrophin-like placental hormone: The human chorionic gonadotropin. Clin Endocrinol 4:1, 1975.
113. Genazzani AR, Felber JP, Fioretti P. Immunoreactive ACTH, immunoreactive human chorionic somatomammotropin and 11-OH steroid plasma levels in normal and pathological pregnancies. Acta Endocrinol (Copenh) 83:800, 1977.
114. Nolten WE, Lindheimer MD, Ruckert PA, et al. Diurnal patterns and regulation of cortisol secretion in pregnancy. J Clin Endocrinol Metab 51:466, 1980.
115. Nolten WE, Ruckert PA. Elevated free cortisol index in pregnancy: Possible regulatory mechanisms. Am J Obstet Gynecol 139:492, 1981.
116. Schulte HM, Weisner D, Allolio B. The corticotropin releasing hormone test in late pregnancy: Lack of adrenocorticotropin and cortisol response. Clin Endocrinol (Oxf) 33:99, 1990.
117. Cousins L, Rigg L, Hollingsworth D, et al. Qualitative and quantitative assessment of the circadian rhythm of cortisol in pregnancy. Am J Obstet Gynecol 145:411, 1983.
118. Goland RS, Stark RI, Wardlaw SL. Response to corticotropin releasing hormone during pregnancy in the baboon. J Clin Endocrinol Metab 70:925, 1990.
119. Goland RS, Wardlaw SL, MacCarter G, et al. Adrenocorticotropin and cortisol response to vasopressin during pregnancy. J Clin Endocrinol Metab 73:257, 1991.
120. Goland RS, Wardlaw SL, Stark RI, et al. High levels of corticotropin releasing hormone immunoreactivity in maternal and fetal plasma during pregnancy. J Clin Endocrinol Metab 63:1199, 1986.
121. Rees LH, Burke CW, Chard T, et al. Possible placental origin of ACTH in normal human pregnancy. Nature 254:620, 1975.

122. Samaan NA, Goplerud CP, Bradbury JT. Effect of arginine infusion on plasma levels of growth hormone, insulin and glucose during pregnancy and the puerperium. Am J Obstet Gynecol 107:1002, 1970.
123. Miyake A, Tanizawa O, Aono T, Kurachi K. Pituitary responses in LH secretion to LHRH during pregnancy. Obstet Gynecol 49:549, 1977.
124. Reyes FI, Winter JSD, Faiman C. Pituitary gonadotropin function during human pregnancy: Serum FSH and LH levels before and after LHRH administration. J Clin Endocrinol Metab 42:590, 1976.
125. Rubinstein LM, Parlow AF, Derzko C, Hershman JM. Pituitary gonadotropin response to LHRH in human pregnancy. Obstet Gynecol 52:172, 1978.
126. De La Lastra M, Llados C. Luteinizing hormone content of the pituitary gland in pregnant and nonpregnant women. J Clin Endocrinol Metab 44:921, 1977.
127. Scheithauer BW, Sano T, Kovacs ST, et al. The pituitary gland in pregnancy: A clinicopathologic and immunohistochemical study of 69 cases. Mayo Clin Proc 65:461, 1990.
128. Hershman JM, Kojima A, Friesen HG. Effect of thyrotropin releasing hormone on human pituitary thyrotropin, prolactin, placental lactogen and chorionic thyrotropin. J Clin Endocrinol Metab 36:497, 1973.
129. Kannan V, Sinha MK, Devi PK, Rastogi GK. Plasma thyrotropin and its response to thyrotropin releasing hormone in normal pregnancy. Obstet Gynecol 42:547, 1973.
130. Glinoer D, de Nayer P, Bourdoux P, et al. Regulation of maternal thyroid during pregnancy. J Clin Endocrinol Metab 71:276, 1990.
131. Harada A, Hershman JM, Reed AW, et al. Comparison of thyroid stimulators and thyroid hormone concentrations in the sera of pregnant women. J Clin Endocrinol Metab 48:793, 1979.
132. Nisula BC, Ketelslegers JM. Thyroid stimulating activity and chorionic gonadotropin. J Clin Invest 54:494, 1974.
133. Silverberg J, O'Donnell J, Sugenoya A, et al. Effect of human chorionic gonadotropin on human thyroid tissue in vitro. J Clin Endocrinol Metab 46:420, 1978.
134. Harada A, Hershman JM. Extraction of human chorionic thyrotropin from term placentas; failure to recover thyrotropic activity. J Clin Endocrinol Metab 47:681, 1978.
135. Musey VC, Collins DC, Musey PI, et al. Long term effects of a first pregnancy on the secretion of prolactin. N Engl J Med 316:229, 1987.
136. Yu MC, Gerkins VR, Henderson BE, et al. Elevated levels of prolactin in nulliparous women. Br J Cancer 43:826, 1981.
137. Kwa HG, Cleton F, Bulbrook RD, et al. Plasma prolactin levels and breast cancer: Relation to parity, weight and height and age at first birth. Int J Cancer 28:31, 1981.
138. Herman V, Fagin J, Melmed S. Clonal origin of pituitary tumors. J Clin Endocrinol Metab 71:1427, 1990.
139. Landis CA, Harsh G. Clinical characteristics of acromegalic patients whose pituitary tumors contain mutant G_s protein. J Clin Endocrinol Metab 71:1416, 1990.
140. Corenblum B, Donovan L. The safety of physiological estrogen plus progestin replacement therapy with oral contraceptive therapy in women with pathological hyperprolactinemia. Fertil Steril 59:671, 1993.
141. Thorner MO. Medical treatment of prolactinomas. J Clin Endocrinol Metab 82:997, 1997.
142. Barbieri RL, Ryan KJ. Bromocriptine: Endocrine pharmacology and therapeutic applications. Fertil Steril 39:727, 1983.
143. McGregor AM, Scanlon MF, Hall R, et al. Effects of bromocriptine on pituitary tumor size. Br Med J 2:700, 1979.
144. Molitch ME, Elton RL, Blackwell RE, et al. Bromocriptine as a primary therapy for prolactin secreting macroadenomas: Results of a prospective multicenter study. J Clin Endocrinol Metab 60:698, 1985.
145. Webster J, Piscitelli G, Polli A, et al. A comparison of cabergoline and bromocriptine in the treatment of hyperprolactinemic amenorrhea. N Engl J Med 331:904, 1994.
146. Raymond JP, Goldstein E, Konopka P, et al. Follow up of children born of bromocriptine treated mothers. Horm Res 22:239, 1985.
147. Bergh T, Nillus SJ, Wide L. Clinical course and outcome of pregnancies in amenorrheic women with hyperprolactinemia and pituitary tumors. Br Med J 1:875, 1978.
148. Konopka P, Raymond JP, Merceron RE, et al. Continuous administration of bromocriptine in the prevention of neurological complications in pregnant women with prolactinomas. Am J Obstet Gynecol 146:935, 1983.
149. Holmgren U, Bergstrand G, Hagenfeldt K, et al. Women with prolactinoma: Effect of pregnancy and lactation on serum prolactin and on tumor growth. Acta Endocrinol (Copenh) 111:452, 1986.
150. Wilson C. The case for initial surgical removal of certain prolactinomas. J Clin Endocrinol Metab 82:999, 1997.
151. Molitch ME. Prolactinoma. *In* Melmed S (ed). The Pituitary. Boston, Blackwell Scientific Publications, 1995, pp 443–477.
152. Molitch M. Pregnancy and the hyperprolactinemic woman. N Engl J Med 312:1364, 1985.
153. Abelove WA, Rupp JJ, Paschkis KE. Acromegaly and pregnancy. J Clin Endocrinol Metab 14:32, 1954.
154. Finkler RS. Acromegaly and pregnancy. Case report. J Clin Endocrinol Metab 14:1245, 1954.
155. Jialal I, Naidoo C, Norman RJ, et al. Pituitary function in Sheehan's syndrome. Obstet Gynecol 63:15, 1984.
156. Barbieri RL, Cooper DS, Daniels GH, et al. Prolactin response to thyrotropin-releasing hormone in patients with hypothalamic-pituitary disease. Fertil Steril 43:66, 1985.
157. Sheehan HL, Whitehead R. The neurohypophysis in postpartum hypopituitarism. J Pathol 85:145, 1965.
158. Whitehead R. The hypothalamus in post-partum hypopituitarism. J Pathol 86:55, 1965.
159. Bakiri F, Benmiloud M, Vallotton MB. Arginine vasopressin in postpartum panhypopituitarism: Urinary excretion and kidney response to osmolar load. J Clin Endocrinol Metab 58:511, 1984.
160. Bakiri F, Benmiloud M. Antidiuretic function in Sheehan's syndrome. Br Med J 289:579, 1984.
161. Asa SL, Bilbao JM, Kovacs K, et al. Lymphocytic hypophysitis of pregnancy resulting in hypopituitarism: A distinct clinicopathologic entity. Ann Intern Med 95:166, 1981.
162. Meichner RH, Riggio S, Manz HJ, Earll JM. Lymphocytic adenohypophysitis causing pituitary mass. Neurology 37:158, 1987.
163. Barron WM, Lindheimer MD. Renal sodium and water handling in pregnancy. Obstet Gynecol Annu 13:35, 1984.
164. Durr JA. Diabetes insipidus in pregnancy. Am J Kidney Dis 9:276, 1987.
165. Iwasaki Y, Oiso Y, Yamauchi K, et al. Neurohypophyseal function in postpartum hypopituitarism: Impaired plasma vasopressin response to osmotic stimuli. J Clin Endocrinol Metab 68:560, 1989.
166. Robertson GL. Posterior pituitary. *In* Felig P, Baxter JD, Broadus AE, Frohman LA (eds). Endocrinology and Metabolism. New York, McGraw-Hill, 1995, pp 338–377.
167. Seki K, Makimura N, Mitsui C, et al. Calcium regulating hormones and osteocalcin levels during pregnancy: A longitudinal study. Am J Obstet Gynecol 161:1248, 1991.
168. Lalau JD, Jans I, El Esper N, et al. Calcium metabolism, plasma parathyroid hormone and calcitriol in transient hypertension of pregnancy. Am J Hypertens 6:522, 1993.
169. Bikle DD, Gee E, Halloran B, Haddad JG. Free 1,25-hydroxyvitamin D levels in serum from normal subjects, pregnant subjects and subjects with liver disease. J Clin Invest 74:1966, 1984.
170. Delvin EE, Arabian A, Glorieux FH, Mamer OA. In vitro metabolism of 25-hydroxycholecalciferol by isolated cells from human decidua. J Clin Endocrinol Metab 60:880, 1985.
171. Seely EW, Brown EM, DeMaggio DM, et al. A prospective study of calcitropic hormones in pregnancy and post partum: Reciprocal changes in serum intact parathyroid hormone and 1,25-dihydroxyvitamin D. Am J Obstet Gynecol 176:214, 1997.
172. Pitkin RM, Reynolds WA, Williams GA, Hargis GK. Calcium metabolism in normal pregnancy: A longitudinal study. Am J Obstet Gynecol 133:781, 1979.
173. Hoskins DJ. Calcium homeostasis in pregnancy. Clin Endocrinol (Oxf) 45:1, 1996.
174. Kovacs CS, Lanske B, Hunzelman JL, et al. Parathyroid hormone related peptide regulates fetal-placental calcium transport through a receptor distinct from the PTH/PTHrP receptor. Proc Natl Acad Sci USA 93:15233, 1996.
175. Gertner JM, Coustan DR, Kliger AS, et al. Pregnancy as a state of physiological absorptive hypercalciuria. Am J Med 81:451, 1986.

176. Gallacher SJ, Fraser WD, Owens IJ. Changes in calcitropic hormones and biochemical markers of bone turnover in normal human pregnancy. Eur J Endocrinol 131:369, 1994.
177. Drinkwater BL, Chestnut CH. Bone density changes during pregnancy and lactation in active women: A longitudinal study. Bone Miner 14:153, 1991.
178. Carella M, Gossain V. Hyperparathyroidism and pregnancy. Case report and review. J Gen Intern Med 7:448, 1992.
179. Ludwig GD. Hyperparathyroidism in relation to pregnancy. N Engl J Med 267:637, 1962.
180. Kelly T. Primary hyperparathyroidism during pregnancy. Surgery 110:1028, 1991.
181. Johnstone RE 2nd, Kreindler T, Johnstone RE. Hyperparathyroidism during pregnancy. Obstet Gynecol 40:580, 1972.
182. Lepre F, Grill V, Martin TJ. Hypercalcemia in pregnancy and lactation associated with parathyroid hormone–related protein. N Engl J Med 328:666, 1993.
183. Pollak M, Chou YH, Marx S, et al. Familial hypocalciuric hypercalcemia and neonatal severe hyperparathyroidism: The effect of mutant gene dosage on phenotype. J Clin Invest 93:1108, 1994.
184. Graham WP, Gordon GS, Loken HF, et al. Effect of pregnancy and of the menstrual cycle on hypoparathyroidism. J Clin Endocrinol Metab 24:512, 1964.
185. Goldberg LD. Transmission of vitamin D metabolite in breast milk. Lancet 2:1258, 1972.
186. Swartz SL, Williams GH, Hollenberg NK, et al. Primacy of the renin-angiotensin system in mediating the aldosterone response to sodium restriction. J Clin Endocrinol Metab 50:1071, 1980.
187. Neufeld M, MacLaren NK, Blizzard RM. Two types of autoimmune Addison's disease associated with different polyglandular autoimmune syndromes. Medicine (Baltimore) 60:355, 1981.
188. Uibo R, Aavik E, Petreson P, et al. Autoantibodies to cytochrome P-450 enzymes in autoimmune polyglandular diseases types I and II and in isolated Addison's disease. J Clin Endocrinol Metab 78:323, 1994.
189. Speckart PF, Nicoloff JT, Behune JE. Screening for adrenocortical insufficiency with cosyntropin. Arch Intern Med 128:761, 1971.
190. Dluhy R, Himathongkam T, Greenfield M. Rapid ACTH test with plasma aldosterone levels. Improved diagnostic discrimination. Ann Intern Med 80:693, 1974.
191. Winkel CA, Simpson ER, Milewich L, Macdonald PC. Deoxycorticosterone biosynthesis in human kidney. Proc Natl Acad Sci USA 77:7069, 1980.
192. Drucker D, Shumak S, Angel A. Schmidt's syndrome presenting with intrauterine growth retardation and postpartum addisonian crisis. Am J Obstet Gynecol 149:229, 1984.
193. Bongiovanni AM, McFadden AJ. Steroids during pregnancy and possible fetal consequences. Fertil Steril 11:181, 1960.
194. Buescher MA, McClamrock HD, Adashi EY. Cushing syndrome in pregnancy. Obstet Gynecol 79:130, 1992.
195. Lindholm J, Schultz-Moller N. Plasma and urinary cortisol in pregnancy and during estrogen-gestagen treatment. Scand J Clin Lab Invest 31:119, 1973.
196. Itsuji Y, Tanaka K, Tanabe T, Takahashi H. Evaluation of urinary excretion of free-cortisol in patients with abnormal pituitary adrenal axis. Rinsho Byori 45:2656, 1997.
197. Lin CL, Wu TJ, Machacek DA, et al. Urinary free cortisol and cortisone determined by high performance liquid chromatography in the diagnosis of Cushing's syndrome. J Clin Endocrinol Metab 82:151, 1997.
198. Freda PU, Wardlaw SL, Bruce JN, et al. Differential diagnosis in Cushing's syndrome. Use of corticotropin releasing hormone. Medicine (Baltimore) 74:74, 1995.
199. Gormley MJJ, Hadden DR, Kennedy TL, et al. Cushing's syndrome in pregnancy—treatment with metyrapone. Clin Endocrinol 16:283, 1982.
200. Close CF, Mann MC, Watts JF, Taylor KG. ACTH-independent Cushing's syndrome in pregnancy with spontaneous resolution after delivery: Control of the hypercortisolism with metyrapone. Clin Endocrinol (Oxf) 39:375, 1993.
201. Hanson TJ, Ballonoff LB, Northcutt RC. Aminoglutethimide and pregnancy. JAMA 230:963, 1974.
202. Aron DC, Schnall AM, Sheeler LR. Cushing's syndrome and pregnancy. Am J Obstet Gynecol 162:244, 1990.
203. Amado JA, Pesquera C, Gonzalez EM, et al. Successful treatment with ketoconazole of Cushing's syndrome in pregnancy. Postgrad Med J 66:221, 1990.
204. Casson IF, Davis JC, Jeffreys RV, et al. Successful management of Cushing's disease during pregnancy by transsphenoidal adenectomy. Clin Endocrinol (Oxf) 27:423, 1987.
205. Pang SY, Wallace MA, Hofman L, et al. Worldwide experience in newborn screening for classical congenital adrenal hyperplasia due to 21-hydroxylase deficiency. Pediatrics 81:866, 1988.
206. Speiser PW, Laforgia N, Kato K, et al. First trimester prenatal treatment and molecular genetic diagnosis of congenital adrenal hyperplasia (21-hydroxylase deficiency). J Clin Endocrinol Metab 70:838, 1990.
207. Pang S, Clark AT, Freeman LC, et al. Maternal side effects of prenatal dexamethasone therapy for fetal congenital adrenal hyperplasia. J Clin Endocrinol Metab 75:249, 1992.
208. Pang S, Pollack MS, Marshall RN, Immken I. Prenatal treatment of congenital adrenal hyperplasia due to 21-hydroxylase deficiency. N Engl J Med 322:111, 1990.
209. Tulchinsky D, Chopra IJ. Estrogen-androgen imbalance in patients with hirsutism and amenorrhea. J Clin Endocrinol Metab 39:164, 1974.
210. Rivarola MA, Forest MG, Migeon CJ. Testosterone, androstenedione and dehydroepiandrosterone in plasma during pregnancy and at delivery. J Clin Endocrinol Metab 28:34, 1968.
211. Bammann BL, Coulam CB, Jiang NS. Total and free testosterone during pregnancy. Am J Obstet Gynecol 137:293, 1980.
212. Saez JM, Forest MG, Morera AM, Bertrand J. Metabolic clearance rate and blood production rate of testosterone and dihydrotestosterone in normal subjects during pregnancy and in hypothyroidism. J Clin Invest 51:1226, 1972.
213. Milewich L, Gomez-Sanchez C, Madden JD, et al. Dehydroepiandrosterone sulfate in peripheral blood of premenopausal, pregnant and postmenopausal women and men. J Steroid Biochem 9:1159, 1978.
214. Gant NF, Hutchinson HT, Siiteri PK, MacDonald PC. Study of the metabolic clearance rate of dehydroisoandrosterone sulfate in pregnancy. Am J Obstet Gynecol 111:555, 1971.
215. McClamrock HD, Adashi EY. Gestational hyperandrogenism. Fertil Steril 57:257, 1992.
216. Norris HJ, Taylor HB. Nodular theca-lutein hyperplasia of pregnancy. Am J Clin Pathol 47:557, 1967.
217. Scully RF. Stromal luteoma of the ovary: A distinctive type of lipoid cell tumor. Cancer 17:769, 1964.
218. Edman CD, Toofanian A, MacDonald PC, Gant NF. Placental clearance rate of maternal plasma androstenedione through placental estradiol formation. Am J Obstet Gynecol 141:1029, 1981.
219. Hensleigh PA, Carter RP, Grotjan HE. Fetal protection against masculinization with hyperreactio luteinalis and virilization. J Clin Endocrinol Metab 40:815, 1975.
220. Roberts JM, Redman CW. Pre-eclampsia, more than just pregnancy induced hypertension. Lancet 342:504, 1993.
221. Gant NF, Daley GL, Chand S, et al. A study of angiotensin II pressor response throughout primigravid pregnancy. J Clin Invest 52:2682, 1973.
222. Muttukrishna S, Knight PG, Groome NP, et al. Activin A and inhibin A as possible endocrine markers for pre-eclampsia. Lancet 349:1285, 1997.
223. Schobel HP, Fischer T, Heuszer K, et al. Preeclampsia—a state of sympathetic overactivity. N Engl J Med 33:1480, 1996.
224. Tabb T, Thilander G, Grover A, et al. An immunochemical and immunocytologic study of the increase in myometrial gap junctions (and connexin 43) in rats and humans during pregnancy. Am J Obstet Gynecol 167:559, 1992.
225. McLean M, Bisits A, Davies J, et al. A placental clock controlling the length of human pregnancy. Nat Med 1:460, 1995.
226. Hillhouse EW, Grammatopoulos D, Milton NGN, Quartero HWP. The identification of a human myometrial corticotropin releasing hormone receptor that increases in affinity during pregnancy. J Clin Endocrinol Metab 76:736, 1993.
227. Petraglia F, Giardino L, Coukos G, et al. Corticotropin releasing factor and parturition. Plasma and amniotic fluid levels and placental binding sites. Obstet Gynecol 75:784, 1990.
228. Jone SA, Challis JRG. Local stimulation of prostaglandin

production by corticotropin releasing hormone in human fetal membranes and placenta. Biochem Biophys Res Commun 159:192, 1989.
229. Benedetto C, Petraglia F, Marozio L, et al. Corticotropin-releasing hormone increases prostaglandin $F_{2\alpha}$ activity on human myometrium in vitro. Am J Obstet Gynecol 171:126, 1994.
230. Challis JRG, Hooper S. Birth: Outcome of a positive cascade. Baillieres Clin Endocrinol Metab 3:781, 1989.

Index

Note: Page numbers in *italics* refer to illustrations; page numbers followed by t refer to tables.